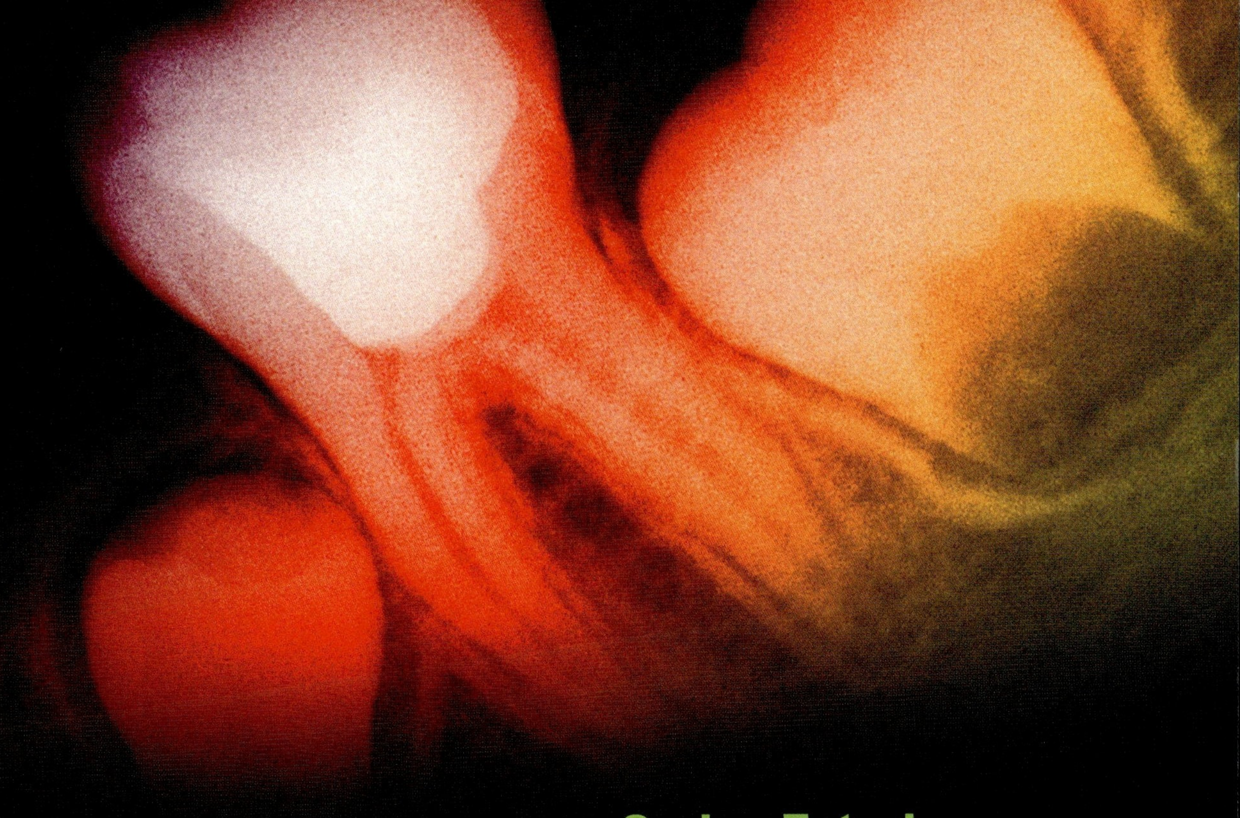

Carlos Estrela

# Endodontic Science

# Endodontic Science

**Carlos Estrela, DDS, MSc, PhD**
Chairman and Professor of Endodontics,
Department of Stomatologic Sciences
Federal University of Goiás, Goiânia, GO, Brazil

Volume 1

2009

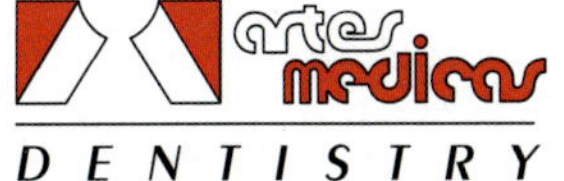

Endodontic Science

ISBN 978-85-367-0083-0



**Publishing Director**

Milton Hecht

**Production Manager**

Fernanda Matajs

**Editorial Production/Cover**

Júnior Bianchi

**Translation Reviewing**

Margery Galbraith

**Printing**

RR Donnelley

Dados Internacionais de Catalogação na Publicação (CIP)
(Câmara Brasileira do Livro, SP, Brasil)

Estrela, Carlos
Endodontic science / Carlos Estrela ; [translation reviewing Margery Galbraith]. - - São Paulo : Artes Médicas, 2009.

Título original: Ciência endodôntica.
Vários colaboradores.
Obra em 2 v.
Bibliografia.
ISBN 978-85-367-0083-0

1. Endodontia I. Título.

08-10697 CDD-617.6342

Índices para catálogo sistemático:

1. Endodontia 617.6342

**Editora Artes Médicas Ltda.**

R. Dr. Cesário Motta Jr, 63 - Vila Buarque - 01221-020 - São Paulo - SP - Brazil

www.artesmedicas.com.br - artesmedicas@artesmedicas.com.br

Tel.: 55 11 3221-9033 - Fax: 55 11 3223-6635

# About the Author

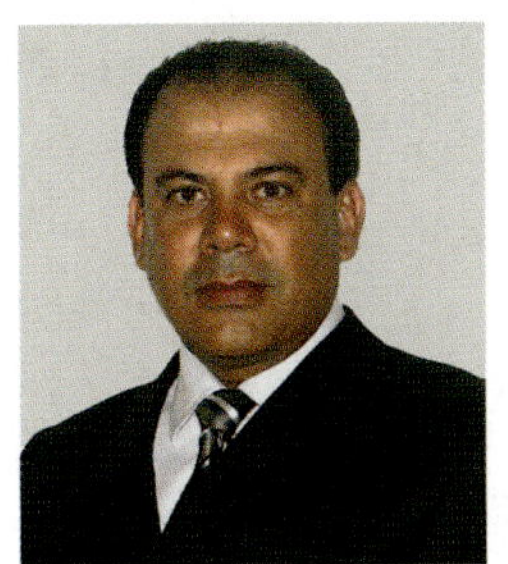


**CARLOS ESTRELA, DDS, MSc, PhD**

Chairman and Professor of Endodontics,
Department of Stomatologic Sciences
Federal University of Goiás, Goiânia, GO, Brazil


Carlos Estrela graduated from Dental School in 1983, in Anápolis, GO, Brazil, and specialized in Endodontics in 1988 from the Brazilian Dental Association in Goiania, GO, Brazil. He completed the MSc Course in Endodontology at the Federal University of Pelotas in 1990. He obtained his PhD in 1994, at the University of São Paulo, Brazil. In 1997 he obtained the position of Free Lecturer from the University of Sao Paulo, in Ribeirao Preto, SP, Brazil. Since 1993 he has taught at the Dental School of the Federal University of Goias, where he has served as Professor and Chairman of Endodontology since 1995. Dr Estrela has been published in the field of Endodontics and Dentistry, having authored 8 books in Dentistry in Portuguese, with 2 translated into Spanish and 1 currently being translated into English. He has published 130 papers in refereed journals and 130 chapters in books. He has lectured extensively in Brazil and Latin America, with more than 300 courses in Endodontics in different countries. He is the Coordinator of the Specialty Course in Endodontology of the Brazilian Dental Association of Goias, Brazil, since 1993. He participates in the Post-graduate Programs in Dentistry at the Masters and PhD levels of the Federal University of Goias and the Federal University of Uberlandia, in Brazil. He is a member of the Editorial Board of several journals in Dentistry, including the prestigious International Endodontic Journal. His areas of interest in research are Oral Microbiology, Endodontic irrigation and medication, Endodontic techniques and imaging related to the root canal system.

# Dedication

To Master Jesus, who showed us the importance of love, the need for faith, hope, charity, essential ingredients for excellence in life.

To all spiritual protectors and friends, for the affection, security, harmony and peace, factors that strengthened our emotions.

To my angels, and loves, gifts from Heaven – Cyntia, Lucas, Matheus, Maria Cristina and Pedro; my parents, Odilon and Maria, indispensable to my life.

To the eternal friend Hildeberto Francisco Pesce, for believing in the possibility of the invisible, coherence of the complex, to see the color of wind and time without space. Here it is my Master, thank you for existing, for walking with me and keeping our commitments.

To all estimated researchers, clinicians and friends who share the same scientific emotions, essential in building this book, my admiration, respect and great affection.

**Roberto Holland, DDS, MSc, PhD**
*Professor of Endodontics, São Paulo State University, Araçatuba, SP, Brazil*

**P. N. Ramachamdran Nair, BVSc, DVM, PhD, Senior Scientist**
*Institute of Oral Biology, Center of Dental and Oral Medicine,University of Zurich, Zurich, Switzerland*

**Carlos Alberto Souza Costa, DDS, MSc, PhD**
*Professor of Oral Pathology, São Paulo State University, Araraquara, SP, Brazil*

**José Antônio Poli de Figueiredo, DDS, MSc, PhD**
*Professor of Endodontics, Pontifical Catholic University of Rio Grande do Sul, Porto Alegre,RS, Brazil*

**Josimery Hebling, DDS, MSc, PhD**
*Professor of Pediatric Dentistry, São Paulo State University, Araraquara, SP, Brazil*

**Ana Helena G. Alencar, DDS, MSc, PhD**
*Professor of Endodontics, Federal University of Goiás, Goiânia, GO, Brazil*

**Sueli Satomi Murata, DDS, MSc, PhD**
*São Paulo State University, Araçatuba, SP, Brazil*

**Cyntia R.A. Estrela, DDS, MSc, PhD**
*Brazilian Dentistry Research and Learning Center, CEPOBRAS, Goiânia, GO, Brazil*

**Mike Reis Bueno, DDS, MSc, PhD**
*Professor of Diagnosis and Radiology, University of Cuiabá, Cuiabá, MT, Brazil*

**Lili Luesche Bammann, DDS, MSc, PhD**
*Professor of Microbiology, Federal University of Pelotas, Pelotas, RS, Brazil*

**Jesus Djalma Pécora, DDS, MSc, PhD**
*Professor of Endodontics, University of São Paulo, Ribeirão Preto, SP, Brazil*

**Paul M.H. Dummer, DDS, MSc, PhD**
*Department of Adult Dental Health, Dental School, Wales College of Medicine, Cardiff University, Cardiff, UK*

**Gilson Blitzkow Sydney, DDS, MSc, PhD**
*Professor of Endodontics, Federal University of Paraná, Curitiba, PR, Brazil*

**Hélio Pereira Lopes, DDS, MSc, PhD**
*Professor of Endodontics, Brazilian Endodontic Association, Rio de Janeiro, RJ, Brazil*

**Carlos Nelson Elias, DDS, MSc, PhD**
*Engeneering Military Institute, Rio de Janeiro, RJ, Brazil*

**Manoel Damião Sousa Neto DDS, MSc, PhD**
*University of São Paulo, Ribeirão Preto, SP, Brazil*

# Collaborators

**Lourdes Esponda, DDS, MSc**

*Professor of Endodontics, University of Mexico, MX, Mexico*

**Álvaro Gonzalez Cruz, DDS, MSc**

*Professor of Endodontics, University of Guadalajara, Jal, Mexico*

**João Carlos Gabrielli Biffi, DDS, MSc, PhD**

*Federal University of Uberlândia, Uberlândia, MG, Brazil*

**Marcelo Sampaio Moura, DDS, MSc, PhD**

*Brazilian Dentistry Research and Learning Center, CEPOBRAS, Goiânia, GO, Brazil*

**Maria Ilma de Souza Côrtes, DDS, MSc, PhD**

*Pontifical Catholic Uniersity of Minas Gerais, Belo Horizonte, MG, Brazil*

**Juliana Vilela Bastos, DDS, MSc, PhD**

*Federal University of Minas Gerais, Belo Horizonte, MG, Brazil*

**Pedro Felício Estrada Bernabé, DDS, MSc, PhD**

*São Paulo State University, Araçatuba, SP, Brazil*

**Elismauro Francisco de Mendonça, DDS, MSc, PhD**

*Professor of Oral Pathology, Federal University of Goiás, Goiânia, GO, Brazil*

**Daniel Almeida Decurcio, DDS, MSc**

*Professor of Endodontics, Federal University of Goiás, Goiânia, GO, Brazil*

**Aleimar Moraes Toledo, DDS, Fellow**

*Postgraduate Student, Federal University of Goiás, Goiânia, GO, Brazil*

**Cláudio Rodrigues Leles, DDS, MSc, PhD**

*Professor of Prosthesis, Federal University of Goiás, Goiânia, GO, Brazil*

**Júlio Almeida Silva, DDS, MSc**

*Professor of Endodontics, Federal University of Goiás, Goiânia, GO, Brazil*

**Luiz Augusto Faitaroni, DDS, Fellow**

*Brazilian Dentistry Research and Learning Center, CEPOBRAS, Goiânia, GO, Brazil*

**Orlando Aguirre Guedes, DDS, MSc**

*Professor of Endodontics, Federal University of Goiás, Goiânia, GO, Brazil*

**Welington Pereira Júnior, DDS, MSc**

*Brazilian Dentistry Research and Learning Center, CEPOBRAS, Goiânia, GO, Brazil*

**Sicknan S. Rocha, DDS, MSc, PhD**

*Professor of Prosthesis, Federal University of Goiás, Goiânia, GO, Brazil*

**João Batista de Souza, DDS, MSc, PhD**

*Professor of Oral Pathology, Federal University of Goiás, Goiânia, GO, Brazil*

**Adair Luiz Stefanello Busato, DDS, MSc, PhD**

*Professor of Operative Dentistry, Luteran University of Canoas, Canoas, RS, Brazil*

# Preface

It is with great satisfaction that we receive the publication of the book Endodontic Science, by Professor Carlos Estrela. His previous books were written either in Portuguese or in Spanish, with enormous impact in Latin America, particularly in Brazil. The book, now in English, makes his valuable knowledge reachable to a much wider readership. For a long time we have been following the scientific evolution of Professor Carlos Estrela. His original research contributions to endodontics and related areas have been extensive as can be judged through the numerous scientific publications appearing in a regular and sustained manner. This book not only draws heavily from his own reserves but also enriches itself through the support and participation of several reputed scientists and clinicians. The given guidelines of endodontic treatment are based on sound scientific works with clinical and histopathological confirmations that confers great strength and validity to the referred procedures. The Endodontic Science organizes the current knowledge on the principles and practice of endodontic treatment in a very didactic mode with the highest available level of evidence. Therefore, we feel very comfortable and confidant to recommend this valuable work in endodontology to students and colleagues who strive for excellence in research, teaching and patient-care.

**Roberto Holland**

*Department of Endodontics, School of Dentistry*
*São Paulo State University São Paulo, Brazil*

**P. N. Ramachandran Nair**

*Institute of Oral Biology School of Dental & Oral*
*Medicine University of Zurich, Switzerland*

Endodontic Science was built from knowledge based on scientific evidences, analyzed from the perspective of reflection, scientific evidence, and a hard work of researchers, clinicians and idealists.

The primary focus of the study was to bring scientific knowledge for the best use of endodontic materials and techniques in different clinical conditions. The magnum regent, the host, was extremely valuable, not only from the perspective of the application of a material or technique for the treatment of the injured tooth, but the context was based on the scientific process of the real state of healing.

The study and understanding of the knowledge of endodontic science transcends the particular knowledge of the material principle, which, in particular, requires the knowledge of the vital principle. Understanding mechanisms of action and reaction is essential to the knowledge of the factors involved in the processes of disease and healing. The biological mechanisms related to the aggression factors and defense of the host, identify the existence of the vital principle, which is the major impetus to the study of endodontic natural structures and their characteristics.

Several challenges have been met with levels of complexity proportional to their sizes. The first dimension (the empirism), involving all new procedures, lack a standard of basic science. The second dimension consisted of images of oral structures in two dimensions. In the third dimension, we move in depth, we began to imagine all the best in several senses. With the fourth dimension we valued even more microscopic structures, allowing more secure procedures. The fifth dimension favored the mysteries of pain, essential to the healing procedures. Well, the sixth dimension is still the challenge, as it rules all the events and the balance of the essential human phenomenon.

The scientific learning should overcome the practical operational limits, besides requiring the privilege of clinical manifestations, the biological aspects that govern them. Clinically we cannot see the microscopic beings (cells, microorganisms) that monitor the organic responses, but it is necessary to understand them for the best treatment.

# Challenges of Endodontic Science

Endodontic Science aims to offer endodontic expressive essence of the knowledge of biological events related to the phenomena of aggression and healing. Therefore, it reflects the incessant search of the most appropriate treatment options for the moment, using biological bases from significant scientific evidences.

Thus, if we knew all the answers of life, the work would make no sense. If we knew fully the science of health, the disease would make no sense. If we knew how to heal the wound, pain would not be felt. The work, the disease and the pain, are strong reasons to struggle for evolution and indicates our limitations in science.

I thank all researchers and teachers who worked in this book, the editor of Artes Medicas, Mr. Milton Hecht, the entire support staff in the person of Renata Bertaco, and their confidence and professionalism in the conduct of this book, which content sought to reflect science.

**Carlos Estrela**

# Contents

# Pulpal Biology

**C. A. S. Costa**
*University of São Paulo State, UNESP, Araraquara, SP, Brazil*

**J. A. P. Figueiredo**
*Pontifical Catholic University of Rio Grande do Sul, PUCRS, Porto Alegre, RS, Brazil*

**J. Hebling**
*University of São Paulo State, UNESP, Araraquara, SP, Brazil*

**C. Estrela**
*Federal University of Goiás, Goiânia, GO, Brazil*

Chapter contents

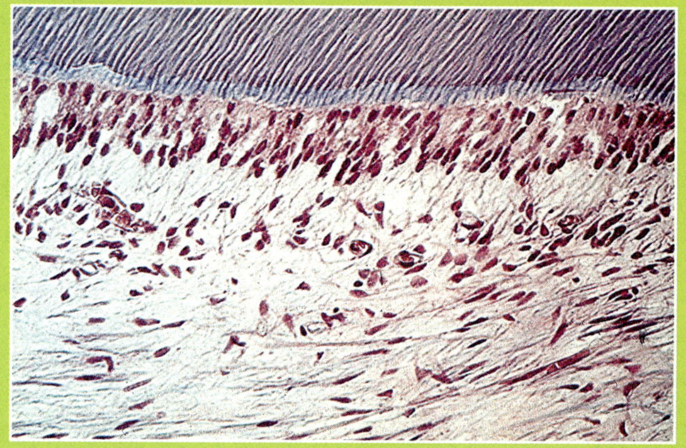

Coronary pulp surrounded by a mineralized dentin wall.

## 1.1 Introduction

The dental pulp can be defined as a specialized loose connective tissue, of mesenchymal origin, surrounded by dentin walls, occupying the pulpal chamber and the root canal. The specialization of the pulp's connective tissue is due to the cells located on its periphery, odontoblasts, which are responsible for the synthesis and deposition of the dentin's organic matrix, which is further mineralized around the pulp tissue. This interdependence of the dentin and pulp indicates that these tissues must be understood and recognized as integrants of the same complex, termed the dentin-pulp complex (Fig. 1.1A-B). Events that happen on the dentin reverberate to the pulp, and vice versa. The existence of a system of dentinal tubules, as well as the signaling that occurs within the pulpal extracellular matrix, influences the formation of dentin by the odontoblasts. These aspects have assumed increasing importance in recent publications involved with this complex.

The dentin-pulp complex is surrounded on the crown by dental enamel and on the root by cementum, periodontal ligament and bone. The harmony of the complex is impaired if the surrounding tissues suffer some kind of injury or change in stasis, that can reach the pulp by the root canal or dentinal tubules. On the other hand, pulpal pathologies of inflammatory or degenerative nature can impair the surrounding tissues. The purpose of this chapter is to educate readers concerning the characteristics of the dentin-pulp complex, its development, structure and function. This education allows for a discussion of the diagnosis of pulpal alterations and the pulpal healing potential against different kind of stimuli, which are presented in future chapters.

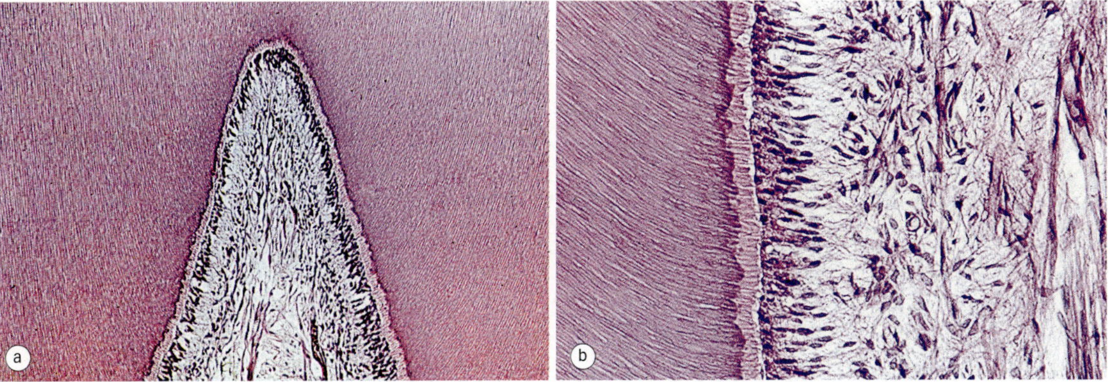


**Figure 1.1** - Dentin-pulp complex. (**A**) Note that the pulpal connective tissue is surrounded by dentin. (**B**) Details of the previous figure (**A**), where the integration of the dentin with the pulp, creating the dentin-pulp complex, is observed.

## 1.2 Formation of the Dentin-Pulp Complex

From the expression of several morphogenetic proteins (among them BMP2 and BMP4) in sites of the oral epithelium that will originate the dental organ, epithelium cells proliferate on the dental lamina (phase of initiation). Around these proliferation sites are condensed ectomesenchymal cells, which are descendant of the neural tube. These cells have an increased ability of proliferation, mobilization and differentiation. The morphogenetic phase involves the stages of sprout, casque (cap) and initial bell phase. During this period, the number of ectomesenchymal cells adjacent to the epithelium increases inside the ectomesenchyma, producing the site of origin for the dental papilla and the dental follicle, which will develop into the dentin-pulp complex and the support tissues of the tooth, respectively. The formation of the enamel knot, during the transition from sprout to cap, marks the start of the crown formation. This is because the cells of the enamel knot do not grow, but serve to signal the cuspid formation pattern, influencing the form of the crown and the development of the dental papilla. During the initial bell phase, the epithelium is modified to characterize the enamel organ, also known as the dental organ. This dental organ is formed into different stratums (internal dental epithelium, intermediate stratum, stellate reticulum and external dental epithelium). Therefore, while cuboidal epithelium cells are organized into one layer to become the external dental epithelium, a unique layer of low cylindrical cells characterizes into the internal dental epithelium. It is also possible to determine the papilla and the dental follicle during this period of development. However, the structure of the dental germ of interest for the formation of the dentin-pulp complex is the internal epithelium of the enamel organ.

The internal epithelium of the enamel organ interacts reciprocally with the undifferentiated mesenchymal cells (also known as embryonic cells) of the dental papilla, characterizing the interaction of epithelium and mesenchyma, which essentially forms the enamel, dentin and pulp. In the internal dental epithelium, the cells related to the future cuspids become highly columnar, starting the late bell stage (phase of cytodifferentiation). This modification of the internal epithelium cells serve as a signal, through the basal membrane, for where the products of secretion of the epithelium cells are released (TGF-(β)1, BMP2, IGF, among others) in such manner that the most peripheral cells of the dental papilla becomes elongated. These cells organized subjacent to the basement membrane are termed odontoblasts. This phenomenon, characterized as differentiation of odontoblasts, has currently been deeply studied, resulting in important advances in the knowledge of pulpal biology related with the mechanisms of reparation of this highly specialized connective tissue.

It is important to know the basic process of differentiation of the superficial undifferentiated mesenchymal cells from the dental papilla by stimuli expressed by cells of the internal dental epithelium. Growth factors, particularly those belonging to the super family TGF(β) are expressed by epithelial cells. While the mesenchymal cells of the most superficial region of the dental papilla acquire competency, the last mitosis of the mother cell positions it adjacent to the basal membrane. The daughter cell remains in a more internal area of the papilla, where it will make part of the cell-rich zone of the pulp. Both mother and daughter cells are then referred to as pre-odontoblasts, because both assume the competency to differentiate in odontoblasts. Among the cells of the internal dental epithelium and the pre-odontoblasts is the basal membrane, which is composed of type I collagen, laminin, heparan sulfate and other proteoglycans. This basal membrane assumes an important role in the reciprocal activation of the epithelium/mesenchyma, resulting in a variety and diversity of epigenetic interactions, determining, in a particular way, the phenotype of the odontoblasts. After the epithelial cells secrete the growth factors of the TGF(β) family, these bioactive proteins remain attached to the basal membrane. The components of the basal membrane activate these TGFs to interact with membrane receptors of the pre-odontoblasts. The translation of these signals results in the activation of the pre-odontoblasts, which start to secrete more growth factors and express the *msxs* genes. During a period of up-regulation of the TGFs, the pre-odontoblasts start to synthesize fibronectin and express the membrane protein 165KDa, which is required to interact with this fibronectin. The *msxs* homeoproteins seem to be involved in the reorganization of the pre-odontoblast cytoskeleton, which play an important role in the process of differentiating into elongated cells, referred to as odontoblasts. Nevertheless, the final differentiation of the pre-odontoblasts to odontoblasts occurs only after the interaction of the fibronectin, which is deposited on the basal membrane, and the 165KDa receptors. The translation of the signals from the 165KDa/fibronectin complex directs the reorganization of the pre-odontoblastic cytoskeleton (microtubules, intermediate filaments and microfilaments), allowing its elongation and nucleus polarization. Then, the nucleus assuming a basal position, while the rough endoplasmic reticulum is relocated parallel to the long axis of the cell. After reorganization, the elongated cells start the synthesis and deposition of the first dentinal matrix, composed principally of type I collagen, proteoglycans (decorin and biglycan), in addition to the secretion of noncollagenous proteins, such as bone sialoprotein, dentin sialoprotein, osteocalcin, phosphorin, osteopontin, osteonectin and others. The functional odontoblasts start to exhibit intercellular junctions. These odontoblasts, during dentinal matrix apposition, moves centripetally to the dental papilla, leaving behind them the cytoplasmic prolongations, which remain inside the dentinal matrix, determining the tubular characteristic of this tissue. The sequence of differentiation of the mesenchymal cells of the dental papilla into odontoblasts until the beginning of the synthesis and deposition of dentinal matrix is demonstrated in Figure 1.2.

It has been reported that odontoblasts synthesize the dentinal organic matrix in two levels: 1) proximal deposition, where the secretion of the matrix occurs adjacent to the cellular body and 2) adjacent to the mineralization *fronts*. The mineralization process is also dependent on the odontoblasts, because these release vesicles containing phospholipids and alkaline phosphatase, from produce the hydroxyapatite crystals. The dentin matrix mineralization is heterogeneous, by globular calcification, resulting in *fronts* of mineralization, or calcospherites. With continuous growth, the crystals (secondary mineralization) tend to fuse themselves, forming a mineralized mass around the odontoblastic prolongations, providing the dentin a tubular aspect (system of dentinal tubules). The portion of the papilla that is involved with dentin becomes the dental pulp. According to Figueiredo & Mezzomo[13], the dentin is a daughter of the pulp, existing interdependently from its origination. The odontoblasts form the dentin, but depend on it to become pulp. The direction of the odontoblasts is towards the center, in relation to the dental pulp, and the decrease of the internal space favors a curved path of these cells. Once the first layer of dentin is formed, the cells of the internal epithelium (pre-ameloblasts) differentiate into ameloblasts and start to produce the enamel organic matrix, which becomes mineralized almost instantaneously. As dentin is formed, the most cervical cells of the internal epithelium of the enamel organ become pre-ameloblasts, an event that occurs from the incisal (or from cuspids) to the cervical area. When the dentin formation approximates the cervical loop, the cells of internal and external epithelium of the enamel organ proliferate from the loop, forming a double layer of cells, also known as Hertwig's epithelial root sheath. The expansion of the sheath is followed by the formation of the radicular dentin. The cells of the dental follicle closer to the external layer of the sheath differentiate into cementoblasts and start to produce the cementum organic matrix; the follicle also produces the periodontal ligament and alveolar bone. There is a free border on the epithelial sheath, the epithelial diaphragm, which closes slowly as the root is formed (Fig. 1.3). The scanning electronic microscopy images below (Fig. 1.4A-F) represent a sequence of roots in different phases of radicular closure.

As long as the apex of the root is not totally formed, there will be dental papilla, composed of ectomesenchymal cells (descendant from the neural tube). This has clinical relevance, because these cells can remain viable, even if there is pulpal necrosis and, in these cases, it is possible to have apexigenesis, or the formation of the radicular apex with dentin. When there is a reduction in the number of ectomesenchymal cells, the tooth can still have apexification, induced by an intracanal dressing that forms a hard tissue through calcic degeneration. Teeth that have undergone induced apexification are less resistant to normal forces and can fracture easier than those that had their apex formed through apexigenesis.



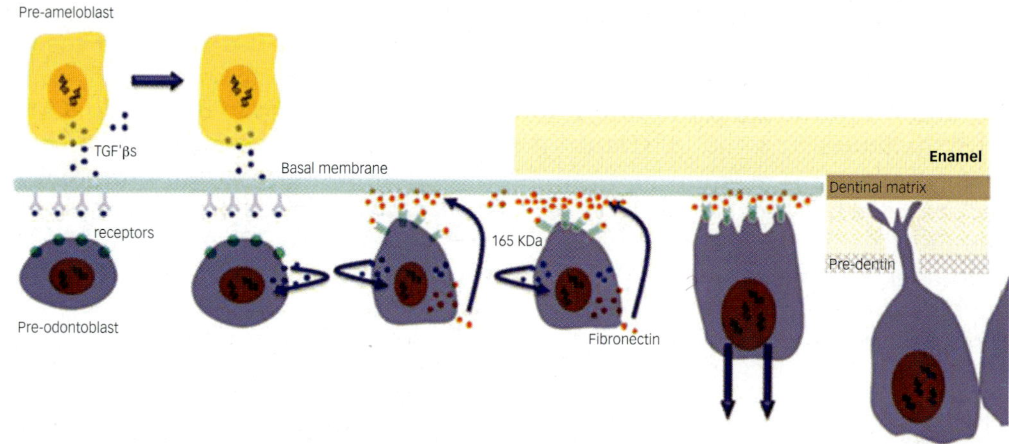


**Figure 1.2** - Mechanism by which the pulpal mesechymal cells present in the periphery of the dental papilla are differentiated in odontoblasts. Adapted from Ruch et al.[22], 1995 (J. Hebling, 2008).

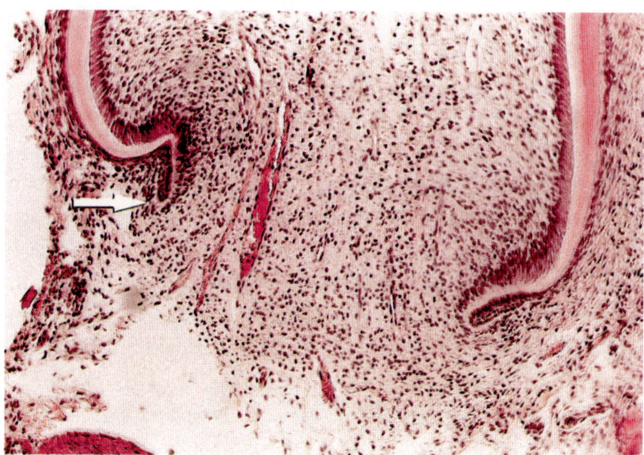

**Figure 1.3** - Histological aspect of the formation of the apex. Hertwig's sheath, involved by ecto-mesenchymal cells of the papilla, can be seen on the left. (Courtesy Prof. Roberto Holland, 2008).

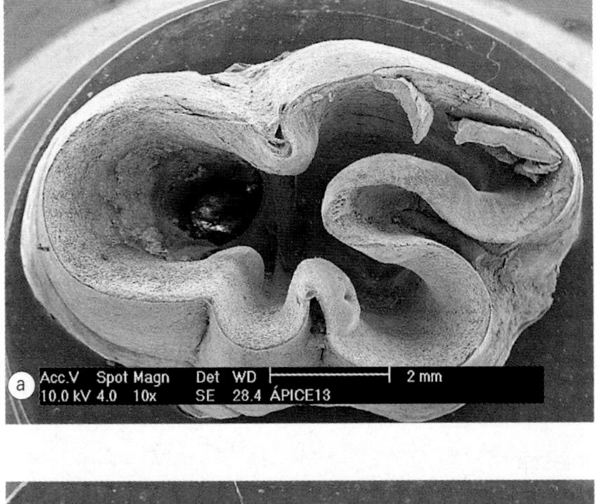


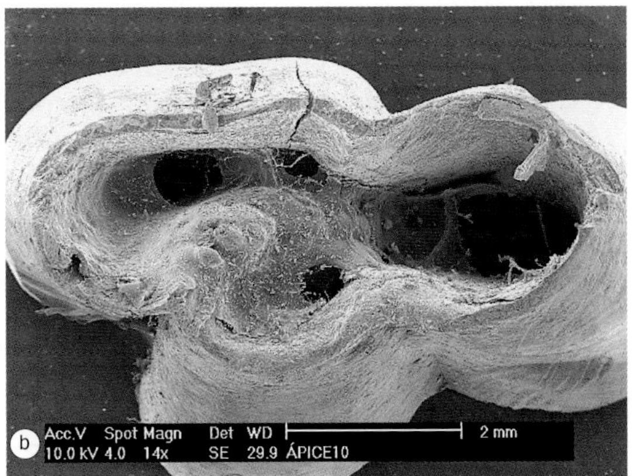


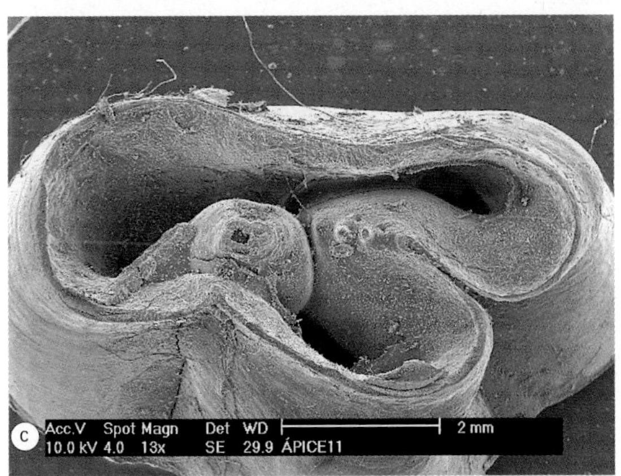


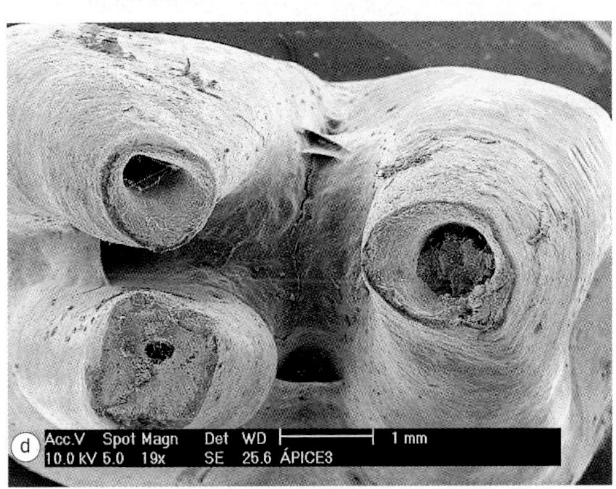


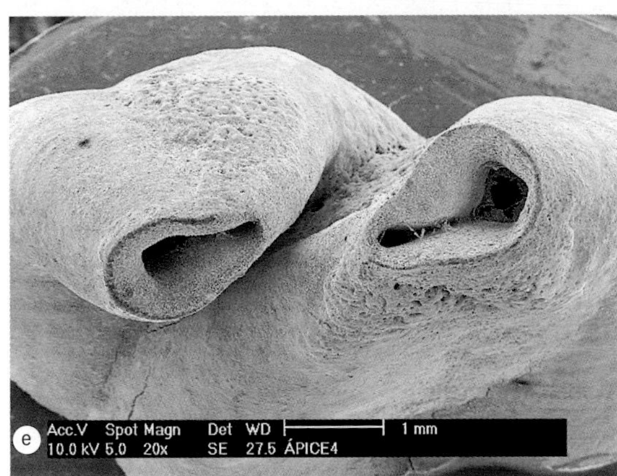


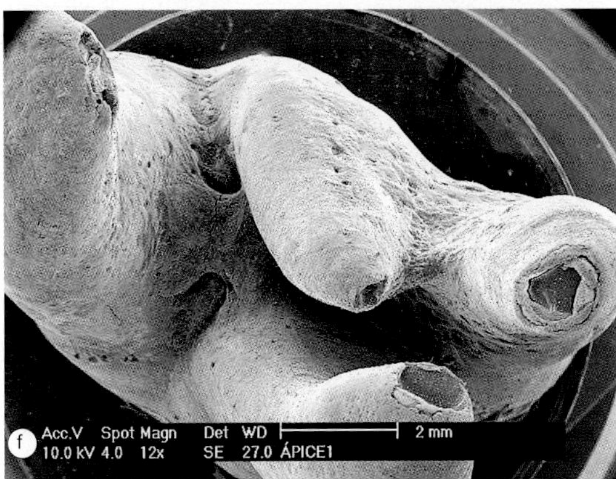


**Figure 1.4** - (**A-F**) Sequence of roots at different phases of radicular closure.

## 1.3 Dental Pulp

Dental pulp is composed of specialized loose connective tissue. What makes dental pulp unique is that it is confined between rigid walls of a tissue that it produced. This development produces the ability of dental pulp to communicate with the external environment of the tooth through apical foramens and foraminas, as well as lateral canals. This provides the pulp with an environment of low tolerance because the nutritional substratum comes from the vascularization that passes through the small foramens and foraminas.

In general, loose connective tissue is distributed throughout the human organism, serving as stroma (nutritional tissue) for organs and functional tissues (parenchyma). In the pulp, this loose connective tissue is stroma and parenchyma at the same time, because this tissue sustains itself and dentin, while also possessing a high functional activity, when producing dentin. With this production of dentin, the pulp encloses itself on the central portion of the tooth, having a coronary portion and a radicular portion (Fig. 1.5A). In monoradicular teeth, coronary pulp and radicular pulp are contiguous. However, in bi- or multiradicular teeth, the floor of the pulp chamber has a more clear distinction. The coronary pulp is richer in cells and extracellular matrix, while the radicular pulp has more fibers and the vascular-nervous sheath is more concentrated, with less anastomosis. According to Avery[1], the pulp chamber acts as a conduction tube that carries the blood to and from the tooth in the direction of the apical canal. The pulp can be divided into four zones: cell-rich, acellular, odontoblastic (a highly organized zone) and central. The central zone contains larger arterioles and venules, the nervous trunks, fibroblasts and the extracellular matrix, which all work to nourish the pulp. At the periphery, there are the cell-rich, acellular, and odontoblastic zones. The odontoblastic zone is a pulp area of high cellular activity which responds to external stimuli. The parietal nerve plexus emits terminations that cross the acellular zone and associate themselves with the odontoblasts (Fig. 1.5B).

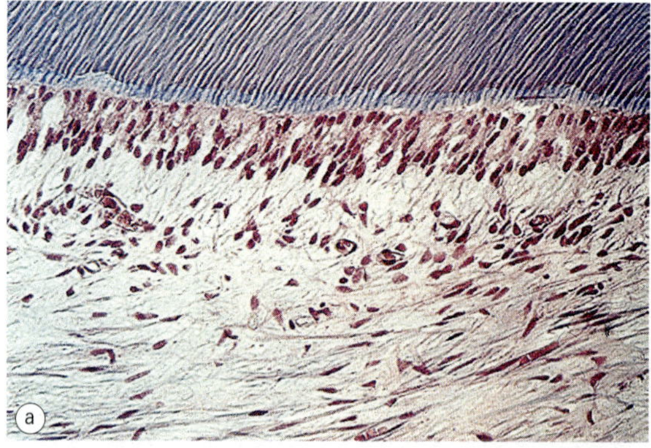


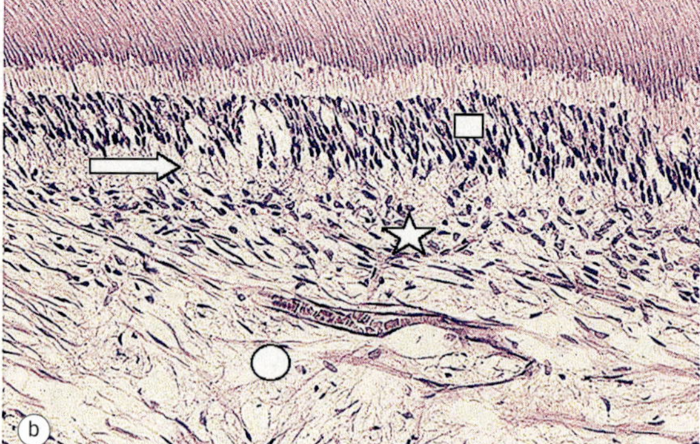


**Figure 1.5** - (**A**) Coronary pulp surrounded by a mineralized dentin wall. (**B**) The dentin, predentin, odontoblastic zone (*), acellular zone (arrow), cell-rich zone (*), and central part of the pulp tissue (*) can be observed.

### 1.3.1 Extracellular matrix of the dental pulp

As early as two decades ago, there was little importance given to the extracellular matrix of the dental pulp. Advances in molecular biology have contributed to the perception that the function of the dental pulp goes beyond its activity of nourishment. The structural proteins of dental pulp actively participate in pulpal events and the expression of dental pulp, either increasing or decreasing, determines its ability to react. The main constituents of this tissue are proteins and the fundamental substance. Collagen is the main organic component of the dental pulp, which is developed from a triple chain of molecules of tropocollagen. The collagen alpha chains represent different compositions and sequences of amino acids. The main types of collagen in pulp are type I and type III. Type I collagen is mainly responsible for the pulpal architecture. It is important to note that the odontoblasts also produce type I collagen; however, the collagen of the pulp is exclusively synthesized by fibroblasts, while the production of the dentinal matrix is the responsibility of the odontoblasts. Type III collagen, the main component of the reticular fibers, is located in the central pulp and serves as a skeleton for the structures that exist there (vessels, nerves etc.). Type III collagen is very well distributed in the cell-rich and acellular zones, providing support and elasticity to these pulp areas. Yet, type V and VI collagen form a mesh on the stroma of the pulpal connective tissue, with type VI being one of the components of the basal membrane of the pulpal capillaries.

Several noncollagenous proteins can be found in the dental pulp. Elastin, produced by fibroblasts and by cells of the vascular smooth muscle and endothelium, has hydrophobic alternated domains, rich in lysine. The elastin molecules connect to form a disorderly spiral that expands and contracts, providing elasticity to tissues. Additionally, the peptides for elastin are chemotactic for monocytes and fibroblasts[23]. Fibronectin is a glycoprotein of the extracellular matrix that presents itself as a protein of the circulating plasma (pFN), where it is produced by hepatocytes, or as a tissue protein (cFN), where it is produced by many cells, such as fibroblasts, epithelial cells and the majority of mesenchymal cells. Fibronectin, a tissue protein, is present in a glycosylated form and is part of the matrix as insoluble fibrils. The most studied role of fibronectin, adhesion to the cellular surface, is performed by a non-glycosylated form that can be phosphorylated and have sulfur added. In the central pulp, fibronectin is distributed as a net and is concentrated closer to the blood capillaries. In the odontoblastic layer, fibronectin is in a spiral form, and seems to mediate the interaction between the odontoblasts and the matrix fibers, in addition to maintaining the specific morphology of these cells. Fibronectin binds cells to the collagen, promotes the migration of embryonic cells and regulates cellular growth and genic expression. It is associated with the repair of the pulpal connective tissue, as well as the formation of repairing dentin. Fibronectin is recognized by most cells through integrins that are receptors for matrix proteins. Laminin and nidogen are proteins related with the organization and structure of the basal membrane. They interact to form non-covalent stable complexes, contributing to intercellular adhesion, mediated by the integrins. Laminin promotes the insertion, migration and proliferation of endothelial cells. Many other proteins of the matrix are observed in the pulp, such as osteonectin, osteopontin, osteocalcin and sialoprotein. The specific functions of these proteins on the pulpal organ are not well defined. It is important to understand the presence of certain proteins and their role in specific areas. In order to have activity of these proteins, mediation of the cell-cell and cell-matrix interactions is necessary. This mediation is performed by the receptors of the cellular surface. Among these receptors, integrins are the most known and studied. They consist of heterodimer proteins, such as alpha and beta sub-units, located on the cellular membranes of mammals. Integrins have a short segment that crosses the cytoplasmic membrane and a long segment that extends into the extracellular space. Cellular signaling by integrins, mediated by ions such as calcium and magnesium, favors several events, like the deposition and maturation of the organic matrix, fibroblastic adhesion, diapedesis and migration of leucocytes, interactions of macrophage-T cells, migration of epithelial cells, coagulation, formation of mineralized tissue, etc.

Glycosaminoglycans and the proteoglycans are other important components of the pulpal extracellular matrix. Glycosaminoglycans, the main carbohydrates that make up proteoglycans, are composed of repeated disaccharide units of uronic acid and hexosamine (except keratan sulfate, which has D-galactose instead of uronic acid). The glycosaminoglycans that compose proteoglycans are all sulfated. Hyaluronic acid is not sulfated and does not bind to proteins. It is synthesized by most of the cells and has several functions, among which are hydration, aggregation with other components of the matrix, cellular migration, development of the tissues and interaction of the cellular surface with the matrix. The ability of hyaluronic acid to bind to calcium is important in making calcium phosphate available during the mineralization of dentin. The other glycosaminoglycans, chondroitin sulphate, dermatan sulphate, heparan sulphate, heparin and keratan sulphate, are distributed in the matrix and act in distinct and coordinated ways. They have affinity to the collagen and influence fibrinogenesis, which occurs prior to mineralization. In addition, these participate in the polarization of odontoblasts. Proteoglycans are extensive glycoproteins, are highly anionic and are present in all of the connective tissues. They are composed of a simple protein nucleus that binds to one or more lateral chains of glycosaminoglycans. Proteoglycans make a portion of the structural component of the matrix and are directly related to hydration, regulation of collagen production, adhesion and maintenance of growth factors, cellular adhesion, cellular growth and differentiation. They are divided into three distinct groups: matrix organizers and tissue space fillers (agrecan, versican, perlecan - larger proteoglycans; biglican, decorin - smaller proteoglycans); proteoglycans of cellular surface that promote the environment necessary for the adhesion of the cells to the matrix (sindecan, CD44); and the intracellular proteoglycans of the hematopoietic cells. Water and mineral salts are the other components of the matrix that participate in the nutrition and diffusion of the elements essential to tissue homeostasis. With the previously mentioned components, the matrix has a gel aspect, with a viscous consistency, serving as a barrier to the dissemination of microorganisms and toxic products[26]. This gel state can be altered with maturing or with etiologic factors of pulpal alterations.

### 1.3.2 Microcirculation of the dental pulp

The vascularization of the dental pulp is better defined as pulpal microcirculation, because the pulp does not have arteries or veins. Arterioles, from the arteries of the apical periodontium, enter the central pulp through the apical foramen and foraminas, as well as the lateral canals. The arterioles form several lateral anastomoses as they get closer to the odontoblastic layer. Each time that the arterioles split, they become smaller, forming a rich surface capillary plexus that provides a rich source of metabolites. In the sub-odontoblastic region, the capillaries are fenestrated, favoring rapid diffusion of nutrients and hormones to the odontoblasts and the cell-rich zone. The return flow of the microcirculation has the capillaries converging to venules that become larger as they leave the central zone of the dental pulp. The venules exit through the apical foramen and foraminas, merging with the veins of the apical periodontium. The pulpal arterioles and venules have very thin walls with their endothelial cells slightly distant one from another. This allows increased microcirculation, with the passage of metabolites from the arterioles to the cells and extracellular matrix and the flow of catabolites from the extracellular environment to the venules. There are arteriovenous anastomoses within the pulp that favor pulpal microcirculation. In addition, these anastomoses remove blood from areas of pulpal injury, where the damage can result in thrombosis or hemorrhage. The terminal arterioles have segments of smooth muscle that serve as pre-capillary sphincters. Under stimuli, such as a response to localized inflammatory process, these can act as functional units that perform localized changes to the blood flow, providing differentiated circulatory conditions to the adjacent regions. In other words, the increase of pressure and the consequent events of a localized lesion do not disseminate for all the pulpal tissue (Fig. 1.6A-B).

The area with the greatest amount of circulatory activity is on the surface of the pulp, through the blood capillaries. These regulate the transportation and diffusion of substances, because the capillary walls work as a semi-permeable membrane. Additionally, as a result to stimuli, the "germination" of capillaries at the site of irritation occurs (Fig. 1.6C-E). This "germination" is the activation of inactive capillaries that were already present, guaranteeing a greater efficiency of the local inflammatory process, propitiating a localized immune response to preserve the residual pulp. The lymphatic circulation follows the route of the venous circulation, except that the lymphatic circulation starts at the pulp's periphery, moves towards the central zone, aiding the venules with draining catabolites. The lymphatic capillaries do not have basal membranes or fenestrations on the endothelial cells. This favors the removal of high molecular weight solutes. In the cellular zone, the lymphatic capillaries are like blind holes, emptying in the periapex, where collecting vessels drain the lymph through the periodontal ligament to the regional lymph nodes.

### 1.3.3 Pulpal innervation

Dental pulp is one of the most innerved tissues. The nerves enter the pulp via the apical foramen, following the arterioles and, similarly, make anastomosis from the center zone to the periphery, resulting in a rich plexus of nerves near the odontoblastic layer. The parietal layer of nerves, also known as the Raschkow plexus, is located near the cell-rich zone. Byers et al.[7] verified that the nerve terminals penetrate the pre-dentin and the deeper layers of dentin. This configuration has importance for the reactions of dentinal sensitivity. It is understood that the pulp is an organ of sensation, able to transmit stimuli for the central nervous system. Independent of the nature of the stimulus, thermal, mechanic, or other, the reaction will be pain, which is the "language" that the pulp uses to manifest alterations in its behavior. The innervation of the pulp is both afferent (sensation), from the trigeminal nerve, or autonomic, regulating microcirculation and the speed of the dentinogenesis.

There are at least six types of afferent neurons that innervate the pulp: A(β), A(δ)-f (fast), polimodal A(δ)-s (slow), C-nociceptive, C - regulated by the neurotrophic factor derived from the glia, C - polimodal nociceptive. These neuron types should be considered as the "state of art" on this area of knowledge, because the nervous fibers are dynamic and continuously adjust their association with the pulp and dentin. Each afferent neuron has a cellular body on the trigeminal ganglion, several central synaptic terminations and a long peripheral axon that is directed to a nerve in the pulpal tissue, where it branches. The terminations of A(β) and A(δ) are myelinated and are the main constituents of the parietal layer of nerves and extend into the acellular zone, odontoblastic layer, pre-dentin and dentin. The A(β) fibers are of medium size and are the most sensitive to hydrodynamic stimuli from the dentin. The A(δ) fibers are of small

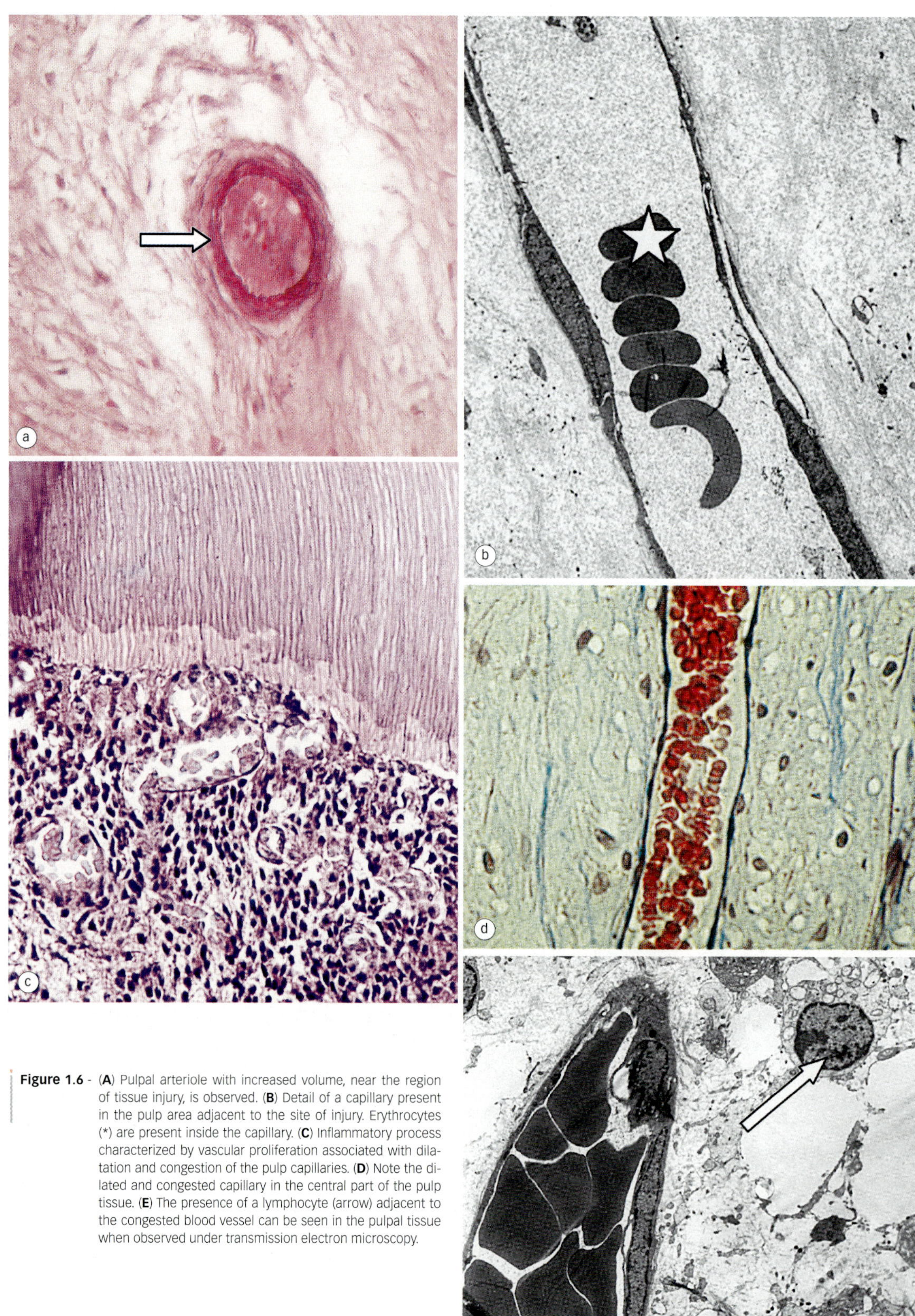

**Figure 1.6** - (**A**) Pulpal arteriole with increased volume, near the region of tissue injury, is observed. (**B**) Detail of a capillary present in the pulp area adjacent to the site of injury. Erythrocytes (*) are present inside the capillary. (**C**) Inflammatory process characterized by vascular proliferation associated with dilatation and congestion of the pulp capillaries. (**D**) Note the dilated and congested capillary in the central part of the pulp tissue. (**E**) The presence of a lymphocyte (arrow) adjacent to the congested blood vessel can be seen in the pulpal tissue when observed under transmission electron microscopy.

size, very numerous on the surface of the coronary pulp, responsible for fast conduction stimuli (except for the A(δ) polimodal fibers, which are slow conducting and are found in a small quantity in the pulp) and are generally related to the hyper-reactive pulpalgias. Type C fibers, found in the central pulp with some branching on the surface, are unmyelinated. They are responsible for slow conduction stimuli and are used in inflammatory events, especially with symptomatic pulpitis.

All of the pulpal nervous fibers have membrane specific receptors for chemical signaling with neighbor cells. Byers[5] reported some of the agents involved in neuro-pulpal interactions:

- neuronal agents that affect the pulpal cells and the blood vessels: sensorial neuropeptides (CGRP, substance P, neuroquinine A, somatostatine, galanine)
- dentinal agents, pulpal vascular or immune agents that affect the function of the dental nerves (specific molecules for odontoblasts) - there are at least 130 classes, including:
  - neurotrophic factors - NGF, BDNF, GDNF
  - inflammation mediators - serotonin, histamine, bradicinin, prostaglandins, cytocins
  - products of the cellular destruction - ATP, cyclooxygenase, oxidative radicals
  - altered pH and its excitation or inhibition of molecular functions
  - shock proteins to heat
  - somatostatin and endocrine factors
  - antinoceptive agents - opioid peptides, canabinoids, adhenosin
  - factors of extracellular matrix - laminin, metalloproteases
  - ionic environment
  - oxygen tension
  - fluid pressures
- neuronal factors that the pulp expresses:
  - neurotensin, nestine, PGP 9.5
  - precursors and receptors for taquinine
  - receptors of neurotrophin - tirosin quinase A, p75
  - neurotrophins - NGF, BDNF, GDNF; nitric oxide

In a recent study[30], nervous fibers and odontoblasts were observed that were mutually influenced for the pulpal activity levels. This interactive environment enables the dentin-pulp complex to react to stimuli, or harm, by using numerous neuronal responses, principally in primary odontoblasts. Thus, as with vascularization, the pulp reacts to the harm from the external environment with the "germination" of nerve terminations after the depletion of neuropeptides that are liberated inside the pulpal tissue. The intensity and duration of the events depend of the severity of the associated lesion.

#### 1.3.4 Cells of the dental pulp

The main pulpal cells can be divided into four groups: defense cells, ectomesenchymal cells, fibroblasts and odontoblasts. The defense cells are elements that migrate to the dental pulp. They are recruited from the bloodstream at the moment that strange agents are found in the pulpal connective tissue. These defense cells interact to create mechanisms that help to defend the tissue from the antigenic invasion. The T lymphocytes are the cells most frequently found in normal pulp. They are predominantly found near the blood vessels of the central pulp, participating in cellular immunity, producing cytotoxins and interacting with other defense cells, when necessary. The B lymphocytes and plasma cells, which participate in the synthesis of immunoglobulins (antibodies), are rare in the normal pulp. Macrophages, constituents of the mononuclear phagocytic system, are found in the pulp as histiocytes, near the blood vessels and capillaries. Macrophages, which contain several lysosomes, participate in processes of phagocythosis of cellular debris and irritants to the pulp, cytotoxins and growth factors while also present antigens for other defense cells. The follicular dendritic cells contribute to the cellular defense by capturing antigens of the pulp and migrating them to the regional lymph nodes, where memory T lymphocytes, specific for the antigen, are produced and taken to the pulp. Upon a subsequent attack of the same antigen, the macrophages and dendritic cells present the antigen to the memory T lymphocytes, initiating the production phase of the immune responses. Neutrophils and eosinophils unite with the other defense cells. Their number increases when the inflammatory process is initiated or when there is a bacterial invasion (Fig. 1.7A-C).

Ectomesenchymal cells are principally in the cell-rich zone of the pulp tissue (Fig. 1.8A-C). Descending from the neural tube, these cells have a great ability for cellular differentiation and mobilization. The cellular types that they differentiate to in the pulp are fibroblasts and odontoblasts. When there is death of odontoblasts, the ectomesenchymal cells support themselves on the dead tracts of dentin and transform into new odontoblasts, referred to as odontoblastoids. The ectomesenchymal cells in the pulp are not replaced, or in other words, once differentiated, their cellular population decreases. This differentiation decreases the regenerative potential of the pulp over time and with repetition of harmful stimuli to the pulp. Fibroblasts are the most numerous cells of the pulp, principally in the central pulp. They are responsible for the formation of the fibers and structural proteins of the extracellular matrix of the dental pulp (Fig. 1.8). Types I and III of collagen and noncollagenous proteins, already described, are among the products secreted by fibroblasts. Depending of the functional state of the pulp, typically with age, fibroblasts change their morphology based on the quantity of cytoplasmic organelles, rough endoplasmic reticulum, Golgi complex and mitochondria. Similar to fibroblasts found in other parts of the human, fibroblasts of the pulp present the ability to degrade collagen. They have lysosomal enzymes specific to collagen fibrils which produce metalloproteases that have the ability to degrade the macromolecules of the matrix, such as the collagen and proteoglycans (Fig. 1.8A-C).

Odontoblasts, specific pulpal cells, are responsible for the synthesis of the organic matrix of dentin. They coat the perimeter of the dental pulp, developing elongations, around which the dentin is formed, with some lateral elongations. They are columnar at the tips of the pulpal horns, decreasing in size as they approach the cervical region, becoming cuboidal on the root and flattened on the radicular apex (Fig. 1.9A-F). The modification of the form ensures the functional activity of the odontoblasts, which are more active on the coronary portion than on the radicular portion. Joined strongly by junctional complexes (occludent zone, *gap* junctions, and intermediate junctions) and desmosomes, the organization of the odontoblasts resembles pseudo-stratified epithelium. The activity of the odontoblasts is variable. They are more active during the initial stages of primary dentin formation and less active when finished with the formation of primary dentin. Prior to a stimulus, these odontoblasts maintain the production of secondary dentin, which is slowly deposited. Non-physiologic stimuli, such as the development of a caries lesion, heat to the dentin due to aggressive cavity preparation, use of toxic materials in deep cavities and others, result in the increase of odontoblast activity, initiating the deposition of tertiary dentin. This tertiary dentin is classified as reactionary and reparative. When active, the odontoblasts exhibit well developed rough endoplasmic reticulum and Golgi complex, many mitochondria and secretory vesicles. The active odontoblasts synthesize type I and III collagen, proteoglycans, bone and dentinal sialoproteins, phosphorin, osteocalcin, osteonectin and osteopontin.

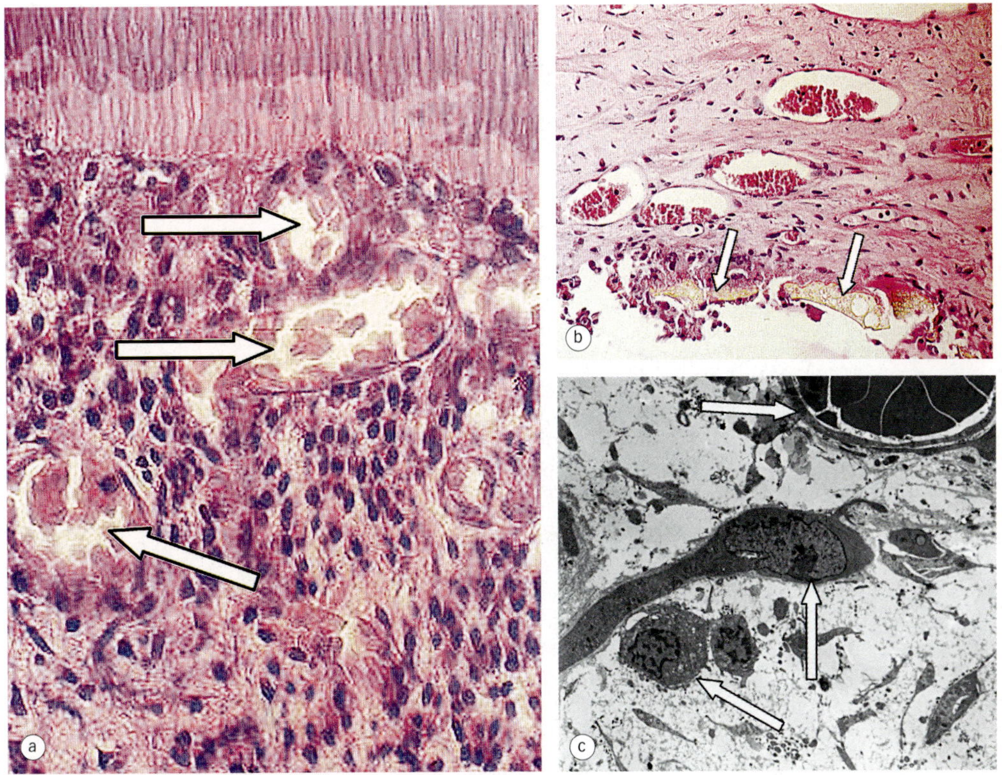

**Figure 1.7** - (**A**) A number of enlarged and congested capillaries (arrows) among mononuclear inflammatory cells are observed adjacent to the dentin. Note the disruption of the odontoblast layer. (**B**) Observe the defense cells initiating a reactionary process against fragments of toxic resinous material (arrows), which was applied over this specialized connective tissue. (**C**) Region of the pulp adjacent to odontoblastic layer. Note the presence of an enlarged and congested capillary (horizontal arrow), a macrophage (oblique arrow) and a dendritic cell (vertical arrow).

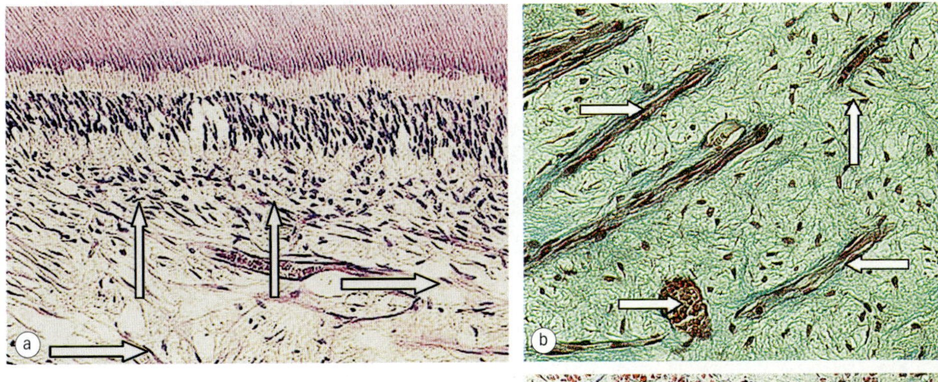

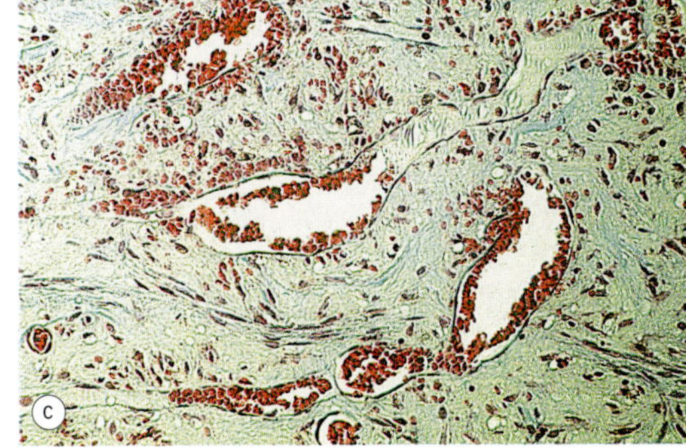

**Figure 1.8** - (**A**) Region of the pulp tissue in which the cell-rich zone (vertical arrows) and fibroblasts (horizontal arrows) are observed. (**B**) Central zone of the pulp tissue. Note the presence of a number of fibroblasts (vertical arrows) and small blood vessels (horizontal arrows). (**C**) Pulp tissue submitted to an injury. Observe the vascular proliferation associated with intense dilatation and congestion of blood vessels. The blood plasma extravasation caused an alteration in the extracellular matrix. Note a number of pulp cells presenting hydropic degeneration.

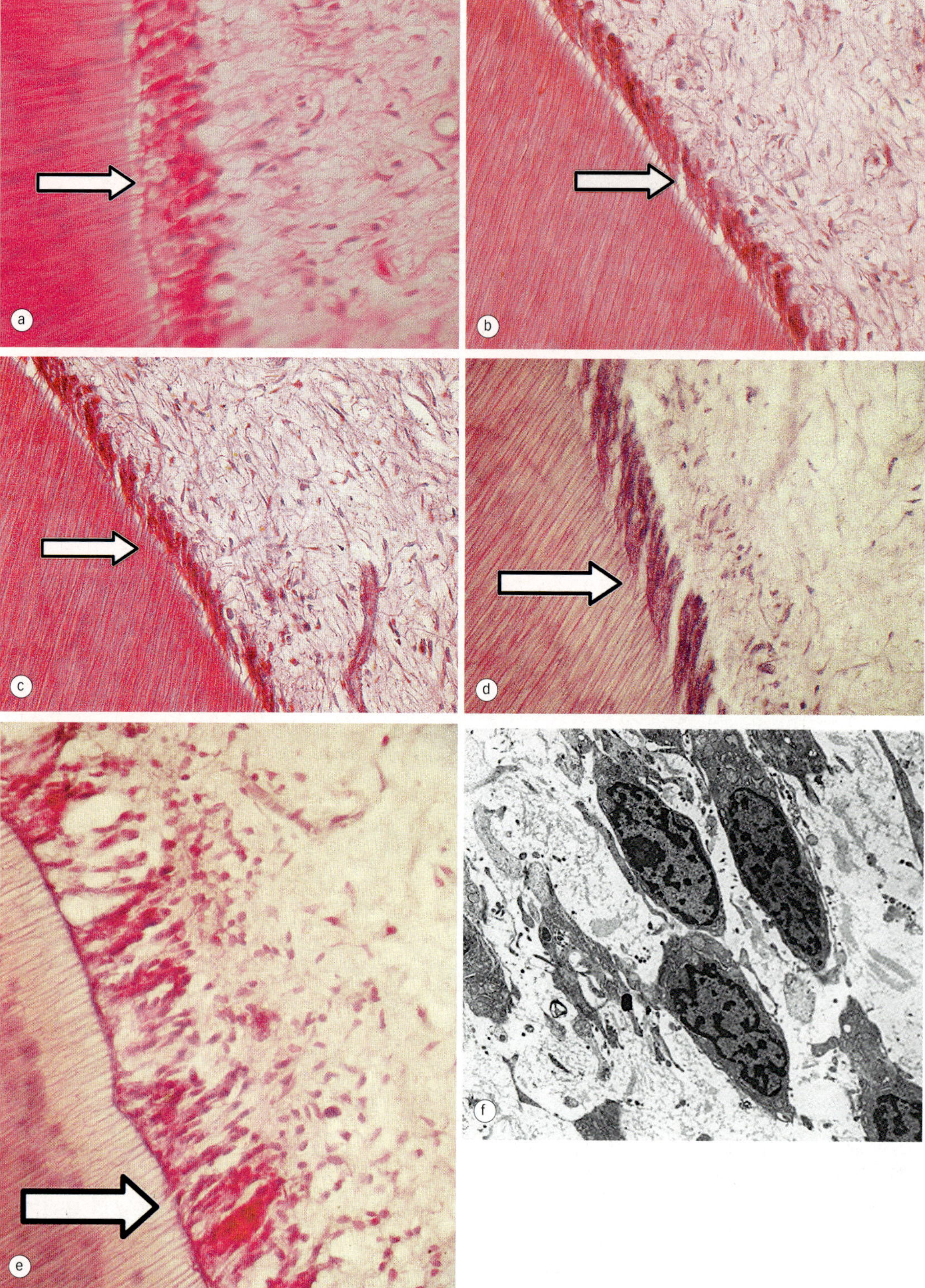

**Figure 1.9** - (**A-E**) Odontoblastic layer. Odontoblasts at different functional states. (**F**) Detail of some odontoblasts, which are characterized as elongated cells. Note the sequence of photomicrographs characterizing the different functional states of the odontoblasts.

They liberate vesicles containing phospholipids that attract calcium for the mineralization *front*, in addition to stimulating alkaline phosphatase, which cleaves pyrophosphate (inhibitor of the additional increase of ions), providing phosphate for the mineralization environment. As mineralization occurs, the odontoblast leaves its extension inside the dentinal tubule. The main component of the extension is a cytoskeleton filled with many microfilaments and microtubules in a structure parallel to its long axis with secretion vesicles (Fig. 1.10A-H).

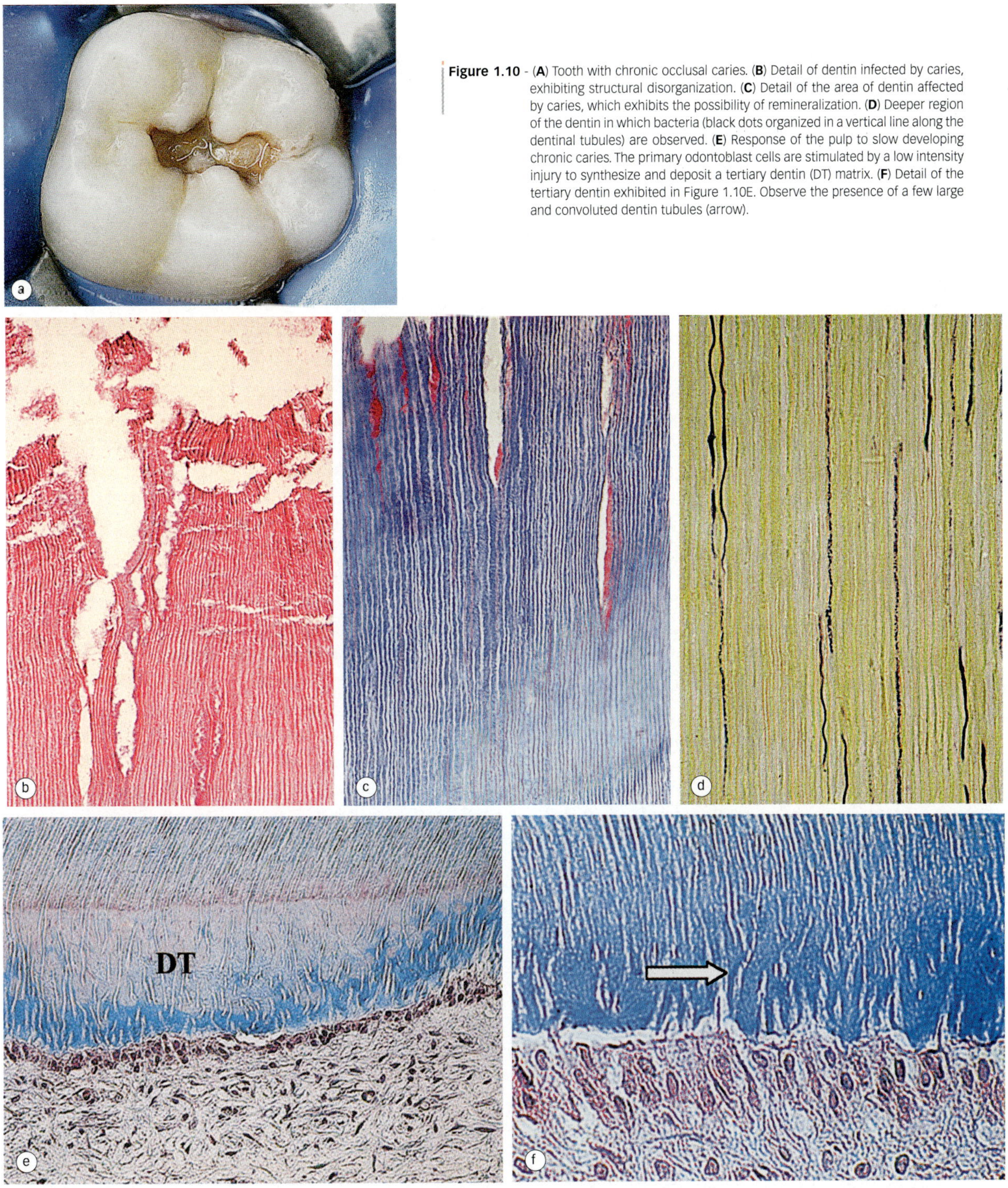

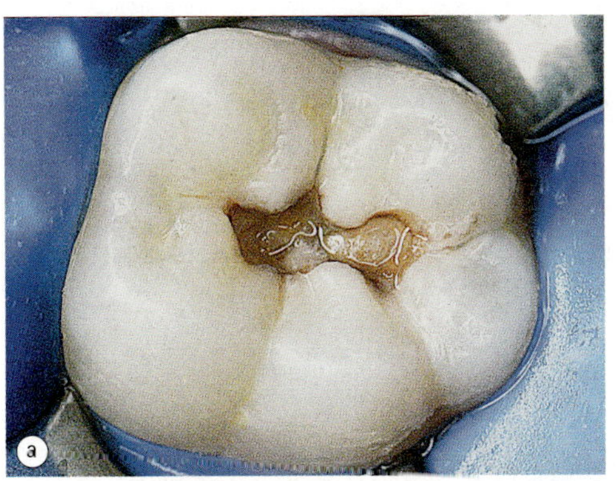

**Figure 1.10** - (**A**) Tooth with chronic occlusal caries. (**B**) Detail of dentin infected by caries, exhibiting structural disorganization. (**C**) Detail of the area of dentin affected by caries, which exhibits the possibility of remineralization. (**D**) Deeper region of the dentin in which bacteria (black dots organized in a vertical line along the dentinal tubules) are observed. (**E**) Response of the pulp to slow developing chronic caries. The primary odontoblast cells are stimulated by a low intensity injury to synthesize and deposit a tertiary dentin (DT) matrix. (**F**) Detail of the tertiary dentin exhibited in Figure 1.10E. Observe the presence of a few large and convoluted dentin tubules (arrow).

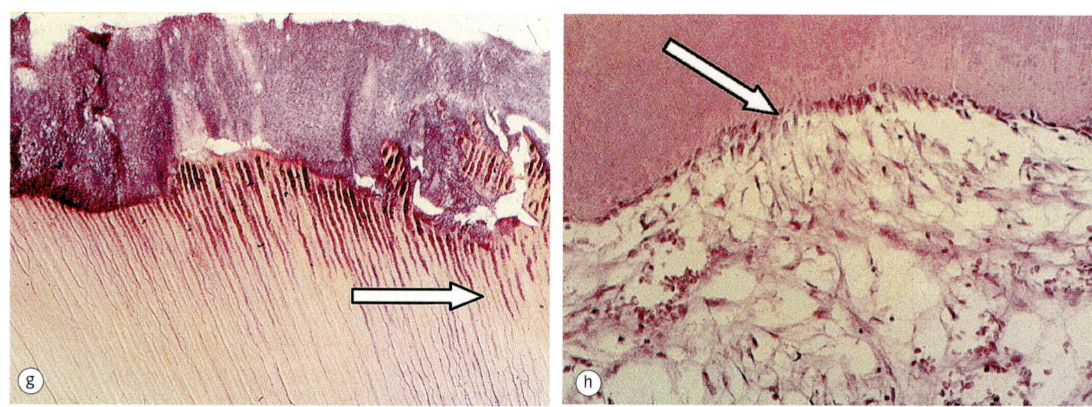

**Figure 1.10** - (**G**) The upper part of the Figure characterizes a caries lesion. This histological section stained with the Brown & Brenn technique exhibits the presence of bacteria inside the dentinal tubules (arrow). (**H**) The odontoblastic layer lining the dentin tissue associated with the caries lesion is disrupted (arrow). Note that the subjacent connective tissue is disorganized and exhibits an area of edema and inflammatory cells.

### 1.3.5 Dentin

Dentin is the most abundant mineral component of teeth. It is composed of 70% inorganic crystals (hydroxyapatite), 20% collagen fibers and other proteins and 10% water (all by %volume). Dentin can be classified as primary, secondary or tertiary, according to the time of development and the histological characteristics of the tissue. Primary dentin is composed of mantle dentin and by circumpulpal dentin that was deposited up to the moment that the tooth erupted and contacted its antagonist. Mantle dentin is the first dentin to be formed. It is deposited along the enamel-dentin or dentin-cementum junction, with a deposition parallel to the tissues that coat it. It is almost totally free of development defects. The odontoblasts, when they are supported by the basal membrane, have several cytoplasmic projections. This results in mantle dentin that is highly branched on the periphery that converges into only one prolongation towards the center of the pulp chamber. Mantle dentin has an approximate thickness of 80 to 100 µm. The circumpulpal dentin is formed after the formation of mantle dentin and constitutes the majority of the dentin. Since the odontoblasts produce the organic matrix of dentin in a direction towards the pulp, a space that becomes increasingly reduced, the orientation of the odontoblasts results in an "S"-shaped curvature in the circumpulpal dentin, which is more pronounced at the crown and more discrete at the root. The phased action of formation and resting of the odontoblasts produces incremental lines, perpendicular to the tubule direction.

Secondary dentin is formed after radicular dentin, maintaining the tubular pattern of the circumpulpal dentin; however this dentin formation is slower and less regular. It is deposited more on the roof and the floor of the pulpal chamber, reducing the pulpal horns and the pulpal chamber in an asymmetrical way. The thickness 1 to 1.5 µm of dentin matrix is incrementally deposited per day inside the pulp chamber. Tertiary dentin is produced in response to stimuli from the external environment, such as caries, attrition, abrasion, restorative procedures, etc. The formation of tertiary dentin occurs adjacent to the stimuli, modifying the pulpal and dentinal architecture. This dentin can be reactionary, when produced by pre-existing odontoblasts termed reparative, which occurs with the replacement of dead odontoblasts by new odontoblasts, or odontoblast-like cells (Fig. 1.11A-B). When low intensity stimuli are applied over odontoblasts, they respond by moving rapidly and centripetally in relation to the central pulp. These cells then deposit a matrix that contains irregular and convoluted tubules. The morphology of recently produced dentinal matrix is characterized as reactionary dentin. On the other hand, when the injury to the odontoblasts is intense, "killing" these specialized pulpal cells, new odontoblasts are differentiated from pre-odontoblasts (mesenchymal cells that were formed during dentinogenesis and remained in the cell-rich zone of the adult pulp). These new odontoblasts deposit a matrix of heterogeneous dentin, which is characteristic as reparative dentin. The process of deposition of reparative dentin is more complex than reactionary dentin, because it occurs by differentiation of the pulpal cells. In this case, undifferentiated reserve mesenchymal cells are used to replace the odontoblasts during the performance of some operative procedures or even during the fast evolution of an acute caries lesion. Consequently, the number of mesenchymal cells (stem cells) decreases in the pulp tissue, creating a reduced potential of healing. Thus, harm to the dentin-pulpal complex should be prevented to allow this integrated structure to maintain its function and natural physiologic metabolism, preventing its aging.



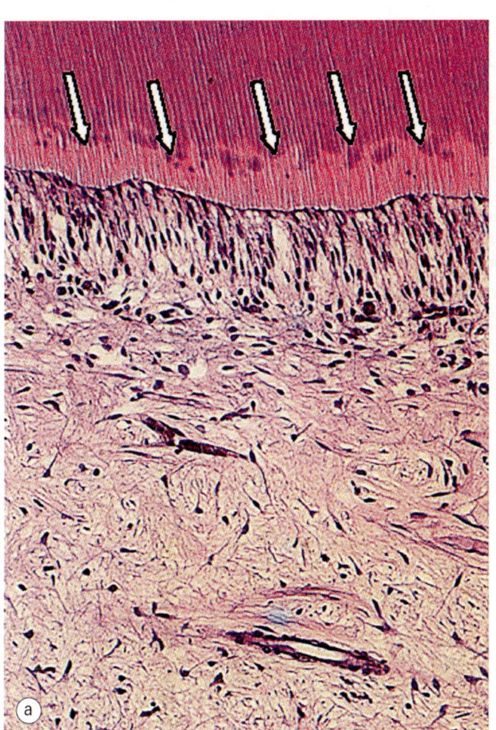


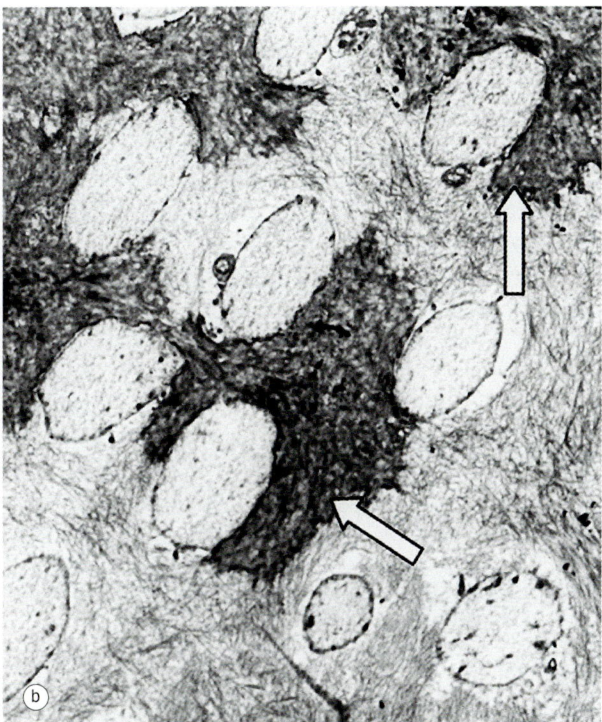


**Figure 1.11** - (**A**) Observe the pre-dentin with fronts of mineralization (arrows). (**B**) Detail of Figure 1.11A in transmission electronic microscopy in which the fronts of mineralization are shown (arrows). Note the collagen fibrils (clear area) of the pre-dentin.

The pre-dentin is a thin layer of dentin matrix recently synthesized by the odontoblasts. As described previously, this non-mineralized dentin matrix presents *fronts* of mineralization, also known as calcospherites (Fig. 1.12).

Failure of the calcospherites to fuse leads to the formation of hypomineralized areas, known as interglobular dentin. These areas are more visible in radicular dentin, where the dentin is produced simultaneously with the eruptive process, and on the most external portion of the coronary dentin, at the limit between mantle dentin and circumpulpal dentin. Pre-dentin principally consists of type I and III collagen, glycoproteins and proteoglycans. Another type of hypocalcification is the Tome's grainy layer that is formed by the terminal loops and branches of the odontoblastic membrane. This membrane configuration is developed during the formation of radicular dentin, giving to the peripheral dentin a grainy appearance.

Dentin is composed of tubules. As the odontoblasts secrete the organic matrix, they emit a projection that is surrounded by liquid, providing the tubular aspect. The tubules have a lightly conical shape, due to the mineralization process of the peritubular dentin that occurs during the life of the tooth. The tubules extend through the entire thickness of dentin, following the sinuous track of the odontoblasts (Fig. 1.13A-B). Although there are variations in the number of dentin tubules per area when different teeth are compared, it has been demonstrated that, at the enamel-dentin junction (superficial dentin), there are approximately 20,000 tubules/mm$^2$, while near the pre-dentin (deep dentin), there are approximately 75,000 tubules/mm$^2$. The dentin that surrounds the periphery of the dentinal tubules is known as peritubular or intratubular dentin. Intertubular dentin is present between dentin tubules. The odontoblast cytoplasmic projections remain within the dentinal tubules (Fig. 1.14A-C). Communications among the dentinal tubules, known as dentinal canaliculus, are frequently observed. The peritubular dentin that constitutes the walls of the dentinal tubules is four times harder than intertubular dentin, since approximately 96% of it is hydroxyapatite crystals. Mild stimuli from the external environment, such as attrition and caries, may cause obliteration of the dentinal tubules, resulting in dentin sclerosis. Intertubular dentin is partially composed of collagen fibrils positioned perpendicularly to the long axis of the tubules, surrounding the tubules (Fig. 1.14B). The conditioning of the dentin substrate with acidic agents, or chelanting substances decreases or removes the peritubular dentin on the surface, leaving a mesh of intertubular collagen exposed to the action of bonding agents or to bacteria from decay (Fig. 1.13B and 1.14B).

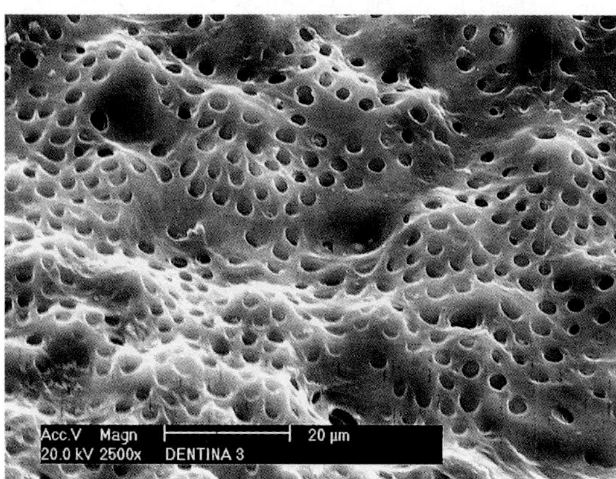


**Figure 1.12** - Calcospherites of the internal dentinal surface, characterizing the irregularity of the continuous mineralization of the dentin.

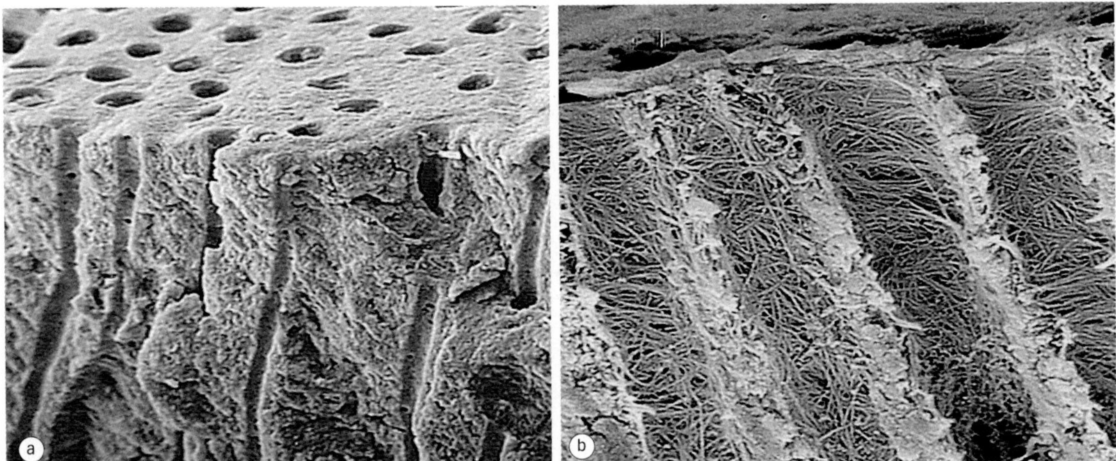

**Figure 1.13** - (**A**) Dentinal tubules in a longitudinal cut. (**B**) Detail of the dentin, exhibiting collagen fibrils that are perpendicular to the dentinal tubules.

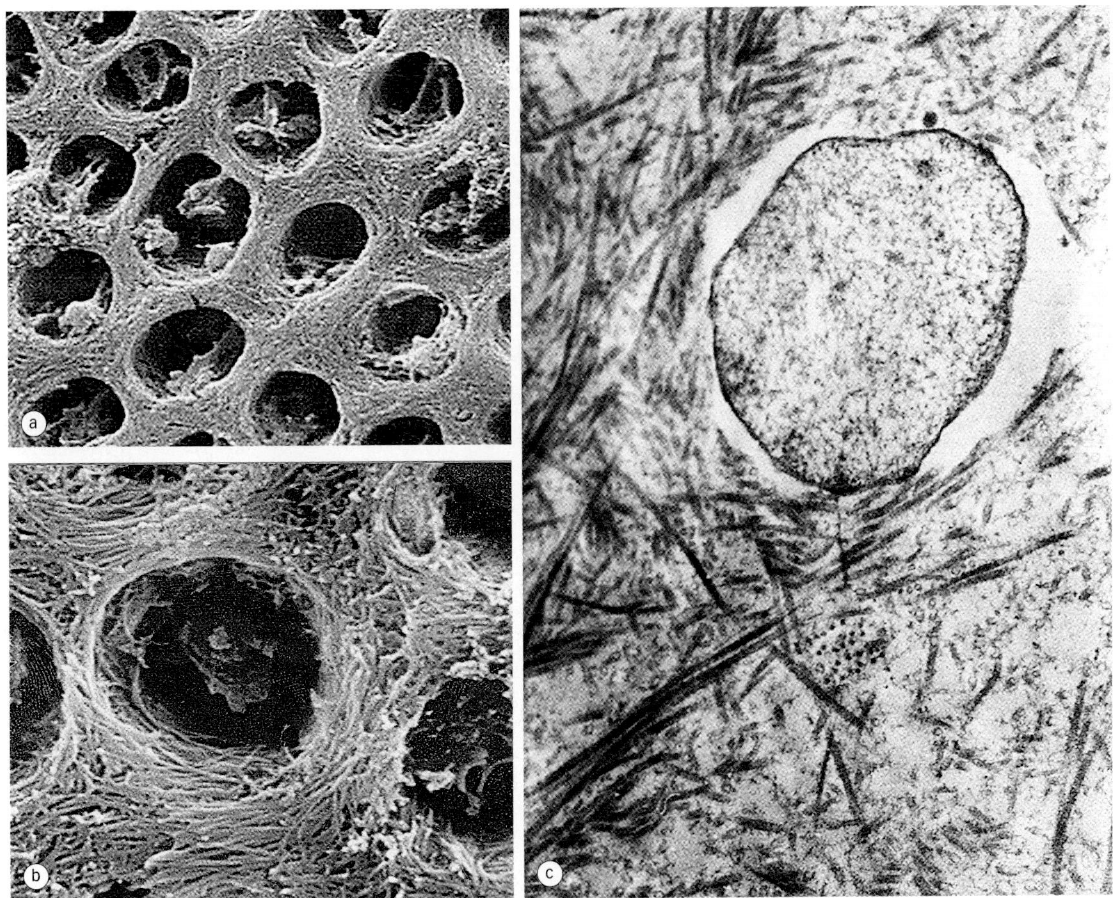

**Figure 1.14** - (**A**) Dentinal tubules in a transverse cut, exhibiting cytoplasmic processes inside them. (**B**) Detail of the rich net of collagen fibrils that surround the dentinal tubules. (**C**) A cytoplasmic process, surrounded by collagen fibrils, is shown using transmission electron microscopy.

## Consulted References and Further Reading


1. Avery JK. Oral development and histology. 3rd ed. Stuttgart: Thieme; 2002. 435p.
2. Bartold PM, Narayanan AS. Biology of the periodontal connective tissue. 1st ed. Chicago: Quintessence; 1998. p.173-195.
3. Brännström MA, Aström A. The hydrodynamics of the dentin: its possible relationship to dentinal pain. Inter Dent J 1972; 22:219.
4. Brew MC, Figueiredo JAP. Histologia geral para a Odontologia. 1st ed. Rio de Janeiro: Guanabara Koogan; 2003. 148p.
5. Byers MR. Dynamic plasticity of dental sensory nerve structure and cytochemistry. Arch Oral Biol 1994; 39:13S-21S.
6. Byers MR, Närhi MVO. Nerve supply of the pulpodentin complex and responses to injury. In: Seltzer and Bender's dental pulp. Hargreaves KM, Goodis HE. 1st ed. Chicago: Quintessence; 2002. p.151-180.
7. Byers MR, Taylor PE, Khayat BG, Kimberly CL. Effects of injury and inflammation on pulpal and periapical nerves. J Endod 1990; 16:78-84.
8. Chiego DJ. Histology of the pulp. In: Oral development and histology. Avery JK. 3rd ed. Stuttgart: Thieme; 2002. p.190-212.
9. Costa CAS, Hebling J, Hanks CT. Current status of Pulp-capping with Dentin adhesive systems: A review. Dent Materials 2000; 16:188-197.
10. D'Souza R. Development of pulpodentin complex. In: Seltzer and Bender's dental pulp. Hargreaves KM, Goodis HE. 1st ed. Chicago: Quintessence; 2002. p.13-40.
11. Estrela C. Dor pulpar. In: Dor odontogênica. Estrela C. 1st ed. São Paulo: Artes Médicas; 2001. p.81-112.
12. Estrela C, Figueiredo JAP. Patologia pulpar. In: Endodontia – princípios biológicos e mecânicos. Estrela C, Figueiredo JAP. São Paulo: Artes Médicas; 1999. p.137-166.
13. Figueiredo JAP, Mezzomo E. Manejo Del complejo dentino-pulpar em los procedimientos protéticos. In: Rehabilitación oral para el clínico. Mezzomo E. Caracas: Actualidades Médico Odontológicas Latinoamérica; 1997. p.121-161.
14. Garant PR. The organization of microtubules within rat odontoblast processes revealed by perfusion fixation with glutaraldehyde. Arch Oral Biol 1972; 17:1047-1058.
15. Garant PR, Szabo G, Nalbandian J. The fine structure of the mouse odontoblast. Arch Oral Biol 1968; 13:857-876.
16. Holland GR. The odontoblast process: form and function. J Dent Res 1985; 64:499-514.
17. Katchburian E, Arana V. Histologia e embriologia oral. Buenos Aires: Panamericana; 1999. 381p.
18. Maas R, Bei M. The genetic control of early tooth development. Crit Rev Oral Biol Med 1997; 8:4-39.
19. Okiji T. Pulp as a connective tissue. In: Seltzer and Bender's dental pulp. Hargreaves KM, Goodis HE. Chicago: Quintessence; 2002. p.95-122.
20. Olgart LM. Neural control of pulpal blood flow. Crit Rev Oral Biol Med 1996; 7:159-171.
21. Pashley D. Pulpodentin complex. In: Seltzer and Bender's Dental Pulp. Hargreaves KM, Goodis HE. Chicago: Quintessence; 2002. p.63-94.
22. Ruch JV, Lesot H, Bègüe-Kirn C. Odontoblast differentiation. Inter J Develop Biol 1995; 39:51-68.
23. Senior RM, Griffen GL, Mechan RP. Chemotactic activity of elastin-derived peptides. J Clin Invest 1980; 304:859.
24. Smith AJ. Dentin formation and repair. In: Seltzer and Bender's dental pulp. Hargreaves KM, Goodis HE. Chicago: Quintessence; 2002. p.41-62.
25. Smith AJ, Lesot H. Induction and regulation of crown dentinogenesis-embryonic events as a template for dental tissue repair. Crit Rev Oral Biol Med 2001; 12:425-437.
26. Smulson MH, Sieraski SM. Histophisiology and diseases of the dental pulps. In: Endodontic therapy. Weine FS. 5th ed. St. Louis: Mosby; 1996. p.84-165.
27. Souza MAL. Biologia pulpar. In: Endodontia – princípios biológicos e mecânicos. Estrela C, Figueiredo JAP. São Paulo: Artes Médicas; 1999. p.1-24.
28. Ten-Cate AR. Histologia bucal. 5th ed. Rio de Janeiro: Guanabara Koogan; 2001. 439p.
29. Trowbridge HO, Kim S. Pulp development, structure and function. In: Pathways of the pulp. Cohen S, Burns RC. 6th ed. St. Louis: Mosby; 1994. p.296-336.
30. Tziafas D, Kolokuris I. Inductive influences of demineralized dentin and bone matrix on pulp cells: an approach of secondary dentinogenesis. J Dent Res 1990; 69:75-81.
31. Woodnutt DA, Wager-Miller J, O'Neill PC, Bothwell M, Byers MR. Neurotrophin receptors and nerve growth factor are differentially expressed in adjacent non-neuronal cells of normal and injured tooth pulp. Cell Tissue Res 2000; 299:225-236.

# Root Development

**J. A. P. Figueiredo**

*Pontifical Catholic University of Rio Grande do Sul, PUCRS, Porto Alegre, RS, Brazil*

**A. H. G. Alencar**

*Federal University of Goiás, Goiânia, GO, Brazil*

**S. S. Murata**

*São Paulo State University, Araçatuba, SP, Brazil*

**C. Estrela**

*Federal University of Goiás, Goiânia, GO, Brazil*

Chapter contents

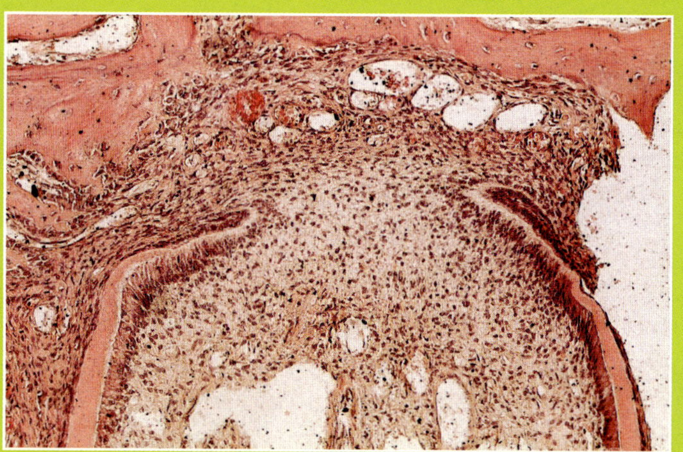

Area in which the apical papilla is present. The apical cell-rich zone would be responsible for the apexogenesis, including dentine formation (Courtesy Prof. Dr. Roberto Holland[39-41]).

## 2.1 Introduction

The knowledge of dental root formation is very important for clinical management of possible dental injuries.

When the teeth emerge in the oral cavity, two thirds of the length of their roots has been formed, and full length will only be complete three years after eruption[9]. In young permanent teeth with incomplete rhizogenesis, histologically the apex of the root does not present the apical dentin covered by cementum, and radiographically the apical end of the root does not reach the stage 10 of Nolla, that is, a complete root apex[9,40,41,61].

Completely formed teeth present the root canal with the approximate shape of the external form of the root, resembling a cone, with the widest base at the pulpal chamber, and the narrowest in the apical third. Next to the apical third, a natural constriction is observed, called cementum-dentin-canal junction (CDC), which limits endodontic procedures and serves as reference so that the filling can be confined inside the dentinal root canal. Teeth with incomplete rhizogenesis have their own characteristics: very wide root canals, and may also have a conical shape, but with the wider base in the apical portion. The apical foramen, still not formed, has a larger diameter than the root canal[62,73].

When root canal treatment is necessary in teeth with incomplete rhizogenesis, these characteristics can make treatment difficult. The thin and fragile walls hinder root canal preparation, and frequently make it impossible. The thin walls prevent any conventional preparation being performed in the root canal. Consequently, the root canal filling is affected, since no "apical stop" can be determined in the root canal preparation, and there is always a risk of overfilling[60-63,73].

The traumatic injuries to the teeth have been one of the reasons for indicating root canal treatment in teeth with incomplete rhizogenesis. Teeth, such as recently erupted first permanent molars that do not have the maximum fluoride incorporated into the enamel become more susceptible to caries. Moreover, due to the great volume of the pulpal chamber in the young teeth, pulpal exposure occurs faster, especially in the presence of decay or while operative procedures are being performed[90].

When the pulp is affected in teeth in the process of root formation, it is of fundamental importance to evaluate the pathological state of the tissues involved in the root completion. The need for performing different procedures in teeth with pulp vitality and in those with pulp necrosis shows the importance diagnosing the state of the pulp[60-63,73].

## 2.2 Root Formation

Starting during the fifth week of intrauterine life, teeth form as the result of a series of specific, reciprocal, and sequential epithelial-mesenchymal signals between the oral epithelium and the underlying neural crest derived ectomesenchyme[45]. Until the twelfth week of intrauterine life, this process is directed by the epithelium, but control subsequently shifts to the ectomesenchymal cells[57].

The tooth bud (sometimes called the tooth germ) is an aggregation of cells that forms a tooth. These cells are derived from the ectoderm of the first branchial arch and the ectomesenchyme of the neural crest. The tooth bud is organized into three parts: the enamel organ, the dental papilla and the dental follicle. Enamel is the only tooth tissue to derive from ectoderm, whilst the dentine-pulp complex and periodontium are derived from ectomesenchyme[82].

The signaling events depend on the participation of BMP2, BMP4 (bone morphogenetic proteins), FGF (fibroblast growth factor), Wnt families, hedgehogs, and the homeobox proteins MSX1 and MSX2[84,92]. There is a progressive restriction of the developmental potential that culminates in the differentiation of the mesenchymal-derived odontoblasts and epithelial-derived ameloblasts, the cells responsible for producing the extracellular matrices that form dentin and enamel, respectively[10,15]. In addition to the known molecular factors, there are other specific signals that cause the terminal differentiation of the odontoblasts and ameloblasts, which culminate in the formation of dentin and enamel, such as enamelin, tubulin, GAD, NeuN, nestin, neurofilament M, NSE, CNPase[31,57,85]. When control is shifted to the ectomesenchyme, the dental papilla is responsible for maintaining the induction of the odontogenic events, more clearly through the bud, cap and bell stages[57].

A sequence of orchestrated events occurs and in human teeth the chronology, although subject to some variations, can be considered predictable. Below (Table 2.1) there is the expected sequence for all tooth groups. Note that root completion is a process that occurs at a much later stage.

**Table 2.1** - A sequence of orchestrated events occurs and in human teeth the chronology

| | Maxillary teeth | | | | | | | |
|---|---|---|---|---|---|---|---|---|
| **Permanent teeth** | **Central incisor** | **Lateral incisor** | **Canine** | **First premolar** | **Second premolar** | **First molar** | **Second molar** | **Third molar** |
| **Initial calcification** | 3 - 4 months | 10–12 months | 4–5 months | 1.5–1.75 years | 2–2.25 years | at birth | 2.5–3 years | 7–9 Years |
| **Crown completion** | 4–5 years | 4–5 years | 6–7 years | 5–6 years | 6–7 years | 2.5–3 years | 7–8 years | 12–16 Years |
| **Root completion** | 10 years | 11 years | 13–15 years | 12–13 years | 12–14 years | 9–10 years | 14–16 years | 18–25 Years |
| | **Mandibular teeth** | | | | | | | |
| **Initial calcification** | 3–4 months | 3–4 months | 4–5 months | 1.5–2 years | 2.25–2.5 years | at birth | 2.5–3 years | 8–10 Years |
| **Crown completion** | 4–5 years | 4–5 years | 6–7 years | 5–6 years | 6–7 years | 2.5–3 years | 7–8 years | 12–16 Years |
| **Root completion** | 9 years | 10 years | 12–14 years | 12–13 years | 13–14 years | 9–10 years | 14–15 years | 18–25 Years |

The first sign of tooth development is a localized thickening of dental epithelium, the dental lamina, which subsequently invaginates into underlying neural-crest-derived ectomesenchyme, forming a bud, after which proliferative mesenchyme condenses around the developing epithelial bud[54,84].

Tooth shape specification occurs early in tooth development, at the dental lamina stage, by homeobox genes, which are specifically expressed in the pre-dental mesenchyme[88,92]. The physical morphological processes begin at the cap stage and are coordinated by enamel knots, via transient signaling centers that lie in the epithelium and which, in some way, are directed by the earlier expression of homeobox genes[44,83,89].

Additional enamel knots appear and pattern the crown. By the late cap stage, enamel knots disappear by apoptosis.[89] After the mesenchyme receives the early odontogenic signals from the epithelium, the ectomesenchyme becomes the source of signals[50]. The epithelium further differentiates into enamel-secreting ameloblasts, whereas the adjacent mesenchyme differentiates into dentine-secreting odontoblasts[92].

At the bell stage, a recognizable tooth germ is formed that consists of an enamel organ, dental papilla and dental follicle. The enamel organ is composed of the outer enamel epithelium, inner enamel epithelium, stellate reticulum and stratum intermedium[44]. These cells give rise to ameloblasts, which produce enamel and the reduced enamel epithelium. The location where the outer enamel epithelium and inner enamel epithelium join is called the cervical loop. The growth of cervical loop cells into the deeper tissues forms Hertwig's epithelial root sheath, which determines the root shape of the tooth[82].

The dental papilla contributes to tooth formation and eventually converts to pulp tissue[18,53,66,67] which is a living connective tissue composed of fibroblasts, blood vessels, nerves, lymphatic ducts and odontoblasts. Odontoblasts are the cells derived from the mesenchymal cells in the dental papilla adjacent to the inner enamel epithelium[82]. Differentiated odontoblasts are postmitotic cells that have withdrawn from the cell-cycle, and cannot proliferate to replace irreversibly injured odontoblasts[66]. Functional odontoblasts show polarized columnar morphology that shift into a resting state and become small and flat after primary dentin formation. However, odontoblasts remain functional throughout their life and can produce secondary dentin if trauma is mild[72,80].

The dental follicle gives rise to three important entities: cementoblasts, osteoblasts, and fibroblasts, and appears as a transient structure when teeth undergo morphogenesis. Cementoblasts form the cementum of a tooth. Osteoblasts give rise to the alveolar bone around the roots of teeth. Fibroblasts develop the periodontal ligaments which connect teeth to the alveolar bone through cementum. In developing teeth, root formation starts as the epithelial cells from the cervical loop proliferate apically and influence the differentiation of odontoblasts from undifferentiated mesenchymal cells and cementoblasts from follicle mesenchyme. This apically extending two-layered epithelial wall (merging with the inner and outer enamel epithelium) forms Hertwig's epithelial root sheath, which is responsible for determining the shape of the root(s) and forms cementum through epithelial-mesenchymal transition[77].

The periodontal ligament functions as a cushion when force is applied, as a source of sensation, and it is regarded as the main impetus for the tooth eruption process. The complex structure that includes the periodontal ligament, adjacent cementum and alveolar bone is called the periodontium. After tooth eruption into the oral cavity, a tooth is clinically divided into two parts: crown and root. Crowns are the visible structures in the oral cavity, whereas roots are the regions that connect the surrounding alveolar bone with the cementum. Anatomically, crowns are the part covered by enamel and lie above the level of the cementoenamel junction; roots are covered with cementum and lie below the junction[92].

There is a lot more knowledge about the way that crowns are formed, than the manner in which roots develop, little being known about the signal mechanisms of root development. Among the factors involved, FGF10 signaling stands out as a candidate for root initiation[93]. A transcription factor NFI-C (nuclear factor I) is essential for root formation[78]. Because the root continues to develop after the bell stage, the location of the dental papilla becomes apical to the pulp tissue. The apical papilla appears to be histologically distinct from the pulp. There is a loose physical connection between apical papilla and pulp, as the papilla can be easily detached from the apex and readily placed next to the pulp[76].

As the differentiated odontoblasts lay down the primary dentine, the dental papilla becomes encased within the dentine structure and develops into pulp tissue. The apical end of the dental papilla, however, has not been discussed much in the literature. It is generally believed that the formation of root dentin is the result of signaling from Hertwig's epithelial root sheath to the adjacent undifferentiated mesenchymal cells, which then turn into odontoblasts that are responsible for the root dentine formation. The anatomic location of these undifferentiated mesenchymal cells has not been clearly elucidated. They may reside either in the pulp or the apical papilla. Dental pulp also harbors undifferentiated mesenchymal cells that are known to be capable of differentiating into new odontoblasts to replace the lost original odontoblasts. The primary odontoblasts are derived from dental papilla during the developing stage and make primary and secondary dentin, whilst the replacement odontoblasts (or odontoblast-like cells) are derived from the dental pulp to replace primary odontoblasts and make tertiary dentin or, more specifically, the reparative dentin. Replacement odontoblasts derive from underlying mesenchymal cells and are located in the cell-rich zone and cell proper, particularly in the perivascular region[28,29,81].

Sonoyama et al.[76] have recently published an elegant study, detecting stem cells of the apical papilla. From histological sections, they verified that there is a cell-rich zone between the pulp and the apical papilla, terming it "apical cell–rich zone." This is important, as the apical papilla appears to contain fewer blood vessels and cellular components than the dental pulp and the apical cell–rich zone, and once the tissues are placed in cultures, cells in the apical papilla start to enter the growth cycle more readily than those in the pulp. With regard to osteo/dentinogenic markers in the apical papilla, DSP, ALP, BSP and OCN were detected only in odontoblasts lined against newly formed dentine, and were not detected in the apical papilla. Dental pulp and apical papilla stem cells express similar osteo/dentinogenic markers and growth factor receptors, but fewer amounts of most of them in the apical papilla. Figure 2.1 demonstrates the area in which the apical papilla is present. The apical cell-rich zone would be responsible for apexogenesis, including the dentine formation.

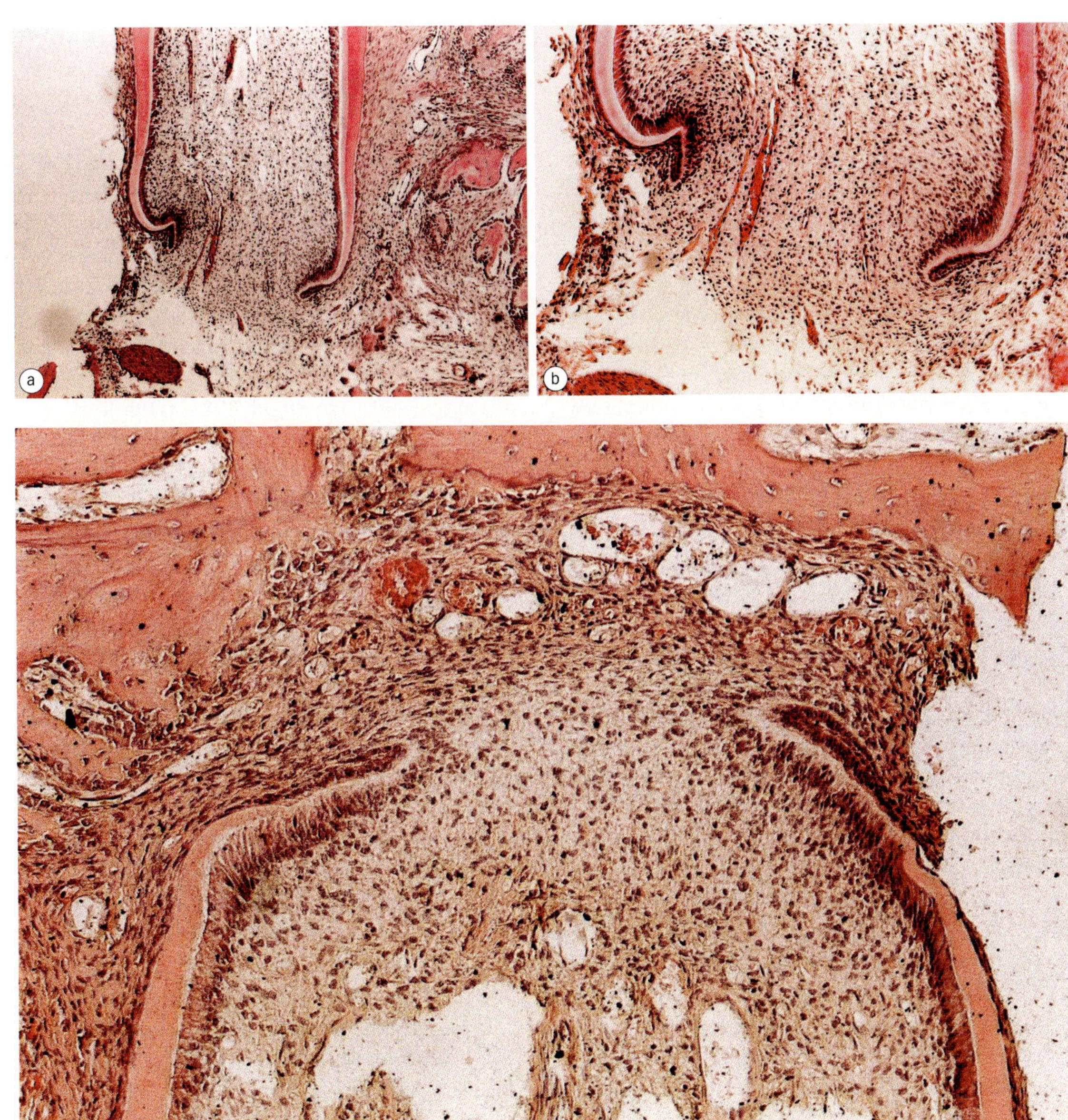


**Figure 2.1** - (**A-C**) Area in which the apical papilla is present. The apical cell-rich zone would be responsible for the apexogenesis, including dentine formation (Courtesy Prof. Dr . Roberto Holland[39-41]).

The stem cells from dental pulp reside in the perivascular and perineural sheath regions[70]. This finding corresponds to one concerning the source of replacement odontoblasts: the perivascular regions where stem/progenitor cells reside. At present, however, it is unknown where the stem cells in the pulp come from. The vascular density in the apical papilla appears to be lower than that of the pulp. However, the proliferation rates of apical papilla stem cells are faster than those of the dental pulp stem cells[76]. This can be explained because adult stem cells generally remain in a non-proliferative, quiescent state until stimulated by the signals triggered by tissue damage and remodeling[74,75]. They are capable of self-renewal and give rise to progenitor cells that eventually differentiate into specialized cells.

The apical papilla is fundamental to root development. If the apical papilla is removed at an early stage of development, despite the pulp tissue being intact, the dental root will not develop. It could be inferred that the stem cells from the apical papilla, and not the dental pulp stem cells, are the cell source for primary odontoblasts that produce root dentine[76]. This would explain why apexogenesis can occur in teeth with open apexes and infected pulp and apical periodontitis or abscesses[5,13,43]. The surviving cells from the apical papilla and the Hertwig's epithelial root sheath would perform the remaining apexogenesis following sanitization of the root canal system.

Pulp tissue in immature teeth with open apices has a rich blood supply and contains a structure at a developing stage that is more potent to regenerate in response to damage. The general consensus for clinical treatment of immature teeth with vital pulps is to preserve the remaining normal vital tissue to allow continued physiological development and complete formation of apexogenesis. Whereas for teeth with nonvital pulps, treatment is to clean and fill the canals with calcium hydroxide, the most commonly used material, to induce the formation of a calcified barrier at the open apex–apexification[63].

After successful apexogenesis teeth develop a normal thickness of dentine and root length. In contrast, those receiving apexification normally gain only an apical hard tissue bridge, not dentin, because of the loss of vital pulp tissues, odontoblasts, and Hertwig epithelial root sheath, needed for complete root development. However, this paradigm has been challenged by recent reports convincingly showing that immature teeth, clinically diagnosed with nonvital pulp and periradicular periodontitis or abscess, can undergo apexogenesis[5,43]. These reports stimulated a new perspective of how we treat these cases. It has been advocated that immature teeth should be treated as conservatively as practical, to allow any possible apexogenesis to occur[91]. After successful apexification, teeth inherit thin and weak roots that are susceptible to fracture. Shifting apexification to apexogenesis even for nonvital pulps with apical periodontitis or abscess would be a clinically beneficial approach for patients if we gathered more clinical experience to help predict the outcome of the treatment. The treatment below is an example of how apexogenesis can occur in the absence of dental pulp vitality. Therefore, the vitality of the apical papilla is the key to the completion of root development (Fig. 2.2AM-2.5AF).

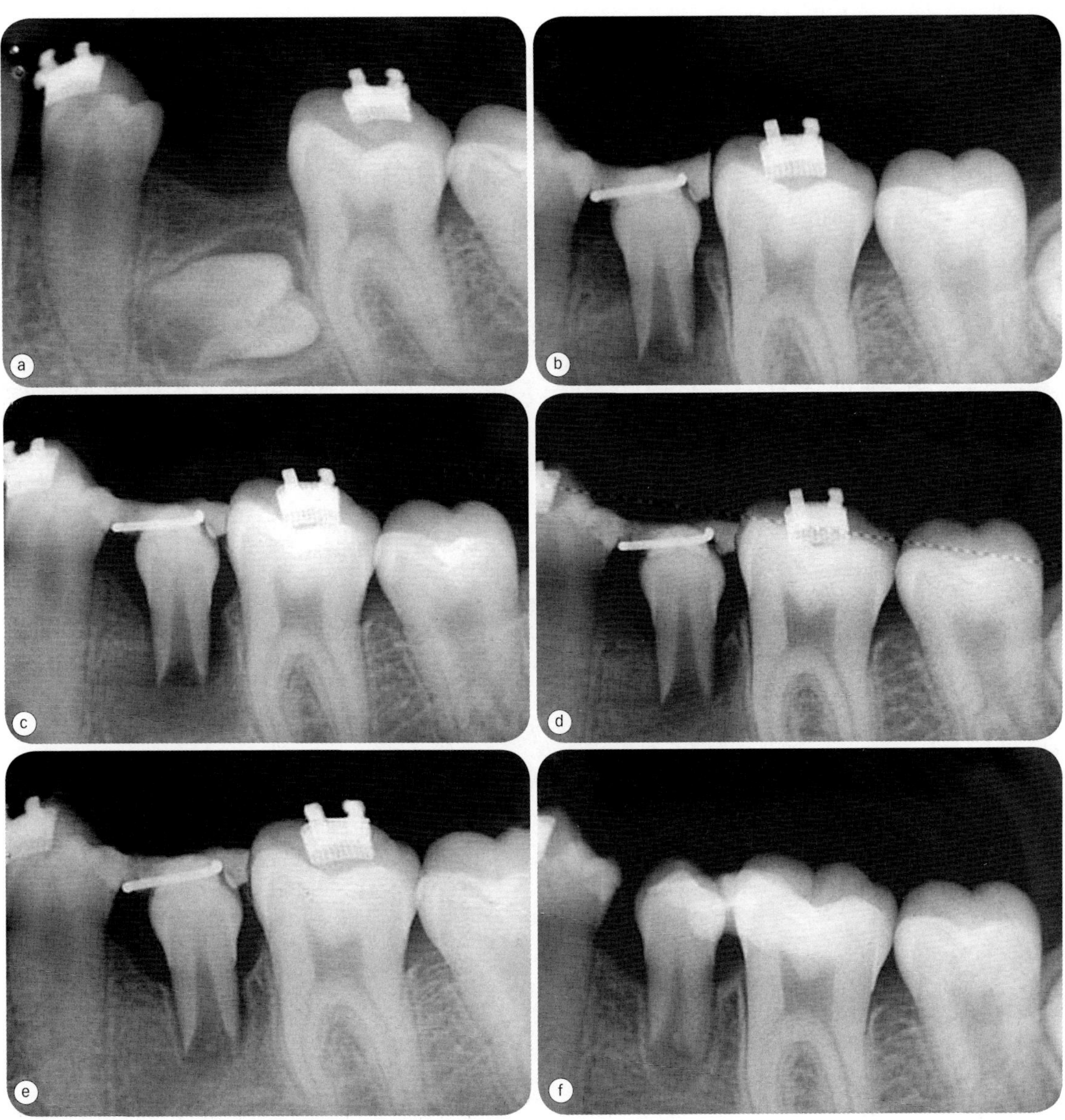


**Figure 2.2** - (**A-F**) Apexogenesis. The maintenance of pulp vitality will make the normal root development possible (Courtesy Prof. Dr. Rinaldo Mattar).

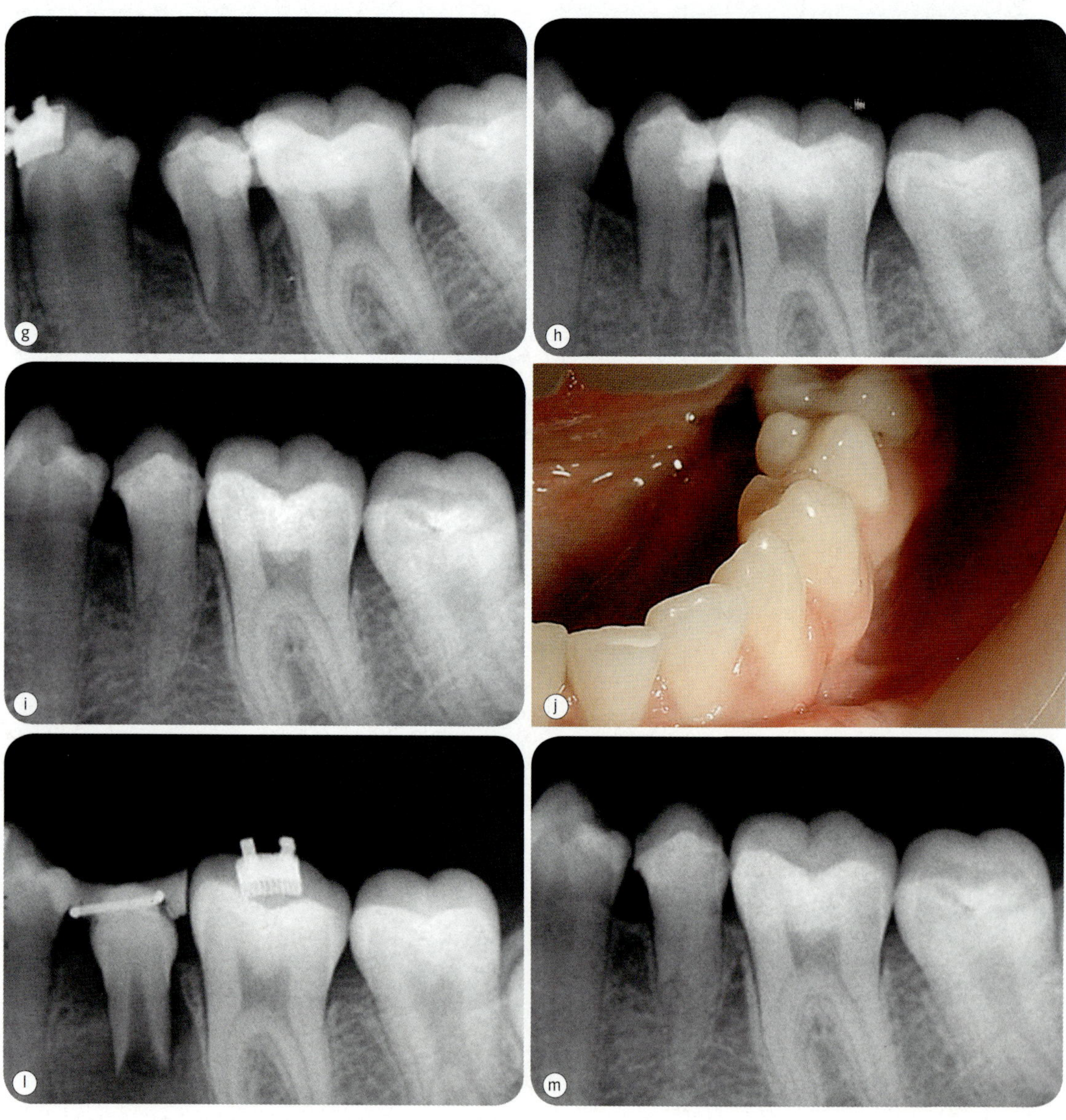

**Figure 2.2** - (**G-M**) Apexogenesis. The maintenance of pulp vitality will make the normal root development possible (Courtesy Prof. Dr. Rinaldo Mattar).

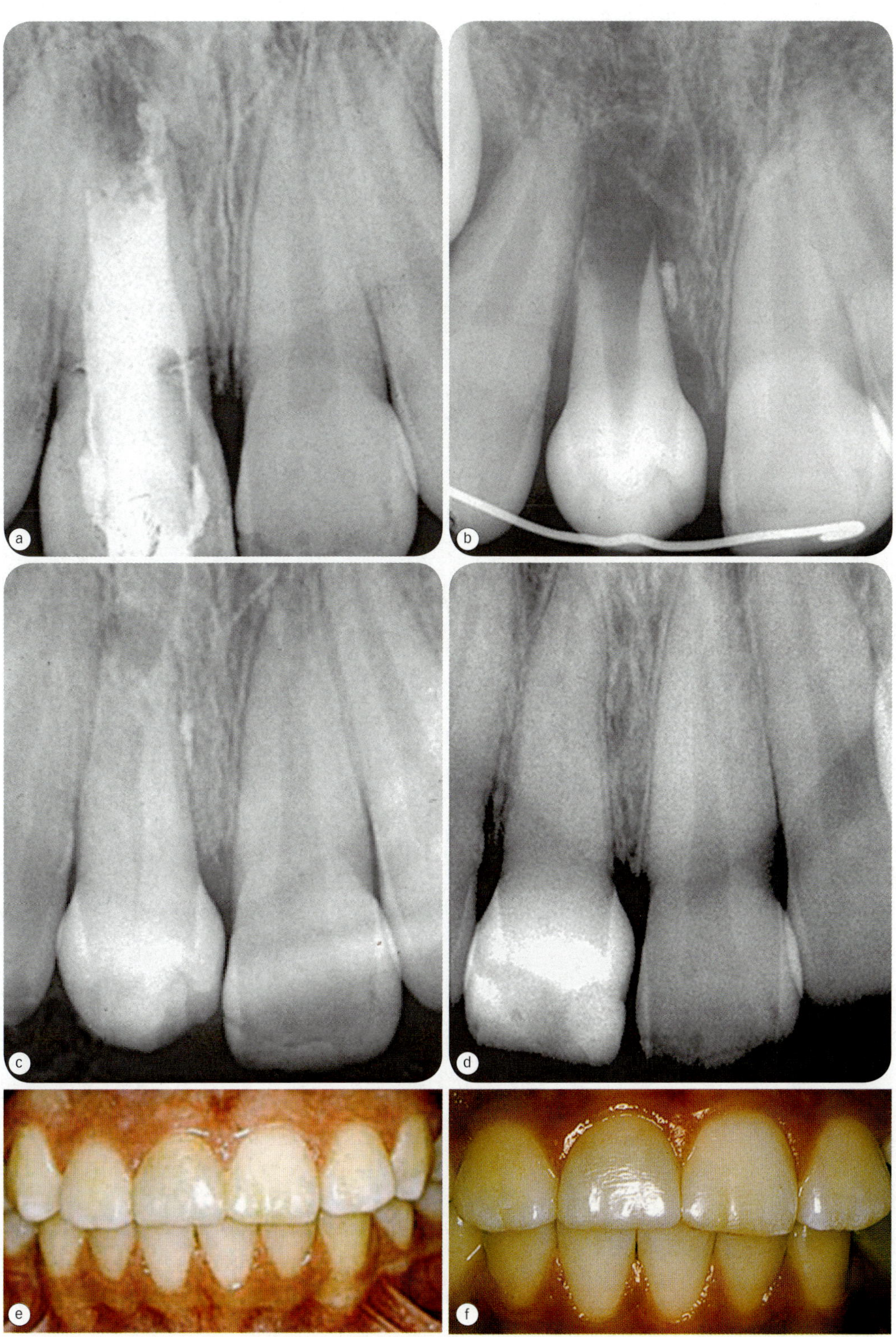


**Figure 2.3** - (**A-F**) Apexogenesis. Dental injury of the right central incisor. First premolar was transplanted for this place. It was observed root developed associated with pulp canal obliteration (Courtesy Prof. Dr. Armelindo Roldi).

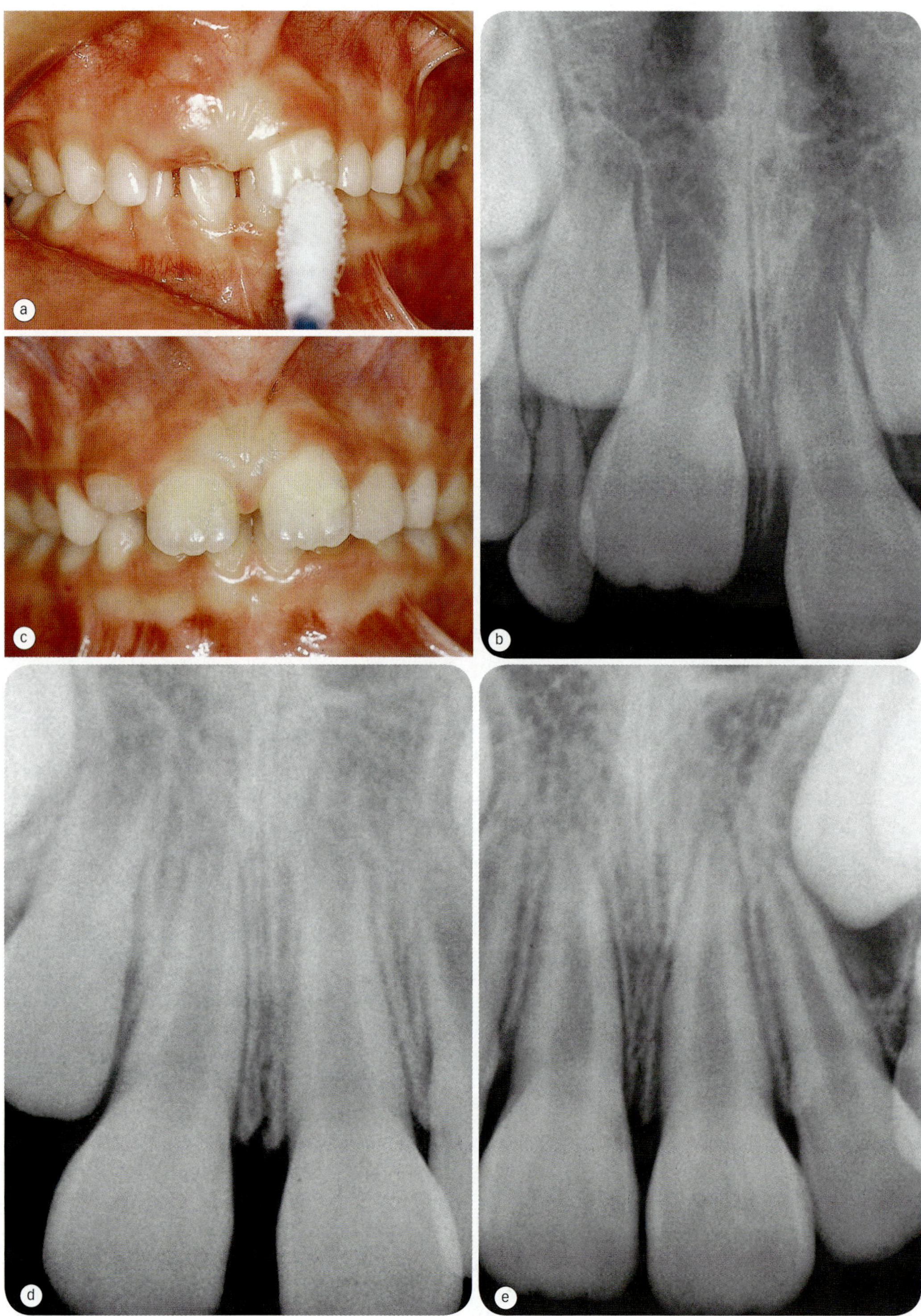


**Figure 2.4** - (**A-E**) Apexogenesis. The maintenance of pulp vitality will make the normal root development possible.

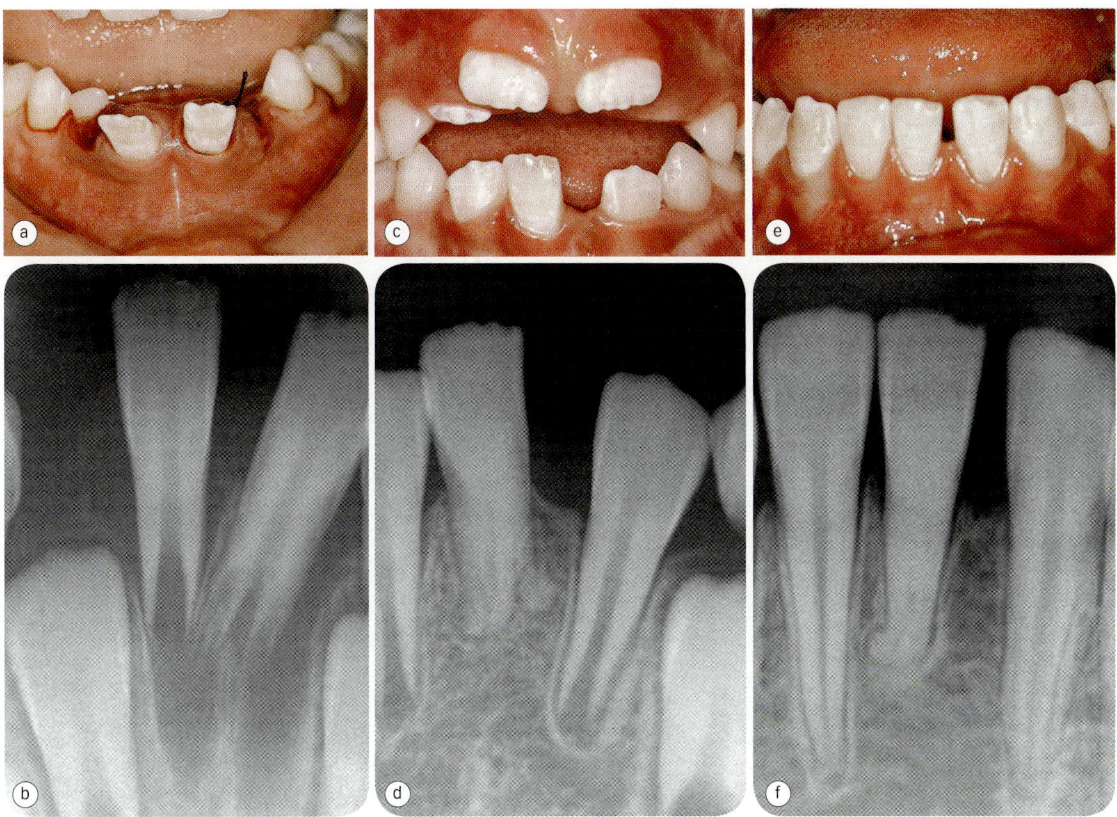

Figure 2.5 - (A-F) Apexogenesis. Root development.

## 2.3 Clinical Managment of Teeth with Incomplete Rhizogenesis

### Diagnosis of the pulpal state

Permanent teeth with incomplete rhizogenesis can receive root canal treatment, under two basic and fundamental conditions: with or without pulp vitality.

The clinical evaluation of the pulpal state requires meticulous anamnesis, physical and radiographic exams. A critical clinical exam and determining the characteristics of pain will help to achieve this diagnosis. The pulp vitality test should also be used, but its results should be interpreted carefully. Two kinds of nerves are observed in the pulp, amyelinic nerves, responsible for the vasoconstriction and vasodilatation, and the myelinic nerves that respond to painful incentives. As the number of myelinic fibers increases with the rhizogenesis of the tooth, teeth with incomplete rhizogenesis have a reduced threshold for electrometrical stimulus, consequently they do not respond to pulp vitality tests in the usual way[8,34,46].

The radiographic exam will provide information about the stage of root development and the condition of the periapical tissues. The radiographic exam should be discerning, because the image of the dental sac, which is an embryonic structure that originates the periodontal tissues and that surrounds the apex of the teeth in formation, is frequently confused with periapical lesion[62,63].

By providing a two-dimensional image, the radiographic exam will, in some cases, be capable of showing the image of a complete root formation, which is not always the reality. Because root formation completes faster in the mesial-distal direction than in the buccal-lingual direction, and due to the proximity of the root walls in this direction, particularly in anterior teeth, the radiographic image presented shows complete root formation[21]. Despite the difficulties presented in determining the extent of apical closure radiographically, it should be emphasized that incorrect evaluation of the stage of the root development can lead to failure.

Unfortunately, it has not been possible to establish a direct relationship between the clinical diagnosis and the histological diagnosis, but combination of the findings of the anamnesis, physical exam and pulp vitality test can lead to improved clinical diagnosis of pulp vitality[63].

In cases with pulp vitality apexogenesis can be indicated. The clinical diagnosis of pulp necrosis leads to treatment for apexification. The success is directly related to correct diagnosis and understanding that the biological process of repair can be facilitated by the treatment performed[63].

## 2.4 Apexogenesis

Whenever pulp vitality is diagnosed, and endodontic intervention is necessary, a conservative treatment should be performed. The maintenance of pulp vitality will make the normal root development possible. This physiologic formation is known as apexogenesis, and is observed in cases of conservative treatment in teeth with incomplete rhizogenesis, when the physiologic process of normal closure of the apex allows the development of root end dentin, as well as the formation of the cementum canal, producing the root canal anatomy, shape and normal length. For the American Association of Endodontics[2], apexogenesis is "the vital pulp therapy procedure, performed to encourage continued physiological development and formation of the root end".

Considering the advantages of apexogenesis, the following can be included[14,33,36,52,56,58,90]:

1. Maintenance of the Hertwig's root sheath, thus the length and the normal shape of the tooth will be maintained, which are important future factors for its resistance and fixation in the dental arch. The favorable crown-root relationship will avoid periodontal disease with bone loss that places the stability of these teeth at an early risk.
2. Maintenance of vital pulp, thus assuring odontoblasts will continue to deposit dentin on the root canal walls and reduce the possibility of root fracture.
3. Complete formation of the root apex, thus creating conditions for future conventional root canal treatment, if necessary (Fig. 2.2-2.5).

When root canal treatment is required in canals with incomplete rhizogenesis, there is little probability of successful root canal filling, therefore teeth in the developmental stage must be treated with a biological focus[90].

In cases of small accidental pulp exposure during cavity preparation, when the pulpal tissue is healthy, direct pulp protection should be the preferred treatment. If there is wide pulp exposure as a result of removing decayed dentin or crown fractures, and other possible conditions, the elected treatment should be pulpotomy.

When the basic principles of pulpotomy are respected, pulp vitality can be proved by the root formation and development of the root walls, as well as by the normal closure of the root apex observed radiographically two years after the pulpotomy, depending on the degree of tooth development at the time of the endodontic intervention[63].

## 2.5 Apexification

One of the main dogmas of endodontics is root canal filling in three dimensions with emphasis on filling the apical third of the root. The filling becomes more predictable when the walls of the root canal converge at the apex, with a final constriction in the cementum-dentin junction. The apical preparation of root canals creates a stop that facilitates the appropriate application of condensation pressure for filling in three dimensions[33,36,52,56,58,64,90].

Although the incidence of caries in young patients has fallen considerably over the last few decades, has been a significant increase in the number of traumatic dental injuries due to the incentive to practice sports, increasing number of automobile accidents and violence[3]. Frequently the incisors are the most affected teeth, and depending on the intensity of the traumatic injury, rupture of the vascular-nerve fibers can occur, causing pulp necrosis and interrupting the completion of the root formation.

Until 1960, non vital permanent teeth with incomplete rhizogenesis were usually treated by conventional methods. However, root canal filling with gutta-percha cones, even when they were rolled or done by the professional, did not have good results, because the apical foramen was usually wider and did not allow condensation. The lack of apical stop frequently led to overfilling the periapical region. It was frequently necessary do apical surgery to remove the excess gutta-percha or do a retrograde filling to obtain the apical seal[35]. Nevertheless, the apical surgery technique associated with retrograde filling was not satisfactory, because of various inconveniences.

The technique of root canal filling with gutta-percha cones under the root apex has shown a low clinical success rate. With incomplete root canal filling, microorganisms can remain in the apical region and healing cannot take place. When the root canal is not infected, but the filling was made underneath, there can be secondary invasion of the unfilled portion by microorganisms coming from the blood stream or from the periodontal ligament, and lead to the development of periapical lesion[59].

Another method also used in the treatment of teeth with pulp necrosis and open apex, is the non surgical condensation of biocompatible material at the extremity of the root canal. The objective is to establish apical stop to enable immediate root canal filling. Although this technique offers the advantage of requiring only a few sessions, the need for retreatment should be considered some time later, if there has been completion of the root. Several biocompatible materials have been proposed, such as calcium hydroxide[40,41,65], resorption ceramic[49], mineral trioxide aggregate (MTA)[19] and others. However, from the clinical point of view, it is difficult to place these materials at apical level only, without leaving residues along the walls of the root canal and without overfilling the periapical area.

Nowadays, authors are unanimous in affirming that the best treatment for teeth with incomplete rhizogenesis and pulp necrosis is to stimulate apical closure, by temporary root canal filling with intracanal dressings (calcium hydroxide paste) until there are anatomical conditions that allow appropriate root filling to be definitively performed [40,41,59,62,63].

Apexification is defined as a method of inducing apical closure by mineralized tissue formation or by continuation of root development of an incompletely formed tooth, whose pulp is not vital. The American Association of Endodontics[2] defines apexification as "a method to induce a calcified barrier in a root with an open apex or the continued apical development of an incomplete root in teeth with necrotic pulp".

The nature of the tissue that contributes to the apical closure has been suggested as being cementum, osteodentin, osteocementum or bone. The apical seal can occur in a hood, barrier or bridge form. With apical sealing, root development may or may not increase the length of the root, but either way, root development is usually irregular, unlike the apexogenesis, which results in a regular apical seal and normal root development[59,63].

Kerekes et al.[47] evaluated the results of root canal treatment in 166 traumatized incisors of patients between 9 and 18 years of age. They observed that the group of teeth treated by apexification produced a success rate of 95% in comparison with the group of teeth treated conventionally, with a rate of 60%.

Apexification has become the most used method of treating teeth with non vital pulp, with incomplete rhizogenesis, because it allows appropriate root canal filling, which would be impossible to treat conservatively, in addition to reducing the possibility of overfilling. With apexification the need for apical surgery is eliminated.[55] Although many materials and methods are proposed for apical barrier formation, calcium hydroxide has had wiser acceptance, due to the high level of clinical success related to its use[32,48,40,42,63]. Chapter 20 discusses the biological and antimicrobial action mechanism of calcium hydroxide medications.

The basic principles of endodontic therapy continue to be of fundamental importance in the treatment of permanent teeth with incomplete rhizogenesis. Thus, some peculiar aspects of this treatment should be emphasized.

## Apexification technique

1. Before operative intervention, periapical radiography should be performed for diagnosis, to evaluate the stage of the root development and the condition of the periapical tissues.

2. The operative field should be isolated with a rubber dam.

3. Conventional coronal opening does not always offer direct or enough access to the root canals and does not allow the instruments to reach all the walls of the root canal in these teeth, frequently resulting in areas not being instrumented. Although coronal openings should be wide, excessive wear of the crown should be avoided.

4. To conclude the coronal opening, the pulp chamber and entrance of the root canal should be irrigated with 1% sodium hypochlorite, always associated with aspiration.

5. Exploration of the root canal should be carefully done. One must consider that in teeth with incomplete rhizogenesis, with the apical portion of the root not completely formed, the radiographic image of the root is not well defined, hindering determination of the length of the tooth, required for exploring the root canal. The presence of pain or hemorrhage during this maneuver indicates the need to keep the exploration instrument at a shorter distance than that of the pre-established length.

6. Preparation of the cervical third.

7. Sanitization process.

8. The real working length should be placed 1 mm short of the radiographic apex. If the patient presents sensitivity, or if there is hemorrhage, the working length should be reevaluated.

9. Emptying the root canal.

10. Root canal preparation in the teeth with incomplete rhizogenesis depends on the anatomical form of the root canal, whose walls can come in three forms: divergent, parallel or convergent to apical.

When the roots present an early stage of rhizogenesis and the root canal is divergent to apical, modeling is hindered since the instruments do not entirely reach the dentinal walls, annulling the file actions and enlargement, so that the objective is only to clean the infected dentinal walls. Quite often the use of third series instruments is necessary, which should exert negative pressure during penetration and positive pressure against all the walls when they are withdrawn.

In these cases, one must remember that because the dental tubules have not yet received the important deposition of intratubular dentin, and the peritubular dentin has not been completely mineralized, the walls become fragile and very thin. Therefore no intense action should be performed against them. Special attention should be paid during the biomechanical preparation, because the absence of an apical stop favors over instrumentation. Another precaution should be the placement of cursors in the irrigation needle, to avoid its excessive penetration, injuring the periapical tissues.

In cases of convergent walls to apical, the action of the K-file instrument during the modeling can be accompanied by an enlarging movement to improve removal of necrotic residues and bacteria from the root canal walls.

11. Drying and application of EDTA.

12. New irrigation and drying of the root canals.

13. Placement of the calcium hydroxide based dressing. The calcium hydroxide placement technique is described under a topic about calcium hydroxide (Chapter 20). Calcium hydroxide placement with a file, absorbent paper points and vertical pluggers presented the lowest frequency of empty spaces in the three thirds of the root canal.

14. Radiography to evaluate the quality of the root canal filling, to check whether it is complete or whether there are radiolucent spaces that show absence of the paste. The presence of spaces in the root canal with calcium hydroxide paste is an indication of the absence of intracanal dressing, which demands more care during placement. When well condensed, the calcium hydroxide will make the lumen of the root canal disappear.

15. Temporary cavity sealing is of fundamental importance to avoid contamination and damage to the reparative process. Dissolution of the intracanal dressing and consequent contamination of the root canal can result in new infection and determine clinical failure.

16. After the placement of the intracanal dressing, it is important to maintain clinical and radiographic control. The clinical condition of the tooth, filling with the calcium hydroxide paste, root and periapical tissue condition should be considered.

There are controversies about whether or not the intracanal dressing should be renewed, and what the ideal interval of time for the performing the renewals would be. Chawla[11] and Chosack et al.[12] suggest the placement of calcium oxide only once until there is radiographic evidence of mineralized tissue barrier formation. They support the clinical application because they believe that the calcium hydroxide is only required to begin the reparative process, and therefore, nothing would be gained by the repeated application, monthly or quarterly.

According to Cvek[17] and Fleiglin[30], every time that clinical-radiographic control demonstrates signs of treatment failure (persistent fistula, tumefaction, increase of the lesion or absence of apical seal) it would be indispensable to reevaluate the treatment performed, to improve the root canal preparation and put back the calcium hydroxide.

Renewal of the calcium hydroxide paste is supported by the statement that when in contact with the carbon dioxide of the tissues, this substance becomes calcium carbonate, altering its inductive capacity of mineralization[32,40,41].

Among the clinical-radiographic controls, the time interval ranges from 30 days, 60 days and 90 days[24-27,71,87,90], depending on the vehicle used in the calcium hydroxide paste, the type of lesion and stage of rhizogenesis. When the apical opening is quite wide, and there is the presence of periapical fluids determining the faster solubilization of the paste, it is necessary to renew the calcium hydroxide after 30 days. Radiolucent (empty) areas in the root canal can be radiographically observed, mainly in the apical third, indicating calcium hydroxide dispersion, and the need for replacing it[17,30].

Abbot[1] emphasizes that the radiographic image of the root canal filling with calcium hydroxide paste is not reliable for determining the presence of calcium hydroxide or to demonstrate whether or not the mineralized tissue barrier is complete. He emphasizes that the regular changes present many advantages, and affirms that the ideal time interval for changes depends on the stage of rhizogenesis at the time of treatment and the size of the apical diameter.

The presence of the patient under treatment for clinical-radiographic control is of fundamental importance. His/her absence can lead to unexpected clinical and radiographic results: partial sealing or periapical recurrence could occur. In the session following after absolute isolation and removal of the temporary restoration, the root canal should be irrigated with saline solution with a needle length ranging from 1 to 2 mm short of the working length.

Using the memory file, the solution should be agitated inside the root canal, which will aid the removal of calcium hydroxide paste. The file should be passed smoothly against the walls of the root canal to remove the intracanal dressing. The root canal should be dried with absorbent paper cones adapted and refilled with calcium hydroxide.

17. In order to detect apical closure in a radiographic exam, after the absolute isolation and removal of the temporary restoration, the root canal should be irrigated with saline solution and the intracanal dressing removed. With the memory instrument, without executing pressure, probe the presence of the apical barrier. Pass the memory instrument again, smoothly against the walls of the root canal, irrigate-aspirate, and dry with absorbent paper cones.

The period necessary for the apical closure can vary from 3 to 18 months[87,90]. Cvek[17] said that the absence or the presence of periapical lesions can be one of the decisive factors at / during this time.

18. Because teeth with incomplete rhizogenesis usually present very wide root canals, they are difficult to fill and there is the need to use resources like: filling, using inverted gutta-percha cones to get a better adaptation in the apical third, molding of the apical third of the root canal, by the superficial plastification with xylol of the selected gutta-percha cone, filling using gutta-percha cones of the third series, or filling using a self-made main gutta-percha cone.

In wide root canals, where even cones #140 are not adjusted to the apical diameter, a gutta-percha cone can be made. Three or more gutta-percha cones of the second series should be heated, uniting them to form a single bunch. After quick heating, the bunch of cones should be rolled between two glass plates forming one homogeneous cone. After cooling and hardening, the cone is in condition to be selected.

In the case of using the classical filling technique with active lateral condensation, a great deal of care should be taken during the condensation maneuvers not to exert excessive pressure on the root canal walls (Fig. 2.6-2.9).

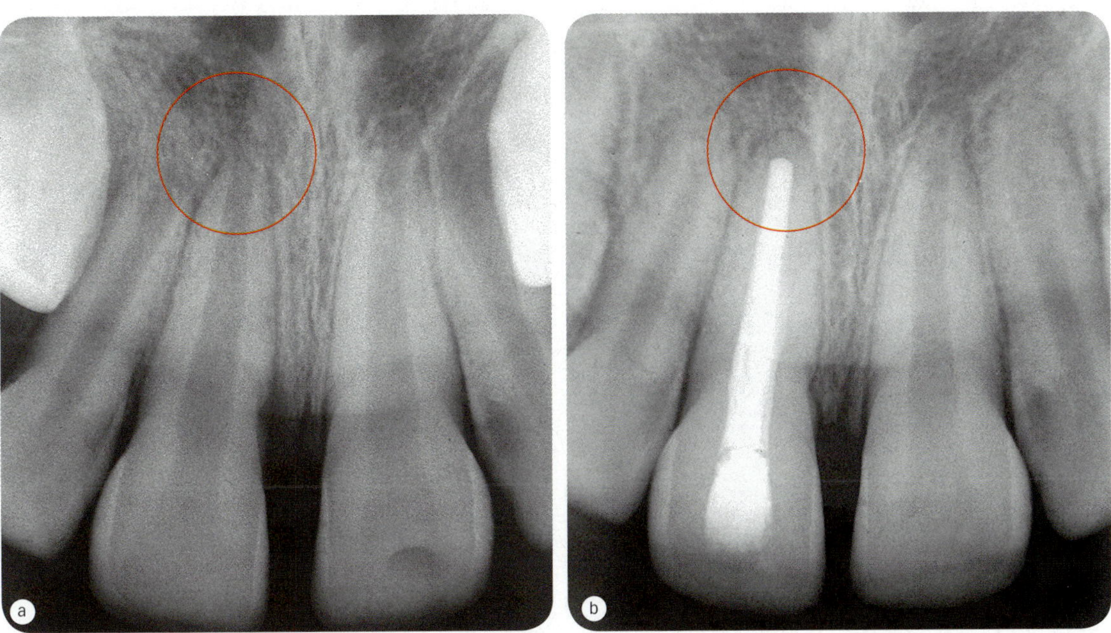

Figure 2.6 - (A-B) Apical closure by mineralized tissue formation of an incompletely formed tooth.

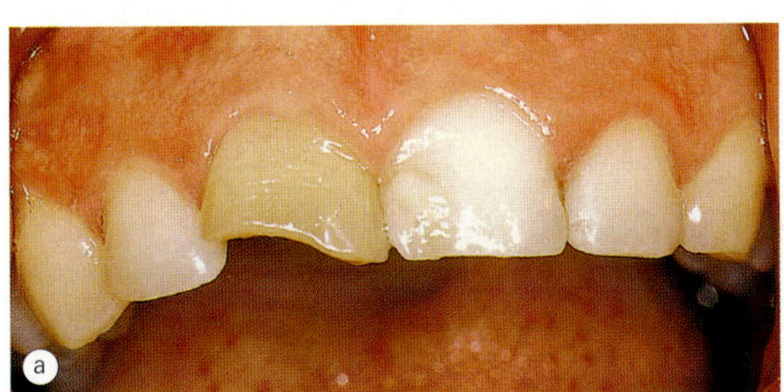

Figure 2.7 - (A-F) Apical closure by mineralized tissue formation of an incompletely formed tooth.

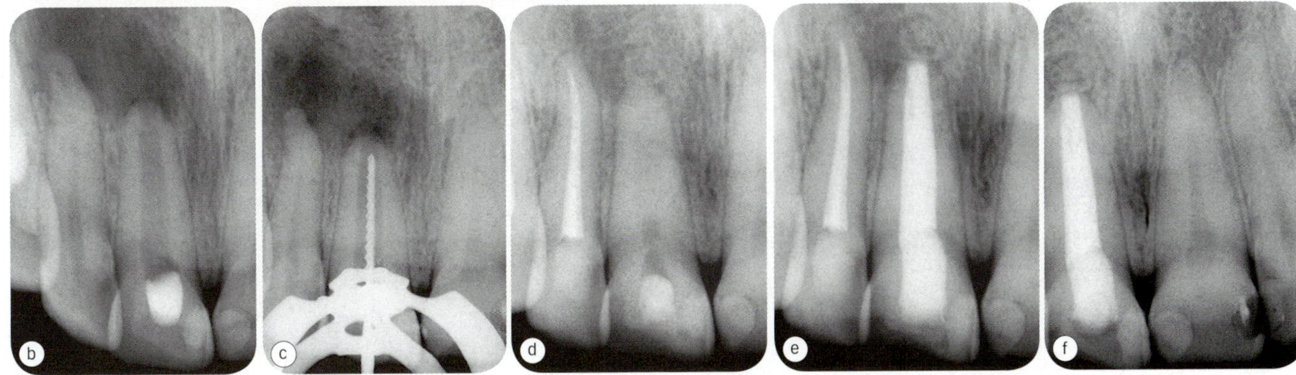

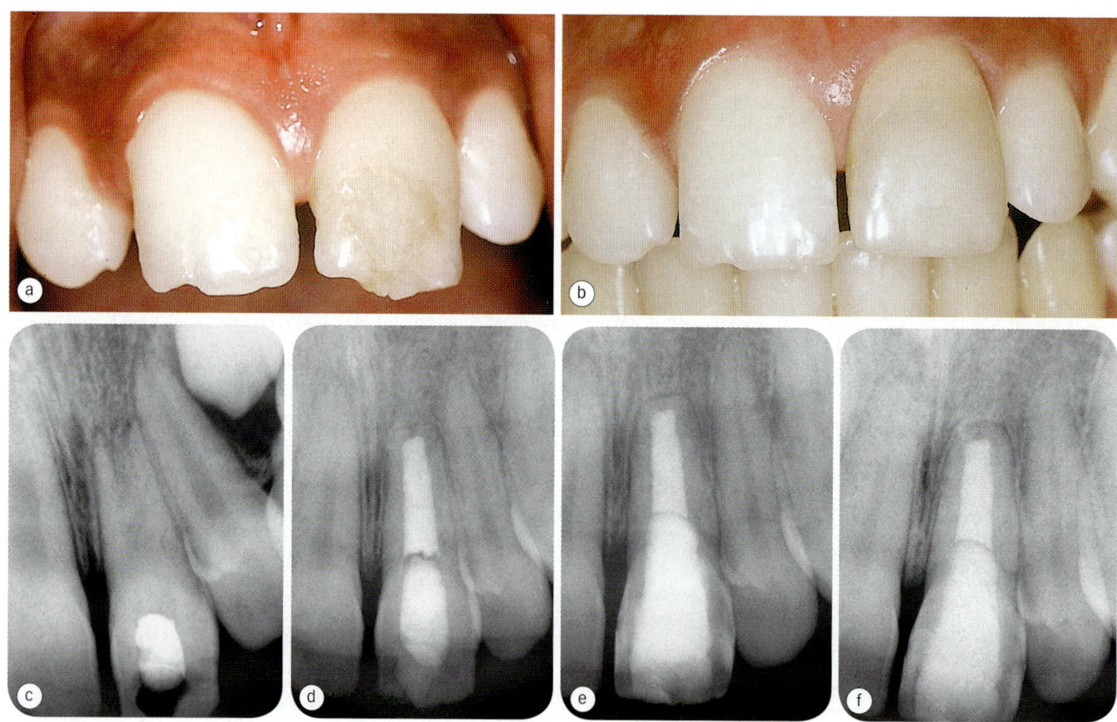


**Figure 2.8** - (**A-F**) Apical closure by mineralized tissue formation of an incompletely formed tooth.

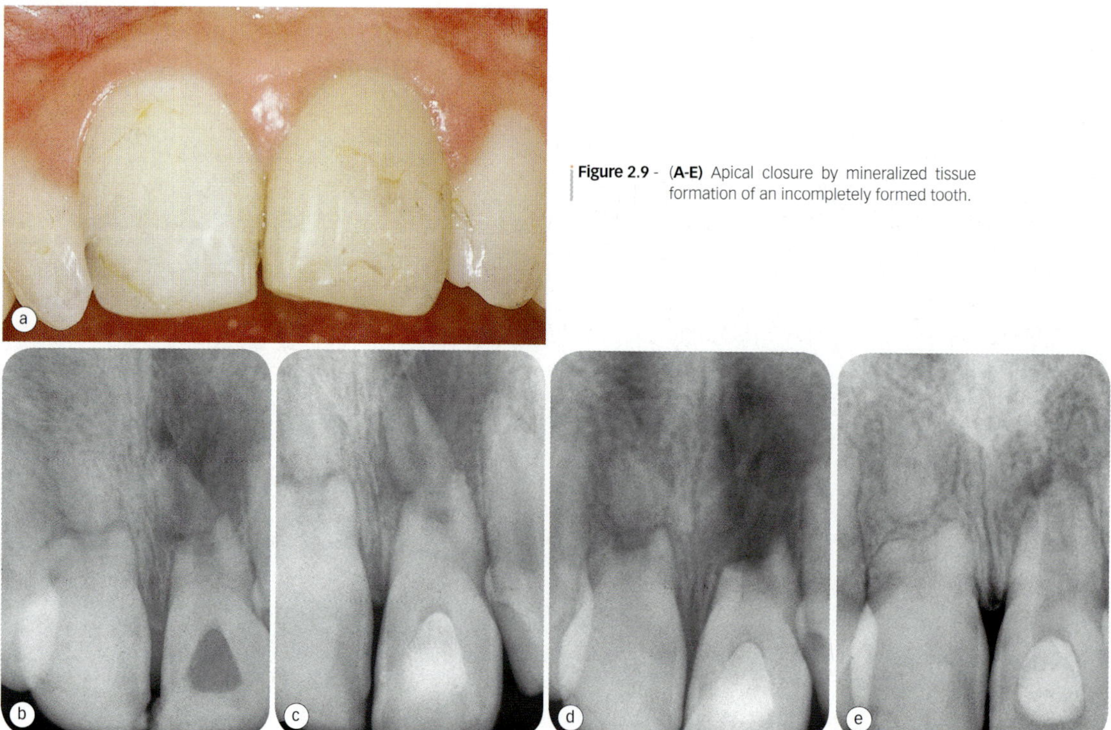


**Figure 2.9** - (**A-E**) Apical closure by mineralized tissue formation of an incompletely formed tooth.

## 2.6 Decisive Factors in Root Development

The process of periapical tissue repair after endodontic treatment has been the object of numerous studies[7,27,39-41,51,60,71,86]. One of the particularities of great interest in this subject concerns teeth with incomplete rhizogenesis and pulp necrosis that have suffered endodontic intervention.

The mechanism of root completion and apical closure post-treatment in teeth with pulp necrosis and incomplete rhizogenesis, still remains obscure. Some authors believe that the dental papilla and the Hertwig's epithelial root sheath stay intact and resume their functions when the infection is eliminated[32,38]. Klein & Levy[48] believe that the cells of the dental follicle around the root keep their genetic codes predisposing them to form cementoblasts, which consequently deposit cementum. Some researchers have suggested that calcium hydroxide stimulates the undifferentiated mesenchymal cells to differentiate into cementoblasts, which begin the cementogenesis in the apex[41].

Holland & Leonardo[39], observed that after root canal treatment, in the reparative process of teeth with incomplete rhizogenesis, root completion occurred exclusively through the deposition of hard tissue, with morphologic characteristics of cementum. Steiner & Van Hassel[79] also demonstrated apical closure with the formation of a mineralized tissue barrier that met the criteria for identification as cementum.

The occurrence of root completion seems to maintain a close relationship with different factors. There are indispensable factors for the occurrence of apical and periapical reparation of teeth with incomplete rhizogenesis, as well as important factors that make it the most organized and closest form of the morphology of a normal apical third. These factors can be related to the pulpal status, stage of root development at the time of endodontic intervention, presence of periapical lesion, intensity of the traumatic injury suffered and endodontic technique used in the treatment.

### Pulpal condition

When the pulp vitality is maintained, through conservative treatment, such as direct pulp protection or pulpotomy, there is greater possibility of complete root formation, by dentin deposition and root cementum[23].

### Stage of root formation

The embryonic structures existent in the apical area of teeth with pulp necrosis and incomplete rhizogenesis can assume an important role in the genesis of the morphologic alterations after root canal treatment[68].

When the dental papilla and Hertwig's epithelial root sheath are preserved, even if disorganized, their cells can differentiate into odontoblasts, to produce dentin formation and root completion[23].

However, when the pulp shows necrosis at an early stage of rhizogenesis, the possibility of complete apical formation becomes reduced, and the result is usually a shortened root. While teeth at more advanced stages of root development can present a reparation process to determine root completion similar to that of normal teeth.

### Presence of periapical lesion

During the physiological process of root completion, the Hertwig's epithelial root sheath begins to disintegrate and follicle cells differentiate into cementoblasts, depositing cementum on the dentin. Since the root does not conclude its normal development, cells of the dental sack close to the open apex, which retain the genetic code, predispose them to differentiate into cementoblasts[69].

Most of the authors have defended that root formation is dependent on the presence of Hertwig's root sheath, which would remain intact even in the presence of periapical lesions[16,38,86].

For Heithersay[38] because it is an epithelium, Hertwig's epithelial root sheath would be more resistant to inflammatory alterations, therefore it would be possible, in cases of teeth with incomplete rhizogenesis, pulp necrosis and periapical lesion, for Hertwig's epithelial root sheath to survive and remain capable of continuing to organize root development when the inflammatory process is eliminated. Andreasen et al.[4] suggest a regenerative potential of Hertwig's epithelial root sheath, where fragments of these remain viable in the face of certain aggressions, with the capacity to recreate a new Hertwig's epithelial root sheath and then to complete root formation.

However, histological studies have not demonstrated the presence of Hertwig's root sheath in the cases of teeth with periapical lesion[22,37,41,42]. Diab & Stallard[20] reported that cementum formation does not depend on the presence or absence of Hertwig's root sheath, and this would explain the root completion, mainly in teeth with periapical lesion.

Esberard et al.[23] related that teeth with incomplete rhizogenesis with periapical lesion tend to have apical and periapical reparation exclusively due to cells originated from the periodontal ligament, only capable of producing hard tissue of the cementoid type. The extent of the lesion can influence this process, because the larger the root involvement of the periapical lesion, the smaller will be the number of cells with the capacity of synthesizing cementoid matrix, migrating to the root apex in order to reconstitute it.

### Intensity of traumatic injury

Hertwig's epithelial root sheath is usually sensitive to the traumatic dental injuries, but because of the vascularization and amount of cells in the apical area, root formation can continue in the presence of pulp inflammation or necrosis[63].

In addition to inducing the inflammatory process in the apical area, associated with pulp necrosis, traumatic injury can disorganize the dental papilla still present in the final phase of the rhizogenesis, as well as disarticulate the components Hertwig's root sheath, fundamental for the formation of the root. The fragmentation of Hertwig's root sheath and the disorganization of the dental papilla are unfavorable conditions for restructuring the normal dental anatomy[23].

## 2.7 Endodontic technique

Some procedures performed during the treatment of these teeth are of considerable importance in root completion: root canal preparation, removal of the necrotic tissue, decrease in the number of microorganisms in the root canal, the intracanal dressing used, and root canal filling.

The inflammatory process presents a vascular-exudative phenomenon, associated with cellular and humoral phenomenon, which interact with the aggressor agent that promotes destructive events in the apical and periapical area. Infection of the root canal of teeth with incomplete rhizogenesis exacerbates these destructive events. The persistence of the infection leads to a progressive destruction of the osteogenic apical structures and periapical remainders, impeding their functions, among them root completion. Infection is always undesirable, and when it is present, the possibility of apical completion, morphologically similar to normality, is reduced; therefore it becomes indispensable to removal all necrotic tissue present in the root canal, by appropriate biomechanical preparation[23,86].

The use of irrigant solutions and medications that are harmful to the apical and periapical tissues, also make the desired apical completion difficult.

Therefore, the factors inherent to the endodontic technique used, which can be decisive in root completion are: absence of infection in the root canal, use of medications or solutions non aggressive to the apical and periapical tissues, biomechanics appropriate to the biology of the remaining tissues, hermetic root canal filling and compatible filling material, and if possible, stimulation of hard tissue matrix synthesis.

## 2.8 Forms of Periapical Repair

The periapical reparation and the formation of hard tissue after treatment with calcium hydroxide occur, in long term, in 79% to 96% of the cases. However, the permanence of these teeth in the buccal cavity is reduced by the potential of cervical fracture due to the thinness of the dental walls[87].

Reconstruction of the apical third in teeth with incomplete rhizogenesis, due to several factors previously discussed, can promote several forms of root completion.[6,32] For Heithersay[38] a greater number of types of mineralized tissue, which can be deposited in the apical area, and varied forms of repair seem to be possible. The periapical environment and its response seem to dictate a particular pattern of repair individually in each case.

### Complete and normal root completion

This completion takes place when the root pulp is preserved in the root canal after a direct pulp protection, pulpotomy or when endodontic intervention is performed in a tooth in which the root was already formed, however, with the apical foramen still open[23].

### Complete and normal root completion, with pulp necrosis

In this form of reparation there is a great formation of mineralized tissue, even with pulp necrosis. This occurs when the apical tissues have not suffered significant damage and the cells in the area have been preserved. In the etiopathogenesis of these cases there is usually a history of light traumatic injury, but sufficient to have caused pulp necrosis, without infection[37,38].

### Root and apical completion with foreshortening of the root

In these cases apical completion is incomplete, because when compared with the homologous tooth, the root is shorter. This condition usually occurs when there is pulp necrosis and the root is at an initial stage of rhizogenesis, with the maximum formation of the medium third[23].

The dental papilla in this condition is wide and its destruction is partial. Thus, elimination of the necrotic pulp offers biological conditions for the remainders of the dental papilla and Hertwig's root sheath to promote the apical completion, but without reestablishing the normal length of the root[23].

### Apical completion with a mineralized tissue barrier

In some cases, the apical closure is a mineralized barrier, but without root development[90]. Complete destruction of Hertwig's root sheath results in cessation of normal root development. Once the dental papilla is destroyed there will be no differentiation of cells into odontoblasts. However, hard tissue can be formed by cementoblasts, which are usually present in the apical area and by fibroblasts of the dental follicle and periodontal ligament, which differentiate into hard tissue producer cells[86].

Radiographic and clinical evidence of the complete formation of the hard tissue barrier, and histological analyses have shown that the barrier is porous, and sometimes partial. However, for the clinical success, a barrier of impermeable material is not necessary[79].

### Absence of apical completion

This clinical condition can occur in teeth in which the apical and periapical area have suffered extensive damage with necrosis of the cells that had the potential to promote the formation of hard tissue. After the harmful agents have been eliminated, none of these cells remain in the apical area of dental papilla or even in periodontal ligament cells, which could favor the formation of hard tissue, even if they were rudimentary and disorganized[23].

## References


1. Abbot P. Apexification with calcium hydroxide – when should the dressing be changed? The case for regular dressing changes. Aust Endod J 1998;24:27-32.
2. American Association of Endodontics. Glossary of endodontics terms. 7th ed. Chicago: American Association of Endodontics, 2003.
3. Andreasen JO, Andreasen FM. Texto e atlas colorido de traumatismo dentário. 3rd ed. Porto Alegre: Artmed, 2001.
4. Andreasen JO, Kristerson L, Andreasen FM. Damage of the Hertwig's epithelial root smeath: effect upon root growth after autotransplantation of teeth in monkeys. Endod Dent Traumatol 1988;4:145-51.
5. Banchs F, Trope M. Revascularization of immature permanent teeth with apical periodontitis: new treatment protocol? J Endod 2004;30:196 –200.
6. Barker, BCN, Mayne JR. Some unusual cases of apexification subsequent to trauma. Oral Surg Oral Med Oral Pathol 1975; 39:144-50.
7. Berbert A. Comportamento dos tecidos apicais e periapicais após biopulpectomia e obturação do canal radicular com AH 26, $Ca(OH)_2$ ou mistura de ambos. Estudo histológico em dentes de cães. (Doctoral thesis), University of São Paulo, 1978.
8. Bernick S. Difference in nerve distribuition between erupted and non-erupted human teeth. J Dent Res 1964;43:406-11.
9. Bhaskar SN. Orban's oral histology and embriology. 11th St. Louis: Mosby-Year Book, 1991.
10. Bosshardt DD, Nanci A. Immunodetection of enamel- and cementum-related (bone) proteins at the enamel-free area and cervical portion of the tooth in rat molars. J Bone Min Res 1997;12:367-79.
11. Chawla HS. Apical closure in a non vital permanent tooth using one calcium hydroxide dressing. J Dent Child 1986;53: 44-7.
12. Chosack A, Sela J, Cleaton-Jones P. A histological and quantitative histomorphometric study of apexification of non vital permanent incisors of vervet monkeys after repeated root filling with calcium hydroxide. Endod Dent Traumatol 1997;13:24-7.
13. Chueh LH, Huang GT. Immature teeth with periradicular periodontitis or abscess undergoing apexogenesis: a paradigm shift. J Endod 2006;32:1205–13.
14. Citrome GP, Kaminski EJ, Hever MA. A comparison study of tooth apexification in the dog. J Endod 1979;5:290-97.
15. Cobourne M, Sharpe P. Tooth and jaw: Molecular mechanisms of patterning in the first branchial arch. Arch Oral Biol 2003;48:1–14.
16. Cooke S, Rowbotham TC. Root canal therapy in non vital teeth with open apices. Br Dent J 1960;108: 147.
17. Cvek M. Treatment of non vital permanent incisors with calcium hydroxide. I – Follow up of periapical repair and apical closure of immature roots. Odonto Revy 1972;28:27-44.
18. D'Souza R. Development of the pulpodentin complex. In: Goodis HE, ed: Seltzer and Bender's Dental Pulp. Carol Stream: Quintessence Publishing Co, Inc; 2002.
19. Darlene RH, Schindler WG, Walker III WA, Thomas DD. The sealing ability and retention characteristics of mineral trioxide aggregate in a model of apexification. J Endod 2002;28:386-90.
20. Diab MA, Stallard RC. A study of the relationship between epithelial root seath and root development. Periodont 1965;3:10-4.
21. Duel RC. Consevative endodontic treatment of the open apex in three dimensions. Dent Clin N Amer 1973; 17:125-35.
22. Dylewski JJ. Apical closures of non-vital teeth. Oral Surg Oral Med Oral Pathol 1971;32:82-9.
23. Esberard RM, Consolaro A, Leonardo RT. Rizogênese incompleta: princípios, técnicas e formas de reparação. (Monografia). Faculdade de Odontologia de Araraquara, Universidade Estadual Paulista; 1993, 12 p.
24. Estrela C, Pesce HF. Chemical analysis of the formation of calcium carbonate and its influence on calcium hydroxide pastes in the presence of connective tissue of the dog. Part II. Braz Dent J 1997;8:49-53.
25. Estrela C, Pesce HF. Chemical analysis of the liberation of calcium and hydroxyl ions of calcium hydroxide pastes in the presence of connective tissue of the dog. Part I. Braz Dent J 1996;7:41-6.
26. Estrela C, Sydney GB, Bammann LL, Felippe-Jr O. Mechanism of the action of calcium and hydroxyl ions of calcium hydroxide on tissue and bacteria. Braz Dent J 1995;6:85-90.
27. Felippe MCS, Felipe WT, Marques MM, Antoniazzi JH. The effect of the renewal of calcium hydroxide paste on the apexification and periapical healing of teeth with incomplete root formation. Int Endod J 2005;38:436-42.
28. Fitzgerald M. Cellular mechanics of dentinal bridge repair using 3H-thymidine. J Dent Res 1979;58:2198-206.
29. Fitzgerald M, Chiego DJ Jr, Heys DR. Autoradiographic analysis of odontoblast replacement following pulp exposure in primate teeth. Arch Oral Biol 1990;35:707-15.
30. Fleiglin B. Differences in apex formation during apexification with calcium hydroxide paste. Endod Dent Traumatol 1985;1:195-9.
31. Fong CD, Hammarström L. Expression of amelin and amelogenin in epithelial root sheath remnants of fully formed rat molars. Oral Surg Oral Med Oral Pathol Oral Radiol Endod 2000;90:218-23.
32. Frank AL. Therapy for the divergent pulpless tooth by continued apical formation. J Am Dent Assoc 1966;72: 87-93.
33. Friend LA. Root canal morphology in incisor teeth in the 6 to 15 – year – old child. J Br Endod Soc 1969;3: 35.

34. Fulling H-J, Andreasen JO. Influence of maturation status and tooth type of permanent teeth upon electrometric and thermal pulp testing. J Dent Res 1976;84:286-90.
35. Gallagher C, Mourino AP. Root end induction. J Am Dent Assoc 1979;98:578-80.
36. Gutmann JL, Heaton JF. Management of the open (Immature) apex 2. Non-vital teeth. Int Endod J 1981;14:173-78.
37. Ham JN, Patterson SS, Mitchel DF. Induced apical closure of immature pulpless teeth in monkeys. Oral Surg Oral Med Oral Pathol 1972;33:438-49.
38. Heithersay GS. Stimulation of root formation in incompletely developed pulpless teeth. Oral Surg Oral Med Oral Pathol 1970;29:620-30.
39. Holland R, Leonardo MR. Processo de reparo de dentes com rizogênese incompleta após tratamento endodôntico - contribuição ao estudo. Rev Bras Odont 1968;154: 570-77.
40. Holland R, Souza V, Russo MC. Healing process after root canal therapy in immature human teeth. Rev Fac Odontol Araçatuba 1973; 2:269-79.
41. Holland R, Souza V, Taglavini RL, Milanezi LA. Healing process of teeth with open apices – histological study. Bull Tokyo Dent Coll 1971;12:333-38.
42. Holland R, Souza V, Nery MJ, Mello W, Bernabé PFE, Otoboni-Filho JA. Effect of the dressing in root canal treatment with calcium hydroxide. Rev Fac Odont Araçatuba 1978;7:39-45.
43. Iwaya SI, Ikawa M, Kubota M. Revascularization of an immature permanent tooth with apical periodontitis and sinus tract. Dent Traumatol 2001;17:185–7.
44. Jernvall J, Kettunen P, Karavanova I, Martin LB, Thesleff I. Evidence for the role of the enamel knot as a control center in mammalian tooth cusp formation: non-dividing cells express growth stimulating FGF-4 gene. Int J Dev Biol 1994;38:463–9.
45. Jernvall J, Thesleff I. Reiterative signaling and patterning during mammalian tooth morphogenesis. Mech Dev 2000;92:19–29.
46. Johnsen DI. Inervation of teeth: qualitative, quantitative and developmental assessment. J Dent Res 1985;64:555-63.
47. Kerekes K, Heide S, Jacobsen I. Follow-up examination of endodontic treatment in traumatized juvenile incisors. J Endod 1980;6:744.
48. Klein SH, Levy BA. Histologic evaluation of induced apical closure of a human pulplesss tooth. Oral Surg Oral Med Oral Pathol 1974;38: 954-59.
49. Koenigs JF, Heller AL, Brilliant JD, Melfi RC, Driskell TD. Induced apical closure of permanent teeth in adult primates using resornable form of tricalcium phosphate ceramic. J Endod 1975; 1:102-6.
50. Kollar EJ, Baird GR. Tissue interactions in embryonic mouse tooth germs. II. The inductive role of the dental papilla. J Embryol Exp Morphol 1970;24:173–86.
51. Leonardo MR, Leal JM, Esberard RM. Tratamiento de los condutos radiculares de dientes con rizogénese incomplieta (Estudo clínico-radiográfico e histológico). Ars Curandi em Odont 1978;5:29-34.
52. Leonardo MR. et al. Histological evaluation of the therapy using calcium hydroxide dressing for teeth with incompletely formed apices and periapical lesions. J Endod 1993;19:348-52.
53. Linde A, Goldberg M. Dentinogenesis. Crit Rev Oral Biol Med 1993;4:679–728.
54. Lumsden AG. Spatial organization of the epithelium and the role of neural crest cells in the initiation of the mammalian tooth germ. Development 1988;103:155-169 (Suppl).
55. Machanowicz JP, Machanowicz AE. A conservative approach and procedure to fill and incompletely formed root using calcium hydroxide as an adjunct. J Am Dent Assoc 1967;34:42-7.
56. Maroto M, Barbería E, Planells P, Vera V. Treatment of non-vital immature incisor with mineral trioxide aggregate (MTA). Dent Traumatol 2003;19:165-9.
57. Mina M, Kollar EJ. The induction of odontogenesis in non-dental mesenchyme combined with early murine mandibular arch epithelium. Arch Oral Biol 1987;32:123–7.
58. Moodnick RM. Clinical correlation of the development of the apex and surrounding structure. Oral Surg Oral Med Oral Pathol 1963;16: 600-7.
59. Morse DR, O'larnic J, Yesilsoy C. Apexification: review of the literature. Quintessence Internacional 1990;21:589-96.
60. Murata SS. Análise histomorfológica de dentes decíduos de cães com rizogênese incompleta, após biopulpectomia e obturação dos canais radiculares com hidróxido de cálcio em diferentes veículos. (Master's Thesis). São Paulo State University, 2006.
61. Nolla CM. The development of the permanent teeth. J Dent Child 1960;27:254-66.
62. Pitt Ford TR. Apexification and Apexogenesis. In: Walton R, Torabinejad M. Principles and Practice of Endodontics. 2nd ed. Philadelphia: Saunders,1996. p. 373-84.
63. Rafter M. Apexification: a review. Dent Traumatol 2005;21:1-8.
64. Rice RT, Rice PL. Endodontic therapy for an open apex - apexification or apexogenesis. Dent Assist 1991;60:13-5.
65. Roberts SC, Brilliant JD. Tricalcium phosphate as an adjunct to apical closure in pulpless permanent teeth. J Endod 1975;1:263-9.
66. Ruch JV. Odontoblast commitment and differentiation. Biochem Cell Biol 1998;76:923–38.
67. Ruch JV, Lesot H, Begue-Kirn C. Odontoblast differentiation. Int J Dev Biol 1995; 39:51– 68.
68. Saad Neto M, Carvalho ACP, Okamoto T. Traumatismo em dentes permanentes com rizogênese incompleta - avaliação radiográfica e histológica em cães. Rev Fac Odont Araçatuba 1978;.7: 95-101.
69. Seltzer S. The root apex. In: Seltzer S. Endodontology: biologic considerations in endodontic procedures. 2nd ed. Philadelphia: Lea & Febiger, 1988. p. 1-30.
70. Shi S, Gronthos S. Perivascular niche of postnatal mesenchymal stem cells in human bone marrow and dental pulp. J Bone Miner Res 2003;18:696 –704.
71. Silva LAB. Tratamento endodôntico de dentes permanentes com rizogênese incompleta. In: Leonardo MR. Endodontia: Tratamento de canais radiculares, princípios técnicos e biológicos. 2nd ed. São Paulo: Arts Médicas, 2005, p. 1216-39.

72. Smith AJ, Lesot H. Induction and regulation of crown dentinogenesis: embryonic events as a template for dental tissue repair? Crit Rev Oral Biol Med 2001;12:425–37.
73. Soares IJ, Goldberg F. Tratamento de dentes com rizogênese incompleta. In: Soares IJ, Goldberg F. Endodontia: técnica e fundamentos. Porto Alegre: Artmed, 2001, p. 252-62.
74. Song L, Webb NE, Song Y, Tuan RS. Identification and functional analysis of candidate genes regulating mesenchymal stem cell self-renewal and multipotency. Stem Cells 2006;24:1707–18.
75. Sonoyama W, Liu Y, Fang D, Yamaza T, Seo BM, Zhang C, Liu H, Gronthos S, Wang CY, Shi S, Wang S. Mesenchymal stem cell-mediated functional tooth regeneration in swine. PLoS ONE 2006;1:79.
76. Sonoyama W, Liu Y, Yamaza T, Tuan RS, Wang S, Shi S, Huang GTJ. Characterization of the apical papilla and its residing stem cells from human immature permanent teeth: a pilot study. J Endod 2008;34:166-71.
77. Sonoyama W, Seo BM, Yamaza T, Shi S. Human Hertwig's epithelial root sheath cells play crucial roles in cementum formation. J Dent Res 2007;86:594 –9.
78. Steele-Perkins G, Butz KG, Lyons GE, Zeichner-David M, Kim HJ, Cho MI, Gronostajski RM. Essential role for NFI-C/CTF transcription-replication factor in tooth root development. Mol Cell Biol 2003; 23:1075-84.
79. Steiner JC, Van Hassel HJ. Experimental root apexification in primates. Oral Surg Oral Med Oral Pathol 1971;31:409-20.
80. Sveen OB, Hawes RR. Differentiation of new odontoblasts and dentine bridge formation in rat molar teeth after tooth grinding. Arch Oral Biol 1968;13:1399-409.
81. Tecles O, Laurent P, Zygouritsas S, Burger AR, Camps J, Dejou J, About I. Activation of human dental pulp progenitor/stem cells in response to odontoblast injury. Arch Oral Biol 2005;50:103-8.
82. Ten Cate AR. Oral Histology: Development, Structure and Function. 6th ed. Amsterdan: Elsevier, 2003.
83. Thesleff I, Keranen S, Jernvall J. Enamel knots as signalling centers linking tooth morphogenesis and odontoblast differentiation. Adv Dent Res 2001;15:14-8.
84. Thesleff I, Sharpe P. Signalling networks regulating dental development. Mech Dev 1997;67:111–23.
85. Tompkins K, Alvares K, George A, Veis A. Two related low molecular mass polypeptide isoforms of amelogenin have distinct activities in mouse tooth germ differentiation in vitro. J Bone Min Res 2005; 20:341-9.
86. Torneck CD, Smith JS, Grindall P. Biologic effects of endodontic procedures on developing incisor teeth. Oral Surg 1973; 34:541-54.
87. Trope M, Chivian N, Sigurdsson A. Traumatic injuries. In: Cohen S, Burns KC. Pathways of the pulp. 7th ed. St. Louis Mosby, 1994, p.552-97.
88. Tucker AS, Matthews KL, Sharpe PT. Transformation of tooth type induced by inhibition of BMP signaling. Science 1998;282:1136–8.
89. Vaahtokari A, Aberg T, Jernvall J, Keranen S, Thesleff I. The enamel knot as a signaling center in the developing mouse tooth. Mech Dev 1996;54:39–43.
90. Webber RT. Apexogenesis versus apexificación. Clin Odont Amer 1984; 28: 657-86.
91. Weisleder R, Benitez CR. Maturogenesis: is it a new concept? J Endod 2003;29:776–8.
92. Yen AH-H, Sharpe PT. Stem cells and tooth tissue engineering. Cell Tissue Res 2008;331:359–72.
93. Yokohama-Tamaki T, Ohshima H, Fujiwara N, Takada Y, Ichimori Y, Wakisaka S, Ohuchi H, Harada H. Cessation of FGF10 signaling, resulting in a defective dental epithelial stem cell compartment, leads to the transition from crown to root formation. Development 2006;133:1359–66.

# Endodontic Treatment Planning


**C. Estrela**

*Federal University of Goiás, Goiânia, GO, Brazil*

**A. H. G. Alencar**

*Federal University of Goiás, Goiânia, GO, Brazil*

**J. A. Silva**

*Federal University of Goiás, Goiânia, GO, Brazil*

**C. R. A. Estrela**

*Brazilian Dentistry Research and Learning Center, CEPOBRAS, Goiânia, GO, Brazil*


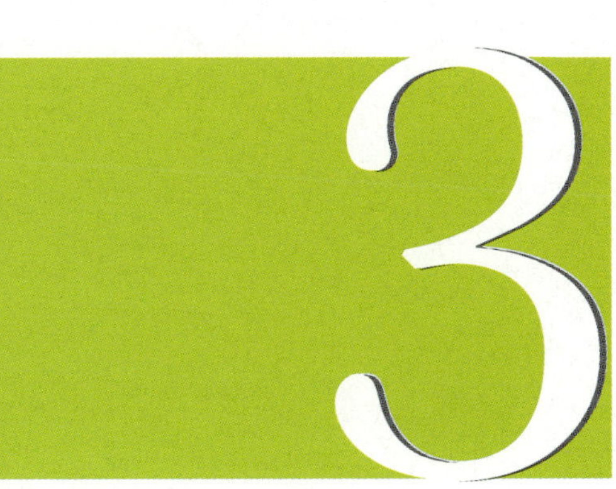

Chapter contents

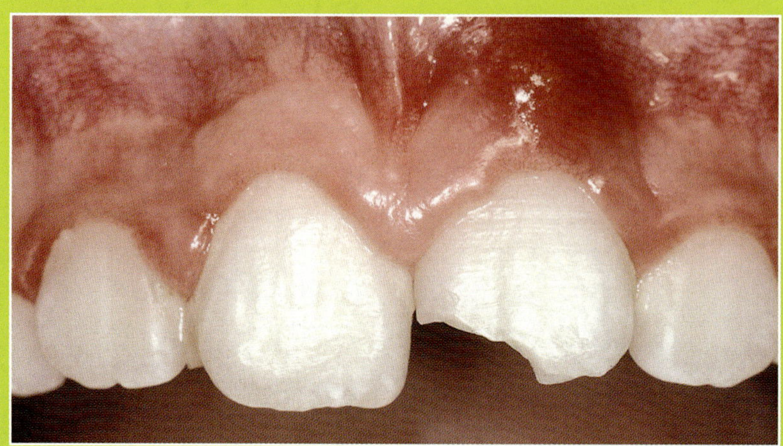

Photograph of the tooth 11 with preserved crown and tooth 21 with crown fracture and fistula.

## 3.1 Introduction

The treatment plan is essential to a successful endodontic procedure. Clear understanding of the diagnosis and organization help facilitate the development of the treatment plan and execution of the procedure.

The percentage of successful endodontic treatments appears to be high. These percentages vary depending on the pulp condition encountered. For teeth with apical asymptomatic periodontitis and endodontic retreatments the values are inferior to those with necrosis under absence of apical periodontitis or pulp vitality. These aspects may not be analyzed separately because they can be influenced by the systemic conditions of the patient.

Several factors contribute to the perfect execution of the endodontic treatment. These include: the correct determination of the diagnosis which represents the essence of the treatment; the case selection which judges the predictability of success of the treatment, the infection control, the organization which will streamline the operational steps, following biological and mechanical principles of root canal preparation, use of biocompatible materials and techniques, adequate restoration of the tooth, and follow-up (Fig. 3.1).

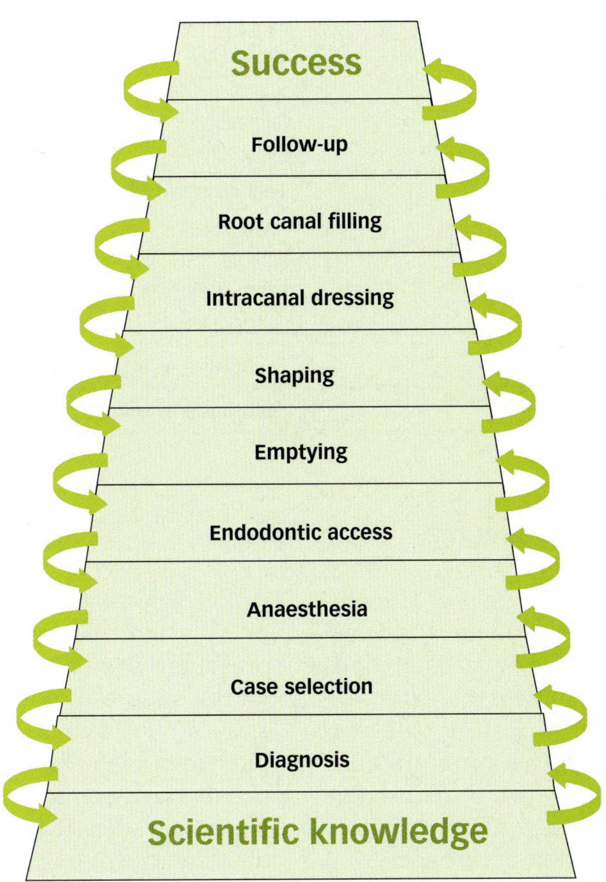


**Figure 3.1** - Endodontic treatment plan.

The present chapter's objective is to present the operational steps, within the systematic parameters of planning for the execution of the endodontic treatment.

## 3.2 Structuring the Diagnosis

The diagnosis begins with an investigation of pulp and periapical alterations. This initial investigation lays the basis of the structure for the diagnosis. The diagnosis is considered as hypothetic, or clinically probable, until the surgical intervention, the microscopic exam, and/or complementary exams. To determine the clinically probable diagnosis of endodontic alterations, representative exams like anamnesis, clinical exam, pulp vitality exam, radiographic exams and the complementary exams are used (Table 3.1).

**Table 3.1** - Semiogenic and Semiotechnique Resources for structuring the diagnosis

| | |
|---|---|
| **Anamnesis** | **Technique of Interrogation**<br>Main Complaint<br>Passed History<br>Current History<br>Medical History/Odontologic Hístory<br>Clinical Pain Characteristics |
| **Clinical Exam** | **Technique of Exploration**<br>Inspection<br>Examination<br>Palpation<br>Percussion |
| **Exam of Pulp Vitality** | **Technique of Stimulation**<br>Heat/Cold Test<br>Electric Test<br>Mechanical Test<br>Other Tests |
| **Exam by Imaging** | **Technique of Interpretation of Images** |
| **Complementary Exams** | **Technique of Investigation** |

## 3.3 Diagnosis of Alterations of the Dental Pulp

The presence of patient pain or discomfort during the initial exam can be an expressive symptom. However the initial exam does not allow to correctly evaluate the extension of the pulp inflammation process nor the possibilities of tissue repair. This symptom does not present a correlation with the microscopic exam. The clinical diagnosis of inflammatory pulp changes structured in accordance with the treatment is described in Table 3.2.

For the treatment of the dental pulp, especially the pulpotomy, Holland & Souza[106] presented some fundamental clinical aspects for the suggestion of this therapeutic option, as shown in Table 3.3. Figure 3.2 shows a sequence of the pathologic pulp and periapical events developing from the microorganisms of dental caries. Figure 3.3 shows a sequence of technique of pulpotomy.

**Table 3.2** - Clinical Classification of Dental Pulp Inflammation

| Clinical Diagnosis | Clinical Characteristics of the Cavity | Symptomatology (pain) |
|---|---|---|
| **Normal pulp** | Closed cavity | Absence of symptoms<br>Positive pulp vitality test (P.V.T.) |
| **Hyper-reactive pulpalgia** | Closed cavity<br>Hyperemia/Hypersensitiveness | Provoked symptom<br>Positive to P.V.T. |
| **Symptomatic pulpitis** | Closed cavity<br>(Pulp inflammation) | Spontaneous symptom<br>Positive to P.V.T. |
| **Asymptomatic pulpitis** | Opened cavity<br>Pulp Hyperplasia/Ulceration | Provoked symptom<br>Little effective to P.V.T. |
| **Pulp necrosis** | Closed cavity<br>Opened cavity | Absence of symptoms<br>Negative P.V.T. |

P.V.T. – Pulp Vitality Test
Observations: Considering a histopathology analysis you can accept the hypothesis of a pulp inflammation under absence of symptomatology.

**Table 3.3** - Fundamental Clinical Aspects for suggestion of Pulpotomy

| Signal | Favoring Factors | Adverse Factors |
|---|---|---|
| **Bleeding** | Normal after cutting the pulp tissue<br>Blood: Red color / alive | Absent<br>Very dark<br>Very clear (yellowish) |
| **Remaining Pulp** | Pulp consistent/body (resistant to a curette action) | |
| **Dental Crown** | Nearly integer or with thin resistant walls | Great dental coronary destruction requiring introduction of intracanal post |

(Holland & Souza[106])

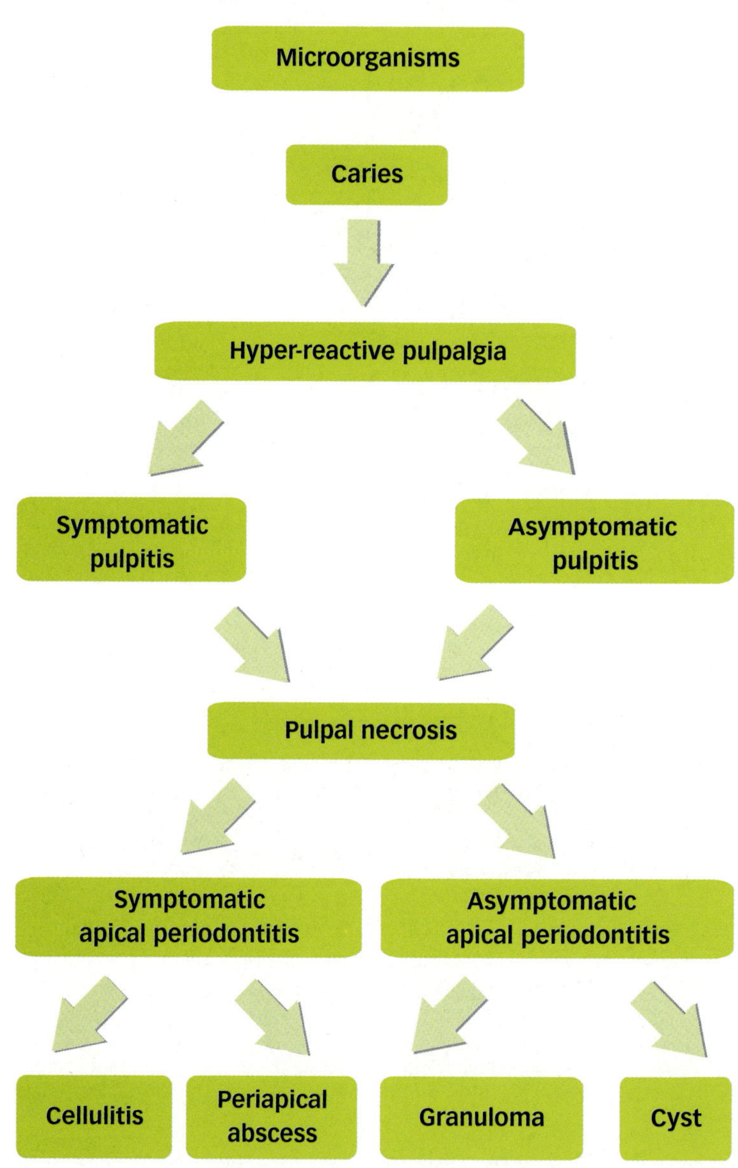


**Figure 3.2** - Sequence of the pathologic pulp and periapical events developing from the microorganisms of dental caries.

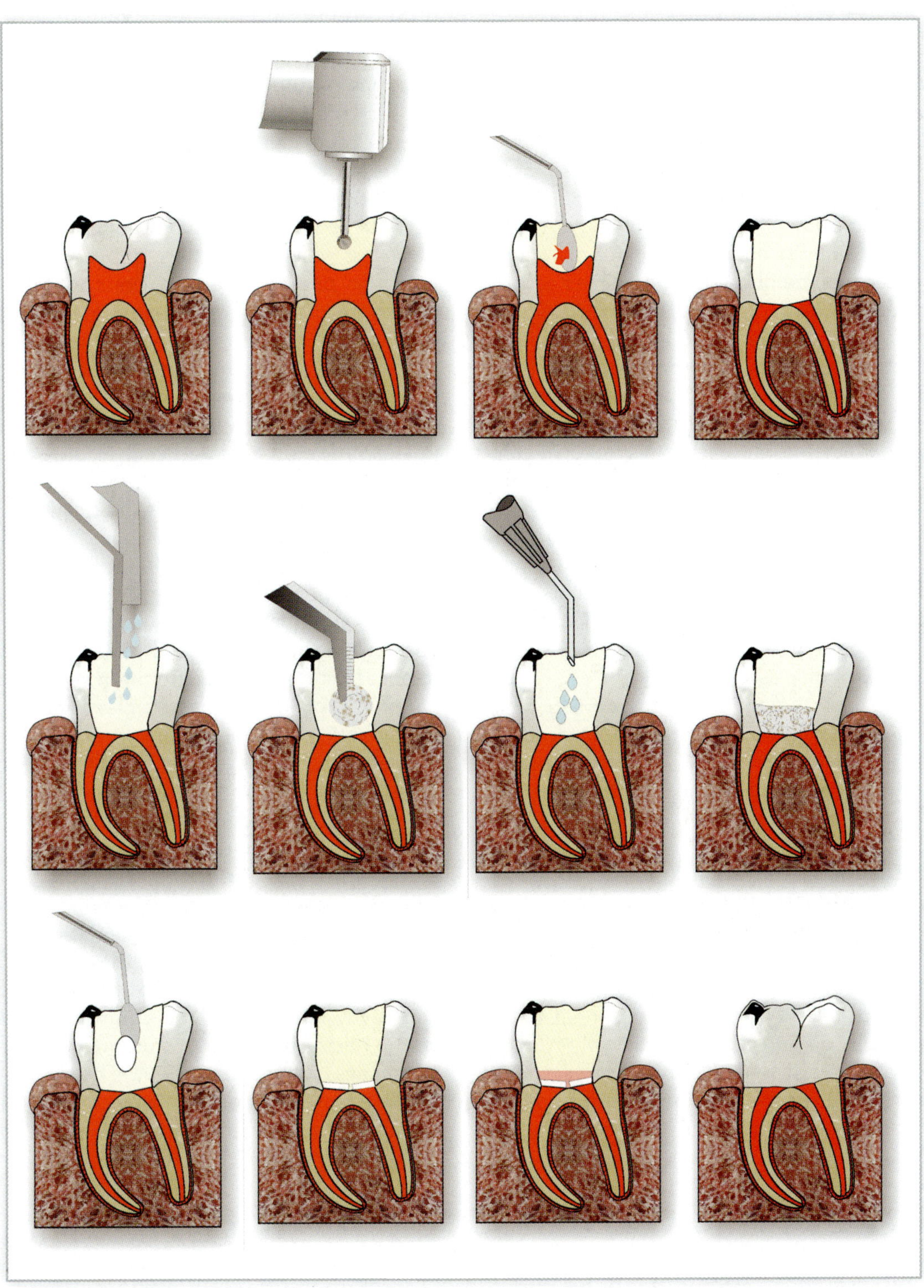

**Figure 3.3** - Sequence of pulpotomy technique.

## 3.4 Diagnosis of Periapical Pathology

The inflammatory pathologies of the periapical area result from invasion and colonization of microorganisms aggressors. These, depending on the specific nature and virulence associated to the host response, characterize the different inflammatory periapical pathologies.

Frequently inflammatory injuries of a chronic nature can be observed, oftentimes accompanied by pain (apical sensitivity to palpation, percussion, swelling etc.). The presence of polymorphonuclear (neutrophil) and mononuclear (macrophage) cells can be also observed. The relation of a pre-existing inflammation, whether acute or chronic, in this region is clinically not exact. When trying to associate the symptomatic characteristics (the presence or absence of pain) with the microscopic characteristics the professional involved may easily make a mistake. In the periapical area the acute phase, as well as the chronic phase, may involve periapical osseous resorption shown by radiographic aspects.

The clinical diagnosis of the periapical alterations has to be structured in accordance with the treatment. The clinical events of the inflammatory periapical pathologies are shown on Figure 3.2.

## 3.5 Diagnosis of the Endodontic-Periodontal Injuries

Understanding the relationship between endodontics and periodontics is important when diagnosing and treating injuries associated to both areas. It is essential to be precise in diagnosis, specifically when coming across extreme situations. From one perspective, there can bean indication of endodontic treatment for a tooth which may not be successful due to serious periodontal problems. An alternative to endodontic therapy may be the extraction of the tooth with subsequent placement of an implant. Under these circumstances a perfect odontological treatment planning has to be discussed between the different specialities.

With regard to a combined injury the following is valid - the more the endodontic etiologic prevails over the periodontal; the better the prognostic of treatment becomes, due to the endodontic environment being better controlled. Once the correct process of cleaning and shaping, intracanal medication and obturation is executed, the injury can have an elevated chance of regress. Nevertheless, for an endoperiodontic injury where periodontal disease is the main factor, the prognosis is less favorable. Regarding molar teeth for example, the access for decontamination of cement and the migration of the junctional to apical epithelium, may form a periodontic pocket in an area difficult to access and subject to frequent recontaminations. Table 3.4 suggests a classification of endodontic-periodontial injury.

Decurcio & Estrela[14] evaluated the efficacy of treatment of endodontic-periodontal injury in longitudinal studies, through a systematic review. Studies found that the success of the treatment of the endodontic-periodontal injuries is related to the brief identification of the etiology, to the control of microbiota, and to the immunological characteristics of the individual. Initial microorganism control in the oral cavity followed by the control of endodontic microorganisms is crucial to the clinical success of the treatment. The patient's immune system is an active participant of the process as component manager (Fig. 3.4).

**Table 3.4** - Classification of Endoperiodontic Injury

|  |
|---|
| **1. Injury of Endodontic Origin** |
| **In patients of risk for periodontal disease** |
| Local risk |
| Systemic risk |
| Both |
| **In patients of no risk for periodontal disease** |
| **2. Injury of Periodontal Origin** |
| Due to local risk factor |
| Due to systemic risk factor |
| Due to local risk factor associated with a systemic risk factor |

(Ruiz et al.[138])

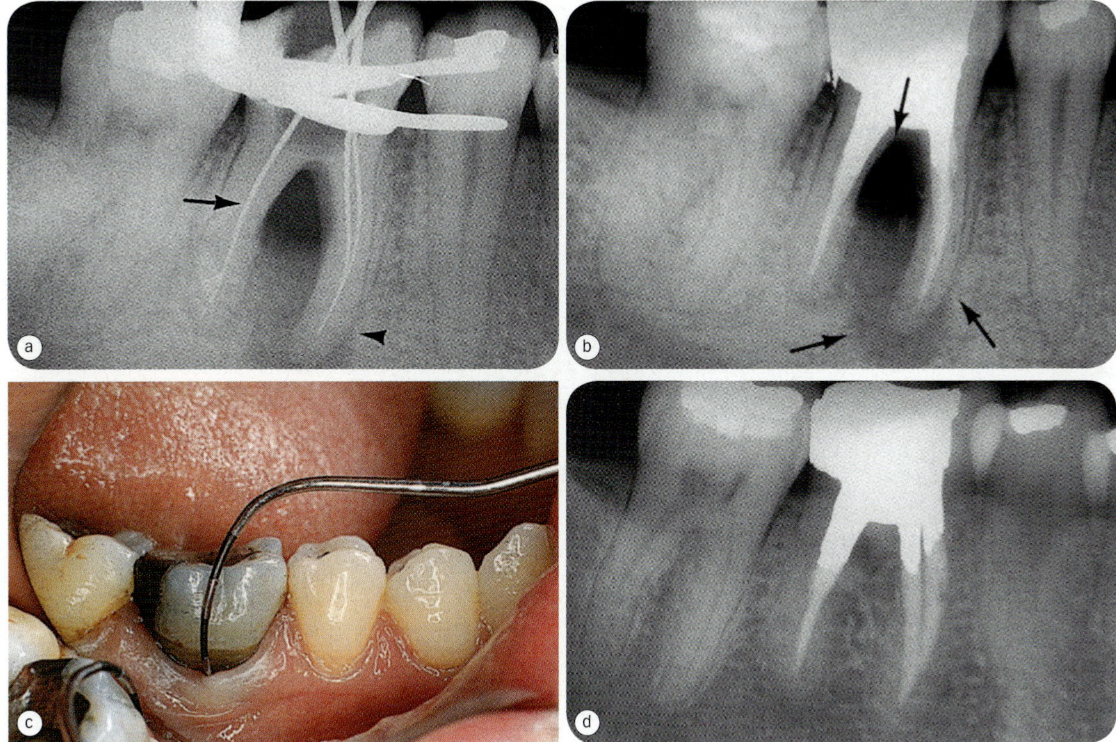

**Figure 3.4** - (**AD**) Follow-up of treatment of endodontic-periodontal injury (Courtesy Prof. Lourdes C. Aguilar de Esponda).

## 3.6 Diagnosis of the Traumatic Injuries

Many efforts have been made over the years to classify traumas. The currently accepted classification is based on the World Health Organization (*Application of International Classification of Diseases to Dentistry and Stomatology*)[4], modified by Andreasen & Andreasen[1] (1993). This classification applies to injuries of the teeth and support structures (Tables 3.5 and 3.6).

Frequency and causes of traumatic injuries vary significantly. This variation is due to a great number of factors including, age, gender, social conditions, and cultural and geographical conditions. In countries where the control of caries is effective, traumatic injuries are the largest problem for oral health care. Epidemiological studies conducted in Denmark revealed an alarming prevalence of 50% of dental trauma among schoolchildren, showing that one of every two children up to 14 years of age had suffered some kind of trauma[3]. Most epidemiological values presented in the literature are probably underestimated, because a large number of children suffer minor injuries, which are not diagnosed or routinely treated by a professional.

**Table 3.5** - Traumatic Injuries to Teeth

| | |
|---|---|
| Enamel infraction | An incomplete fracture (crack) of the enamel without loss of tooth substance |
| Enamel fracture | (Uncomplicated crown fracture). A fracture with loss of enamel only |
| Enamel-dentin fracture | (Uncomplicated crown fracture). A fracture with loss of enamel and dentin, but not involving the pulp |
| Complicated crown fracture | A fracture involving enamel and dentin, and exposing the pulp |
| Crown-root fracture | A fracture involving enamel, coronal and radicular dentin, and cementum |
| Root fracture | A fracture involving radicular dentin, cementum, and the pulp. Root fractures can be further classified according to displacement of the coronal fragment (see luxation injuries) |
| Luxation injuries | Concussion: An injury to the tooth-supporting structures without abnormal loosening or displacement of the tooth, but with increased reaction to percussion |
| | Subluxation (loosening): An injury to the tooth supporting structures with abnormal loosening, but without displacement of the tooth |
| | Extrusive luxation (peripheral dislocation, partial avulsion): Partial displacement of the tooth out of its socket |
| | Lateral luxation: Displacement of the tooth in a direction other than axially. This is accompanied by comminution or fracture of the alveolar socket |
| | Intrusive luxation (central dislocation): Displacement of the tooth into the alveolar bone. This injury is accompanied by comminution or fracture of the alveolar socket |
| | Avulsion (exarticulation): Complete displacement of the tooth out of its socket |

(Bakland & Andreasen[5])

**Table 3.6** - Soft Tissue and Bony Injuries

| | |
|---|---|
| Laceration of gingiva or oral mucosa | A shallow or deep wound in the mucosa resulting from a tear; usually produced by a sharp object |
| Contusion of gingiva or oral mucosa | A bruise usually produced by impact with a blunt object and not accompanied by a break in the mucosa, usually causing submucosal hemorrhage |
| Abrasion of gingiva or oral mucosa | A superficial wound produced by rubbing or scraping of the mucosa, leaving a raw, bleeding surface |
| Fracture of the mandibular or maxillary alveolar socket wall | A fracture of the alveolar process which involves the alveolar socket (see lateral luxation) |
| Fracture of the mandibular or maxillary alveolar process | A fracture of the alveolar process that may or may not involve the alveolar socket |

(Bakland & Andreasen[5])

Treating dental trauma is a common practice of most endodontists. However, knowledge of dental trauma for emergency treatment or long term treatment is not universal among these professionals. Since many traumatic injuries require both immediate and follow-up attention, a correct diagnosis can determine the success or failure of the treatment.

As traumatic injuries occur randomly, often the time for examination, diagnosis, and treatment is limited. It should be understood, however, that an incomplete examination could lead to an inaccurate diagnosis and an unsuccessful treatment. A diagnosis based on a proper clinical examination, with written documentation, radiographs and often, photographs, can eliminate many questions and lead to appropriate treatment. It should be considered that many later complications are a consequence of failures in the initial diagnosis.

Although traumatic injuries often present a complex picture, the majority of these injuries can be separated into several smaller components (Figs. 3.5-3.7). Information obtained from well conducted exams will help the professional to define treatment priorities. The procedures for diagnosis can be summarized as follows: Identification of the patient, medical history, recording of extra-oral injuries and face palpation, recording of injuries to the oral mucosa or the gums, examination of the teeth crowns, recording of teeth displacements, verification of occlusion and abnormal teeth mobility, sensitivity to percussion and reaction to the tests of pulp vitality.

The ability of the patient to provide information regarding name, age, and residence can assist in the evaluation of his general mental state. The medical history is essential to provide information about various conditions that could influence the actual state of emergency as well as subsequent treatments.

Andreasen & Andreasen[2] affirms that three factors are important for the diagnosis during the evaluation of the patient: when, where, and how the injury occurred. The time lapse (when) between the trauma itself and the first attendance by a professional can significantly affect the treatment and success of repair of coronary and bone fractures. Knowing the location (where) of the accident allows the professional to assess the degree of contamination of the affected structures and to assess the need to indicate a prophylaxis against tetanus. The nature of the accident can provide information on the type of trauma to be expected. For example: A blow on the chin often causes condyle fractures, as well as fractures of the posterior teeth. It is crucial that the face and oral cavity of the patient are properly cleaned to enable a correct assessment. Extra-oral injuries are commonly present and must be addressed.

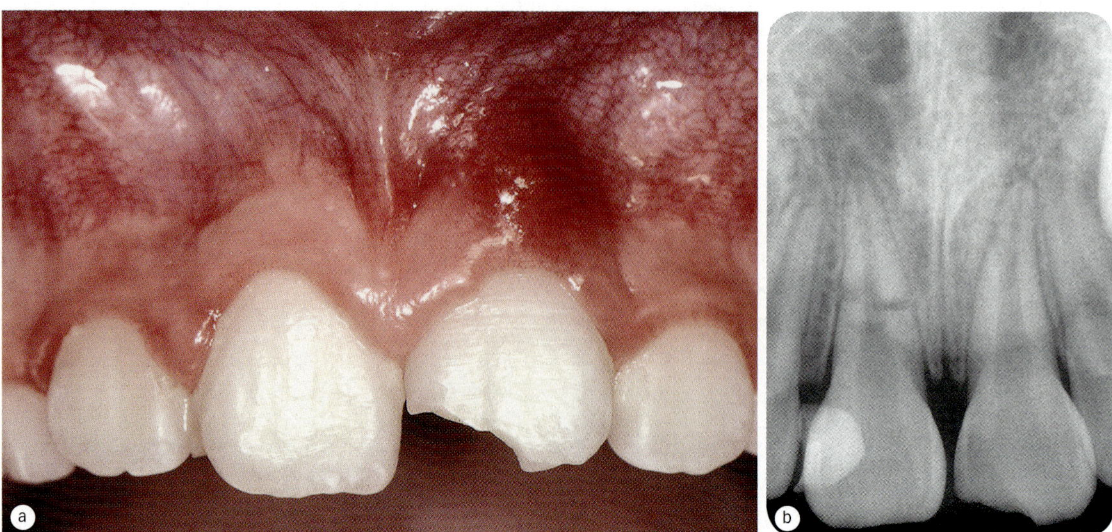

**Figure 3.5** - (**A**) Photograph of the tooth 11 with preserved crown and tooth 21 with crown fracture and fistula. (**B**) Radiography of the tooth 11 with root fracture of the medium third.

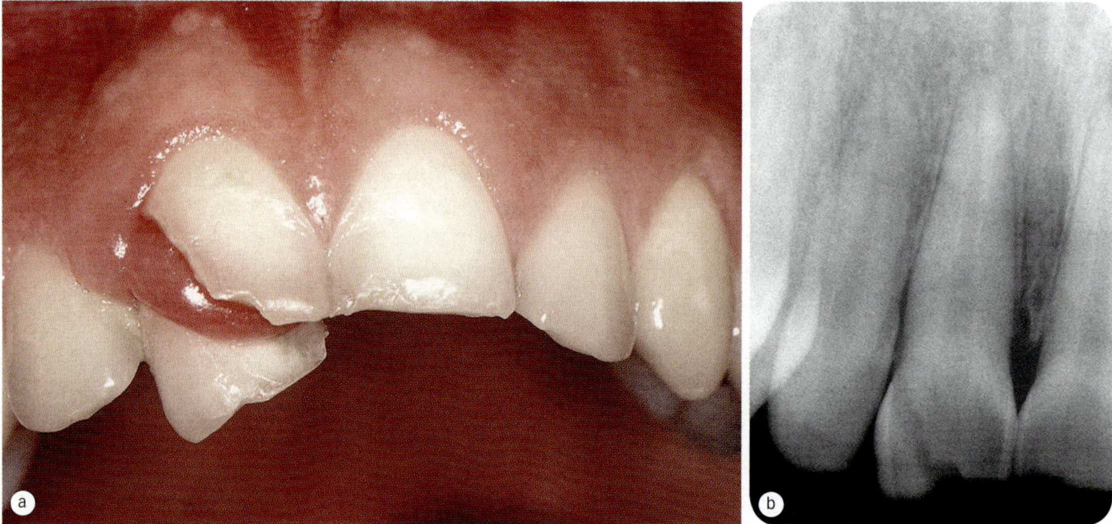

**Figure 3.6** - (**A**) Photograph of the tooth 11 with crown-root fracture (3 months after the traumatic injury). (**B**) Radiography of the tooth 11 with crown-root fracture.

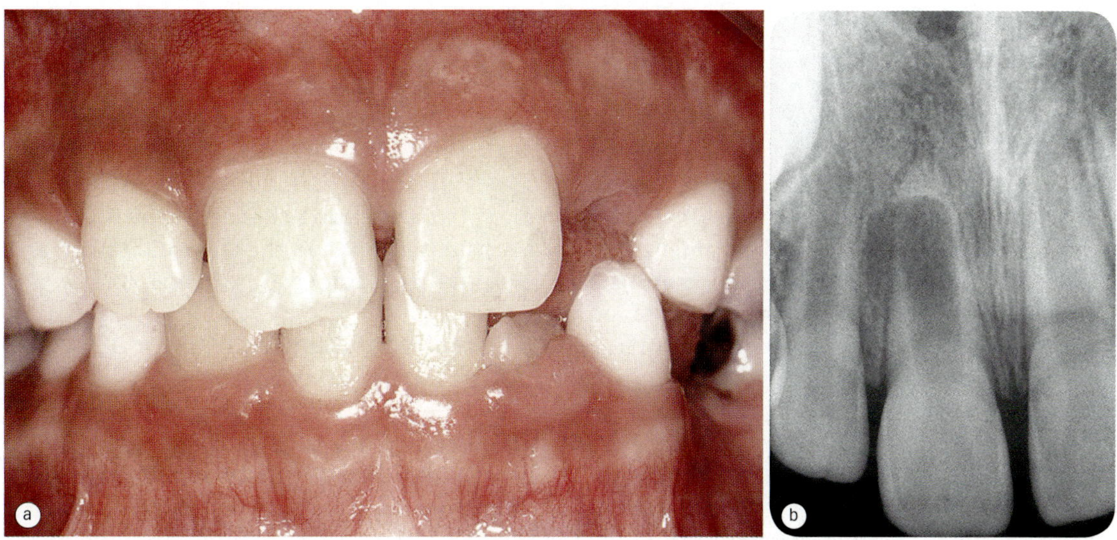


**Figure 3.7** - (**A**) Photograph of the tooth 11 and 21 with intact crowns after concussion injury. (**B**) Radiography of the tooth 21 showing communicating resorption.

The examination must be detailed and thorough, taking into consideration swelling, bruising, cuts, abrasions, and contusions, to ensure success of the treatment, all information about location, extent, form, and depth of the injuries should be recorded. Traumas to the oral mucosa or the gingiva also have to be recorded.

Wounds that compromise the entire thickness of the lip should be observed due to possibility of dental fragments displaced into the soft tissues. Gingival lacerations may often be associated with dental displacement. It is also important to be aware of bleeding, noninjured marginal gums, which can indicate damage to the periodontal ligament

Before examining the traumatized teeth, the crowns should be cleaned of blood and debris. Fragments of enamel should be located and recorded. In examining crown fractures it is important to note whether they are limited to enamel or involve bonding. Crown-root fractures should be expected in cases of indirect trauma and with similar fractures in the opposite arch.

The color of the teeth should be recorded, because changes may occur in the post-traumatic period. Displacement of teeth, usually, is evident in the visual examination, however minor abnormalities can be difficult to be detect. Abnormalities of occlusion may indicate fracture of mandibles, or the alveolar process.

The palpation of the facial skeleton can reveal bone fractures. Irregular forms felt during the palpation of the alveolar process also may indicate bone fracture. Another sign of alveolar fracture is the mobility of a group of teeth when the mobility of a single tooth is tested. All teeth should be tested for abnormal mobility, both vertically and horizontally. A positive reaction to percussion is indicative of damage to the periodontal ligament.

The periodontal ligament injury results in pain. At the time of examination, the percussion test with the finger may precede the test with the handle of the mirror. The test should be initiated on a non-traumatized tooth to ensure a reliable response from the patient.

The testing of pulp vitality during emergency treatment is not possible. This would require the full cooperation of a relaxed patient to avoid false reactions. Instead, the radiographic examination is more valuable to the clinical diagnosis. All traumatized teeth have to be radiographed. This examination reveals the stage of root development and the injuries that affect the root portion and the structures of support. Most root fractures are revealed by radiographic examinations only.

Another important reason for radiography is to examine the presence of foreign bodies that may possibly have penetrated the wounds of soft tissue. Bone fractures usually are discernible in intra-oral radiographs. If fracture of the maxilla is suspected then extra-oral radiographs should be taken.

Multiple radiographs from various angles provide valuable information. One auxiliary method may be tomography, which allows the evaluation of the entire extent of root surface, leading to a more precise diagnosis of fractures and resorption.

The diagnosis and treatment of traumatic injuries also include post-treatment monitoring (follow-up) in order to complete or confirm the diagnosis, to assess the response to treatment, to determine the need for additional treatment or change the treatment plan, and evaluate any complications (Table 3.7).

## 3.7 Treatment Plan

Once the diagnosis of the actual alteration is defined, the following phase consists of executing the surgical steps. One has to be aware of the fact that some clinical situations deserve special care, which means that priorities need to be established, weighing the trade-off between the risk of treatment against the benefit of the eventual outcome. Thus certain factors related to the selection of cases for the endodontic treatment deserve considerations.

**Table 3.7** - Follow-up of dental traumatisms

| | | |
|---|---|---|
| 1 week | After 7-10 days | To remove contention, pulp vitality test and to begin endodontic treatment if indicated. |
| 3-4 weeks | 30 days | To remove contention, clinical exam, radiography to analysis of possible resorption and pulp vitality test. |
| 6-8 weeks | 60 days | Clinical and radiographic exams can show pulp necrosis and resorption. |
| 3-6 months | 90-180 days | Assessments to diagnosis of healing or complications. |
| 1 to 5 years | | The minimum time for follow-up of traumatic injuries is a year, although some kind of trauma may require a long time of observation. |

## Case selection

Different factors can influence the professional performance during endodontic treatment.

To help ensure the success of a given treatment it is necessary to take into consideration some of the following factors: a calm, reassuring setting for the patient, sufficient time for the execution of the planned treatment; adequate technical and scientific understanding of the treatment; and training for the execution of surgical techniques. With regard to the patient, systemic and local factors have to be considered. Some local factors can maintain the doubtful prognosis and/or constitute an impediment for the correct execution of the endodontic technique. The following are some examples of these local factors. A – Anatomic-pathologic factors such as, modifications of the internal anatomy, excessive dilacerations, and calcification of the pulp cavity; B – factors resulting from endodontic accidents. This includes the loss of working length – step, root perforation, fracture of endodontic instrument; C– endodontic retreatments such as the presence of extensive posts, obturations with sealers, or only with glass ionomer.

## Control of infection in endodontics

Infection control in the health sector, especially after the first reports of Acquired Immune Deficiency Syndrome (AIDS), that establish a series of measures which were adopted to avoid cross contamination. The fear of contamination the human immunodeficiency virus (HIV) resulted in studies with the purpose to better clarify the mechanisms of the pathogenicity of the virus and establish more effective measures needed to prevent transmission.

The endodontist frequently comes in contact with potentially contaminated body fluids. For this reason it is imperative that all members of the oral health team wear individual protection equipment (IPE) – long sleeved aprons, caps, masks, protection glasses and gloves. This is essential for the control of cross contamination.

## Relation radiology and endodontics relation

Since their discovery in 1895 by Röntgen, x-rays have made an unprecedented difference in the world of health care, allowing imaging of internal areas of the body that would otherwise remain unseen. In the past, the images interpreted by the x-rays were in only two planes. Today, cone beam computed tomography allows a visualization of a three-dimensional image, where a new plane is added, depth. Due to its high accuracy, computed tomography is used in all the areas of dental specialty – surgery, dental implantology, orthodontics, endodontics, periodontology, and temporomandibular joint (TMJ) dysfunctions – to aid in diagnosis.

Estrela et al.[20] analyzed the accuracy in 1.508 images made by cone beam tomographs, periapical and panoramic radiographs for detection of apical periodontitis. The results showed that the CBCT images presented elevated accuracy, compared to the conventional methods. Apical periodontitis was correctly identified in 54.5% using periapical radiographs (sensibility 0.55) and in 27.8% with panoramic radiography (sensibility 0.28). The accuracy of the periapical radiographs was more significant than of the panoramic ones. The apical periodontitis was correctly identified with conventional methods only when observed in a severe condition (Fig. 3.8).

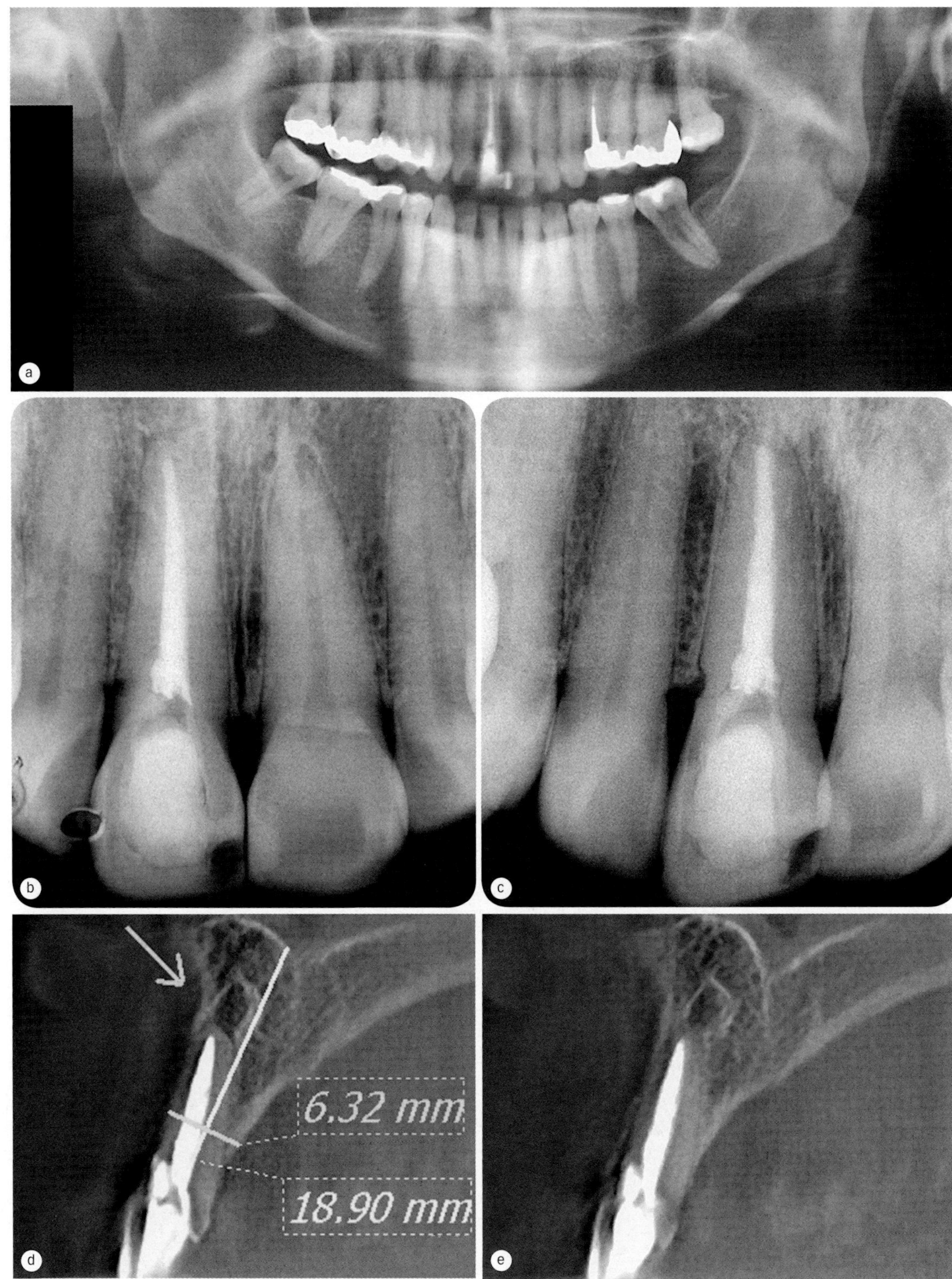


**Figure 3.8** - (**A**) Panoramic and (**B,C**) periapical radiographs shows normal periapical area of the upper right incisor. AP can be seen in the CBCT (**D,E**).

### Anaesthesia

The collaboration between patient and dental surgeon is fundamental for the success of the endodontic treatment. One of the principal aspects for successful treatment is the control of pain. This is done through anaesthesia. In order for the anaesthesia to work correctly, various factors need to be taken into consideration. Some of these factors include, the anxiety control of the patient, the knowledge of the pathologies which provoke an intensive pain (symptomatic pulpitis, symptomatic apical periodontitis, periapical abscess without fistula), the knowledge of the anatomic structures and anaesthesia techniques, and the effect and complications of the anaesthetics. For any endodontic treatment the patient's sense of pain must be controlled, because the worst remembrance is the memory of pain present during treatment.

### Isolation with rubber dam

The maintenance of the aseptic environment during the endodontic treatment is compulsory in all clinical situations. One of the ways to guarantee complete sterility during a surgical procedure is to use a rubber dam. Isolation with a rubber dam also minimizes cross infection. Other justifications for its use include the prevention of surgical accidents (like aspiration and deglutition of endodontic instruments), protection of the patient against medicinal substances (such as sodium hypochlorite), ergonomics and time economy (against several changes of the cotton rolls).

### Endodontic access

The endodontic access is the first surgical step which forms the basis of the endodontic trinity – crown opening, sanification/shaping and obturation of the canal, providing the instrument with the free access to the pulp cavity. The success of cleaning, shaping and obturation is dependent upon the manner of the endodontic access. As a consequence the endodontic access has to allow enough space for the endodontic instrument to act freely and directly in the entire length of the work. Difficulties resulting from internal abnormal morphologies require the preparation of the atypical cavities for the crown approach.

### Root canal sanitization

The root canal emptying is the procedure to eliminate the organic remains from the pulp cavity. This is executed in cases of live pulp (sound or inflamed), remains of necrotic pulp material, or remains of obturation material or fragments of endodontic instruments in the case of endodontic retreatment. The emptying and shaping of the root canal is achieved by means of a joint mechanical action between the endodontic instruments and the physical-chemical action of the irrigating solution. Sodium hypochlorite, despite its properties (antimicrobial capacity, dissolution, and tissue tolerance), is the most used irrigating solution.

The root canal emptying allows the identification of the entry orifice of the canal, its diameter (caliber), and the direction of the curvature. It also allows identification of obstacles not visualized by radiography, passage for the insertion of additional instruments. The exploration instrument has to be of small caliber and of curved tip, as it allows an easier transport of pulp remains found in the root canal. The explorer also penetrates easier the entire working length, reduces the possibility of extrusion of microorganisms and contaminated dentin debris. It also aids in greater precision planning of canal preparation with regards to lateral limits of instrumentation and detecting obstacles or obstructions.

The root canal emptying is executed before shaping. During the process of exploring the root canal, which can involve pulpectomy, disinfection, disobturation and/or disobstruction, the essential moment of the sanitization process is being developed. Thus, it is important to consider that the endodontic treatment normally is indicated for clinical situations which involve an inflammation and/or an infection. Figures 3.9 and 3.10 exhibit a sequence of surgical steps related to pulpectomy and sanitization process.

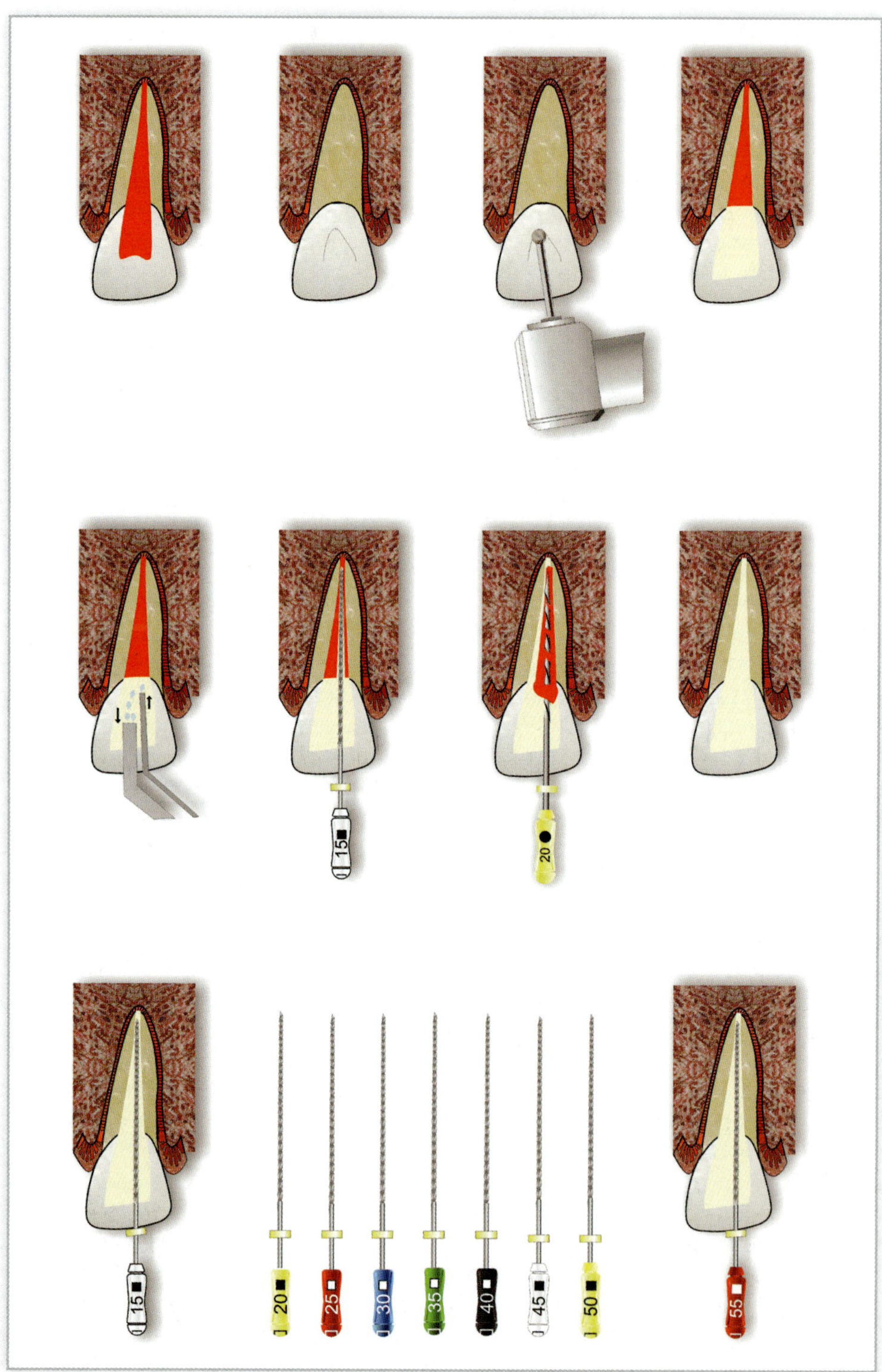


**Figure 3.9** - Sequence of steps related to pulpectomy.

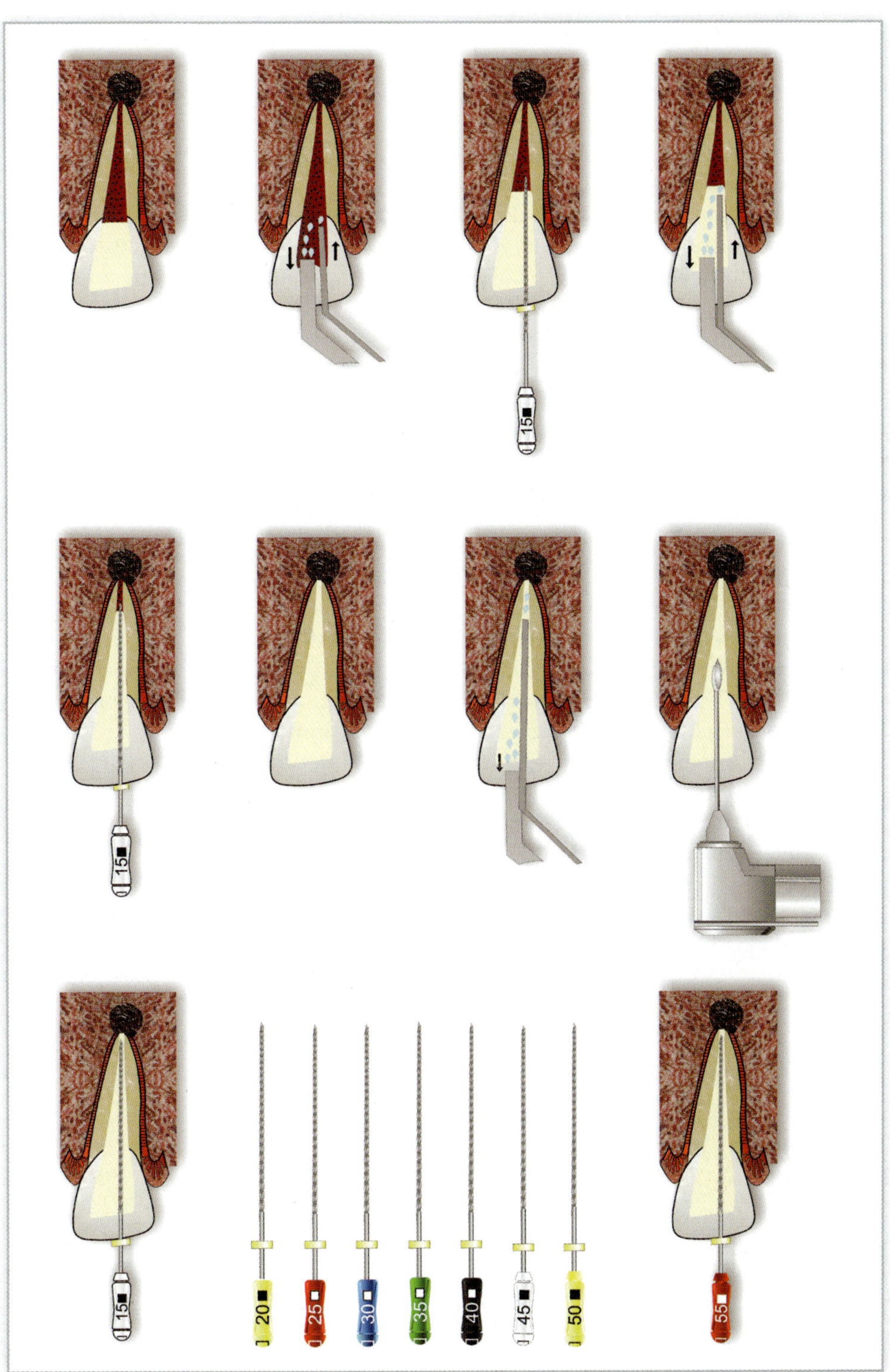


**Figure 3.10** -Sequence of steps related to sanitization process.

## Biological and mechanical parameters

The process of cleaning and shaping requires free access to the entire pulp cavity. Together, biological and mechanical parameters provide a perfect foundation for the modern concept of root canal preparation. During shaping, a direct relation between the walls of the root canal and the endodontic instruments impose standards which have to be well guided. Especially with regard to the individuality of the root canal, which does not tolerate misapplication or mismanagement of instruments. As a consequence we highlight, as biological and mechanical parameters which have to be monitored during root canal preparation, the complete emptying, the longitudinal shaping and the transversal shaping.

## Root canal preparation

The step of endodontic treatment which has received, during recent years, special attention from new technologies is the shaping of the root canal. The essential principles and the fundamental elements for the root canal preparation are maintained as follows: to empty, to enlarge, disinfect, and fill. Success in root canal shaping has come from the development of flexible instruments and new rotating systems.

The root canal preparation, if possible, has to be started and concluded during the same visit. Nevertheless, the root canal obturation depends upon the pathological pulp state, or in other words if the pulp is either alive or necrotic. In the cases of the pulp being alive it does not make any difference whether the obturation is done in one or two visits, the best option usually being treatment in one visit. In situations of pulp necrosis, with or without presence of periapical bone rarefaction, the best option is to enhance the process of sanitization begun during root canal preparation, using an intracanal medication.

Figures 3.11 to 3.12 show the operative sequence of the preparation techniques (manual preparation with stainless steel files and preparation with nickel-titanium instruments.

## Intracanal medication

The employment of intracanal medication in endodontics is justified in the following situations: maintenance of the sanitization reached during root canal preparation in a tooth with live pulp, control of microrganisms in teeth with pulp necrosis, persistent exudates, apexcification, dental resorptions, perforations, and large apical periodontitis.

In situations of pulp vitality, where it is impossible to finish an obturation in only one visit, one should make an intracanal medication on the basis of calcium hydroxide. In situations of pulp necrosis, with or without periapical bone rarefaction, the recommended intracanal medication is a calcium hydroxide paste. Table 3.8 presents the enzymatic qualities of calcium hydroxide.

**Table 3.8** - Enzymatic qualities of calcium hydroxide (Estrela[49], 1994)

| **Antibacterial Effect** |
|---|
| (Inactivation Bacterial Enzymes) |
| Reversible enzymatic inactivation |
| Irreversible enzymatic inactivation |
| **Mineralization Effect** |
| (Activation Tissue Enzymes) |

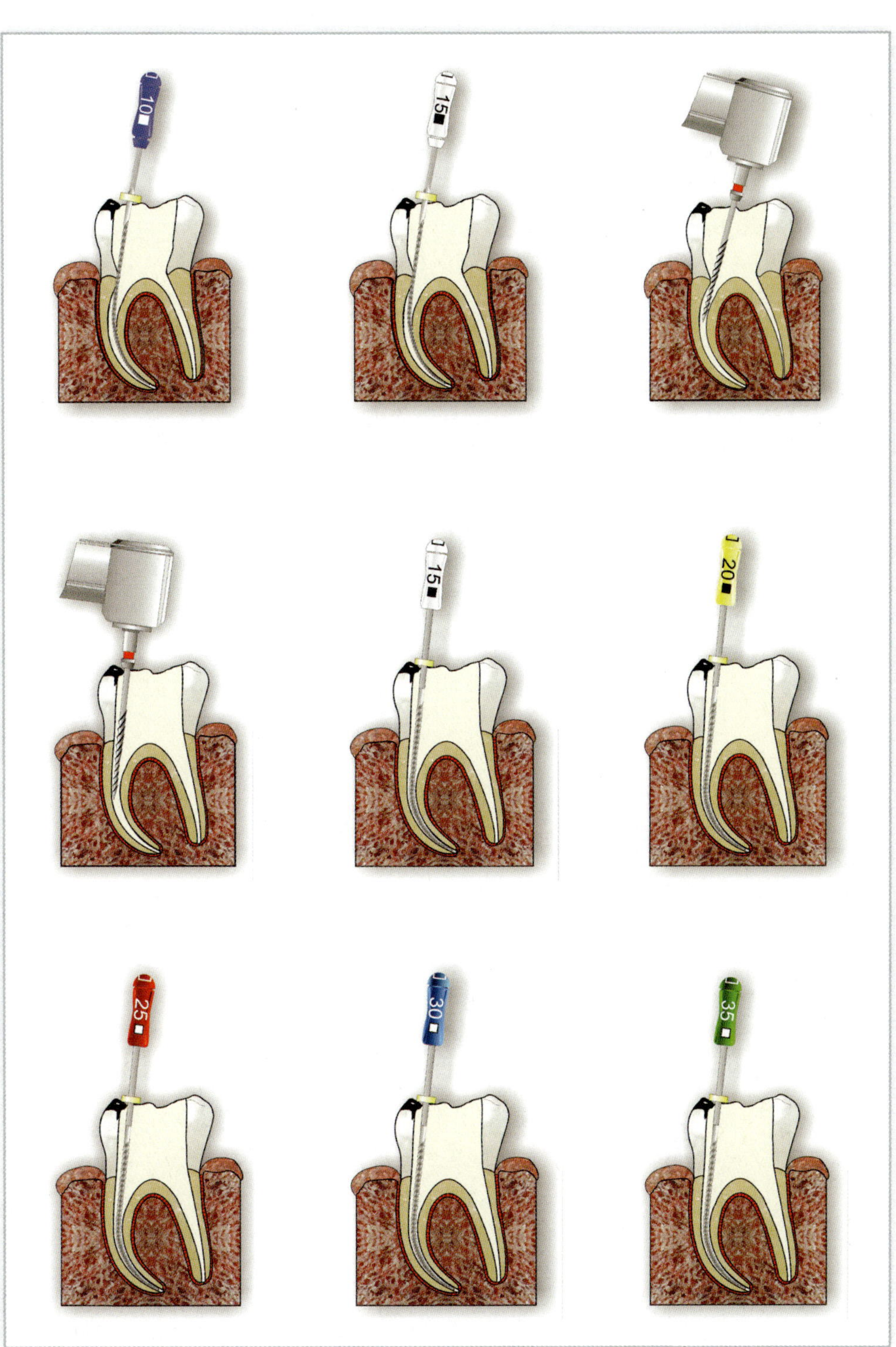


**Figure 3.11** - Operative sequence of the preparation with stainless steel files.

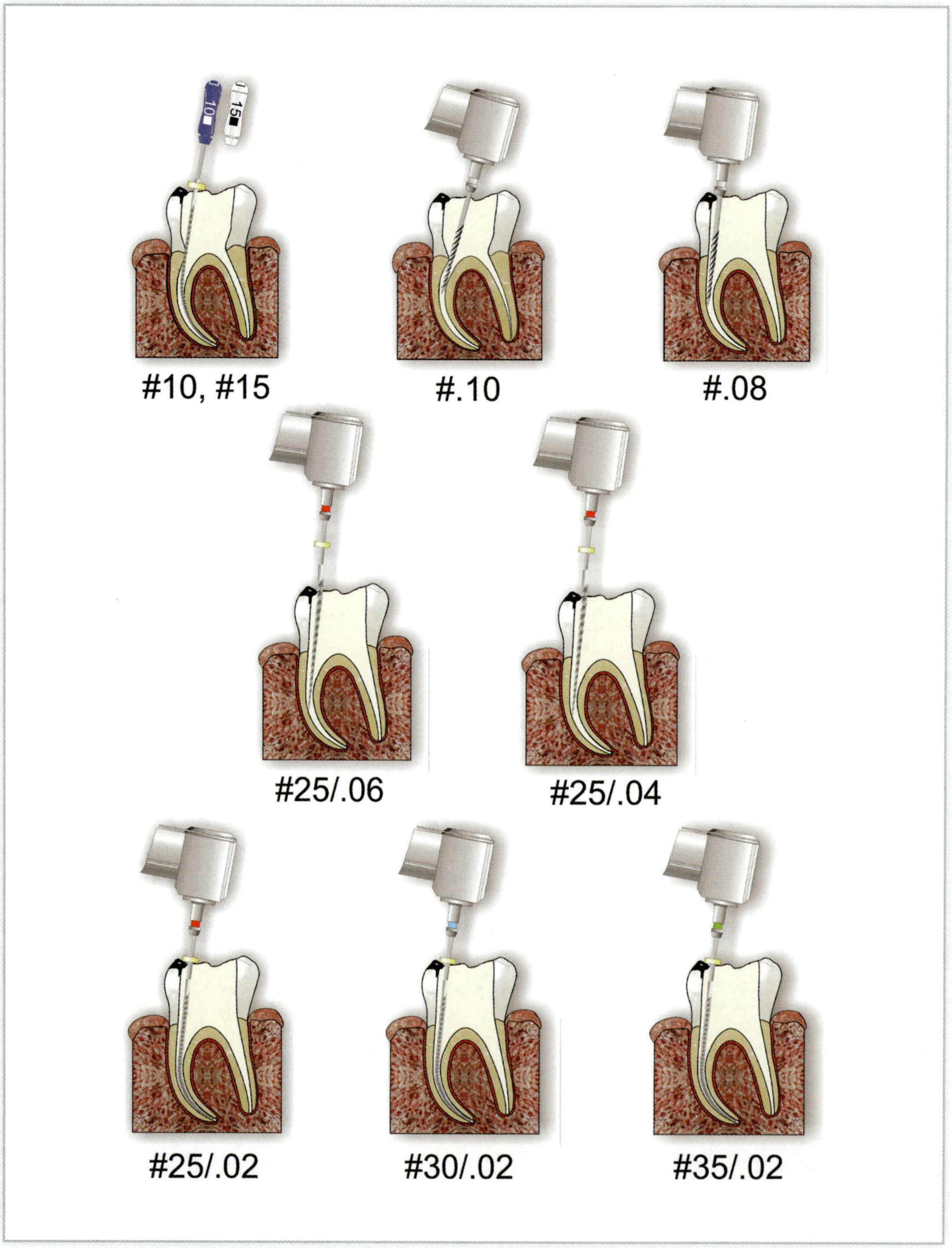

#10, #15

#.10

#.08

#25/.06

#25/.04

#25/.02

#30/.02

#35/.02

**Figure 3.12** -Operative sequence of the preparation with nickel-titanium instruments driven by electric motor with continuous rotation.

## Root canal obturation

The root canal obturation is the end of the endodontic trinity (crown opening, sanitization/shaping and obturation of the root canal), highlighting the importance of eliminating empty spaces inside the pulp cavity. In this sense it promotes tissue repair, by offering healing for the periapical tissues, which in turn allows repairing of the periodontal ligament and the reintegration of the hard tissue, by formation of osteocement. The idea of biological obturation is a goal that is yet to be attained by modern endodontics. A commonly accepted technique in endodontics is the obturation technique with lateral condensation of gutta-percha (Fig. 3.13).

## Endodontic retreatment

Endodontic retreatment, once failure has been confirmed, is a complex maneuver and requires special care. Once the factors responsible for the failure have been discussed, the professional may begin planning the operative execution to repair the failed treatment. Endodontic retreatment requires much attention and refined skills. Retreatment is achieved by using the same surgical phases as the initial treatment. Many difficulties and complications are present in the retreatment, thus resulting in oftentimes a grim prognosis. Table 3.9 shows the reasons responsible for endodontic failures. Figure 3.14 show a technical sequence of the endodontic retreatment and the main situations of endodontic failures. Table 3.10 highlights the technical difficulties encountered in all steps of the endondontic treatment.

**Table 3.9** - Causes responsible for endodontic failures

| **Causes of Microbial Origin** |
|---|
| Intra-radicular Factor<br>Bacteria<br>Fungi<br><br>Extra-radicular Factor<br>Actinomicosis |
| **Causes of Non-Microbial Origin** |
| Exogenous factors (reaction type: foreign body)<br>Obturation material<br>Paper tips<br><br>Endogenous factors<br>Cyst<br>Crystal of cholesterol |

(Nair[122])

**Table 3.10** - Operative factors which may interfere with endodontic success or failure

**1. Endodontic Access**

*Technical Difficulties*

- Inadequate access
- Perforation
- Instrument fracture
- Presence of restoration material

*Anatomic difficulties*

- Calcification
- Anatomical alterations

**2. Root Canal Preparation**

*Technical Difficulties*

- Location of canal
- Weakness of dental structure
- Presence of additional canal
- Loss of work length - step
- Deviation
- Foramen transport
- Exaggerated enlargement
- Perforation
- Fracture of endodontic instrument
- Over-instrumentation

*Anatomic Difficulties*

- Canal calcification
- Canal dilaceration
- Tooth out of position

**3. Root Canal Obturation**

*Technical Difficulties*

- Excessive instrumentation
- Over-obturation
- Spacer fracture (Lentulo)
- Fast binding cement

*Post-surgical pain*

**4. Endodontic Retreatment**

*Technical Difficulties*

- Presence of paste
- Presence of cement
- Gutta-percha point and cement
- Silver point and cement
- Presence of intracanal posts

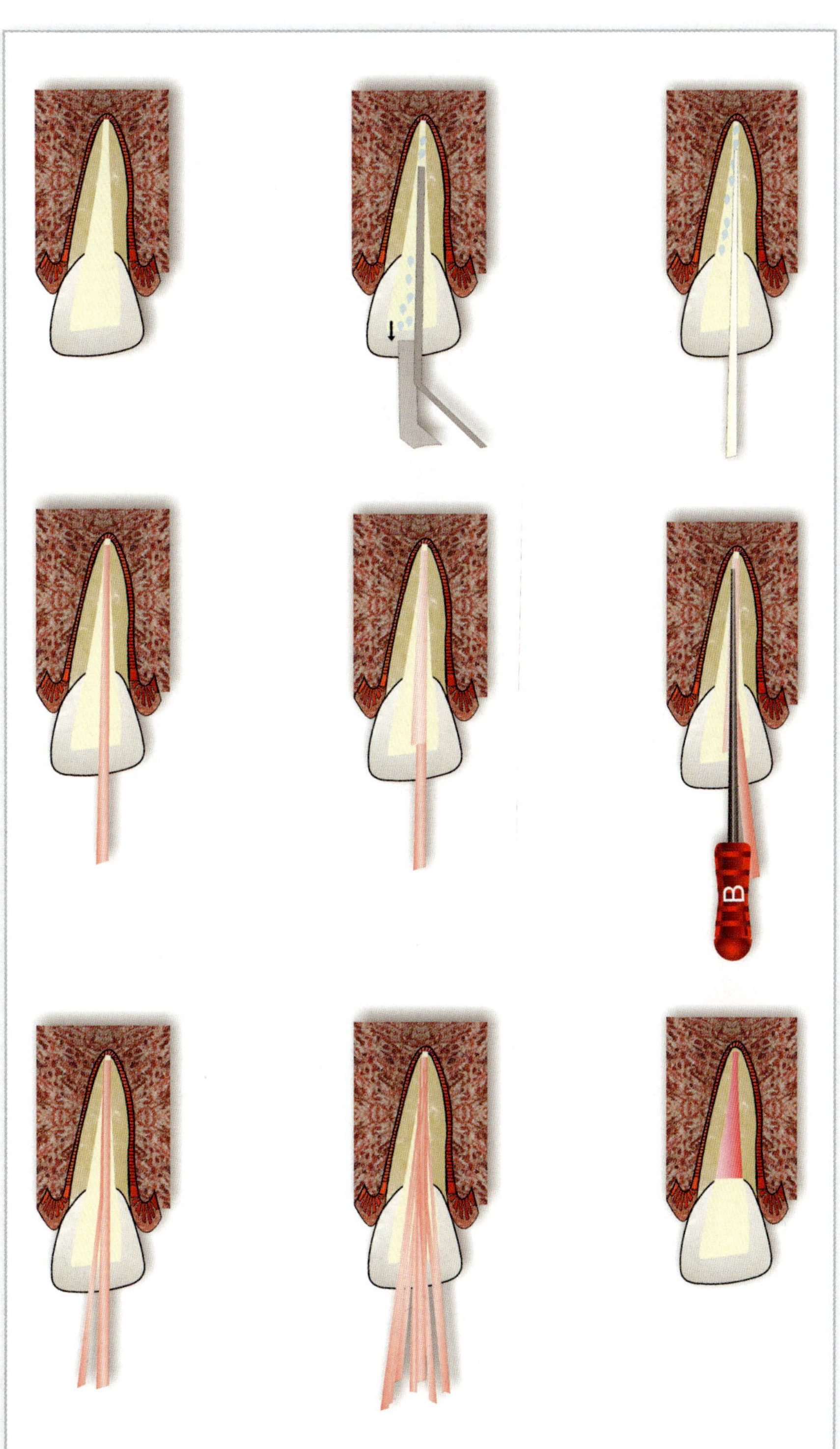


Figure 3.13 - Sequence of obturation technique.

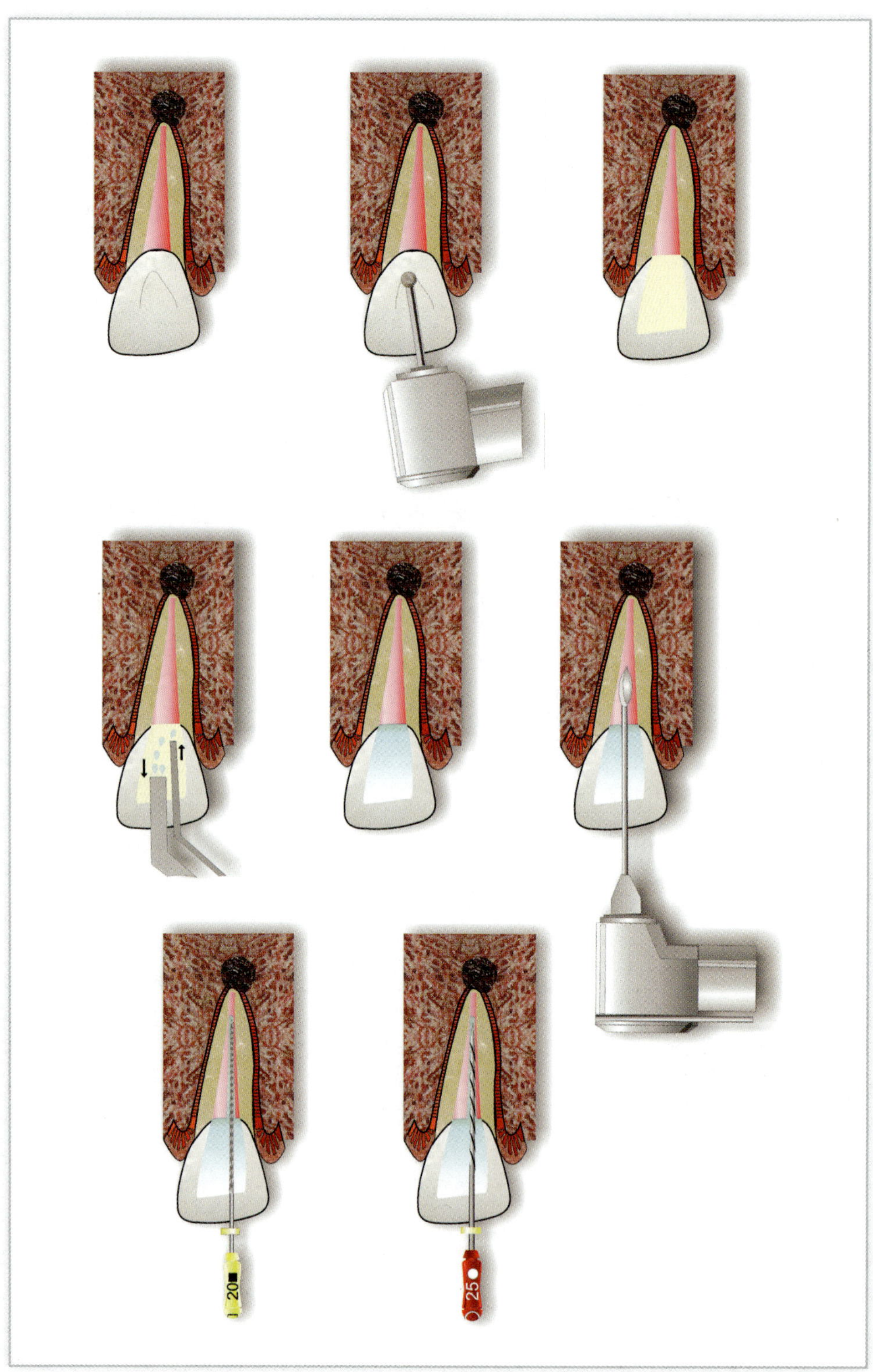


**Figure 3.14** -Sequence of endodontic retreatment.

## Follow-up

The final result of an endodontic treatment depends on the factor time. The preservation of the endodontic treatments carried out on teeth with live pulp has to be made after a time period of 6 months to one year. However, under conditions with pulp necrosis with or without periapical bone rarefaction, the preservation should be executed 2 to 5 years after the treatment. It's important to note that the image of a root canal obturation gives only an incomplete picture of the sanitization and shaping process of the canal because it represents a three-dimensional image represented in only two dimensions.

Recently, cone beam computed tomography (CBCT) introduced the third dimension into dentistry. CBCT images present high accuracy for detecting apical periodontitis.

### References and Further Reading


1. Andrease JO, Ravn J J. Epidemiology of traumatic injuries to primary and permanent teeth in a Danish population sample. Int J Oral Surg 1972;1: 235-9.
2. Andreasen JO, Andreasen FM. Classification, etiology and epidemiology of traumatic dental injuries. In: Textbook and color atlas of traumatic injuries to the teeth. 3rd ed., Copenhagen: Musksgaard; 1993; p.151-77.
3. Andreasen JO, Andreasen FM. Texto e atlas colorido de traumatismo dental. 3rd ed., Porto Alegre: Artmed, 2001.
4. Application of the International Classification of Diseases to Dentistry and Stomatology IDC-DA, 3rd ed., Geneva: WHO, 1995.
5. Bakland LK, Andreasen JO. Dental traumatology: essencial diagnosis and treatment planning. Endodontic Topics 2004;7:14-34.
6. Bender IB, Seltzer S. The effect of periodontal disease on the pulp. Oral Surg Oral Med Oral Pathol 1972;33:458-74.
7. Bergenholtz G, Hasselgren G. Endodontia e Periodontia. In: Lindhe J, Karring T, Lane NP. Tratado de Periodontia Clínica e Implantologia Oral. 4th ed. Rio de Janeiro: Guanabara Koogan; 2005. p.309-41.
8. Bergenholtz G, Lindhe J. Effect of experimentally induced marginal periodontitis and periodontal scaling on dental pulp. J Clin Periodontol 1978;5:59-73.
9. Bramante CM, Berbert A, Bernadineli N. Recursos técnicos radiográficos aplicados à endodontia. Rev Bras Odontol 1980;37:8-24.
10. Bramante CM, Berbert A. Recursos radiográficos no diagnóstico e no tratamento endodôntico. São Paulo: Pancast, 1991. 103p.
11. Bueno MR. Pesquisa na Internet. In: Estrela C. Metodologia Científica. 2nd ed. São Paulo: Artes Médicas; 2005. p.679-701.
12. Bueno MR, Estrela C, Azevedo B, Brugnera Júnior A, Azevedo JR. Tomografia computadorizada cone beam: revolução na odontologia. Rev Assoc Paul Cir Dent 2007; 61:354-363.
13. Clark CA. A method of ascertaining the relative position of unerupted teeth by means of film radiographs. Royal Soc Med Transactions 1909; 3:87-9.
14. Decurcio RA, Estrela C. Avaliação em estudos longitudinais sobre a eficácia do tratamento da lesão endodôntica-periodontal: uma revisão sistemática. Scientific- A 2007;1:17-27.
15. Estrela C, Bammann LL, Estrela CRA, Silva RS, Pécora JD. Antmicrobial and chemical study of MTA, Portland cement, calcium hydroxide paste, Sealapex and Dycal. Braz Dent J 2000;11:3-9.
16. Estrela C, Bammann LL, Lopes HP, Moura J. Análise comparativa da ação antibacteriana de três cimentos obturadores contendo hidróxido de cálcio. Rev Ass Bras Odontol Nac 1995;3:185-7.
17. Estrela C, Bammann LL, Pimenta FC, Pécora JD. Control of microorganism in vitro by calcium hydroxide pastes. Int Endod J 2001;34:416-8.
18. Estrela C, Bammann LL, Sydney GB, Moura J. Efeito antibacteriano de pastas de hidróxido de cálcio sobre bactérias aeróbias facultativas. Rev Fac Odontol Bauru 1995; 3:109–14.
19. Estrela C, Bammann LL. Efeito enzimático do hidróxido de cálcio. Rev Ass Bras Odontol Nac 1999; 7:32-42.
20. Estrela C, Bueno MR, Azevedo B, Azevedo JR, Pécora JD. A New Periapical Index Based on Cone Beam Computed Tomography. J Endod 2008; 34:1325-31.
21. Estrela C, Bueno MR, Leles CR, Azevedo B, Azevedo JR. Accuracy of cone beam computed tomography and panoramic ad periapical radiography for detection of apical periodontitis. J Endod 2008; 34:273-9.
22. Estrela C, César OVS, Leles CR, Pimenta FC, Alencar AHG. Avaliação em estudos longitudinais da eficácia do hidróxido de cálcio sobre o *Enterococcus faecalis* em infecções endodônticas - Revisão Sistemática. Rev Bras Odontol. 2007;64:117-28.
23. Estrela C, Estrela CRA, Bammann LL, Pécora JD. Two methods to evaluate the antimicrobial action of calcium hydroxide paste. J Endod 2001;27:720–3.
24. Estrela C, Estrela CRA, Barbin EL, Spanó JCE, Marchesan MA, Pécora JD. Mechanism of action of sodium hypochlorite. Braz Dent J 2002;13:113–7.
25. Estrela C, Estrela CRA, Decurcio DA, Hollanda ACB, Silva JA. Antimicrobial efficacy of ozonated water, gaseous ozone, sodium hypochlorite and chlorhexidine in infected human root canals. Int Endod J 2007;40:85-93.

26. Estrela C, Estrela CRA, Hollanda ACB, Decurcio DA, Pécora JD. Iodoform effect on antimicrobial potential of intracanal medicament. Braz Endod J 2002;6:11–7.
27. Estrela C, Estrela CRA, Pécora JD. A study of the time necessary for calcium hydroxide to eliminate microorganism in infected canals. J Applied Oral Science 2003;11:133-7.
28. Estrela C, Estrela CRA, Silva RS, Pécora JD. Molar conductivity of calcium hydroxide solutions. Braz Endod J 2001;5:13–7.
29. Estrela C, Estrela CRA, Silva RS, Pécora JD. Surface tension of calcium hydroxide associated at different substances. Braz Endod J 2002;6:23-5.
30. Estrela C, Guedes OA, Brugnera Júnior A, Estrela CRA, Pécora JD. Dor pós-operatória em dentes com infecções endodônticas secundárias: Revisão Sistemática. Rev Ass Paul Cir Dent 2007; 61:185-202.
31. Estrela C, Guedes OA, Brugnera Júnior A, Estrela CRA; Pécora JD. Dor pós-operatória em dentes com infecções endodônticas primárias: Revisão sistemática. Rev Gaúcha Odontol 2008;56:353-9.
32. Estrela C, Guedes OA, Pereira-Jr W, Bueno MR. Terapêutica do abscesso periapical sem fístula: Revisão sistemática. Rev Bras Odontol 2008 (in press).
33. Estrela C, Leles CR, Hollanda ACB, Moura MS, Pécora JD. Prevalence and risk factors of apical periodontitis in endodontically treated teeth in a selected population of Brazilian adults. Braz Dent J 2008;19:28-34.
34. Estrela C, Lopes HP, Felippe-Jr O, Sydney GB. Chemical analysis of calcium carbonate present in various calcium hydroxide samples. Braz Endod J 1997;2:7-9.
35. Estrela C, Mamede-Neto I, Estrela CRA, Pécora JD. Evaluation of density of calcium hydroxide pastes in dog's mandible. Braz Endod J 1998;3:24-30.
36. Estrela C, Mamede-Neto I, Lopes HP, Estrela CRA, Pécora JD. Root canal filling with calcium hydroxide using different techniques. Braz Dent J 2002;13:53-56.
37. Estrela C, Marcelo VC, Sabino GA. Trabalho Científico. In: Estrela C. Metodologia Científica. São Paulo: Artes Médicas; 2005. p.151-83.
38. Estrela C, Pécora JD, Silva RS. pH analyse of vehicles and calcium hydroxide pastes. Braz Endod J 1998;3:41-47.
39. Estrela C, Pécora JD, Sousa-Neto MD, Estrela CRA, Bammann LL. Effect of vehicle on antimicrobial properties of calcium hydroxide paste. Braz Dent J 1999;10:63-72.
40. Estrela C, Pesce HF. Chemical analysis of the formation of calcium carbonate and its influence on calcium hydroxide pastes in the presence of connective tissue of the dog. Part II. Braz Dent J 1997; 8:49-53.
41. Estrela C, Pesce HF. Chemical analysis of the liberation of calcium and hydroxyl ions of calcium hydroxide pastes in the presence of connective tissue of the dog. Part I. Braz Dent J 1996;7:41-46.
42. Estrela C, Pimenta FC, Estrela CRA. Testes microbiológicos aplicados à pesquisa odontológica. In: Metodologia Científica: Ensino e Pesquisa em Odontologia. Estrela C. São Paulo: Artes Médicas; 2001. 500p.
43. Estrela C, Pimenta FC, Ito IY, Bammann LL. Antimicrobial evaluation of calcium hydroxide in infected dentinal tubules. J Endod 1999; 26:416-418.
44. Estrela C, Pimenta FC, Ito IY, Bammann LL. In vitro determination of direct antimicrobial effect of calcium hydroxide. J Endod 1998; 24:15-17.
45. Estrela C, Ribeiro RG, Estrela CRA, Pécora JD, Souza-Neto MD. Antmicrobial effect of 2% sodium hypochlorite and 2% chlorhexidine tested by different methods. Braz Dent J 2003; 14:58–62.
46. Estrela C, Siqueira RMG, Resende EV, Silva S, Silva FAC. Influência da substância química, do cimento obturador e do número de sessões na incidência de pericementite traumática. Rev Odontol Brasil Central 1996; 6:9–13.
47. Estrela C, Sydney GB, Bammann LL, Felippe-Jr O. Mechanism of the action of calcium and hydroxyl ions of calcium hydroxide on tissue and bacteria. Braz Dent J 1995; 6:85-90.
48. Estrela C, Sydney GB, Bammann LL, Fellipe-Jr O. Estudo do efeito biológico do pH na atividade enzimática de bactérias anaeróbias. Rev Fac Odontol Bauru 1994;2:31-8.
49. Estrela C, Sydney GB, Pesce HF, Felippe-Jr O. Dentinal diffusion of hydroxil ions of various calcium hydroxide pastes. Braz Dent J 1995;6:5-9.
50. Estrela C, Sydney GB. EDTA effect on root dentin pH after exchange of calcium hydroxide paste. Braz Endod J 1997;2:20-3.
51. Estrela C, Toledo AM, Brugnera Júnior A, Decurcio RA; Pécora JD. Dor pós-operatória em dentes com inflamação pulpar: Revisão sistemática. Robrac; 2006, 15:34-45.
52. Estrela C. Análise química de pastas de hidróxido de cálcio, frente à liberação de íons de cálcio, de íons hidroxila e ação do carbonato de cálcio na presença de tecido conjuntivo de cão. (Doctoral Thesis). University of São Paulo, 1994.
53. Estrela C. Ciência Endodôntica. São Paulo: Artes Médicas; 2004. 1010p.
54. Estrela C. Eficácia antimicrobiana de pastas de hidróxido de cálcio. (Livre-Docência Thesis). University of São Paulo, 1997.
55. Estrela CRA, Estrela C, Reis C, Bammann LL, Pécora JD. Control of microorganisms in vitro by endodontic irrigants. Braz Dent J 2003; 11:133-7.
56. Estrela CRA. Eficácia antimicrobiana de soluções irrigadoras de canais radiculares. (Master's Thesis) Goiânia: Federal University of Goiás; 2000.
57. Evans M, Davies JK, Sundqvist G, Fidgor D. Mechanism involved in the resistance of *Enterococcus faecalis* to calcium hydroxide. Int Endod J 2002; 35:221-8.
58. Fabricius L, Dahlén G, Öhman AE, Möller AJR. Predominant indifenous oral bacteria isolated from infected root canals after varied times of closure. Scand J Dent Res 1982; 90:134-44.
59. Gift H C, Bhat M. Dental visits for orofacial injury: defining the dentist's role. J AM Dent Assoc 1993;124: 92-8.

60. Glenny AM, Esposito M, Coulthard P, Worthington HV. The assessment of systematic reviews in dentistry. Eur J Oral Sci 2003;111:85-92.
61. Hiatt WH. Pulpal periodontal disease. J Periodontol 1977;48:598-609.
62. Holland R et al. Diffusion of corticosteroid-antibiotic solutinos through human dentine. Rev Odontol UNESP 1991;20:17-23.
63. Holland R, Cruz AG, Nery MJ, Souza V, Otoboni-Filho JA, Bernabé PFE. Efecto de los medicamentos colocados en el interior del conducto, hidrosolubles y no hidrosolubles en el proceso de reparación de dientes de perro con lesión periapical. Endodoncia 1999;17:90-100.
64. Holland R, Ingle JI, Valle GF, Taintor JF. Influence of bony resorption on Endodontic treatment. Oral Surg Oral Med Oral Pathol 1983; 55:191-203.
65. Holland R, Maisto OA, Souza V, Maresca BM, Nery MJ. Acción y velocidad de reabsorción de didtintos materiales de obturación de conductos radiculares em el tejido periapical. Rev Assoc Argentina 1981;69:7-17.
66. Holland R, Mello W, Nery MJ, Bernabé PFE, Souza V. Reaction of human periapical tissue to pulp extirpation and immediate root canal filling with calcium hydroxide. J Endod 1977;3:63-7.
67. Holland R, Mello W, Nery MJ, Souza V, Bernabé PFE, Otoboni-Filho JA. The influence of the sealing material in the healing process of inflamed pulps capped with calcium hydroxide or zinc oxide-eugenol cement. Acta Odontol Pediatr 1981;2:5-9.
68. Holland R, Mello W, Souza V, Nery MJ, Bernabé PFE, Otoboni-Filho JA. Reacción de la pulpa y tejidos periapicales de dientes de perros, com forámenes incompletamente formados, posteriormente a la pulpotomia y protección com hidróxido de cálcio o formocresol: estudo histologico a distância. Endodoncia 1983;1:33-8.
69. Holland R, Murata SS, Souza V, Lopes HP, Salia O. Análise do selamento marginal obtido com cimentos à base de hidróxido de cálcio. Rev Ass Paul Cir Dent 1996;50:61-4.
70. Holland R, Nery MJ, Mello W, Souza V, Bernabé PFE, Otoboni-Filho JA. Root canal treatment with calcium hidroxide I – Effect of overfilling and refilling. Oral Surg Oral Med Oral Pathol 1979;47:87-92.
71. Holland R, Nery MJ, Mello W, Souza V, Bernabé PFE, Otoboni-Filho JA. Root canal treatment with calcium hydroxide II – Effect of instrumentation beyond the apices. Oral Surg Oral Med Oral Pathol 1979; 47:93-6.
72. Holland R, Nery MJ, Mello W, Souza V, Bernabé PFE, Otoboni-Filho JA. Root canal treatment with calcium hydroxide III – Effect of debris and pressure filling. Oral Surg Oral Med Oral Pathol 1979; 47:185-8.
73. Holland R, Nery MJ, Souza V, Mello W, Bernabé PFE, Otoboni-Filho JA. The effect of corticosteroid-antibiotic dressing in the behaviour of the periapical tissue of dog's teeth after instrumentation. Rev Odontol UNESP 1981;10:21-5.
74. Holland R, Nery MJ, Souza V, Mello W, Bernabé PFE, Otoboni-Filho JA. The effect of the filling material in the tissue reactions following a prool plugging of the root canal with dentin chips. A histologic study in monkey's teeth. Oral Surg Oral Med Oral Pathol 1983;53:398-401.
75. Holland R, Otoboni-Filho JA, Bernabé PFE, Nery MJ, Souza V, Berbert A. Effect of root canal status on periodontal healing after surgical injury in dogs. Endod Dent Traumatol 1994;10:77-82.
76. Holland R, Otoboni-Filho JA, Souza V, Mello W, Nery MJ, Bernabé PFE, Dezan-Jr E. Calcium hydroxide and corticosteroid-antibiotic association as dressings in cases of biopulpectomy. A comparative study in dogs teeth. Braz Dent J 1998;9:67-76.
77. Holland R, Otoboni-Filho JA, Souza V, Nery MJ, Bernabé PFE, Dezan-Jr E. Reparação dos tecidos periapicais com diferentes formulações de $Ca(OH)_2$ – Estudo em cães. Rev Ass Paul Cir Dent 1999;53:327-31.
78. Holland R, Otoboni-Filho JA, Souza V, Nery MJ, Bernabé PFE, Dezan-Jr E. A comparison of one versus two appointment endodontic therapy in dogs' teeth with apical periodontitis. J Endod 2003;29:121-5.
79. Holland R, Otoboni-Filho JA, Souza V, Nery MJ, Bernabé PFE, Dezan-Jr E.Tratamiento endodôntico en una o en dos visitas. Estudio histológico en dientes de perros con lesión periapical. Endodoncia 2003;21:20-27.
80. Holland R, Pinheiro CE, Mello W, Nery MJ, Souza V. Histochemical analysis of the dog's dental pulp after pulp capping with calcium, barium and strontium hydroxides. J Endod 1982;8:444-7.
81. Holland R, Soares IJ, Soares IM. Influence of irrigation and intracanal dressing on the healing process of dog's teeth with apical periodontitis. Endod Dent Traumatol 1992;8:223-9.
82. Holland R, Souza V, Mello W, Nery MJ, Bernabé PFE, Mello W, Otoboni-Filho JA. Emprego da associação corticosteróide antibiótico durante o tratamento endodôntico. Rev Paul Endod 1980;1:4-7.
83. Holland R, Souza V, Mello W, Nery MJ, Bernabé PFE, Otoboni-Filho JA. Healing process of dog's dental pulp after pulptomy and protection with calcium hydroxide. Rev Odontol Unesp 1979/1980; 8:67-73.
84. Holland R, Souza V, Mello W, Nery MJ, Bernabé PFE, Otoboni-Filho JA. Manual de Endodontia - Faculdade de Odontologia de Araçatuba – UNESP; 1978/1979.
85. Holland R, Souza V, Mello W, Russo MC. Healing process of the pulp stump and periapical tissues in dog teeth. II. Histological findings following root filling with zinc oxide-eugenol. Rev Fac Odontol Araçatuba 1977;6:59-67.
86. Holland R, Souza V, Mello W, Russo MC. Healing process of the pulp stump and periapical tissue in dog teeth. III – Histopathological findings following root filling with calcium hydroxide. Rev Fac Odontol Araçatuba 1978;7:25-30.
87. Holland R, Souza V, Milanezi LA. Behaviour of pulp stump and periapical tissues to some drugs used a root canal dressings. A morphological study. Rev Bras Pesq Med Biol 1969; 2:13-23.
88. Holland R, Souza V, Milanezi LA. Estudo morfológico do coto pulpar e tecidos periapicais frente à alguns materiais empregados nas obturações dos canais radiculares. Ciência e Cultura 1968;20:355.
89. Holland R, Souza V, Milanezi LA. Resposta do coto pulpar e tecidos periapicais a algumas pastas empregadas na obturação dos canais radiculares. Arq Cent Est Fac Odontol 1971; 8:189-97.

90. Holland R, Souza V, Murata SS, Nery MJ, Bernabé PFE, Otoboni-Filho JA, Dezan-Jr E. Healing process of dog dental pulp after pulpotomy and pulp covering with mineral trioxide aggregate or portland cement. Braz Dent J 2001; 12:109-13.
91. Holland R, Souza V, Nery MJ, Bernabé PFE, Mello W, Otoboni-Filho JA. The effect of calcium hydroxide in dentine. Rev Fac Odontol Araçatuba 1978;7:177-80.
92. Holland R, Souza V, Nery MJ, Bernabé PFE, Otoboni-Filho JA, Dezan-Jr E. Agregado de trióxido mineral y cemento Portland en la obturación de conductos radiculares de perro. Endodoncia 2001; 19:275-80.
93. Holland R, Souza V, Nery MJ, Bernabé PFE, Otoboni-Filho JA, Dezan-Jr E, Murata SS. Calcium salts deposition in rat connective tissue after the implantation of calcium hydroxide – contaming sealers. J Endod 1979;28:173-76.
94. Holland R, Souza V, Nery MJ, Faraco-Jr IM, Bernabé PFE, Otoboni-Filho JA, Dezan-Jr E. Reaction of Rat Connective Tissue to Implanted Dentin Tube Filled with Mineral Trioxide Aggregate, Portland Cement or Calcium Hydroxide. Braz Dent J 2001; 12:3-8.
95. Holland R, Souza V, Nery MJ, Faraco-Jr IM, Bernabé PFE, Otoboni-Filho JA, Dezan-Jr E. Reaction of rat connective tissue to implanted dentin tubes filled with a white mineral trioxide aggregate. Braz Dent J 2002; 13:23-6.
96. Holland R, Souza V, Nery MJ, Mello W, Bernabé PFE, Otoboni-Filho JA. Comportamento dos tecidos periapicais de dentes de cães com rizogênese incompleta após obturação dos canais radiculares com diferentes materiais obturadores. Rev Bras Odontol 1992;49:49–53.
97. Holland R, Souza V, Nery MJ, Mello W, Bernabé PFE, Otoboni-Filho JA. Effect of the dressing in root canal treatment with calcium hydroxide. Rev Fac Odontol Araçatuba 1978;7:39-45.
98. Holland R, Souza V, Nery MJ, Mello W, Bernabé PFE, Otoboni-Filho JA. Root canal treatment of pulpless teeth with calvital or zinc oxide-eugenol, in one or two sittings. Histological study in dog. Rev Fac Odontol Araçatuba 1978;7:47-53.
99. Holland R, Souza V, Nery MJ, Mello W, Bernabé PFE, Otoboni-Filho JA. A histological study of the effect of calcium hydroxide in the treatment of pulpless teeth of dogs. J Brit Endod Soc 1979; 12:15-23.
100. Holland R, Souza V, Nery MJ, Mello W, Bernabé PFE, Otoboni-Filho JA. Effect of the dressing in root canal treatment with calcium hydroxide. Rev Fac Odontol Araçatuba 1980;7:39-45.
101. Holland R, Souza V, Nery MJ, Mello W, Bernabé PFE, Otoboni-Filho JA. Tissues reactions following apical plugging of the root canal with infected dentin chips. Oral Surg Oral Med Oral Pathol 1980;49:366-9.
102. Holland R, Souza V, Nery MJ, Melo, W, Bernabé PFE. Root canal treatment with calcium hydroxide. Effect of an oil water soluble vehicle. Rev Odontol Unesp 1983;12:1-6.
103. Holland R, Souza V, Nery MJ, Melo, W. Resposta ao tecido conjuntivo subcutâneo do rato ao implante de alguns materiais obturadores de canal. Rev Fac Odontol Araçatuba 1973; 2:217-25.
104. Holland R, Souza V, Nery MJ, Otoboni-Filho JA, Bernabé PFE, Dezan-Jr E. Reaction of rat connective tissue to implanted dentin tubes filled with mineral trioxide aggregate or calcium hydroxide. J Endod 1999; 25:161-6.
105. Holland R, Souza V, Otoboni-Filho JA. Root canal treatment with calcium hydroxide. I – Effect of overfilling and refilling. Oral Surg Oral Med Oral Pathol 1979;47:87-92.
106. Holland R, Souza V, Otoboni-Filho JA. Root canal treatment with calcium hydroxide. II – Effect of instrumentation beyond the apices. Oral Surg Oral Med Oral Pathol 1979;47:93-96.
107. Holland R, Souza V, Tagliavini RL, Milanezi LA. Healing process of teeth with open apices: histological study. Bull Tokyo Dent Coll 1971; 12:333-8.
108. Holland R, Souza V. Ability of a new calcium hydroxide root canal filling material to induce hard tissue formation. J Endod 1985; 11:535-43.
109. Holland R, Souza V. Considerações clínicas e biológicas sobre o tratamento endodôntico. 1 - Tratamento endodôntico conservador. Rev Ass Paul Cirur Dent 1977; 31:152-62.
110. Holland R, Souza V. Resposta da conjuntiva do olho de coelho a algumas substâncias empregadas na desinfecção dos canais radiculares. APUD: Souza V, Holland R, Nery MJ, Mello W. Emprego de medicamentos no interior dos canais radiculares. Ação tópica e a distância de algumas drogas. Ars Curandi 1978;5:4-15.
111. Holland R. Emprego tópico de medicamentos no interior de canais radiculares. Odonto Máster – Endodontia 1994; 1:1-13.
112. Holland R. Histochemical response of amputed pulps to calcium hydroxide. Rev Bras Pesq Med e Biol 1971;4:83-95.
113. Holland R. Processo de reparo da polpa dental após pulpotomia e proteção com hidróxido de cálcio. (Doctoral Thesis). Araçatuba: São Paulo State University; 1966.
114. Holland R. Processo de reparo do coto pulpar e dos tecidos periapicais após biopulpectomias e obturação de canal com hidróxido de cálcio ou óxido de zinco e eugenol. Estudos histológicos em dentes de cães. (Livre-Docência Thesis) Araçatuba: São Paulo State University; 1975.
115. Kerekes K, Olsen I. Similarities in the microfloras of the canals and deep periodontal pockets. Endod Dent Traumatol. 1990;6:1-5.
116. Kojima K, Inamoto K, Nagamatsu K, Hara A, Nakata K, Morita I, Nakagaki H, Nakamura H. Sucess rate of endodontic treatment of teeth with vital and nonvital pulps. A meta-analysis. Oral Surg Oral Med Oral Pathol Oral Radiol Endod 2004;97:95-9.
117. Kurihara H, Kobayashi Y, Francisco IA, Isoshima O, Nagai A, Murayama Y. A microbiological and immunological study of endodontic-periodontic lesions. J Endod 1995;21:617-21.
118. Law A, Messer H. An evidence-based analysis of the antibacterial effectiveness of intracanal medicaments. J Endod 2004;30:689-94.
119. Leles CR, Freire MCM. Odontologia Baseada em Evidências. In: Estrela C. Metodologia Científica. 2 ed. São Paulo: Artes Médicas; 2005. p.475-488.
120. Marinho V. Revisões sistemáticas e Metanálise. In: Crivello-Jr O. Fundamentos de odontologia – Epidemiologia da Saúde Bucal. Rio de Janeiro: Guanabara Koogan; 2006. p.422-33.

121. Nair PNR, Sjögren U, Kahnerg KE, Sundqvist G. Intraradicular bacteria and fungi in root - files, assymtomatic human teeth with therapy-resistant periapical lesions: A long-term light and electron microscopic follow-up study. J Endod 1990; 16:580-88.
122. Nair PNR, Sjögren U, Schumacher E, Sundqvist G. Radicular cyst affecting a root-filled human tooth: a long-term post-treatment follow-up. Int Endod J 1993;26:225-33.
123. Nair PNR. Apical periodontitis: a dynamic encounter between root canal infection and host response. Periodontology 2000 1997; 13:29-39.
124. Nair PNR. Light and electrom microscopic studies on root canal flora and periapical lesions. J Endod 1987; 13:29-39.
125. Nair PNR. Pathobiology of the periapex. In: Pathways of the pulp. Cohen S, Burns RC. 8th edn. St. Louis: Mosby; 2002.
126. Paiva JG, Antoniazzi JH. Endodontia – bases para a prática clínica. São Paulo: Artes Médicas; 1984.
127. Pécora JD, Barbin EL, Spanó JC, Silva RS. In vitro analysis of gas released using different concentrations of sodium hypochlorite with 3% hydrogen peroxide. Braz Endod J 1997; 2:16-8.
128. Pécora JD, Guerisoli DMZ, Silva RS, Vansan SP. Shelf-life of 5% sodium hypochlorite solutions. Braz Endod J 1997; 2:43-5.
129. Pécora JD, Guimarães LF, Savioli RN. Surface tension of several drugs used in Endodontics. Braz Dent J 1991; 2:123-7.
130. Pécora JD, Murgel CAF, Guimarães LFL, Costa WF. Verificação do teor de cloro ativo de diferentes marcas de líquido de Dakin encontrados no mercado. Rev Odont Univ São Paulo 1988; 2:10-13.
131. Pécora JD, Murgel, CAF, Savioli RN, Costa WF, Vansan LP. Estudo sobre o shelf life da solução de Dakin. Rev Odont Univ São Paulo 1987; 1:3-7.
132. Pécora JD, Souza-Neto MD, Estrela C. Soluções auxiliares do preparo do canal radicular. In: Endodontia: princípios biológicos e mecânicos. Estrela C, Figueiredo JAP. São Paulo: 1st ed. Artes Médicas; 1999. p.553-69.
133. Pécora JD, Souza-Neto MD, Guerisoli DMZ, Marchesan MA. Effect of reduction of the surface tension of different concentrations of sodium hypochlorite solutions on radicular dentine permeability. Braz Endod J 1998; 3:38-40.
134. Pécora JD, Souza-Neto MD, Saquy PC,. Silva RG, Cruz-Filho AM. Effect of Dakin's and EDTA solutions on dentin permeability of root canals. Braz Dent J 1993; 4:79-84.
135. Pécora JD. Contribuição ao estudo da permeabilidade dentinária radicular. Apresentação de um método histoquímico e análise morfométrica. (Master's Thesis). Ribeirão Preto: University of São Paulo; 1985. 110p.
136. Pécora JD. Efeito das soluções de Dakin e de EDTA, isoladas, alternadas e misturadas, sobre a permeabilidade da dentina radicular. (Livre-Docência Thesis).University of São Paulo, 1993.
137. Pécora JD. Estudo da permeabilidade dentinária do assoalho da câmara pulpar dos molares inferiores humanos, com raízes separadas. (Doctoral Thesis). University of São Paulo, 1990.
138. Petitti DB. Metanalysis, decision analysis, and cost-effectiveness analysis: methods for quantitative synthesis in medicine. New York: Oxford University Press; 2000.
139. Rotsein IS, Simon JH. The endo-perio lesion: a critical appraisal of the disease condition. Endodontic Topics 2006:13:34-56.
140. Ruiz LFN, Mendonça JA, Estrela C. Inter-relações entre a endodontia e a periodontia. In: Estrela C, Figueiredo JAP. Endodontia: princípios biológicos e mecânicos. São Paulo: Artes Médicas; 1999: p.248-91.
141. Sacks HS, Berrier J, Reitman D, Ancona-Berk VA, Chalmers TC. Meta-analyses of randomized controlled trials. N Engl J Med 1987;316:450-1.
142. Sathorn C, Parashos P, Messer H. Antibacterial efficacy of calcium hydroxide intracanal dressing: a systematic review and meta-analysis. Int Endod J 2007;40:2-10.
143. Seltzer S, Bender IB, Ziontz M. The interrelationship of pulpal and periodontal disease. Oral Surg Oral Med Oral Pathol 1963;16:1474-90.
144. Simon JH, Glick DH, Frank AL. The relationship of endodontic-periodontic lesions. J Periodontol 1972;43:202-8.
145. Simon P, Jacobs D. The so-called periodontal pulpal problem. Dent Clin N Amer. 1969;13:45-52.
146. Siwek J, Gourlay ML, Slawson DC, Shaughnessy AF. How to write an evidence-based clinical review article. Am Fam Physician 2002;65:251-8.
147. Socransky SS, Haffajee AD, Cugini MA, Smith C, Kent-Jr RL. Microbial complexes in subgingival plaque. J Clin Periodontol 1998;25:134-44.
148. Socransky SS, Haffajee AD. Microbiologia da doença periodontal. In: Lindhe J, Karring T, Lang NP. Tratado de Periodontia Clínica e Implantodontia Oral. 4th ed. Rio de Janeiro: Guanabara Koogan; 2005: p.105-47.
149. Socransky SS, Haffajee AD. The bacterial etiology of destructive periodontal disease: current concepts. J Periodontol. 1992;63:322-31.
150. Tanner ACR, Visconti RA, Haldeman LV, Sundqvist G, Socranscky SS. Similarity of Wolinella recta strains isolated from periodontal pockets and root canals. J Endod. 1982;8:294-300.
151. Taubman MA. Immunological aspects of periodontal diseases. In: Slots J, Taubman MA. Contemporary Oral Microbiology and Immunology. 1st ed. St Louis: Mosby; 1992. p.542-54.
152. Vakalis SV, Whitworth JM, Ellwood RP, Preshaw PM. A pilot study of treatment of periodontal-endodontic lesions. Int Dent J. 2005;55:313-8.

# Endodontic Diagnosis Planning

**C. Estrela**

*Federal University of Goiás, Goiânia, GO, Brazil*

**C. R. A. Estrela**

*Brazilian Dentistry Research and Learning Center, CEPOBRAS, Goiânia, GO, Brazil*

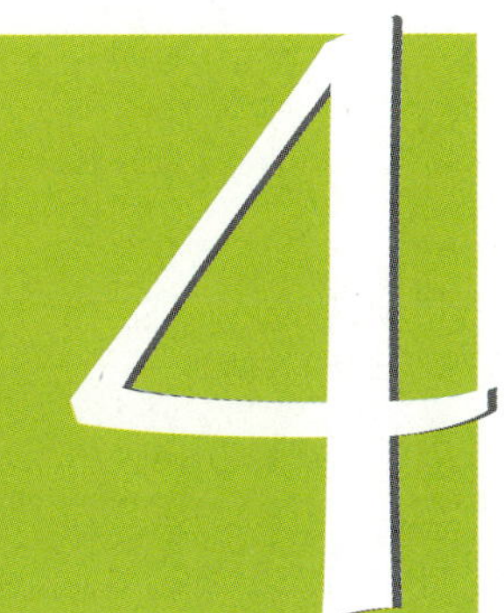

Chapter contents

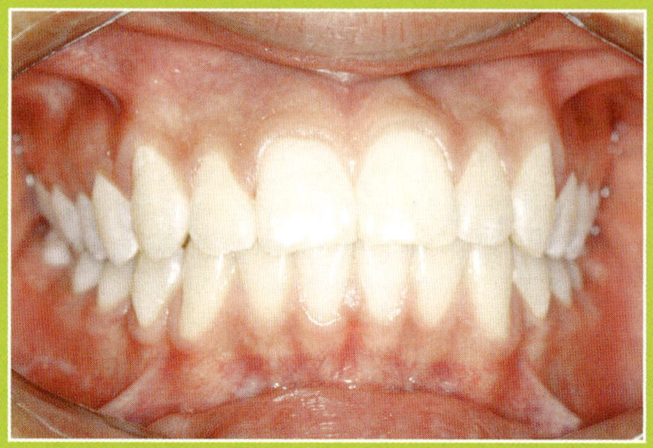

Inspection of a healthy oral cavity.

## 4.1 Introduction

Diagnosis represents the basis for structuring dental treatment, especially when the patient's chief complaint is related to pain. Odontogenic pain is the most frequent reason that obliges a person to seek dental treatment. The great challenge is to recognize the etiological factor responsible for the origin of the pain process in oral structures, and distinguishes this stage of diagnosis as fundamental and most important within the context of dental treatment.

When verifying the etiological agent of pain, it is important for the investigator to make an elaborate analysis; collect, tabulate, identify and interpret the signs and symptoms that characterize a possible alteration in the tissue structure.

Diagnosis of odontogenic pain consists of different stages, as follows: semiogenesis – the genesis of signs and symptoms; semiotechnique – the resources for collecting the signs and symptoms; and the propaedeutic stage, consisting of analysis, study and interpretation of the collected data.

The semiological technique used for structuring the diagnosis requires the knowledge and the study of the states of normality; that is, the health of tissues related to the problem, so that a hypothesis of the identity of the pathology can be determined in an organized way. From a systematic record of the collected and tabulated data, the alteration can be interpreted and identified.

To identify the origin and interpret the type of odontogenic pain, biological and functional knowledge of the tissue or organ is mandatory. Careful analysis depends on the criteria of knowing how to listen, see, feel, observe and structure information. Some pathologies can present preclinical signs and symptoms, or they can show pathognomonic characteristics – typical and evident aspects that allow them to be differentiated from one another. In other situations, however, antagonistic signs and symptoms, or inconsistent responses to the semiotechnique resources used can be evidenced, which can make it difficult to recognize the pathology. Differential diagnosis is based on the comparison of similar signs and symptoms among several pathologies, and exclusion analysis frequently leads to diagnosis by elimination of similar signs and symptoms[1,7,8,13-16,29-31,34,52-55]. Table 4.1 describes the different stages of structuring the diagnosis.

**Table 4.1** - Stages of diagnosis

**Semiogenic Stage**
- Analysis of the appearance/onset of signs and symptoms (Questioning the Patient)

**Semiotechnique**
- Resources for collecting the signs and symptoms (Exploratory clinical exam)

**Propaedeutic Stage (Preliminary)**
- Analysis, study and interpretation of the collected data (Structuring the diagnostic hypothesis)

Successful treatment depends on determining the diagnosis perfectly and this is only complete when it is done in a rational and intelligent manner, with the goal of solving the patient's problem, and not exclusively and essentially the problem of the tooth. To solve the pathologic problem affecting the person, all efforts must always be directed towards holistic treatment – the person as a whole, and not restricted to trying to understand the disease in an isolated way. It is important to understand the consequences of the potential alteration to other body parts, as well as the contrary. However, the professional must be very well prepared for this important mission and be conscious of the extent it represents.

The semiotechnique resources are also useful as an aid to achieve the diagnostic hypothesis of the alterations responsible for odontogenic pains. The exact interpretation of the results obtained leads to determining the clinical state. It should be pointed out that the investigator must know how to listen to and observe the patient, and have a great deal of patience and interest in solving his/her symptomatic problem. In many situations, the patient does not transmit the real significance of his/her chief complaint to the dentist, and it is the Dentist's responsibility to use his ability and skill to discover this and indicate the treatment options.

Filgueiras et al.[29] do not believe that it is possible to learn the art of examining the sick, as one learns any other art, from books. Study provides essential rules, however this is not enough. The art of examining demands several highly refined attributes of the senses; the ability to observe, analyze, discern, deduce, and use good sense and basic knowledge and particularly, experience.

Cohen & Liewehr[14] related that diagnostic testing of some common complaints may produce classical results; occasional testing will produce inconsistent or incomplete results that need to be carefully interpreted by the astute and curious clinician to resolve discrepancies. Accurate diagnoses can only result from the synthesis of scientific knowledge, clinical experience, intuition, and common sense. The process is thus both an art and a science.

Above all, one must remember something that frequently happens when performing the anamnesis and clinical exams:

*"quite often we look at our patients,*
*but we do not see;*
*we listen, but we do not hear"*

so, the outstanding requirement for achieving a diagnosis is to really see the patient and hear what he/she has to say.

## 4.2 Semiologic Exam

Structuring the semiologic exam is the first stage in planning the endodontic treatment, in which systematic examination is necessary to encourage the professional to develop the habit of following protocols to reach the correct diagnosis, inducing him to know the characteristics of tissues in their normal state, as well as their variations. In many situations, this knowledge allows several pathologies to be diagnosed at an early stage, which eliminates complications and sequelae, particularly those related to symptomatic cases.

The diagnosis of the odontogenic pain is complex and difficult because of different peculiarities involved in this phenomenon. The subjective factors related to pain, such as emotional factors, favor personal reactions that characterize different sensations in response to the same problem[15,21].

One of the difficulties the professional faces when structuring a diagnosis that involves a pain condition, results from a mechanical vision of the illness. A significant and basic factor in diagnosis must be understood: not all pains are somatic; neuropathic and psychogenic pains may occur[43-45].

The methodology to develop for structuring the diagnosis consists of fundamental stages, as follows: anamnesis – a subjective exam, clinical exam – an objective exam, pulp vitality test involving stimulation by semiotechnique resources, imaging exam providing the radiographic aspect, and when necessary, requesting complementary exams that are part of the systemic investigation). Table 4.2 characterizes the stages and basis for structuring odontogenic pain diagnosis.

**Table 4.2** - Semiogenic and semiotechnique resources for structuring the diagnosis

| | |
|---|---|
| **1. Anamnesis** | • **Questioning Technique**<br>Chief complaint<br>Past History<br>Current History<br>Medical history<br>Dental history<br>Clinical characteristics of Pain |
| **2. Clinical Exam** | • **Explorative Technique**<br>Inspection<br>Exploration<br>Palpation<br>Percussion |
| **3. Pulp Vitality Exam** | • **Stimulation Technique**<br>Thermal Test<br>Electrical Test<br>Mechanical Test<br>Other Tests |
| **4. Imaging Exam** | • **Interpretation Technique** |
| **5. Complementary Exams** | • **Investigation Technique** |



## Anamnesis

Anamnesis represents the subjective exam carried out by the technique of questioning the patient, which directs the investigation to the appearance of signals and symptoms involved in the pathological process. The clinical history must be collected and recorded in a guided and controlled manner, through defined questions, to the point of including detailed and dynamic explanations. Anamnesis involves analyzing the data obtained separately, and interpreting it in an associated way, to compose part of the diagnostic process. It is composed of the chief complaint, current and past history of the illness in question, thus establishing the dental history. General information contained in the medical history, however, is essential to facilitate planning and structuring of the diagnosis, as well as forecasting the prognosis.

Frequently, the patient informs that he is a carrier of a disease, which obliges the professional to use the necessary knowledge to perform the correct therapies. In other situations, the patient does not know that he is carrier of a certain disease, and during the health inventory, supplementary questions become necessary which, through signs and symptoms, can also favor recognition of a systemic disease.

The anamnesis retrieves from the patient's memory, aspects that favor identification of the agents responsible for the pain or pathological condition, which enable one to find evidence that will make it easier to differentiate significant aspects for determining the problem. With the clinical exam, a better definition of the pathological condition is obtained, which frequently helps to verify and confirm the data obtained through the anamnesis.

Many systemic conditions require special care, as the patient sometimes does not know of their existence. Outstanding among them are: hepatitis, tuberculosis, AIDS, diabetes, anemia, and so on.

## 4.3 Chief Complaint

The chief complaint represents the reason why the patient required treatment, normally because of presenting pain. This must be written down in the patient's own words, in answer to correct and well directed questions:

- What made you seek treatment?
- When did the pain appear?
- Where is the pain?
- Which factor stimulates or lessens the pain?
- How frequent is the pain?
- How intense is the pain?
- What is the pain like?

The treatment must preferably not be started before the probable clinical diagnosis has been established.

The subjective exam, obtained by the questioning technique includes the medical and dental history, as well as characterization of the chief complaint. The dental history is undoubtedly an essential stage in the diagnostic process, establishing a list of fundamental conditions for patient-professional interaction, in order to solve the problem. The good investigator requires some special attributes, such as; knowledge, intuition, curiosity, patience, good sense. Skills such as, organization, interpretation, understanding the language of pain, synthesis, action and experience are also required[5,12-14,31,32,34,49].

## 4.4 Clinical Characteristics of the Pain

Pain is the most related symptom during the anamnesis to describe the chief complaint. It is derived from pathological processes of inflammatory origin, often not represented by a simple discomfort, but by complex experiences within the scope of tissue, psychological and social factors. This experience can be described by different feelings (acute, chronic, pulsating, throbbing, twinging, burning pains, shock) and is expressed in various forms.

The literature records[36-40] different ways to describe aspects of pain experience, among them, sensitive, affective, evaluative and various other forms are mentioned.

Ingle & Glick[34] related that some modalities of pain can give clues for diagnosis, such as the following characteristics: burning, penetrating and spasmodic visceral pains, hammering headaches, complaints of rheumatism and menstrual colic.

With regard to the phenomenon of the pain with pulpitis, it can be inferred that pain is the only language the dental pulp has to reveal structural alterations, but it says little of the real extent of the pathological process[14,20]. Some clinical characteristics of the odontogenic pain help to establish the diagnostic hypothesis. Among them, we can point out the place, appearance, duration, frequency and intensity.

The patient identifying the location of the pain does not allow one to affirm its exact origin, and it is left to the investigator to ascertain the correct location. The pain location indicates a locality of perception or possible extension or diffusion to other regions. When the symptoms radiate, or when the pain is secondary, one tries to observe its direction and extent. There is great possibility of a mistaken diagnosis in situations of referred pain, which leads to mistakes in treatment. Thus, the goal is to identify the true origin of the symptom – the primary pain, from the signs coming from the affected tooth, in order to establish the correct treatment of the affected tooth.

Okeson[45] reports that there are many theories that seek to explain the phenomenon of referred pain. The most prevalent theory is the one of convergence, documented in the sensitive nuclear complex on the encephalic trigeminus, since the oral and interpolar subnucleus receive extensive convergence of the muscle afferent impulses of the orofacial muscle. The afferent impulses from deep structures converge to a greater degree than the afferent impulses from cutaneous structures, which allow one to admit that the pain of deep structures is felt in a more diffuse and less located way than the pain felt in cutaneous structures, which makes it difficult for the patient to pinpoint its location. The convergent impulse can result in other effects, such as secondary hyperalgesia, increased response to stimulation in the pain area, in the absence of local cause[57]. It is convenient to clarify that hyperalgesia is referred to as the increase in sensitivity by stimulation in the area of pain, and that primary hyperalgesia occurs as result of a diminished threshold in the peripheral structures (presence of algogenic substances, such as bradykinin, potassium, histamine and serotonin).

Referred (heterotopic) pain from pulp is felt in a place that normally is not its true origin. Glick[30] relates referred pain to the excess of afferent stimulations of the pain that penetrates into a "*pool*" of sensitive neurons, in which there are superimpositions of deep and cutaneous neurons. In referred pain, the consequence to other teeth and regions can be observed[30].

Among the criteria for diagnosis[31], the following can be pointed out:

a) It is not accentuated by the stimulation of the place of the referred pain.
b) It is not alleviated by anesthesia of the place of the referred pain.
c) It is accentuated by anesthesia of the place of the referred pain.
d) It is alleviated by analgesic that blocks the original pain.

As regards the pathways of referred pain, the following can be considered; maxillary canines reflect the pain to the 1st or 2nd maxillary premolar and also to the 1st and 2nd mandibular premolar. The maxillary premolars can reflect the pain to the mandibular premolars. The inverse can also occur. The mandibular incisors, canines and 1st premolars can reflect the pain to the mentum area. The mandibular 2nd premolar can reflect the pain to the mentum region or the middle of the ascendant ramus. The mandibular 1st and 2nd premolars can reflect the pain to the maxillary molars. The mandibular molars can promote referred pain to the anterior region (mandibular premolars). The maxillary incisors can reflect the pain to the frontal area. The maxillary canine and the maxillary 1st premolar can reflect the pain to the nasolabial area and to the orbit. The maxillary 2nd premolar and 1st molar can reflect the pain the jaw and backwards, to the temporal area. The maxillary 2nd and 3rd molars can reflect the pain to the mandibular molar area and, occasionally, to the ear. The mandibular 1st and 2nd molar can, commonly, reflect the pain to the ear and mandibular angle. The mandibular 3rd molar can reflect the pain to the ear and, occasionally, to the upper region of the larynx.[30,34] The appearance of provoked or spontaneous pain can determine the type of stimulation as a function of the degree of pulp involvement. The beginning and development of the painful process help to establish the diagnosis. It is common in situations of dentin tubule exposure (as a result of dental caries, gingival recession, fracture or restoration leakage, or for other reasons) for provoked pain to appear, mainly caused by thermal stimulations, such as the cold, sweet foods, ingestion of acid foods. These stimulations promote vascular alterations, from changes in the movement of the intratubular fluids, which stimulate the afferent and myelinic nerve fibers present in the peripheral zone of the dental pulp, and cause symptomatic clinical situations. Deep caries or marginal leakage in restored teeth lead to symptoms of pain with provoked appearance, either because of temperature changes (cold/hot) or by the ingestion of foods (sweet/ acid). In this situation, pulp involvement also demonstrates similar clinical characteristics to those of dental hypersensitivity, and normally characterizes previous evidence of establishment of an inflammatory process in the pulp. They are clinical situations of pain, although, suggesting pulp involvement, they never determine the histopathological condition and the extent of pulp involvement[12,15].

Quite often dental pain suggests valuable information, because depending on the etiological agent and the intensity of the aggression, by eliminating the factor that sets off the pain, there is the possibility that the symptoms may disappear. In a situation of deep caries, fractured restoration, or gingival recession, when the aggressive agent and/or pain stimulant is eliminated, protection can be provided without direct pulp intervention, and the tooth can be restored (in this case the suggested diagnosis is hyper-reactive pulpalgia). The appearance of spontaneous pain suggests inflammatory alterations in the pulp, however, without being indicative of the need for radical treatment of the dental pulp (pulpectomy). It is fitting to evaluate the clinical conditions of the pulp tissue (consistency and bleeding) to define the best option (pulpotomy or pulpectomy). Other important aspects to analyze at the point of pain appearance, are the agents that stimulate the pain (sugar, masticatory pressure, heat) and those that attenuate it, such as cold.

Holland & Souza[32] conducted a histopathological study in 28 human teeth, in which the patients complained of spontaneous nocturnal pains. The results of the histopathological analyses showed that in all cases there was the presence of an inflammatory process that varied in intensity (from moderate neutrophilic infiltrate; microabscesses and to even more voluminous abscesses), which compromised almost all the coronal pulp. No radically compromised pulp was observed in any case. The inflammatory process was located exclusively in the coronal pulp. Thus, pulpotomy can be performed in teeth with spontaneous pains, since the pulp remainders show characteristics of vitality.

The appearance of any symptom or clinical aspect associated with the painful process must be well observed and recorded (either at ocular, muscular, cutaneous, nasal, hearing, smell or taste level). On the other hand, there are factors that can influence the development of pain, such as a paraxystic condition. The factors that influence the aggravation or stimulation of pain (such as face movements, deglutition, act of brushing teeth, shaving the beard, head position, presence of noise or crepitus while opening the mouth) deserve to be pointed out when recording information. At a personal level, the presence of other diseases, stress, emotional tension, and the use of medicine can significantly affect the pain condition.

The duration of the painful phenomenon can be related to different factors, for instance, the difference between a momentary pain, that lasts seconds, and long a drawn out pain, that remains for hours or days; this as well as the relationship between the duration and the intensity must be investigated and well evaluated.

According to Bell[4], the term *acute pain* is related to the pain of short duration, whereas *chronic pain* involves a pain that has persisted for longer than 6 months. Pain of shorter duration can denote less involvement than that of extensive duration. The same applies to the frequency of the pain, and similar conditions must be established from the aspect of whether it is continuous or intermittent.

On the other hand, microscopic analysis of acute inflammation indicates the presence of polymorphonuclear cells (mainly neutrophils) and evident exudative processes; whereas in chronic inflammation the mononuclear cells predominate (lymphocytes, plasmocytes and macrophages), distinguishing the proliferative processes.

The intensity of pain is another very variable clinical characteristic, described with much subjectivity, and related not only to the pathological involvement and pain threshold of the patient, but also to the emotional and psychological aspect. The attempt to quantify pain by setting zero degrees as the absence of pain, and ten for intense pain, helps to characterize the conditions that increase or diminish the symptomatic condition, such as the relationship with stimulation that affects the tooth. Among these stimulators are heat, cold, sweet or acidic foods, chewing or the emotional state. These factors can facilitate diagnosis, and after treatment has been established, can express involvement, maintenance or development of an initial pathological condition. The symptom usually only has meaning when the professional, apart from hearing about it, knows how to interpret it and how to associate it with a possible pathological condition.

In view of the clinical characteristics and the different aspects that are related to orofacial pains, it is up to the investigator to define the possibilities of structuring the diagnosis, formulating at least one hypothesis (probable clinical diagnosis). An initial aspect to be pointed out, although one of variable character is in the observation of the category of pain proposed by Bell[4], as is demonstrated in Table 4.3. Once characterized, the direction of the orofacial pain diagnosis points to the definition of the probable diagnosis of the disease in question, with regard to the specific area of occurrence of the odontogenical pain, such as, for example: pulp pain, periodontal pain, pain resulting from temporomandibular dysfunction. Table 4.4 indicates fundamental aspects to be investigated within the clinical characteristics of pain. Table 4.5 describes questions directed towards facilitating identification of temporomandibular dysfunctions.

**Table 4.3** - Pain categories

1. **Somatic, neuropathic or psychogenic pain**

- Clinical characteristics of neuropathic pain
  Sensation of burning, spontaneous pain, intermittent or constant; pain disproportionate to the stimulation; pain followed by neurologic symptoms; pain started or accentuated by efferent sympathetic activity at the area

- Clinical characteristics that support the suspected influence of psychological factors associated with the pain
  Progressive emotional and/or physical alteration; anxiety; change in sleep pattern; concern or obsession about the painful condition; depression; progressive non-physiological behavior of pain.

2. **Acute or chronic pain (pain with duration exceeding 6 months)**
3. **Primary or secondary pain (related pain or secondary hyperalgesia)**
4. **Superficial or deep pain**
5. **Visceral or muscle-skeletal pain**
6. **Inflammatory or non-inflammatory pain**

(Bell[4])

**Table 4.4** - Clinical Characteristics of Pain

| | |
|---|---|
| **Place**<br>(Where is the pain?) | • **Located**<br>• **Diffuse** |
| **Appearance**<br>(How did the pain appear?)<br>(Which factor stimulates or attenuates the pain?) | • **Provoked**<br>• **Spontaneous** |
| **Duration**<br>(How long has the pain been there?) | • **Short**<br>• **Long** |
| **Frequency**<br>(How often does the pain occur?) | • **Intermittent**<br>• **Continuous** |
| **Intensity**<br>(How intense is the pain?) | • **Light (0 to 3 degrees)**<br>• **Moderate (4 to 7 degrees)**<br>• **Severe (8 to 10 degrees)** |

**Table 4.5** - Clinical characteristics of tempormandibular disturbances

1. Pain or difficulty during mouth opening
2. Irregular displacement of the mandible
3. Locking (or immobilization) of the mandible
4. Noise at the temporomandibular joint
5. Earache, headache, neckache, toothache.
6. Traumatism in the head, temporomandibular joint or mandible
7. Pain in the chewing muscles

## 4.5 Clinical Exam (Exploration Technique – Objective Exam)

### Inspection

The clinical examination represents the objective analysis of signs that characterize a certain disease in a particular way. The visual observation, physical inspection, extra and intraoral examination of the soft tissues determine many aspects of tissue conditions (asymmetry, coloring, edema, fistula, ulcerations, hyperplasias) and dental structure conditions (coronal integrity, restoration quality, coloring, periodontal pockets) constituting fundamental aspects to be analyzed. The inspection must be very critical, detailed and very well recorded. Minute observation of the aspect of restorations and prosthesis with functional problems, together with the absence of teeth can be responsible for occlusal disturbances and muscle overload. The presence of noises in the temporomandibular joints can indicate alterations in it.

Table 4.6 demonstrates the biophysical dental characteristics important in the diagnostic process applied to endodontic pain. Table 4.7 expresses the clinical and radiographic criteria for the diagnosis of periodontal lesions.

**Table 4.6** - Biophysical dental characteristics important in endodontic diagnosis

| | |
|---|---|
| **Pulp Cavity** | • Open (Pulp Exposure)<br>• Closed (Without Exposure) |
| **Rhizogenesis** | • Complete<br>• Incomplete |
| **Pulp Vitality Test** | • Positive to cold<br>• Negative to cold<br>• Positive to heat<br>• Negative to heat |

**Table 4.7** - Clinical and radiographic criteria for the diagnosis of periodontal lesions

| Diagnosis | Criteria (Radiographic analysis) | Variations |
|---|---|---|
| **Gingivitis** | • Without loss of support tissue | • Bleeding on probing |
| **Slight Periodontitis** | • Horizontal loss of support tissue < 1/3 of the root length | • Bleeding on probing |
| **Serious Periodontitis** | • Horizontal loss of the support tissues > 1/3 of the root length | • Bleeding on probing |
| **Serious and complicated Periodontitis** | • Angle osseous defect (infrabony pocket, interdental osseous crater), furcation involvement Degree 2, 3. | |

(Nyman & Lindhe[41])

## Exploration

Exploration constitutes of a sequence of inspections, in which it can be observed the presence of dental cavities, periodontal pockets, fistulous passages, coronal and root fractures. In this examination, probing (physical exploration), translighting (passage of light through dental structure or tissue), and radiography with contrast is often used. A dental microscope can also be used for a better view in this type of exam.

## Palpation

By tactile perception (tact/ light pressure) palpation determines the consistency and texture of the tissues, adherence, mobility and smoothness; in addition to characterizing painful responses to this type of stimulation. Lymph node involvement can be verified by palpation. In periapical abscesses without fistula, palpation can also verify the stage of development, and analyze whether it presents a fluctuation point (initial stage; in development, developed). At this stage, this procedure must be extended beyond the oral cavity, reaching the nodes next to the masticatory muscles and temporomandibular joint region, etc.

**Percussion**

Percussion is not an exact resource for establishing diagnosis, but it can sometimes indicate the tooth involved in chewing pain through bite or premature contact. To test this, we can stimulate the tooth, by asking the patient to bite on a plastic and flexible point, for example, the saliva ejector. This can also be established with quick and moderate stimulations with a finger or instrument, to verify the symptoms, for example, of periapical inflammatory alterations, and/or sound responses, e.g., dental traumatism – ankylosis, metallic sound). In the situations of symptomatic apical periodontitis and periapical abscess without fistula, percussion is painful.

Vertical percussion can be associated with periapical inflammation, whereas horizontal percussion is associated with periodontal alterations[2,34].

Kerr et al.[38] reported that despite the fundamental similarity of structure in all patients, individual variations do occur. Almost everyone is familiar with the differences in musculature and other anatomic features of the various races. The clinical or physical examination of the patient should include the exposed parts of the body and the structures of the mouth. A logical and orderly scheme of examination should be practiced. Even though the physical examination may consist of only an examination of the affected part as determined by the chief complaint, only a thorough and complete examination can one expect to produce a high yield of unsuspected disease or even the obvious disease.

Figures 4.1 to 4.12 characterize determining signs of a healthy oral cavity and clinical and radiographic evidences of pathological alterations caused by dental caries. Figures 4.13 to 4.22 express representative clinical and radiographic aspects when establishing the diagnosis of dental alterations. Figures 4.23 to 4.28 demonstrate periodontal alterations, while Figures 4.29 and 4.30 show perforated internal resorption.

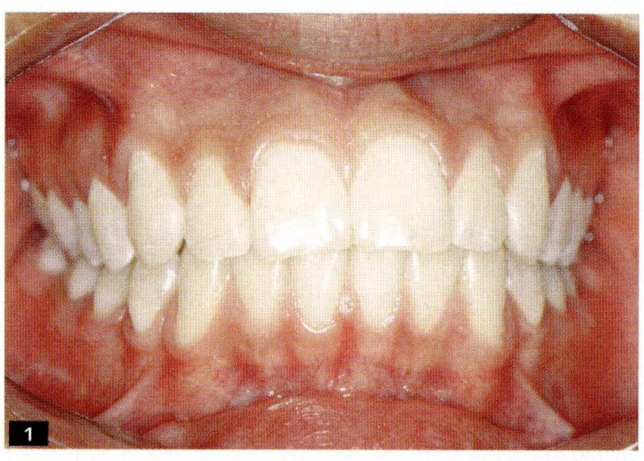


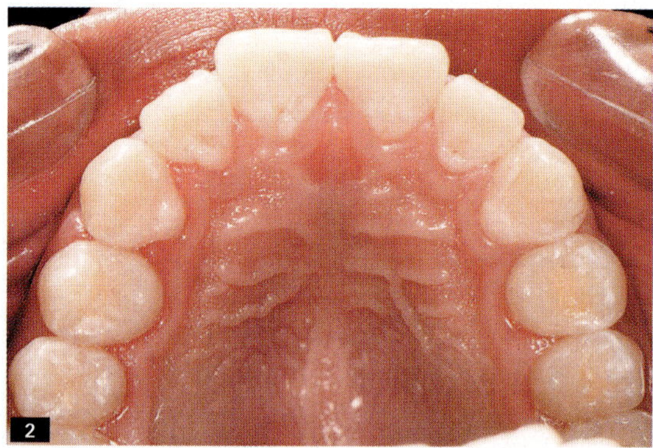


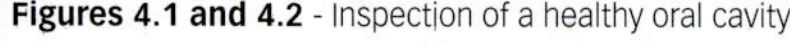
**Figures 4.1 and 4.2** - Inspection of a healthy oral cavity.

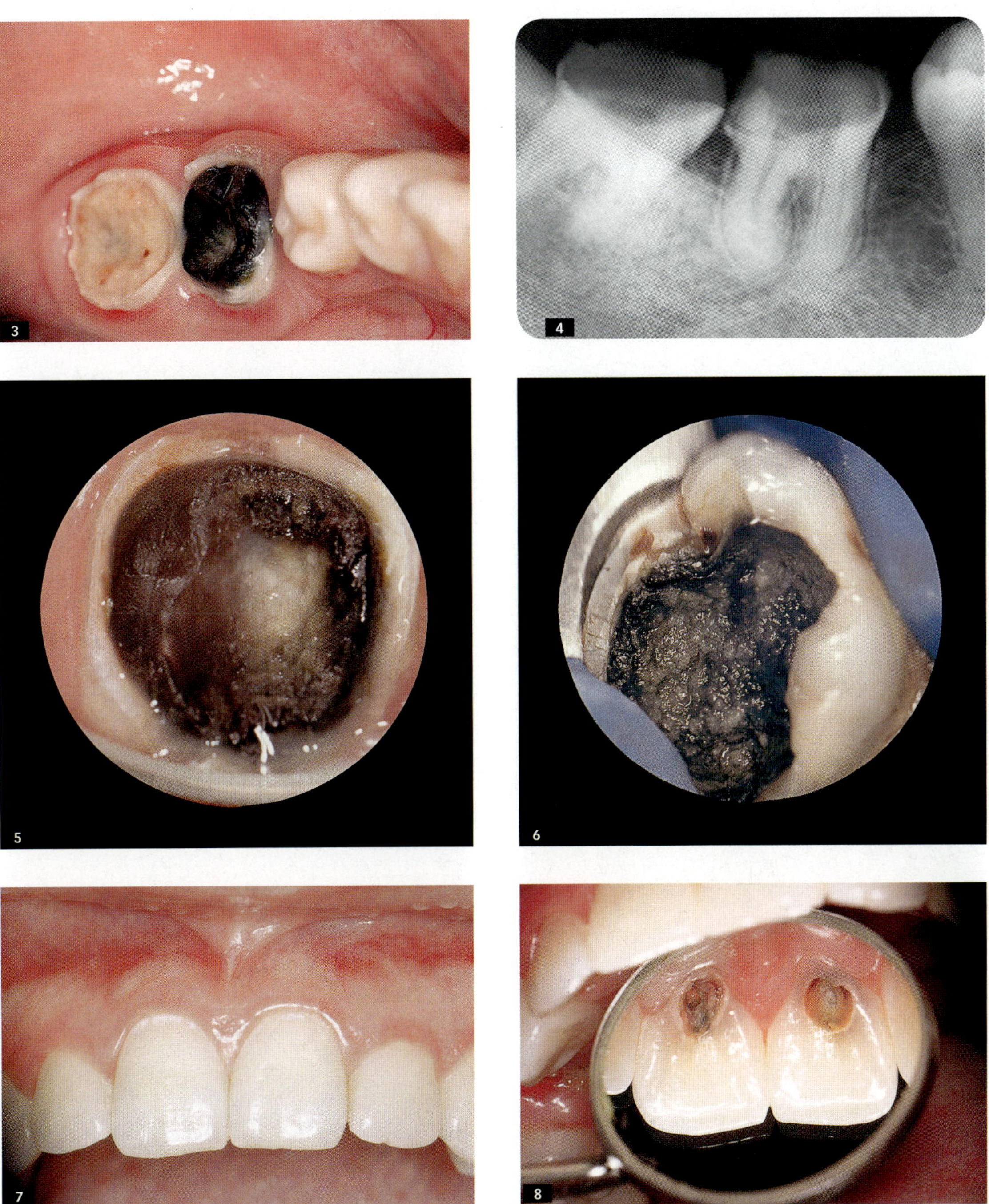

**Figures 4.3 to 4.8** - Clinical and radiographic evidences of pathological alterations caused by dental caries.

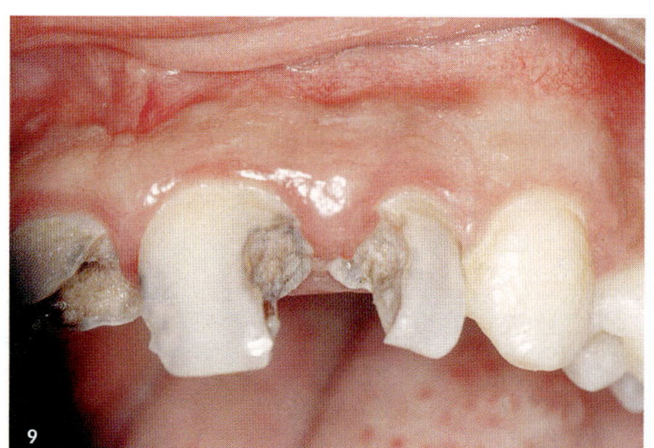

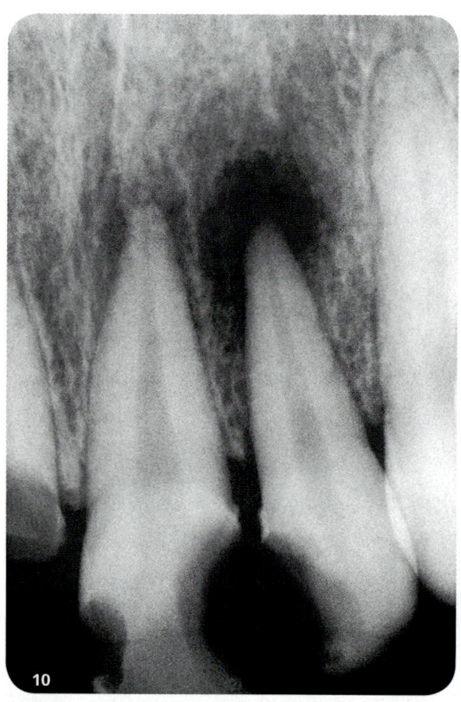

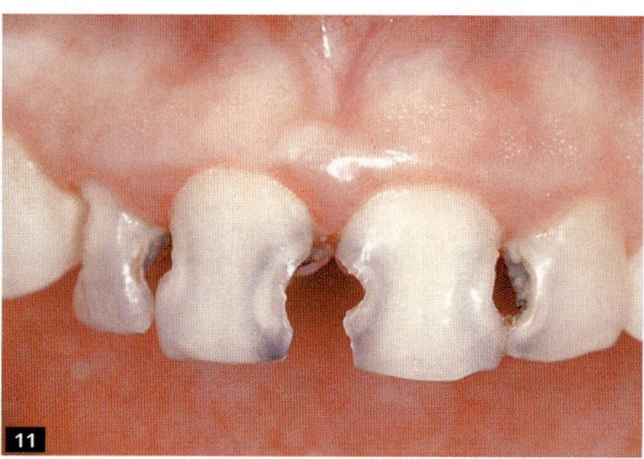

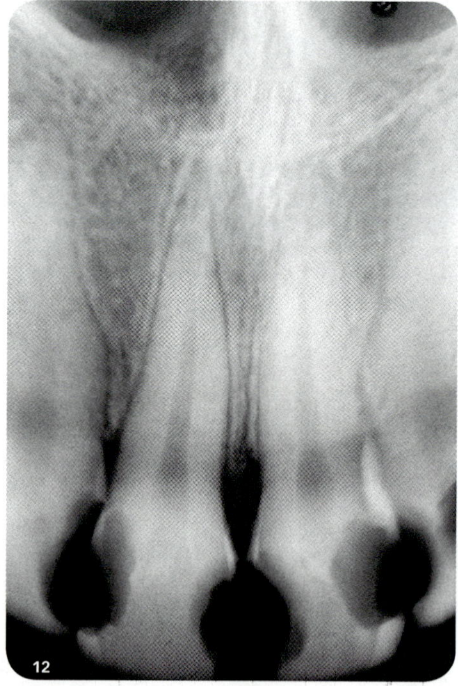

**Figures 4.9 to 4.12** - Clinical and radiographic evidences of pathological alterations caused by dental caries.

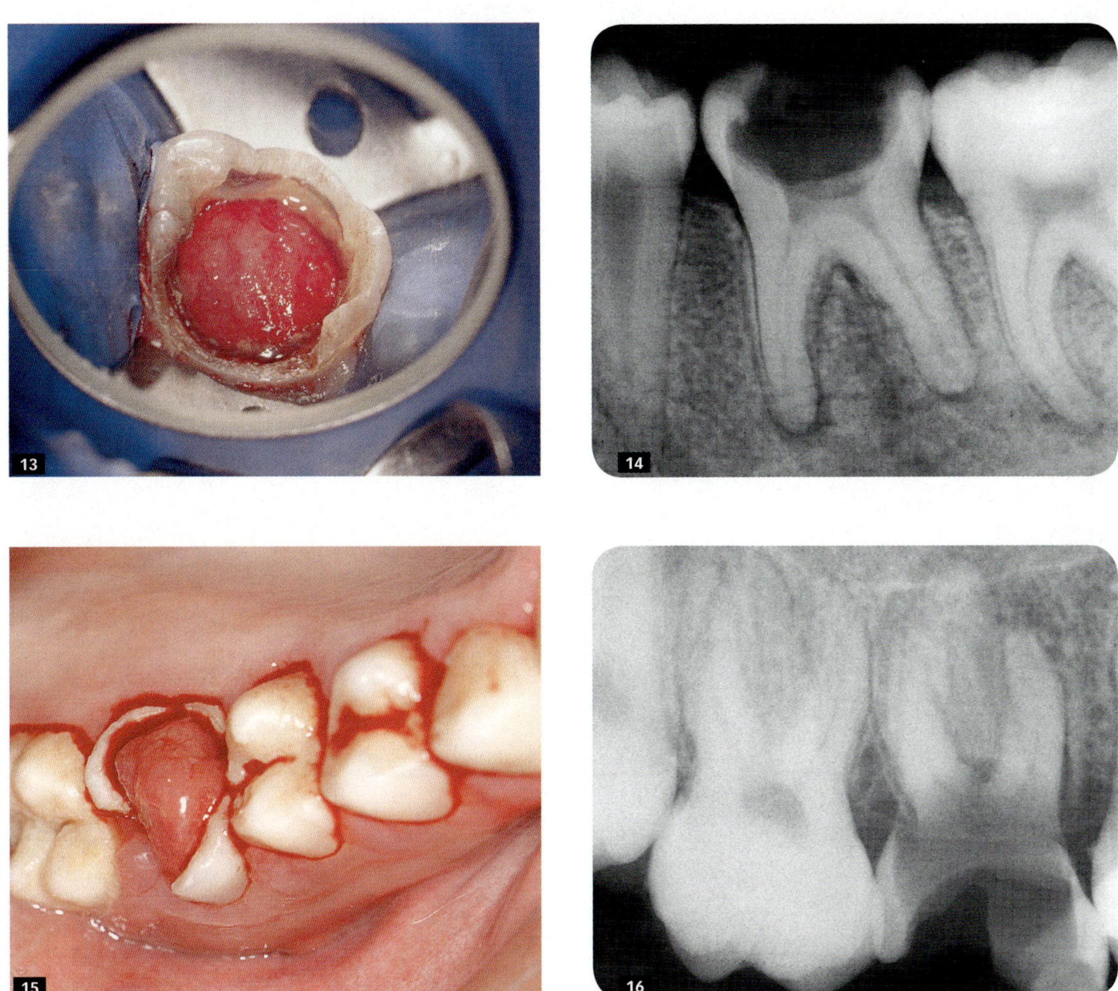


**Figures 4.13 to 4.16** - Asymptomatic Pulpitis.

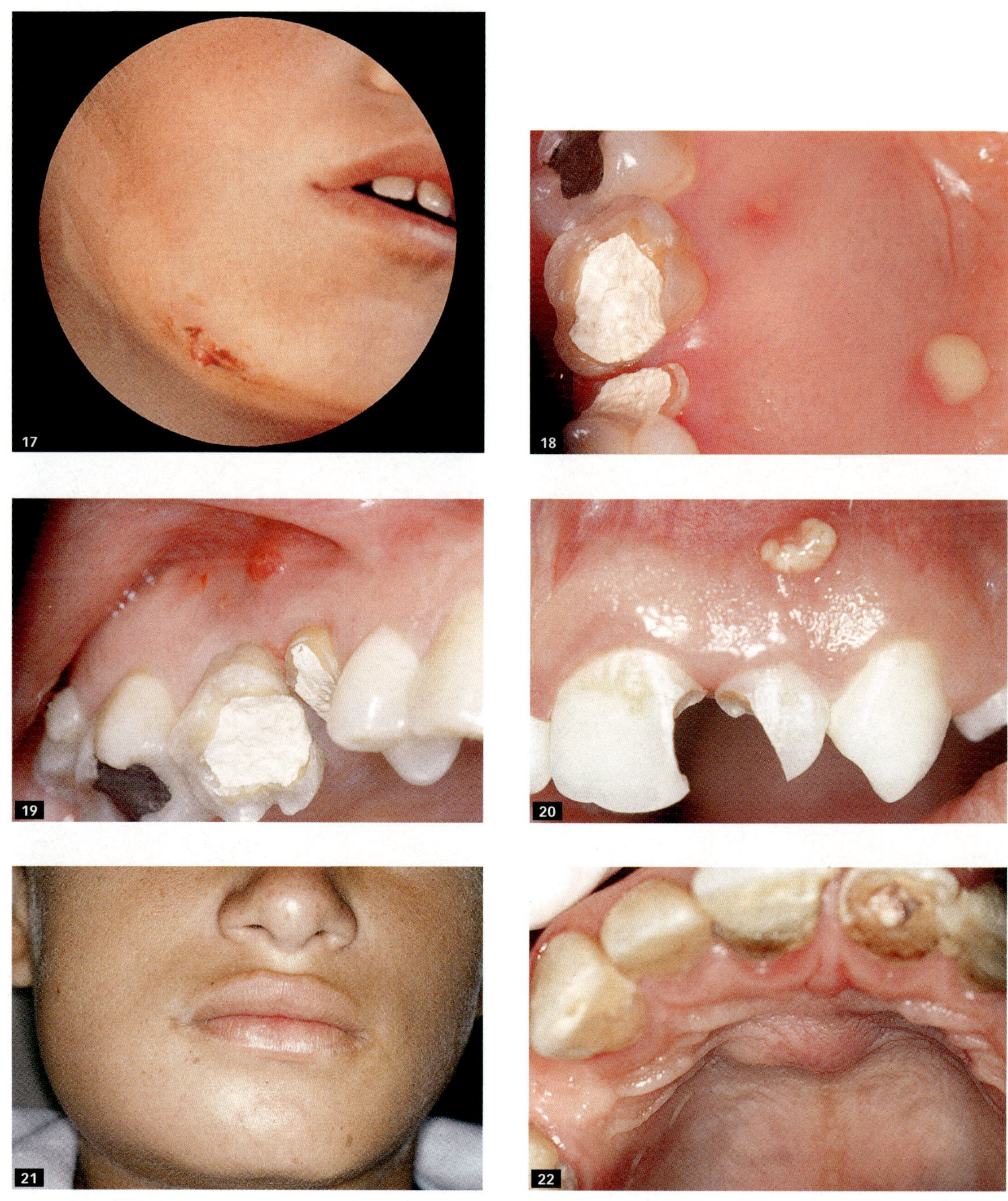

**Figures 4.17 to 4.22** - Extra and intraoral fistula, extra and intraoral edema.

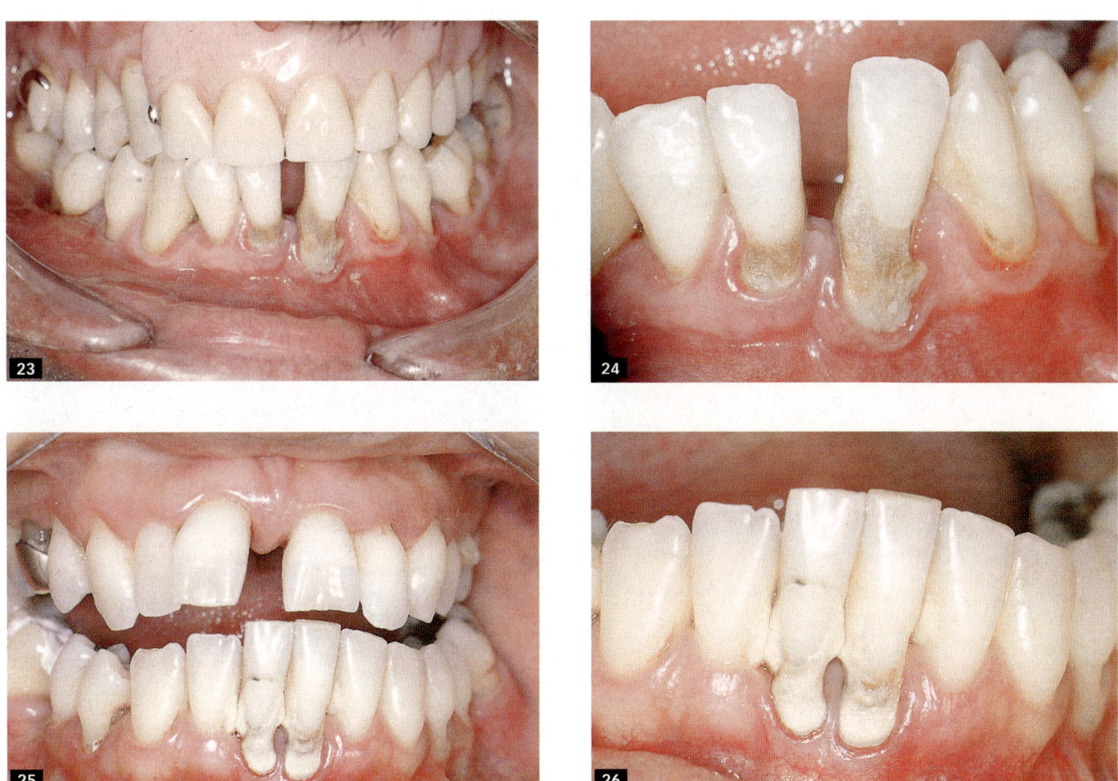

Figures 4.23 to 4.26 - Teeth with periodontal alterations.

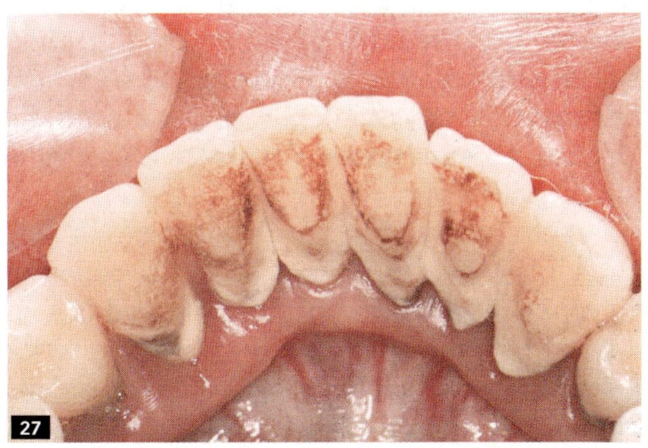

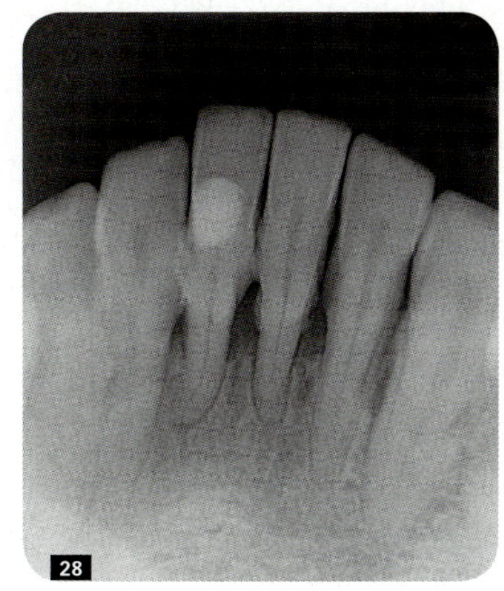

Figures 4.27 to 4.28 - Teeth with periodontal alterations.

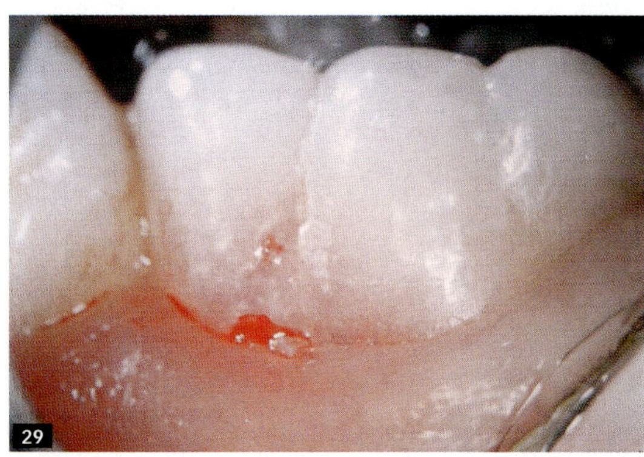

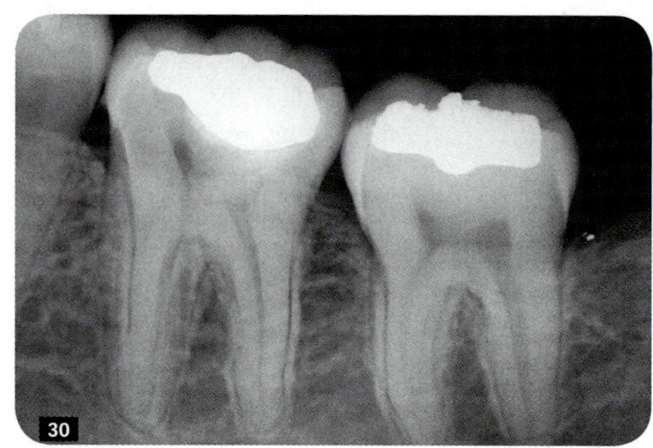

**Figures 4.29 to 4.30** - Teeth with perforated internal resorption.

## 4.6 Pulp Vitality Test

Pulp vitality tests are extremely useful for structuring the clinical diagnosis, being efficient to test the status of normality, inflammation and pulp necrosis. Since it is agreed that the pulp inflammatory alterations are related to vascular alterations, such as changes in the internal pulp pressure, agents that produce changes, such as vasoconstriction or vasodilatation, are significant resources able to induce stimulation on nerve terminals, denoting a possible clinical tissue state, either inflammatory or healthy, but vital. However, other agents are able to stimulate sensitivity in nerve terminals, which does not necessarily certify that the tooth is vital. The nerve fibers are the last to degenerate, and in teeth with pulp necrosis sensitivity can occur when the nerve fibers are stimulated.

Pain, a frequent symptom in situations of inflamed dental pulp, can be stimulated, either exaggerated or attenuated by thermal, electrical and mechanical tests. Pulp response to thermal stimulations provides valuable information about the pulp health status when establishing vascular alterations in dental pulp. In innumerable clinical cases the symptomatology is the first indication of a tooth that presents pathological alteration and needs treatment. However, in other situations this may not occur, as it is a problem or doubt that requires tests to determine pulp vitality[15-25].

With regard to the application of any type of pulp vitality test, it is advisable to inform to the patient of the type and the intensity of the stimulation that is going to be used, because of the degree of sensitivity that could be caused.

It is difficult and complex to measure and interpret the pain produced by different pulp stimulations, because in a characteristic state of normality, the perception of pain, represented by the quantity of stimulation applied to induce it, differs from patient to patient, and is influenced by several factors.

## Thermal Stimuli – Heat and Cold Testing

Thermal stimulation with cold can be done with an ice baton (ice tubettes made in empty Carpules that can be kept for this purpose), ethyl chloride, a refrigerant gas – dichlorodifluoromethane, or carbon dioxide, known as carbonic snow[2-4,6,7,12-14,17-26,34,40,43,47-49]. These agents produce different reductions in intrapulp temperature, stimulating pulp nerve terminals as a result of vascular alterations – vasoconstriction. The greater the temperature reduction, the more the stimulation.

Augsburger & Peters[2] measured the intrapulp temperature produced by carbonic snow, dichlorodifluoromethane and ice, in human mandibular molars. In integral teeth, the carbonic snow produced a temperature reduction around 15.6°C (4.01F), the dichlorodifluoromethane around 8.24°C (2.06F) and the ice around 4.2°C (1.05F), even considering that at the source, the temperature of the carbonic snow was –78°C (-108F). In addition to the low temperatures, carbonic snow has shown that it does not produce alteration to the dental structures.

Barletta & Pesce[3] analyzed the use of the carbonic snow baton to determine its degree of trustworthiness as regards pulp vitality, its refrigerant capacity and possible damages to the enamel and dental pulp structures. The carbonic snow baton showed a high degree of trustworthiness, and caused quick and significant decrease in intrapulp temperature, which does not indicate damage to the pulp tissue structure.

The use of dry ice (carbon dioxide) or gaseous refrigerant allows us to obtain reliable and uniform responses of pulp vitality. There is a bigger difference between the responses in the teeth with complete prosthetic crowns and caries when using the tests that have a greater ability to cool the healthy or restored dental surface.

When applying this cold test, one must use relative isolation, the test being done first on the lateral teeth or even in an analog tooth, from posterior to anterior, on the vestibular face, and lastly performing it on the target tooth. The examination time of the test is approximately 1 to 2 seconds, being repeated again after 5 minutes have elapsed. The absence of pain response, after removing the thermal stimulation can indicate that the dental pulp is necrotic, since positive response is indicative of pulp vitality[20].

In the thermal test performed with heat, a gutta-percha baston is heated by fire until it becomes bright or the baston starts to bend. In this test, it is difficult to control the temperature and application time exactly. It is important to lubricate the tooth before application, so that the gutta-percha will not adhere to the tooth surface. Care must be taken not to overheat. The method using hot water is inconvenient, because the heat spreads to unintended regions[15].

One should remember that the cold test does not complicate the situation of normal or inflamed dental pulp. Whereas this is not the case with the heat test, which is not suggested as routine for normal pulp. Preferably use the cold test, which is more reliable, quick and effective, and does not cause pulp damage as heat does. The heat test is used in situations in which one needs to establish a differential diagnosis. Because heat promotes vasodilation, the painful response to heat in teeth with symptomatic pulp inflammation, or even pulp necrosis, is immediate and intense. With cold stimulus on normal dental pulp the response is immediate, while with heat the response is delayed, so the time lapse with cold is shorter. The pulp responses normally obtained when using thermal tests in normal and inflamed situations are shown in Table 4.8.

Among the different researches that evaluated pulp vitality tests, the applicability of the cold test with refrigerant gas is noted, because it is technically simple to perform. This exam is essential for the clinical diagnosis of endodontic pathologies[1-63].

Estrela et al.[22] evaluated pain and pulp vitality tests to diagnose pulp inflammation. Faced with several difficulties in correctly establishing the clinical diagnosis, one can ask whether the pain characteristics and the radiographic exam allow one to achieve a high ratio of targets/objectives for determining reversible or irreversible processes in inflamed dental pulp and, whether these processes are part of the diagnosis or the prognosis. It has been observed, however, that it is most complex to evaluate the extent of the inflammatory process through the clinical characteristics of the pain and responses to the vitality tests, and precisely establish the clinical diagnosis.

Based on these responses and pain characteristics, one is unable to establish the histopathological diagnosis, all one can determine is whether or not there is pulp vitality.

The periodontal exam can also distinguish lesions of periodontal origin from those of endodontic origin. But the pulp vitality test using cold, facilitates the differential diagnosis between the symptomatic periapical abscess and the acute periodontal abscess.

**Table 4.8** - Pulp responses to thermal tests

| Stimulus | Normal Pulp | Inflamed Pulp |
|---|---|---|
| **Cold** | • vasoconstriction<br>• decrease in internal pressure<br>• Pain (immediate response) | • vasoconstriction<br>• decrease in internal pressure<br>• relief of pain<br>• sometimes "stimulate the pain" |
| **Heat** | • vasodilatation<br>• increase in internal pressure<br>• Pain (delayed response)<br>• C Fibers (tissue damage) | • vasodilatation<br>• increase in internal pressure<br>• Pain (immediate response) |

## Electrical Test

The electrical test allows a pulp response to electrical stimulation of the dental pulp nerve fibers. The electrical test suggests whether or not the pulp tissue is vital, as a result of sensitivity due to neural response. This test does not provide information about the blood pulp supply, a determinant factor of the pulp vitality, but, its goal is to stimulate sensitivity.

Some clinical situations can lead to false interpretations when the pulp vitality test is used. Although the dental pulp sometimes responds to the test, this tissue could be necrotic, generating a false-positive response, for example, in extensive metal restorations (fixed denture), when pulp necrosis in a liquefied phase due to isolation and imprecise drying. In situations of vital pulp, the absence of response to the electrical test can also denote a false-positive action, such as in cases of traumatized teeth, calcifications in the root canal, incomplete rhizogenesis, and in patients that have used analgesic/ataractic medicines, or as a result of defects in the test unit itself.[10-12,49]

## Mechanical Test (Cavity)

The cavity is a good mechanical test. Without anesthesia, a stimulus is induced on the tooth with a small spherical drill, reaching the amelodentinal junction or a little under it, which can trigger acute symptoms. This test is used as an appeal to exclusion, after inconclusive results of the thermal test performed with cold.

### Other Tests to Vitality Exams (Laser, Doppler Flowmetry, Pulse Oximetry)

In difficult situations, such as referred pain, the anesthesia test helps to identify the tooth responsible for the origin of the pain, by blocking nerve conduction. Frequently, the anesthesia testis a valuable aid as an exclusion test.

Biting on the plastic dental pump or rubber disc held between the tooth cusps can, by visualization of the separated cusps and / or the pain stimulus, raise the suspicion of a coronal or even a root fracture.

Other attempts to evaluate the degree of pulp vitality, such as quantification of the blood flow have been performed by using a flowmeter with Doppler laser, used in Medicine[35,49,51,59]. This method is hardly ever applied in clinical endodontic routine however, the preference being to evaluate the condition of pulp tissue. Cohen & Liewehr[14] reported that Laser Doppler Flowmeter (LDF) is complicated because the laser beam must interact with the moving blood cells within the pulpal vasculature, but when equipment costs decrease and clinical application improves, this technology could be useful in patients that are unable to communicate effectively, or whose responses may not be reliable. Pitt Ford & Patel[49] related that for the pulp of many teeth, testing can easily be undertaken using current thermal or electrical tests, such as the modern refrigerants or electric pulp testers. In a minority of cases, these tests are inconclusive and something more effective is needed. LDF is the most promising alternative as it measures blood flow rather than nerve conduction, and produces data that can be re-examined at a later time. Diagnosis of the dental pulp status is frequently given insufficient attention by many dentists, and where doubt exists, root canal treatment is too often performed, even though it is a costly procedure, and may reduce the prognosis for the restored tooth.

Pulse oximetry is another diagnostic method for determining pulp vitality, being studied at present[49].

Schnettler & Wallace[52] investigated the potential of the pulse oximeter to detect vascular integrity within the human tooth. Forty-nine young adults were evaluated for the vitality of their maxillary central incisors utilizing thermal, electrical, and oximetric techniques. The pulse oximeter was found to indicate a pulse rate and oxygen saturation reading for the vital teeth and no readings for the teeth that had previously been endodontically treated. The accuracy of this diagnostic method supports the need for additional study in the use of the pulse oximeter to interpret the pathological processes of the pulp.

Kahan et al.[37] studied the present routine methods for assessing pulp vitality, which rely on stimulation of A-$\alpha$ nerve fibers and give no direct indication of blood flow within the pulp. Recent articles have suggested that pulse oximeters may be used to diagnose pulp vitality by blood flow detection. In this study, an optimized pulse oximeter probe for teeth was designed, built, and tested using the Biox 3740 Oximeter (Ohmeda, Louisville, CO). Following preliminary in vitro tests, the probe was tested clinically. Pulse waveforms from maxillary and mandibular anterior teeth were noted. Simultaneous readings from the subject's finger were used as controls. Pulse wave readings from the teeth were found to be synchronous with the finger probe, but not consistently. It was easier to maintain continuous readings from mandibular incisors than from maxillary incisors. The average percentage synchronization with the pulse was 28.95% for maxillary incisors and 50.28% for mandibular incisors. The overall accuracy of the commercial instrument was disappointing, and in its present form it is not considered to have a predictable diagnostic value.

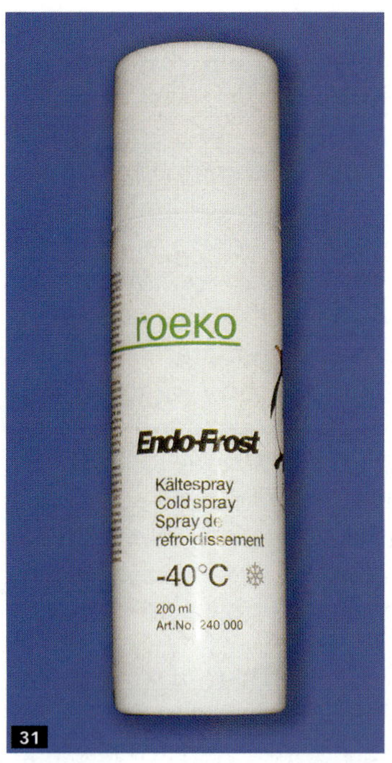


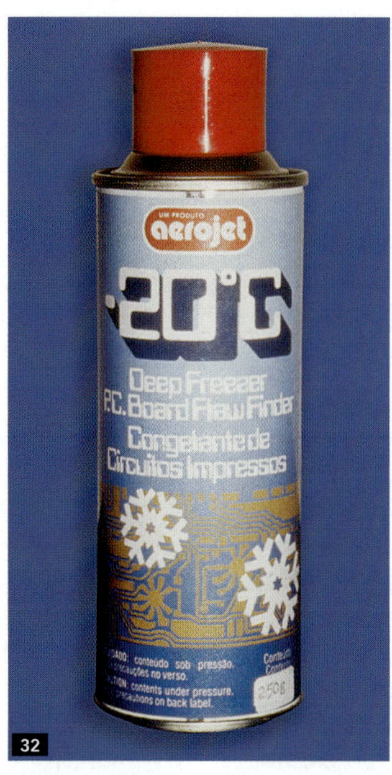


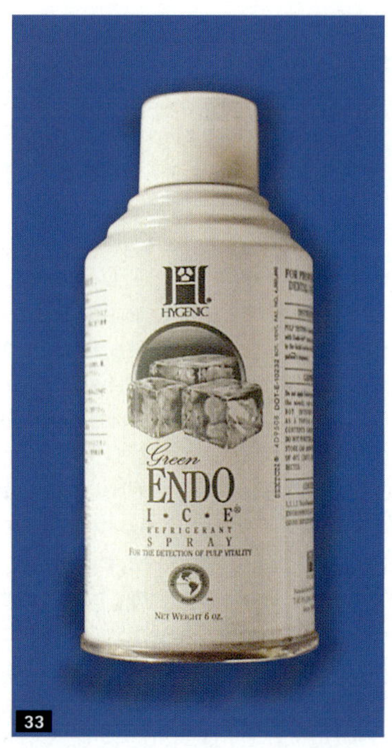


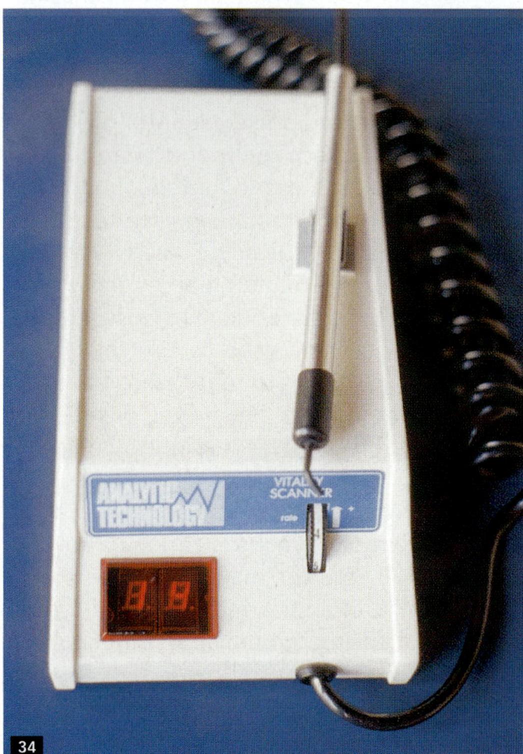


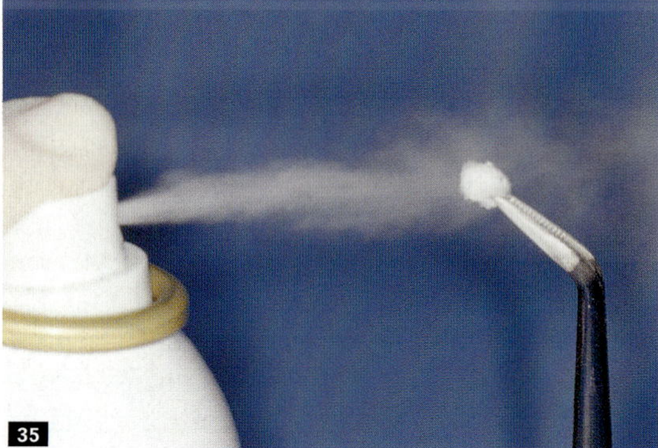


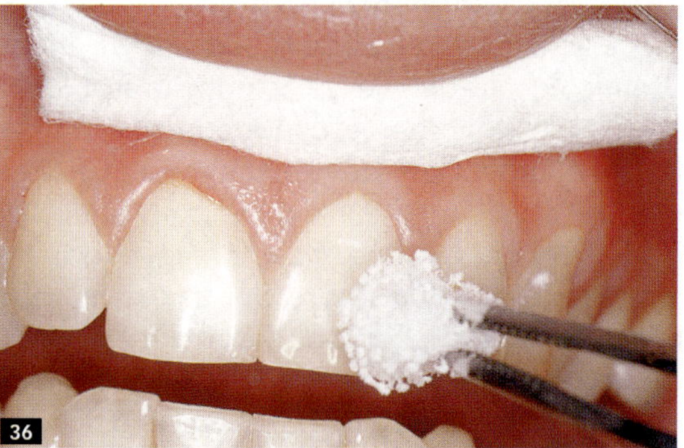


**Figures 4.31 to 4.36** - Shows the agents used in the vitality tests (Cold test, Electrical test).

Rodrigues & Estrela[51] discussed based on a case report the importance of the correct diagnosis to establish the appropriate therapeutic. The traumatic bone cyst is a pseudocyst, usually asymptomatic found by a routine radiographic exam. Unicystic radiolucency is almost always observed, which can involve the periapical area of teeth, simulating an inflammatory periapical lesion of endodontic origin. Differential diagnosis can involve other pathologies, such as: odontogenic keratocyst, central giant cell granuloma and unicystic ameloblastoma. Its etiology and pathogenesis are not yet definitely established. In the present study, after anamnesis, clinical and radiographic exam of teeth #41-43 (pulpal vitality test showed positive), the hypothesis of diagnosis was traumatic bone cyst. The planning was excisional biopsy. After surgical exposition it was observed only one small blood clot in the intraosseous socket, which was carefully curetted and filled with blood. Clinical and radiographic exams after 6 months showed apical formation and pulpal vitality preserved (Figs. 4.37 to 4.39).

## 4.7 Radiographic Image Analysis

After tabulation of data related to signs and symptoms (anamnesis, clinical exam, pulp vitality exam), observation and interpretation of radiographic aspects can favor the clinical diagnosis, and from a certain aspect, suggest consistent images of dental and bone destruction[1-63]. Nevertheless, radiographs are incapable of properly reflecting the real conditions of the teeth and surrounding bone, and are of help only as complementary exams.

Certainly, one of the great problems that Endodontics faces is the poor visualization of the operating field, because the image offered is a partial one.

The clinical protocol to determine the diagnosis, treatment planning and follow-up of endodontic infection treatment usually requires periapical or panoramic radiography. Therefore, it is interesting to understand the importance and at the same time, the limitations of images obtained by radiography for identifying evidence of periapical pathology, observed only from the aspect of radiolucence. This radiographic image corresponds to a two-dimensional aspect of a three-dimensional structure.

Nowadays, several advanced radiographic techniques for detecting lesions in bone are used in Dentistry, as follows: digital radiography, densitometry methods, cone beam computed tomography, magnetic resonance imaging, ultrasound, and nuclear techniques. Cone beam computed tomography has been used in Endodontics with several objectives (Fig. 4.40), such as: the anatomic study of root canals, external and internal macromorphology in 3D-reconstruction of the teeth, evaluation of root canal preparation and obturation, re-treatment, coronal microleakage, detection of lesions in bone and in application of experimental endodontology[10,16,17,33,47,49].

A few studies have compared the different image interpretations of apical periodontitis, using conventional periapical radiographs, digital radiography or cone beam computed tomography. The results were promising for cone beam computed tomography to detect apical periodontitis with more precision.

The acceptance of endodontic therapeutic protocol to treat a disease has routinely been based on pathological and clinical characteristics frequently helped by radiographic exam. The diagnostic aid method most used in endodontic treatment, is the radiographic image.

It has been observed that distortions of radiographic images constitute a serious inconvenience during endodontic treatment. To resolve this problem, the technique of choice should be the long cone paralleling technique, which may increase the exactness of diagnosis, an accurate radiograph with minimal distortion and high level reproducibility.

Therefore, considering some limitations on traditional radiographic methods for the detection of periapical bone lesions, and the possible analysis produced by advanced imaging methods, such as cone beam computed tomography, the quality of treatment planning, diagnosis and consequently the prognosis, can be increased.

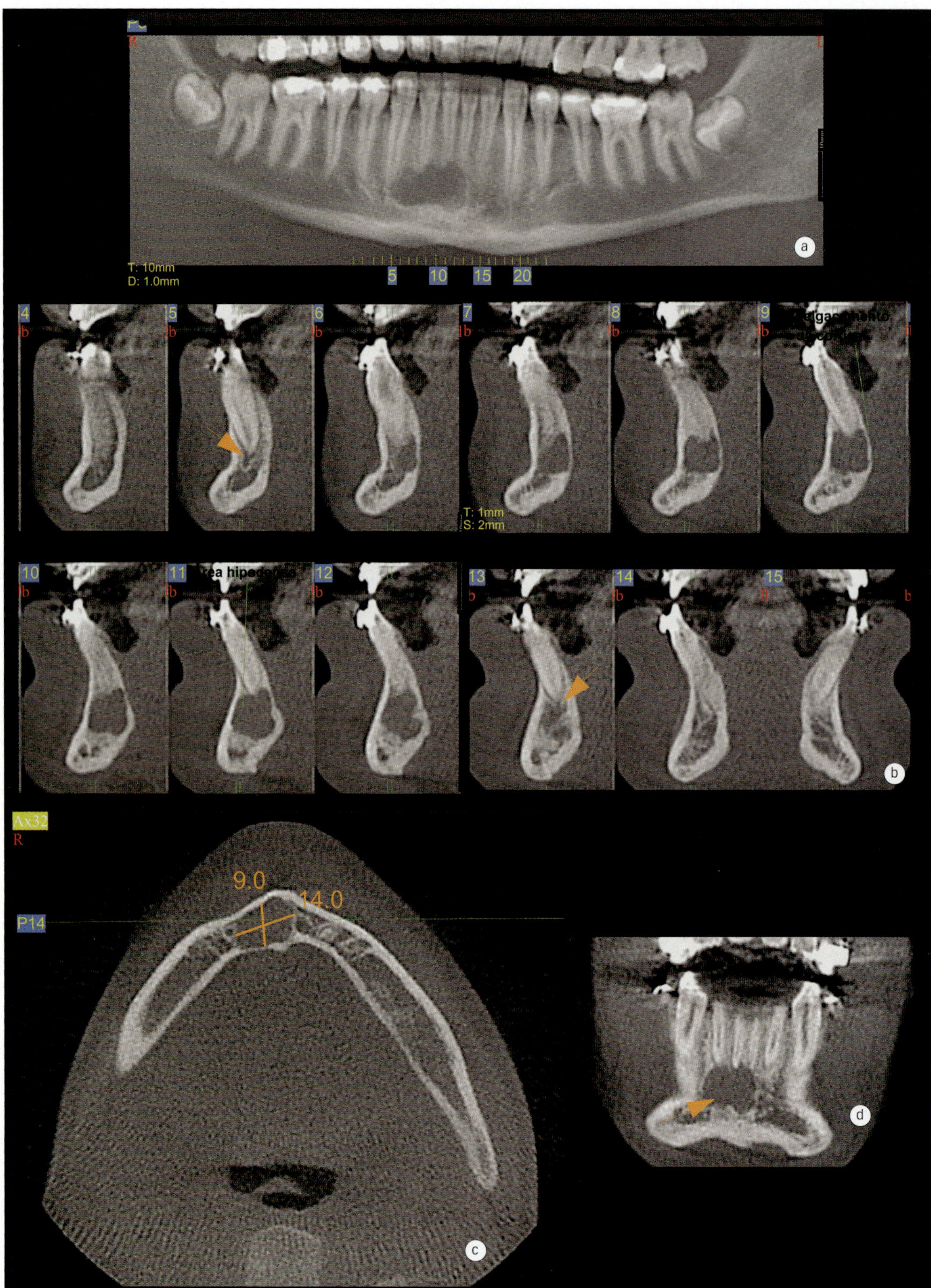

Figure 4.37 - Cone beam computerized tomography, (A) Panoramic image, (B) Transaxiais; (C) Axial; (D) Coronal.

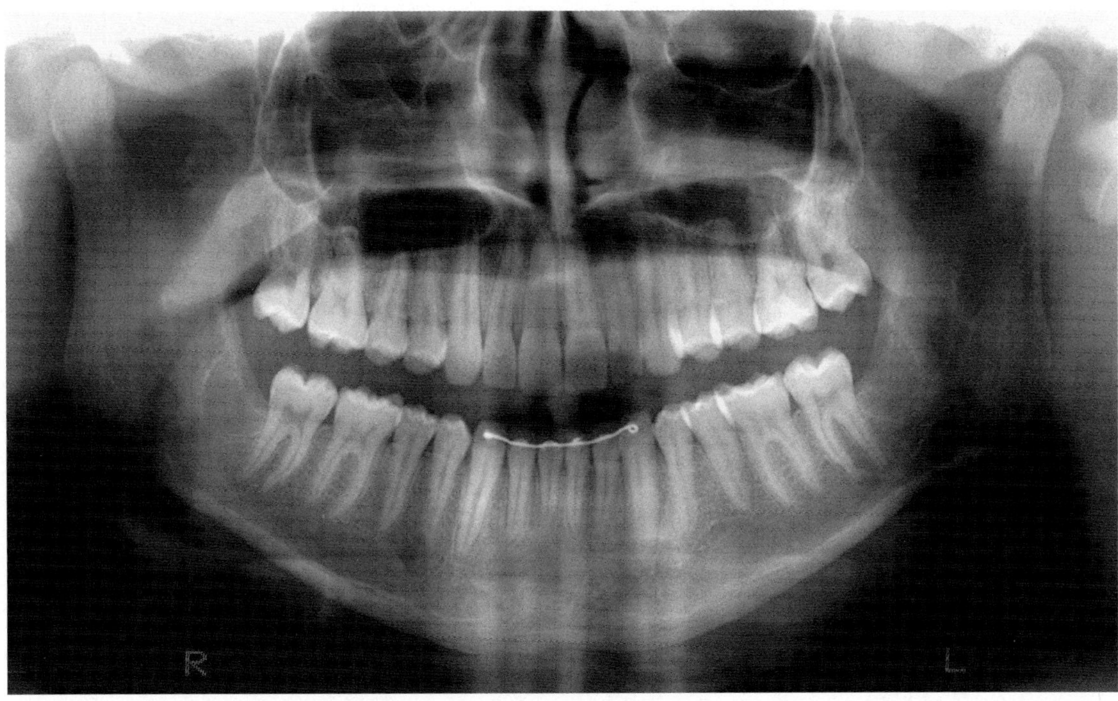


**Figure 4.38** - Panoramic image showing normal aspect on periapical area of teeth # 41-43, 6 months after surgery.

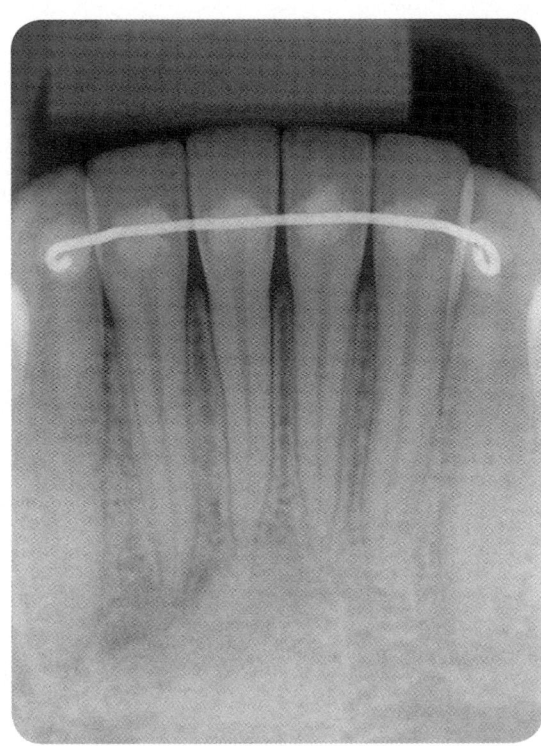

**Figure 4.39** - Periapical radiography presenting normal aspect on periapical area of teeth # 41-43, remaining only small radiolucid adjacent area to the apex of tooth # 42, 6 months after surgery.

Estrela et al.[17] analyzed the accuracy in 1.508 images made by cone beam computed tomography, periapical and panoramic radiographs for apical periodontitis detection. The prevalence of AP was significantly higher using CBCT, in comparison with periapical and panoramic radiographs. AP was correctly identified in 54.5% of the cases using periapical radiographs and in 27.8% of the cases using panoramic radiographs. Minor changes in sensitivity were found for the different tooth groups, except for incisors in panoramic radiographs. ROC analysis suggests that AP is correctly identified with conventional methods, when in an advanced stage. CBCT was shown to be an accurate diagnostic method to identify AP.

Estrela et al.[16] suggested a new periapical index based on cone beam computed tomography for identification of apical periodontitis (AP). The periapical index proposed in this study (CBCTPAI) was developed based on criteria established from measurements corresponding to periapical radiolucency interpreted on CBCT scans. Radiolucent images suggestive of periapical lesions were measured using the working tools of Planimp® software on CBCT scans in three dimensions: buccopalatal, mesiodistal and diagonal. The CBCTPAI was determined by the largest lesion extension. A 6-point (0-5) scoring system was used with addition of two variables: expansion of bone cortical and destruction of cortical bone (Table 4.9). A total of 1,014 images (periapical radiographs and CBCT scans) originally taken from 596 patients were evaluated by 3 observers using the CBCTPAI criteria. AP was identified in 39.5% and 60.9% of cases by radiography and CBCT, respectively. The CBCTPAI offers an accurate diagnostic method for use with high-resolution images, which can reduce the incidence of false-negative diagnosis, minimize observer interference and increase the reliability of epidemiological studies, especially those referring to AP prevalence and severity.

Bueno et al.[10] emphasized that CBCT is a great contemporary revolution in dentistry that will certainly benefit uncountable diagnostic and planning activities. Different applications of these benefits and applications in different specialties are shown in the following clinical cases. Cone beam computer tomography allows the best results to be obtained in evaluations of hard tissue examinations of the oral cavity in three dimensions. Chapter 5 discusses endodontic diagnosis aided by cone beam computed tomography.

**Table 4.9** - Cone Beam Computed Tomography Periapical Index (CBCTPAI) Scores[16]

| Score | Quantitative bone alterations in mineral structures |
|---|---|
| **0** | Intact periapical bone structures |
| **1** | Diameter of periapical radiolucency > 0.5-1mm |
| **2** | Diameter of periapical radiolucency > 1-2mm |
| **3** | Diameter of periapical radiolucency > 2-4mm |
| **4** | Diameter of periapical radiolucency > 4-8mm |
| **5** | Diameter of periapical radiolucency > 8mm |
| **Score (n) + E*** | Expantion of periapical cortical bone |
| **Score (n) + D*** | Destruction of periapical cortical bone |

* The variables E (expansion of bone cortical) and D (destruction of cortical bone) were added to each score, if either of these conditions was detected in the CBCT analysis.

## 4.8 Diagnosis Hypothesis

Once the phases of the semiologic process have been analyzed and interpreted, the data signal a probable diagnosis (or diagnostic hypothesis). However, the clinical, microscopic and radiographic aspects must be differentiated with regard to the designations and classifications of the existent pathologies, particularly within the context of the diagnosis, prognosis and therapeutic options. The pathological classification must follow the parameters used to obtain it. It is pointed out that within the clinical parameters, the diagnosis must follow the clinical aspects of tissue modifications, without attempts to correlate them with the microscopic characteristics, since most of the time there could be absence of any correlation.

Thus, it is important to use nomenclature that better approaches the clinical condition studied, since the diagnosis is clinical. As there are current classifications that better define and clinically associate the pathologies with the therapeutical options, it is correct to use them and leave some of the philosophical values behind in the past when they were used. It is always time to change when you have a more appropriated option.

Tables 4.10 and 4.11 show the clinical classification of dental pulp and periapical tissue inflammations. Tables 4.12 to 4.14 describe the pain situations involved in Pedodontics, Periodontology and Surgery. Table 4.15 shows the urgent situations in dental traumatism.

**Table 4.10** - Clinical Classification of Pulp Pathologies

| Pulp Pathologies |
|---|
| • **Normal pulp response** |
| • **Hyper-reactive Pulpalgia** |
| • **Symptomatic Pulpitis** |
| • **Asymptomatic Pulpitis** |
| • **Pulp Necrosis** |

**Table 4.11** - Clinical Classification of Periapical Pathologies

| Periapical Pathologies |
|---|
| **Symptomatic Apical Periodontitis**<br>• Traumatic<br>• Infectious |
| **Asymptomatic Apical Periodontitis** |
| **Periapical Abscess without Fistula**<br>• Phase I - Initial Stage<br>• Phase II - In Development Stage<br>• Phase III - Developed Stage |
| **Periapical Abscess with Fistula** |

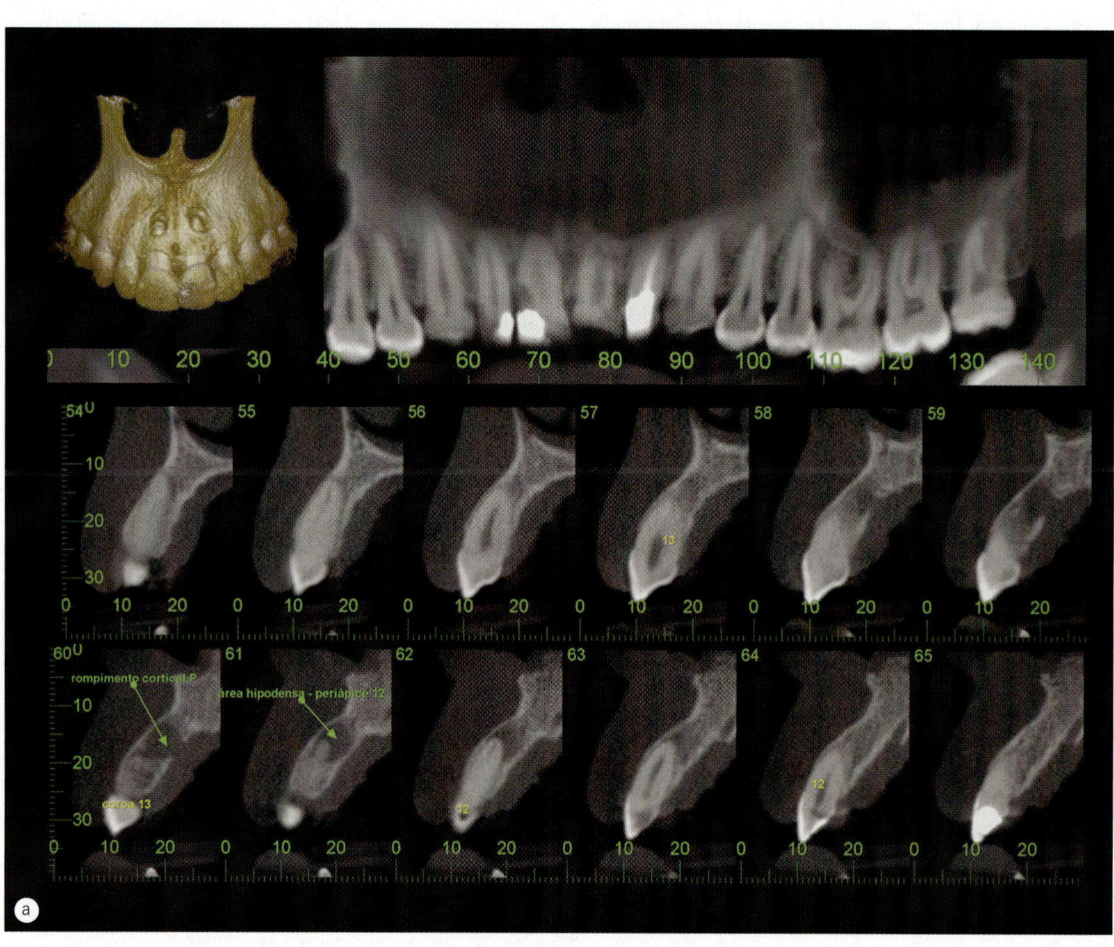


**Figure 4.40** - (**A-C**) Cone beam computerized tomography.

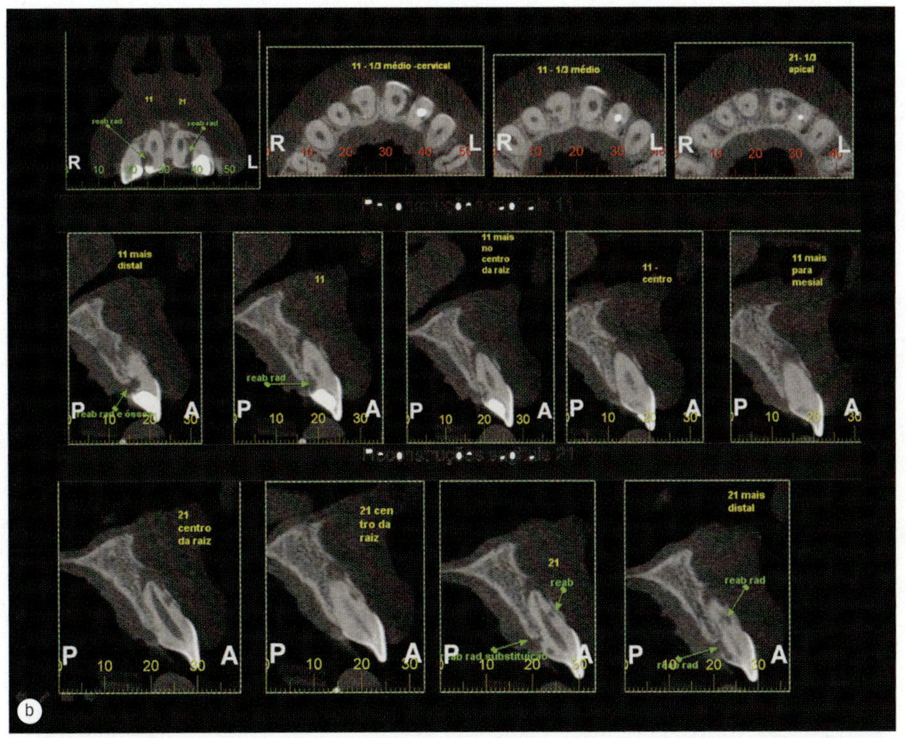

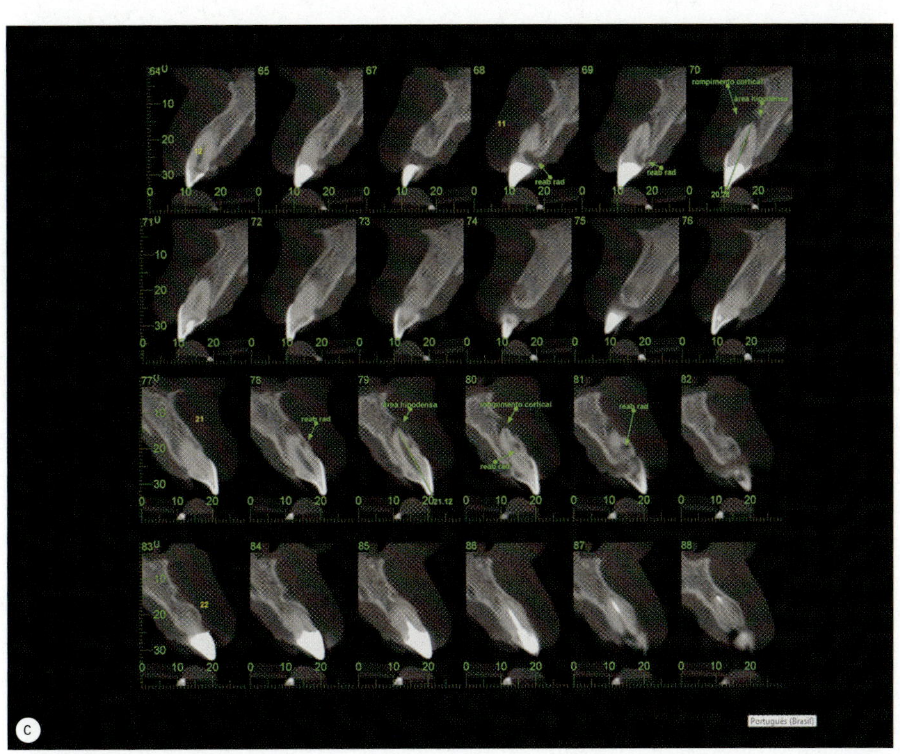

**Table 4.12** - Symptomatic Conditions related to Pedodontics

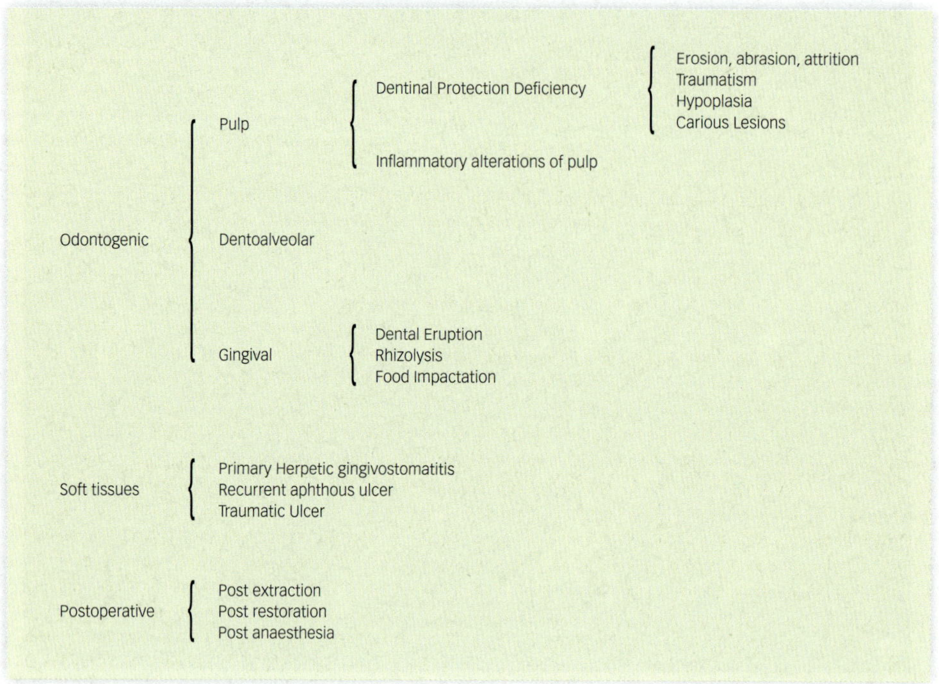

- Odontogenic
  - Pulp
    - Dentinal Protection Deficiency
      - Erosion, abrasion, attrition
      - Traumatism
      - Hypoplasia
      - Carious Lesions
    - Inflammatory alterations of pulp
  - Dentoalveolar
  - Gingival
    - Dental Eruption
    - Rhizolysis
    - Food Impactation
- Soft tissues
  - Primary Herpetic gingivostomatitis
  - Recurrent aphthous ulcer
  - Traumatic Ulcer
- Postoperative
  - Post extraction
  - Post restoration
  - Post anaesthesia

**Table 4.13** - Symptomatic Conditions related to Periodontics

- Acute Necrotizing Ulcerative Gingivitis
- Acute Herpetic Gingivostomatitis
- Pericoronaritis
- Periodontal Abscess

**Table 4.14** - Symptomatic Conditions related to Post Surgery Complications

| Complications From Trauma | Complications from Infection |
|---|---|
| • Muscular Lesion by anaesthesia needle<br>• Consequences of traumatic surgery technique<br>• Myalgia after prolonged effort<br>• Luxation of neighboring teeth during extraction | • Alveolitis<br>• Cellulitis and Postoperative Abscesses<br>• Subperiosteal Abscess<br>• Ludwig's Angina |

**Table 4.15** - Urgencies in Dental Trauma Injuries

| | |
|---|---|
| • Coronal Fracture of enamel and dentin | • Subluxation |
| • Coronal Fracture with pulp exposure | • Extrusive Luxation |
| • Corono-radicular Fracture | • Lateral Luxation |
| • Radicular Fracture | • Avulsion |

## 4.9 Dental Case History

The diagnosis of endodontic disease consists of several analyses that involve a synthesis of history, clinical and imagiological examination, and pulp vitality tests. Decisions on treatment based on limited information obtained from the patient may be contradictory and require caution. Well structured diagnosis with important clinical details must be carefully recorded. Today, contemporary endodontics offers resources for registering all the information obtained during the clinical examinations of patients, especially involving the digital technology. Thus, the use an electronic dental chart is important because of various factors. Table 4.16 shows the model of a dental case record.

**Table 4.16** - Dental Case Record

## 1. Identification

Name: ______________________________________________

Date of birth: ____/____/____ Gender: ______________ Age: ____________ Weight: ______________

Stature: ________ Marital status: ______________ Blood Type: ______________________

Occupation: ______________________________________________

Name of the Physician in charge: ______________________ Telephone: ______________________

Address: ______________________________________________

Home phone: ______________________ Business Phone: ______________________

Reference/Name: ________________ Telephone: __________ E-mail: ______________________

Indication: ______________________________________________

## 2. Medical History

Are you in good health? ______________________________________________

Are you under medical care? ________ Why? ______________________________________

Date of the last medical appointment: ______________________________________

Are you taking any medicine? ________ Which? ______________________________________

Do you have any medicine allergy? ______________________________________

Have you ever been hospitalized in recent years? ______________________________________

Blood pressure: ______________________________________________

Do you have fever? ______________________________________________

**Patient Habits**

Do you smoke? ________ How long? ______________________________________

Do you drink alcohol regularly? ________ Which drink? ______________________________________

Daily consumption? ______________ Other habits: ______________________________________

**Check the past or present diseases:**

| | | | |
|---|---|---|---|
| ☐ Heart Disease | ☐ Enphysema | ☐ Labyrinthitis | ☐ Allergy/Urticaria |
| ☐ Attack | ☐ Migraine | ☐ Liver/Kidney | ☐ Anemia |
| ☐ Surgery | ☐ Epilepsy | ☐ Nervous Probl. | ☐ Angina Pectoris |
| ☐ Weight Gain | ☐ Rheumatic Fever | ☐ Respiratory Probl. | ☐ Arthritis |
| ☐ Hypertension | ☐ Glaucoma | ☐ Sinusitis | ☐ Cancer |
| ☐ Insufficiency | ☐ Hepatitis | ☐ Gastric Ulcer | ☐ Frequent Headache |
| ☐ Pacemaker | ☐ Hemophilia | ☐ Others | ☐ Drug Dependence |
| ☐ Murmur | ☐ Herpes | ☐ Diabetes | ☐ Chagas Disease |
| ☐ Jaundice | ☐ Nervous Disorder | ☐ Congenital Disease | ☐ Immunodeficiency |

**Other information about health:**

______________________________________________

______________________________________________

## 3. Dental History

### 3.1 Anamnesis (Subjective Exam/Interrogation Technique)

**A. Chief Complaint**

________________________________________

What made you seek treatment? ____________________

Have you ever had an unusual reaction to the dental anaesthesia? ____________________

Have you ever had any medical-dental treatment trauma? ____________________

Where is the pain located? ____________________

How does the pain appear? ____________________

Which factor stimulates or decreases the pain? ____________________

How long ago did the pain appear? ____________________

How often is the pain? ____________________

How intense is the pain? ____________________

Have you ever been submitted to endodontic treatment? ____________________

Have you ever had any dental traumatism? ____________________

What is your expectation considering the treatment you will undergo? ____________________

Which tooth or region is bothering you? ____________________

**B. Clinical Characteristics of Pain/Tooth**

| | | | |
|---|---|---|---|
| Seat | ☐ location | ☐ diffuse | |
| Forthcoming | ☐ provoked | ☐ spontaneous | |
| Duration | ☐ short | ☐ long | |
| Frequency | ☐ intermittent | ☐ continuous | |
| Intensity | ☐ light (0-3) | ☐ moderate (4-7) | ☐ severe (8-10) |

## 3.2. Physical Exam (Exploration Technique)

### A. Inspection (Visual Observation)

- Hard Tissues:

Teeth: ______________________ Region: ______________________

| | | | | |
|---|---|---|---|---|
| Dental Structure | ☐ Complete | ☐ Decayed | ☐ Restored | ☐ Fractured |
| Dental Coloring | ☐ Normal | ☐ Modified | | |
| Tissue Coloring | ☐ Normal | ☐ Modified | | |
| Edema | ☐ Local | ☐ Diffuse | ☐ Intraoral | ☐ Extraoral |
| Fistula | ☐ Mucosa | ☐ Cutaneous | | |

- Soft Tissue: Irrespective of the chief complaint, the patient must be routinely evaluated on the integrity of the oral tissues through a careful, systematic and complete physical exam. The aim is to detect, in a general manner, any type of alteration of normality standard that could be present, irrespective of symptomatology. These alterations must be evaluated relating the location, size, coloring, consistency, presenting clinical form, tissue attachment, presence of mobility, regional lymphadenopathy, occlusion disorders, and analysis of temporomandibular joint.

Observations:

______________________________________________

______________________________________________

______________________________________________

### B. Exploration

| | Shallow | Medium | Deep |
|---|---|---|---|
| **Caries (Depth)** | | | |
| Protective Material | Absent | Present | Type: |
| Restorative Material | Amalgam | Resin | Others: |
| Dental Pulp Exposure | Absent | Present | |
| Dental Trauma | Enamel | Enamel/dentin | Enamel/dentin/pulp |
| Periodontal Pocket | Absent | Present | Depth: |
| Hygiene | Good | Regular | Bad |

## C. Palpation/ Percussion

| | | |
|---|---|---|
| Coronal | Presence of pain | Absence of pain |
| Periapical | Presence of pain | Absence of pain |
| Edema | Developing | Developed |
| Mobility | Absent | Present |
| Vertical | Absence of pain | Presence of pain |
| Horizontal | Absence of pain | Presence of pain |
| TMJ | Absence of pain | Presence of pain |
| Mouth Opening | Absence of pain | Presence of pain |
| Deviation of midline | Yes? | No? |

## 3.3. Pulp Vitality Exam (Pain stimulation technique)

| Thermal Tests | | |
|---|---|---|
| Cold (refrigerant gas/ Carbonic Snow) | Relief | Stimulus |
| Heat (Heated gutta-percha) | Relief | Stimulus |
| Electrical Test | Relief | Stimulus |
| Mechanic Test (Cavity) | Presence of pain | Absence of pain |
| Anaesthesia test | Presence of pain | Absence of pain |

## 3.4 Analysis of Radiographic Aspect

| Pulp Chamber | Root Canal | Periapical Region |
|---|---|---|
| Normal | Normal | Normal Periodontal ligament space |
| Ample | Ample | Reamed Periodontal ligament space |
| Atresic | Atresic | Hypercementosis |
| Calcification | Internal Resorption | Periapical bone resorption |
| Calculus | External Resorption | Diffuse bone resorption |
| Obturated | Totally obturated | Surrounding bone rarefaction |
| Decayed | Partially obturated | Condensing osteitis |
| | Incomplete Rhizogenesis | |
| | Osteosclerosis | |

Observations:

_______________________________________________

_______________________________________________

_______________________________________________

_______________________________________________

_______________________________________________

**4 . Probable Clinical Diagnosis**

______________________________________________
______________________________________________
______________________________________________

**5. Treatment Planning**

______________________________________________
______________________________________________
______________________________________________

**6. Description of the Treatment Performed**

______________________________________________
______________________________________________
______________________________________________
______________________________________________

**7. Revealing Term**

(It is essential to provide the patient with a detailed description, clarifying all the treatment to be performed, explaining the benefits, risks, possible accidents, material and technique used).

______________________________________________
______________________________________________
______________________________________________

**8. Informed Consent**

(It is fundamental to obtain a term relating that the patient received clarification about all the procedures involved in the treatment, risks, benefits, material and technique used, and that he/she is fully in favor of developing the treatment).

______________________________________________
______________________________________________
______________________________________________

**9. Clinical-Radiographic Control:**

Treatment conclusion: ______________________________________________
Return to control: 30 days after the end of the treatment
Date: ___/___/_____ Goiânia, ___/___/_____

**10. Control**

______________________________________________
______________________________________________
______________________________________________
______________________________________________

1. Alling CC. História e exame do paciente. In: Diagnóstico diferencial das lesões bucais. Wood NK, Goaz PW. 2nd ed. Rio de Janeiro: Guanabara Koogan; 1983. p.4-16.
2. Augsburger RA, Peters DD. In vitro effects of ice, skin refrigerant, and $Co_2$ snow on intrapulpar temperature. J Endod 1981;7:110-6.
3. Barletta FB, Pesce HF. Avaliação in vitro dos efeitos na superfície do esmalte dentário humano utilizando-se bastão de neve carbônica. Rev Odontol Univ São Paulo 1994;8:111-15.
4. Bell WE. Orofacial Pains: Classifications, diagnosis, management. Chicago: Boca Raton; 1989.
5. Bellizi R, Hartwell GR, Ingle JI, Georig AC, Neaverth EJ, Marshall FJ, Kransny RM, Frank AL, Gaum C. Procedimento para el diagnóstico. 4th ed. México: McGraw-Hill, Interamericana; 1996.
6. Beveridge EE, Brown AC. The measurement of human dental intrapulp pressure and its response to clinical variables. Oral Surg Oral Med Oral Pathol 1965;19:655-68.
7. Boraks S. Considerações preliminares. In: Diagnóstico Bucal. São Paulo: Artes Médicas; 1996.
8. Bueno MR, Carvalhosa AAC, Castro PHS, Pereira KC, Borges FT, Estrela C. Mesenchymal chondrosarcoma mimicking apical periodontitis. J Endod 2008;34:1415-19.
9. Bueno MR, Estrela C. Prevalência de tratamento endodôntico e periodontite apical em várias populações do mundo, detectados por radiografias panorâmicas, periapicais e tomografias computadorizadas cone beam. Rev Bras Odontol Brasil Central 2008;17:79-90.
10. Bueno MR, Estrela C, Azevedo BC, Brugnera-Jr. A, Azevedo JR. Tomografia computadorizada Cone Beam: Revolução na odontologia. Rev Ass Paul Cir Dent 2007;61:325-8.
11. Castro AL. Estomatologia. 1st ed. São Paulo: Santos; 1992.
12. Chambers E. The role and methods of pulp testing in oral diagnosis: a review. Int Endod J 1982;15:1-15.
13. Cohen S, Burns RC. Caminhos da polpa. 7th ed. Rio de Janeiro: Guanabara Koogan; 2000.
14. Cohen S, Liewehr F. Diagnostic procedures. Pathways of the pulp. 8th ed. St Loius:Mosby; 2002; p.1-30.
15. Estrela C. Dor Odontogênica. São Paulo: Artes Médicas; 2001. 296p.
16. Estrela C, Bueno MR, Azevedo B, Azevedo JR, Pécora JD. A New Periapical Index Based on Cone Beam Computed Tomography. J Endod 2008; 34:1325-31.
17. Estrela C, Bueno MR, Leles CR, Azevedo B, Azevedo JR. Accuracy of cone beam computed tomography and panoramic and periapical radiography for detection of apical periodontitis. J Endod 2008;34:273-9.
18. Estrela C, César OVS, Sydney GB, Lopes HP, Pesce F. Incidência de dor frente ao tratamento da inflamação periapical aguda e crônica. Rev Bras Odontol 1996;53:21-25.
19. Estrela C, Estrela CRA, Dirceu RF, Mamede Neto I. Considerações sobre a periodontite apical assintomática com extensa rarefação óssea. Rev Fac Odontol UFG 1998; 2:25-30.
20. Estrela C, Decúrcio DA, Silva JA, Mendonça EF, Estrela CRA. Persistent apical periodontitis associated with calcifying odontogenic. Int Endod J 2009 (in press). doi:10.1111/J.1365-2591.2008.01477.x
21. Estrela C, Lopes HP. Conceitos atuais no diagnóstico em endodontia. In: Odontologia Integrada. Rio de Janeiro: Pedro Primeiro; 2001.
22. Estrela C, Lopes HP, Resende EV, Alencar AH. Avaliação da dor e de teste de vitalidade para o diagnóstico da inflamação pulpar. Rev Odontol Brasil Central 1995; 5:4-8.
23. Estrela C, Pesce HF, Silva MT, Fernandes JMA, Silveira HP. Análise da redução da dor pós-tratamento da hipersensibilidade dentinária. Rev Odontol Brasil Central 1996; 6:4-10.
24. Estrela C, Tormin FC, Araújo CR, Barleta FB. Prevalência de pulpite aguda e necrose pulpar frente a diferentes agentes etiológicos. Rev Fac Odontol UFG 1997; 1:15-20.
25. Estrela C, Zina O, Borges AH, Santos ES, Resende EV. Correlação entre o diagnóstico clínico da polpa dental inflamada e o reparo após a pulpotomia. Rev Odontol Brasil Central 1996; 6:4-8.
26. Eversole LR. Endodontia e dor facial de natureza não odontogênica: síndromes dolorosas dos maxilares que simulam odontalgia. In: Caminhos da polpa. Cohen S, Burns RC. 7th ed. Rio de Janeiro: Guanabara Koogan; 2000.
27. Faillace RR. Hemograma - manual de interpretações. 2nd ed. São Paulo: Artes Médicas; 1991.
28. Figueiredo MAZ, Estrela C, Figueiredo JAP. Métodos de diagnóstico em endodontia. In: Estrela C, Figueiredo JAP. Endodontia: princípios biológicos e mecânicos. São Paulo: Artes Médicas, 2003. Cap. 2.p.24-49.
29. Filgueiras J, Bevilacqua S, Mello C. Endodontia Clínica. Rio de Janeiro: Científica; 1962.
30. Glick DH. Locating referred pulpal pains. Oral Surg Oral Med Oral Pathol 1962; 15:613.
31. Gluskin AH, Cohen S, Brown DC. Emergência em dor orofacial de natureza odontogênica: diagnóstico e tratamento endodôntico. In: Caminhos da polpa. Cohen S, Burns RC. 7th ed. Rio de Janeiro: Guanabara Koogan; 2000.
32. Holland R, Souza V. O problema do diagnóstico clínico e indicação de tratamento da polpa dental inflamada. Rev Assoc Paul Cirur Dent 1970;24:188-93.
33. Huumonen S, Ørstavic D. Radiological aspects of apical periodontitis. Endod Topics 2002;1:3-25.
34. Ingle JI, Glick DH. Diagnostico diferencial y tratamiento del dolor dental. In: Endodoncia. Ingle JI, Bakland LK. 4thed. México: McGraw; 1996. p.548-75.
35. Ingolfsson AER, Tronstad L, Hersh E, Riva CE. Efficacy of laser Doppler flowmetry in determining pulp vitality of human teeth. Endod Dent Traumatol 1994;10:83-87.
36. Jaeger B. Diagnóstico diferencial y tratamiento Del dolor craneofacial. In: Endodoncia. Ingle JI, Bakland LK. 4th ed. México: McGraw; 1996. p.576-636.
37. Kahan RS, Gulabivala K, Snook M, Setchell DJ. Evaluation of a pulse oximeter and customized probe for pulp vitality testing. J Endod 1996;22:105-9.

38. Kerr DA, Ash MM, Millard HD. Oral diagnosis. St. Louis:Mosby, 1978.
39. Melzack R. The McGrill pain questionnaire: major properties and scoring methods. Pain 1975; 1:277-99.
40. Mistak EJ, Loushine RJ, Primak PD, West LA, Runyan DA. Interpretation of periapical lesions comparing conventional, direct digital, and telephonically transmitted radiographic images. J Endod 1998; 24:262-66.
41. Nyman S, Lindhe J. Exames em pacientes com doença periodontal. In: Tratado de periodontia clínica e implantologia oral. Lindhe J, Karring T, Lang NP. 3rd ed. Rio de Janeiro: Guanabara Koogan; 1997.
42. Okada H, Kassai Y, Kida T. T-lynphocyte substes in the inflamed gingiva of human adult periodontitis. J Dent Res 1984; 19:595-598.
43. Okeson JP. Dores orofaciais de Bell. 5th ed. São Paulo:Quintessense; 1998.
44. Okeson JP. Dor orofaciais: guia de avaliação, diagnóstico e tratamento. São Paulo: Quintessense; 1998.
45. Okeson JP. Tratamento das desordens temporomandibulares e oclusão. 4th ed. São Paulo: Artes Médicas; 2000. 500p.
46. Paiva JG, Antoniazzi JH. Endodontia - bases para a prática clínica. 1st ed. São Paulo: Artes Médicas; 1984.
47. Patels, Dawood A, Pitt Ford T, Whaites E. The potencial applications of cone beam computed tomography in the management of endodontic problems. Int Endod J 2007;40:818-23.
48. Pesce HF. Diagnóstico diferencial das odontalgias. In: Atualização na clínica odontológica. São Paulo: Artes Médicas; 1992. p.146.
49. Pitt Ford TR, Patel S. Technical equipament for assessment of dental pulp status. Endod Topics 2004;7:2-13.
50. Reeh ES, Eldeeb E. Referred pain of muscular origin resembling endodontic involvement. Oral Surg Oral Med Oral Pathol 1991; 71:223-227.
51. Rodrigues CD, Estrela C. Traumatic bone cyst suggestive of large apical periodontitis. J Endod 2008;34:484-9.
52. Schnettler JM, Wallace JA. Pulse oximetry as a diagnostic tool of pulpal vitality. J Endod 1991;17:488-90.
53. Shafer W, Hine M, Levy B. Tratado de Patologia Bucal. 5th ed. Rio de Janeiro: Guanabara Koogan; 1987. 837p.
54. Sonis S, Fazio R, Fang L. Medicina Oral. 1st ed. Rio de Janeiro: Interamericana; 1985.
55. Sonis S, Fazio R, Fang L. Princípios e prática de medicina oral. 2nd ed. Rio de Janeiro: Guanabara Koogan; 1996. 491p.
56. Tommasi AF. Diagnóstico em patologia bucal. 2nd ed. São Paulo: Pancast; 1989. 637p.
57. Tovo MF, Vono BG, Tavano O, Pavarini A. Estudo comparativo do método radiográfico utilizando filmes de diferentes sensibilidades e o sistema digital Digora, no diagnóstico de lesões de cárie em superfície proximal de molares decíduos. Rev Fac Odontol Bauru 1999; 7:23-30.
58. Treede RD, Cole JD. Dissociates secondary hyperalgesia in a subject with a large – fibre sensory neuropathy. Pain 1993;53:169-174.
59. Vandre RH, Webber RL. Future trends in dental radiology. Oral Surg Oral Med Oral Pathol 1995; 80:471-78.
60. White SC, Atchison KA, Hewlett ER, Flack VF. Efficacy of FDA guidelines for prescribing radiographs to detect dental and intraosseous conditions. Oral Surg Oral Med Oral Pathol Oral Radiol Endod 1995;80:108-14.
61. White SC, Pharoah MJ. Oral radiology: principles and interpretation. 5th ed. St. Louis: Mosby, 2004.
62. Wildersmith PEEB. A new method for the noninvasive measurement of pulpal blood flow. Int Endod J 1988;21:307.
63. Wood NK, Goaz PW. Differential diagnosis of oral and maxillofacial lesions. 3rd ed. St Louis, MO: Mosby, 1985.

# Cone Beam Computed Tomography in Endodontic Diagnosis

**M. R. Bueno**
*University of Cuiabá, MT, Brazil*

**C. Estrela**
*Federal University of Goiás, Goiânia, GO, Brazil*

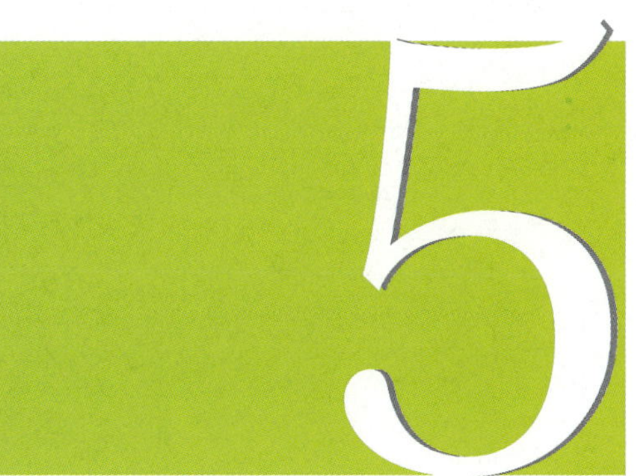


Chapter contents

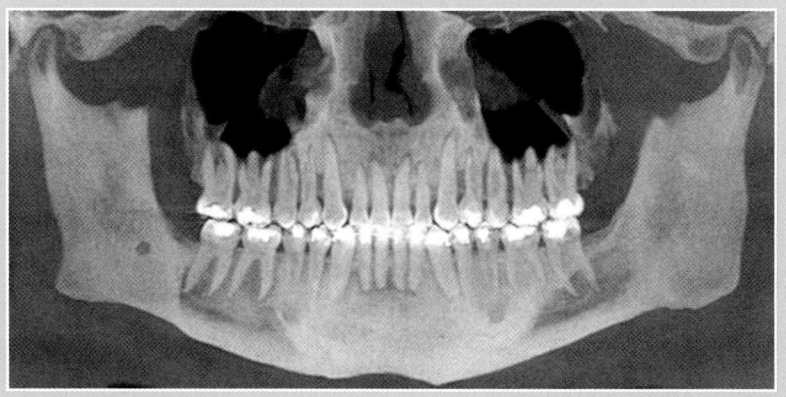

Reconstruction of three dimensional image from panoramic view (I-Cat).

## 5.1 Introduction

Continual changes can be observed in paradigms and dogmas in different sectors of society. The industrial revolution changed the way of living of many nations. The contemporary world is witnessing one of the agents responsible for the revolution of the moment: computer science, which has brought benefits, especially to the health care sector. The application of the benefits and their relationship with the separate health sectors has allowed important time saving as well as influencing the quality of life. Biotechnology has revolutionized today's way of thinking.

Since the discovery of X-rays by Roentgen, in 1895, radiology has witnessed a constant revolution. New technologies open other horizons. The angle variations proposed by Clark and the development of panoramic radiography by Paatero pointed to different applications in endodontics.

At the moment, the majority of dentistry professionals still maintain the clinical and radiographic methods as the standard for evaluating the outcome of endodontic treatment[6-8,16-19,24,33,38,43,44], despite all the limitations that the two-dimensional projection of three-dimensional structures represent[11,17]. Conventional radiographs (periapical, bitewing, occlusal and panoramic) continue to constitute important resources that favor diagnosis, structure, treatment and follow-up in endodontic practice.

Huumonem & Ørstavik[28] emphasized that radiographic diagnosis of chronic apical periodontitis is a complex task, which is confounded by several anatomical and biological variables. Between the extremes of well-defined, normal periapical structures and pathognomonic radiolucencies, detection and grading of radiographic signs of chronic apical periodontitis may be difficult. In view of these aspects, systems for training and calibrating observers may be used to improve diagnostic performance, and digital manipulations have great potential for detecting subtle changes indicating disease.

Recently, cone beam computed tomography (CBCT) introduced the third dimension into dentistry[1-5,9-23,25-32,34-37,39-43,45-65], being of benefit to specialties which, up to this time had not used the advantages of medical CT, due to lack of specificity.

CBCT allows visualization of a three dimensional image, in which a new plane has been added: depth. Its clinical application allows high accuracy and is directed towards nearly all areas of dentistry - surgery, implant dentistry, orthodontics, endodontics, periodontics, temporomandibular dysfunction, image diagnosis, etc. The real view of associating these indicators with the clinical aspects, projects a fourth dimension, marked by the requirement of time and space.

Several studies have shown important indications and applications for CBCT[1-5,9-23,25-32,34-37,39-43,45-65]. Thus, this new technology certainly represents a new benchmark in contemporary dentistry.

## 5.2 Medical Computed Tomography

Tomography is a generic term meaning an image of a section of the human body. Medical computed tomography was developed in the UK in 1972 by Hounsfield & Comark[10,49], and represented one of the biggest scientific revolutions of our time, earning them the Nobel Prize for Medicine in 1979. Medical computed tomography is an important tool for three dimensional visualization of anatomic structures and pathological processes.

To undergo computed tomography (CT), the patient lies down on a table that glides through an opening called gantry. The gantry contains the X-ray tube and the sensors (scintillation crystals), coupled to a support in a ring shape. Traditional medical tomography uses a collimated fan-shaped radiation beam, which is captured by the sensors (Fig. 5.1). During every 360° spin around the patient, slices are captured and transferred to the computer, which identify the variations in mitigation of tissues and use complex mathematical calculations to form an image[21,32]. The new generation CT apparatuses have synchronized the movements of the table and the X-ray tube, which enables the X-ray beam to flow in the form of a spiral, thus reducing the exposure time and improving the image quality. Today's technology is the *multislice* system, with several detector rings and a bigger area per rotation of the gantry[29].

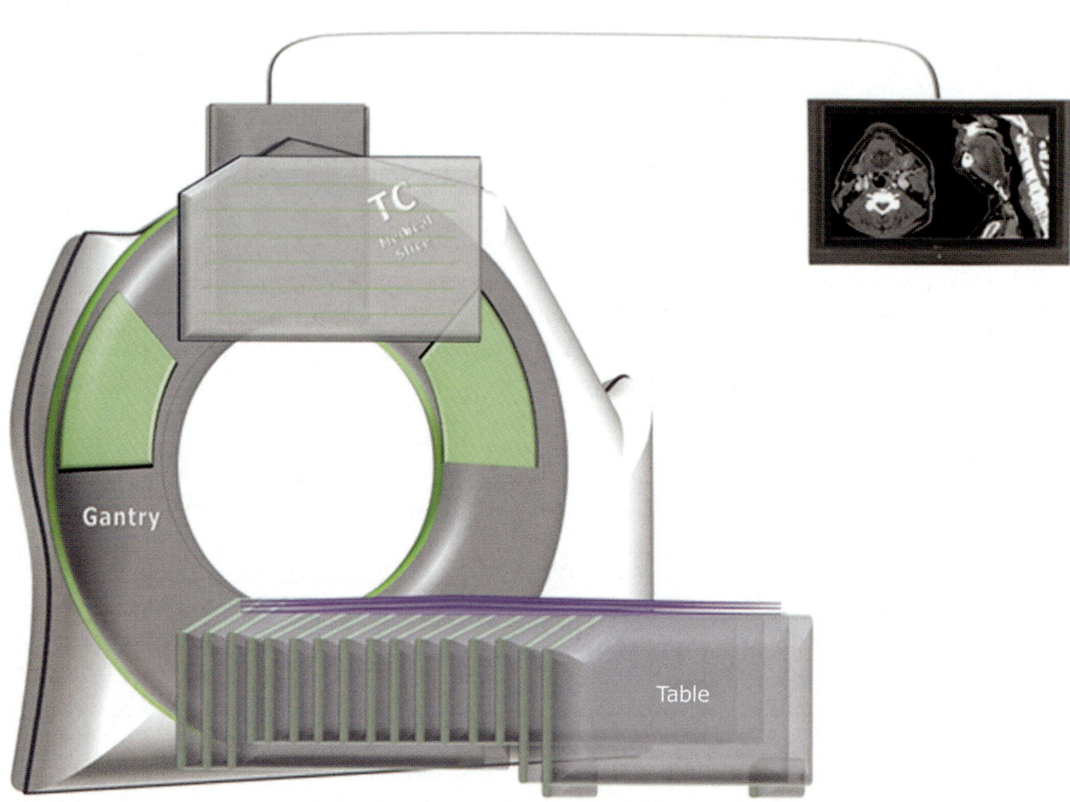


**Figure 5.1** - Schematic representation of traditional medical tomography.

Medical computed tomography was not widely used in dentistry despite the technological progress, due to a series of limitations such as[25,49]: high X-ray doses to patients, low resolution for dentistry, height of the equipment and the need for a special room for performing the exam, high equipment cost and consequently, of the exam itself, limitation of specific dentistry protocols, and difficult professional communication between doctors and dentists.

### 5.3 Cone Beam Computed Tomography

Cone beam tomography provides a lower dose of radiation and a higher image quality than medical tomography does, with distinction of the delicate structures, such as the enamel, dentin, pulp cavity and alveolar cortical[13].

Cone beam tomography was used in a restricted way in the medical area. Arai et al.[1-4], considered the father of cone beam tomography in dentistry, was the pioneer in improving this technique for dentistry developed in Japan (Nihon University,1997). The prototype developed, consists of a high resolution tomography, modifying Scanora equipment (*Soredex Corporation, Helsinki, Finland*), called ortho-ct. Afterwards, Mozzo et al.[42] were responsible for the first commercial tomography (Newton - 9000). Among the main models on the world market, one can find: *I-Cat (Imaging Sciences-Kavo)* (Fig. 5.2); *New-Tom 3G (NewTom Dental); 3D Accuitomo (J. Morita MFG Corp., Kyoto, Japan); ProMax 3D (Planmeca); CB MercuRay (Hitachi), Iluma (Imtec Imaging); PreXion (TeraRecon); Galileos (Sirona); Picasso (Ewoo).*



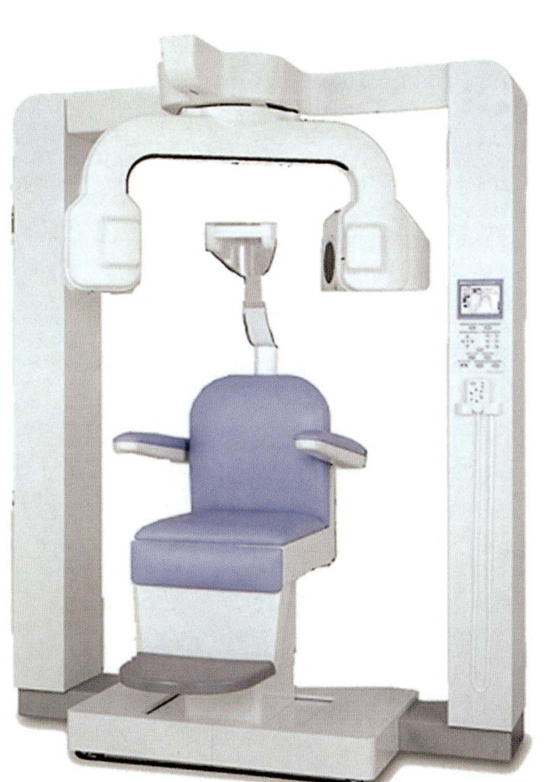

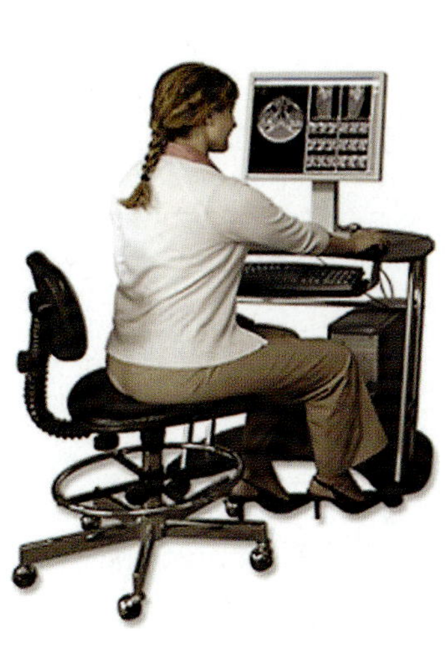

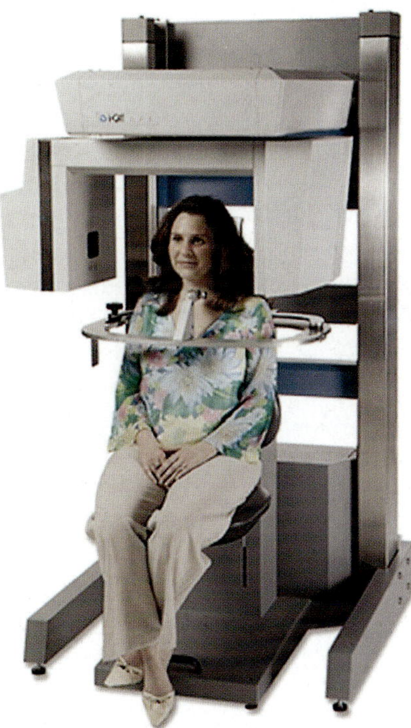

**Figure 5.2** - Commercially available tomography models- *3D Accuitomo, I-Cat.*

## 5.4 Mechanical Components of the Cone Beam Equipment

Cone beam tomographs are compact, when compared with medical tomographs. The patient can remain standing, sitting or in a supine position depending on the model used. Tomography consists of a tube that emits pulsatile X-rays in form of conical beam and a sensor joined by an arm, similar to the panoramic equipment. A motorized chair or table with support systems for mandible and head, complete the equipment, which is connected to a normal computer, not requiring a specific work station.

There are two types of sensors for the cone beam technology: Image intensifier and Flat Panel. The first generation of cone beam volumetric tomography used the intensifier system of 8 bits. As the equipment developed the Flat Panel sensor became the one most used, due to the advantages offered. The Flat panel sensor produces distortion-free images, with less noise, is not sensitive to magnetic fields and does not require frequent calibrations[42]. Nowadays, the Flat Panel sensors work with 12 to 16 bits. The higher the number of bits, the higher the number of grey tones.

**Image acquisition**

The arm containing the sensor and the X-ray tube turns around the patient, acquiring multiple two-dimensional images from different projections. The number of projections varies between 250 and 600 images acquired within a turn of 180 to 360 degrees. The time for performing an exam is generally 8 to 40 seconds, but as the X-ray is pulsatile[55], the exposure time is much shorter. The cone beam system is very sensitive to movements of the patient's head; therefore he/she has to remain motionless during image acquisition. Equipment with an adequate contention system helps to keep the patient motionless.

**Image volume and processing**

The images obtained by multiple exposures generate a cylindrical volume and the computer performs the primary reconstruction. Afterward, for working purposes, a secondary reconstruction of the image is performed according to requirements and the attendance protocols. In addition to the cuts, based on the cone beam tomography, plane or three dimensional images can be generated (Fig. 5.3) from the panoramic radiographs in real size 1:1, as well as lateral and frontal teleradiography images, and many other exams with a much higher sharpness than that delivered by the conventional exams[39,55].

Digital images are formed by little dots which are small squares with identical lateral measurements, width (x) and height (y). The smallest unit of these dots is a called pixel. Because tomography is a three dimensional volume, a new dimension is added, the depth (z); therefore it no longer consists of a square, but of a cube, called voxel (Fig. 5.4). Cone beam tomography has isometric[20] voxels (voxel with identical dimensions of height, width and depth) and isomorph voxels, increasing the capacity of sharper and clearer reproduction of details of hard than the medical tomograms (which do not have isometric voxels), especially of delicate structures, such as, for example the alveolar bone. Theoretically the smaller the size of the voxel, the sharper the image usually becomes, however, other factors like quality of the sensor, design of the equipment, stability of the patient and software, interfere in the final sharpness.

In the medical CT, the exam is processed by a high cost dedicated server computer. In cone beam tomography a conventional high performance computer is used. This aspect brings advantages due to the advances in today's processors with dual core, cheaper RAM memory and more affordable hard disc (HD) prices for high capacity storage.

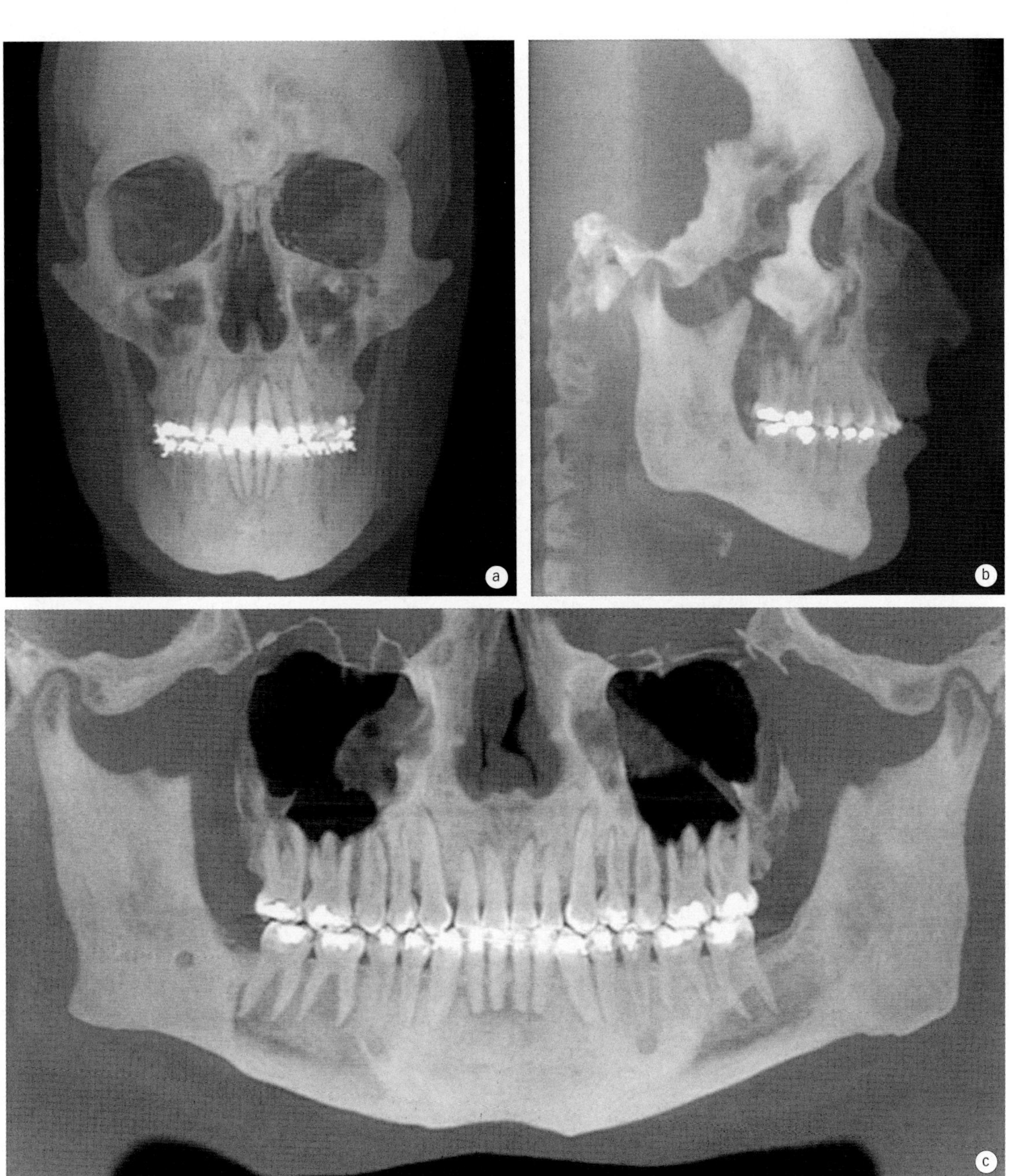

**Figure 5.3** - (**A-C**) Reconstruction of three dimensional images from frontal, lateral and panoramic views (I-Cat).

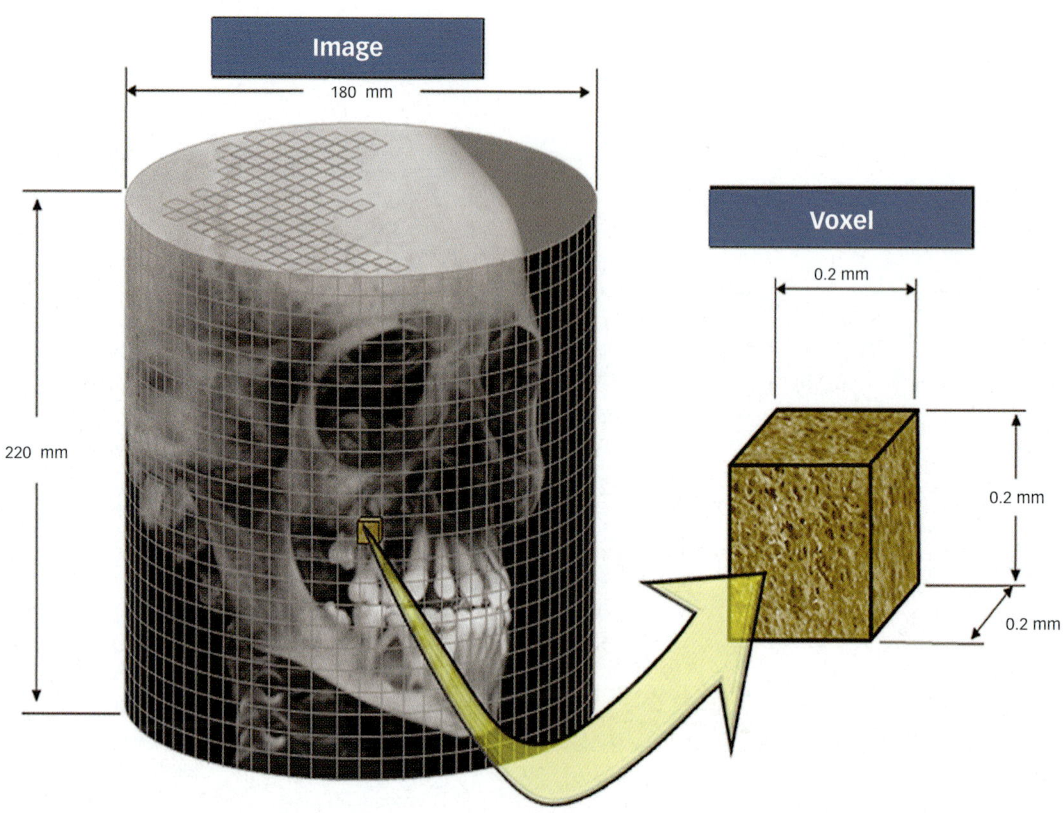


**Figure 5.4** - Schematic representation of formation of voxels by acquired volume.

As in the traditional medical tomography, in the cone beam system it is also possible to export the images as a *Dicom* file (*Digital Imaging and Communications in Medicine*). The Dicom file has been especially developed for the medical area with the idea of integrating and visualizing different modalities of images in one digital filing system only. The Dicom system can store technical data starting with acquisition of the exam, date, clinical information of the patient etc. The Dicom images can only be opened with specific software. These files can then be converted into STL format for making three dimensional models.

## 5.5 Cone Beam Equipment Types

Items of cone beam CT equipment have their own characteristics and differ with respect to sensor type, size of image field (Field of View – FOV), resolution and software. These differences make certain equipment more indicated for certain specialties like endodontics, where a high resolution image is necessary, differently from orthodontics, which requires a more wide-ranging area of larger volume. It is possible to classify the cone beam tomographs by the size of their fields of view (FOV). 1. Small volume Equipment; 2. Large volume Equipment; 3.Large volume and small volume Equipment.

### Small volume equipment

The small volume tomographs (Fig. 5.5) have a field of view (FOV) up to 8x8 cm. The advantage of this acquisition is to be able to evaluate areas of interest only, in high resolution, without exposing the patient unnecessarily to radiation in areas of no interest. Occasionally, when a major field of image is required, two or more volumes can be acquired to complement the exam. In dentistry the great majority of exam requirements are limited to specific areas of the mouth. It is a highly adequate exam for evaluating dental and adjacent bone tissue structures. The small volume is the adequate choice in cases where high resolution is required, such as in endodontics, re-absorptions, and implants of some elements, ATM and pathologies.

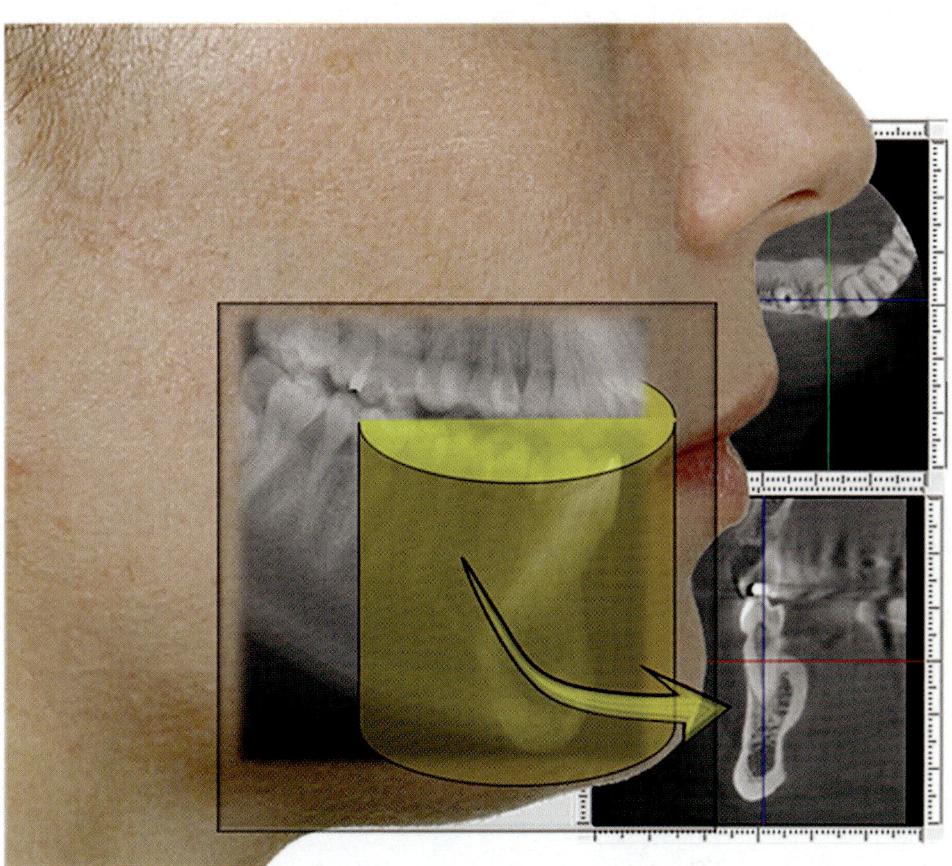

**Figure 5.5** - Representation of image acquired with small volume equipment.

## Large volume equipment

Large volume tomographs (Fig. 5.6) acquire an image volume of over 8x8 cm, generally 12x12cm to 18x22cm. Their radiation dose is higher and their image quality is inferior when compared with the small volume equipment. It is worth stressing that the radiation dose is higher than for the small volume, however much lower than that of medical tomography. The large volume tomograms can generate multilayer reconstructions with two and three dimensional visions, like lateral, frontal and axial teleradiographs, as well as panoramic radiographs with virtually no distortions. These aspects help in special requirements, where a big area has to be analyzed, like multiple implants, extensive pathologies, orthodontics and traumatology.

Patel et al.[51], while discussing the absorbed radiation dose, reported that the effective doses from CBCT scanners differ, but can be almost as low as those from panoramic dental X-ray units and considerably less than that from medical CT scanners. *The higher effective doses from certain makes of CBCT scanners is, in part, due to the larger size of the field of view (FOV) and the type of image receptor used. As is to be expected, the small volume scanners, such as the 3D Accuitomo and Planmeca Promax 3D, which are specifically designed to capture information from a small region of the maxilla or mandible, deliver a very low effective dose and are therefore best suited for endodontic imaging of only one tooth or two neighboring teeth, the FOV is similar in size to that of a conventional periapical radiograph. Indeed, the effective dose of the 3D Accuimoto has been reported to be of the same order of magnitude as 2-3 standard periapical radiograph exposures[1], whilst the effective dose for a full mouth series of periapical radiographs has been reported to be of an order of magnitude comparable with the effective dose of a large volume CBCT scan[15,23].*

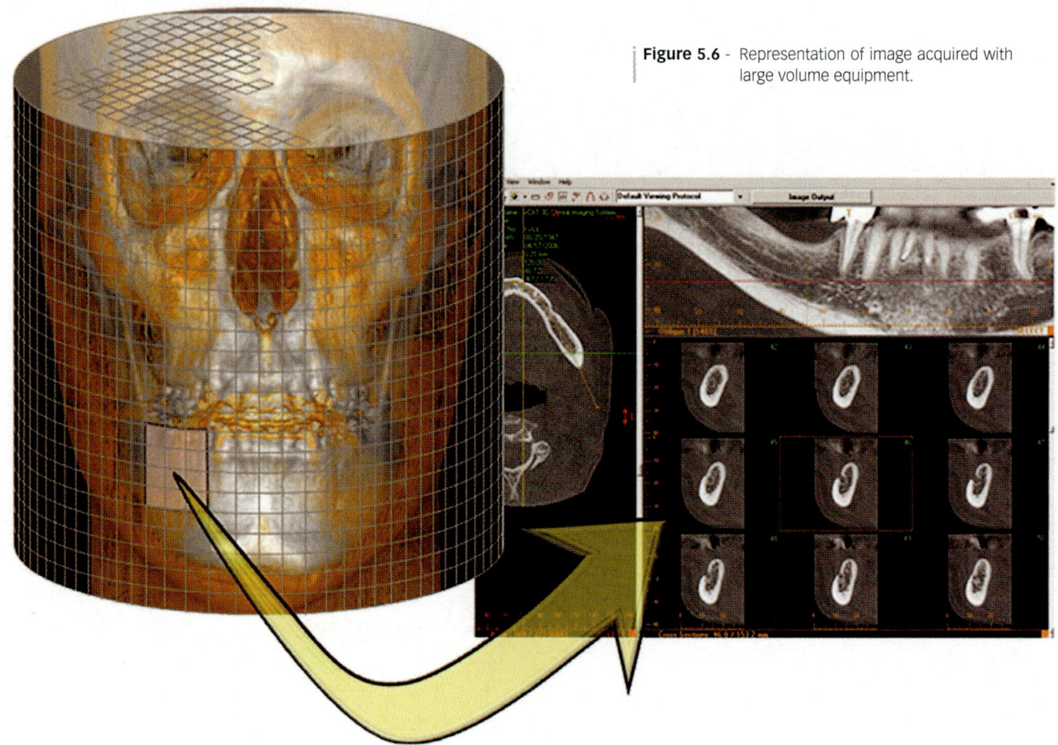

**Figure 5.6** - Representation of image acquired with large volume equipment.

**Large and small volume equipment**

New generations of tomographs are being developed with the idea of uniting large and small volume. The radiation dose of a cone beam exam depends on the brand and the model of the equipment, configurations of k-voltage (KV), milli-amperage (MA), exposure time and range of volume of the exam[36,49]. The dose from cone beam tomography of the main models sold in Brazil is on an average, almost equivalent to a periapical exam of the whole mouth with film[26] or 4 to 15 panoramic[55] images and only 1.3% to 6.4% of the exposure to one medical face tomography[5,36,42,46,55].

## 5.6 Main Advantages of Cone Beam Tomography over Traditional Medical Tomography

1. More compact equipment;
2. Higher resolution (isotropic and isomorphic voxel) resulting in sharper images;
3. Small FOV - makes it possible to have images of only the area of interest;
4. Fewer metal devices;
5. For most equipment the patient is in a sitting position, and in not lying down, as in the medical CT, increasing comfort and acceptance by patients. Temporomandibular Joint (TMJ) and maxillary sinus exams are more precise with the patient in a vertical position;
6. Less exposure time and lower radiation dose when compared with medical CT.

## 5.7 Traditional Radiographic Exams versus Cone Beam Tomography

The extra and intraoral radiographs are exams of great value in dentistry. Many professionals recognize that despite the benefits, these exams have major limitations, mainly due to the superimposition of images. Other present limitations involve the requirement of extensive bone loss, between 30 to 50%, before the rarefaction image starts to show up in radiographic periapical exams[6-8]. Cone beam tomography allows better and higher accuracy[12,27,31,41] compared with other imaging methods, distinction between the gray tones for tissues with density difference of 0.5% whereas with conventional radiography, this limit is between 5 and 10%[49]. Therefore tomography is between 10 to 20 times more sensitive than the conventional exam, when verifying tone variations.

Many of the other limitations inherent to conventional radiographs are; fractured teeth, hidden apical periodontitis, reabsorptions and others.

Trope et al.[59] analyzed periapical lesions on 60 human cadavers. Periapical radiolucencies were seen in conjunction with 33 teeth. The computerized tomography examination of the lesions was correlated to the histopathology. Seven of the 8 periapical lesions studied were histologically shown to be granulomas. In the computed tomography these lesions had a cloudy appearance with a density similar to each other and to the surrounding soft tissues of the lips and nose. A cyst could be differentiated from periapical granulomas by computerized tomography because of a marked difference in density between the content of the cyst cavity and granuloma tissue.

Simon et al.[56] compared the differential diagnosis of large periapical lesions (granuloma versus cyst) with that of traditional biopsy using cone beam computed tomography (CBCT, NewTom 3G). Seventeen large periapical radiolucencies were scanned using the CBCT-scan machine to determine densities. The lesions were then removed surgically after cleaning, shaping, and filling the canals and sent for histopathological examination. Thirteen out of 17 had the same diagnosis, with both the CBCT-scan and biopsy; four out of 17 had a split diagnosis. All four were labeled "cyst" by the CBCT-scan and chronic apical periodontitis by the oral pathologist. In evaluating the last four lesions, it was found that the CBCT-scan *may* be clinically more precise and more useful than the biopsy. Thus, the CBCT may provide a more accurate diagnosis than biopsy and histology, providing a diagnosis without invasive surgery and/or waiting for year to see whether nonsurgical therapy is effective.

On the other hand, Laux et al.[33] evaluated the reliability of routine X-rays in detecting apical root reabsorptions, correlating the radiographic diagnosis with the histologic findings. Specimens were collected with a diagnosis of apical periodontitis, radiographically with apical radiolucence. After extraction, the teeth were processed and histological layers made, using 114 histological specimens in this study. When the histological and radiographic data were combined, a total of 104 histological/radiographic pairs were available for analysis. Of the 104 radiographs, 51% were periapical films and 49% orthopantomograms. In the first part of the study, the 124 radiographs were analyzed by an endodontist, who had no knowledge of the histological diagnosis. The teeth were examined with respect to absence or presence of root reabsorptions in the apical third; in the second part of the study, histological sections were analyzed by means of microscopy. Histologically two types of root reabsorptions could be diagnosed: 1) Faults which were repaired with cement and 2) unrepaired gaps. Only the reabsorptions without repair received histological evaluation. During the third stage, the relationship between the radiographic diagnosis and histological findings was analyzed. Root reabsorptions were radiographically diagnosed in 19% of the evaluated teeth, whereas in histological examination this change was observed in 81% of the specimens. The evaluation correlating the radiographic diagnosis with the histological findings revealed a match in 7% of the specimens, with no correlation in 76% of cases.

A disadvantage of the cone beam tomography in comparison with conventional radiograph exams is the shape of artifacts (much more visible in medical tomography) principally close to high density objects, like the metal artifacts (intracanal posts, crowns and metal restorations)[30,34]. This effect is called *"beam hardening"*. Beam hardening can happen in a discrete way, due to the presence of very thick enamel, such as the occlusal surfaces of pre-molar and molar teeth, with projection of a dark, radiolucent image in a neighboring tooth, resembling caries. For this reason complementary interdental or periapical radiographs may be required.

The radiologist has to be prepared to identify the shape of this effect, which forms an image according to the characteristics of neighboring objects, through three dimensional tracking. These artifacts tend to diminish with more sophisticated software and sensors.

## 5.8 Request and Reception of a Cone Beam Computed Tomography Exam

To request tomographic exams is very easy and direct. It is sufficient to include the area of interest that led to this indication and the more significant clinical conditions. Examples:

1. Tomography of retained tooth #23 - verify integrity of roots of neighboring teeth;
2. Tomography in the area of tooth #36 (absent) - verify bone height and thickness; evaluate position of mandibular canal.
3. Bilateral tomography of the TMJ - difficulty of opening the mouth and presence of pain.
4. Tomography of maxilla - complete evaluation for implants.
5. Tomography of teeth #21 and #22 - suspected root fracture;
6. Tomography for three dimensional cephalometry.

The dental surgeon receives the expertise together with the images, which can be printed on photographic paper or film, with the more representative cuts and three dimensional reconstructions. Today, digital radiology is a reality. An exam is accompanied by a CD or DVD with all cuts obtained from the original volume. Software to visualize the three dimensional exams can be installed in the dentist's or dental surgeon's computer, to perform simulation with the patient's images. Thus the dentist has access to browse in the three dimensions of space, X-Y-Z (Fig. 5.7). It is an extraordinary tool because the professional can navigate through volume, use zoom, make his own measurements, explain the treatment plan to the patient, perform virtual surgeries and consult colleagues via internet.

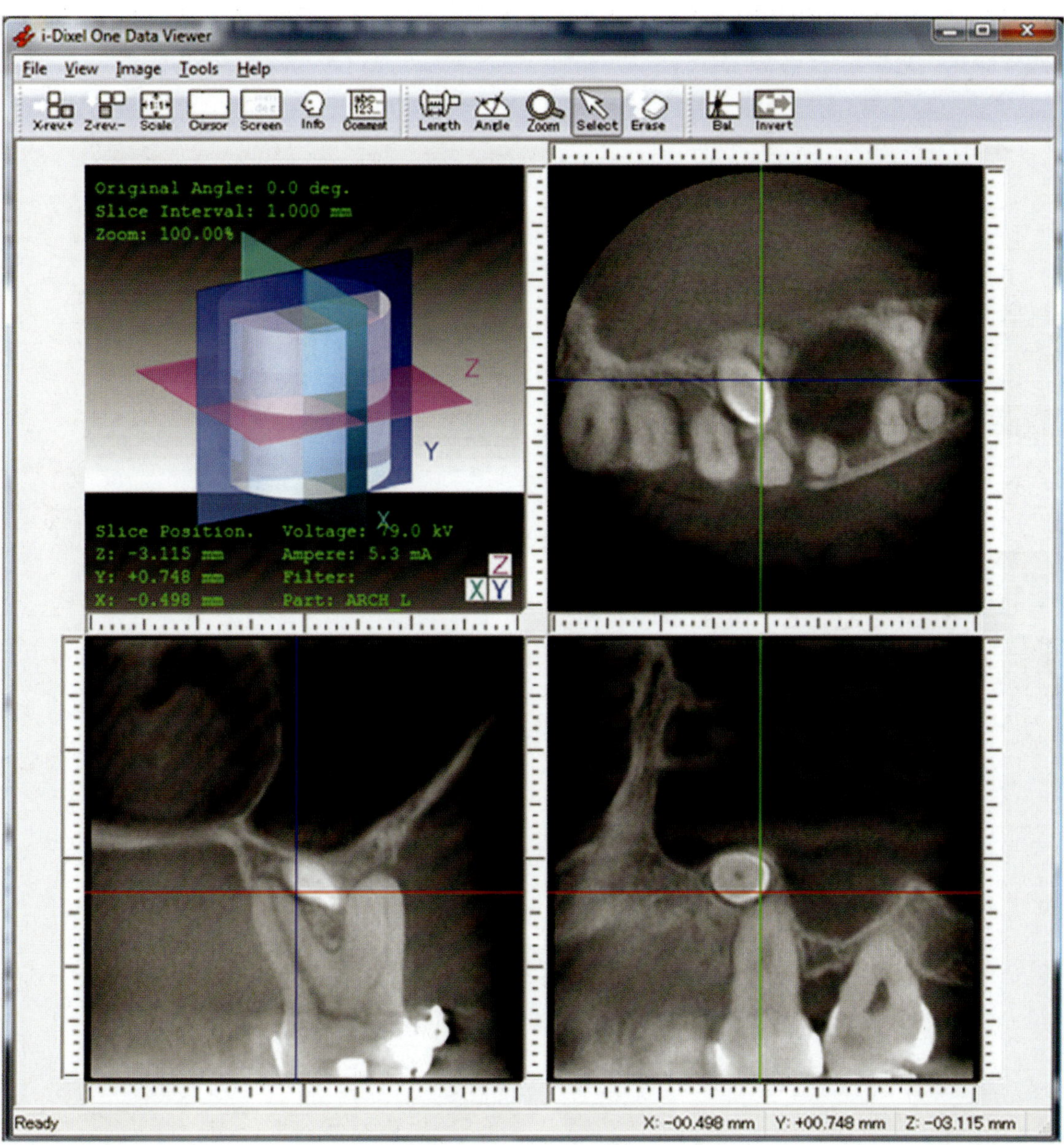


**Figure 5.7** - Computer Tomography showing different cuts of one tooth (supernumerary), with navigation in three planes of space with the software view i-Dixel of high resolution cone beam tomography equipment Accuitomo (J.Morita MFG Co., Kyoto, Japan).

## 5.9 Interpretation of the Exam

When one receives the exam, one first needs to interpret the origin of the cuts, which usually come with a numerical indexation in an easily recognizable image, such as a panoramic view or segments of it (Fig. 5.8). These indexation images are obtained by the cone beam exam itself and also serve as a means of diagnosis. There are other forms of indexation, like synchronized navigation in the three planes of space (Fig. 5.9).

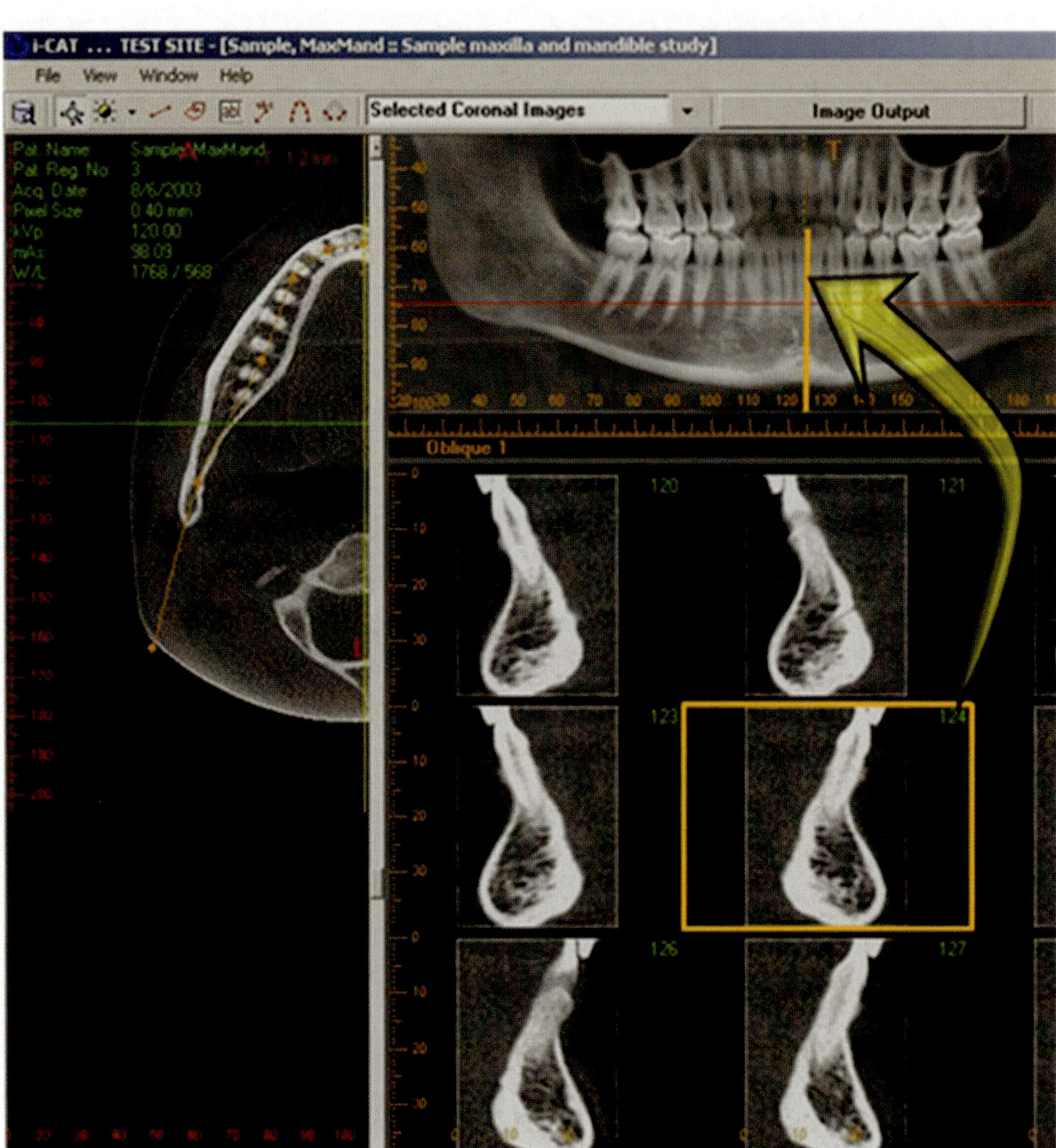


**Figure 5.8** - CBCT I-Cat showing possibilities of synchronized navigation.

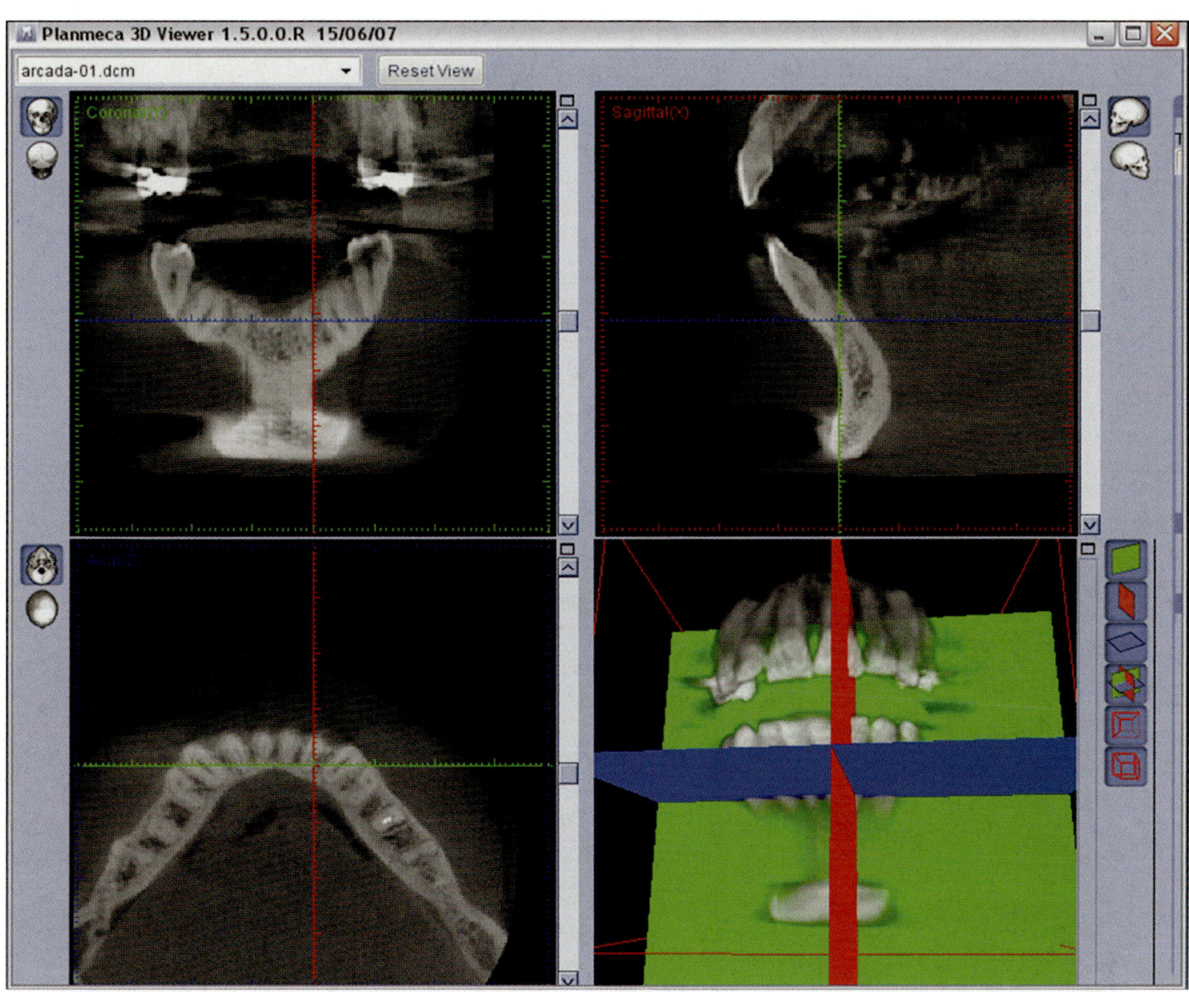


**Figure 5.9** - CBCT Planmeca ProMax 3D presenting possibility of synchronized navigation in the three planes of space.

The dental surgeon/radiologist has to be very well prepared scientifically, to analyze the tomographic exams and interpret the images in the three planes of space: Axial, sagittal and coronal. The expert has to include the information of the entire volume and not only the area of major interest in the exam, shown in the radiographic request. When a dental surgeon accepts a partial expert report he/she is responsible for the areas that were not described in the expert report by the radiologist.

## 5.10 Planning the use of Cone Beam Tomography

Cone beam images require more planning than conventional exams. Bjerklin & Ericson[9] showed that 43.7% of retained planning cases of maxillary canine teeth have been changed after the patient undergoes cone beam tomography.

The Adobe Photoshop CS3 Medical, launched by the Adobe Company has excellent filters for the fine interpretation of *Dicom* images, as well as for preparing the exam. There already is good and sophisticated software for planning, such as *Dolphin* in the orthodontic area, *Implant /* and *Nobel Biocare* for the implant area, DentalSlice for the surgical planning area (DentalSlice of Bioparts - Fig. 5.10), among others.

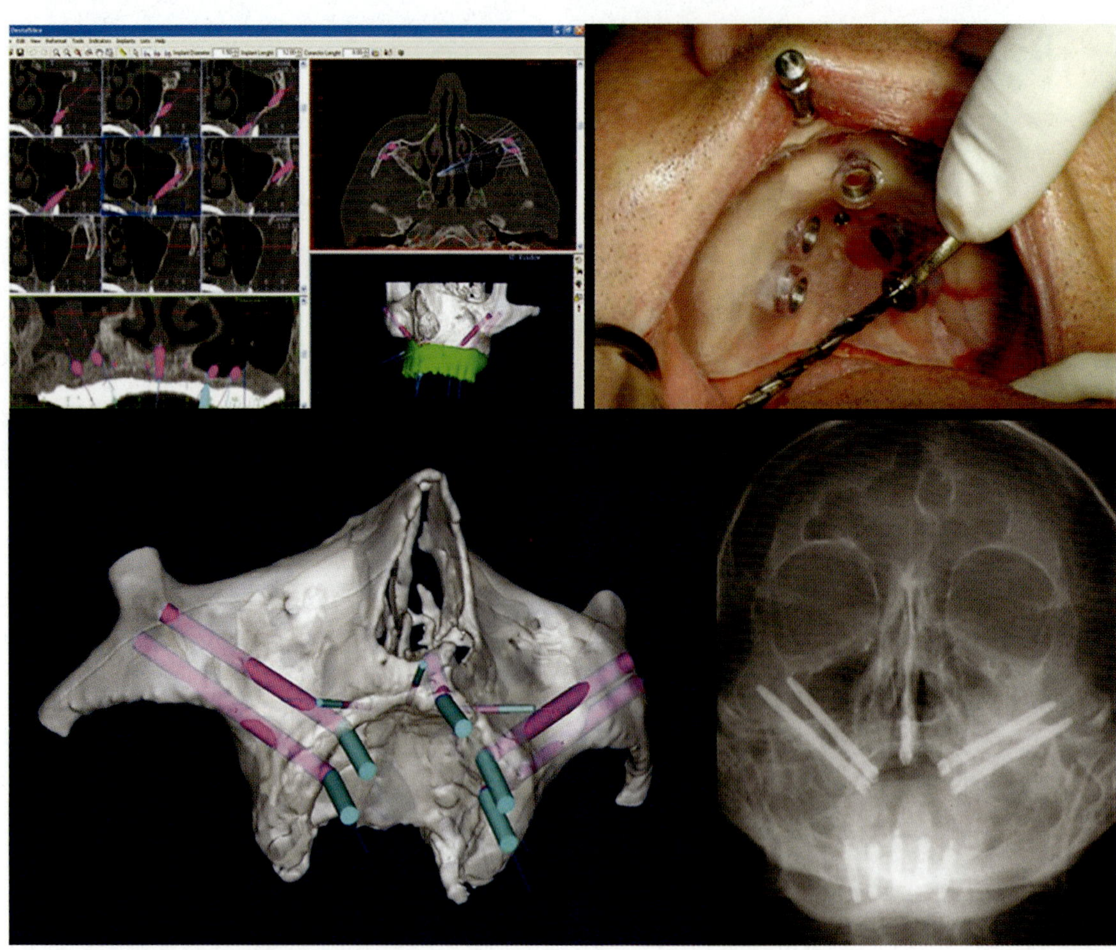

**Figure 5.10** - Virtual planning with preparation of a surgical guide as prototype and placement of a zygomatic implant with *DentalSlice* software from Bioparts.

*Dolphin* (Fig. 5.11) developed a photographic image capture system, also three dimensional, in which images are included as variable transparencies in reconstructions of the tomographic images, and the whole set can be turned so that the image can be observed from various angles.

As cone beam tomographs export images in *Dicom* standard format, it is possible to send the data to a prototype laboratory to have a solid, physical model made of the precisely represented, tactile and three dimensional parts of the patient's anatomy. They are used specially in cases involving planning of complex approaches.



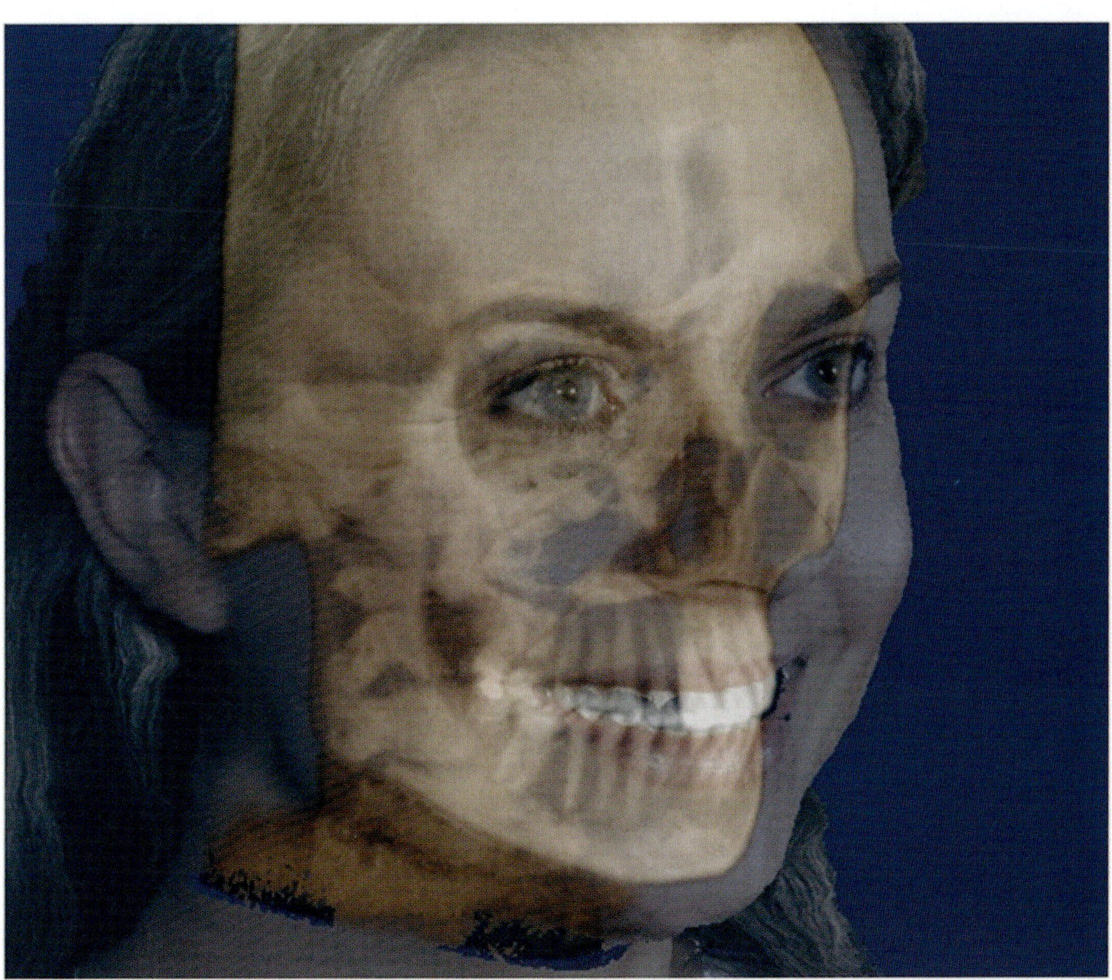

**Figure 5.11** - Application of a photographic image in the form of transparencies in three dimensional reconstructions (Dolphin).

## 5.11 Endodontic Clinical Applications and Accuracy of Cone Beam Computed Tomography

The search for the ideal system to control a person's health has made it possible to develop many innovative systems, among them, cone beam computed tomography.

The diagnosis of apical periodontitis (AP) represents an essential strategy to determine the selection of an effective therapeutic protocol for endodontic infection control. Apical periodontitis is a consequence of root canal system infection, which can involve progressive stages of inflammation and changes in periapical bone structure, resulting in resorption, identified as radiolucencies in radiographs[44].

Some studies have shown that a periapical lesion from endodontic infection may be present without being visible radiographically. The radiographic image corresponds to a two-dimensional aspect of a three-dimensional structure[6-8,60,64]. Artificial lesions produced in cadavers can be detected by conventional radiography only if there is perforation, extensive destruction of the bone cortex on the outer surface or erosion of the cortical bone from the inner surface. Lesions confined within the cancellous bone cannot be detected, while lesions with buccal and lingual cortical involvement produce distinct radiographic areas of rarefaction. In order to be visible radiographically, the periapical radiolucency of mineral bone loss should reach nearly 30% to 50%[6-8]. Other conditions, such as morphological variations in the apical region, surrounding bone density, X-ray angulations and radiographic contrast, also influence radiographic interpretation[24]. An experimentally induced lesion may or may not be detected, depending on its location. A periapical lesion of a certain size can be detected in a region covered by a thin cortex, whereas the same size lesion will not be seen in a region covered by a thicker cortex. Lesion locations in different types of bone influence radiographic visualization[28].

A large number of studies using different diagnostic methods have evaluated the type and incidence of periapical lesions[33,44,56,59]. There is scientific consensus that apical periodontitis is accurately identified by histological analysis[33]. On the other hand, it has been demonstrated that CT can determine the difference in density between the cystic cavity content and granulomatous tissue, favoring the choice of a noninvasive diagnosis[56,59].

Several advanced radiographic techniques to detect bone lesions have been used in dentistry, namely digital radiography, densitometry methods, CBCT, magnetic resonance imaging, ultrasound, nuclear techniques[1-5,11,13,14,28,43,47,60-65]. CBCT has been successfully used in endodontics with different goals, including study of root canal anatomy, external and internal macromorphology in 3D-reconstruction of the teeth, evaluation of root canal preparation, obturation, re-treatment, coronal microleakage, bone lesion detection and experimental endodontology[1-5,11,13,28,34,43,45,52,60-65].

Few studies have compared the differences in AP image interpretation using CBCT, conventional periapical radiography or digital radiography. CBCT has provided promising results with more accurate apical periodontitis detection[14,34,45,61]. The therapeutic protocol to treat diseases of endodontic origin has routinely been based on evaluating pathological and clinical characteristics, frequently complemented by radiographic findings. Radiographic imaging is the most commonly used diagnostic resource in endodontic diagnosis and treatment and image distortions constitute a serious inconvenience. In addition, it is important to emphasize the limited number of endodontic epidemiological studies. The knowledge of prevalence and severity of apical periodontitis is often based on periapical radiography, whose accuracy is questionable.

Therefore, considering some of the limitations of conventional radiography for detecting periapical bone lesions, advanced imaging methods, such as CBCT, may add benefits to endodontics and offer a higher quality of diagnosis, treatment planning and prognosis.

Estrela et al.[17] analyzed the accuracy of 1.508 images made by cone beam computed tomography, periapical and panoramic radiographs for detecting apical periodontitis. Imaging exam records of 888 consecutive patients (59% women, mean age 50 ± 12 years) including periapical and panoramic radiographs and CBCT, were selected from the Dental and Radiological Institute of Brasília databases (IORB, Brasília, DF, Brazil). Exams performed between May, 2004 and August, 2006 were obtained. All patients had at least one tooth with a history of secondary and primary endodontic infections, confirmed by clinical examination. Table 5.1 shows the prevalence of AP in both endodontically treated and untreated teeth, as identified by periapical and panoramic radiographs and dental CBCT. The high discrepancy between imaging methods for detecting apical periodontitis indicated the possibility of false negative diagnoses when using conventional radiography.

Overall sensitivity was 0.55 and 0.28 for periapical and panoramic radiographs, respectively, which indicates that AP was correctly identified in 54.5% of the cases using periapical radiographs and in 27.8% of the cases using panoramic radiographs. Minor changes in sensitivity were found for the different tooth groups, except for incisors in panoramic radiographs (0.16). High specificity values were found for all tooth groups, ranging from 0.96 to 1.00. Predictive values showed high probability of a positive diagnosis indicating that a tooth actually had AP (PPV range from 0.96 to 1.00). Negative predictive values (NPV) were significantly lower, ranging from 0.35 to 0.65. This means a rather low probability of a negative diagnosis, indicating an actual absence of periapical lesion, particularly in incisors and molars using panoramic radiographs (0.35 and 0.35, respectively). Overall accuracy was 0.70 and 0.54 for periapical and panoramic radiographs. Accuracy of periapical radiographs was significantly higher than that of panoramic radiographs ($p<0.05$), which means that periapical radiographs were shown to be more accurate than panoramic to correctly identify or exclude the presence of a periapical lesion[17].

The findings of the present investigation[17] demonstrated that the CBCT images present high accuracy for detecting AP. CBCT images tend to offer higher scores than periapical and panoramic radiographs, suggesting that diagnosis of the AP score when using conventional images is frequently underestimated. AP was correctly identified in 54.5% of the cases using periapical radiographs (sensitivity 0.55) and in 27.8%, using panoramic radiographs (sensitivity 0.28). Accuracy of periapical radiographs was significantly higher than that of panoramic radiographs. Apical periodontitis was correctly identified with conventional methods when a severe condition was present.

The likelihood of apical periodontitis existing and not being identifiable by periapical or panoramic radiographs is considerably high (Fig. 5.12). The difficulty of accurately detecting apical periodontitis has been mentioned elsewhere. An important aspect to consider is that there must be approximately 30% to 50% of mineral loss in order to visualize apical periodontitis[6-8]. Morphologic variations in the apical region, bone density, X-ray angulations, radiographic contrast and actual location of the periapical lesion will influence the radiographic interpretation[28]. The limitations of radiographic assessment as a study method should not be overlooked, mainly to reduce false negative results[17].

In view of the limitations of periapical radiography to visualize AP, a review of epidemiological studies should be undertaken, considering the quality of periapical aspects offered by CBCT images. In addition, it will certainly reduce the influence on radiographic interpretation, with less possibility of false negative diagnosis. In the present study, apical periodontitis prevalence in endodontically treated teeth, when comparing the panoramic and periapical radiographs and CBCT images was 17.6%, 35.3% and 63.3%, respectively. One can observe a considerable discrepancy among the imaging methods used to identify AP.

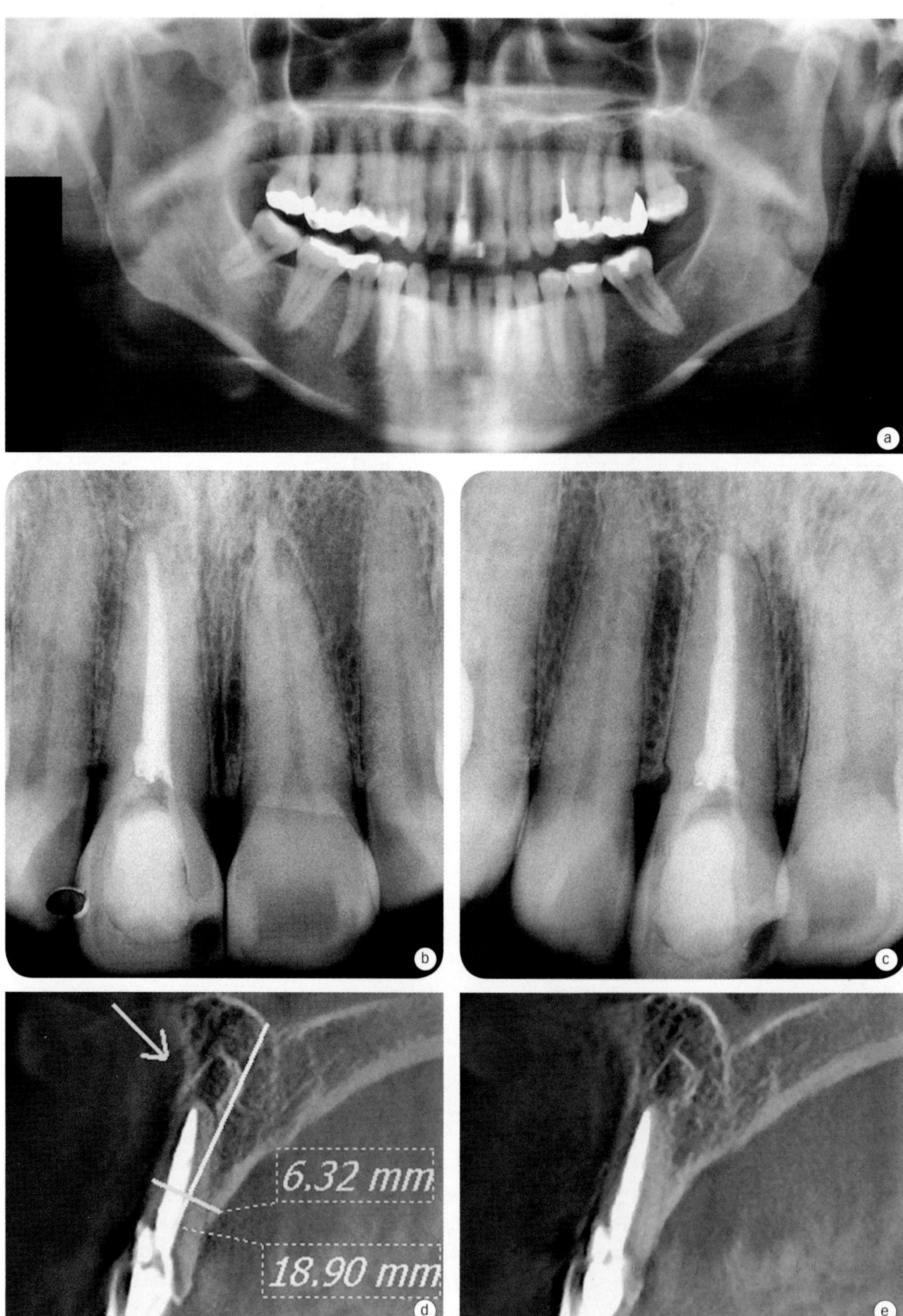


**Figure 5.12** - (**A**) Panoramic and (**B, C**) periapical radiographs show normal periapical area of the upper right incisor. AP can be seen in the CBCT (**D, E**).

Another aspect to consider is that irrespective of the method used to obtain the radiographic image, care should be taken to avoid misinterpretation. As regards CBCT images, the presence of a metal intracanal post may lead to mistaken interpretations due to artifact formation. Lofthag-Hansen et al.[34] reported that, when metal objects are present in either the tooth of interest or an adjacent one, artifacts can pose difficulties when analyzing Accuitomo images. In these cases, periapical radiographs are helpful to complement the diagnosis.

The truth is that most dentists do not have a CBCT equipment in their dental offices. Thus, during endodontic treatment, it is important to choose a radiographic technique that minimizes image distortions, such as the cone parallel technique, in order to obtain a high level of reproducibility and increase the diagnostic accuracy of the imaging method.

The feasibility and cost-effectiveness of CBCT images in clinical routine should be weighed, considering the caution with radiation doses, as it is not in accordance with the standard dose recommended in some countries. It is important to remember that this study was conducted based on databases from a radiological institute.

Care should be taken when using conventional radiographic images to detect apical periodontitis, because of the high possibility of false negative diagnosis. A great advantage of using CBCT in endodontics is its usefulness for aiding identification of periapical lesions, and in a differential diagnosis with a highly accurate, non-invasive technique.



**Table 5.1** - Prevalence of AP in endodontically treated and untreated teeth, identified by panoramic, periapical and cone beam computed tomography (CBCT) images (n=1508)

| | Panoramic | Periapical | CBCT | P-value* |
|---|---|---|---|---|
| **Treated teeth** (n=1425) | | | | |
| Presence of AP | 251 (17.6%) | 503 (35.3%) | 902 (63.3%) | P<0.001 |
| Absence of AP | 1174 (82.4%) | 922 (64.7%) | 523 (36.7%) | |
| **Non treated teeth** (n=83) | | | | |
| Presence of AP | 18 (21.7%) | 30 (36.1%) | 62 (74.7%) | P<0.001 |
| Absence of AP | 65 (78.3%) | 53 (63.9%) | 21 (25.3%) | |

* Chi-square test

Lofthag-Hansen et al.[34] compared intraoral periapical radiography with 3D images (3D Accuitomo) for diagnosing periapical pathology in 36 patients (46 teeth). When the two diagnostic methods were analyzed by all observers, they agreed that the Accuitomo images provided clinically relevant additional information not found in the periapical radiographs. Stavropoulos & Wenzel[57] evaluated the accuracy of CBCT (New Tom 3G), intraoral digital and conventional film radiography in mechanically created periapical defects in pig jaws. The results showed that the New Tom 3G has a higher sensitivity, PPV and diagnostic accuracy than intraoral radiography (digital - Dixi2 or conventional radiography). No difference was observed between the two periapical (digital vs. conventional) radiographs. Rohlin et al.[53] evaluated the diagnostic accuracy of panoramic and periapical radiography and verified that for sclerotic lesions and all the lesions on maxillary premolars and mandibular molars, periapical radiography was significantly superior.

The precision of CBCT to identify AP compared with panoramic and periapical radiographs indicate the need for taking care, particularly when one wants to obtain high quality in endodontic treatment planning, with diagnosis and its consequences, such as the prognosis. There is considerably higher probability of the existence of AP and it not being discernible by periapical or panoramic radiographies (Fig. 5.12). Therefore, a common difficulty with interpreting the radiographic aspects of AP occurs in endodontically treated teeth, when the periapical lesion found seems to be in the process of healing, stable or in expansion[13,14,17,28,43,44,51].

Velvart et al.[61], using another design study, correlated the information gathered from standard dental radiography and high resolution CBCT scans with the findings obtained during surgery, as regards the presence of the endodontic lesion in fifty patients. All 78 lesions diagnosed during surgery were also visible in the CBCT scan. In contrast, only 61 (78.2%) of the lesions were noted by conventional radiographs. The mandibular canal could be identified in 31 cases in dental radiographs, whereas in the oblique cuts of the corresponding CBCT scans the mandibular canal was detected in all the patients. The amount of cortical and cancellous bone and the bone thickness as well as the three-dimensional extent of the lesion could only be adequately interpreted in CBCT scans.

A study by von Stechow et al.[62] determined whether a 3-D volumetric quantification of periradicular bone resorption could be achieved and how this would correlate with two-dimensional lesion area by histology. The results showed a significant correlation between lesion void volume and two-dimensional lesion area by histology, as well as high correlations between void volume and void thickness and standard deviation of the void thickness, but no relationship with void surface. These results show that three-dimensional analysis of CBCT images is highly correlated with two-dimensional cross-sectional measures of periradicular lesions. Nevertheless, CBCT allows additional microstructural features, as well as subregional analysis of lesion development to be assessed.

With regard to the gold standard in diagnosis, there are continuous signs that in addition to the need for confirming findings by images, microscopic identification is also required. Undoubtedly, the advances in the field of diagnosis have been astounding, especially by providing better accuracy associated with a lower degree of tissue invasion, however, one should be cautious about extrapolations and excesses should always be thoroughly measured.

One must consider the numerous advantages associated with the use of CBCT in endodontic diagnosis, but it is emphasized that one must be careful with regard to artifacts (much more evident in medical tomography) in the presence of metal objects.

Cone beam computed tomography allows the best results to be obtained in evaluations of hard tissue examinations of the oral cavity in three dimensions.

This technology increasingly spreads in the major urban centers of Brazil, to the benefit of patients and dentist surgeons, in order to prepare more appropriate treatment plans and consequently achieve better results for the patients.

Some reviews on endodontic applications, advantages and limitations of CBCT were recently discussed[11,13,14,38,43,51].

It will be possible to resolve several challenges and difficult situations in endodontics, with the aid of images obtained by CBCT (apical periodontitis, differential diagnosis, fracture of endodontic instrument, perforation, overfilling, and evaluation of endodontic treatment outcome, among others). Another significant aspect is being able to visualize the relationship between anatomic structures prior to endodontic surgery, and to evaluate the pattern and content of the lesions. Certainly, CBCT will be universally considered a useful complement to conventional radiology examination[13].

Cotton et al.[14] reported that CBCT technology helps with diagnosing endodontic disease and canal morphology, assessing root and alveolar fractures, analyzing resorptive lesions, identifying disease of non-endodontic origin, and pre-surgical assessment before root-end surgery. When compared with medical CT, CBCT has increased accuracy, provided higher resolution images, and also reduced scan time, radiation doses and costs to the patient. Compared with conventional periapical radiography, CBCT eliminates superimposition of surrounding structures, providing additional clinically relevant information.

Nair et al.[43] related that CBCT will continue to be explored for more applications in endodontics. However, it is imperative for the data thus acquired, using large area sensors, to be read by a board-certified radiologist. Occult pathology and incidental findings in adjacent regions are easily missed or not recognized if the evaluator has not received specific training in interpretation of regional anatomy. Additional imaging may be necessary if such pathology is discovered, including magnetic resonance imaging, nuclear medicine studies, or even medical CT for evaluation of soft tissues with and without the use of contrast agents. The advent of 3D imaging has provided the endodontist with tools that were not available to the clinician before, and facilitated interactive image manipulation and enhancement to visualize the area of interest as a 3D volume. Lack of distortion, magnification, artifacts associated with conventional radiography, and the relatively low radiation dose in comparison with medical-grade CT will result in more clinicians adopting this technology to enable accurate diagnoses and treatment planning, in addition to long-term follow-up and evaluation of healing.

Patel et al.[51] described that traditional radiographic examinations are usually limited to two-dimensional views captured using radiographic film or digital sensors. Crucially, essential information about the three-dimensional anatomy of the tooth/teeth and adjacent structures is obscured, and even with the best intentions and paralleling techniques, distortion and superimposition of dental structures in periapical views is unavoidable. A major advantage of CBCT that has been reported is the three-dimensional geometric accuracy when compared with conventional radiographs. Sagittal, coronal and axial CBCT images eliminate the superimposition of anatomical structures.

Estrela et al.[16] suggested a new periapical index based on cone beam computed tomography for identification of apical periodontitis (AP). The periapical index proposed in this study (CBCTPAI) was developed based on criteria established from measurements corresponding to periapical radiolucency interpreted on CBCT scans. Radiolucent images suggestive of periapical lesions were measured using the working tools of Planimp® software on CBCT scans in three dimensions: buccopalatal, mesiodistal and diagonal. The CBCTPAI was determined by the largest lesion extension. A 6-point (0-5) scoring system was used with addition of two variables: expansion of cortical bone and destruction of cortical bone (Table 5.2). A total of 1,014 images (periapical radiographs and CBCT scans) originally taken from 596 patients were evaluated by 3 observers using the CBCTPAI criteria. AP was identified in 39.5% and 60.9% of cases by radiography and CBCT, respectively ($p<0.01$). The CBCTPAI offers an accurate diagnostic method for use with high-resolution images, which can reduce the incidence of false-negative diagnosis, minimize observer interference and increase the reliability of epidemiological studies, especially those referring to AP prevalence and severity. Figures 5.13 to 5.19 show the schematic representation and clinical cases of groups of mandibular and maxillary teeth corresponding to CBCTPAI.

**Table 5.2** - Cone beam computed tomography periapical index (CBCTPAI) scores[17]

| Score | Quantitative bone alterations in mineral structures |
|---|---|
| 0 | Intact periapical bone structures |
| 1 | Diameter of periapical radiolucency > 0.5-1mm |
| 2 | Diameter of periapical radiolucency > 1-2mm |
| 3 | Diameter of periapical radiolucency > 2-4mm |
| 4 | Diameter of periapical radiolucency > 4-8mm |
| 5 | Diameter of periapical radiolucency > 8mm |
| Score (n) + E* | Periapical bone cortical expansion |
| Score (n) + D* | Periapical bone cortical destruction |

* The variables E (expansion of bone cortical) and D (destruction of cortical bone) were added to each score, if either of these conditions was detected in the CBCT analysis.

Bueno et al.[11] emphasized that CBCT is a great contemporary revolution in dentistry that will certainly benefit uncountable diagnostic and planning activities. Different applications of these benefits in different specialties are shown in the following clinical cases. Cone beam computed tomography allows the best results to be obtained in evaluations of hard tissue examinations of the oral cavity in three dimensions.

One of the discoveries responsible for the world revolution is informatics. The application of its benefits in the different health sectors has provided significant help with diagnosis, therapies, science, time saving, in addition to influencing the quality of life. Biotechnology continues to revolutionize current thinking. Since their discovery by Roentgen in 1895, the images interpreted by X-rays in only two planes have spanned almost a century. Today, computerized cone beam tomography allows a three-dimensional image to be visualized, with the addition of a new plane: depth. Its clinical applications are directed towards all of the areas of dentistry-surgery, implant dentistry, orthodontics, endodontics, periodontology, temporomandibular joint (TMJ) dysfunctions and diagnosis by highly accurate images. The real vision of the association of these indicators with clinical aspects projects the fourth dimension, marked by the need for time and space.

CBCT is a great contemporary revolution in dentistry that will certainly benefit uncountable diagnostic and planning activities. Different applications of these benefits and applications in different specialties are shown in the following clinical cases (Fig. 5.20 to 5.29).

## Acknowledgements

We thank the manufacturers of cone beam tomographs, software companies and the Radiology Dentistry Institute of Brasília-DF (IORB) for permission to use the some images in this publication.



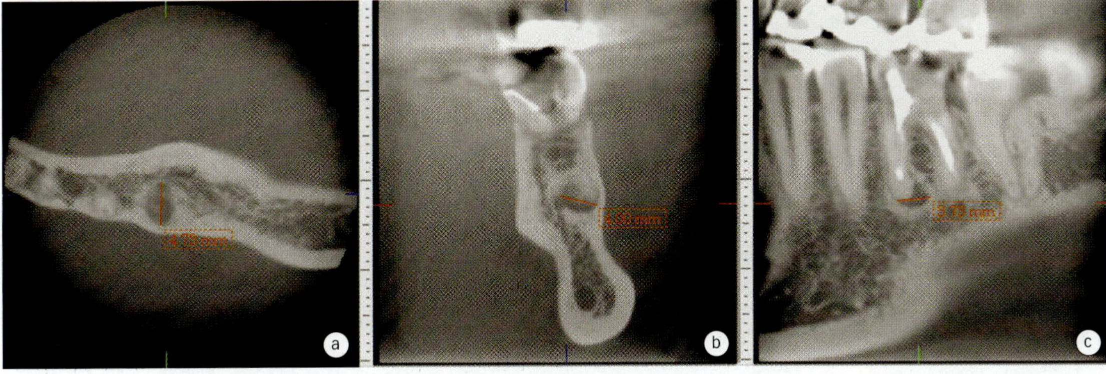


**Figure 5.13** - Clinical case of mandible molar showing the axial (**A**), sagital (**B**) and coronal (**C**) planes. The CBCTPAI was determined by the largest extension of the lesion.

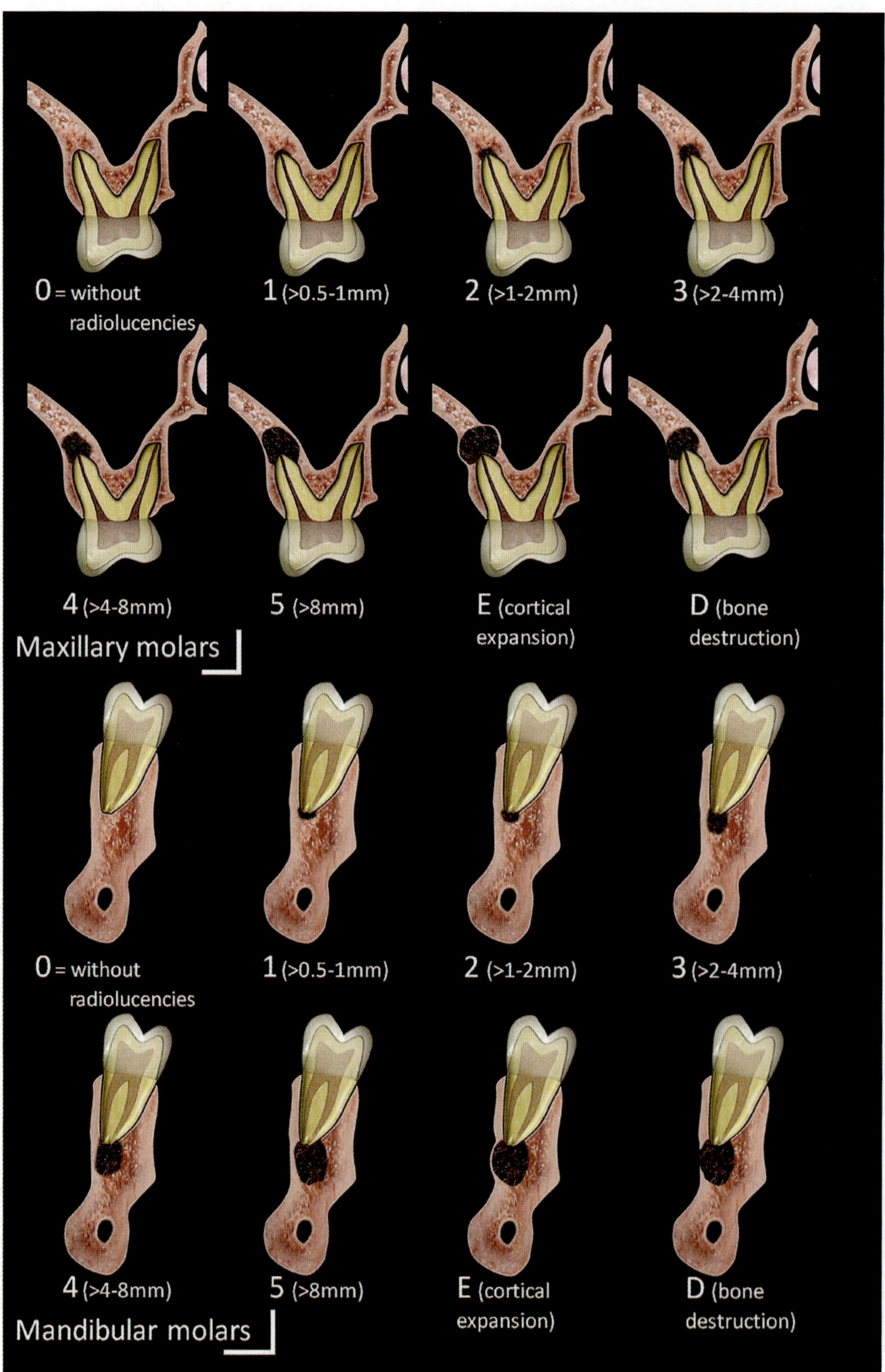


**Figure 5.14** - Schematic representation of molars CBCTPAI.

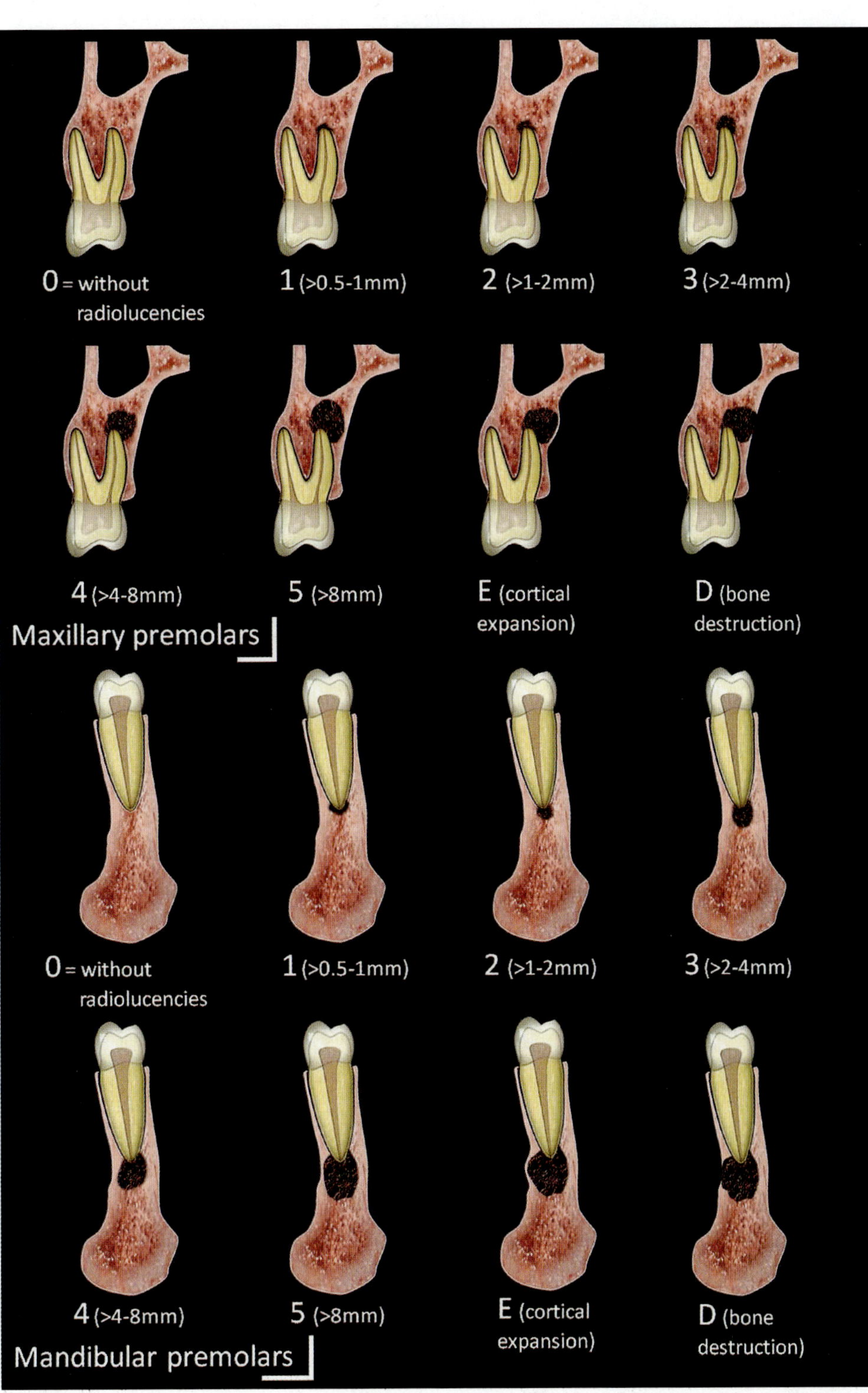


**Figure 5.15** - Schematic representation of premolars CBCTPAI.

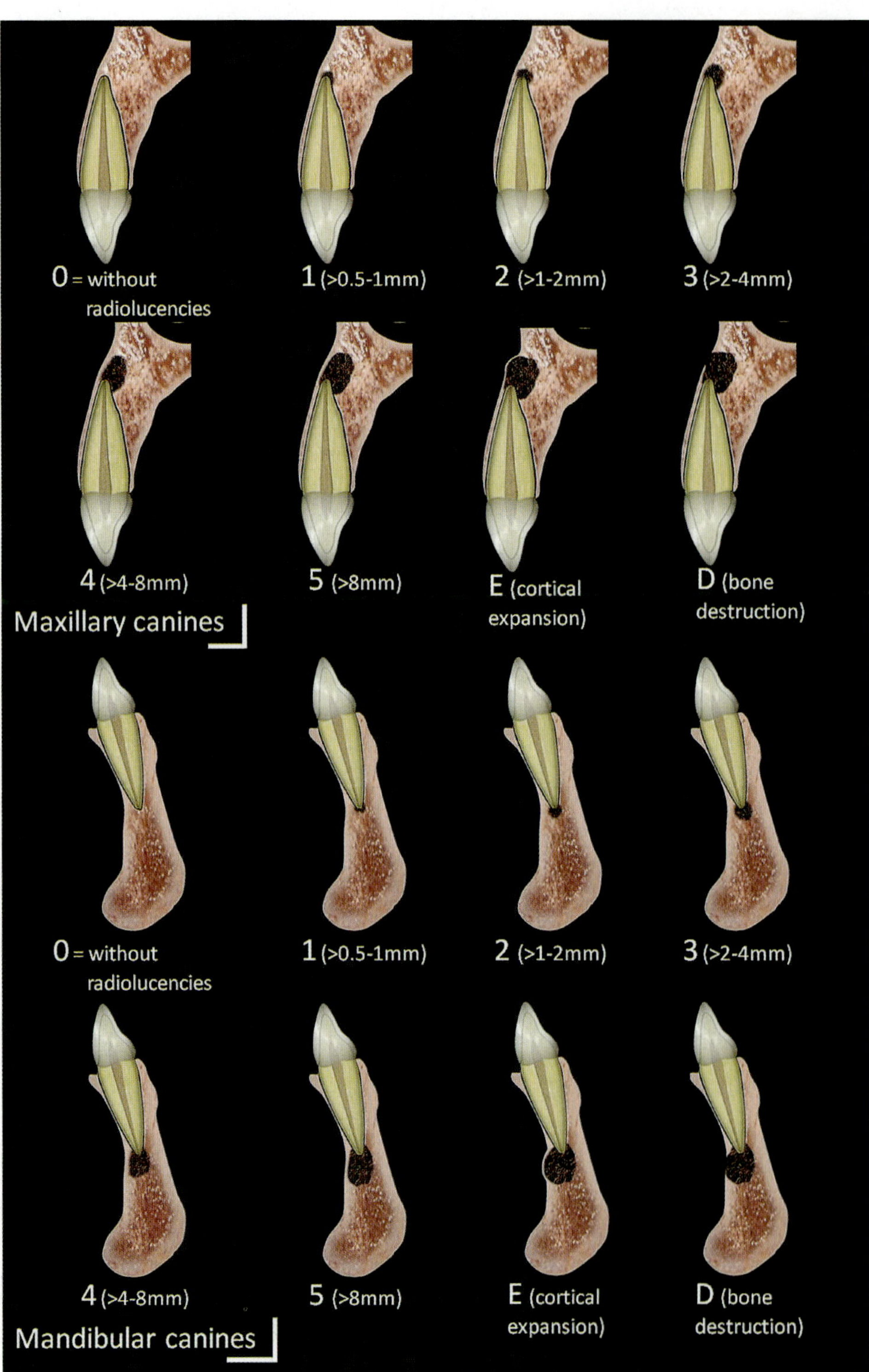


**Figure 5.16** - Schematic representation of canines CBCTPAI.

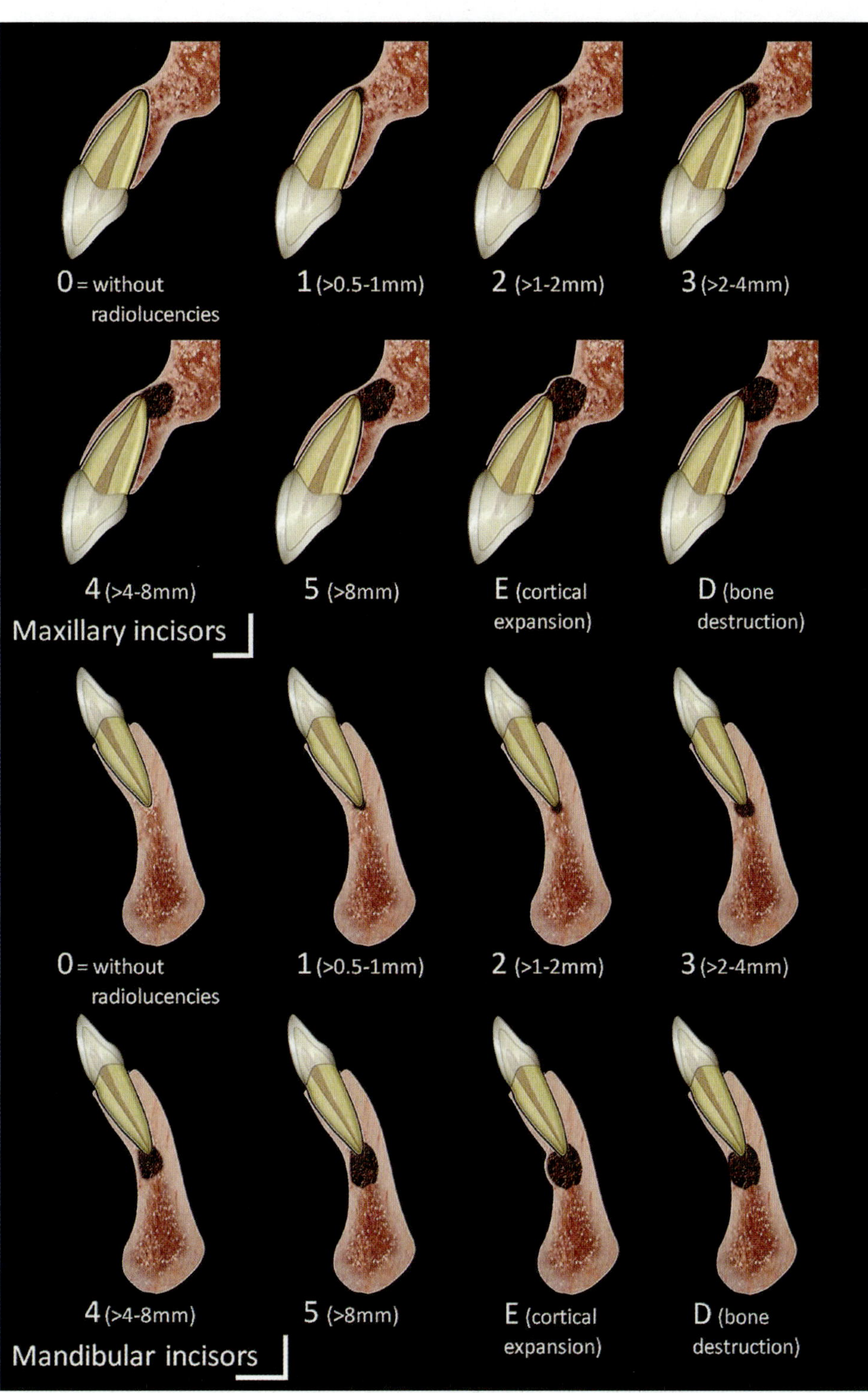


**Figure 5.17** - Schematic representation of incisors CBCTPAI.

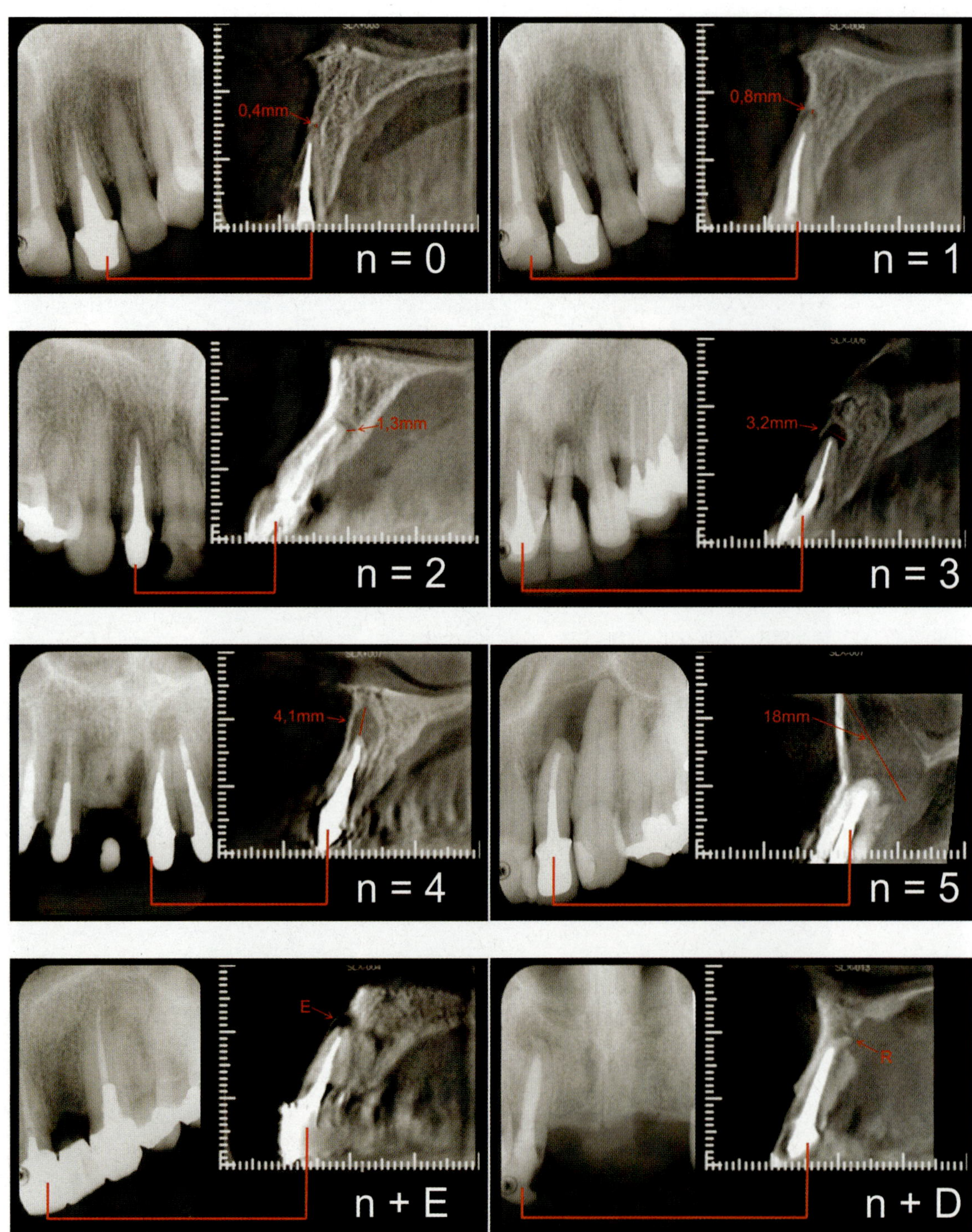


**Figure 5.18** - Clinical cases of maxillary incisors to CBCTPAI showing all the scale with two variables (expansion of cortical bone and destruction of cortical bone).

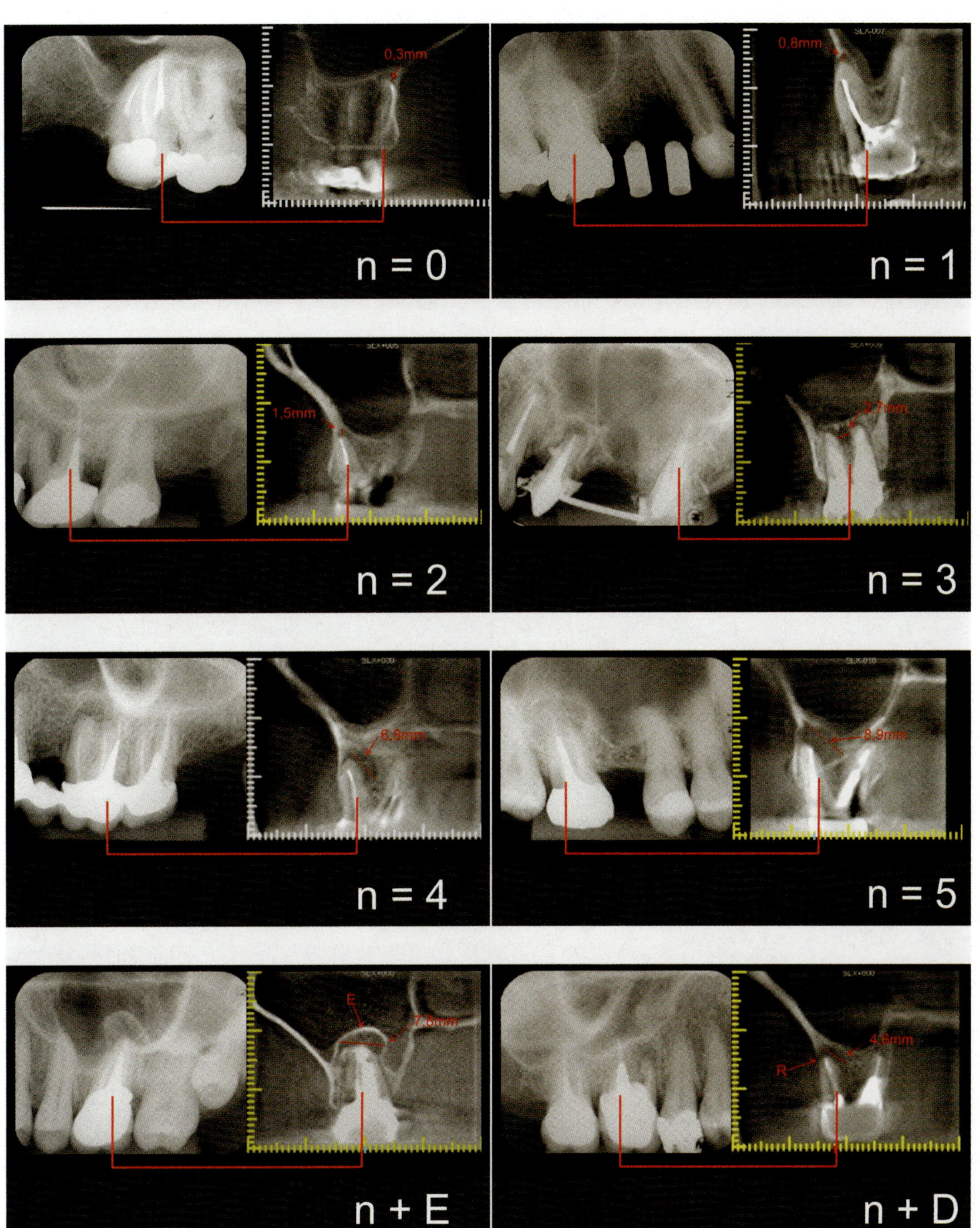


**Figure 5.19** - Clinical cases of maxillary molars to CBCTPAI showing all the scale with two variables (expansion of cortical bone and destruction of cortical bone).

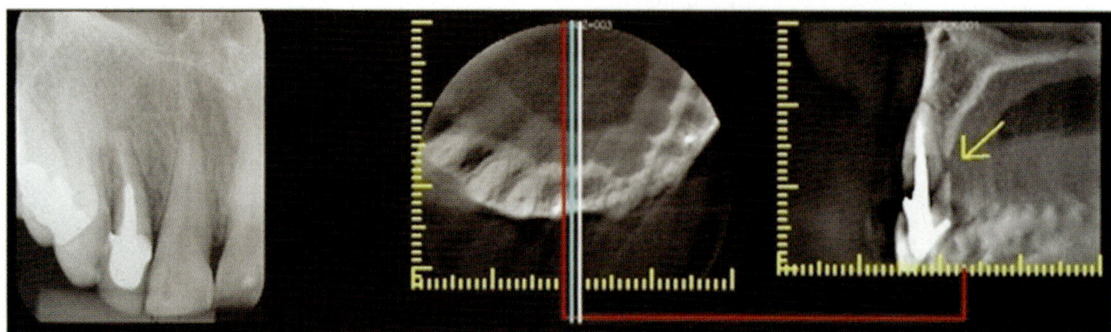

**Figure 5.20** - Periapical Radiography: Radiographic aspect of tooth #12 with mild bone rarefaction in the mesial root, and radiographic absence of traces of fracture. Tomography: Oblique fracture line with separation of fragments.

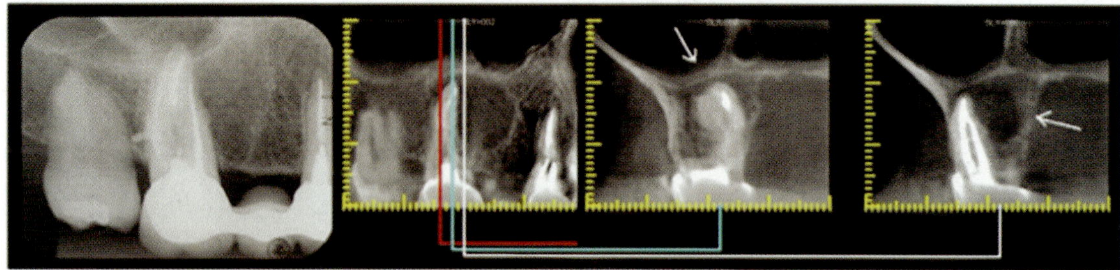

**Figure 5.21** - Periapical Radiography: Discrete change in the trabecular pattern in the mesial portion of the mesio buccal root of tooth #17. Tomography: Extensive periapical bone rarefaction in tooth #17.

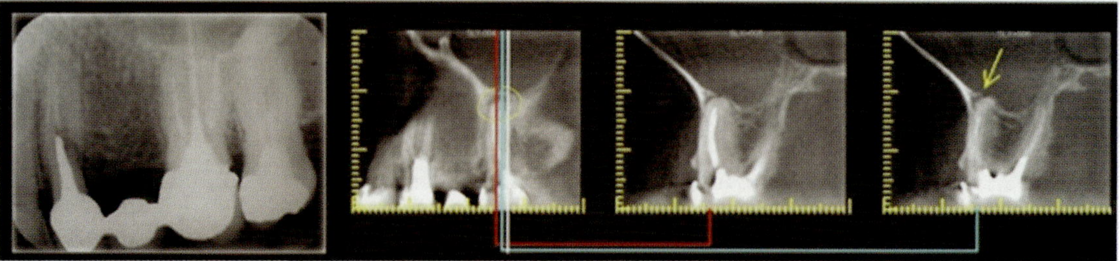

**Figure 5.22** - Periapical Radiography: Does not present evidence of apical periodontitis in buccal roots of tooth #27. Tomography: Presence of apical periodontitis in mesiobuccal root of tooth #27, with disruption of the maxillary sinus floor.

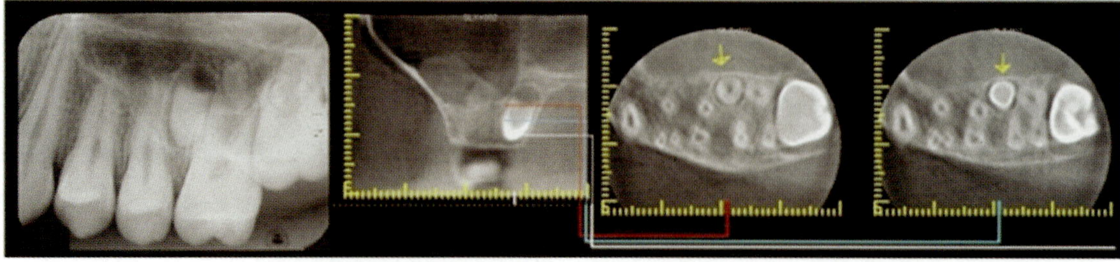

**Figure 5.23** - Periapical Radiography: Presence of supernumerary element between teeth #25 and #26. Tomography: Space evaluation of the supernumerary element in the alveolar ridge and the relationship of proximity to the roots of the neighboring teeth.

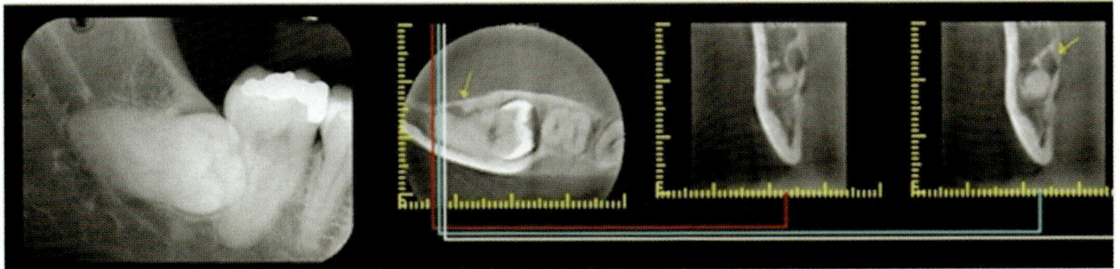

**Figure 5.24** - Periapical Radiography: Tooth #48 included, with apex overlaid by the mandible canal. Tomography: Mandible canal lingually positioned, on the side and above the curved root of tooth #48.

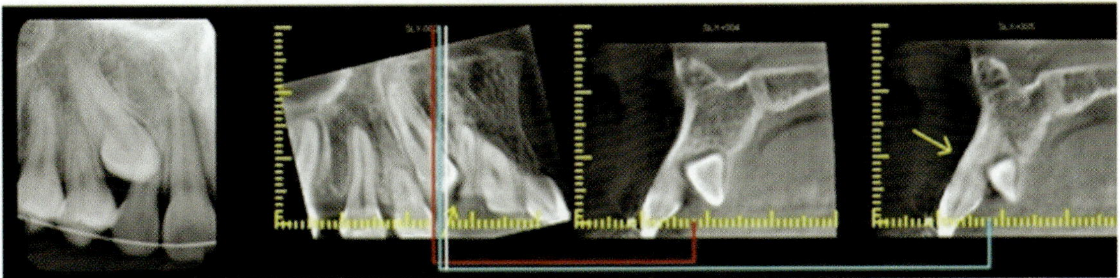

**Figure 5.25** - Periapical Radiography: Tooth #13 retained and impacted in a mesial position, overlaid on tooth #12. It is not possible to assess the presence of reabsorptions in this image. Tomography: Tooth #6 located in palatine direction in relation to tooth #13. Tooth #13 with root resorptions.

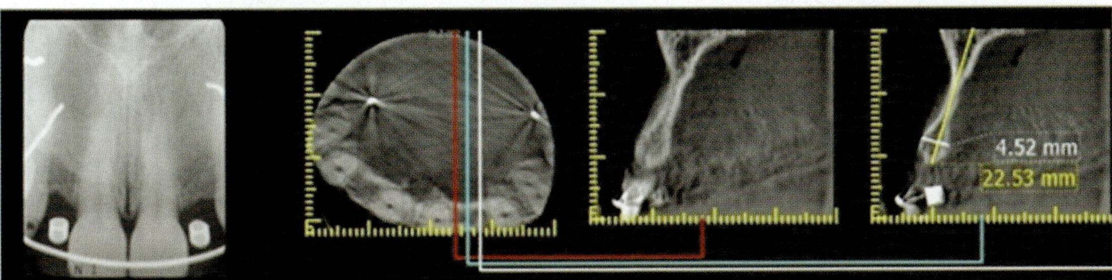


**Figure 5.26** - Periapical Radiography: Absence of lateral maxillary incisors. Tomography: The lower portion of the ridge with sufficient thickness for implant placement. Middle portion of the alveolar ridge with insufficient thickness. Bone graft required.

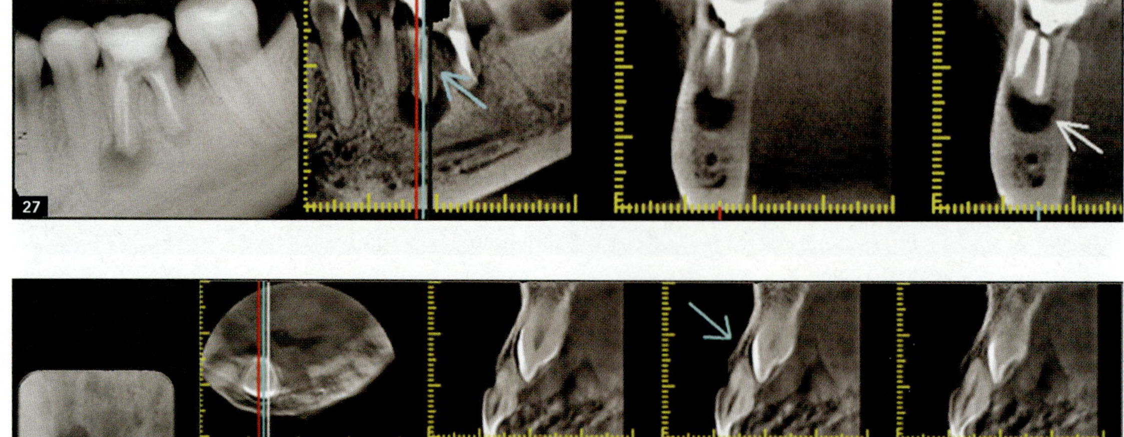

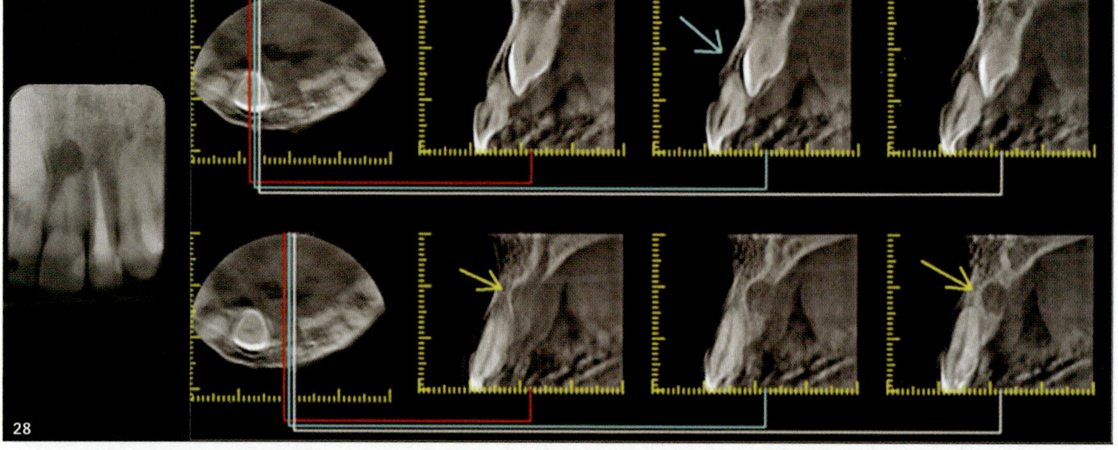

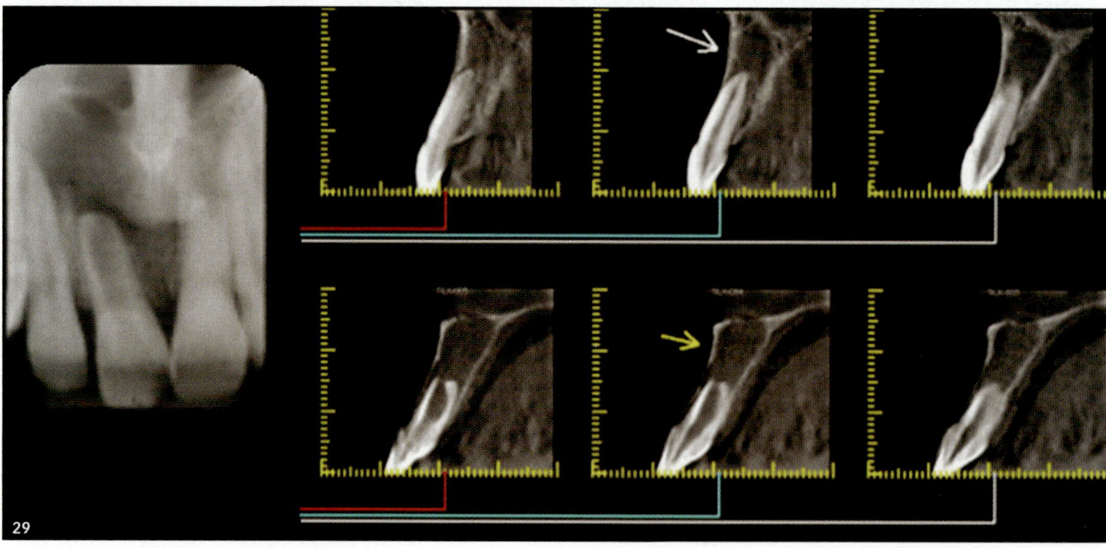

**Figures 5.27 to 5.29** - The precision of CBCT to identify AP compared with periapical radiographs from endodontic and non-endodontic origin.

## References


1. Arai Y, Honda K, Iwai K, Shinoda K. Practical model "3DX" of limited cone-beam X-ray CT for dental use. In: Lemke HU, Vannier MW, Inamura K, Farman AG, Doi K, editors. Computer assisted radiology and surgery. Amsterdam: Elsevier; 2001. p.713-18.
2. Araki K, Maki K, Seki K, et al. Characteristics of a newly developed dentomaxillofacial X-ray cone beam CT scanner (CB MercuRay): system configuration and physical properties. Dentomaxillofac Radiol 2004;33:51-9.
3. Arai Y, Tammisalo E, Iwai K, Hashimoto K, Shinoda K. Development of a compact computed tomographic apparatus for dental use. Dentomaxillofac Radiol 1999;28:245-8.
4. Arai Y, Tammisalo E, Iwai K, Hashimoto K, Shinoda K. Development of Ortho Cubic Super High Resolution CT (Ortho-CT). Car'98 Computed Assisted Radiolo Surg 1998;8:780-5.
5. Baba R, Ueda K, Okabe M. Using a flat panel detector in high resolution cone beam CT for dental imaging. Dentomaxillofac Radiol 2004;33:285-90.
6. Bender IB. Factors influencing the radiographic appearance of bony lesions. J Endod 1982,8:161-70.
7. Bender IB, Seltzer S. Roentgenographic and direct observation of experimental lesions in bone I. J Amer Dent Ass1961;62:152-60(a).
8. Bender IB, Seltzer S. Roentgenographic and direct observation of experimental lesions in bone II. J Amer Dent Ass1961;62:708-16(b).
9. Bjerklin K, Ericson S. How a computerized tomography examination changed the treatment plans of 80 children with retained and ectopically positioned maxillary canines. Angle Orthod Appleton 2006;76:43-51.
10. Brooks SL. Computed tomography. Dent Clin North Am Dent 1993;37:575-90.
11. Bueno MR, Estrela C, Azevedo BC, Brugnera-Jr. A, Azevedo JR. Tomografia computadorizada Cone Beam: Revolução na odontologia. Rev Ass Paul Cir Dent 2007;61:325-8.
12. Cevidanes LH et al. Superimposition of 3D cone-beam CT models of orthognathic surgery patients. Dentomaxillofac Radiol 2005;34:369-75.
13. Cotti E, Campisi G. Advanced radiographic techniques for the detection of lesions in bone. Endodontic Topics 2004;7:52-72.
14. Cotton TP, Geisler TM, Holden DT, Schwartz SA, Schindler WG. Endodontic applications of cone-beam volumetric tomography. J Endod 2007;33:1121-32.
15. Danforth RA, Clarke DE. Effective does from radiation absorbed during a panoramic examination with a new generation machine. Oral Surg Oral Med Oral Pathol Oral Radiol Endod 2000;89:236-43.
16. Estrela C, Bueno MR, Azevedo B, Azevedo JR, Pécora JD. A New Periapical Index Based on Cone Beam Computed Tomography. J Endod 2008; 34:1325-31.
17. Estrela C, Bueno MR, Leles CR, Azevedo B, Azevedo JR. Accuracy of cone beam computed tomography and panoramic and periapical radiography for detection of apical periodontitis. J Endod 2008;34:273-9.
18. Estrela C, Bueno MR, Sousa-Neto MD, Pécora JD. Method for determination of root curvature radius using cone beam computed tomography images. Braz Dent J 2008;19:114-8.
19. Estrela C, Leles CR, Hollanda ACB, Moura MS, Pécora JD. Prevalence and risk factors of apical periodontitis in endodontically treated teeth in a selected population of Brazilian adults. Braz Dent J 2008;19: 34-39.
20. Farman AG, Scarfe WC. Development of imaging selection criteria and procedures should precede cephalometric assessment with cone-beam computed tomography. Am J Orthod Dentofacial Orthop 2006;130:257-65.
21. Frederiksen NL. Specialized radiographic techniques. In: Goaz PW, White SC. Oral radiology: principles and interpretation. 3rd ed. St. Louis: Mosby; 1994. p.266-90.
22. Garib D, Raymundo R, Raymundo MV, Raymundo DV, Ferreira SN. Tomografia computadorizada de feixe cônico (cone beam): entendendo este novo método de diagnóstico por imagem com promissora aplicabilidade na Ortodontia. R Dental Press Ortodon Ortop Facial 2007;12:129-38.
23. Gibbs SJ. Effective does equivalent and effective dose: comparison for common projections in oral and maxillofacial radiology. Oral Surg Oral Med Oral Pathol Oral Radiol Endod 2000;90:538-45.
24. Halse A, Molven O, Fristad I. Diagnosing periapical lesions - disagreement and borderline cases. Int Endod J 2002;35:703-9.
25. Hashimoto K, Arai Y, Iwai K, Araki M, Kawashima S, Terakado M. A comparison of a new limited Cone Beam computed tomography machine for dental use with a multidetector row helical CT machine. Oral Surg Oral Med Oral Pathol Oral Radiol Endod 2003;95:371-7.
26. Hatcher DC, Aboudara CL. Diagnosis goes digital. Am J Orthod Dentofacial Orthop 2004;125:512-5.
27. Hilgers ML et al. Accuracy of linear temporomandibular joint measurements with cone beam computed tomography and digital cephalometric radiography. Am J Orthod Dentofacial Orthop 2005;128:803-11.
28. Huumonen S, Ørstavik D. Radiological aspects of apical periodontitis. Endodontic Topics 2002;1:3-25.
29. Hu H, He HD, Foley WD, Fox SH. Four multidetector-row helical CT: image quality and volume coverage speed. Radiology 2000;215:55-62.
30. Katsumata A, Hirukawa A, Noujeim M, Okumura S, Naitoh M, Fujishita M, Ariji E, Langlais RP. Image artifact in dental cone-beam CT. Oral Surg Oral Med Oral Pathol Oral Radiol Endod 2006;101:652-7.
31. Kobayashi K, Shimoda S, Nakagawa Y, Yamamoto A. et al. Accuracy in measurement of distance using limited cone-beam computerized tomography. Int J Oral Maxillofac Implants 2004;19: 228-31.
32. Langlais RP, Langland OE, Nortjé CJ. Decision making in dental radiology. In: Diagnostic imaging of the jaws. Baltimore: Williams & Wilkins; 1995. p. 1-17.

33. Laux M, Abbott PV, Pajarola G, Nair PNR. Apical inflammatory root resorption: a correlative radiographic and histological assessment. Int Endod J 2000;33:483-93.
34. Lofthag-Hansen S, Huumonen S, Gröndahl K, Gröndahl H-S. Limited cone beam CT and intraoral radiography for the diagnosis of periapical pathology. Oral Surg Oral Med Oral Pathol Oral Radiol Endod 2007;103:114-9.
35. Ludlow JB, Davies-Ludlow LE, Brooks SL, Howerton B. Dosimetry of 3 CBTC units for oral and maxillofacial radiology. International Congress of the International Association of Dentomaxillofacial Radiology; 2005.
36. Ludlow JB, Davies-Ludlow LE, Brooks SL. Dosimetry of two extraoral direct digital imaging devices: NewTom Cone Beam CT and Orthophos Plus DS panoramic unit. Dentomaxillofacial Radiology 2003;32:229-34.
37. Ludlow JB. et al. Dosimetry of 3 CBCT devices for oral and maxillofacial radiology: CB Mercuray, NewTom 3G and i-CAT. Dentomaxillofacial Radiology 2006;35:219-26.
38. Ørstavik D, Kerekes K, Eriksen HM. The periapical index: a scoring system for radiographic assessment of apical periodontitis. Endod Dent Traumatol 1986;2:20-4.
39. Maki K, Inou N, Takanishi A, Miller AJ. Computer-assisted simulations in orthodontic diagnosis and the application of a new Cone Beam X-ray computed tomography. Orthod Craniofac Res 2003;6:95-101.
40. Marmulla R. et al. Geometric accuracy of the NewTom 9000 Cone Beam CT. Dentomaxillofac Radiol 2005;34:28-31
41. Misch KA, Yi ES, Sarment DP. Accuracy of Cone Beam computed tomography for periodontal defect measurements. J Periodontol 2006;77:1261-66.
42. Mozzo P, Procacci C, Taccoci A, Martini PT, Andreis IA. A new volumetric CT macine for dental imaging based on the cone-beam technique: preliminary results. Eur Radiol 1998;8:1558-64.
43. Nair MK, Nair UP. Digital and advanced imaging in endodontics: a review. J Endod 2007;33:1-6.
44. Nair PNR, Pajarola G, Schroeder HE. Types and incidence of human periapical lesions obtained with extracted teeth. Oral Surg Oral Med Oral Pathol Oral Radiol Endod 1996;81:93-102.
45. Nakata K, Naitoh M, Izumi M, Inamoto K, Ariji E, Nakamura. Effectiveness of dental computed tomography in diagnostic imaging of periradicular lesion of each root of a multirooted tooth: a case report. J Endod 2006 32:583-7.
46. Ngan DC, Kharbanda OP, Geenty JP, Darendeliler MA. Comparison of radiations levels from computed tomography and conventional dental radiographs. Aust Orthod J 2003;19:67-75.
47. Nielsen RB, Alyassin AM, Peters DD, Carnes DL, Lancaster J. Microcomputed tomography: an advanced system for detailed endodontic research. J Endod 1995;21:561-8.
48. Papaiz EG, Carvalho PL. Métodos recentes de diagnóstico através da imagem. In: Freitas, A, Rosa JE, Faria e Souza I. Radiologia odontológica. 4th ed. São Paulo: Artes Médicas; 1998.
49. Parks ET. Computed tomography applications for dentistry. Dent Clin North Am 2000;44:371-94.
50. Patel S, Dawood A. The use of cone beam computed tomography in the management of external cervical resorption lesions. Int Endod J 207:40:730-7.
51. Patel S, Dawood A, Pitt Ford T, Whaites E. The potential applications of cone beam computed tomography in the management of endodontic problems. Int Endod J 2007;40:818-3.
52. Peters OA, Schönenberger K, Laib A. Effects of four NiTi preparation techniques on root canal geometry assessed by micro computed tomography. Int Endod J 2001;34:221-30.
53. Rohlin M, Kullendorff B, Ahlquist M, Henrikson CO, Hollender L, Stenstrom B. Comparison between panoramic and periapical radiography in the diagnosis of periapical bone lesions. Dentomaxillofac Radiol 1989;18:151-5.
54. Rohlin M, Kullendorff B, Ahlqwist M, Stenstrom B. Observer performance in the assessment of periapical pathology: a comparison of panoramic with periapical radiography. Dentomaxillofac Radiol 1991;20:127-31.
55. Scarfe WC, Farman AG, Sukovic P. Clinical applications of Cone-Beam computed tomography in dental practice. J Can Dent Assoc 2006;72:75-80.
56. Simon JHS, Enciso R, Malfaz JM, Rogers R, Bailey-Perry M, Patel A. Differential diagnosis of large periapical lesions using cone-beam computed tomography measurements and biopsy. J Endod 2006;32:833-7.
57. Stavropoulos A, Wenzel A. Accuracy of Cone Beam dental CT, intraoral digital e conventional fi lm radiography for detection of periapical lesions. An ex vivo study in pig jaws. Clin Oral Invest 2007;11:101-6.
58. Stheeman SE, Mileman PA, van't Hof MA, van der Stelt PF. Diagnostic confidence and the accuracy of treatment decisions for radiopaque periapical lesions. Int Endod J 1995;28:121-8.
59. Trope M, Pettigrew J, Petras J, Barnett F, Tronstad L. Differentiation of radicular cyst and granulomas using computerized tomography. Endod Dent Traumatol 1989;5:69-72.
60. Van der Stelt PF. Experimentally produced bone lesions. Oral Surg Oral Med Oral Pathol Oral Radiol Endod 1985;59:306-12.
61. Velvart P, Hecker H, Tillinger G. Detection of the apical lesion and the mandibular canal in conventional radiography and computed tomography. Oral Surg Oral Med Oral Pathol Oral Radiol Endod 2001;92:682-8.
62. von Stechow D, Balto K, Stashenko P, Müller R. Three-dimensional quantitation of periradicular bone destruction by micro-computed tomography. J Endod 2003;29:252-6.
63. Weiger R, Hitzler S, Hermle G, Löst C. Periapical status, quality of root canal fillings and estimated endodontic treatment needs in an urban German population. Endod Dent Traumatol 1997;13:69-74.
64. White SC, Atchison KA, Hewlett ER, Flack VF. Efficacy of FDA guidelines for prescribing radiographs to detect dental and intraosseous conditions. Oral Surg Oral Med Oral Pathol Oral Radiol Endod 1995;80:108-14.
65. Yajima A, Otonari-Yamamoto M, Sano T, Hayakawa Y, Otonari T, Tanabe K, Wakoh M, Mizuta S, Yonezu H, Nakagawa K, Yajima Y. Cone beam CT (CB Throne) applied to dentomaxillofacial region. Bull Tokyo Dent Coll 2006;47:133- 41.

# Inflamed Dental Pulp Diagnosis

**C. Estrela**
*Federal University of Goiás, Goiânia, GO, Brazil*

**R. Holland**
*São Paulo State University, Araçatuba, SP, Brazil*

Chapter contents

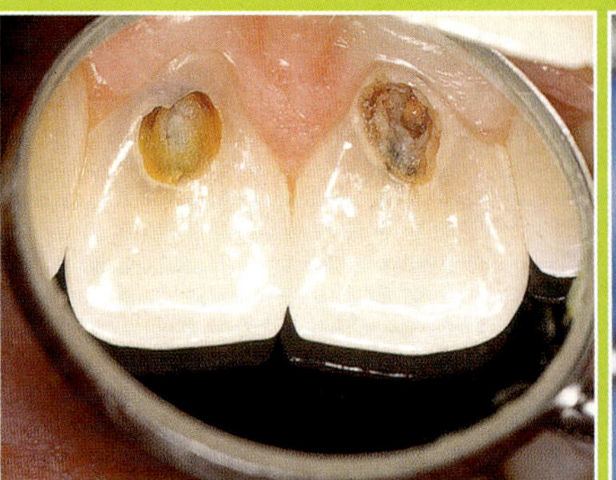

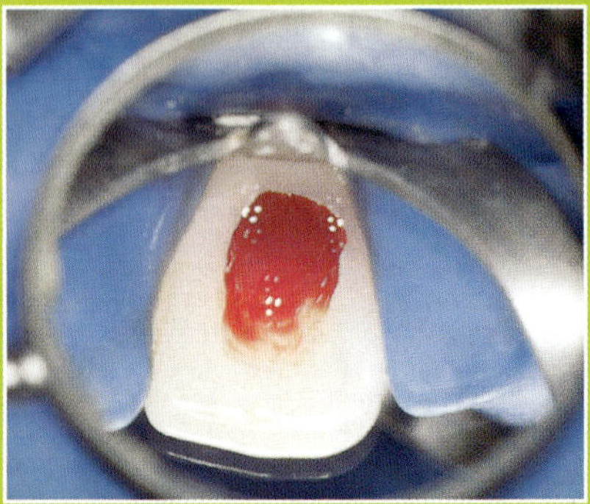

Symptomatic Pulpitis.

## 6.1 Introduction

Cellular and molecular biology investigations have provided significant results in the study of the pulp biology and pathology. The knowledge of factors involved in the etiology of pulp diseases enables a more accurate diagnosis. These factors contribute to increasing the success of conservative treatments of healthy or inflamed dental pulps.

Modern concepts for the reconstruction of dental tissues involve operative procedures, new restorative materials and treatments for traumatic dental injury. These concepts involve many important factors in the study of responses to pulp injury. Thus, during root canal therapy, attention is directed to the dental pulp, since it is the main target of injuries and the source of pain.

The commonest reason why an individual consults a dentist is pulp pain, an unpleasant experience generally due to pulp inflammation. However, systemic therapy alone does not definitively resolve pain, and local intervention is necessary.

Dental pulp is located in the pulp cavity, protected by a mineralized structure (dentin). The inflammatory phenomena results in vascular alterations, such as vasodilation and an increase in permeability. Chemical inflammatory mediators can stimulate pain reception, due to nociceptive nerve endings. The dental pulp has one of the highest internal pressures in the body, and during the inflammatory process, this internal pressure increases. In order to diminish it and relieve pain, the injurious agent needs to be removed, and this usually requires preparation of an access cavity and partial or complete removal of the dental pulp. The inflammatory events that caused this pain in the dental pulp do not differ from the events that occur in other tissues[16].

The general dental practitioner and endodontic specialist frequently diagnose and treat diseases of pulpal origin. The success of this treatment (pulpotomy or pulpectomy) depends on knowledge of the physiology and pathology of the pulpodentin complex, in order to correctly diagnose and treat the pulp tissue alterations.

## 6.2 Dental Pulp Structures

The dental pulp consists of connective tissue similar that in other parts of the body of the same embryonic origin (ectomesenchymal), with identical physiological and pathological reactions. The anatomical location of the pulp tissue alters its physiological reactions that are primarily conditioned by this tissue being surrounded by mineralized dentin. The intimate relationship between the odontoblasts, cells present at the pulp surface, which are responsible for dentin formation, and the dentin can be referred to as the pulpodentin complex. As the pulp is protected by mineralized tissue, it has a limited capacity to increase in volume or to expand during vasodilation.

Among the structural components of the dental pulp, are: progenitor cells (fibroblast, odontoblast, and undifferentiated mesenchymal cells), defense cells (lymphocytes, plasmocytes and macrophages), amorphous interstitial substance (proteoglycans and glycoprotein) and fibrous interstitial substance (collagen fibers).

It should be noted that the progenitor cells are capable of synthesis and differentiation. Fibroblasts are effective in synthesizing collagen and some glycoproteins, mainly fibronectin. The fibronectin is present in high concentrations in the extracellular matrix, blood vessel walls and basal membranes, as it is responsible for cellular adhesion. The chemical components of the amorphous fundamental substance involve a complex of carbohydrates and proteins (mucopolysaccharide) and glycosaminoglycans (glycoprotein)[75,90]. There are two types of mucopolysaccharides in the dental pulp: a non-sulfated type, the commonest being hyaluronic acid (acid mucopolysaccharide); and the sulfated type, chondroitin sulfuric acid. Hyaluronic acid, which is hydrophobic, varies from a slightly viscous liquid to a gelatinous form. The mucopolysaccharide molecules are highly polymerized (firmly united), allowing a viscous consistency. Any change in the nature or quality of the fundamental substance (in the polymerization state) directly influences the spread of inflammation and infection. The viscous fundamental substance acts as a barrier against the spread of microorganisms and toxic products. These can spread due to hyaluronidase, an enzyme that acts to dissolve the substance and enables faster invasion[65,75,86,90].

The fibroblasts are located mainly in the cell-rich zone and are found equally in the coronal and root pulp. The odontoblasts are differentiated cells responsible for dentin formation. They present a direct extension of the cell body, called an odontoblastic process, which occupies most of the dentinal tubules. Stanley[94] considers the odontoblast a post-mitotic cell, without the capacity to divide (they do not undergo terminal mitosis). Seltzer & Bender[85] reported that morphologic variations are common in odontoblasts: in the crown of the tooth they are high columnar cells, halfway along the root they are low columnar; and in the root portion they are shorter and cuboidal. At the apex, odontoblasts become flat and seem like fibroblasts. In the coronal pulp, odontoblasts are more columnar and they produce dentin in the tubules; in the middle third, the tubules are fewer in number and less regular; while, in the apical third they are less differentiated and the dentin is less tubular and more amorphous. The undifferentiated mesenchymal cells are capable of differentiating into odontoblasts and fibroblasts and are located in the central cell-rich zone. The odontoblasts are physically close together and communicate through numerous junctional complexes. Therefore, when one odontoblast is attacked, others are affected. A cross-section of dentin exposes 30,000 to 75,000 tubules per mm$^2$. Odontoblasts extend their cytoplasmic membranes into the tubules, with the remaining tubule filled by dentinal fluid[90].

The central area of the pulp is composed of undifferentiated mesenchymal cells and fibroblasts, considered reserve cells. In the peripheral area, the sub-odontoblastic layer (Weil's zone) presents a poor population of cells. The arterioles and venules that enter and leave the pulp cavity through the apical foramen and apical ramifications, which are accompanied by nerves, constitute the rich vascular and nervous supply of the dental pulp.

The dental pulp has four recognized functions: formation, nutrition, nervous and defense. The formation function is essential, because there is dentin formation throughout the life of the tooth. Pulp nutrition is provided by the rich vascularization, with nutrients and oxygen entering through the vessels and the removal of tissue metabolites. The nervous function is characterized by the capacity of the pulp to respond to pain from different injuries, through the myelinated and unmyelinated nerve fibers. The defense function can be observed when the pulp defends itself against injuries by forming peritubular dentin, also called dental sclerosis, the first defense barrier against dental caries. The second defense is tertiary dentin formation in the coronal chamber.

Kim[53], studying the microcirculation of healthy and pathological dental pulp, reported that the diameter of the arterioles is 100 µm or less. As the arterioles pass into the coronal pulp, disperse towards the dentin, decrease in size and produce a capillary network that is the source of nutrients to the odontoblasts. The diameter of the venules does not exceed 200 μm. Capillary blood circulation in the coronal portion is approximately 2 times that of the root portion. Among the oral tissues, this blood flow is the largest volume of blood circulation; however, this volume is substantially smaller than that found in the main visceral organs. The intravascular speed of pulp vessels is approximately the same as the flow speed of the typical arterioles and venules of other tissues, between the low flow of skeletal muscles and the high flow of the brain or kidney[100]. The dental pulp has three unique vascular characteristics: arterio-venous anastomoses, venule-venule anastomoses and the arterioles that form a U-turn. As the intrapulp pressure increases (reducing the blood flow) during the inflammatory process, the vessels in anastomoses can open up in an effort reduce the intrapulp pressure and maintain the normal blood flow[53]. It is believed that this system exists to maintain the pulp circulation in the event of certain injuries. The primary function of microcirculation is to transport nutrients and remove the metabolic residues from the tissues[51]. Kramer[54] points out that there is absence of a subodontoblastic capillary plexus in areas of naturally occurring secondary dentin. Bernick[7], observing the difference between the lymphatic drainage of decayed pulps and restored teeth, emphasized that the lymphatic vessels in decayed teeth constitute a medium for removing the inflammatory fluid to reduce the pressure and to resolve the initial inflammation.

The liquid pressure of dental pulp varies, and is considered high when compared with the pressure of other organs. The rhythmic fluctuation in the pulp pressure in response to the heart beat usually happens, and for a certain period of time, the tissue pressure of the pulp can follow the blood pressure. It is noted, however, that local trauma can cause hyperemia, because the trauma does not require initial dilation of the capillaries inside the tissue[65,75]. Beveridge & Brown[8] indicated that in punctures in the crown and close to the pulp surface, the intrapulp pressure was around 10 mmHg, a value found among the means of critical areas, such as the cerebrospinal fluid that varies from 5 to 14 mmHg. Van Hassel[101] reported that in moderate inflammation, the intrapulp pressure can reach 13 mmHg (which is considered reversible). When pulp pressure reaches 35 mmHg, the damage caused is irreversible.

It should be stressed that as the intratubular liquid is in communication with the pulp vessels, substances put directly onto the pulp or on dentin diffuse to the interstitial liquid and pass directly into the blood stream.

Pulp innervation follows the path of the blood vessels, being constituted of unmyelinated and myelinated sensory nerve fibers from the trigeminal nerve branches. Of the nerves that enter through the apical foramen, 90% go to the coronal portion and approximately 10% remain in the root portion. Most of the pulp nerves finish in the subodontoblastic plexus (Raschkow's plexus). Nerves leave this plexus and penetrate into the pre-dentin (intratubular nerves with medium course of 100 μm), loop around, and re-enter the plexus[65,75].

Pain in the pulp results from the inflammatory response. The vascular alterations of the inflammatory process are manifested in different ways: vasodilation, an increase in vascular permeability and the release of chemical mediators, capable of maintaining inflammation and stimulating pain. Among the agents that produce pain is bradykinin. These agents stimulate the C fibers (non-myelinated, peripheral nociceptives). The cellular body of the neuron contains synthesized neurotransmitters (neuropeptides). In association with tissue injuries or stimulus of the neuron, these neurotransmitters are released and can affect vasodilation, increase vascular permeability and transmit pain sensation. In the presence of stimulus, the nerve fibers release neuropeptides and produce a neurogenic inflammatory reaction. The main neuropeptides are: P substance, A neurokinin and K neuropeptides, as well as the calcitonin gene-related peptide (CGRP). Pulp pain is considered a deep visceral somatic pain[34,65,70,75,98,99].

Närhi[70] reported that irrespective of the type of stimulus applied to the tooth, pain is the only sensation induced in response to activation of the pulpal sensory nerves. "*The functional properties of the two pulp nerve fiber groups may explain the changes in the quality of pain symptoms during pulpitis: from rather sharp or shooting and quite well localized, to dull and lingering. The type and duration of the symptoms in patients with pulpal inflammation are of diagnostic value and may give some indication of the pulp condition. It must be underlined again that the correlation between the symptoms and histopathological changes in pulpitis is poor and determination of the type and extent of the inflammatory changes on the basis of the symptomology is inaccurate*".

## 6.3 Etiological Factors of Pulp Alterations

The pulpodentin complex reaction to injury can be observed in several ways, depending on the type and the intensity. The pulp response associated with pain is usually due to the inflammatory process.

Table 6.1 relates the main etiological and physiologic factors of pulp alterations.

The alterations of the pulpodentin complex in response to different injuries (microbial, physical, chemical and other), determine the various degrees of response. The dental pulp attempts to block these injurious agents through: dentinal sclerosis, formation of tertiary dentin and pulp inflammation.

One of the most important agents injurious to dental pulp is dental caries, caused by oral microorganisms. Dental caries is considered an infectious and contagious disease, characterized by degradation of the dentin/dental minerals. Caries originates as a result of organic acids from the metabolism of carbohydrates by oral bacteria denaturing dentin collagen, and selecting other microorganisms that are capable of surviving and growing in acidic conditions, and also metabolize denatured collagen. Therefore, specific microorganisms and cariogenic diet represent important and indispensable factors in the etiology of the dental caries process[58].

**Table 6.1** - Etiological factors of pulp alterations

| **Etiological Factors** | | |
|---|---|---|
| 1. Bacterial | • Toxins and enzymes of microorganisms associated with dental caries | |
| 2. Physical | • Mechanical<br>• Iatrogenics<br>• Pathological<br>• Thermal | • Crown fractures<br>• Cavity opening<br>• Attrition, abrasion, erosion, periodontal scaling<br>• Heat due to cavity preparation or restorative materials |
| 3. Chemical | • Agents of the adhesive system (primers), materials originating from resin restorations<br>• Chemical irrigators used to wash the pulp tissue | |
| 4. Physiological Factors | • Dimensional alterations of the pulp cavity (dentin tubule diameter, dentinal sclerosis, dead tracts) | |
| 5. Aging | • Structural alterations of the dental pulp (cells, fibers, vascularization and innervation, calcification) | |

Orland[74], using germ free animals in an experimental study of dental caries, studied the emergence of dental caries based on the presence of microorganisms. Some of the germ-free mice did not develop dental caries when fed a cariogenic diet for 90 days. However, animals with oral microorganisms, which received the same diet, developed dental caries.

Among the main microorganisms that lead to the onset of dental caries are *Streptococcus mutans*, *Lactobacilos sp.* and *Actinomyces sp.*

Some observations based on studies using laboratory animals suggest that *S. mutans* can be involved in the initiation of the carious lesion, while caries progression depends on *Lactobacilos sp. S. mutans* is capable of synthesizing extracellular polysaccharides from saccharose, which is responsible for the mechanism of adhesion that guarantees the fixation of microorganisms to the dental structures. Another function of *S. mutans* is the capacity to produce intracellular polysaccharides that serve as a reserve substratum, that will enable the production of acid in periods where nutrients are not available[58,97]. Furthermore, toxic substances are able to diffuse through the dentinal tubules. The extension of the pulp irritation is characterized by the depth of toxin penetration into the dentinal tubules.

Estrela[25] identified *Streptococcus mutans*, *Enterococcus faecalis*, *Porphyromonas gingivalis* and *Prevotella intermedia* and determined their prevalence in 30 patients with chronic periodontitis. Samples of saliva and plaque from different buccal tissues: tongue dorsum, buccal mucosa, supragingival and subgingival plaques, were collected. After DNA extraction, the samples were analyzed using multiplex PCR. The results indicated the prevalence of *S. mutans* in 70% of the saliva samples (Fig. 6.1); 60% of the samples collected from the tongue dorsum; 50% of the samples collected on the buccal mucosa; 56.66% in the supragingival plaques and 53.33% in the subgingival plaques. The prevalence of *E. faecalis* was 3.33% in the saliva samples; 13.33% in the samples collected from the tongue dorsum; 3.33% in the samples collected on the buccal mucosa; 6.66% in the supragingival plaque and 6.66% in the subgingival plaque. *P. gingivalis* presented in 23.33% of the saliva samples and samples collected on the tongue dorsum; 30% of the samples collected on the buccal mucosa; 40% in the supragingival plaque and 53.33% in the subgingival plaque. For *P. intermedia*, a prevalence of 23.33% was observed in the saliva samples; 33.33% in the samples collected from the tongue dorsum; 26.66% in the samples collected on the buccal mucosa; 33.33% in the supragingival plaque and 30% in the subgingival plaques. All of the microorganisms analyzed in this study were identified in the patients with chronic periodontitis, in saliva and in the other sample collection sites. *S. mutans* showed a higher prevalence in all the microenvironments. There was no statistically significant difference between saliva and the other sample collection locations.

Estrela et al.[18] studied the prevalence and risk factors of pulpal and periapical pain. A cross-section study was carried out evaluating patients who had experience of pulpal or periapical pain associated to inflammation and/or infection and to search treatment in the Faculty of Dentistry (Urgency Dental Service, Federal University of Goiás, GO, Brazil), during the years of 2005 and 2006. The sample consisted of 1,765 patients (675 male, 1090 female) with history of endodontic pain without dental trauma. The higher prevalence of odontogenic pain was symptomatic pulpitis and symptomatic apical periodontitis of infectious origin. The risk factor for pulpal pain of more expression was caries lesion, and for periapical pain was open cavity.

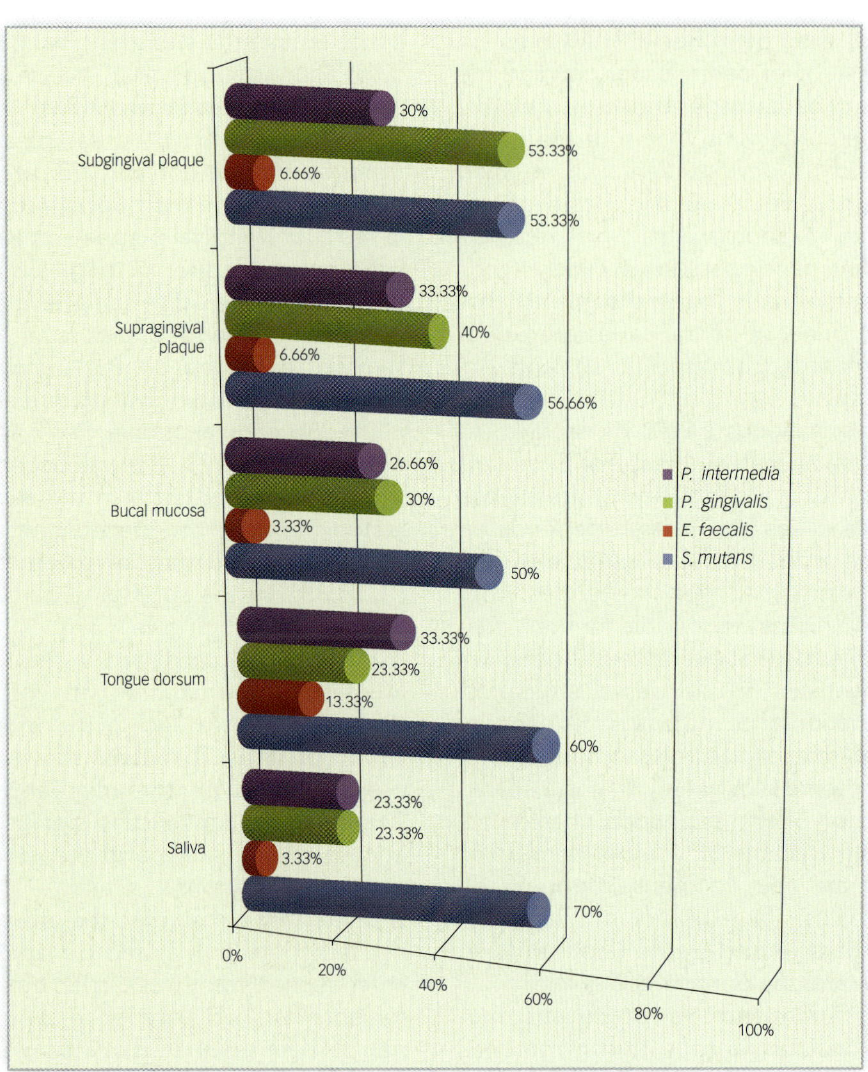


**Figure 6.1** - Prevalence of *S. mutans*, *E. faecalis*, *P. gingivalis* and *P. intermedia* in different buccal microenvironments as determined by using Multiplex PCR[25].

In this relationship of attack and defense, the dental pulp is able to react to reduce the effect of microbial toxins by reducing dentinal permeability through dentinal sclerosis, or by filling the tubules with calcium ions (apatite)[92]. Another attempt to obstruct the progress of dental caries is the formation of tertiary dentin in the coronal chamber, at the same rate as that of primary dentin destruction.

The progression of dental caries can influence the pulp response. Rapid progression of acute dental caries prematurely exposes pulp, which elicits a response unlike the one to chronic dental caries[100]. Tubules with thick walls are found at the border between primary and tertiary dentin, which was developed with a material similar to that of peritubular dentin, less permeable than normal dentin, to form a barrier against the entry of bacteria and their products[83]. This new dentin is structurally organized with the rhythm of formation, with dentinal tubules that are fewer in number, regularly distributed, and with irregular diameter and length[66,100].

However, when there is rapid progression of dental caries lesions, mainly in young teeth, a more intense aggression to the pulp is observed, destroying the odontoblast projections, allowing increased dentinal permeability and the formation of dead tracts in the dentin. Nevertheless, the pulp can react by depositing tertiary dentin.

Pulp inflammation originating from dental caries presents chronic instead of acute lesion, with low intensity injuries. After the pulp has been invaded by microbes, the characteristics of acute lesion become evident, describing the entire pulp inflammatory process.

Kakehashi et al.[48], studying the effect of mechanical exposure of the dental pulp in conventional laboratory mice (with typical microbiota) and in mice with absence of microorganisms (germ-free), demonstrated that one of the decisive factors for pulp survival is the presence or absence of bacterial irritation. In the group of animals with absence of microorganisms, in spite of the accumulation of foods, there was formation of a mineralized barrier after pulp exposure. While, in the group of mice that lived under in normal laboratory conditions, the presence of pulp necrosis, formation of abscesses and apical granulomas could be observed.

Dental caries bacteria are the etiological agents that more frequently cause injuries to the dental pulp, and are responsible for infecting it and forming periapical lesions. Reeves & Stanley[81], analyzing the correlation of bacterial penetration and pulp pathology of decayed teeth, reported that if the proximity of the dental caries bacteria to the pulp is 1 mm or more, the pathological alterations to the pulp will be insignificant, in terms of inflammatory cell infiltration, congestion, capillary dilation and formation of tertiary dentin. However, the responses are more significant when the proximity to the dental pulp reaches 0.5 mm.

Another important injurious agent of the pulp is cavity opening, heat being outstanding as the agent responsible for the most severe injuries. Factors associated with this aggression are the extent of the cavity preparation and its depth. It is opportune to remember that the dentinal thermal conductivity is low.

Kim[53], analyzing the alterations in dental pulp blood circulation in response to procedures and dental materials, reported that in total crown preparation without cooling in dog' teeth, with 1 mm of remaining dentin, a drastic reduction in the pulp blood flow was verified, and in 1 hour after the end of the preparation, irreversible damage could be observed. However, when water cooling is used, little alteration in the pulp blood flow is noted. Langeland[55], studying the pulp reactions to cavity preparation and dentin heating, reports that in preparations without cooling, irreversible damage to the pulp was observed in 11 seconds, and complete disintegration can occur. The heat and pressure can kill millions of odontoblasts[56].

Dental traumatisms (such as crown fractures) that affect the support and the hard tissues are responsible for extensive inflammation and pulp necrosis.

Restorative materials (temporary or definitive) contribute to pulp injuries. The materials used in prosthesis cementation, such as resinous and zinc phosphate cements, are some of the agents injurious to the pulpodentin complex. Chemical aggression can be observed in the agents that constitute the adhesive systems and in restorations containing resins. The use of these adhesive systems on the pulp tissue caused irreversible injuries, due to their high toxicity. Adhesive system (primers) particles spread into the pulp tissue and were detected inside the macrophages and multinucleated giant cells. They are transported to other locations, and with the death of the macrophages they can bring undesirable consequences, such as the pulp necrosis[9,13-15,35,43,57,66,78].

Within the group of agents injurious to dental pulp, it should be pointed out that there is cumulative injury; initially there are injuries from the action of microorganisms, then as a result of cavity preparation and lastly from the protective and restorative material. The individual's organic conditions (host response) should also be considered. Busato et al.[9], analyzing the biocompatibility of the pulpodentin complex protective materials, related that over the last few years, dentistry has observed the emergence of new restoratives techniques and materials that require accurate longitudinal evaluations before they are considered suitable for routine use by dentists. Among the new formulations, dentin adhesive systems are pointed out. However, one of the criteria for evaluating the result of the restorative treatment is its physical integrity, absence of marginal leakage and the response to biological compatibility with the pulpodentin complex. As the properties of and problems inherent to the use of calcium hydroxide are known and have been demonstrated, its indication as an ideal material for pulp exposures and very deep cavities, followed by the restorative system should be emphasized. Hebling et al.[35] analyzed the pulpodentin complex response to the application of an adhesive system in deep cavities with or without pulp exposure, in experimental periods of 7, 30 and 60 days. Histopathological evaluation demonstrated that the adhesive system All Bond 2 was more irritating to the pulpodentin complex than the materials made of calcium hydroxide, especially when applied directly on the pulp tissue. The adhesive system did not allow the formation of a dentin bridge, and hydropic degeneration of the pulp cells and hyalinization of the interstice associated with the inflammatory reaction of varied intensity persisted until the last experimental period. Holland et al.[43], analyzing the behavior of the dental pulp of dog's teeth after pulp exposure or pulpotomy and direct pulp protection with the system All Bond 2, after 60 days observed that the dental pulps came inflamed or necrosed, the results of the pulpotomy being worse than those of pulp capping. No case of a hard tissue bridge was observed. Faraco & Holland[27] used the histomorphological method to evaluate the response of the pulp of dog teeth submitted to pulp capping with an adhesive system, calcium hydroxide cement and two types of mineral trioxide aggregate. The results showed that the dental pulps capped with the adhesive system were inflamed or necrosed. No case of repair and bridge formation was observed. The pulps capped with calcium hydroxide cement exhibited repair with complete hard tissue bridges in 33.3% of cases, allied to the absence of inflammatory infiltrate in only 20%. Repair with hard tissue bridge formation was noted with the two types of mineral trioxide aggregate.

In view of so much evidence, the use of a technique that has been contraindicated in different well conducted researches, [9,12-14,35,43,57,66,77,78,93,95], to the point of allowing the use of an injurious agent capable of inducing inflammation and pulp necrosis to continue, is not justified[12-14,43].

In a clinical study, Estrela et al.[24] analyzed the prevalence of acute pulpitis and pulp necrosis as regards the use of agents injurious to the pulpodentin complex: dental caries, restorative material and dental trauma. An analysis was made of 380 teeth, considering the cavity characteristics (opened/closed), presence of symptomatology, response to pulp vitality tests and radiographic aspect of the pulp cavity, to establish the probable clinical diagnosis. They considered the etiological agents, injuries to the pulpodentin complex, presence of dental caries, type of the restorative material (amalgam, composite resin, other – metal-plastic restorations, metal-ceramics, cast metal), and dental trauma (among these, crown fractures - involving enamel/shallow cavity; involving enamel and dentin/medium cavity; involving enamel, dentin and pulp/deep cavity). Among the etiological agents, interactive factors, such as: the depth of the cavity (shallow, medium and deep); the presence or absence of protecting material; the dental group (anterior teeth, premolar and molars) and the patient's age (Group I - 12 to 25 years; Group II - 25 to 40 years; Group III - 40 to 60 years) were verified. Subsequent to surveying and tabulating the data, the analysis proceeded, and the following results could be observed: a) in 206 teeth the clinical diagnosis was symptomatic pulpitis, 104 (50.5<%) were linked to restored teeth, 66 teeth (32%) to processes of dental caries and 36 teeth (17.5%) to teeth with crown fractures; b) in 174 teeth with pulp necrosis, 80 teeth (46%) were linked with restored teeth, 73 teeth (42%) with dental caries and 21 teeth (12%) with crown fractures; c) the restorative material that lead to the highest rate of symptomatic pulpitis and pulp necrosis was the resin composite without pulp protection, 76% and 78%, respectively. Figures 6.2 to 6.7 show dental caries as the main etiological factor of pulp inflammation.





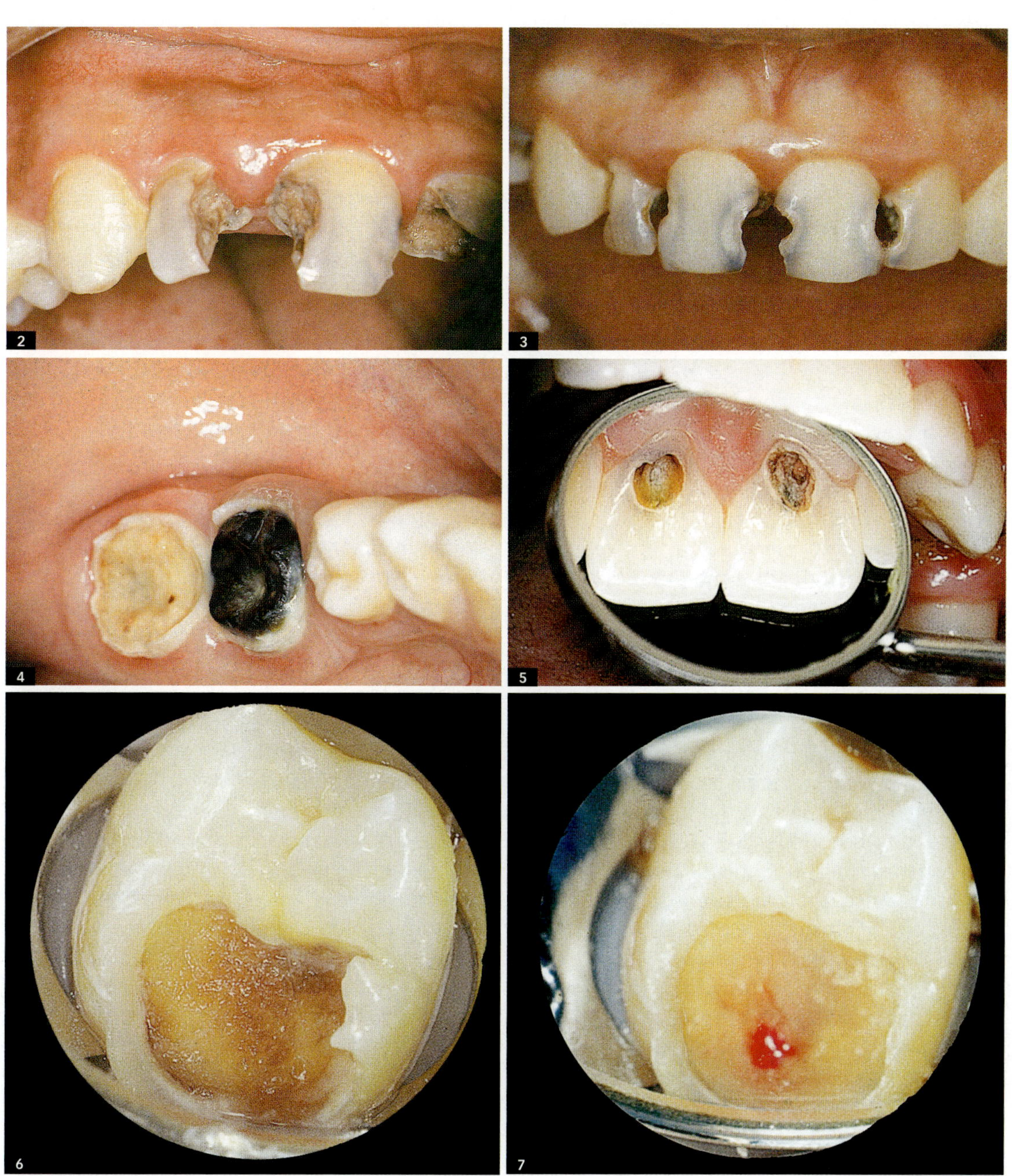


**Figures 6.2 to 6.7** - Etiological factors of pulp inflammation – dental caries.

## 6.4 Pain and Pulp Inflammation

Odontogenic pain is a response that signals tissue alteration with complex sensorial characteristics. The symptom pain links to the somatic structure, and to neuropathic and psychogenic aspects. The individual and special character of the phenomenon pain make it difficult to imagine and to evaluate the subjective context, in which the experimental and personal meaning of pain stands out, the intensity of which varies from a simple discomfort to an incommensurable suffering.

Odontogenic pain can be defined as the result of stimulation of specialized nerve endings capable of producing an uncomfortable experience, variable in intensity and extent, which represents a significant alert and protection mechanism[6].

The international association for the study of pain, according to Merskey[64], refers to pain as an unpleasant sensorial and emotional experience, associated with real or potential harm to the tissue, or still described in terms of such damages. Historically, several concepts were attributed to pain, in which there was an attempt to place value, not only on the biological factors, but the emotional and the affective factors as well[62].

Okeson[72] states that although pain is recognized as being more of an experience than a sensation, it presents a sensorial dimension that records the nature of the stimulus, involving quality, intensity, location and duration. It also includes other dimensions: cognitive (understanding the meaning of the experience), emotional (generated feelings) and motivational (initiative to exterminate it). In this sense, pain represents a subjective psychological state more than an activity induced only by noxious stimulus. Thus, pain and the lesion can be coincident only when attention is addressed to the lesion.

Frequently, the professional is asked to solve problems that affect the oral cavity, especially evidenced by pain, and a significant percentage of the problems originate from factors involving the inflammatory process (related to alterations in the pulpodentin complex, periodontal tissues, dental trauma, oral mucosa, occlusal dysfunctions and other complications).

Many studies[1-104] have endeavored to investigate the different mechanisms involved in the phenomenon of pain, considering the most varied parameters.

Furthermore, considering the breadth and complexity of the theme, the aim at this time is to present and discuss the factors that are most commonly related to pain of endodontic origin, for which it is necessary to establish the perfect diagnosis and safe and immediate treatment.

### Nerve structures

The primordial function of the nervous system is to process the information it receives, in order to provide the appropriate responses. The nervous system has an integrator function, and it emphasizes the role of the synapses (point of connection between one neuron and the next) in controlling the transmission of signals[34]. Essential areas can be mentioned, such as the core of the spinal cord, reticular formation, thalamus, hypothalamus, limbic structures and the cortex. The thalamus monitors the communications among the encephalic trunk, cerebellum and brain. As the pulses arrive in the thalamus they are appraised and addressed to the appropriate areas for the purpose of objective interpretation and response[73].

Over the last few years, several changes have observed as regards the neurophysiology of pain (a sensation transmitted by the peripheral and central nervous system until it is finally interpreted by the cortex)[12].

The brain has specific characteristics at each of the functional levels: spinal medulla (protecting reflexes), limbic structures around the superior portion of the medulla (emotions and instinctive initiatives, control of balance) and the cerebral cortex (capacity to reason and process thought)[33,72].

The cortex is where pain is noted, as a result of an accumulated pulse. The presence or absence of the nociceptive stimulus is not always entirely related to pain. It is at this level that the meaning and the consequence of pain is understood[33,72].

The nervous system is divided into: the peripheral nervous system (responsible for dealing with information of the musculoskeletal and cutaneous structures), the autonomous nervous system (responsible for regulating the blood flow, breathing and digestion), and is subdivided into the sympathetic and parasympathetic and the central nervous system (main controlling system, composed of the cerebral peduncle and cortex - considered the cerebral computer)[33].

The somatic nerve impulses that originate in the oral structures do not enter the spinal medulla through the spinal nerves, but are transmitted by the trigeminal nerve, and the cell bodies of the afferent neurons are located in the trigeminal ganglion. The pulses transmitted by the trigeminal nerve enter directly into the encephalic trunk and synapse with the trigeminal spinal core.

The trigeminal nerve (largest cranial nerve, V pair) is constituted of mixed, sensorial and motor somatic nerves, being composed of thick branches, the ophthalmic nerve, maxillary nerve and mandibular nerve. Figure 6.8 shows a schematic representation of the trigeminal nerve ramifications.

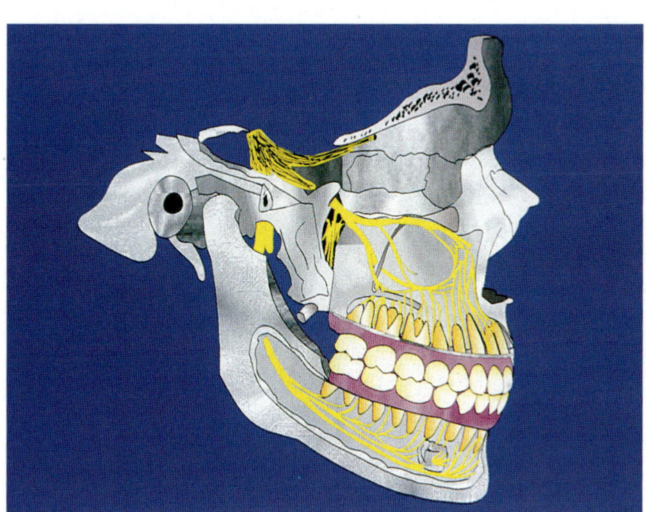

**Figure 6.8** - Schematic representation of the trigeminal nerve ramifications.

## 6.5 Odontogenic Pain

Odontogenic pain starts in the peripheral nervous system. A tissue lesion that causes inflammatory response induces the release of chemical substances (prostaglandins and bradykinin - they increase the local vasodilation and the vascular permeability) that stimulate pain receptors (peripheral nociceptors). The alteration in sensitivity and receptivity promotes depression of the pain threshold, making the nociceptors and mechanoceptors more sensitive to uncounted stimulus (hyperalgesia). The primary afferent nociceptors are constituted of δ-delta fibers (myelinics) and C fibers (amyelinics)[3,47]. The δ-delta fiber responds to mechanical stimulation[3]. These fibers transmit the nerve impulses, which transmit them to the second order neurons that are modulated and projected in specialized areas (thalamus, cerebral cortex), to evidence pain to the cerebral cortex[47].

The tooth is constituted of a visceral tissue (dental pulp), contained inside a cavity composed of mineralized tissue and maintained in the dental alveolus by the periodontal tissue (that works as a musculoskeletal structure). The sensorial responses at pulp and periodontal level have visceral and musculoskeletal characteristics. Pain of odontogenic origin, based on the classification proposed by Bell[6], has characteristics that allow the origin tissue to be identified. Dental pain is a somatic pain (it involves noxious stimulus and a compatible response). In addition to being somatic, it is reported to be deep, because it originates in internal structures. Deep somatic pain can also be subdivided into visceral pain (that arises in blood vessels, glands, gastrointestinal tract, organs and dental pulp) and musculoskeletal pain (that arises in bones, joints, muscles and the periodontal ligament - biomechanics functions). In addition to the somatic pain, neuropathic pain is observed (morphologically altered nerve tissue - trigeminal neuralgia) and the psychogenic pain.

There are many characteristics involved in the pain process, such as: acute pain, chronic pain, clinical pain, experimental pain, primary pain, secondary pain, provoked pain, spontaneous pain, somatic pain, neuropathic pain, superficial pain, deep pain, visceral pain, musculoskeletal pain, inflammatory pain, non-inflammatory pain [6,72].

According to Bell[6], acute pain refers to pains of short duration (related to the somatic tissue alterations at the time of diseases, traumas). Chronic pain is linked to pains of long duration, with different a therapeutic meaning (pain lasting longer than 6 months - pain that continues beyond the normal time of repair).

The terms acute pain (pain of short duration) and chronic pain (pain of long duration) are associated with the time of permanence of the pain process. In pulp and periapical diseases, as the inflammatory nature prevails, they are classified clinically starting from different aspects of pain, presence or absence of symptoms, biophysical tooth characteristics and responses to the pulp vitality test[16].

The nerve consists of a filamentous structure capable of transmitting chemical and electric stimuli. Some nerve fibers present a layer of greasy nervous tissue (called myelin sheath- medullar sheath or white substance of Schwan). The constrictions are called Ranvier nodules and they occur in the myelinated nerves, about 1mm. The myelin acts as insulation in the nerves, so that the action potential of the transfer impulse is expressed only at the level of the Ranvier nodule. The myelin exacerbates the transport speed of the nerve fiber[34,72].

The nerve fibers are classified as regards diameter and transport speed into A fibers ($\alpha,\beta,\gamma,\delta$), B fibers and C fibers. The A fibers ($\alpha,\beta,\gamma,\delta$) induce tactile and proprioceptive reactions (they supply information to the musculoskeletal structures, relative to the presence, position and movement of the body), but not pain. The A-$\delta$ and C fibers transmit pain, although they are not specifically for pain. The A-$\delta$ myelinic fibers are from 2 to 5 µm in diameter, speed from 12 to 30 m/s, they respond to mechanical and thermal stimulus (pain quickly felt - pinprick sensation, sting); while the C, amyelinic fibers, have smaller diameters, less than 2µm, speed from 0.5 to 2 m/s and they respond to mechanical, thermal and chemical stimulus (slow pain - burn sensation). Only 13% of the nerve fibers that enter the human premolar are myelinated; of these, 93% are A-$\delta$ fibers and the remaining 7% are A-$\beta$ fibers. Of the remaining nerve fibers, 87% that enter the human premolar are the type C fibers[68,69]. Nair[67], analyzing the neural elements of the dental pulp and of the dentin, classified the nerve fibers of mammals showing the type, diameter, speed and function, as shown in Table 6.2.

**Table 6.2** - Classification of the nerve fiber in Mammals

| Type | Diameter | Speed | Function |
|---|---|---|---|
| Aα (A-alpha) | 12-22 μm | 70-120 m/s | motor |
| Aβ (A-beta) | 5-12 μm | 30-70 m/s | sensory |
| Aγ (A-gamut) | 3-6 μm | 15-30 m/s | motor |
| Aδ (A-delta) | 2-5 μm | 12-30 m/s | sensory |
| B | < 3 μm | 3-15 m/s | autonomous pre-ganglion |
| C | < 2 μm | 0.5-2 m/s | sensory (autonomous post-ganglion) |

(Nair[67], 1995)

## Physiological aspects of pain perception

The neuron is the central unit of the nervous system, composed of a cell body and serves for one or more processes. The cell bodies can be located in the spinal cord (gray substance of the central nervous system) and out of the central nervous system (contained in the ganglions). The protoplasmatic processes of the nerve cell body are called dendrites (a ramified process that transmits impulses in the direction of the cell body) and neuraxon (central structure that forms the essential conductive portion of the nerve fiber, being the extension of the cytoplasm of the cell). The neural impulses are led from the dendrites to the neuraxon to the pathway of a membrane potential of action. The potential action links the physiochemical property of the cellular membrane of the neuron. To transport a nerve impulse, one observes that sodium ions penetrate into the neuraxon. The neurons can be denominated afferents (receptors or sensitive - they transmit the nerve impulse of the receptor organs to the central nervous system) and efferents (motor - they transmit the impulse towards periphery to produce the effects). The first sensitive neuron is called a primary neuron (first order); the second or third order neurons are internuncial. These internuncial neurons (or interneurons) are located only in the central nervous system (formed by the encephalon and spinal cord). The nerve impulses are transmitted from one neuron to the other in by synapses that are located inside the gray substance of the central nervous system. The stimulus of the tissues must be transferred into the central nervous system and to the superior centers (encephalic trunk and cortex) to interpret and to evaluate them. When they arrive there, the response is sent in impulses to the spinal medulla and in turn to the periphery, so that the efferent organ performs the desired action[34,72].

Certain stimulus (physical) is converted in nerve impulses through sensorial receptors, among them there are the exteroceptors, interoceptors and propioceptors[72].

The description of the neurophysiological mechanism of pain can summarized, based on the transduction, transmission, modulation and perception processes[29].

The nerve impulses are led from the dendrites to the neuraxon to the pathway of an action potential[33], with alteration in the permeability of the neuron membrane and with the action of the cell sodium-potassium pump. When the nerve fiber comes to rest, the sodium ions with positive (Na+) load are more concentrated in the extracellular tissue than in the cytoplasm of the nerve itself. At the same time, the potassium ions with positive (K+) load are more concentrated in the cytoplasm than in the extracellular matrix. The surface of the cellular membrane is loaded in a slightly negative way (rest state - polarized). Due to unequal ionic concentration, the fibers are polarized, that is, the interior of the membrane becomes negative in comparison with the exterior. The depolarization of the membrane is necessary for the propagation of the nerve impulse along the neuraxon. When the membrane is depolarized (permeable to the sodium ions), a large number of sodium ions are allowed to flow into the interior of the neuraxon. In the face of the release of excitatory neurotransmitters in the synaptic gap, the impulse begins, and is led to the neuraxon. If the chemical agent stays in the synapse, the neuron is more quickly depolarized, which causes sensitization (result of the decrease in the threshold). When a neural signal is transported, the action potential moves along the nerve fiber until it reaches its extremity[72,89].

In the synapses the signs are transmitted from one neuron to the other, being composed of electrical (found in flat and heart muscles) and chemical (nervous system) signals. In the pre-synaptic terminals there are synaptic vesicles (that contain transmitter substances which, when released, inhibit or excite the post-synaptic neuron) and the mitochondria (they supply the adenosine triphosphate - ATP, for the synthesis of new transmitters). In the post-synaptic neuron membrane there are a large number of receptor proteins that are projected into the synaptic gap and also inside the post-synaptic neuron. The part projected into the gap acts as connection area for released neurotransmitters, while the one that extends into the neuron, leads the neurotransmitters that influence the cellular activity. The ions involved with the ionic canal receptors are sodium (the neurotransmitters that open the sodium canals are excitatory), potassium and chloride (opening of the potassium canals and chloride are inhibitory transmitters)[33,72].

The neurotransmitters are neurochemical substances responsible for the transmission of the impulses through the synaptic gap, action of small molecules (fast action - acute response) or larger molecules (slow action - chronic response).

Among the fast acting neurotransmitters (small molecule) with effects on the post-synaptic neurons are: acetylcholine (excitatory effect), norepinephrine (excitatory effect), glutamate (excitatory effect), serotonin (algogenic agent), gamut-aminobutyric acid (inhibitory effect), glycine (inhibitory effect) and dopamine (inhibitory effect). Among the neurotransmitters of larger molecules are the neuropeptides (produced in the ribosomes of the neuronal body and not in the pre-synaptic terminal), lead to the periphery through the axonal flow until their release in the nerve terminal after a tissue aggression[102]. Important neuropeptides that act as neurotransmitters should be emphasized: P substance, A neurokinin, K neuropeptide and the peptide related to the calcitonin gene (CGRP). The P substance acts as an excitatory neurotransmitter for nociceptive impulses, and is also involved in neurogenic inflammatory phenomena; it takes part in the inflammatory process starting from the induction of increased vascular permeability, with plasma extravasation and formation of edema[2,11,103].

Bradykinin constitutes an endogenous polypeptide released as part of the inflammatory reaction, and is characterized as a potent vasodilator. It generates the increase in vascular permeability and acts as algogenic agent capable of exciting all of the types of receptors.

It is emphasized that the primary sensorial neurons that innervate the dental pulp have their cell bodies in the trigeminal ganglion. Some of these cell bodies contain the P substance, which is transported by the terminals, and it is located in the C fibers (non myelinated), affecting the code of pain[2]. Other neuropeptides originating from the ganglion of the trigeminus found in the dental pulp are the peptides related to the calcitonin gene and A neurokinin [2,52].

Pain involves various aspects with respect to its interpretation. The physiological mechanisms for understanding pain are very complex. Melzack & Wall[63] studied an explanation for the mechanism of pain, called the theory of gate control, in the sense of knowing the modulation of pain better. In this sense, it was observed that in three systems of the spinal column the nerve impulses are lead when there is a noxious stimulation of the skin: 1. cells of the gelatinous substance, located in the dorsal cornu; 2. fibers of the dorsal column, that are projected towards the brain; 3. cells of main central transmission, in the dorsal cornu. This theory suggests that the gelatinous substance can modulate the afferent impulses (as a gate control system) before they influence the transmission cells[6].

Thus, the transmission of the nerve impulses could be altered. Later, Wall[103], analyzing the theory of gate control, reported that painful experience is much more complex than the simple mechanism of perception and reaction. The concepts of the theory are valid, although its original presentation cannot be maintained.

Okeson[72] reported that the modulation concept is very important to understand the patient's experience, since the neural impulses are sent to painful centers, the transmission pathway could be altered (increase of the pulse - facilitation; decrease of the pulse - inhibition). With the modulation, it can be explained why in some circumstances there is pain without any apparent cause, and in another lesion no pain is induced.

In another part, there are pain modulation mechanisms: the system of analgesia (endorphin, serotonin) must be related; thus the presence of exciting modulators (anxiety and fear) and inhibiting modulators (serenity, trust, safety)[6].

In view of all the forms of explaining the neurophysiological mechanism of pain, it can be summarized based on the transduction, transmission, modulation and perception processes. Transduction can be characterized by the transformation of noxious incentives to electrical activity in the sensitive nerve endings (activation of the sensitive receptor). Transmission refers to the events that lead the nociceptive impulses to the central nervous system for processing. Modulation consists of control of the transmitter neurons before they reach the cortex, identifying the impulses, and exacerbating or reducing them. Perception occurs when the impulse reaches the thalamus, the limbic structures and the cortex, where the interaction and subjective experience of pain begin[34,70,72,84].

Considering the neurophysiological process of pain, it is observed that in the dental clinic, a factor that triggers off odontogenic pain is the inflammatory process. Thus, the inflammatory response should be understood as a protective factor in which the repair process is sought. In this sense, understanding the most significant events than develop in the inflammatory response, helps one to know about the action of some drugs that favor the control of inflammatory pain[33,34,70,72,84].

## 6.6 Inflammatory Process

Pain of inflammatory origin presents as potent inductors to the action of chemical mediators on the nociceptive receptors, with special prominence of bradykinin, prostaglandin and the neuropeptides. These chemical mediators act jointly to increase local vasodilation and capillary permeability, being capable of altering the sensitivity and stimulation of the sensorial nerve receptors.

In local inflammation, various inflammatory agents are observed, such as bradykinin, histamine, serotonin, prostaglandins, and a host of vasoactive agents released from the cells and tissues. It has been shown that the pulp has higher healing potential. Inflammation is an important protective reaction of the body. Some clinical aspects of inflammation identify phenomena characterized as cardinal signs, among them, the following should be emphasized: pain, rubor, heat, tumor and altered function.

The events of vascular response to injuries do not follow an accurate sequence, as chronologically, they can happen simultaneously, or in an interactive way[26,37].

In this sense, tissue physiology depends on the circulatory process of transport, and compensatory mechanisms (homeostatic) can occur in circulatory alterations. The arterioles (50 μm in diameter), capillary (8 to 10 μm in diameter) and venula are the main microcirculation vessels, and can respond in equal proportion to functional variations of the tissues. The main function of microcirculation is transcapillary exchange, which includes the transport of nutrients and oxygen to the tissues and elimination of the products of the metabolism[26,32,99]. The inflammatory process is a consequence of the alteration in microcirculation caused by tissue injuries, capable of altering blood flow, vascular permeability and establishing the exit of cellular components from the blood.

The movement of vascular fluid in and out of the arterioles, capillaries and venula is governed by the balance among four pressures: 1. hydrostatic vascular pressure; 2. vascular osmotic pressure; 3. hydrostatic tissue pressure; 4. osmotic tissue pressure. These are regulated by exchanges that take place through diffusion, and the combination of filtration and absorption and micropinocytosis. Under conditions of normality, the highest pressure is in the arterial capillary, which favors filtration, while the largest drop is in the venula, which facilitates fluid absorption. The fall in filtration pressure occurs as the blood flows along the capillary, and when it arrives in the veined part, it has a lower value than the osmotic pressure of the plasma[26,32,99].

Starling's Law regulates the balance between filtration pressure and reabsorption. The first forces the fluid out of the vessels, which reduces the pressure at venular level and facilitates the fluid return to circulation, regulated by hydrodynamic forces. The moment proteins leave the vessels, more fluid leaves the tissues and the osmotic tissue pressure increases[26,99].

In acute inflammation the filtration pressure (hydrostatic pressure) of the capillary rises due to vasodilation, while the reabsorption pressure (osmotic pressure), decreases due to the increase in vascular permeability, with more extravasation of proteins and increase in plasmatic exudation being observed[32].

The regulation of the blood flow is controlled by nervous and humoral activity. Vasomotor control can be promoted by the innervation of arterioles, which generates muscular contraction in the vascular wall, and it regulates the amount of blood circulating. Another regulatory mechanism can be observed by the vasoconstriction stimulated by adrenaline, and the vasodilation obtained by the release of the acetylcholine[99].

The first sign of inflammation is hyperemia. When there are tissue injuries (microbial, physics or chemistry) vasoconstriction is verified, and in a few seconds the vascular flow is re-established and vasodilation appears. With vasodilation and increased permeability, stages developed simultaneously, essential vascular events occur, such as plasmatic exudation and cellular transmigration[82].

These fundamental events of the inflammatory process (increased permeability and polymorphonuclear activation) are directly influenced by some chemical substances formed or released at the site of the lesion, which act as inflammatory chemical mediators, responsible for the ordered progression of the events, and appear in defined stages and have a specific role. These chemical mediators formed at the site of the lesion are in the form of inactive precursors in the plasma or they are sequestered in the cell. Subsequent to tissue lesion, loss of endothelial cell integrity is observed, liquid, plasma, platelet, erythrocyte and leucocytes leave the vessels and go into the extravascular space.

In the inflammatory process, vascular permeability can be characterized by the immediate phase, subdivided into two phases. 1 – initial - not linked to any chemical mediator (nonspecific), 2 - mediated by histamine (histamine dependent), and the late phase, the most important, since it assures vascular permeability for a long time. This phase is influenced by different chemical mediators, responsible for cellular transmigration and chemotaxis[9]. The contact of the extravased plasma with the biochemically altered conjunctive tissue triggers the inflammatory mechanism.

Several chemical mediators are related to the inflammatory process. Important biochemical systems should be emphasized, such as the vessel-active amines, kinins system, complementary system and the arachidonic acid metabolites[26,32,47,50]. Table 6.3 shows the most important chemical mediators of the inflammatory process.

Once present in the tissue, the vessel-active amines lead to capillary vasodilation and increase in venular permeability. Among the vessel-active amines, histamines and serotonin must be emphasized. Histamine appears in the initial events of the acute inflammatory process, being one of the first mediators to act. It is present in the granules of the mast cells located in the conjunctive tissue. The connection of the histamine with the specific receptor in the endothelial vascular cells favors the emergence of intracellular spaces (vasodilation)[32].

In the face of tissue injuries, the activated Hageman's factor (factor XII of the coagulation system) activates several plasmatic proteins and sets off the beginning of a cascade of events. The Hageman's factor converts the plasminogen (inactive precursor) into plasmin, which is capable of degrading fibrin, with release of polypeptides (fibrinopeptides) that act to induce vascular permeability during the inflammatory reaction. The plasmin also acts on the kininogen to form kinins. Added to these events, the plasmin can cleave components of the complementary system and generate metabolically active products, such as C3a and C5a anaphylatoxins [26,32,82,89,99].

The anaphylatoxins can induce the release of histamine from the mast cell. Once activated the complementary system, in addition to mediating the vascular response with histamine release, is capable of promoting cell lyses if the cascade in the cellular membrane is activated; increasing phagocytosis through the interaction of the complementary receptors on surfaces of the phagocytic cells; increasing permeability and acting as a chemotactic factor for granulocytes and macrophages[26,99].

The complementary system is constituted of a group of 20 plasmatic proteins capable of interacting among themselves and with other systems, constituting a source of vessel-actives mediators and are an essential part of the immunological system, with an important role in the host's defense against bacterial infection. Activation of the complementary system involves a complex cascade, with two forms of activation: 1 – the classical way - the complementary system is an important mechanism of the specific immunological response - activation is begun by complexes of antigen-antibodies; 2 – the alternative way - direct interaction of some components of the system occurs with complexes at the surfaces of the cellular walls of microorganisms[26,99]. Chart 6.1 illustrates the main biochemical systems related to the inflammatory process.

**Table 6.3** – Chemical inflammation mediators

| Origin | Chemical Mediators | |
|---|---|---|
| Plasmatic | Clotting Cascade | (Hageman's Factor) |
| | Fibrinolytic System | (Plasmin) |
| | Kinin System | (Bradykinin) |
| | Complementary System | (C3a, C5a, C5,6,7) |
| Tissue | Vessel-Actives Amines | (Histamine, serotonin) |
| | Arachidonic Acid Derivative | (Prostaglandins PGE PGF, leukotrienes and thromboxanes) |
| | Lipid acids | (Substance of slow action of anaphylaxis – SRS-A) |
| | Platelet Activator Factor | (Histamine, serotonin) |
| | Neuropeptides | (P Substance, CGRP, A Neurokinin) |

**Chart 6.1** - Biochemical systems related to the inflammatory process

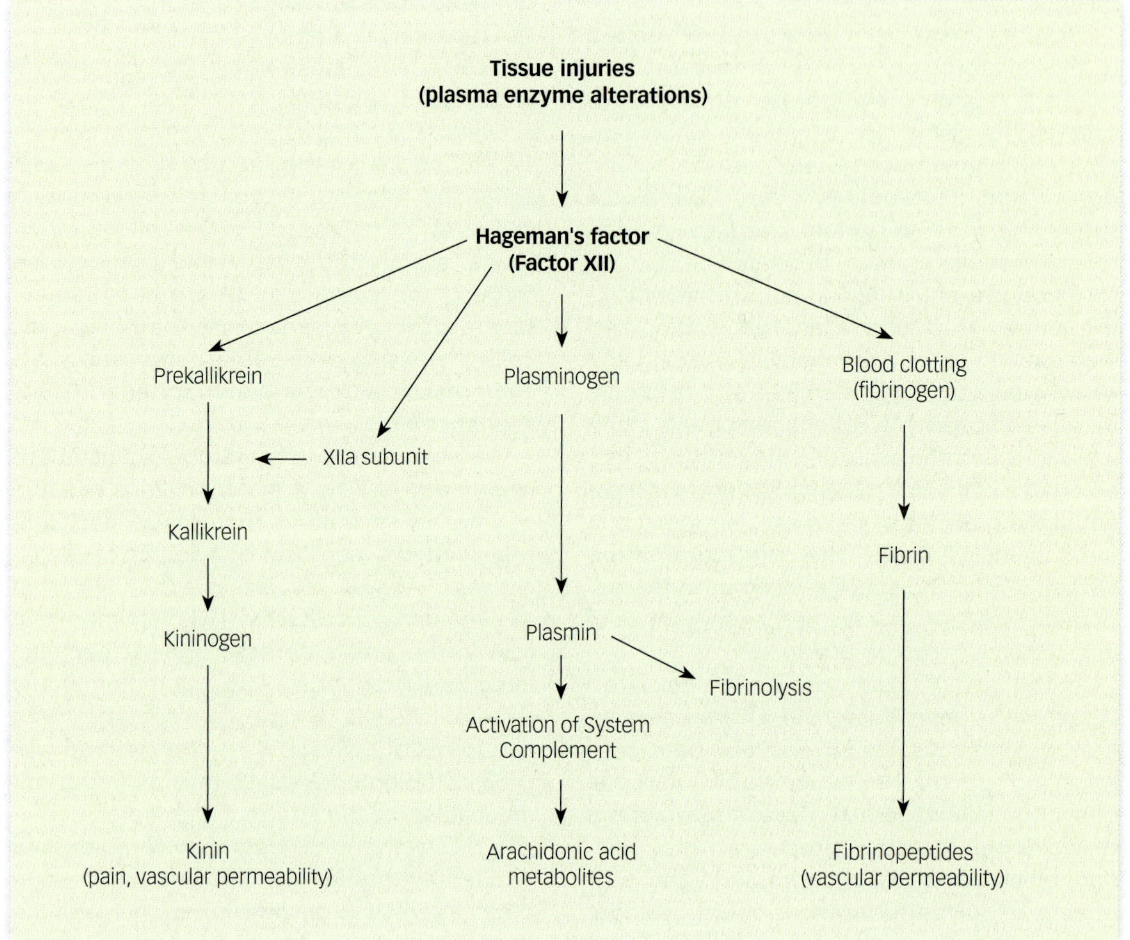


Different mechanisms are observed in the regulation of the complementary system: spontaneous fall of the individual complexes; proteolytic inactivity of specific components through inhibitors present in the plasma; connection of active components through specific proteins of the plasma[26].

The vascular response is influenced by other mediators produced by inflammatory cells and injured tissues, derived from the phospholipids and fatty acids. The action of $A_2$ phospholipase (lysosomal enzyme of the neutrophil activated during the inflammatory process) on the phospholipids of the cellular membrane produces eicosanoids derived from arachidonic acid. Arachidonic acid metabolism can take place through the cyclooxygenase and lipoxygenase (oxidation of the arachidonic acid) pathways, released from the lipids of the cellular membranes[26,89]. Through the cyclooxygenase pathway, prostaglandins ($PGE_2$, $PGF_2$), thromboxanes and prostacyclin ($PGI_2$) are produced; while, through the lipoxygenase pathway, leukotrienes are formed. The $PGI_2$ and $PGE_2$ produce vasodilator effects and increase permeability; $A_2$thromboxane (potent vasoconstrictor) is responsible for platelet aggregation. $B_4$ leukotriene causes adherence of the neutrophil to the post-capillary venula endothelium, and it is chemotatic for the neutrophil, in addition to increasing the permeability. The mixture of three leukotrienes ($LTC_4$, $LTD_4$, $LTE_4$) characterizes the substance of slow action of the anaphylaxis (SRA-A) responsible for vasoconstriction, bronchospasm and increase in vascular permeability[26,89,99]. Chart 6.2 illustrates arachidonic acid metabolism.

The late and lingering phase of the vascular permeability is due to the action of the prostaglandins and leukotrienes. The prostaglandins act jointly with the histamine and bradykinin causing vasodilation and increase in vascular permeability[26,32,82,89]. In addition to these inflammatory mediators, other also act, and among them is the platelet activator factor that releases histamine and serotonin starting from the platelet[99].

Pain is a consequence of the increased pressure in the tissues due to the hyperemia, edema and release of inflammatory algogenic agents (that produce pain), such as bradykinin. These agents stimulate the amyelinic type C fibers. Neuropeptides are synthesized in the cell body of the neuron, usually subsequent to a tissue aggression or stimulation of the neuron itself. As biological effects, neuropeptides can present vasodilation, increase in vascular permeability and transmission of the pain sensation. In the presence of stimulus, the nerve fibers release neuropeptides (proteins) and produce a neurogenic inflammatory reaction. The main neuropeptides are P substance, A neurokinin and K neuropeptide and the peptide related to the calcitonin gene (CGRP)[50,52,82,84,85,87,89,96,98,99,102].



**Chart 6.2** - Arachidonic acid metabolism

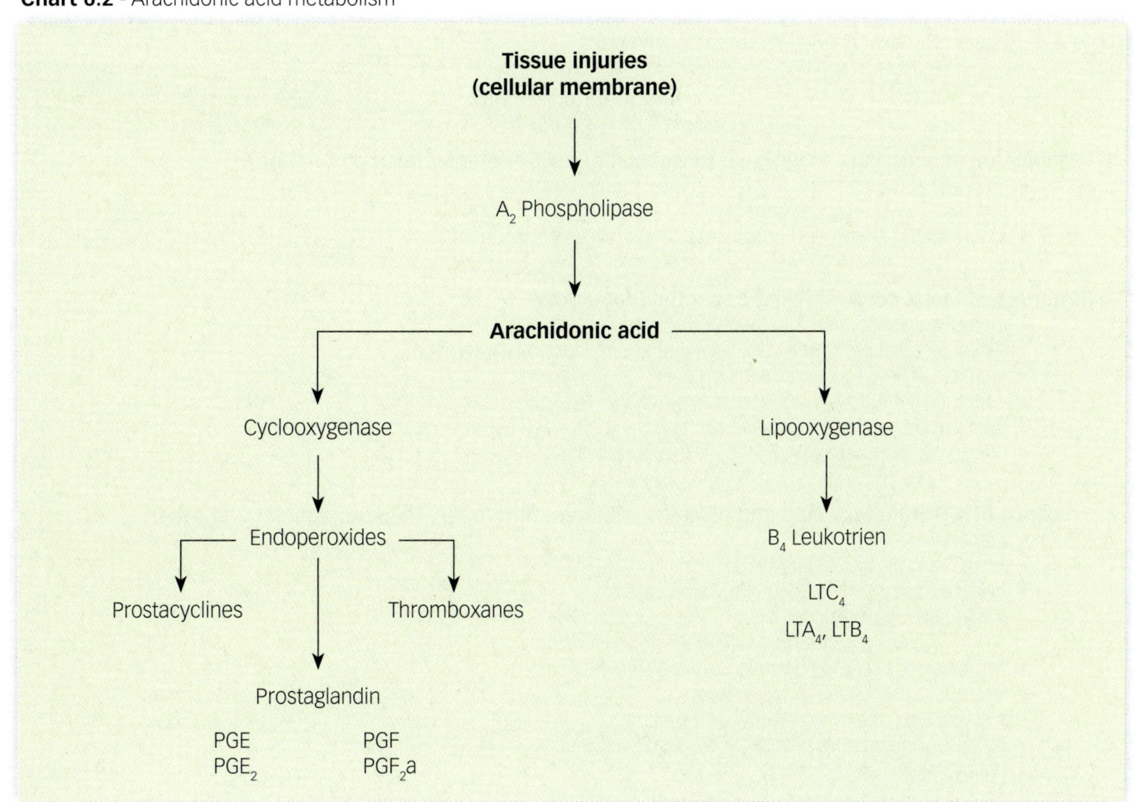

Trowbridge & Emling[99], discussing the events that take place during the inflammatory process, characterized the exit of leukocytes (mainly the phagocytes - neutrophil and monocyte) from the blood stream, enumerating them in the following way: 1- Margination (getting in touch with the vessel wall); 2- Adhesion (adhesion to the endothelial surface); 3- Migrating (leaving the blood stream); 4- Chemotaxis (moving towards the target); 5- Opsonization (recognizing and attacking the objective); 6- Phagocytosis (swallowing the target); 7- Degranulation (unloading the granules in the phagosome); 8- Degradation or death (destroying the target).

Consequently, the chemical mediators already emerge sequentially in stages already mentioned. The first stage of inflammation (amine stage) occurs when small preformed biological amines are released as a result of the tissue lesion. The second stage (polypeptide) takes place when the serum proteins are converted into vasoactive and neuroactive peptides by blood enzymes. The third stage is associated with the release of intracellular enzymes that begin to attack the tissue remains, and one of these enzymes is $A_2$ phospholipase that releases acid lipids from the cell membrane, which are converted into prostaglandins and leukotrienes. The last stage involves the lymphocytic phase of cleaning and repairing the lesion[26,32,82,99]. Table 6.4 enumerates and summarizes the sequence of events of the inflammatory process.

Byers & Närhi[10] reported that researches conducted over the last two decades greatly increased understanding of dentinal innervation and sensitivity, efferent signals from sensory nerve fibers that affect pulp cells, the neurophysiology of pulp nociceptors, neuroanatomical and functional responses to injury, pulpal neuro-inflammatory interactions, and the relationship of all these different features with dental pain.

**Table 6.4** - Sequence of events of the inflammatory process

| Inflammatory events |
|---|
| **1. Vasodilation and increase in vascular permeability (exit of fluids / microcirculation)**<br>• increase in the filtration pressure (hydrostatic pressure)<br>• increase in vascular permeability<br>• increase in reabsorption pressure (osmotic) (active hyperemia) |
| **2. Retention of blood cells - slowing down the blood flow**<br>• increase in blood viscosity (hemoconcentration)<br>• leukocytes adhere to the venula endothelium (leucocyte migration)<br>• increase in resistance of the blood flow<br>• decrease in blood flow to complete stagnation (vascular stasis/probably occurs in the post-capillary venula / influence of histamine) (passive hyperemia)<br>• due to the increase in permeability the fluid loss is greater |
| **3. Presence of inflammatory fluid and proteins (albumin, fibrinogen, immunoglobulin and other)**<br>• diapedesis<br>• increase in plasmatic exudation<br>• larger exit of proteins (globulins / fibrinogen)<br>immediate phase - unspecific<br>histamine dependent phase<br>• activation of tissue collagenases (proteases / lipases)<br>• late phase (histamine independent)<br>• it guarantees the permeability for long time<br>• cellular transmigration (kinins and prostaglandins)<br>• chemotaxis |

Hargreaves[34] related that in the inflamed dental pulp, the terminals of primary afferent nociceptors detect the presence of inflammatory mediators with receptors that are synthesized in the afferent fiber cell body and then transported to the periphery. *If the mediator reaches a concentration in the inflamed tissue sufficient to activate the receptor, the nociceptive neuron could become activated (ie, the membrane would be conducted to the central nervous system or sensitized.*

Knowledge of the essential factors related to the nerve structures and inflammatory process favors understanding of the pain phenomenon within its magnificent complexity.

### 6.7 Inflamed Dental Pulp Diagnosis

Diagnosis of alterations in the pulp determines the need for a clear concept of inflammation, the primordial purposes of which are to address the injuries, (metabolically altered cells, microorganisms, strange particles and antigens) eliminate and promote the repair of the damage caused to the tissues. Inflammation is characterized by vascular reactions in microcirculation, observed by the movement of liquids and leukocytes from the blood to the extravascular tissues. The action of chemical mediators induces the nerve fibers to produce pain. When the inflammatory reaction begins, the sequence of the fundamental physiological and morphological alterations is always the same, however, factors relative to the host and the injurious agent can modify the final nature, extent, and severity of the tissue alterations.

For long period, the dental pulp might have been attacked by several etiological agents (dental caries, periodontitis), traumatisms (occlusal trauma, knock), and by the restorative treatment (restorative materials - resins, ionomer, amalgam, cements) ending in succumbing, hurting or simply in silence, as it became necrosed because it was stressed.

The dental pulp reaction to different injuries can be manifested by inflammation which, irrespective of its nature, results in fundamental vascular alterations, such as vasodilation and increase in capillary permeability, transmigration and chemotaxis.

Kim[51] studied healthy and pathological dental pulp microcirculation. The author emphasized that the well-being of this tissue depends on appropriate microcirculation. Alterations in microcirculatory functions, such as the blood flow, intravascular and extravascular pressure, blood volume and capillary permeability play an important role in the onset of pulp disorders and in the contribution to the pathophysiological process. The pulp blood flow is ranked in an intermediate position between the blood flow of the skeletal muscles, which is low, and that of the brain or kidney, which is high. The pressure of the pulp tissue liquid varies from 20 to 30 mmHg, being considered high when compared with that of one of the other organs[100].

Based on a review, Hargreaves[34] discussed the mechanisms of pulpodentinal pain and various clinical implications. Dentinal pain is primarily due to the myelinated fibers that innervate dentinal tubules, in which fluid movement is detected and signaled back to the brain. Therapeutic reductions of dentinal fluid movement or neuronal activation can reduce dentinal hypersensitivity. Inflammation is detected by receptors expressed in pulpal nociceptors; the binding of inflammatory mediators to these receptors can activate or sensitize these nociceptors. Drugs that reduce tissue levels of inflammatory mediators (e.g., NSAIDs) relieve pain by reducing the activation of these altered pain states and provide the biologic basis for the endodontic diagnostic test. Hyperalgesia and allodynia can occur by both peripheral and central mechanisms, and may persist beyond the dental appointment. Thus, patients with preoperative pain have an increased risk of experiencing postoperative pain. Referred pain is partly due to convergence of multiple sensory fibers onto the same central projection neuron. Pulp testing, using either electrical or thermal stimuli, requires an appreciation of the conditions of both the tooth and patient, and to minimize potential confusion due to false positive or false negative results.

Thermal agents are capable of altering pulp vascular and tissue pressures, producing vasoconstriction or vasodilation. Among these agents, the stick of ice, compressed spray, carbon dioxide snow, and warm gutta-percha are used. It has been noted, however, that in cold tests, the greater the decrease in temperature on the tooth surface, the better the conditions for determining pulp vitality. Interpretation of the responses obtained to the different stimuli applied (cold, heat, electrical) on the dental crown, is essential for obtaining the correct diagnosis.

The cold thermal test is the stimulus more frequently used, the heat test being for use in situations of differential diagnosis[18]. Table 6.5 describes the pulp responses to the thermal agents.

Van Hassel[101] points out tissue pressure as a critical factor during the inflammatory process. With the exit of exsudate from the vessels there is an increase in pressure that can lead to collapse of the veined part of microcirculation, which interrupts the blood transport system, and tissue hypoxia and anoxia can occur at the site, which leads to necrosis. The products originated from of the necrosed tissues contribute to the extension of inflammation.

The anatomical location of the dental pulp, contained within hard and inelastic walls, associated with the lack of collateral circulation are the cause of the difficulty of pulp expansion that is observed, starting with the increase in blood flow (vasodilation) and vascular permeability, which results in the increase in the hydrostatic pressure of the pulp[18].

In vascular congestion, part of the interstitial liquid is forced out of the pulp, in order to accommodate the increase in blood flow. At first, there is the increase in arterial flow (arterial or active hyperemia) and in the subsequent stage, a decrease in the veined flow (veined or passive hyperemia) is noted, with the appearance of plasmatic exudation and cellular transmigration, which characterizes acute inflammation. Trowbridge & Kim[100] explained that if the tissue pressure increases to the point of being equal to the intravascular pressure, the venula with thin walls would be compressed, thus increasing vascular resistance and reducing the pulp blood circulation.

Clinically it is impossible to distinguish the increase in arterial flow from the decrease in veined flow. Based on these responses and on the clinical characteristics of pain, the histopathological diagnosis cannot be defined, but it can simply affirm whether or not the pulp is diseased.

**Table 6.5** - Normal and inflamed pulp response to thermal tests

| Stimulus | Normal Pulp | Inflamed Pulp |
|---|---|---|
| Cold | • vasoconstriction<br>• reduces the internal pressure<br>• pain (imediate response) | • vasoconstriction<br>• reduces the internal pressure<br>• relief of pain<br>• sometimes "stimulates pain" |
| Heat | • vasodilation<br>• increases the internal pressure<br>• pain (late response) | • vasodilation<br>• increases the internal pressure<br>• pain (imediate response) |

Within the context of clinical diagnosis of the pulp pain, acute or chronic symptoms should be distinguished from acute or chronic inflammation. Acute inflammation has been characterized by exudative vascular events, while, in chronic inflammation, proliferative processes are observed. The presence of polymorphonuclear leucocytes in the acute process and of lymphocytes and cell plasma in the chronic process, together with the characteristics of the exudate are important factors in the histopathological classification of pulp diseases.

According to Bell[6], acute and chronic pain are linked to the time of pain duration; acute (pain of short duration), chronic (pain of long duration - longer than 6 months).

Pain does not favor assessment of the real conditions of pulp tissue health, and the diagnosis applied in endodontics at present is imprecise for accurately informing the state of the pulp. It is indispensable to analyze the types of pain, however, it is also necessary to interpret it very well, since it is a subjective experience, associated with somatic, neuropathic and psychogenic factors.

In general, pulp diseases of inflammatory origin have been classified in different ways[18, 30-32,39,41,46,49,59,61,76,80,85,90,91,104] according to histopathological and clinical characteristics. The correlation between the symptoms and histopathological changes in pulpitis is poor, and to determine the type and extent of inflammatory changes on the basis of symptomology is inaccurate[70]. Basically, the histopathological classifications of pulp diseases most frequently used are shown in Table 6.6. In Table 6.7, except for regressive pulp alterations, various classifications show the status of pulp disease.

It is evident that all of the mentioned histopathological events were observed in different stages of pulp inflammation, which established a scientific basis for the different classifications of pulp diseases that have been proposed.

**Table 6.6** - Histopathological classifications of the diseases of the dental pulp

| | | |
|---|---|---|
| **A** - | 1. Pulp Hyperemia | |
| | 2. Acute Pulpitis | • Serous<br>• Purulent |
| | 3. Chronic Pulpitis | • Ulcerative<br>• Hyperplastic |
| | 4. Pulp Necrosis | |
| **B** - | 1. Closed Pulpitis | • Pulp Hyperemia<br>• Infiltrative Pulpitis<br>• Abscessed Pulpitis |
| | 2. Open Pulpitis | • Ulcerous traumatic Pulpitis<br>• Ulcerous non-traumatic pulpitis<br>• Hyperplastic Pulpitis |
| | 3. Pulp Necrosis | |
| **C** - | 1. Reversible Pulpitis | |
| | 2. Pulpitis in the Transition period | |
| | 3. Irreversible Pulpitis | |
| | 4. Pulp Necrosis | |

Table 6.7 - Different classifications of the status of pulpal diseases





| Organization/Author | Normal pulp | Pulpitis |
|---|---|---|
| World Health Organization | • Normal Pulp (not mentioned) | • Initial Pulpitis (hyperemia)<br>• Acute Suppurative (pulpal abscess) |
| Grossman | • Normal pulp (not mentioned) | • Hyperemia<br>• Pulpitis<br>• Acute pulpitis |
| Ingle | • Normal pulp | • Hyper-reactive pulpalgia<br>• Hypersensitivity<br>• Hyperemia<br>• Acute pulpitis (Incipient, Moderate, Advanced) |
| Seltzer & Bender | • Normal pulp (not mentioned) | • Pulpitis<br>• Incipient form of chronic pulpitis<br>• Acute pulpitis |
| Weine | • Normal pulp (not mentioned) | • Hyperalgesia (reversible pulpitis)<br>• Hypersensitive dentin<br>• Hyperaemia<br>• Painful pulpitis<br>• Acute pulpalgia (acute pulpitis) |
| Cohen & Burns | Within normal limits:<br>• Normal pulp<br>Calcifie metamorphosis | • Reversible pulpitis<br>• Irreversible pulpitis Asymptomatic<br>• Irreversible pulpitis |
| Tronstad | • Healthy pulp | • Asymptomatic<br>• Symptomatic |
| Bergenholtz | • Healthy Pulp | • Pulpitis |
| Abbott | • Clinically normal pulp | • Reversible pulpitis<br>• Acute<br>• Chronic<br>• Irreversible pulpitis<br>• Acute Chronic<br>• Necrobiosis |
| Paiva & Antoniazzi | • Normal pulp (not mentioned) | • Reversible pulpitis<br>• Irreversible pulpitis |
| Stock | • Normal pulp | • Concussed pulp<br>• Reversible pulpitis<br>• Irreversible pulpitis |
| Walton & Torabinejad | • Normal pulp (not mentioned) | • Reversible pulpitis<br>• Irreversible pulpitis |
| Sapp, Eversole & Wysocki | • Normal pulp (not mentioned) | • Reversible pulpitis<br>• Irreversible pulpitis |
| Estrela | • Normal pulp response | • Hyper-reactive pulpalgia<br>• Symptomatic |

(Figure modificated from Abbot & Yu[1], 2007).

| Pulpitis | Necrosis |
|---|---|
| • Chronic pulpitis<br>• Chronic ulcerative<br>• Chronic hyperplastic (pulpal polyp)<br>• Other unspecified pulpitis<br>• Unspecified Pulpitis | • Pulp Necrosis |
| • Chronic ulcerative pulpitis<br>• Chronic hyperplastic pulpitis | • Necrosis |
| • Chronic pulpalgia<br>• Hyperplastic pulposis | • Pulp necrosis –liquefaction, Sicca |
| • Chronic partial pulpitis with partial necrosis<br>• Chronic total pulpitis with partial liquefaction necrosis<br>• Chronic partial pulpitis (hyperplasic form) | • Pulp necrosis |
| • Chronic pulpalgia (Subacute pulpitis)<br>• Nonpainful pulpitis<br>• Chronic ulcerative pulpitis<br>• Chronic pulpitis (no caries)<br>• Chronic hyperplastic pulpitis (pulp polyp) | • Pulp necrosis |
| • Hyperplastic pulpitis<br>• Internal resorption<br>• Canal calcification<br>• Asymptomatic<br>• Symptomatic<br>• Symptomatic<br>• Irreversible pulpitis | • Necrosis partial/complete |
| | • Necrotic pulp |
| | • Pulp Necrosis |
| | • Pulp necrosis (No sign of infection) Infected |
| | • Pulpal necrosis |
| | • Pulpal necrosis |
| | • Pulpal necrosis |
| • Hyperplastic pulpitis | • Pulpal necrosis |
| • Asymptomatic | • Pulpal necrosis |

Clinical diagnosis and indication for the treatment of inflamed dental pulp was verified by Holland & Souza[40], who reported that the most important thing is to define whether the tooth has inflamed pulp. Through histopathological analysis of 28 human teeth presenting spontaneous pain at night, they observed the presence an inflammatory process of varied intensity (moderate neutrophilic infiltrate and microabscess to bulkier abscesses that affected the entire coronal pulp). In none case the root pulp was compromised. The pulp inflammation is a reversible process, similar to inflammation in other sites in body, provided that appropriate treatment is instituted.

Aydos[5], analyzing different aspects of inflamed dental pulp treatment, argues that it is clinically impossible to accurately establish the histopathological condition of pulp tissue. The coincidence of the clinical diagnosis with the histopathological condition would only be laboratory verification, which does not evaluate the potential of the pulp to recover and does not allow one to foresee whether the pulp lesion is reversible or irreversible.

Estrela et al.[19] when evaluating pain and performing vitality tests to diagnose inflamed dental pulp, affirmed that due to countless difficulties with correctly establishing the clinical diagnosis, pain characteristics, the vitality test and the radiographic exam do not allow one to reach a precise determination of whether the processes of the inflamed dental pulp are reversible or irreversible. Thus, the characteristics of reversible or irreversible processes should be included in the prognosis and not in the diagnosis. Pulp inflammation is a reversible process, of which the essential purposes are to eliminate the injuries and to promote tissue repair. The clinical diagnosis does not reveal, or allow one to foresee with accuracy whether the pulp lesion is reversible or irreversible. To establish the diagnosis of an inflamed pulp is easy, the complex matter is to accurately evaluate the extent of the inflammatory process by means of the clinical characteristics of pain and the responses to the vitality tests. Furthermore, it is necessary to know the differences between acute and chronic inflammation, and acute and chronic symptoms.

Pain is an important clinical symptom in the context of the diagnosis, however, it does not allow the extent of pulp inflammation and the possibilities of repair to be established. On the other hand, the clinical characteristics of pain in pulp injuries responsible for the formation of tertiary dentin, pulp hyperemia and inflammation are not exact. The intensity and duration of the injuries, together with the dental pulp resistance signal several types of pulp diseases. When considering the concept and the purposes of inflammation (to eliminate the injuries and to promote the cure process), it is interpreted that inflammation should be considered a reversible process. However, some factors of the pulp cavity anatomy can modify the inflammatory response, such as: the presence of a closed or opened cavity, and radiographic evidence of complete or incomplete rhizogenesis. These factors influence the vascular alterations in the pulp.

The complaint of pulp pain in different clinical situations is shown to have different characteristics appearance (spontaneous or provoked), duration (long or short), frequency (continuous or intermittent), site (localized or diffuse), intensity (severe, moderate or light), however it does not explain the true histopathological conditions of the dental pulp.

Pulp pain analysis with a view to successful treatment should be guided on the basis of the requirements for structuring the clinical diagnosis; that it is composed of the anamnesis, clinical exam, pulp vitality test and radiographic exam. In this sense, logical reasoning demands knowledge of the clinical characteristics of pain, verified during the anamnesis (site, appearance conditions, duration, frequency, intensity), the physical alterations of the tooth obtained through the clinical exam (opened or closed cavity) and the pulp responses provided by thermal stimulus (pulp vitality test). The signs and symptoms present during the pulp exam allow one to reach a clinical diagnostic hypothesis. Nevertheless, it is known that clinical evidences do not present correlations with the microscopic discoveries of the pulp alterations.

Consequently, the pulp pain diagnosis should be made on the basis of the real clinical evidences, signs and symptoms, such as: biophysical characteristics of the tooth (signs that denote the cavity - opened - exposed pulp; closed - absence of pulp exposure); symptomatology presented (presence or absence of pain / appearance of pain - provoked or spontaneous); pulp vitality test (positive response - it suggests presence of a live pulp; negative response - it suggests presence of pulp necrosis). In the impossibility of direct inspection of the dental pulp, semiotechnical resources allow one to reach the probable diagnosis of the pulp pain (a diagnostic hypothesis). Thus, it only leaves the analysis of signs and the patient's clinical symptoms, without correlation with possible histopathological events (their occurrence only being supposed), increasing the chances of a higher percentage of successful clinical diagnosis.

The intensity of pain is an extremely variable clinical characteristic, described with a great deal of subjectivity and related not only to the pathological involvement and the patient's pain threshold, but also to the emotional and psychological aspect. The attempt to quantify pain, by determining the degree 0 (zero - pain absence) to 10 (ten - intense pain), aids the characterization of conditions that increase or reduce the symptomatological aspects, such as the relationship with stimuli that affect the tooth. Among these one can list heat, cold, sweet and/or acid foods, mastication, and the emotional state. These factors can facilitate diagnosis, and after treatment has been established, can express the involvement, maintenance or development of the initial pathology. The symptom is usually significant when, in addition to hearing about it, the professional knows how to interpret it and associate it with the possible pathologies.

The pulp hyperemia and reversible pulpitis are considered speculative terms, because they do not describe clinical entities, or the clinical-pathological process[85].

The clinical characteristics of pulp pain in the situation when its appearance was provoked, present responses suitable to dentinal hypersensitivity, or reversible pulp alterations (hyperemia). Considering the conditions of the symptoms similar to these clinical situations (provoked pains) and the responses to the pulp vitality tests (positive), the clinical exam allows one to make the distinction.

However, for these clinical conditions, the best option for denominating the clinical diagnosis would be hyper-reactive pulpalgia[18,85,89].

Among the clinical characteristics of pulp pain due to hyper-reaction, dentinal hypersensitivity or hyperemia ("reversible pulpitis"), provoked pain, of short duration, localized, responding positively to the pulp vitality test are observed. On the other hand, it is opportune remember that historically, inflammation has been considered acute and/or chronic, depending on the persistence of the lesion, characteristics of the exudate, symptomatology and nature of the inflammatory response. The clinical diagnosis of symptomatic pulpitis is applied to situations of pulp pain, present in a closed cavity, with spontaneous appearance, and positive response to the pulp vitality test. This is the most appropriate denomination and can best be applied to the clinical diagnosis. However, the hypothesis of pulpitis should be admitted in the absence of symptomatology in a closed cavity. The term asymptomatic pulpitis is applied to situations of provoked symptom, usually with an open cavity (hyperplasia or pulp ulceration), in which the pulp vitality test is shown to be less effective. For the situation considered to be pulp necrosis, there are no reports of current complaints of pain, the pulp vitality test is negative, and the cavity can be open or closed. Apart from the above-mentioned situations, the clinical diagnosis of inflammatory pulp alterations should be formulated considering the treatment, in which the dental pulp or the root canal is treated.

Table 6.8 shows the characteristics of the cavity, symptomatology and responses to the pulp vitality test present in pulp diseases, in agreement with the clinical classification of the pulp inflammation. Figures 6.9A-F and 6.10A-F show clinical situations of symptomatic and asymptomatic pulpitis. Chart 6.3 illustrates the pathological events and therapeutic options for pulp.

**Table 6.8** - Clinical Classification of Inflamed Dental Pulp

| Clinical Diagnosis | Clinical Characteristics of the Cavity | Symptomatology (pain) |
|---|---|---|
| **Normal pulp** | • Closed cavity | • Absence of symptoms<br>• Positive pulp vitality test |
| **Hyper-reactive pulpalgia** | • Closed cavity<br>Hyperemia/Hypersensitivity | • Provoked symptom<br>• Positive to P.V.T. |
| **Symptomatic pulpitis** | • Closed cavity<br>(Pulp inflammation) | • Spontaneous symptom<br>• Positive to P.V.T. |
| **Asymptomatic pulpitis** | • Open cavity<br>Pulp Hyperplasia/Ulceration | • Provoked symptom<br>• Little effectiveness of P.V.T. |
| **Pulp necrosis** | • Closed cavity<br>• Open cavity | • Absence of Symptoms<br>• Negative P.V.T. |

P.V.T. - Pulp vitality test

Observations: Considering the histopathological condition the hypothesis of pulp inflammation without symptomatology can be admitted

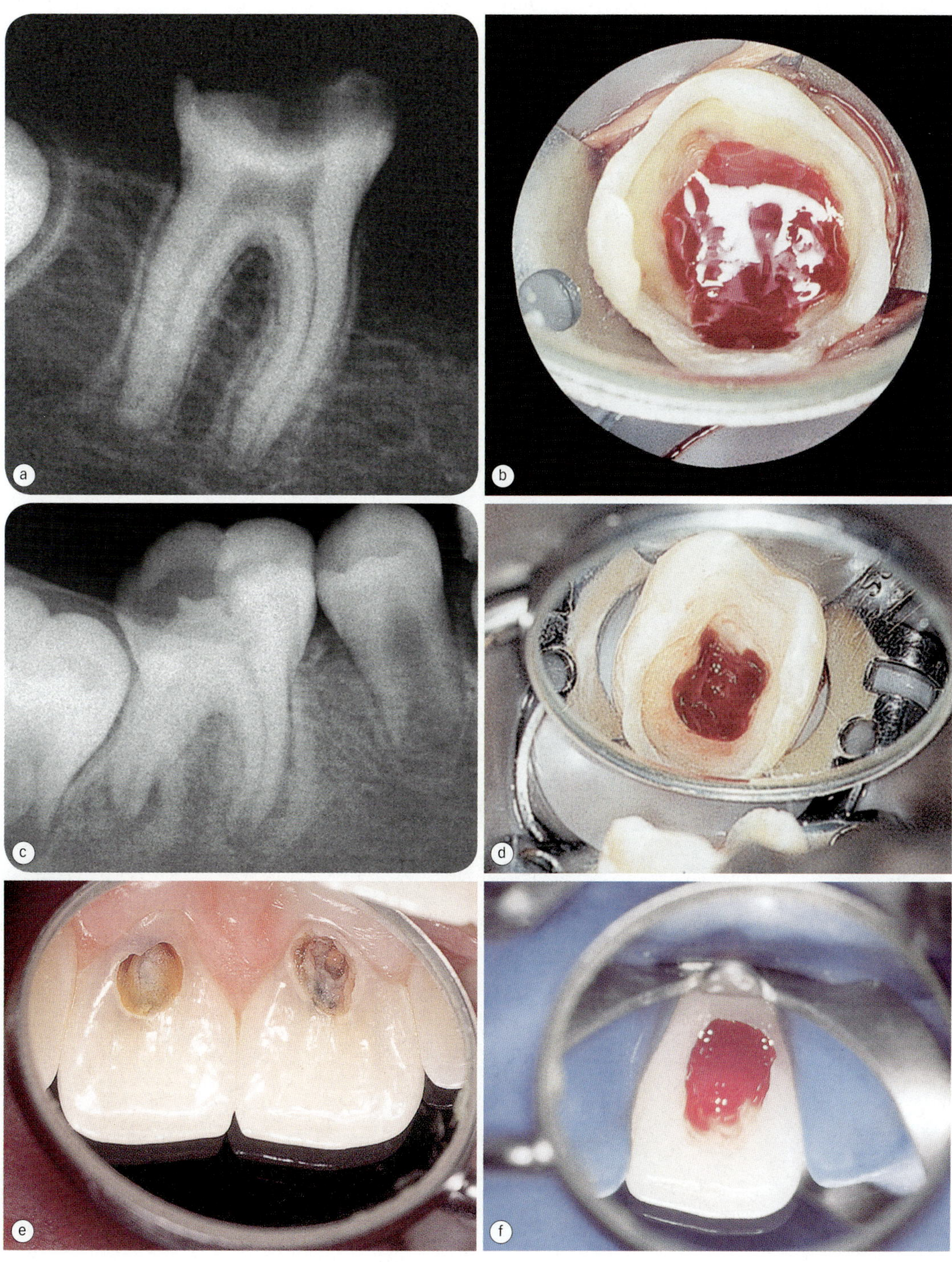

**Figure 6.9** - (**A-F**) Symptomatic Pulpitis.

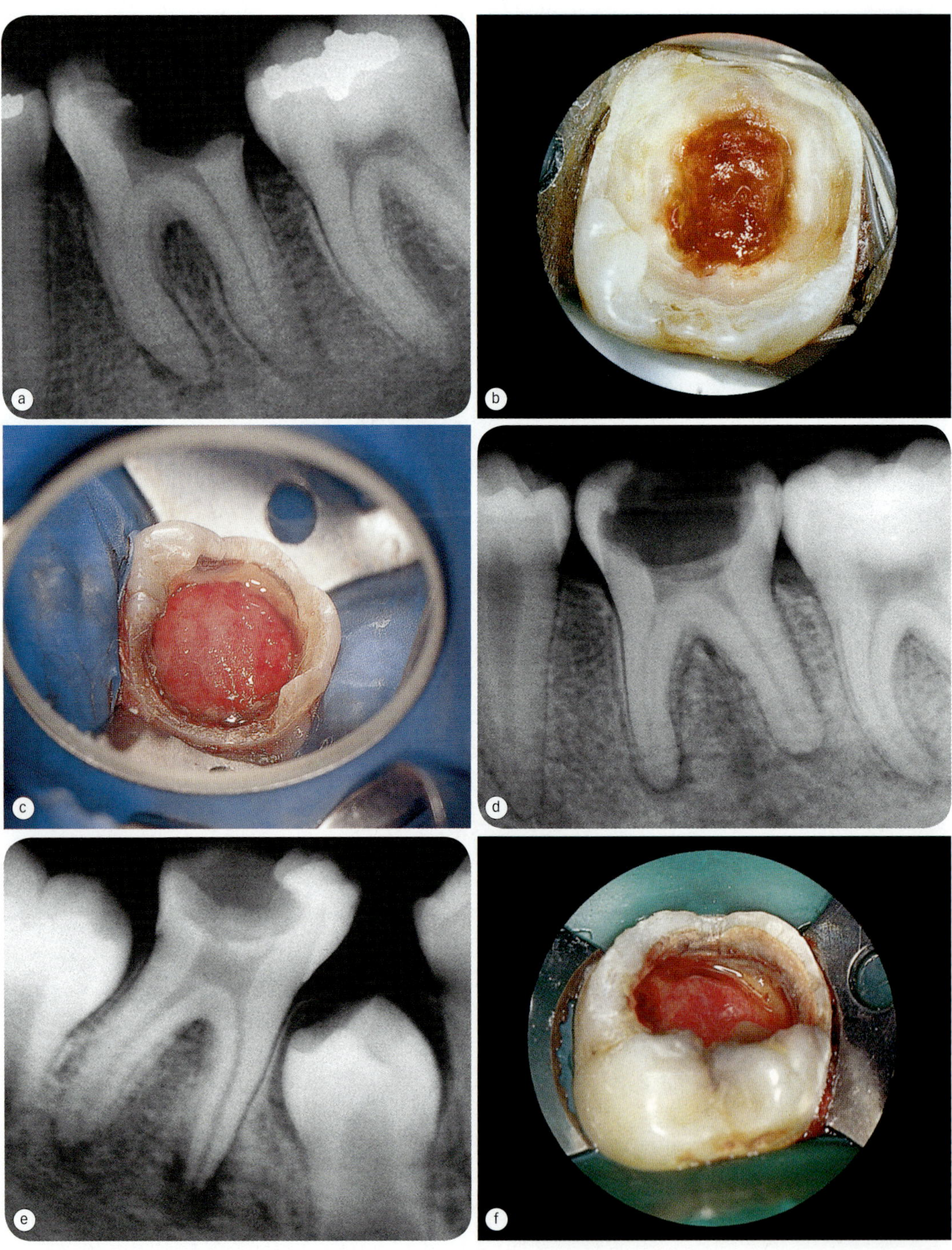


**Figure 6.10** - (**A-F**) Asymptomatic Pulpitis.

**Chart 6.3** - Pulp pathological events and therapeutic options

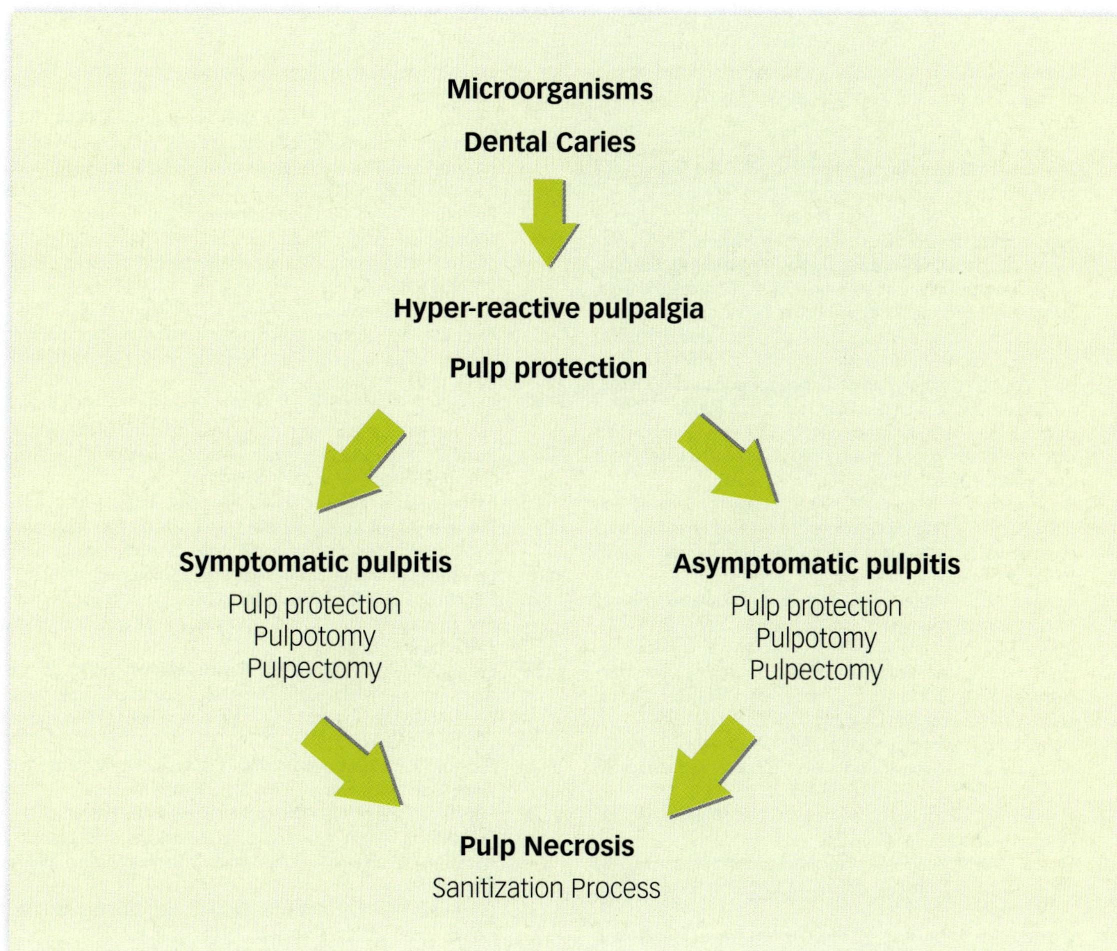

## References


1. Abbot PV, Yu C. A clinical classification of the status of the pulp and the root canal system. Aust Dent J 2007;52:17-31.
2. Ahlquist ML, Frazén OG. Encoding of the subjective intensity of sharp dental pain. Endod Dent Traumatol 1994; 10:153.
3. Ahlquist ML, Frazén OG. Inflammation and dental pain in man. Endod Dent Traumatol 1994; 10:201-9.
4. Avery JK, Rapp R. An investigation of the mechanism of neural impulse transmission in human teeth. Oral Surg Oral Med Oral Pathol 1959; 12:190-8.
5. Aydos JH. Tratamento da polpa dental inflamada. Rev Fac Odontol Porto Alegre 1985; 27:153-71.
6. Bell WE. Orofacial Pains: Classifications, diagnosis, management. Chicago. London: Boca Raton; 1989.
7. Bernick S. Vascular and nerve changes associated with the healing of human pulp. Oral Surg Oral Med Oral Pathol 1972; 33:983-1000.
8. Beveridge EE, Brown AC. The measurement of human dental intrapulpal pressure and its response to clinical variables. Oral Surg Oral Med Oral Pathol 1965;19:655-68.
9. Busato ALS, Costa CAS, Estrela C. Biocompatibility of restorative materials. Braz Endod J 1997; 2:14-22.
10. Byers MR, Närhi MVO. Nerve supply of the pulpodentin complex and responses to injury. In: Hargreaves KM, Goodis HE. Seltzer and Bender dental pulp. Quintessence: Chicago, 2002. P.151-179.
11. Byers MR, Taylor PE, Khayat BG, Kimberly CL. Effects of injury and inflammation on pulpal and periapical nerves. J Endod 1990; 16:78-84.
12. Cailliet R. Dor: mecanismos e tratamento. Porto Alegre: Artmed; 1999. 312p.
13. Costa CAS, Mesas NA, Hebling J. Pulp response to direct capping with an adhesive system. Amer J Dent 2000; 13:81-7.
14. Costa CAS, Montano TCP, D'Abreu MCF, Hebling J, Gonzaga HFS. Avaliação histológica da capacidade de reparação do tecido conjuntivo pulpar de rato capeado com o sistema adesivo Scothbond MP e o cimento de óxido de zinco e eugenol. Rev Paul Odontol 1997; 29:26-32.
15. Costa CAS, Nascimento ABL, Teixeira HM, Fontana UF. Response of human pulps capped with a self-etching adhesive system. Dent Mat 2001; 17:230-40.
16. Estrela C. Dor Pulpar. In: Estrela C. Dor odontogênica. Artes Médicas Ltda: São Paulo, 2001.
17. Estrela C, Bammann LL, Estrela CRA, Silva RS, Pécora JD. Antimicrobial and chemical study of MTA, Portland cement, calcium hydroxide paste, Sealapex and Dycal. Braz Dent J 2000; 11:19-27.
18. Estrela C, Guedes OA, Leles CR, Decurcio DA, Silva JA. Prevalence and risk factors of pulpal and periapical pain. 2008 (studdy submitted).
19. Estrela C, Lopes HP, Resende EV, Alencar AH. Avaliação da dor e de testes de vitalidade para o diagnóstico da inflamação pulpar. Rev Odontol Brasil Central 1995; 5:4-8.
20. Estrela C, Pécora JD, Souza-Neto MD, Estrela CRA, Bammann LL. Effect of vehicle on antimicrobial properties of calcium hydroxide pastes. Braz Dent J 1999; 10:63-72.
21. Estrela C, Pesce HF, Silva MT, Fernandes JMA, Silveira HP. Análise da redução da dor pós-tratamento da hipersensibilidade dentinária. Rev Odontol Brasil Central 1996; 6:4-10.
22. Estrela C, Sydney GB, Bammann LL, Felippe-Jr O. Mechanism of action of calcium and hydroxyl ions of calcium hydroxide on tissue and bacteria. Braz Dent J 1995; 6:85-90.
23. Estrela C, Tormin FC, Araújo CR, Barleta FB. Prevalência de pulpite aguda e necrose pulpar frente a diferentes agentes etiológicos. Rev Fac Odontol UFG 1997; 1:15-20.
24. Estrela C, Zina O, Borges AH, Santos ES, Resende EV. Correlação entre o diagnóstico clínico da polpa dental inflamada e o reparo após a pulpotomia. Rev Odontol Brasil Central 1996; 6:4-8.
25. Estrela CRA. Pimenta FC, Alencar AHG, Ruiz LFN. Prevalence of selected bacterial species in intraoral sites associates with chronic periodontitis using multiplex polymerase chain reaction. 2008 (submitted).
26. Fantone JC, Ward PA. Inflamação. In: Patologia. Rubin E, Farber JL. 1st ed. Rio de Janeiro: Interlivros; 1990. p. 32-58.
27. Faraco-Jr IM, Holland R. Response of the pulp of dogs to capping with Mineral Trioxide Aggregate or a calcium hydroxide cement. Dent Traumatol 2001;17:163-166.
28. Fidgor D. Pain of dentinal and pulpal origin. Ann Roy Aust Coll Dent Surg 1994;12:131-42.
29. Fields HL. Pain. New York: McGraw-Hill; 1987.
30. Fristad I. Dental innervations: functions and plasticity after peripheral injury. Acta Odontol Scand 1997; 55:236-54.
31. Grossman LI. Endodontia Prática. 8th ed. Rio de Janeiro: Guanabara Koogan; 1976. p.26-67.
32. Guimarães SAC. Patologia básica da cavidade bucal. Rio de Janeiro: Guanabara Koogan, 1982; p.197-281.
33. Guyton AC. Fisiologia humana e mecanismos das doenças. 5th ed. Rio de Janeiro: Guanabara Koogan; 1993. 574 p.
34. Harvegreaves KM. Pain mechanisms of the pulpdentin complex. In: Hargreaves KM, Goodis HE. Seltzer and Bender dental pulp. Quintessence: Chicago, 2002. p.181-203.
35. Hebling J, Giro EMA, Costa CAS. Biocompatibility of an adhesive system applied to exposed human dental pulp. J Endod 1999;25:676-682.
36. Holland R. Histochemical response of amputed pulps to calcium hydroxide. Rev Bras Pesq Med Biol 1971; 4:83-95.
37. Holland R, Otoboni-Filho JA, Souza V, Mello W, Nery MJ, Bernabé PFE, Dezan-Jr E. Calcium hydroxide and corticosteroid-antibiotic association as dressings in cases of biopulpectomy. A comparative study in dogs' teeth. Braz Dent J 1998; 9:67-76.
38. Holland R, Souza V. Ability of a new calcium hydroxide root canal filling material to induce hard tissue formation. J Endod 1985; 11:535-43.

39. Holland R, Souza V. Considerações clínicas e biológicas sobre o tratamento endodôntico. I – Tratamento endodôntico conservador. Rev Ass Paul Cir Dent 1977; 31:152-62.
40. Holland R, Souza V. O problema do diagnóstico clínico e indicação de tratamento da polpa dental inflamada. Rev Ass Paul Cir Dent 1970; 24:188-93.
41. Holland R, Souza V. Quando e como o clínico geral deve realizar o tratamento conservador pulpar. In: Atualização em Odontologia Clínica. Bottino MA, Feller C. São Paulo: Artes Médicas; 1984. p.89-117.
42. Holland R, Souza V. Tratamento conservador da polpa dentária. Ars Curandi 1975; 2:3-17.
43. Holland R, Souza V, Mauro SJ, Dezan-Jr E, Otoboni-Filho JA, Bernabé PFE, Nery J. Comportamento da polpa dental do cão diante da exposição pulpar ou pulpotomia e proteção direta com o sistema All Bond 2. Rev Ciência Odontol 1998; 1:75-80.
44. Holland R, Souza V, Nery MJ, Faraco-Jr IM, Bernabé PFE, Otoboni-Filho JA, Dezan-Jr E. Reaction of Rat Connective Tissue to Implanted Dentin Tube Filled with Mineral Trioxide Aggregate, Portland Cement or Calcium Hydroxide. Braz Dent J 2001; 12:3-8.
45. Holland R, Souza V, Nery MJ, Otoboni-Filho JA, Bernabé PFE, Dezan-Jr E. Reaction of rat connective tissue to implanted dentin tubes filled with mineral trioxide aggregate or calcium hydroxide. J Endod 1999; 25:161-166.
46. Ingle JI, Taintor JF. Endodontia. 3rd ed. Rio de Janeiro: Guanabara Koogan; 1989. 737 p.
47. Jaeger B. Diagnostico diferencial y tratamiento del dolor craneofacial. In: Endodoncia. Ingle JI, Bakland LK. 4th ed. México: McGriw-Hill; 1996. p.576-637.
48. Kakehashi S, Stanley HR, Fitzgerald RJ. The effects of surgical exposures of dental pulps in germ free and conventional laboratory rats. Oral Surg Oral Med Oral Pathol 1965; 2:340-9.
49. Kantorowicz A. Escuela Odontológica Alemana. Editorial Labor S. América; 1937.
50. Kettering JD, Torabinejad M. Microbiologia e Imunologia. In: Caminhos da polpa. Cohen S, Burns RC. 7th ed. Rio de Janeiro: Guanabara Koogan; 1998. p.347-448.
51. Kim S. Microcirculation of the dental pulp in hearth and disease. J Endod 1985; 11:467-71.
52. Kim S. Neurovascular interactions in the dental pulp in health and inflammation. J Endod 1990; 16:48-53.
53. Kim S. Regulation on pulpal blood flow. J Dent Res 1985; 64:590-96.
54. Kramer IR. The distribution of blood vessels in the human dental pulp. In: Biology of the dental pulp organ: a symposium. Finn SB. University of Alabama Press; 1968.
55. Langeland K. Pulp reactions to cavity preparation and to burns in the dentin. Odont Tskr 1960; 68:463-70.
56. Langeland K, Langeland K. Pulp reactions to crown preparation, impression, temporary crown fixation and permanent cementation. J Prosthet Dent 1965; 15:129.
57. Lanza L. Avaliação clínica e microscópica de um sistema adesivo aplicado em proteções pulpares diretas de dentes humanos. (Doctoral Thesis). University of São Pauloo; 1997.
58. Loesche WJ. Cárie Dental – Uma infecção tratável. Rio de Janeiro: Cultura Médica; 1993. 349p.
59. Lopes HP, Estrela C, Elias CN. Comparative study of the hard tissue bridge after pulpotomy with calcium hydroxide associated of various vehicles. Braz Endod J 1996; 1:43-6.
60. Madeira MC. Anatomia da face: bases anátomo-funcionais para a prática odontológica. São Paulo: Sarvier; 1995. 174p.
61. Maisto OA. Endodoncia. Buenos Aires: Mundi; 1967. 355p.
62. Melzac R. The McGrill Pain Questionnaire: Major properties and scoring methods. Pain 1975; 1:277-299.
63. Melzack JD, Wall PD. Pain mechanisms: A new theory. Science 1965; 150:971-79.
64. Merskey H. Pins terms. A list with definitions and notes on usage. Pain 1979; 6:249-252.
65. Mjor IA, Fejerskow O. Embriologia e Histologia Oral Humana. São Paulo: Panamericana; 1990.
66. Mondelli J. Proteção do complexo dentinopulpar. Artes Médicas: São Paulo; 1988. 316p.
67. Nair PNR. Neural elements in dental pulp and dentin. O Surg O Med O Pathol 1995; 80:710-719.
68. Nair PNR, Luder HU, Schroeder HE. The number and size-spectra of myelinated nerves in human premolars. Anat Embryol 1992; 92:123-8.
69. Nair PNR, Schoeder HE. Number and size-spectra of nom-myelinated nerves in human premolars. Anat Embryol 1995; 192:35-41.
70. Närhi MVO. Dentinal and pulpalpain. In: Bergenholtz G et al. Textbook of Endodontology. Oxford: Blackwell, 2003. p.43-56. The characteristics of intradental sensory units and their responses to stimulation. J Dent Res 1985; 64:564-71.
71. Närhi MVO. The characteristics of intradental sensory units and their responses to stimulation. J Dent Res 1985; 64:564-71.
72. Okeson JP. Dores orofaciais de Bell. 5th ed. São Paulo: Quintessence; 1998. 500p.
73. Okeson JP. Tratamento das desordens temporomandibulares e oclusão. 4th ed. São Paulo: Artes Médicas; 2000. 500p.
74. Orland FJ. Use of the germfree animal technique in the study of experimental dental caries. J Dent Res 1954; 33:147-74.
75. Osborn JW, Ten Cate AR. Histologia Dental Avançada. 4th ed. São Paulo: Quintessence Books; 1988. 231p.
76. Paiva JG, Antoniazzi JH. Endodontia – bases para a prática clínica. São Paulo: Artes Médicas; 1988. 886p.
77. Pameijer CH, Stanley HR. The disastrous effects of the total etch technique in vital pulp capping in primates. Am J Dent 1998; 11:45-54.
78. Pereira JC, Segala AD, Costa CAS. Human pulpal response to direct pulp capping with an adhesive system. Am J Dent 2000; 13:139-47.
79. Pesce HF. Diagnóstico diferencial das odontalgias. In: Atualização na clínica odontológica – o dia a dia do clínico geral. São Paulo: Artes Médicas; 1992. p.143-53.
80. Pucci FM, Reig R. Conductos Radiculares: anatomia, patología y terapia. Montevideo: Barreiro y Ramos; 1945.
81. Reeves R, Stanley HR. The relationship of bacterial penetration and pulpal pathosis in caries teeth. Oral Surg Oral Med Oral Pathol 1966; 22:59-65.

82. Robins SL, Angell M, Kumar V. Patologia Básica. São Paulo: Atheneu ed.; 1986. p.32-68.
83. Scott JN, Weber DF. Microscopy of the junctional region between human coronal primary and secondary dentin. J Morphol 1977; 154:133.
84. Seltzer S. Pain. In: Endodontology: biologic considerations in Endodontic procedures. ______. 2nd ed. Philadelphia: Lea & Feibiger; 1988. p.471-499.
85. Seltzer S, Bender IB. Inervacion pulpar y percepcion del dolor. In: Pulpa Dental. _____. 3rd ed. México: Manual Moderno; 1987. p.124-142.
86. Seltzer S, Bender IB. Pulpa Dental. 3rd ed. Moderno: México; 1987. 427p.
87. Sesse BJ. Recent developments in pain research: central mechanisms of orofacial pain and its control. J Endod 1986; 12:435-517.
88. Shuttleworth CA, Berry L, Bloxsome C, Wilson NHF. Synthesis of sulfated glycominoglycans by rabbit dental pulp fibroblasts in culture. Arch Oral Biol 1982; 27:645.
89. Smulson MH, Hagen JC, Ellens SJ. Patologia pulpoperiapical e considerações imunológicas. In: Tratamento Endodôntico. Weine FS. 5th ed. São Paulo: Santos; 1998. p.166-202.
90. Smulson MH, Sieraski SM. Histophysiology and diseases of the dental pulps. In: Endodontic therapy. Weine FS. 4 th ed. St. Louis: Mosby; 1989. p.74-153.
91. Soares IA. Resposta pulpar ao MTA - Agregado de trióxido mineral - Comparada ao hidróxido de cálcio, em pulpotomia. Histológico em dentes de cães. (Thesis). Florianópolis; 1996.
92. Souza V, Holland R. Treatment of the inflamed dental pulp. Aust Dent J 1974; 19:191-96.
93. Stanley HR. Criteria for standarding and increasing credibility of direct pulp capping studies. Am J Dent 1998; 11:17-34.
94. Stanley HR. The cells of the dental pulp. Oral Surg Oral Med Oral Pathol 1962; 15:849-58.
95. Stanley HR, Pameijer CH. Dentistry's friends: calcium hydroxide. Oper Dent 1997; 22:1-3.
96. Torabinejad M, Eby WC, Naidorf IJ. Inflammatory and imunogical aspects of the pathogenesis of human periapical lesions. J Endod 1985; 11:479-88.
97. Torriani DD. Cárie dental. In: Dentística: Restaurações em dentes posteriores. Busato ALS. São Paulo: Artes Médicas; 1996. p.23-32.
98. Trowbridge HO. Review of dental pain – histology and physiology. J Endod 1986; 12:445-452.
99. Trowbridge HO, Emling RC. Inflamação. 4th ed. São Paulo: Quintessence Books; 1996. 172p.
100. Trowbridge HO, Kim S. Pulp development, structure and function. In: Pathways of the pulp. Cohen S, Burn R. 6th ed. St. Louis: Mosby; 1994. p.296-334.
101. Van Hassel HJ. Physiology of the human dental pulp. Oral Surg Oral Med Oral Pathol 1971; 32:126.
102. Wakisaka S. Neuropeptides in the dental pulp: distribution, origins and correlation. J Endod 1990; 16:67-69.
103. Wall PD. The gate control theory of pain mechanisms: A reexamination and restatement. Brain 1978; 101:1-18.
104. Weine FS. Endodontic therapy. 4th ed. St. Louis: Mosby; 1989. 752p.

# Inflamed Dental Pulp Treatment

**C. Estrela**

*Federal University of Goiás, Goiânia, GO, Brazil*

**R. Holland**

*São Paulo State University, Araçatuba, SP, Brazil*

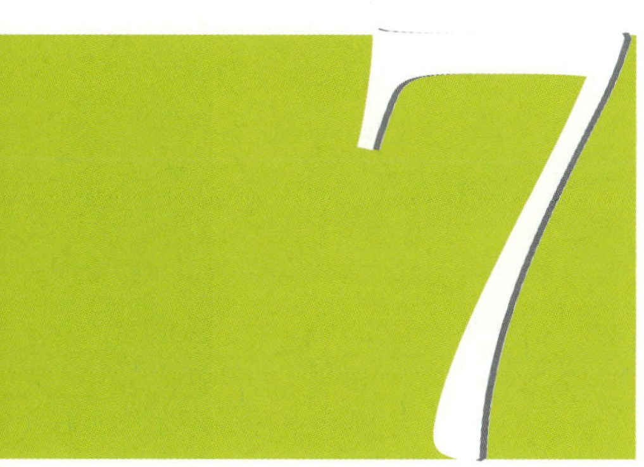


Chapter contents

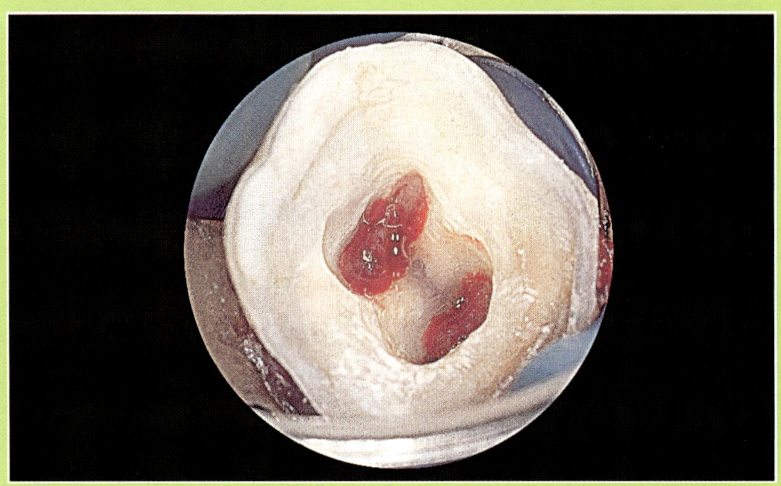

Teeth with symptomatic pulpitis
(Pulp tissue with structural resistance).

## 7.1 Introduction

The dentin-pulp complex is covered by dental enamel on the crown, by cementum on the root, and surrounded by periodontal ligament and bone. The harmony of the complex is impaired if the surrounding tissues suffer any type of aggression that can reach the pulp through the root canal or dentinal tubule systems. Dental caries is a microbial disease that affects the calcified tissues of the teeth and consequently the dental pulp. A main etiologic factor for pulp inflammation is the invasion of bacteria or their by-products into the dental pulp, although dental procedures and traumatic injuries can also contribute[134].

Due to countless difficulties involved in correctly establishing the clinical diagnosis and pain characteristics, the use of pain and vitality tests and radiographic exams to diagnose inflamed dental pulp do not allow reversible or irreversible processes of the inflamed dental pulp to be precisely determined. Thus, the characteristics of reversible or irreversible processes should be included in the prognosis and not in the diagnosis. The pulp inflammation is a reversible process whose essential purposes are to eliminate the injuries and to promote tissue repair. The clinical diagnosis does not reveal or allow one to foresee with accuracy, whether the pulp lesion is reversible or irreversible. To establish the diagnosis of an inflamed pulp is easy; the complex task is to accurately evaluate the extent of the inflammatory process by the clinical characteristics of the pain, and the responses to the vitality tests. The diagnostic resources for determining the extent of pulp inflammation under a caries lesion are very imprecise.

When indicating treatment, the prevailing goal should always be to maintain the organs of the human body in their normal physiological conditions. Among the group of agents injurious to the dental pulp, it should be clear that there is cumulative injury, initially through the action of microorganisms, then as a result of the cavity preparation, and lastly by the protective and restorative material. The individual's organic conditions (host response) should also be considered.

The presence of odontogenic pain, due to pulp inflammation, dental caries or accidental exposure, should receive special attention during the anamnesis and the clinical exam, to enable the conservation of this tissue. It is a myth that inflamed or exposed pulp always requires radical root canal treatment. Many clinicians are afraid to expose the dental pulp, because this could result in condemning it. These professionals should know and master the conservative techniques, diagnostic methods that identify the different pulp problems, as well as the safe and precise indication of the treatment. To condemn exposed or inflamed pulp presenting spontaneous pain is unjustifiable nowadays. It requires knowledge and special skills to perform radical root canal treatment of good quality, and this frequently demands the attention of a specialist.

The discussion about whether or not to preserve the inflamed dental pulp, or whether to extract the tooth, is well defined and directed towards conservative treatment, whenever convenient[1-143]. The social view calls for pulp preservation as a first option, in preference to other treatments. Therefore, it is understood that from the social or any other aspect, the goal is always to maintain healthy pulp conditions. Either the general clinician or the specialist must master the diagnosis methods that allow different clinical problems to be identified, as well as the conservative treatment techniques, which will certainly assure the precise indication of treatment.

The famous phrases – inflamed pulp is lost pulp, or exposed pulp is lost pulp, have no scientific basis to support them. It is practically impossible to analyze the capacity of pulp reparation based only on the clinical characteristics of the pain. It is essential to consider the limitations of the clinical diagnosis of pulp inflammation. The intensity, length and the type of pulp aggression are important aspects to consider in precise clinical evaluations. For example, in aggression due to a cavity preparation with pulp exposure, reparation normally develops with adequate treatment. Another question that has no scientific backing, and still distresses those that have not learned the biological, clinical, technical and social meaning of conservative treatment, is the issue of the importance of retaining the pulp remainder in a patient of over thirty years of age. It is opportune to clarify that there is no physiopathological justification for not maintaining the pulp remainder after the age of thirty years. These and other famous statements are clarified over the course of time, which exposes many myths and philosophic dogmas that are not scientific. Science is certainly self-corrected in time, but until the mistakes are corrected, the cost is high.

Inflammation should be understood as an essential defense reaction of the living being, essential to the maintenance of life, even considering the factors that modify the inflammatory responses to the pulp environment, such as the presence of an open or closed cavity, complete or incomplete rhizogenesis.

## 7.2 Inflamed Dental Pulp Diagnosis

Dental pulp is a connective tissue, similar to other parts of the organism, with identical reaction to physiological and pathological conditions. The anatomic location and the presence of cells specialized to form dentin, represent significant differences to the other connective tissues. Due to its geographic position, the pulp has critical moments, because it has limited capacity to increase in volume or expand during vessel-dilatation and increase in vascular permeability, which makes the edema (although not very exuberant) increase the internal pressure to unbearable limits.

Some previously mentioned factors are responsible for modifying the pulp inflammatory response, among them the presence or absence of pulp exposure, the complete or incomplete rhizogenesis. These factors alter the blood flux of an inflamed pulp, modifying the internal pulp pressure.

Determining the correct clinical diagnosis of the injured dental pulp represents an essential factor for the success of the treatment.

Several etiologic agents can be responsible for injuries to the pulp tissue, and among these are dental caries, cavity preparation, protective agent etc. The intensity of the aggression influences the pulp response. Different studies[5,15-17,30,44,80,89,105,126-128,130] showed the negative effects of the use of adhesive systems, applied directly over dental pulps.

The microscopic limits during the development of the pulp inflammatory response are frequently imprecise during the clinical evaluation. Based on scientific evidences, this demonstrates clearly the absence of correlation between the clinical and microscopic findings.

Pain is an important clinical symptom in the context of the clinical diagnosis, however it does not allow the precise extent of the pulp inflammation and the possibilities of reparation to be established. The clinical characteristics of pain, among which are pulp aggression, responsible for the formation of reparative dentin, pulp hyperemia and inflammation, are not exact. The intensity and the duration of the aggression, the pulp resistance and the factors that modify its response, point to several types of pulp diseases[21].

As discussed in the chapter 6 about diagnosis of the alterations in dental pulp, for the treatment to succeed, the analysis of the pulp pain should be based on requirements of the clinical structure of the diagnosis, based on the anamnesis, clinical exam, pulp vitality exam and the radiographic exam. Thus, the logic of the thought requires knowledge of the clinical characteristics of pain, verified during anamnesis (conditions of appearance, duration, frequency, location, intensity), physical alterations of the tooth found in the clinical exam (open or closed cavity), and pulp responses provided by the thermal stimuli (pulp vitality exam). The sign and symptoms presented during the semiological pulp exam allow one to obtain a hypothesis of clinical diagnosis[21].

Consequently, the diagnosis of the pulp pain must be performed from real clinical evidences, of the signs and symptoms, such as: biophysical characteristics of the tooth (signs that denote the cavity – open – exposed pulp; closed – absence of pulp exposure); symptomatology presented (presence or absence of pain / onset of pain – provoked or spontaneous); pulp vitality exam ( positive response – suggests presence of vital pulp; negative response – suggests presence of pulp necrosis). As direct inspection of the dental pulp is almost impossible, the semiotechnical resources allow a probable diagnosis of the pain (a diagnosis hypothesis). Thus, only the analysis of the clinical signals and the symptoms of the patient are supported, without correlation with possible histopathological events, whose occurrence is only presumed). The intensity of the pain is a very variable clinical characteristic, subjectively described and related not only to the pathological involvement and patient's pain threshold, but also to the emotional and psychological aspect. An attempt to quantify pain, by determining the degree 0 (zero – absence of pain) to 10 (ten – intense pain), helps to characterize the conditions that increase or decrease the symptomatology, in relation to stimuli that affect the tooth, among which are heat, cold, sweet and/or acidic food, chewing and the emotional state. These factors can aid diagnosis, and after treatment has been established, express the involvement, maintenance or development of the initial pathological state. The symptom normally presented is significant when the professional, in addition to hearing it, knows how to interpret it and associate it with the possible pathological state[21].

Zerlotti[143] investigated the pulps of 68 teeth with caries or painful pulpitis and periapical normality. After the histopathological interpretation of the results, the presence of cells that characterize acute and chronic inflammatory responses, could be observed in different areas of the pulp lesion. When the inflammation was confined to small areas, the remainder of the pulp tissue did not present evident alterations. In the situations that the inflammation was extended to the entire coronal pulp, the root pulp presented almost no damage. Thus, it can be pointed out that the behavior of the pulp tissue is very similar to that of other connective tissues described. Holland & Souza[60] analyzed the problem of clinical diagnosis and indication of treatment of inflamed dental pulp. After the histopathological analysis of 28 human dental pulps, with spontaneous nocturnal pain, they observed the presence of an inflammatory process that varied in intensity (from moderate neutrophilic infiltrate and microabscesses to even more voluminous abscesses that compromised almost all the coronal pulp). In no case was the root pulp compromised. In view of the results, they emphasized that teeth with spontaneous pain could be treated with pulpotomy, if the root remainders present signs of vitality, such as abundant bleeding (intense red) and consistency (resistance to cutting).

Pulp inflammation is a reversible process, similar to what happens in other locations in the body, if adequate treatment is given. The Table 7.1 presents the fundamental clinical aspects for indicating conservative treatment (pulpotomy) (Fig. 7.1 to 7.10). The success rates depend on the correct visual clinical diagnosis of the dental pulp, and the technically correct performance of the pulpotomy[59,60,61].

The literature reports several studies[4,5,7,8,14,29-31,45,60,94,102,103,110,112,121] that showed high success rates after pulpotomies in teeth with inflamed dental pulps.

**Table 7.1** - Fundamental clinical aspects for indicating pulpotomy

| Signs | Favorable Aspects | Unfavorable Aspects |
|---|---|---|
| **Bleeding** | Normal after cutting the pulp tissue<br>Blood: intense red | Absent<br>Too dark<br>Too clear (yellowish) |
| **Pulp Remainder** | Consistent pulp (resistance to the action of the curette) | Pulp without consistence that is easily degraded<br>Pasty / liquid aspect |
| **Dental Crown** | Almost intact or with thick and resistant walls | Great coronal destruction needing placement of intracanal retention |

(Holland & Souza[60])

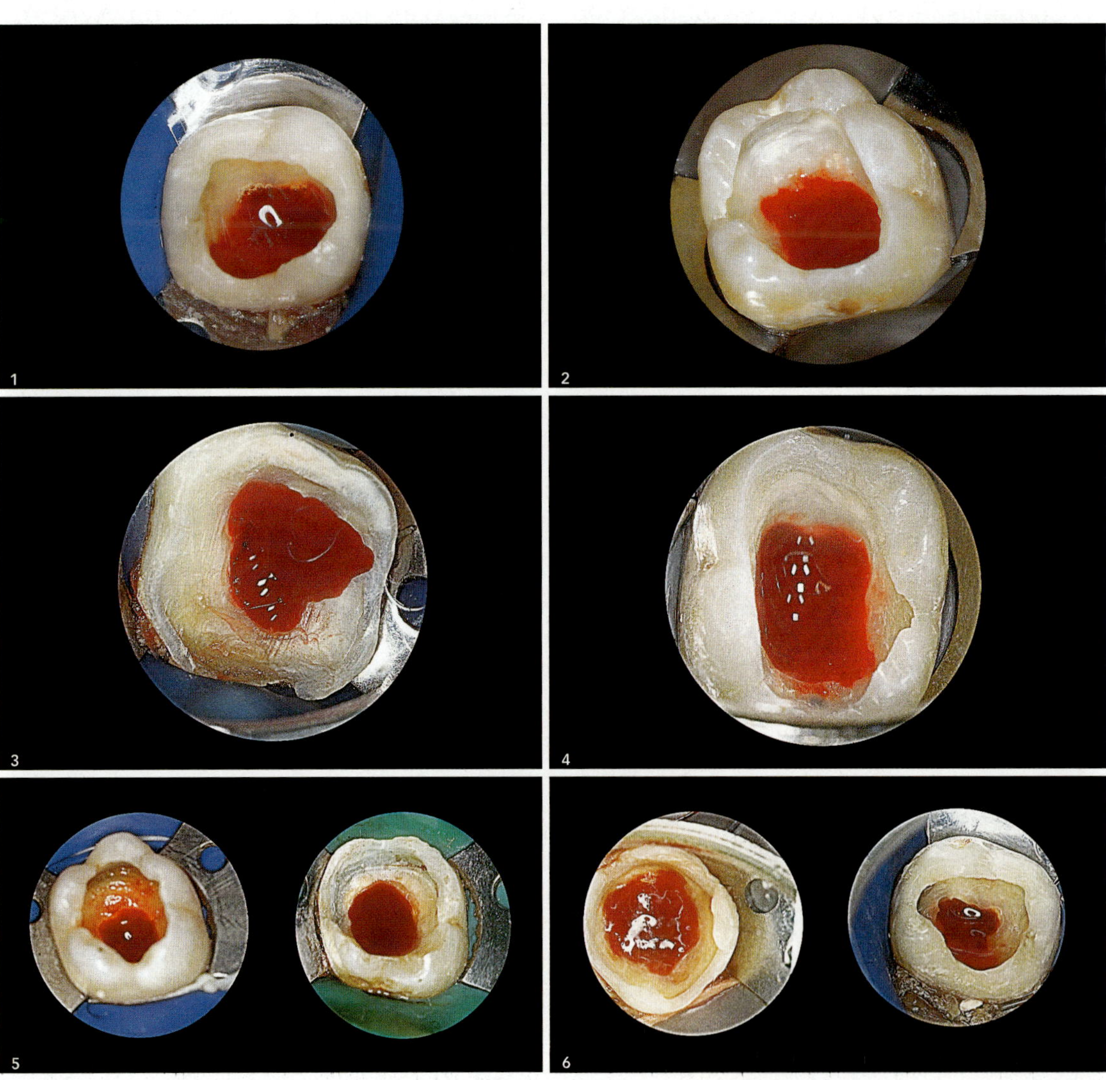


**Figures 7.1 to 7.6** - Teeth with symptomatic pulpitis (normal and red bleeding).

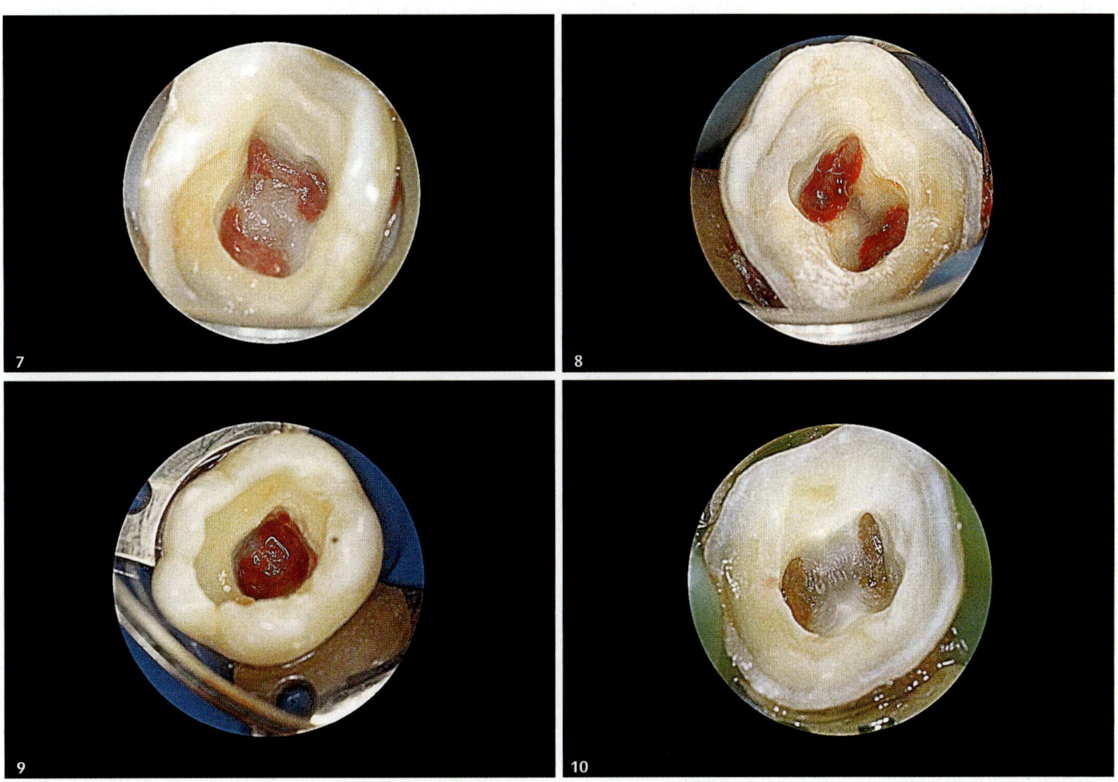

**Figures 7.7 to 7.10** - Teeth with symptomatic pulpitis (Pulp tissue with structural resistance).

## 7.3 Pulp Protective Materials

The literature presents different materials that have been proposed for application over the dentin-pulp complex, which led to many studies to test the biologic compatibility of thesematerials[5-7,15-17,20,24-28,30-31,34,38,41,42,44,45-90,92-94,97,99-103,105-111, 114, 116-118,123-126,129,130,132,133,134,143].

The use of materials without known biocompatibility has been questioned and discussed a great deal[5,15-17,30,31,89,127]. It is known that among the pulp aggressors, microorganisms, pulp heating and toxicity of some dental materials are always in evidence. The ideal substance for pulp capping presents functions directly related to the health of the tissue, capable of maintaining a biocompatible behavior and at the same time allows perfect neutralization of several types of aggressors (thermal, mechanical and chemical).

Calcium hydroxide, introduced to dentistry by Hermann[41], in 1920, has become the chosen material to protect the pulp tissue.

For a long time, however, it was believed that calcium hydroxide acted well on healthy pulp but was precarious on the inflamed pulp. Thus, when corticosteroid was used, it would improve the pulp inflammation, which would allow satisfactory action of the calcium hydroxide. Nevertheless, even after the application of the corticosteroid on dental pulp, it was verified that the area remained inflamed for a long time.

Souza & Holland[121] studied the treatment of inflamed dental pulp. Dog anterior teeth, whose pulps were experimentally exposed to oral the environment for 48 hours, had their crowns removed for histopathological examination of the pulp tissue. The root pulps were capped with antibiotic-corticosteroid and calcium hydroxide; these drugs were used alone or in combinations. After 90 days, a histological examination was done. The authors observed a relationship between the status of the coronal pulp tissue: the capped root pulps were submitted to pulpotomy and protected with calcium hydroxide, with or without a previous dressing of antibiotic or corticosteroid. As the inflammatory reaction of the coronal pulp intensified, success decreased. The treatment that attained the highest success rate was when a corticosteroid-antibiotic dressing applied for 48 hours was replaced by calcium hydroxide.

Holland et al.[66] comparatively analyzed the techniques of curettage and pulpotomy, whether a corticosteroid dressing was used or not. The pulps of 120 dog's teeth were exposed to the oral environment for 24 hours before the treatment. The dental pulps were submitted to curettage or pulpotomy and then either dressed with prednisolone acetate for 10 minutes, or not. The pulp remnants were protected with calcium hydroxide in distilled water or in corticosteroid. Thirty days later the animals were sacrificed and the specimens prepared for histological study. The data analysis showed that the pulpotomy technique produced better results than curettage. The use of a corticosteroid seemed to have no influence on the results of the treatment. This suggests that the topical application of corticosteroid for such a short time, or its addition to calcium hydroxide is an unnecessary procedure.

In another study, Holland et al.[65] evaluated the use of corticosteroid and antibiotic association during endodontic treatment. Thirty root canals of a young mongrel dog, were treated and dressed with the following corticosteroid-antibiotic associations: Otosporin, Otosynalar and Panotil. Forty-eight hours after the treatment, the animal was sacrificed and the specimens prepared for histological analyses, in the routine way. The results obtained with Otosporin were better than those obtained with the other medicaments. Otosporin preserved the pulp stump vitality and controlled the intensity and extent of the inflammatory reaction, which usually occurs after pulpectomy. In view of these results it was concluded that Otosporin can be used as a root canal dressing in cases of vital pulp extirpation, when one wishes to control the inflammatory reaction. In addition to this study, Otosporin has clinically been the most indicated and tested medicament in several investigations[59-61], showing satisfactory results in moderation of the inflammatory process. Thus, these evidences clarify the importance and the need for the use of a corticosteroid-antibiotic between the pulpotomy appointments.

Various options of traditional procedures for conservative dental pulp treatment are found, which include: pulp capping, pulp curettage and dental pulpotomy. In all these therapeutic options, the most important factor is adequate protection of the living pulp exposed to the oral environment, with the purpose of preserving its vitality.

In the last few years, Dentistry has observed the appearance of new restorative techniques and materials, which deserve accurate longitudinal evaluations before they are considered suitable for routine use by professionals. The appearance of several materials and restorative techniques[5-20,30,31,34,37,39,41-50,72-79,92-94,97-103,106-109,112,113,119,120,125,133-143] shows that throughout several different eras, there was the expectation that the discovery of new products could solve the functional, aesthetic and biologic problems. Nevertheless, some of the criteria for evaluating the result of the restorative treatment are the physical integrity, absence of marginal leakage, and the response of biological compatibility with the pulp dentin complex. Since the properties shown by calcium hydroxide, and the inherent problems of its use are known, its indication as an ideal material for pulp exposures and very deep cavities should be emphasized, followed by the restorative system.

The selection of the biologic capping to be used over the pulp remainder and its influence on the reparation process deserves in depth discussion. Several materials have been tested as pulp protectors, and among the most studied at present[1-143] are: calcium hydroxide, mineral trioxide aggregate (MTA), Portland cement, zinc oxide and eugenol, glass ionomer, the dentinal adhesive systems etc.

Calcium hydroxide, introduced by Hermann[41], in 1920, was a great milestone in conservative dentistry. A variety of materials have been proposed for conservative dental pulp treatment, but calcium hydroxide is still the gold standard against which new materials are tested, particularly in human teeth. This material has shown capacity to induce the formation of a mineralized barrier over the pulp tissue, proved by several researches[45-90].

Calcium hydroxide has been researched for many years. Herman[38] in 1920 suggested calcium hydroxide for the treatment of dental pulp. The formula (Calxyl-Otto & CO; Frankfurt, Germany) was considered to be the pioneer in the use of calcium hydroxide, with addition of other substances. For Stanley[115] a new era had begun. Calcium hydroxide encourages the deposition of a hard tissue bridge that usually protects the dental pulp[41,42,45-90]. The ability to stimulate mineralization associated with its antimicrobial effectiveness has at present made it successful as an endodontic medication.

A few minutes after the pulp tissue comes into contact with calcium hydroxide, the formation of necrotic areas begins[45] Right at the limit between the live and necrotic tissue there is deposition of calcium salts, whereas dentin is observed about 15 days after treatment[45]. In direct contact with conjunctive tissue, calcium hydroxide initiates a zone of necrosis, altering the physic-chemical status of intercellular substance which, through rupture of glycoproteins seems to determine protein denaturation[45]. Mineralized tissue formation was observed from the 7th to the 10th day after the calcium hydroxide came into contact with the conjunctive tissue[45]. Holland[45], studying the healing process of dental pulp after pulpotomy with calcium hydroxide, verified the existence of massive granulation in the superficial granulosis zone interposed between the necrosis zone and the deep granulosis zone. He went on to report that these structures are made up of calcium salts and calcium-protein complexes. They were shown to be birefringent to polarized light, reacting positively to chloramilic acid and to von Kossa's method, proving that part of the calcium ions come from the protective material. Below the deep granulation zone, there are the cellular proliferation zone and the normal pulp (Fig. 7.11 to 7.16 ). Similar results were obtained by Seux et al.[116,] who studied odontoblast-like cytodifferentiation of human dental pulp cells in vitro in the presence of a calcium hydroxide-containing cement. The cement produced microcrystals of calcite by reaction with the culture medium supplemented with calf serum. Human dental pulp cells seeded on such a substrate preferentially adhered to and aggregated around the microcrystals. Immunofluorescence and immunogold labeling revealed a high affinity of serum fibronectin molecules for the calcite crystals. At 4 weeks in culture, the cells had various features of differentiated odontoblasts, notably nuclear polarization, typical appearance of the Golgi apparatus, synthesis of type I collagen and absence of type III, and apical accumulation of actin and vimentin. These cells also elaborated a collagenous extracellular matrix which did not mineralize.

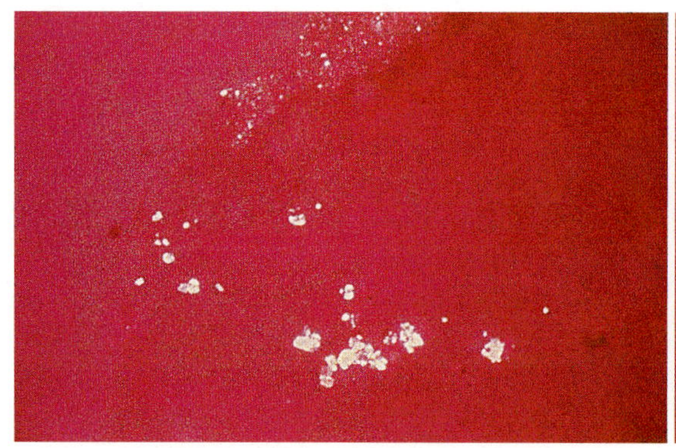

**Figure 7.11** - Calcium hydroxide. Granulations 2 hours after pulpotomy. Note granulations of birefringent calcite (Holland[45]).

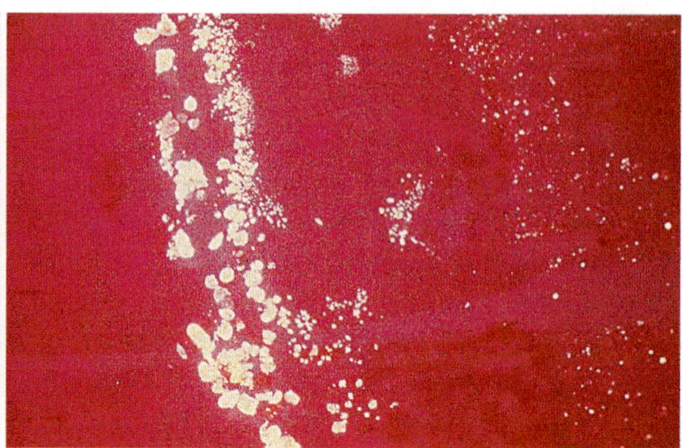

**Figure 7.12** - Calcium hydroxide. Granulations 48 hours after pulpotomy. Note granulations of birefringent calcite (Holland[45]).

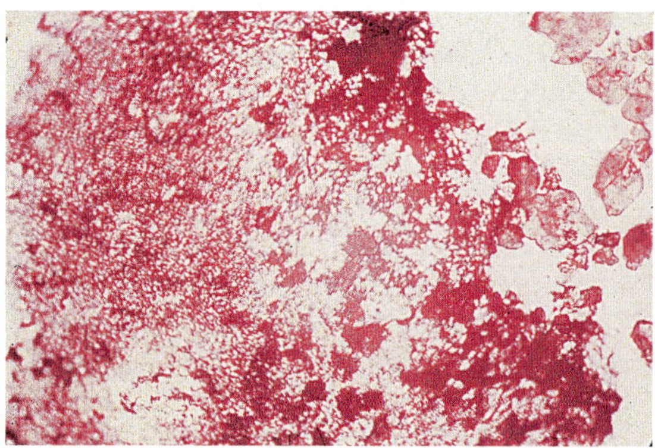

**Figure 7.13** - Calcium hydroxide. Granulations 48 hours after pulpotomy. Von Kossa's reaction showing granulations of calcite and dystrophic calcification area (Holland[45]).

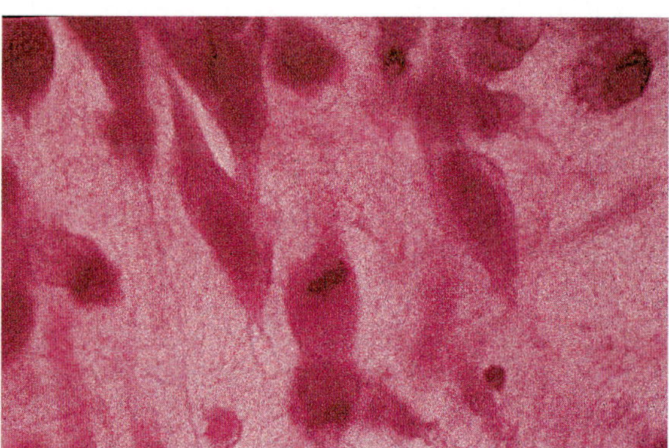

**Figure 7.14** - Calcium hydroxide. 48 hours after pulpotomy. Area of cellular proliferation (Holland[45]).

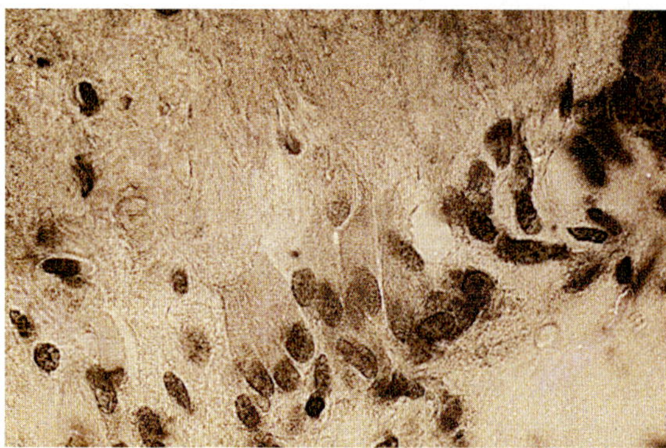

**Figure 7.15** - Calcium hydroxide. 7 days after pulpotomy. Deep granular area. Some young odontoblasts (Holland[45]).

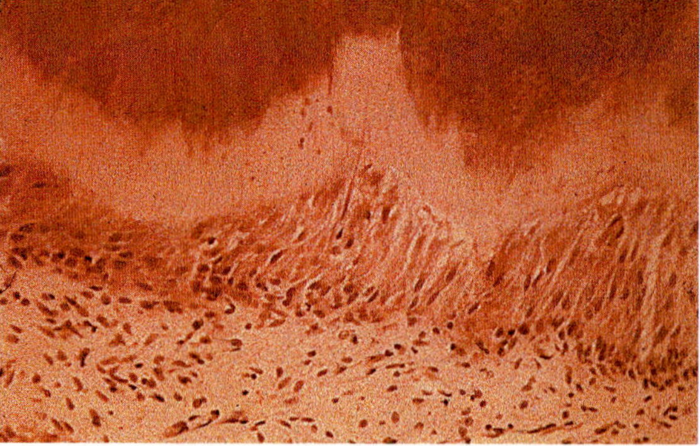

**Figure 7.16** - Calcium hydroxide. 30 days after pulpotomy. Complete odontoblastic layer (Holland[45]).

Sciaky & Pisanti[114] and Pisanti & Sciaki[108] did not observe that any of the calcium ions in the mineralized barrier came from the calcium hydroxide used in the protection of exposed dog's pulp and which contained radioactive calcium ($Ca^{45}$) or from the intravenous injection in dogs of a solution containing radioactive calcium. Probably, it occurred due to the methodology used, since the authors used auto radiographies. Holland et al.[56] preceded a histochemical analysis of dog dental pulp after pulp capping with calcium, barium, and strontium hydroxides. The dental pulps of dogs were capped with one of the hydroxides, and 48 hours after treatment, all pulps had a layer of large carbonate granulations that were von Kossa positive, birefringent to polarized light, and located mainly in the area between the necrotic and the living pulp tissue. In the pulps treated with barium or strontium hydroxide, the histochemical analyses showed that the metal of these granulations came from the capping material. These data suggest that the calcium from calcium hydroxide may participate in the composition of the birefringent granulations observed in the calcium hydroxide group (Fig. 7.17 to 7.24).

Experimental studies proved that when the dental pulp was cut at different levels, it reacts to the treatment with calcium hydroxide with a hard tissue bridge deposition, recommended for dental pulp and root canal treatment[59].

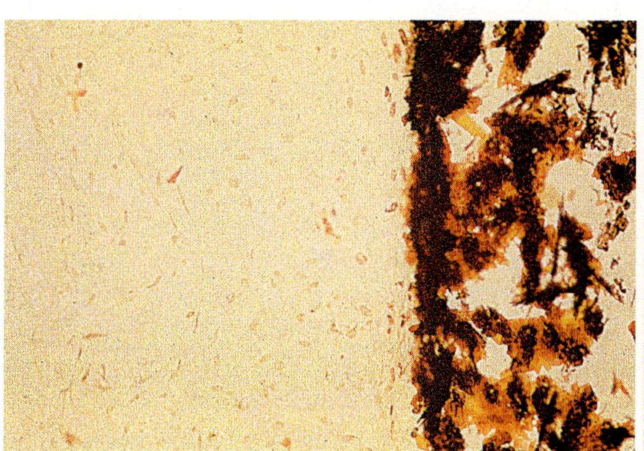

**Figure 7.17** - Strontium hydroxide. Pulpotomy and protection after 48 hours. Sodium rhodizonate staining that proves the presence of strontium (Holland et al.[56]).

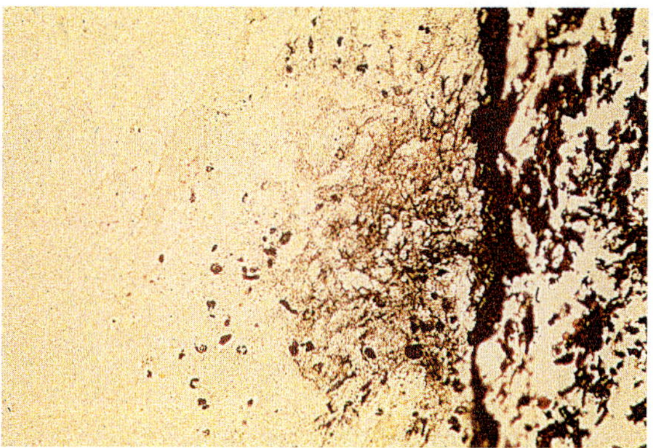

**Figure 7.18** - Strontium hydroxide. Pulpotomy and protection after for 48 hours. Von Kossa's staining shows the presence of calcium salts under the granulations of strontium carbonate (Holland et al.[56]).

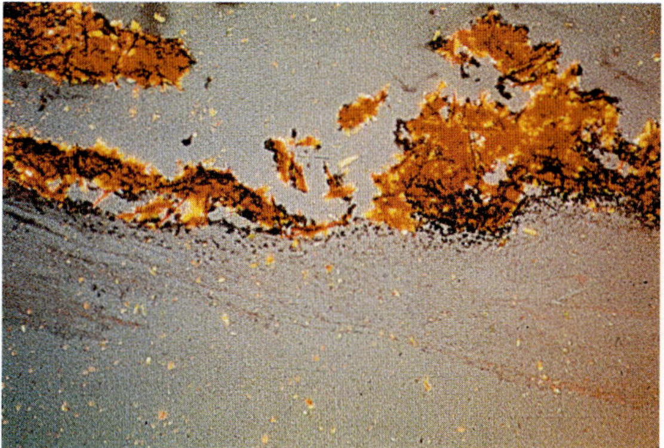

**Figure 7.19** - Strontium hydroxide. Pulpotomy and protection after 48 hours. Cut stained with sodium rhodizonate (Holland et al.[56]).

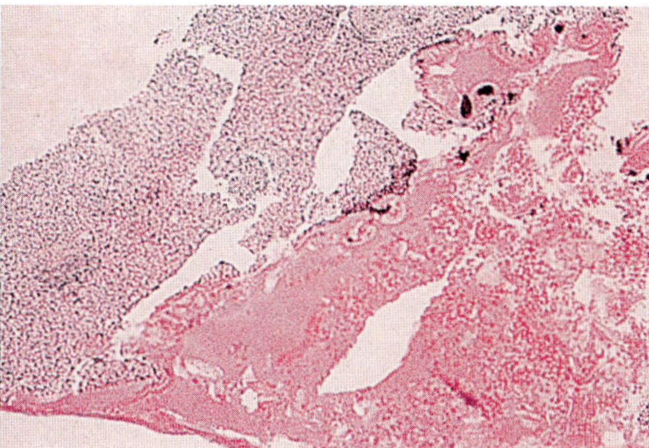

**Figure 7.20** - Barium hydroxide. Pulpotomy and protection after 48 hours. Barium hydroxide and area of necrosis are observed (after 30 days)(Holland et al.[56]).

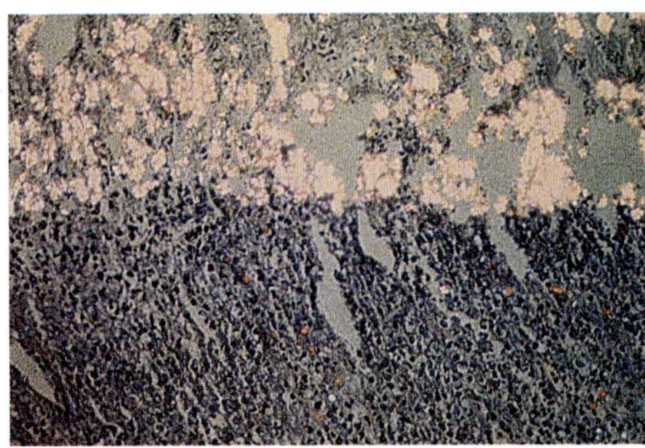

**Figure 7.21** - Granulations of barium carbonate birefringent to polarized light and Von Kossa positive (after 2 days) (Holland et al.[56]).

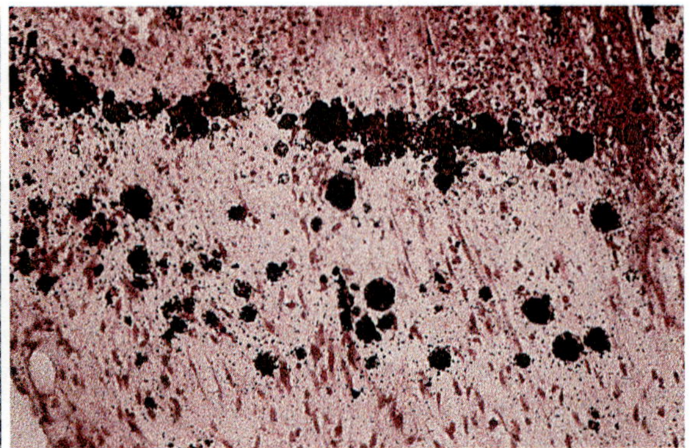

**Figure 7.22** - Granulations of barium carbonate birefringent to polarized light and Von Kossa positive (after 2 days) (Holland et al.[56]).

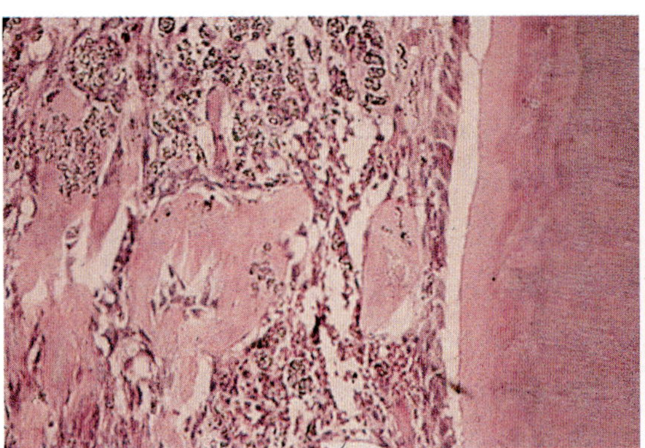

**Figure 7.23** - Calcifications below the granulations of barium carbonate (after 30 days). (Holland et al.[56]).

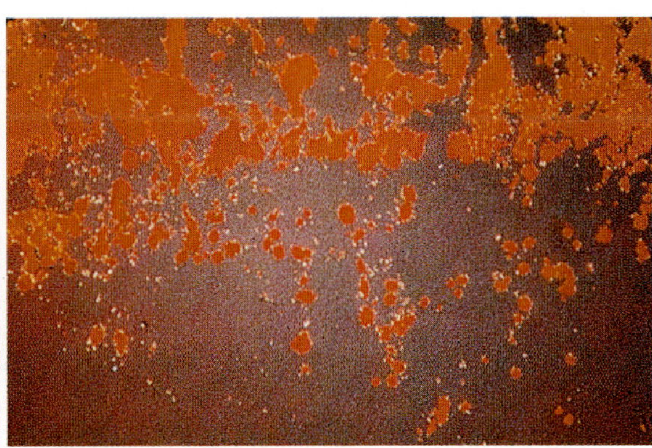

**Figure 7.24** - Positive granulations of barium carbonate to the sodium rhodizonate (after 30 days) (Holland et al.[56]).

Holland et al.[51] evaluated the healing process of the dental pulp of 40 dogs after pulpotomy and pulp covering with calcium hydroxide in powder or paste form. The results were analyzed histologically 30 days after the treatment. No differences were observed between the two experimental groups. Almost 90% of the specimens showed a complete hard tissue bridge protecting a vital and noninflamed dental pulp (Fig. 7.25-7.26).

Stanley & Lundy[129] observed Dycal therapy for pulp exposures. Teeth were intentionally subjected to pulp exposure and capped with Dycal for eventual microscopic evaluation. Peculiar to Dycal, is that the new bridge forms directly against the layer of Dycal, because of the action of macrophages in removing the chemically cauterized tissue. The size and thickness of the pulp tissue at the site of exposure determine whether a pulp-capping procedure or a pulpotomy is the treatment of choice. A re-evaluation of the criteria for pulp-capping procedures is in order.

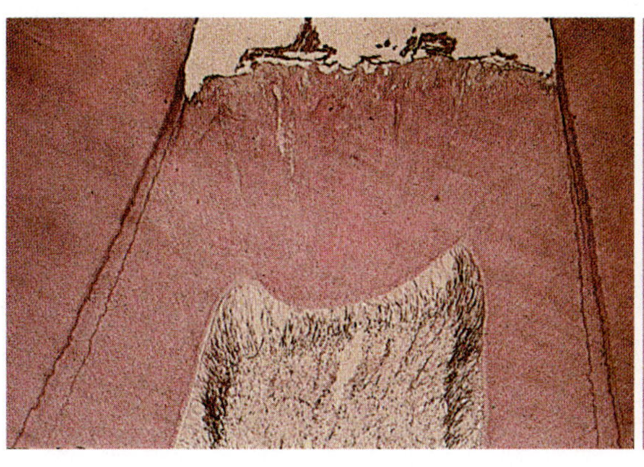

**Figure 7.25** - Calcium hydroxide in paste form. Complete hard tissue bridges and absence of inflammation (H.E.) (Holland et al.[51]).

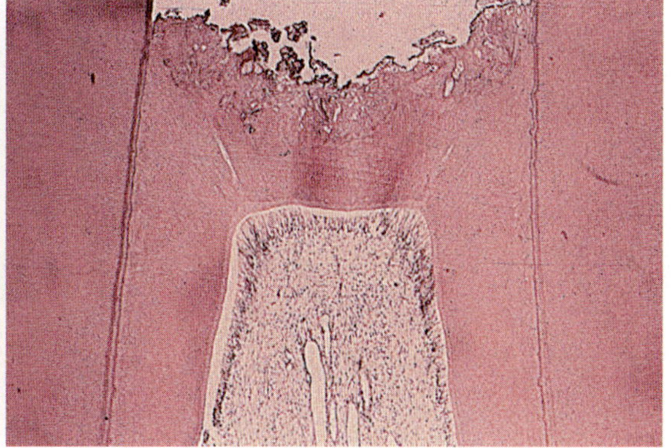

**Figure 7.26** - Calcium hydroxide in powder form. Complete hard tissue bridges and absence of inflammation (H.E) (Holland et al.[51]).

Tronstad & Mjor[133] studied the healing properties of the inflamed pulp of a monkey following exposure and capping with calcium hydroxide or zinc oxide and eugenol. Calcium hydroxide was found not to have any beneficial effect on the healing of the exposed inflamed pulp. The results with zinc oxide and eugenol were more favorable. Holland et al.[77] studied the healing process of dog's dental pulp after pulpotomy and protection with calcium hydroxide or Dycal. The histological results suggested that the mechanism of repair is the same in the pulps protected with calcium hydroxide or Dycal. The percentage of success, however, was smaller in the group of teeth treated with Dycal (Fig. 7.27 to 7.34).

Holland et al.[64] histologically evaluated the permeability of the hard tissue bridge formed after pulpotomy with calcium hydroxide. Pulpotomy and pulp capping with calcium hydroxide were performed in single-rooted teeth of five adult monkeys. After 30 days, some of the sealed teeth were opened and the hard tissue bridge was protected with silicate or zinc phosphate cement. Some teeth were left open and others, unopened, were used as controls. The more effective protection is directly related to the coronal surface of the hard tissue bridges. As the coronal surface has no or few dentinal tubules, it is more difficult for the irritating agent to come into contact with the odontoblast processes. Analysis of these results shows that complete hard tissue bridges, in addition to occurring with great frequency, produce satisfactory pulp protection. In a case in which the barrier is incomplete, some future clinical problems may result as an incomplete barrier does not offer adequate protection, as shown by the chronic inflammatory reaction in the remaining pulp tissue.

Holland et al.[50] studied the influence of the sealing material in the healing process of inflamed pulps capped with calcium hydroxide or zinc oxide-eugenol cement. Thus, dog dental pulps were experimentally inflamed and capped with these materials. Half of the specimens capped with calcium hydroxide had their coronal openings sealed with amalgam and the other half with zinc oxide-eugenol cement. The results were analyzed histologically ninety days after the treatment. Better results were obtained in the specimens treated with calcium hydroxide and with coronal openings sealed with zinc oxide eugenol cement.

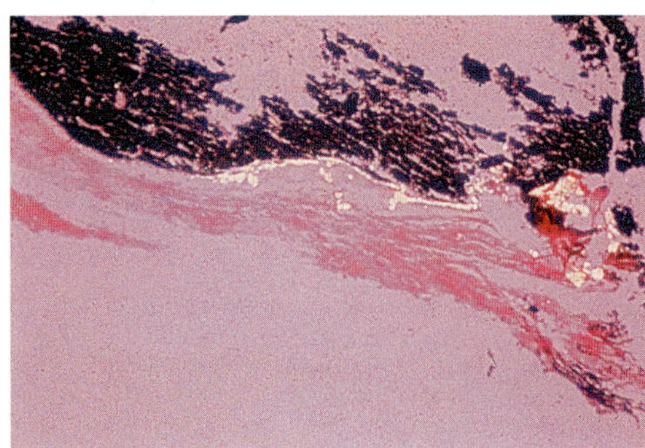

**Figure 7.27** - Calcite granulations in intimate contact with Dycal. Absence of necrosis area (2 days)(Holland et al.[67]).

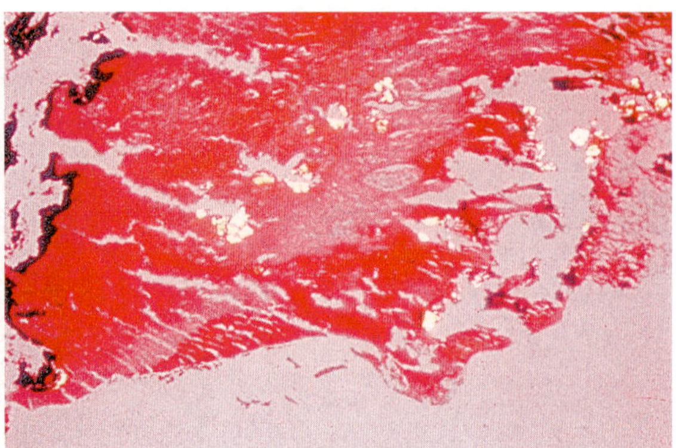

**Figure 7.28** - Calcite granulations distant from the material (Dycal). Presence of necrosis area (2 days) (Holland et al.[67]).

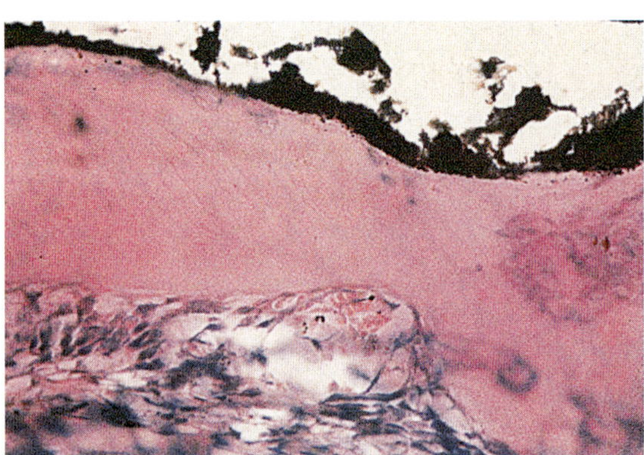

**Figure 7.29** - When a case such as the one in Figure 7.27 occurs, the dentin bridge is deposited in contact with Dycal (Holland et al.[67]).

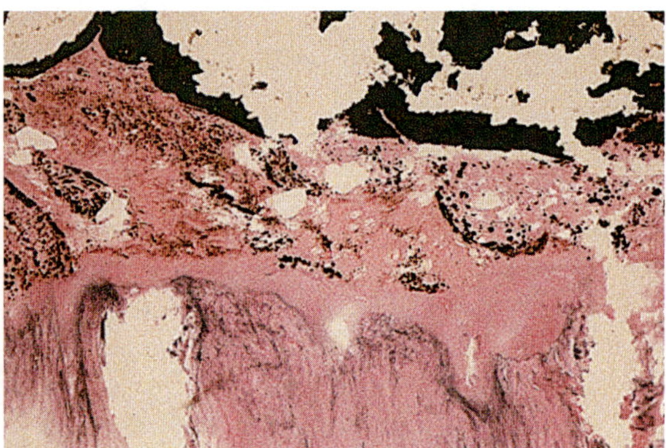

**Figure 7.30** - When a case such as the one in Figure 7.28 occurs, there is presence of necrosis between Dycal and the hard tissue bridge (Holland et al.[67]).

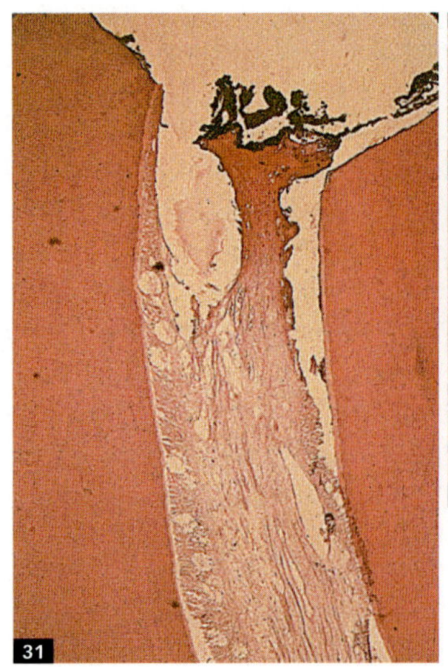


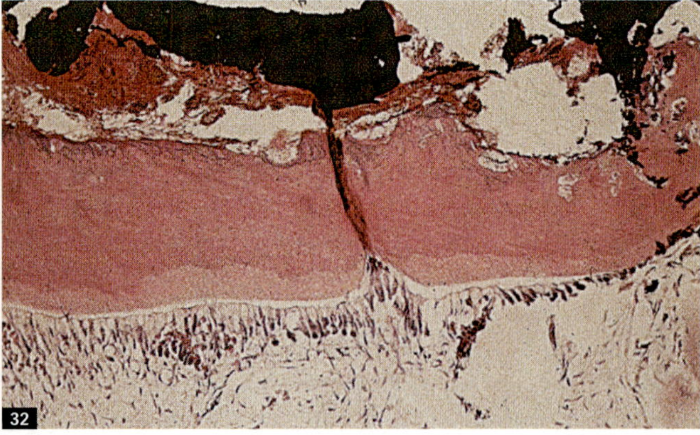


**Figure 7.31** - Necrosed pulp. Proportion established by the manufacturer (H.E.) (Holland et al.[77]).

**Figure 7.32** - Repair with formation of hard tissue. Paste with larger amount of catalyst (H.E.)(Holland et al.[77]).

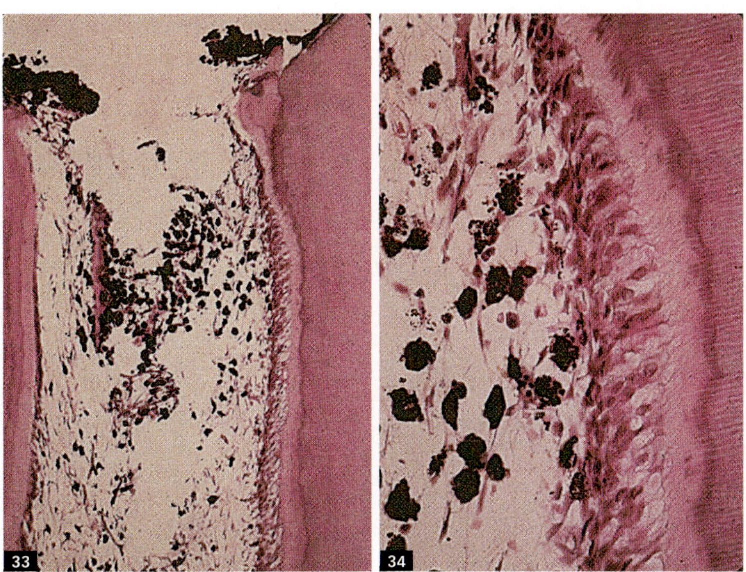

**Figure 7.33** - Paste with larger amount of base. Absence of hard tissue bridge and inflamed pulp (H.E.) (Holland et al.[77]).

**Figure 7.34** - Magnification of Figure 7.33 – Note; macrophages with particles of Dycal in their cytoplasm (H.E.)(Holland et al.[77]).

Mello et al.[103] analyzed the dental pulp response to calcium hydroxide and to zinc oxide eugenol paste, handled in two different consistencies. Pulp exposures 0.4 mm in diameter were performed in the vestibular surfaces of 42 dog's anterior teeth. The exposed tissue was then protected with the above mentioned materials. After 30 days, the histological examination showed that the dental pulp response to the zinc-oxide eugenol was an inflammatory infiltration in addition to the absence of healing. The polymorphonuclear leukocytes were the predominant cells close to the exposure site, and at some distance the infiltration was constituted of lymphocytes, plasma cells and macrophages. This result was seen in all pulps capped with zinc oxide eugenol, but there was less severity and spreading of the reactions when the capping cement was zinc oxide. This greater proportion of power was also related to a higher frequency of hard tissue deposition, mainly near dentin fragments proceeding from the operating procedure, but they never completely closed the exposed area. In all specimens, capping with calcium hydroxide was related to a dentin bridge scaling off the area of tissue under the experimental exposure. Occasional lymphocytes were seen in a few cases.

Mello et al.[102] conducted a histological study of the reaction of the inflamed dental pulp of dog's teeth after pulpotomy or pulp-curettage, and covering with calcium hydroxide. The dental pulps of the single root teeth of 8 young mongrel dogs were exposed to the oral environment for 7 days. The teeth of one animal were taken as control to evaluate dental pulp inflammation.

Pulpotomy or curettage was performed in the teeth of 7 dogs and 50% of these immediately had their pulp remainder protected with calcium hydroxide. The other 50% received a dressing of 2.5% prednisolone associated with Furacin oto-solution, in equal amounts, for 48 hours before being protected with calcium hydroxide. The crown openings of all the treated teeth were sealed with zinc oxide-eugenol cement. Thirty days after the treatment, the teeth were extracted, fixed and decalcified. Serial sections 6 microns thick were stained with hematoxylin and eosin. The pulps with total hard tissue barrier and no inflammatory reaction were considered as successful cases. The results obtained suggest the following conclusions:

1. The pulpotomy technique was better than pulp-curettage for the treatment of inflamed dental pulp;
2. The best results were obtained in the pulpotomy group in which a glucocorticoid dressing was used for 48 hours before pulp protections with calcium hydroxide;
3. The glucocorticoid dressing was not effective in the pulp-curettage group (Fig. 7.35 to 7.39).

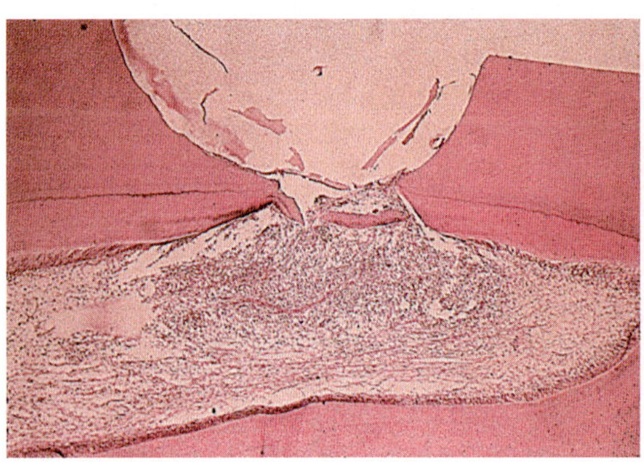

**Figure 7.35** - Zinc Oxide and eugenol. Absence of repair and intense inflammatory infiltrate (30 days, H.E., X40)(Mello et al.[103]).

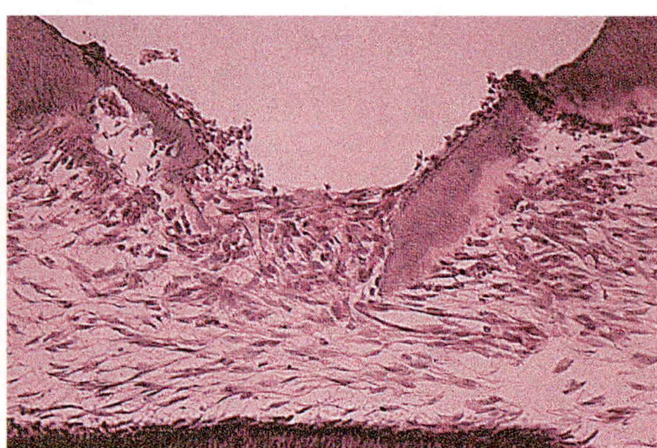

**Figure 7.36** - Magnification of Figure 7.35 (Mello et al.[103]).

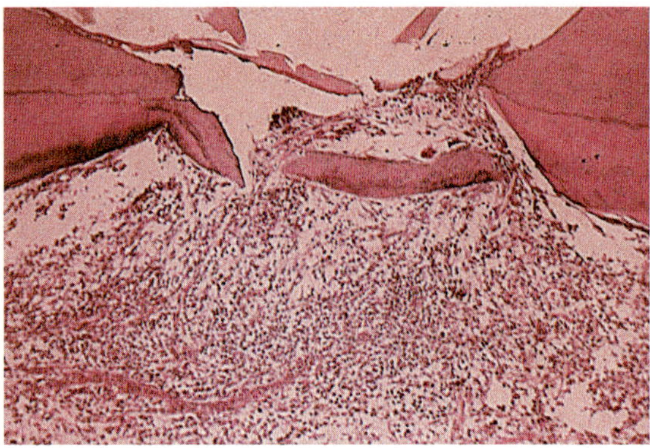

**Figure 7.37** - Consistent zinc oxide and eugenol, with less eugenol. Dental pulp with less intensely and extensively infiltrated (30 days, H.E., X40)(Mello et al.[103]).

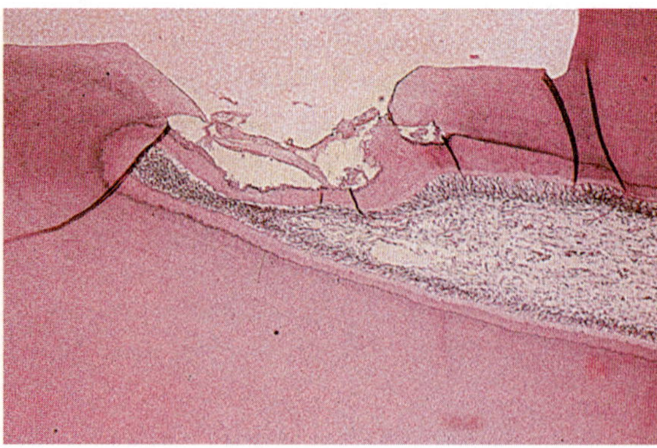

**Figure 7.38** - Calcium hydroxide. Pulp capping. Complete hard tissue bridge and absence of inflammation (H.E.)(Mello et al.[103]).

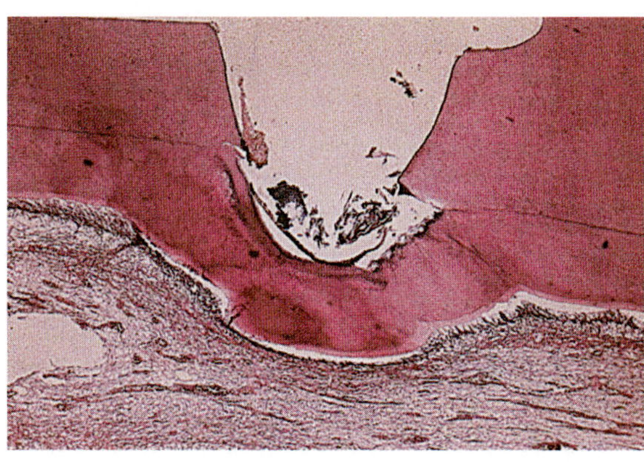

**Figure 7.39** - Calcium hydroxide. Pulp capping. Complete hard tissue bridge and absence of inflammation (H.E.) (Mello et al.[103]).

Hollland et al.[63] analyzed the effect of dentin fragments on the healing of the exposed dental pulp, in two stages. In the first, 20 dog's teeth were submitted to pulpotomy and the pulp tissue remainder was capped with dentin fragments, which were obtained from the treated tooth. Inflammatory reaction in different degrees and hard tissue deposition over some dentin fragments, located inside the dental pulp, was usually observed. In the second stage, 38 dog's teeth were analyzed from another experiment, in which the teeth had already been submitted to pulpotomy or pulp capping with calcium hydroxide. Dentin fragments were shown in the pulp tissue remainder, which disturbed healing so that the formation of dentin bridges was partial or defective, and the dental pulp was inflamed. The results suggested that: 1) there are no favorable results in pulp capping with dentin fragments; 2) the presence of dentin fragments on the pulp surface disturbs or inhibits the healing process after pulp capping with calcium hydroxide.

The pulpotomy technique is indicated for the conservative treatment of inflamed dental pulp. Some researchers, however, criticize the quality of the hard tissue bridge formed with calcium hydroxide, saying it may have tunnel defects, which can compromise the protective efficiency of the bridge. Recently, an experimental research in monkey's teeth demonstrated that the change of calcium hydroxide, after the formation of the hard tissue bridge, can promote new hard tissue deposition that efficiently repairs the tunnel defects on the bridge, if there are any[90].

Aydos[4] clinically and radiographically evaluated the behavior of the inflamed dental pulp, subjected to pulpotomy, corticoid-antibiotic action and afterwards to calcium hydroxide. As in the case of diagnostic and prognostic data, the visual clinical aspect of the pulp is exclusively considered. The success was 94.3%. Santini[113] tested the efficacy of calcium hydroxide in combination with a corticosteroid-antibiotic as a pulp dressing in contra-lateral pairs of human permanent premolars and molars with mature apices. All the teeth had been diagnosed as having a chronic pulpitis associated with a painful active carious lesion. In 100 patients, a total of 200 teeth radiographically shown to have mature apices, were treated. Assessment of bridge formation at the exposure site and direct inspection for an associated vital pulp was carried out. One tooth of each contralateral pair in each group was randomly selected and assessed after 2 years (Group 1) and 5 years (Group 2). Success rates to the order of 65% were obtained in both groups when a vital pulp associated with hard tissue formation at the exposure site was taken as the criterion of pulp wound healing. The results suggested that pulpotomy can be used in pediatric practice as an interim procedure pending routine endodontic treatment, especially suited for the young or nervous patient, unaccustomed to prolonged dental procedures. Caliskan[8] studied the success of pulpotomy in the management of hyperplasic pulpitis. In the study, 24 permanent teeth of individuals, aged 10–22 years and diagnosed as hyperplastic pulpitis were treated by pulpotomy using an atraumatic surgical technique with calcium hydroxide alone. The treatment was successful in 22 teeth, according to the following criteria: absence of clinical symptoms, absence of any intraradicular or periradicular radiographic pathological changes, presence of dentin bridge detected by clinical examination and sometimes observed radiographically, and sensitivity to electrical stimulation. The follow-up examination ranged from 12 to 48 months. The high frequency of clinical healing in this study appears to justify recommending pulpotomy as the treatment regime in selected cases of chronic hyperplastic pulpitis.

Lopes et al.[97] studied the calcified bridge after pulpotomy and the application of calcium hydroxide associated with saline, propylene glycol 400, and glycerin. In nine premolars, diagnosed for extraction for orthodontic reasons, pulpotomy was performed and calcium hydroxide was applied. The above mentioned items were associated in the treatment of 3 pairs of teeth. The teeth were extracted and radiographed after 60 days. The dental bridges formed were analyzed from a protective material and a dental pulp perspective, using a scanning electron microscopy. The calcified bridge surfaces showed agglutinates of calcospherites, existence of numerous circular and oval orifices and a smaller number of dentinal tubules (Fig. 7.40 to 7.49). Ulmansky et al.[135] evaluated calcium hydroxide induced bridges by scanning electron microscopy. The observation that the defects on the coronal surface are larger than those on the apical surface suggests that the quality of the bridge improves, as the odontoblasts migrate apically with the apposition of dentin. Goldberg et al.[38] studied the characteristics of the hard tissue bridge formed after pulpotomies and the dressing of the pulp wound with a calcium hydroxide camphorated p-monochlorophenol paste in 13 young premolars, with the use of a scanning electron microscopy and methylene blue dye. The coronal surface of the bridge showed the presence of crystals of different sizes and shapes. The pulp surface of the bridge was formed by the coalescence of calcospherites, showing the existence of numerous circular or oval holes approximately 20 to 250 µm in diameter. The permeability of the bridge was evaluated with the use of 2% methylene blue dye, showing intense dye leakage through the aforementioned orifices.

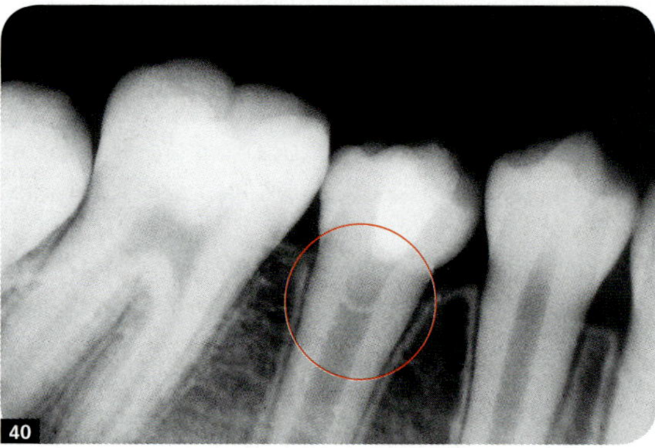


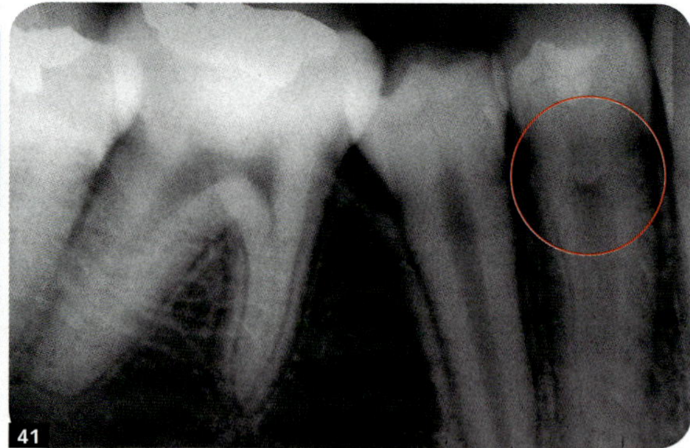


**Figures 7.40 and 7.41** - Radiographies of human first premolar after the pulpotomy, showing the formation of mineralized barrier after 60 days.

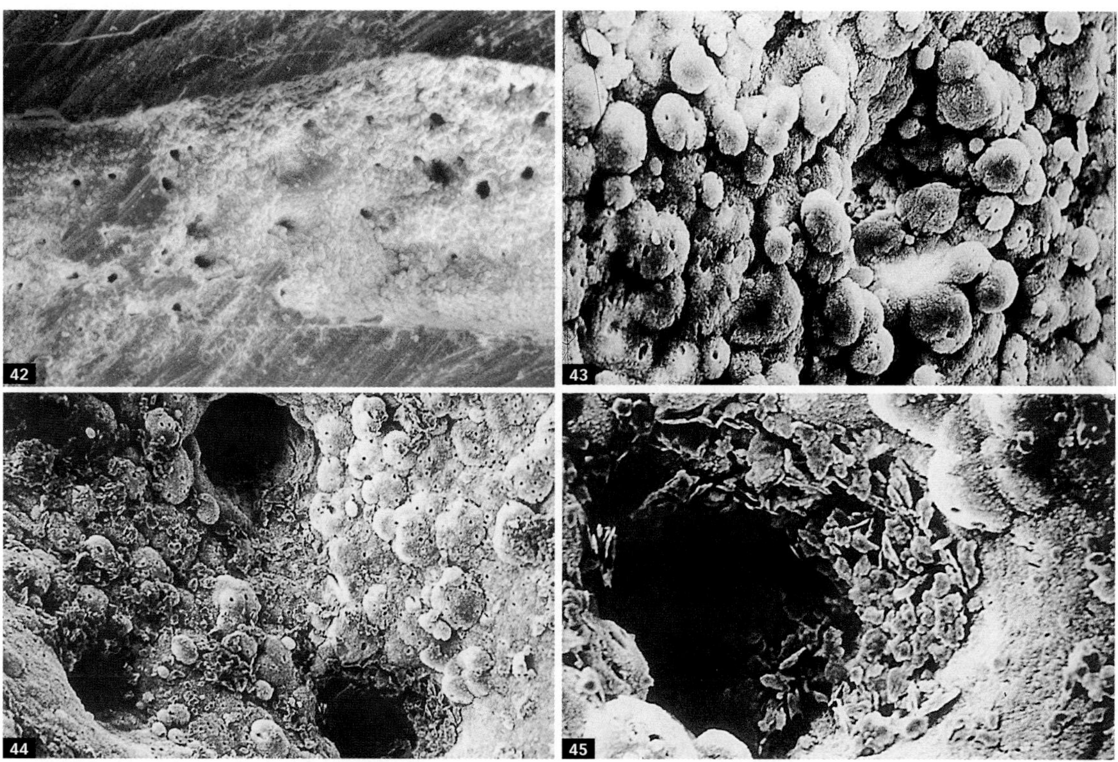

**Figures 7.42 to 7.45** - Pulp surfaces of the mineralized barrier visualized by Scanning Electron Microscopy, showing calcospherite agglutinations with reduced number of dental tubules and orifices of small dimensions.

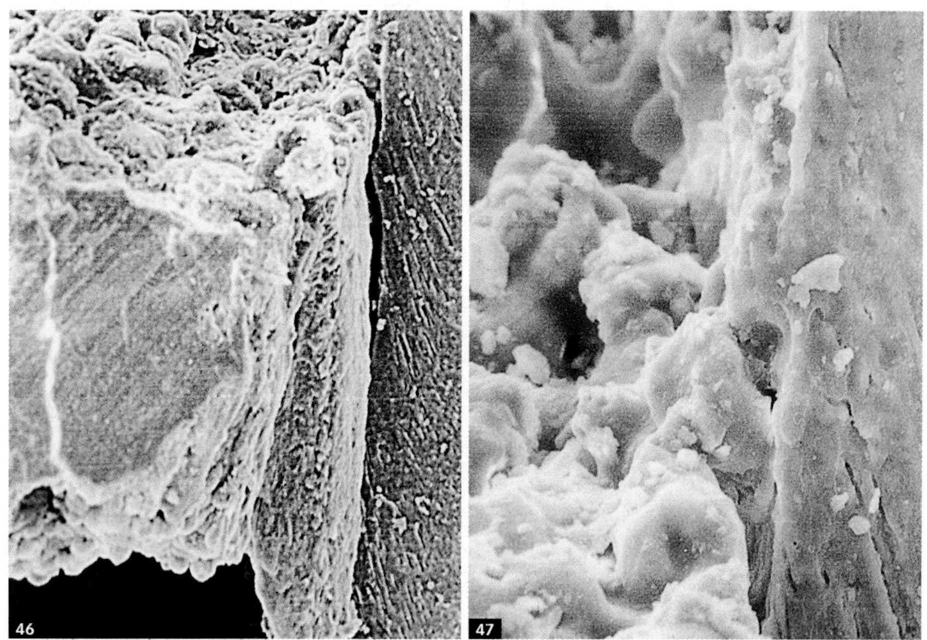

**Figures 7.46 and 7.47** - Buccal-lingual surface of the union areas between the mineralized barrier and the surrounding dentin of the walls of the root canal by through SEM.

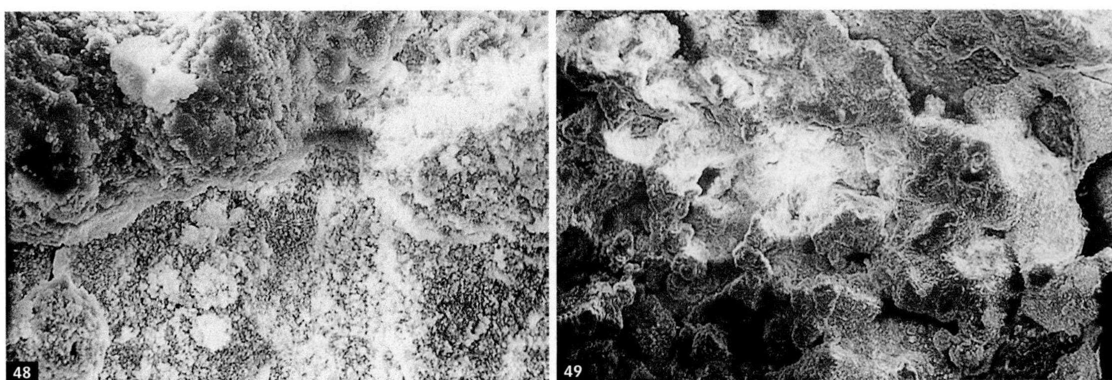

**Figures 7.48 and 7.49** - Crown surface of the mineralized barrier examined by SEM, showing mineralized structures with amorphous morphologies and absences of orifices.

In the last few years, dentistry has observed the appearance of new materials and new techniques that deserve precise, longitudinal and serious evaluations, before being indicated for use in routine treatment, and substituting those materials that have demonstrated satisfactory results in the process of tissue repair. It is opportune to emphasize that of these new materials, some have stimulated explanations and defined new conduct, and others are waiting on the natural development of the facts, scientific evidences and greater improvement. Among the materials that have been applied on dental pulp, the appearance of the adhesive systems, mineral trioxide aggregate and dentinogenic proteins have been noted.

Adhesive systems certainly represent important developments, however, the way they have been divulged and indicated have aroused huge speculation, principally when their direct application on the dental pulp was indicated. There is no doubt about the importance and development achieved with the appearance of the adhesive system, however, the location of application and the form of divulgation were the subject of surprise to some endodontists. The definition of parameters for certain investigations that were being revealed caused several researches on pulp biology to be questioned, which made Stanley[127] discuss and present criteria for standardizing and increasing the credibility of the studies about direct pulp capping.

There are many skeptics who condemn pulp capping, but like to keep an eye on the research progress being made. Considerable literature emphasizes the negative aspects of vital pulp therapy and discourages its practice. Some clinicians and investigators continue to condemn pulp capping therapy for the same reasons reported in the literature 80 years ago, despite the advances made in pulp biology. Clinicians are well aware of the immediate and long-term success rates after root canal therapy, but are less certain of the success of pulp capping. The research data on pulp capping is at times inadequate, confusing, misleading or even incorrect, and diminishes the confidence of the practitioner in performing pulp capping[127,128].

One of the important factors for the evaluation of the success in the result of restorative treatment is the physical integrity, absence of marginal leakage and the good biologic behavior of the material towards the dentin-pulp complex. There has been a great deal of discussion as regards the use of the adhesive system directly over the dental pulp, as noticed in several previously described studies. When particles of the primers of adhesive systems come into contact with the pulp tissue, it leads to irreversible aggressions, because in attempting to solve the problem, macrophages and giant cells move to another location and die, making the lesion persist[5,15-17,30,44,89,105,106,126,127].

In the group of the pulp aggressors represented by the restorative materials, it must be made clear that these aggressors range from the action of the microorganisms in the caries process to the consequences of cavity preparation, protective and restorative material. Moreover, the host's response should never be underestimated.

In different studies conducted by Lanza[94], Hebling et al.[44], Holland et al.[89], Costa et al.[15], poor results of the application of the adhesive system directly over the pulp tissue could be observed.

Hebling et al.[44] studied the biocompatibility of an adhesive system applied to exposed human dental pulp. Human pulp tissue was directly capped with All Bond 2, or calcium hydroxide and evaluated 7, 30, or 60 days after the procedures. Histological analysis was performed to assess the inflammatory cell response, tissue disorganization, dentin bridging, and the presence of bacteria. With All Bond 2 capping, at 7 days there was a large area of neutrophilic infiltrate underlying the pulp capping material, and the death of adjacent odontoblasts, was observed. With time, however, the neutrophic reaction was replaced by fibroblastic proliferation, with macrophages and giant cells surrounding globules of resin scattered in the coronal pulp tissue. The persistent inflammatory reaction and hyaline alteration of extracellular matrix inhibited complete pulp repair or dentin bridging. Whereas, at 7 days, the pulp tissue capped with calcium hydroxide exhibited odontoblast-like cells organized underneath coagulation necrosis. Pulp repair developed into apparently complete dentin bridge formation at 60 days. All Bond 2 did not appear to allow any pulp repair and does not appear to be indicated for direct pulp capping of human teeth. Costa et al.[15] evaluated the pulp response following direct pulp capping with an adhesive system and a zinc-oxide eugenol (ZOE) cement on pulp exposures in rat molar teeth. Both pulp capping materials allowed pulp repair, characterized by reorganization of a new odontoblast cell layer underlying the dentin bridge formation. The adhesive, however, promoted a large zone of cell-rich fibrodentin matrix deposition between the pulp capping material and the dentin bridge, which was deposited far from the pulp exposure site. On the other hand, pulps capped with ZOE showed dentin bridging immediately subjacent to the pulp capping material. In the samples in which microleakage occurred between dental material and cavity walls, there was a persistent inflammatory reaction and lack of complete pulp repair. Costa et al.[17] investigated the biocompatibility of two current adhesive resins and a calcium hydroxide cement. At 7 days, both adhesive resins elicited a moderate/intense inflammatory reaction that decreased over time. Fibrous capsules surrounding the tubes were observed at 30 days. Half of the samples in Groups 1 and 2 showed thin fibrous capsule formation containing macrophages, capillaries, lymphocytes, fibroblasts, and collagen fibers. Connective tissue healing was observed even though many specimens exhibited a persistent inflammatory reaction mediated by macrophages and giant cells at the 60-day evaluation. Dycal allowed complete healing at 30 days with only a thin fibrous capsule. In conclusion, all experimental materials were successfully walled off by the connective tissue of the rat. The adhesive resins, however, may release particles that may in turn, induce a persistent local inflammatory reaction. Consequently, under this specific condition, these materials cannot be regarded as biocompatible. Dycal was less irritating than the adhesive resins and was better tolerated by the connective tissue.

Pameijer & Stanley[106] discussing the disaster effects of the technique of total acid attack on pulp capping in primates, concluded that until a modification or new technique or material that exceeds the success produced by calcium hydroxide appears, the use of acid etching and application of the adhesive system in pulp capping is contraindicated.

Holland et al.[89] conducted research to observe whether the tunnel defects in dentin bridges are exclusively due to the use of the calcium hydroxide. Thus, human teeth indicated for extractions for orthodontic reason, had their pulps exposed experimentally and protected directly with the adhesive system Prime & Bond (Dentsply). One hundred and fifty days later, the teeth were extracted and processed for histomorphologic analysis. Tunnel defects that allowed communication between the surface of the dentin bridge formed and pulp tissue, were detected. As also admitted by Stanley & Pameijer[130], it was concluded that the tunnel defects were not related to the pulp protector material used, but to the number and size of blood vessels present (Fig.7.50 to 7.55). Figures 7.56 to 7.69 show a study published by Holland et al.[89], which analyzed the pulp capping and the pulpotomy in monkey's teeth, using the adhesive system All Bond 2.

Using optic microscopy, Faraco-Jr & Holland[30] analyzed the effect of a dentin bonding agent on the dental pulp of dogs. Fifteen permanent teeth from 8-month-old dogs were used. Class V cavities were prepared on the labial surfaces and the pulps were exposed. The dentinal adhesive system (Single Bond) was applied on the pulp and the cavities were sealed with composite resin. The animals were sacrificed 60 days after the treatment and the teeth were prepared according to the usual histological techniques. Serial sections were stained with hematoxylin and eosin as well as by the Brown and Breen method. No dentinal bridge formation could be observed in any of the specimens, while inflammatory infiltrate or necrosis of the dental pulp was observed in all cases (Fig. 7.70 to 7.73).

Holland et al.[47] studied the tunnel defects in dentin bridges and their relationship with calcium hydroxide use. Human teeth indicated for extraction for othodontic reasons were used in this research. Their pulps were experimentally exposed and directly protected with the adhesive system Prime & Bond 2.1. One hundred and fifty days after the treatment the teeth were extracted and prepared for histomorphological analysis. There were numerous tunnel defects in the neoformed dentin bridges, allowing communication between the top surfaces of the bridges and the pulp tissue. As admitted by Stanley & Pameijer[106], it was concluded that the tunnel defects observed in dentin bridges are not related to the material used in direct pulp protection, but to number and size of the vessels in this portion of the tissue (Fig.7.74 to 7.76).

Accorinte et al.[2] evaluated the response of human pulps capped with a calcium hydroxide cement after bleeding control with 2 hemostatic agents. Pulps were exposed on the occlusal floor, and the bleeding was controlled either with saline solution or 2.5% sodium hypochlorite. After that, the pulp was capped with calcium hydroxide cement and restored with resin composite. After 30 and 60 days, the teeth were extracted and processed with hematoxylin-eosin and categorized in a histologic score system. As regards dentin bridge formation, an inferior response of the sodium hypochlorite group (60 days) was observed when compared with saline (in 60 days). The response of the sodium hypochlorite in the 30 days group generally was similar to that of the groups treated with saline solution. Nevertheless, after 60 days, 2.5% sodium hypochlorite showed a trend toward an inferior response. Using saline solution as a hemostatic agent before pulp capping with calcium hydroxide cement resulted in a significantly better histomorphologic response than using 2.5% sodium hypochlorite for this purpose.

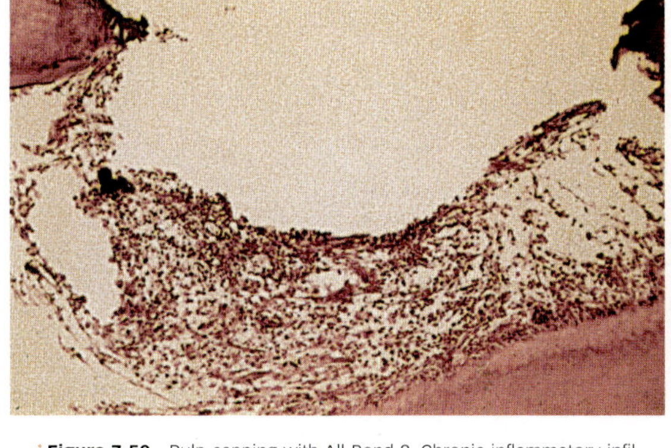

**Figure 7.50** - Pulp capping with All Bond 2. Chronic inflammatory infiltrate 60 days after the treatment. Absence of hard tissue bridge (H.E., X40) (Holland et al.[89]).

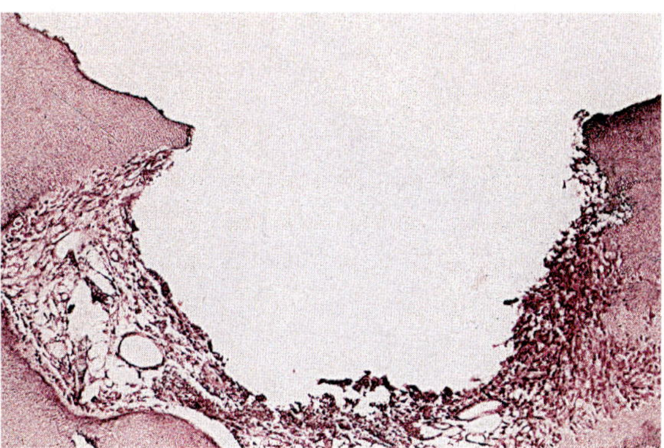

**Figure 7.51** - Pulp capping with All Bond 2. Chronic inflammatory infiltrate 60 days after the treatment. Absence of hard tissue bridge (H.E., X40) (Holland et al.[89]).

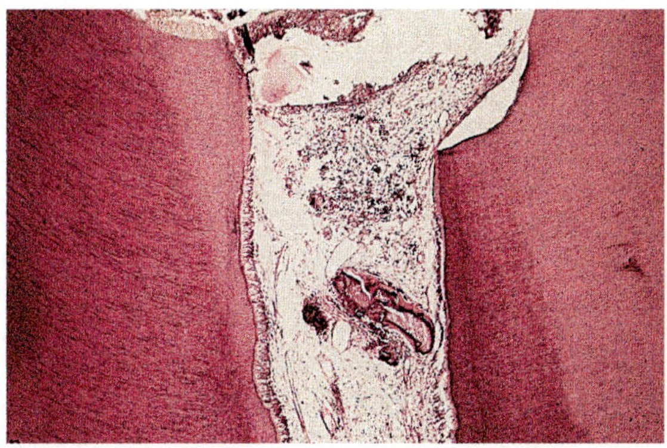

**Figure 7.52** - Pulpotomy with All Bond 2. Chronic inflammatory infiltrate 60 days after the treatment. Absence of hard tissue bridge (H.E., X40) (Holland et al.[89]).

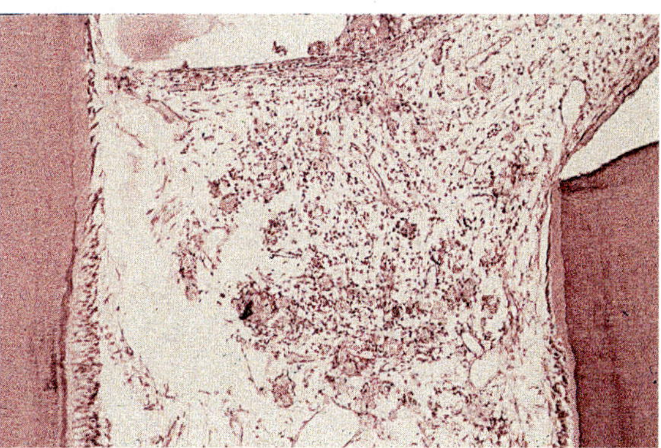

**Figure 7.53** - Magnification of Figure 7.52 (Holland et al.[89]).

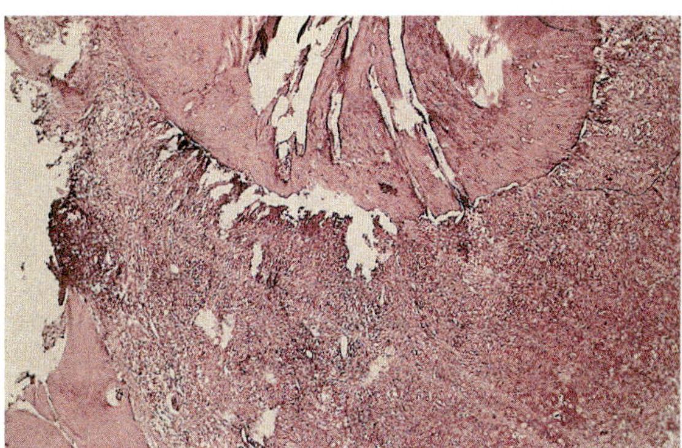

**Figure 7.54** - Pulpotomy with All Bond 2. Necrotic pulp and periapical lesion (H.E., X40) (Holland et al.[89]).

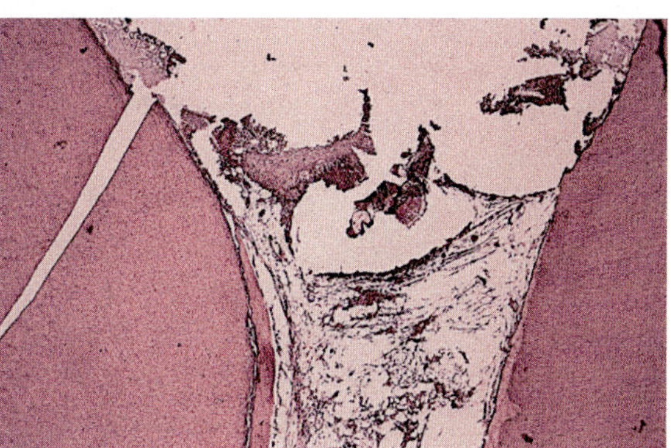

**Figure 7.55** - Pulpotomy with the All Bond 2. Chronic inflammatory infiltrate 60 days after the treatment. Absence of hard tissue bridge (H.E., X40) (Holland et al.[89]).

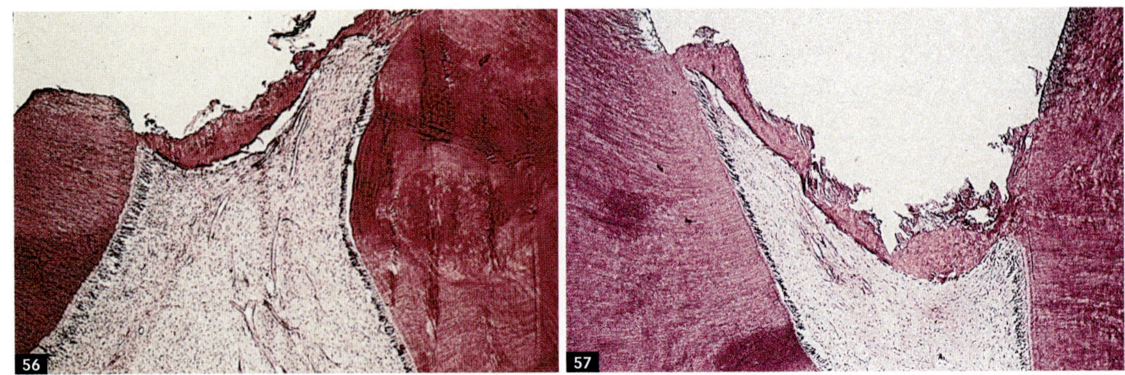


**Figures 7.56 and 7.57** - Pulp capping with $Ca(OH)_2$. Presence of hard tissue bridge. Monkey's pulp (90 days) (H.E., X40) (Holland et al.).

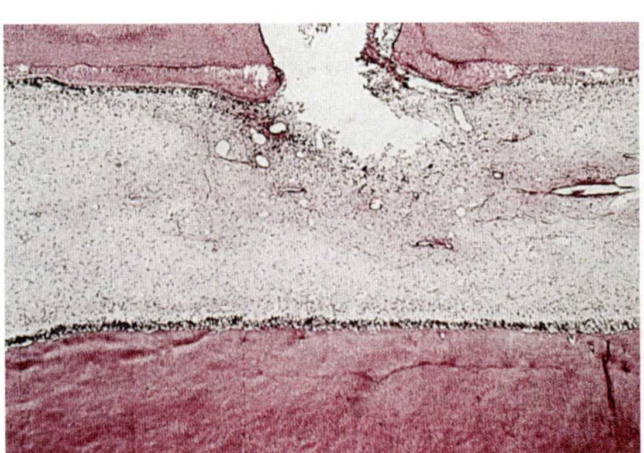

**Figure 7.58** - Pulp capping with All Bond 2. Absence of repair and alteration of the intercellular substance. Monkey pulp (90 days)(H.E., X40) (Holland et al.).

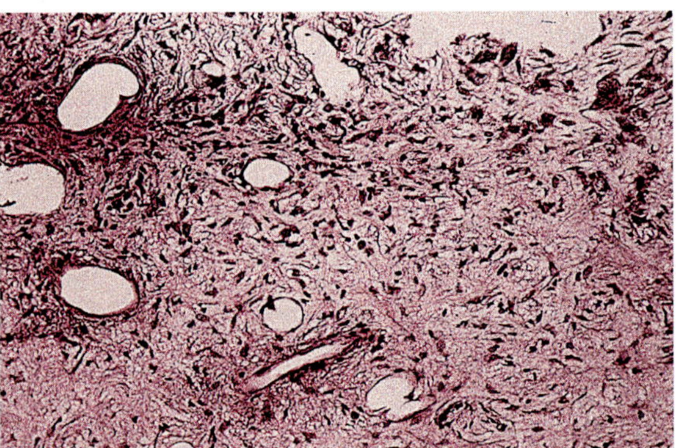

**Figure 7.59** - Magnification of Figure 7.58 (Holland et al.).

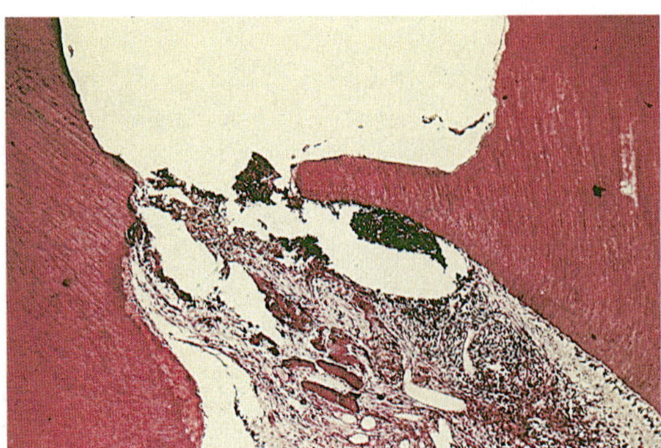

**Figure 7.60** - Pulp capping with All Bond 2. Absence of repair. Monkey pulp. (90 days) (H.E. X40) (Holland et al.).

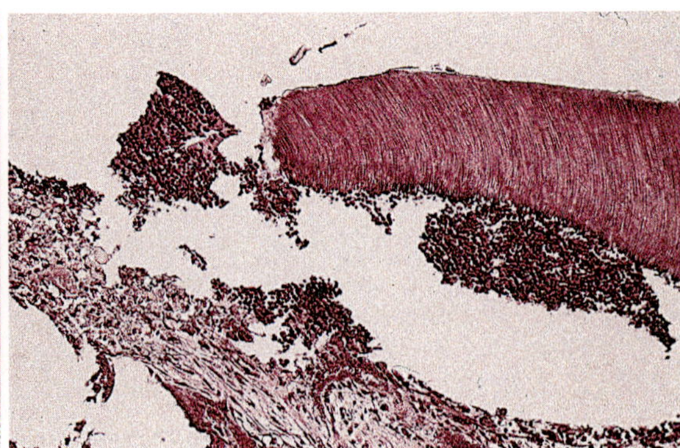

**Figure 7.61** - Magnification of Figure 7.60 (Holland et al.).

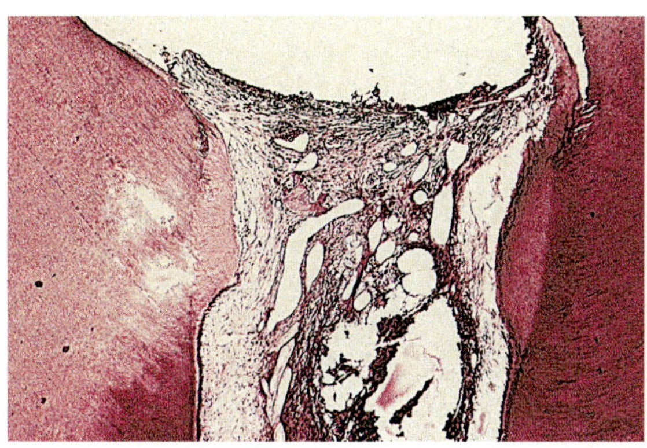

**Figure 7.62** - Pulpotomy with All Bond 2. Absence of repair and chronic inflammation. Monkey pulp. (90 days)(H.E., X40) (Holland et al.).

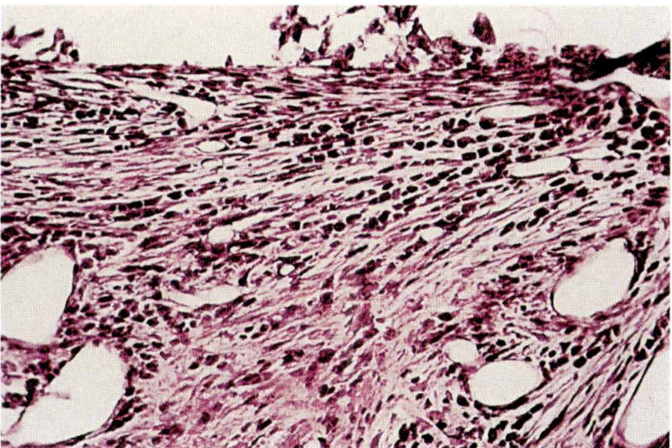

**Figure 7.63** - Magnification of Figure 7.62 (Holland et al.).

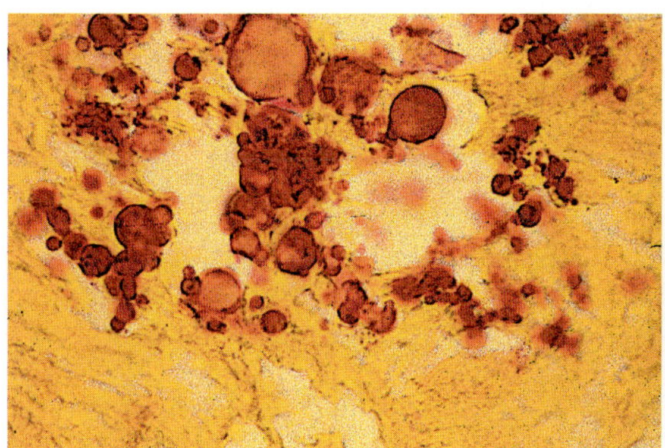

**Figure 7.64** - Particles of primer inside the pulp, see with the of Brown and Brenn stain.

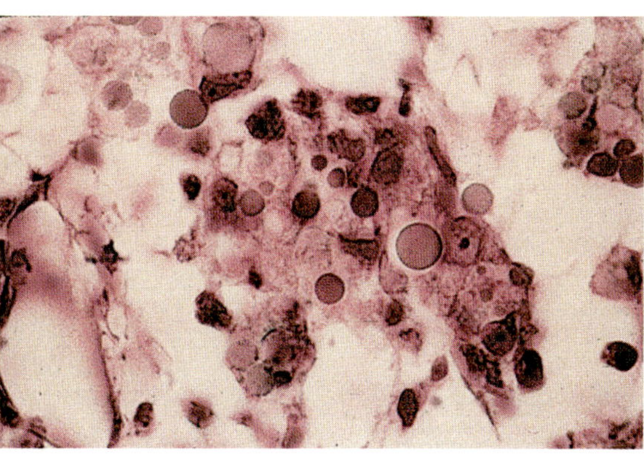

**Figure 7.65** - Particles of primer inside the pulp, see with the H.E stain (X40) (Holland et al.).

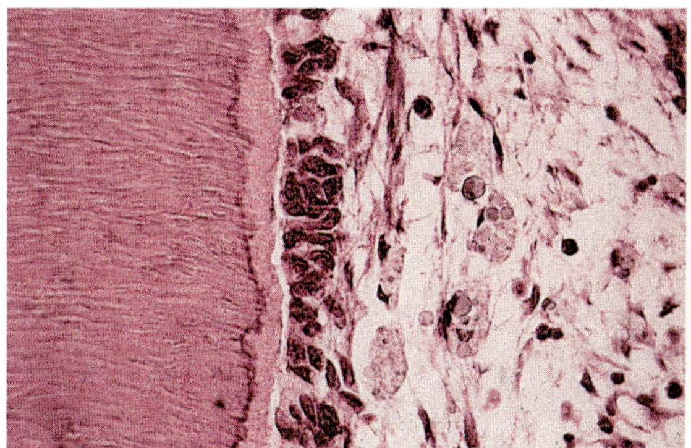

**Figure 7.66** - Residues of primer in depth, close to the odontoblastic layer in the root pulp. Monkey's pulp (H.E., X40) (Holland et al.).

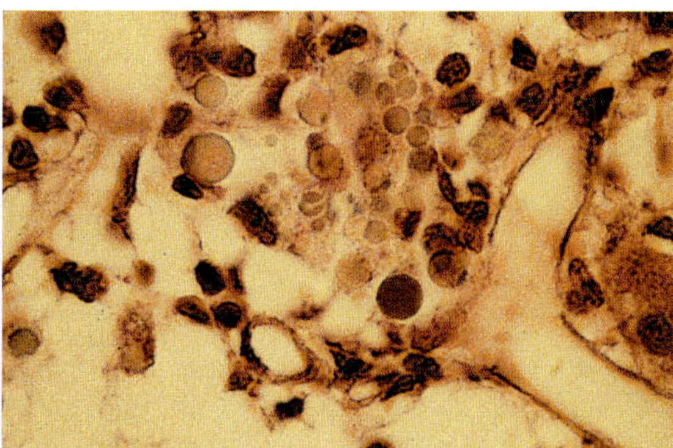

**Figure 7.67** - Particles of Primer inside the Monkey pulp (H.E., X40) (Holland et al.)

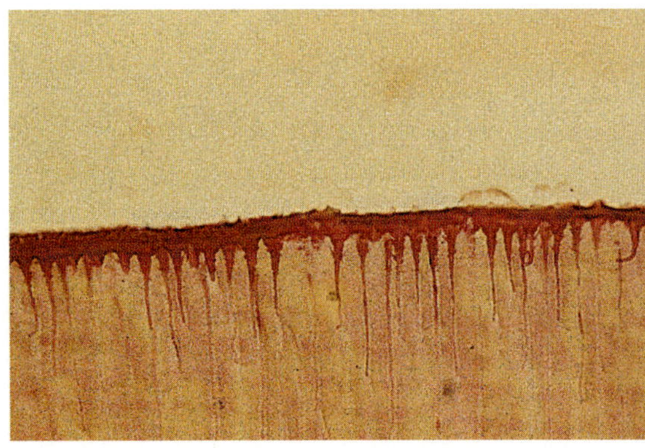

**Figure 7.68** - Human dentin - Primer inside the dental tubules (Holland et al.).

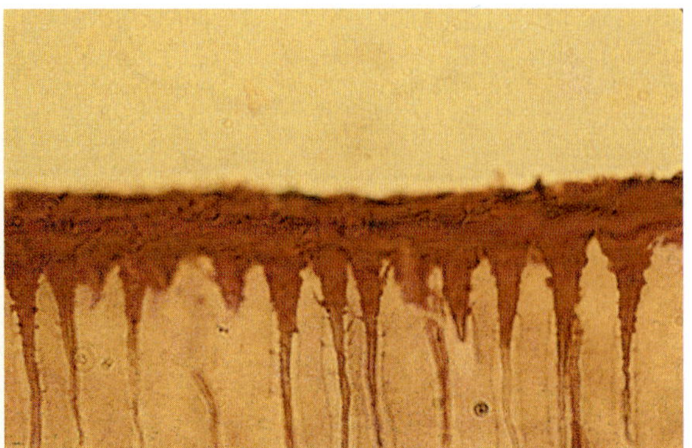

**Figure 7.69** - Human dentin - Primer inside the dental tubules. Magnification (Holland et al.).

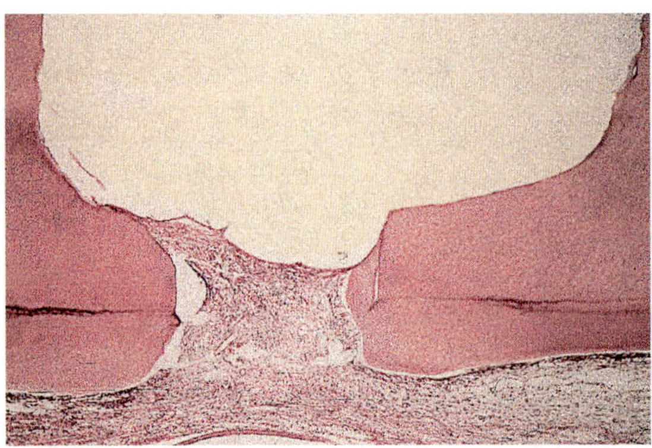

**Figure 7.70** - Pulp capping with Single Bond. Absence of hard tissue bridge (60 days, H.E., X40) (Faraco & Holland[30]).

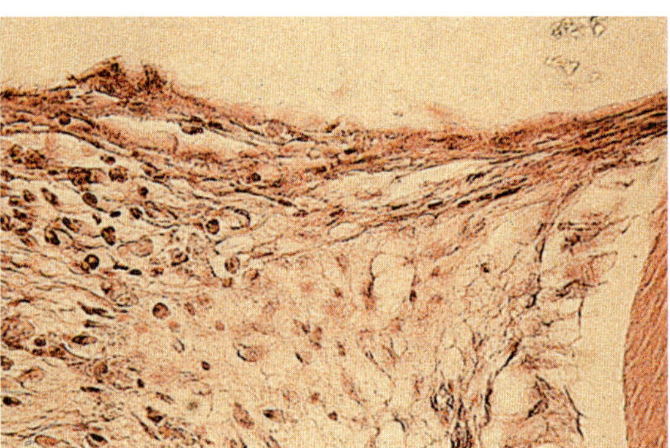

**Figure 7.71** - Magnification of Figure 7.70. Chronic inflammatory infiltrated. (H.E., X200) (Faraco & Holland[30]).

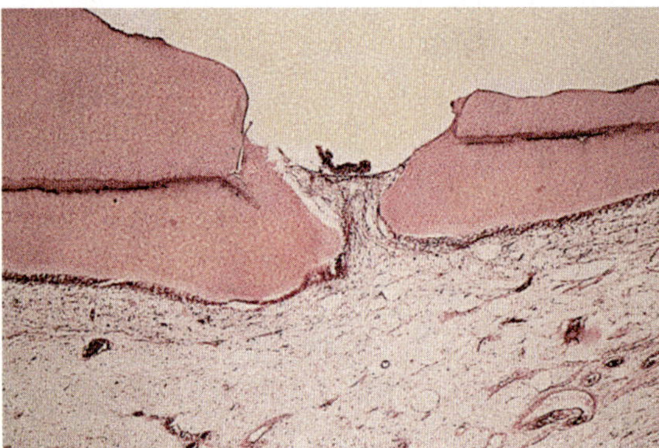

**Figure 7.72** - Single Bond. Absence of hard tissue bridge - Presence of neoformed dentin in the lateral teeth (H.E., X40) (Faraco & Holland[30]).

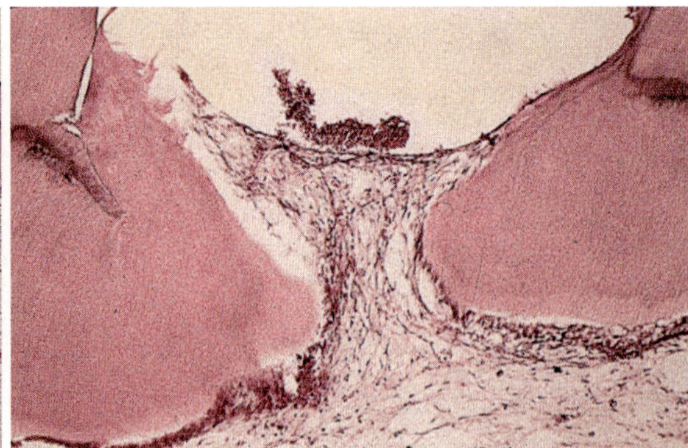

**Figure 7.73** - Magnification of Figure 7.72. Neoformed dentin and pulp with small infiltrated inflammatory chronic (H.E., X200) (Faraco & Holland[30]).

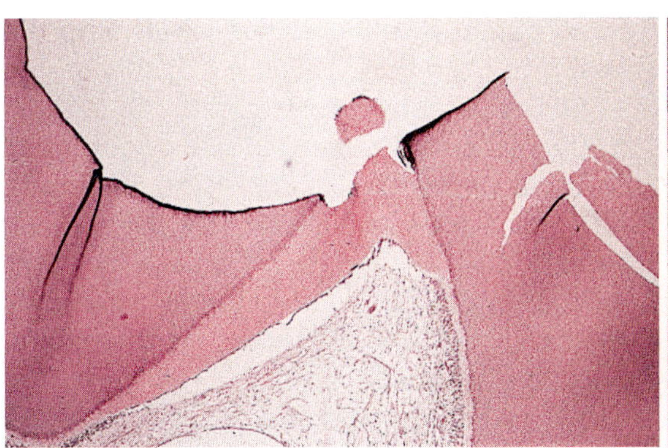

**Figure 7.74** - Pulp capping with Single Bond in human tooth. Dentin bridge with appearance of integrity (H.E., X40) (Holland et al.[47]).

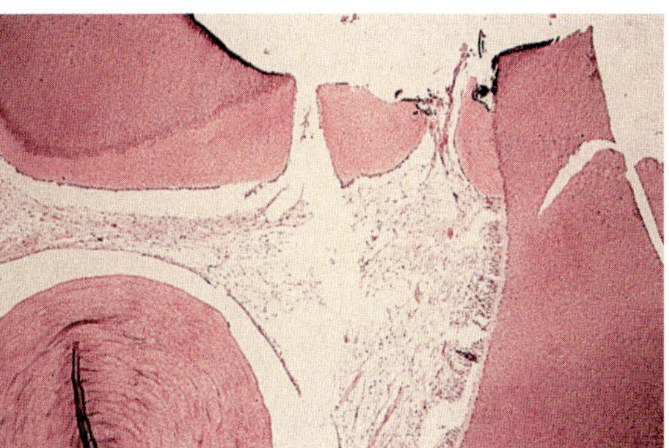

**Figure 7.75** - Pulp capping with Single Bond in human tooth. Deeper Cut of Figure 7.74, shows that the bridge is not complete (H.E., X40) (Holland et al.[47]).

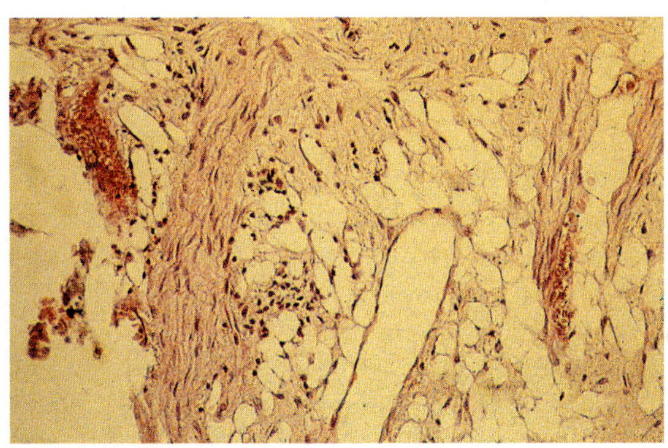

**Figure 7.76** - Pulp capping with Single Bond in human tooth. Hydropic degeneration of the pulp and chronic inflammatory infiltrate (H.E.) (Holland et al.[47]).

Another material that has been much studied lately, and that presents excellent capacity of stimulating the mineralization is the Mineral Trioxide Aggregate. This material was developed by the University of Loma Linda (United States) with the purpose of sealing communications between the tooth and the external surfaces[95,131]. Several investigations were performed, in vivo and in vitro[3,6,7,22,31,73,75,78,79,81,93,104,112,118].

Soares[118] analyzed the pulp response to the mineral trioxide aggregate (MTA) compared with calcium hydroxide, in pulpotomies performed in dog teeth. The authors observed the formation of the hard tissue barrier in 91.66% and 96.43% of the teeth treated with calcium hydroxide and MTA, respectively. There was no significant statistical difference between the reparative phenomena or between the adverse effects on reparation among the tested materials, except as regards continuity of the dentin barrier, in relation to cracks, where it was significant, evidencing the similarity of behavior of the pulp tissue towards both materials.

Various studies[6,22,75,79,81,112] discussed the main properties and clinical applications of MTA and Portland cement in pulp treatment. Holland et al.[81] observed the rat subcutaneous connective tissue reaction to the implanted dentin tubes filled with calcium hydroxide or mineral trioxide aggregate. The animals were sacrificed after 7 and 30 days, and the specimens were prepared for morphological study. Some undecalcified specimens were prepared for histological analysis for calcium with polarized light and Von Kossa technique. The results were similar for both studied materials. At the tube openings, there were Von Kossa-positive granules that were birefringent to polarized light. Next to these granulations, there was an irregular tissue like a bridge, which was Von Kossa-positive. The dentin walls of the tubes exhibited a structure in the tubules, highly birefringent to polarized light, usually like a layer and at different depths. It is possible that there is some similarity between the mechanism of action of the two materials (Fig.7.77 to 7.86).

Wucherpfenning & Green[140] studied the similarity of Mineral Trioxide Aggregate and Portland Cement (PC). The major ingredients of MTA – calcium, phosphate and silica as matched by Koh et al.[92], match the primary ingredients of Portland Cement. Macroscopically, microscopically and by x-ray defraction analysis, both substances seem almost identical. Both are mixed with water, and take up water while they go into the solid phase. In order to explore the biocompatibility of Portland Cement, osteoblast-like cells were cultured in the presence of PC and MTA. Four and six week cultures showed that both substances support matrix formation in a similar fashion. In vivo experiments in adult rats, where PC and MTA were used as direct pulp capping materials after sterile pulp exposure on maxillary molar, confirmed that both materials have a very similar effect on the pulp cells. Apposition of reparative dentin was seen in some cases, as early as two weeks after injury, with both materials.

Estrela et al.[22] investigated the antimicrobial action of mineral trioxide aggregate, Portland cement, calcium hydroxide paste (CHP), Sealapex and Dycal. The chemical elements of MTA and two Portland cements were also analyzed. Four standard bacterial strains: *S. aureus*, *E.faecalis*, *P.aeruginosa*, *B.subtilis*, one wild fungus, *C.albicans*, and one mixture of these were used. Analyses of chemical elements present in MTA and in two samples of Portland cement were performed with a fluorescence spectrometer x-ray. The results showed that the antimicrobial activity of CHP was superior to those of MTA, Portland cement, Sealapex and Dycal, for all microorganisms tested, presenting inhibition zones of 6-9.5 mm and diffusion zones of 10-18 mm. MTA, Portland cement, and Sealapex presented only diffusion zones and among these, Sealapex produced the largest zone. Dycal did not show inhibition or diffusion zones. Portland cements contain the same chemical elements as MTA except that MTA also contains bismuth.

Holland et al.[73] analyzed the behavior of dog dental pulp after pulpotomy and direct pulp protection with Mineral Trioxide Aggregate or Portland Cement. After pulpotomy, the pulp stumps of 26 roots of dog's teeth were protected with MTA or Portland Cement. Sixty days after treatment, the animal was sacrificed and the specimens removed and prepared for histomorphological analysis. There was a complete tubular hard tissue bridge in almost all specimens. In conclusion, MTA and Portland Cement show similar comparative results when used in direct pulp protection after pulpotomy (Fig.7.87 to 7.93).

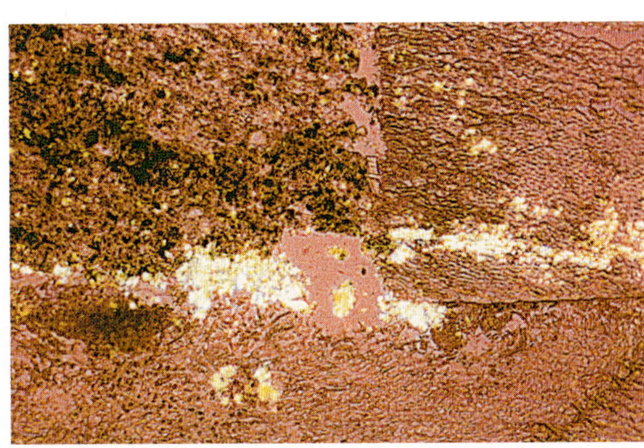

**Figure 7.77** - MTA – 7 days. Polarized light, calcite granulations close to the material (Holland et al.[81]).

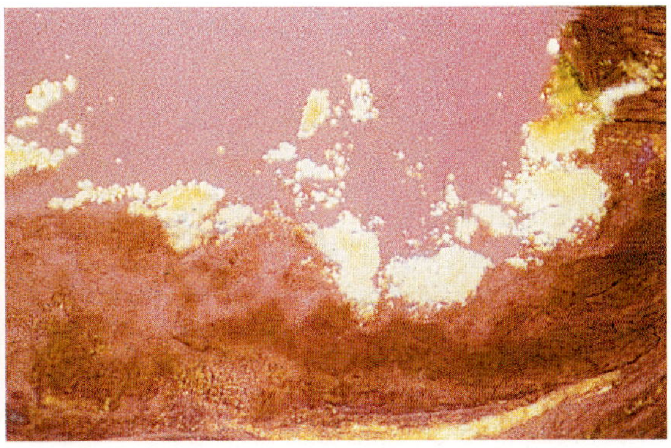

**Figure 7.78** - $Ca(OH)_2$–30 days. Polarized light, calcite granulations (Holland et al.[81]).

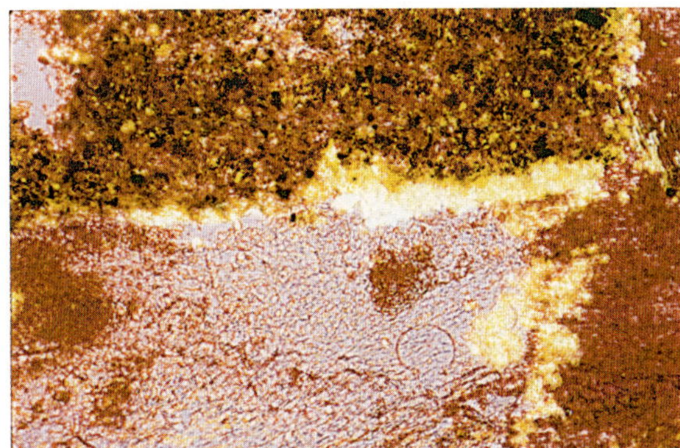

**Figure 7.79** - MTA – 30 days. Polarized light, calcite granulations close to the material (Holland et al.[81]).

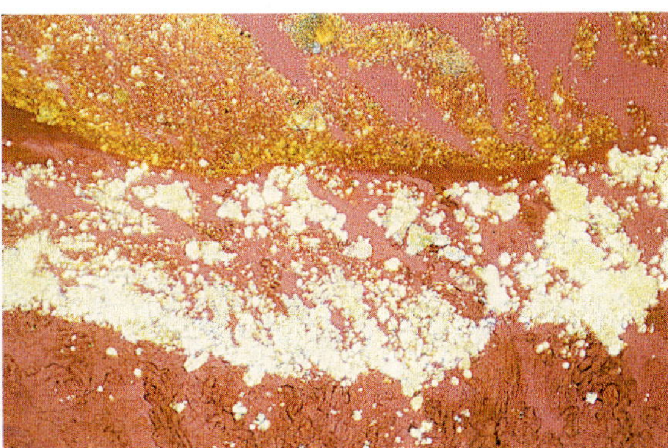

**Figure 7.80** - $Ca(OH)_2$ – 7 days. Polarized light, calcite granulations (Holland et al.[81]).

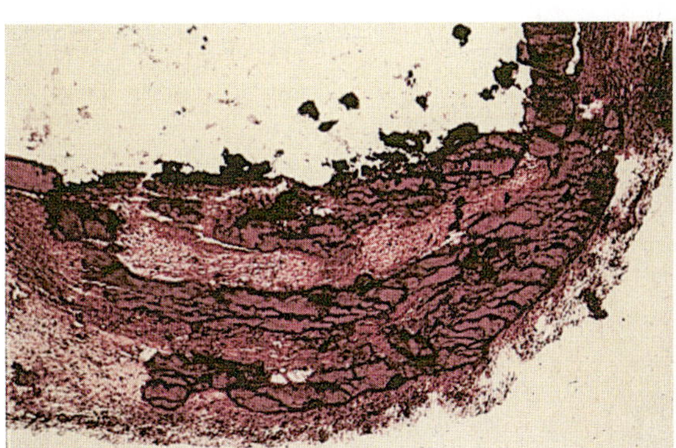

**Figure 7.81** - MTA – 7 days. Positive von Kossa material close to the light of the tubes (Holland et al.[81]).

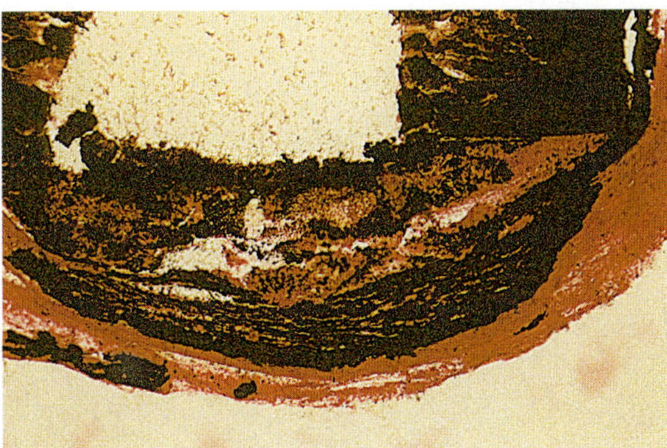

**Figure 7.82** - $Ca(OH)_2$ – 7 days. Positive von Kossa bridge close to the light of the tubes. (Holland et al.[81]).

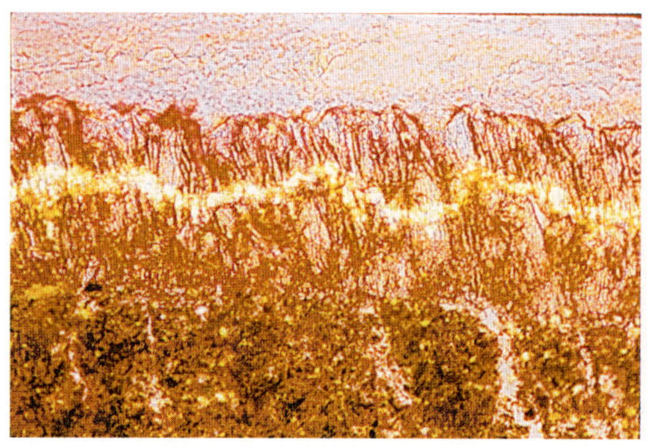

**Figure 7.83** - MTA – 7 days. Polarized light. Calcite granulations in the tubules of the dentin wall (Holland et al.[81]).

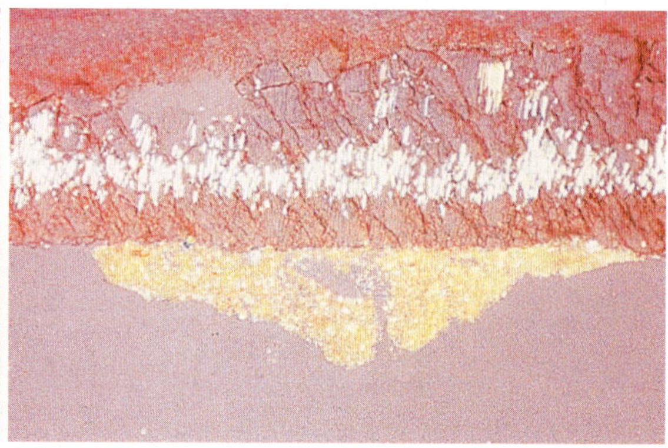

**Figure 7.84** - $Ca(OH)_2$ – 7 days. Polarized light. Calcite granulations in the tubules of the dentin wall (Holland et al.[81]).

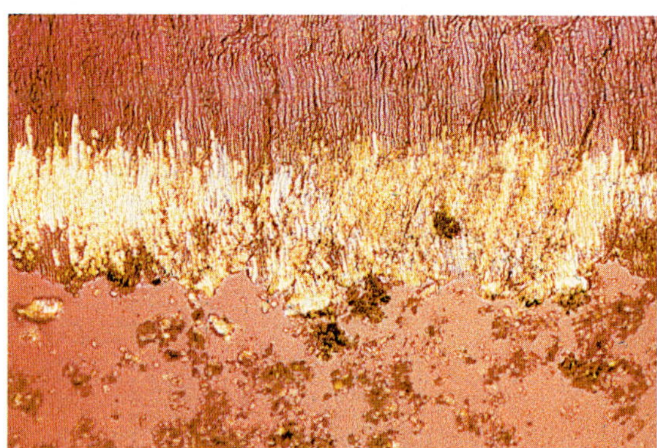

**Figure 7.85** - MTA – 30 days. Polarized light. Calcite granulations in the tubules of the dentin wall (Holland et al.[81]).

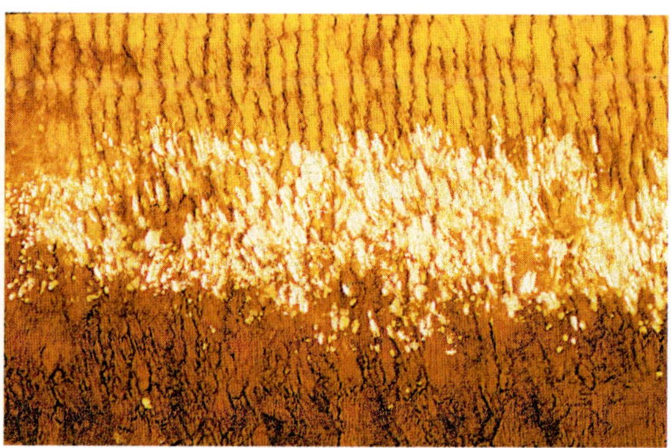

**Figure 7.86** - $Ca(OH)_2$ – 30 days. Polarized light. Calcite granulations in the tubules of the dentin wall (Holland et al.[81]).

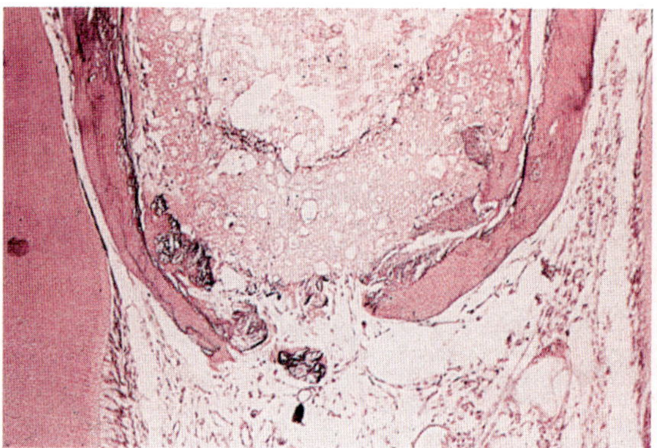

**Figure 7.87** - MTA - 60 days. Partial bridge with eosinophile structure to the center. (H.E., X40) (Holland et al.[73]).

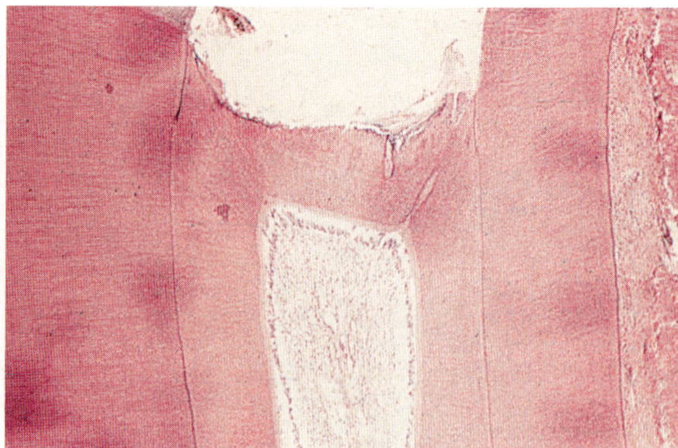

**Figure 7.88** - MTA – 60 days. Complete hard tissue bridge and dental pulp with absence of inflammatory reaction (H.E., X 40) (Holland et al.[73]).

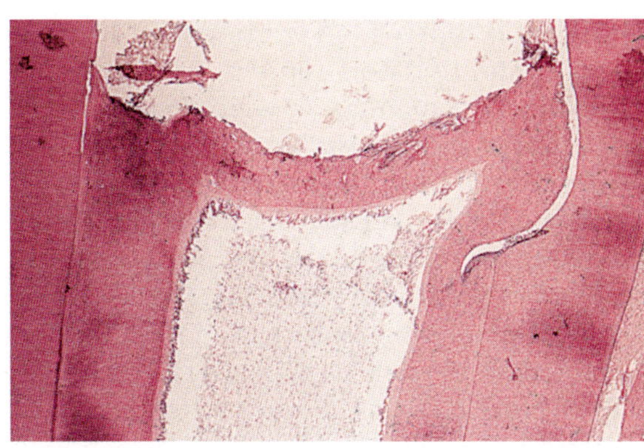

Figure 7.89 - MTA – 60 days. Complete hard tissue bridge and dental pulp with absence of inflammatory reaction (H.E., X 40) (Holland et al.[73]).

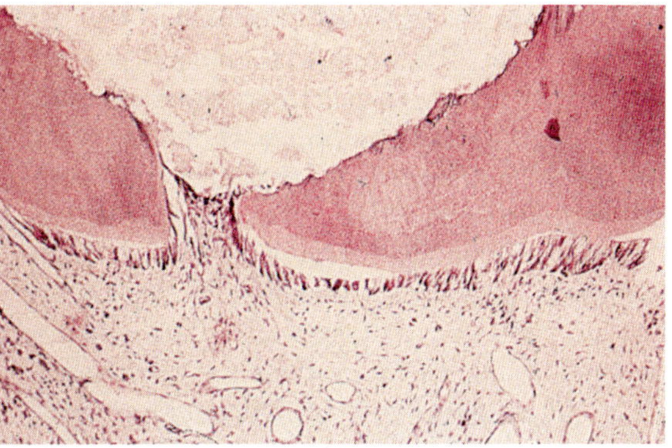

Figure 7.90 - Portland cement– 60 days. Partial bridge and chronic inflammatory process (H.E., X 40) (Holland et al.[73]).

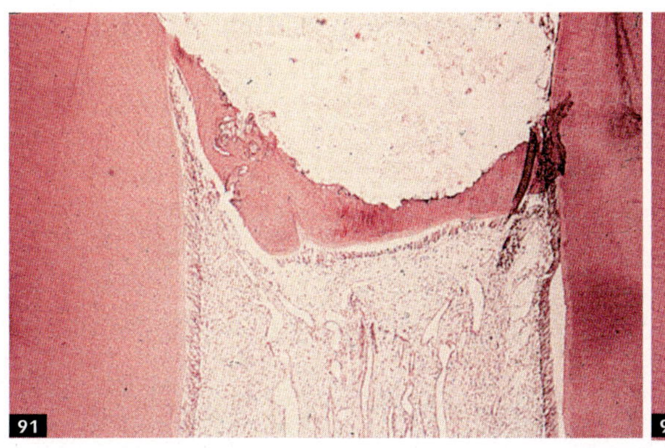

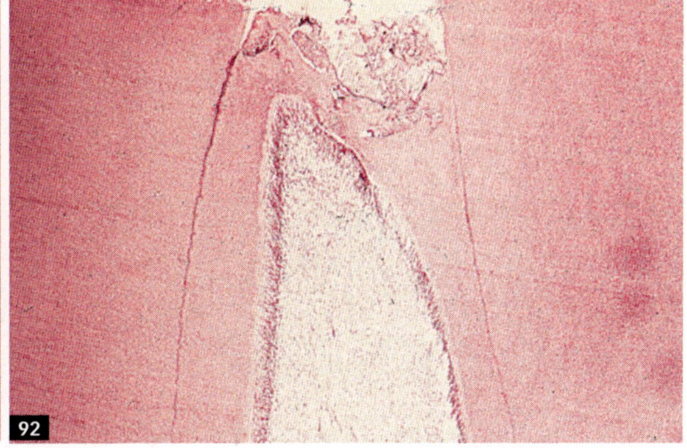

Figures 7.91 and 7.92 - Portland cement – 60 days. Complete hard tissue bridge, and pulp without inflammation (H.E., X40) (Holland et al.[73]).

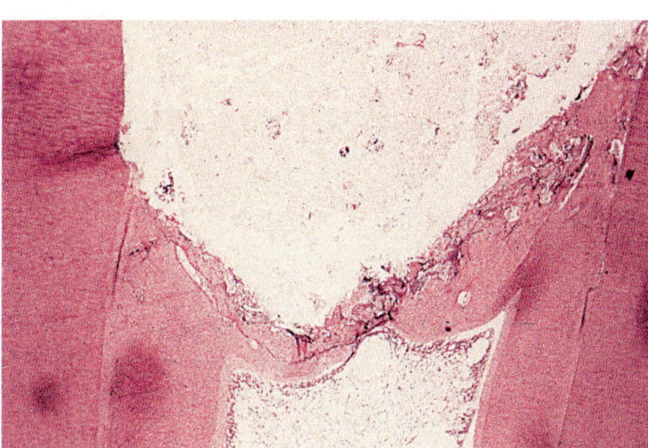

Figure 7.93 - Portland cement–60 days. Complete hard tissue bridge, and pulp without inflammation (H.E., X40) (Holland et al.[73]).

Faraco-Jr & Holland[78] evaluated the response of dog's dental pulp to mineral trioxide aggregate and a calcium hydroxide cement when used as pulp capping materials. After the pulps of 30 teeth were exposed, they were capped with either MTA or a calcium hydroxide cement. Histological analysis was performed 2 months after treatment. Results showed a healing process with complete tubular dentin bridge formation and no inflammation in any of the pulps capped with MTA. On the other hand, only five specimens from the calcium hydroxide cement group formed a complete dentin bridge. In this experimental group, pulp inflammation was observed in all but three cases. In conclusion, MTA exhibited better results than the calcium hydroxide cement for the capping of the pulp in dog teeth (Fig. 7.94 to 7.99).

Holland et al.[79] studied the rat's subcutaneous connective tissue reaction to implanted dentin tubes filled with mineral trioxide aggregate, Portland cement or calcium hydroxide. The animals were sacrificed after 7 or 30 days and the undecalcified specimens were prepared for histological analysis with polarized light and von Kossa technique for mineralized tissues. The results were similar for the studied materials. At the tube openings, there were von Kossa-positive granules that were birefringent to polarized light. Next to these granulations, there was an irregular tissue like a bridge that was von Kossa-positive. The dentin walls of the tubes exhibited a highly birefringent structure to polarized light in the tubules, usually like a layer, and at different depths. The mechanism of action of the studied materials has some similarities (Fig.7.100 to 7.113).

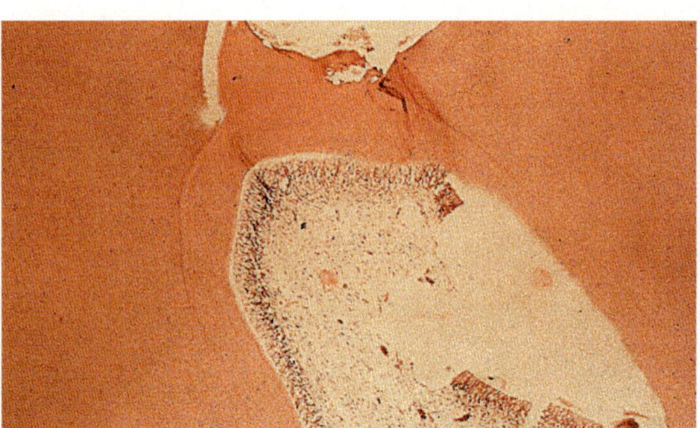

**Figure 7.94** - 60 days after capping with grey MTA. Complete hard tissue bridge and pulp without inflammation (H.E., X40) (Faraco & Holland[31]).

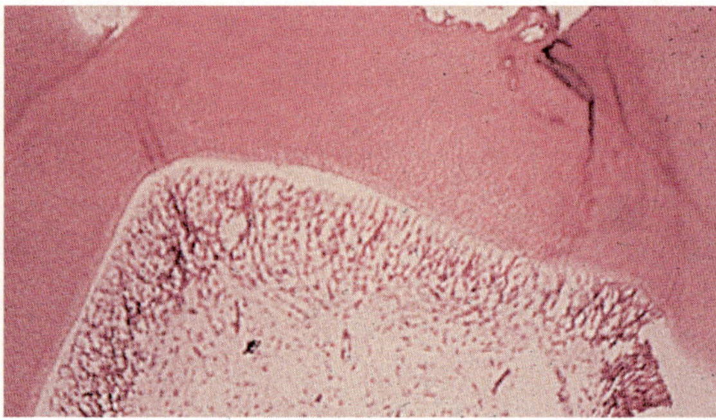

**Figure 7.95** - Magnification of the Figure 94 (H.E., X100) (Faraco & Holland[31]).

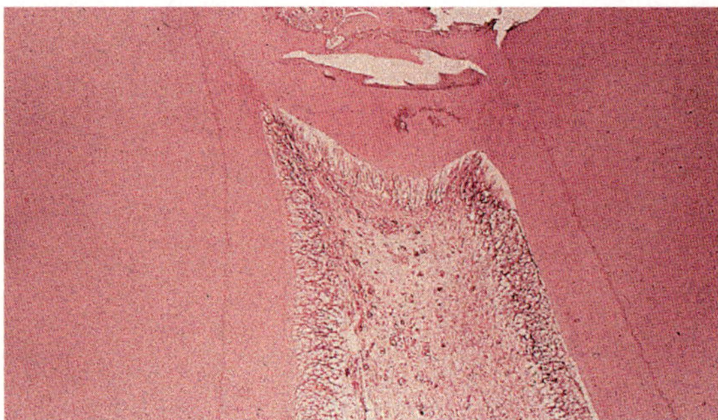

**Figure 7.96** - 60 days after capping with grey MTA. Complete hard tissue bridge and pulp without inflammation (H.E., X40) (Faraco & Holland[31]).

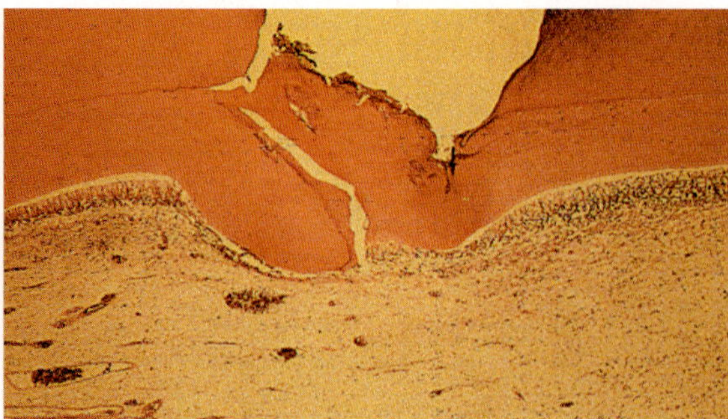

**Figure 7.97** - Barrier with dentin fragment (displacement during the histological processing) (H.E., X40) (Faraco & Holland[31]).

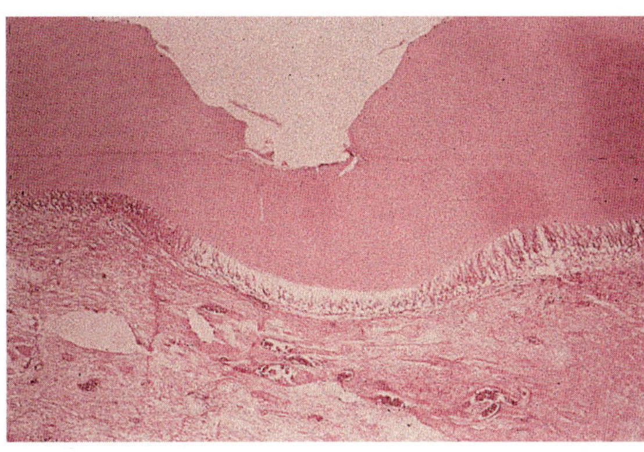

**Figure 7.98** - 60 days after capping with grey MTA. Complete hard tissue bridge and pulp without inflammation (H.E., X40) (Faraco & Holland [31]).

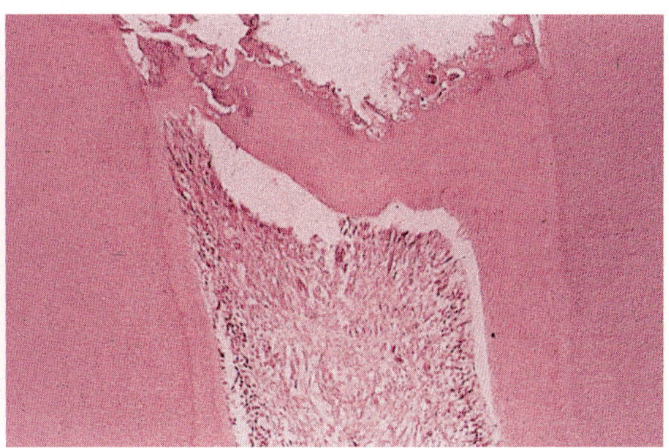

**Figure 7.99** - 60 days after capping with grey MTA. Complete hard tissue bridge and pulp without inflammation (H.E., X40)(Faraco & Holland [31]).

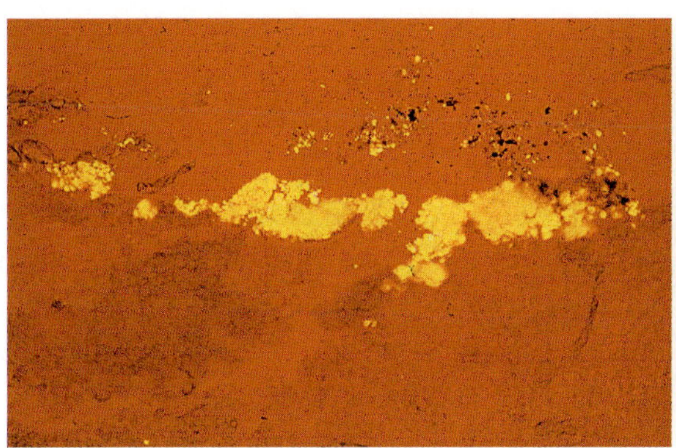

**Figure 7.100** - MTA – 7 days. Under polarized light, note calcite granulations close to the implanted material (Holland et al.[78]).

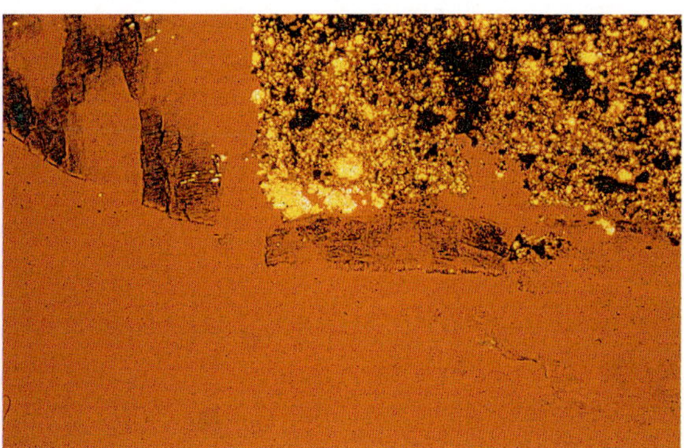

**Figure 7.101** - Portland cement – 7 days. Under polarized light, note calcite granulations close to the implanted material (Holland et al.[78]).

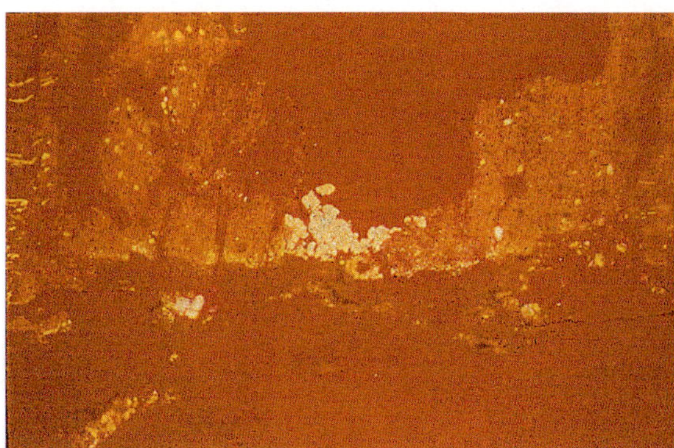

**Figure 7.102** - MTA – 7 days. Under polarized light, note calcite granulations close to the implanted material (Holland et al.[78]).

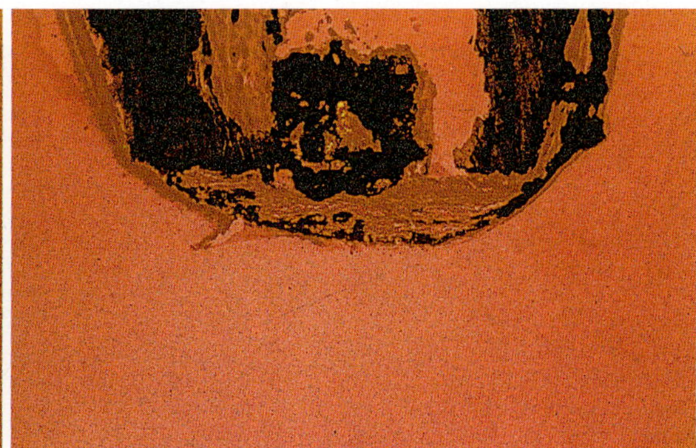

**Figure 7.103** - MTA – 7 days. von Kossa stain. Note strait von Kossa positive deposited close to the light of the tube. (Polarized light) (Holland et al.[78]).

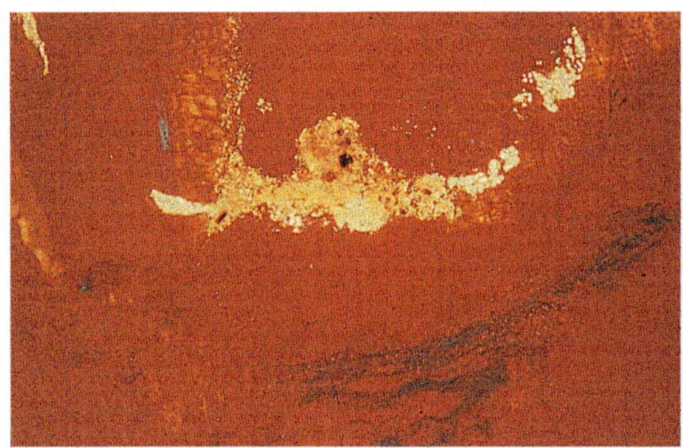

**Figure 7.104** - Portland cement –7 days. Calcite granulations. (Polarized light) (Holland et al.[78]).

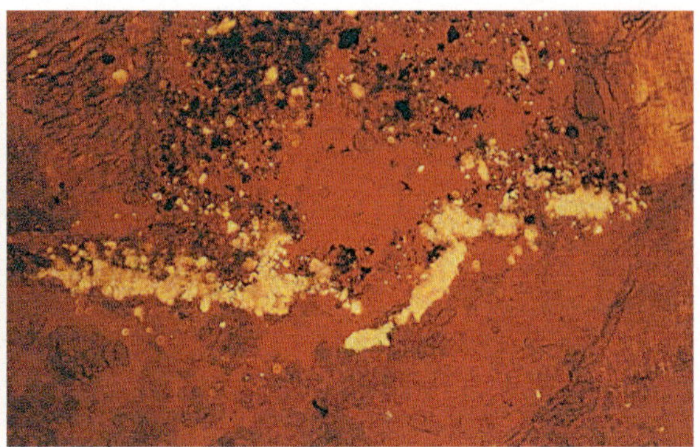

**Figure 7.105** - MTA – 7 days. Calcite granulations close to the implanted material. (Polarized light) (Holland et al.[78]).

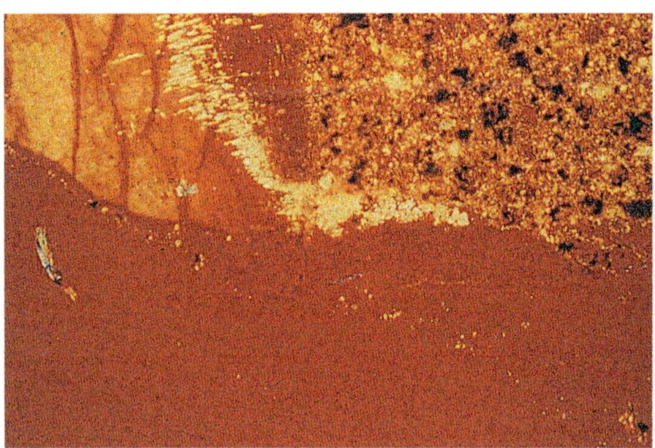

**Figure 7.106** - MTA - 7 days. Calcite granulations close to the implanted material. (Polarized light) (Holland et al.[78]).

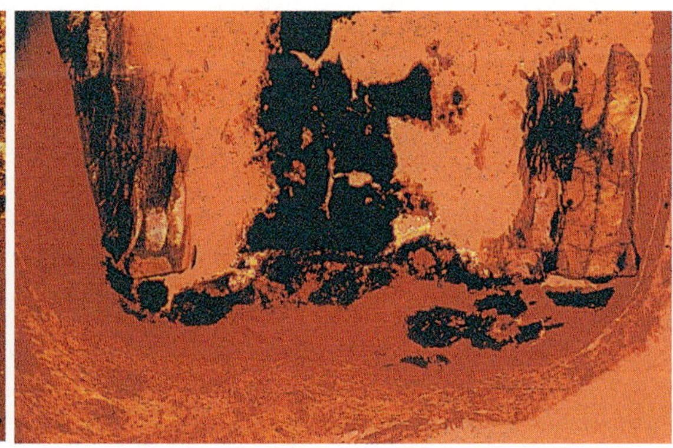

**Figure 7.107** - MTA – 30 days. Deposition of von Kossa positive material. (Polarized light) (Holland et al.[78]).

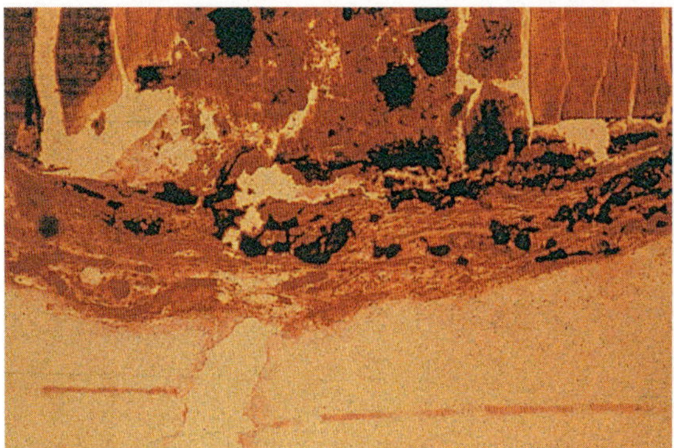

**Figure 7.108** - Portland cement - 7 days. Deposition of Von Kossa positive material. (Polarized light) (Holland et al.[78]).

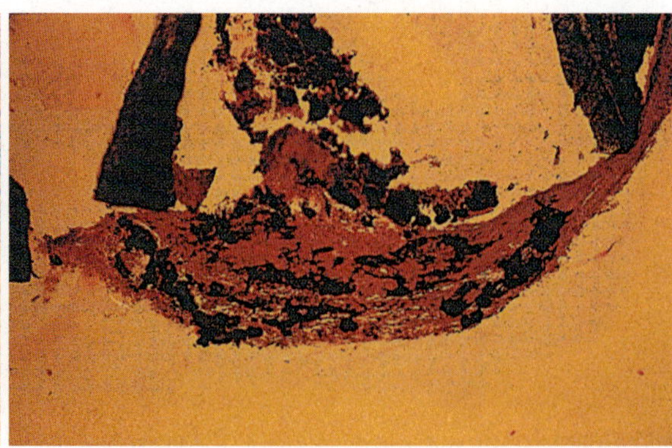

**Figure 7.109** - MTA – 7 days. Deposition of von Kossa positive material. (Polarized light) (Holland et al.[78]).

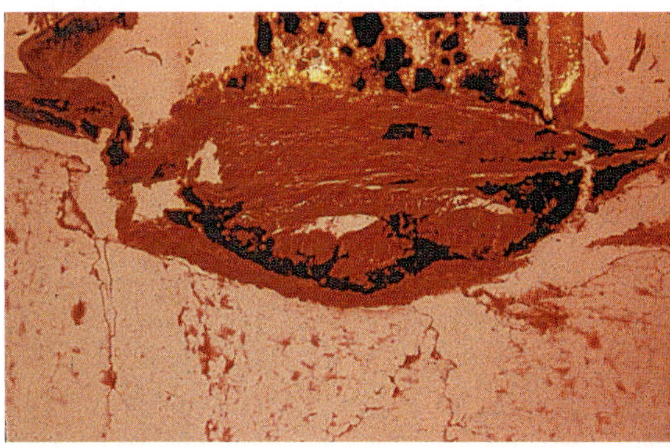

**Figure 7.110** - Portland cement - 7 days. Deposition of Von Kossa positive material. (Polarized light) (Holland et al.[78]).

**Figure 7.111** - Portland cement–7 days. Calcite deposition inside the dental tubules. (Polarized light) (Holland et al.[78]).

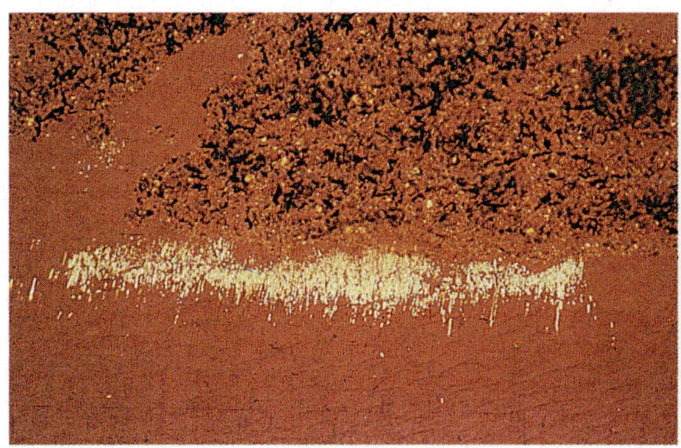

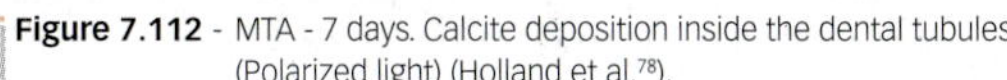

**Figure 7.112** - MTA - 7 days. Calcite deposition inside the dental tubules. (Polarized light) (Holland et al.[78]).

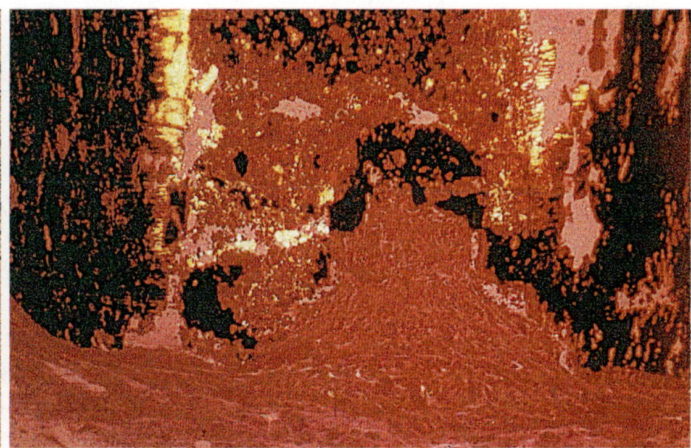

**Figure 7.113** - Portland cement – 30 days. Calcite deposition inside the dental tubules. Structure von Kossa positive. (Polarized light) (Holland et al.[78]).

Holland et al.[79] studied the reaction of rat's subcutaneous connective tissue to the implantation of dentin tubes filled with white mineral trioxide aggregate, a material that will be marketed. The tubes were implanted into rat subcutaneous tissue and the animals were sacrificed after 7 and 30 days. The undecalcified pieces were prepared for histological analysis with polarized light and von Kossa's technique for mineralized tissues. Granulations birefringent to polarized light and an irregular structure like a bridge were observed next to the material; both were von Kossa positive. Also, in the dentin wall tubules a layer of birefringent granulations was observed. The results were similar to those reported for gray MTA, indicating that the mechanisms of action of the white and gray MTA are similar (Fig. 7.114 to 7.115). The Figures 7.116 to 7.122 showed histological aspects of pulpotomy and pulp protection using calcium hydroxide and MTA.

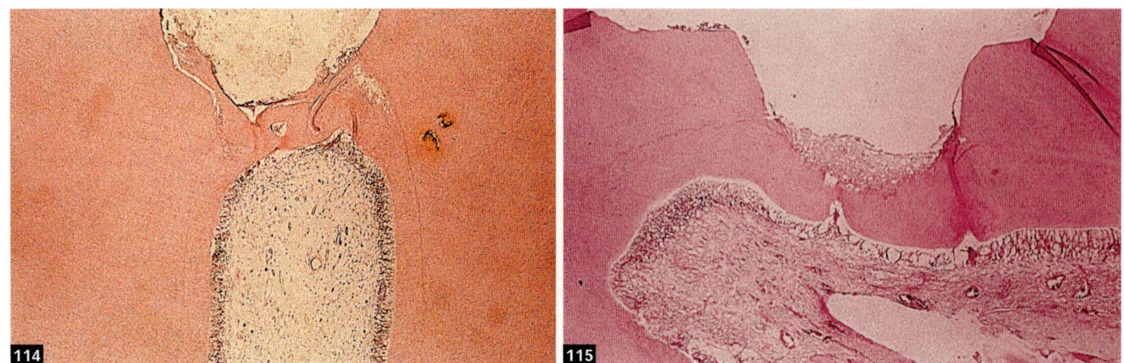


**Figures 7.114 and 7.115** - White MTA – 60 days. Complete hard tissue bridge, without inflammation (H.E., X40) (Faraco & Holland[31]).

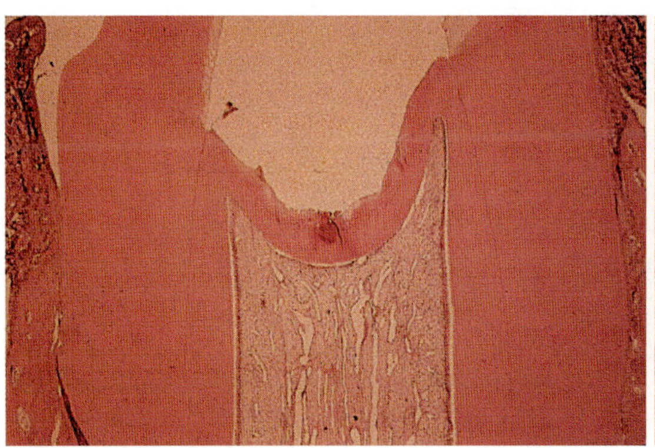

**Figure 7.116** - $Ca(OH)_2$ – 60 days. Complete hard tissue bridge, without inflammation (H.E., X40).

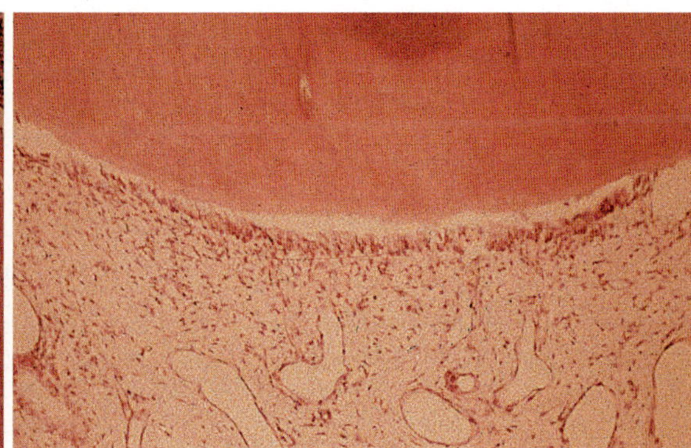

**Figure 7.117** - Magnification of Figure 7.116 (Holland, 2003).

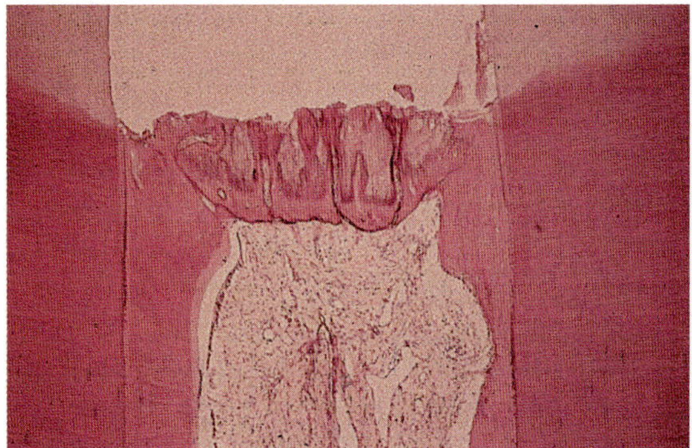

**Figure 7.118** - $Ca(OH)_2$ – 60 days. Complete hard tissue bridge, without inflammation (H.E. X40) (Holland, 2003).

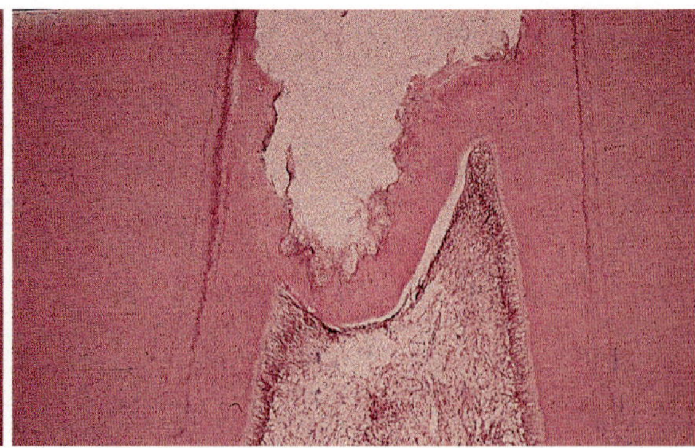

**Figure 7.119** - Defects in tunnel form, which are sealed in the most coronary portion (H.E., X40) (Holland, 2003).

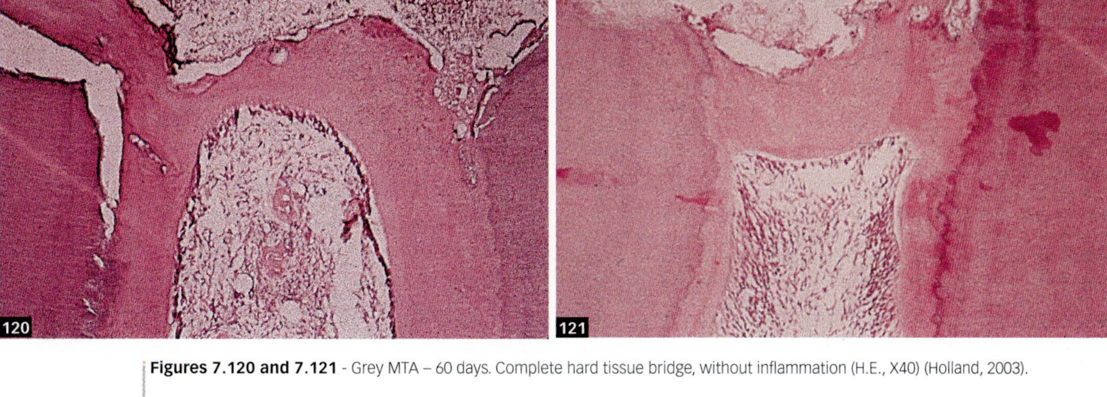


**Figures 7.120 and 7.121** - Grey MTA – 60 days. Complete hard tissue bridge, without inflammation (H.E., X40) (Holland, 2003).

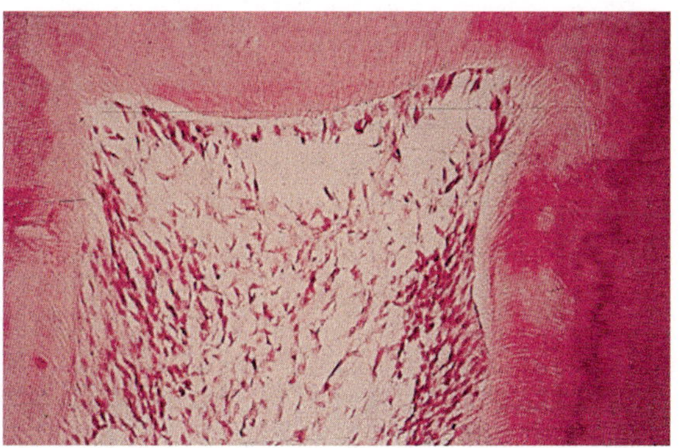

**Figure 7.122** - Grey MTA – 60 days. Complete hard tissue bridge, without inflammation. Magnification of the Figure 7.121 (H.E., X40) (Holland, 2003).

Saidon et al.[112] compared the cytotoxic effect in vitro and the tissue reaction of MTA and Portland cement in bone implantation in the mandibles of guinea pigs. There was no difference in cell reactions in vitro. Bone healing and minimal inflammatory response were observed adjacent to ProRoot and PC implants in both experimental periods, suggesting that both materials are well tolerated. MTA and PC show comparative biocompatibility when evaluated in vitro and in vivo. The results support the idea that PC has the potential to be used in clinical situations similar to those in which MTA (ProRoot) is being used. Although the results are very encouraging, further studies in human beings need to be conducted before unlimited clinical use can be recommended.

Camilleri & Pitt Ford[6] reviewed the literature on the constituents and biocompatibility of mineral trioxide aggregate. A Medline search was conducted. The first publication on the material was in November 1993. The Medline search identified 206 articles published from November 1993 to August 2005. Specific searches on constituents and biocompatibility of mineral trioxide aggregate, however, yielded few publications. Initially all abstracts were read to identify which fitted one of the two categories required for this review, constituents or biocompatibility. Relatively few articles addressed the constituents of MTA, whilst cytological evaluation was the most widely used biocompatibility test. In the past 10 years, 13 studies have been published on the constituents, while 53 studies have been published on the biocompatibility of MTA: 27 studying the material to host interactions at a cellular level and 26 using histological methods to study host tissue reactions. Collectively, these studies have shown that MTA is biocompatible. There has, however, been a lack of knowledge and understanding about the constituents of the material and its interaction with the surrounding tissues. Recent studies on the material constituents have clarified that MTA is a silicate cement rather than an oxide mixture.

Nair et al.[104] investigated the pulp response to direct pulp capping in healthy human teeth with mineral trioxide aggregate in comparison with calcium hydroxide cement (Dycal). A total of 35 teeth from 23 patients were included in the study, of which 33 were histomorphologically processed. Iatrogenic / pulp wounds treated with MTA were mostly free of inflammation after 1 week and became covered with a compact, hard tissue barrier of steadily increasing length and thickness within 3 months following capping. Control teeth treated with Dycal® revealed distinctly less consistent formation of a hard tissue barrier that had numerous tunnel defects. The presence of pulp inflammation up to the longest observation period (3 months) after capping, was a common feature in Dycal® specimens. The MTA was clinically easier to use as a direct pulp–capping agent and resulted in less pulp inflammation and more predictable hard tissue barrier formation than Dycal®. Therefore, MTA or equivalent products should be the material of choice for direct pulp capping procedures instead of hard setting calcium hydroxide cements.

Accorinte et al.[2] evaluated the histomorphologic response of human dental pulps capped with mineral trioxide aggregate and calcium hydroxide cement (CH). The pulp was capped either with calcium hydroxide cement Life® or MTA (Pro-root®) and restored with composite resin. After 30 and 60 days, teeth were extracted and processed for histologic exam and categorized by a histologic score system. All groups performed well in terms of hard tissue bridge formation, inflammatory response, and other pulp findings. A lower response of calcium hydroxide cement (30 days) was observed for the dentin bridge formation, however, when compared with MTA (30 days) and MTA (60 days) groups. The pulp healing with calcium hydroxide was slower than it was with MTA, both materials were successful for pulp capping in human teeth.

Iwamoto et al.[33] analyzed the clinical, radiographic and histologic findings in human third molars in which mechanical pulp exposures were capped with white ProRoot mineral trioxide aggregate (WMTA). Forty-eight human third molars, caries-free or with incipient caries, scheduled for extraction were used and randomly divided into two groups: Group A – (n=24) received WMTA and control Group B – (n=24) received chemical set calcium hydroxide Dycal®. The teeth were isolated with a rubber dam and Class I cavities prepared. Pulp exposure was performed using a sterile diamond bur and confirmed by frank bleeding. A sterile cotton pellet dipped in saline solution was placed over the exposure for 60 seconds. The preparation was then lightly rinsed with water and gently air-dried. WMTA or CH was placed over the exposure site followed by a small amount of a light polymerized compomer and resin composite. Evaluations were performed by phone after 7 days and clinically at $30 \pm 5$ and $136 \pm 24$ days, using standardized tests and radiographs. The teeth were extracted after $136 \pm 24$ days and processed for routine histological evaluation. No significant differences in post-operative sensitivity between the two materials were reported after 7 days. Clinical examination demonstrated no significant differences at $30 \pm 5$ and $136 \pm 24$ days. Histological findings: 45 of 48 teeth were suitable for microscopic evaluation (22 with WMTA and 23 with CH). Twenty from the WMTA and 18 from the CH group had developed a bridge. A statistically significant difference was found for the diameter of exposure between WMTA ($x=0.35 \pm 0.19$ mm) and CH ($x=0.25 \pm 0.09$mm). Only a minimal association between clinical and histological findings could be established for either material.

Chacko & Kurikose[7] studied the histologic changes in the dental pulp following pulpotomy with mineral trioxide aggregate (MTA) and calcium hydroxide cement. The study included 31 non carious premolars scheduled for extraction for orthodontic reasons from 10 children in the 11-14 year-old age group. The coronal pulp tissue was scooped using a spoon excavator and the chamber was washed with saline to clear out the debris. Once hemostasis was obtained, the root pulp was capped with either MTA or calcium hydroxide cement and restored with IRM. The cotton pellet provided the moisture MTA required for proper setting. The teeth were extracted at 4 and 8 week intervals. Longitudinal sections were then prepared and viewed under a light microscope. At the end of 4 and 8 weeks, the pulps capped with MTA showed dentin bridge formation which was more homogenous and continuous with the original dentin when compared with the pulps capped with calcium hydroxide cement. The pulp inflammation was also less in the MTA group, in comparison with the calcium hydroxide group, at the end of 4 and 8 weeks.

Aeinehchi et al.[3] compared mineral trioxide aggregate (MTA) with calcium hydroxide cement when used as pulp-capping materials in human teeth. Eleven pairs of intact maxillary third molars free of restorations, which required extraction, from subjects between 20 and 25 years of age were selected. They were subsequently isolated with rubber dam and a conventional Class I cavity of approximately 1mm width was prepared on the occlusal surface. A standard exposure of 0.5 mm diameter was created in the pulp with a high-speed handpiece and round bur, by an operator who did not have prior knowledge of the pulp-cap agent to be used. No salivary contamination was allowed. Homeostasis was gained by irrigating the cavity with sterile saline and application of small pieces of cotton before capping with calcium hydroxide (Dycal®) or MTA (ProRoot®) on the contralateral third molars of the same subject. Zinc oxide eugenol (ZOE) cement at a thickness of 2 mm was used over both materials. Amalgam served as the filling material. A total of 14 teeth were extracted after periods of 1 week (two molars), 2 months (three molars), 3 months (five molars), 4 months (two molars) and 6 months (two molars). Every sample was also evaluated for severity, type and site of inflammation, presence of necrosis, hyperemia, calcification other than in the area of the bridge and odontoblastic layer. Histological evaluation demonstrated less inflammation, hyperemia and necrosis plus thicker dentinal bridge and more frequent odontoblastic layer formation with MTA than with calcium hydroxide.

The results favor the use of MTA, further studies with larger samples and a longer follow up are suggested.

Other perspectives for the treatment of dental pulps have permitted advanced studies in the fields of biology and genetics, such as the formation of tissues (bone, dentin). The use of the osteogenic protein (OP-1) or bone morphogenetic protein (BMP) is being investigated because it is related to de cellular differentiation, tissue morphogenesis, regeneration and reparation. These non-collagenic proteins are known as transformation growth factor β (TGB-β) and among their properties; they present the capacity of inducing the formation of osteodentin and tubular dentin when used as pulp protectors[34,94,112].

Holland & Consolaro (work not published) analyzed the action of the osteogenic protein after pulpotomies in mandibular incisors of dog. Thirty days after the pulpotomies, the coronal sealing in some teeth was removed and left open for 30 more days, with the objective of verifying the degree of protection obtained. The teeth with sealing showed new hard tissue formed, whereas in the teeth whose seals had been removed dental pulp necrosis occurred (Fig. 7.123 to 7.130).

Certainly, there is a constant and necessary search for new pulp treatment alternatives in the scientific world, full of promising expectations. Nevertheless, for the moment, until there are new feasible alternatives, based on serious scientific evidences, calcium hydroxide continues to be the chosen material for the pulp capping.

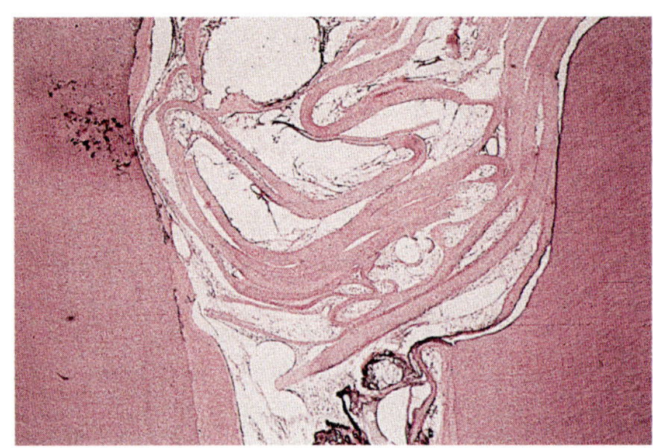

**Figure 7.123** - Pulpotomy and osteogenetic protein. Neoformation of hard tissue (H.E., X40) (Holland & Consolaro, 2003).

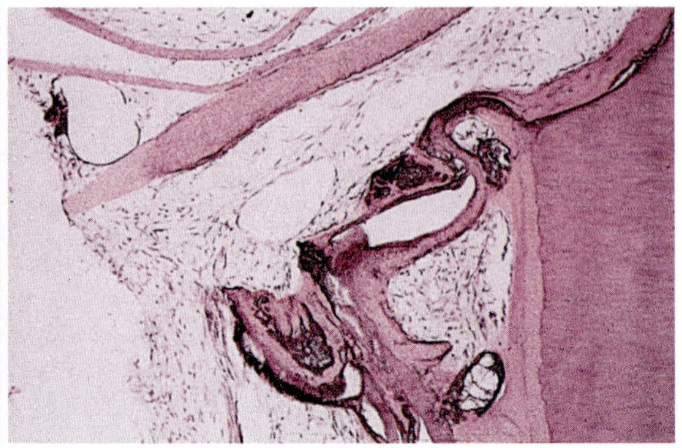

**Figure 7.124** - Magnification of the Figure 7.123 (X100) (Holland & Consolaro, 2003).

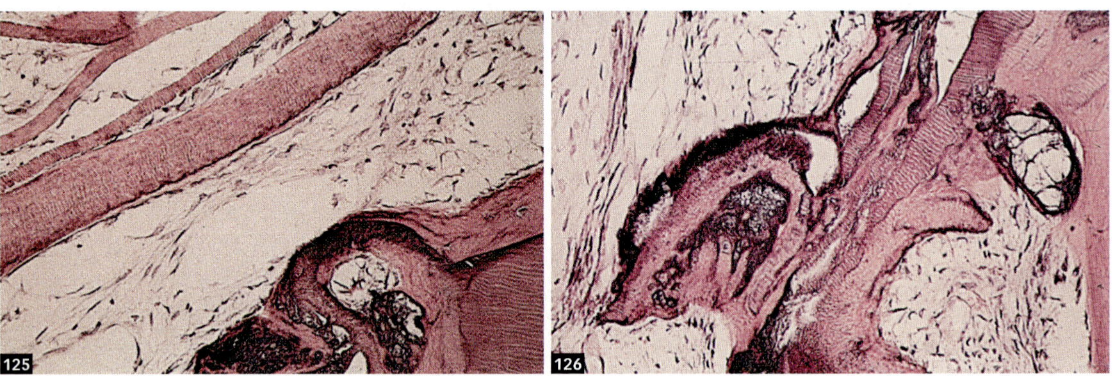

**Figures 7.125 and 7.126** - Magnifications of Figure 7.124 (Holland & Consolaro, 2003).

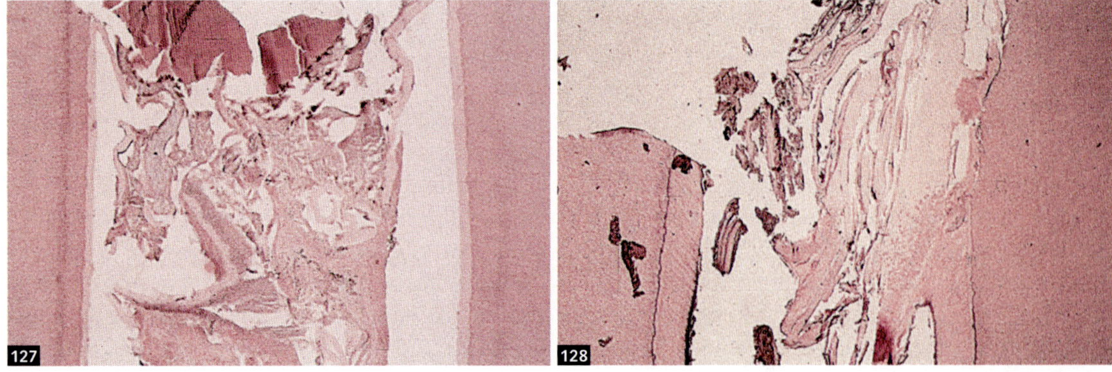

**Figures 7.127 and 7.128** - Tooth from which crown sealing was removed at 30 days. Note pulp necrosis (H.E., X40) (Holland & Consolaro, 2003).

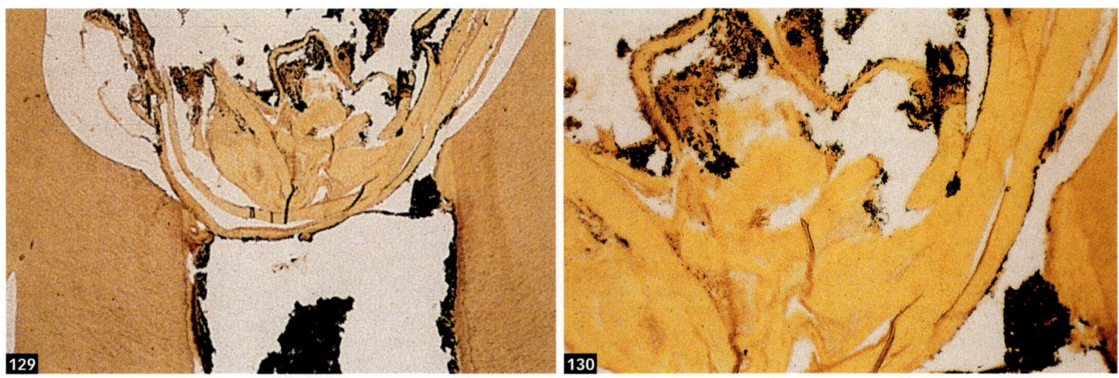

**Figures 7.129 and 7.130** - Brown and Brenn stain shows Gram-positive microorganisms close to the dentin slices and root canal walls. The neoformed hard tissue did not adequately seal the communication between the pulp and the outside, at least until 30 days, in the same way that calcium hydroxide does (Holland & Consolaro, 2003).

## 7.4 Treatment of Inflamed Dental Pulp

The conservative treatment of inflamed dental pulp involves direct pulp protection, pulp curettage and pulpotomy.

Direct pulp protection is indicated in clinical situations of pulp exposure due to cavity preparation, when the pulp tissue is healthy.

The pulp curettage is a clinical conduct that can be indicated for situations of accidental pulp exposures (coronal fractures), or exposures in which there were dentinal caries remainders (pulp exposure by caries). Holland & Souza[59] analyzed some clinical and biologic considerations on conservative endodontic treatment. In pulp curettage, although it is indicated for cases in which there is doubt about the health of the last layer of dentin that covers the dental pulp, some lesions can be present in areas not reached by the surgical maneuvers, and thus the removal of the coronal pulp by pulpotomy would allow higher chance of success.

Holland et al.[66] investigated the process of dental pulp reparation after pulpotomy or pulp curettage and protection with calcium hydroxide, and the influence of the use of corticosteroid. Therefore, dog's teeth were exposed to the oral environment for 24 hours. Later they were subjected to pulpotomy or curettage. Pulp protection with calcium hydroxide was performed, with the teeth distributed into the following experimental groups: 1. 10 minutes of prednizolone before the calcium hydroxide protection; 2. protection with calcium hydroxide manipulated with corticosteroid; 3. protection with calcium hydroxide and distilled water. After 30 days the animals were sacrificed. The best results were obtained with pulpotomy, and the use of corticosteroid did not alter the results (Fig. 7.131-7.136).

In view of the above-mentioned considerations, one notes that when in doubt about the precision of determining the extent of the inflammatory process, the more coherent and better clinical approach to apply is pulpotomy.

Nevertheless, in cases indicated for performing direct protection of the dental pulp accidentally exposed during cavity preparation, as well as in coronal traumatisms, the choice could be pulp curettage of the accidentally exposed area. The correct performance of the technique is as fundamental as the perfect selection of the biologic pulp capping material.

Determining the clinical success achieved in the conservative treatment should not be based exclusively on the formation of the mineralized barrier, but in addition to the clinical absence of symptomatology, the integrity of the space of the periodontal ligament should be observed. If possible, the response to the pulp vitality exam must be positive.

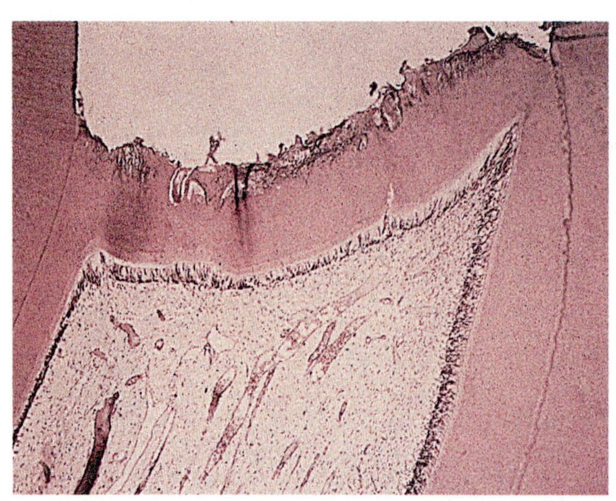

**Figure 7.131** - Pulpotomy, corticosteroid for 10 minutes and $Ca(OH)_2$ and distilled water. Complete hard tissue bridge and absence of inflammation (H.E., X40) (Holland et al. [66]).

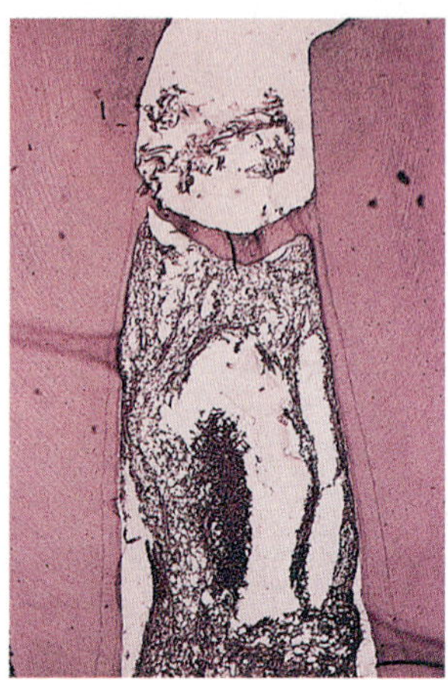

**Figure 7.132** - Curettage, $Ca(OH)_2$ and corticosteroid. Note serious pulp alterations (H.E., X40) (Holland et al. [66]).

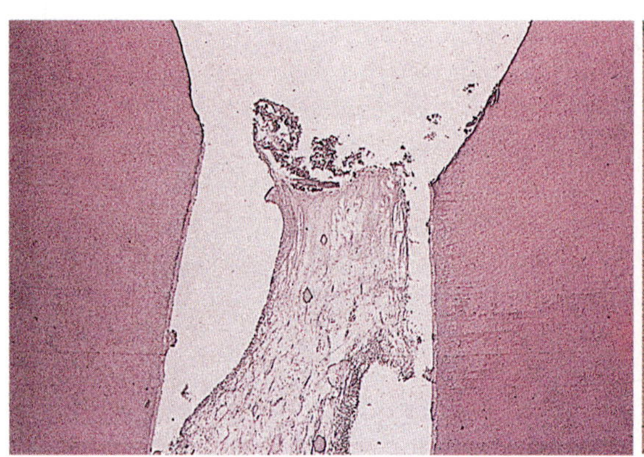

**Figure 7.133** - Curettage, $Ca(OH)_2$ and distilled water. Necrosed pulp (Holland et al. [66]).

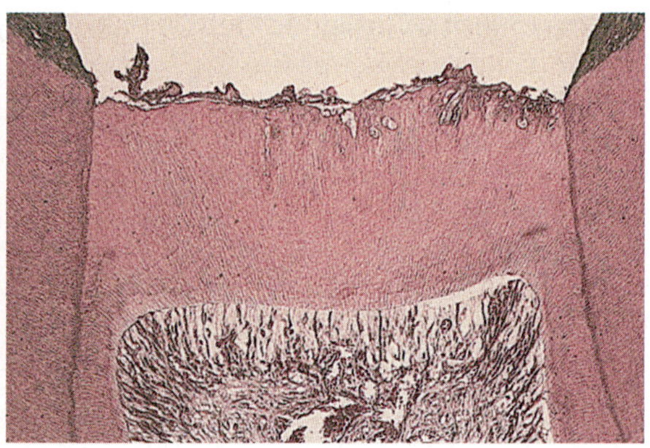

**Figure 7.134** - Pulpotomy, corticosteroid for 10 minutes, $Ca(OH)_2$ and distilled water. Complete hard tissue bridge and absence of inflammation (H.E.) (Holland et al. [66]).

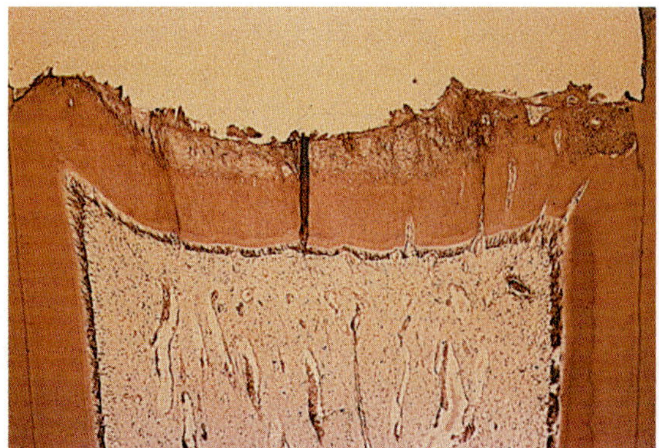

**Figure 7.135** - Pulpotomy, $Ca(OH)_2$ with corticosteroid. Complete hard tissue bridge and absence of inflammation (H.E., X40) (Holland et al. [66]).

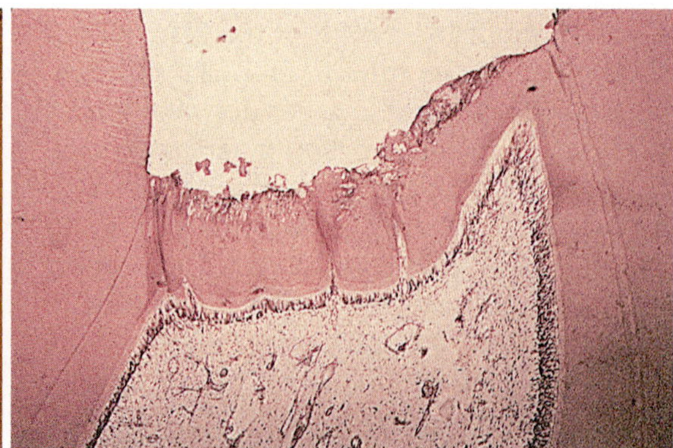

**Figure 7.136** - Pulpotomy, $Ca(OH)_2$ with corticosteroid. Complete hard tissue bridge and absence of inflammation (H.E.) (Holland et al. [66]).

Holland et al.[63] evaluated the effect of dentin fragments on the healing process of the exposed dental pulp from 20 dog's teeth. The remaining pulp tissue was capped with dentin fragments obtained from the treated tooth. The results suggested that capping the pulp with dentin fragments did not produce a favorable outcome; the presence of dentin fragments on the pulp surface disturbed or inhibited the healing process after pulp capping with calcium hydroxide (Fig. 7.137-7.142).

Russo et al.[109] observed the effects of the calcium hydroxide dressing under pressure, on pulp healing in pulpotomized human teeth. Twenty human first bicuspids were submitted to pulpotomy and calcium hydroxide application. Ten teeth received the capping material under pressure, while in the other teeth, the material was gently applied on the tissue surface. The microscopical analysis showed that: 1. no difference was observed between the groups; 2. a hard tissue bridge was found in all teeth; 3. two failures (incomplete bridges over inflamed pulps) could not be related to pressure application, but to the presence of dentin fragments in the pulp tissue; 4. as some discomfort may arise after application of a dressing under pressure, the capping material must be gently brought into contact with the pulp tissue (Fig. 7.143-7.150).

One of the arguments that question the validity of performing pulpotomies concerns the occurrence of internal resorptions. It is opportune to remember that this occurrence should not be linked to the pulpotomy, since this lesion can be observed in different circumstances. Russo et al.[110], based on the success obtained with pulpotomies in permanent teeth, and on reports in the literature, which emphasized that the capping material would be responsible for the internal resorptions after pulpotomies and the use of calcium hydroxide, histologically evaluated internal resorptions in primary teeth with no treatment. When comparing their results with the incidence of resorptions as a result of pulpotomy reported by other authors, they observed that the analysis of these authors probably represented the progression of alterations that were already existent when the pulp treatment was instituted.

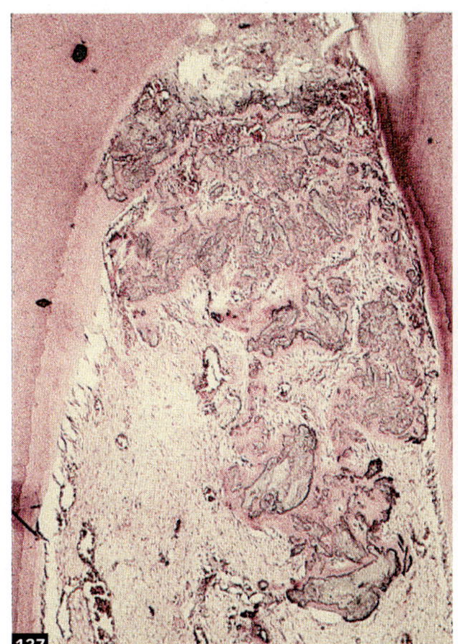

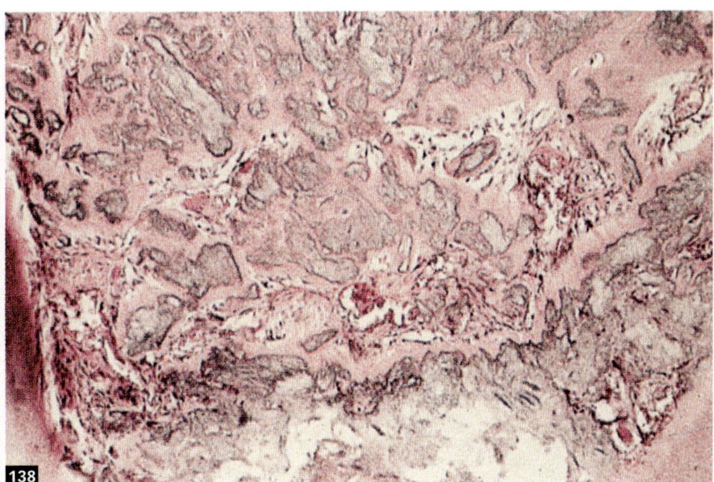

**Figure 7.137** - 30 days. Pulp protected with dentin chips (H.E., X40) (Holland et al.[63]).

**Figure 7.138** - Magnification of the Figure 7.137. Dentin chips are being surrounded by neoformed hard tissue (H.E.) (Holland et al.[63]).

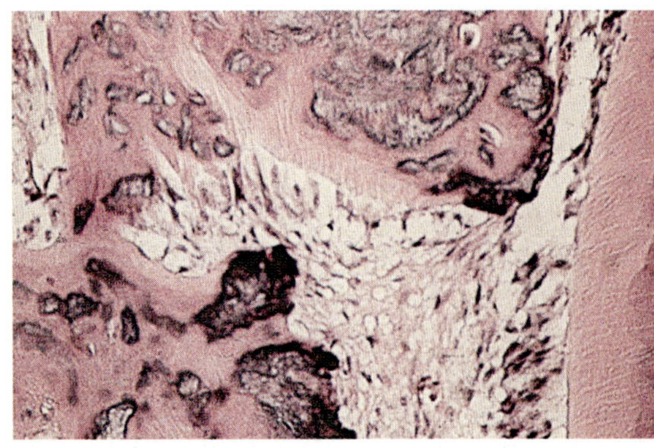

**Figure 7.139** - 30 days. Neoformed odontoblast and dentin deposit close to the dentin chips (H.E., X100) (Holland et al.[63]).

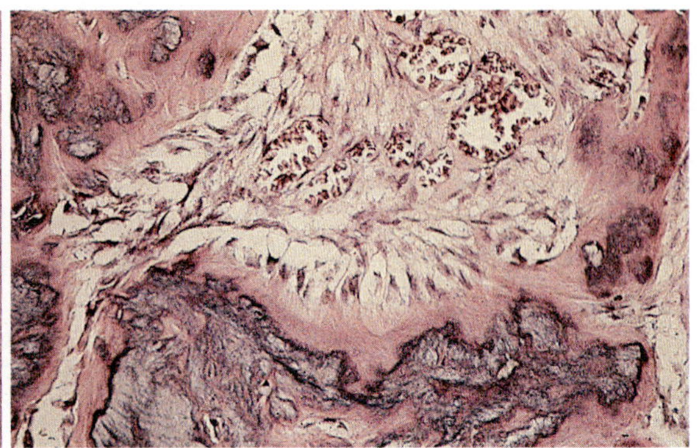

**Figure 7.140** - Magnification of the Figure 7.139 (H.E., X100) (Holland et al.[63]).

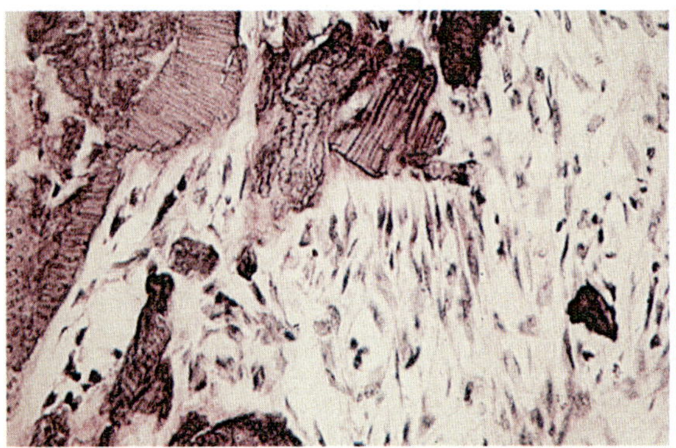

**Figure 7.141** - 30 days. Neoformed odontoblast and dentin deposit close to the dentin chips (H.E., X100)(Holland et al.[63]).

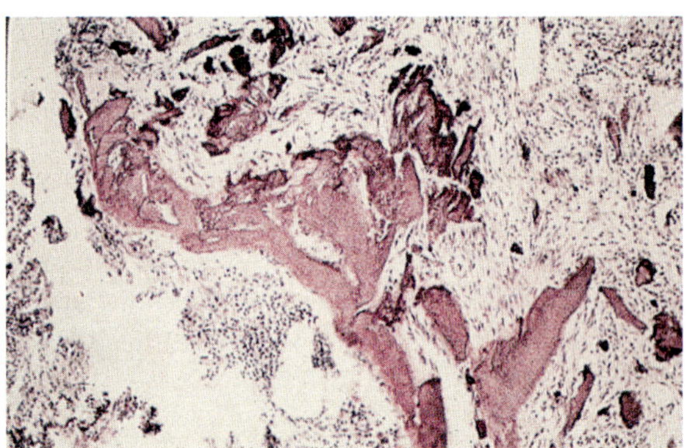

**Figure 7.142** - The pulp tissue close to the dentin chips exhibit inflammatory process (H.E., X100)(Holland et al.[63]).

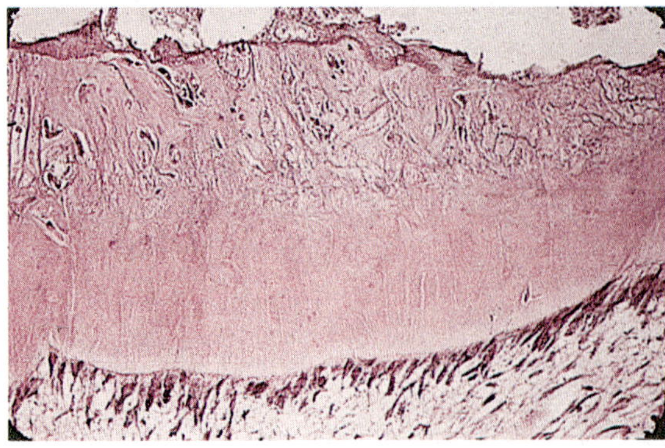

**Figure 7.143** - 30 days. Pulpotomy in human teeth and placement of $Ca(OH)_2$ with pressure (H.E., X200) (Russo et al.[109]).

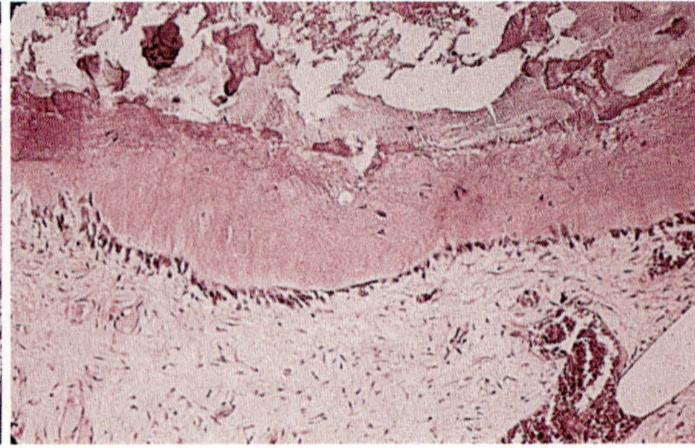

**Figure 7.144** - 30 days. Pulpotomy in human teeth and placement of $Ca(OH)_2$ with pressure (H.E., X100)(Russo et al.[109]).

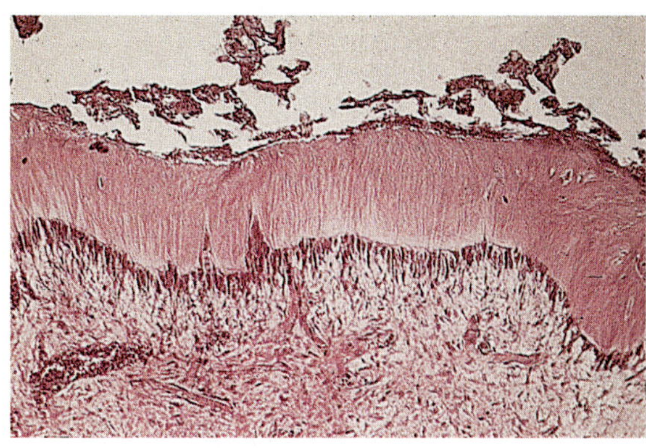

**Figure 7.145** - 30 days. Pulpotomy in human teeth and placement of $Ca(OH)_2$ with pressure. A cellular bridge (H.E., X100) (Russo et al.[109]).

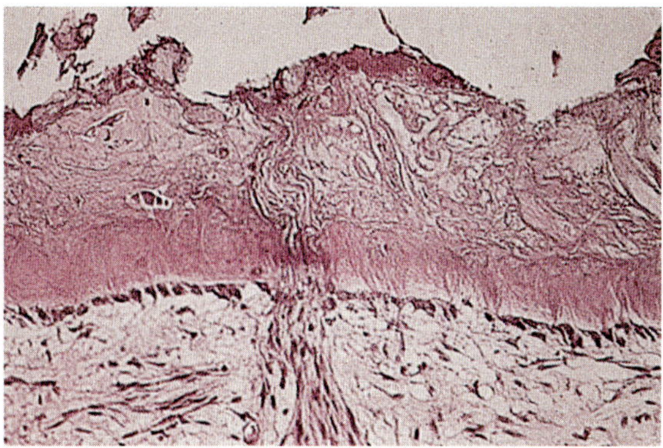

**Figure 7.146** - 30 days. Pulpotomy in human teeth and placement of $Ca(OH)_2$ with pressure. Bunch of nerve fibers surrounded by the hard tissue bridge (H.E., X200) (Russo et al.[109]).

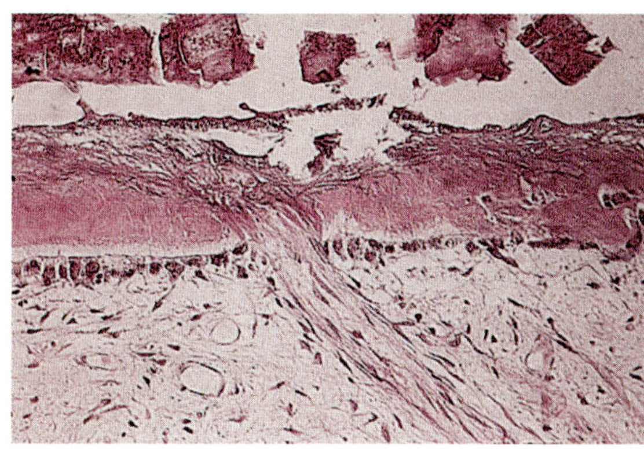

**Figure 7.147** - 30 days. Pulpotomy in human teeth and placement of $Ca(OH)_2$ with pressure. Bunch of nerve fibers involved by the hard tissue bridge (H.E., X200) (Russo et al.[109]).

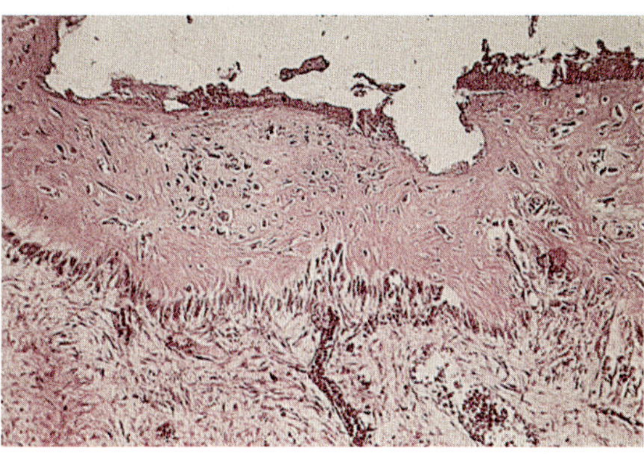

**Figure 7.148** - 30 days. Pulpotomy in human teeth and placement of $Ca(OH)_2$ with pressure. Hard tissue bridge. Cellular dentin (H.E., X100) (Russian et al.[109]).

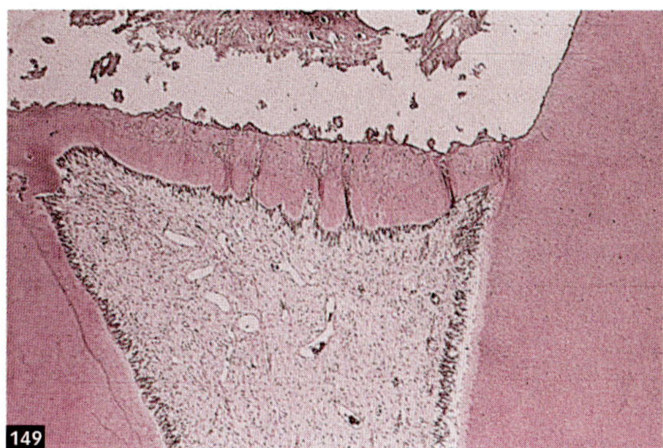



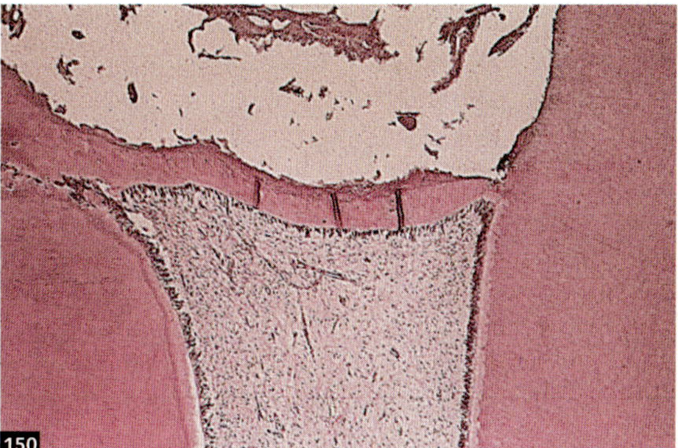



**Figures 7.149 and 7.150** - 30 days. Pulpotomy in human teeth and placement of $Ca(OH)_2$ with pressure. Complete hard tissue bridge and absence of the inflammation (H.E., X40)(Russo et al.[109]).

### 7.4.1 Technique for direct pulp protection after accidental exposure

The technique for performing direct protection of the dental pulp after accidental exposure, requires the immediate use of rubber dam isolation. Next, the exposed pulp surface is abundantly irrigated-aspirated with saline solution. The exposed area is dried with sterilized cotton pellets and a cotton pellet imbibed in corticosteroid-antibiotics (Otosporin®) is kept on it for a period of 5 minutes. It is dried again, and calcium hydroxide is applied, covering the exposure completely. Over this material, a layer of calcium hydroxide cement is applied (i.e. Dycal or Life). Later the lateral walls of the cavity are completely cleaned, since these procedures normally dirty these walls. After this, a protective base of glass ionomer is placed and the tooth is restored, preferably during the same session.

When performing conservative treatment in which biologic pulp capping is calcium hydroxide, one can choose to insert it in the form of a paste (associated with the saline solution or distilled water) or powder (pro-analysis calcium hydroxide).

In the clinical situation of pulp exposure due to coronal fractures, pulp curettage is indicated .

### 7.4.2 The pulp curettage technique

The technical procedures of pulp curettage start with a perfect and efficient anesthesia. Next, isolation is performed, copiously irrigating the exposed cavity with saline solution or whitewash water, drying it with a sterilized cotton pellet. Later, part of the pulp tissue is cut, preferably with very sharp curettes. In some situations, it is difficult to perform curettage of this small portion of exposed tissue with curettes, making it necessary to use cooled, high speed spherical burs, followed by copious irrigation with saline solution. This technique is very common when there is fracture with small exposure, in which the fracture fragment will be bonded. After these procedures, a cotton pellet, imbibed with corticosteroid-antibiotics, should be applied over the exposed cavity for 5 minutes (Otosporin). The cavity is then dried with sterilized cotton pellets and calcium hydroxide placed, covering the cavity with a thin layer of calcium hydroxide cement. After this, the tooth fragment will be bonded or the tooth restored, preferably, during the same session. Figure 7.151 diagrammatically illustrates the sequence of the pulp curettage technique.

Although one is aware that fragments of dentin can produce small calcifications under conditions of exposure during pulp curettage, it sometimes becomes opportune to use spherical burs, as mentioned before.

Holland et al.[50] analyzed the influence of the sealing material on the healing process of inflamed pulps capped with calcium hydroxide or zinc oxide-eugenol cement. The results were analyzed histologically ninety days after the treatment and showed that better results were obtained in the specimens treated with calcium hydroxide and with coronal openings sealed with zinc oxide-eugenol cement (Fig. 7.152-7.162).

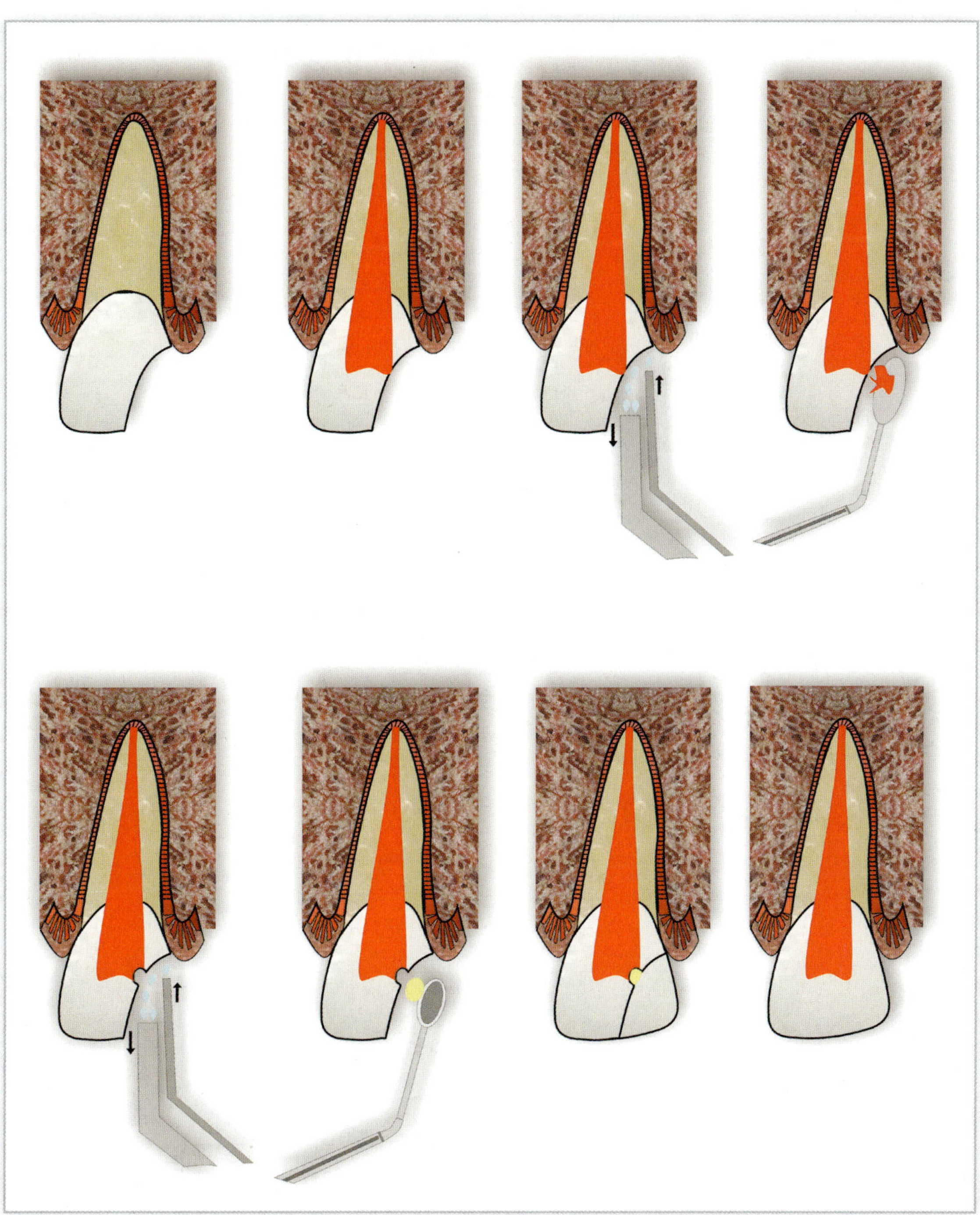

**Figure 7.151** - Schematic representation of the pulp curettage; coronal fracture with pulp exposure; pulp curettage with very sharp curette; use of high speed spherical bur; copious irrigation of the pulp remainder; application of the calcium hydroxide; pulp remainder covered with calcium hydroxide paste and cement ; restoration of the fractured tooth.

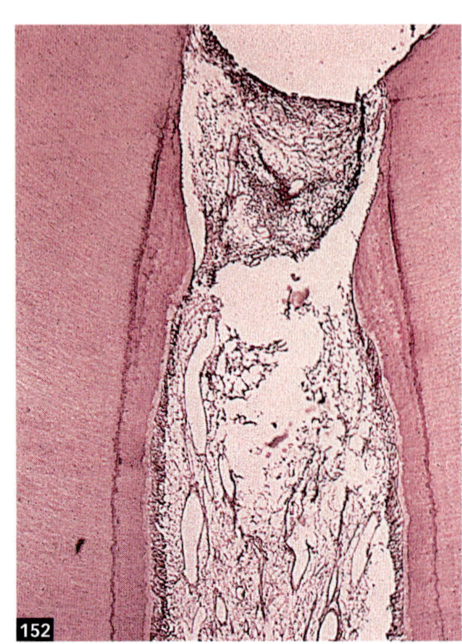


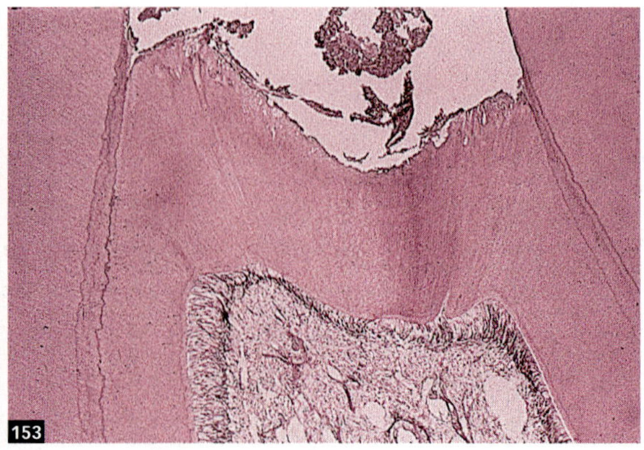


**Figure 7.152** - Sealing with amalgam. Absence of hard tissue bridge and inflamed dental pulp (H.E., X40) (Holland et al.[50]).

**Figure 7.153** - Sealing with zinc oxide and eugenol. Note complete hard tissue bridge, absence of inflammation (H.E., X40) (Holland et al.[50]).

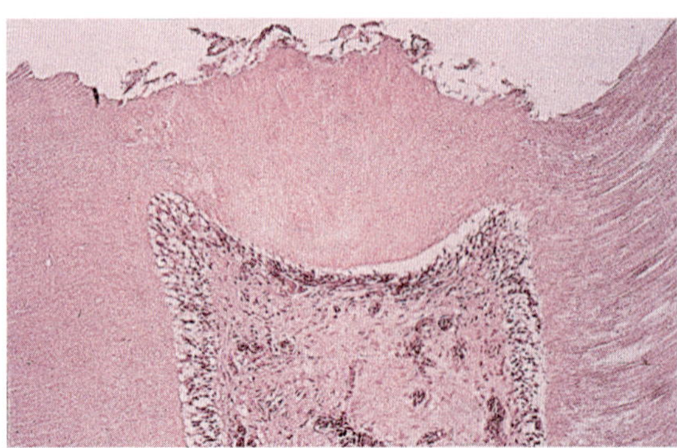

**Figure 7.154** - Complete hard tissue bridge without inflammation. Group without change of $Ca(OH)_2$ and without pulp exposure (H.E., X40) (Holland et al.[72]).

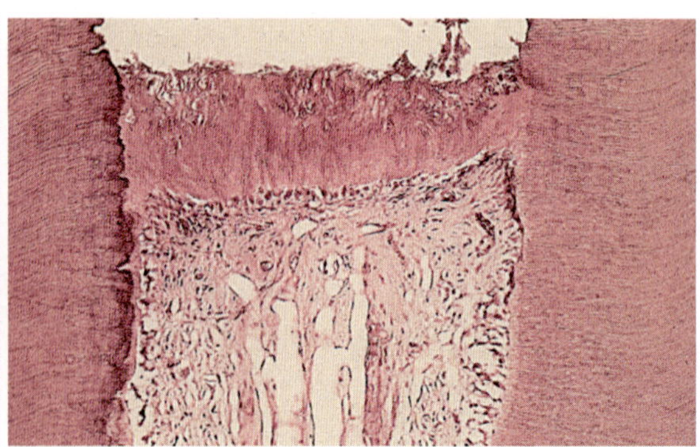

**Figure 7.155** - Complete hard tissue bridge without inflammation. Group without change of $Ca(OH)_2$ and without pulp exposure (H.E., X40) (Holland et al.[72]).

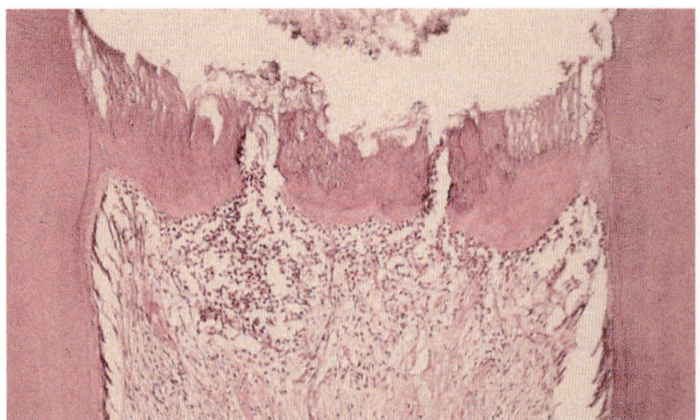

**Figure 7.156** - Hard tissue bridge with defects and with consequent inflammation after exhibition to the oral environment. Group without change of $Ca(OH)_2$ and with pulp exposure (H.E., X40)(Holland et al.[72]).

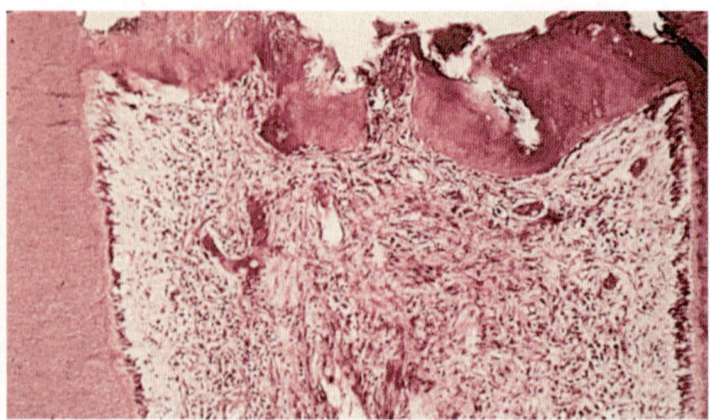

**Figure 7.157** - Hard tissue bridge with defects and with consequent inflammation after pulp exposure to the oral enviroment. Group without change of $Ca(OH)_2$ and with pulp exposure (H.E., X40)(Holland et al.[72]).

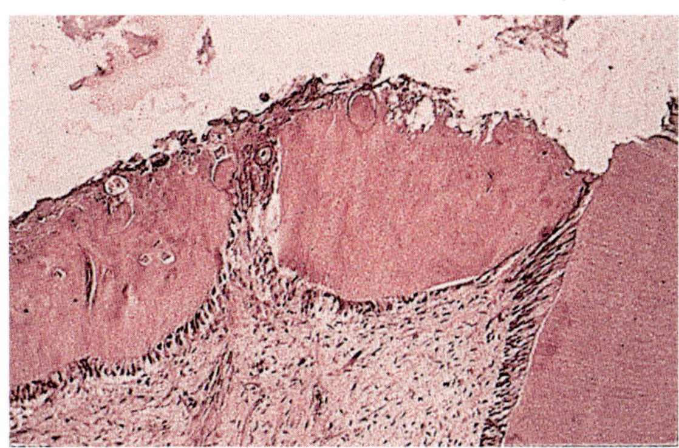

**Figure 7.158** - Group with change of $Ca(OH)_2$ and with pulp exposure. Note that the change of $Ca(OH)_2$ repaired the failure of the bridge in the correct way, and did not lead to inflammation after pulp exposure (H.E., X40) (Holland et al.[72]).

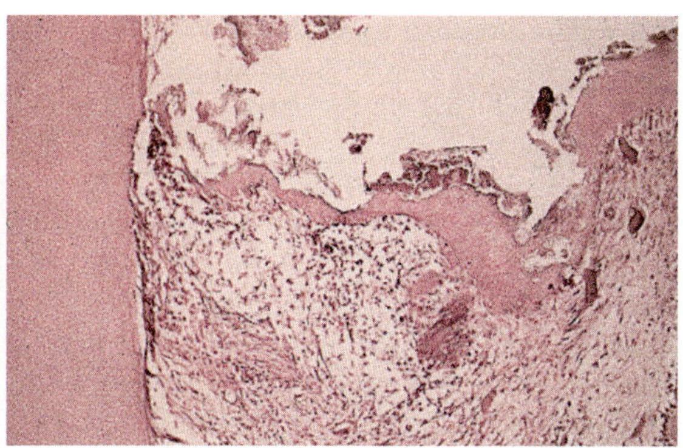

**Figure 7.159** - Group without change of $Ca(OH)_2$ and with pulp exposure. The absence of change lead to the failure remaining inflammation after the after pulp exposure (H.E., X40) (Holland et al.[72]).



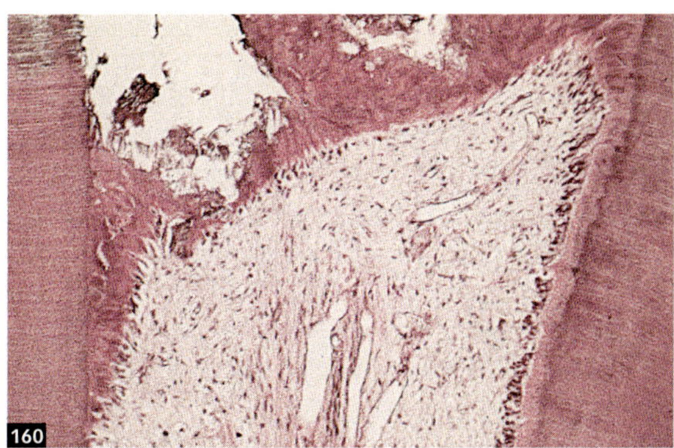

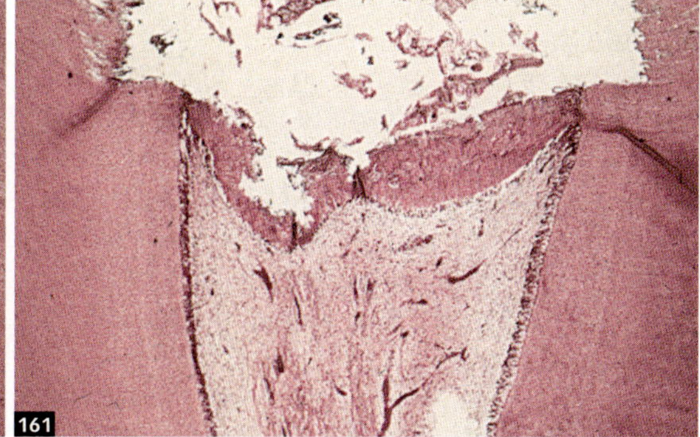

**Figures 7.160 and 7.161** - Group with change of $Ca(OH)_2$ and with after pulp exposure. Note that the change of $Ca(OH)_2$ repaired several types of failures and allowed appropriate protection after pulp exposure (H.E., X40) (Holland et al.[72]).

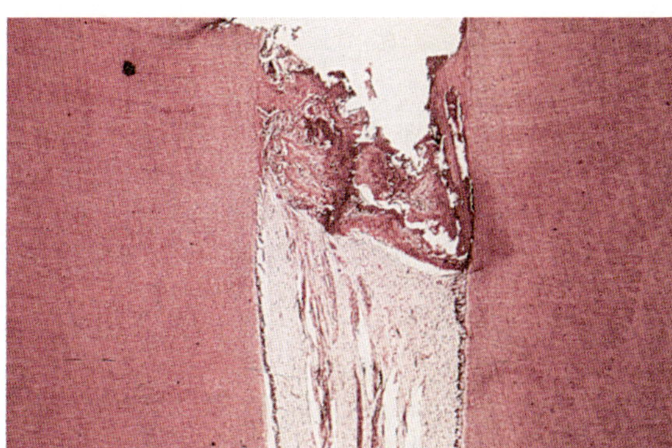

**Figure 7.162** -Group with change of $Ca(OH)_2$ and with pulp exposure. Note that the change of $Ca(OH)_2$ repaired several types of failures and allowed appropriate protection after pulp exposure (H.E., X40) (Holland et al.[72]).

### 7.4.3 The pulpotomy technique

Pulpotomy fits in with conservative treatment, as the goal is to remove the live coronal pulp completely, whether it is healthy or inflamed, and to maintain the root portion viable. The sequence of the technique is described (Fig. 7.163). Figure 7.164A-B presents a schematic representation of pulpotomy.

In clinical attendances, when it is impossible to arrange a second appointment, or when there is uncertainty as regards correct coronal cavity sealing, pulpotomy is performed in one session. In this case, corticosteroid antibiotics are applied over the pulp remainder for five minutes, and calcium-hydroxide is placed later, taking all the necessary care. A higher success rate is, however, reached when the pulpotomy is performed in two sessions. Conservative treatment should be considered definitive and not temporary.

Francischone[32] analyzed the results of the pulpotomies in 77 human teeth with spontaneous pain, intermittent or pain caused by thermal stimuli, and in cases in which the clinical exam presented wide pulp exposure. Between appointments, a mixture of prenizolone (deltacortril) and a nitrofuranic compound (furacin Oto-solution), was used, and, after 48 hours, this dressing was replaced by calcium hydroxide paste. The percentage of success of the pulpotomies in the patients aged between 8 and 15 years was 100% and, from 15 to 42 years, it was 84.37%. Vieira[138], evaluating pulpotomies performed in 120 patients between 10 and 60 years of age, with pulp exposures as a result of caries, or spontaneous pains, reported a success rate of 93.4%. Santini[113] studied the efficacy of calcium hydroxide combined with corticosteroid (Ledermix) in 200 teeth with chronic pulpitis associated with acute caries. The author recommended pulpotomy in pediatric dentistry as a routine procedure before the root canal treatment, specially in young or nervous patients, not used to long dental procedures. Lopes & Costa-Filho[96], analyzing 112 cases of pulpotomy as a clinical procedure, with the technique proposed by Holland & Souza[60], emphasized its low cost and time spent in relation to conventional root canal treatment, and placed a high socio-economic value on pulpotomy for attending the population. Aydos[4] based on clinical and radiographic exams, verified the treatment of 52 teeth with inflamed dental pulps, subjected to pulpotomies, performed in 2 appointments, using corticosteroid-antibiotics and calcium hydroxide, in patients between the ages of 12 and 40 years. After the post-operative control of 18 months, he observed success in 94.3% of the cases (49 teeth). The author considers some of the possible causes of failure, such as the loss of coronal sealing, possible presence of extra-pulp coagulum, and the previous use of analgesic medication on the pulp to control the pain (chemical aggression). Estrela et al.[29] studied the correlation between the clinical diagnosis of inflamed dental pulp and repair after pulpotomy. Forty maxillary and mandibular molars presenting pulp inflammation with enlarged periodontal membrane space were used. Pulpotomy was performed in two sessions, using corticosteroid-antibiotic and calcium hydroxide, associated with saline. Sixty days after pulpotomy, the teeth were opened and a clinical test (exploration) was performed directly over the calcified bridge, as well as the vital test and radiographies. After 180 days, the teeth were again evaluated clinically a radiographically. Of the 40 teeth analyzed, 97.5% had a positive response to the vital test applied directly over the hard tissue bridge and showed the integrity of the hard barrier.

A systematic review[105] showed few studies in humans, according the inclusion criteria, involving the pulp capping. Olsson et al.[105] evaluated the evidence on the formation of a hard tissue barrier after pulp capping in humans. A PubMed and CENTRAL literature search with specific indexing terms, and a manual search, were made. The authors assessed the level of evidence of each publication as high, moderate or low. Based on this, the evidence grade of the conclusions was rated as strong, moderately strong, limited or insufficient. The initial search process resulted in a total of 171 publications. After reading the abstracts, and manually searching the reference lists of the retrieved publications, 107 studies were retrieved in full-text and interpreted. After the interpretation, 21 studies remained and were included in the systematic review of evidence: one study had moderate, and 20 studies had a low level of evidence. There was heterogeneity between the studies, therefore, no meta-analysis was performed. The majority of studies on pulp capping using calcium hydroxide-based materials reported formation of hard tissue bridging, studies on other pulp capping materials such as bonding agents presented inferior results. The evidence grade was insufficient. Insufficient evidence grade does not necessarily imply that there is no effect of a pulp capping procedure, or that it should not be used. Rather, insufficient evidence supports the need for high-quality studies in humans.

Figures 7.167 to 7.172, present cases of mineralized tissue barriers protecting the pulp remainder without inflammation, after pulpotomy in the teeth of dogs, monkeys and humans. Figures 7.173 to 7.205 show clinical cases of pulpotomies performed in teeth with symptomatic pulpitis and asymptomatic pulpitis.



| | **Pulpotomy Technique** |
|---|---|
| **1.** | Anesthesia, rubber dam isolation and asepsis of the operative field. |
| **2.** | Coronal opening, with complete removal of the pulp chamber roof. |
| **3.** | Removal of the coronal pulp with long to intermediate and very sharp curettes. |
| **4.** | Copious irrigation-aspiration of the pulp chamber with saline solution. |
| **5.** | Pulp decompression for 5 minutes. |
| **6.** | Irrigation-aspiration with saline solution, dry with sterilized cotton pellets and exam of the pulp remainder surface, which should present the already mentioned characteristics. |
| **7.** | Application of corticosteroid-antibiotics (Otosporin®), maintaining a sterilized cotton pellet imbibed in this medicament. |
| **8.** | Double Seal with gutta-percha and cement. |
| **9.** | After 2 to 7 days, remove the seal and the dressing, irrigate copiously with saline solution, removing any coagulum. |
| **10.** | With slight pressure on the pulp remainder, place the Pro-Analysis calcium hydroxide paste with saline solution, in a thin layer, adapted by sterilized cotton pellet. Remove the excess of paste from the lateral walls and insert a biologic capping of a thin layer of calcium hydroxide cement over it (Dycal, Life), to protect it. |
| **11.** | Then, place the glass ionomer as protector base for the restoration or directly perform the coronal sealing, checking the occlusion. |

**Figure 7.163** - The Pulpotomy Technique.

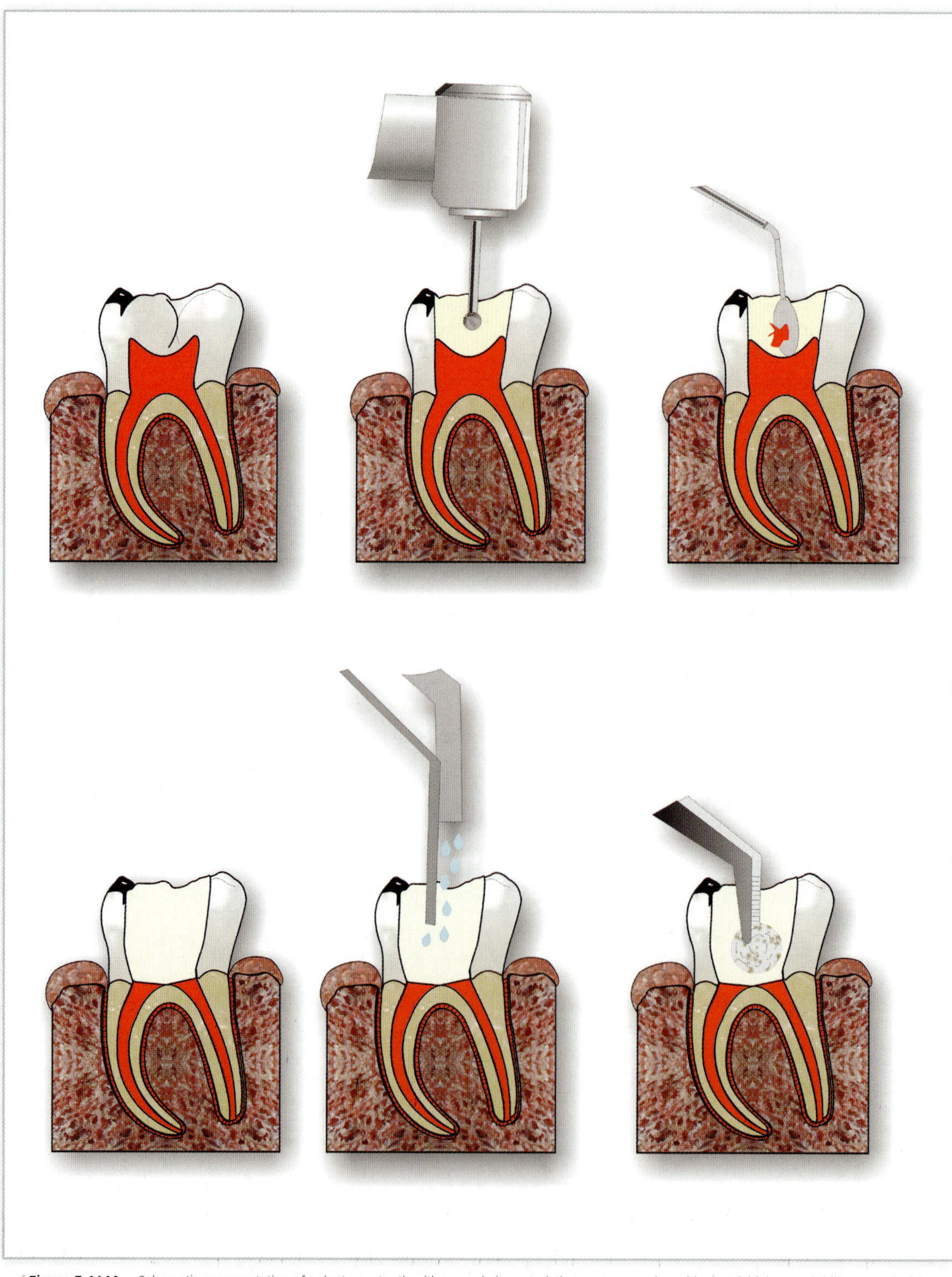

**Figure 7.164A** - Schematic representation of pulpotomy; tooth with normal characteristics; crown opening with round, high speed drill; removal of the crown dental pulp with very sharp curettes; remainder of the root dental pulp; abundant irrigation-aspiration with saline solution; drying of the cavity with sterilized cotton pellets; placement of corticosteroid-antibiotic; insertion of calcium hydroxide paste and of a fine layer of calcium hydroxide cement; placement of a protecting base and restoration of the tooth.

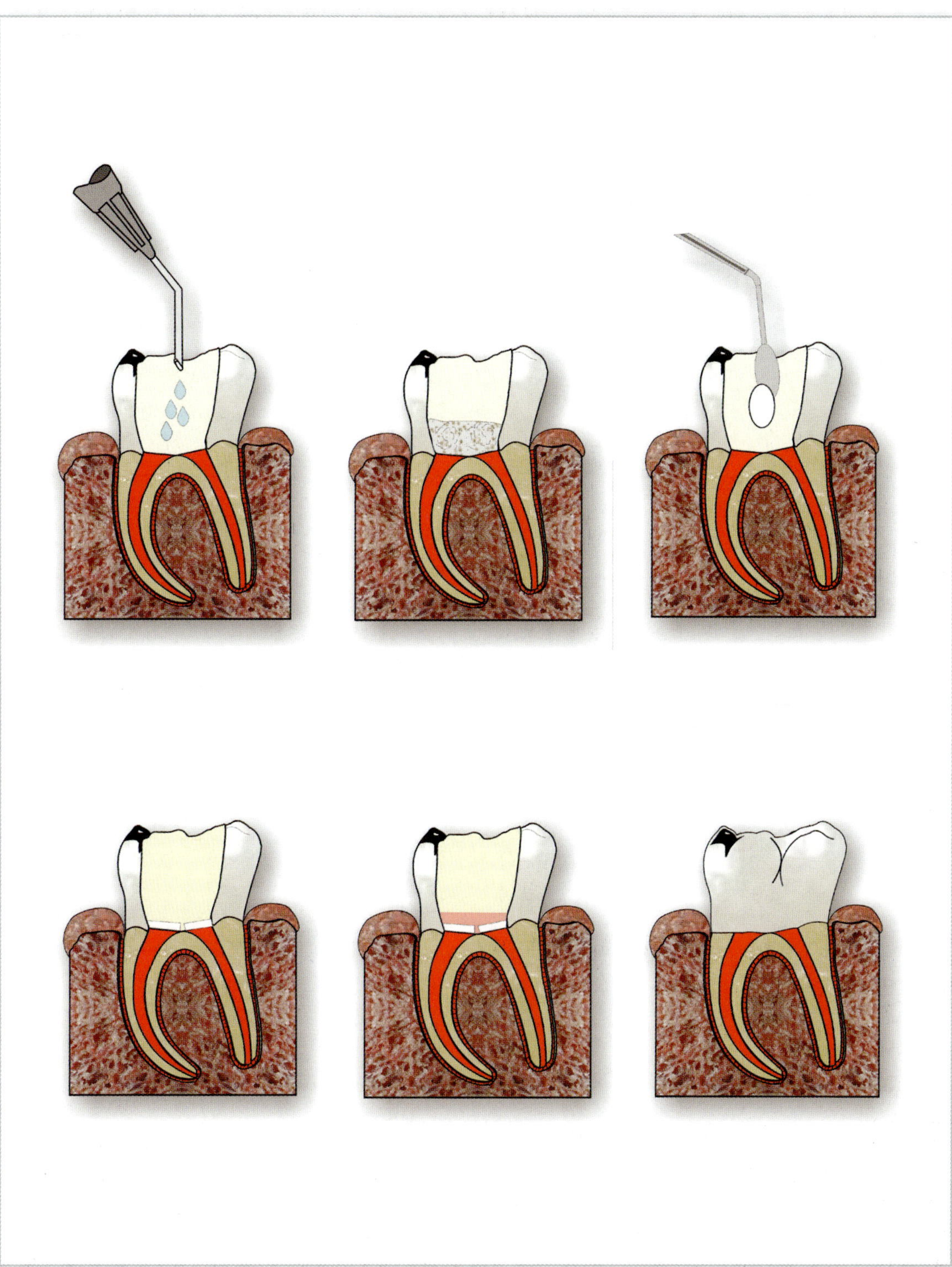

**Figure 7.164B** - Schematic representation of pulpotomy; tooth with normal characteristics; crown opening with round, high speed drill; removal of the crown dental pulp with very sharp curettes; remainder of the root dental pulp; abundant irrigation-aspiration with saline solution; drying of the cavity with sterilized cotton pellets; placement of corticosteroid-antibiotic; insertion of calcium hydroxide paste and of a fine layer of calcium hydroxide cement; placement of a protecting base and restoration of the tooth.

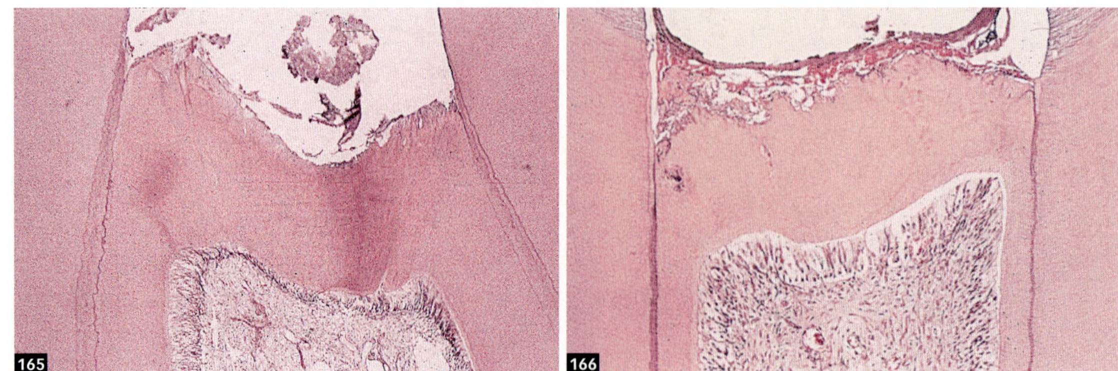


**Figures 7.165 and 7.166** - Mineralized tissue bridge protecting the pulp remainder without inflammation, after pulpotomy with calcium hydroxide in dog's teeth (H.E., X40) (Holland, 2003).

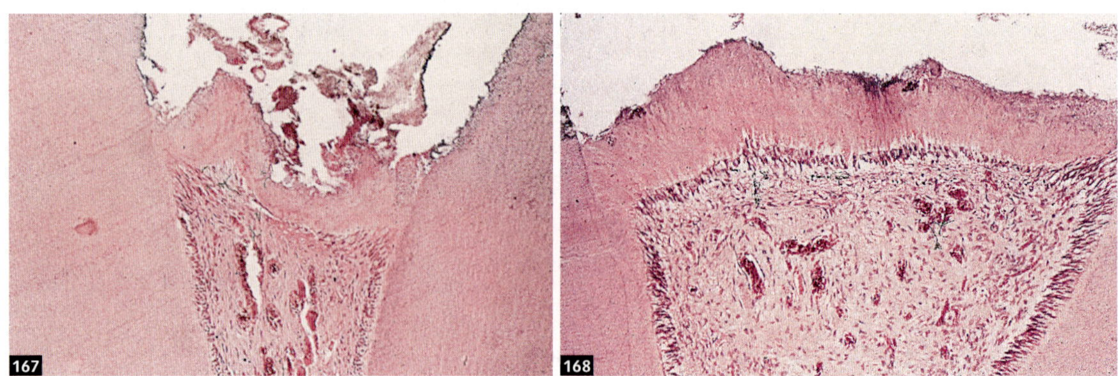


**Figures 7.167 and 7.168** - Mineralized tissue bridge protecting the pulp remainder without inflammation, after pulpotomy with calcium hydroxide in monkey's teeth (H.E., X40) (Holland, 2003).

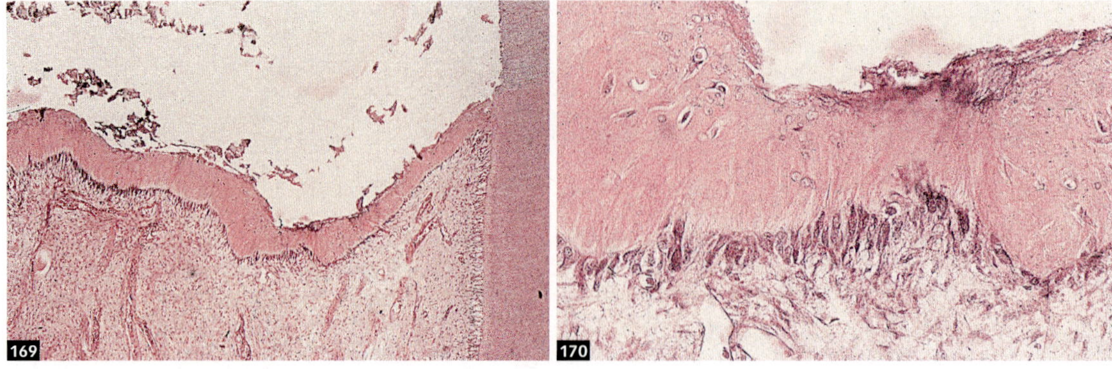


**Figures 7.169 and 7.170** - Mineralized tissue bridge protecting the pulp remainder without inflammation, after pulpotomy with calcium hydroxide in human teeth (H.E.) (Holland, 2003).

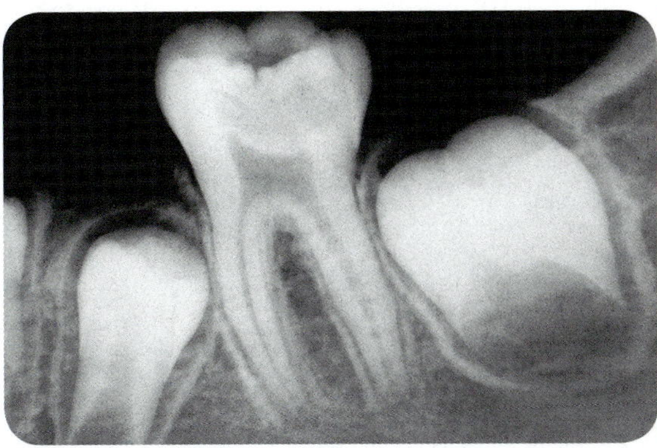

**Figure 7.171** - Radiographic aspect of tooth #36, with deep decay and thickness of the periodontal membrane space.

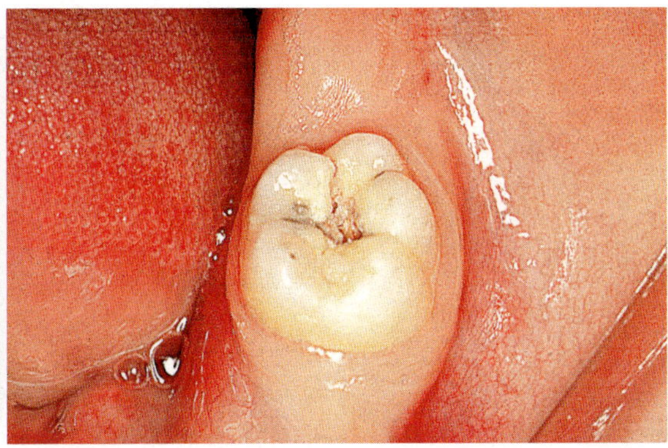

**Figure 7.172** - Clinical aspect of deep decay, tooth #36 with symptomatic pulpitis.

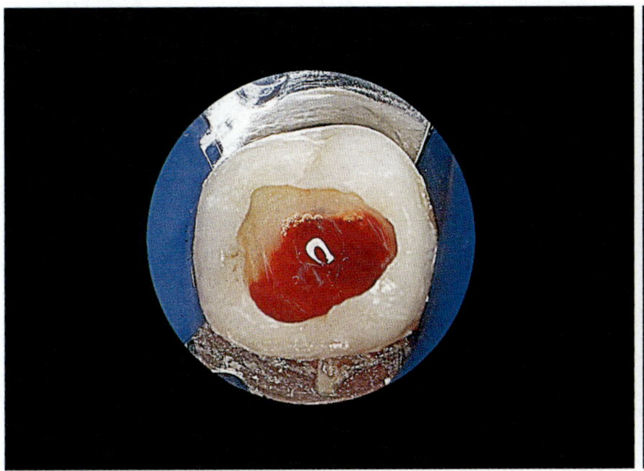

**Figure 7.173** - Clinical aspect demonstrating abundant livid red-colored bleeding, tooth #36.

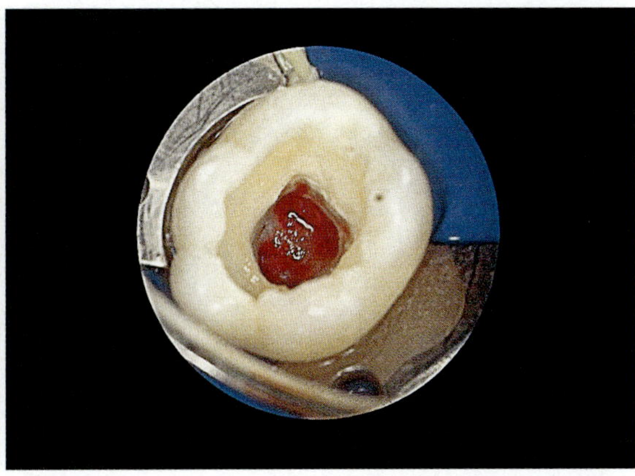

**Figure 7.174** - Clinical aspect demonstrating of the pulp remainder, tooth #36.

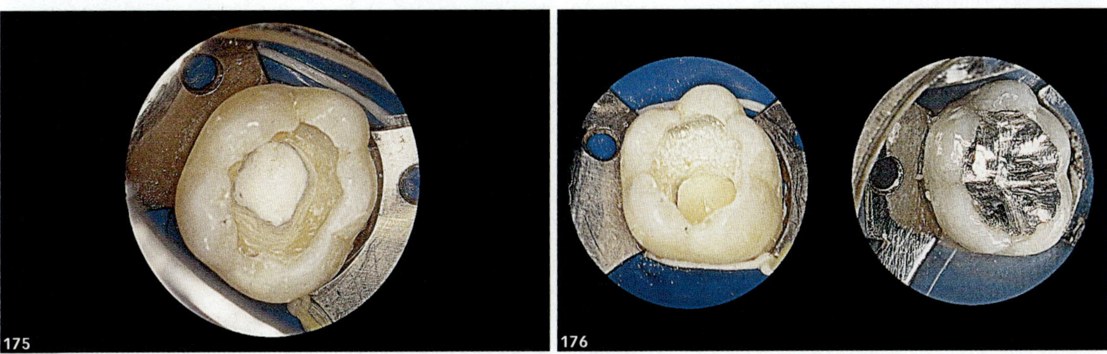


**Figures 7.175 and 7.176** - Placement of the biological capping (calcium hydroxide paste with saline solution) on the pulp remainder. Calcium hydroxide cement over the paste. Restored tooth.

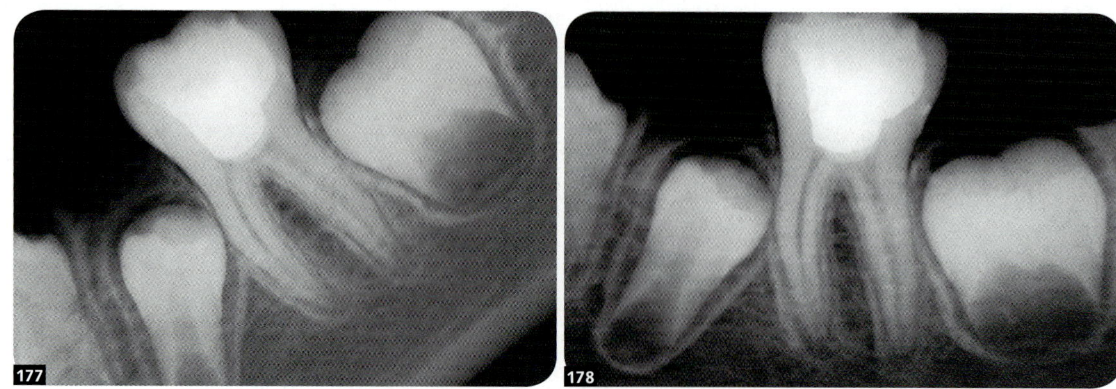


**Figures 7.177 and 7.178** - Radiographic aspect on the day of the pulpotomy and 180 days after, showing integrity of the lamina dura.

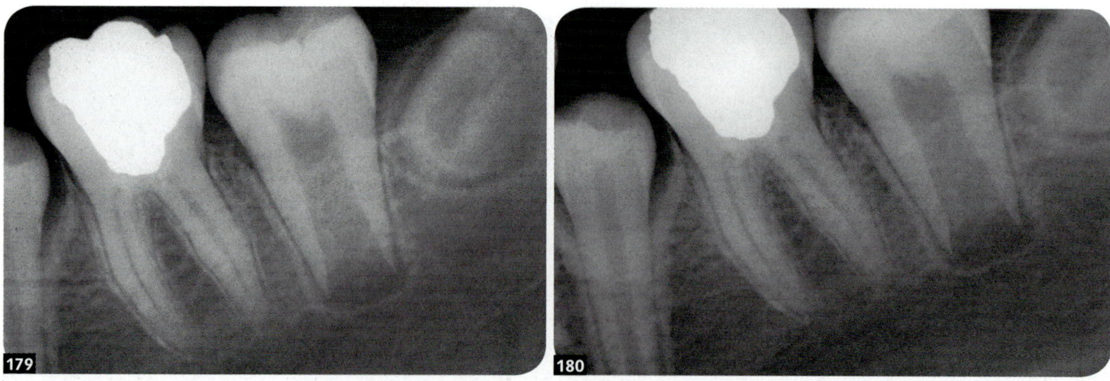


**Figures 7.179 and 7.180** - Radiographic aspects 360 and 480 days after the pulpotomy, demonstrating integrity of the lamina dura, tooth #36.

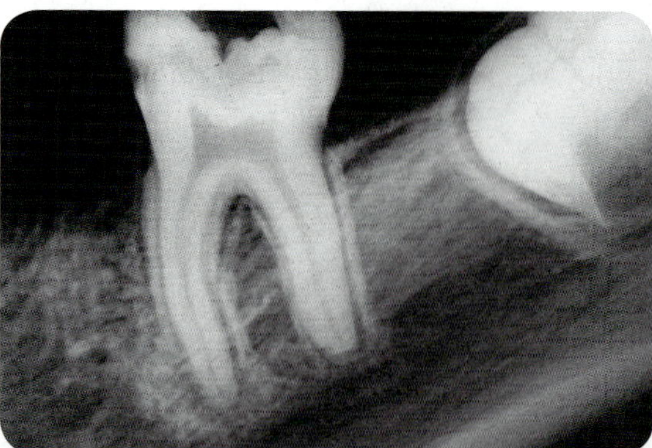

**Figure 7.181** - Radiographic aspect demonstrating chronic and deep caries, thickness of the periodontal membrane space, tooth #37.

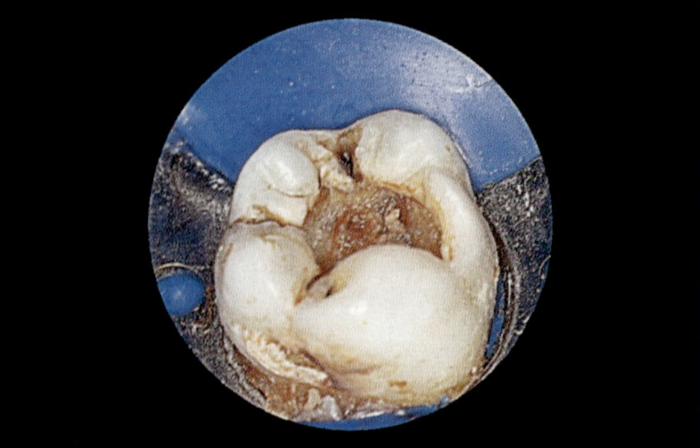

**Figure 7.182** - Clinical aspect of deep caries, tooth #37 with symptomatic pulpitis.

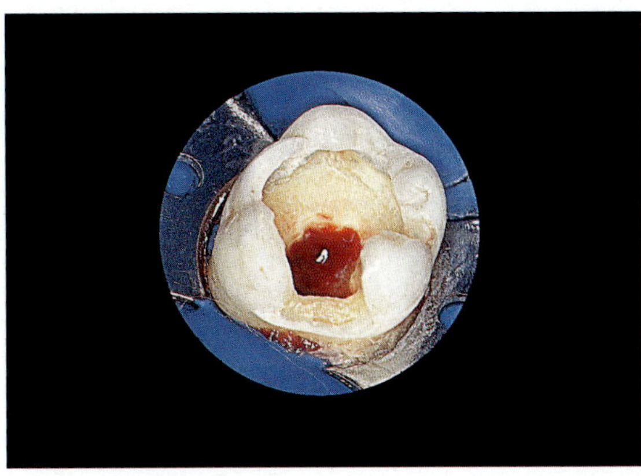

**Figure 7.183** - Clinical aspect demonstrating livid red-colored bleeding, tooth #37.

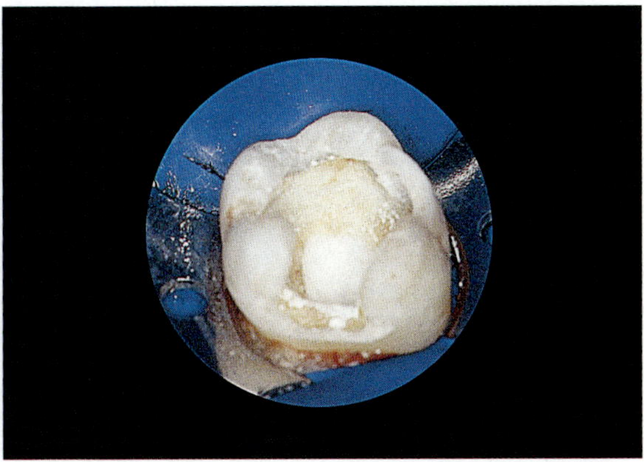

**Figure 7.184** - Placement of the biological covering calcium hydroxide paste with saline solution) on the pulp remainder, tooth #37.

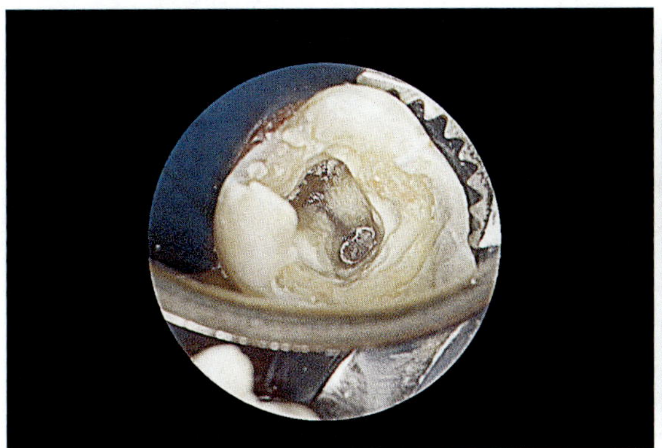

**Figure 7.185** - Mineralized bridge, 90 days after the pulpotomy, tooth 37.

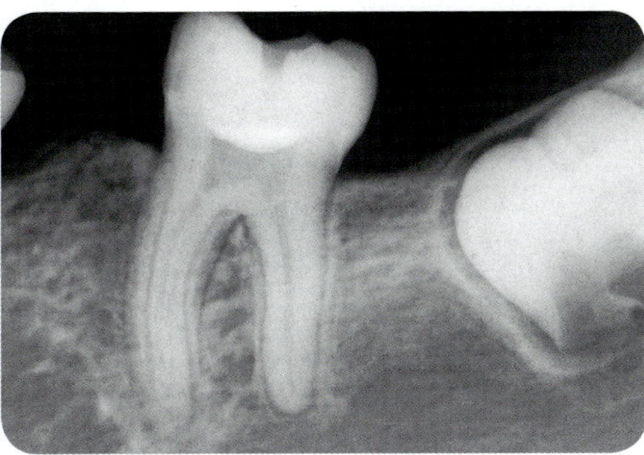

**Figure 7.186** - Radiographic aspect of the mineralized bridge, 90 days after the pulpotomy, tooth #37.

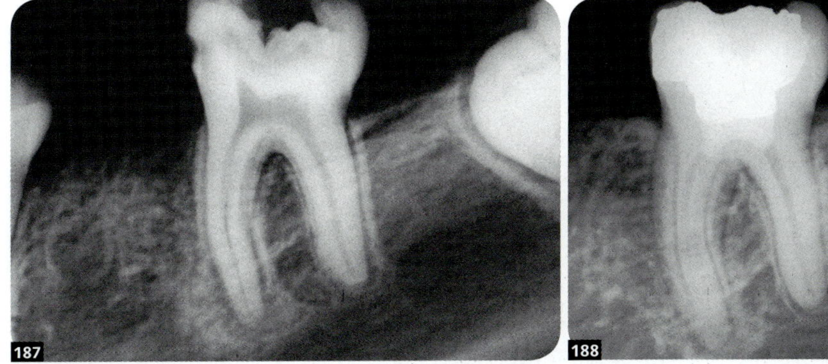


**Figures 7.187 and 7.188** - Radiographic aspect of the periapical area, before and after the pulpotomy, demonstrating integrity of the lamina dura, tooth #37.

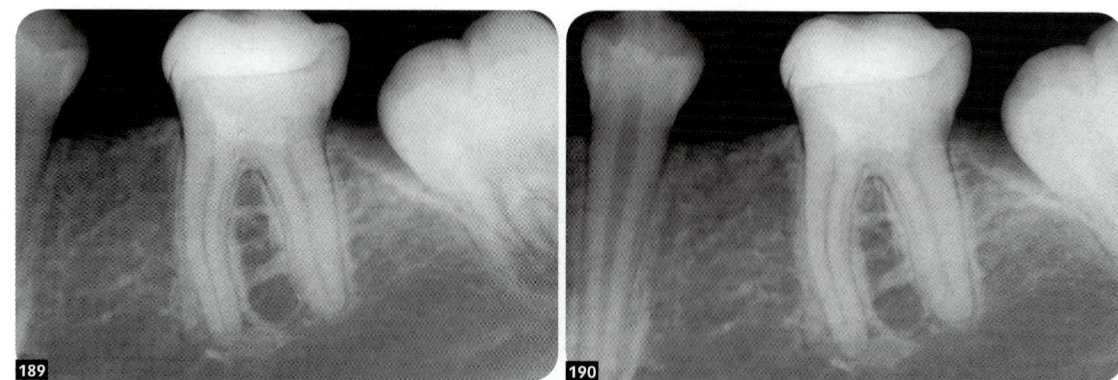


**Figures 7.189 and 7.190** - Radiographic aspects 360 and 480 days after the pulpotomy, demonstrating integrity of the lamina dura, tooth #37.

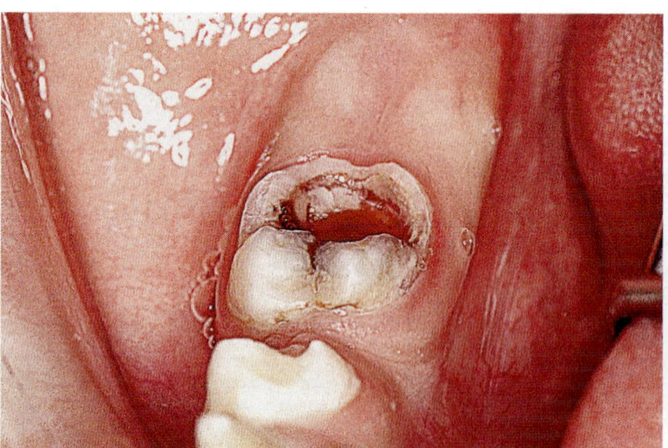

**Figure 7.191** - Clinical aspect showing open cavity, presence of pulp polyp, tooth #46 with asymptomatic pulpitis.

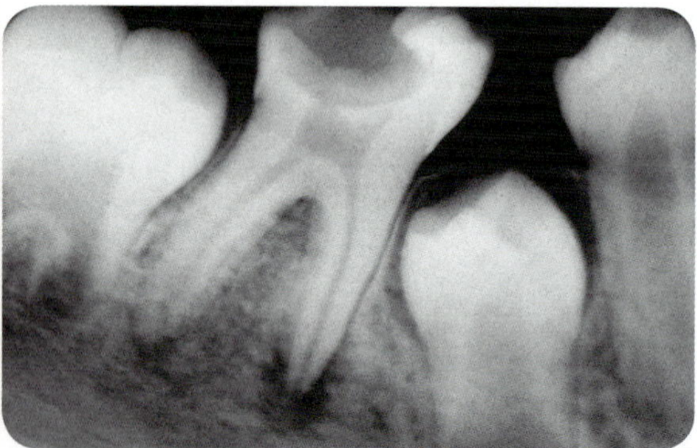

**Figure 7.192** - Radiographic aspect of deep decay with pulp exposure and periapical bony rarefaction tooth #46.

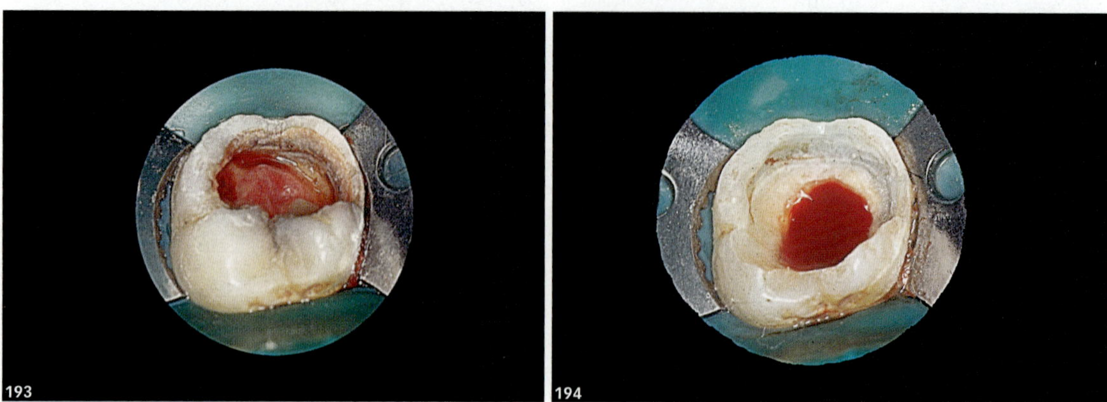


**Figures 7.193 and 7.194** - Clinical aspect of infected cavity, pulp polyp; Clinical aspect, tooth #46 with livid red-colored bleeding.

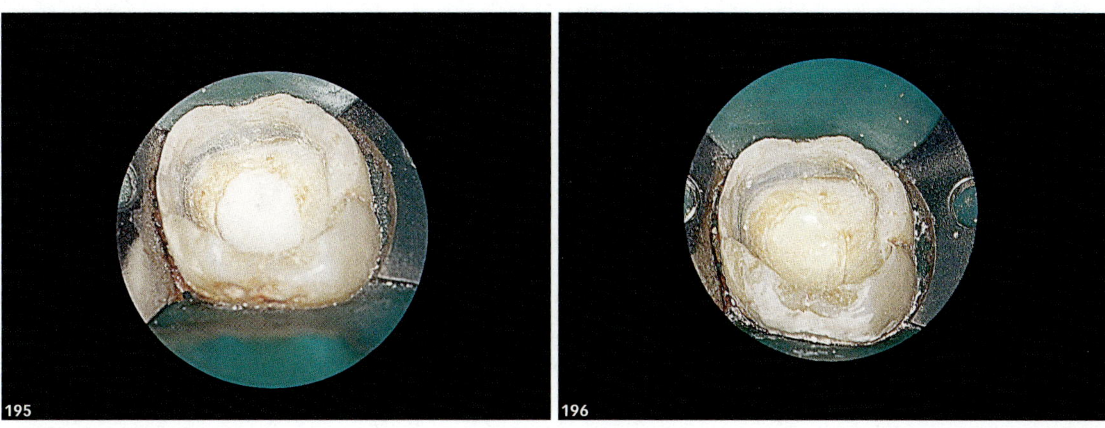


**Figures 7.195 and 7.196** - Placement of the biological covering (calcium hydroxide paste with saline solution) on the pulp remainder; calcium hydroxide cement over the paste.

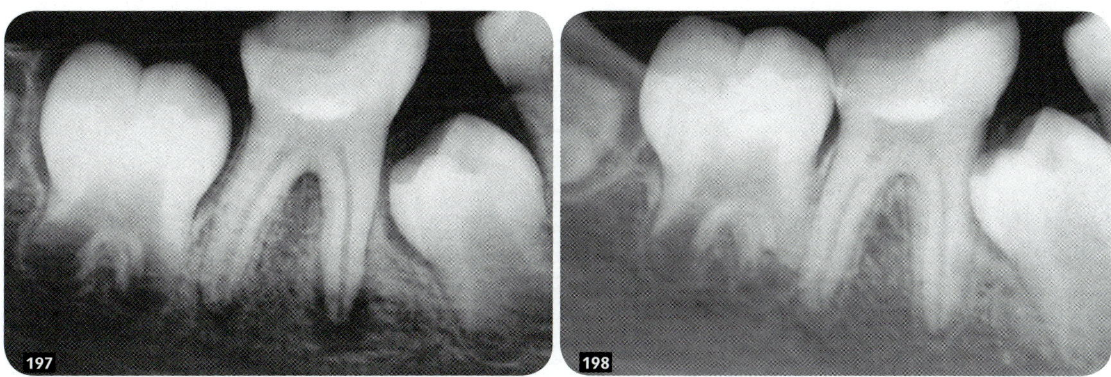


**Figures 7.197 and 7.198** - Radiographic aspects of the day of the pulpotomy and 180 days after demonstrating disappearance of the periapical bony rarefaction and integrity of lamina dura tooth #46.

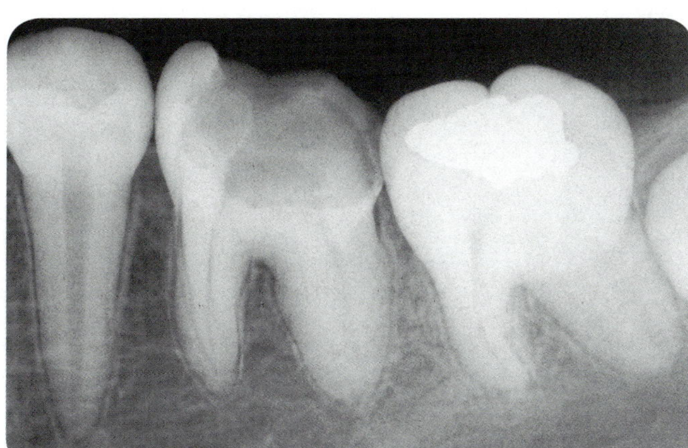

**Figure 7.199** - Radiographic aspect demonstrating deep decay, tooth #36 with symptomatic pulpitis.

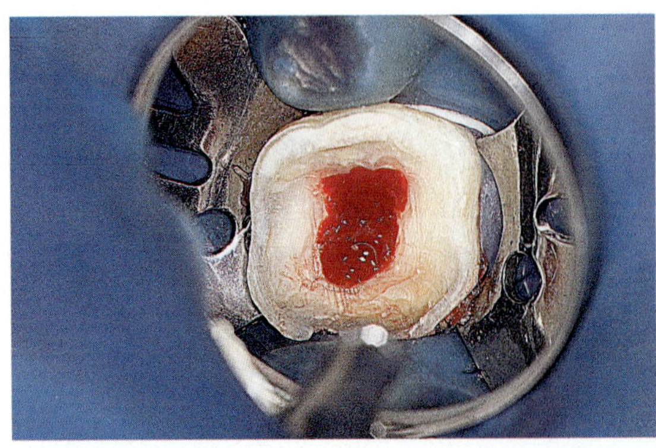

**Figure 7.200** - Clinical aspect of the tooth #36, evidencing pulp with abundant livid red-colored bleeding.

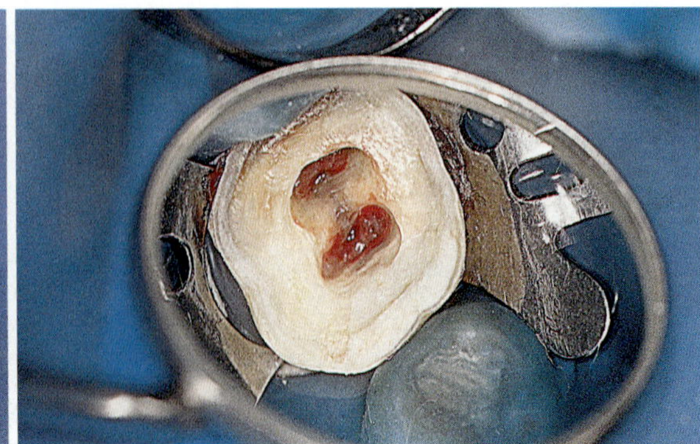

**Figure 7.201** - Clinical aspect demonstrating the pulp remainder of tooth #36, with consistency and structures.

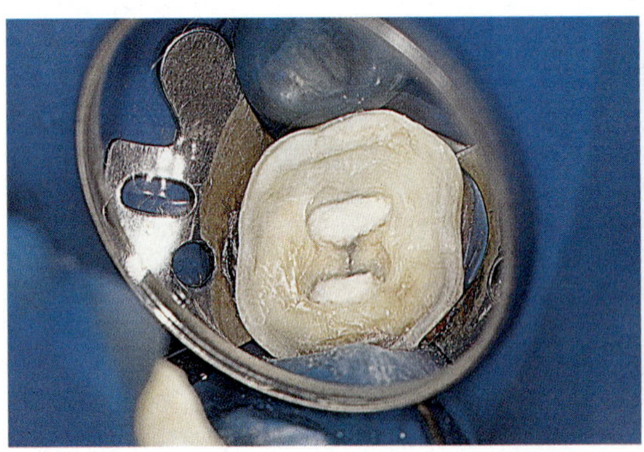

**Figure 7.202** - Placement of the biological covering (calcium hydroxide paste with saline solution) on the pulp remainder, tooth #36.

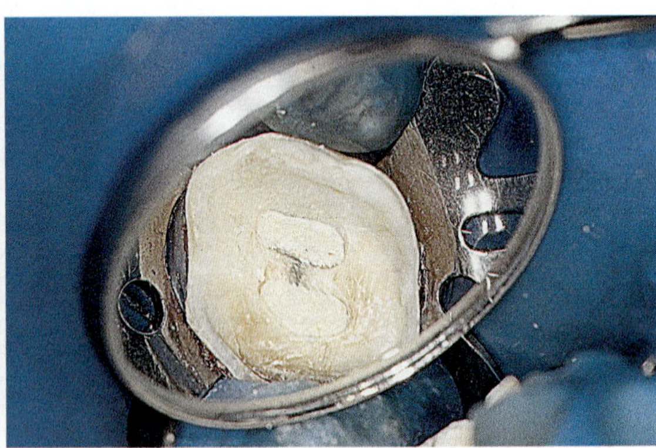

**Figure 7.203** - Calcium hydroxide cement over the paste, tooth #36.

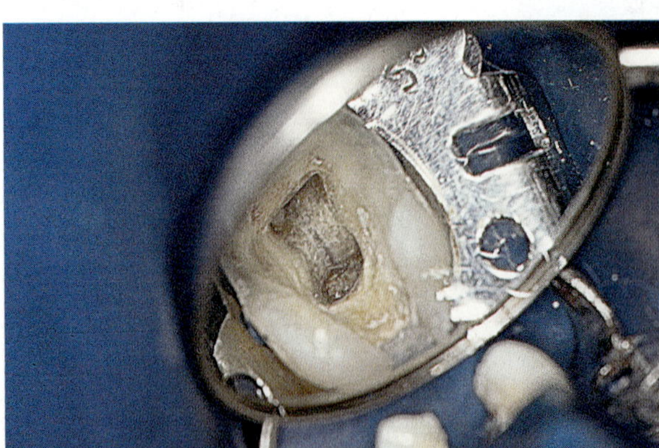

**Figure 7.204** - Mineralized bridge, 90 days after the pulpotomy, tooth #36.

1. Abbot PV, Yu C. A clinical classification of the status of the pulp and the root canal system. Aust Dent J 2007;52:17-31(Suppl).
2. Accorinte MLR, Holland R, Reis A, Bortoluzzi MC, Murata SS, Dezan Jr E, Souza V, Alessandro LD. Evaluation of Mineral Trioxide Aggregate and calcium hydroxide cement as pulp-capping agents in human teeth. J Endod 2008;34:1– 6.
3. Aeinehchi M, Eslami B, Ghanbariha M, Saffar AS. Mineral Trioxide Aggregate (MTA) and calcium hydroxide as pulp-capping agents in human teeth: a preliminary report. Int Endod J 2003;36:225-231.
4. Aydos JH. Tratamento da polpa dental inflamada. Rev Fac Odontol Porto Alegre 1985;27:153-171.
5. Busato ALS, Costa CAS, Estrela C. Dental restorative material biocompatibility Braz Endod J 1997;2:14-22.
6. Camilleri J, Pitt Ford TR. Mineral trioxide aggregate: a review of the constituents and biological properties of the material. Int Endod J 2006;39:747-754.
7. Chacko V, Kurikose S. Human response to mineral trioxide aggregate (MTA): a histologic study. J Clin Pediatr Dent 2006;30:203-210.
8. Caliskan MK. Success of pulpotomy in the management of hyperplastic pulpitis. Int Endod J 1993;26:142-148.
9. Castagnolla L, Negro V. L'esame della vitalitá pulpare mello pratica. Mondo Odontostomat 1972;14:919-31.
10. Castagnolla L, Orlay HG. Direct capping of the pulp and vital amputation. Brit Dent J 1950;16:324-30.
11. Chain M, Chain JB, Cox CC. Hidróxido de cálcio: uma revisão crítica. Rev Bras Odontol 1997;54: 306-11.
12. Clarke NG. The corticosteroid-antibiotic dressing as a capping for inflamed dental pulps. Aust Dent J 1971;16:71-76.
13. Consolaro A. Ácidos e sistemas adesivos sobre a polpa dentária: uma abordagem crítica. Rev Bras Odontol 1997;54:198-203.
14. Costa CA, Mesas AN, Hebling J. Pulp response to direct capping with an adhesive system. Am J Dent 2000;13:81-87.
15. Costa CA, Hebling J, Hanks CT. Current status of pulp capping with dentin adhesive systems: a review. Dent Mat 2000;16:188-197.
16. Costa CAS, Hebling J, Teixeira MF. Estudo preliminary da compatibilidade biológica dos adesivos dentinários All-Bond 2 e ScotchBond MP – Avaliação histológica de implantes subcutâneos em ratos. Rev Odontol USP 1997;11:11-18.
17. Costa CAS, Teixeira HM, Nascimento ABN, Hebling J. Biocompatibility of two current adhesive resins. J Endod 2000;26:512-516.
18. Cox CF. Effects of adhesive resins and various dental cements on the pulp. Oper Dent 1992;17:165-176.
19. Cox CF, Subay RK, Ostro E, Suzuki S, Sizuki SH. Tunnel defects in dentin bridges: their formation following direct pulp capping. Oper Dent 1996;21:4-11.
20. Eda S. Histochemical Análisis on the mechanism of dentin formation in dog's pulp. Bull Tokio Dent Coll 1961;2:59-88.
21. Estrela C. Diagnóstico da dor odontogênica. In: Dor Odontogênica. Artes Médicas: São Paulo; 2001.
22. Estrela C, Bammann LL, Estrela CRA, Silva RS, Pécora JD. Antimicrobial and chemical study of MTA, Portland cement, calcium hydroxide paste, Sealapex and Dycal. Braz Dent J 2000;11:19-27.
23. Estrela C, Lopes HP, Resende EV, Alencar AH. Avaliação da dor e de testes de vitalidade para o diagnóstico da inflamação pulpar. Rev Odontol Brasil Central 1995;5:4-8.
24. Estrela C, Lopes HP, Sydney GB, Felippe-Jr O. Chemical study of calcium carbonate present in various calcium hydroxide samples. Braz Endod J 1997;2:7-9.
25. Estrela C, Pesce HF. Chemical analysis of the liberation of calcium and hydroxyl ions of calcium hydroxide pastes in connective tissue of the dog – Part I. Braz Dent J 1996;7:41-46.
26. Estrela C, Pesce HF. Chemical analysis of the formation of calcium carbonate and its influence on calcium hydroxide pastes in connective tissue of the dog – Part II. Braz Dent J 1997;8:45-53.
27. Estrela C, Sydney GB, Bammann LL, Felippe-Jr O. Mechanism of action of calcium and hydroxyl ions of calcium hydroxide on tissue and bacteria. Braz Dent J 1995;6:85-90.
28. Estrela C, Sydney GB, Pesce HF, Felippe-Jr O. Dentinal diffusion of hydroxyl ions on various calcium hydroxide pastes. Braz Dent J 1995;6:5-9.
29. Estrela C, Zina O, Borges AH, Santos ES, Resende EV. Correlação entre o diagnóstico clínico da polpa dental inflamada e o reparo após a pulpotomia. Rev Odontol Brasil Central 1996;6:4-8.
30. Faraco-Jr IM, Holland R. Comportamento da polpa dentária diante do capeamento com o sistema adesivo Single Bond. Rev Ass Paul Cir Dent 2000;54:282-287.
31. Faraco-Jr IM, Holland R. Response of the pulp of dogs to capping with Mineral Trioxide Aggregate or a calcium hydroxide cement. Dent Traumatol 2001;17:163-166.
32. Francischone CE. Avaliação clínica e radiográfica feita a curto e longo prazo de uma técnica de pulpotomia, em função da idade do paciente, do grupo de dentes e da propedêutica pré-operatória. (Doctoral Thesis). University of São Paulo; 1978.
33. Francischone CE. Comportamento da polpa dental após pulpotomia e aplicação de trifosfato de adenosina, hidróxido de cálcio e combinação de ambos. Estudo histológico em dentes humanos. (Livre Docência Thesis). University of São Paulo, 1983.
34. Gao Y et al. The inductive effect of bone morphogenetic protein (BPM) on human periodontal fibroblast-like cells in vitro. J Osaka Dent Univ 1995;29:9-17.

35. Giasante-Jr S, Holland R. Pulpotomia em 3 sessões. J Braz Endo/Perio 2001;2:343-349.
36. Giasante-Jr S, Holland R. Pulpotomia em Saúde Pública: avaliação da técnica empregada nos serviços odontológicos da região administrativa da DIRVI "SUS" de Araçatuba. J Bras Endod 2002;3:55-61.
37. Glass RL, Zander HA. Pulp healing. J Dent Res 1949;28:97-107.
38. Goldberg F, Massone EJ, Spielberg C. Evaluation of the dentinal bridge after pulpotomy and calcium hydroxide dressing. J Endod 1984;10:318-320.
39. Grossman LI. Endodontic Pratice. 8th ed. Lea & Febiger: Philadelphia; 1976. p. 26-67.
40. Hallet GEM, Porteous JR. Fracture incisors treated by vital pulpotomy. Br Dent J 1963;115:279-87.
41. Hermann BW. Calciumhydroxyd als mittel zurn behandel und füllen von xahnwurzelkanälen. (Doctoral Thesis) Würzburg; 1920. 50p.
42. Hermann BW. Dentinobliteration der wurzel-kanalen nach behandlung mit calcium. Zahn Rundschau 1930;39:888-899.
43. Hess W. Pulp amputation as a method of treating root canals. Items Int 1929;51:596.
44. Hebling J, Giro EMA, Costa CAS. Biocompatibility of an adhesive system applied to exposed human dental pulp. J Endod 1999;25:676-682.
45. Holland R. Histochemical response of amputed pulps to calcium hydroxide. Rev Bras Pesq Méd Biol 1971;4:83-95.
46. Holland R. Processo de reparo do coto pulpar e dos tecidos periapicais após biopulpectomias e obturação de canal com hidróxido de cálcio ou óxido de zinco e eugenol. Estudos histológicos em dentes de cães. (Livre Docência Thesis). Araçatuba, São Paulo State University;1975.
47. Holland R, Delgado RJM, Souza V. Defeitos em forma de túnel em pontes de dentina são características exclusivas do emprego do hidróxido de cálcio? Rev Ciências Odontol 2001;4:51-56.
48. Holland R, Maisto OA, Souza V, Maresca BM, Nery MJ. Acción y velocidad de reabsorción de distintos materiales de obturación de condutos radiculares en el tejido conectivo periapical. Rev Asoc Odontol Argent 1981;69:7-17.
49. Holland R, Mello W, Nery MJ, Bernabé PFE, Souza V. Reaction of human periapical tissue to pulp extirpation and immediate root canal filling with calcium hydroxide. J Endod 1977;3:63-67.
50. Holland R, Mello W, Nery MJ, Souza V, Bernabé PFE, Otoboni-Filho JA. The influence of the sealing material in the healing process of inflamed pulps capped with calcium hydroxide or zinc oxide-eugenol cement. Acta Odontol Pediatr 1981;2:5-9.
51. Holland R, Mello W, Nery MJ, Souza V, Bernabé PFE, Otoboni-Filho JA. Healing process of dog's dental pulp after pulpotomy and pulp covering with calcium hydroxide in powder or paste form. Acta Odontol Pediatr 1981;2:47-51.
52. Holland R, Mello W, Nery MJ, Souza V, Bernabé PFE, Otoboni-Filho JA. O Endogel no tratamento conservador da polpa dental. Rev Bras Odontol 1986;48:14-18.
53. Holland R, Mello W, Souza V, Nery MJ, Bernabé PFE, Otoboni-Filho JA. Reacción de la pulpa y tejidos periapicales de dientes de perros, com forâmenes incompletamente formados, posteriormente a la pulpotomia y protección com hidróxido de cálcio o formocresol: estudo histologico a distância. Endodoncia 1983;1:33-38.
54. Holland R, Nery MJ, Souza V, Mello W, Bernabé PFE, Otoboni-Filho JA. The effect of corticosteroid-antibiotic dressing in the behaviour of the periapical tissue of dog´s teeth after overinstrumentation. Rev Odontol UNESP 1981;10:21-25.
55. Holland R, Otoboni-Filho JA, Souza V, Nery MJ, Bernabé PFE, Dezan-Jr E. Calcium hydroxide and corticosteroid-antibiotic association as dressing in cases of biopulpectomy. A comparative study in dog´s teeth. Braz Dent J 1998;9:67-76.
56. Holland R, Pinheiro CE, Mello W, Nery MJ, Souza V. Histochemical analysis of the dog's dental pulp after pulp capping with calcium, barium and strontium hydroxides. J Endod 1982;8:444-47.
57. Holland R, Soares IJ, Soares IML, Dias NV. The effect of the dressing in the tissue reactions following apical plugging of the root canal of dog´s pulpless teeth with dentin chips. Rev Odontol UNESP 1989;18:101-108.
58. Holland R, Souza V. Ability of a new calcium hydroxide root canal filling material to induce hard tissue formation. J Endod 1985;11:535-543.
59. Holland R, Souza V. Considerações clínicas e biológicas sobre o tratamento endodôntico. 1 – Tratamento endodôntico conservador. Rev Ass Paul Cirur Dent 1977;31:152-62.
60. Holland R, Souza V. O problema do diagnóstico clínico e indicação de tratamento da polpa dental inflamada. Rev Assoc Paul Cirur Dent 1970;24:188-93.
61. Holland R, Souza V. Quando e como o clínico geral deve realizar o tratamento conservador pulpar. In: Bottino MA, Feller C. Atualização em Odontologia Clínica. Artes Médicas: São Paulo; 1984. p-89-117.
62. Holland R, Souza V, Mello W. Processo de reparo da polpa dental pós pulpotomia e proteção com Formagen. Rev Fac Odontol Araçatuba 1974;3:77-81.
63. Holland R, Souza V, Mello W, Nery MJ, Bernabé PFE. Influência dos fragmentos de dentina no resultado do tratamento conservador da polpa dental exposta ou inflamada. Rev Gaúcha Odontol 1978;26:98-102.
64. Holland R, Souza V, Mello W, Nery MJ, Bernabé PFE, Otoboni-Filho JA. Permeability of the hard tissue bridge formed after pulpotomy with calcium hydroxide: a histologic study. J Amer Dent Ass 1979;99:472-75.
65. Holland R, Souza V, Mello W, Nery MJ, Bernabé PFE, Mello W, Otoboni-Filho JA. Emprego da associação corticosteróide antibiótico durante o tratamento endodôntico. Rev Paul Endod 1980;1:4-7.
66. Holland R, Souza B, Mello W, Nery MJ, Pannain R, Bernabé PFE, Otoboni-Filho JA. Healing process of dental pulp after pulpotomy or curettage and calcium hydroxide protection. Effect of corticosteroid dressing. Rev Fac Odont Araçatuba 1978;7:153-61.

67. Holland R, Souza V, Mello W, Nery MJ, Bernabé PFE, Otoboni-Filho JA. Healing process of dog's dental pulp after pulpotomy and protection with calcium hydroxide or dycal. Rev Odontol UNESP 1979;8/9:67-72.
68. Holland R, Souza V, Mello W, Russo MC. Healing process of the pulp stump and periapical tissues in dog teeth. I. Histopathological findings following pulp extirpation. Rev Fac Odontol Araçatuba 1977;6:1-2.
69. Holland R, Souza V, Mello W, Russo MC. Healing process of the pulp stump and periapical tissues in dog teeth. III. Histopathological findings following root filling with calcium hydroxide. Rev Fac Odontol Araçatuba 1978;7:25-37.
70. Holland R, Souza V, Milanezi I. Behaviour of pulp stump and periapical tissues to some drugs used as root canal dressings. A morphological study. Rev Bras Pesq Méd 1969;2:13-23.
71. Holland R, Souza V, Milanezi LA, Mello W. Comportamento da polpa dental após pulpotomia e aplicação tópica de alguns fármacos empregados na terapêutica conservadora. Rev Bras Odontol 1971;28:33-36.
72. Holland R, Souza V, Murata SS. Técnica da pulpotomia com troca de hidróxido de cálcio. Rev Ciência Odontol 1999;2:7-12.
73. Holland R, Souza V, Murata SS, Nery MJ, Bernabé PFE, Otoboni-Filho JA, Dezan-Jr E. Healing process of dog dental pulp after pulpotomy and pulp covering with mineral trioxide aggregate or Portland cement. Braz Dent J 2001;12:109-113.
74. Holland R, Souza V, Nery MJ, Bernabé PFE, Otoboni-Filho JA. Behaviour of the human periapical tissue to root canal filling with Caulk guta-percha cones. Rev Fac Odontol Araçatuba 1978;7:163-167.
75. Holland R, Souza V, Nery MJ, Bernabé PFE, Otoboni-Filho JA, Dezan-Jr E. Agregado de trióxido mineral y cemento Portland en la obturación de conductos radiculares de perro. Endodoncia 2001;19:275-280.
76. Holland R, Souza V, Nery MJ, Bernabé PFE, Mello W, Otoboni-Filho JA. The effect of calcium hydroxide in dentine. Rev Fac Odont Araçatuba 1978;7:177-180.
77. Holland R, Souza V, Nery MJ, Bernabé PFE, Mello W, Otoboni-Filho JA. Healing process after pulpotomy and covering with calcium hydroxide, Dycal or MPC. Histological study in dog teeth. Rev Fac Odont Araçatuba 1978; 7:185-191.
78. Holland R, Souza V, Nery MJ, Faraco-Jr IM, Bernabé PFE, Otoboni-Filho JA, Dezan-Jr E. Reaction of rat connective tissue to implanted dentin tube filled with mineral trioxide aggregate, Portland cement or calcium hydroxide. Braz Dent J 2001;12:3-8.
79. Holland R, Souza V, Nery MJ, Faraco-Jr IM, Bernabé PFE, Otoboni-Filho JA, Dezan-Jr E. Reaction of rat connective tissue to implanted dentin tubes filled with a white mineral trioxide aggregate. Braz Dent J 2002;13:23-26.
80. Holland R, Souza V, Nery MJ, Mello W, Bernabé PFE, Otoboni-Filho JA. Effect of the dressing in root canal treatment with calcium hydroxide. Rev Fac Odontol Araçatuba 1978;7:39-45.
81. Holland R, Souza V, Nery MJ, Otoboni-Filho JA, Bernabé PFE, Dezan-Jr E. Reaction of rat connective tissue to implanted dentin tubes filled with mineral trioxide aggregate or calcium hydroxide. J Endod 1999;25:161-166.
82. Holland R, Souza V, Nery MJ, Otoboni-Filho JA, Bernabé PFE. Comportamento da polpa de dentes de cães após capeamento e pulpotomia com o Sankin tipo II. Rev Ciência Odontol 1999;2:41-46.
83. Holland R, Souza V, Otoboni-Filho JA, Nery MJ, Bernabé PFE, Dezan-Jr E, Garlipe O. Comportamento dos tecidos periapicais de dentes de cães a obturação de canal com o cimento experimental Sealer Plus. Rev Bras Odontol 2000; 57:114-116.
84. Holland R, Souza V, Russo MC. Healing process after root canal therapy in immature human teeth. Rev Fac Odontol Araçatuba 1973;2:269-273.
85. Holland R, Souza V, Russo MC. Tratamento conservador da polpa dentária. ARS Curandi 1975;2:3-17.
86. Holland R, Souza V, Tagliavini RL, Milanezi LA. Healing process of teeth with open apices: histological study. Bull Tokyo Dent Coll 1971;12:333-338.
87. Holland R, Takayama S, Komatsu J, Souza V. Pulpal response to high speed cavit preparation using water or air spray as coolants. J Nihon Univ Sch Dent 1972;14:16-21.
88. Holland R et al. Diffusion of corticosteroid-antibiotic solutions through human dentine. Rev Odontol UNESP 1991;20:17-23.
89. Holland R et al. Comportamento da polpa dental do cão diante da exposição pulpar ou pulpotomia e proteção direta com o sistema All Bond 2. Rev Ciencia Odontol 1998;1:75-80.
90. Holland R et al. Recambio del hidroxido de cálcio despues de la pulpotomia y su influencia em la reparacion. Estudio histologico em dientes de monos. Endodoncia 1999;17:35-45.
91. Kakehashi S, Stanley HR, Fitzgerald RJ. The effects of surgical exposures of dental pulps in germ free and conventional laboratory rats. Oral Surg Oral Med Oral Pathol 1965;2:340-49.
92. Koh ET, Torabinejad M, Pitt Ford TR, Brady K, McDonald F. Mineral Trioxide Aggregate stimulates a biological response in human osteoblasts. J Biomed Materials Res 1997;37:432-9.
93. Iwamoto CE, Adachi E, Pameijer CH, Barnes D, Romberg EE, Jefferies S. Clinical and histological evaluation of white ProRoot MTA in direct pulp capping. Am J Dent 2006;9:85-90.
94. Lanza L. Avaliação clínica e microscópica de um adesivo aplicado em proteções pulpares diretas de dentes humanos. (Doctoral Thesis). Bauru; University of São Paulo.1997.
95. Lee SJ, Monsef M, Torabinejad M. Sealing ability of a mineral trioxide aggregate for repair of lateral root perforations. J Endod 1993;19:541-544.
96. Lopes HP, Costa-Filho A. A pulpotomia como opção no atendimento ambulatorial – Estudo preliminar. Rev Bras Odontol 1987;44:50-56.
97. Lopes HP, Estrela C, Elias CN. Comparative study of the hard tissue bridge after pulpotomy with calcium hydroxide associated of various vehicles. Braz Endod J 1996;1:43-46.

98. Markowitz K, Moynihan M, Liu M, Kim S. Biologic properties of eugenol and zinc oxide-eugenol. Oral Surg Oral Med Oral Pathol 1992;73:729-37.
99. Massone JE, Goldberg F, Barros RE. Histological evaluation of the effect of intrapulpal anesthesia in pulpotomies. Endod Dent Traumatol 1987;3:259-262.
100. Mello W. Comportamento da polpa dental inflamada após pulpotomia ou curetagem pulpar e proteção com hidróxido de cálcio e a influência de curativo com agente antiflogístico. (Master's Thesis). Bauru, Universidade de São Paulo; 1979.
101. Mello W. Reações histopatológicas após pulpotomias em dentes de cães. (Doctoral Thesis). Bauru, University of São Paulo; 1984.
102. Mello W, Holland R, Berbert A. Estudo histopatológico da polpa dental inflamada de dentes de cães após pulpotomia ou curetagem pulpar e proteção com hidróxido de cálcio – Efeito de um agente antiflogístico. Rev Odont UNESP 1983;12:7-19.
103. Mello W, Holland R, Souza V. Capeamento pulpar com hidróxido de cálcio ou pasta de óxido de zinco e eugenol. Rev Fac Odontol Araçatuba 1972;1:33-44.
104. Nair PNR, Duncan HF, Pitt Ford TR, Luder HU. Histological, ultrastructural and quantitative investigations on the response of healthy human pulps to experimental capping with mineral trioxide aggregate: a randomized controlled trial. Int Endod J 2008;41:128-150.
105. Olsson H, Petersson K, Rohlin M. Formation of a hard tissue barrier after pulp cappings in humans. A systematic review. Int Endod J 2006;39:429-442.
106. Pameijer CH, Stanley HR. The disastrous effects of the total etch technique in vital pulp capping in primates. Am J Dent 1998;11:S45-S54.
107. Pereira JC, Stanley HR. Pulp capping, influence of the exposure site on pulp healing. Histologic and radiographic study in dog's pulp. J Endod 1981;7:213-223.
108. Pisanti S, Sciaky I. Origin of calcium hydroxide in their repair wall after pulp exposure in the dog. J Dent Res 1964;43:641-44.
109. Russo M, Souza V, Holland R. Effects of the dressing with calcium hydroxide under pressure on the pulpal healing of pulpotomized human teeth. Rev Fac Odontol Araçatuba 1974;3:303-306.
110. Russo M, Holland R, Souza V. Radiographic and histological evaluation of the treatment of inflamed dental pulps. Int Endod J 1982; 15:137-142.
111. Rutherford RB et al. Induction of reparative dentine formation in monkeys by recombinant human osteogenic protein-1. Archs Oral Biol 1993;38:571-576.
112. Saidon J, He J, Zhu Q, Safavi K, Spångberg LSW. Cell and tissue reactions to mineral trioxide aggregate and Portland cement. Oral Surg Oral Med Oral Pathol 2003;95:483-9.
113. Santini A. Long-term clinical assessment of pulpotomies with calcium hydroxide containig Ledermix in permanent premolars and molars. Acta Odontol Pediatr 1986;7:45-50.
114. Sciaky I, Pisanti S. Localization of calcium placed over amputed pulps in dog's teeth. J Dent Res 1960;39:1128-32.
115. Seltzer S, Bender IB. Some influences effecting repair of the exposed pulps of dogs teeth. J Dent Res 1958; 37:678-87.
116. Seux D, Couble ML, Hartmann DJ, Gauthier JP, Magloire H. Odontoblast – Like cytodifferentation of a calcium hydroxide – containing cement. Arch Oral Biol 1991;136:117-128.
117. Soares IML. Efeito imediato de diferentes instrumentos rotatórios e curetas utilizadas na pulpotomia. (Doctoral Thesis). Florianópolis, Federal University of Santa Catarina;1984.
118. Soares IML. Resposta pulpar ao MTA – Agregado de trióxido mineral – Comparada ao hidróxido de cálcio, em pulpotomia. Histológico em dentes de cães. (Thesis). Florianópolis; 1996.
119. Souza V. Reação entre quadros inflamatórios das polpas dentais coronárias e os resultados do emprego do cloridrato de tetraciclina, acetato de hidrocortisona e hidróxido de cálcio, na terapêutica de polpas dentais inflamadas submetidas à pulpotomia. Estudo histológico efetuado em dentes de cães. (Master's Thesis). Araçatuba, São Paulo State University; 1969.
120. Souza V. Reação ao tecido conjuntivo do rato ao implante de tubos de dentina, com aberturas de diferentes diâmetros, preenchidos com algumas pastas à base de hidróxido de cálcio. Estudo histológico. (Doctoral Thesis). Araçatuba, São Paulo State University; 1976.
121. Souza V, Holland R. Treatment of the inflamed dental pulp. Aust Dent J 1974;19:191-96.
122. Souza V, Holland R, Hyzatugu R. Evaluation of X-rays examination in the diagnosis of pulp response to conservative treatment. N York J Dent 1971;41:206-213.
123. Souza V, Holland R, Holland-Jr C, Nery MJ. Estudo morfológico do comportamento da polpa dentária após pulpotomia e proteção com óxido de magnésio ou hidróxido de cálcio. O Incisivo 1972;1:18-21.
124. Souza V, Holland R, Mello W, Nery WJ. Reaction of rat connective tissue to the implant of calcium hydroxide pastes. Rev Fac Odontol Araçatuba 1977;6:69-76.
125. Soviero VM, Souza IPR, Gama FVA. Proteínas dentinogênicas: uma nova tendência para a realização de pulpotomia. Rev Bras Odontol 1998;5:314-317.
126. Stanley HR. Calcium hydroxide and vital pulp therapy. In: Hargreaves KM, Goodis HE. Seltzer and Bender's dental pulp. Qintessence books: Chicago; 2002. 309-324.
127. Stanley HR. Criteria for standardizing and increasing credibility of direct pulp capping studies. Am J Dent 1998;11:S1-S63.
128. Stanley HR. Pulp capping: conserving the dental pulp. Can it be done. Is worth it. Oral Surg Oral Med Oral Pathol 1989;68:628-639.

129. Stanley HR, Lundy T. Dycal therapy for pulp exposures. Oral Surg Oral Med Oral Pathol 1972;34:818-827.
130. Stanley HR, Pameijer CH. Dentistry's friend: calcium hydroxide. Operat Dent 1997; 22:1-3.
131. Torabinejad M, Watson TF, Pitt-Ford TR. Sealing ability of a mineral trioxide aggregate when used as a root end filling material. J Endod 1993;19:591-595.
132. Tronstad L. Reation of the exposed pulp to Dycal treatment. Oral Surg Oral Med Oral Pathol 1974;38:945-53.
133. Tronstad L, Mjor IA. Capping the inflamed pulp. Oral Surg Oral Med Oral Pathol 1972; 34:477-85.
134. Trowbridge HO. Histology of pulpal inflammation. In: Hargreaves KM, Goodis HE. Seltzer and Bender's dental pulp. Qintessence books: Chicago; 2002. p.227-245.
135. Ulmansky M, Sela J, Sela M. Scanning electrom microscopy of calcium hydroxide induced bridges. J Oral Pathol 1972;1:244-8.
136. Van Hassel HJ. Physiology of the human dental pulp. Oral Surg Oral Med Oral Pathol 1971;32:126.
137. Van Hassel HJ, MacHugh JW. Effect of prednisolone on intra-pulpal pressure. J Dent Res 1972;51:172 (Abstract).
138. Vieira MS. Pulpotomia em duas sessões na clínica de endodontia da Marinha. Rev Naval de Odontol 1985; 1:37.
139. Wakabayashi H, Horikawa M, Funato A, Onodera A, Matsumoto K. Biomicroscopical observation of dystrophic calcification induced by calcium hydroxide. Endod Dent Traumatol 1993;9:165-70.
140. Wucherpfennig AL, Green DB. Mineral trioxide vs Portland cement: two biocompatible filling materials. J Endod 1999;25:308 (Abstract).
141. Zander HA. Reaction of the pulp to calcium hydroxide. J Dent Res 1939;18:373-79.
142. Zander HA, Law DB. Pulp management in fractures of young permanent teeth. J Amer Dent Ass 1942;29:737-41.
143. Zerlotti E. Histochemical changes in the connective tissue of the dental pulp during inflamation. Oral Surg Oral Med Oral Pathol 1969;27:664-677.

# Microbiological Aspects in Endodontics

**L. L. Bammann**
*Federal University of Pelotas, Pelotas, RS, Brazil*

**C. Estrela**
*Federal University of Goiás, Goiânia, GO, Brazil*

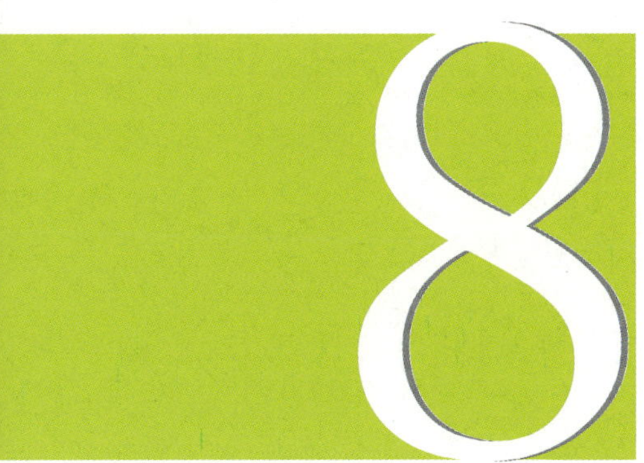

Chapter contents

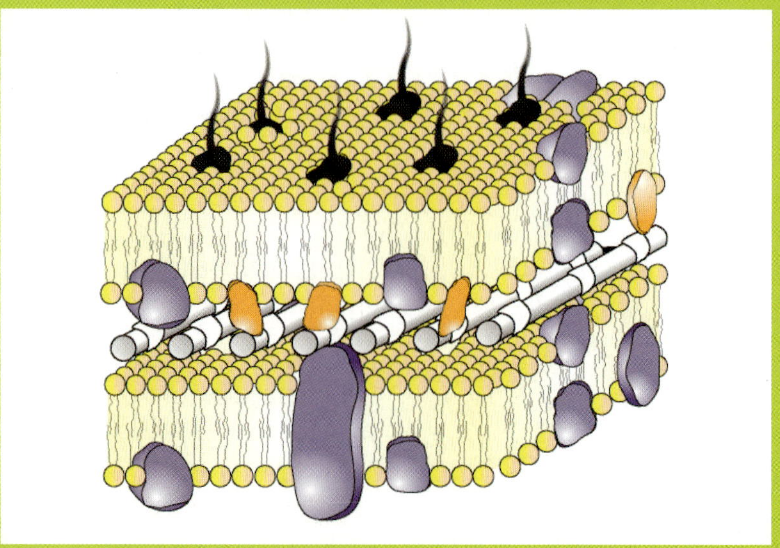

Diagram of the envelope of a Gram-negative cell (adjusted Tortora et al.[62]).

## 8.1 Introduction

Microbiology is a specialized area of the science of Biology that studies organisms of very small sizes - microorganisms, comprising bacteria, whose dimensions fall within the range of micrometers (μm = $10^{-3}$ mm), fungi, which are bigger than bacteria, protozoa, that can reach 5 mm, and also unicellular or multicellular algae, which are able to perform photosynthesis; the viruses, which are also studied in Microbiology, are non-cellular entities considered the smallest infectious agents, whose dimensions are between 15 and 300 nm and, actually, not much bigger than a large molecule.

The origin of microorganisms, especially as regards bacteria, dates from approximately four billion years ago, making them the ancestors of all life forms.

Although they are ancient, the first careful observation of these organisms were made in the 17th century, in the 1670's, thanks to the skill and curiosity of Anton van Leeuwenhoek (1632-1723), a Dutch salesman whose hobby was lens construction. Leeuwenhoek was self-made in biological science, which makes his findings more valuable, and he was also the first person to survey and travel through this fascinating Old-New World, describing and drawing its forms with perfection.

In spite of the enhancement of microscopic techniques, it was only after the advent of electronic microscopy, during the 1930's, that ultra-structural studies were done, establishing microorganisms present a prokaryotic cell structure – rough, rustic, primitive – or an eukaryotic cell structure – refined, sophisticated, evolved – depending on the microorganism considered. Bacteria belong to the first group and fungi, protozoa and algae are included in the second, while viruses are not included in this classification, since they are considered as acellular entities.

Among their superlative properties, these organisms are ubiquitous and, consequently, they are also detected in man, constituting the human microbiota. The microbial population that has the human body as its "home" is "fantastic"; in fact, the number of microorganisms is ten times higher than the number of cells that compose the human body, thus, "man is 10% human and 90% microbial".

Under healthy conditions, however, the human organism is sterile before birth, from a microbiological point of view. Nevertheless, during birth the process of contact between human being and microorganisms begins and the establishment of the infectious process occurs – considering infection as the entry into and colonization of the host by microorganisms, which does not necessarily mean disease.

To the human being, the maternal genital tract, oral cavity and upper respiratory tract of the mother, father and others represent sources of microorganisms, as well as food and environment. These microorganisms, stressed by complex ecological determinants, start colonizing certain areas of the human body, which normally harbors numerous and complex microbial populations, while other areas present a discreet number of microorganisms, usually transient, and some tissues and organs are usually sterile from a microbiological point of view.

The oral cavity is one of the septic environments of organism, supporting a complex microbiota, from either the qualitative or quantitative approach; this complexity becomes perfectly characterized by the presence of Gram-negative and Gram-positive bacteria, fungi, protozoa and viruses, distributed, sometimes in significant concentrations depending on the microorganism group considered, in the four major oral ecosystems[40]

– oral epithelium, upper side of the tongue, dental surface, dental and epithelial subgingival surfaces – and also in saliva, which does not have its own microbiota, but it expresses, at least in part, that which exists in oral sites.

## 8.2 Microorganism Biology

Many of microorganisms that colonize the oral cavity, as well as those present in other areas of the human body, in significant numbers establish a relationship of amphibiosis with their host, according to Rosebury's concepts[38], and for that reason they are called amphibiotic. This relationship between host and parasite is extremely dynamic, presenting mutual, bilateral cooperation between micro and macro organisms involved; therefore, generally, amphibiosis is a beneficial interaction. However, from this aspect, it is worth emphasizing that amphibiotic microorganisms have pathogenic potential and, in their formidable biologism, can cause damage to the host through different strategies, leading to a relationship of antibiosis, which is a synonym of disease.

As regards oral microorganisms, bacteria are the most important among pathogenic agents, being responsible for the etiology of diseases such as dental caries, periodontal diseases, pulp and periapical pathology, considering those which most demand the attention, skill and knowledge of dental professionals.

The biological role of bacteria, particularly the one related to aggression mechanisms and the host reaction they induce, can only be understood through the knowledge of cellular structure, ultra-structure and energetic metabolism.

### 8.2.1 Bacteria structure and ultra-structure

From a structural point of view, a bacterial cell consists of:

1. **Cell envelope**: in most bacteria, it is composed of a cell wall and cytoplasmic membrane (some authors consider a third component, the glycocalyx, as a constituent of the cell envelope).
2. **Internal structures:** cytoplasm, genetic material and endospore;
3. **External structures:** glycocalyx, flagella, pilus (fimbria) and fibrillar structures.

Cell envelope, as the name suggests, involves bacterial body on the outside, presenting a complex ultra-structure[4].

#### Cell Wall

The composition of the cell wall must be studied according to the reactivity of the bacteria to Gram staining; it is the difference in the structure of this component that allows the bacterial world to be classified into two groups – the group of Gram-positive bacteria and the one of Gram-negative bacteria. The bacterium is called Gram-positive when its wall, after exposure to alcohol-ketone – the differentiation agent - becomes impermeable, retaining the violet crystal + iodine complex and appearing deep violet in color during microscopic observation. Oppositely, it is called Gram-negative when its wall becomes permeable after exposure to the differentiation agent, losing the complex referred; thus, the Gram-negative cells will appear stained with the red dye – diluted fuchsin or safranin -, the contrast stain.

The Gram-positive cell wall is formed by a polymer called peptidoglycan, a gigantic molecule, which is composed of glycan strands plus short peptides, and corresponds to 40 to 80% of the dry weight of the cell wall (Fig. 8.1).

The glycan strands of peptidoglycan are formed by N-acetylglucosamine and N-acetylmuramic acid, derived from glucose, which alternate in its disposition on the macromolecule structure and are linked by β1-4 glycosidic bonds. The peptide component is always bound to the residue of N-acetylmuramic acid, comprising a chain of four amino acids, positioned in L and D forms, respectively. The glycan and peptide residues comprise the blocks of which peptidoglycan are made

These blocks of peptidoglycan appear in several layers. To form a rigid framework around the cells, the tetrapeptides on one peptidoglycan chain are cross-linked with

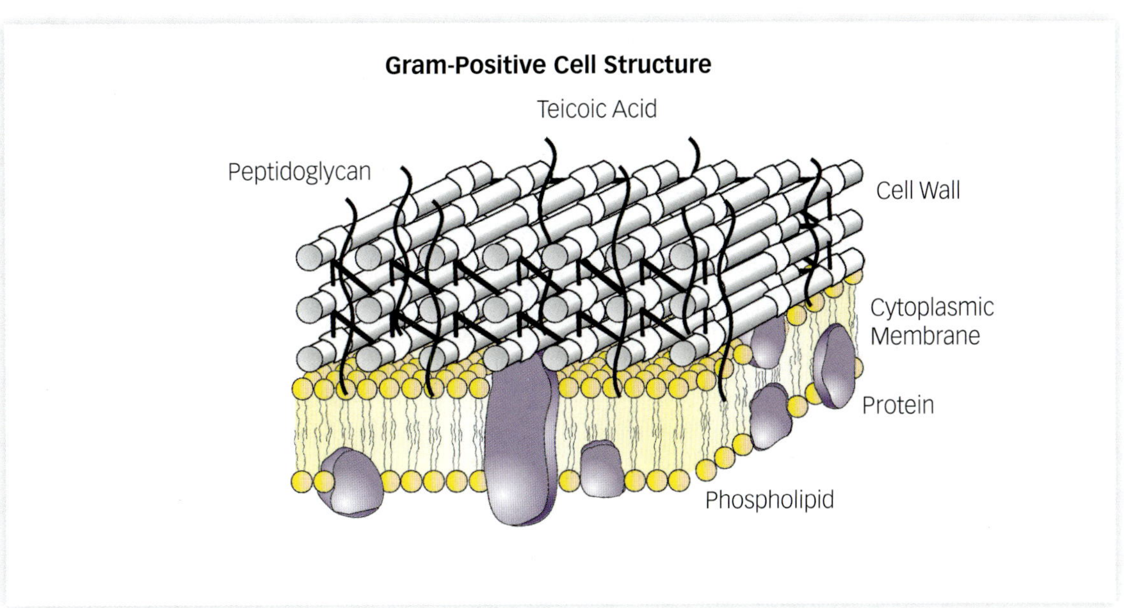


**Figure 8.1** - Diagram of the envelope of a Gram – positive cell (adjusted from Tortora et al. [62]).



those of adjacent chain. Although there is a remarkable degree of constancy in the composition of glycan strands, different groups of bacteria show some variation in the composition of the interpeptide bridges and, to a lesser extent, in the peptide subunits, in positions 3 and 2.

In addition to peptidoglycan, teichoic acids, composed of ribitol or glycerol phosphates, are also part of this structure. As regards these polymers, there are some associated with peptidoglycan (either glycerol or ribitol-type) and those covalently linked to the glycolipids of the cytoplasmic membrane level (glycerol-type); furthermore, transient teichoic acids can be found, released from the membrane. Teichoic acids related to membrane are known as lipoteichoic acids. These polymers are situated perpendicularly to the bacterial body, and one of its ends surpasses the outer limit of the cell. Their topographical location, in the *front* of the cell unit, gives them a privileged situation in the performance of their biological role, with special reference to adherence phenomenon.

Polysaccharides and proteins can also be present in the cell wall, and their importance is related to the bacterium involved.

The cell walls of Gram-negative bacteria are considerably more complex than those of the Gram-positive bacteria. The peptidoglycan layer, which corresponds to 5 to 10% of this wall, presents the basic structure described previously, with its intrinsic peculiarities, and it is located in the periplasmic space, an area limited externally by an outer membrane, and internally by the cytoplasmic membrane. In this space, hydrolytic enzymes named hydrolases are also concentrated, as well as binding proteins that participate in nutritive mechanisms of the cell under consideration (Fig. 8.2).

The outer membrane, another structural component of this wall, is similar in many aspects to the cytoplasmic membrane (which will be described later). When compared with the cytoplasmic membrane, however, it presents a distinctive component, lipopolysaccharide (LPS).

Lipopolysaccharide, the typical constituent of the Gram-negative cell wall, is located exclusively in the outer leaflet of the membrane bilayer. LPS is composed of three covalently linked segments: Lipid A, Core and Antigen O (Fig. 8.3).

Lipid A is firmly embedded in the outer membrane, and consists of an unusual glycolipid composed of disaccharides to which are attached short-chains fatty acids and phosphate groups. Lipid A is the endotoxin of the Gram-negative bacteria, and is liberated not only when the bacterium disintegration occurs, but also during its growth and multiplication[33] and, as a consequence, expressing its toxic potential and inducing complex organic reactions.

Core and *O* antigen have a polysaccharide nature. The first is composed of short sugar chains, whose structure is more or less common among Gram-negative bacteria, while the second one comprises long carbohydrate chains, up to 40 sugars in length, which are specific to the bacterial species being considered, and for this reason the *O* antigen is responsible for antigenic characteristics of Gram-negative bacteria.

Strategically, the outer membrane also presents hollow protein molecules, called porines, which constitute real canals through which the diffusion of simple nutritive components is provided, such as sugars, amino acids and some ions. Enclosing the bacterial body, the outer membrane together with the peptidoglycan, to which it is bound by lipoprotein molecules, provides the bacterial cell integrity.

The third component of the Gram-negative cell wall is a lipoprotein compound, a molecule composed of both a lipid and a protein, and is embedded in the outer membrane and bound covalently to peptidoglycan. Its main function, according to studies conducted with mutant strains, is to stabilize the outer membrane.

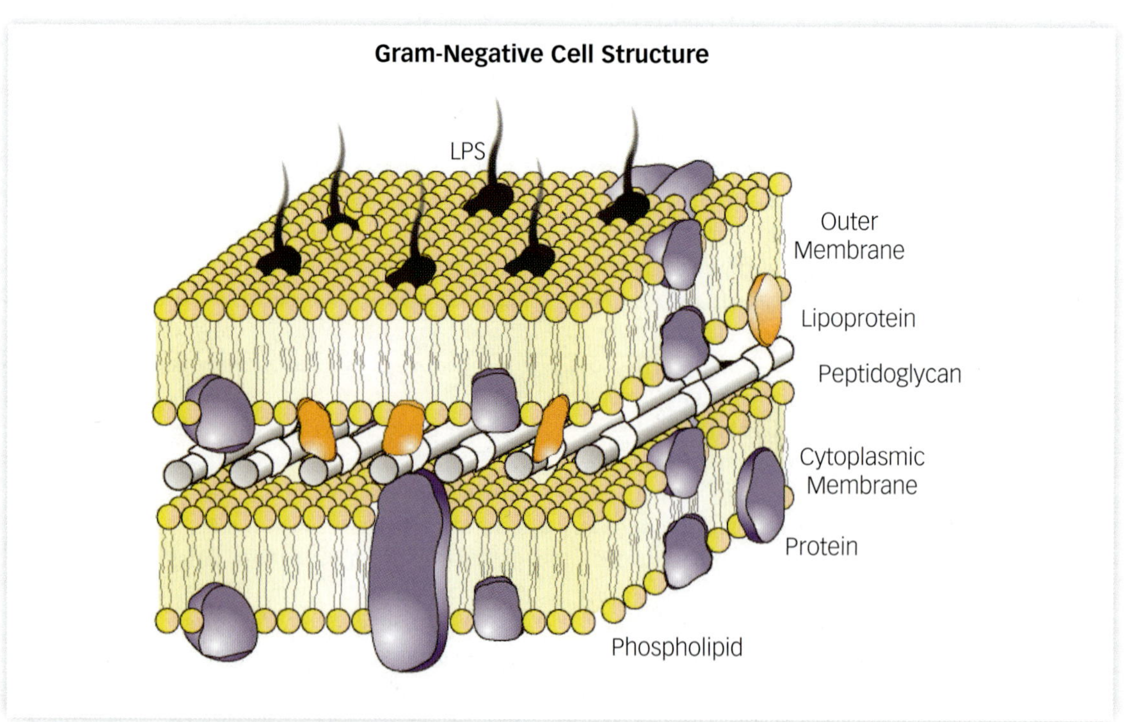


**Figure 8.2** - Diagram of the envelope of a Gram–negative cell (adapted from Tortora et al.[62]).

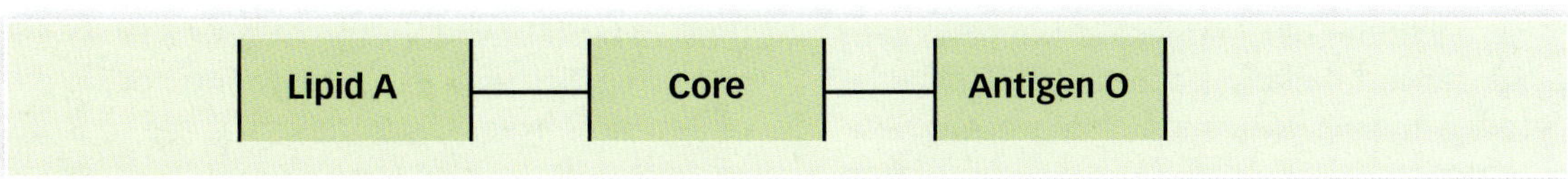


**Figure 8.3** - Lipopolysaccharide structure.

The cell wall accounts for important bacterial characteristics, such as shape, Gram reaction, division and cell protection from osmotic shock; the relatively rigid, protective quality of this macromolecule relies on chemical composition and structure of peptidoglycan. The superlative biological role of cell wall explains why ß-lactam agents, like penicillins, that inhibit the last reactions of peptidoglycan synthesis, are mostly use when the clinical findings of an endodontic infection require a supplementary therapy.

### Cytoplasmic Membrane

Cytoplasmic membrane, called plasma membrane as well, is located beneath the cell wall, and appears similar in composition and structure to other biological systems.

It consists of amphipathic phospholipids disposed in two adjacent layers, forming a bilayer. Polar head – the phosphate end –, which is negatively charged, is hydrophilic (water-loving) and is strategically located on the outer and inner double-layer surfaces, therefore can interact with the watery environment; the nonpolor tail – hydrocarbon end – is not charged, is hydrophobic (water-fearing) and is located between the outer and inner double – layer surfaces, forming a proper barrier between the cell and its environment. In addition, functional and structural proteins, which also present amphipathic properties, are embedded in the membrane, giving it a phospholypoprotein composition. With regard to its chemical composition, the bacterial membrane does not contain sterols, which are a characteristic of bacterial species of *Mycoplasma* and eukaryotic cells.

Cytoplasmic membrane has essential functions, which causes some authors to characterize it as a "very busy place" in the bacterial cell. This structure is the main site of basic oxidative metabolism reactions; it contains specific carrier proteins called permeases that regulate most movements of the materials through the cell by three main transport mechanisms: carrier –mediated diffusion, that does not require the input of metabolic energy; transport linked to phosphorylation and active transport, that require the input of metabolic energy; finally, it concentrates expressive biosynthetic intermediates, assisting DNA replication and participating in cell division. The mesosomes, which are typical invaginations of the cytoplasmic membrane of Gram-positive bacteria, enhance the biological role of this cell structure by expanding their surfaces.

Considering its biological functions, it is easy to understand the effectiveness of certain antimicrobial substances, which target the structures or enzymatic system of the cytoplasmic membrane. This is the mechanism of antimicrobial action of polymyxins, a classic chemotheraupeutic group, of polyenes, which are famous for their antifungal potential, and also of calcium hydroxide, a renowned intracanal medication[12,13,35].

## Internal Structures

### Cytoplasm

Cytoplasm must be considered as a gel, a semi fluid substance composed of approximately 80% of water, and also of substances such as enzymes and other proteins, carbohydrates, lipids, nucleic acids and a variety of inorganic ions. Complex chemical reactions, of catabolic and anabolic nature, take place in cytoplasm.

In addition, ribosomes are found in cytoplasm and, in many bacteria, the so-called cytoplasmic inclusions are also present.

Ribosomes are structures constituted of approximately 60% of ribonucleic acid (RNA) and 40% of protein. Some of them are found free in cytoplasm, while others, especially those involved with synthesis of secreted proteins, are associated with the inner surface of the cytoplasmic membrane. In a prokaryotic cell, these structures are composed of two subunits, a smaller one – 30S, and a bigger one – 50S ("S" expresses a sedimentation speed unit, and is derived from Svedberg, the name of the Swedish scientist who developed the ultracentrifuge). During protein synthesis, these two subunits become associated to form a complete, working ribosome 70S. It is important to emphasize that the speed of the sedimentation depends on the form and size of the structure, so arithmetical precision cannot be applied to this biological phenomenon.

Since these structures represent the site where protein synthesis occurs, the property of some substances to adhere specifically to ribosome subunits interferes in the construction of these macromolecules. This phenomenon is the basis of useful antimicrobial substances used in dental practice, like tetracyclines, helpful as an adjuvant in the treatment of periodontal diseases, lincomycin/clindamicyn, clarithromycin and azithormycin, which are important in Endodontics.

Inclusions, in general, are insoluble, since they present heavily condensed substances. Their chemical nature varies according to the microorganism considered, but, here, those formed of glucose polymers are more expressive, especially in dental caries mechanisms.

The storage property of these substances has been observed in many bacteria isolated from dental plaque and decayed dentine[2,17]. Since these inclusions represent nutritive storage material, those that are glucose polymers ascertain the residual production of lactic acid, a potent tissue aggressor, through their catabolization in the absence of exogenous carbohydrate. Considering these parameters, it is easy to understand the reasons why these inclusions are reduced or absent in starvation periods.

### Genetic Material

As mentioned at the beginning of this Chapter, the prokaryotic structure of bacteria does not support a proper nucleus. Nuclear material, also named nucleoid, is composed basically of deoxyribonucleic acid (DNA), but has also some RNA and proteins. Therefore, DNA is the main component of the characteristic single and circular chromosome, and concentrates all the genetic information of the cell. Its structure was formerly determined by Watson & Crick[64], who described this macromolecule as a double-helix, made up of building blocks called nucleotides. Each nucleotide is composed of one molecule of a nitrogenous base, one molecule of the pentose sugar, deoxyribose, and one molecule of phosphate; the nitrogenous bases are the purines (adenine and guanine) and pyrimidines (thymine and cytosine), which are complementary among them – adenine links to thymine and guanine links to cytosine, through hydrogen bonds.

Some bacteria also have small and, mostly, circular molecules of DNA that are not part of the chromosome. These structures are called plasmids or extrachromosomal DNA, and replicate independently of the chromosome.

Plasmids have occupied a superlative importance in cellular biology due to their genes, codifying the following general functions:

1. They carry genes that provide bacterial resistance to different antimicrobials;
2. They codify the synthesis of ecological determinants;
3. They determine the synthesis of pathogenicity factors;
4. They direct the synthesis of proteins that self-assemble into sex pili;
5. They can cause tumors in plants.

Plasmids can be transmitted by genetic phenomena from one bacterium to another; some resistance plasmids can readily transfer antibiotic-resistance genes to other bacterial cells.

**Endospore**

This typical and characteristic structure of bacteria of the genera *Bacillus* and *Clostridium* is also known as endospore, but it must not be confused with those described in fungi. In the prokaryotic world, in general, a cell originates an endospore in the sporulation cycle, and an endospore reverts to a fully active vegetative cell, through a phenomenon known as germination.

In the current concept, this process is a protective strategy by which some bacteria prepare themselves to resist adverse condition and facilitating survival, and not a reproduction mechanism. Spore resistance to physical and chemical agents is characteristic and is related to its chemical composition – very low water content and the presence of dipicolinic acid and a large quantity of calcium ions – and to the complexity of its structure, respectively.

**External Structures**

Glycocalyx, flagella, pili or fimbriae and fibrillar structures must be considered as accessory structures, since they are not essential to cellular biology, and with the exception of glycocalyx, they are not necessarily present in all bacteria.

**Glycocalyx**

Bacterial glycocalyx, which seems to be present, at least, in all the wild strains, is a viscous material that externally surrounds the cell wall, and depending on its thickness and/or organization, is called capsule or slime layer.

The capsule envelopes a single bacterial cell, is organized into a defined structure and is attached firmly to the cell wall; mostly has a polysaccharide nature, but it can also be a polypeptide. The slime layer does not have any definite shape and is a loosely-bound material that surrounds groups of cells; extracellular polysaccharides synthesized by species from the "*mutans streptococci*" group are prototypes of the slime layer.

As a result of its topographic situation and chemical composition, glycocalyx generally plays a significant role in bacterial nutrition, as well as in protecting the cell from physical and chemical agents; it also stimulates the immune response and plays an important role in mechanisms of bacterial pathogenicity.

**Flagella**

Flagella are filamentous structures characteristically present in rod-shaped or spiral forms. They are significantly longer than the size of bacteria, are composed of contractile protein subunits named flagellin and are embedded in the cell through a basal body, which is of a protein nature.

These appendixes are responsible for bacterial motility, and are able to perform chemotaxis, which consists of directing bacteria to ecologically favorable environments.

Corckscrew-shaped bacteria called spirochetes, such as *Treponema denticola*, show an unusual wriggly mode of locomotion caused by two or more long, coiled threads, the axial filament. Because it is indeed a type of modified flagellum, an axial filament consists of a long, thin microfilm inserted into a hook; unlike flagella, however, the entire structure is enclosed in space between the outer and cytoplasmic membranes; for this reason it is also known as periplasmic flagellum or endoflagellum. *Treponema denticola*, a spirochete, exhibits this type of flagellum.

**Pili or Fimbriae**

Classically, the term pili – or fimbriae – refer to another type of filamentous structure, typical of Gram-negative bacteria. These cell constituents are formed by protein subunits, known as pilin; they are rigid, and also shorter and thinner than flagella.

There are two types of pili – sex and somatic. The first type establishes the physical contact between donor and receptor cells, allowing the passage of genetic material, and is responsible for the transference of this material between bacterial cells; somatic pili represent pathogenicity factors, specifically as regards adherence and colonization of microorganisms.

**Fibrillar Structures**

These structures form a fibrillar layer around the bacterial body and are present, especially, in Gram-positive cells. Their chemical composition is variable, depending on the bacterium involved and, comparatively, they correspond to somatic pili of Gram-negative cells from a functional point of view. In the oral cavity, there are several bacterial species that adhere to oral surfaces by using these structures.

### 8.2.2 Energetic Metabolism

All living cells require energy. Microorganisms of dental and/or medical interest obtain this energy from the use of organic compounds and, at the same time, they use organic sources of carbon. That is why these microorganisms are called chemoheterotrophic.

Classically, in biologic systems energy is generated from oxidation reactions that are linked to reduction reactions. Thus, during catabolism (the breakdown of nutrients or chemical substrates) of energetic substrates, there is liberation of energy that is captured and stored by certain metabolic intermediates, and when necessary, used in anabolic or biosynthetic cellular processes (the synthesis or construction of cell constituents). Several kinds of high-energy compounds occur in cells, but the major energy storing mechanism resides in the synthesis of adenosine triphosphate (ATP). In fact, ATP is by far the most important trapping-energy intermediate, which links the generation and consumption energy reactions of metabolism.

The energetic balance of a microorganism depends on its enzymatic equipment. Thus, those bacteria that can use inorganic compounds as terminal acceptors of electrons, like molecular oxygen – aerobic respiration –, sulfate or nitrate – anaerobic respiration –, will have a great energy gain; oral facultative microorganisms use $0_2$ as final electron acceptor in an aerobic environment. However, those that use organic substances as terminal acceptors of electrons – fermentation – will present, comparatively, a discrete energetic gain; most of endodontopathogens are included in this group.

As regards bacteria sensibility to molecular oxygen, they are classified into five respiratory types (Fig. 8.4).

Thus, taking into account the above considerations, at one extreme are strict aerobic bacteria that require the presence of free oxygen and use it as a final acceptor of electrons, forming water and carbon dioxide; generally speaking, the oral cavity does not support the presence of strict aerobic bacteria and, in positive cases, their presence is discrete and brief. At the other extreme, anaerobic bacteria are those that are inhibited by the oxygen concentration present in atmospheric air and, therefore, they do not use $O_2$ in their energetic mechanisms. Loesche[23], studying the sensitivity of various anaerobic bacteria to air atmosphere, which contains 21% of oxygen, classified them into two groups. Moderate anaerobic bacteria tolerate oxygen levels as high as 2-8%, while strict anaerobic bacteria do not concretize their metabolism in environments presenting a concentration greater than 0.5% oxygen. Important endodontopathogens belong to the moderate anaerobic group, capable of tolerating around two hours of exposure to external environment, which facilitates their manipulation in the laboratory, but spirochetes are classified among strict anaerobic microorganisms.

There are other respiratory groups between these extremes. Thus, facultative bacteria are those that live in environments with or without molecular oxygen, having the ability to choose, depending on environmental conditions, between aerobic metabolism and fermentation pathway. Aerotolerant cells have a similar behavior to facultative cells, since they tolerate environments with or without molecular oxygen, but they always follow

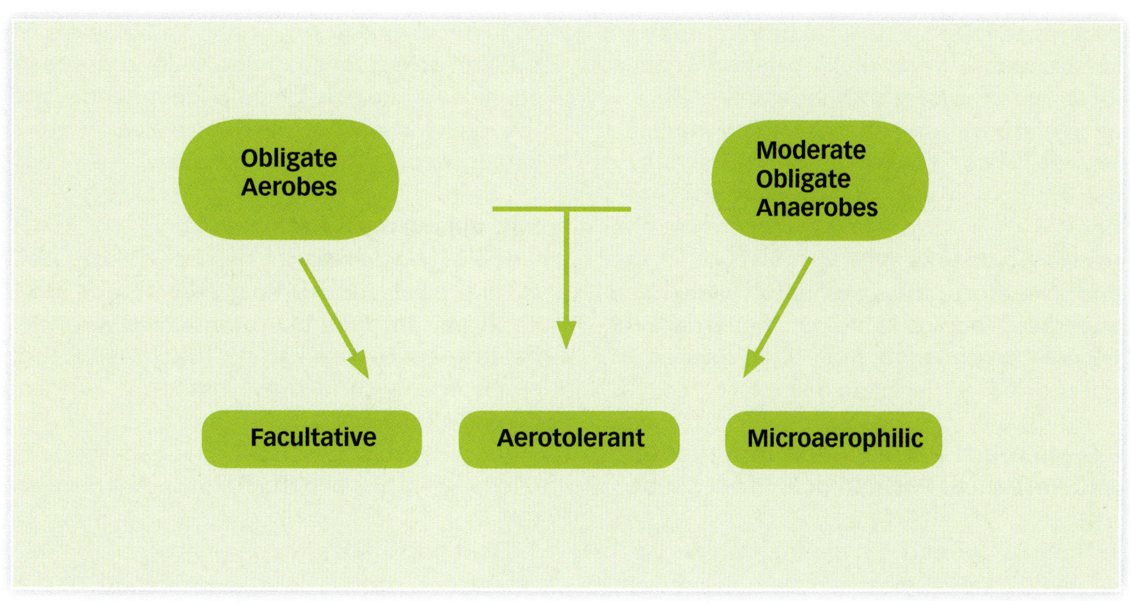


**Figure 8.4** - Bacterial classification, considering the effect of $O_2$ on their metabolism.

fermentative metabolism. Microaerophilic bacteria are inhibited by the atmospheric tension of oxygen and are favored by its intermediate levels, apparently below 12%.

As regards the characterization and significance of anaerobic bacteria in oral processes, it is pertinent to stress the reasons why oxygen is toxic to them. During their metabolism, a superoxide radical is formed due to univalent reduction of $O_2$ as in the following reaction:

**1.** $O_2 + e^- \rightarrow O_2^{\cdot -}$

**Oxygen + electron → Superoxide Radical**

This radical is extremely toxic to cells. In their protective mechanism against this radical, oxygen-resistant microorganisms produce the enzyme superoxide dismutase, which assures its neutralization as follows:

**2.** $2O_2^{\cdot -} + 2H^+ \rightarrow O_2 + H_2O_2$

In addition, the radical superoxide reacts with hydrogen peroxide, giving rise to the radical hydroxyl, as in the following chemical reaction:

**3.** $O_2^{\cdot -} + H_2O_2 + Fe \rightarrow O_2 + OH^- + OH^{\cdot}$

However, hydrogen peroxide, formed in equation 2, has a damaging effect on bacterial compounds, and the hydroxyl radical, generated in equation 3, is a potent cellular poison, even presenting an effect on genetic material. The complete conversion of superoxide ion requires the effectiveness of another chemical reaction, showed in equation:

**4.** $H_2O_2 + H_2O_2 \xrightarrow{\text{catalase}} 2H_2O + O_2$

Aerotolerant bacteria, such as *Streptococcus* species, do not have catalase, but produce superoxide dismutase or peroxidase (enzymes that reduce hydrogen peroxide to two water molecules, in charge of organic substrates with reduction capacity). Thus, fragile oxygen microorganisms are sensitive to superoxide radical because they lack the enzyme superoxide dismutase, while oxygen resistant ones have protective mechanisms against this and other oxygen derived compounds, and since they elaborate superoxide dismutase (reaction 2), catalase (reaction 4) or peroxydases, they guarantee their viability in environments containing molecular oxygen. Thus, it seems that the presence of these enzymes, in higher or lower concentration, or their absence, may determine their resistance or sensitivity to molecular oxygen and, therefore, their respiratory type. Strict anaerobic microorganisms, which are extremely sensitive to molecular oxygen, do not produce superoxide dismutase[16].

## 8.3 Microbial Participation in Endodontic and Periapical Pathological Processes

Pulp is formed by undifferentiated connective tissue of mesenchymal origin, which is extremely vascularized, enervated and comprise immunological cells. Its anatomical location, limited by non-elastic walls, guarantees its isolation from the septic environment of the oral cavity, but at same time this makes pulp a fragile structure when exposed to biological, physical and/or chemical aggressors. Irrespective of the agent, pulp responds with an inflammatory reaction that may show an acute or chronic form.

Microorganisms are the main aggressor agents associated with the pulp cavity and periapex pathology.

The role of oral microorganisms in the etiology of local and systemic diseases was studied in depth by W. D. Miller, in the last decade of the nineteenth century. In his anthological work – *The Micro-Organisms of the Human Mouth* -, Miller[27] discusses the ecological aspects of pulp and periapex, and shows quantitative results from necrotic pulps, as well as investigates the pathogenic potential of some microorganisms.

Using an *in vivo* model of study, Kakehashi, Stanley and Fitzgerald[21] proved the role of microorganisms in pathological processes in endodontics. In this investigation, the pulp of germ-free and conventional rats was surgically exposed to the oral environment. At the end of the experimental period, an osteodentin formation was observed in the first group, while, in the second group of animals, a process of pulp destruction and the development of periapical lesion were established.

### Microbial Access Pathways

Pulp and periapical tissues, as opposed to oral cavity, are a host area that is sterile, from the microbial point of view, under healthy conditions. Thus, the presence of microorganisms in these tissues is suggestive of disease.

In order to colonize the root canal system, microorganisms use the following pathways:

#### 1. Dentinal tubules

After a carious lesion, or during dental procedures, microorganisms may use this pathway in a centripetal direction to reach the pulp. This is the most commonly used pathway, and carious lesion is the most frequent source of infection. Observations suggest that bacteria have access to the pulp when the dentin distance, between the border of the carious lesion and pulp, is 0.2 mm, and is gradually guaranteed by a process of cell division, occasionally favored by the mechanical effect of chewing[10,44].

#### 2. Open cavity

Direct pulp exposure of traumatic origin, such as in coronal fracture, or that of iatrogenic nature due to operative procedures, breaks the physical barrier imposed by dental structures and leaves pulp in contact with the septic oral environment, as described previously.

#### 3. Periodontal membrane

Microorganisms from gingival sulcus may reach the pulp chamber through the periodontal membrane, using a lateral channel or the apical foramen as a pathway. This pathway may, for example, become available to microorganisms during a dental prophylaxis, due to dental luxation and, more significantly, as a result of the migration of epithelial insertion to the establishment of periodontal pockets.

Regarding this strategy, it is pertinent to consider that the motility of certain periodontopathogens, such as *Selenomonas*, provides it with ecological conditions for reaching the pulp and eventually colonizing it[10].

4. Bloodstream

The use of this pathway depends on the occurrence of bacteremia and septicemia. The suffix *emia* is derived from Greek and means blood. Thus, bacteremia consists of the presence of viable microorganisms in the bloodstream; it is a transient phenomenon that lasts no longer than 30 minutes[36], and most of the time, it is not a complication for the patient. Septicemia, on the other hand, is a pathological systemic manifestation, associated with the presence and multiplication of microorganisms in the blood.

According to some researchers, when this access is used, pulp colonization is favored by a phenomenon known as anachoresis, which means the colonization of microorganisms in host areas that previously presented lowered resistance, enhancing the mechanisms of the aggressor. Thus, Gier and Mitchell[18], after causing damage of varying natures and intensities in dog teeth, injected certain bacteria into the bloodstream of these animals and further detected that the inflammatory reaction was proportional to the damage. Using the same hypothetical line, other researchers[1], after inoculating aerotolerant and aerobic microorganisms into pulpectomized teeth, were able, after 28 to 120 days of the study, to isolate them from non-infected teeth that had been previously pulpectomized. During this study, a transport mechanism, that justified the results obtained, was proposed, according to which bacteria from the experimental canal (infected area) would enter the bloodstream, pass through the heart and then be colonized in the control root canal (non-infected area).

Nevertheless, other studies do not admit anachoresis as a phenomenon that offers conditions for pulp colonization. Möller et al[30], using monkeys as experimental models, analyzed the possibility of necrotic pulp tissue remaining sterile for a period of six to seven months. The authors concluded that even considering the hematogenic pathway (bloodstream), the risk of infection of the root canals was very low. In another study, completely prepared but not obturated root canals were incapable of attracting microorganisms from the bloodstream, even when experimentally injected with a suspension of *Streptococcus sanguis* over a long period of time; infection occurred in cases in which periapical tissues were intentionally traumatized[11].

Therefore, in spite the fact that the anachoresis phenomenon has been demonstrated by some researches, its importance in the establishment of infectious process in humans instigates many doubts.

5. Extent

In this case, microorganisms reached the principal and/or lateral canals migrating from an infected tooth to a healthy pulp as a consequence of the contiguousness of the tissues. In this clinical possibility, the microbial reservoir is the infection of an adjacent tooth.

## 8.4 Endodontic Microbiota

### Ecological determinants

Up to present time it is estimated that about 500 microbial species inhabit the human oral cavity. In principle, it is possible for all of these species to reach the root canal system. However, based on cultural studies, a very small number of bacteria, between one and more than 12 species (10 to 50 bacterial species by molecular genetic methods), have been detected in endodontic infectious - an average of four to six species -, in varying concentrations, commonly from $< 10^2$ to $> 10^8$ bacterial cells, according to data reported by Sundqvist[56,58]

When analyzing these data, it is easy to admit the occurrence of ecological determinants at the levels of the pulp cavity and periapex, responsible for the selective pressure that determines which microorganisms will be able to colonize the area.

Studies on the dynamics of endodontic infections support the consideration of the following ecological determinants[56,58]:

1. Oxidation-reduction potential;
2. Nutrient availability;
3. Microbial interactions – synergism or antagonism.

### Oxidation-reduction potential

One of the main defense mechanisms of the host, when exposed to potentially anaerobic microorganisms, is represented by the positive Eh of tissues. Thus, just before the onset of an infectious process, the conditions of the pulp cavity favor microorganisms that tolerate the presence of oxygen, which are the first pulp colonizers. However, the metabolism of these microorganisms, the development of the infectious process and, consequently, the deficiency in blood supply, lower the Eh potential, due to the consumption of oxygen and its products. The succession of these factors ensures that more anaerobic microorganisms gradually become established; therefore, this respiratory group of microorganisms is considered the second invader of root canal and periapex.

### Nutrient availability

In general, nutrition is the process through which chemical substances, called nutrients, are taken from the endogenous or exogenous (diet) environments and used in vital activities, such as biosynthetic processes and function of cell components. As regards basic nutritive requirements, microorganisms rarely differ in comparison with each other or with the cells of other biological systems. All cells require carbon, nitrogen, oxygen, hydrogen, phosphorous, sulphur, iron, sodium, calcium, magnesium and water sources. Other nutrients are required in extremely low amounts, and therefore are called trace nutrients. This is the case of zinc, copper, manganese, molybdenum and cobalt, which act as enzymatic activators.

The input control of these components is the responsibility of the cytoplasmic membrane, as mentioned before.

Iron is essential to all living cells metabolism, therefore, its acquisition mechanisms are worthy of attention. In general, bacteria can use two main iron uptake mechanisms – 1) Under aerobic conditions, iron is not readily accessible to cells in humans because it is bound to body proteins, as a complex; thus, strict aerobe and facultative bacteria excrete small quantities of compounds, called siderophores, that form chelated complexes with iron, the iron-siderophore compound is taken up by specific receptors on the cell surface and then the essential nutritive molecule is released inside the bacteria. However, in an anaerobiosis environment, iron is highly soluble and is used as other metal ions 2) Another possible iron acquisition strategy of pathogenic bacteria is based on the production of hemolysins which lyse erytrocytes, resulting in the liberation of hemoglobin that represents a potential source of iron for bacterial metabolism; hemolysins have been reported to be produced by *Porphyromonas gingivalis* and *T. denticola*, for example.

As regards this parameter, nutritive variables depend upon the origin of a specific substance, its chemical form and the amount required by a specific microorganism. These characteristics determine whether colonization occurs or not. In the root canal system, nutrients are taken from tissue fluids and disintegrated pulp tissues. Substances that are similar to those present in serum, represent significant sources of nutrients.

Using as reference the experiments conducted by Ter Steeg & Van der Hoeven[61], in relation to the development of subgingival microbiota in culture medium with serum, it may be considered that, in bacterial colonization of root canal, there are also three nutritive phases[56]. In the first phase, carbohydrates would be used, with the production of lactic and formic acids; further, some proteins would be hydrolyzed and some amino acids would be fermented, and the remaining carbohydrates, derived from serum glycoproteins, would be mobilized; finally, in the third phase, progressive protein degradation would occur, with extensive fermentation of amino acids.

Thus, the availability of nutrients – carbohydrates, proteins, glycoproteins and amino acids – supports the succession of events which gradually replaces saccharolytic by proteolytic microbiota. This characterizes the dynamism of infectious process at root canal level.

### Microbial interactions

In addition to physical and chemical factors directly or indirectly imposed by environment, the relationship between microorganisms significantly determine the composition of the microbiota.

In general, synergistic interactions comprise those in which a microorganism, through its metabolism, guarantees the source of a special nutrient that is required, but not synthesized, by other members of the microbial population. This is the reason why many authors prefer to study these microbial interactions in the previous topic. Some compounds, such as lactate, vitamin K, carbon dioxide ($CO_2$), hydrogen sulfide ($H_2$), ammonia ($NH_4$), formate, succinate and acetate[56], establish the connection between the primary (producer microorganism) and the secondary (consumer microorganism) feeders. Hemin is another substance required by endodontic pathogens, and it can be supplied by microorganisms, such as *Campylobacter rectus*, which produces a factor related to this substance, but can also be a product of hemoglobin disintegration[19,44,58].

Sundqvist[55,56,58] characterized root canal microbiota from teeth with periapical lesions according to its frequency and proportion, and analyzed the association among the species detected. In these studies, a positive correlation was shown among, *F. nucleatum, Peptostreptococcus micros, Porphyromonas endodontalis, Selenomonas sputigena* and *C rectus; Prevottela intermedia, P. micros; Peptostreptococcus anaerobius* and *Eubacterium species; Eubacterium species* and *Peptrostreptococcus species; P. endodontalis, F. nucleatum, Eubacterium alactolyticum* and *C. rectus*. Observation of these interactions allowed the author to relate the high prevalence of these microorganisms in root canal to the synergistic phenomenon.

Bacterial aggregation (co-aggregation) is another parameter of significant importance to consider on root canal ecology[56]. It also has implications at the gingival sulcus level..

The identification of receptors on the bacterial cell and the specific interactions between complementary surface molecules on the partner cells culminate in aggregation phenomenon, which has metabolic and/or protective functions.

In the complex and dynamic endodontic environment, negative interactions simultaneously occur. The interactions of microbial antagonism depend on the production of substances produced by the catabolism of a microorganism. Through "*cide*" or "*static*" mechanisms, these substances inactivate another microorganism present in the same habitat. This potential gives the former microorganism an ecological advantage.

As examples of these substances, there are: lactate, ammonia, hydrogen peroxide, short chain fatty acids and sulphur-containing compounds[44,56]. It is pertinent to stress that antimicrobial expression of these catabolites depends on the moment of their production, their concentration and also of the target microorganism under consideration. Thus, lactate derived from carbohydrate metabolism, which has the ability of lowering the pH, may influence the phase in which this substrate is mobilized, acting on acid-sensitive microorganisms and selecting the acid-resistant ones; however, it is important to remember that this catabolite is used as a carbon source by *Veillonella* species, which are unable to use glucose. Depending on its concentration, ammonia derived from amino acids presents antimicrobial potential; on the other hand, it may be used as a nutrient by some microorganisms. For the reasons previously mentioned, hydrogen peroxide is toxic to anaerobic bacteria, which do not have the protective mechanism; short chain fatty acids and sulphur amino acids derived from fermentation processes may have a controlling function on some microorganisms, having implication on their colonization.

In general, species of *Streptococcus*, *Propionibacterium*, *Capnocytophaga* and *Veillonella* do or do not present a negative correlation with other bacteria[54,58].

Another important group of antimicrobial determinants with recognized repercussions on root canal ecology is comprised of the bacteriocins or bacteriocin-like substances.

The production of bacteriocins can depend on plasmids, in which certain genes codify their formation. The mentioned substances are classified as low molecular weight polypeptides. Typically, they present toxicity over those species closely related to the producer strain, but there are some bacteriocins that are broad spectrum, inhibiting species belonging to several Gram-positive and Gram-negative bacteria. Their mechanism is complex, since some of them have DNA as a target, others interfere in protein synthesis, destroying some molecules in this process, and others act on the cytoplasmic membrane level, inhibiting transport mechanisms or increasing the cytoplasmic membrane permeability to ions. Up to now, bacteriocins have not shown therapeutic effects but are considered important ecological determinants.

Microorganisms that present high prevalence in endodontic microbial infections are bacteriocin-positive, and, therefore, they are potentially able to interfere with growth and multiplication of microorganisms that compete for the same ecological niche. In this context, it was observed that *P. endodontalis* is able to inhibit "*in vitro*" species of *Prevotella*, which may explain the negative correlation between them when analyzing the root canal microbiota[56,63].

## Composition

Root canal and periapex infectious diseases are of a mixed and endogenous nature, since they result from the interaction of several bacterial species, which are members of the amphibiotic microbiota of the host.

Studies on endodontic microbiota published several years ago stressed the occurrence of facultative and/or aerotolerant microorganisms, consisting mainly of alpha and gamma streptococci and enterococci, and less frequently, coagulase-positive staphylococci and β-hemolytic streptococci. Thus, at that time, it was assumed that streptococci were the most prevalent bacteria in infected pulps, although their activity was not compatible with the histopathology of pulpal and periapical infections and the organisms did not contemplate Koch's postulates[14]. It is convenient to point out that these postulates, regardless of some restrictions today, can be useful in establishing the etiology of a disease.

With the improvement of bacteriological technique, aseptic sample collection procedures, meticulous transportation methods to protect oxygen-sensitive microorganisms, culture media rich in nutrients and processing and incubation in absence of molecular oxygen, began to be applied in Endodontics. Thus, after the classical works of Möller[31] and Sundqvist[55], the presence and significance of anaerobic microorganisms in endodontic and periapical infections was recognized. Based on culture analysis, teeth presenting necrotic pulp and periapical pathologies may present a average ranging from > 70 to < 90% of anaerobic microorganisms, depending on the conditions of the tooth considered[6,33,66], that is, if it is a noncarious or carious tooth.

According to Nair[33], the composition of microbiota varies considerably. Using microscopic and cultural techniques as a reference, this author stresses the following genera as important in endodontic infections (Table 8.1).

*Porphyromonas* and *Prevotella*, bacterial genera that comprise asaccharolytic and saccharolytic species respectively, were removed from the *Bacteroides* genus, produce protoheme or protoporphyrin pigments, which give their colonies grown on blood agar surface a black color; this is why these microorganisms belong to the group of black-pigment producer bacteria (BPPB). In specialized literature, there are several references that relate their activity to signs and symptoms of root

**Table 8.1.** Microorganisms of Endodontic Importance *

| Anaerobic | | Facultative-Aerotolerant-Microaerophilic | |
|---|---|---|---|
| Gram+ Cocci | *Peptostreptococcus* | Gram+ Cocci | *Streptococcus*<br>*Enterococcus* |
| Gram+ Rods | *Actinomyces*<br>*Eubacterium*<br>*Propionibacterium* | Gram+ Rods | *Actinomyces*<br>*Lactobacillus*<br>*Corynebacterium* |
| Gram- Cocci | *Veillonella* | Gram- Cocci | *Neisseria* |
| Gram- Rods | *Porphyromonas*<br>*Prevotella*<br>*Fusobacterium*<br>*Selenomonas* | Gram- Rods | *Capnocytophaga*<br>*Eikenella*<br>*Campylobacter* |
| Spirochetes | *Treponema* | Yeast | *Candida* |

*Modificated from Nair[33].

canal and periapex infections[20,44,53,55]. Specifically concerning *P. endodontalis*, this species has been found in acute infections, but is absent in chronic infections[32]. Interestingly, this microbial species has frequently been detected in the subgingival plaque of patients with periodontitis, but was not observed in healthy patients[34].

The genus *Treponema*, generally known as spirochetes, comprises amphibiotic species in the mouth, intestinal and genital tracts in humans and animals. Oral spirochetes may be small, medium or large sized and are difficult to cultivate, which certainly complicates their study. Using dark-field and scanning electron microscopy, Dahle et al.[9] described a spirochete isolated from a root canal that is seven times larger and five times thicker than those known to date. The absence or presence of spirochetes, according to previous publications[14], may be indicative of endodontic or periodontal abscesses, but their detection in root canal infections[8,33,43] and their intense proteolytic activity suggests that these microorganisms are not a consequence of infection, but participate in its etiology.

*Enterococcus* species play a significant role in endodontic microbiota. If not controlled, these bacteria, which present an inherent resistance to antimicrobial agents and other pathogenicity factors, may be favored by the alteration in ecological conditions of the root canals and establish an infectious process that is hard to treat. Recently, *E. faecalis,* the most important species of the genus, has been related to failure in endodontic treatment[28,52].

Some investigators consider microorganisms of the genus *Candida,* which are cells with eukaryotic structure, to be contaminants, without taking into account their frequency in infected root canal or their pathogenic potential[10]. However, Sen et al.[42], with the application of scanning electron microscopy, observed root canals with necrotic pulp and periapical lesions densely colonized by yeasts, in spherical or oval forms, ranging from 4 – 6 μm in diameter. Waltimo et al.[64] found a high prevalence of yeasts in samples collected from root canals with persistent endodontic infections, most of them belonging to the genus *Candida*. These findings, in addition to those in which a strain of *Candida albicans* was found to resist a 25% citric acid solution, after 15 minutes of *in vitro* exposure[26], suggest that yeasts, and particularly those of genus *Candida*, may be significant in cases of endodontic pathology that is resistant to conventional treatment.

More recently, studies conducted with non-microscopic and non-cultural techniques, using molecular biology approaches, have revealed a great diversity in the microbiota of endodontic infections, an uncommon finding in different aspects. Thus, endodontic microbiota of teeth presenting carious lesions, necrotic pulp and bone resorption showed a predominance of *Bacteroides forsythus* (presently *Tanerella forsythensis*), *Haemophilus aprhrophilus, Corynebacterium matruchotii, P. gingivalis* and *T. denticola*[43]; it is important to compare this spectrum to the participation of red complex – *P. gingivalis, T. forsythia* and *T. denticola* – in the etiopathogeny of periodontal disease. Likewise, samples collected from teeth presenting chronic apical periodontitis[32] confirm the mentioned magnitude of endodontic microbiota and indicate, for example, the presence in the five cases studied, of a new species from the genus *Dialister*.

## 8.5 Aggressive Microbial Mechanisms

Endodontic microbiota, in general, present pathogenic potential, because when they are tested using different animal models, they are able to induce inflammatory lesions in laboratory animals.

A classic study that documents this ability is the work by Sundqvist et al[50], in which combinations of bacteria isolated from infected root canals with necrotic pulp and periapical bone destruction were tested as regards their ability to induce abscess formation and guarantee the transmission of infection, when inoculated subcutaneously in guinea pigs. At this time, it was verified that combinations, obtained from teeth with purulent apical inflammation, that supported the transmission of the lesion and prevented its resolution, contained strains of *B. melaninogenicus* (presently *Prevotella melaninogenica*) or *B. asaccharolyticus* (currently *Porphyromonas asaccharolytica*). However, with one exception, the strains required the support of additional microorganisms in order to express their pathogenicity; *P. micros* appears to be also essential. In another publication, Sundqvist[57], using pathogenic bacterial mixtures, containing specific bacteria combinations, emphasizes the need of the presence of *P. intermedia, P. endodontalis* and *P. gingivalis,* with the aid of other microorganisms, to express their endodontic pathogenic potential. Other experiments, using distinct experimental models have supported the ability of endodontopathogens to induce pathological alterations[3,44].

Collectively, the above observations, that some microbial combinations are required for the establishment, intensity, maintenance and transmission of endodontic processes, can be comparable to those published by MacDonald et al.[25], studying the pathogenesis of mixed bacterial anaerobic infections of mucous membranes; the data obtained by the authors provide significance to ecological variables, in the specific case of synergistic type, that also occur in the root canal system and periapex.

Microorganisms, most of them simple and rustic, use sophisticated strategies to damage the host. Since the infectious process is dynamic, it is not unilateral and should not be evaluated only from a microbiological point of view. The host response, which effectively represents a two-edged sword, must also be considered; it is able to protect the human host, but it is also capable of causing tissue damage (Fig. 8.5).

### Adherence and colonization

Irrespective of the area of the organism, the crucial event for the expression of microorganism pathogenicity is its ability to adhere to host surfaces. Thus, the bacterial structures, especially the cell wall, glycocalyx, pili and fibrillar structures, have a paramount biological role. Once this adherence is assured, the next step is colonization, and in this chapter, it is assumed to be the accumulation of microorganisms in the area; concerning this mechanism, it is a complex phenomenon that involves surface microbial structures, interaction among microorganisms and host components. As soon as the

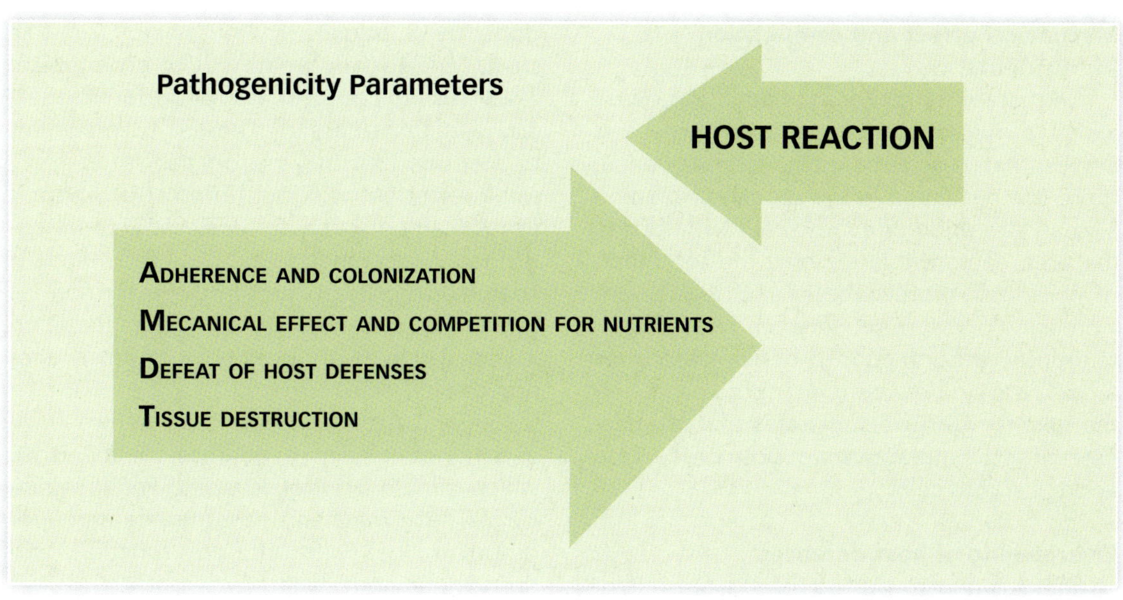


**Figure 8.5** - Pathogenicity Parameters.

colonization occurs, microorganisms are able to express their pathogenic potential, invade tissues and, therefore, assure propagation of the infection.

The importance of adherence in bacterial aggressive strategy is documented in the work of Love[24], whose purpose was to identify a mechanism for the participation of *E. faecalis* in root canal treatment failures. At this time, the author mainly studied two parameters *in vitro*: 1- the ability of the studied microorganism to adhere to immobilized collagen in the wells of micro plates; 2- the ability of this microorganism to invade the dentinal tubules of single-rooted teeth. The research was conducted comparing cells of *S. gordonii* and *S. mutans* with an *E. faecalis* strain.

In the first proposal, adherence was investigated under standard and experimental conditions – microbial cells, in pure culture, suspended in a buffer solution, collagen and serum. Thus, it was noted that the presence of free collagen in the mixture significantly inhibited the adherence of the analyzed bacterial species, while the serum prevented the adherence of *S. gordonii* and *S. mutans* strains, and significantly enhanced the adherence of *E. faecalis*. To assess the invasion potential of dentin, microorganisms were propagated under three cultural conditions: in a referential medium, in the same medium plus collagen and in the control medium plus serum. Microscopic exam of the preparations, using Brown & Brenn stain, revealed that the presence of collagen interfered negatively in the invasive ability of the selected strains, while the presence of serum prevented the infiltration of the *Streptococcus* species and inhibited, but did not block, the invasion of dentinal tubules by *E. faecalis*.

Thus, based on the data obtained, Love[24] hypothesized that the presence of serum favors the adherence of enterococci cells to immobilized collagen, making dentinal invasion possible and assuring bacterial viability inside the tubules, which, among other factors, justifies *E. faecalis* association with therapeutic failures; *in vivo* situation, nutritional support would be provided by interstitial fluid originating from alveolar bone and periodontal attachment, which seems to have a similar composition to serum.

### Mechanical effect and competition for nutrients

The establishment of an infectious process exerts a mechanical pressure on veins and nerves that reach the pulp. Consequently, there is a reduction in the blood supply and also an alteration of ecological conditions in the area, factors that support the formation of a gradually more complex microbiota, with increasing pressure on nerve endings. Simultaneously, the infection process establishes a competition between microorganisms and the host for nutritive substrates that are necessary for the metabolism of both prokaryote and eukaryote cells.

### Overcoming of host defenses

While trying to protect itself from microbial aggression, the host mobilizes its nonspecific defenses that target microorganisms in general, and also the specific defenses that target a particular pathogen. On the other hand, aggressive agents use different and complex mechanisms while trying to overcome these defenses, through their cellular constituents and metabolic activity.

The capsule, which is hydrophilic and also present, for example, in *P. gingivalis, P. endodontalis* and *P. intermedia* strains, may prevent the action of leucocytes and, therefore, prevent or make the phagocytosis of these microorganisms difficult[47,51]. Thus, it is important to point out that capsulated bacteria are more capable of inducing abscesses. As an example of the importance of surface components, it has been observed that strains of *Eubacterium yurii* subspecies *margaretiae,* isolated from root canal and periodontal pockets, have an extracellular material that can mask the reactive sites that participate in phagocytosis, making this phenomenon dependant on antibodies or serum components[22,58].

Cellular aggregation seems to protect microorganisms from the action of phagocytes. The species *Actonomyces israelii* is difficult to control in periapical lesions, according to bacteriological and histological observations done by Sundqvist & Reuterving[59], in this study, endodontic treatment of a periapical lesion using conventional endodontic therapy was unsuccessful. Thus, it is important to mention that this microorganism is easily phagocyted *in vitro*, but not *in vivo*, where it forms filamentous and ramified bacterial aggregates, immersed in extracellular matrix. It seems that cells present in these formations overcome the destruction and elimination associated with the unspecific defense phenomenon[15].

Several proteins present in serum have a paramount role in defense mechanisms, which aim to control invading microorganisms. These mechanisms comprise immunoglobulins (Igs), with antibody function, and the complement system.

Immunoglobulins are synthesized and secreted by plasma cells resulting from maturation and specific differentiation of B cells derived from the bone marrow; this is why plasma cells are considered real "factories" of these protein molecules of humoral immunity. There are five classes of Igs – IgG, IgM, IgA, IgE and IgD. The complement system is constituted of almost 20 interactive serum proteins[35], and plays an important role in resistance against infection; it is the principal mediator of the inflammatory response. Complement activation, which may occur in the presence – classic pathway – or in the absence – alternative pathway – of antibodies, gives rise to several peptides, which have important biological roles: to attract phagocytes to the infection site by a chemotactic effect; enhance the blood supply and vessel permeability where the infectious process is taking place, causing the output of plasma molecules; and also damage the microorganisms, viruses and cells that activated the system.

As regards endodontic infectious processes, Sundqvist et al.[49] with the aid of immunochemical methods, investigated the ability of Gram-negative microorganisms, that produce black pigments, to destroy human serum proteins. In this study, it was verified that *P. endodontalis* (at that time *B. endodontalis*), *P. gingivalis* (at that time *B. gingivalis*) and *P. intermedia* (at that time *B. intermedius*) strains, isolated from the root canals, have enzymatic activity and are respectively able to inactivate IgG and C3, IgG, IgM, C3 and C5, and IgG and C3, respectively; a *Prevotella loescheii* (then *B. loescheii*) strain, taken from gingival sulcus, showed proteolytic activity only on IgG. These data support previous investigation done by Sundqvist et al[48], in which a pathogenic strain of *P. gingivalis* was able to degrade *in vivo* the C3 fraction of guinea-pig complement.

Therefore, considering that IgG presents a complex antibacterial effectiveness; that IgM presents an effective mechanism in fixing complement; and that the complement interferes in phagocytosis through deposition of a protein – C3b - on the microbial surface, which originates from the cleavage of the fraction C3, and interacts with specific receptors on the surface of the phagocyte, optimizing the defense process; and that the component C5b, derived from the fragmentation of the component C5, starts the generation of a lytic complex, which results in destruction of the target cell, it is easy to understand the participation of microbial proteases, that destroy Igs and complement fractions, in the strategies of microbial aggression against the host.

Further, Gram-negative microorganisms, which have an important role in endodontic pathogenesis, release cell constituents, such as membrane components and soluble reactive antigens, which react with protective antibodies. This bacterial strategy consumes the antibodies and makes them unavailable for reaction with the microorganism itself, compromising the specific resistance of the host[33].

Another option to overcome the action of antibodies is the antigenic variation of the microbial agent, which has been observed in *Streptococcus* species[5] and has consequences on the specificity of immune response.

**Tissue Destruction**

Histolytic enzymes, such as collagenase, hyaluronidase and fibrinolysin, which have host tissue components as substrate, are produced by microorganisms present in the root canal, such as *Porphyromonas, Prevotella, Fusobacterium, Peptostreptococcus, Streptococcus* and *Enterococcus*, favoring microbial dissemination in tissues. Collagenase is a type of metalloproteinase that is produced by several types of cells[37] and has the ability to hydrolyze collagen, the main component of connective tissue. Hyaluronidase hydrolyzes hyaluronic acid, a mucopolysaccharide that is a component of the extracellular matrix from the epithelial and connective tissues; this is why the enzyme is considered a microbial spreading factor. Fibrinolysin transforms serum plasminogen into plasmin, a proteolytic enzyme that is able to digest fibrin, which normally delimits inflammatory reaction. In addition to these enzymes, chondroitinase, glucuronidase, deoxyribonuclease, acid phosphatase and lipase can also be mentioned, since they are also significant when microbial aggressive mechanisms are under consideration.

Another mechanism is the one that depends on the production of substances derived from microbial catabolism, which have a remarkably destructive effect on human cells. Among these by-products ammonia, hydrogen sulfide, amines, fatty acids and organic acids must be considered. Microorganisms of endodontic importance – such as the species of genera *Porphyromonas, Prevotella, Fusobacterium, Veillonella* and *Peptostreptococcus* - are, in general, producers of these catabolic products.

Also, toxins are important inducers of tissue damage. Hemolysin targets erythrocytes which, once destroyed, release hemoglobin, an important iron source, and, therefore, it presents an enhancing effect, since, in addition to damaging the host, it favors bacterial nutrition. Fibroblast-inhibiting toxin has a remarkable role in periodontal disease, because it interferes in the synthesis and turnover of collagen, which results in the loss of this connective tissue constituent[45]. Extrapolating this effect to endodontic field, it is possible that the above toxic substance is also significant in the etiopathogeny of infectious processes in pulp and periapex, since endodontic microorganisms, like *P. gingivalis* and *P. intermedia*, are able to produce this specific toxin.

Undoubtedly, the LPS, which have endotoxic potential, has to be considered among the tissue aggressors and, together with other components of the cell envelope, has a superlative biological role.

The LPS of Gram-negative bacteria, peptidoglycan from the cell walls of both Gram-positive and Gram-negative bacteria, as also lipoteichoic acid, the surface structure of Gram-positive bacteria, due to their chemical composition, play a significative role in processes of host damage, stimulating complex organic reactions.

Thus, LPS stimulates infiltrating mononuclear cells, with the consequent production of molecular mediators, such as cytokines and prostaglandins. Cytokines are low weight polypeptides, derived mainly from macrophages and T cells, but can also be produced by a wide variety of cells involved in the inflammatory response. They seem to be of paramount importance in the development of apical periodontitis. Considering all the cytokines, the most prominent are interleukins 1β and 1α (IL-1β and IL-1α) and tumor necrosis factor alpha (TNFα), which are produced by activated macrophages, and tumor necrosis factor beta (TNFβ), which is also called lymphotoxin, released by activated T cells. These molecular mediators are osteoclast-activating factors (OAFs) and participate in bone resorption that has a significant future in the development of periapical lesions[33,41,46].

Further, LPS, IL-1β and IL-1α have the ability to stimulate the production of prostaglandin $E_2$ ($PGE_2$) by fibroblasts, osteoblasts and macrophages. This mediator is an arachidonic acid metabolite, and is an important osteoclast activator. Arachidonic acid is a polyunsaturated fatty acid extensively present in cell membranes[33,41,46].

On the other hand, LPS and bone resorption inducing cytokines may cause bone resorption by interfering in the coupling reaction regulated by osteoclasts and osteoblasts; thus, by inhibiting the stimulating effects of growth factors on osteoblasts, the considered cellular component of Gram-negative cells and cytokines block bone repair at the inflammatory site[46].

The biological role of peptidoglycan and lipoteichoic acid is detailed and recognized in specialized literature[14,44]. Peptidoglycan is active in the induction of molecular mediators as IL-1β, IL-6 and GM-CSF (granulocyte-macrophage colony stimulating factor), M-CSF (macrophage colony stimulating factor), and is also capable of activating the complement and stimulating B cells. Lipoteichoic acid, by binding to macrophages through its lipidic component, induces the release of cytokines - IL-1β, IL-6, IL-8 and TNFα, and is also able to activate the complement.

In addition, bacteria and their by-products enhance the antigen-antibody complex formation in the periapical area, which activates the complement, generates chemotactic factors C3a end C5a and causes the influx of polymorphonuclear neutrophils, which are a source of lysosomal enzymes.

These different and complex mechanisms of microbial aggression, together with the host response, are responsible for the pathogenesis of endodontic infections at root canal and periapical area.

## 8.6 Microbiological Examination

As mentioned elsewhere in this chapter, the microbiological conditions of root canals have been studied and determined by different study techniques, consisting of the microscopic observation of the material, culture of microorganisms present in the clinical sample and, more recently, by application of molecular biology techniques. Data obtained from these studies are important to enhance the biological principles of Endodontics.

In Dentistry, since the majority of pulp disturbances are of an infectious nature, the purpose of endodontic treatment is to create adverse conditions for the presence and proliferation of microorganisms in root canal system. Considering the anatomy of the root canal system, the above-mentioned therapy is referred to as sanitization - the process that consists of reducing the microbial population to levels compatible with tissue repair, as schematized below (Fig. 8.6).

However, recognizing the impressive role of microorganisms in the establishment and maintenance of the root canal infectious processes, the microbiological examination, used as a tool for evaluating the therapeutic effect, is not routinely used in endodontic clinics and academic institutions[28,44,57]. Supporting this fact, the following arguments seem pertinent – microscopy is restricted, since it is unable to differentiate a variety of microorganisms; microbiological procedures, such as sampling, transport, manipulation, culture and incubation, with the aim of preserving and propagating anaerobic microorganisms, are not very practical for use by the professional, in addition to being expensive and time-consuming; genetic techniques present restrictions as regards practice and clinical evaluation; the negative result may express a lack of sensitivity of the technique; the use of efficient antimicrobial substances during chemical and mechanical treatment, as well as in intracanal medication, optimize microbial control. Thus, the cost-benefit ratio must be taken in account by the clinician; the decision, as to when it is convenient to fill the canal relies on clinician expertise and "feeling" – today, the use of appropriate endodontic techniques supports a predictably clinical success.

At the present time, although it has limitations, the microbiological test, based on the culture of microorganisms from the root canal seems to be a valuable laboratory tool in endodontics, being pertinent to teaching, research and as an auxiliary resource in the treatment of persistent clinical cases, resistant to conventional therapy[57,60]. When indicated under these circumstances, this examination has a pedagogic function, since it represents a reference for the assessment

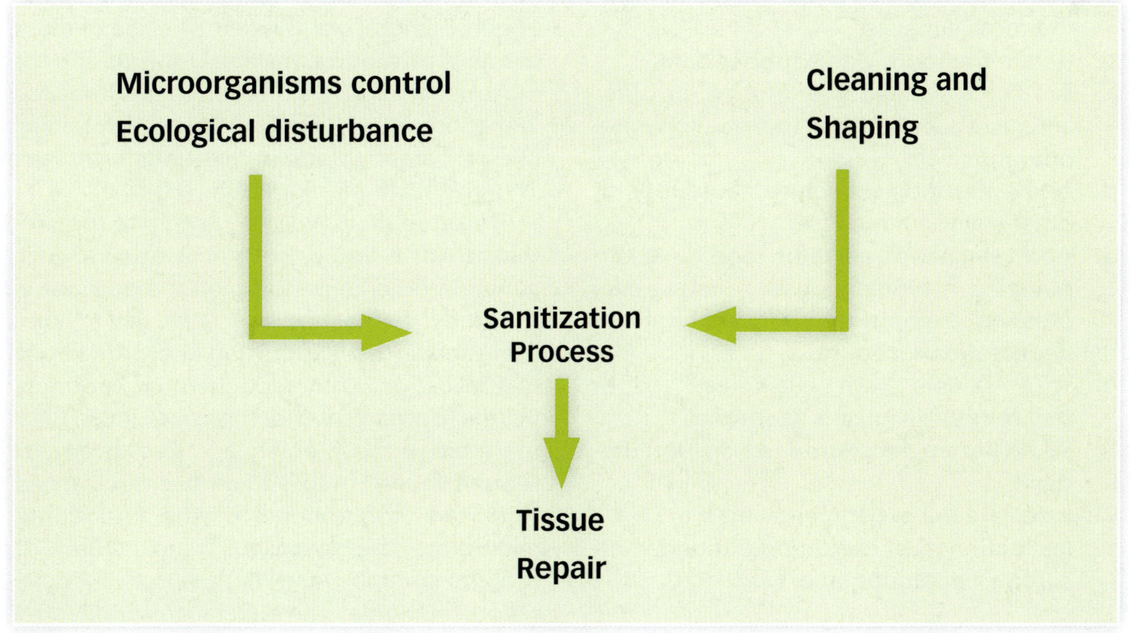


**Figure 8.6** - Purposes of endodontic therapy.

and enhancement of aseptic and endodontic techniques used by students during treatment. It has great significance, in research, making it possible to study the etiopathogeny of the process; it supports the estimation of the antimicrobial effectiveness of substances used during the treatment and, consequently, contributes to the development of the endodontic technique. Finally, the microbiological examination of root canals is helpful for evaluating and following-up recurrent cases, since it allows the isolation of *Enterococcus, Streptococcus, Actinomyces* and *Propionibacterium* (formerly *Arachnia*) and *Candida*, for example, frequently associated with these cases[15,28,29,52,59], making it possible to identify them and determine their sensitivity to antimicrobial agents; thus, laboratory tests helps to determine the etiopathogeny, apply efficient therapies and prevent future complications.

The following recommendations and procedures are generally accepted for microbiological examination of root canal samples (adapted from Dahlén & Möller[10]):

a. Remove all hard and soft deposits from the tooth surfaces.
b. Isolate the tooth with a rubber dam.
c. Apply 5 or 10% iodine tincture, or other antimicrobial chemical agent, all over the operation field.
d. Apply the iodine tincture neutralizer or other specific neutralizer.
e. Add sampling solution and execute pumping movements with a coarse file, pressing it against the root canal walls.
f. Repeat the procedure.
g. Take sample with charcoaled paper points until all liquid is absorbed.
h. All points are transferred to transport medium.
i. Inoculate the experimental media.
j. Incubation must be carried out under anaerobic conditions, at 37° C.

When abscess, osteomyelitis or other infection in the periapical region must be investigated, sampling through the root canal offers least risk of contamination because the procedure can be fairly well controlled[10].

It is important to stress that the considered assay must be conducted under aseptic conditions, preventing microorganisms not present in the root canal from interfering in the results. Further, it is mandatory to apply neutralization procedures to prevent the carry-over of the antimicrobial agents, used during the endodontic procedures, into the experimental medium, in order to neutralize the post-treatment interference of these substances that may cause a false-negative result; the neutralizers must be used in step d and also added to sampling solution and/or to microbiological media used. Table 2 lists some antimicrobial substances and their reactive neutralizers, as well as their recommended concentrations

The aim of the transport media is to protect the microorganisms that may be in the sample during the interval between obtaining the microbial sampling and culturing in the laboratory. According to their formula and characteristics they preserve the microbiota viability, maintain the original proportions of bacteria and protect them against the toxic effects of molecular oxygen. The use of these media is currently a universal tool; among the most used transport media are the Reduced Transport Fluid (RTF), Viability-Maintaining Microbiostatic Medium III (VMGA III) and Thioglycollate Medium USP (THM)[7,10,44].

The step that involves the culture requires the use of a liquid, solid and/or semi-solid culture media, depending on the purpose of the study. These media must be rich in nutritive substances, supporting the growth and multiplication of the spectrum of endodontic microorganisms, comprising those with more biosynthetic ability and also those that require more complex nutritive substances; significant components of the endodontic microbiota are fastidious, and, therefore, require complex and high nutritive bacteriological media. The substances applied for medium enhancement are hemin (final concentration, 5 μg/mL) and vitamin K (final concentration, 0.1 μg/mL for liquid medium and

10 µg/mL for semi-solid or solid medium); complementarily, defibrinated sheep, horse or rabbit blood must be added to solid medium (final concentration, 5%).

Among the liquid media, Trypticase Soy Broth (TSB) and Brain Heart Infusion (BHI) can be mentioned. When semi-solid media are used, the choice can be THM - in fact, this medium is useful for transport and for culture of microorganisms from infected root canals, as well -, or other enriched media containing 0.075 - 0.15% of agar. The solid medium most used is Brucella Agar Base[10], which supports the isolation of the main endodontic pathogens, when it is enriched , as the another ones, with the above mentioned supplements.

Taking in consideration that the endodontic microbiota is virtually devoid of strict aerobes, the incubation procedure must give priority to anaerobic microorganisms. There are three major incubation systems for isolation of anaerobes: 1) The roll tube system, which uses prereduced anaerobically sterilized media, and the oxygen-free atmosphere of the tubes is kept by inoculation under a stream of oxygen-free gas. 2) The anaerobic chamber, in which all bacteriological manipulations are conducted in an atmosphere without molecular oxygen. 3) Anaerobic jars, GasPak, BBL for example, in which the anaerobic environment can be set up by two methods. The easiest one uses a commercially available hydrogen and $CO_2$ generator envelope that is placed in the jar with the inoculated plates/tubes, 10 mL of water are added and, then, the anaerobiosis is achieved by a catalytic reaction between the hydrogen-containing gas mixture and the oxygen. Alternatively, anaerobiosis can be obtained by evacuation of the air inside the jar and replace it with an oxygen-free gas mixture, consisting of 80% $N_2$, 10% $H_2$ and 10% $CO_2$. The incubation period ranges between 3, 6 and 14 days, with daily observation, due to the size of the inoculum used, which is frequently small, and the time needed for growth and multiplication of microorganisms, which need a long incubation time.

In liquid or semisolid media, the reading shows the presence or lack of turbidity, indicative of whether microbial growth and multiplication occur or not. The solid medium allows microorganisms to be isolated, to detect hemolysis, as well as to obtain a pure culture. After a pure culture is obtained, others studies can be done like morphological, physiological, antigenic and/or genetic characterization. When necessary, an antimicrobial susceptibility test can also be performed.

Finally, it seems pertinent to stress that microbial control at levels compatible with health, whether or not proved by a microbial examination, favors the success of the noble mission of healing, and optimizes the prevention of future complications[12].

**Table 8.2.** Antimicrobial substances and their neutralizers (Adjusted from Russel[39]).

| Substance | Neutralizer | Concentration |
|---|---|---|
| Phenolic compounds | Tween 80 | 1% |
| Mercury compounds | Sodium Thioglycollate | 0.05 – 0.1% |
| Ammonium quaternary compounds | Lecithin + Tween 80 | 0.5% + 1.0% |
| Chlorhexidine | Lecithin + Tween 80 | 0.5% + 1.0% |
| Hypochlorites | Sodium thiosulphate | 1% |
| Iodine | Sodium thiosulphate | 1% |

## References

1. Allard U, Nord C, Sjöberg L, Strömberg T. Experimental infections with *Staphylococcus aureus, Streptococcus sanguis, Pseudomonas aeruginosa,* and *Bacteroides fragilis* in the jaws of dogs. Oral Surg Oral Med Oral Pathol 1979;48:454-66.
2. Bammann LL, Araújo WC. Espectro microbiano da cárie profunda de dentina. Arq Cent Est Cur Odont 1976;13:7-32.
3. Baumgartner JC, Falkler-Júnior WA, Beckerman T. Experimentally induced infection by oral anaerobic microorganisms in a mouse model. Oral Microbiol Immunol 1992;7:253-6.
4. Black JG. Microbiology: principles and applications. Englewood Cliffs: Prentice-Hall Inc.;1993.
5. Bratthall D, Köhler B. *Streptococcus mutans* serotypes: some aspects of their identification, distribution, antigenic shifts and relationship to caries. J Dent Res 1976;55:C15-C21.
6. Byström A, Sundqvist G. Bacteriological evaluation of the efficacy of mechanical root canal instrumentation in endodontic therapy. Scand J D Res 1981;89:321-8.
7. Carlsson J, Sundqvist G. Evaluation of methods of transport and cultivation of bacterial specimens from infected dental roots. Oral Surg Oral Med Oral Pathol 1980;49:451-4.
8. Dahle UR, Tronstad L, Olsen I. Observation of an unusually large spirochete in endodontic infection. Oral Microbiol Immunol 1993;8:251-3.
9. Dahle UR, Tronstad L, Olsen I. Spirochaetes in oral infections. Endod Dent Traumatol 1993;9:87-94.
10. Dahlén G, Möller AJR. Microbiology of endodontic infections In: Contemporary Oral Microbiology and Immunology. Slots J, Taubman MA. St. Louis: Mosby Year Book Inc.;1991. p.444-55.
11. Delivanis PD, Fan VSC. The localization of bloodborne bacteria in instrumented unfilled and overinstrumented canals. J Endod 1984;10:521-4.
12. Estrela C, Sydney GB, Bammann LL, Felippe-Júnior O. Mechanisms of action of calcium and hydroxyl íon of calcium hydroxide on tissue and bacteria. Braz Dent J 1995;6:85-90.
13. Estrela C. Eficácia antimicrobiana de pastas de hidróxido de cálcio. (Livre- Docência Thesis). University of São Paulo; 1997.
14. Farber PA, Seltzer S. Endodontic Microbiology. I. Etiology. J Endod 1988;14:363-71.
15. Figdor D, Sjögren U, Sörlin S, Sundqvist G, Nair PNR. Pathogenicity of *Actinomyces israelii and Arachnia propionica:* experimental infection in guinea pigs and phagocytosis and intracellular killing by human polymorphonuclear leukocytes *in vitro.* Oral Microbiol Immunol 1992;7:129-36.
16. Finegold SM. Anaerobic bacteria in human disease. NewYork: Academic Press; 1977. pp.1- 40.
17. Gibbons RJ, Kapsimalts P. Synthesis of intracellular iodophilic olysaccharide by *Streptococcus mitis.* Archs Oral Biol 1963;8:319-29.
18. Gier RE, Mitchell DF. Anachoretic effect of pulpitis. J Dent Res 1968;47:564-70.
19. Grenier D, Mayrand D. Nutriotional relationships between oral bacteria. Infect Immun 1986;53:616-20.
20. Griffee MB, Patterson SS, Miller CH, Kafrawy AH, Newton CW. The relationship of *Bacteroides melaninogenicus* to symptoms associated with pulpal necrosis. Oral Surg Oral Med Oral Pathol 1980;50:457-61.
21. Kakehashi S, Stanley HR, Fitzgerald RJ. The effects of surgical exposures of dental pulps in germ-free and conventional laboratory rats. Oral Surg Oral Med Oral Pathol 1965;20:340-9.
22. Kerosuo E, Haapasalo M, Lounatmaa K. *Eubacterium yurii* subspecies *margaretiae* is resistant to nonopsonic phagocytic ingestion. Scand J Dent Res 1993;101:304-10.
23. Loesche WJ. Oxygen sensitivity of various anaerobic bacteria. Appl Microbiol 1969;18:723-7.
24. Love RM. *Enterococcus faecalis* – a mechanism for its role in endodontic failure. Int Endod J 2001;34:399-405.
25. MacDonald JB, Socransky SS, Gibbons RJ. Aspects of the pathogenesis of mixed anaerobic infections of mucous membranes. J Dent Res 1963;42:529-44.
26. Menin MF. Atividade antimicrobiana de fármacos coadjuvantes da instrumentação de canais radiculares. (Master´s Thesis). University of Pelotas; 1993.
27. Miller WD. Micro-organisms of the human mouth, Philadelphia: The S.S. White Dental MFG. Co.; 1890.
28. Molander A, Reit C, Dahlén G, Kvist T. Microbiological status of root-filled teeth with apical periodontitis. Int Endod J 1998;31:1-7.
29. Molander A, Reit C, Dahlén G. Microbiological root canal sampling: diffusion of a technology. Int Endod J 1996;29:163-7.
30. Möller AJR, Fabricius L, Dahlén G, Ohman AE, Heyden G. Influence on periapical tissues of indigenous oral bacteria and necrotic pulp tissue in monkeys. Scand J Dent Res 1981;89:475-84.
31. Möller AJR. Microbiological examination of root canals and periapical tissues of human teeth. (Thesis). Göteborg Akademiförlaget: University of Göteborg; 1966.
32. Munson MA, Pitt-Ford T, Chong B, Weighman A, Wade WG. Molecular and cultural of the microflora associated with endodontic infections. J Dent Res 2002;8:761-6.
33. Nair PNR. Apical periodontitis: a dynamic encounter between root canal infection and host response. Periodontology 2000 1997;13:121-48.
34. Paster BJ, Boches SK, Galvin JL, Ericson RE, Lau CN, Levanos VA, Sahasrabudhe A, Dewhirst FE. Bacterial Diversity in Human Subgingival Plaque. J Bacteriol 2001;183:3770-83.
35. Pelczar-Jr MJ, Chan ECS, Krieg NR. Microbiology: concepts and applications. NewYork: McGraw-Hill, Inc.; 1993.
36. Petersdorf RG. Antimicrobial prophylaxis of bacterial endocarditis. Am J Med 1978;65:220-3.
37. Reynolds JJ, Meikle MC. Mechanisms of connective tissue matrix destruction in periodontitis. Periodontology 2000 1997;14:144-57.

38. Rosebury T. Microorganisms Indigenous to Man. New York: McGraw-Hill Book Company, Inc.; 1962.
39. Russell AD. Neutralization procedures in the evaluation of bactericidal activity. In: Disinfectants. Their use and evaluation of effectiveness. Collins CH, Allwood MC, Bloomfield SF, Fox A. London: Academic Press; 1981. p.45-59.
40. Schonfeld SE. Oral Microbial Ecology. In: Contemporary Oral Microbiology and Immunology. Slots J, Taubman MA. St Louis: Mosby Year Book Inc.; 1991. p.267-74.
41. Schwartz Z, Goultschin J, Dean DD, Boyan BD. Mechanisms of alveolar bone destruction in periodontitis. Periodontology 2000 1997;14:158-72.
42. Sen BH, Piskin B, Demirci T. Observation of bacteria and fungi in infected root canals and dentinal tubules by SEM. Endod Dent Traumatol 1995;11:6-9.
43. Siqueira-Jr JF, Roças IN, Souto R, Uzeda M, Colombo AP. Checkerboard DNA-DNA hybridization analysis of endodontic infections. Oral Surg Oral Med Oral Pathol 2002;80:744-8.
44. Siqueira-Jr JF. Tratamento das infecções endodônticas. Rio de Janeiro: MEDSI Editora Médica e Científica Ltda; 1997.
45. Slots J, Rams TE. Microbiology of periodontal disease In: Contemporary Oral Microbiology and Immunology. Slots J, Taubman MA. St Louis: Mosby Year Book Inc.; 1982. p.425-43.
46. Stashenko P. Immunological aspects of pulpal infection In: Contemporary Oral Microbiology and Immunology Slots J, Taubman MA. St Louis: Mosby Year Book Inc.; 1991. p.555-60.
47. Sundqvist G, Bloom G, Enberg K, Johansson E. Phagocytosis of *Bacteroides melaninogenicus* and *Bacteroides gingivalis* in vitro by human neutrophils. J Periodontol 1982;17:113-21.
48. Sundqvist G, Carlsson J, Herrmann BF, Hofling JF, Väätäinen A. Degradation *in vivo* of the C3 protein of guinea-pig complement by a pathogenic strain of *Bacteroides gingivalis*. Scand J Dent Res 1984;92:14-24.
49. Sundqvist G, Carlsson J, Herrmann BF, Tärnvik A. Degradation of human immunoglobulins G and M and complement factors C3 and C5 by black-pigmented *Bacteroides*. J Med Microbiol 1985;19:85-94.
50. Sundqvist G, Eckerbom MI, Larsson AP, Sjögren UT. Capacity of anaerobic bacteria from necrotic dental pulps to induce purulent infections. Infec Immun 1979;25:685-93.
51. Sundqvist G, Figdor D, Hänström L, Sörlin S, Sandström G. Phagocytosis and virulence of different strains of *Porphyromonas gingivalis*. Scand J Dent Res 1991;99:117-29.
52. Sundqvist G, Figdor D, Persson S, Sjögren UT. Microbiologic analysis of teeth with failed endodontic treatment and the outcome of conservative re-treatment. Oral Surg Oral Med Oral Pathol 1998;85:86-93.
53. Sundqvist G, Johansson E, Sjögren UT. Prevalence of black-pigmented *Bacteroides* species in root canal infections. J Endod 1989; 15:13-9.
54. Sundqvist G. Associations between microbial species in dental root canal infections. Oral Microbiol Immunol 1992;7:257-62.
55. Sundqvist G. Bacteriological studies of necrotic dental pulps. (Thesis). Umea: University of Umea; 1976.
56. Sundqvist G. Ecology of the root canal flora. J Endod 1992; 18:427-30.
57. Sundqvist G. Microbiología endodontológica. In: Endodoncia. Guldener PA, Langeland K. Barcelona: Springer-Verlag Ibérica S.A.; 1995.
58. Sundqvist G. Taxonomy, ecology, and pathogenicity of the root canal flora. Oral Surg Oral Med Oral Pathol 1994;78:522-30.
59. Sundqvist GK, Reuterving CO. Isolation of *Actinomyces israelii* from periapical lesion. J Endod 1980;6:602-6.
60. Teixeira JIL, Stumpf M, Paz MHP. Exame bacteriológico dos canais radiculares. Rev Odontol 1980;2:36-42.
61. Ter Steeg PF, Van DER, Hoeven JS. Development of periodontal microflora on human serum. Microbial Ecol Health Dis 1989;2:1-10.
62. Tortora GJ, Funke BR, Case CL. O Mundo Microbiano e Você. Microbiologia. In: Tortora GJ, Funke BR, Case CL. 8th ed. Porto Alegre, Artmed, 2005. pp.1-25.
63. Van Winkelhoff AJ, Kippuw NDE, Graaff J. Cross inhibition between blackpigmented *Baceteroides* species. J Dent Res 1987;66:1663-7.
64. Waltimo TMT, Sirén EK, Torkko HLK, Olsen I, Haapasalo M. Fungi in therapy-resistant apical periodontitis. Int Endod J 1997;30:96-101.
65. Watson JD, Crick FHC. The structure of DNA, Cold Spring Harbor Symp. Quant Biol 1953;18:123-31.
66. Williams BL, Shoenknecht FD. Bacteriology of dental abscesses of endodontic origin. J Clin Microbiol 1983;18:770-4.

# Biology and Pathology of Apical Periodontitis

**P. N. R. Nair**

*Institute of Oral Biology, Center of Dental and Oral Medicine, University of Zurich, Zurich, Switzerland*

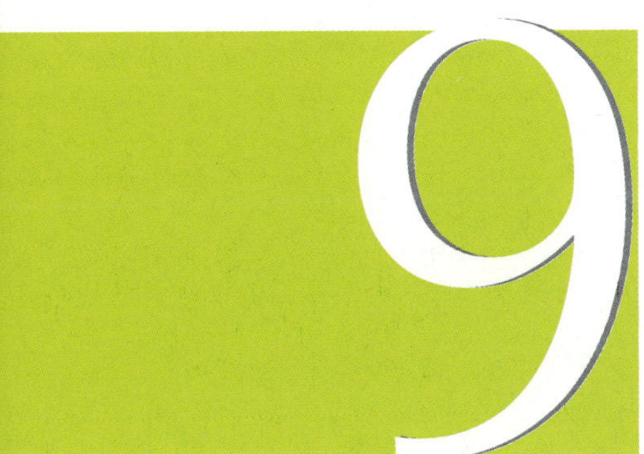


Chapter contents

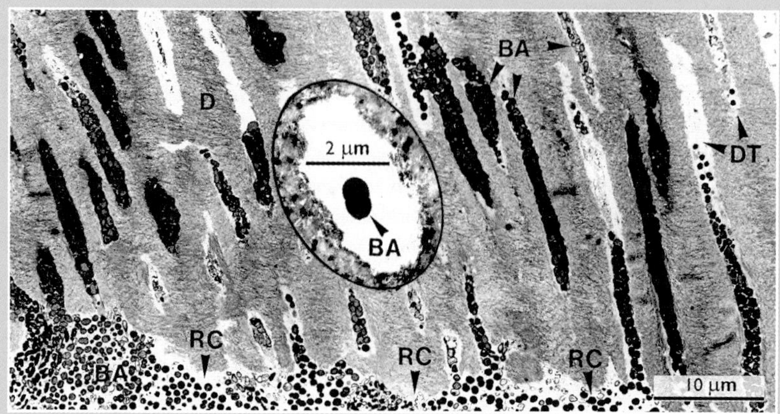


Bacteria (BA) in dentinal tubules (DT) in the apical part of human root dentin (D). The bacteria invade the tubules from the infected root canal (RC). The presence of dividing forms (inset) is a clear sign of vitality of the microorganisms at the time of fixation (x2480; inset, x9600).

## 9.1 Introduction

Contemporary advances in the microbiology have far reaching influence on the understanding of the etiology, pathogenesis and treatment of chronic inflammatory diseases of persistent infections. Single, specific etiological agents cause classical infectious diseases such as tuberculosis and tetanus. But there are several diseases that are caused by a consortium of microbial species living together in ecologically ordered form of survival, known as biofilms[51]. Apical periodontitis belongs to this category of diseases. It is an inflammatory disorder of periradicular tissues caused by irritants of endodontic origin, mostly of persistent microbes living in the root canal system of the affected tooth[119, 299]. The necrotic pulp provides a selective habitat for the endodontic flora[73] that grows in adhesive biofilms, aggregates, coaggregates, and as planktonic cells suspended in the fluid phase of the canal[182]. A biofilm[51] is an extracellular matrix-embedded community of microorganisms that adheres to each other and/or to a moist surface as against planktonic organisms, which are free-floating single microbial cells in an aqueous environment. Microorganisms are protected in biofilms where they have the ability to resist microbicides several hundred times that of the same organisms in planktonic form[49, 348]. Essentially apical periodontitis is the body's defence response to the destruction of the tooth-pulp and microbial settlement of the root canal system[134]. The microbes residing in the root canal can advance or their products can egress into the periapex. In response, the body mounts an array of defence consisting of several classes of cells, of intercellular messengers, of chemical weapons and of effector molecules. In spite of the formidable defence, the body cannot get rid of the microbes, mostly well entrenched as biofilms, in the sanctuary of the necrotic root canal. Therefore, the apical periodontitis is not self-healing. The microbial factors and host defence clash, strike an equilibrium that allows the persistence of microbes in the root canal and limited host response leading to the formation of different categories of apical periodontitis lesions[183].

## 9.2 Nomenclature and Classification

Being an inflammatory disorder, apical periodontitis can be classified on several bases such as the etiology, symptoms and histopathological features. The World Health Organization (WHO)[347] classified apical periodontitis into various categories (Table 9.1). It is clinically a very useful classification but does not take into account the structural aspects of the lesions. As the structural components of the lesion form the basis for an understanding of the pathological process, a histopathological classification is followed in this chapter (Fig. 9.1). The criteria for classification include the distribution of various cell populations within the lesion, the presence or absence of epithelial cells, whether the lesion has been transformed into a cyst and the relationship of the cyst-cavity to the root canal of the affected tooth[183, 194].

### Acute Apical Periodontitis

This is acute inflammation at the periapex. An *incipient* or *primary* acute apical periodontitis is inflammation of transient nature initiated within a healthy periapex in response to irritants (Fig. 9.1A). If the irritation is due to microbial infection this response may develop into a primary abscess. A secondary acute apical periodontitis (Fig. 9.1B) is an acute inflammatory response occurring in an already existing chronic apical periodontitis lesion. Such a response is often clinically referred to as periapical flare-up, acute exacerbation, 'phoenix abscess' or secondary abscess. Depending on the presence or absence of epithelial cells the secondary acute apical periodontitis may be further subdivided into epithelialized or non-epithelialized lesions. The PMN response may be restricted to a small area in the periapex forming a micro abscess or may engulf the whole periapical area when it is referred to as dento-alveolar abscess which may "point" and open to the exterior by formation of a sinus tract or fistula.

### Chronic Apical Periodontitis

This is periapical inflammation extending to a long period of time and characterized by the presence of a granulomatous tissue predominantly infiltrated with lymphocytes, plasma cells and macrophages (Fig. 9.1C). These lesions may be epithelialized or non-epithelialized.

### Periapical True Cyst

This is an apical inflammatory cyst (*Kystis* = bladder) with a distinct pathological cavity completely enclosed in an epithelial lining so that no communication to the root canal exists (Fig. 9.1D).

**Table 9.1** - WHO classification of diseases of periapical tissues

| Code N° | Category |
|---|---|
| K04.4 | Acute apical periodontitis |
| K04.5 | Chronic apical periodontitis (Apical granuloma) |
| K04.6 | Periapical abscess with sinus (Dentoalveolar abscess with sinus, Periodontal abscess of pulpal origin) |
| K04.60 | Periapical abscess with sinus to maxillary antrum |
| K04.61 | Periapical abscess with sinus to nasal cavity |
| K04.62 | Periapical abscess with sinus to oral cavity |
| K04.63 | Periapical abscess with sinus to skin |
| K04.7 | Periapical abscess without sinus (Dental abscess without sinus, Dentoalveolar abscess without sinus, Periodontal abscess of pulpal origin without sinus) |
| K04.8 | Radicular cyst (Apical periodontal cyst, Periapical cyst) |
| K04.80 | Apical and lateral cyst |
| K04.81 | Residual cyst |
| K04.82 | Inflammatory paradental cyst |

(Names in parenthesis denote given synonyms and conditions that are included in the category)

### Periapical Pocket Cyst

This is an apical inflammatory cyst containing a sac-like, epithelium-lined cavity that is open to and continuous with the root canal (Fig. 9.1E).

## 9.3 Primary Apical Periodontitis

### 9.3.1 A microbial disease

Antony van Leeuwenhoek is generally credited with the first description of microorganisms ("animalcules") in the necrotic root canals of diseased human teeth. In one of his celebrated letters to the Royal Society of London, England, he wrote on the 10th of September 1697: "...one of the back teeth in my mouth got loose again, and bothered me much in eating. So I decided to press it hard on the side with my thump ... so as to get rid of the tooth, which I succeeded in doing. ... The crown of the tooth was nearly all decayed while the root consisted of two branches; so that the very roots were uncommon hollow and the holes in them were stuffed with a soft matter. I took this stuff out of the hollows of the roots, and mixed it with clean rain water, and set it before the magnifying glass so as to see if there were so many living creatures as I had aforetime discovered in such material: and I must confess that the whole stuff



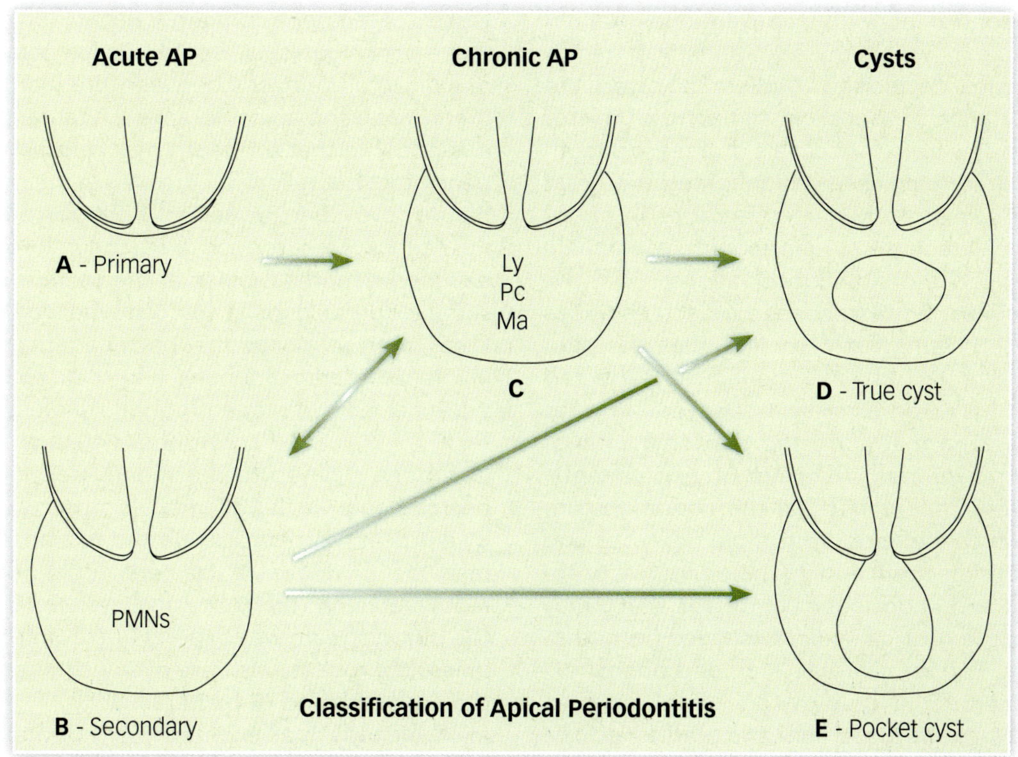


**Figure 9.1** - Pathogenesis of acute (**a**, **b**), chronic (**c**) and cystic (**d**, **e**) apical periodontitis (AP) lesions. The acute lesion may be primary (**a**) or secondary (**b**) and is characterized by the presence of a focus of neutrophils (PMNs). The major components of chronic lesions (**c**) are lymphocytes (Ly), plasma cells (Pc) and macrophage (Ma). Periapical cysts can be differentiated into true cysts (**d**) with completely enclosed lumina and pocket cysts (**e**) with cavities open to the root canal. Arrows indicate the direction in which the lesions can change.

seemed to be alive ... the number of these *animalcules* was so extraordinarily great"[64]. It took another 200 years when Miller[165] demonstrated again the presence of several types of bacteria in the necrotic dental. Nevertheless, the role of microorganisms in the causation of apical periodontitis remained uncertain for several decades thereafter. Only bacteria found within intact solid lesions, within phagocytic cells, were considered genuine[99] because of the problem of microbial contamination. As bacteria were detected only in a small fraction of the lesions, apical periodontitis was considered to be caused not only by microbial infection alone but also by other independent factors such as the necrotic pulp[138, 288], stagnant tissue fluid[227] or root canal fillings. In 1965 Kakehashi et al.[119] reported that no apical periodontitis developed in gnotobiotic rats when their molar-pulps were kept exposed to the oral cavity as compared with control rats with a conventional oral microflora in which massive periapical radiolucencies developed. Möller[169] showed the importance of asepsis in sampling of microorganisms from root canals of diseased teeth for culture-studies and highlighted the great significance of obligate anaerobes in endodontic infections. Independent researchers confirmed the latter observations[23, 120, 352]. In the 1970s, advanced anaerobic techniques enabled Sundqvist[299] to find that the root canals of 18 out of 19 periapically affected teeth harbored a mixture of several species of bacteria that consisted predominantly of strict anaerobes. A series of experimental studies[71] determined: (a) the conditions under which the endodontic flora develops and establishes itself, and (b) the biological properties and endodontic conditions which may favor the root canal flora to become pathogenic. Further clinical[66, 127, 310] and animal experimental[170, 330] studies conclusively showed that stagnant tissue fluid and sterile necrotic pulp tissue do not cause sustaining inflammation at the periapex. The application of the precise technique of correlative light and transmission electron microscopy enabled the ultrastructural visualization of intracanal microbial biofilms and their strategic location in the apical root canal system[182]. These studies provide a chain of evidence on the essentiality of microorganisms in the development of apical periodontitis.

### 9.3.2 Routes of pulpal infection

The possible routes through which microorganisms can reach the dental pulp are many. Breaches in the hard tissue wall, resulting from caries, clinical procedures, fractures and cracks are the frequent portals of pulpal infection. Microbes have also been isolated from teeth with necrotic pulps and crowns appearing 'intact' to naked eye[19, 21, 33, 45, 69, 153, 169, 299, 352]. Necrosis of the pulp precedes endodontic infections of such teeth. Microbes from the gingival sulci or periodontal pockets have also been suggested to reach the root canals of these teeth through severed blood vessels of the periodontium[93]. But, it is unlikely that microorganisms would survive the immunological defenses between the marginal gingiva and the apical foramen. Alternatively, it is possible that the teeth may clinically appear intact but reveal microcracks in their hard tissues, providing portals of entry for bacteria. Pulpal infection can also occur through exposed dentinal tubules at the cervical root surface due to gaps in the cemental coating. It has been proposed that bacteria remaining in infected dentinal tubules (Fig. 9.2) can be a potential reservoir for endodontic reinfection[8, 151, 179, 182, 216, 222, 267, 336]. Microbial infection has also been claimed to reach and seed in the necrotic pulp via the general blood circulation by a process sometimes referred to a anachoresis[6, 38, 89, 230]. However, bacteria could not be recovered from the root canal systems when the blood stream was experimentally infected unless the root canals were over instrumented during the period of bacteremia[6, 38, 63, 89, 230]. In another study[170], all experimentally devitalised pulps (n=26) in monkeys remained sterile for more than six months. Therefore, pulpal exposure to the oral cavity mainly as a result of caries is the pathway of endodontic infections.

### 9.3.3 Root canal flora

On necrosis of the dental pulp the pulpal space provides a selective habitat for the infecting oral microflora[73]. The endodontic flora consists of a mixed population of cocci, rods, spirochetes and filamentous organisms. Numerous dividing forms of cocci, rods and yeast cells are generally identifiable by transmission electron microscopy[182, 200] which is a clear sign of vitality of the organisms at the time of cell fixation. The root canal microbes exist as aggregates of one microbial type (Fig. 9.3A-C), co-aggregates (Fig. 9.4) of several forms[182] and also as planktonic cells, suspended in the fluid phase of the infected and necrotic root canal. The undisturbed intracanal flora of an infected tooth with apical periodontitis is mostly organized as a matrix-embedded collection of multi-species of organisms that are immobilized on the dentinal wall (Fig. 9.3 to 9.5)[182, 183, 200]. Apical periodontitis, therefore, is caused by an intraradicular growth of certain microorganisms that are organized into protected adhesive biofilms[49, 51] composed of cells embedded in a hydrated exopolysaccharide-complex that cannot be eradicated by host defenses and/or chemotherapy alone.

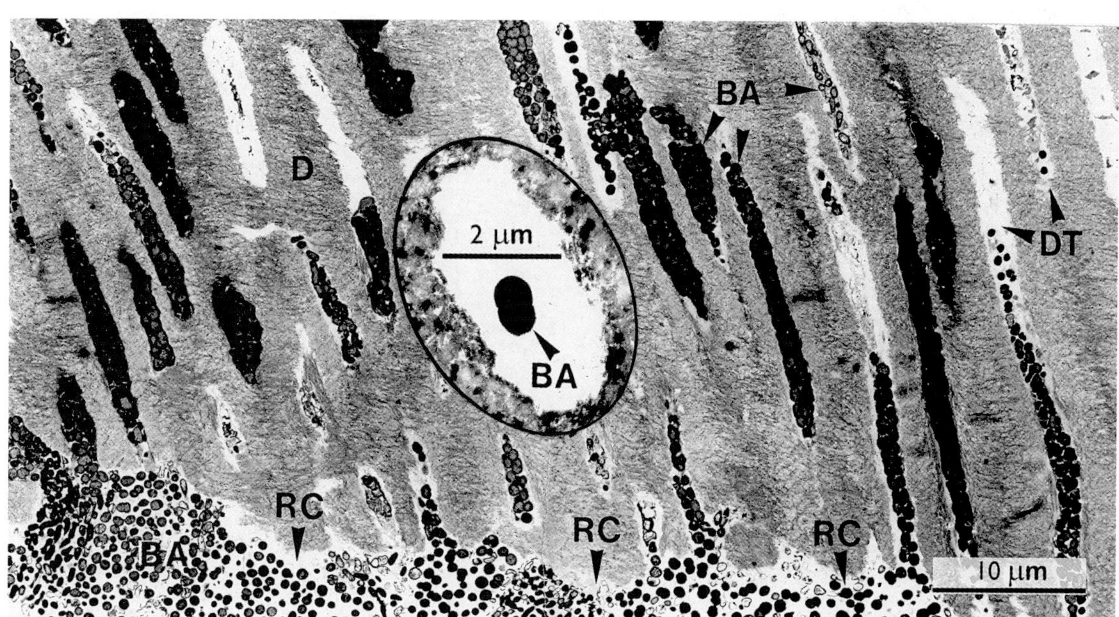


**Figure 9.2** - Bacteria (BA) in dentinal tubules (DT) in the apical part of human root dentin (D). The bacteria invade the tubules from the infected root canal (RC). The presence of dividing forms (inset) is a clear sign of vitality of the microorganisms at the time of fixation (x2480; inset, x9600).

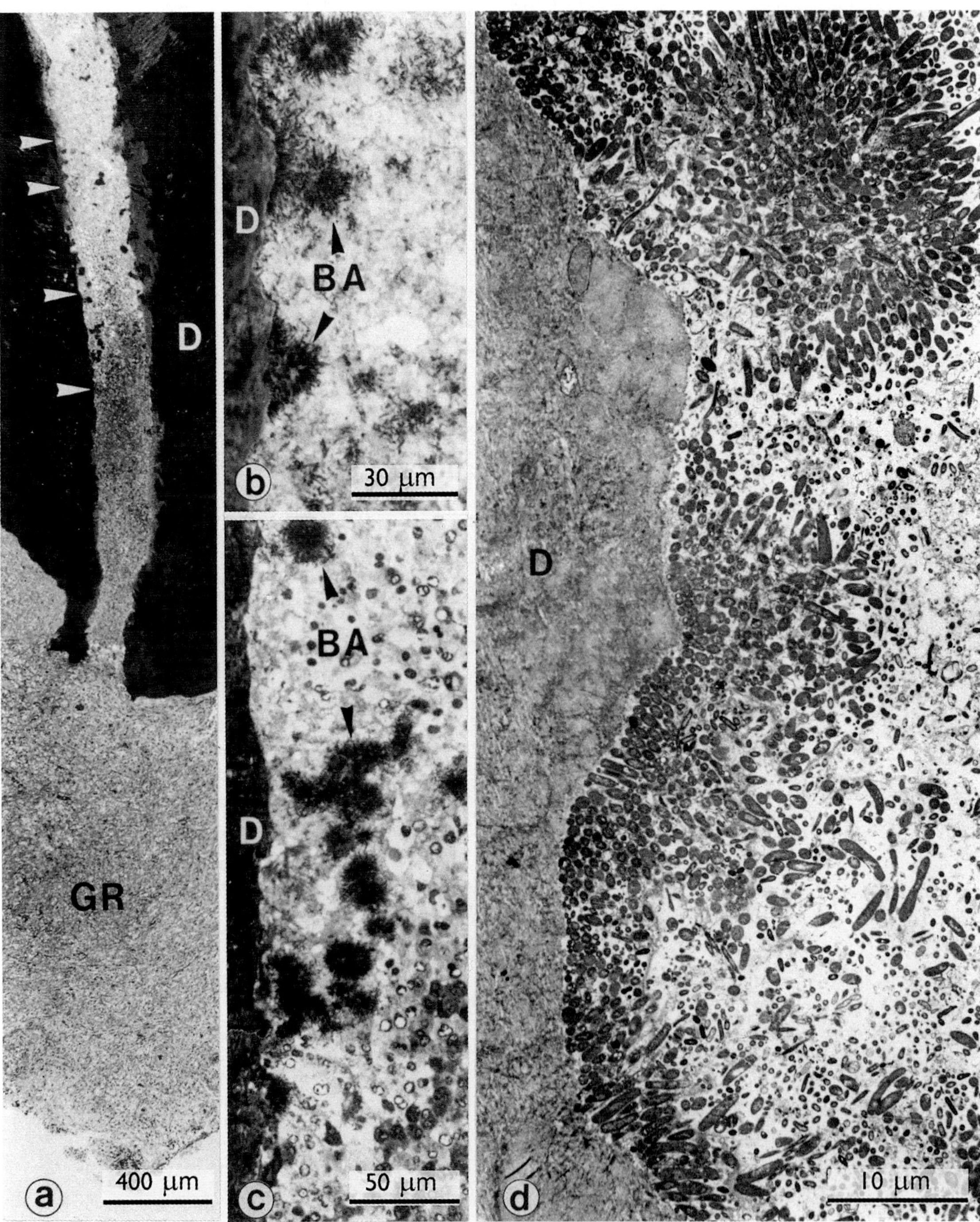


**Figure 9.3** - Axial view endodontic microbial biofilm of a human tooth with apical periodontitis (GR) and previously untreated root canal in axial view. The areas within the axial section of the tooth (**A**) in between the upper two and the lower two arrowheads in are magnified in (**B**, **C**), respectively. Note the biofilm as dense bacterial aggregates (BA) sticking (**B**) to the dentinal (**D**) wall and also remaining suspended among neutrophilic granulocytes in the fluid phase of the root canal (**C**). A transmission electron microscopic view (**D**) of the pulpo-dentinal interface shows bacterial condensation on the surface of the dentinal wall forming sessile biofilm. Magnifications: **A** x46; **B** x600; **C** x370; **D** x2350 (From Nair[183]).

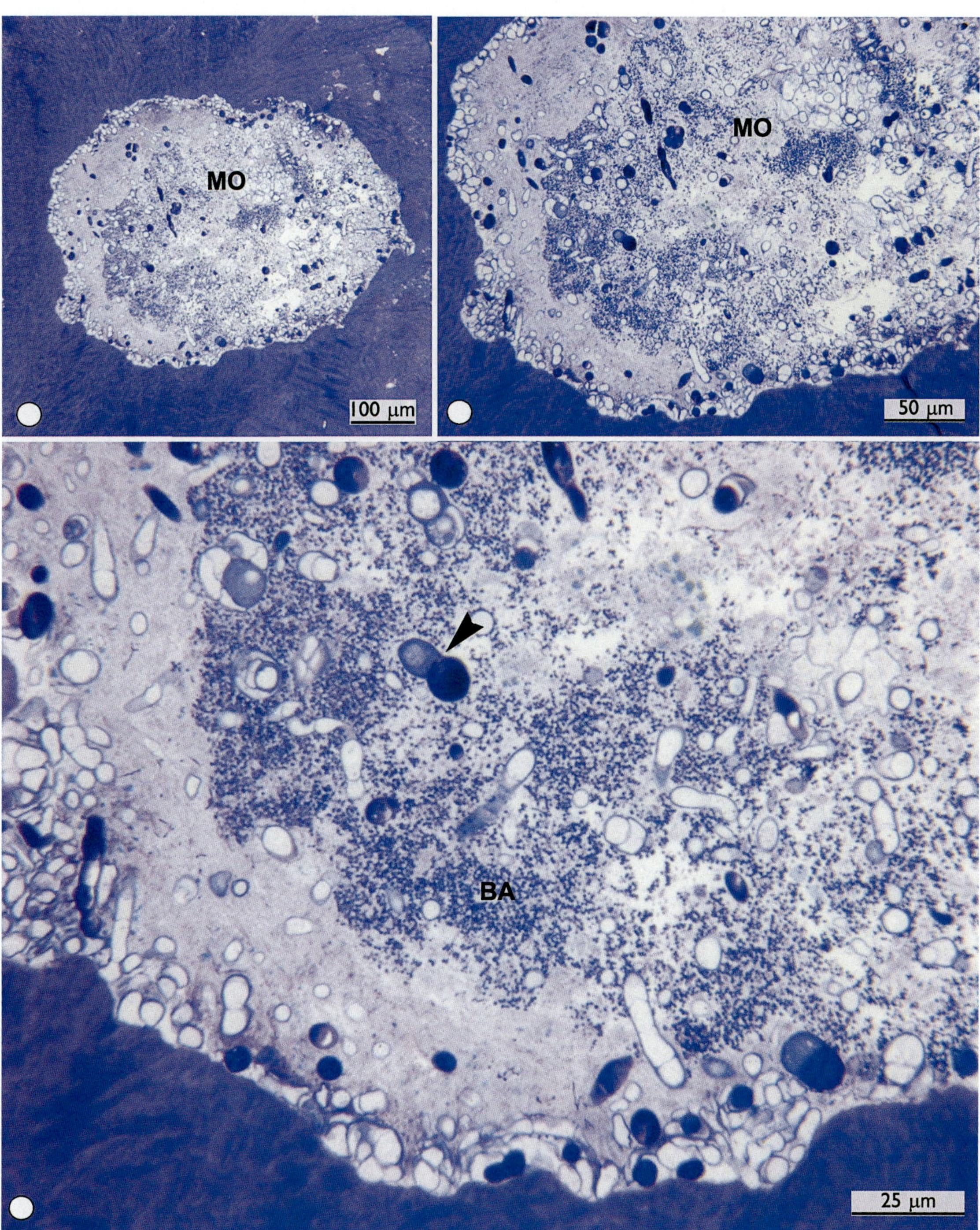


**Figure 9.4** - Horizontal view of endodontic biofilm within the apical root canal system of a human tooth with apical periodontitis and previously untreated root canal. Stage-wise magnifications of a ramified segment of the canal system (**A**-**C**) . Note the segment of the canal system is filled with microorganisms (MO) of varying morphological forms. The small dot-like bacteria (BA in **C**) and the large pleomorphic organisms showing filamentous and dividing forms (arrow head) seem to be yeast stage of fungi. Original magnifications: **A** x100, **B** x280, **C** x800 (From Nair et al.[200]).

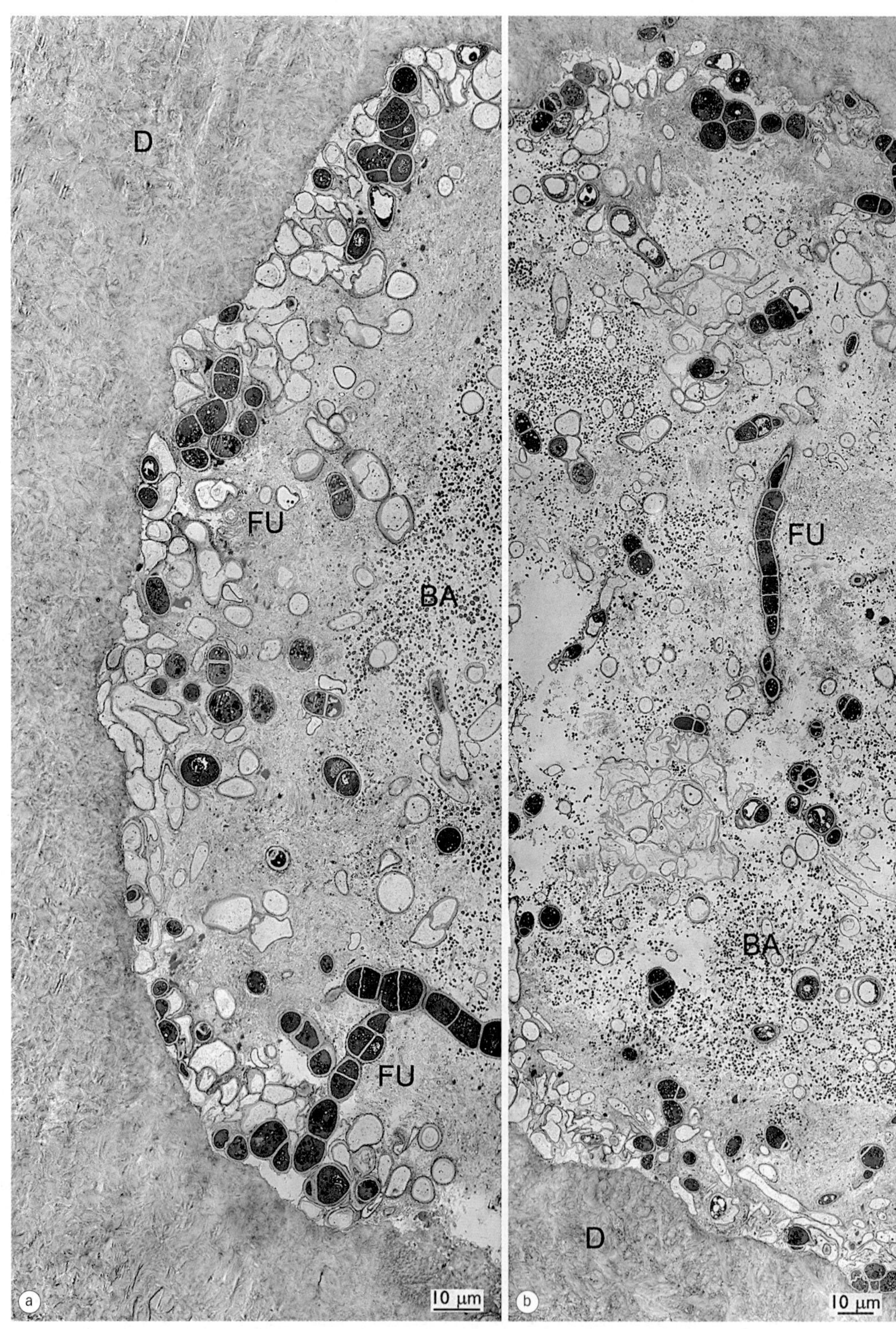


**Figure 9.5** - Composite transmission electron micrographs show the presence of bacteria (BA) and fungi (FU) in the accessory canal illustrated in Figure 14. Note the distinct electron lucent cell wall and the larger size of fungal organisms in comparison to that of the bacteria (BA). The fungus (FU) shows several dividing forms some of which form chains. The organisms marked FU are further magnified in Figure 14. Original Magnifications: **A** x750, **B** x600 (From Nair et al.[200]).

### Cultivable Microbes

The database on the taxonomy of the endodontic flora of infected root canals that has been built-up during the latter half of the 20th century has been based on the application of advanced microbial culture techniques. The onset of the new millennium was marked by the application of molecular genetic methods in endodontic microbiology[178, 234] with the consequence that this database is being re-evaluated and widened. The results of early endodontic microbial culture studies have become largely irrelevant due to the difficulty of avoiding bacterial contamination from the oral surroundings[25, 169, 350] and to the absence of appropriate anaerobic methods for root canal sampling and cultivation of fastidious organisms. In order to recover such microorganisms from the necrotic pulp, stringent anaerobic sampling and cultivation techniques are necessary. These methods have been developed and refined only during the latter half of the 20th century[110]. The two most significant advances in anaerobic technology have been (i) the innovative use of an anaerobic glove-box[235, 282] in which bacteria are protected from oxygen during isolation and cultivation, and (ii) the development of pre-reduced, anaerobically sterilized culture media for transport and growth[114, 174]. Obligate anaerobes were believed to be killed by brief exposure to atmospheric $O_2$, but they can survive for several hours in media supplemented with hemolysed blood[43]. The enzyme, catalase, present in hemolysed blood, breaks down the toxic $H_2O_2$ in the medium to non-toxic $O_2$ and $H_2O$. Advances in anaerobic techniques have enabled the isolation and characterization of obligate anaerobes from the root canal systems of periapically affected teeth and facilitated the study of their pathogenic properties[59, 60, 71-73, 120, 169, 170, 299, 309, 352].

A characteristic feature of the endodontic microflora is the few number of species that are usually isolated from root canals of teeth with necrotic and infected pulp. Application of advanced anaerobic techniques helped to establish that the root canal flora of teeth with clinically intact crowns but having necrotic pulps and diseased periapices is dominated (>90%) by obligate anaerobes[39, 94, 299, 306] usually belonging to the genera *Fusobacterium*, *Porphyromonas* (formerly *Bacteroides*[261]), *Prevotella* (formerly *Bacteroides*[262]), *Eubacterium* and *Peptostreptococcus*. However, the composition of the microflora, even in the apical third of the root canal of periapically diseased teeth with pulp canals exposed to the oral cavity by caries is not only different but also less dominated (<70%) by strict anaerobes[17]. Spirochetes have been found in necrotic root canals using microbial culture techniques[55, 95, 120], dark-field[33, 54, 318], transmission electron microscopy[182] and molecular techniques[18, 231, 270]. Spirochetes are motile invasive pathogens (Fig. 9.6) that are associated with certain marginal periodontitis[147] and suspected etiological agents of acute narcotizing ulcerative gingivitis (ANUG)[148]. Their etiological role in apical periodontitis remains to be clarified. Culture studies, application of correlative light and transmission electron microscopy[200] (Figs. 9.4 and 9.5) and scanning electron microscopy[260] revealed the presence of *fungi* in canals of teeth with primary apical periodontitis[341]. The presence of intraradicular *viruses* has so far been shown only in non-inflamed dental pulps of patients infected with human immunodeficiency virus[90]. Viruses can replicate themselves only by infecting a host cell. They cannot reproduce on their own and do not survive in a necrotic root canal without living cells to host them. Therefore, virus may not play an etiological role in primary apical periodontitis.

### Culture-Difficult Microbes and Microbial Remnants

Several methods contributed to the advancement of endodontic microbiology, such as conventional histology, correlative light and electron microscopy, scanning confocal laser microscopy, microbial culturing, biochemical, and molecular techniques. All these methods have varying degrees of limitations with respect to sensitivity, specificity, and etiological relevance. The advent of molecular genetic methods revolutionized biological sciences with huge impact on oral and endodontic microbiology. Among the DNA based methods, the polymerase chain reaction (PCR)[177] has enabled detection of microbes by amplification of their DNA, when PCR has been targeted at 16S rRNA gene sequences for taxonomic identification. There are several aspects to be considered in the useful application of molecular methods in endodontic microbiology such as: (1) PCR is a very sensitive technology, (2) molecular genetic approaches are of great scientific value, (3) PCR can be applied to identify as-yet-uncultivable species, (4) such species of microbes may in the future become cultivable, (5) molecular genetic methods detect dead microbes, (6) molecular techniques have been successfully applied to recover many-hundred-year-old DNA, (7) contamination of microbial samples is a very serious concern, (8) application of molecular methods in endodontic research keeps pace with change[74], (9) culture techniques remain important in microbiology.

**Contamination problem.** The molecular genetic methods have confirmed the microbial species that have been previously detected by culture methods[178, 234] and also facilitated the identification of "as-yet-culture-difficult"[178] endodontic organisms. The PCR replicates and amplifies the DNA. The importance and advantages of the molecular genetic methods cannot be over emphasized. But understanding the importance and application of the technology is not sufficient on its own. Research that utilizes this technology, or any technology, must be performed with a methodological rigor and scientific standards that allow safe and justifiable conclusions. In the absence of a valid scientific procedure the resulting data has only very limited etiological relevance.

For example, controls for microbial contamination were shown to be essential for culture studies in order to get authentic results. The procedures for taking microbial samples from infected root canals have been well established by Möller[169]. It is essential that the tooth and surrounding area be thoroughly cleaned and disinfected before preparation of the access cavity. After gaining access and before reaching the pulp chamber, a second cleaning, disinfection and inactivation are essential. This must be followed by a control for contamination of samples to check that no contaminating species remain at the surface before entry to the pulp chamber. That a second decontamination step is essential was shown in a classic work more than 35 years ago in which bacteria were found to thrive under restorations[31]. These methods are well established for culture studies, yet most molecular studies contain none or inadequate molecular contamination procedures and controls.

To the author's knowledge, only one study has applied these steps: a first and second cleaning, disinfection and oligonucleotide decontamination followed by sampling for contamination control[202]. They found that use of pumice, hydrogen peroxide and iodine resulted in contaminating DNA recovered from 45% of investigated teeth. Furthermore, cleaning by pumice, hydrogen peroxide and sodium hypochlorite (NaOCl), yielded 13% of samples that were positive for contaminating DNA. Thus, the study[202] showed the importance of a second round of cleaning, greater effectiveness of NaOCl as against iodine and the challenge of achieving a contamination-free surface before entry to the pulp chamber. The point was confirmed again in a more recent study[253] in which the initial cleaning and decontamination procedures were done using pumice, hydrogen peroxide and NaOCl but was not followed by the second round of cleaning procedures. The result was that contamination controls showed[253] contaminating "... bacterial DNA in all ... samples".

These findings illustrate an essential step for valid isolation of microbial species from the root canal, namely accurate recovery without contamination. More than 40 years ago, this lesson was learnt and applied for culture work[169], yet studies using highly sensitive molecular methods appear to have ignored this valuable lesson of the past. In brief: while research should keep pace with change, the lessons learnt previously and from other scientific approaches must not be discarded when it comes to applying molecular tools for the study of the endodontic microbial flora.

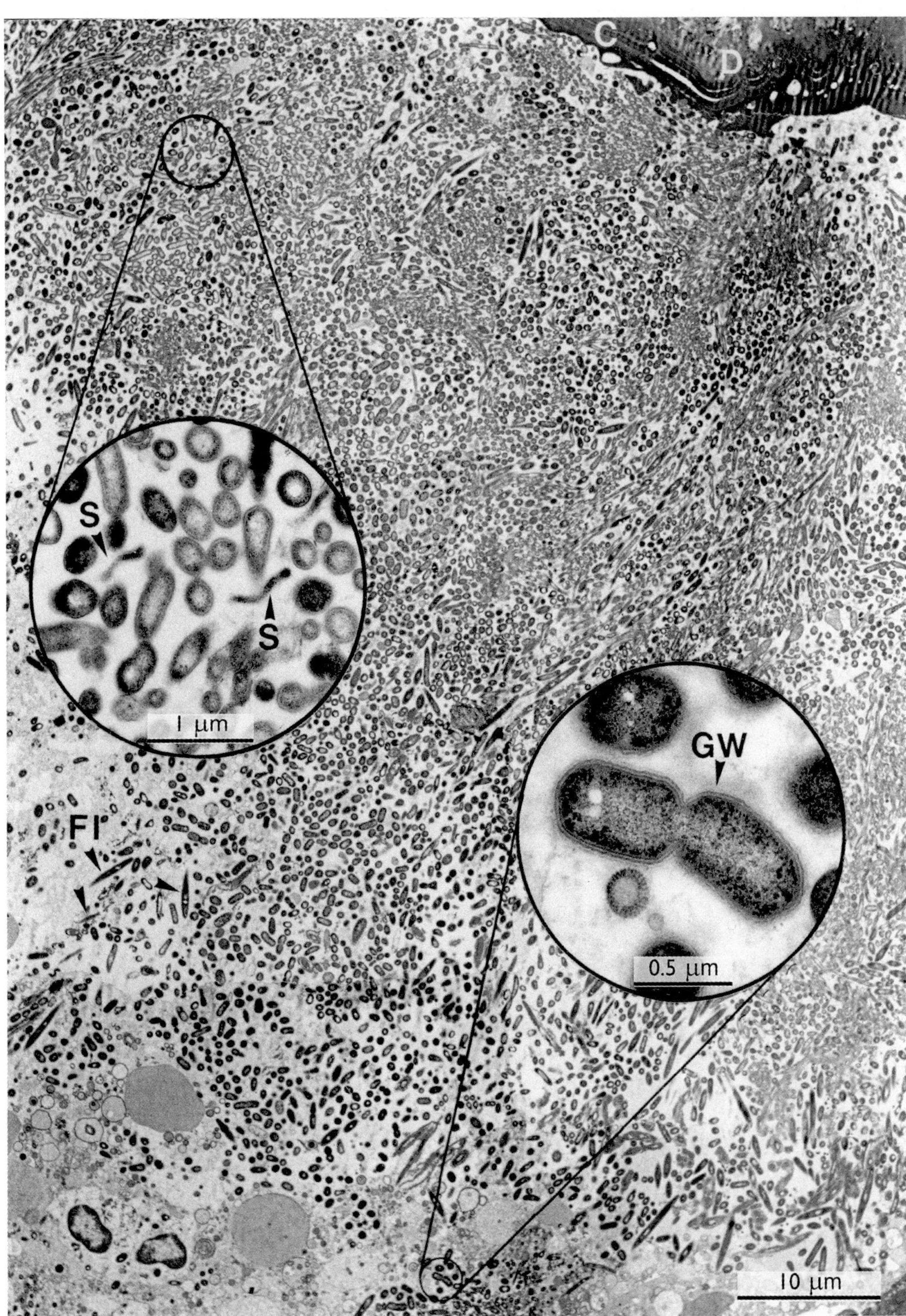


**Figure 9.6** - A microbial biofilm at the root-tip of a human tooth with secondary acute apical periodontitis of endodontic origin. The mixed bacterial flora consists of numerous dividing cocci, rods (lower inset), filaments (FI) and spirochetes (S, upper inset). Rods often reveal a gram negative cell wall (GW, lower inset). C, cementum; D, dentin. Magnifications: x2' 680; upper inset x 19' 200; lower inset x 36' 400 (Adapted from Nair[182]).

**Non-viability problem.** Apart from the possible contamination of samples, the molecular technique does not differentiate between viable and non-viable organisms, but can pick up a minuscule amount of microbial DNA that is amplified using the PCR[177] resulting in an exponential accumulation of several million copies of the original DNA fragments. An estimated 700 or more different species of microorganisms live in a healthy human mouth. Theoretically speaking, all of them have equal opportunity to gain access into and establish themselves in the exposed pulp space. But, for each pulp diseased tooth, only a very limited number of microbial species has been found to do so. Even with the highly sensitive molecular genetic methods the number of identified intracanal species remains low. This disparity between the potential and actual number of species in infected canals is due to the selective environment of the root canal. Obviously, a large majority of the microbial species die off, leaving behind cellular remnants including the DNA. Vital pulp may contain host nucleases that may degrade free microbial DNA. But the necrotic root canal, with many pockets of dry areas, is a favorable place for persistence of bacterial remnants particularly DNA. This is particularly so with root canal treated and obturated teeth. There is no evidence yet that all such free microbial DNA, particularly those located in the drier parts of necrotic root canals, are degraded by nucleases released from microbes living and/or dying in the root canal. *How long DNA from dead microorganisms may persist in the root canal is unknown*[272, 305]. It may be pointed out that application of PCR methods enabled to detect and amplify DNA fragments of *Mycobacterium tuberculosis* from hundreds of year-old human remains[78, 129, 248] and from that of an "extinct bison dated 17,000 years before the present"[236]. Detection of 400-year-old *Yersinia pestis* DNA in human dental pulp helped to diagnose ancient septicaemia and deaths in humans[65]. These research findings on the detection of ancient DNA cannot be dismissed as instances of contamination. The data derived from the molecular technique, therefore, require very careful interpretation in the light of the technique's many advantages and numerous limitations. The DNA based molecular method is superior for microbial sensitivity and specificity, but it is prone to false positive results due to detection of dead organisms and/or contaminants. Refinements or adjustments in molecular methods, such as the application of real time PCR, using larger primers and targeting rRNA or mRNA may mitigate some of the 'high sensitivity' and 'non-viablity' problems.

**Taxonomical data.** Another aspect is the identification of microbial species in infected root canals[305]. There is absolutely no doubt about the usefulness of molecular tools for the precise taxonomical identification of the microbes. But the validity of the 'newly identified' organisms as the authentic residents of infected root canals to be considered as the etiological agents of pulpal and apical disease remains unaddressed. While it is true that some species that are culture difficult or not-yet-culturable have been detected by molecular approaches, most of the 'new' species are merely re-classified or split off from other genera. It may be pointed out that in principle any metabolically active microorganism living in sufficient numbers in an infected root canal can participate in inflammation of the periradicular tissues. That means all viable microbes in root canal are 'candidate pathogens' for endodontic disease. Therefore, it is important to show that the microbial DNA detected by molecular methods really originates from viable root canal microbes.

Sound understandings on the etiology of microbial diseases is under threat of erosion or even reversal[189] by writings such as: "In the event DNA from dead cells is detected, the results by no means lack significance with regard to participation in disease causation"[272]. Apparently some researchers avoid meeting the basic tenets that are required to relate a pathogen to a disease and provide robust evidence for their conclusions. It is obvious that a mere detection of already known microbes or 'discovering' new microbes, cultured or "as-yet-culture-difficult"[178] at disease sites using any technology is the most preliminary and relatively simple of the stringent requirements needed today to implicate the organisms in question to causation of diseases. A mere observation of the presence of certain microbial remnants in necrotic root canals of pulp diseased teeth is not sufficient to implicate the organisms in question as etiological agents of endodontic diseases. Therefore, the onus is on the researchers, particularly those using DNA-based methods in endodontic microbiology, to provide proof for causation of pulpal and periapical disease in the contemporary sense.

### 9.3.4 Virulence factors

Pathogenicity is the capacity of a microbe to produce disease and virulence is the relative capacity (degree of pathogenicity) of a microbe to cause injurious damage in a host[349]. The term virulence is derived from the Latin word *virulentus* meaning "full of poison". Any metabolically active microbe living in the root canal has the potential to participate in the inflammation of periradicular tissues. However, certain differentiation is essential between a mere presence and the ability of the microbe to induce the disease or comparable pathology in susceptible experimental animals. This is particularly important in infectious diseases in which the organisms have to be present within the body milieu of the host. In apical and marginal periodontitis the microbes, living in biofilm, are located in the necrotic pulp or periodontal pocket, which are outside the body milieu. Viable, metabolically active microbes, situated at those locations release antigenic and other molecules that irritate periodontal tissues, both at the apical and marginal sites to cause inflammation, irrespective of them living there with or without virulence and tissue invasiveness. Individual species in the endodontic flora may be of low virulence, but their survival in the necrotic root canal and pathogenic properties are influenced by a combination of several factors. These include, (i) the ability to build biofilms, interact with other microorganisms in the biofilm and develop synergistically beneficial partners, (ii) the capability to interfere with and evade host defenses (iii) the release of lipopolysaccharides (LPS) and other microbial modulins, and (iv) the synthesis of enzymes that damage host tissues.

#### Biofilm Formation

The ability to form biofilms, depending on several properties such as adhesion and colonization, has to be considered as a virulence factor for disease producing organisms. The importance of a mixed endodontic microflora in the development of apical periodontitis has long been recognized through carefully planned studies[72, 73, 309]. There is clear evidence that interaction among various microbial species[42, 73, 142, 149] play a significant role in the ecological regulation and eventual development of an endodontic habitat-adapted polymicrobial flora[300, 301, 305] that live in biofilms. Biofilms are matrix-embedded microbial populations adherent to each other and/or to surfaces or interfaces[50]. Current understanding of biofilms has been based on diverse research approaches that particularly include the application novel scanning confocal laser microscopy, molecular methods to determine gene expression, cell signaling, and culture-independent methods that identify (gene amplification and sequencing) and localize (fluorescent *in situ* hybridization (FISH)) biofilm components. These methods have shown that biofilms are well structured with diverse microbial species existing as organized symbiotic communities in a protective extracellular matrix and traversed by a network of fluid channels reminiscent of a very primitive circulatory system[50]. The ability to organize and live in biofilms with an open architecture has provided several biological advantages to the microbes such as gene transfer, novel gene expression, co-ordinated gene expression, population size dependent (quorum sensing) and independent cell signaling, limiting physical hazards (dehydration), protection from host defenses, increased resistance to biocides and enhanced virulence.

### Microbial Interference

The ability of certain microbes to shirk and interfere with the host defenses has been well elaborated[302]. The LPS can signal the endothelial cells to express leukocyte adhesion molecules that initiate extravasation of leukocytes into the area of the infection. It has been reported that *Porphyromonas gingivalis*, an important endodontic and periodontal pathogen, and its LPS do not signal the endothelial cells to express E-selectin. *P. gingivalis* therefore has the ability to block the initial step of inflammatory response, 'hide' from the host and multiply. The antigenicity of LPS occurs in several forms that include mitogenic stimulation of B-lymphocytes so as to produce non-specific antibodies. Gram-negative organisms release membrane particles (blebs) and soluble antigens which may 'mop up' effective antibodies so as to make them unavailable to act against the organism itself[166]. *Actinomyces israelii*, a recalcitrant periapical pathogen, is easily killed by PMN *in vitro*[77]. In tissues, *A. israelii* aggregate to form large cohesive colonies that cannot be killed by host phagocytes[77].

### LPS and Other Microbial Modulins

LPS, erroneously known as endotoxin, form an integral part of the outer membrane of Gram-negative cell walls. They are released during disintegration of bacterial cells after death and also during multiplication and growth. The patho-biological effects of LPS are due to its interaction with endothelial cells and macrophages. LPS signal the endothelial cells to express adhesion molecules and activate macrophages to produce a number of cytokines such as the tumor necrosis factor$_{-a}$ (TNF-$\alpha$) and interleukins (IL)[11]. Administarion of exogenous TNF-$\alpha$ into experimental animals induce a lethal shock that is indistinguishable from that caused by LPS. The latter signal the presence of Gram-negative bacteria in the neighbourhood. The impact of LPS in tissues has been aptly stated[320]. "When we sense LPS, we are likely to turn on every defense at our disposal; we will bomb, defoliate, blockade, seal off and destroy all tissues in the area". The presence of LPS has been reported in samples taken from the root canal[57, 251] and the pulpal dentinal wall of periapically involved teeth[112]. The Gram-negative organisms living in the root canal multiply and die, thereby releasing LPS that egresses through the apical foramen into the periapex[354], where it initiates and sustains apical periodontitis[56, 58].

In addition to LPS, there are number bacterial degradation products that can induce mammalian cells to produce cytokines. Several proteins, carbohydrates and lipids of bacterial origin form a novel class of 'modulins' that induce the formation of cytokine networks and host tissue pathology[106]).

### Enzymes

Microbes living in the necrotic pulp and root canal produce many enzymes, that are not directly toxic but aid in the spread of the organisms in host tissues. Collagenase, hyaluronidase, fibrinolysins and several proteases are examples. Some of these enzymes can degrade plasma proteins that are involved in blood coagulation and other body defenses. The ability of certain *Porphyromonas* and *Prevotella* species to break down plasma proteins, particularly IgG, IgM[125], and the complement factor $C_3$[307] is of particular significance as these molecules are opsonins necessary for both humoral and phagocytic host defenses.

## 9.4 Host Defense

Apical periodontitis is the defense response of the body to the threat of microbial invasion from the root canal. The host defense consist of cells, intercellular mediators, metabolites, effector molecules and antibodies.

### 9.4.1 Cells

The radiographic and histologic changes taking place at the periapex in the form of hard tissue resorption and infiltration of inflammatory cells in the area have long been recorded[24, 82, 161, 319, 356]. The presence of neutrophils, lymphocytes, plasma cells and macrophages was initially visualized only as a defense maneuver against the microbes, but their role in the destruction of the periapical tissues was not initially recognised. Most of the early information came from data on periodontal diseases[210]. Major roles were assigned to defense cells and immune-reactions in the tissue destruction associated with marginal periodontitis, and by de *facto* in apical periodontitis. The immune system itself was regarded as the 'culprit' for the disease process[325]. This resulted in sidelining the central role of microorganisms in the disease process. Subsequent investigations on apical periodontitis provided a molecular basis for the disease as a dynamic interaction between microbial invaders and the body defense at the tooth-apex[12, 52, 163, 245, 289, 313, 316, 329, 343]. Several classes of cells participate in periapical defence. Majority of them are recruited from the defense systems. They include neutrophils, lymphocytes, plasma cells and monocyte/macrophages (Fig. 9.7). The importance of neutrophils and monocyte derivatives in apical periodontitis has been experimentally shown[291]. The intensity of induced murine pulpitis and apical periodontitis can be suppressed by treating the animals with a biological response-modifying drug, PGG glucan, that enhances the number and ability of circulating neutrophils and monocytes. In addition, structural cells such as fibroblasts, osteoblasts and epithelial remnants of the enamel organ (rests of Malassez)[155] also play particular roles.

**Polymorphonuclear leukocytes (PMN)**

The PMN are the non-specific fighting force and the hallmark of acute inflammation. Their function is to find and destroy microorganisms intruding into the body. PMN are phagocytes and are well equipped to attack with weapons already stored within them or quickly assembled by them. These weapons consist of various cytoplasmic granules that are classified into primary, secondary and tertiary groups. The primary granules or azurophilic granules, contain lysosomes, myeloperoxidase, cationic proteins and neutral proteinases. The secondary or specific granules are marked by lactoferrin and vitamin $B_{12}$ binding protein. The tertiary or secretory granules are released into the tissues in response to stimuli[337].

The PMN extravasate (Fig. 9.8), in great numbers at the site of tissue injury where they seek the targets by chemotaxis. They move in the direction of an ascending gradient of the chemotactic molecules so as to congregate at the site of maximum concentration which coincides with the site of microbial presence. In the meantime the microbes are generally opsonized. Opsonins are complement factors or antibodies that coat the surface of microbes and facilitate phagocytosis. The microbes are ingested and isolated in membrane bound phagosomes. Depending on the availability of oxygen ($O_2$) the PMN are provided with two pathways for intracellular killing of the microbes. During the early stages of inflammation there is generally plenty of oxygen in the tissues and the PMN follow an aerobic route, commonly known as the "respiratory burst", in which the enzyme NADPH oxidase situated on the phagosome-membrane converts molecular $O_2$ into oxygen-derived free radicals, also known as reactive oxygen species (ROS). They are very small, highly reactive molecules due to the presence of unpaired valence shell electrons.

Being highly unstable and reactive they literally 'rob' electrons from other molecules thereby damaging them. Speroxide ($O_2$-) is formed when NADPH oxidase acts on stable $O_2$. A pair of $O_2$- can interact to form a molecule of hydrogen peroxide ($H_2O_2$). Both the $O_2$- and $H_2O_2$ are mildly microbicidal. But the latter in the presence of the enzyme myleoperoxidase oxidises halides ions (eg.,$Cl^-$) to form hypochlorous acid (HOCl) which is highly bactericidal. It is important to realize that clinicians reproduce this process by using sodium hypochlorite (NaOCl) for endodontic irrigation. This antimicrobial pathway is known as the *$H_2O_2$-halide-myeloperoxidase system*. Under hypoxic conditions (abscess) PMN shift the intracellular killing process to the anaerobic pathway in which the phagosomes fuse with primary or secondary granules containing powerful enzymes that can kill and digest the microbes.

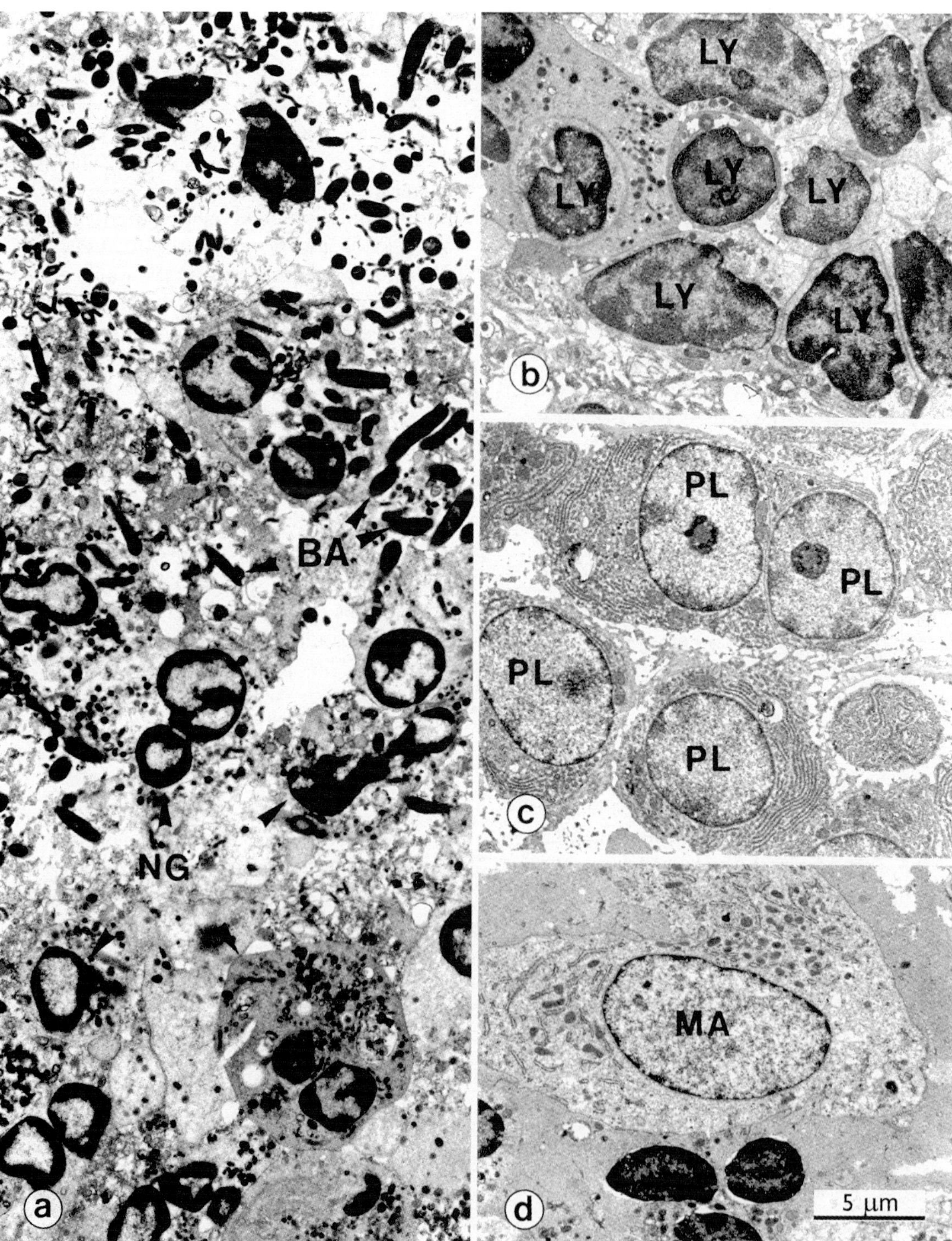


**Figure 9.7** - The primary body cells involved in the pathogenesis of apical periodontitis. Neutrophils (NG in **A**) in combat with bacteria (BA) in a secondary acute apical periodontitis. Lymphocytes (LY in **B**) are the major components of chronic apical periodontitis but their subpopulations cannot be identified on a structural basis. Plasma cells (PL in **C**) form a significant component of chronic asymptomatic lesions. Note the highly developed rough endoplasmic reticulum of the cytoplasm and the localized condensation of heterochromatin subjacent to the nuclear membrane which gives the typical 'cart wheel' appearance in light microscope. Macrophages (MA in **D**) are voluminous cells with elongated or U-forming nuclei and cytoplasm with rough endoplasmic reticulum. (Magnifications: **A**,**B**,**C**,**D** x3900).

Although the PMN are to kill microorganisms (Fig. 9.7A), they also cause severe damage to the host tissues. The cytoplasmic granules of PMN contain scores of enzymes which on release can degrade the components of tissue cells and extracellular matrices. The zinc-dependent enzymes which are responsible for the breakdown of most of the extracellular matrices are classified under the family of enzymes known as the matrix metalloproteinases (MMP)[180]. However, the PMN-derived weapons (super oxide, hydrogen peroxide and hypochlorous acid) do not discriminate between hostile microbes and own tissues[337]. In the tissues the PMN live only for about 3 days and die in great numbers at acute inflammatory sites[240]. It is the high concentration of PMN-derived myeloperoxidase that gives purulence its creamy white appearance. Irrespective of the cause of PMN mobilization, the accumulation and rapid death of neutrophils is a major cause for tissue breakdown in acute apical periodontitis.

## Lymphocytes

Lymphocytes belong to the special fighting force of the defense system. They play several roles in apical periodontitis. There are three major classes of lymphocytes designated as T-lymphocytes (T cells), B-lymphocytes (B cells) and the natural killer (NK) cells. The primary function of NK cells is to monitor and destroy neoplastic and virus infected cells. Therefore, they may not be of significance in apical periodontitis. But the T- and B-cells are of particular importance. The three classes of lymphocytes originate from bone-marrow stem cells, but undergo different pathways of growth and differentiation. Nevertheless, they are morphologically identical (Fig. 9.7B) and cannot be distinguished by conventional microscopical examination and require special immunohistochemical or *in situ* hybridization techniques for identification. Lymphocytes and other leukocytes are phenotyped on the basis of surface receptors using monoclonal antibodies (mAbs) against the latter.



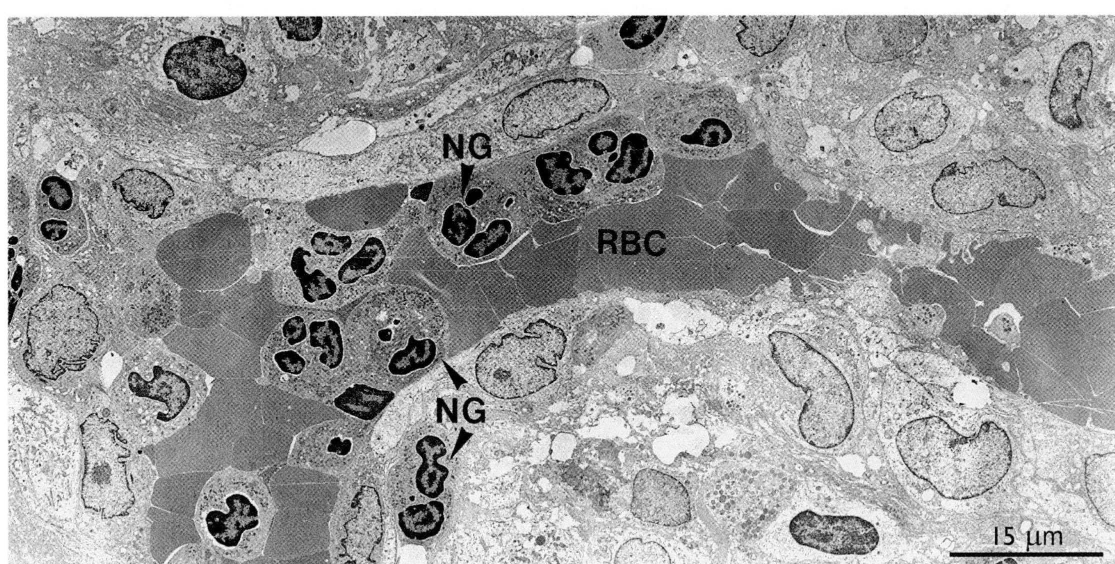


**Figure 9.8** - Intravascular neutrophilic granulocytes (NG) marginating, adhering to the endothelial cells, and transmigrating across the blood vessel wall into the inflamed periapical tissues. RBC, Red blood cells (x1650).

Cells so identified are given a *cluster of differentiation* (CD) number. The CD nomenclature was established in the 1st International Workshop and Conference on Human Leukocyte Differentiation Antigens (HLDA), held in Paris in 1982. The CD system was intended for the classification of the many mAbs generated by different laboratories around the world against certain surface molecules of leucocytes. Its use has been expanded to include many other cell types. So far more than 320 CD clusters have been identified. The proposed surface molecule is assigned a CD number once two specific mAb are shown to bind to the molecule.

**T-lymphocytes.** The thymus-derived lymphocytes are known as T-cells. Originating from the bone-marrow stem cells, the pre-T-cells migrate to the thymus and undergo further differentiation, immunological specialization and stringent selection before, the 'successful candidates' are released into general circulation. T-cells constitute about 60 to 70% of circulating lymphocytes. They also concentrate in the para-cortical areas of lymph nodes and other lymphoid organs. T-cells are multifunctional with certain division of labor so that the various functions are performed by their subpopulations. The nomenclature of T-cells can be confusing. Traditionally, they have been designated after their effect or functions, as for instance the T-cells working with B-cells have long been known as T-helper/inducer ($T_{h/i}$) cells and those with direct toxic and suppressive effects on other cells have been named T-cytotoxic/suppressive ($T_{c/s}$) cells. The $T_{h/i}$ cells are $CD_4^+$; and the $T_{c/s}$ cells are $CD_8^+$. The $CD_4^+$ cells differentiate further into two types known as $T_{h1}$ and $T_{h2}$ cells. The former produce IL-2 and interferon-γ (IF-γ), and control the cell mediated arm of the immune system. The $T_{h2}$ cells secrete IL-4, -5, -6 and -10 so as to control the humoral immune responses by regulating the production of antibodies by the plasma cells.

**B-lymphocytes.** They are the bursa-equivalent (B) cells directly responsible for antibody production. The B-cells were originally discovered in chicken in which their early differentiation was found to take place in a gut-associated organ called the bursa of Fabricius. Humans do not have this structure. The origin and differentiation of B-cells in man occur in bone marrow itself[233]. The differentiated B-cells enter the blood circulation where they constitute about 10 to 20% of the lymphocyte population. They also accumulate and proliferate in and around the germinal centers of extrathymic lymphoid tissues. On receiving signals from antigens and the $T_{h2}$-cells some of the B-cells transform into large ***plasma cells*** (Fig. 9.7C) with characteristic nuclei of "cartwheel" appearance and extensive rough endoplasmic reticulum. Plasma cells are the only cells that can manufacture and secrete antibodies, the specific chemical weapons of the immune system.

### Macrophages

Macrophages[164] (Greek = big eaters) are cells within the tissues that originate from blood monocytes. Macrophages are phagocytes acting in both nonspecific and specific defenses. They are large mononuclear phagocytes (Fig. 9.7D) that represent the major differentiated element of the *mononuclear phagocytic system*[211, 338], previously known as the *reticuloendothelial system*. This system consists of closely related cells of bone marrow origin that comprise blood monocytes and tissue macrophages. The latter are diffusely distributed throughout the body. Depending on their location, they have been known by various names such as the macrophages of connective and lymphoid tissues, alveolar macrophages of the lung, Kupfer cells of the liver, Langerhan's cells of the integument, microglial cells of the brain and fusion-macrophages that produce various types of multinucleated giant cells such as osteoclasts, dentoclasts, and foreign body giant cells.

Monocytes begin to migrate relatively early in inflammation. Extravasation of monocytes is governed by the same factors that are involved in PMN emigration. On reaching the extravascular tissue monocytes undergo transformation into large phagocytic cells, the macrophages (Fig. 9.7D). Unlike PMN, macrophages are long living (months) and slow-moving cells. Once they arrive, the macrophages can persist at the inflammatory site for several months to years. If the first wave of PMN-defense has failed to exterminate the enemy the process becomes a chronic inflammation. Thus, macrophages form a major component of the inflammatory cells in later stages of inflammation. They move by chemotaxis and are activated by microorganisms, their products (LPS), chemical mediators or foreign particles. Activated macrophages become larger, show numerous lysosomal and other cytoplasmic granules and a greater affinity for phagocytosis and intracellular killing of microorganisms. They possess the same biochemical weapons for killing of microbes as the PMN do and can attach to foreign objects[273]. Among the various molecular mediators that are secreted by macrophages, the cytokines IL-1, TNF-$\alpha$, interferons (IFN) and growth factors are of particular importance in apical periodontitis. They also release other metabolites such as prostaglandins and leukotrienes that are important in inflammation.

The functions of macrophages include (i) phagocytic killing of microorganisms, (ii) scavenging of dead cells and tissue components, (iii) removal of small foreign particles, (iv) immunological surveillance by antigen capture, (v) processing and presentation of antigens to immune competent cells and (vi) secretion of wide variety of biologically active molecules and their regulation.

**Osteoclasts**

Osteoclasts (Greek = bone and broken) are bone resorbing cell. Histologically it is characterised by high expression of tartrate resistent acid phosphatase (TRAP) and cathepsin K. One of the major pathological events of apical periodontitis is bone resorption. Osteoclasts are the effector cells in this process. There are extensive reviews on the origin[203], structure[88], regulation[105] and 'coupling'[225] of these cells with osteoblasts. Bone marrow stem-cells provide the progenitor-cells of osteoclasts. The pro-osteoclasts migrate through blood as monocytes to the periradicular tissues and attach themselves to the surface of bone. They remain dormant till signaled for further changes and activity. In the physiological state those signals, involving several cytokines and other mediators, are given by osteoblasts and other cells. It is known that osteoclast formation requires the presence of RANK ligand (receptor activator of nuclear factor $\kappa\beta$) and M-CSF (macrophage colony stimulating factor). These membrane bound proteins and cytokines are produced by neighbouring stromal cells and osteoblasts; thus requiring direct contact between these cells and osteoclast precursors. During apical periodontitis these mediators are also released by several other cells which stimulate the pre-osteoclasts. As a result, the latter begin to proliferate and several daughter cells fuse to form multinucleated osteoclasts which spread over injured and exposed bone surface. The cytoplasmic border of the osteoclasts facing the bony surface becomes ruffled as a result of extensive infolding of the plasma membrane. Bone resorption take place beneath this ruffled border known as the subosteoclastic resorption compartment. At the periphery, the cytoplasmic clear-zone is a highly specialized area which regulates the biochemical activities involved in breaking down the bone. The bone destruction happens extracellularly at the osteoclast/bone interface and involves, (i) demineralization of the bone by solubilizing the mineral phase in the resorption compartment as a result of ionic lowering of pH in the microenvironment and (ii) enzymatic dissolution of the organic matrix. In the process the enzyme-families cystineproteinases and MMPs are involved. Root cementum and dentin are also resorbed in apical periodontitis by fusion macrophages designated as odontoclasts. However, they belong to the same cell population as osteoclasts in view of their ultrastructural and histochemical similarities[246].

### Epithelial cells

About 50% of all apical lesions contain proliferating epithelium[82, 139, 194, 258, 268, 284, 319, 356]. The cell rests of Malassez[155] are believed to be stimulated by cytokines and growth factors released during apical inflammation to undergo division and proliferation. These cells participate in the pathogenesis of periapical cysts by serving as the source of epithelium. However, ciliated epithelial cells are also found in periapical lesion[196, 264] particularly in lesions affecting maxillary molars. The maxillary sinus-epithelium was suggested to be a source of those cells[193, 196].

### 9.4.2 Molecular mediators

The pathogenesis of apical periodontitis is the result of interaction among the cells described above and several molecular mediators belonging to *cytokines*[47], *eicosanoides*, *effector-molecules* and *antibodies.*

### Cytokines

They are low molecular weight (< 30 kDa) polypeptides or glycoproteins, secreted transiently by activated source-cells under various stimuli[71]. Cytokines are produced by a variety of haematopoietic and structural cells, having pleotropic effects on target cells in the regulation of immunological defense, inflammatory response, cellular growth and differentiation, tissue remodelling and repair. They act on multiple target cells with numerous effects (ambiguity of action) and structurally dissimilar cytokines may have overlapping spectrum of actions (redundancy). They function in a net-work fashion so as to increase or decrease the production of other cytokines. Most of the cytokines have functions with synergistic or antagonistic effects on the source-cell (autocrine) or other target cells (paracrine) in the nearby tissue. Spill over into general circulation with effects on distant cells (endocrine) are exceptional. One endocrine example is the role of IL-1 in the production of fever due to a bacterial infection. Cytokines are effective in very low concentrations (pg/ml) as they produce their actions by binding to high affinity cell surface receptors.

**Terminology.** The current knowledge on cytokines is evolved from various independent sources of research in immunology, virology, cell and molecular biology. Consequently, a unifying concept of cytokines has been slow-emerging and the terminology has been in a state of flux and confusion. Four decades ago when early evidence for the existence of intercellular mediators in supernatants of antigen-sensitized lymphocytes in culture were reported, they were designated on the basis of their biological effects. The terms *lymphokines* and *monokines* have been used to denote the products of lymphocytes and macrophages respectively. A decade later a plethora of eponyms existed for the monocyte and lymphocyte-derived activities. It also became evident that a large number of designations existed for the same biochemical molecule. This motivated a group of investigators at the Second International Lymphokine Workshop held at Interlaken/Switzerland in 1979 to propose the term *interleukin* (IL) to describe the molecular messengers acting between leukocytes. The names IL-1 and IL-2 were introduced for the two important molecules which until then had been known under various names. But IL is a restrictive term to designate the signal-molecules among leukocytes. A number of IL are, however, not only produced by non-haematopoietic cells but also affect the functions of diverse cells. Therefore, after a long period of negligence the term *cytokine*[47] has become the preferred collective designation for the cell regulatory proteins. Nevertheless, many cytokines continue to be designated as IL and many others remain to be known by their old designations based on historical names (interferons) or biological effects (cytotoxic factors, colony stimulating factors and certain growth factors).

**Proinflammatory & chemotactic cytokines.** They include interleukin (IL)-1, -6, -8 and tumor necrosis factors (TNF)[208]. The systemic effects of IL-1 are identical to those observed in toxic shock. Local effects include enhancement of leukocyte adhesion to endothelial walls, stimulation of lymphocytes, potentiation of neutrophils, activation of the production of prostaglandins and proteolytic enzymes, enhancement of bone resorption and inhibition of bone formation. IL-$1_{\beta}$ is the predominant form found in human periapical lesions and their exudates[13, 14, 143, 160]. IL-$1_{\alpha}$ is primarily involved in apical periodontitis in rats[313, 343]. IL-6 is produced by both lymphoid and non-lymphoid cells under the influence of IL-1, $TNF_{-\alpha}$ and IFN-γ [108]. It down-regulates the production and counters some of the effects of IL-1. IL-6 has been demonstrated in human periapical lesions[62] and in inflamed marginal periodontal tissues[355]. IL-8 is a family of chemotactic cytokines[61]. They are produced by monocyte/macrophages and fibroblasts under the influence of IL-$1_{\beta}$ and $TNF_{-\alpha}$. Massive infiltration of neutrophils is a characteristic of the acute phases of apical periodontitis for which IL-8 and other chemo-attractants such as bacterial-peptides, plasma-derived complement split-factor $C_{5a}$ and leukotriene $B_4$ are important. TNF has direct cytotoxic effects and general debilitating effects in chronic disease. In addition, the macrophage-derived $TNF_{-\alpha}$[332] and the T-lymphocyte-derived $TNF_{-\beta}$[239], formerly *lymphotoxin*, have numerous systemic and local effects similar to those of IL-1. The presence of $TNF_{-\alpha}$ has been reported in human apical periodontitis lesions and root canal exudates of teeth with apical periodontitis[12, 13, 245].

**Interferon (IFN).** It was originally described as an antiviral agent and is now classified as a cytokine. There are three distinct IFN designated as -α, -β and -γ molecules. The antiviral protein is the IFN-γ produced by virus-infected cells and normal T-lymphocytes under various stimuli whereas the $IFN_{-\alpha/\beta}$ proteins are produced by a variety of normal cells particularly macrophages and B-lymphocytes.

**Colony Stimulating Factors (CSF).** Another major group of cytokines that regulate the proliferation and differentiation of haematopoietic cells are the colony stimulating factors (CSF). The name originates from the early observation that certain polypeptide molecules promote the formation of granulocyte or monocyte colonies in semisolid medium. Three distinct proteins of this category have been isolated, characterized and designated as cytokines. They are (i) Granulocyte-Macrophage Colony Stimulating Factor (G-MCF), (ii) Granulocyte Colony Stimulating Factor (G-CSF) and (iii) Macrophage colony Stimulating Factor (M-CSF). In general, CSF stimulate the proliferation of neutrophil and osteoclast precursors in the bone marrow. They are also produced by osteoblasts[225] thus providing one of the communication links between osteoblasts and osteoclasts in bone resorption.

### Growth Factors

The term 'growth factor' refers to a naturally occurring signal protein capable of stimulating cellular proliferation and differentiation. Growth factor is often used interchangeably with the term cytokine. It is already stated that the latter is associated with hematopoitic and immune cells. This is logical for the circulatory system and bone marrow in which cells occur in a liquid suspension and not generally tied up in solid tissue, necessitating to communicate by soluble, circulating molecules. However, as research in various fields converged, it became clear that some of the same signaling proteins of the hematopoietic and immune systems are also used by all sorts of body cells, during growth and in maturity. Generally 'growth factor' implies a positive effect on cell division and 'cytokine' is a neutral term with respect to whether a molecule affects cell proliferation. Some cytokines can be growth factors as in the cases of G-CSF and GM-CSM. However, some other cytokines have an inhibitory effect on cell growth or proliferation. Certain other cytokines, such as the 'Fas ligand' signals programmed cell death or apoptosis.Therefore, growth factors are proteins that regulate the growth and differentiation of non-haematopoietic cells. *Transforming Growth Factors* (TGF) are produced by normal and neoplastic cells that were originally identified by their ability to induce non-neoplastic, surface adherent colonies of fibroblasts in soft agar cultures. This process appears to be similar to neoplastic transformation of normal to malignant cells and therefore the name TGF. Based on their structural relationship to the Epidermal Growth Factor (EGF) family, they are classified into $TGF_{-\alpha}$ and $TGF_{-\beta}$. The former is closely related to EGF in structure and effects but are produced primarily by malignant cells and therefore is not significant in apical periodontitis. But $TGF_{-\beta}$ is synthesized by a variety of normal cells and platelets and is involved in the activation of macrophages, proliferation of fibroblasts, synthesis of connectives tissue fibers and matrices, local angiogenesis, healing and down regulation of numerous functions of T-lymphocytes. Therefore, $TGF_{-\beta}$ is important to counter the adverse effects of inflammatory host response.

#### Eicosanoids

Eicosanoids are signalling molecules derived from injured cell membranes. Outer membranes of mammalian cells contain phospholipids. Some of these are polyunsaturated essential fatty acids, particularly arachidonic acid. In response to a variety of inflammatory signals, the arachidonic acid is cleaved out of the phospholipid to release free fatty acids. They are then oxygenated (by one of two pathways), further modified, to yield the eicosanoids or $C_{20}$ compunds (Greek: eicosi = twnty). The eicosanoides are thought of as paracrine mediators with physiological effects at very low concentrations. They mediate inflammatory response, regulate blood pressure, induce blood clotting, pain and fever, and control several reproductive functions such as ovulation and induction of labor. Prostaglandins (PG) and leukotrienes (LT)[250] are two major groups of eicosanoids involved in inflammation.

**Prostaglandins.** The name prostaglandin derives from the prostate gland. When prostaglandin was first isolated from human semen in 1935 by the Swedish physiologist Ulf von Euler, it was believed to be part of the prostatic secretions. It was later found that many other tissues secrete prostaglandins for various functions. Prostaglandins (e.g. $PGE_2$, $PGD_2$, $PGF_{2a}$, $PGI_2$) are formed when arachidonic acid is metabolized via the cyclooxygenase pathway. The $PGE_2$ and $PGI_2$ are potent activators of osteoclasts. Much of the rapid bone loss in marginal and apical periodontitis happens during episodes of acute inflammation when the lesions are dominated by PMN, which are an important source of $PGE_2$. High levels of $PGE_2$ have been shown to be present in acute apical periodontitis lesions[163]. Apical hard tissue resorption can be suppressed by parenteral administration of indomethacin, an inhibitor of cyclooxygenase[328].

**Leukotrienes.** Leukotrienes (e.g. $LTA_4$, $LTB_4$, $LTC_4$, $LTD_4$ and $LTE_4$) are formed when arachidonic acid is oxidized via the lipoxygenase pathway. LTB4 is a powerful chemotactic agent for neutrophils[207] and causes adhesion of PMN to the endothelial walls. $LTB_4$[329] and $LTC_4$[52] have been detected in apical periodontitis with a high concentration of the former in symptomatic lesions[329].

### 9.4.3 Effector-molecules

Degradation of extracellular matrices is one of the earliest histopathological changes that take place in apical periodontitis. The destruction of the matrices is caused by enzymatic effector-molecules. Four major degradation pathways have been recognized: (1) osteoclastic, (2) phagocytic, (3) plasminogen-dependent and (4) metallo-enzymes regulated.(27) These are are zinc-dependent endopeptidases belonging to the super family of enzymes called the matrix metalloproteinases (MMP). They degrade all kinds of extracellular matrix proteins. MMP are responsible for the degradation of much of the tissue matrices built on collagen, fibronectin, laminin, gelatin and proteoglycan-core-proteins. The biology of MMP has been extensively researched and reviewed[28, 29]. MMP have also been reported in apical periodontitis lesions[266, 316].

### 9.4.4 Antibodies

They are specific weapons of the body that are produced solely by plasma cells. Different classes of immunoglobulins have been found in plasma cells[118, 135, 176, 224, 279, 293] and extracellularly[135, 159, 181, 331] in human apical periodontitis.

The concentration of IgG in apical periodontitis was found to be nearly five times of that in non-inflamed oral mucosa[92]. Immunoglobulins have also been shown in plasma cells residing in the periapical cyst-wall[224, 281, 293, 324] and in the cyst-fluid[255, 278, 324, 359]. Their concentration in the cyst fluid was several times higher than that in blood[255, 278]. The specificity of the antibodies present in apical periodontitis may be low as LPS may act as antigens or mitogens. The resulting antibodies may be a mixture of both mono- and polyclonal varieties. The latter are non-specific to its inducer and therefore ineffective. However, the specific monoclonal component may participate in the antimicrobial response and may even intensify the pathogenic process by forming antigen-antibody complexes[328]. Intracanal application of an antigen against which the animal was immunized before resulted in the induction of a transient apical periodontitis[326].

## 9.5 Pathogenesis

The 'dynamic encounter' between the microbial and host factors at the periapex results in different categories of apical pathology (Fig. 9.1). The histological picture and the cellular composition of the lesions are determined at any particular time by the equilibrium at the periapex between the microbial and host factors.

### 9.5.1 Initial apical periodontitis

Sustaining inflammation of the periapex (apical periodontitis) is generally initiated by intracanal biofilms and microbes invading from the apical root canal into the periapical tissues (Fig. 9.6). It can also be induced by trauma, injury from instrumentation or irritation from chemicals and endodontic materials, each of which can provoke an intense tissue-response of short duration. The process is accompanied by pain, tooth elevation and tenderness to pressure on the tooth. Such initial, symptomatic lesions are viewed as the primary *acute apical periodontitis* (Fig. 9.1A). The tissue response is generally limited to the apical periodontal ligament and the neighboring spongiosa. They are initiated by typical neuro-vascular response of inflammation resulting in hyperaemia, vascular congestion, and edema of the periodontal ligament and extravasation of neutrophils. The latter are attracted to the area by chemotaxis, induced initially by tissue-injury, bacterial products (LPS) and complement-factor $C_{5a}$. As the integrity of bone, cementum and dentin has not yet been disturbed, the periapical changes at this stage are undetectable radiographically. If non-infectious irritants have induced inflammation, the lesion may subside and the structure of the apical periodontium may be restored[9].

If microbial infection has initiated the inflammation, the PMN not only attack the microbes (Fig. 9.7A) but also release leukotrienes and prostaglandins. The former ($LTB_4$) attracts more neutrophils and macrophages into the area and the latter activate osteoclasts. In a few days time the bone surrounding the periapex can be resorbed and a radiolucent area may become detectable at the periapex[289]. This initial rapid bone resorption can be prevented by indomethacin[326, 328] that inhibits cyclooxygenase, thus suppressing prostaglandin synthesis. Neutrophils die at the inflammatory site (Fig. 9.7A) and release enzymes from their cytoplasmic granules that cause destruction of the extracellular matrices and cells. The self-induced destruction of the tissues prevents the spread of infection to other parts of the body and provides space for the infiltration of specialized defense cells. During the acute phase, macrophages also appear at the periapex. Activated macrophages produce a variety of mediators among which the proinflammatory (IL-1, -6 and TNF-$\alpha$) and chemotactic (IL-8) cytokines are of particular importance. These cytokines intensify the local vascular response, osteoclastic bone resorption, effector-mediated degradation of the extracellular matrices and can place the body on a general alert by endocrine action so as to raise the output of acute phase proteins by hepatocytes[141]. They also act in concert with IL-6 to up-regulate the production of hematopoietic colony stimulating factors, which rapidly mobilize the neutrophils and the pro-macrophages from bone marrow. The acute response can be intensified, particularly in later stages, by the formation of antigen-antibody complexes[326, 328]. The acute primary apical periodontitis has several possible outcomes such as; spontaneous healing, intensification and spreading into the bone (alveolar abscess) or open to the exterior (fistulation or sinus tract formation). The lesion usually becomes chronic.

### 9.5.2 Development of chronic apical periodontitis (Granuloma)

Persistence of microbial irritants leads to a shift in the PMN-dominated lesion to a macrophage, lymphocyte and plasma cell rich one, encapsulated in a collagenous connective tissue. Such asymptomatic, radiolucent lesion can be visualized as a 'lull phase' following an intense phase in which PMN die *en mass*, the foreign intruders have been temporarily beaten and held back in the root canal (Fig. 9.9). The macrophage-derived proinflammatory cytokines (IL-1, -6; TNF-$\alpha$) are powerful lymphocyte stimulators. The quantitative data on the various types of cells residing in chronic periapical lesions may not be representative. Nevertheless, investigations based on monoclonal antibodies suggest a predominant role for T-lymphocytes and macrophages. Activated T-cells produce a variety of cytokines that down-regulate the output of proinflammatory cytokines (IL-1, -6 and TNF-$\alpha$), leading to the suppression of osteoclastic activity and reduced bone resorption. On the other hand, the T-cell derived cytokines may concomitantly up-regulate the production of connective tissue growth factors (TGF-$\beta$), with stimulatory and proliferative effects on fibroblasts and the microvasculature. $T_{h1}$ and $T_{h2}$ cell populations may participate in this process[290]. The option to down-regulate the destructive process explains the absence or retarded bone resorption and rebuilding of the collagenous connective tissue during the chronic phase of the disease. Consequently, the chronic lesions can remain 'dormant' and symptomless for long periods of time without major changes in the radiographic status. But the delicate equilibrium prevailing at the periapex can be disturbed by one or more factors that may favor the microorganisms stationed within the root canal. The microbes may advance into the periapex (Fig. 9.6) and the lesion spontaneously becomes acute with clinical manifestations (*Secondary acute apical periodontitis, Periapical exacerbation, Phoenix abscess*). As a result, microorganisms can be found extraradicularly during these acute episodes with rapid enlargement of the radiolucent area. This radiographic feature is due to apical bone resorption occurring rapidly during the acute phases with relative inactivity during the chronic periods. The progression of the disease, therefore, is not continuous, but happens in discrete leaps after periods of 'stability'.

Asymtomatic chronic apical periodontitis is also referred to as solid dental or periapical granuloma. Histopathologically the lesion consists of a granulomatous tissue with infiltrate cells, fibroblasts and a well-developed fibrous capsule. Serial sectioning shows[194] that about 45% of all chronic periapical lesions are epithelialized. When the epithelial cells begin to proliferate, they may do so in all directions at random forming an irregular epithelial mass in which vascular and infiltrated connective tissue becomes enclosed. In some lesions the epithelium may grow into the entrance of the root canal forming a plug-like seal at the apical foramen[156, 192, 284]. The epithelial cells generate an 'epithelial attachment' to the root surface or canal wall which in TEM reveals a basal lamina and hemidesmosomal structures[192]. In random histological sections the epithelium in the lesion appears as arcades and rings. The extraepithelial tissue predominantly consists of small blood vessels, lymphocytes, plasma cells and macrophages. Among the lymphocytes T-cells are likely to be more numerous than B-cells[53, 130, 204, 327] and $CD4^+$ cells may outnumber $CD8^+$ cells[14, 152, 158, 219] in certain phases of the lesions. The connective tissue capsule of the lesion consists of dense collagenous fibers that are firmly attached to the root surface so that the lesion may be removed *in toto* with the extracted tooth.

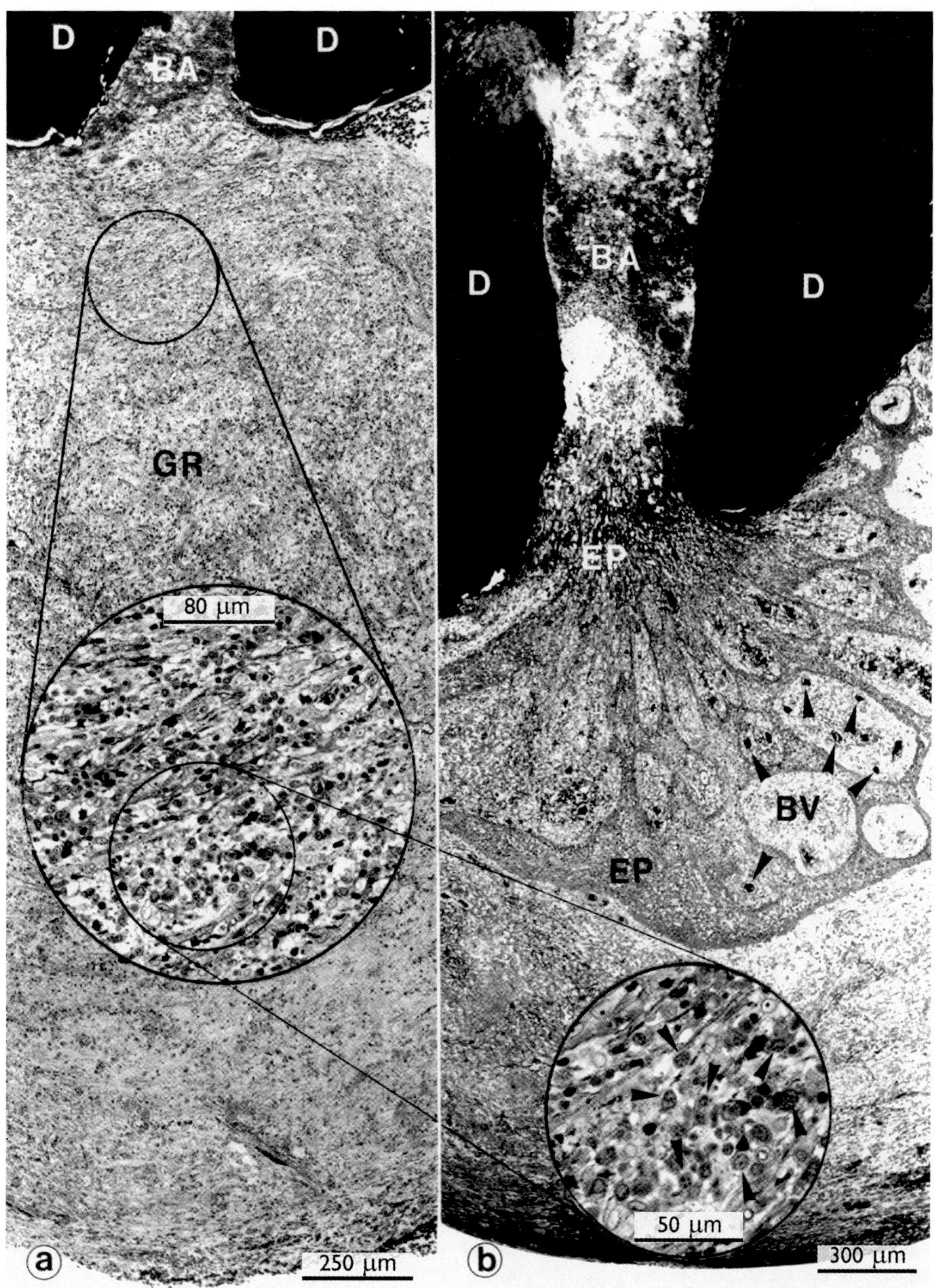


**Figure 9.9** - Chronic asymptomatic apical periodontitis without (**A**) and with (**B**) epithelium (EP). The root canal contains bacteria (BA in **A** and **B**). The lesion in (**A**) has no acute inflammatory cells, even at the mouth of the root canal with visible bacteria at the apical foramen (BA). Note the collagen-rich maturing granulation tissue (GR) infiltrated with plasma cells and lymphocytes (insets in **A** and **B**, D, Dentin; BV, blood vessels (**A** x80; **B** x60; inset in **A**, x250; inset in **B**, x400) (From Nair[183]).

### 9.5.3 Cystic transformation of apical periodontitis (Radicular cysts)

Periapical cysts are a sequel to chronic apical periodontitis. However, every chronic lesion does not develop into a cyst. Although the reported prevalence of cysts among apical periodontitis lesions varies from 6 to 55%[184] investigations based on meticulous serial sectioning and strict histopathological criteria[194, 268, 284] show that the actual prevalence of the cysts may be well below 20%. There are two distinct categories of radicular cysts namely, those containing cavities completely enclosed in epithelial lining (Fig. 9.10) and those containing epithelium-lined cavities that are open to the root canals (Fig. 9.11)[194, 268]. The latter was originally described as 'bay cysts'[268] and has been newly designated as 'periapical pocket cysts'[194]. More than half of the cystic lesions are apical true cysts and the reminder is apical pocket cysts[194, 268]. In view of the structural difference between the two categories of cysts, the pathogenic pathways leading to the formation of them may differ in certain respects.

#### True cyst

Many authors attempted to explain the pathogenesis of apical true cysts[86, 154, 232, 263, 315, 319, 325]. The formation of true cyst has been discussed as taking place in three stages[264]. During the first phase the dormant epithelial cell-rests [155, 156] are believed to proliferate, probably under the influence of growth factors[85, 145, 317] that are released by various cells residing in the lesion. During the second phase an epithelium-lined cavity comes into existence. The two long-standing theories regarding the formation of the cyst cavity are: (i) the 'nutritional deficiency theory' is based on the assumption that the central cells of the epithelial strands get removed from their source of nutrition and undergo necrosis and degeneration. The products in turn attract neutrophilic granulocytes into the necrotic area. Such microcavities containing degenerating epithelial cells, infiltrating leukocytes and tissue exudate coalesce to form the cyst cavity lined by stratified squamous epithelium, (ii) the 'abscess theory' postulates that the proliferating epithelium surrounds an abscess formed by tissue necrosis and lysis because of the innate nature of epithelial cells to cover exposed connective tissue surfaces. During the third phase, the cyst grows, the exact mechanism of which has not yet been adequately clarified. Theories based on osmotic pressure[117, 322, 323] have receded to the background in favor of a molecular basis for the cystogenesis[26, 36, 100, 101, 316]. The fact that apical pocket cyst (Fig. 9.11), with a lumen open to the necrotic root canal, can grow would eliminate osmotic pressure as a potential factor in the development of radicular cysts[183, 194]. Although no direct evidence is yet available, the tissue dynamics and the cellular components of radicular cysts suggest possible molecular pathways for cyst expansion. The neutrophils that die in the cyst lumen provide a continuous source of prostaglandins[79], which can diffuse through the porous epithelial wall[264] into the surrounding tissues. The cell population residing in the extraepithelial area contains numerous T-lymphocytes[327] and macrophages produce a battery of cytokines particularly the IL-$1_{\beta}$. The prostaglandins and the inflammatory cytokines can activate osteoclasts culminating in bone resorption. The presence of effector molecules (MMP-1 and -2) has also been reported in human periapical cysts[316].

#### Pocket cyst

The development of periapical pocket cyst is not yet well understood. It has been suggested to be initiated by the accumulation of PMN around the apical foramen in response to the microbial presence in the apical root canal[183, 194]. The microabscess can get enclosed by the proliferating epithelium, which on coming in contact with the root-tip forms an epithelial collar with 'epithelial attachment'[192]. The latter seals off the infected root canal with the microabscess from the periapical tissue milieu. When the externalized neutrophils die and disintegrate, the space occupied by them becomes a microcyst.

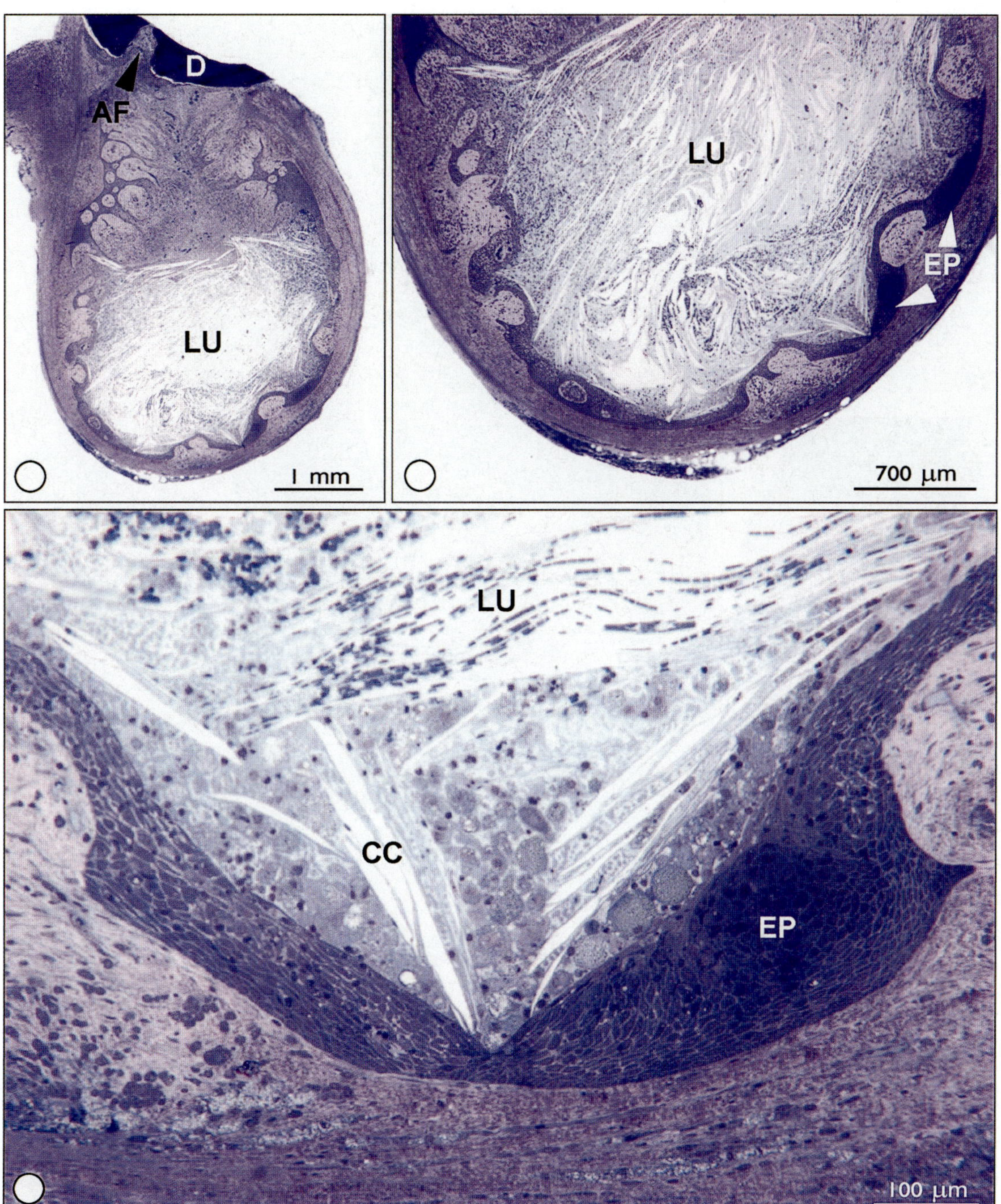


**Figure 9.10** - Structure of an apical true cyst. (**A**), Photomicrograph of an axial section passing through the apical foramen (AF). The lower half of the lesion and the epithelium (EP in **B**) are magnified in (**B** and **C**), respectively. Note the cystic lumen (LU) with cholesterol clefts (CC) completely enclosed in epithelium (EP), with no communication to the root canal. (**A** x15; **B** x30; **C** x180) (From Nair[187]).

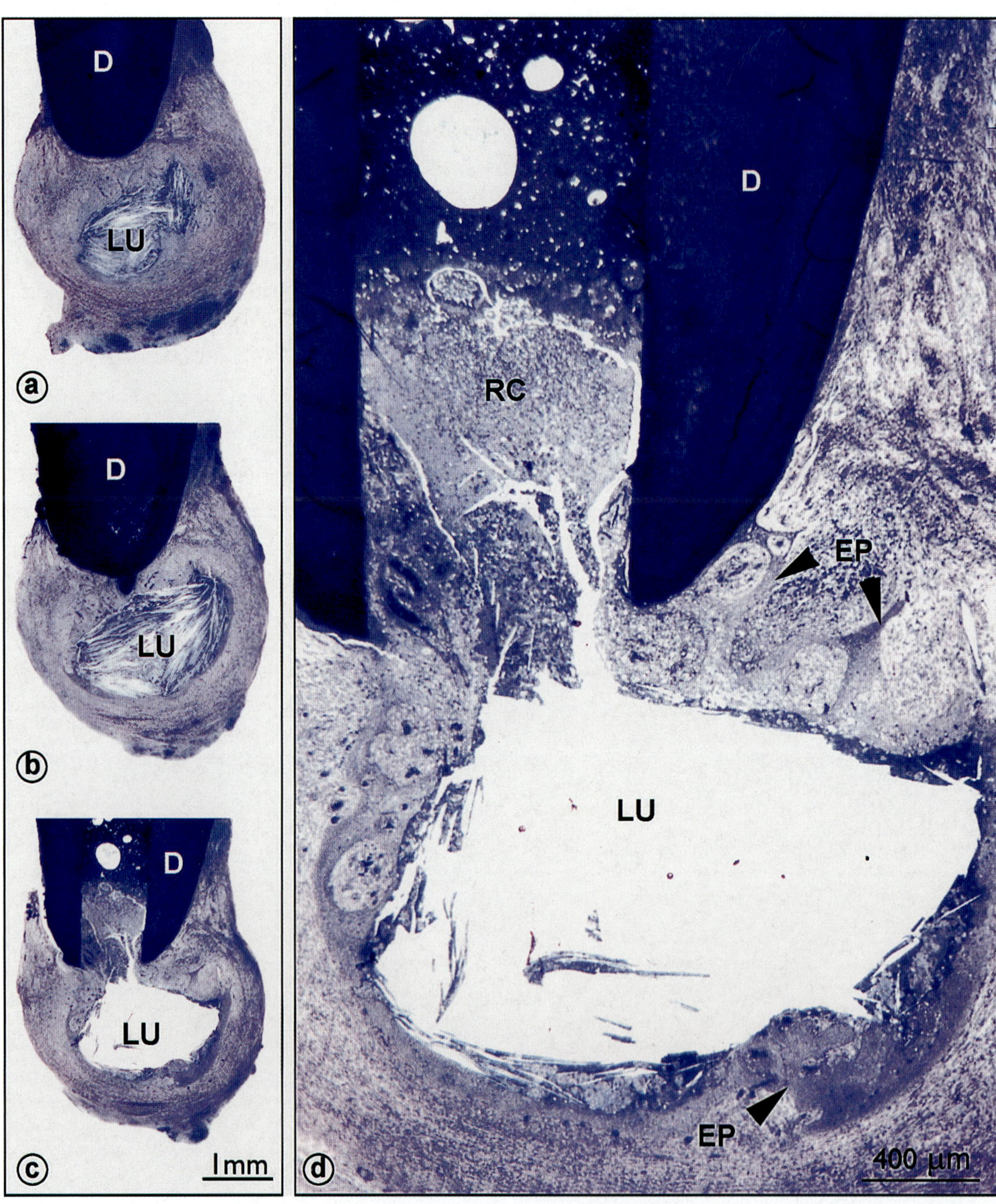


**Figure 9.11** - Structure of an apical pocket cyst. (**A** and **B**) Axial sections passing peripheral to the root canal give the false impression of a cystic lumen (LU) completely enclosed in epithelium. Sequential section (**C**) passing through the axial plane of the root canal clearly reveals the continuity of the cystic lumen (LU) with the root canal (RC in **D**). The apical foramen and the cystic lumen (LU) of the section (**C**) are magnified in (**D**). Note the pouchlike lumen (LU) of the pocket cyst, with the epithelium (EP) forming a collar at the root apex. D, Dentin. (**A-C** x15; **D** x50) (From Nair[187]).

The presence of biofilm in the apical root canal, their products and the necrotic cells in the cyst-lumen, attract more PMN by a chemotactic gradient. Because the pouch-like lumen is biologically outside the periapical milieu it acts as a 'death trap' to the transmigrating PMN. As the necrotic cells accumulate, the sac-like lumen enlarges and may form a voluminous diverticulum of the root canal space extending into the periapical area[183, 194]. Bone resorption and degradation of the matrices that are essential for the enlargement of the pocket cyst follow a similar molecular pathway as in the case of the true cyst[194]. From the pathogenic, structural, tissue dynamic and host-benefit points of view the pouch-like extension of the root canal space has much similarities with a periodontal pocket. These similarities are sufficient to justify the name of periapical pocket cyst[194].

## 9.6 Persistent Apical Radiolucencies (Endodontic failures)

Because intraradicular microorganisms are the essential etiological agents of apical periodontitis[119, 299], the treatment of apical periodontitis consists of eradicating the root canal microbes or substantially reducing the microbial load and preventing re-infection by orthograde obturation[200]. When root canal treatment is done properly, healing of the periapical lesion usually occurs with hard tissue regeneration, which is characterized by a gradual resolution of the radiolucency[91, 124, 171, 172, 257, 275, 276, 295, 296, 308]. Nevertheless, a complete healing of the periapex or reduction of the apical radiolucency may not occur in all root canal treated teeth. Such cases of non-resolving post-treatment periapical radiolucencies usually occur when treatment procedures have not reached a satisfactory standard for the control and elimination of infection. Inadequate aseptic control, poor access cavity preparation, missed canals, insufficient instrumentation, and leaking temporary or permanent fillings are common problems that may lead to post-treatment apical periodontitis[304]. Even when most careful clinical procedures are followed, apical periodontitis may persist in certain cases. This is because of the anatomical complexity of the root canal system[107, 217] with regions that cannot be debrided and obturated with existing technology[200]. In addition, there are causative factors located beyond the root canal system[77, 186, 187, 191, 199, 274], within the inflamed periapical tissue, that can interfere with post-treatment healing of the lesion, including compromising host factors associated with certain systemic disease such as diabetes[80].

### 9.6.1 Microbial causes

#### *9.6.1.1 Intraradicular and apical biofilm*

Microscopic investigation of periapical tissues removed by surgery has been a method to detect potential etiological agents of failures in root canal treated teeth. Historical investigations[10, 30, 139, 144, 259] of apical biopsies had several limitations such as the use of unsuitable specimens, inappropriate methodology and criteria of analysis. Therefore, these studies did not yield relevant information about the reasons for apical periodontitis persisting as asymptomatic radiolucencies even after proper orthograde root canal treatment.

A histological analysis[259] of apical specimens of failed cases, there was not even a mention of persisting microbial infection as a potential cause of the failures. An investigation[10], using serial step sectioning and special bacterial stains, found bacteria in the root canals of 14% of the[66] specimens examined. Two other studies[30, 139] analysed 230 and 35 endodontic surgical specimens, respectively, by routine paraffin histology. Although bacteria were found in 10% and 15% of the respective biopsies, only in a single specimen, in each study, intraradicular infection was detected. In the remaining biopsies in which bacteria were found, the data also included those specimens in which bacteria were found as "contaminants on the surface of the tissue". In yet another study[144] "bacteria and or debris" was found in the root canals of 63% of the 86 endodontic surgical specimens, although it is obvious that 'bacteria and debris' cannot be equated as etiological agents in endodontic treatment failures. The reported low incidence of intraradicular infections in these studies is mainly due to a methodological inadequacy as microorganisms often go undetected when the investigations are based on random paraffin sections alone. This has been convincingly demonstrated[182, 201]. Consequently, early studies on teeth with non-healing apical lesions did not consider residual intracanal infection as a major factor that prevented healing.

For the identification of the etiological agents of persistent apical periodontitis by microscopy, the cases must be selected from teeth that have had the best possible orthograde root canal treatment and the radiographic lesions remain asymptomatic till surgical intervention. The specimens must be anatomically intact block-biopsies that include apical portion of the roots and the inflamed soft tissue of the lesions. Such specimens should undergo meticulous investigation by serial or step-serial sections that are analyzed using correlative light and transmission electron microscopy. A study that met these criteria and also did microbial monitoring before and during treatment[201] *revealed intracanal microorganisms in six of the nine block biopsies* (Fig. 9.12). The finding conclusively show that the majority of root canal treated teeth evincing asymptomatic apical periodontitis harbor persistent infection in the apical portion of the complex root canal system. However, the proportion of failed cases with intraradicular infection is likely to be much higher in routine endodontic practice than the two third of 9 cases reported[201] because of several reasons. At the light microscopic level it was possible to detect bacteria in only one of the six cases[201]. Microorganisms were found as biofilm located within small canals of apical ramifications of the root canal (Fig. 9.12) or in the space between the root fillings and the canal wall. Obviously conventional paraffin technique is inadequate to detect infections in apical tissue specimens.

Whether the apical root canal system contain microbes immediately after orthograde endodontic treatment has been of great interest. In a very recent study, it has been shown that 14 of the 16 instrumented and root canal-treated mandibular molars showed residual infection of mesial roots when the treatment was completed in one-visit during which instrumentation, irrigation with NaOCl and obturation were done. The infectious agents were mostly located in the uninstrumented recesses of the main canals, isthmus communicating them and accessory canals. The microbes in such untouched locations existed primarily as biofilms that were not removed by instrumentation and irrigation with NaOCl. In view of the great anatomical complexity of the root canal system, particularly of molars[107, 217], and the ecological organization of the flora into protected sessile biofilms[49, 51] composed of microbial cells embedded in a hydrated exopolysaccharide-complex in micro-colonies[182], it is very unlikely that an absolutely microorganism-free canal-system can be achieved by any of the contemporary root canal preparation, cleaning and root filling procedures. Then the question arises as to why a large number of apical lesions heal after conventional root canal treatment. It has been shown that some periapical lesions heal even when infection persists in the canals at the time of root filling[276]. Although this may imply that the organisms may not survive post-treatment, it is more likely that the microbes may be present in quantities and virulence that may be sub-critical to sustain the inflammation of the periapex[200]. In some cases the residual microbes can delay or prevent periapical healing as was probably was the case with six of the nine biopsies studied[201].

Based on the ultrastructure, only Gram-positive bacteria were found (Fig. 9.13), an observation fully in agreement with the results of purely microbiological investigations of root canals of previously root filled teeth with persisting periapical lesions. Of the six specimens that contained intraradicular infections, four had one or more morphologically distinct types of bacteria and two revealed yeasts (Fig. 9.14).

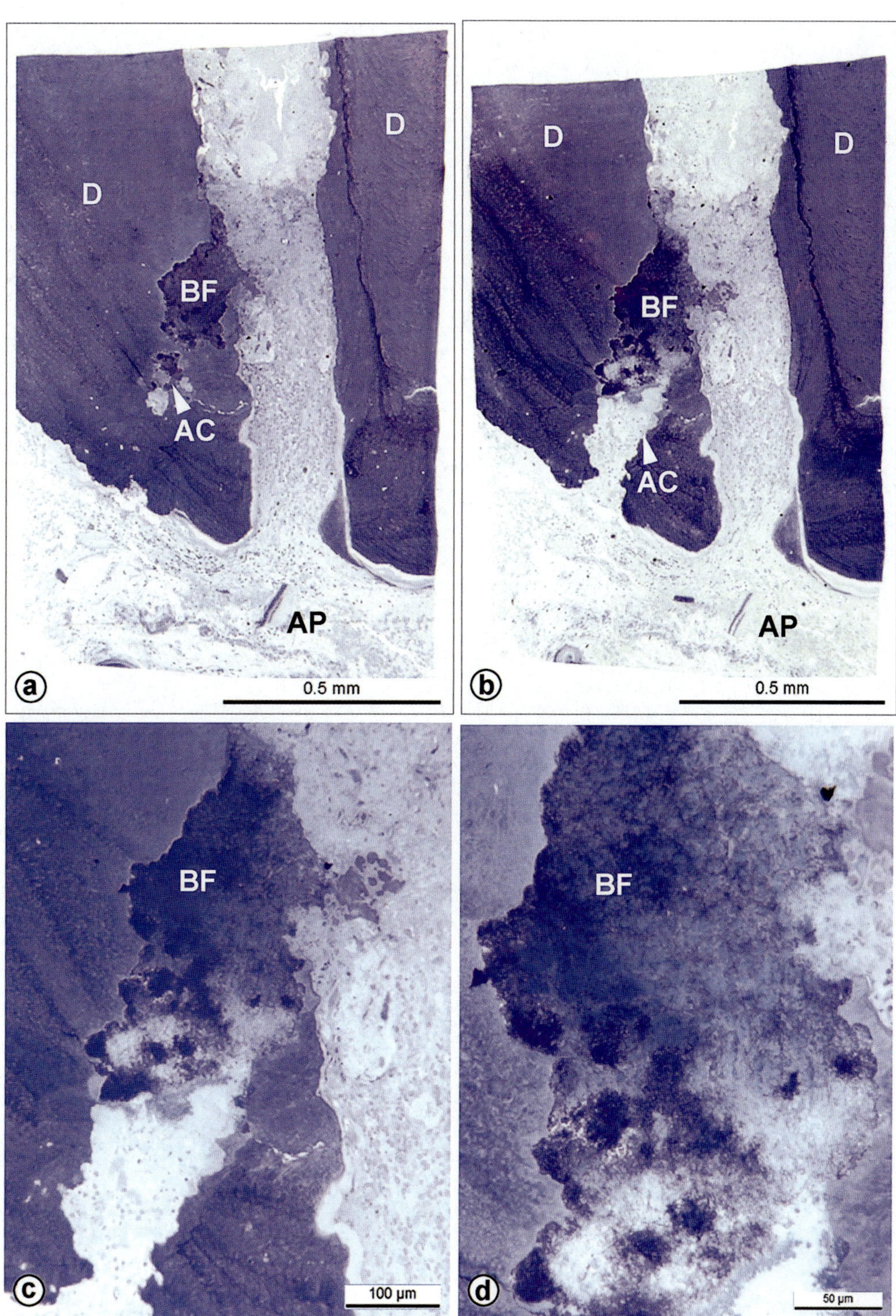


**Figure 9.12** - Photomicrographs of axial semithin sections through the surgically removed apical portion of the root with a persistent apical periodontitis. Note the adhesive biofilm (BF) in the root canal. Consecutive sections (**A** to **B**) reveal the emerging widened profile of an accessory canal (AC) that is clogged with the biofilm. The AC and the biofilm are magnified in (**C** and **D**) respectively. Magnifications: **A** x75, **B** x70, **C** x110, **D** x300 (Adapted from Nair et al. [201]).

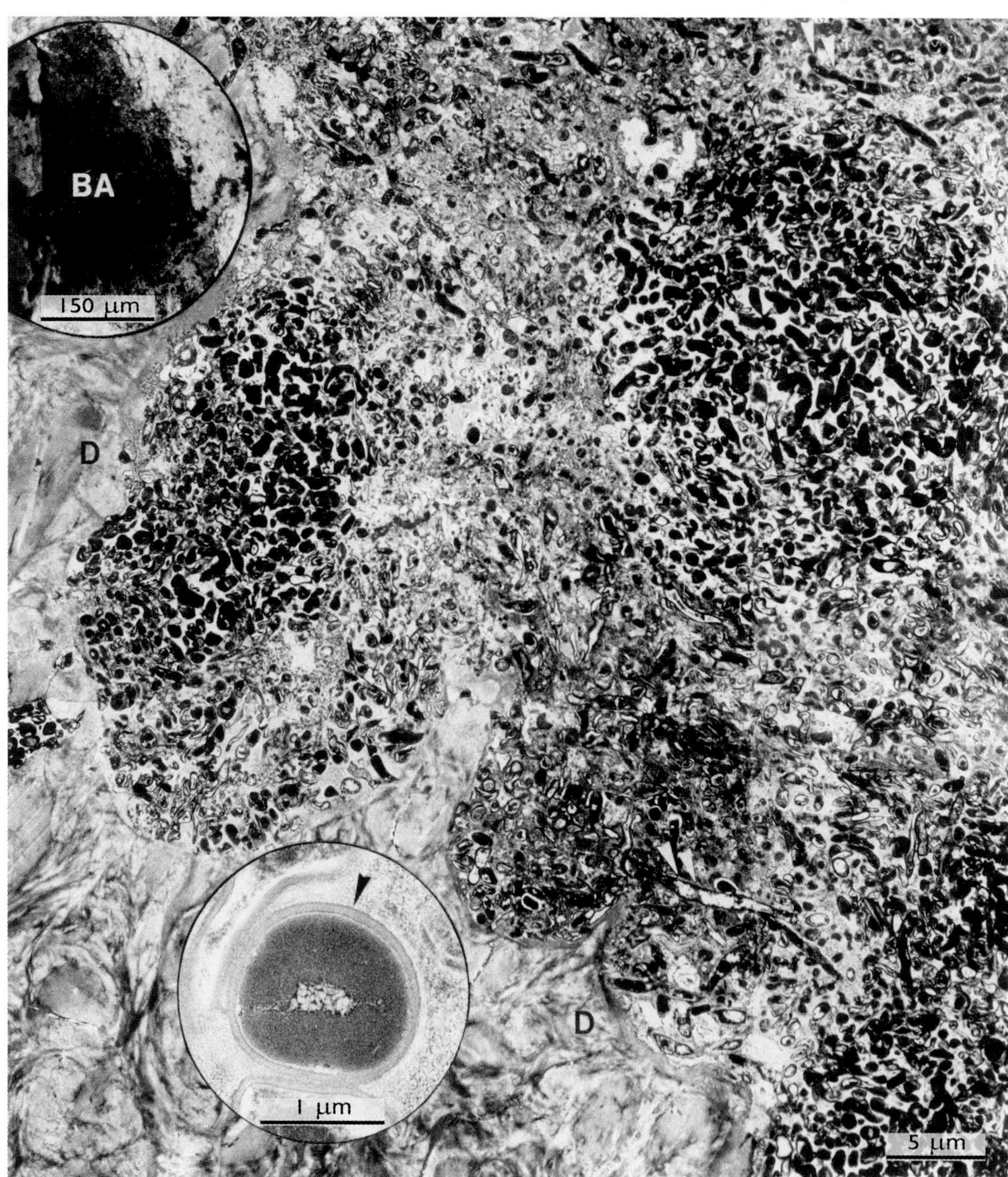


**Figure 9.13** - Composite transmission electron micrographs of the biofilm (BA, upper inset) illustrated in Figure 9.12. The bacterial population is composed of only Gram-positive, filamentous organisms (arrowhead in lower inset). Note the distinctive Gram-positive cell wall. The upper inset is a light microscopic view of the biofilm (BA). Magnifications: x3400; insets: upper x135, lower x21,300 (From Nair et al.[201]).

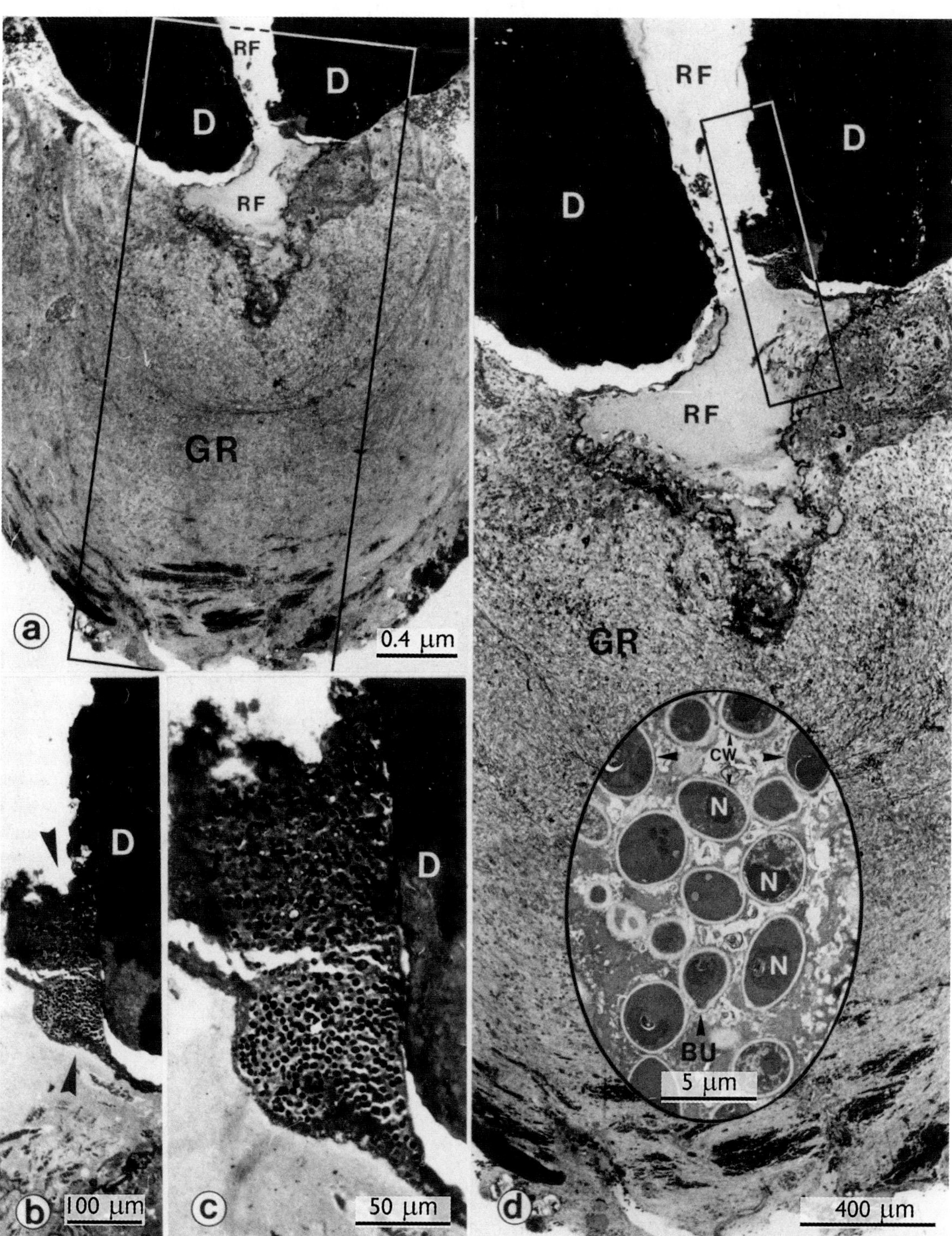


**Figure 9.14** - Fungi as a potential cause of endodontic failures. (**A**). Low-power overview of an axial section of a root-filled (RF) tooth with a persisting apical periodontitis lesion (GR). The rectangular demarcated areas in **A** and **B** are magnified in **C** and **D**, respectively. Note the two microbial clusters (arrowheads in **B**) further magnified in **C**. The oval inset in D is a transmission electron microscopic view of the organisms. Note the electron-lucent cell wall (CW), nuclei (N) and budding forms (BU). Magnifications: **A** x35, **B** x130, **C** x330, **D** x60, oval inset x3400 (Adapted from Nair et al.[201]).

The presence of intracanal fungi in root treated teeth with apical periodontitis was also confirmed by microbiological techniques[214, 340]. These findings clearly associate *intraradicular fungus* as a potential non-bacterial, microbial cause of endodontic failures.

It has been suggested that infection can also remain within dentinal tubules that serves as a reservoir for endodontic reinfection that might interfere with periapical healing[150, 151, 179, 218, 267, 336]. It must be pointed out that the idea provides disproportionate importance to tubular microbes as against those in the complex canal system. Tubular infection is restricted to the inner third of radicular dentine. A substantial portion of the tubular microbes are removed by instrumentation and irrigation. Further, dentinal tubules are far less numerous in apical parts of the root dentine and are also mostly occluded in mature and aging patients. On the other hand, the canal system in the apical area, particularly of posterior teeth, is very complex. Most of the microbes remaining in the complex canal system are not only inaccessible to conventional instrumentation[200] but also for medicaments and devices such as endodontic lasers.

The microbiology of treated canals is lesser understood than that of untreated infected necrotic dental pulps. This may be due to the search for non-microbial causes of a purely technical nature for the failure of root canal treatments[304]. Only a small number of species has been found in the root canals of teeth that have undergone proper endodontic treatment that, on follow-up, revealed persisting, asymptomatic periapical radiolucencies. The bacteria found in these cases are predominantly Gram-positive cocci, rods and filaments. By culture-based techniques, species belonging to the genera *Actinomyces*, *Enterococcus* and *Propionibacterium* (previously Arachnia) are frequently isolated and characterized from such root canals[84, 96, 97, 168, 169, 220, 274, 303, 308]. The presence of *Enterococcus faecalis* in cases of post-treatment apical periodontitis is of particular interest because it is rarely found in infected but untreated root canals[304] *E. faecalis* is the most consistently reported organism from former cases, with a prevalence ranging from 22% to 77% of cases analyzed[81, 96, 168, 169, 213, 220, 271, 308]. The organism is resistant to most of the intracanal medicaments, and can tolerate[40] a pH up to 11.5, which may be one reason as to why this organism survives antimicrobial treatment with calcium hydroxide dressings[22]. The latter is probably by virtue of its ability to regulate internal pH with an efficient proton pump[70]. E. faecalis can survive prolonged starvation[76]. It can grow as monoinfection in treated canals in the absence of synergistic support from other bacteria[72]. Therefore, *E. faecalis* is held to be a very recalcitrant microbe among the potential etiological agents of post-treatment apical periodontitis. However, the presence of *E. faecalis* in cases of post-treatment apical periodontitis is not a universal observation. This is because one microbial culture[44] and a molecular based[234] study, in which the presence of *E. faecalis* in such cases was investigated, failed to detect the organism. Further, the prevalence of *E. faecalis* is found to be 22% and 77% respectively of cases analyzed by two molecular techniques[81, 271]. In this context the long reported correlation between the prevalence of enterococci in root canals of primary and retreatment cases and that in other oral sites, such as gingival sulcus and tonsils, of the same patients, is worth noting[68]. It has been suggested that enterococci may be opportunistic organisms that populate exposed root-filled canals from elsewhere in the mouth[81]. Therefore, in spite of the current focus of attention, it still remains to be shown, in controlled studies, that *E. faecalis* is the pathogen of significance in most cases of failing endodontic treatment[188].

Conventional microbiological methods[169, 340] and correlative electron microscopic[201] studies have shown the presence of yeasts (Fig. 9.14) in canals of root filled teeth with non-healing apical lesions. *Candida albicans* is the frequently identified fungus from root filled teeth with apical periodontitis[168, 308].

**Apical biofilm (Periapical plaque)** It is biofilm adherent to the root tip of pulp infected teeth with apical lesions. In an anatomical and semantic sense it is extraradicular in location and has been confused with the presence of microbes within the inflamed periapical tissue[229, 333] commonly referred to as extraradicular microbes (see further below). Biologically, those two conditions are different entities and should be distinguished from each other. The periapical plaque is an outgrowth or extension of intraradicular microbes spreading as adhesive biofilm around the root tip. Therefore, it is biologically part of the intraradicular flora. The apical biofilm or plaque, being tooth-adherent, is also protected from host defences. Presence of such apical biofilm (apical plaque) is fully compatible with the concepts of (1) intraradicular microbes as the major etiological agent of persisting apical periodntitis and (2) microbes do not generally live and propagate within solid granulomas (exception: actinomycosis).

#### *9.6.1.2 Extrararadicular microbes*

##### *9.6.1.2.1 Actinomycosis*

Actinomycosis is a chronic, granulomatous, infectious disease in humans and animals caused by the genera *Actinomyces* and *Propionibacterium*[162]. The etiological agent of bovine actinomycosis, *Actinomyces bovis*, was the first species to be identified[103]. The disease in cattle, known as 'lumpy jaw' or 'big head disease', is characterized by extensive bone rarefaction, swelling of the jaw, suppuration and fistulation. The causative agents were described as non-acid fast, non-motile, Gram-positive organisms revealing characteristic branching filaments that end in clubs or hyphae. Because of the morphological appearance these organisms were considered fungi and the taxonomy of *Actinomyces* remained controversial for more than a century. The intertwining filamentous colonies are often called "sulphur granules" because of their appearance as yellow specks in exudates. On careful crushing, the tiny clumps of branching microorganisms with radiating filaments in pus, give a "starburst appearance" which prompted Harz[103] to coin the name *Actinomyces* or 'ray fungus'. Four years later *Actinomyces israelii* was isolated from humans in pure culture, characterized and its pathogenicity in animals demonstrated[353]. Many researchers, nevertheless, considered the human and bovine isolates as identical. However, *A. bovis* and *A. israelii* are now classified as two distinct bacterial species and in natural infections the former is restricted to animals and the later to humans.

Human actinomycosis is clinically divided into cervicofacial, thoracic and abdominal forms. About 60% of the cases occur in the cervicofacial region, 20% in the abdomen and 15% in the thorax[121, 209]. The most species isolated from humans is *A. israelii*[353], which is followed by *Propionibacterium propionicum*[37], *Actinomyces naeslundii*[321], *Actinomyces viscosus*[113] and *Actinomyces odontolyticus*[15] in descending order.

Periapical actinomycosis (Fig. 9.15) is a cervicofacial form of actinomycosis. The endodontic infections are generally a sequel to caries. *A. israelii* is a commensal of the oral cavity and can be isolated from tonsils, dental plaque, periodontal pockets and carious lesions[303]. Most of the publications on periapical actinomycosis are case reports and have been reviewed[35, 157, 191, 247, 249, 345]. Although periapical actinomycosis is considered to be rare[191], it may not be so infrequent[115, 173, 247]. The data on the frequency of periapical actinomycosis among apical periodontitis lesions are scarce. A microbiological control study revealed actinomycotic involvement in 2 of the 79 endodontically treated cases[41]. A histological analysis showed the presence of characteristic actinomycotic colonies (Fig. 9.15) in two of the 45 investigated lesions[191]. An identification and etiological association of the species involved can be established only through laboratory culturing[303] of the organisms, molecular techniques and by experimental induction of the lesion in susceptible animals[77]. However, the strict growth requirements of *A. israelii* make isolation in pure culture difficult. A histopathological diagnosis has generally been reached on the basis of demonstration of typical colonies[191] and by specific immunohistochemical staining of such colonies[98, 303]. Today, an unequivocal identification of the organism can be achieved by molecular methods. The characteristic light microscopic feature of an actinomycotic colony is the presence of an intensely dark staining, Gram and PAS positive, core with radiating peripheral filaments (Fig. 9.15) that gives the typical "star burst" or "ray fungus" appearance. Ultrastructurally[77, 191], the center of the colony consists of a very dense aggregation of branching filamentous organisms held together by an extracellular matrix (Fig. 9.15). Several layers of PMN usually surround an actinomycotic colony.

Because of the ability of the actinomycotic organisms to establish extraradicularly, they can perpetuate the inflammation at the periapex even after orthograde root canal treatment. Therefore, periapical actinomycosis is important in endodontics[97, 98, 191, 199, 274, 303]. *A. israelii* and *P. proprionicum* are consistently isolated and characterized from the periapical tissue of teeth, which did not respond to proper conventional endodontic treatment[97, 274]. A strain of *A. israelii*, isolated from a case of failed endodontic treatment and grown in pure culture, was inoculated into subcutaneously implanted tissue cages in experimental animals. Typical actinomycotic colonies were formed within the experimental host tissue. This would implicate *A. israelii* as a potential etiological factor of failed endodontic treatments. *Actinomyces* have been shown to posses hydrophobic cell surface property, Gram-positive cell wall surrounded by a fuzzy outer coat through which fimbriae-like structures protrude[75]. These may help the cells to aggregate into cohesive colonies[77]. The properties that enable these bacteria to establish in the periapical tissues are not fully understood, but appear to involve the ability to build cohesive colonies that enables them to escape host defense system[77]. *P. propionicum* is known to be pathogenic and associated with actinomycotic infections. But the mechanism of pathogenicity of the organism has not yet been explained.

##### *9.6.1.2.2 Non-actinomyces microbes in inflamed periapical tissue*

Periapical inflammation has been viewed as a defense enclosure against invasion of microorganisms into periradicular tissues[134, 183]. It is, therefore, possible that microorganisms invade extraradicular tissues during expanding and exacerbating phases of the disease. Based on histological investigations[99] there has been a consensus of opinion that 'solid granuloma' may not harbor infectious agents within the inflamed periapical tissue. Nevertheless, microbes are consistently detected in the periapical tissue of cases with clinical signs of exacerbation, abscesses and draining sinuses. This has been substantiated by modern correlative light and transmission electron microscopic techniques[182].

Two decades ago, there was some renewed interest in the idea of extraradicular microbes in apical periodontitis[116, 333, 334, 344] with the suggestion that extraradicular infections are the cause of many failed endodontic treatments. It was further argued that such cases would not be amenable to orthograde root canal treatment and would need apical surgery and/or systemic medications. Several species of bacteria have been reported to be present at extraradicular locations of lesions described as "asymptomatic periapical inflammatory lesions...refractory to endodontic treatment"[334]. However, 5 of the 8 patients had "long-standing fistulae to the vestibule..."[334], a clear sign of abscessed apical periodontitis draining by fistulation. Obviously the microbial samples were obtained from periapical abscesses that always contain microbes and not from asymptomatic periapical lesions persisting after proper endodontic treatment. Other publications also show serious problems. In one[116], the 16 periapical specimens studied were collected "during normal periapical curettage, apicectomy or (during the procedure of) retrograde filling".

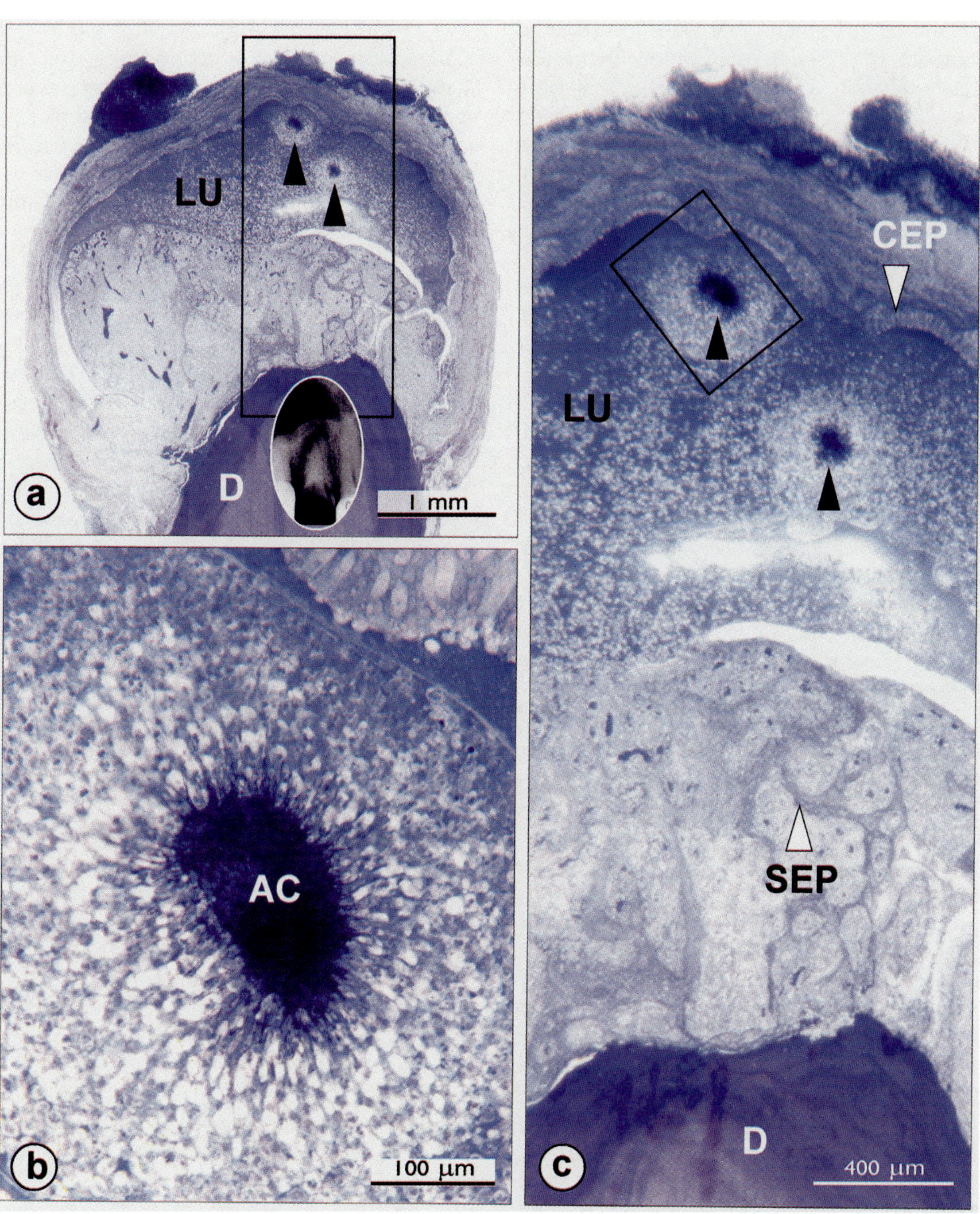


**Figure 9.15** - An actinomyces infected periapical pocket cyst affecting a human maxillary first premolar (radiographic inset). The cyst is lined with ciliated columnar (CEP) and stratified squamous (SEP) epithelia. The rectangular block in (**A**) is magnified in (**C**). The typical "ray-fungus" type of actnomycotic colony (AC in **B**) is a magnification of the one demarcated in (**C**). Note the two black arrow-headed, distinct actinomycotic colonies (AC in **C**) within the lumen (LU). Original magnifications: **A** x20, **B** x60, **C** x210 (From P.N.R. Nair et al. Oral Surg Oral Med Oral Pathol Oral Radiol Endod 94: 485-493, 2002).

Of the 58 specimens that were investigated in another[344], "29 communicated with the oral cavity through vertical root fractures or fistulas". Further, the specimens were obtained during routine surgery and were "submitted by seven practitioners". An appropriate methodology is essential and in these studies[116, 334, 344] unsuitable cases were selected for investigation or the sampling was not performed with the utmost stringency needed to avoid bacterial contamination[169].

Contamination of periapical samples is generally considered to occur from the oral cavity and other extraneous sources. Even if such 'extraneous contaminations' are avoided, contamination of periapical tissue samples with microbes from the infected root canal remains a serious problem. This is because microorganisms generally live at the apical foramen of teeth affected in both the primary[182, 221, 342] and post-treatment apical periodontitis[199, 201]. Microbes can be easily dislodged from this location during apical surgery and the sampling procedures. Tissue samples so contaminated with *intraradicular* microbes may be reported positive for the presence of an *extraradicular* infection. This is most likely the reason for the repeated reporting of microbes in the periapical tissue of asymptomatic post-treatment lesions by culture[2, 297] and molecular techniques[87, 298] even if strict aseptic sampling procedures could have been used.

As discussed before, the molecular techniques, in spite of the sophistication and high sensitivity, are less suitable to solve the problem of extraradicular infection[189, 190]. Apart from the unavoidable contamination of the samples with intraradicular microbes, molecular genetic analysis: (1) does not differentiate between viable and non-viable organisms, (2) does not distinguish between microbes and their structural elements in phagocytes from extracellular microorganisms in periapical tissues and (3) exaggerates the findings by PCR amplification.

#### *9.6.1.2.3 Viruses*

A virus (Latin: virus = toxin or poison) is an ultramicroscopic particle that infect and live in the cells of a biological organism. It can replicate only by infecting a host cell and cannot reproduce on its own. Lately several publications[241-244] reported the presence of certain viruses in inflamed periapical tissues with the suggestion of an etio-pathogenic relationship to apical periodontitis. The claims about possible viral involvement in endodontic failures were quickly consolidated in a review article even before some of the original works appeared in print[280]. Understandably the investigations were not supported by proper controls because it is almost impossible to provide controls for such observations. This is because the reported viruses are present in almost all humans from previous primary infections. Therefore, the possibility that such latent viruses may be activated by periapical inflammatory process cannot be excluded.

In conclusion, extraradicular infections occur in: (i) exacerbating apical periodontitis lesions[182], (ii) periapical actinomycosis[97, 98, 191, 274, 303] (iii) association with pieces of infected root dentine that may be displaced into the periapex during root canal instrumentation[111, 360] or having been cut off from the rest of the root by massive apical resorption[140, 336] and (iv) infected periapical cysts, particularly in periapical pocket cysts with cavities open to the root canal[182, 194, 199]. These situations are compatible[22, 183] with the long-standing and still valid idea that solid granuloma generally do not harbor microorganisms. Therefore, the aim of treatment of persistent apical periodontitis should be the biofilms[200] located in the complex apical root canal system.

### 9.6.2 Non-microbial causes

#### *9.6.2.1 Cystic lesions*

The issue of healing of periapical cysts after conventional root canal treatment has been long-standing. Surgeons are of opinion that cysts do not heal and have to be removed by surgery. Many endodontists, hold the view that majority of cysts heals after root canal treatment. This controversy is probably an outcome of the reported high prevalence of cysts among apical lesions and the reported high 'success rate' of root canal treatments. There have been several studies on the prevalence of radicular cysts among human apical periodontitis (Table 9.2). The prevalence of cysts among apical lesions varies from 6% to 55%. Apical periodontitis cannot be differentially diagnosed into cystic and non-cystic lesions based on radiographs alone[16, 24, 136, 146, 175, 223, 228, 339]. A correct histopathological diagnosis of periapical cysts is possible only through serial sectioning or step-serial sectioning of the lesions removed *in toto* as has been convincingly shown in a recent study correlating the presence of a radiopaque lamina with histological findings[228]. The vast discrepancy in the reported prevalence of periapical cysts is probably due to the difference in the interpretation of the sections. Histopathological diagnosis based on random or limited number of serial sections, usually leads to wrong categorization of epithelialized lesions as radicular cysts. This was clearly shown in a study using meticulous serial sectioning (194) in which an overall 52 % of the lesions (n = 256) were found to be epithelialized but only 15% were actually periapical cysts. In routine histopathological diagnosis, the structure of a radicular cyst in relation to the root canal of the affected tooth



**Table 9.2** - The prevalence of radicular cysts among apical periodontitis lesions

| Reference | Cysts | Granuloma | Others | Total lesions |
|---|---|---|---|---|
| | % | % | % | n |
| Sommer & Kerr (1966)[283] | 6 | 84 | 10 | 170 |
| Block et al. (1976)[30] | 6 | 94 | - | 230 |
| Sonnabend & Oh (1966)[284] | 7 | 93 | - | 237 |
| Winstock (1980)[351] | 8 | 83 | 9 | 9804 |
| Linenberg, et al. (1964)[146] | 9 | 80 | 11 | 110 |
| Wais (1958)[339] | 14 | 84 | 2 | 50 |
| Patterson et al. (1964)[212] | 14 | 84 | 2 | 501 |
| Nair et al. (1996)[194] | 15 | 50 | 35 | 256 |
| Simon (1980)[268] | 17 | 77 | 6 | 35 |
| Stockdale & Chandler (1988)[294] | 17 | 77 | 6 | 1108 |
| Lin et al.(1991)[144] | 19 | - | 81 | 150 |
| Nobuhara & Del Rio (1993)[205] | 22 | 59 | 19 | 150 |
| Baumann & Rossman (1956)[16] | 26 | 74 | - | 121 |
| Mortensen et al. (1970)[175] | 41 | 59 | - | 396 |
| Bhaskar (1966)[24] | 42 | 48 | 10 | 2308 |
| Spatafore et al. (1990)[287] | 42 | 52 | 6 | 1659 |
| Lalonde & leubke (1968)[137] | 44 | 45 | 11 | 800 |
| Seltzer et al. (1967)[259] | 51 | 45 | 4 | 87 |
| Priebe et al. (1954)[223] | 55 | 45 | - | 101 |

has not been taken into account. As apical biopsies obtained by curettage do not include root-tips of the diseased teeth, structural reference to the root canals of the affected teeth is not possible. Histopathological diagnostic laboratories and publications based on retrospective reviewing such histopathological reports sustain the notion that nearly half of all apical periodontitis are cysts.

A 'success rate' of 85 to 90% has been reported by endodontic investigators[124, 275, 292]. But, the histological status of a radiographic lesion at the time of treatment is unknown to the clinician who is also unaware of the differential diagnosis of the 'successful' and 'failed' cases. Nevertheless, a great majority of the cystic lesions should heal to account for the 'high success rate' after endodontic treatment and the reported 'high histopathological incidence' of radicular cysts. As orthograde endodontic treatment removes much of the infectious material from the root canal and prevents reinfection by obturation, a periapical pocket cyst (Fig. 9.11) may heal after conventional endodontic therapy[194, 198, 268]. But a true cyst (Fig. 9.10) is *self-sustaining*[198] by virtue of its tissue dynamics and independence of the presence or absence of irritants in the root canal[268].

The structural difference between apical true cysts and pocket cysts has therapeutic significance. The aim of the root canal treatment is the elimination of canal-infection and prevention of reinfection by root filling. Periapical pocket cysts, particularly the smaller ones, may heal after root canal therapy[268]. A true cyst is *self-sustaining* as the lesion is no longer dependent on the presence or absence of root canal infection[194, 268]. Therefore, the true cysts, particularly the large ones, are less likely to be resolved by non-surgical root canal treatment. This has been reported in a long-term radiographic follow-up (Fig. 9.16) of a case and subsequent histological analysis of the surgical block-biopsy[198].

It can be argued that the prevalence of cysts in post-treatment apical periodontitis should be substantially higher than that in primary apical periodontitis. However, this remains to be clarified by research based on a statistically reliable number of specimens. Limited investigations[198, 199, 201] on 16 histologically reliable block biopsies of post-treatment apical periodontitis revealed 2 cystic specimens (13%), which is well above the 9% of true cysts observed in a large study[194] on mostly primary apical periodontitis lesions. The two distinct histological categories of periapical cysts and the low prevalence of cystic lesions among apical periodontitis would *question the rationale* of certain diagnostic and therapeutic practices such as: (i) routine histopathological examination of periapical lesions removed by curettage which may not provide relevant diagnostic information (neoplasia?) but only satisfies certain health-care formalities, (ii) application of apical surgery based on unfounded radiographic diagnosis of apical lesions as cysts, and (iii) the notion that majority of cysts heal after root canal treatment. As cysts can sustain post-treatment apical periodontitis, the option of apical surgery should be considered, particularly when previous attempts at orthograde retreatment have not resulted in healing[187].

#### *9.6.2.2 Cholesterol crystals*

Cholesterol[314] is a steroid lipid that is present in all animal cells. Excess blood level of cholesterol is suspected to play a role in arteriosclerosis as a result of its deposition in the vascular walls[357, 358]. Deposition of cholesterol crystals in tissues and organs can cause ailments such as otitis media and the "pearly tumor" of the cranium[7]. Cholesterol clefts have long been observed to in apical periodontitis lesions. But the etiological significance of the observation to failed root canal treatment has not been fully appreciated[185]. Accumulation of cholesterol crystals in apical lesions[24, 34, 198, 263, 335] has clinical significance in endodontics[184, 198]. In histopathological sections, such deposits of cholesterol appear as narrow elongated clefts because the crystals dissolve in fat solvents used for the tissue processing and leave behind the spaces they occupied as clefts (Fig. 9.17).

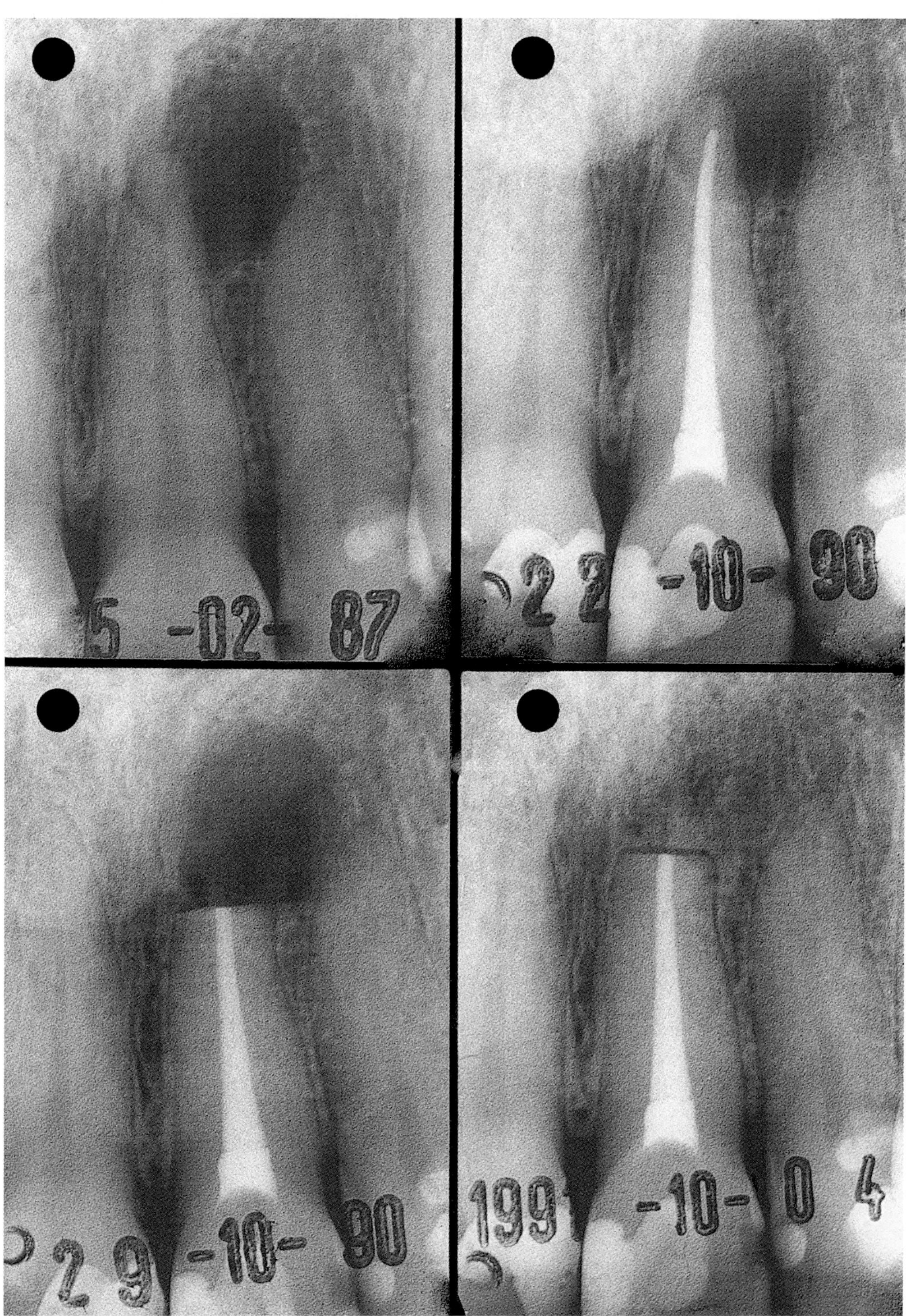


**Figure 9.16** - Longitudinal radiographs (**A**-**D**) of a periapically affected central maxillary incisor of a 37 year old woman for a period of 4 years and 9 months. Note the large radiolucent asymptomatic lesion before (**A**), 44 months after root-filling (**B**), and immediately after periapical surgery (**C**). The periapical area shows distinct bone healing (**D**) after 1 year post-operatively. Histopathological examination of the surgical specimen by modern tissue processing and step-serial sectioning technique confirmed that the lesion was a true radicular cyst that also contained cholesterol clefts (Selected radiographs from Nair et al.[198]).

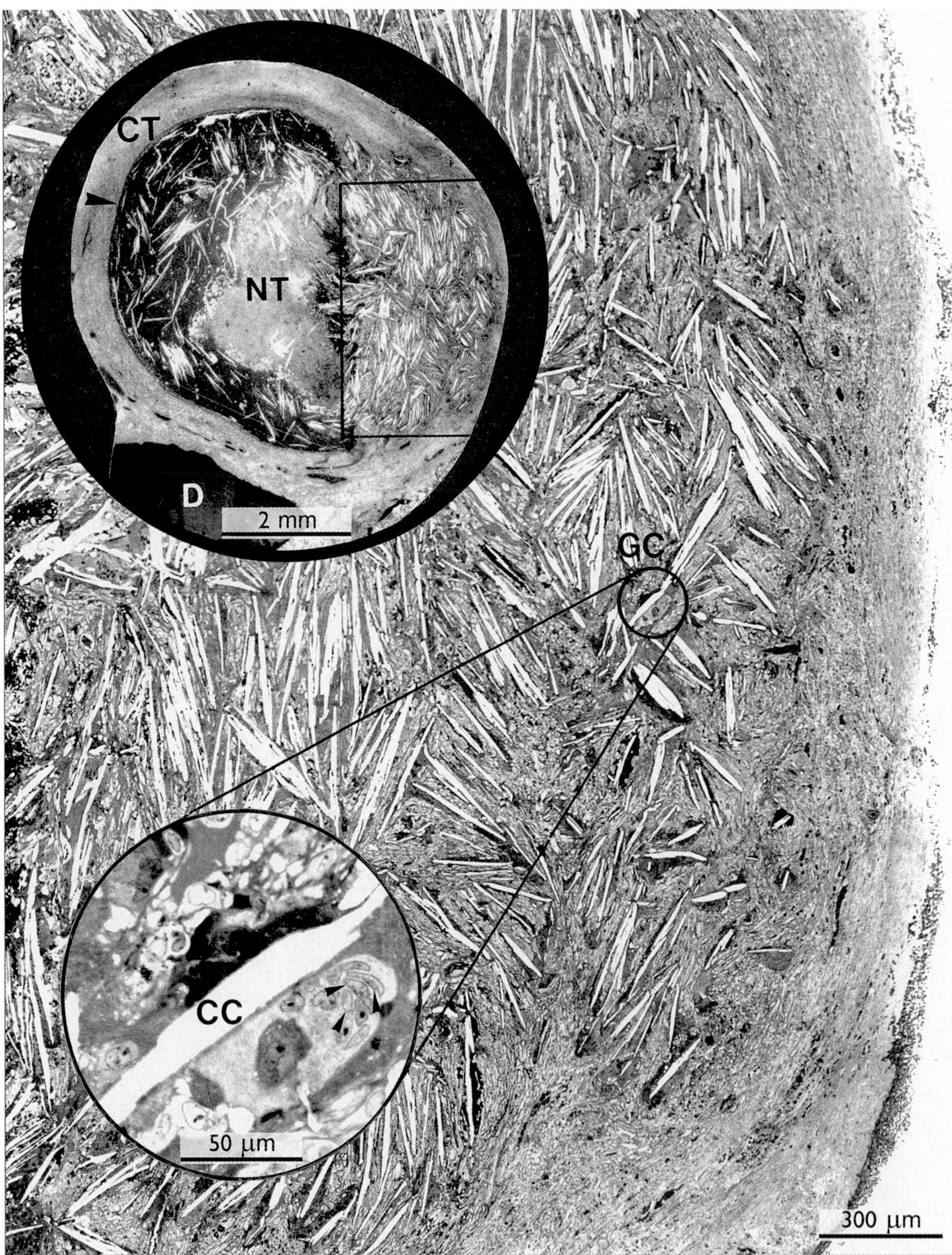


**Figure 9.17** - Cholesterol crystals and cystic condition of apical periodontitis as potential causes for endodontic failures. Overview of a histological section (upper inset) of an asymptomatic apical periodontitis that persisted after conventional root canal treatment. Note the vast number of cholesterol clefts (CC) surrounded by giant cells (GC) of which a selected one with several nuclei (arrowheads) is magnified in the lower inset. D = dentine, CT = connective tissue, NT = necrotic tissue. Magnifications: x68; upper inset x11; lower inset x412 (From Nair[185]).

The incidence of cholesterol clefts in apical periodontitis varies from 18% to 44% of such lesions[34, 263, 335]. The crystals are believed to be formed from cholesterol released by, (i) disintegrating erythrocytes of stagnant blood vessels within the lesion[34], (ii) lymphocytes, plasma cells and macrophages which die in great numbers and disintegrate in chronic periapical lesions, and (iii) the circulating plasma lipids[263]. All these sources may contribute to the concentration and crystallization of cholesterol in periapical area. Nevertheless, locally dying inflammatory cells may be the major source of cholesterol as a result of its release from disintegrating membranes of such cells in long-standing lesions[198, 256].

Cholesterol crystals are hydrophobic and intensely sclerogenic[1, 20]. They induce granulomatous lesions in dogs[46], mice[1, 4, 5, 20, 286] and rabbits[109, 285, 286]. In an experimental study that investigated the association of cholesterol crystals and non-resolving apical periodontitis lesions[195], pure cholesterol crystals were placed in Teflon cages that were implanted subcutaneous in guinea pigs. The cage contents were retrieved after 2, 4 and 32 weeks of implantation and processed for light and electron microscopy. The cages revealed delicate soft connective tissue that grew in through perforations on the cage wall. The crystals were densely surrounded by numerous macrophages and multinucleate giant cells forming a well circumscribed area of tissue reaction (Fig. 9.18). The cells, however, were unable to eliminate the crystals during an observation period of eight months. The accumulation of macrophages and giant cells around cholesterol crystals suggests that the crystals induced a typical foreign-body reaction[48, 197, 273].

Although macrophages and giant cells surround cholesterol crystals, they are not only unable to degrade the crystalline cholesterol. Further these cells are major sources of apical inflammatory and bone resorptive mediators. Bone resorbing activity of cholesterol-exposed macrophages due to enhanced expression of IL-$1_{\alpha}$ has been experimentally shown[277]. Accumulation of cholesterol crystals in apical periodontitis lesions (Fig. 9.17) can adversely affect post-treatment healing of the periapical tissues as has been shown in a long-term longitudinal follow-up of a case in which it was concluded that "the presence of vast numbers of cholesterol crystals ... would be sufficient to sustain the lesion indefinitely"[198]. The evidence from the general literature reviewed[185] is clearly in support of that assumption. Therefore, accumulation of cholesterol crystals in apical periodontitis lesions can prevent healing of periapical tissues after conventional root canal treatment. This is because root-filling retreatment cannot remove the tissue irritating cholesterol crystals within the inflamed periapical tissues.

### *9.6.2.3 Foreign bodies*

Foreign materials trapped in periapical tissue during and after endodontic treatment[131, 197] can perpetuate apical periodontitis persisting after root canal treatment. Endodontic clinical materials[131, 197] and certain food particles[269] can reach the periapex, induce a foreign body reaction that appears radiolucent and remain asymptomatic for several years[197].

#### Gutta-percha

Gutta-percha cone is the most frequently used root canal sealant in orthograde obturation of root canals. It is widely held to be biocompatible and well tolerated by human tissues. That view, however, is not consistent with the clinical observation that extruded gutta-percha is associated with delayed healing of the periapex[124, 197, 257, 275, 296]. It has been experimentally shown in guinea pigs that large pieces of gutta-percha are well encapsulated in collagenous capsules, but fine particles of gutta-percha induce an intense, localized tissue response (Fig. 9.19), characterized by the presence of macrophages and giant cells[273]. The congregation of macrophages around the fine particles of gutta-percha is important for the clinically observed impairment in the healing of apical periodontitis when teeth are root filled with excess.

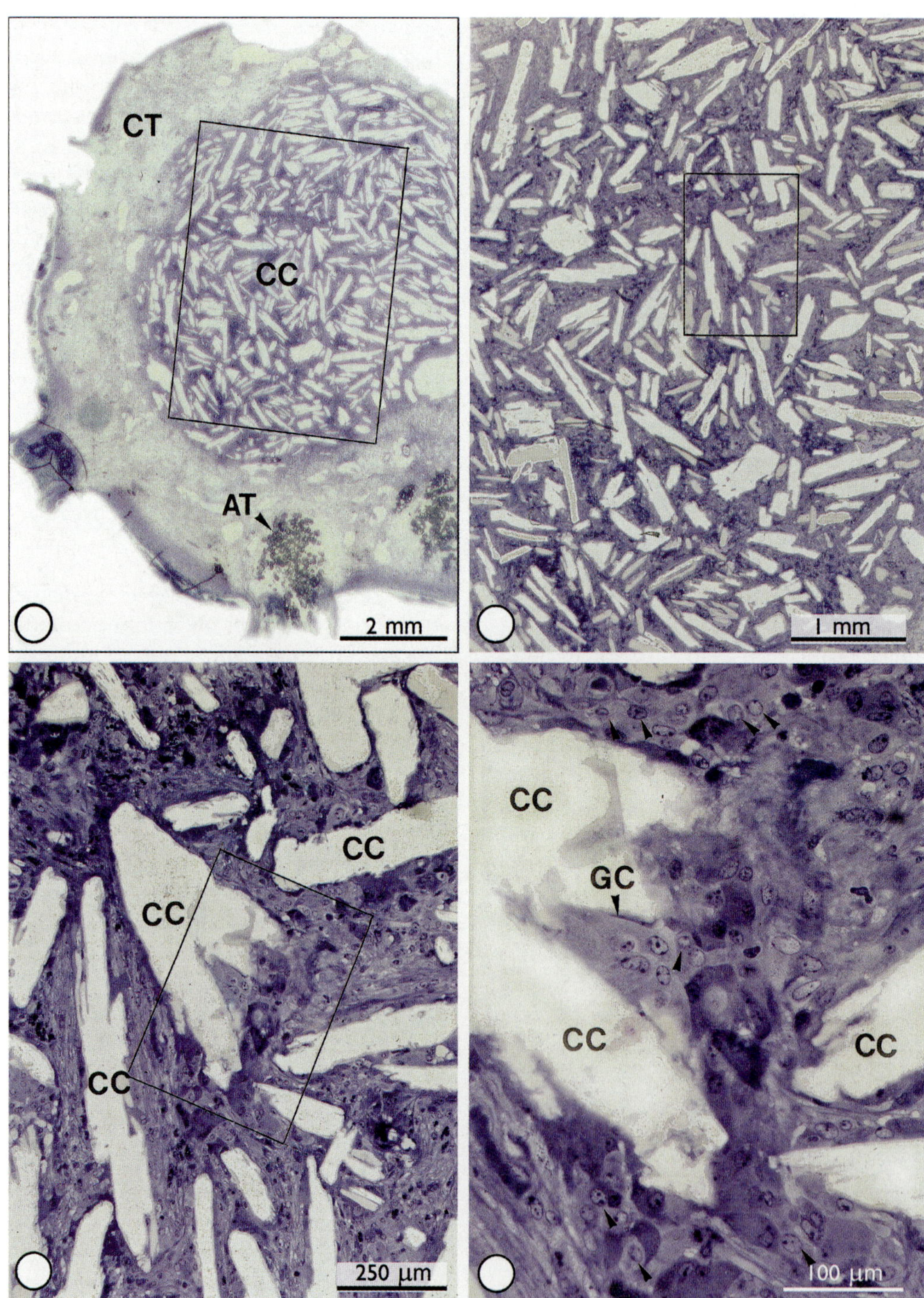


**Figure 9.18** - Photomicrograph (**A**) of guinea pig tissue reaction to aggregates of cholesterol crystals after an observation period of 32 weeks. The rectangular demarcated areas in **A**, **B** and **C** are magnified in **B**, **C** and **D** repectively. Note that rhomboid clefts left by cholesterol crystals (CC) surrounded by giant cells (GC) and numerous mononuclear cells (arrowheads in **D**). AT = adipose tissue, CT = connective tissue. Magnifications: **A** x10, **B** x21, **C** x82 and **D** x220 (From Nair.[185]).

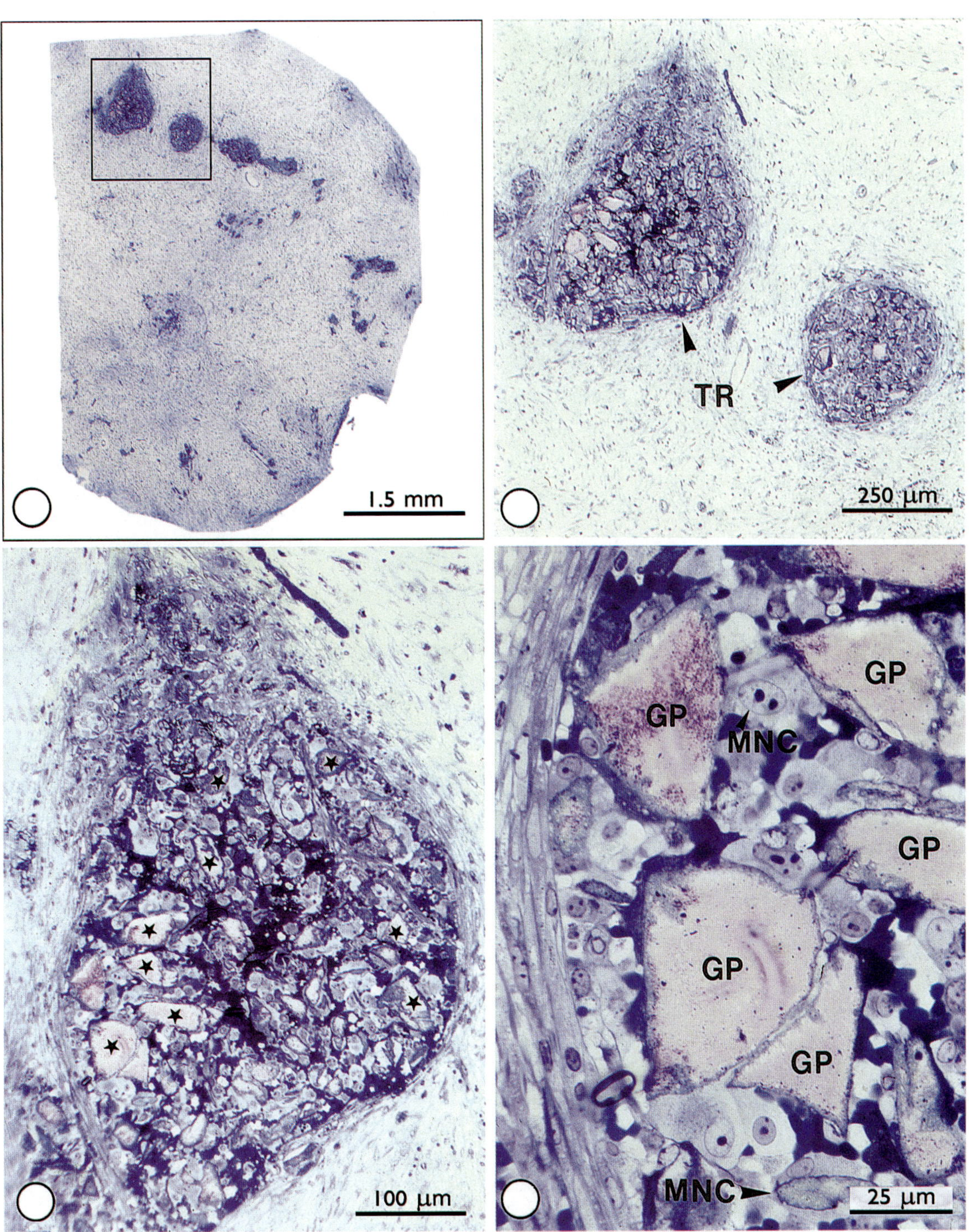


**Figure 9.19** - Disintegrated gutta-percha as potential cause of post-treatment apical periodontitis. As clusters of fine particles (**A**) they induce intense circumscribed tissue reaction (TR) around. Note that the fine particles of gutta-percha (* in **C**, GP in **D**) are surrounded by numerous mononuclear cells (MNC). Original magnifications: **A** x20, **B** x80, **C** x200, **D** x750 (From Nair.[186]).

Gutta-percha cones contaminated with tissue irritating materials can induce a foreign body reaction at the periapex. In an investigation on nine asymptomatic apical periodontitis lesions that were removed as surgical block biopsies and analyzed by correlative light and electron microscopy, one biopsy revealed the involvement of contaminated gutta-percha[197]. The radiolucency grew in size but remained asymtomatic for a decade of post-treatment follow-up. The lesion was characterized by the presence of vast numbers of multinucleate giant cells with birefringent inclusion bodies (Fig. 9.20). In transmission electron microscope the birefringent bodies were highly electron dense. An X-ray microanalysis of the inclusion bodies using scanning transmission electron microscope (STEM) revealed the presence of magnesium and silicon. These elements are presumably the remnants of a talc-contaminated gutta-percha that protruded into the periapex and had been resorbed during the follow-up period.

### Other plant materials

Food particles of plant origin such as leguminous seeds (pulses), and endodontic clinical materials of plant origin can get lodged in the periapical tissue before and/or during endodontic treatment and cause treatment failures. *Oral pulse granuloma* is a distinct histopathological entity[126]. The lesions are also referred to as the giant cell hyaline angiopathy[67, 126], vegetable granuloma[102] and food-induced granuloma[32]. Pulse granuloma has been reported in lungs[104], stomach walls and peritoneal cavities[265]. Experimental lesions have been induced in animals by intratracheal, intraperitonial and submucous introduction of leguminous seeds[128, 311]. Periapical pulse granuloma are associated with teeth damaged by caries and with the antecedence of endodontic treatment[269, 312]. Pulse granuloma are characterized by the presence of intensely iodine and PAS positive hyaline rings or bodies surrounded by giant cells and inflammatory cells[167, 269, 311, 312]. Leguminous seeds are the most frequently involved vegetable food material in such granulomatous lesions. This indicates that certain components in pulses such as antigenic proteins and mitogenic phytohaemaagglutinins may be involved in the pathological tissue response[128]. The pulse granuloma are clinically significant because particles of vegetable food materials can reach the periapical tissue via root canals of teeth exposed to the oral cavity by trauma, carious damage or by endodontic procedures[269].

**Cellulose granuloma** are apical periodontitis developing against particles of predominantly cellulose-containing materials that are used in endodontic practice[132, 133, 254, 346]. The cellulose in plant materials is a granuloma-inducing agent[128]. Endodontic *paper points* (Fig. 9.21) are utilized for microbial sampling and drying of root canals. Sterile and medicated *cotton wool* has been used as an apical seal. Particles of these materials can dislodge or get pushed into the periapical tissue[346] so as to induce a foreign body reaction at the periapex. The resultant clinical situation may be a "prolonged, extremely troublesome and disconcerted course of events"[346]. Presence of cellulose fibers in periapical biopsies with a history of previous endodontic treatment has been reported[132, 133, 254]. The endodontic paper points and cotton wool consists of cellulose that cannot be degraded by human body cells. They remain in tissues for long periods of time[254] and induce a foreign body reaction around them. The particles, in polarized light, are birefringent due to the regular structural arrangement of the molecules within cellulose[133]. Infected paper points can protrude through the apical foramen (Fig. 9.21) and allow a biofilm to grow around it. This will sustain and even intensify the apical periodontitis post-treatment.

### Other foreign materials

Amalgam, endodontic sealants and calcium salts derived from periapically extruded $Ca(OH)_2$ are often found in persitent apical lesions. In a histological and X-ray microanalytical investigation of 29 apical biopsies 31% of the specimens were found to contain materials compatible with amalgam and endodontic sealer components[131].

#### 9.6.2.4 Periapical scar

Persistent apical radiolucencies may occasionally be due to healing of the lesion by scar tissue[24, 199, 215, 259] that may be misdiagnosed as a radiographic sign of failed endodontic treatment (Fig. 9.22). The tissue dynamics of periapical healing after conventional root canal treatment and periapical surgery is unknown. However, the data available on normal healing and guided regeneration of the marginal periodontium suggest that several types of cells participate in the healing process. The pattern of healing depends on two decisive factors. They are the regeneration potential and the speed with which the tissue cells bordering the defect react[122, 123, 206, 252]. A scar healing is likely to follow when precursors of soft connective tissue colonize both the root tip and periapical tissue. If such cell seeding happens before the appropriate cells with the potential to restore various structural components of the apical periodontium, scar tissue development occurs at the periapex[199].

## 9.7 Persistent Post-surgical Radiolucencies

Radiolucencies can persist after surgical treatment of the disease. Apical surgery covers various procedures. It can include one or a combination of periapical curettage, apicectomy and retrograde filling. However, before apical surgery is attempted on a tooth with persistent apical lesions, a careful consideration of the potential causes is necessary. Teeth wit persistence of radiolucencies associated with substandard endodontic procedures respond well with proper retreatment of the root canal. However, for cases in which a root canal retreatment is unlikely to result in periapical healing, or such treatment may not be possible, periapical surgery should be the preferred clinical procedure to follow. Works on the outcome of apical surgery have been extensively reviewed[83, 226]. The reported success rates of apical surgery range from 25% to 95%[226, 361]. This disparity is attributed to differences in methods and criteria for evaluation of success[226]. Methods include several aspects such as selection of appropriate cases, surgical procedures, period of follow-up, sample size and so on. It is recognized that a large number periapical surgery is performed on cases in which such treatment is not justified[3]. Well-defined case selection and skilled application of 'state of the art' surgical techniques resulted in a success rate of 91% after periapical surgery[361]. Nevertheless, a small % of surgically treated cases may not show hard tissue healing of the periapex even after proper case selection and skilled surgical procedures. Albeit the classical histological attempts of the pioneers[237, 238], the reasons for post-surgically persistent radiographic lesions are currently unknown. In order to identify the potential causative agents of asymptomatic post-surgical apical radiolucencies by microscopy, the cases must be selected from teeth that have had proper orthograde root canal treatment, good coronal restoration, the best possible surgical treatment and the radiographic lesions remain asymptomatic. Further, the surgical specimen must be anatomically intact (block-biopsies) that include certain length of the apical portion of the previously surgerized roots and the radiolucent lesions. Only such specimens should be selected and undergo investigation. Meticulous serial or step-serial sections should be prepared and analyzed using correlative light and transmission electron microscopy as has been done for apical lesions persisting after conventional root canal treatment[201]. Studies meeting these criteria is not yet available.

In brief, to identify the reasons for post-surgical failures in endodontics, the problem must be investigated in a scientific manner. Evaluating radiographs, analysis of literature on prognostic studies, or surveying epidemiological type of investigations are unlikely to yield meaningful results. Rigorous analysis denotes investigating well-documented cases by careful and painstaking correlative light and transmission electron microscopy.

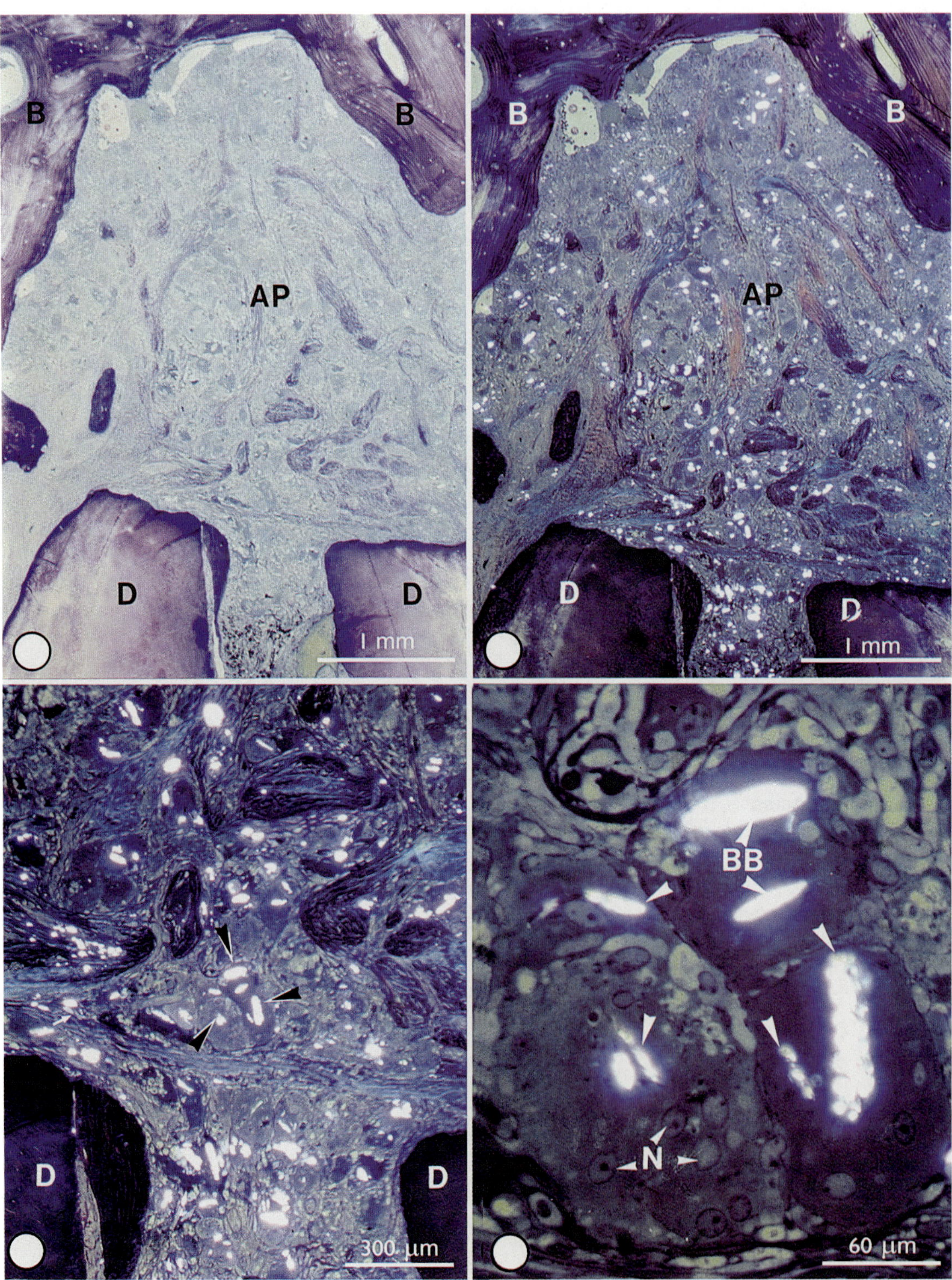


**Figure 9.20** - Talc contaminated gutta percha as a potential cause of endodontic failure. Note the apical periodontitis (AP) characterized by foreign-body giant cell reaction to gutta-percha cones contaminated with talc (**A**). The same field when viewed in polarized lights (**B**). Note the birefringent bodies distributed throughout the lesion (**B**). The apical foramen is magnified in (**C**) and the dark arrow-headed cells in (**C**) are further enlarged in (**D**). Note the birefringence (BB) emerging from slit-like inclusion bodies in multinucleated (N) giant cells. B, bone; D, dentin. (Magnifications: **A**, **B** x25; **C** x66; **D** x300).

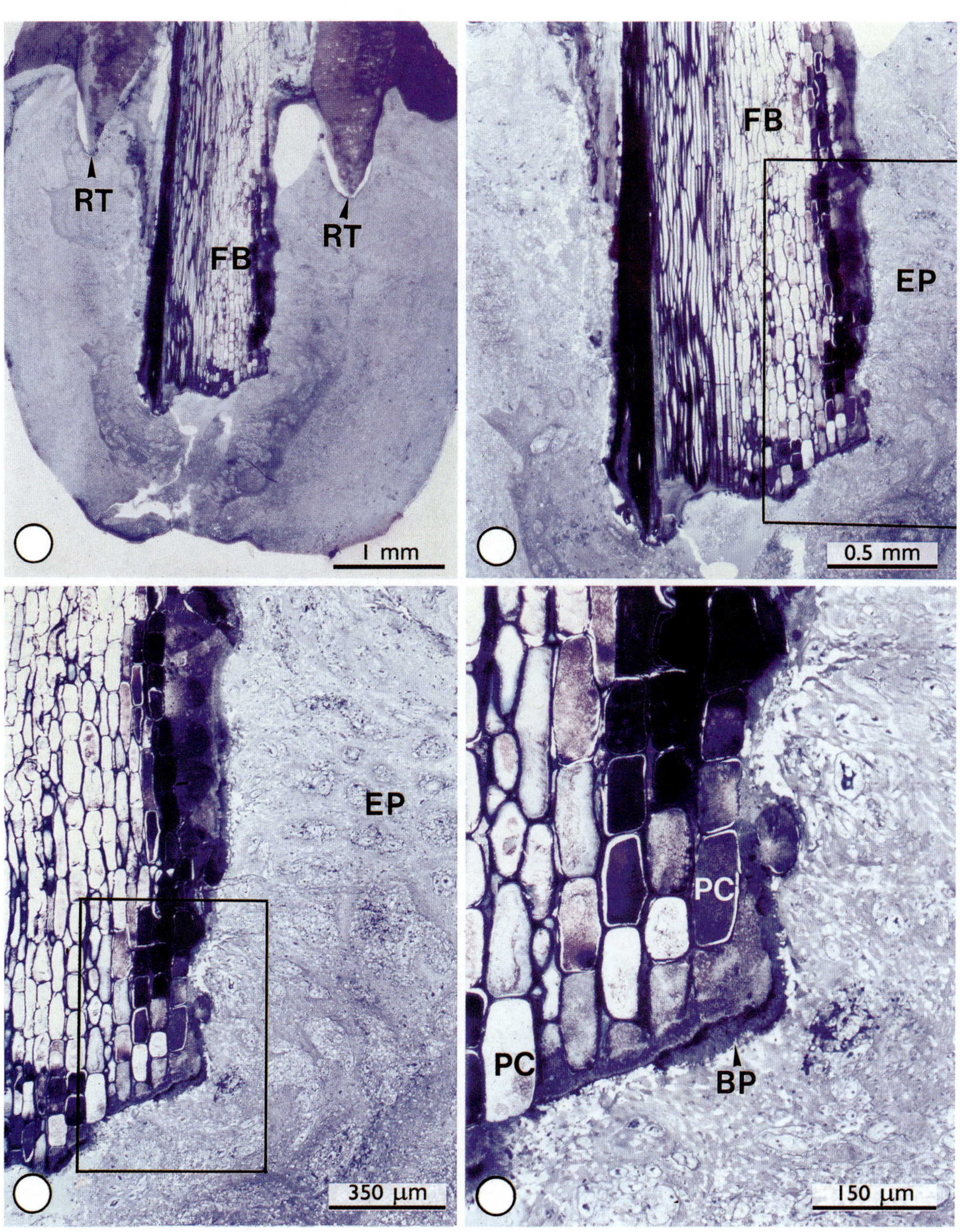


**Figure 9.21** - A massive paper-point granuloma affecting a root-canal-treated human tooth (**A**). The demarcated area in (**B**) is magnified in (**C**) and that in the same is further magnified in (**D**). Note the tip of the paper point (FB) projecting into the apical periodontitis lesion and the bacterial plaque (BP) adhering to the surface of the paper point. RT, root tip; EP, epithelium; PC, plant cell. (Magnifications: **A** x20, **B** x40, **C** x60, **D** x150).

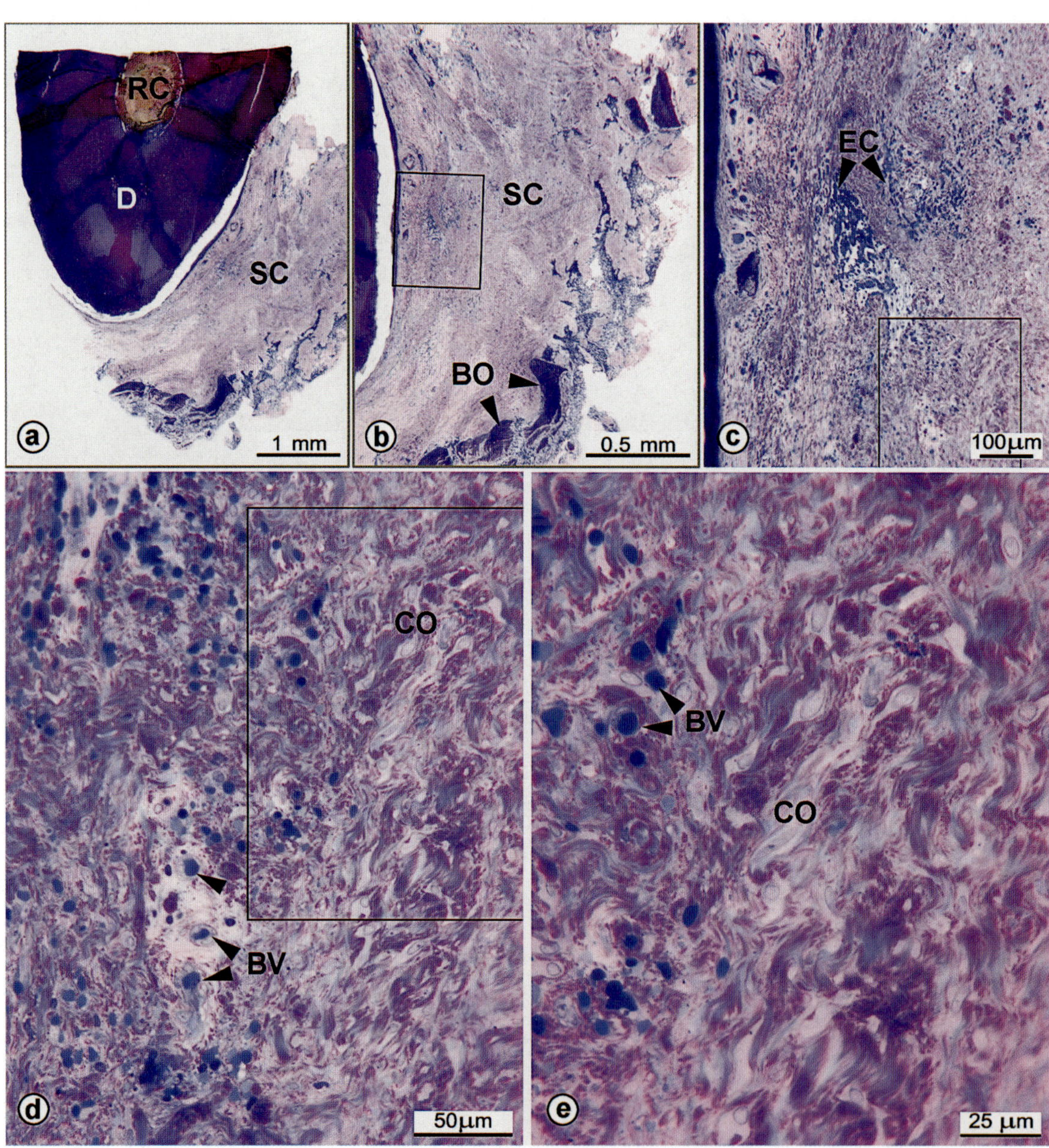


**Figure 9.22** - Periapical scar (SC) of a root canal (RC) treated tooth after 5-year follow-up and surgery. The rectangular demarcated areas in (**B**-**D**) are magnified in (**C**-**E**) respectively. The scar tissue reveals bundles of collagen fibers (CO), blood vessels (BV) and erythrocytes due to haemorrhage. Infiltrating inflammatory cells are notably absent. Original magnifications: **A** x14, **B** x35, **C** x90, **D** x340, **E** x560 (Partially adapted from Nair et al.[199]).

### 9.8 Concluding Remarks

The primary apical periodontitis is caused by the presence of infection within the root canal system. The purpose of endodontic treatment is to eliminate intracanal infection or to reduce the microbial load of the root canal and to prevent re-infection by root filling[188, 200]. The complexity of the canal system[107, 217] and the organization of the microbes into biofilms[49, 51] make it unlikely that a microbe-free root canal can be achieved by current treatment procedures[200] Therefore, radiolucent lesions of periapices may not heal in all root canal treated teeth.

The cause of post-treatment apical periodontitis is more complex than that of teeth with primary apical periodontitis. The etiological agents of persistent apical periodontitis include: (1) infection persisting in the apical root canal system; (2) extraradicular infection, mostly in the form of periapical actinomycosis; (3) root filling or other exogenous materials that cause a foreign body reaction; (4) accumulation of cholesterol crystals that irritate periapical tissues; (5) cystic transformation of lesions, and (6) healing of the periapex by scar tissue. *Among them, infection persisting in the root canal system is the major cause of post-treatment apical periodontitis.* Actinomycosis, true cysts, foreign-body reaction and periapical scar are of rare occurrence. Recognizing the importance of intracanal infection in persistent apical periodontitis[201], the main target of treatment should be the biofilm residing within the root canal system.

Apical periodontitis persisting due to non-microbial causes are not dependent on the presence or absence of biofilm in the root canal system. Initiation of a foreign body reaction in periapical tissues and/or cystic transformation of the lesion delay or prevent post-treatment healing. In well root canal treated teeth with adequate root filling, an orthograde retreatment is unlikely to solve the problem, as it does not remove the offending agents or pathology that exist beyond the root canal[131, 133, 197-199, 201]. A differential diagnosis for the existence of the extraradicular agents of persistent apical periodontitis is not yet available. Although, the great majority of persistent apical periodontitis are caused by residual infection in the complex apical root canal system[107, 217], it is not guaranteed that retreatment of an otherwise well root canal treated tooth can eradicate the residual intracanal infection. Therefore, with cases of asymptomatic, persistent, periapical radiolucencies, it is worth removing the extraradicular factors by an apical surgery[361], in order to improve the long-term outcome of treatment. A periapical surgery not only enables to remove the extraradicular factors that sustain the apical radiolucency post-treatment but also simultaneously allows a retrograde access to potential infection in the apical portion of the root canal system that can also be removed or sealed within the canal by a retrograde root-end filling[186].

### Acknowledgement

The author is indebted to Mrs. Margrit Amstad-Jossi for skilful technical assistance.

## References


1. Abdulla YH, Adams CWM, Morgan RS. Connective tissue reactions to implantation of purified sterol, sterol esters, phosphoglycerides, glycerides and free fatty acids. J Pathol Bacteriol 1967;94:63-71.
2. Abou-Rass M and Bogen G. Microorganisms in closed periapical lesions. Int Endod J 1997;31:39-47.
3. Abramovitz I, Better H, Shacham A, Shlomi B, Metzger Z. Case selection for apical surgery: A retrospective evaluation of associated factors and rational. J Endod 2002;28:527-30.
4. Adams CWM, Morgan RS. The effect of saturated and polyunsaturated lecithins on the resorption of 4-14C-cholesterol from subcutaneous implants. J Pathol Bacteriol 1967;94:73-6.
5. Adams CWM, Bayliss OB, Ibrahim MZM, Webster MW. Phospholipids in atherosclerosis: The modification of the cholesterol granuloma by phospholipid. J Pathol Bacteriol 1963;86:431-6.
6. Allard U, Nord CE, Sjöberg L, Strömberg T. Experimental infections with *Staphylococcus aureus, Streptococcus sanguis, Pseudomonas aeruginosa*, and *Bacteroides fragilis* in the jaws of dogs. Oral Surg Oral Med Oral Pathol 1979;48:454-62.
7. Anderson WAD. Pathology. 5th ed, St. Louis: CV Mosby, 1996. p.777-1404.
8. Ando N, Hoshino E. Predominant obligate anaerobes invading the deep layers of root canal dentine. Inter Endod J 1990;23:20-7.
9. Andreasen FM. Transient apical breakdown and its relation to color and sensibility changes after luxation injuries to teeth. Endod Dent Traumatol 1985; 2:9-19.
10. Andreasen JO, Rud J. A histobacteriologic study of dental and periapical structures after endodontic surgery. Int J Oral Surg 1972;1:272-81.
11. Arden LA. Revised nomenclature for antigen nonspecific T cell proliferation and helper factors. J Immunol 1979;123:2928-9.
12. Artese L, Piattelli A, Quaranta M, Colasante A, Musiani P. Immunoreactivity for interleukin 1$\beta$ and tumor necrosis factor-$\alpha$ and ultrastructural features of monocytes/macrophages in periapical granulomas. J Endod 1991;17:483-7.
13. Ataoglu T, Üngör M, Serpek B, Haliloglu S, Ataoglu H, Ari H. Interleukin-1$\beta$ and tumour necrosis factor-$\alpha$ levels in periapical exudates. Int Endod J 2002;35:181-5.
14. Barkhordar RA, Hussain MZ, Hayashi C. Detection of Interleukin-1 beta in human periapical lesions. Oral Surg Oral Med Oral Pathol 1992;73:334-6.
15. Batty I. *Actinomyces odontolyticus*, a new species of actinomycete regularly isolated from deep carious dentine. J Pathol Bacteriol 1958;75:455-9.
16. Baumann L, Rossman SR. Clinical, roentgenologic and histologic findings in teeth with apical radiolucent areas. Oral Surg Oral Med Oral Pathol 1956;9:1330-6.
17. Baumgartner JC, Falkler WA. Bacteria in the apical 5 mm of infected root canals. J Endod 1991;17:380-3.
18. Baumgartner JC, Khemaleelkul SU, Xia T. Identification of spirochetes (treponemas) in endodontic infections. J Endod 2003;29:794-7.
19. Baumgartner JC, Watkins BJ, Bae K-S, Xia T. Association of black-pigmented bacteria with endodontic infections. J Endod 1999;25:413-5.
20. Bayliss OB. The giant cell in cholesterol resorption. Br J Exper Pathol 1976;57:610-8.
21. Bergenholtz G. Micro-organisms from necrotic pulp of traumatized teeth. Odontol Revy 1974;25:347-58.
22. Bergenholtz G, Spångberg L. Controversies in endodontics. Crit Rev Oral Biol Med 2004;15:99-114.
23. Bergenholtz G, Lekholm U, Liljenberg B, Lindhe J. Morphometric analysis of chronic inflammatory periapical lesions in root filled teeth. Oral Surg Oral Med Oral Pathol 1983;55:295-301.
24. Bhaskar SN. Periapical lesion - types, incidence and clinical features. Oral Surg Oral Med Oral Pathol 1966;21:657-71.
25. Birch RH, Melville TH, Neubert EW. A comparison of root-canal and apical lesion flora. Br Dent J 1964;116:350-2.
26. Birek C, Heersche D, Jez D, Brunette DM. Secretion of bone resorbing factor by epithelial cells cultured from porcine rests of Malassez. J Period Res 1983;18:75-81.
27. Birkedal-Hansen H. Role of matrix metalloproteinases in human periodontal diseases. J Periodontol 1993, 64:474-484.
28. Birkedal-Hansen H, Werb Z, Welgus HG, Van Wart HE. Matrix metalloproteinases and inhibitors. Stuttgart: Gustav Fischer Verlag, 1992.
29. Birkedal-Hansen H, Moore WG, Bodden MK, Windsor LJ, Birkedal-Hansen B, Decarlo A, Engler JA. Matrix metalloproteinases: A review. Crit Rev Oral Biol Med 1993;4:197-250.
30. Block RM, Bushell A, Rodrigues H, Langeland K. A histopathologic, histobacteriologic, and radiographic study of periapical endodontic surgical specimens. Oral Surg Oral Med Oral Pathol 1976;42:656-78.
31. Brännström M, Nyborg H. The presence of bacteria in cavities filled with silicate cement and composite resin materials. Swed Dent J 1971;64:149-55.
32. Brown AMS, Theaker JM. Food induced granuloma - an unusual cause of a submandibular mass with observations on the pathogenesis of hyalin bodies. Br J Maxillofac Surg 1987;25:433-6.
33. Brown-Jr LR, Rudolph-Jr CE. Isolation and identification of microorganisms from unexposed canals of pulp-involved teeth. Oral Surg Oral Med Oral Pathol 1957;10:1094-9.
34. Browne RM. The origin of cholesterol in odontogenic cysts in man. Arch Oral Biol 1971;16:107-13.
35. Browne RM, O'Riordan BC. Colony of Actinomyces-like organism in a periapical granuloma. Br Dent J 1966;120:603-6.
36. Brunette DM, Heersche JNM, Purdon AD, Sodek J, Moe HK, Assuras JN. In vitro cultural parameters and protein and prostaglandin secretion of epithe-

lial cells derived from porcine rests of Malassez. Arch Oral Biol 1979;24:199-203.
37. Buchanan BB, Pine L. Characterization of a propionic acid producing actinomycete, Actinomyces propionicus, sp nov. J Gen Microbiol 1962;28:305-23.
38. Burke GWJ, Knighton HT. The localization of microorganisms in inflamed dental pulps of rats following bacteremia. J Dent Res 1960;39:205-14.
39. Byström A, Sundqvist G. Bacteriologic evaluation of the efficacy of mechanical root canal instrumentation in endodontic therapy. Scand J Dent Res 1981;89:321-8.
40. Byström A, Claeson R, Sundqvist G. The antibacterial effect of camphorated paramonochlrophenol, camphorated phenol and calcium hydroxide in the treatment of infected root canals phenol. Endod Dent Traumatol 1985;1:170-5.
41. Byström A, Happonen RP, Sjögren U, Sundqvist G. Healing of periapical lesions of pulpless teeth after endodontic treatment with controlled asepsis. Endod Dent Traumatol 1987;3:58-63.
42. Carlsson J. Microbiology of plaque associated periodontal disease. In: Lindhe J. Textbook of clinical periodontology. Munksgaard: Copenhagen, 1990. p.129-52.
43. Carlsson J, Frölander F, Sundqvist G. Oxygen tolerance of anaerobic bacteria isolated from necrotic dental pulps. Acta Odontol Scand 1977;35:139-45.
44. Cheung GS, Ho MW. Microbial flora of root canal-treated teeth associated with asymptomatic periapical radiolucent lesions. Oral Microbiol Immun 2001;16:332-7.
45. Chirnside IM. A bacteriological and histological study of traumatised teeth. N Z Dent J 1957;53:176-91.
46. Christianson OO. Observations on lesions produced in arteries of dogs by injection of lipids. Arch Pathol 1939;27:1011-20.
47. Cohen S, Bigazzi PE, Yoshida T. Similarities of T cell function in cell- mediated immunity and antibody production. Cell Immun 1974;12:150-9.
48. Coleman DL, King RN, Andrade JD. The foreign body reaction: a chronic inflammatory response. J Biom Mat Res 1974;8:199-211.
49. Costerton JW, Stewart PS. Biofilms and device-related infections. In: Nataro PJ, Balser MJ, Cunningham-Rundels S. Persistent bacterial infections. ASM Press: Washington D.C. 2000. p.423-39.
50. Costerton JW, Lewandowski DE, Caldwell DE, Krober DR, Lappin-Scott H. Microbial Biofilms. Annual Rev Microbiol 1995;49:711-45.
51. Costerton W, Veeh R, Shirtliff M, Pasmore M, Post C. The application of biofilm science to the study and control of chronic bacterial infections. J Clin Investig 2003;112:1466-77.
52. Cotti E, Torabinejad M. Detection of leukotriene C4 in human periradicular lesions. Int Endod J 1994;27:82-6.
53. Cymerman JJ, Cymerman DH, Walters J, Nevins AJ. Human T-lymphocyte subpopulations in chronic periapical lesions. J Endod 1984;10:9-11.
54. Dahle UR, Tronstad L, Olsen I. Observation of an unusually large spirochete in endodontic infection. Oral Microbiol Immun 1993;8:251-3.
55. Dahle UR, Tronstad L, Olsen I. Characterization of new periodontal and endodontic isolates of spirochetes. Eur J Oral Sci 1996;104:41-7.
56. Dahlén G. Studies on lipopolysaccharides from oral Gram-negative anaerobic bacteria in relation to apical periodontitis. Dr. Odont Thesis, University of Göteborg, Sweden, 1980.
57. Dahlén G, Bergenholtz G. Endotoxic activity in teeth with necrotic pulps. J Dent Res 1980;59:1033-40.
58. Dahlén G, Magnusson BC, Möller Å. Histological and histochemical study of the influence of lipopolysaccharide extracted from *Fusobacterium nucleatum* on the periapical tissues in the monkey Macaca fascicularis. Arch Oral Biol 1981;26:591-8.
59. Dahlén G, Fabricius L, Holm SE, Möller ÅJR. Circulating antibodies after experimental chronic infection in the root canal of teeth in monkeys. Scand J Dent Res 1982;90:338-44.
60. Dahlén G, Fabricius L, Heyden G, Holm SE, Möller ÅJR. Apical periodontitis induced by selected bacterial strains in root canals of immunized and nonimmunized monkeys. Scand J Dent Res 1982;90:207-16.
61. Damme JV. Interleukin-8 and related chemotactic cytokines. In: Thomson AW. The cytokine handbook. Academic Press: London, 1994. p.185-221.
62. De Sá AR, Pimenta FJGS, Dutra WO, Gomez RS. Immunolocalization of Interleukin 4, interleukin 6, and lymphotoxin $\alpha$ in dental granuloma. Oral Surg Oral Med Oral Pathol Oral Radiol Endod 2003;96:356-60.
63. Delivanis PD, Fan VSC. The localization of blood-borne bacteria in instrumented unfilled and overinstrumented canals. J Endod 1984;10:521-4.
64. Dobell C. Antony van Leeuwenhoek and his little animals. New York: Dover Publications, 1960. p.252-3.
65. Drancourt M, Aboudharm G, Signoli M, Dutour O, Raoult D. Detection of 400-year-old Yersinia pestis DNA in human dental pulp: An approach to the diagnosis of ancient septicemia. Proceed National Acad Sci USA 1998;95:12637-40.
66. Dubrow H. Silver points and gutta-percha and the role of root canal fillings. J Am Dent Assoc 1976;93:976-80.
67. Dunlap CL, Barker BF. Giant cell hyalin angiopathy. Oral Surg Oral Med Oral Pathol 1977;44:587-91.
68. Engström B. The significance of enterococci in root canal treatment. Odontol Rev 1964;15:87-106.
69. Engström B, Frostell G. Bacteriological studies of the non-vital pulp in cases with intact pulp cavities. Acta Odontol Scand 1961;19:23-39.
70. Evans M, Davies JK, Sundqvist G, Figdor D. Mechanisms involved in the resistance of *Enterococcus faecalis* to calcium hydroxide. Int Endod J 2002;35:221-8.
71. Fabricius L. Oral bacteria and apical periodontitis. An experimental study in monkeys. Dr. Odont. Thesis, Göteborg, Sweden, University of Göteborg, 1982.
72. Fabricius L, Dahlén G, Holm SC, Möller ÅJR. Influence of combinations of oral bacteria on periapical tissues of monkeys. Scand J Dent Res 1982;90:200-6.
73. Fabricius L, Dahlén G, Öhman AE, Möller ÅJR. Predominant indigenous oral bacteria isolated from infected root canal after varied times of closure. Scan J Dent Res 1982;90:134-44.

74. Farman AG. Technology continually transitions ... research should keep pace with change. Oral Surg Oral Med Oral Pathol Oral Radiol Endod 2007;104:149-50.
75. Figdor D, Davies J. Cell surface structures of Actinomyces israelii. Aust Dent J 1997;42:125-8.
76. Figdor D, Davies JK, Sundqvist G. Starvation survival, growth and recovery of *Enterococcus faecalis* in human serum. Oral Microbiol Immun 2003;18:234-9.
77. Figdor D, Sjögren U, Sorlin S, Sundqvist G, Nair PNR. Pathogenicity of *Actinomyces israelii* and *Arachnia propionica*: experimental infection in guinea pigs and phagocytosis and intracellular killing by human polymorphonuclear leukocytes in vitro. Oral Microbiol Immun 1992;7:129-36.
78. Fletcher HA, Donoghue HD, Holton J, Pap I, and Spigelman M. Widespread occurrence of Mycobacterium tuberculosis DNA from 18th-19th century Hungarians. Am J Physiol Anthropol 2003;120:144-52.
79. Formigli L, Orlandini SZ, Tonelli P, Giannelli M, Martini M, Brandi ML, Bergamini M, Orlandini GE. Osteolytic processes in human radicular cysts: morphological and biochemical results. J Oral Pathol Med 1995;24:216-20.
80. Fouad AF, Burleson J. The effect of diabetes mellitus on endodontic treatment outcome: data from an electronic patient record. J Am Dent Assoc 2003;134:43-51.
81. Fouad AF, Zerella J, Barry J, Spangberg LS. Molecular detection of *Enterococcus species* in root canals of therapy-resistant endodontic infections. Oral Surg Oral Med Oral Pathol Oral Radiol Endod 2005;99:112-8.
82. Freeman N. Histopathological investigation of dental granuloma. J Dent Res 1931;11:176-200.
83. Friedman S. Treatment outcome and prognosis of endodontic therapy. In: Ørstavik D, Pitt Ford TR. Essential Endodontology. Blackwell: Oxford, 1998. p.368-401.
84. Fukushima H, Yamamoto K, Hirohata K, Sagawa H, Leung KP, Walker CB. Localization and identification of root canal bacteria in clinically asymptomatic periapical pathosis. J Endod 1990;16:534-8.
85. Gao Z, Flaitz CM, Mackenzie IC. Expression of keratinocyte growth factor in periapical lesions. J Dent Res 1996;75:1658-63.
86. Gardner AF. A survey of periapical pathology: Part I. Dent Digest 1962;68:162-7.
87. Gatti JJ, Dobeck JM, Smith C, Socransky SS, Skobe Z. Bacteria of asymptomatic periradicular endodontic lesions identified by DNA-DNA hybridization. Endod Dent Traumatol 2000;16:197-204.
88. Gay CV. Osteoclast ultrastructure and enzyme histochemistry: functional implications. In: Rifkin BR, Gay CV. Biology and physiology of the osteoclasts. CRC Press: Boca Raton FL, 1992. p.129-50.
89. Gier RE, Mitchell DF. Anachoretic effect of pulpitis. J Dent Res 1968;47:564-70.
90. Glick M, Trope M, Bagasra O, Pliskin ME. Human immunodeficiency virus infection of fibroblasts of dental pulp in seropositive patients. Oral Surg Oral Med Oral Pathol Oral Radiol Endod 1991;71:733-6.
91. Grahnén H, Hansson L. The prognosis of pulp and root canal therapy: a clinical and radiographic follow-up examination. Odontol Revy 1961;12:146-65.
92. Greening AB, Schonfeld SE. Apical lesions contain elevated immunoglobulin G levels. J Endod 1980;12:867-9.
93. Grossman LI. Origin of microorganisms in traumatized, pulpless, sound teeth. J Dent Res 1967;46:551-3.
94. Haapasalo M. Bacteroides spp in dental root canal infections. Endod Dent Traumatol 1989;5:1-10.
95. Hampp EG. Isolation and identification of spirochetes obtained from unexposed canals of pulp-involved teeth. Oral Surg Oral Med Oral Pathol 1957;10:1100-4.
96. Hancock H, Sigurdsson A, Trope M, Moiseiwitsch J. Bacteria isolated after unsuccessful endodontic treatment in a North American population. Oral Surg Oral Med Oral Pathol 2001;91:579-86.
97. Happonen RP. Periapical actinomycosis: a follow-up study of 16 surgically treated cases. Endod Dent Traumatol 1986;2:205-9.
98. Happonen RP, Söderling E, Viander M, Linko-Kettungen L, Pelliniemi LJ. Immunocytochemical demonstration of *Actinomyces species* and *Arachnia propionica* in periapical infections. J Oral Pathol 1985;14:405-13.
99. Harndt E. Histo-bakteriologische Studie bei Parodontitis chronika granulomatosa. Korrespondent-Blatt für Zahnärzte 1926;50:330-5, 365-70, 399-404, 426-33.
100. Harris M, Goldhaber P. The production of a bone resorbing factor by dental cysts in vitro. Br J Oral Surg 1973;10:334-8.
101. Harris M, Jenkins MV, Bennett A, Wills MR. Prostaglandin production and bone resorption by dental cysts. Nature 1973;145:213-5.
102. Harrison JD, Martin IC. Oral vegetable granuloma: ultrastructural and histological study. J Oral Pathol 1986;23:346-50.
103. Harz CO. Actinomyces bovis, ein neuer Schimmel in den Geweben des Rindes. Deutsche Zeitschrift für Thiermedizin Leipzig 1879;5(2 Supplement):125-40.
104. Head MA. Foreign body reaction to inhalation of lentil soup: giant cell pneumonia. J Clin Pathol 1956;9:295-9.
105. Heersche JN. Systemic factors regulating osteoclast function. In: Rifkin R, Gay CV. Biology and physiology of the osteoclasts. CRC Press: Boca Raton, 1992. p.151-70.
106. Henderson B, Poole S, Wilson M. Bacterial modulins: a novel class of virulence factors which cause host tissue pathology by inducing cytokine synthesis. Microbiol Rev 1996;60:316-41.
107. Hess W. Formation of root canal in human teeth. J Nat Dent Assoc 1921;3:704-34.
108. Hirano T. Interleukin-6. In: Thomson AW. The cytokine handbook. Academic Press: London, 1994. p.145-68.
109. Hirsch EF. Experimental tissue lesions with mixtures of human fat, soaps and cholesterol. Arch Pathol 1938;25:35-9.
110. Holdeman LV, Cato EP, Moore WEC. Anaerobe laboratory manual. Blacksburg: Virginia Polytechnique Institute and State University, 1977.
111. Holland R, De Souza V, Nery MJ, de Mello W, Bernabé PFE, Filho JAO. Tissue reactions following apical plugging of the root canal with infected dentin chips. Oral Surg Oral Med Oral Pathol 1980;49:366-9.

112. Horiba N, Maekawa Y, Matsumoto T, Nakamura H. A study of the detection of endotoxin in the dental wall of infected root canals. J Endod 1990;16:331-4.
113. Howell A, Jordan HV, Georg LK, Pine L. Odontomyces viscosus gen nov spec nov. A filamentous microorganism isolated from periodontal plaque in hamsters. Sabouraudia 1965;4:65-7.
114. Hungate RE. The anaerobic mesophilic cellulolytic bacteria. Bacteriol Rev 1950;14:1-49.
115. Hylton RP, Samules HS, Oatis GW. Actinomycosis: is it really rare? Oral Surg Oral Med Oral Patol 1970;29:138-47.
116. Iwu C, MacFarlane TW, MacKenzie D, Stenhouse D. The microbiology of periapical granulomas. Oral Surg Oral Med Oral Pathol 1990;69:502-5.
117. James WW. Do epithelial odontomes increase in size by their own tension? Proceed Royal Soc Med 1926;19:73-7.
118. Jones OJ, Lally ET. Biosynthesis of immunoglobulin isotopes in human periapical lesions. J Endod 1980;8:672-7.
119. Kakehashi S, Stanley HR, Fitzgerald RJ. The effects of surgical exposures of dental pulps in germ-free and conventional laboratory rats. Oral Surg Oral Med Oral Pathol 1965;20:340-9.
120. Kantz WE, Henry CA. Isolation and classification of anaerobic bacteria from intact pulp chambers of non vital teeth in man. Arch Oral Biol 1974;19:91-6.
121. Kapsimalis P, Garrington GE. Actinomycosis of the periapical tissues. Oral Surg Oral Med Oral Pathol 1968;26:374-80.
122. Karring T, Nyman S, Lindhe J. Healing following implantation of periodontitis affected roots into bone tissue. J Clin Periodontol 1980;7:96-105.
123. Karring T, Nyman S, Gottlow J, Laurell L. Development of the biological concept of guided tissue regeneration - animal and human studies. Periodontol 2000 1993;1:26-35.
124. Kerekes K, Tronstad L. Long-term results of endodontic treatment performed with standardized technique. J Endod 1979;5:83-90.
125. Killian M. Degradation of human immunoglobulins A1, A2 and G by suspected principal periodontal pathogens. Infec Immun 1981;34:57-65.
126. King OH. "Giant cell hyaline angiopathy": Pulse granuloma by another name? Presented at the 32nd Annual Meeting of the American Academy of Oral Pathologists, Fort Lauderdale. 1978.
127. Klevant FJH, Eggink CO. The effect of canal preparation on periapical disease. Int Endod J 1983 ;16:68-75.
128. Knoblich R. Pulmonary granulomatosis caused by vegetable particles. So-called lentil pulse granuloma. Am Rev Resp Diseases 1969;99:380-9.
129. Konomi N, Lebwohl E, Mowbray K, Tattersall I. Detection of mycobacterial DNA in Andean mummies. J Clin Microbiol 2002;40:4738-40.
130. Kopp W, Schwarting R. Differentiation of T-lymphocyte subpopulations, macrophages, HLA-DR-restricted cells of apical granulation tissue. J Endod 1989;15:72-5.
131. Koppang HS, Koppang R, Stølen SØ. Identification of common foreign material in postendodontic granulomas and cysts. J Dent Assoc South Africa 1992;47:210-6.
132. Koppang HS, Koppang R, Solheim T, Aarnes H, Stølen SØ. Identification of cellulose fibers in oral biopsies. Scan J Dent Res 1987;95:165-73.
133. Koppang HS, Koppang R, Solheim T, Aarnes H, Stølen SØ. Cellulose fibers from endodontic paper points as an etiologic factor in post-endodontic periapical granulomas and cysts. J Endod 1989;15:369-72.
134. Kronfeld R. Histopathology of the teeth and their surrounding structures. Philadelphia: Lea & Febiger, 1939. p.210-1.
135. Kuntz DD, Genco RJ, Guttuso J, Natiella JR. Localization of immunoglobulins and the third component of complement in dental periapical lesions. J Endod 1977;3:68-73.
136. Lalonde ER. A new rationale for the management of periapical granulomas and cysts. An evaluation of histopathological and radiographic findings. J Am Dent Assoc 1970;80:1056-9.
137. Lalonde ER Luebke RG. The frequency and distribution of periapical cysts and granulomas. Oral Surg Oral Med Oral Pathol 1968;25:861-8.
138. Langeland K. Erkrankungen der Pulpa und des Periapex. In: Guldener PHA, Langeland K. Endodontie. Georg Thieme: Stutgart, 1993. p.59-70.
139. Langeland MA, Block RM, Grossman LI. A histopathologic and histobacteriologic study of 35 periapical endodontic surgical specimens. J Endod 1977;3:8-23.
140. Laux M, Abbott P, Pajarola G, Nair PNR. Apical inflammatory root resorption: a correlative radiographic and histological assessment. Int Endod J 2000;33:483-93.
141. Lerner UH. Regulation of bone metabolism by the kallikrein-kinin system, the coagulation cascade, and acute phase reactions. Oral Surg Oral Med Oral Pathol 1994;78:481-93.
142. Lew M, Keudel KC, Milford AF. Succinate as a growth factor for Bacteroides melaninogenicus. J Bacteriol 1971;108:175-8.
143. Lim CG, Torabinejad M, Kettering J, Linkhardt TA, Finkelman RD. Interleukin 1β in symptomatic and asymptomatic human periradicular lesions. J Endod 1994;20:225-7.
144. Lin LM, Pascon EA, Skribner J, Gängler P, Langeland K. Clinical, radiographic, histologic study of endodontic treatment failures. Oral Surg Oral Med Oral Pathol 1991;71:603-11.
145. Lin LM, Wang S-L, Wu-Wang C, Chang K-M, Leung C. Detection of epidermal growth factor in inflammatory periapical lesions. Int Endod J 1996;29:179-84.
146. Linenberg WB, Waldron CA, DeLaune GF. A clinical roentgenographic and histopathologic evaluation of periapical lesions. Oral Surg Oral Med Oral Pathol 1964;17:467-72.
147. Listgarten MA. Structure of the microflora associated with periodontal health and disease in man. A light and electron microscopic study. J Periodontol 1976;47:1-18.
148. Listgarten MA, Lewis DW. The distribution of spirochetes in the lesion of acute necrotizing ulcerative gingivitis: an electron microscopical and statistical study. J Periodontol 1967;38:379-86.

149. Loesche WJ, Gusberti F, Mettraux G, Higgins T, Syed S. Relationship between oxygen tension and subgingival bacterial flora in untreated human periodontal pockets. Infec Immun 1983;42:659-67.
150. Love RM, Jenkinson HF. Invasion of dentinal tubules by oral bacteria. Critic Rev Oral Biol Med 2002;13:171-83.
151. Love RM, McMillan MD, Jenkinson HF. Invasion of dentinal tubules by oral Streptococci is associated with collagen regeneration mediated by the antigen I/II family of polypeptides. Infec Immun 1997;65:5157-64.
152. Lukic A, Arsenijevic N, Vujanic G, Ramic Z. Quantitative analysis of the immunocompetent cells in periapical granuloma: Correlation with the histological characteristcs of the lesion. J Endod 1990;16:119-22.
153. Macdonald JB, Hare GC, Wood AWS. The bacteriologic status of the pulp chambers in intact teeth found to be nonvital following trauma. Oral Surg Oral Med Oral Pathol 1957;10:318-22.
154. Main DMG. The enlargement of epithelial jaw cysts. Odontol Revy 1970;21:29-49.
155. Malassez ML. Sur l'existence de masses épithéliales dans le ligament alvéolodentaire chez l'homme adulte et à l'état normal. Comptes Rendus des Séauces de la Société de Biologie et de ses filiales 1884 ;36:241-44.
156. Malassez ML. Sur le role débris épithélaux paradentaris: In: Travaux de L'année 1885, Laboratorie d'histologie du Collége de France; Paris ed. Masson, G: Librairie de l'Académie de Médicine, 1885. p.21-121.
157. Martin IC, Harrison JD. Periapical actinomycosis. Br Dent J 1984;156:169-70.
158. Marton IJ, Kiss C. Characterization of inflammatory cell infiltrate in dental periapical lesions. Int Endod J 1993;26:131-6.
159. Matsumoto Y. Monoclonal and oligoclonal immunoglobulins localized in human dental periapical lesion. Microbiol Immun 1985;29:751-7.
160. Matsuo T, Ebisu S, Nakanishi T, Yonemura K, Harada Y, Okada H. Interleukin-1$\alpha$ and interleukin-1$\beta$ in periapical exudates of infected root canal: Correlations with the clinical findings of the involved teeth. J Endod 1994;20:432-5.
161. McConnell G. The histopathology of dental granulomas. J Nat Dent Assoc 1921;8:390-8.
162. McGhee JR, Michalek SM, Cassel GH. Dental microbiology. Philadelphia: Harper & Row, 1982. p.416-38.
163. McNicholas S, Torabinejad M, Blankenship J. The concentration of prostaglandin E2 in human periradicular lesions. J Endod 1991;17:97-100.
164. Metchinkoff E. Lectures on the comparative pathology of inflammation. New York: Dover Publications, 1968. p.1-224.
165. Miller WD. The micro-organisms of the human mouth. Philadelphia: White Dental MFG Co, 1890. p.96.
166. Mims CA, Dimmock N, Nash A, Stephen J. Mims' pathogenesis of infectious disease. 4th ed, London: Academic Press, 1995. p.152-78.
167. Mincer HH, McCoy JM, Turner JE. Pulse granuloma of the alveolar ridge. Oral Surg Oral Med Oral Pathol 1979;48:126-30.
168. Molander A, Reit C, Dahlén G, Kvist T. Microbiological status of root filled teeth with apical periodontitis. Int Endod J 1998 ;31:1-7.
169. Möller ÅJR. Microbiological examination of root canals and periapical tissues of human teeth, Thesis, Akademiförlaget, Göteborg, Sweden, University of Göteborg, 1966.
170. Möller ÅJR, Fabricius L, Dahlén G, Öhman AE, Heyden G. Influence on periapical tissues of indigenous oral bacteria and necrotic pulp tissue in monkeys. Scan J Dent Res 1981;89:475-84.
171. Molven O. The frequency, technical standard and results of endodontic therapy. Norske Tannlaegeforenings Tidende 1976;86:142-7.
172. Molven O, Halse A. Success rates for gutta-percha and Klorperka N-Ø root fillings made by undergraduate students: radiographic findings after 10-17 years. Int Endod J 1988;21:243-50.
173. Monteleone L. Actinomycosis. J Oral Surg Anest Hosp Dent Serv 1963;21:313-8.
174. Moore WEC. Techniques for routine culture of fastidious anaerobes. Int J Syst Bacteriol 1966;16:173-90.
175. Mortensen H, Winther JE, Birn H. Periapical granulomas and cysts. Scan J Dent Res 1970;78:241-50.
176. Morton TH, Clagett JA, Yavorsky JD. Role of immune complexes in human periapical periodontitis. J Endod 1977;3:261-8.
177. Mullis KB, Faloona FA. Specific synthesis of DNA in vitro via a polymerase-catalyzed chain reaction. Meth Enzymol 1987;155:335-50.
178. Munson MA, Pitt-Ford T, Chong B, Weightman A, Wade WG. Molecular and cultural analysis of the microflora associated with endodontic infections. J Dent Res 2002;81:761-6.
179. Nagaoka S, Miyazaki Y, Liu HJ, Iwamoto Y, Kitano M, Kawagoe M. Bacterial invasion into dentinal tubules in human vital and nonvital teeth. J Endod 1995;21:70-3.
180. Nagase H, Barrett AJ, Woessner-Jr JF. Nomenclature and glossary of the matrix metalloproteinases. In: Birkedal-Hansen H et al. Matrix metalloproteinases and inhibitors. Gustav Fischer Verlag: Stuttgart, 1992. p.421-4.
181. Naidorf IJ. Immunoglobulins in periapical granulomas: a preliminary report. J Endod 1975;1:15-7.
182. Nair PNR. Light and electron microscopic studies of root canal flora and periapical lesions. J Endod 1987;13:29-39.
183. Nair PNR. Apical periodontitis: a dynamic encounter between root canal infection and host response. Periodontol 2000 1997;13:121-48.
184. Nair PNR. New perspectives on radicular cysts: do they heal? Int Endod J 1998;31:155-60.
185. Nair PNR. Cholesterol as an aetiological agent in endodontic failures - a review. Aust Endod J 1999;25:19-26.
186. Nair PNR. Non-microbial etiology: Foreign body reaction maintaining post-treatment apical periodontitis. Endod Topics 2003;6:96-113.
187. Nair PNR. Non-microbial etiology: Periapical cysts sustain post-treatment apical periodontitis. Endod Topics 2003;6:114-34.
188. Nair PNR. Pathogenesis of apical periodontitis and the causes of endodontic failures. Critic Rev Oral Biol Med 2004;15:348-81.

189. Nair PNR. Abusing technology? Culture-difficult microbes and microbial remnants. Oral Surg Oral Med Oral Pathol Oral Radiol Endod 2007.
190. Nair PNR. Strength of evidence in current endodontic microbial research. Oral Surg Oral Med Oral Pathol Oral Radiol Endod 2007.
191. Nair PNR, Schroeder HE. Periapical actinomycosis. J Endod 1984;10:567-70.
192. Nair PNR, Schroeder HE. Epithelial attachment at diseased human tooth-apex. J Period Res 1985;20:293-300.
193. Nair PNR, Schmid-Meier E. An apical granuloma with epithelial integument. Oral Surg Oral Med Oral Pathol 1986;62:698-703.
194. Nair PNR, Pajarola G, Schroeder HE. Types and incidence of human periapical lesions obtained with extracted teeth. Oral Surg Oral Med Oral Pathol 1996;81:93-102.
195. Nair PNR, Sjögren U, Sundqvist G. Cholesterol crystals as an etiological factor in non-resolving chronic inflammation: an experimental study in guinea pigs. Eur J Oral Sci 1998;106:644-50.
196. Nair PNR, Pajarola G, Luder HU. Ciliated epithelium lined radicular cysts. Oral Surg Oral Med Oral Pathol Oral Radiol Endod 2002;94:485-93.
197. Nair PNR, Sjögren U, Krey G, Sundqvist G. Therapy-resistant foreign-body giant cell granuloma at the periapex of a root-filled human tooth. J Endod 1990;16:589-95.
198. Nair PNR, Sjögren U, Schumacher E, Sundqvist G. Radicular cyst affecting a root-filled human tooth: A long-term post-treatment follow-up. Int Endod J 1993;26:225-33.
199. Nair PNR, Sjögren U, Figdor D, Sundqvist G. Persistent periapical radiolucencies of root filled human teeth, failed endodontic treatments and periapical scars. Oral Surg Oral Med Oral Pathol 1999;87:617-27.
200. Nair PNR, Henry S, Cano V, Vera J. Microbial status of apical root canal system of human mandibular first molars with primary apical periodontitis after 'one-visit' endodontic treatment. Oral Surg Oral Med Oral Pathol Oral Radiol Endod 2005;99:231-52.
201. Nair PNR, Sjögren U, Kahnberg KE, Krey G, Sundqvist G. Intraradicular bacteria and fungi in root-filled, asymptomatic human teeth with therapy-resistant periapical lesions: A long-term light and electron microscopic follow-up study. J Endod 1990;16:580-8.
202. Ng Y-L, Spratt D, Sriskantharaja S, Gulabivala K. Evaluation protocols for field decontamination before bacterial sampling of root canals for contemporary microbiology techniques. J Endod 2003;29:317-20.
203. Nijweide PJ, De Grooth R. Ontogeny of the osteoclast. In: Rifkin BR, Gay CV. Biology and physiology of the osteoclast. CRC Press: Boca Raton, 1992. p.81-104.
204. Nilsen R, Johannessen A, Skaug N, Matre R. In situ characterization of mononuclear cells in human dental periapical lesions using monoclonal antibodies. Oral Surg Oral Med Oral Pathol 1984;58:160-5.
205. Nobuhara WK, Del Rio CE. Incidence of periradicular pathoses in endodontic treatment failures. J Endod 1993;19:315-8.
206. Nyman S, Lindhe J, Karring T, Rylander H. New attachment following surgical treatment of human periodontal disease. J Clin Periodontol 1982;9:290-6.
207. Okiji T, Morita I, Sunada I, Murota S. The role of leukotriene B4 in neutrophil infiltration in experimentally induced inflammation of rat tooth pulp. J Dent Res 1991;70:34-7.
208. Oppenheim JJ. Foreword. In: Thomson AW. The cytokine handbook. Academic Press: London, 1994. p.xvii-xx.
209. Oppenheimer S, Miller GS, Knopf K, Blechman H. Periapical actinomycosis. Oral Surg Oral Med Oral Pathol 1978;46:101-6.
210. Page RC, Schroeder HE. Periodontitis in man and other animals. Basel, Switzerland: Karger, 1982. p.22-41,251-271.
211. Papadimitriou JM, Ashman RB. Macrophages: current views on their differentiation, structure and function. Ultrastructural Pathol 1989;13:343-72.
212. Patterson SS, Shafer WG, Healey HJ. Periapical lesions associated with endodontically treated teeth. J Am Dent Assoc 1964;68:191-4.
213. Peciuliene V, Balciuniene I, Eriksen H, Haapasalao M. Isolation of *Enterococcus faecalis* in previously root filled canals in a Lithuanian population. J Endod 2000;26:593-5.
214. Peciuliene V, Reynaud A, Balciuniene I, Haapasalo M. Isolation of yeasts and enteric bacteria in root-filled teeth with chronic apical periodontitis. Int Endod J 2001;34:429-34.
215. Penick EC. Periapical repair by dense fibrous connective tissue following conservative endodontic therapy. Oral Surg Oral Med Oral Pathol 1961;14:239-42.
216. Perez F, Calas P, de Falguerolles A, Maurette A. Migration of a *Streptococcus sanguis* through the root dentinal tubules. J Endod 1993;19:297-301.
217. Perrini N, Castagnola L. W. Hess & O. Keller's anatomical plates: Studies on the anatomical structure of root canals in human dentition by a method of making the tooth substance transparent (1928). Lainate (MI), Italy: Altini Communicazioni Grafiche, 1998.
218. Peters LB, Wesselink PR, Moorer WR. The fate and the role of bacteria left in root dentinal tubules. Int Endod J 1995;28:95-9.
219. Piattelli A, Artese L, Rosini S, Quarenta M, Musiani P. Immune cells in periapical granuloma: Morphological and immunohistochemical characterization. J Endod 1991;17:26-9.
220. Pinheiro ET, Gomes BPFA, Ferraz CCR, Sousa ELR, Teixeira FB, Souza-Filho FJ. Microorganisms from canals of root filled teeth with periapical lesions. Int Endod J 2003;36:1-11.
221. Pitt Ford TR. The effects of the periapical tissues of bacterial contamination of the filled root canal. Int Endod J 1982;15:16-22.
222. Poertzel E, Petschelt A. Bakterien in der Wurzelkanalwand bei Pulpagangrän. Deutsche Zahnärztliche Zeitschrift 1986;41:772-7.
223. Priebe WA, Lazansky JP, Wuehrmann AH. The value of the roentgenographic film in the differential diagnosis of periapical lesions. Oral Surg Oral Med Oral Pathol 1954;7:979-83.
224. Pulver WH, Taubman MA, Smith DJ. Immune components in human dental periapical lesions. Arch Oral Biol 1978;23:435-43.

225. Puzas JE and Ishibe M. Osteoblast/osteoclast coupling. In: Rifkin BR, Gay CV. Biology and physiology of the osteoclast. 1992. p.337-56.
226. Rahbaran S, Gilthorpe MS, Harrison SD, Gulabivala K. Comparison of clinical outcome of periapical surgery in endodontic and oral surgery units of a teaching dental hospital: A retrospective study. Oral Surg Oral Med Oral Pathol Oral Radiol Endod 2001;91:700-9.
227. Rickert UG and Dixon CM. The controlling of root surgery. In: Transactions of the Eighth International Dental Congress, Paris. Section IIIa, 1931.
228. Ricucci D, Mannocci F, Pitt Ford TR. A study of periapical lesions correlating the presence of a radiopaque lamina with histological findings. Oral Surg Oral Med Oral Pathol Oral Radiol Endod 2006;101:389-94.
229. Ricucci D, Martorano M, Bate AL, Pascon EA. Calculus-like deposit on the apical external root surface of teeth with post-treatment apical periodontitis: report of two cases. Int Endod J 2005;38:262-71.
230. Robinson HBG, Boling LR. The anachoretic effect in pulpitis. Bacteriologic studies. J Am Dent Assoc 1941;28:268-82.
231. Rôças I, Siqueira-Jr J, Rade A, Uzeda M. Polimerase chain reaction detection of *Treponema denticola* in endodontic infections within root canals. Int Dent J 2003;34:280-4.
232. Rohrer A. Die Aetiologie der Zahnwurzelzysten. Deutsche Monatszeitschrift für Zahnheilkunde 1927;45:282-94.
233. Roitt I. Essential Immunology. Oxford: Blackwell Scientific Publications, 1994. p.147.
234. Rolph HJ, Lennon A, Riggio MP, Saunders WP, MacKenzie D, Coldero L, Bagg J. 2001) Molecular identification of microorganisms from endodontic infections. J Clin Microbiol 2001, 39(9):3282-3289.
235. Rosebury T, Reynolds JB. Continuous anaerobiosis for cultivation of spirochetes. Proceed Soc Exper Biol Med 1964;117:813-5.
236. Rothschild BM, Martin LD, Lev G, Bercovier H, Bar-Gal GK, Greenblatt C, Donoghue H, Spiegelman M, Britain D. *Mycobacterium tuberculosis* complex DNA from an extinct bison dated 17'000 years before the present. Clin Infec Diseases 2001;33:305-11.
237. Rud J, Andreasen JO. A study of failures after endodontic surgery by radiographic, histologic and stereomicroscopic methods. Int J Oral Surg 1972;1:311-28.
238. Rud J, Andreasen JO, Möller-Jensen JE. Radiographic criteria for the assesment of healing after endodontic surgery. Int J Oral Surg 1972;1:195-214.
239. Ruddle NH. Tumour necrosis factor-beta (Lymphotoxin-alpha). In: Thomson AW. The cytokine handbook. Academic Press: London, 1994. p.305-19.
240. Ryan GB, Majno G. Acute inflammation. Am J Pathol 1977;86:185-276.
241. Sabeti M, Slots J. Herpesviral-bacterial coinfection in periapical pathosis. J Endod 2004;30:69-72.
242. Sabeti M, Simon JH, Slots J. Cytomegalovirus and Epstein-Barr virus are associated with symptomatic periapical pathosis. Oral Microbiol Immun 2003;18:327-8.
243. Sabeti M, Simon JH, Nowzari H, Slots J. Cytomegalovirus and Epstein-Barr virus active infection in periapical lesions of teeth with intact crowns. J Endod 2003;29:321-3.
244. Sabeti M, Valles Y, Nowzari H, Simon JH, Kermani-Arab V, Slots J. Cytomegalovirus and Epstein-Barr virus DNA transcription in endodontic symptomatic lesions. Oral Microbiol Immun 2003;18:104-8.
245. Safavi KE, Rossomando ER. Tumor necrosis factor identified in periapical tissue exudates of teeth with apical periodontitis. J Endod 1991;17:12-4.
246. Sahara N, Okafugi N, Toyoki A, Ashizawa Y, Deguchi T, Suzuki K. Odontoclastic resorption of the superficial nonmineralized layer of predentine in the shedding of human deciduous teeth. Cell Tissue Res 1994;277:19-26.
247. Sakellariou PL. Periapical actinomycosis: report of a case and review of the literature. Endod Dent Traumatol 1996;12:151-4.
248. Salo WL, Aufderheide AC, Buikstra J, Holcomb TA. Identification of *Mycobacterium tuberculosis* DNA in a pre-Columbian Peruvian mummy. Proceed Nat Acad Sci USA 1994;91:2091-4.
249. Samanta A, Malik CP, Aikat BW. Periapical actinomycosis. Oral Surg Oral Med Oral Pathol 1975;39:458-62.
250. Samuelsson B. Leukotrienes: Mediators of immediate hypersensitivity reactions and inflammation. Sci 1983;220:268-75.
251. Schein B, Schilder H. Endotoxin content in endodontically involved teeth. J Endod 1975;1:19-21.
252. Schroeder HE. The Periodontium. Handbook of Microscopic Anatomy. Berlin: Springer-Verlag, 1986.
253. Sedgley C, Buck G, Appelbe O. Prevalence of *Enterococcus faecalis* at multiple oral sites in endodontic patients using culture and PCR. J Endod 2006;32:104-9.
254. Sedgley CM, Messer H. Long-term retention of a paper-point in the periapical tissues: a case report. Endod Dent Traumatol 1993;9:120-3.
255. Selle G. Zur Genese von Kieferzysten anhand vergleichender Untersuchungen von Zysteninhalt und Blutserum. Deutche Zahnärztliche Zeitschrift 1974;29:600-10.
256. Seltzer S. Endodontology. 2nd ed, Philadelphia: Lea & Febiger, 1988. p.223-4.
257. Seltzer S, Bender IB, Turkenkopf S. Factors affecting successful repair after root canal treatment. J Am Dent Assoc 1963;67:651-62.
258. Seltzer S, Soltanoff W, Bender IB. Epithelial proliferation in periapical lesions. Oral Surg Oral Med Oral Pathol 1969;27:111-21.
259. Seltzer S, Bender IB, Smith J, Freedman I, Nazimov H. Endodontic failures - An analysis based on clinical, roentgenographic, histologic findings. Parts I and II. Oral Surg Oral Med Oral Pathol 1967;23:500-30.
260. Sen BH, Piskin B, Demirci T. Observation of bacteria and fungi in infected root canals and dentinal tubules by SEM. Endod Dent Traumatol 1995;11:6-9.
261. Shah HN, Collins MD. Proposal for classification of *Bacteroides asaccharolyticus*, *Bacteroides gingivalis*, and *Bacteroides endodontalis* in a new genus, *Porphyromonas*. Int J Syst Bacteriol 1988;38:128-31.
262. Shah HN, Collins MD. *Prevotella*, a new genus to include *Bacteroides melaninogenicus* and related species formerly classified in the genus *Bacteroides*. Int J Syst Bacteriol 1990;40:205-8.
263. Shear M. The histogenesis of dental cysts. Dent Practitioner 1963;13:238-43.

264. Shear M. Cysts of the oral regions. 3rd ed. Oxford: Wright, 1988. p.136-70.
265. Sherman FE, Moran TJ. Granulomas of stomach. Response to injury of muscle and fibrous tissue of wall of human stomach. Am Clin Pathol 1954;24:415-21.
266. Shin S-J, Lee J-I, Baek S-H, Lim S-S. Tissue levels of matrix metalloproteinases in pulps and periapical lesions. J Endod 2002;28:313-5.
267. Shovelton DS. The presence and distribution of microorganisms within non-vital teeth. Br Dent J 1964;117:101-7.
268. Simon JHS. Incidence of periapical cysts in relation to the root canal. J Endod 1980;6:845-8.
269. Simon JHS, Chimenti Z, Mintz G. Clinical significance of the pulse granuloma. J Endod 1982;8:116-9.
270. Siqueira-Jr J, Rôças I. PCR-based identification of *Treponema maltophilum, T. amylovorum, T. medium* and *T. lecithinolyticum* in primary root canal infections. Arch Oral Biol 2003;48:495-502.
271. Siqueira-Jr JF, Rôças IN. Polymerase chain reaction-based analysis of microorganisms associated with failed endodontic treatment. Oral Surg Oral Med Oral Pathol Oral Radiol Endod 2004;97:85-94.
272. Siqueira-Jr JF, Rôças IN. Exploiting molecular methods to explore endodontic infections: Part 1 - Current molecular technologies for microbiological diagnosis. J Endod 2005;31:411-23.
273. Sjögren U, Sundqvist G, Nair PNR. Tissue reaction to gutta-percha of various sizes when implanted subcutaneously in guinea pigs. Eur J Oral Sci 1995;103:313-21.
274. Sjögren U, Happonen RP, Kahnberg KE, Sundqvist G. Survival of *Arachnia propionica* in periapical tissue. Int Endod J 1988;21:277-82.
275. Sjögren U, Hägglund B, Sundqvist G, Wing K. Factors affecting the long-term results of endodontic treatment. J Endod 1990;16:498-504.
276. Sjögren U, Figdor D, Persson S, Sundqvist G. Influence of infection at the time of root filling on the outcome of endodontic treatment of teeth with apical periodontitis (Published erratum appears in Int Endod J 1998;31:148). Int Endod J 1997;30:297-306.
277. Sjögren U, Mukohyama H, Roth C, Sundqvist G, Lerner UH. Bone-resorbing activity from cholesterol-exposed macrophages due to enhanced expression of interleukin-1$\alpha$. J Dent Res 2002;81:11-6.
278. Skaug N. Proteins in fluids from non-keratinizing jaw cysts: 4. Concentrations of immunoglobulins (IgG, IgA and IgM) and some non-immunoglobulin proteins: Relevance to concepts of cyst wall permeability and clearance of cyst proteins. J Oral Pathol 1974;3:47-61.
279. Skaug N, Nilsen R, Matre R, Bernhoft C-H, Christine A. In situ characterization of cell infiltrates in human dental periapical granulomas 1. Demonstration of receptors for Fc region of IgG. J Oral Pathol 1982;11:47-57.
280. Slots J, Sabeti M, Simon JH. Herpes virus in periapical pathosis: An etiopathologic relationship? Oral Surg Oral Med Oral Pathol Oral Radiol Endod 2003;96:327-31.
281. Smith G, Matthews JB, Smith AJ, Browne RM. Immunoglobulin-producing cells in human odontogenic cysts. J Oral Pathol 1987;16:45-8.
282. Socransky S, Macdonald JB, Sawyer S. The cultivation of *Treponema microdentium* as surface colonies. Arch Oral Biol 1959;1:171-2.
283. Sommer RF, Ostrander F, Crowley M. Clinical Endodontics. 3rd ed, Philadelphia: W. B. Saunders Co, 1966. p. 409-11.
284. Sonnabend E, Oh C-S. Zur Frage des Epithels im apikalen Granulationsgewebe (Granulom) menschlicher Zähne. Deutsche Zahnärztliche Zeitschrift 1966;21:627-643.
285. Spain D, Aristizabal N. Rabbit local tissue response to triglycerides, cholesterol and its ester. Arch Pathol 1962;73:94-7.
286. Spain DM, Aristizabal N, Ores R. Effect of estrogen on resolution of local cholesterol implants. Arch Pathol 1959;68:30-3.
287. Spatafore CM, Griffin JA, Keyes GG, Wearden S, Skidmore AE. Periapical biopsy report: An analysis over a 10-year period. J Endod 1990;16:239-41.
288. Spinner JR. Vom Chemismus der Pulpagangrän. Ein akutes Problem der konservierenden Zahnheilkunde. Zahnärztliches Welt 1947;2:305-13.
289. Stashenko P, Yu SM, Wang C-Y. Kinetics of immune cell and bone resorptive responses to endodontic infections. J Endod 1992;18:422-6.
290. Stashenko P, Teles R, D'Souza R. Periapical inflammatory responses and their modulation. Critic Rev Oral Biol Med 1998;9:498-521.
291. Stashenko P, Wang CY, Riley E, Wu Y, Ostroff G, Niederman R. Reduction of infection-stimulated periapical bone resorption by the biological response modifier PGG glucan. J Dent Res 1995;74:323-30.
292. Staub HP. Röntgenologische Erfolgstatistik von Wurzelbehandlungen. Dr. med. dent. Thesis, University of Zurich, Switzerland, 1966.
293. Stern MH, Dreizen S, Mackler BF, Levy BM. Antibody producing cells in human periapical granulomas and cysts. J Endod 1981;7:447-52.
294. Stockdale CR, Chandler NP. The nature of the periapical lesion - a review of 1108 cases. J Dent 1988;16:123-9.
295. Storms JL. Factors that influence the success of endodontic treatment. J Can Dent Assoc 1969;35:83-97.
296. Strindberg LZ. The dependence of the results of pulp therapy on certain factors. An analytic study based on radiographic and clinical follow-up examinations. Acta Odontol Scand 1956;14(Suppl 21):1-175.
297. Sunde PT, Olsen I, Debelian GJ, Tronstad L. Microbiota of periapical lesions refractory to Endodontc therapy. J Endod 2002;28:304-10.
298. Sunde PT, Tronstad L, Eribe ER, Lind PO, Olsen I. Assessment of periradicular microbiota by DNA-DNA hybridization. Endod Dent Traumatol 2000;16:191-6.
299. Sundqvist G. Bacteriological studies of necrotic dental pulps. Dr. Odont. Thesis, Umeå, Sweden, 1966.
300. Sundqvist G. Ecology of the root canal flora. J Endod 1992;18:427-30.
301. Sundqvist G. Associations between microbial species in dental root canal infections. Oral Microbiol Immunol 1992;7:267-72.
302. Sundqvist G. Taxonomy, ecology and pathogenicity of the root canal flora. Oral Surg Oral Med Oral Pathol 1994;78:522-30.

303. Sundqvist G, Reuterving CO. Isolation of *Actinomyces israelii* from periapical lesion. J Endod 1980;6:602-6.
304. Sundqvist G, Figdor D. Endodontic treatment of apical periodontitis. In: Ørstavik D, Pitt Ford TR. Essential Endodontology. Blackwell: Oxford, England, 1998. p.242-77.
305. Sundqvist G, Figdor D. Life as an endodontic pathogen: Ecological differences between the untreated and root-filled root canals. Endod Topics 2003;6:3-28.
306. Sundqvist G, Johansson E, Sjögren U. Prevalence of black pigmented Bacteroides species in root canal infections. J Endod 1989;15:13-9.
307. Sundqvist G, Carlsson J, Herrman B, Tärnvik A. Degradation of human immunoglobulins G and M and complement factor C3 and C5 by black pigmented Bacteroides. J Med Microbiol 1985;19:85-94.
308. Sundqvist G, Figdor D, Persson S, Sjögren U. Microbiologic analysis of teeth with failed endodontic treatment and the outcome of conservative re-treatment. Oral Surg Oral Med Oral Pathol 1998;85:86-93.
309. Sundqvist GK, Eckerbom MI, Larsson AP, Sjögren UT. Capacity of anaerobic bacteria from necrotic dental pulps to induce purulent infections. Infec Immun 1979;25:685-93.
310. Szajkis S, Tagger M. Periapical healing in spite of incomplete root canal debridement and filling. J Endod 1983;9:203-9.
311. Talacko AA, Radden BG. The pathogenesis of oral pulse granuloma: an animal model. J Oral Pathol 1988;17:99-105.
312. Talacko AA, Radden BG. Oral pulse granuloma: clinical and histopathological features. Int J Oral Maxillofac Surg 1988;17:343-6.
313. Tani-Ishii N, Wang C-Y, Stashenko P. Immunolocalization of bone-resorptive cytokines in rat pulp and periapical lesions following surgical pulp exposure. Oral Microbiol Immun 1995;10:213-9.
314. Taylor E. Dorland's illustrated medical dictionary. 27th ed, Philadelphia: W.B. Saunders Co, 1988. p.324.
315. Ten Cate AR. Epithelial cell rests of Malassez and the genesis of the dental cyst. Oral Surg Oral Med Oral Pathol 1972;34:956-64.
316. Teronen O, Salo T, Laitinen J, Törnwall J, Ylipaavainiemi P, Konttinen Y, Hietanen J, Sorosa T. Characterization of interstitial collagenases in jaw cyst wall. Eur J Oral Sci 1995;103:141-7.
317. Thesleff I. Epithelial cell rests of Malassez bind epidermal growth factor intensely. J Period Res 1987;22:419-21.
318. Thilo BE, Baehni P, Holz J. Dark-field observation of bacterial distribution in root canals following pulp necrosis. J Endod 1986;12:202-5.
319. Thoma KH. A histo-pathological study of the dental granuloma and diseased root apex. J Nat Dent Assoc 1917;4:1075-90.
320. Thomas L. The lives of a cell. Toronto: Bantam Books Inc, 1994. p.92.
321. Thompson L, Lovestedt SA. An actinomyces-like organism obtained from the human mouth. Proceed Staff Meet Mayo Clin 1951;26:169-75.
322. Toller PA. Experimental investigations into factors concerning the growth of cysts of the jaw. Proceed Royal Soc Med 1948;41:681-8.
323. Toller PA. The osmolarity of fluids from cysts of the jaws. Br Dent J 1970;129:275-8.
324. Toller PA, Holborow EJ. Immunoglobulins and immunoglobulin-containing cells in cysts of the jaws. Lancet 1969;2:178-81.
325. Torabinejad M. The role of immunological reactions in apical cyst formation and the fate of the epithelial cells after root canal therapy: a theory. Int J Oral Surg 1983;12:14-22.
326. Torabinejad M, Kriger RD. Experimentally induced alterations in periapical tissues of the cat. J Dent Res 1980;59:87-96.
327. Torabinejad M, Kettering J. Identification and relative concentration of B and T lymphocytes in human chronic periapical lesions. J Endod 1985;11:122-5.
328. Torabinejad M, Clagett J, Engel D. A cat model for evaluation of mechanism of bone resorption; induction of bone loss by simulated immune complexes and inhibition by indomethacin. Calc Tissue Int 1979;29:207-14.
329. Torabinejad M, Cotti E, Jung T. Concentration of leukotriene B4 in symptomatic and asymptomatic periapical lesions. J Endod 1992;18:205-8.
330. Torneck CD. Reaction of rat connective tissue to polyethylene tube implants. Part I. Oral Surg Oral Med Oral Pathol 1966;21:379-87.
331. Torres JOC, Torabinejad M, Matiz RAR, Mantilla EG. Presence of secretory IgA in human periapical lesions. J Endod 1994;20:87-9.
332. Tracey KJ. Tumour necrosis factor-alpha. In: The cytokine handbook. Thomson AW. Academic Press: London, 1994. p.289-304.
333. Tronstad L, Barnett F, Cervone F. Periapical bacterial plaque in teeth refractory to endodontic treatment. Endod Dent Traumatol 1990;6:73-7.
334. Tronstad L, Barnett F, Riso K, Slots J. Extraradicular endodontic infections. Endod Dent Traumatol 1987;3:86-90.
335. Trott JR, Chebib F, Galindo Y. Factors related to cholesterol formation in cysts and granulomas. J Can Dent Assoc 1973;38:76-8.
336. Valderhaug J. A histologic study of experimentally induced periapical inflammation in primary teeth in monkeys. Int J Oral Surg 1974;3:111-23.
337. Van Dyke TE, Vaikuntam J. Neutrophil function and dysfunction in periodontal disease. In: Williams RC, Yukna RA, Newman MG. Current Opinion in Periodontology. Current Science: Philadelphia, 1994. p.19-27.
338. Van Furth R, Cohn ZA, Hirsch JG, Humphry JH, Spector WG, Langevoort HL. The mononuclear phagocyte system: A new classification of macrophages, monocytes and their precursors. Bull World Health Organization 1972;46:845-52.
339. Wais FT. Significance of findings following biopsy and histologic study of 100 periapical lesions. Oral Surg Oral Med Oral Pathol 1958;11:650-3.
340. Waltimo TMT, Siren EK, Torkko HLK, Olsen I, Haapasalo MPP. Fungi in therapy-resistant apical periodontitis. Int Endod J 1997;30:96-101.
341. Waltimo TR, Sen BH, Meurman JH, Orstavik D, Haapasalo MPP. Yeasts in apical periodontitis. Critic Rev Oral Biol Med 2003;14:128-37.
342. Walton RE and Ardjmand K. Histological evaluation of the presence of bacteria in induced periapical lesions in monkeys. J Endod 1992;18:216-21.

343. Wang CY, Stashenko P. The role of interleukin-1α in the pathogenesis of periapical bone destruction in a rat model system. Oral Microbiol Immun 1993;8:50-6.
344. Wayman BE, Murata M, Almeida RJ, Fowler CB. A bacteriological and histological evaluation of 58 periapical lesions. J Endod 1992;18:152-5.
345. Weir JC, Buck WH. Periapical actinomycosis. Oral Surg Oral Med Oral Pathol 1982;54:336-40.
346. White EW. Paper point in mental foramen. Oral Surg Oral Med Oral Pathol 1968;25:630-2.
347. WHO. Application of the international classification of diseases to dentistry and stomatology. 3rd ed, Geneva: WHO, 1995. p.66-67.
348. Wilson M. Susceptibility of oral bacterial biofilms to antimicrobial agents. J Med Microbiol 1996;44:79-87.
349. Wilson M, McNab R, Henderson B. Bacterial disease mechanisms: An introduction to cellular microbiology. Cambridge: Cambridge University Press, 2002.
350. Winkler TF. Review of the literature: A histologic study of bacteria in periapical pathosis. Pharm Therap Dent 1975;2:157-81.
351. Winstock D. Apical disease: an analysis of diagnosis and management with special reference to root lesion resection and pathology. Ann Royal Coll Surg Engl 1980;62:171-9.
352. Wittgow-Jr WC, Sabiston-Jr CB. Microorganisms from pulpal chambers of intact teeth with necrotic pulps. J Endod 1975;1:168-71.
353. Wolff M, Israel J. Ueber Reinkultur des Actinomyces und seine Ubertragbarkeit auf Thiere. Archives der Pathologishe Anatomie Physiologie und Klinishe Medizin. 1891;126:11-59.
354. Yamasaki M, Nakane A, Kumazawa M, Hashioka K, Horiba N, Nakamura H. Endotoxin and Gram-negative bacteria in the rat periapical lesions. J Endod 1992;18:501-4.
355. Yamazaki K, Nakajima T, Gemmell E, Polak B, Seymour GJ, Hara K. IL-4 and IL-6-producing cells in human periodontal disease tissue. J Oral Pathol Med 1994;23:347-53.
356. Yanagisawa W. Pathologic study of periapical lesions. I. Periapical granulomas: Clinical, histologic and immunohistopathologic studies. J Oral Pathol 1980;9:288-300.
357. Yeagle PL. The biology of cholesterol. Boca Raton: CRC Press, 1988.
358. Yeagle PL. Understanding your cholesterol. San Diego: Academic Press, 1991. p. 35-51.
359. Ylipaavalniemi P. Cyst fluid concentrations of immunoglobulins α2-macroglobulin and α1-antitrypsin. Proceed Finnish Dent Soc 1977;73:185-8.
360. Yusuf H. The significance of the presence of foreign material periapically as a cause of failure of root treatment. Oral Surg Oral Med Oral Pathol 1982;54:566-574.
361. Zuolo ML, Ferreira MOF, Gutmann JL. Prognosis in periradicular surgery: a clinical prospective study. Int Endod J 2000;33:91-8.

# Epidemiology and Therapy of Apical Periodontitis

**C. Estrela**
*Federal University of Goiás, Goiânia, GO, Brazil*

**M. R. Bueno**
*University of Cuiabá, MT, Brazil*

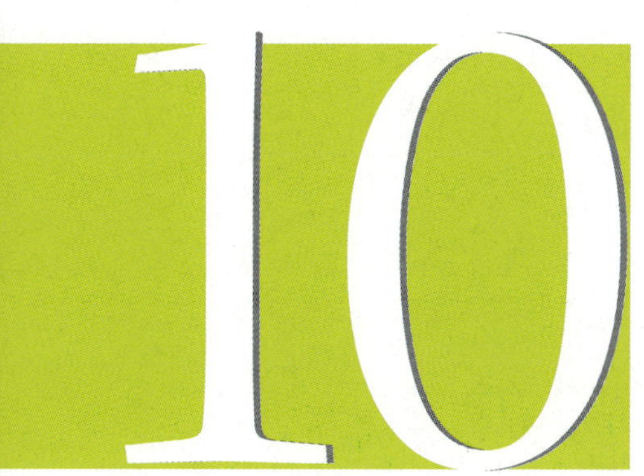


Chapter contents

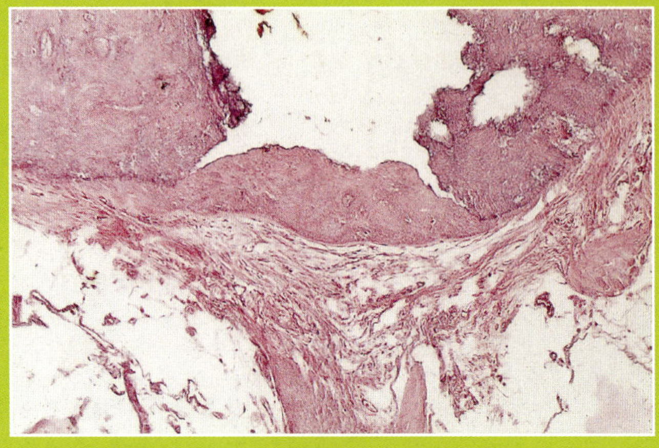

$Ca(OH)_2$ – Sealapex – Biologic closure main foramen (H.E., X 100) (Holland et al.[162], 1998).

## 10.1 Introduction

The periapical inflammation represents a biological answer of natural defense, caused by several etiologic agents (microbial, chemical, physical and others). The model of the inflammatory response is similar to other parts of the organism.

The inflammatory and / or infectious condition involved on the periapical alteration modulates the diagnosis and the treatment option. The traumatic or infectious injury on the dental pulp is capable to produce harmful consequences on the periapical region. The infection of the dental pulp mobilizes microorganisms to develop on apical direction, invade and colonize the periapical tissues. It is unpredictable the period of time to occur an infection process. The microorganisms with different characteristics (structural, metabolic and pathogenic) when arrive at the periapical region stimulate the inflammatory and immunologic response. The organic defenses and the degree of virulence of the microorganisms establish several types of periapical alterations.

## 10.2 Epidemiology of Apical Periodontitis

Apical periodontitis (AP) often appears as a response to intraradicular or extraradicular infection. The acceptance of endodontic therapeutic protocol to treat a disease has usually been based on pathological and clinical characteristics aided frequently by radiographic exam.

The modern knowledge has shown that the logical clinical experience is not sufficient to show the best manner to establish preventive and therapeutic conducts. Several parameters are essential to study a disease, including its distribution, prevalence, severity and risk factors. Epidemiological studies in different populations contribute with scientific observations of factors associated with the disease at issue, such as treatment and outcomes[97]. According to Eriksen et al.[97], the results from analytical epidemiology together with the knowledge from experimental and clinical studies indicate the quality of root canal filling as a key prognostic factor.

Some studies[163,182,271,347] have correlated different factors with the prevalence of AP, especially the quality of root canal filling and coronal restoration and the presence of intracanal post. Ray & Trope[271] examined the radiographs of 1,010 endodontically treated teeth and observed absence of periapical pathology in 61.07% of the cases. These authors concluded that the technical quality of the coronal restoration was significantly more important than the technical quality of the endodontic treatment for apical periodontal health. Kirkevang et al.[182] evaluated the radiographs of 773 root-filled teeth to investigate the quality of endodontic treatments and coronal restorations as well as its association with the periodontal status and reported an AP prevalence of 52.3%. Inadequate root canal filling and coronal restoration were associated with an increased AP incidence. Tronstad et al.[347] examined the radiographs of 1,001 root-filled teeth and found a success rate of 67.4%. Technical quality of endodontic treatment was found to be more important than the technical quality of the coronal restoration. Hommez et al.[164] reported that the technical quality of coronal restorations and root fillings influenced the periapical health.

Estrela et al.[111] assessed the prevalence and risk factors of apical periodontitis in endodontically treated teeth in a selected population of Brazilian adults. This cross-sectional study was based on a fullmouth radiographic survey of randomly selected endodontically treated teeth (except third molars) of patient charts from the

Brazilian Dentistry Association (Postgraduate Course in Endodontics, Goiânia, GO, Brazil). The sample consisted of 1,372 endodontically treated teeth observed by periapical radiographs taken using the parallelism technique and all films being developed by a specialized radiological clinic. The inclusion criteria comprehended selection of radiographs from patients attending the clinic of a Postgraduate Course in Endodontics and having endodontic treatments performed within the last 10 years by postgraduate students. The prevalence of AP associated with adequate endodontic treatment was only 16.5%. In the present study, 61.8% of the teeth with poor root canal filling and adequate coronal restoration had AP. When both unfavorable conditions were present (poor root canal filling and poor coronal restoration), AP prevalence increased to 71.7%. When both favorable conditions were combined (i.e., adequate endodontic and coronal sealing), the rate of AP was remarkably lower (12.1%) (Table 10.1, Fig. 10.1).

This is a low rate compared to those found in other epidemiological studies, ranging from 20 to 52%[50,86-89,94-97,101,111,163,164,180-185,264-266,271,347]. The discrepancies observed between the results of different studies might be explained by the following aspects: 1. lack of homogeneity of the populations being compared; 2. lack of standardization of the methods of radiographic assessment; 3. use of teeth or individuals as referential; 4. quality of endodontic treatment rated by either general dentists or endodontists; and 5. different levels of endodontic practice and infection control in the different populations.

Explanations for the results obtained in the current study[111], which led to positive estimates, should be clarified. The time interval included in this investigation provided a good estimative of quality of endodontic treatment and indicated that root canal fillings and coronal restorations had been done according to modern scientific, biological and technological knowledge. These factors contribute to enhance the estimation of endodontic treatment prognosis and may justify the lower rate of AP found in the current investigation. Another factor that influenced these results was the good technical quality of the postgraduate students that performed the endodontic treatments.

**Table 10.1** - Prevalence of apical periodontitis as influenced by the quality of the endodontic treatment and coronal restoration, and the presence of intracanal post (n=1,372) (Selected population of Brazilian adults)[111]

| Factor | n (%) | Prevalence of apical periodontitis n (%) | *p** | OR (CI 95%) |
|---|---|---|---|---|
| Endodontic treatment | | | | |
| Adequate | 781 (56.9) | 129 (16.5) | 0.000 | 9.96 (7.66 – 12.95) |
| Poor | 591 (43.1) | 392 (66.3) | | |
| Coronal Restoration | | | | |
| Adequate | 881 (64.2) | 265 (30.1) | 0.000 | 2.53 (2.00 – 3.20) |
| Poor | 491 (35.8) | 256 (52.1) | | |
| Intracanal Post | | | | |
| Absent | 768 (56.0) | 305 (39.7) | 0.134 | 0.85 (0.67 – 1.06) |
| Present | 604 (44.0) | 216 (35.8) | | |
| **Combined endodontic treatment and coronal restoration** | | | | |
| Adequate endodontic treatment (n=781) | | | | |
| Adequate coronal restoration | 562 (72.0) | 68 (12.1) | 0.000 | 2.80 (1.87 – 4.22) |
| Poor coronal restoration | 219 (28.0) | 61 (27.9) | | |
| Poor endodontic treatment (n=591) | | | | |
| Adequate coronal restoration | 319 (54.0) | 197 (61.8) | 0.011 | 1.57 (1.09 – 2.25) |
| Poor coronal restoration | 272 (46.0) | 195 (71.7) | | |

* Chi-square test

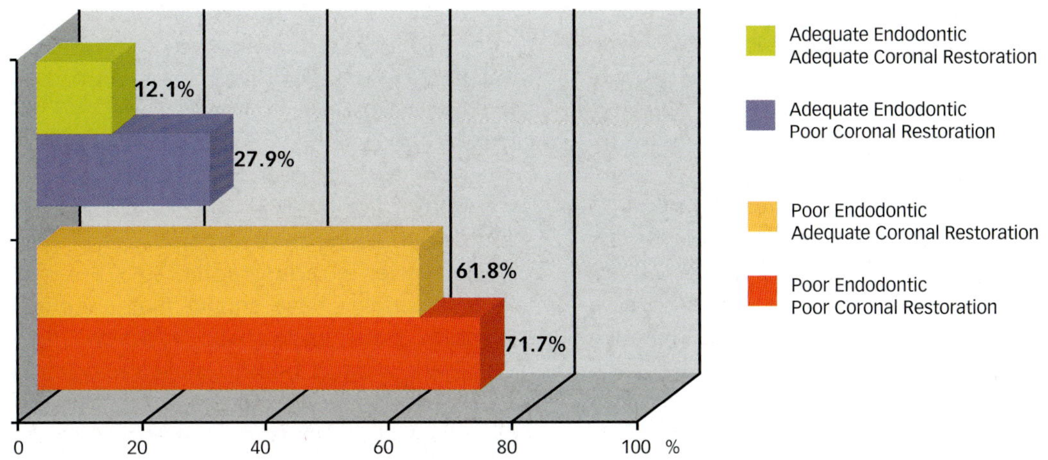


**Figure 10.1** - Prevalence of apical periodontitis as determined by the combination of endodontic treatment and coronal restoration (Selected population of Brazilian adults)[111].

The prevalence of endodontically treated teeth in the Brazilian adult population evaluated recently[163] was higher than that observed in epidemiological studies conducted in other countries. Of 29,467 teeth evaluated, 6,313 (21.4%) were treated endodontically.

Endodontic epidemiological studies conducted with different populations worldwide have shown that the periapical health status is related to factors like quality of root canal filling, coronal restoration and presence of intracanal post[50,86-89,94-97,101,111,163,164,180-185,264-266,271,347]. Therefore, root canal obturation represents an important phase of endodontic treatment, which is completed with the placement of an adequate coronal restoration.

It has also been demonstrated that higher rates of endodontic treatment failures are related to inadequate root canal obturation[164,182,347]. Hence, the best strategy to significantly reduce the number of microorganisms in endodontic infections requires a combination of steps that include effective root canal preparation and sanitization, use of proper intracanal medication and three-dimensional filling of the entire root canal system and coronal chamber. All these factors enhance the prognosis of AP treatment.

Some aspects relative to AP should be taken into consideration. By definition, AP consists in the inflammation of the periodontal tissues at the root apex and presents distinct pathological stages of development. Nair et al.[231], observing 256 human periapical lesions, found that 35% of them were diagnosed as periapical abscess, 50% as granuloma and 15% as cysts (9% apical true cysts, 6% apical pocket cysts). The pocket cysts may heal after root canal treatment, but true cysts are less likely to be eliminated by conventional root canal therapy. The etiological factors involved in AP include intrarradicular and extraradicular infection, as well as foreign-body reactions.

The critical factor for endodontic success is the elimination of microorganisms from the root canal system by means of the association of procedures, i.e., cleaning, enlarging, shaping, use of antimicrobial intracanal medications and quality of root canal filling and coronal restoration. Previous studies have reported high success rates of endodontic treatment depending on the preoperative status of the pulp and periapical tissues[190,310]. Sjögren et al.[310] evaluated the factors that would affect the long-term outcomes of root canal therapy 8 to 10 years after the treatment.

The success rate for cases with vital or nonvital pulps, but having no periapical radiolucency, exceeded 96%, whereas 86% of the cases with pulp necrosis and periapical radiolucency showed apical healing. From all periapical lesions present on previously root-filled teeth, only 62% healed after retreatment. Kojima et al.[190] analyzed by cumulative meta-analysis the success rate of root canal filling as well as the effect of underextension, overextension and flush filling on outcome. The cumulative success rate for treatment of teeth with vital pulp was higher than that of teeth with nonvital pulp, which might be related to the fact that the pulp space of nonvital teeth is often infected. There was higher success rate with flush filling, as confirmed by the radiographic examination of both vital and nonvital teeth. Schaeffer et al.[288] determined the relation of success/failure of different obturation lengths. The meta-analysis indicated that a better success rate is achieved when treatment includes obturation short of the apex.

It is important to be aware of the limitations of radiographic assessment as a study method. One of these limitations involves the evaluation of the quality of root canal filling and coronal restoration based on a two-dimensional image of three-dimensional structures. The radiographic appearance of the filled root canal space has been considered a method to evaluate its quality of sealing. Radiographic images have been used to indicate the presence of periapical infection or coronal leakage, consisting of an important diagnostic resource. Previous studies have also employed periapical radiographs with the same purpose of this study[164,182,271,347]. Extrapolation of these data must be done with caution, considering all methodological implications and limitations.

The findings of the present investigation[111] showed that the prevalence of AP was low when associated with high technical quality of root canal treatment. Poor coronal restoration increased the risk of AP even when endodontic treatment was adequate. The presence of intracanal posts had no influence on the risk of AP.

The diagnosis of apical periodontitis (AP) represents an essential strategy to determine the selection of an effective therapeutic protocol for endodontic infection control. AP is a consequence of root canal system infection, which can involve progressive stages of inflammation and changes of periapical bone structure, resulting in resorption identified as radiolucencies in radiographs[235].

Some studies have shown that a periapical lesion from endodontic infection might be present without being visible radiographically. The radiographic image corresponds to a 2-dimensional aspect of a 3-dimensional structure[27-29,358,371]. Artificial lesions produced in cadavers can be detected by conventional radiography only if perforation, extensive destruction of the bone cortex on the outer surface, or erosion of the cortical bone from the inner surface is present. Lesions confined within the cancellous bone cannot be detected, whereas lesions with buccal and lingual cortical involvement produce distinct radiographic areas of rarefaction. To be visible radiographically, a periapical radiolucency should reach nearly 30%–50% of bone mineral loss[28,29]. Other conditions, such as apical morphologic variations, surrounding bone density, X-ray angulations, and radiographic contrast, also influence radiographic interpretation[152]. An experimentally induced lesion might or might not be detected, depending on its location. A periapical lesion of a certain size can be detected in a region covered by a thin cortex, whereas the same size lesion will not be seen in a region covered by a thicker cortex. Lesion location in different types of bone influences the radiographic visualization[169].

A large number of studies with different diagnostic methods have evaluated the type and incidence of periapical lesions[193,231,298,351]. Scientific consensus has been reached to the fact that AP is accurately identified by histologic analysis[193]. On the other hand, it has been demonstrated that cone beam computed tomography (CBCT) can determine the difference in density between the cystic cavity content and the granulomatous tissue, favoring the choice for a noninvasive diagnosis[298,351].

Several advanced radiographic techniques for the detection of bone lesions have been used in dentistry, namely digital radiography, densitometry methods, CBCT, magnetic resonance imaging, ultrasound, and nuclear techniques[65,66,169,230,251]. CBCT has been successfully used in endodontics with different goals, including study of root canal anatomy, external and internal macromorphology in 3-dimensional reconstruction of the teeth, evaluation of root canal preparation, obturation, retreatment, coronal microleakage, detection of bone lesions, and experimental endodontology[65,66,169,199,230,247,257,359].

Few studies have compared the differences in AP image interpretation by using CBCT, conventional periapical radiography, or digital radiography. CBCT has provided promising results with a more accurate detection of AP[66,199,247,359]. The therapeutic protocol to treat diseases of endodontic origin has routinely been based on the evaluation of pathologic and clinical characteristics frequently complemented by radiographic findings. Radiographic imaging is the most commonly used diagnostic resource in endodontic diagnosis and treatment, and image distortions constitute a serious inconvenience. In addition, it is important to emphasize the limited number of endodontic epidemiologic studies. The knowledge of prevalence and severity of AP is often based on periapical radiography, whose accuracy is questionable. Therefore, considering some limitations on conventional radiography for detection of periapical bone lesions, advanced imaging methods such as CBCT might add benefits to endodontics and offer a higher quality on diagnosis, treatment planning, and prognosis.

Estrela et al.[102] determined the accuracy of CBCT imaging and panoramic and periapical radiographs on detection of AP. Imaging exam records of 888 consecutive patients (59% female; mean age, 50 ± 12 years) including periapical and panoramic radiographs and CBCT were selected from databases from the Dental and Radiological Institute of Brasília. Exams were obtained between May 2004 and August 2006. All patients had at least 1 tooth with history of secondary and primary endodontic infections. A total of 1508 teeth were selected for the study, 523 molars, 597 premolars, 154 canines, and 234 incisors, and 94.5% of the sample had been treated endodontically. Three calibrated examiners performed visual analysis of all digital images, and the periapical index (PAI) by Ørstavik et al.[257] was used to determine the periapical status as follows: 1, normal periapical structures; 2, small changes in bone structure; 3, changes in bone structure with some mineral loss; 4, periodontitis with well-defined radiolucent area; 5, severe periodontitis with exacerbating features.

The prevalence of AP in both endodontically treated and untreated teeth, as identified by periapical and panoramic radiographs and dental CBCT, is shown in Table 10.2.

**Table 10.2** - Prevalence of AP in endodontically treated and untreated teeth, identified by panoramic, periapical and cone-beam computed tomography (CBCT) images (n=1508)

| | Panoramic | Periapical | CBCT | p-value* |
|---|---|---|---|---|
| **Treated teeth** (n=1425) | | | | |
| Presence of AP | 251 (17.6%) | 503 (35.3%) | 902 (63.3%) | p<0.001 |
| Absence of AP | 1174 (82.4%) | 922 (64.7%) | 523 (36.7%) | |
| **Non treated teeth** (n=83) | | | | |
| Presence of AP | 18 (21.7%) | 30 (36.1%) | 62 (74.7%) | p<0.001 |
| Absence of AP | 65 (78.3%) | 53 (63.9%) | 21 (25.3%) | |

* Chi-square test

The findings of the present investigation[102] demonstrated that the CBCT images present high accuracy for the detection of AP. CBCT images tend to offer greater scores than periapical and panoramic radiographs, suggesting that diagnosis of the graduation of AP with conventional images is frequently underestimated. AP was correctly identified in 54.5% of the cases with periapical radiographs (sensitivity, 0.55) and in 27.8% with panoramic radiographs (sensitivity, 0.28). Accuracy of periapical radiographs was significantly higher than that of panoramic radiographs. AP was correctly identified with conventional methods when a severe condition was present.

The likelihood of AP to exist and not to be identifiable by periapical or panoramic radiographs is considerably high (Fig. 10.2). The difficulty to accurately detect AP has been mentioned elsewhere[28,29,169,257]. One important aspect to be considered is that it is necessary to have approximately 30%–50% of mineral loss to visualize AP[28,29]. Morphologic variations of the apical region, bone density, x-ray angulations, radiographic contrast, and actual location of the periapical lesion will influence the radiographic interpretation[152,153,225]. The limitations of radiographic assessment as a study method should not be overlooked, mainly to reduce false-negative results.

In view of the limitations of periapical radiography to visualize AP, *a review of epidemiologic studies should be undertaken considering the quality of periapical aspects offered by CBCT images*. In addition, it will certainly reduce the influence on radiographic interpretation, with minor possibility of false-negative diagnosis. In the present study, AP prevalence in endodontically treated teeth, when comparing the panoramic and periapical radiographs and CBCT images, was 17.6%, 35.3%, and 63.3%, respectively. A considerable discrepancy can be observed among the imaging methods used to identify AP.

The truth is that most dentists do not have CBCT equipment in their dental offices. Thus, during endodontic treatment, it is important to choose a radiographic technique that minimizes image distortions, such as cone parallel technique, to obtain a high level of reproducibility and increase the diagnostic accuracy of the imaging method.

The use of conventional radiographic images for detection of AP should be done with care because of the high possibility of false-negative diagnosis. A great advantage of using CBCT in endodontics refers to its usefulness in aiding in the identification of periapical lesions and in a differential diagnosis with a noninvasive technique with high accuracy.

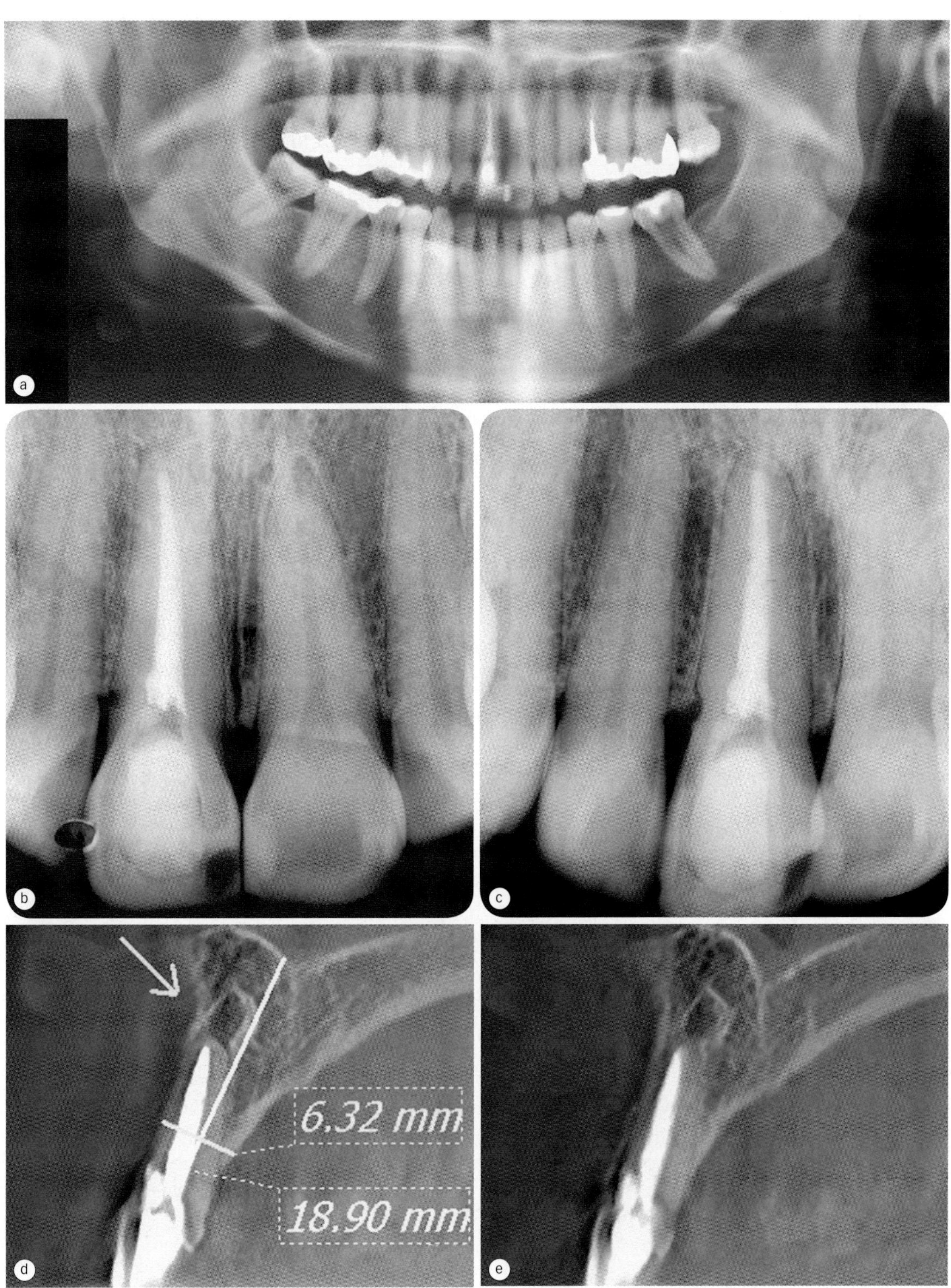


**Figure 10.2** - (**A-E**) Panoramic and periapical radiographs show normal periapical area of the upper right incisor. AP can be seen in the CBCT[102].

## 10.3 Periapical Index Based on Cone Beam Computed Tomography

With the great technological advances of recent years, new imaging modalities have been added to dental radiology as viable diagnostic tools. CBCT has been used for several clinical and investigational purposes in Endodontics [10,66,251,260,374].

Previous studies[47,257,273] have referred to the periapical index (PAI) as a scoring system for radiographic assessment of apical periodontitis. The PAI represents an ordinal scale of five scores ranging from no disease to severe periodontitis with exacerbating features, and is based on reference radiographs with confirmed histological diagnosis originally published by Brynolf[47]. Ørstavik's et al.[257] applied the PAI to both clinical trials and epidemiological surveys, and may be transformed into success and failure criteria by defining cut-off points on the scale for a dichotomous outcome assessment[169].

Given the limitations of conventional radiography for detection of AP and the availability of new emerging three-dimensional imaging modalities, the development of new periapical index seems to be a necessity. The purpose of this discussion was to evaluate a new periapical index based on CBCT for identification of AP.

Estrela et al.[101] evaluated a new periapical index based on CBCT for identification of apical periodontitis. The periapical index proposed in this study (CBCTPAI) was developed based on criteria established from measurements corresponding to periapical radiolucency interpreted on CBCT scans. Radiolucent images suggestive of periapical lesions were measured using the working tools of Planimp® software on CBCT scans in three dimensions: buccopalatal, mesiodistal and diagonal. The CBCTPAI was determined by the largest lesion extension. A 6-point (0-5) scoring system was used with two additional variables: expansion of cortical bone and destruction of cortical bone (Fig. 10.3 to 10.9). A total of 1,014 images (periapical radiographs and CBCT scans) originally taken from 596 patients were evaluated by 3 observers using the CBCTPAI criteria. AP was identified in 39.5% and 60.9% of cases by radiography and CBCT, respectively (Table 10.3). The CBCTPAI offers an accurate diagnostic method for use with high-resolution images, which can reduce the incidence of false-negative diagnosis, minimize observer interference and increase the reliability of epidemiological studies, especially those referring to AP prevalence and severity.

The accuracy of CBCT scans compared to periapical radiographic images are in accordance with the findings of previous studies[66,102,199,251,260,287,298,351]. Lofthag-Hansen et al.[199] compared intraoral periapical radiography and a 3D imaging system (3D Accuitomo) for the diagnosis of apical pathology in 36 patients (46 teeth). When both diagnostic methods were analyzed by all observers, they agreed that the CBCT images provided clinically relevant additional information not found in the periapical films. The capacity of computer tomography to evaluate a region of interest in three dimensions might benefit both novice and experienced clinicians alike. The advantages include increased accuracy, higher resolution, scan-time reduction and lower radiation dose[66].

The use of conventional radiography for detection of AP should be done with care because of the great possibility of false-negative diagnosis. The benefits of using CBCT in endodontics refer to its high accuracy in detecting periapical lesions even in its earliest stages and aiding in differential diagnosis as a non-invasive technique[102].

Simon et al.[298] compared the differential diagnosis of large periapical lesions (granuloma versus cyst) to traditional biopsy using CBCT. Seventeen large periapical radiolucencies (equal to or greater than 1 cm x 1 cm) were scanned to determine densities and a preoperative CBCT diagnosis was made. The lesions were then removed surgically and sent for histopathological examination. In 13 out of 17 cases, the biopsy report and CBCT diagnosis coincided. In 4 out of 17 cases, the CBCT read cyst, while the oral pathologist's diagnosis was chronic apical periodontitis. These results suggest that CBCT may provide a faster method to differentially diagnosis a solid from a fluid filled lesion or cavity, without invasive surgery and/or waiting a long time to see if nonsurgical therapy is effective.

The CBCTPAI proposed hereby has some advantages for clinical applications. CBCTPAI scores are calculated by analysis of the lesion in three dimensions, with CT slices being obtained in mesiodistal, buccopalatal and diagonal directions. The measurement of lesion depth contributes significantly to the diagnosis and consequently to improve case prognosis. The addition of the variables *expansion* of *cortical bone* and *destruction of cortical bone* to CBCTPAI scoring system permits the analysis of two possible sequels to AP that may be missed by periapical radiography. Detection of these conditions will alter the diagnostic hypothesis and the treatment plan. The goal of this new index is therefore to offer a method based on the interpretation of high-resolution images that can provide a more precise measurement of AP extension, minimizing observer interference and increasing the reliability of research results.

The PAI index as indicated by Ørstavik's et al.[257] range from health to severe periodontitis, based on the interpretation of two-dimensional radiographic images, while CBCTPAI scores have been established according to the interpretation of three dimensional CBCT scans. These two periapical indices have thus different scoring systems due to the characteristics of each target image (conventional periapical radiograph or CBCT scan). The scope of the present study is to evaluate a new periapical index that is based on an imaging modality that allow detection of lesions that are not visible radiographically. Considering the clinical history, the relation between health and disease in CBCTPAI can be begun by stage 1, without to detect cortical bone expansion or destruction of the cortical bone (Tables 10.3-10.4).

**Table 10.3** - Cone beam computed tomography periapical index (CBCTPAI) scores[101]

| Score | Quantitative bone alterations in mineral structures |
|---|---|
| **0** | Intact periapical bone structures |
| **1** | Diameter of periapical bone structure loss > 0.5-1mm |
| **2** | Diameter of periapical bone structure loss > 1-2mm |
| **3** | Diameter of periapical bone structure loss > 2-4mm |
| **4** | Diameter of periapical bone structure loss > 4-8mm |
| **5** | Diameter of periapical bone structure loss > 8mm |
| **Score (n) + E*** | Expansion of periapical cortical bone |
| **Score (n) + D*** | Destruction of periapical cortical bone |

*The variables E (expansion of cortical bone) and D (destruction of cortical bone) were added to each score, if either of these conditions was detected in the CBCT analysis.

**Table 10.4** - AP prevalence in endodontically treated teeth as determined by periapical radiography and cone beam computed tomography (CBCT) (n=1,014)[101]

| | Periapical radiography | CBCT | *p* value* |
|---|---|---|---|
| **Presence of AP** | 401 (39.5%) | 618 (60.9%) | p<0.001 |
| **Absence of AP** | 613 (60.5%) | 396 (39.1%) | |

* Chi-square test.

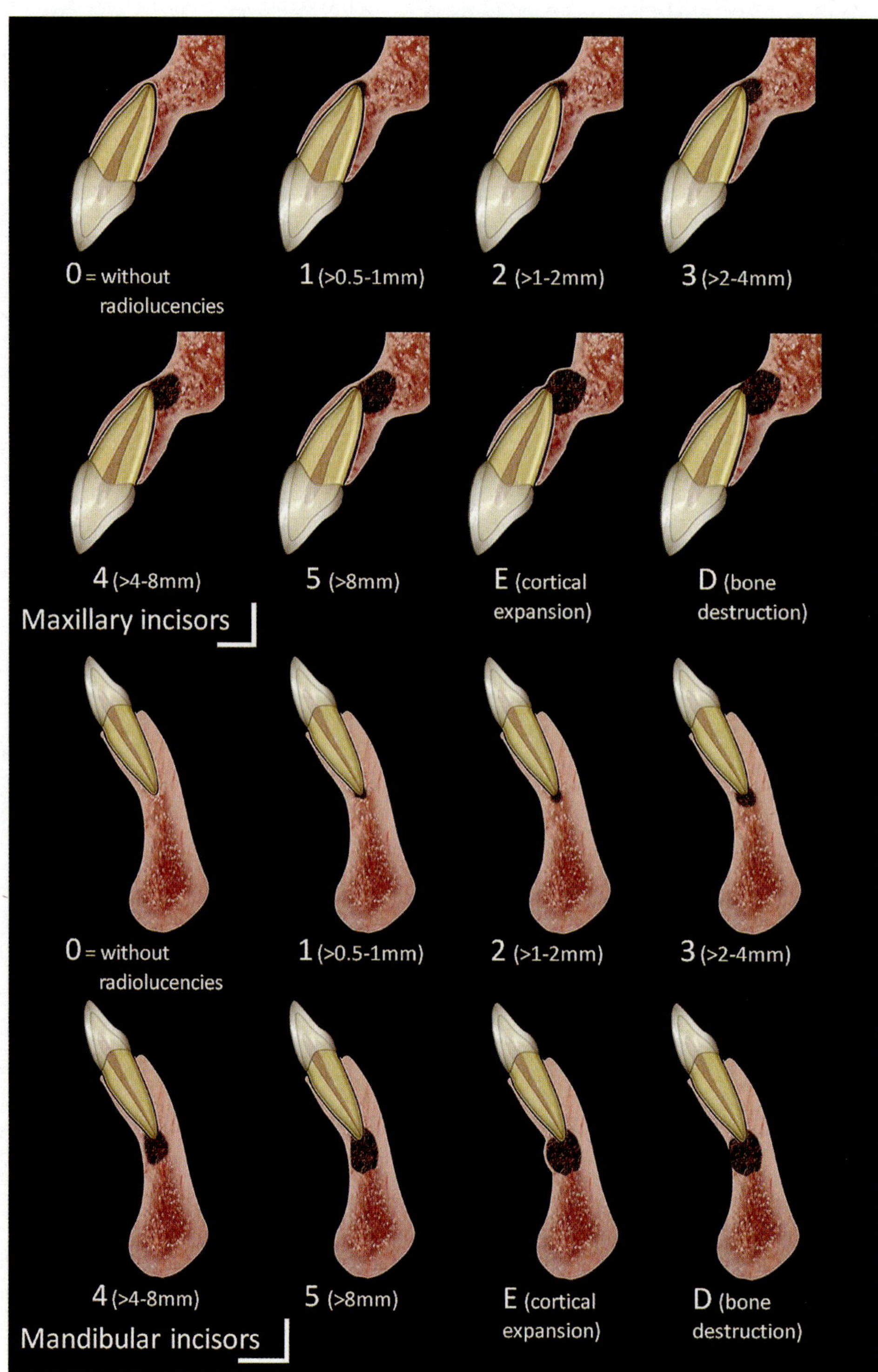


**Figure 10.3** - Schematic representations of incisors CBCTPAI[101].

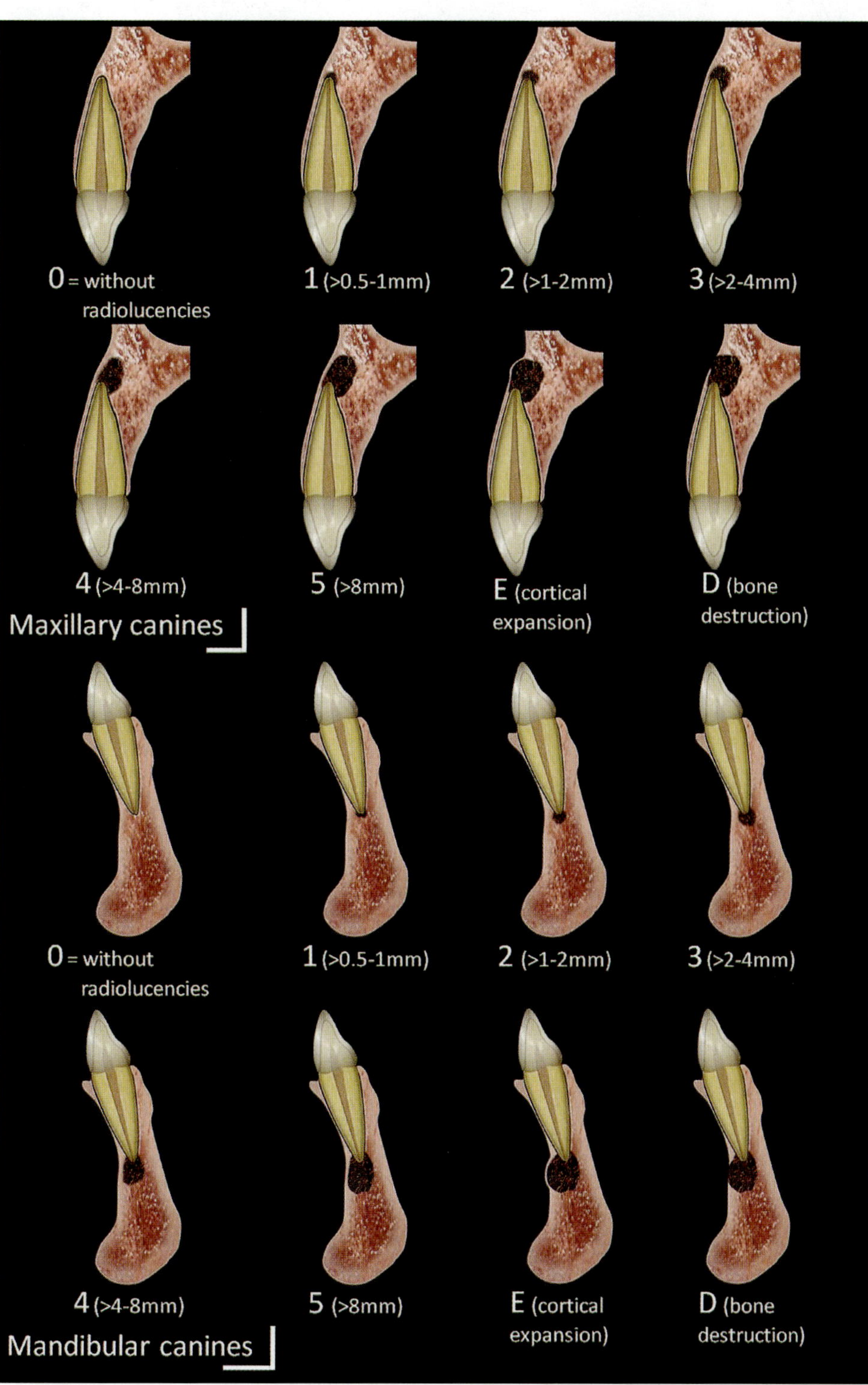


**Figure 10.4** - Schematic representations of canines CBCTPAI[101].

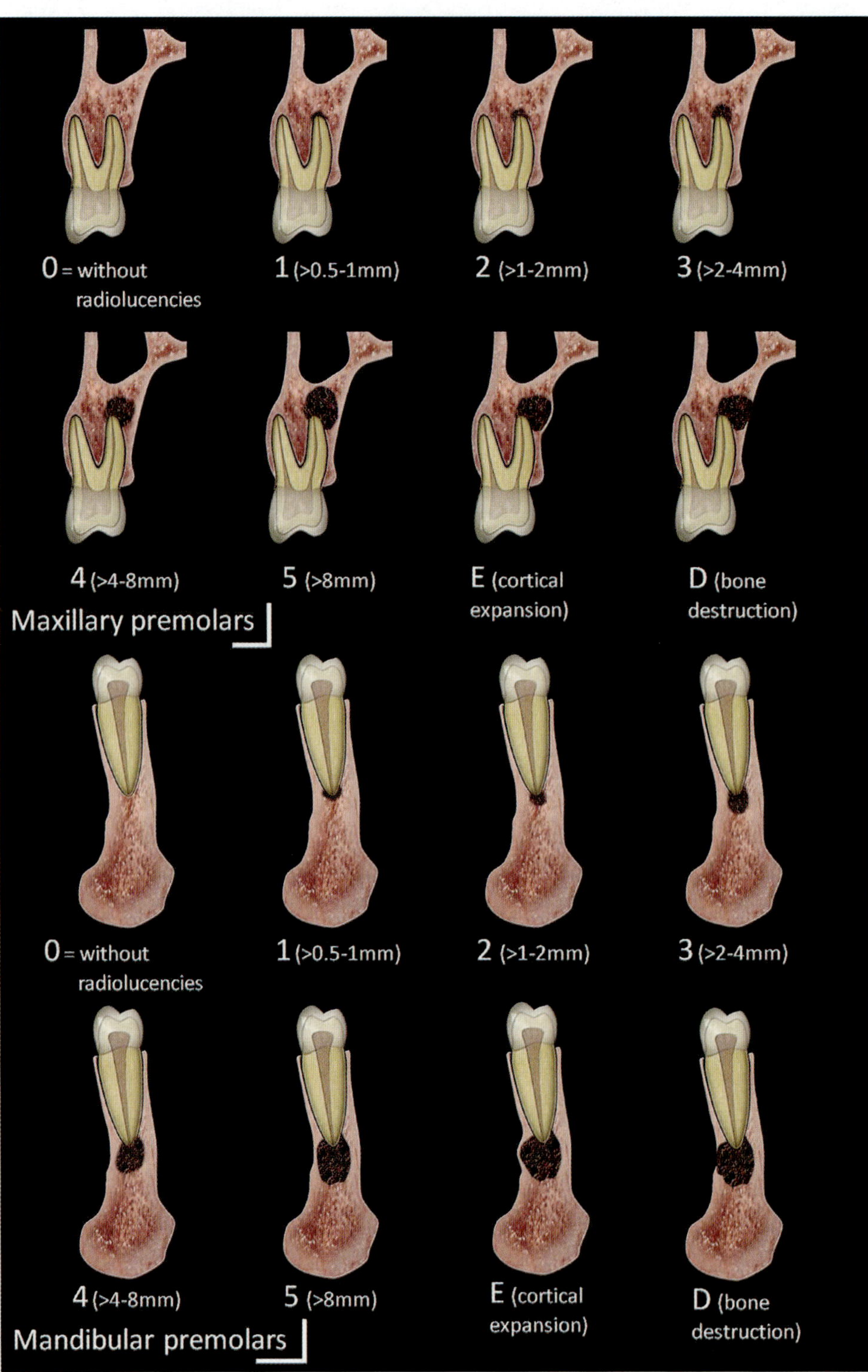


**Figure 10.5** - Schematic representations of premolars CBCTPAI[101].

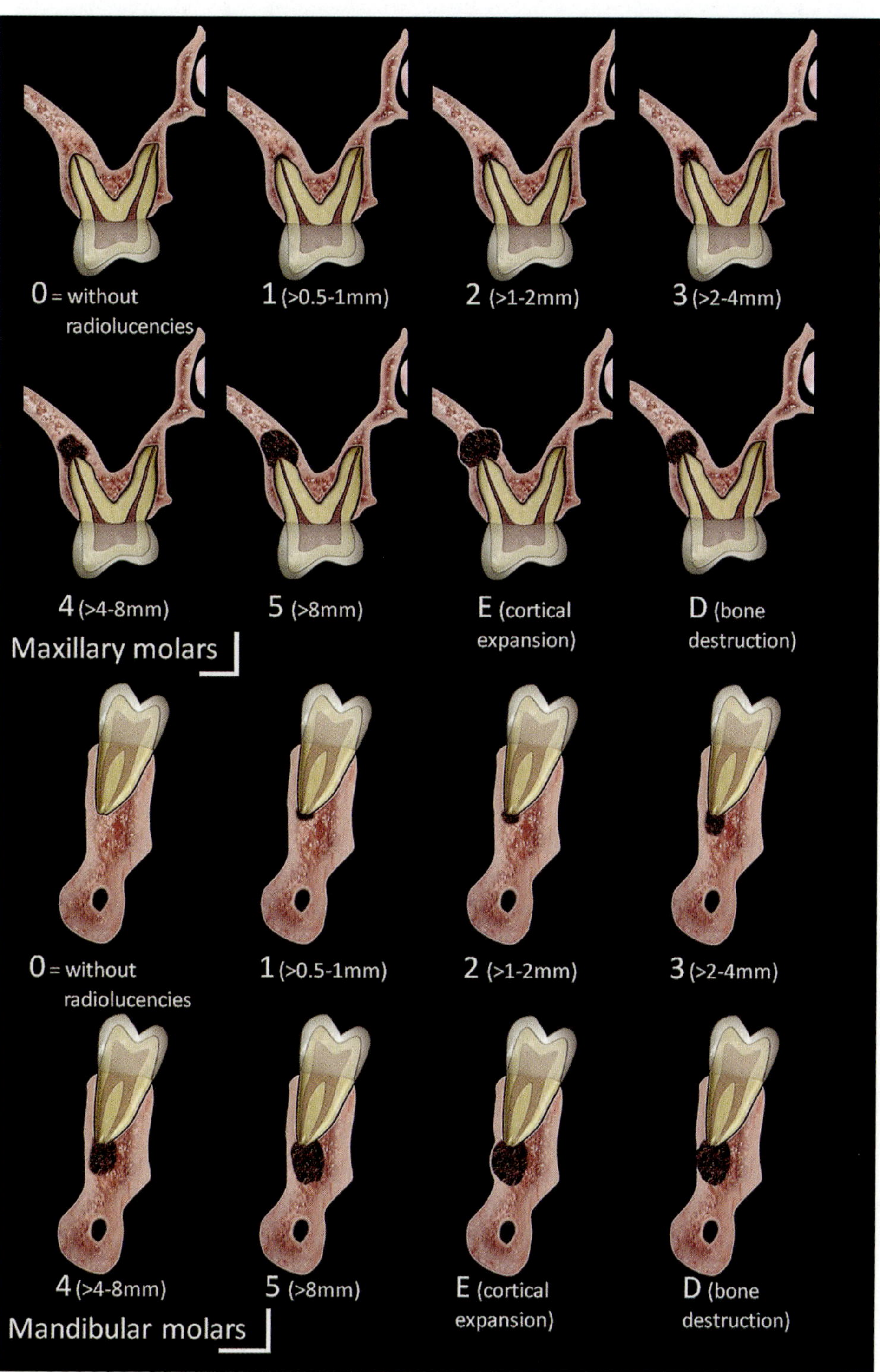


**Figure 10.6** - Schematic representations of molars CBCTPAI[101].

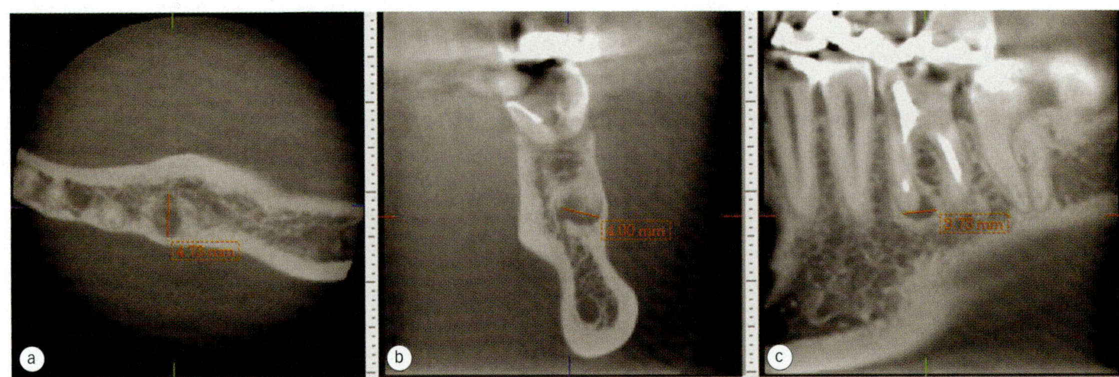


**Figure 10.7** - Clinical case of mandibular molar showing the axial (A), sagital (B) and coronal (C) planes. The CBCTPAI was determined by the largest extension of the lesion[101].

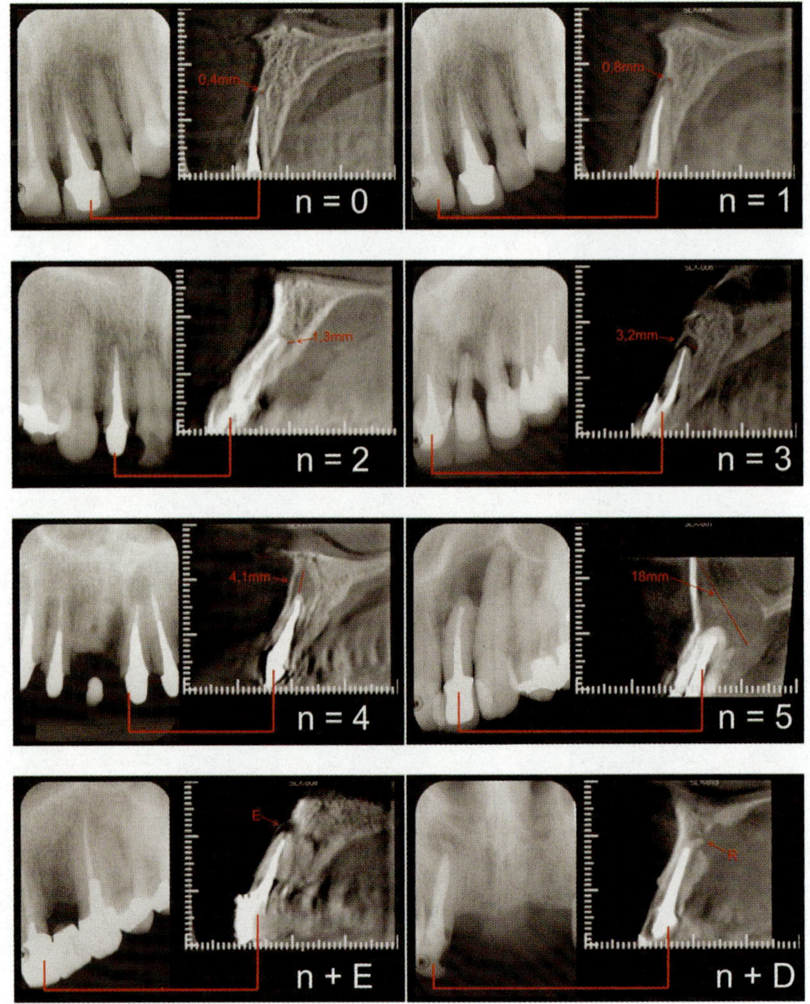


**Figure 10.8** - Clinical cases of maxillary incisors CBCTPAI showing all scores used and two additional variables (expansion of cortical bone and destruction of cortical bone)[101].

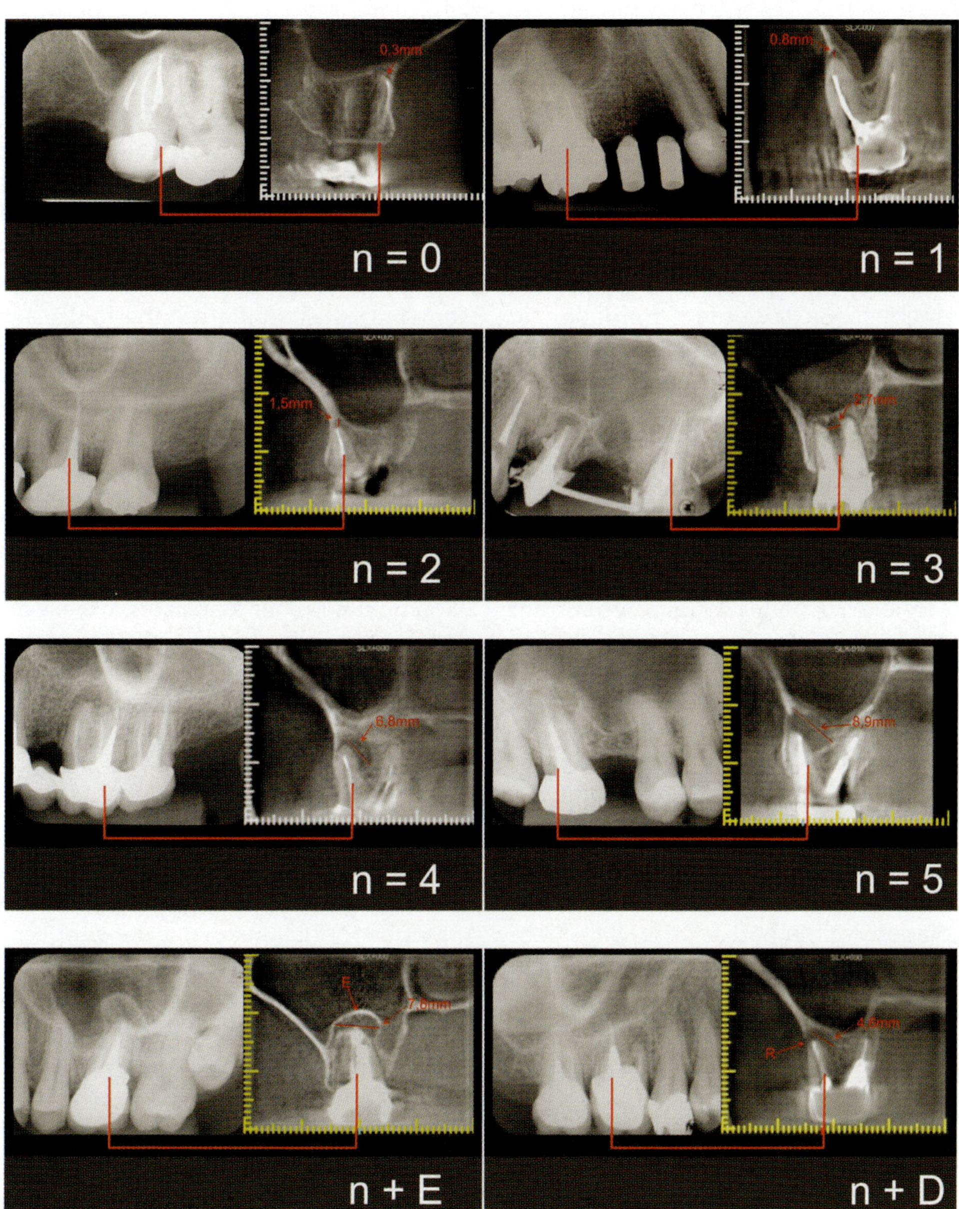


**Figure 10.9** - Clinical cases of maxillary molars CBCTPAI showing all scores used and two additional variables (expansion of cortical bone and destruction of cortical bone)[101].

The limitations of periapical radiography to identify AP support the need to review the epidemiological studies conducted in different populations worldwide. A considerable discrepancy among the imaging methods used to diagnose AP, especially with a new baseline value certainly may reduce the influence of radiographic interpretation and the possibility of false negative diagnosis.

In spite of the dental imaging technique, care should be taken to avoid misinterpretation. The presence of intracanal metallic posts, for example, may lead to equivocated interpretations due to artifact formation in CBCT images. Metallic objects can be present in either the tooth of interest or an adjacent one, and hinder the analysis of CBCT images[199], though in current days the influence of this artifact has been reduced. This artifact has been found to be closely related to the type of tissue or object (i.e., CT value) and the x-ray energy applied[177].

Biotechnology has brought important changes to today thinking and the contemporary world has witnessed the benefits brought by computer-based sciences to several fields of knowledge and health sciences, including dental specialties.

It may be concluded that AP detection was considerably higher using CBCT than periapical radiography. The periapical index proposed in this study (CBCTPAI) offers an accurate diagnostic method for use with high-resolution images, which can reduce the incidence of false-negative diagnosis, minimize observer interference and increase the reliability of epidemiological studies, especially those referring to AP prevalence and severity.

## 10.4 Therapy of Apical Periodontitis

### 10.4.1 Periapical biology

The periapical region is composed by the cementum, periodontal ligament and alveolar bone. The cementum is constituted of avascular and mineralized connective tissue, that covers the tooth's root surface. The thickness of the cementum on the apical region (150 a 200 μm) is larger than on the medium and cervical regions (50 μm); it is a cellular type (cementocytes), due to the reparative capacity, maintaining the deposition process, on which new layers can substitute the aged ones. The fibers of the periodontal ligament that penetrate the cementum (Sharpey fibers) are produced by the fibroblasts and are incorporated to this cementum, as it occurs the increase of the thickness. The periodontal ligament is formed by connective tissue (containing cells, fibers, fundamental substance, vessels and nerves). The periodontal ligament acts as element of sustentation of the tooth, and presents the fibroblast as predominant cell (contains yet osteoblasts and cementoblasts) and epithelial cells near the cementum (epithelial rests of Malassez). The epithelial net impedes the alveolar bone of uniting to the cementum structure. On the apical foramen it follows with the dental pulp. The index of renewing and remodeling of the collagen on the periodontal ligament is higher than in any other part of the body. The vascular supply of the periodontal ligament is abundant. The net of capillaries is more developed near the alveolar bone than near to the radicular surface. The lymphatic drainage follows the path of the blood vessels. There are myelinic and amyelinic nervous fibers. Proprioceptive nervous terminations, sensible to pressure (percussion), are also seen. It is highlighted, among the main functions of the periodontal ligament, the support, sensorial, nutritive, synthesis and resorption. This tissue is found on continuous state of physiologic activity, which promotes the maintenance and adaptation of the support structures. On the radiographic aspect, it is observed a radiolucent space correspondent to the periodontal ligament. On this local it is found cells of the connective tissue (fibroblasts, cementoblasts and osteoblasts); epithelial rests of Mallassez (forming interlaced net on the periodontal ligament, instituting the residual epithelial of Hertwig, that is distributed near the cementum); defense cells (macrophages, mastocytes, eosinophils and cells associated to neuromuscular elements)[37,218,259,342].

The alveolar bone (lamina dura composed of compact bone) covers the dental alveolus, being perforated by several canals (Volman's canals) which contain blood vessels and supply the periodontal ligament. Between the lamina dura and the cortical bone (external to the alveolar process) it is found the spongy bone. The radiographic aspect is composed of radiopaque line distributed without interruption [37,218,259,342].

**10.4.2 Pulpal necrosis**

The periapical reaction is observed by the apical extension of the pulpal aggressor agents. With the progression of the inflammation of the pulpal tissue, it can be observed the tissue's dissolution (autolysis of tissue's proteins), due to the action of proteolytic enzymes of the lysosomes. The infiltration of polymorphonuclears favors the liquefaction of the necrotic tissue, by the conjunct action of autolysis and heterolysis. The liquefaction necrosis results from the action of hydrolytic, bacterial and endogenous enzymes (neutrophils). Another situation occurs when there is the development of the phenomenon of the proteic denaturation, predominating over the autolysis, impeding the total dissolution of the cells. The pulpal tissue looses water without decomposing, demonstrating firm consistency, from the coagulation, characterizing other form of necrosis. Usually, it is observed this kind of necrosis on the traumatic lesions, when there was tissue's ischemia. It is found yet, other clinical situation on which the pulpal cavity is empty. Probably, there was liquefaction necrosis with additional loss of liquid, remaining only rests[57,147,368].

After the pulpal necrosis, the environment of the pulpal cavity becomes propitious and ideal to the factors that influence the microbial growth and colonization (nutrients, low tension of oxygen, carbonic gas and the existent interactions). These factors are connected to the aggressions and to the responses, because are related with the microbial pathogenicity and virulence[122,147,216,217,231-258,276,301-337].

The presence and distribution of the microorganisms in infected root canals and its influence as expressive precursors of the inflammatory reactions of the dental pulp and of the periapical tissues established an important association of cause and effect, better defining some parameters of responses to different aggressor agents[61]. The dynamic existent between microorganism, virulence and organic response motivated the development of researches that propitiated more comprehensible and convincing explications and definitions about the intimate relation between microbiology and pathology. The microorganisms represent an important role on the establishment of the periapical lesion. Among the bacterial pathogenic mechanisms on the periapical disease, there are: invasion; production of exotoxins; cellular constituents (endotoxins, surface components, capsules); production of enzymes (collagenase, hialuronidase, acid phophatase, fibrinolysin, coagulase, protease, enzyme degrading fibronectin); products of the microbial metabolism (greasy acids – propionic, butyric, acetic acid; ammonia, sulphurated composts ($H_2S$), indol); evasion of the immunologic responses of the host. The combination of the direct (enzymes, toxins, metabolic products) and indirect (stimulation of the liberation of mediators, as the cellular constituents – lipopolysaccharide, peptideoglycan, lipoteicoic acid) bacterial effects influences the host's defense and determines the periapical response. The most frequent path of microbial invasion in the root canal and periapical tissues is by the coronary path – dental caries and debility on the coronary sealing.

The microorganisms when infect the root canal present the potential of stimulating the periapical inflammation. The virulence and pathogenicity of individual species vary considerably and can be affected by other microorganisms. Although isolated species of the endodontic microbiota are of low virulence, in association (due to combination of factors) it can be pathogenic. Among the factors, there are: interactions with other microorganisms in the root canal (benefic synergism); liberation of endotoxins; synthesis of enzymes that damage host's tissues; ability to interfere and evade host's defenses[246]. The microbial aggregations represent a valuable resource for the feasibility of determined microorganisms. Nevertheless, some microorganisms present capacity to avoid the host's defenses, blocking the first important step of the inflammatory response[246,336,337].

The mechanism of formation of the periapical lesion is complex. Bacteria, as the Gram-negative anaerobic, presenting the lipopolysaccharide (LPS) as constituent of the cellular wall, plays an important role on this mechanism.

Thus, it is evidenced the extension of the inflammatory and/or infectious processes of the dental pulp to the periapical tissues. In the pulpal cavity the microorganisms proliferate protected of the organism's defense elements, that are conducted by the blood vessels present in the periapical region. When the microorganisms cross the apical foramen, the defense cells try to block its advance. The response of the battle between aggressor and the defense characterizes the periapical pathologic stage. Thus, two factors should be considered on the nature of the periapical lesion: the virulence of the microorganisms and the organic resistance. Considering that the Chapter 9 discussed the biology and pathology of the apical periodontitis, on the present topic it will be discussed clinical aspects relative to the epidemiology and therapy of the apical periodontitis. The Figure 10.10 show schematic representation of microbial injuries factors influent on the development of apical periodontitis.

## 10.5 Inflammatory Pathologies of the Periapex

The inflammatory pathologies of the periapical region are influenced by the pathogenic characteristics, by the number of aggressor microorganisms (gifted with the respective virulence armory) that invade this area, associate with the dynamic of responses of the host. This interaction between the microorganisms and the host's responses determines the different types of periapical alterations. It is frequently observed inflammatory lesions of chronic nature accompanied or not of the presence of symptom (periapical pain to palpation, percussion, localized edema). The presence of polymorphonuclears (neutrophils) and mononuclear cells (macrophages) can be observed. Clinically, the relation of the occurrence of inflammation of acute and/or chronic nature on this region is imprecise. The professional trying to associate the symptomatology characteristics (presence or absence of pain) with microscopic observations, can misinterpret, because there can be neutrophils and no symptomatology. Either the acute or the chronic phase of the inflammation on the periapical region can involve periapical osseous resorption.

However, it should be noticed the fact that these microorganisms, besides being pathogenic to the periapical tissues, can invade and attack other regions. The odontogenic infections can disseminate to facial spaces, becoming more problematic to the treatment alternatives and requiring more attention and special care handling the patient. The Figures 10.11 express the most frequent dissemination paths of the odontogenic infections.

The World Health Organization[373] classifies the periapical inflammation in five categories: acute apical periodontitis (K04.4), chronic apical periodontitis (K04.5), periapical abscess without fistula (K04.7), periapical abscess with fistula (K04.6) and periapical cyst (K04.8)[241].

The diagnosis of the periapical alterations adopted on the clinical context will be structured according to the treatment. This topic was excellently discussed on the previous chapter, and following the same parameters previously adopted, however with a clinical perspective the diagnosis adopted on the present chapter uses the classification exhibited on Figure 10.12. Thus, the Figure 10.13 presents a sequence of pulpal and periapical pathologic events.

| Direct Action | |
|---|---|
| **Microorganisms** | |
| | ⇒ Periodontal Ligament<br>⇒ Alveolar Bone |
| **Enzymes** | |
| | ⇒ Collagenase<br>⇒ Hialuronidase<br>⇒ Acid Phosphatase<br>⇒ Other enzymes |
| **Toxins** | |
| | ⇒ Lipopolysaccharide<br>⇒ Teicoic/Lipoteicoic Acid<br>⇒ Peptideoglycan |
| **Metabolic Products** | |
| | ⇒ Greasy acid, butyric acid, acetic acid, ammonia, sulphurated compounds, indol |
| **Indirect Action** | |
| **Lipopolysaccharide (LPS)** | |
| | **Cytocins**<br>⇒ Interleukin 1 $\alpha$<br>⇒ Interleukin 1 $\beta$<br>⇒ Tumoral Necrosis Factor $\alpha$<br>⇒ Factor of migration of macrophages<br>⇒ Factor of activation of osteoclasts<br>⇒ Metabolic products of the aracdonic acid<br>⇒ Prostaglandin $E_2$ |

**Figure 10.10** - Schematic representation of microbial aggression factors influent on the development of the apical periodontitis.

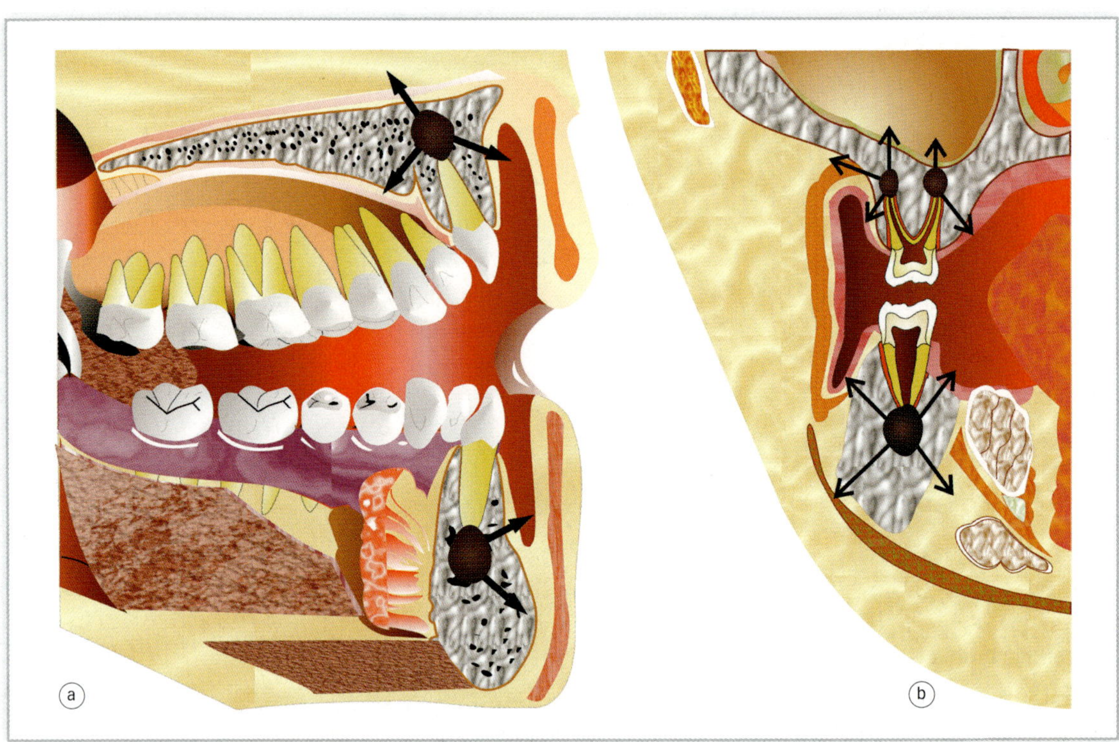


**Figures 10.11AB** - Dissemination paths of the odontogenic infections.

| Clinical Classification of the Periapical Inflammation |
|---|
| **Symptomatic Apical Periodontitis** |
| → Traumatic |
| → Infectious |
| **Asymptomatic Apical Periodontitis** |
| **Periapical Abscess Without Fistula** |
| → Phase I – Initial |
| → Phase II – Evolving |
| → Phase III – Evolved |
| **Periapical Abscess With Fistula** |

**Figure 10.12** - Clinical classification of the periapical inflammation.

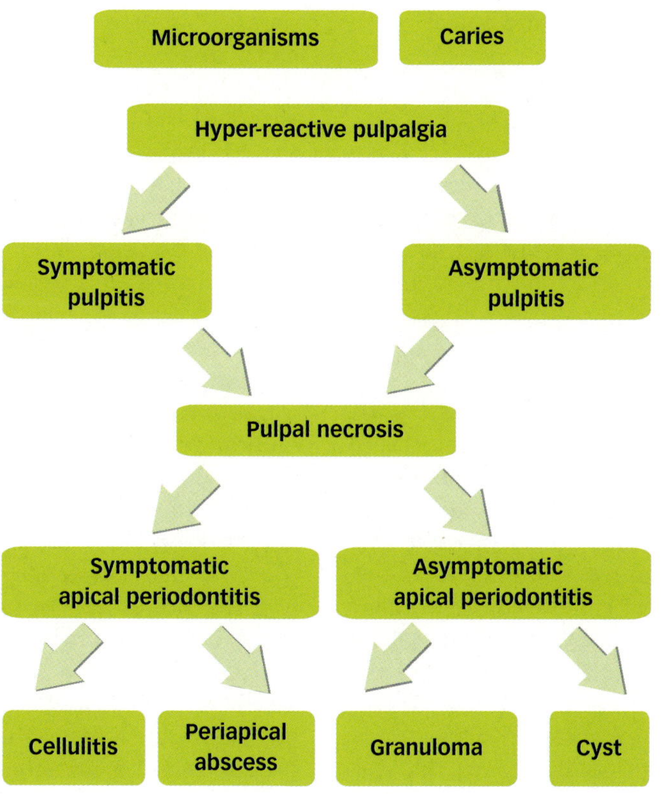


**Figure 10.13** - Sequence of pulpal and periapical pathological events.

## 10.6 Symptomatic Apical Periodontitis

The symptomatic apical periodontitis is an inflammation that occurs in the apical periodontium in consequence to traumatic irritations (occlusal trauma, over-instrumentation), chemical (over-irrigation, over-medication), physical (over-fillings or rests of materials that are extruded) and microbial (invasion of microorganisms, dissemination of toxins and enzymes, metabolic products, cellular components), which determine inflammatory and immunologic responses.

This localized inflammation in the apical periodontal ligament is characterized by acute exuding reaction, composed of polymorphonuclear cells, leukocytes and some dispersed mononuclear cells. Besides the edema, on these traumatic situations occurs focus of hemorrhage. The pain is present and it is pathognomonic, because the external pressure compresses nervous fibers, what maintains the tooth painful until the bone suffer resorption and accommodate the edema. On this situation of infection with severe aggression, the final result can be the formation of periapical abscess.

Thus, it can be established two sub-classifications: the symptomatic apical periodontitis of traumatic nature and the symptomatic apical periodontitis of infectious nature. The first is observed after the treatment of tooth with vital pulp, while the second with necrotic pulp. Due to the characterization of the etiological factors it is not difficult to distinguish neither identifies them.

### 10.6.1 Traumatic symptomatic apical periodontitis

Clinical and therapeutic aspects

The traumatic symptomatic apical periodontitis is an inflammatory manifestation that can occur either after a restoration, which remains a premature contact, or after the instrumentation and filling of a tooth with pulpal vitality. The process usually evolves to the cure with the removal of the etiologic agent.

The appearance of pain after the root canal treatment on teeth with pulpal vitality occurs due to the installation of inflammatory process in the periodontal ligament. The periapical pain is a reality present and experimented by the patient, that seeks the solution with the root canal treatment (relief of pain, of the sequels of the inflammatory process and the reestablishment of the referred tooth). Different etiologic factors can be responsible for the present aggression, such as: the act of the pulpectomy, the apical limit of instrumentation, the irrigating chemical substance, the intracanal dressing, the filling material, the instrumentation technique, among others. The correct execution of the operative stages, of the biological and mechanic principles of the preparation and filling of the root canal should lead to high number of success on the treatment, identified either by the absence of postoperative symptomatology or by tissue's reparation.

Crump[67] emphasizes that although the preparation and filling of the root canal apparently look satisfactory (obeyed the adequate diagnosis and operative technique), it can persist clinical signals and symptoms that characterize possible failures on the executed treatment. The analysis of systemic factors is important during the anamnesis and the clinical exam, because the decrease of the organic resistance makes possible that the alterations caused by the disease exceed the host's potential of reparation, maintaining persistent the painful frame.

The establishment of criteria for the measurement of painful responses, on the comparative analysis of agents used on the root canal treatment is questionable, due to the difficulties on the reproduction and quantification of the values obtained. Several scales of responses and evaluations of the pain have been used; however, they are subjective data, but acceptable, because at the moment it is what can be used[112].

During the root canal treatment it is complex and difficult to distinguish fully the aggressor agent responsible for the postoperative pain, since there is a sum of factors triggering the inflammatory process (instrumentation technique, apical limit, chemical substance, intracanal dressing, systemic condition associated).

Estrela et al.[116] studied the influence of the chemical substance, of the filling sealer and the number of sessions on the prevalence of the traumatic symptomatic apical periodontitis. It was analyzed 160 teeth with pulpal vitality indicated for radical root canal treatment. After the diagnosis, it was proceeded the anesthesia, absolute isolation and coronary opening. The apical limit of instrumentation adopted was of 1 to 1.5 mm beneath the radiographic apex vertex. For the large canals, the pulpectomy was performed by pulpal excision using a modified Hedströem file, while for the atresic canals it was performed together with the preparation (fragmentation). The root canal preparation was made using two principles of the crown down technique[113]. The minimum lateral limit of enlargement adopted was the following: single root teeth – file # 35, mesial roots of lower molars and buccal of upper molars – file # 30, distal roots of lower molars and lingual of upper molars – file # 40. During the preparation of the root canal it was performed at each change of file abundant irrigation-aspiration with 1% sodium hypochlorite. On the last two files used, the root canal was dried and completely filled with 17% trisodic EDTA, maintained for a period of 3 minutes, followed of irrigation-aspiration with 1% sodium hypochlorite. From the 160 teeth used on the present study, 82 were filled on one session and 78 on two sessions. The teeth treated on two sessions remained with calcium hydroxide associated to saline solution, which paste had the consistency of a toothpaste, filling totally the prepared canal. For the filling maneuvers, it was used the active lateral condensation of gutta-percha. On 84 teeth, it was used the Sealapex sealer, while on 76 it was used the sealer based of zinc oxide and eugenol (Grossman sealer, Fill-Canal). Passed 24 hours of execution of the definitive treatment, the patients returned for postoperative evaluation, when it was registered the presence or absence of postoperative pain, according to the following criteria: absent, when the patient did not report any symptomatology; mild, when the patient reported the not constant use of analgesic for pain relief; and severe, when the use of analgesic was constant by the patient and the pain was not relieved. Nevertheless, independently of the degrees of pain mild and severe, it was tabulated only as symptomatology present. The teeth filled with Sealapex showed a percentage of 87.5% and 88.6% of absence of pain after the root canal treatment, performed on one and two sessions, respectively. When the sealer used was the FillCanal®, the percentage of absence of pain with the treatment on one or two sessions was 85.7% and 82.3%, respectively. On all groups it was used the 1% sodium hypochlorite alternated on the two last irrigations with EDTA and instrumented with the cervical preparation technique. Facing the analysis of the number of sessions, it is noticed high percentage of absence of postoperative pain, independently of the number of sessions, one or two, having no significant differences between them. It should be considered, besides the number of sessions, the influence of factors inherent to the therapy itself.

The number of sessions (one or two) for the execution of the root canal treatment, histologically seems not to show expressive differences, if it is adopted an atraumatic root canal preparation technique, and used a filling material biologically compatible.

Facing situations of traumatic apical periodontitis, Holland et al.[162] analyzed on dog's teeth the biologic effects of the calcium hydroxide and the corticosteroid-antibiotics (Otosporin), as intracanal dressing in pulpectomies, after over-instrumentation, using two filling materials – the zinc oxide and eugenol and the Sealapex. After 180 days, the interpretations of the results allowed the following conclusions (Fig. 10.14-10.19):

1. Using the Otosporin® as intracanal dressing, the biologic closure of the main apical foramen was observe on 73.35% of the cases when the filling material was the Sealapex (Fig. 10.15) and 20% with the zinc oxide and eugenol;
2. Using the calcium hydroxide as dressing the biologic closure of the apical foramen was observed on 80% of the canals filled with Sealapex (Fig. 10.16-10.17) and 40% with zinc oxide and eugenol (Fig. 10.18-10.19);
3. Using the calcium hydroxide as dressing, it was not observed differences in relation to the small accessory canals between the two filling sealers;
4. When the dressing was the Otosporin, the accessory canals showed high incidence of closure when the filling material was the Sealapex;
5. When particles of Sealapex reached the periodontal ligament, they caused mild inflammatory reaction, characterized mainly by macrophage reaction. On the absence of biologic closure the zinc oxide and eugenol frequently produced mild chronic inflammatory reaction.

The advantages for the execution of the root canal treatment in teeth with pulpal vitality on one session are obtained with the reduction of the possibilities of contamination between the appointments, with the professional's technical advantages, observed with the familiarization of the anatomy and due to economic factors involved on the number of appointments.

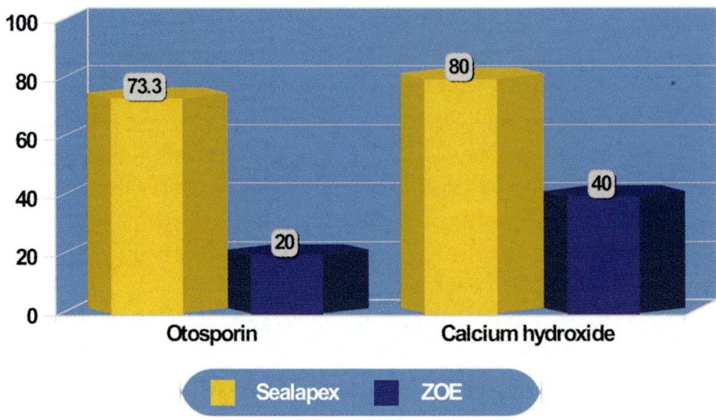


**Figure 10.14** - Biologic closure observed on the experimental groups (Holland et al.[162], 1998).

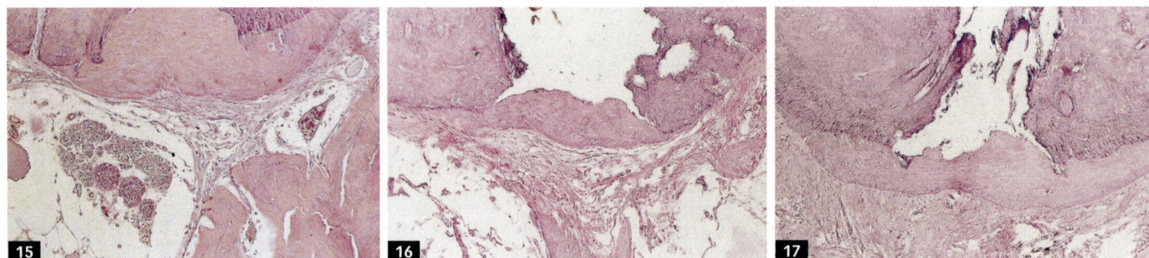


**Figure 10.15** - Otosporin – Sealapex – Biologic closure of the main foramen (H.E., X 100) (Holland et al.[162], 1998).
**Figure 10.16** - $Ca(OH)_2$ – Sealapex – Biologic closure of the main foramen (H.E., X 100) (Holland et al.[162], 1998).
**Figure 10.17** - $Ca(OH)_2$ – Sealapex – Biologic closure of the of the main foramen (H.E., X 100) (Holland et al.[162], 1998).

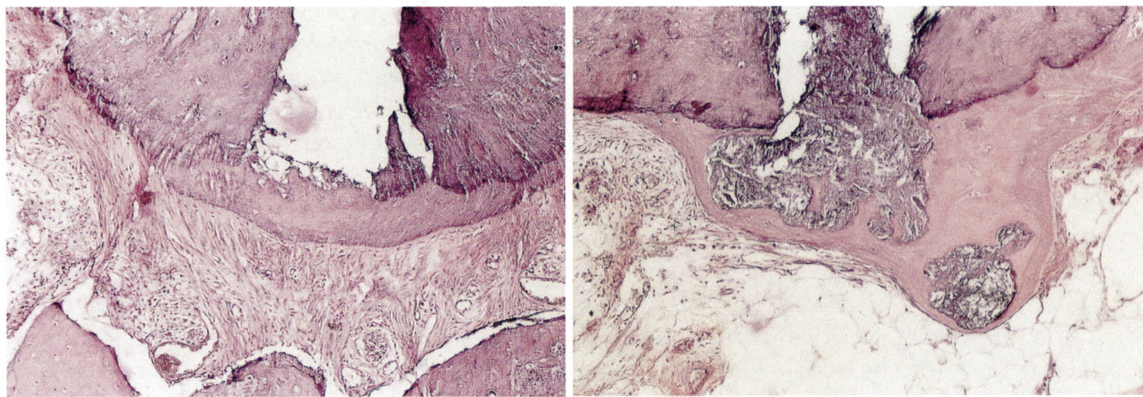

**Figure 10.18** - $Ca(OH)_2$ – zinc oxide and eugenol. Biologic closure of the main foramen (H.E., X 100) (Holland et al.[162], 1998).

**Figure 10.19** - $Ca(OH)_2$ – zinc oxide and eugenol. Biologic closure of the main foramen. Presence of dentinal scraps (H.E., X100) (Holland et al.[98], 1998).

Marion[208] analyzed the in vivo effect of using or not a corticosteroid-antibiotic (Otosporin) dressing on the healing process of dogs' teeth after biopulpectomy and root canals filling with Sealapex or MTA with propylene glycol. Were used forty roots of incisives and pre-molars of two young adult mongrel dogs' from the same litter aging about 2 years old. The teeth were biomechanically prepared by reverse mixed technique. After that the cementary barrier was perforated and enlarged up to file K#25, originating a main foramen. Twenty canals received a dressing with Otosporin for 7 days aiming to allow the neo-formation of a pulp stump. Each root canal was then filled by the lateral condensation technique with gutta-percha points and one of the studied materials. The remaining 20 canals were filled in just one session using the same root canal filling technique and materials, but without the use of Otosporin dressing. After 90 days, the animals were sacrificed by an overdose of anesthetic, the jaws were removed the teeth were prepared for histomorphological and histomicrobiological analysis. The materials presented similar results independently of the use of the Otosporin. The Otosporin dressing favored the healing process with both studied filling material. In conclusion, the root canal filling with Sealapex or MTA with propylene glycol preceded by the Otosporin dressing improved the healing process (Fig. 10.20A-D).

The prevalence of symptomatic apical periodontitis, of traumatic origin, depends not only of the professional's ability, but also is admitted the possibility of suffering influences of the chemical substance, the filling sealer, the number of appointments and the systemic conditions of the patient[116] (Fig. 10.21A-D).

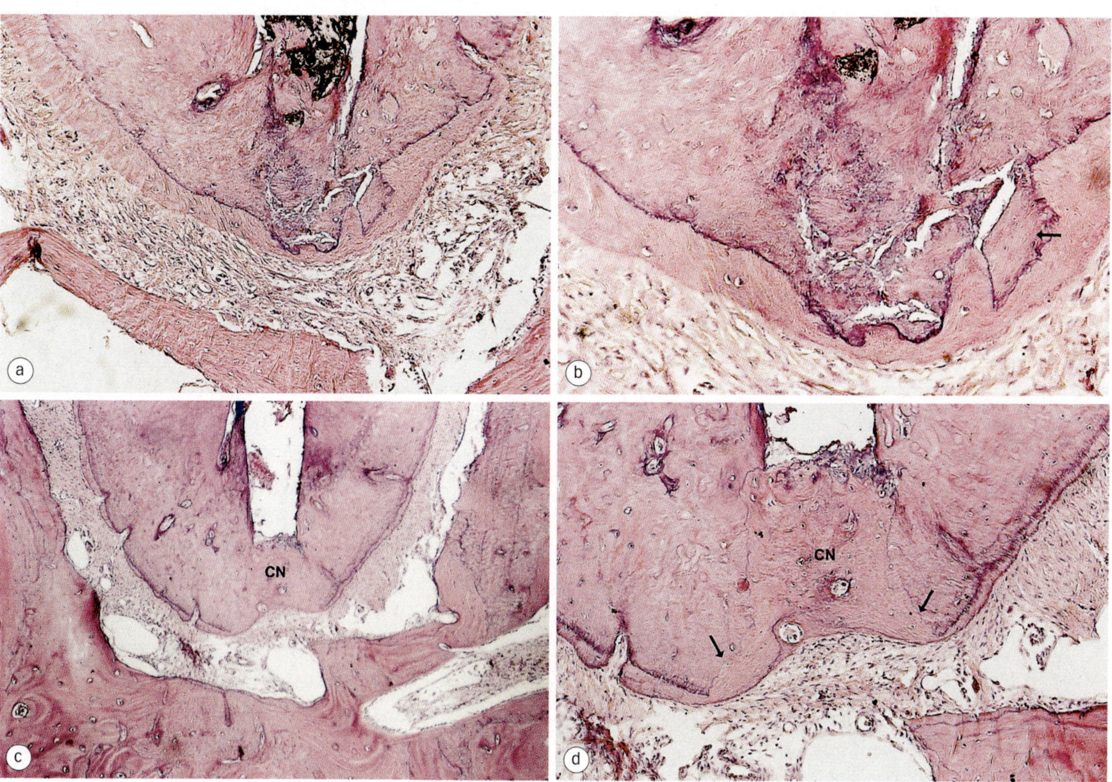


**Figure 10.20** - (**A**) Sealapex with Otosporin. Biological closure of the main root canal (H.E. X100). (**B**) Biological closure of the main root canal (H.E. X200). (**C**) MTA with Otosporin. Biological closure of the main root canal (H.E. X40). (**D**) Biological closure of the main root canal (H.E. X100) (Marion & Holland et al.[208]).

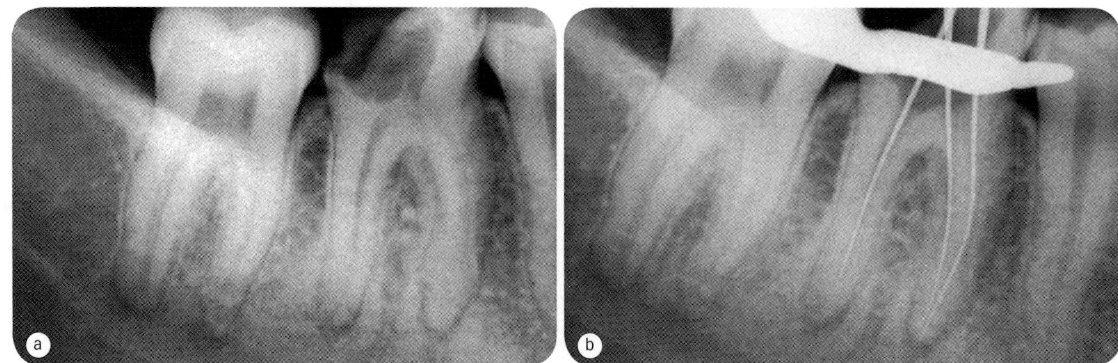

**Figure 10.21** - (**A-B**) Symptomatic pulpitis.

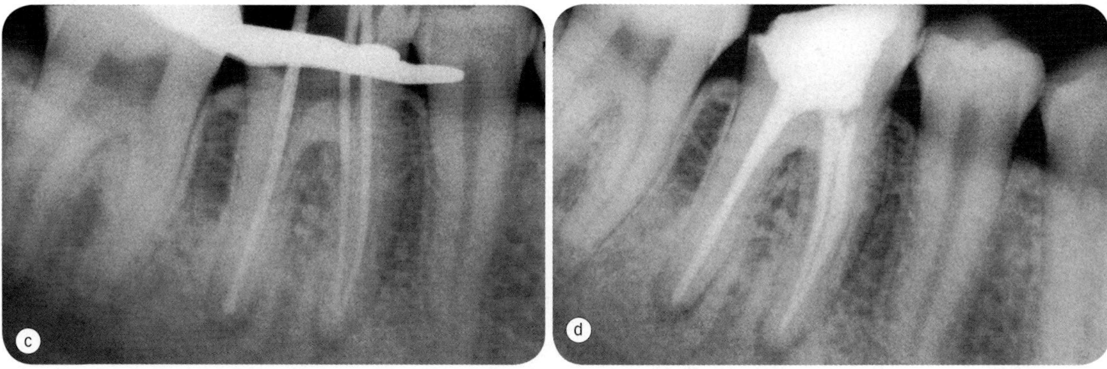

**Figure 10.21** - (**C-D**) Traumatic Symptomatic Apical Periodontitis.

The use of the 1% sodium hypochlorite during the root canal preparation, associated with EDTA on the final irrigations, conjunct with the use of an atraumatic instrumentation, conducts to low indexes of postoperative pain on the root canal treatments of teeth with pulpal vitality.

Some clinical characteristics collaborate for the establishment of the diagnosis of the traumatic symptomatic apical periodontitis, such as:

1. Pain after the preparation of root canal with vital pulp (inflamed or healthy);
2. Presence of pain to palpation and percussion;
3. Feeling of extruded tooth after restoration, with pain at touch;
4. Premature contact.

The radiographic aspect is not a determinant factor, because the space correspondent to the periodontal membrane can vary from normal to a slight enlargement.

The treatment of the traumatic symptomatic apical periodontitis usually is directed to the adoption of systemic measure to control the pain and inflammation. The etiologic agent is due to a chemical, physical or traumatic aggression on a clinical situation of pulpal vitality, which is presumed absence of microorganisms. When the case is executed by the own professional, in which the option was the treatment on one appointment, or on two appointments (if maintained intracanal dressing based on calcium hydroxide), well conducted, it is waited the postoperative control of the systemic medication prescribed. When the case was executed by other professional, on one appointment, the root canal treatment is evaluated, and when considered satisfactory, maintain it and wait the effect of the systemic medication. If there is continuity of the pain or doubt about the quality of treatment, it is chosen the retreatment (emptying of the canal, placement of intracanal dressing), and waited the disappearance of the symptomatic condition for new filling. On the cases of treatment on two appointments which it is not known which were the conditions of preparation of the root canal, the chemical substance and the intracanal dressing used, the tooth is again opened, the root canal is cleaned, the intracanal dressing is used filling the root canal (calcium hydroxide paste), and waited the control of the pain and the effect of the local and systemic medication, to finalize the root canal treatment. The Figure 10.21 exhibit a clinical case of symptomatic pulpitis, executed on one appointment, that after the endodontic treatment developed a frame of traumatic symptomatic apical periodontitis. The therapeutics adopted, considering as possible etiologic agent a traumatism due to clinical maneuvers, was only systemic medication to control the pain and inflammation.

Estrela et al.[118] evaluated longitudinal studies about the pain after use of intracanal medicaments in treatment of inflamed pulp, using systematic review. A MEDLINE search strategy was developed to identify articles using the following search terms: *Chlorhexidine and Periapical pain or Symptom or Flare-up or Endodontic Post-treatment or Inter-appointment / Calcium hydroxide and Periapical pain or Symptom or Flare-up or Endodontic Post-treatment or Inter-appointment / Sodium Hypochlorite and Periapical pain or Symptom or Flare-up or Endodontic Post-treatment or Inter-appointment / Intracanal dressing and Periapical pain or Symptom or Flare-up or Endodontic Post-treatment or Inter-appointment / Intracanal medicament and Periapical pain or Symptom or Flare-up or Endodontic Post-treatment or Inter-appointment / Paramonochlorophenol and Periapical pain or Symptom or Flare-up or Endodontic Post-treatment or Inter-appointment.* The search included articles from the MEDLINE (http://www.pubmed.gov), from 1966 to May 17th of 2007. 64 articles were selected, but only 2 studies[135,255] satisfied the inclusion criteria. Considering the success estimative of analyzed studies, it could be observed evidence about the higher rate of absence of pos-treatment pain, when it was used an adequate sanitization process and a rational use of intracanal medicament in endodontic treatment of teeth with pulpal inflammation.

### 10.6.2 Infectious symptomatic apical periodontitis

#### Clinical and therapeutic aspects

The importance of microorganisms in the root canal has been the object of discussion for many years[1-379]. In clinical situations, endodontic treatment aims to eliminate microorganisms from the root canal system by means of the various of procedures, i.e., biomechanical preparation, irrigation with different solutions and the use of intracanal dressings and a three-dimensional filling.

The success of endodontic treatment is directly influenced by the control of microorganisms in infected root canals. It is therefore important to consider the type of infection occurring. The primary root canal infection is associated with endodontic microbiota generally composed of Gram-negative anaerobic bacteria. In root-filled teeth, the microorganisms can persist and maintain the apical periodontitis. Microorganisms present in secondary root canal infection are those that were resistant to the first treatment or penetrated after the root canal filling and coronal sealing. Sundqvist et al.[329] determined what microbial flora was present in teeth after failed root canal therapy and established the outcomes of conservative re-treatment. The microbial flora was mainly composed of single species mostly of Gram-positive organisms. The most commonly recovered isolates were bacteria of the species *E. faecalis*. The overall success rate of re-treatment was 74%. The microbial flora in canals after failed endodontic therapy differed markedly from the flora found in untreated teeth. The infection at the time of root filling and the size of the periapical lesion were factors that had a negative influence on the prognosis. Three of four endodontic failures were successfully managed by retreatment. Sundqvist & Figdor[330] in a discussion on the life of endodontic pathogens concluded that root canal infection is not a random event. The type and the combination of the microbial flora developed in response to the surrounding environment. Factors that influence whether species shall die or survive are the particular ecological niche, nutrition, anaerobiosis, pH and competition with other microorganisms.

The invasion of microorganisms on the periapical region, descendant of the extension of the infection of the root canal (or extrusion of microorganisms during the instrumentation) permits the triggering of the inflammation. The infectious symptomatic apical periodontitis is clinically characterized by the presence of pain, after the preparation of teeth with pulpal necrosis, pain to palpation and percussion, or pain independently of previous treatment. The radiographic aspect can vary from normal, to enlargement of the space correspondent to the periodontal membrane and periapical osseous rarefaction. The clinical frame of infectious symptomatic apical periodontitis is very near to the frame of periapical abscess without fistula on the initial phase (phase 1). The clinical limit between one and other, many times is imprecise, however, microscopically it is observed on the periapical abscess the presence of purulent collection, what can implicate on edema and dental mobility.

The predominant bacteria on the mixed infections of the root canal, Gram-negative anaerobic, exert effects of biological activation on the organic defense, and results on the increase of the inflammatory response with the presence of painful periapical lesions.

Several studies[1-9,11-26,30-36,42-46,52-61,69-84,105-108,116,118,131-142,149,150,154-161,164,165,173-176,179,189,201,202,211-224,227-229,293,294,301-313,328-341,343,362-379] demonstrated the intimate relation between bateria in infected root canals and clinical symptoms present on periapical inflammation.

Sundqvist[335] observed anaerobic bacteria in pulpal necrosis, and on the acute exacerbations of the periapex it was isolated the *Bacteroides meleninogenicus* combined with other bacteria *(Peptostreptococcus, Fusobacterium, Lactobacillus* and others). Griffee et al.[44], also found the *Bacteroides meleninogenicus* in pulpal necrosis associated to clinical symptoms. Yoshida et al.[379], evaluating the correlation between clinical symptoms and microorganisms isolated from root canals of teeth with periapical pathology, concluded that the mixture of potent anaerobic bacteria *(Bacteroides* and *Peptococcus* species*)* is vigorously related to the presence of these clinical symptoms.

Other works[1-9,11-26,30-36,42-46,52-61,69-84,105-108,116,118,131-142,149,150,154-161,165,166,173-176,179,189,201,202,211-224,227-229,293,294,301-313,328-341,343,362-379] showed several factors that can be involved on the incidence of pain that characterizes the periapical inflammation during and after the root canal treatment.

Among the etiologic factors the acute manifestations before and during the root canal treatment, Seltzer & Naidorf[293] emphasized: alteration of the local adaptation syndrome, changes on the periapical tissue's pressure, microbial factors, effects of chemical mediators, manifestations of the cyclic nucleotides, immunologic phenomena and psychological factors.

However, the chronic periapical inflammation (asymptomatic apical periodontitis) can suffer induction to the symptomatic exacerbation, principally with the increase of the microorganisms' virulence, added to the diminution of the organic defenses. This fact can be noted by the extrusion, through the apical foramen, of bacteria and its sub-products, of contaminated dentinal scrapes and certain medications.

Estrela et al.[104] evaluated the prevalence of pain with the treatment of the acute and chronic periapical inflammation. It was evaluated on the study, 176 teeth with pulpal necrosis, that on the radiographic exam presented absence of periapical osseous rarefaction, diffuse osseous rarefaction or circumscribed osseous rarefaction. From these analyzed teeth, 62 were symptomatic (pain – slight, mild or severe), with no apparent edema, and 114 were asymptomatic (total absence of pain). The pain was considered slight when the patient did not report the use of analgesic; mild, not constant use; severe when the use was constant. From the symptomatic cases, 23 were evaluated as severe pain, 6 with necrosis without osseous rarefaction, 7 with necrosis and diffuse rarefaction, and 10 with circumscribed rarefaction. The rest varied from slight to mild pain. After the coronal opening, it was performed careful sanitization process, using the 1% sodium hypochlorite as irrigating solution. The apical limit of emptying was the radiographic apex, enlarging until the file # 20 (total emptying of the root canal). It was detected in some symptomatic cases the presence of exudation, that initially, was established the drainage. Next, it was performed the complete root canal preparation on the same appointment, 1 mm short of the radiographic apex, using the principles adopted by the cervical preparation technique[113]. The minimum limit of lateral enlargement, adopted during the preparation of different groups was: single root teeth, file # 35; mesial roots of lower molars and buccal of upper molars, # 30; distal roots of lower molars and lingual of upper molars, file # 40. After the preparation, the root canal was dried and filled with 17% trisodic EDTA, kept for 5 minutes. There was recapitulation with the file # 20 until the radiographic apex, followed of new irrigation-aspiration with 1% sodium hypochlorite. The canal was again dried and filled with calcium hydroxide paste. On the situations of symptomatic teeth, with mild pain, it was prescribed the analgesics. Past 48 hours, all the patients returned for a second appointment, when it was registered the presence or absence of postoperative pain, according to the following criteria: absent, slight-mild and severe. On the cases of severe pain the second appointment required anticipation to 24 hours, when it was instituted the antibiotic therapy (penicillin, cephalosporin). On the other situations, after the complete disappearance of the symptomatology, it was removed the intracanal dressing an proceeded the final filling. It was observed that on the situations of pulpal necrosis with diffuse and circumscribed rarefaction presenting previous symptomatology, there was total absence of postoperative pain in 64.3%, 68.2% and 61.5%, respectively. When the preoperative was asymptomatic, the maintenance of the asymptomatic postoperative was of 87%, 82.4% and 84%, and the appearance of severe pain had the percentage of 2%, 13.6% and 15.4%, respectively according to the radiographic aspects. With these results it can be concluded that: 1. On the clinical cases with pulpal necrosis (symptomatic, asymptomatic), independently of the radiographic aspect, it can be performed on the first appointment the complete root canal preparation, filling of the root canal with calcium hydroxide paste and the coronal sealing; 2. The incidence of apical periodontitis of infectious origin was low, and on decreasing order it is: necrosis with diffuse rarefaction – 8%, pulpal necrosis without rarefaction – 6.5%, and necrosis with circumscribed rarefaction – 6% (Fig. 10.22A-B).

Considering as reference the presented study, Estrela et al.[103] also verified the prevalence of postoperative pain on 184 teeth that needed endodontic retreatment. The absence of postoperative pain on the endodontic retreatments of the asymptomatic teeth was high, 83.3%, 82.8% and 82%, according to the radiographic aspect present, absence of periapical osseous rarefaction, diffuse and circumscribed osseous rarefaction, respectively. On the clinical situations that the periapical inflammatory process was developing (symptomatic situations) the absence of postoperative pain was of 59%, 50% and 54.5%, corresponding respectively to the radiographic aspects previously described (Fig. 10.23A-B).

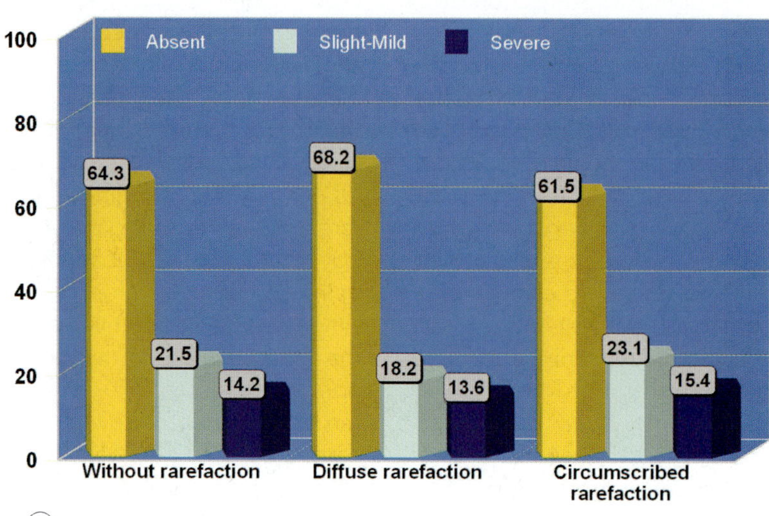


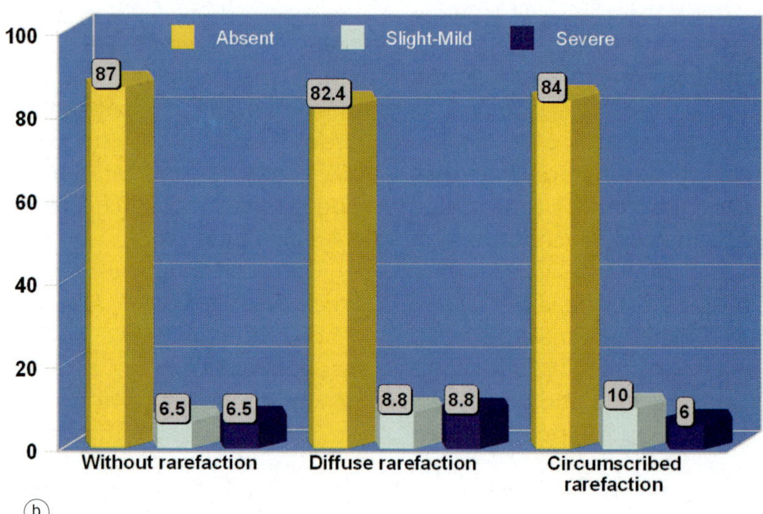


**Figure 10.22** - (**A-B**) Prevalence of postoperative pain – symptomatic and asymptomatic teeth[104].

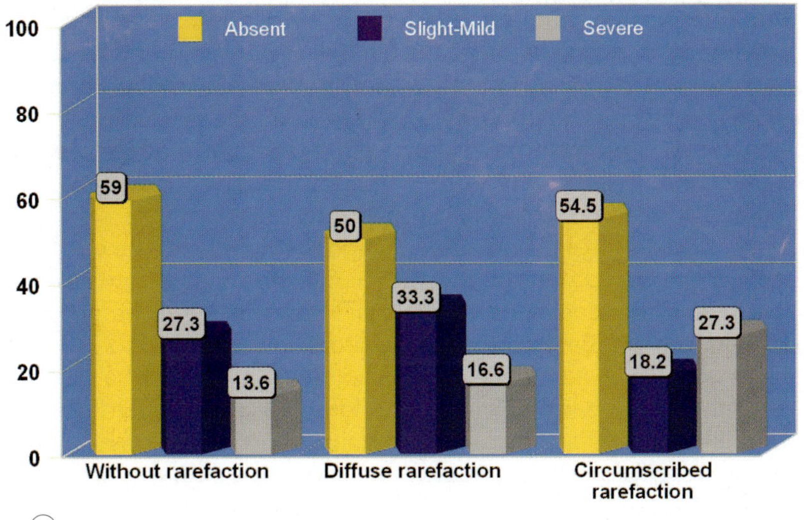


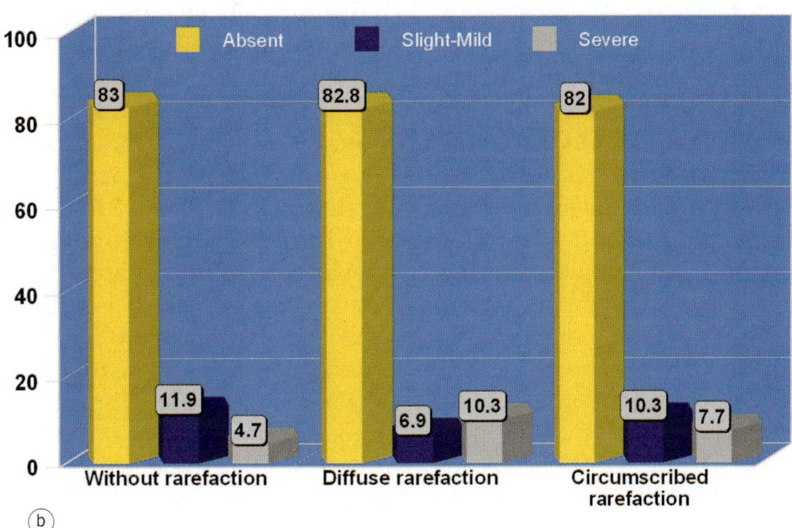


**Figure 10.23** - (**A-B**) Prevalence of postoperative pain endodontic retreatments – symptomatic and asymptomatic teeth[103].

The pain descendant of the periapical infection, after the acute exacerbation with the treatment of the chronic and asymptomatic inflammatory process, puts in risk the reputation of the responsible professional. On these situations, the chronic inflammatory lesion can be adapted to the irritant, and when the treatment is performed, new aggressor agents (microorganisms, infected dentin, medications, irrigation solutions, tissue's proteins chemically altered) can be introduced in the lesion, promoting a violent reaction, constituting an alteration of local adaptation. Besides this, a decrease on the host's organic resistance can represent the beginning of the symptomatic process. The exteriorization of a sub-clinical asymptomatic phase is unpredictable. Thus, the patient should always be clarified and informed about a possible situation of symptomatic postoperative, impossible to predict.

Sundqvist et al.[328] analyzed the ability of bacteria descendant of the pulpal necrosis induce purulent infections. They defended, however, that certain acute exacerbations are caused by polymicrobial infections, in which important special microorganisms achieve the pathogenicity by synergism, what can explain why it does not occur more frequently. Notoriously, the postoperative pain constitutes a serious problem for the good pace of the root canal treatment. The complete cleaning and shaping of the root canal on the first appointment constitutes a good therapeutic option front to the elimination of the injury agent responsible for the pain, although, it can also occur an undesired situation of pain.

Several studies [11,12,25,42-45,52-56,100-119,157-161,227-229,309-313,328-337,343-346,365-368,374,379] evaluated the different alternatives for treatment of infectious apical periododntitis.

Balaban et al.[14] did not find statistic differences comparing the incidence of the acute exacerbations front to these two options of treatment: pre-medication or complete cleaning on the first session. Trope[352], comparing the effect of three intracanal dressings (Formocresol, Ledermix and calcium hydroxide) on the incidence of post-instrumentation flare-up, reports that its incidence is independent of the medication used, and that occurred on the teeth with radiographic signs of apical periodontitis. Gatewood et al.[132], verifying changes on the clinical conducts on the treatment of the endodontic emergency in United States, (from 1977 until 1988), observed that there was increase on the defenders of the complete instrumentation, indifferent to the condition of the emergency. It was also noticed an increase of the defenders who let the teeth closed in pulpal necrosis associated to pain, and the diminution of the use of the camphorated monoclorophenol with increase of the use of the calcium hydroxide paste.

Morse et al.[227] compared the periapical instrumentation with intracanal instrumentation in asymptomatic teeth pulpal necrosis and associated periapical radiolucent lesions. One hundred six patients (55 male patients and 51 female patients) were treated in one visit. The teeth involved included 55 mandibular, 51 maxillary, 10 anterior, and 96 posterior teeth. Periapical radiographs were taken of all of involved teeth bay means of long cone technique. The periapical radiolucencies were divided on the basis of diameter in four categories: (1) small, 2 to 8mm; (2) medium, 9 to 15mm; (3) large, 16 to 22mm and (4) very large, 23mm and greater. The cases of intracanal instrumentation the instrumentation was confined to the root canal system. For the cases of periapical instrumentation, after access preparation, R-C prep was placed on a small file (#10 to #25) and the file was carefully inserted until the apex followed by complete periapex preparation (#25 to #70) without instrumentation into the lesion. Copious irrigation with 0.5% sodium hypochlorite was then done. After the thorough root canal debridement, filing (with the last file being from size #25 to #35) was then continued into approximate center of the periapical lesion. With each use of the file, a pull motion was performed. To avoid and control possible swelling, flare-ups and pain, systemic medication was given to the patients. The patients were evaluated after 1 day, 1week and 2 months. A 6.6% incidence of flare-up as found with no significant difference between intracanal instrumentation (30.2%) and periapical instrumentation (24.5%). No significant correlation was found between the goups and any other factor. Walton & Fouad[366] determined the incidence of flare-ups correlated it with: the age, gender, pulpal and periapical diagnosis, pain as well as it level, presence and the nature of the swelling, use of medications, general health conditions, endodontic treatment and group executioner of the treatment. Data were collected at root canal treatment appointments on demographics, pulp/periapical diagnoses, presenting symptoms, treatment procedures, and number of appointments. Patients that then experienced a flare-up (a severe problem requiring an unscheduled visit and treatment) had the correlating factors examined. The operator concluded the treatment when it was possible. No intracanal medicaments were used among the sessions, not being also accomplished the oclusal adjustment. At the end of the consultation the patients received postoperative orientations. In the presence of problems the patients were called to return the clinic immediately where the most suitable treatment was accomplished. Nine hundred forty-six visits resulted in an incidence of 3.17% flare-ups. Flare-ups were positively correlated with more severe presenting symptoms, pulp necrosis with painful apical pathosis, and patients on analgesics. Fewer flare-ups occurred in undergraduate patients and following obturation procedures. There was no correlation between patient demographics or systemic conditions, number of appointments, treatment procedures, or taking antibiotics. Al-Negrish & Habahbeh[8] determined the flare up rate related to root canal treatment of asymptomatic non vital maxillary central incisor teeth performed in one and two appointments and the relationship, between pain and number of treatment visits. A total of 120 patients (66 female and 54 males) with only one asymptomatic necrotic central incisor without any evidence of periapical radiolucent lesion in the periapical radiograph were included in the study. Out of the 112 patients involved in the study, 54 patients had been treated in a one visit and 58 patients had been treated in two visits. The flare up rate (percentage of patients experiencing moderate to severe pain) after 2 days was 9.2% for the one visit, 13.8% for the two visit and 11.6% for both procedures. After 7 days the flare up rate was 1.8% for the one visit, 5.2% for the two visit and 3.6% for both procedures. Mattscheck et al.[213] studied the factors associated with posttreatment pain in patients receiving root canal retreatment (RCR) and in those receiving initial root canal treatment (IRCT). Eighty four patients scheduled for RCR or IRCT completed questionnaires on pretreatment pain levels (Visual Analogue Scale, 0-100) and demographics data, tooth number, pulpal diagnosis (ie, reversible pulpitis, irreversible pulpitis, necrosis, or previously treated), and periapical diagnosis (ie, normal, chronic apical periodontitis, acute apical periodontitis, or acute apical abscess) were recorded. In RCR cases, the type of previous obturating material (gutta-percha, silver point, or paste) was also recorded. The treatment procedures for cases were routine, the root canals were irrigated with 2.6% NaOCl and some patients were seen in single visits, and others were seen in multiple visits. At 4, 8, 12, 24, 48, 72, 96, and 120 hours, patients recorded posttreatment pain levels. Seventy one patients returned completed questionnaires. There was no significant difference in posttreatment pain with respect to patients undergoing RCR and patients undergoing IRCT, type of original obturating material, or pretreatment diagnosis. Posttreatment pain levels were significantly increased at 4, 8, and 12 hours after treatment. Patients reporting higher levels of pretreatment pain (Visual Analogue Scale > 20) had significantly increased posttreatment pain up to 24 hours after the procedure. Yoldas et al.[378] evaluated the incidence and the level of postoperative pain in retreatment cases in 1- or 2-visit root canal therapy. Two hundred eighteen cases that required retreatment were included. Obturated and unfilled canal space and the status of periapical tissues were evaluated according to the PAI index. 68 patients had symptomatic teeth (mild or moderate pain) and 159 had asymptomatic teeth (no pain before the treatment). Thirty-five of symptomatic teeth and 80 of asymptomatic teeth were treated in 1 visit; the remaining patients were treated in 2 visits. No systemic medication was prescribed and the patients were instructed to take mild analgesics if they experienced pain. One week after the initial appointment, patients were asked about the occurrence of postoperative pain. The level of discomfort was rated as no pain, mild pain, moderate pain, or severe pain (flare-up). Eight patients from the 1-visit group and 2 patients from the 2-visit group had flare-ups. The overall incidence of flare-ups was 4.6%. There was a statistical difference between the groups. The authors found that two-visit root canal treatment with an intracanal medication (calcium hydroxide paste), reduces postoperative pain in endodontically retreated symptomatic teeth and decreases the number of flare-ups in all retreatment cases compared to 1-visit endodontic retreatment.

On the other hand, in relation to the prophylactic administration of the penicillin, to prevent the flare-up or other undesirable sequels after the treatment of infected root canals, Walton & Chiappinelli[365] reported that after study in 80 patients with diagnosis of pulpal necrosis and asymptomatic apical periodontitis, its use was not related to the incidence of the severity of the post-operative symptoms. They argued, however, against the prophylactic prescription of antibiotics on the described situations, due to its ineffectiveness for pre-existent contamination.

The perfect emptying with the complete preparation on the first session in root canal with pulpal necrosis associated or not to the presence of pain, did not favor the increase of the chances of acute exacerbation. Contrarily, the elimination of the endodontic microbiota with the removal of several factors of bacterial virulence (endotoxins, substrates, possible interactions of these microorganisms) constitutes, certainly, a promising conduct, due to the proper cleaning and sanitization of the infected root canal. Another favorable point is the local and direct combat of the microorganisms there situated, by the action of the chemical substances (sodium hypochlorite, calcium hydroxide), due to the antimicrobial effect, the biological action, and yet by acting as temporary sealing (physical filling of the root canal, as observed with the calcium hydroxide paste)[52-56,98-120,162,229,294,340].

The fact of the maintenance of the tooth closed only contributes to the control of possible superinfection or re-infection, what absolutely conducts to unpleasant consequences. Thus, these local procedures and the possible adoption of general procedures, such as the use of systemic medication, contribute efficiently for the post-operative results of symptomatic teeth with pulpal necrosis, which root canals are instrumented on the first visit.

However, when establishing the clinical treatment, there are defenders of the pre-medication (aldehydes, phenolic derivates) and defenders of the complete cleaning and shaping on the first session, objecting minimize the incidence of acute exacerbations after the initial treatment of these teeth with pulpal necrosis and periapical pathologies. Another polemic is perceived front to the conduct of maintaining the tooth open or closed on the treatment of acute periapical inflammations (infectious symptomatic apical periodontitis and apical abscess without fistula).

Although until today there are defenders of the pre-medication, it is believed that for the elimination of any aggressor agent, specially of microbial origin, the first conduct should be directed to promote its complete destruction, that occurs by the sanitization process, emptying and preparation of the root canal, when it is also observed the action of the antimicrobial irrigants. The maintenance of the microbial control occurs with the permanence of the intracanal dressing. When the clinical situation is symptomatic and is associated to the presence of infection, besides the local conducts, it should be adopted general measures, such as the systemic microbial control. Thus, it can be minimized the evolution of an undesirable infectious state.

It has been reported also bacteremia associated to the root canal treatment. Debelian et al.[56], analyzing the bacteremia during and after the root canal treatment in teeth with asymptomatic apical periodontitis, compared microorganisms isolated from the root canal and the blood by different phenotypic characteristics. From biochemical tests and antimicrobial sensibility of the microorganisms isolated from the root canals and the blood, that showed the same profiles, it was possible to suggest that the microorganisms isolated from the blood had as origin source the root canal.

In relation to the selection of the intracanal dressing, the calcium hydroxide has been the best option, due to its excellent antimicrobial (inactivation of bacterial enzymes) and biological (activation of tissue's enzymes) properties[109,110,117]. Nevertheless, there are situations which the impossibility of enlargement of the root canal impedes its placement. On other moments, it can be noticed until impediment of the adoption of local procedures, as in the periapical abscess without fistula (on the presence of trismus). It should be understood that the treatment here developed occurs in urgency situation, a special action for the relief of pain and control of odontogenic infection.

The treatment of the infectious symptomatic apical periodontitis should be established based on two conditions of appearance: asymptomatic or symptomatic previous phase.

On the first situation, it can be characterized the previous phase that is asymptomatic (pulpal necrosis or asymptomatic apical periodontitis) and occurred the beginning of the infectious symptomatic apical periodontitis during the treatment. On the initial root canal treatment it was performed the sanitization process, with the emptying of the root canal until the radiographic apex, the preparation of the canal 1 mm beneath, the placement of intracanal dressing (calcium hydroxide paste) and the coronal sealing. When the patient returns with pain on the tooth being treated, it should be evaluated the conducts performed and, with the certitude of having obeyed all the procedures compatible with the modern endodontic therapy, performed by the same professional, it is maintained the tooth closed and prescribed systemic medication, analgesic and antibiotics. If it persists the symptomatology, the tooth is opened, the root canal is emptied, evaluated the presence or absence of exudate and it is placed again the intracanal dressing (calcium hydroxide paste) and the tooth is maintained closed. The use of the calcium hydroxide is conditioned to the enlargement of the root canal, fact that not always is possible.

On the second situation, the patient looks for urgency attendance with symptomatology, when the diagnosis was infectious symptomatic apical periodontitis (the pain is already installed). On the former state, the previous treatment was made by the own professional. On this situation, the patient arrived with infection and presence of pain, or was previously attended by other professional and arrived for a new attendance complaining of pain. The tooth should be opened, emptied associated to the sanitization process. There can be presence or absence of exudates, being unusual on this stage. It should be emptied the root canal until the instrument # 20 (on the molars), or until the # 25 (on the anterior teeth). If it is added more 2-4 instruments, of superior caliber, it is practically concluded the preparation of the root canal. At the end, when possible, it is placed the intracanal dressing (calcium hydroxide paste), and the tooth is maintained closed. As systemic procedure, it is prescribed antibiotics and analgesic. If there is maintenance of the painful state, it is repeated the conduct of opening again the tooth and evaluate it after new emptying. The systemic procedures are maintained, as the prescription of antibiotics and analgesic. It should always be considered the specificity of the microorganism, the spectrum of action of the antibiotics administered and the organic resistance. Some diseases of general order favor the maintenance of the inflammatory / infectious state, with necessity of being investigated, diagnosed and, also, treated or indicated for treatment, favoring, thus, the resolution of the problem. The systemic medication prescribed has function of aid altering the course of infection.

It should be emphasized that these conducts are special, constituting treatments that require urgency on relief of the pains and of the infectious processes. Not all the locals of public health attendance have material conditions and specialized professionals to intervene locally, what makes that only the general procedures (or systemic) are adopted; or simply the tooth is opened for possible relief of the pain or to drain the abscess.

It is clear that when there is possibility of adopting an ideal therapeutics (more effective) this should constitute the desired option. Another complex point is the use of an intracanal dressing. When it is not concluded the canal preparation, or its enlargement is not sufficient for the adequate placement of the intracanal dressing, it will not be reached the desired effects, once the medication will not enter in contact or will not fill the entire canal. The important of this urgency local intervention is the emptying of the canal, neutralizing the aggressor agents.

Estrela et al.[107] evaluated longitudinal studies about the pain after endodontic treatment in teeth with primary infection, using a systematic review. A MEDLINE search strategies was developed to identify articles using the following uniterms: *endodontic(s)* and *pulpal pain*, *endodontic(s)* and *periapical pain*, *endodontic(s)* and *symptom*, *endodontic(s)* and *flare-ups*, *endodontic(s) pain* and *post-treatment*, *endodontic(s)* and *inter-appointment / interappointment*. The search included articles from the MEDLINE (http://www.ncbi.nlm.nih.gov/PubMed), from 1966 to February 23th of 2007. 351 articles were selected (6 articles about epidemiological studies, 16 about literature review, 55 cases reports. Concerning to pain associated with apical limit were verified 10 articles; irrigants solutions, 12 articles; intracanal medicaments, 29 articles; root canal filling, 9 articles and pain interappointment, 24 articles. Only 9 studies satisfied the inclusion criteria. The success estimative of evaluated studies shows that the sanitization process and rational use of intracanal medicaments lead to high rate (88%) of absence of post-treatment pain in treatment of teeth with primary endodontic infections. In other systematic review, Estrela et al.[106] analyzed in longitudinal studies about the post endodontic pain treatment with secondary infection, using a systematic review. A Medline search strategy was developed to identify articles using the following uniterms: endodontic(s) and pulpal pain, endodontic(s) and periapical pain, endodontic(s) and symptom, endodontic(s) and flare-ups, endodontic(s) pain and post-treatment, endodontic(s) and inter-appointment/interappointment. The search included articles from the Medline (http://www.ncbi.nlm.nih.gov/PubMed), from 1966 to February 23th of 2007. 351 articles were selected, but only 5 studies satisfied the inclusion criteria. Considering the exiting estimative of analyzed studies, it could be observed evidence about the higher rate of absence of pos-treatment pain.

Tsesis et al.[355] determined the frequency of flare-ups and evaluated factors that affect it by using meta-analysis of results of previous studies. The search covered all articles published in dental journals in English from 1966–May 2007, and the relevancy of 119 selected articles was evaluated by reading their titles and abstracts, from which 54 were rejected as irrelevant and 65 were subjected to a suitability test. Six studies that met all the above mentioned criteria were included in the study. Flare-up frequency was 8.4% on the basis of 982 patients from 6 studies that defined flare-up as strong pain with or without swelling that occurred after the initiation or continuation of root canal treatment and estimated within 48 hours after the procedure. The relatively high frequency of flare-ups should be considered in planning root canal therapy.

The sequence of the technique of the sanitization process is described next. The Figures 10.24 and 10.25 show the sanitization technique and schematic representation the sequence of the emptying in pulpal necrosis.

1. Anesthesia, absolute isolation and antisepsis of the operative field;
2. Coronary opening with complete removal of the pulp chamber's roof;
3. Copious irrigation-aspiration with 1-2.5% sodium hypochlorite, followed of eventual removal of the pulpal cavity's content with curettes of long intermediate;
4. Filling of the coronary chamber with 1-2.5% sodium hypochlorite;
5. Introduction of an instrument of small diameter (files #08 to #15), depending of the diameter of the root canal, with progressive movement of penetration and removal (forwards and backwards), dislocating the organic rests, followed of its neutralization with sodium hypochlorite. It is observed the complete removal of the coronary chamber's roof through an explorer and, if necessary, complement the coronary opening;
6. The neutralization of the septic content is made in steps, working in small longitudinal amplitudes, what allows the action of the chemical substance over the necrotic residuals released from the walls of the root canals, through the mechanic action of the files;
7. On the exploration, the working length adopted is based on the determination made only with an initial radiography and the average length of the tooth. The complete emptying and the sanitization process are executed after the preparation of the entrance orifice, preparation of the cervical third and length determination;
8. After the accomplishment of theses operative steps, complete the sanitization process and empty it until the radiographic apex. Copious irrigation-aspiration with sodium hypochlorite should be done, frequently, looking towards the complete removal of the possible necrotic rests and / or automatically, promote its neutralization;
9. After the sanitization process, execute the root canal preparation and place the intracanal dressing (calcium hydroxide paste) (Fig. 10.25).

**Figure 10.24** - Sanitization Technique (Emptying in Pulpal Necrosis).

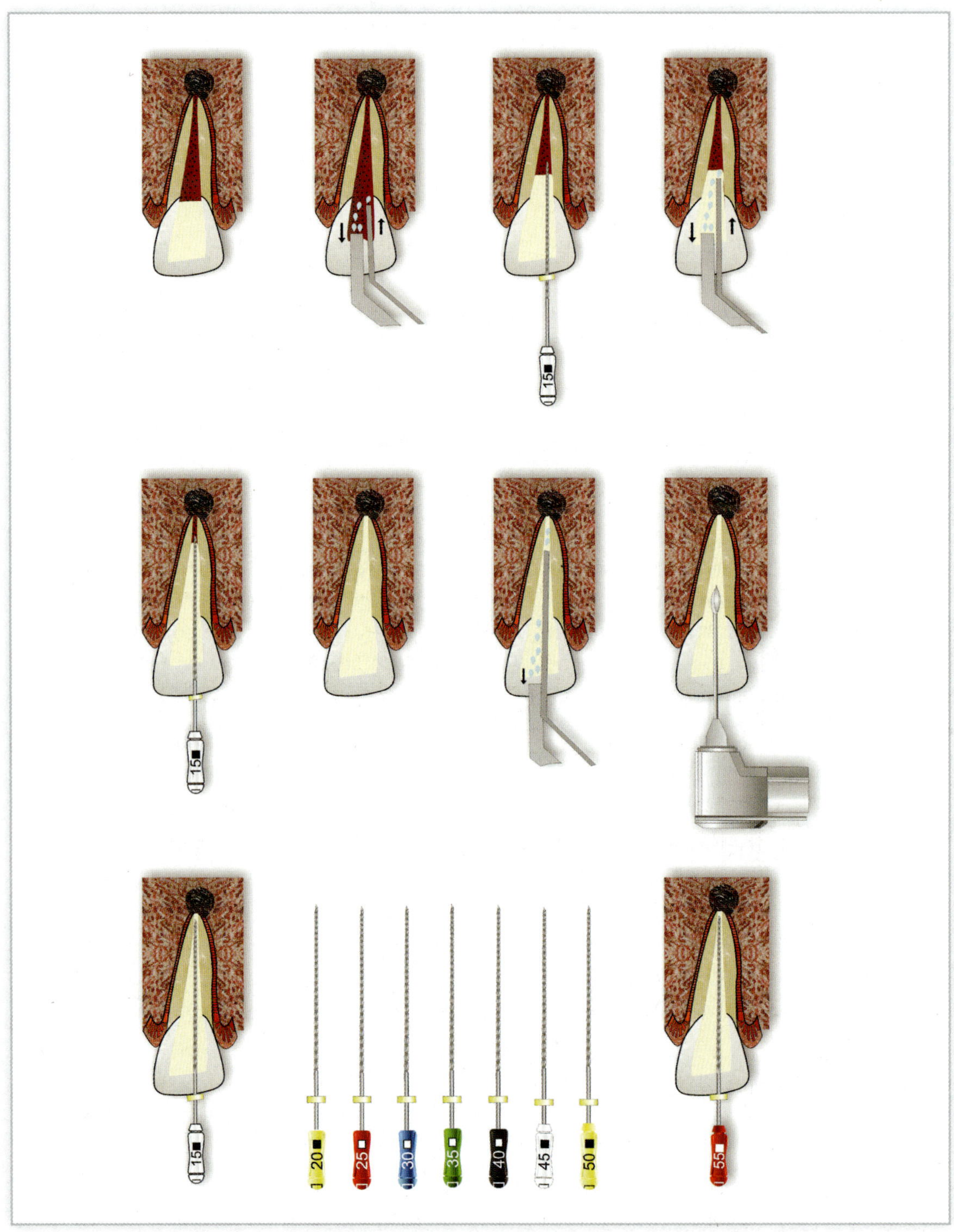


**Figure 10.25** - Squematic representation of the sanitization process.

## 10.7 Asymptomatic Apical Periodontitis

The asymptomatic apical periodontitis is characterized by chronic inflammation, of long lasting, which the radiographic aspect varies of small enlargement of the space of the periodontal membrane to resorption of the lamina dura and the periapical bone.

Frequently, apical periodontitis is associated with periapical granuloma or cyst. The safer way to differentiate the granuloma from the periapical cyst, with similar radiographic aspects, is by histopathological exam (microscopic analysis). The periapical granuloma is constituted of inflammatory tissue, with domain of macrophages infiltrated, lymphocytes, plasmocytes, polimorphonuclears and giant cells. It presents several capillaries, fibroblasts, connective fibers, and can be epitheliated or not epitheliated. The granuloma represents the first attempt of the organism for healing the lesions. The formation of the periapical cyst occurs from inflammatory stimuli over the epithelial rests of Malassez[205], which proliferate, increase the size and form on epithelial island inside the granuloma. The enlargement of the epithelium makes the most central cells become distant of its nutrition sources, located in the granulation tissue, what results on its degeneration and central cavity. With the liquefaction of the mortified cells, it is formed the cavity and the cystic liquid[38,64,342].

Besides this theory of the formation of the cyst, there are others. Campos[57] reports that the true cyst presents three constant elements: the internal coating epithelium, a capsule of fibrous connective tissue, that serves as support tissue and source of nutrition to the epithelium, and the content, that can be liquid or semiliquid (containing epithelial desquamated cells, inflammatory cells, cholesterol crystals).

On the chronic inflammatory reaction (macrophages, lymphocytes, plasmocytes) it is also observed immunologic response, presented with the purpose of neutralize, inactivate or destruct the stimulus (antigen or microorganisms). The neutralization can be direct, of the stimulus by the bonding to the antibody, and/or destruction of the stimulus by the sensitized lymphocytes, or by activation of biochemical and cellular mediators that act destructing the antigen[299,300].

Nair et al.[231] determined the types and incidences of the periapical lesions obtained of 156 extracted human teeth. It was observed that from the 256 analyzed lesions, 127 (50%) were granulomas, 69 (55%) not epitheliated and 58 (45%) epitheliated. A total of 39 (15%) of periapical cysts, 24 (61%) of true cysts and 15 (39%) periapical pocket cyst (small lumen and appearance of an extension of the space of the root canal in the periapical region). The authors discuss from these findings, that the prevalence of cyst among other periapical lesions observed by other authors, denoted that almost half was cyst, and that the incidence varied from 6% to 55%. The discrepancy between the reported incidences of periapical cysts is due to the differences of microscopic interpretations that characterized inappropriately certain periapical lesions as cysts. This possibility is strongly supported by the information that shows that 52% of the lesions were epitheliated and that only 15% were truly periapical cysts. Simon[299], analyzing the incidence of periapical cyst reported that this is low for true cysts (8.6%). The author defines the epitheliated granuloma as apical proliferative inflammatory lesion, with presence of epithelium, but absence of recognizable cavity; pocket cyst as apical inflammatory lesion with epithelial wall in cavity, but, interrupted by the dental apex projected inside the cavity; true cyst as apical inflammatory cyst with complete epithelial wall and closed cavity without connection with the apical foramen or root canal. It is observed that the true cyst is independent of the root canal system, and the endodontic therapy would not have effect over it.

These works support the idea that the high success rate (85 to 90%) achieved exclusively with the root canal treatment of teeth porting periapical lesions is due to the prevalence of true cysts lower than 10% as demonstrated by Simon[299] and Nair et al.[231]. Souza et al.[321] observed that the non surgical treatment of teeth with periapical lesions, using as intracanal dressing the paste of calcium hydroxide, conducted to the percentage of 94% of success with clinical-radiographic following for a minimum period of 1 year after the definitive filling. The relation of treated or non treated teeth, with the non surgical regression, of periodontal apical cysts was studied by microscopy and immunohistochemic by Rocha[279]. After the elimination of this antigenic source, the organism has conditions to stimulate the immunologic system to direct it not anymore for a variety of antigen, but for more specific and uniform antigens, that certainly are found on the surface of the cells, or as constituent of the cellular membrane of the own epithelial cells. On an individual who presents an efficient immunologic system, the non surgical regression can occur. When there is alteration of this system, or if it is precarious, the natural evolution of the cystic lesion happens.

Front to the works discussed and the existent controversies, and knowing that radiographic and clinically it is impossible to differentiate the granuloma from the periapical cyst, it can be observed that the first clinical therapeutic option on the situations of asymptomatic apical periodontitis is the non surgical root canal treatment. The clinical-radiographic control for a period over 2 years is what can determine the final result of the treatment performed, needing or not a surgical complementation.

Sjögren et al.[310], verifying the factors that affect the result of the root canal treatment, after the period of 8 to 10 years of treatment, found in relation to the pre-operative state of the pulp and periapical tissues, 96% of success when there was no periapical lesion, 86% when there was periapical lesion, 98% of success on the retreatment cases without periapical lesion and 62% of success on the cases of retreatment that presented periapical lesion. On the teeth with pre-operative apical periodontitis, when the instrumentation and root canal filling remained 2 mm beneath the apex, the prognosis was significantly better that on the cases of overfilling, or when the filling was more than 2 mm from the apex.

Nair et al.[236] observed that on the absence of microbial factors, filling materials that contain irritant substances can evoke strange body reaction in the periapical region, leading to the development of asymptomatic periapical lesions that can remain refractory to the endodontic therapy. Nair & Sundqvist[240] induced inflammatory cysts in an animal model so as to test the hypothesis that radicular cysts develop via the abscess pathway. *This was a prospective, hypothesis-driven, experimental investigation that resulted in successful induction of inflammatory cysts in a murine model. The outcome provides strong evidence in support of the "abscess theory" of development of radicular cysts. The results of this study allow the conclusion that inflammatory cysts are most likely induced by the initiation of an acute inflammatory focus (abscess/necrosis) that gets enclosed and delimited by a proliferating epithelium. This finding provides strong experimental evidence in support of the "abscess theory" of development of inflammatory periapical cysts.*

The Figures 10.26 and 10.27 show the radiographic aspects of root canal treatment of asymptomatic periapical periodontitis, with regression of the periapical lesion.

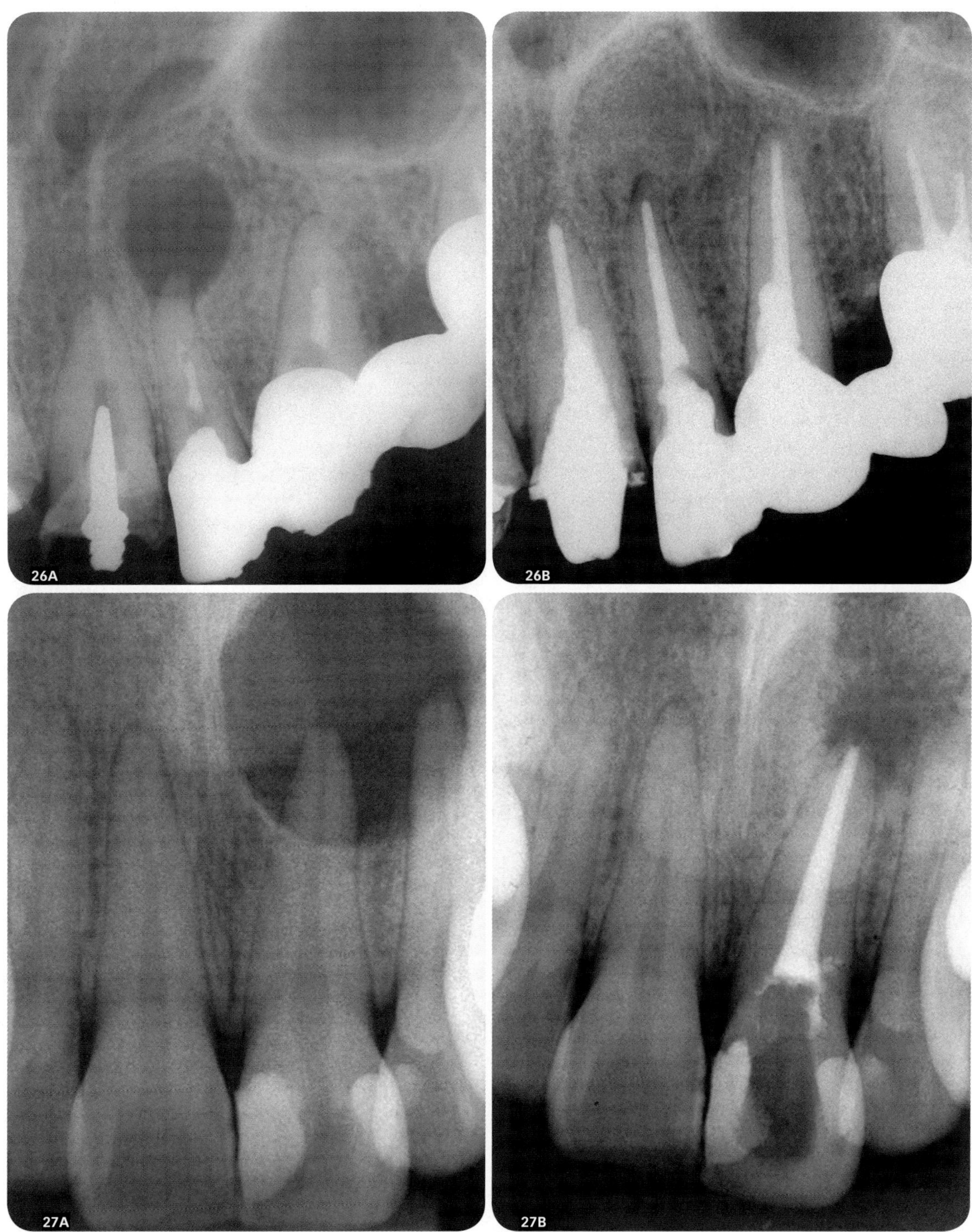


**Figures 10.26 and 10.27** - (**A-B**) Radiographic aspects of root canal treatment of tooth with asymptomatic apical periodontitis with regression of periapical lesion.

## 10.8 Periapical Abscess without Fistula

The periapical abscess without fistula constitutes an periapical inflammatory alteration associated to purulent collection, composed by the tissue´s disintegration and characterized by the presence of exudates inside the lesion. This alteration appears when occurs low organic resistance of the host, concomitant to the increase of the number and virulence of the microorganisms, what denotes the intensity of the inflammatory process.

The knowledge of the microbiota of the periapical abscess becomes important at the moment that it is necessary to institute a local and systemic treatment. On the Figure 10.28, there is information related by Dahlén & Möller[74] in different studies about the microbiota of the odontogenic infection.

Brook et al.[43] analyzed the anaerobic and aerobic microflora of the periapical abscess. It was analyzed 39 samples collected from periapical abscesses, processed and analyzed with adequate methodology. From these cases collected, it was recovered microorganisms in 32 cases. A total of 78 isolated bacteria (55 anaerobic and 23 aerobic and facultative) were found. The isolated bacteria that predominated were *Bacteroides sp.* (23 isolated, 13 *Bacteroides melaninogenicus),* anaerobic coccus (18 isolated) and *Fusobacterium sp.* (9 isolated). The production of Beta-lactamase was detected in 8 isolated bacteria *(Bacteroides fragilis, Bacteroides melaninogenicus, Bacteroides intermedius, Bacteroides asaccharolyticcus e Staphyloccus aureus).* The resistance of the bacteria *Staphylococcus aureus* and *Bacteroides fragilis* is known for a long time. The authors emphasized that although the therapy of surgical drainage is a first clinical conduct, the administration of the antibiotics therapeutic is an essential part of the handling of the patient with periapical abscesses and its complications.

Generally the histological aspect of acute answer (exudative) evidences the presence of neutrophils polimorphonuclear leukocytes that from the liberation of lysossomic enzymes on the tissue´s space and its degradation originates the abscess. On the central region with liquefaction it is found degraded neutrophils, cellular rests surrounded by macrophages, lymphocytes and some plasmocytes. The pressure of the exudates over the lamina dura and the spongy bone can result on periapical bone resorption. However, not always the radiographic aspect of the periapical region evidences visible bone destruction. On some situations it is observed enlargement of the space of the periodontal membrane, although it can occur interruption of the alveolar lamina dura. On the chronic process, it is observed diffuse or circumscribed apical radiolucency.

The etiologic factors responsible for the appearance of the periapical abscess are commonly involved with microorganisms, that by the evolution of the dental caries resulted on pulpal necrosis, that later evolutes to infectious apical periodontitis. Other maneuvers during the preparation of the root canal of teeth with pulpal necrosis can conduct microorganisms to this region, with increase of the number and virulence, facilitated by the microbial interactions and debility of the organic resistance. The same way, the asymptomatic apical periodontitis can become acute and lead to the periapical abscess.

Among the characteristic clinical aspects, it is found the presence of intense pain, localized, pain to palpation, percussion and dental mobility. The accumulation of exudates on the space of the periodontal ligament promotes compression of the lamina dura, determining the dental extrusion, the compression of the nervous fibers, besides the action of several mediators, intensifying the state of pain. The grade of tumefaction is variable, depending of the extension, evolution and diffusion of the abscess. Besides the pain and the edema, it can appear fever and debility. The periapical abscess can be evaluated in 3 different phases of evolution (initial abscess, abscess in evolution and advanced abscess), what better characterizes the diagnosis and favors the treatment.

| Bacterial Group | % | | Bacterial Group | % | |
|---|---|---|---|---|---|
| Aerobics | | | Anaerobics | | |
| *Streptococcus α-Hemolitic* | 13.9 | | *Streptococcus* | 7.6 | |
| *Streptococcu β-Hemolitic* | 2.0 | | *Peptostreptococcus* | 18.0 | |
| *Enterococcus* | 1.1 | | *Veillonella* | 8.0 | |
| *Staphylococcus aureus* | 1.0 | | *Propionibacterium* | 1.1 | |
| *Staphylococcus epidermidis* | 1.5 | | *Actinomyces* | 2.7 | |
| *Neisseria* | 0.6 | | *Arachnia* | 0.1 | |
| *Corynebacterium* | 0.6 | | *Eubacterium* | 3.8 | |
| *Eikenella corrodens* | 0.4 | | *Lactobacillus* | 3.5 | |
| *Haemophilus* | 0.6 | | *Bifidobacterium* | 0.9 | |
| *Enterobacterium* | 0.1 | | *Prevotella or Porphyromonas* | 26.0 | |
| *Capnocytophaga* | 0.9 | 24.0 | *Fusobacterium* | 4.5 | |
| | | | *Spirochetes* | 0.7 | 76.0 |

(Dahlén & Möller[74] - Information of different studies)

**Figure 10.28** - Distribution of bacterial genders of 289 periapical abscesses.

## 10.8.1 Periapical abscess without fistula (initial phase)

The clinical-radiographic characteristics of the abscess on initial phase can be grouped in: intense pain, spontaneous, pulsing, continuous and localized, pain to apical palpation and percussion, feeling of grown tooth; negative answer to the pulpal vitality exam. Considering that at this moment the purulent collection is confined in the space of the periodontal ligament, promoting compression of the dental apex and the alveolar lamina dura, it is common the dental mobility. The radiographic aspect of periapical destruction is little evident, varying from normality to increase of the space of the periodontal ligament. The therapeutic conduct adopted on this initial phase is divided in local and systemic.

Again, it should be emphasized that the conducts for this clinical situation are special and of urgency for the relief of pain and control of the infectious process. Not always the opportunity permits the better option of local treatment, what imposes a general control (systemic).

### Local and systemic therapeutics

1. Anesthesia, absolute isolation and cleaning of the operative field;
2. Occlusal relief;
3. Coronal opening;
4. Abundant irrigation-aspiration with 1 to 2.5% sodium hypochlorite;
5. Emptying of the content of the root canal, with consequent sanitization process, aided by thin instrument and 1% sodium hypochlorite. The apical foramen is enlarged until the file #20-25 (type K-file), depending of the tooth, being passed by 1 mm;

6. Considering that with more 2 or 3 instruments it can be concluded the canal´s preparation, thus, more effective will be the sanitization process and easy the insertion of the intracanal dressing. Concluded the preparation of the root canal, it is retaken the last instrument used on the emptying and performed the recapitulation. On some cases due to the pain, mobility and disturbance and resistance of the patient, this conduct is practically impossible;
7. Front to these procedures, it is analyzed the occurrence or not of drainage. When present, many times, it is insignificant;
8. On the cases that occur drainage it is common the immediate relief of the pain. Independent of the exudates, if the root canal is dry, it is convenient to maintain the tooth closed and with intracanal dressing;
9. With the local therapeutics described, it is presumed that the problem is no longer situated inside the root canal, what induces the use of systemic therapeutics, with antimicrobial and analgesic;
10. It should be given special and constant attention for the patient until the end of all the urgency state.

### 10.8.2 Periapical abscess without fistula (phase in evolution)

The clinical-radiographic characteristics of the abscess in evolution involve: spontaneous pain, with lower intensity than on the initial phase, pulsing, localized, evident edema without fluctuation point and volumetric increase of the injured area, negative answer to the pulpal vitality test. The radiographic aspect, although it´s not applicable, in some situations is characterized by enlargement of the apical periodontal space. The purulent collection crossed the alveolar lamina dura, invaded the medullar spaces (bone trabecules) reaching the sub-periosteum region. It can be observed situations of inflammation with edema without formation of purulent collection, promoting tumefaction and facial asymmetry. On some situations of abscess in evolution, as the facial edema increases, the symptoms decrease. On this phase, some clinical characteristics should be well analyzed, such as: consistency of the edema (capsulated, hard), previous treatment with antibiotics and interruption (but not advanced), trismus and fever. It should be considered this phase as one of the most critical of the abscesses, and that requires safe and constant vigilance of the patient, principally when occurs presence of fever. The Figures 10.29 to 10.38 demonstrate a clinical case of periapical abscess without fistula.

#### Local and Systemic Therapeutics

1. Anesthesia, absolute isolation and cleaning of the operative field;
2. Occlusal relief;
3. Coronal opening;
4. Abundant irrigation-aspiration with 1 to 2.5% sodium hypochlorite;
5. Emptying of the content of the root canal, with consequent sanitization process aided by thin instrument and 1% sodium hypochlorite. The apical foramen is enlarged until the file # 20-25 (type K-file), depending of the tooth, being passed by 1 mm;
6. With the enlargement of the apical foramen and the passage in 1 mm of the file, it is expected the drainage, however, not always occurs drainage via canal. Many times it is discrete or absent, the same way that on the periapical abscess in initial phase.
7. It is analyzed the presence or absence of drainage of the abscess via canal, and it is difficult its elimination via apical foramen. On the situations which there are drainage, the process walks faster to involution. It is convenient that, between appointments, the tooth remains closed and preferably with intracanal dressing.

8. Some situations can be associated at this moment of the abscess, requiring special and constant vigilance, such as cases of debility, fever, presence of trismus, capsulated abscess, which the patient was subjected previously to therapeutics with antibiotics. On the case of trismus, the local procedures are difficult to be performed, however, it should be applied hot water bag, mouth wash with hot water and salt, systemic medication with anti-inflammatory (muscular relaxing) and antibiotics. For the patient with hardened abscess which there was previous antibiotics medication, it is performed the local procedures described previously, when possible, added of prescription of antibiotic. The patient with fever deserves special care, requiring control of the fever (anti-thermal) and antibiotics therapy. The alternative of surgical drainage on this phase is complicated and painful, when it is not found the focus of the purulent collection.
9. Special attention and complete assistance for the patient until the end of all the urgency state.



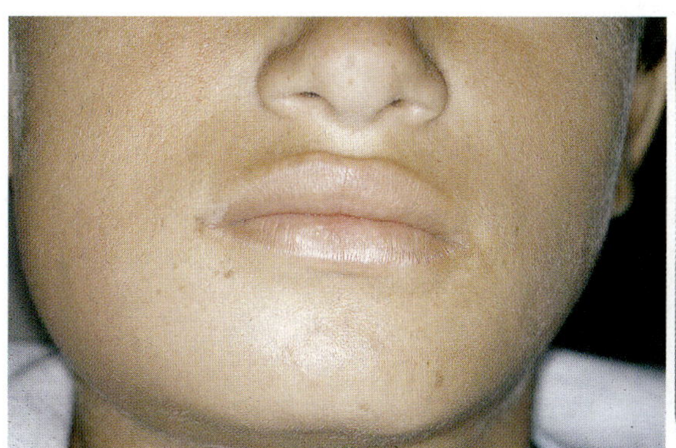

**Figure 10.29** - Facial edema on the region of mandibular molars.

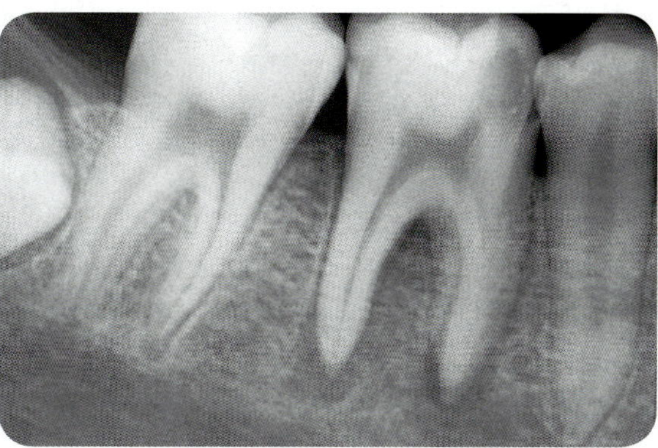

**Figure 10.30** - Radiographic aspect of the caries on mesial region of tooth 46, and diffuse periapical bone rarefaction.

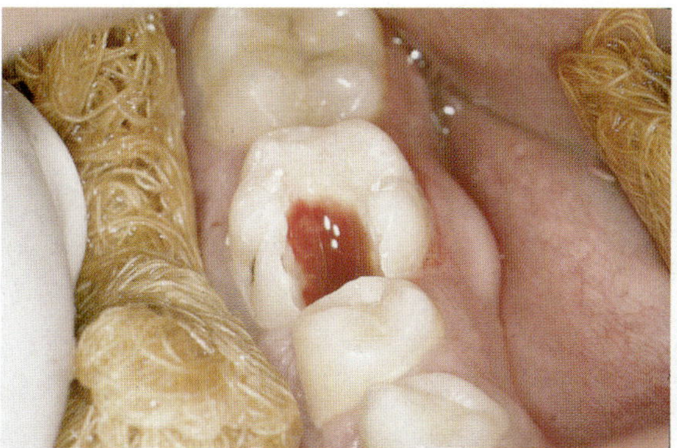

**Figure 10.31** - Clinical aspect of coronal drainage of tooth 46.

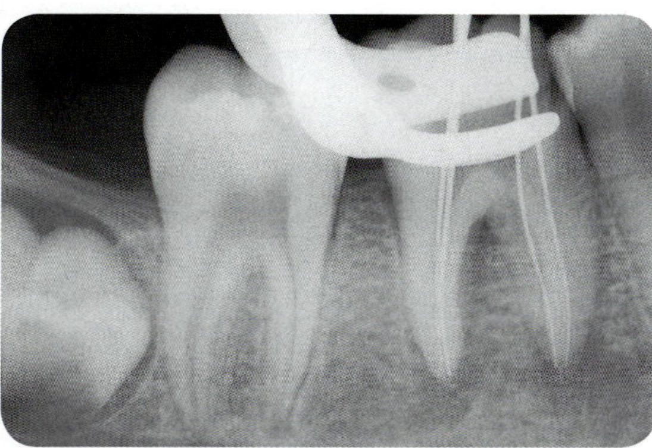

**Figure 10.32** - Emptying and preparation of root canals of tooth 46.

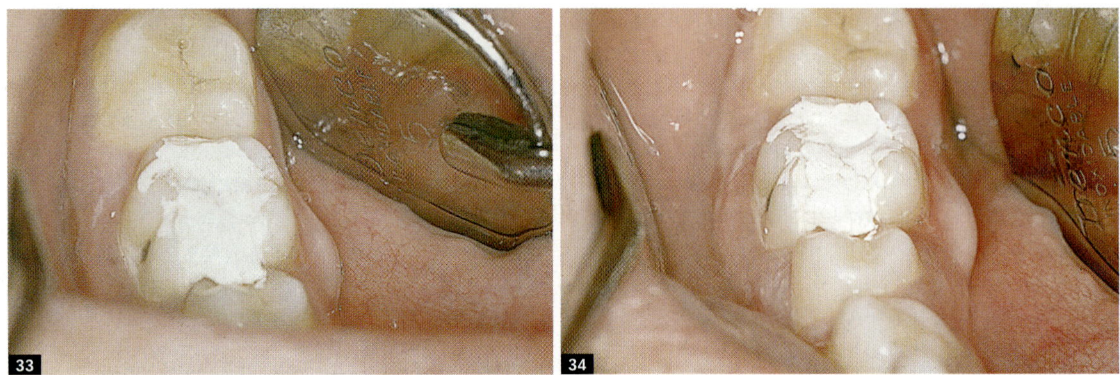

**Figures 10.33 and 10.34** - Occlusal relief of tooth 46.

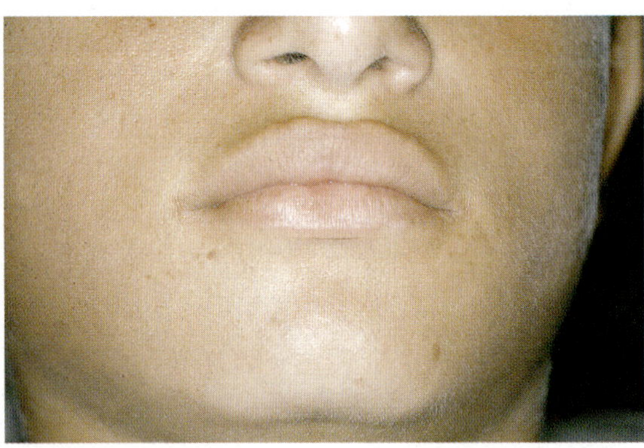

**Figure 10.35** - 7 days after attendance, disappeared the facial edema.

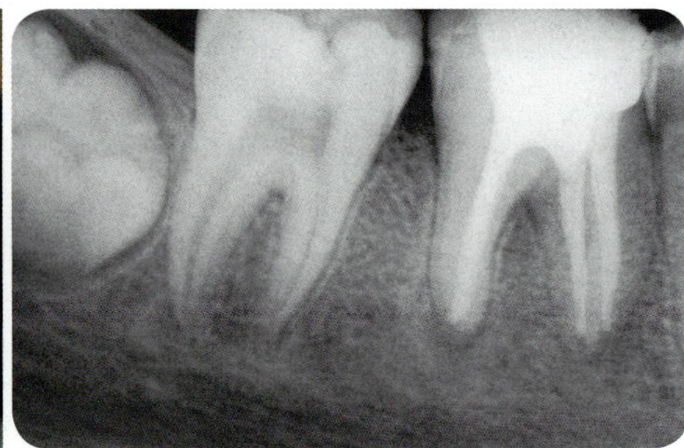

**Figure 10.36** - Filling of the canal after 30 days. The tooth was maintained with calcium hydroxide paste.

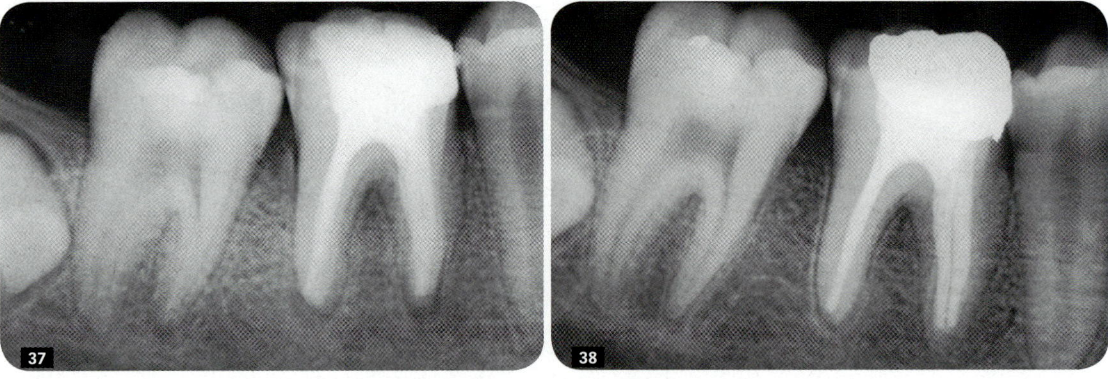

**Figures 10.37 and 10.38** - Clinical and radiographic control on the period of 3 to 6 months. Radiographic aspect with characteristics of disappearing the diffuse periapical rarefaction.

### 10.8.3 Periapical abscess without fistula (advanced)

The clinical-radiographic characteristics of the advanced abscess, characterizing the final stage, involves: spontaneous pain, with lower intensity than on the initial phase, pulsing, localized, evident edema with fluctuation point and volumetric increase of the injured area, negative answer at the pulpal vitality exam. The area of tumefaction shows certain consistency, nevertheless, with little resistance (local of the purulent collection). The radiographic aspect although it is not applicable, on some situations characterizes enlargement of the apical periodontal space and diffuse periapical bone rarefaction. The purulent collection crossed the alveolar lamina dura, invaded the medullar spaces (bone trabecula), won the sub-periosteum region and installed on the sub-mucosal region. Tumefaction and facial asymmetry are commonly observed, besides the region is reddish. It is common the patient showing debility, and even presence of fever. The Figures 10.39 to 10.43 exhibit cases of advanced periapical abscess without fistula. The Figures 10.39A-H shows a case of extra-oral drainage of advanced periapical abscess without fistula.

#### Local and systemic therapeutics

1. Anesthesia, absolute isolation and cleaning of the operative field.
2. Occlusal relief.
3. Coronal opening.
4. Abundant irrigation-aspiration with 1 to 2.5% sodium hypochlorite.
5. Emptying of the content of the root canal, with consequent sanitization process aided by thin instrument and 1% sodium hypochlorite. The foramen is enlarged until the file # 20-25 (type K-file), depending of the tooth, passing 1 mm.
6. With the enlargement of the apical foramen and passing 1 mm with the file, not always occurs drainage via canal. Many times it is discrete, the same way that on the periapical abscess on initial phase. It is difficult for the purulent collection return completely for drainage via root canal.
7. The pain is disturbing and constant, making necessary the fastest possible the opening of a pathway for the drainage of the formed pus. Special care with the patient with fever, and advanced debility.
8. At this moment, it is established the intra-oral drainage, close to the region of the tooth, and fluctuation point. With a scalpel over the fluctuation point, it is incised the surface, and with the scissor of thin tip it is made the dilatation, achieving the area of necrosis and pus, allowing its exit. It can yet be pressed the region with edema with gauze favoring a bigger drainage. The extra-oral drainage made with scalpel on the region of fluctuation of the skin should be directed following the anatomic lines, avoiding, thus, the formation of a future scar. Once determined the drainage of the purulent collection, it is prepared a drain favoring the maintenance of the incision's opening, maintaining the drainage for a larger period. This drain can be made of a part of the rubber dam, maintained for an average period of 48 to 72 hours.
9. The area of the incision can be protected with the application of antiseptic pomade, assisting the microbial control, and on the easy removal of the drain and protector gauze.
10. As systemic procedure it is important the utilization of systemic medication.
11. Special attention and complete assistance for the patient until the end of all the urgency state.

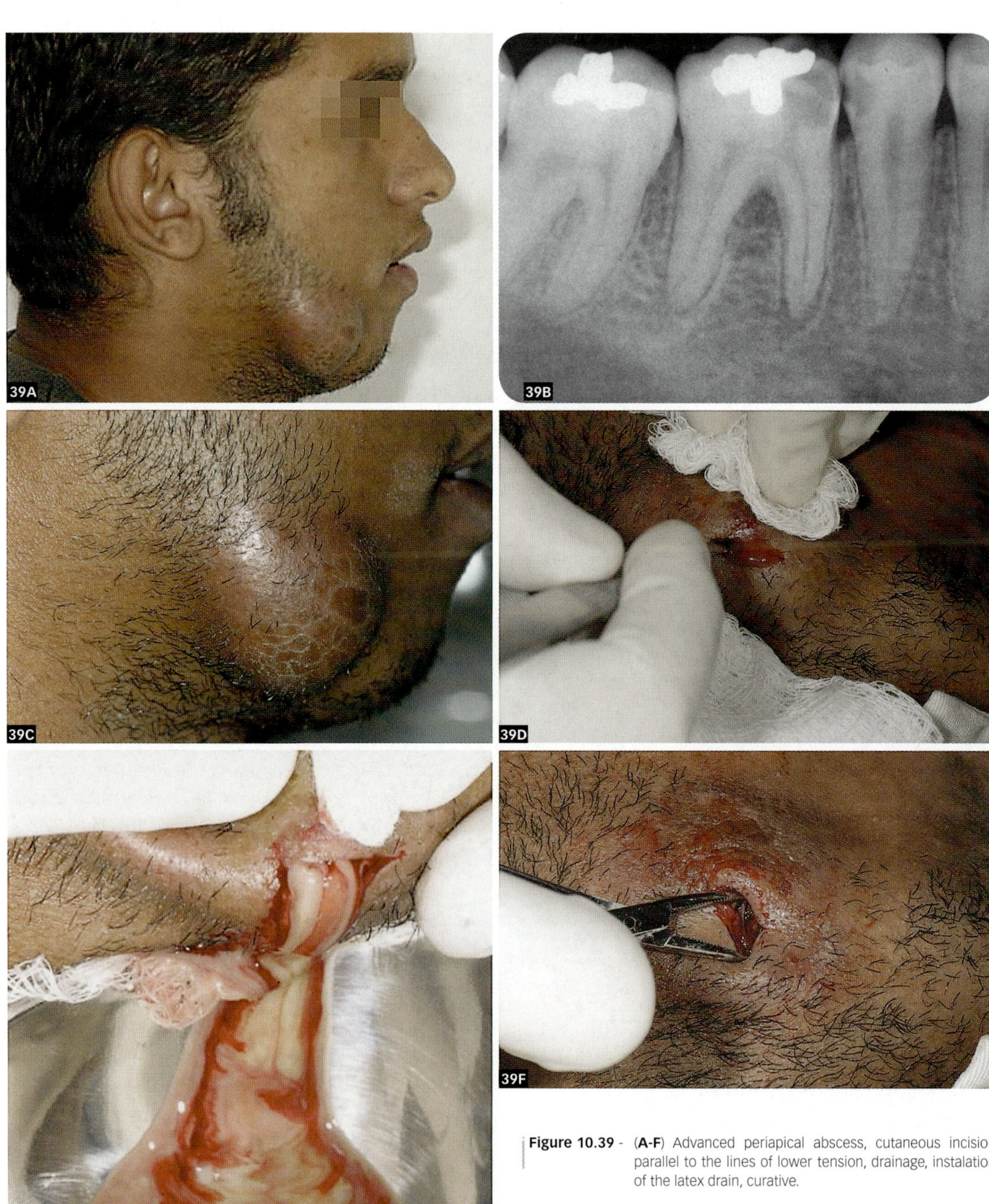


**Figure 10.39** - (**A-F**) Advanced periapical abscess, cutaneous incision parallel to the lines of lower tension, drainage, instalation of the latex drain, curative.

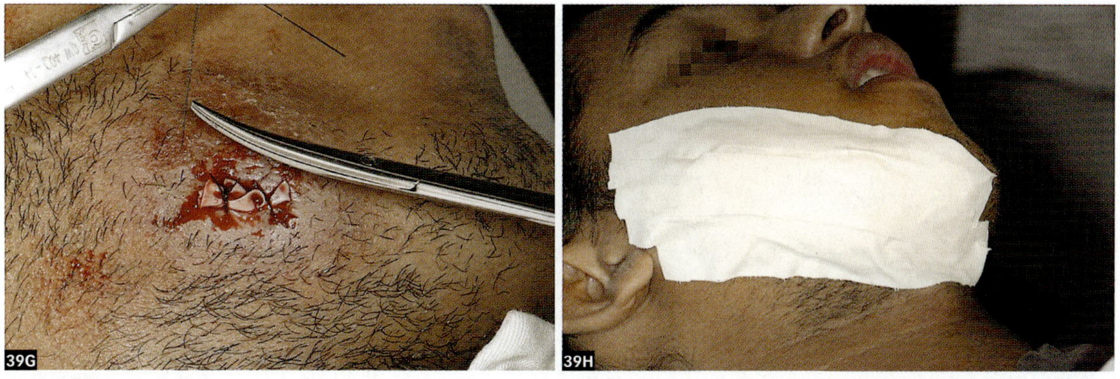


Figure 10.39 - (G-H) Advanced periapical abscess, cutaneous incision parallel to the lines of lower tension, drainage, instalation of the latex drain, curative.

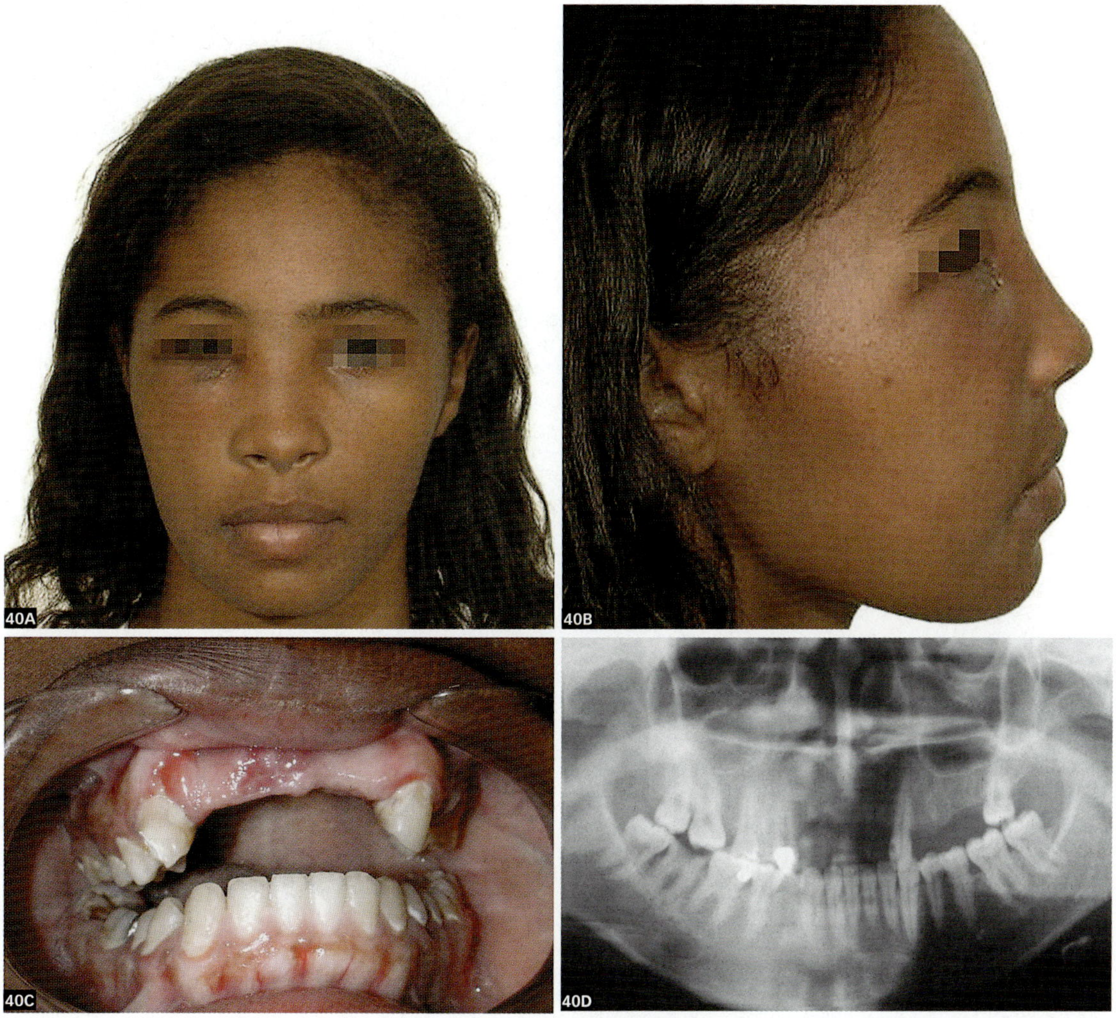

Figure 10.40 - (A-D) Advanced periapical abscess.

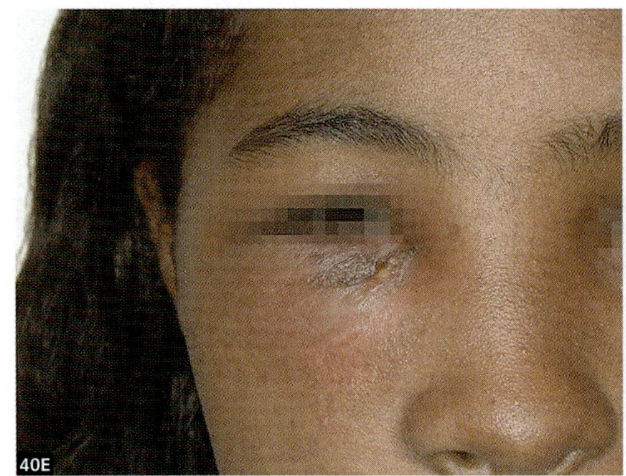


Figure 10.40 - (E-F) Advanced periapical abscess.

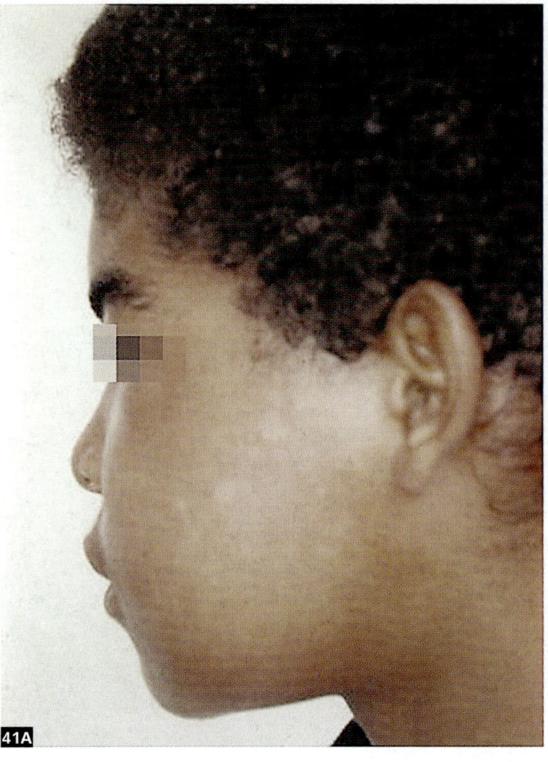


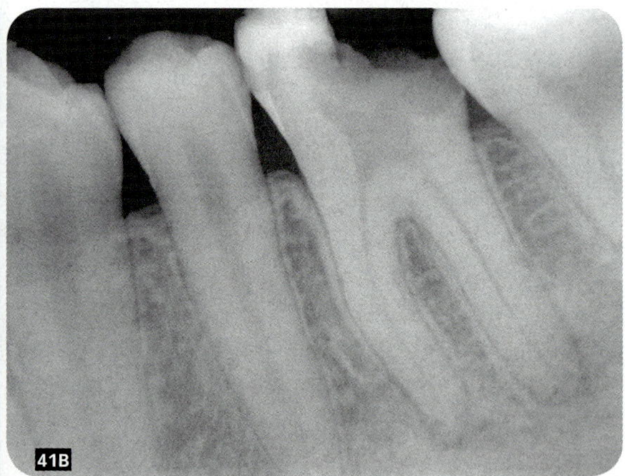


**Figure 10.41** - (**A-B**) Advanced periapical abscess.

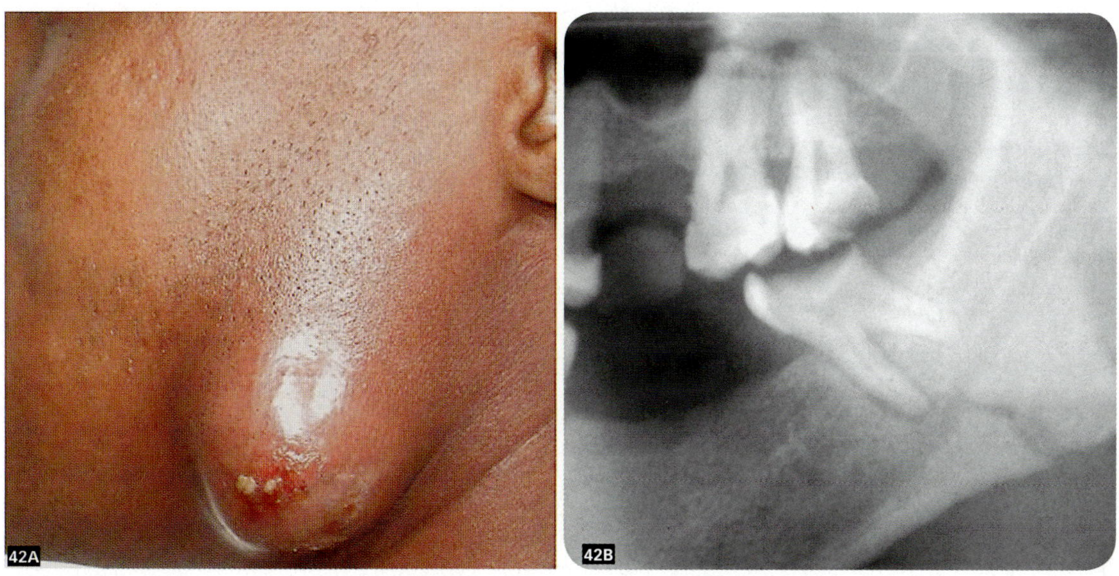

**Figure 10.42** - (**A-B**) Advanced periapical abscess.

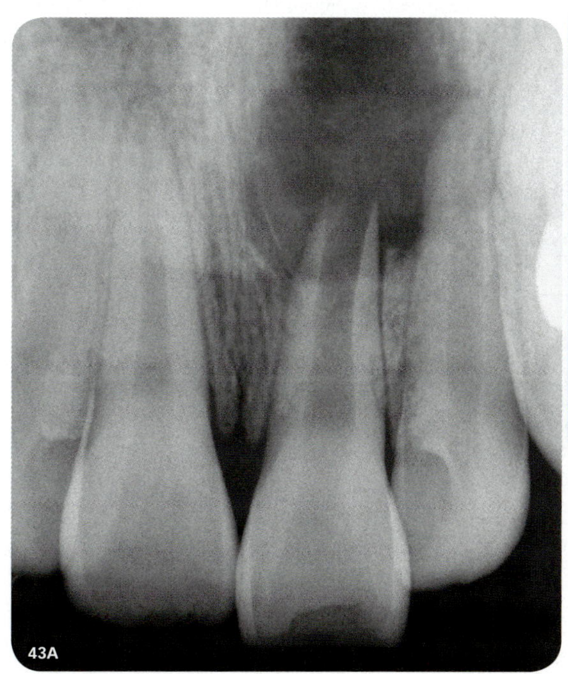

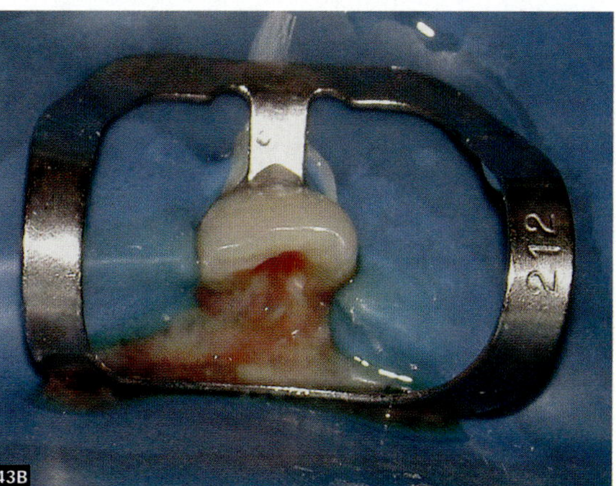

**Figure 10.43** - (**A-B**) Advanced periapical abscess, drainage (Prof. Dr. Luzi Augusto Faitaroni).

Estrela et al.[105] evaluated longitudinal studies about the treatment of periapical abscess without fistula, using a systematic review. A MEDLINE search strategy was developed to identify articles using the following uniterms: *Endodontic(s) and Alveolar Abscess, Endodontic(s)and Acute Apical Periodontitis, Endodontic(s) and Periapical Abscess, Endodontic(s) and Dento-Alveolar Abscess, Endodontic(s) and Acute Abscess, Endodontic(s) and Acute Periapical Abscess* The search included articles from the MEDLINE (http://www.ncbi.nlm.nih.gov/PubMed), from 1952 to August 29th of 2007. From 543 studies (Fig. 10.44), 1 article satisfied the inclusion criteria. The analysis of the found studies, observed that the local and systemic microbial control (with neutralization of the virulence arsenal) aid the defenses of the host and favor the reduction of the course of the infectious process. Whenever possible should take the emptying and enlargement of the root canal, drainage of the purulent collection, local and systemic medication and to maintain the closed tooth.

Fouad et al.[128] assessed the effect of penicillin supplementation on the reduction of symptoms and the course of recovery of the localized acute apical abscess after emergency endodontic treatment. Patients with pulp necrosis and periapical pain and/or swelling diagnosed with acute apical abscess were considered for the study. After local anesthesia, the offending tooth was accessed, the working length determined, and cleaning and shaping of the canals was either partially or completely done (depending on the availability of time) with copious irrigation with 2.6% sodium hypochlorite. Canals were dried, medicated with calcium hydroxide paste, and then temporized with Cavit or IRM. When indicated, a localized intraoral swelling was incised for drainage with a drain inserted for 24 to 48 hours. In a double-blind design, the patients were then randomly assigned to one of three groups: (1) penicillin group: Penicillin (Phenoxymethyl) VK 500 mg, two tablets at the conclusion of the visit followed by 1 tablet four times daily for 7 days; (2) placebo group; placebo tablets according to the same regimen; (3) neither medication group; these patients received neither penicillin nor the placebo. All participating patients were given 600 mg ibuprofen immediately before treatment and were maintained on this medication four times daily for 24 hours, and then as needed. The assignment was done according to a double-blind protocol. Each patient was given an envelope labeled A, B, or C with the medications (or placebo) and instructions for use. Neither patient nor practitioner knew whether they received penicillin, the placebo, or only the analgesics. Each patient was also given a stamped self addressed posttreatment card and instructed to mark their pain and swelling experience before treatment, as well as at 6, 12, 24, 48, and 72 hours after treatment. Based on a visual analog scale (VAS) on the posttreatment card, pain experience was rank ordered into four categories that were given scores as follows: pain of no clinical significance (0 to 25)= 0; mild pain (25 to 50)= 1; moderate pain (50 to 75) = 2; and severe pain (75 to 100) = 3. Swelling experience was ranked into five categories and given the following scores: no swelling = 0; significant reduction in swelling = 1; slight decrease in swelling = 2; same size swelling as before treatment = 3; and an increase in the size of swelling = 4. All patients who had preoperative swelling or who reported reduction in swelling from the preoperative state were given a score of 3 for preoperative swelling; otherwise patients received a score of 0 for preoperative swelling. Resolution was fairly rapid in most patients. Statistical analysis of the scores of 32 respondents revealed no significant differences between the three groups in course of recovery or symptoms at any time period. Patients with localized periapical pain or swelling generally recovered quickly with local treatment. The data did not show a demonstrable benefit from penicillin supplementation.

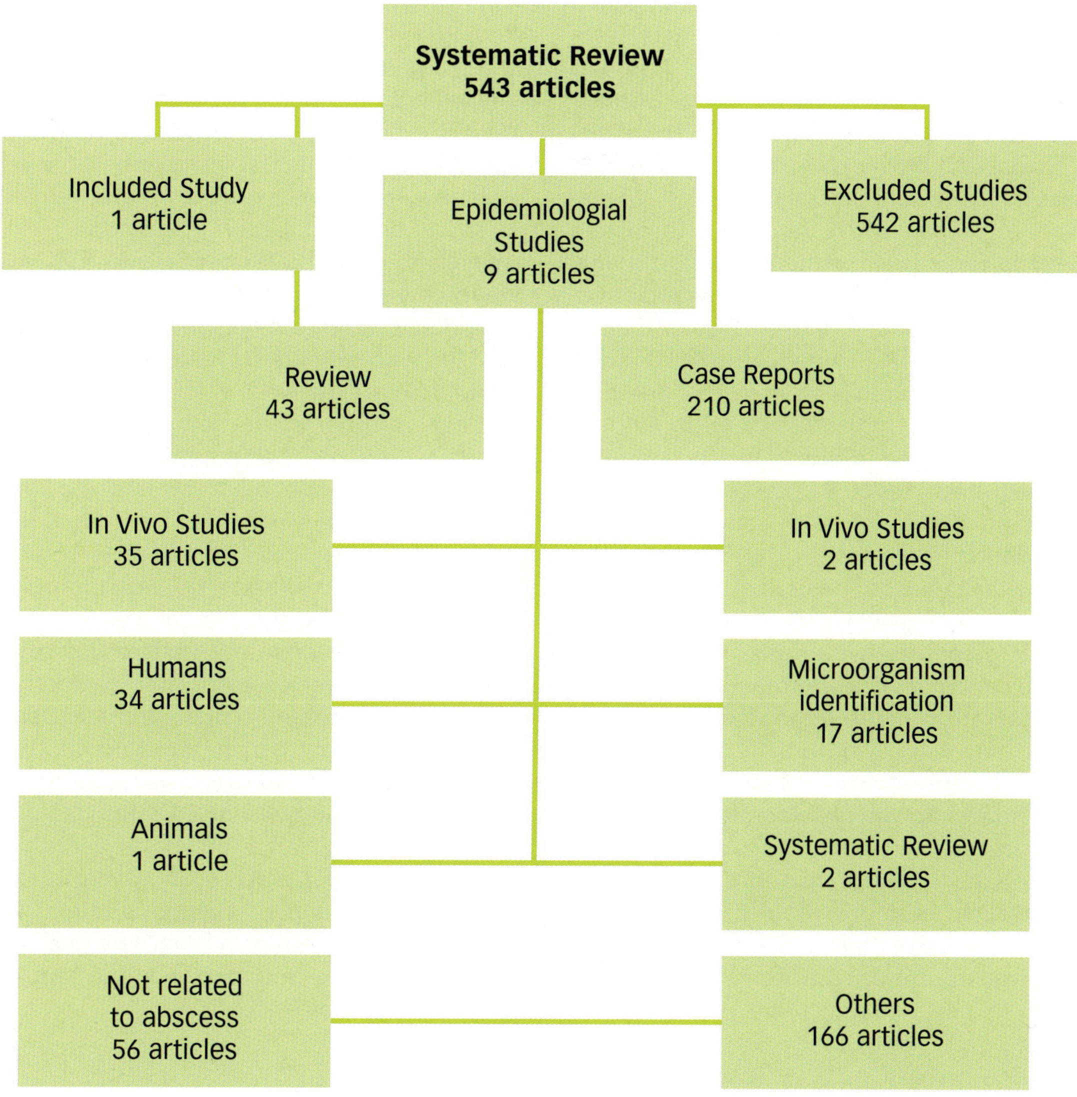


**Figure 10.44** - Squematic representation of longitudinal studies about the pain after endodontic treatment in teeth with periapical abscess.

Estrela et al.[108] (work not published) studied the prevalence and risk factors of pulpal and periapical pain. A cross-section study was carried out evaluating patients who had experience of pulpal or periapical pain associated to inflammation and/or infection and to search treatment in the Faculty of Dentistry (Urgency Dental Service, Federal University of Goiás, GO, Brazil), during the years of 2005 and 2006. The sample consisted of 1,765 patients (675 male, 1090 female) with history of endodontic pain without dental trauma. These individuals were from low socioeconomic background. The mean age of the patients was 32 years. Among the teeth studied were associated with mandible (n=889), maxillary (876), molars (n=974), premolars (n=399), canines (n=95) and incisors (n=203); between these teeth, 94 present endodontic treatment and 1,671 teeth showed absence endodontic treatment.

The analysis of the pulpal and periapical pain was based on guidelines from the clinical diagnosis hypothesis of pulpal and periapical diseases (hyperreactive pulpalgia, symptomatic pulpitis, asymptomatic pulpitis, pulpal necrosis, symptomatic apical periodontitis (traumatic or infection origin), asymptomatic apical periodontitis, periapical abscess without fistula, periapical abscess with fistula). In clinical situations that pain did not involved pulp or periapex, it was including into the others type of pain. The structure of clinical exam was composed by the anamnesis (medical and dental history; the clinical characteristics of the pain verified during the anamnesis were: how appeared-provoked or spontaneous, duration, frequency, seat, intensity); the clinical exam; the pulpal vitality and the radiographic exam. To determine the prevalence, it was used the clinical classification of the pulp and periapical disease describe previously. The characteristics analyzed about risk factors involved: 1. for pulpal pain – patient's gender (male, female), position of tooth (anterior, posterior), arch (maxillary, mandible), intact crown (no, yes), open cavity (no, yes), caries lesion (no, yes), amalgam restoration (yes, no), resin restoration (no, yes), temporary restoration (no, yes), crown fracture (no, yes); 2. for periapical pain-patient's gender (male, female), position of tooth (anterior, posterior), arch (maxillary, mandible), endodontic treatment (no, yes), intact crown (no, yes), open cavity (no, yes), caries lesion (no, yes), amalgam restoration (no, yes), resin restoration (no, yes), temporary restoration (no, yes), crown fracture (no, yes); restoration with post (no, yes). In this study, the dental urgencies associated with others symptomatic problems, like traumatic dental injuries, periodontal pain, temporomandibular pain, it were included in others categories. The results are shown in the Tables 10.5-10.8. The higher prevalence of odontogenic pain was symptomatic pulpitis and symptomatic apical periodontitis of infectious origin. The risk factor for pulpal pain of more expression was caries lesion, and for periapical pain was open cavity (Tables 10.6-10.7).

**Table 10.5** - Prevalence of pulpal and periapical pain (n=1765)[108]

| Types of Urgencies | Frequency | Percentage |
|---|---|---|
| Symptomatic Pulpitis | 499 | 28.3% |
| Symptomatic Apical Periodontitis of Infectious origin | 466 | 26.4% |
| Hyperreactive Pulpalgia | 255 | 14.4% |
| Periapical Abscess without Fistula - phase I | 83 | 4.7% |
| Periapical Abscess with Fistula | 68 | 3.9% |
| Asymptomatic Apical Periodontitis | 66 | 3.7% |
| Periapical Abscess without Fistula - phase II | 39 | 2.2% |
| Pulpal Necroses | 31 | 1.8% |
| Periapical Abscess without Fistula - phase III | 24 | 1.4% |
| Asymptomatic Pulpitis | 23 | 1.3% |
| Periapical Abscess without Fistula | 18 | 1.0% |
| Symptomatic Apical Periodontitis of Traumatic origin | 11 | 0.6% |
| Others Categories | 172 | 9.7% |
| Total | 1765 | 100.0 |

**Table 10.6** - Risk factors for pulpal pain (n=1765)

| Factor | n | Pulpal pain | | $\chi2$ | p | OR (95% CI) |
|---|---|---|---|---|---|---|
| | | Yes (n=809) | No (n=956) | | | |
| Patient's gender | | | | | | |
| Male | 675 (38.2) | 312 | 363 | 0.066 | 0.798 | 1 |
| Female | 1090 (61.8) | 497 | 593 | | | 0.97 (0.80 – 1.18) |
| Position of tooth | | | | | | |
| Anterior | 303 (17.2) | 77 | 226 | 61.46 | 0.000 | 1 |
| Posterior | 1462 (82.8) | 732 | 730 | | | 2.94 (2.23 – 3.89) |
| Arch | | | | | | |
| Maxillary | 876 (49.6) | 390 | 486 | 1.212 | 0.271 | 1 |
| Mandibular | 889 (50.4) | 419 | 470 | | | 1.11 (0.92 – 1.34) |
| Intact Crown | | | | | | |
| Yes | 102 (5.8) | 27 | 75 | 16.35 | 0.000 | 1 |
| No | 1663 (94.2) | 782 | 881 | | | 2.47 (1.57 – 3.87) |
| Open Cavity | | | | | | |
| No | 1477 (83.7) | 796 | 681 | 236.70 | 0.000 | 1 |
| Yes | 288 (16.3) | 13 | 275 | | | 0.04 (0.02 – 0.07) |
| Caries lesion | | | | | | |
| No | 473 (26.8) | 141 | 332 | 66.85 | 0.000 | 1 |
| Yes | 1292 (73.2) | 668 | 624 | | | 2.52 (2.01 – 3.16) |
| Amalgam restoration | | | | | | |
| No | 1391 (78.8) | 576 | 815 | 51.81 | 0.000 | 1 |
| Yes | 374 (21.2) | 233 | 141 | | | 2.34 (1.85 – 2.96) |
| Resin restoration | | | | | | |
| No | 1663 (94.2) | 775 | 888 | 6.82 | 0.009 | 1 |
| Yes | 102 (5.8) | 34 | 68 | | | 0.57 (0.38 – 0.87) |
| Provisional restoration | | | | | | |
| No | 1657 (93.9) | 765 | 892 | 1.203 | 0.273 | 1 |
| Yes | 108 (6.1) | 44 | 64 | | | 0.80 (0.54 – 1.19) |
| Coronal fracture | | | | | | |
| No | 1720 (97.5) | 793 | 927 | 1.97 | 0.161 | 1 |
| Yes | 45 (2.5) | 16 | 29 | | | 0.65 (0.35 – 1.20) |

**Table 10.7** - Risk factors for periapical pain (n=1765)[108]

| Factor | n | Periapical pain Yes (n=774) | Periapical pain No (n=991) | χ2 | p | OR (95% CI) |
|---|---|---|---|---|---|---|
| Patient's gender | | | | | | |
| Male | 675 (38.2) | 285 | 390 | 1.180 | 0.277 | 1 |
| Female | 1090 (61.8) | 489 | 601 | | | 1.11 (0.92 – 1.35) |
| Position of tooth | | | | | | |
| Anterior | 303 (17.2) | 169 | 134 | 21.12 | 0.000 | 1 |
| Posterior | 1462 (82.8) | 605 | 857 | | | 0.56 (0.44 – 0.72) |
| Arch | | | | | | |
| Maxillary | 876 (49.6) | 416 | 460 | 9.34 | 0.002 | 1 |
| Mandibular | 889 (50.4) | 358 | 531 | | | 0.75 (0.62 – 0.90) |
| Endodontic treatment | | | | | | |
| Yes | 93 (5.3) | 87 | 6 | 98.47 | 0.000 | 1 |
| No | 1672 (94.7) | 687 | 985 | | | 0.05 (0.02 – 0.11) |
| Intact Crown | | | | | | |
| Yes | 102 (5.8) | 12 | 90 | 45.27 | 0.000 | 1 |
| No | 1663 (94.2) | 762 | 901 | | | 6.34 (3.45 – 11.67) |
| Open cavity | | | | | | |
| No | 1477 (83.7) | 503 | 974 | 352.87 | 0.000 | 1 |
| Yes | 288 (16.3) | 271 | 17 | | | 30.87 (18.69 – 50.98) |
| Caries lesion | | | | | | |
| No | 473 (26.8) | 176 | 297 | 11.58 | 0.001 | 1 |
| Yes | 1292 (73.2) | 598 | 694 | | | 1.45 (1.17 – 1.81) |
| Amalgam restoration | | | | | | |
| No | 1391 (78.8) | 673 | 718 | 54.71 | 0.000 | 1 |
| Yes | 374 (21.2) | 101 | 273 | | | 0.40 (0.31 – 0.51) |
| Resin restoration | | | | | | |
| No | 1663 (94.2) | 716 | 947 | 7.44 | 0.006 | 1 |
| Yes | 102 (5.8) | 58 | 44 | | | 1.74 (1.16 – 2.61) |
| Provisional restoration | | | | | | |
| No | 1657 (93.9) | 711 | 946 | 9.80 | 0.002 | 1 |
| Yes | 108 (6.1) | 63 | 45 | | | 1.86 (1.26 – 2.76) |
| Coronal fracture | | | | | | |
| No | 1720 (97.5) | 745 | 975 | 7.95 | 0.005 | 1 |
| Yes | 45 (2.5) | 29 | 16 | | | 2.37 (1.28 – 4.40) |
| Restoration with post | | | | | | |
| No | 1753 (99.3) | 763 | 990 | 11.22 | 0.001 | 1 |
| Yes | 12 (0.7) | 11 | 1 | | | 14.27 (1.84 – 110.79) |

**Table 10.8** - Logistic regression analysis for each explanatory variable for pulpal, periapical and periodontal pain in odontogenic urgencies (n=1765)[108]

| Explanatory variable | Logistic regression analysis | |
|---|---|---|
| | OR (95% CI) | P-value |
| Pulpal Pain | | |
| Position of tooth | 1.68 (1.22 – 2.32) | 0.002 |
| Caries lesion | 3.60 (2.80 – 4.63) | 0.000 |
| Amalgam restoration | 1.81 (1.39 – 2.36) | 0.000 |
| Open Cavity | 0.03 (0.02 – 0.06) | 0.000 |
| Periapical Pain | | |
| Open Cavity | 26.73 (16.02 – 44.62) | 0.000 |
| Intact Crown | 4.41 (2.34 – 8.32) | 0.000 |
| Provisional restoration | 2.57 (1.69 – 3.90) | 0.000 |
| Resin restoration | 1.87 (1.20 – 2.93) | 0.006 |
| Endodontic Treatment | 0.09 (0.04 – 0.21) | 0.000 |
| Position of tooth | 0.63 (0.46 – 0.86) | 0.004 |
| Amalgam restoration | 0.67 (0.51 – 0.90) | 0.007 |
| Periodontal Pain | | |
| Periodontal Pocket | 23.57 (13.85 – 40.11) | 0.000 |
| Intact Crown | 0.10 (0.06 – 0.17) | 0.000 |
| Caries Lesion | 0.10 (0.10 – 0.17) | 0.000 |

## 10.9 Periapical Abscess with Fistula

The periapical abscess with fistula can be developed from the infectious symptomatic (acute) apical periodontitis, asymptomatic (chronic) apical periodontitis, periapical abscess without fistula, originated from the process of infection of the root canal. This abscess can be characterized as proliferative chronic inflammatory process, with focus of suppuration localized near the periapical region with nutrition from the root canal with pulpal necrosis. The cellular population is represented by neutrophils, lymphocytes, plasmocytes and macrophages. The quantity of mononuclear cells is always higher than on the acute process. On this chronic phase, the abscess shows areas of bone resorption varying from diffuse to circumscribed aspect, and can be mapped radiographically by the introduction of a gutta-percha cone through the fistula and radiograph, allowing to identify the dental apex responsible for the infection. The process is asymptomatic and, normally, the correct root canal treatment is enough to disappear with this state.

It is clear that it cannot be discarded the refractory lesions. The fistula can represent a pathway of entrance of microorganism from the oral cavity to internal tissues, specially fungi. The vertical fracture, radicular fracture by pressure of the intra-radicular post, endo-periodontal involvement, secondary infection constitute common situations of presence of fistula which treatment should be very well advised and conducted. It should be considered that the treatment of teeth with fistula, due to failure of the initial root canal treatment should not be faced as a simple case and of easy solution. The Figures 10.45A-B demonstrate clinical cases of periapical abscess with fistula.

## 10.10 Condensing Osteitis

The grade of virulence of the microorganisms associated to the resistance of the host determines the type of periapical lesion. The aggression of low intensity, long duration can determine a chronic periapical inflammation, denominated condensing osteitis. Among the characteristics generally found, it is observed the excessive synthesis of periapical bone, localized around the dental apexes, what demonstrates, with the radiographic aspect – the increase of the bone density (opacity and accentuated evidencing of the bone trabecullas, circumscribed by active osteoblasts), instead of the transparency of the resorbed bone. The pathognomonic signal is the radiopaque area circumscribed around one or all the tooth's roots. Clinically, the tooth is asymptomatic and, after the root canal treatment, usually the radiopaque alterations return to normal. The Figures 10.46A-B demonstrate radiographic aspects characteristic of condensing osteitis, on the periapical region of molars.

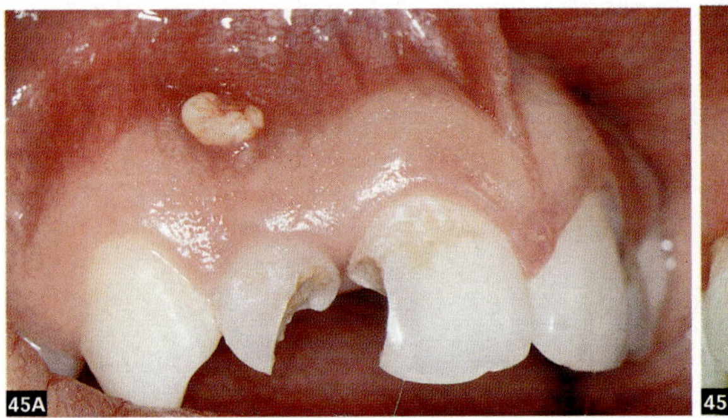


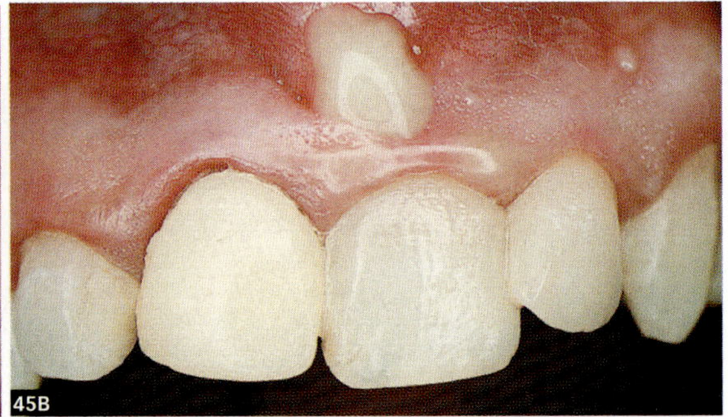


**Figure 10.45** - **(A-B)** Periapical Abscess with Fistula.

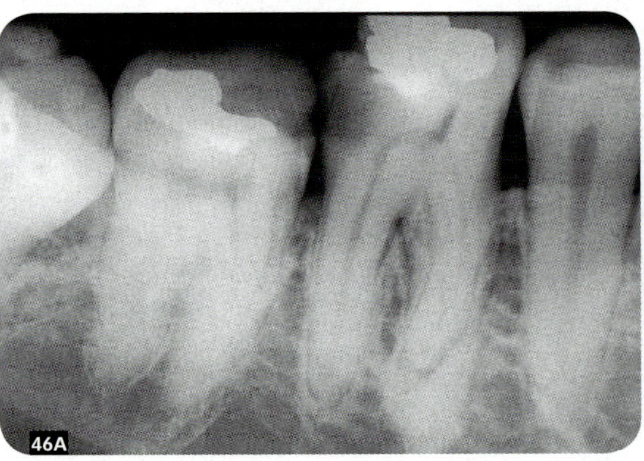


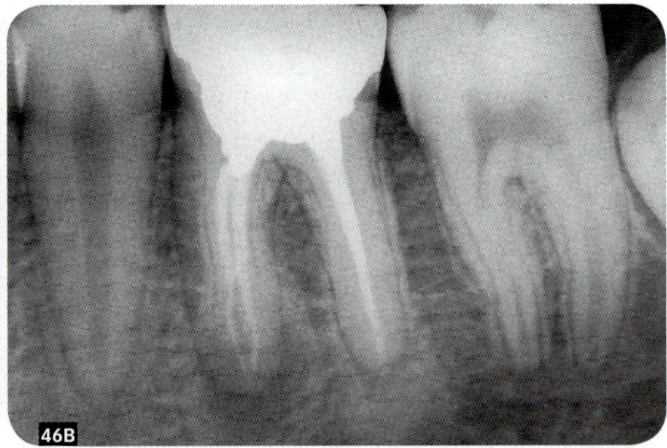


**Figure 10.46** - **(A-B)** Condensing osteitis. Radiographic aspect of condensing osteitis on the mesial root of tooth 46 and on distal root of tooth 36.

1. Abou-Rass M, Bogen G. Microorganisms in closed periapical lesions. Int Endod J 1998;31:39-47.
2. Alaçam T, Tinaz AC. Interappointment emergencies in teeth with necrotic pulps. J Endod 2002;28:375-77.
3. Alaçam T. Incidence of postoperative pain following the use of different sealers in immediate root canal filling. J Endod 1985;11:135-37.
4. Albashaireh ZS, Alnegrish AS. Postobturation pain after single- and multiple-visit endodontic therapy. A prospective study. J Dent 1998;26:227-32.
5. Aleksejuniene J, Eriksen HM, Sidaravicius B, Haapasalo M. Apical periodontitis and related factors in an adult Lithuanian population Oral Surg Oral Med Oral Pathol Oral Radiol Endod 2000;90:95-101.
6. Allard U, Palmqvist S. A radiographic survey of periapical conditions in elderly people in a Swedish county population. Endod Dent Traumatol 1986;2:103–08.
7. Allen RK, Newton CW, Brown CE. A statiscal analysis of surgical and nonsurgical endodontic retreatment cases. J Endod 1989;15:261-66.
8. Al-Negrish AR, Habahbeh R. Flare up rate related to root canal treatment of asymptomatic pulpally necrotic central incisor teeth in patients attending a military hospital. J Dent 2006;34:635-40.
9. Ando N, Hoshino E. Predominant obligate anaerobis invading the deep layers root canal dentine. Int Endod J 1990;23:20-27.
10. Arai Y, Tammisalo E, Iwai K, Hashimoto K, Shinoda K. Development of a compact computed tomographic apparatus for dental use. DentMaxillofac Radiol 1999;28:245-48.
11. August DS. Managing the abscessed tooth: instrument and close? Part 1. J Endod 1977;3:316-18.
12. August DS. Managing the abscessed tooth: instrument and close? Part 2. J Endod 1977;8:364-66.
13. Baker PT, Evans RT, Slots J, Genco RJ. Antibiotic susceptibility of anaerobic bacteria from the human oral cavity. J Dent Res 1985;64:1233-44.
14. Balaban FS, Skidmore AE, Griffin JA. Acute exacerbations following initial treatment of necrotic pulps. J Endod 1984;10:78-81.
15. Barbakow FH, Cleaton JPE. Treatment of teeth with periapical radiolucent areas in general dental practice. Oral Surg Oral Med Oral Pathol 1981;51:552-59.
16. Barnett F, Axelrod P, Tronstad L, Graziani A, Slots J, Talbott G. Ciprofloxacin treatment of periapical *Pseudomonas aeruginosa* infection. Endod Dent Traumatol 1988;4:132-37.
17. Barnett F, Tronstad L. The prevalence of flare-ups following endodontic treatment. J Dent Res 1989;68:1253.
18. Batista A, Sydney GB, Estrela C. Uma análise da conduta de urgência de origem endodôntica. Scientific-A 2007;1:56-67.
19. Baumann L, Rossman SK. Clinical, roentgenologic, and histologic findings in teeth with apical radiolucent areas. Oral Surg Oral Med Oral Pathol 1956;9:1330-36.
20. Baumgartner JC, Falkler WA. Bacteria in the apical 5mm of the infected root canals. J Endod 1991;17:380-83.
21. Baumgartner JC, Heggers JP, Harrison JW. Incidence of bacteremias related to endodontic procedures. II. Surgical endodontics. J Endod 1977;3:399-402.
22. Baumgartner JC, Huter JW. Endodontic microbiology and treatment of infections. In: Pathways of the pulp. Cohen S, Burns RC. St. Louis: Mosby;2001.
23. Baumgartner JC, Watkins BJ, Bae KS, Xia T. Association of black-pigmented bacteria with endodontic infection. J Endod 1999;25:413-15.
24. Baumgartner JC, Xia T. Antibiotic susceptibility of bacteria associated with endodontic abscesses. J Endod 2002;29:44-47.
25. Baumgartner JC. Microbiologic and pathologic aspects of endodontics. Current Opinion in Dentistry 1991;1:737-43.
26. Beck JD, Offenbacher S, Williams R, Gibbs P, Garcia R. Periodontitis: a risk factor for coronary heart disease? Ann Periodontol 1998;3:127.
27. Bender IB, Seltzer S. Combination of antibiotics and fungicides used in treatment of the infected pulpless tooth. J Amer Dent Ass 1952;45:293-300.
28. Bender IB, Seltzer S. Roentgenographic and direct observation of experimental lesions in bone I. J Am Dent Ass 1961;62:152-60.
29. Bender IB, Seltzer S. Roentgenographic and direct observation of experimental lesions in bone II. J Am Dent Ass 1961;62:708-16.
30. Bergenholtz G, Lekholm U, Liljenberg B, Lindhe J. Morphometric analysis of chronic inflammatory periapical lesions in root-filled teeth. Oral Surg Oral Med Oral Pathol 1983;55:295-301.
31. Bergenholtz G, Lekholm U, Milthon R, Engström B. Influence of apical overinstrumentation and overfilling on re-treated root canals. J Endod 1979;5:310-14.
32. Bergenholtz G, Lekholm U, Milthon R, Heden G, Odesjo B, Engström B. Retreatment of endodontic fillings. Scand J dent Res 1979;87:217-24.
33. Bergenholtz G, Malmcrona E, Milthon R. Endodontisk behandling och periapikalstatus. Tandläkartidningen 1973;65:64–73.
34. Bergenholtz G. Effect of bacterial products on inflammatory reaction in the dental pulp. Scand J Dent Res 1977;85:122-29.
35. Bergenholtz G. Micro-organisms from necrotic pulp of traumatized teeth. Odont Revy 1974;25:347-58.
36. Bergström J, Eliasson S, Ahlberg KF. Periapical status in subjects with regular dental care habits. Comm Dent O Epidemiol 1987;15:236-39.
37. Bhaskar SN. Histologia e Embriologia Oral de Orban. Artes Médicas: São Paulo;1978.
38. Bhaskar SN. Periapical lesion: types, incidence, and clinical features. Oral Surg Oral Med Oral Pathol 1966;21:657-71.
39. Block RM, Bushell A, Rodrigues H, Langeland K. A histologic, histobacteriologic, and radiographic study of periapical endodontic surgical specimens. Oral Surg Oral Med Oral Pathol 1976;42:656-78.
40. Bohórquez Avila SP, Rocha RSS, Consolaro A. Avaliação da presença e localização de bactérias nos canais radiculares e nas lesões periapicais crônicas pelo método de coloração de Brown e Brenn. Rev Fac Odontol Bauru 1995;3:25-31.

41. Boucher Y, Matossian L, Rilliard F, Machtou P. Radiographic evaluation of the prevalence and technical quality of root canal treatment in a French subpopulation. Int Endod J 2002;35:229-38.
42. Brook I, Frazier E. Clinical features and aerobic and anaerobic microbiological characteristics of cellulites. Arch Surg 1995;130:786-92.
43. Brook I, Frazier EH, Gher ME. Aerobic and anaerobic microbiology of periapical abscesses. Oral Microbiol Immunol 1991;6:123-25.
44. Brook I, Frazier EH, Gher ME. Microbiology of periapical abscesses and associated maxillary sinusitis. J Periodontal 1996;67:608-10.
45. Brook I. Microbiology and management of endodontic infections in children. J Clin Pediatr Dent 2003;28:13-17.
46. Brown JH, Brenn L. A method for the differential staining Gram-positive and Gram-negative bacteria in tissue section. Bull J Hork Hosp 1931;48:69-73.
47. Brynolf I. A histologic and roentgenologic study of the periapical region of human upper incisors. Odontol Revy 1967;18:171-76.
48. Buckley M, Spångberg LS. The prevalence and technical quality of endodontic treatment in an American subpopulation. Oral Surg Oral Med Oral Pathol Oral Radiol Endod 1995;79:92–100.
49. Bueno MR, Estrela C. Prevalência de tratamento endodôntico e periodontite apical em várias populações do mundo, detectada por radiografias panorâmicas, periapicais e tomografias computadorizadas cone beam. Rev. Odontol Brasil Central 2008;17:79-90.
50. Bueno MR, Estrela C, Azevedo BC, Brugnera-Jr. A, Azevedo JR. Tomografia compoutadorizada Cone Beam: Revolução na odontologia. Rev Ass Paul Cir Dent 2007;61:325-28.
51. Burnett GW, Schuster GS. Microbiologia Oral e Enfermidades infecciosas. Panamericana: Buenos Aires;1982. p.31-70.
52. Byström A, Claesson R, Sundqvist G. The antibacterial effect of camphorated paramonochlorophenol, comphorated phenol and calcium hydroxide in the treatment of infected root canals. Endod Dent Traumatol 1985;1:170-75.
53. Byström A, Happonen RP, Sjögren U, Sundqvist G. Healing of periapical lesions of pulpless teeth after endodontic treatment with controlled assepsis. Endod Dent Traumatol 1987;3:58-63.
54. Byström A, Sundqvist G. Bacteriologic evaluation of the effects of 0,5% sodium hypochlorite in endodontic therapy. Oral Surg Oral Med Oral Pathol 1983;55:307-12.
55. Byström A, Sundqvist G. Bacteriologic evaluation of the efficacy of mechanical root canal instrumentation in endodontic therapy. Scand J Dent Res 1981;89:321-28.
56. Byström A, Sundqvist G. The antibacterial action of sodium hypoclorite and EDTA in 60 cases of endodontic therapy. Int Endod J 1985;18:35-40.
57. Campos GM. Patologia Bucal. Ribeirão Preto;1978. (Apostila).
58. Caplan DJ, Chasen JB, Krall EA, Cai J, Kang S, Garcia RI, Offenbacher S, Beck JD. Lesions of endodontic origin and risk of coronary heart disease. J Dent Res 2006;85:996-1000
59. Chazel J-C, Valcarcel J, Tramini P, Pelissier B, Mafart B. Coronal and apical lesions, environmental factors: study in a modern and an archeological population. Clin Oral Invest 2005;9:197-202.
60. Chen C-Y, Hasselgren G, Serman N, Elkind M S V, Desvarieux M, Engebretson S P. Prevalence and quality of endodontic treatment in the northern manhattan elderly. J Endod 2007;33:230-34
61. Cheung GSP. Endodontic failures – changing the approach. Int Dent J 1996;46:131-38.
62. Consolaro A. Reabsorções dentárias. Maringá: Dental Press, 2002. 447p.
63. Cortezi W. Infecção Odontogênica Oral e Maxillofacial. Rio de Janeiro, Pedro Primeiro Ltda., 1995.226p.
64. Costa CAS, Pamplona FC. Mecanismos de formação de lesões periapicais – granuloma e cistos. Rev Odontol Brasil Central 2002;11:34-41.
65. Cotti E, Campisi G. Advanced radiographic techniques for the detection of lesions in bone. Endod Topics 2004;7:52–72.
66. Cotton TP, Geisler TM, Holden DT, Schwartz SA, Schindler WG. Endodontic applications of cone beam volumetric tomography. J Endod 2007;33:1121-32.
67. Crump MC. Diagnóstico diferencial del fracasso endodontica. Clin Odontol Amer Norte 1979;4:613-31.
68. Cymbler DM, Ardakani P. Sodium hypochlorite injection into periapical tissues. Dent Update. 1994;21:345-46.
69. Dahle UR, Tronstad L, Olsen I. Observation of an unusually large spirochete in endodontic infection. Oral Microbiol Immunol 1993;8:251-53.
70. Dahlén G, Fabricius L, Heydem G, Holm SE, Möller AJR. Apical periodontitis induced by selected bacterial strains in root canals of immunized and non immunized monkeys. Scand J Dent Res 1982;90:207-16.
71. Dahlén G, Haapasalo M. Microbiology of apical periodontitis. In: Essential endodontology. Ørstavik D, Pitt-Ford TR. Oxford: Black Well;1998.
72. Dahlén G, Hofstad T. Endotoxic activities of lipopolysaccharide of microorganisms isolated from an infection root canal in Macaca cynomolus. Scand J Dent Res 1977;85:272-78.
73. Dahlén G, Magnusson BC, Möller AJR. Histological and histochemical study of the influence of lipopolysaccharide extracted from *Fusobacterium nucleatum* on the periapical tissues in the monkey *Macaca fascicularis*. Arch Oral Biol 1981;26:591-98.
74. Dahlén G, Möller AJR. Microbiology of endodontic infections. In: Slots J, Taubman MA. Contemporary microbiologigy and immunology. St Louis: Mosby, 1992. p.444-75.
75. Dahlén G. Studies on lipopolysaccharides from oral Gram-negative anaerobic bacteria in relation to apical periodontitis. (Doctoral Thesis). Götemborg: University of Götemborg, Sweden;1980.
76. Dahlén H, Bergenholtz G. Endotoxic activity in teeth with necrotic pulps. J Dent Res 1980;59:1233-40.
77. Daum RS et al. A model of *Staphylococcus aureus* bacteremia, septic arthritis, and osteomyelitis in chickens. J Orthop Res 1990;8:804-13.
78. De Cleen MJH, Schuurs AHB, Wesselink PR, Wu M-K. Periapical status and prevalence of endodontic treatment in an adult Dutch population. Int Endod J 1993;26:112-19.

79. De Moor RJ, De Witte AM. Periapical lesions accidentally filled with calcium hydroxide. Int Endod J 2002;35:946-58.
80. De Moor RJG, Hommez GMG, De Boever JG, Delmé KIM, Martens GEI. Periapical health related to the quality of root canal treatment in a Belgian population. Int Endod J 2000;33:113-20.
81. Debelian GJ, Olsen I, Tronstad L. Bacteremia in conjuction with endodontic therapy. Endod Dent Traumatol 1995;11:142-49.
82. Debelian GJ, Olsen I, Tronstad L. Profiling of *Propionibacterium acnes* recovered from root canal and blood during and after endodontic treatment. Endod Dent Traumatol 1992;8:248-54.
83. Debelian GJ. Bacteremia and fungenia in pacients undergoing endodontic therapy. (Doctoral Thesis). Oslo: University of Oslo, Norway;1997.
84. Dugas NN, Lawrence HP, Teplitsky PE, Pharoah MJ, Friedman S. Periapical health and treatment quality assessment of rootfilled teeth in two Canadian populations. Int Endod J 2003;36:181-92.
85. Dziak R. Biochemical and molecular mediators of bone metabolism. J Periodontol 1993;65:407-15.
86. Eckerbom M, Andersson J-E, Magnusson T. A longitudinal study of changes in frequency and technical standard of endodontic treatment in a Swedish population. Endod Dent Traumatol 1989;5:27-31.
87. Eckerbom M, Andersson J-E, Magnusson T. Frequency and technical standard of endodontic treatment in a Swedish population. Endod Dent Traumatol 1987;3:245-48.
88. Eckerbom M, Flygare L, Magnusson T. A 20-year follow-up study of endodontic variables and apical status in a Swedish population. Int Endod J 2007;40:940-48.
89. Eckerbom M, Magnusson T, Martinsson T. Prevalence of apical periodontitis, crowned teeth and teethwith posts in a Swedish population. Endod Dent Traumatol 1991;7:214-20.
90. Ehrmann EH, Messer HH, Adams GG. The relationship of intracanal medicaments to postoperative pain in endodontics. Int Endod J;2003, 36:868-75.
91. Ehrmann EH, Messer HH, Clark RM. Flare-ups in endodontics and their relationship to various medicaments. Aust Endod J, 2007;33:119-30.
92. Engström B, Frostell G. Experiences of bacteriological root canal control. Acta Odontol Scand 1964;22:43-69.
93. Engström B. The significance of *Enterococci* in root canal treatment. Odontologisk Revy 1964;15:87-106.
94. Eriksen HM, Berset GP, Hansen BF, Bjertness E. Changes in endodontic status 1973–1993 among 35-year-olds in Oslo, Norway. Int Endod J 1995;28:129-32.
95. Eriksen HM, Bjertness E, Ørstavik D. Prevalence and quality of endodontic treatment in an urban adult population in Norway. Endod Dent Traumatol 1988;4:122–26.
96. Eriksen HM, Bjertness E. Prevalence of apical periodontitis and results of endodontic treatment in middle-aged adults in Norway. Endod Dent Traumatol 1991;7:1–4.
97. Eriksen HM, Kirkevang L-L, Petersson K. Endodontic epidemiology and treatment outcome: general considerations. Endodontic Topics 2002;2:1–9.
98. Estrela C. Análise química de pastas de hidróxido de cálcio, frente à liberação de íons de cálcio, de íons hidroxila e ação do carbonato de cálcio na presença de tecido conjuntivo de cão. (Doctoral Thesis). University of São Paulo, 1994. 140p.
99. Estrela C. Dor Odontogênica. São Paulo: Artes Médicas, 2001.
100. Estrela C, Bammann LL, Pimenta FC, Pecora JD. Control of microorganisms in vitro by calcium hydroxide pastes. Int Endod J 2001;34:341-45.
101. Estrela C, Bueno MR, Azevedo B, Azevedo JR, Pécora JD. A New Periapical Index Based on Cone Beam Computed Tomography. J Endod 2008; 34:1325-31.
102. Estrela C, Bueno MR, Leles CR, Azevedo BC, Azevedo JR. Accuracy of cone beam computed tomography, panoramic and periapical radiographic for the detection of apical periodontitis. J Endod 2008;34:273-79.
103. Estrela C, Camapum FF, Lopes HP. Prevalência de dor nos retratamentos endodônticos. Rev Bras Odontol 1998;55:18-24.
104. Estrela C, César OVS, Sydney GB, Lopes HP, Pesce HF. Incidência de dor frente ao tratamento da inflamação periapical aguda e crônica. Rev Bras Odontol 1996;53:21-25.
105. Estrela C, Guedes OA, Brugnera Júnior A, Estrela CRA; Pécora JD. Terapêutica do abscesso periapical sem fístula. Rev Bras Odontol 2008; (in press).
106. Estrela C, Guedes OA, Brugnera Júnior A, Estrela CRA;Pécora JD. Dor pós-operatória em dentes com infecções endodônticas secundárias: Revisão sistemática. Rev Assoc Paul Cir Dent 2007;61:185-92.
107. Estrela C, Guedes OA, Brugnera Júnior A, Estrela CRA;Pécora JD. Dor pós-operatória em dentes com infecções endodônticas primárias: Revisão sistemática. Rev Gaúcha Odontol 2008;56:353-9.
108. Estrela C, Guedes AO, Leles CR, Decurcio DA, Silva JA. Prevalence and risk factors of pulpal and periapical pain. 2008 (study not published).
109. Estrela C, Holland R. Calcium Hydroxide: study based on scientific evidences. J Appl Oral Sci 2003;14:269-83.
110. Estrela C, Holland R. Hidróxido de Cálcio. In: Estrela C. Ciência Endodôntica. São Paulo: Artes Médicas; 2004. p.457-38.
111. Estrela C, Leles CR, Hollanda ACB, Moura MS, Pécora JD. Prevalence and risk factors of apical periodontitis in endodontically treated teeth in a selected population of Brazilian adults. Braz Dent J 2008;19:34-39.
112. Estrela C, Pesce HF, Silva MT, Fernandes JMA, Silveira HP. Análise da redução da dor pós-tratamento da hipersensibilidade dentinária. Rev Odontol Brasil Central 1996;6:4-9.
113. Estrela C, Pesce HF, Stephan IW. Proposição de uma técnica de preparo do terço cervical para canais radiculares curvos. Rev Odontol Brasil Central 1995;2:21-24.

114. Estrela C, Pimenta FC, Ito IY, Bammann LL. Antimicrobial evaluation of calcium hydroxide in infected dentinal tubules. J Endod 1999;26:416-18.
115. Estrela C, Ribeiro RG, Estrela CRA, Pécora JD, Souza-Neto MD. Antmicrobial effect of 2% sodium hypochlorite and 2% chlorhexidine tested by different methods. Braz Dent J 2003;14:58 – 62.
116. Estrela C, Siqueira RM, Resende EV, Silva SA, Silva FC. Influência da substância química, do cimento obturador e do número de sessões na prevalência de pericementite traumática. Rev Odontol Brasil Central 1996;6:9-13.
117. Estrela C, Sydney GB, Bammann LL, Fellipe-JR O. Mechanism of action of calcium and hydroxil ions of calcium hydroxide on tissue and bacteria. Braz Dent J 1995;6:85-90.
118. Estrela C, Toledo AM, Brugnera-JR A, Decurcio RA;Pécora JD. Dor pós-operatória em dentes com inflamação pulpar: Revisão sistemática. Rev Odontol Brasil Central 2006;15: 34-45.
119. Estrela C, Tormin FC, Araújo CR, Barleta FB. Prevalência de pulpite aguda e necrose pulpar frente a diferentes agentes etiológicos. Rev Fac Odontol UFG 1997;1:15-20.
120. Estrela CRA, Estrela C, Reis C, Bammann LL, Pécora JD. Control of microorganisms in vitro by endodontic irrigants. Braz Dent J 2003;14:187-92.
121. Evans M, Davies JK, Sundqvist G, Fidgor D. Mechanism involved in the resistance of *Enterococcus faecalis* to calcium hydroxide. Int Endod J 2002;35:221-28.
122. Faber PA, Seltzer S. Endodontic microbiology – I – Etiology. J Endod 1988;14:363-71.
123. Fabricius L, Dahlén G, Öhman AE, Möller AJR. Influence of combinations of oral bacteria on periapical tissues of monkeys. Scand J Dent Res 1982;90:200-206.
124. Fabricius L, Dahlén G, Öhman AE, Möller AJR. Predominant indigenous oral bacteria isolated from infected root canals after varied times of clousure. Scand J Dent Res 1982;90:134-44.
125. Fava LR. Acute apical periodontitis: incidence of post-operative pain using two different root canal dressings. Int Endod J 1998;31:343-47.
126. Figdor D, Sjögren U, Sorlin S, Sundqvist G, Nair PNR. Pathogenicity of *Actinomyces israelii* and *Arachnia propionica*: experimental infection in guinea pigs and phagocytosis and intracellular killing by human polymorphonuclear leukocyties in vitro. Oral Microbiol Immunol 1992;7:129-36.
127. Figueiredo CRLV, Santos JN, Albuquerque-Jr RLC. Mecanismos imunopatológicos de formação e expansão do cisto radicular: uma abordagem atual. Rev Pos Grad 1999;6:180-87.
128. Fouad AF, Rivera E.M, Walton R.E. Penicillin as a supplement in resolving the localized acute apical abscess. Oral Surg Oral Med Oral Pathol Oral Radiol Endod 1996;81:590-95.
129. Fox J, Atkinson JS, Dinin AP, Greenfield E, Hechtman E, Reeman CA, Salkind M, Todaro CJ. Incidence of pain following one-visit endodontic treatment. Oral Surg Oral Med Oral Pathol 1970;30:123-30.
130. Frisk F, Hakeberg M. A 24-year follow-up of root filled teeth and periapical health amongst middle aged and elderly women in Göteborg, Sweden. Int Endod J 2005;38:246–54.
131. Fukushima H, Yamamoto K, Sagawa H, Leung KP, Walker CB. Localization and identification of root canal bacteria in clinically asymptomatic periapical pathosis. J Endod 1990;11:534-38.
132. Gatewood RS, Himel VT, Dorn SO. Treatment of the endodontic emergency: A decade later. J Endod 1990;16:284-91.
133. Genet JM, Hart AAM, Wesselink PR, Thoden van Velzen SK. Preoperative and operative factors associated with pain after the first endodontic visit. Int Endod J 1987;20:53-64.
134. Georgopoulou MK, Spanaki-Voreadi AP, Pantazis N, Kontakiotis EG. Frequency and distribution of root filled teeth and apical periodontitis in a Greek population. Int Endod J 2005;38:105–11.
135. Gesi A, Hakeberg M, Warfvinge J, Bergenholtz G. Incidence of periapical lesions and clinical symptoms after pulpectomy-a clinical and radiographic evaluation of 1- versus 2-session treatment. Oral Surg Oral Med Oral Pathol Oral Radiol Endod 2006;101:379-88.
136. Ghoddusi J, Javidi M, zarrabi MH, bagheri H. Flare-up incidence and severity after using calcium hydroxide as intracanal dressing. N Y State Dent J 2006;72:24-28.
137. Glenny AM, Esposito M, Coulthard P, Worthington HV. The assessment of systematic reviews in dentistry. Eur J Oral Sci 2003;111:85-92.
138. Goldman M, Pearson AH, Darzenta N. Reliability of radiographic interpretations. Oral Surg Oral Med Oral Pathol 1974;38:287-93.
139. Gomes BPFA, Drucker DB, Lilley JD. Association of endodontic signs and symptoms with particular combinations of specific bacteria. Int Endod J 1996;29:69-75.
140. Gomes BPFA, Drucker DB, Lilley JD. Association of specific bacteria with some endodontic signs and symptoms. Int Endod J 1994;27:291-98.
141. Gomes BPFA, Drucker DB, Lilley JD. Clinical significance of dental root canal microflora. J Endod 1996;24:47-55.
142. Gomes BPFA, Lilley JD, Drucker DB. Variations in the susceptibilities of components of the endodontic microflora to biomechanical procedures. Int Endod J 1996;29:235-41.
143. Greenhalgh T. How to read a paper: the basics of evidence based medicine. 2nd ed. London: BMJ Books;2001.
144. Griffee MB, Patterson SS, Miller, Kafrawy A, Newton CW. The relation of *Bacteroides melaninogenicus* to symptoms associated to pulpal necrosis. Oral Surg Oral Med Oral Pathol 1980;50:457-61.
145. Grossman LI, Sheprd LI, Pearson LA. Roentgenologic and clinical evaluation of endodontically treated teeth. Oral Surg Oral Med Oral Pathol 1964;17:368-74.
146. Grossman LI. Endodontic Failures. Dent Clin North Amer 1972;16:59-70.
147. Guimarães SAC. Patologia básica da cavidade bucal. Guanabara Koogan: Rio de Janeiro;1982. 419p.
148. Gulsahi K, Gulsahi A, Ungor M, Genc Y. Frequency of root-filled teeth and prevalence of apical periodontitis in an adult Turkish population. Int Endod J 2008, 41:78–85.

149. Haapasalo M. The genus *Bacteroides* in human dental root canal infections. (Dissertation – Master). Finland: University of Helsinki;1986. 87p.
150. Haapasalo M, Ørstavik D. In vitro infection and disinfection of dentinal tubules. J Dent Res 1987;66:1375-79.
151. Hales JJ, Jackson CR, Everett AP, Moore SH. Treatment protocol for the management of a sodium hypochlorite accident during endodontic therapy. Gen Dent 2001;49:278-81.
152. Halse A, Molven O, Fristad I. Diagnosing periapical lesions – disagreement and borderline cases. Int Endod J 2002;35:703-09.
153. Halse A, Molven O. A strategy for the diagnosis of periapical pathosis. J Endod 1986;12:534-38.
154. Hancock HH, Sigurdsson A, Trope M, Moiseiwitsch J. Bacteria isolated after unsuccessful endodontic treatment in a North American population. Oral Surg Oral Med Oral Pathol 2001;5:579-86.
155. Hansen BF, Johansen JR. Oral roentgenologic findings in a Norwegian urban population. Oral Surg Oral Med Oral Pathol 1976;41;261-66.
156. Happonen RP. Periapical actinomycosis: a follow-up study of 16 surgically treated cases. Endod Dent Traumatol 1986;2:205-09.
157. Harrison JW, Baumgartner C, Svec TA. Incidence of pain associated with clinical factors during and after root canal therapy. Part 2. Postobturation pain. J Endod 1983;9: 434-38
158. Harrison JW, Baumgartner JC, Svek TA. Incidence of pain associated with clinical factors during and after root canal therapy. Part 1. Interappointment Pain. J Endod 1983;9:384-87.
159. Harrison JW, Baumgartner JC, Zielke DR. Analysis of interappointment pain associated with the combined use of endodontic irrigants and medicaments. J Endod 1981;7:272-76.
160. Hashioka K, Suzuki K, Yoshida T, Nakame A, Horiba N, Nakamura H. Relationship between clinical symptoms and enzyme-producing bacteria isolated from infected root canals. J Endod 1994;20:75-77.
161. Hashioka K, Yamasaki W, Nakane A, Horiba N, Nakamura H. The relationship between clinical symptoms and anaerobic bacteria from infected root canals. J Endod 1992;18:558-61.
162. Holland R, Otoboni-Filho JA, Souza V, Mello W, Nery MJ, Bernabé PFE, Dezan Jr. E. Calcium hydroxide and corticosteroid-antibiotic association as dressing in cases of biopulpectomy. A comparative study in dog's teeth. Braz Dent J 1998;9:67-76.
163. Hollanda ACB, Alencar AHG, Estrela CRA, Bueno MR, Estrela C. Prevalence of endodontically treated teeth in a Brazilian adult population. Braz Dent J 2008;19:313-17.
164. Hommez GMG, Coppens CRM, DeMoor RJG. Periapical health related to the quality of coronal restorations and root fillings. Int Endod J 2002;35:680-689.
165. Horiba N, Maekawa Y, Ito M, Matsumoto T, Nakamura H. Correlations between endotoxin and clinical symptoms or radiolucent areas in infected root canals. Oral Surg Oral Med Oral Pathol 1991;71:492-95.
166. Hoshino E, Ando N, Sato M, Kota K. Bacterial invasion of nonexposed dental pulp. Int Endod J 1992;25:2-5.
167. Hugoson A, Koch G. Oral health in 1000 individuals aged 3–70 years in the community Jönköping, Sweden. Swed Dent J 1979;3:69-87.
168. HülsmannM, LorchV, Franz B. Untersuchung zurHaufigkeit und qualitat von Wurzelfullungen. Eine Auswertung von Orthopantomogrammen. Deutsch Zahnärztliche Zeitschrift 1991;46:296-99
169. Huumonen S, Ørstavik D. Radiological aspects of apical periodontitis. Endod Topics 2002;1:3-25.
170. Imfeld TN. Prevalence and quality of endodontic treatment in an elderly urban population of Switzerland. J Endod 1991;17:604–07.
171. Imura N, Zuolo ML. Factors associated with endodontic flareups: perspective study. Int Endod J 1995;28:261-65.
172. Iwu C, MacFarlane TW, Mackenzie D, Stenhouse D. The microbiology of periapical granulomas. Oral Surg Oral Med Oral Pathol 1990;69:502-05.
173. Jacinto RC, Gomes BPFA, Chia HN, Ferraz CC, Zaina AA, Souza Filho FJ. Quantification of endotoxins in necrotic root canals from symptomatic and asymptomatic teeth. J Med Microbiol 2005;54:777-83.
174. Jacinto RC, Gomes BPFA, Ferraz CC, Zaia AA, Souza Filho FJ. Microbiological analysis of infected root canals from symptomatic and asymptomatic teeth with periapical periodontitis and the antimicrobial susceptibility of some isolated anaerobic bacteria. Oral Microbiol Immuno 2003, 18: 285-92.
175. Kabak Y, Abbott PV. Prevalence of apical periodontitis and the quality of endodontic treatment in an adult Belarusian population. Int Endod J 2005;38:238–45.
176. Kakehashi S, Stanley HR, Fitzgerald RJ. The effects of surgical exposures of dental pulps in germ-free and conventional laboratory rats. Oral Surg Oral Med Oral Pathol 1965;20:340-49.
177. Katsumata A, Hirukawa A, Noujeim M, Okumura S, Naitoh M, Fujishita M, Ariji E, Langlais RP. Image artifact in dental cone-beam CT. Oral Surg Oral Med Oral Pathol Oral Radiol Endod 2006;101:652-57.
178. Keenan JV, Farman AG, Fedorowicz Z, Newton JT. Antibiotic use for irreversible pulpitis. *Cochrane Database of Systematic Reviews* 2005, Issue 2.
179. Kettering JD, Torabinejad M. Presence of natural killer cells in human chronic periapical lesions. Int Endod J 1993;26:344-47.
180. Kirkevang L-L, Hörsted-Bindslev P, Ørstavik D, Wenzel A. A comparison of the quality of root canal treatment in two Danish subpopulations examined 1974–75 and 1997–98. Int Endod J 2001;34:607–12.
181. Kirkevang L-L, Hörsted-Bindslev P, Ørstavik D, Wenzel A. Frequency and distribution of endodontically treated teeth and apical periodontitis in an urban Danish population. Int Endod J 2001;34:198–205.
182. Kirkevang L-L, Krstavik D, Hörsted-Bindslev P,Wenzel A. Periapical status and quality of root fillings and coronal restorations in a Danish population. Int Endod J 2000;33:509-15.
183. Kirkevang L-L, Ørstavik D, Hörsted-Bindslev P, Wenzel A. Periapical status and quality of root fillings and coronal restorations in a Danish population. Int Endod J 2000;33:509–15.
184. Kirkevang L-L, Væth M, Hörsted-Bindslev P, Wenzel A. Longitudinal study of periapical and endodontic status in a Danish population. Int Endod J 2006;39:100-7.

185. Kirkevang L-L, Wenzel A. Risk indicators for apical periodontitis. Commun Dent Oral Epidemiol 2003;31:59–67.
186. Kiryu T, Hoshino E, Iwaku M. Bacteria invading periapical cementum. J Endod 1994;20:169-72.
187. Kiryu T, Tronstad L. Long term results of endodontic treatment perfomed with a standardized technique. J Endod 1979;5:83-90.
188. Klausen B, Helbo M, Dabelsteen E. A differential diagnostic approach to the symptomatology of acute dental pain. Oral Surg Oral Med Oral Pathol 1985;59:297-301.
189. Koch F, Breil P, Marroquín BB, Gawehn J, Kunkel M. Abscess of the orbit arising 48h after root canal treatment of a maxillary first molar. Int Endod J 2006;39:657-64.
190. Kojima K, Inamoto K, Nagamatsu K, Hara A, Nakata K, Morita I, Nakagaki H, Nakamura H. Success rate of endodontic treatment of teeth with vital and nonvital pulps. A meta-analysis. Oral Surg Oral Med Oral Pathol Oral Radiol Endod 2004;97: 95-99.
191. Landis JR, Koch GG. The measurement of observer agreement for categorical data. Biometrics 1977;33:159-74.
192. Laurell L, Holm G, Hedin M. Tandhälsan hos vuxna i Gävleborgs län. Tandlaekartidningen 1983: 75:759–77.
193. Laux M, Abbott P, Pajarola G, Nair PNR. Apical inflammatory root resorption: a correlative radiographic and histological assessement. Int Endod J 2000;33:483-93.
194. Lavstedt S. Behovet av tandhälsovård och tandsjukvård hos en normalpopulation. Tandläkartidningen 1978;70: 971–91.
195. Law A, Messer H. An evidence-based analysis of the antibacterial effectiveness of intracanal medicaments. J Endod 2004;30:689-94.
196. Lewis M, McGowen D. Antibiotic susceptibilities of bacteria isolated from acute dentoalveolar abscesses. J Antimicrob Chemother 1989;23:69-77.
197. Lim CG, Torabinejad M, Kettering J, Linkhardt TA, Finkelman RD. Interleukin 1$\alpha$ in symptomatic and asymptomatic human periradicular lesions. J Endod 1994;20:225-27.
198. Lin ML, Pascon EA, Skribner J, Gängler P, Langeland K. Clinical, radiographic and histologic study of endodontic treatment failures. Oral Surg Oral Med Oral Pathol 1991;11:603-11.
199. Lofthag-Hansen S, Hummonen S, Gröndahl K, Gröndahl H-G. Limited cone-beam CT and intraoral radiography for the diagnosis of periapical pathology. Oral Surg Oral Med Oral Pathol Oral Radiol Endod 2007;103:114-19.
200. Loftus JJ, Keating AP, McCartan BE. Periapical status and quality of endodontic treatment in an adult Irish population. Int Endod J 2005;3: 81–86.
201. Love MR. *Enterococcus faecalis* – a mechanism for its role in endodontic failure. Int Endod J 2001;34:399-405.
202. Love MR, McMillan MD, Jenkinson HF. Invasion of dentinal tubules by oral *Streptococci* is associated with collagen regeneration mediated by the antigen I-II family of polypeptides. Infect Immun 1997;65:51-57.
203. Lupi-Pegurier L, Bertrand M-F, Muller-Bolla M, Rocca JP, Bolla M. Periapical status, prevalence and quality of endodontic treatment in an adult French population. Int Endod J 2002;35:690-97.
204. Maddox DL, Walton RE, Davis CO. Incidence of post treatment endodontic pain related to medicaments an other factors. J Endod 1977;3:447-52.
205. Malassez ML. Sur L'existence de masses épitheliales dans le ligament alveolodentaire. Compt Rend Soc Biol 1884;36:241-44.
206. Marinho V. Revisões sistemáticas e Metanálise. In: Crivello-Jr O. Fundamentos de odontologia – Epidemiologia da Saúde Bucal. Rio de Janeiro: Guanabara Koogan;2006. p.422-33.
207. Marques MD, Moreira B, Eriksen HM. Prevalence of apical periodontitis and results of endodontic treatment in an adult Portuguese population. Int Endod J 1998;31:161-65.
208. Marrion JJ. Processo de reparo de dentes de cães após biopulpectomia e obturação dos canais radiculares com os cimentos Sealapex ou MTA manipulado com propilenoglicol, associados ao efeito do emprego ou não de um curative de corticosteróide-antibiótico. (Master's of Thesis). University of Masrília, São Paulo, 2008.
209. Marshall JG, Liesinger AW. Factors associated with endodontic post-treatment pain. J Endod 1993;19:573-75.
210. Martin IC, Harrison JD. Periapical actinomycosis. Br Dent J 1984;156:169-70.
211. Mata E, Koren LZ, Morse DR, Sinai IH. Prophylactic use of penicillin V in teeth with necrotic pulps and asymptomatic periapical radiolucencies. Oral Surg Med Oral Pathol 1985;60:201-07.
212. Matthews D.C, Sutherland S, Basrani B. Emergency management of acute apical abscesses in the permanent dentition: a systematic review of the literature. J Can Dent Assoc 2003;69:660-60i.
213. Mattscheck DJ, Law AS, Noblett C. Retreatment versus initial root canal treatment: factors affecting posttreatment pain. Oral Surg Oral Med Oral Pathol Oral Radiol Endod 2001;92:321-24
214. McIntosh HM, Woolacoot NF, Bagnall AM. Assessing harmful effects in systematic Reviews. BMC Medical Research Methodology. 2004;4:1-6.
215. Michelich VJ, Schuster GS, Pashley DH. Bacterial penetration of human dentin in vitro. J Dent Res 1980;59:1398-403.
216. Miller WD. An introduction to the study of the bacteriopathology of the dental pulp. Dental Cosmos 1894;36:505-28.
217. Miller WD. The microorganisms of the human mounth. S.S.White Dental Mfgo. CO.: Philadelphia;1890.
218. Mjor IA, Fejerskov O. Embriologia e Histologia Oral Humana. Panamericana: São Paulo;1990.
219. Molander A, Lundquist P, Papapanou PN, Dahlén G, Reit C. A protocol for polymerase chain reaction detection of *Enterococcus faecalis* and *Enterococcus faecium* from the root canal. Int Endod J 2002;35:1-6.
220. Molander A, Reit C, Dahlen G, Kvist T. Microbiological status of root-filled teeth with apical periodontitis. Int Endod J 1998;31:1-7.

221. Molander A, Reit C, Dahlén G. Microbiologic evaluation of clindamycim as root canal dressing in teeth with apical periodontitis. Int Endod J 1990;23:113-18.
222. Möller AJR, Fabricus L, Dahlén G, Öhman AE, Heyden G. Influence on periapical tissues of indigeneous oral bacteria and necrotic pulp tissue in monkeys. Scand J Dent Res 1981;89:475-84.
223. Möller AJR. Microbiological examination of root canals and periapical tissues of human teeth. Odontologisk Tidskrift 1966;74:1-38.
224. Möller O, Möller AJR. Some methodological considerations for anaerobic cultivation. Acta Pathol Microbiol Scand 1961;51:245-47.
225. Molven O, Halse A, Fristad I. Long-term reliability and observer comparisons in the radiographic diagnosis of periapical disease. Int Endod J 2002;35:142-47.
226. Mor C, Rotstein I, Friedman S. Prevalence of interappointment emergency associated with endodontic therapy. J Endod 1992;18:509-11.
227. Morse DR, Furst M, Belott R, Lefkowitz R, Spritzer I, Sideman B. Infections flare-up and serious sequelae following endodontic treatment: a prospective randomizes trial efficacy of antibiotic prophylaxis in cases of asymptomatic pulpal-periapical lesions. Oral Surg Oral Med Oral Pathol 1987;64:96-109.
228. Morse DR, Koren LZ, Eposito SV, Goldberg JM, Belott RM, Sinai IH, Furst MC. Infections flare-ups: induction and prevention. Int J Psychsom 1986;33:5-17.
229. Morse DR. Endodontic flare-ups: prevention and treatment. Hawaii Dent J 1987;18:10-13.
230. Nair MK, Nair UP. Digital and advanced imaging in endodontics: a review. J Endod 2007;33:1-6.
231. Nair PNR, Pajarola G, Schroeder HE. Types and incidence of human periapical lesions obtained with extracted teeth. Oral Surg Oral Med Oral Pathol 1996;81:93-102.
232. Nair PNR, Schmid-Meier E. An apical granuloma with epithelial integument. Oral Surg Oral Med Oral Pathol 1986;62:698-703.
233. Nair PNR, Schroeder HE. Epithelial attachment at diseased human tooth-apex. J Periodontol Res 1985;20:293-300.
234. Nair PNR, Schroeder HE. Periapical Actinomycosis. J Endod 1984;10:567-70.
235. Nair PNR, Sjögren U, Fidgor D, Sundqvist G. Persistent periapical radiolucencies of root-filled human teeth, failed endodontics treatments, and periapical scars. Oral Surg Oral Med Oral Pathol 1999;87:617-27.
236. Nair PNR, Sjögren U, Krey G, Kahnberg KE, Sundqvist G. Intraradicular bacteria and fungi in rootfilled, asymptomatic human teeth with therapy-resistant periapical lesions: A long-term light and electron microscopic follow-up study. J Endod 1990;16:580-88.
237. Nair PNR, Sjögren U, Krey G, Sundqvist G. Therapy- resistant foreign body giant cell granuloma at the periapex of a root-filled human tooth. J Endod 1990;16:589-95.
238. Nair PNR, Sjögren U, Schumacher E, Sundqvist G. Radicular cyst affecting a root-filled human tooth: a long-term post-treatment follow-up. Int Endod J 1993;26:225-33.
239. Nair PNR, Sjögren U, Sundqvist G. Cholesterol crystals as an etiological factor in non-resolving chronic inflammation: an experimental study in guines pigs. Eur J Oral Sci 1998;106:644-50.
240. Nair PNR, Sundqvist G, Sjögren U. Experimental evidence supports the abscess theory of development of radicular cysts. Oral Surg Oral Med Oral Pathol Oral Radiol Endod 2008;106:294-303.
241. Nair PNR. Apical periodontitis: a dynamic encounter between root canal infection and host response. Periodontology 2000 1997;13:29-39.
242. Nair PNR. Cholesterol as an aetiological agent in endodontic failures – a review. Australian Endod J 1999;25:19-26.
243. Nair PNR. Light and electron microscopic studies on root canal flora and periapical lesions. J Endod 1987;13:29-39.
244. Nair PNR. New perspectives on radicular cysts: do they heal? Int Endod J 1998;31:155-60.
245. Nair PNR. Pathobiology of the periapex. In: Pathways of the pulp. Cohen S, Burns RC. St. Louis: Mosby;2001.
246. Nair PNR. Pathology of apical periodontitis. In: Essential Endodontology. Ørstavik D, Pitt-Ford DR. Oxford: Black Well;1998.
247. Nakata K, Naitoh M, Izumi M, Inamoto K, Ariji E, Nakamura H. Effectiveness of dental computed tomography in diagnostic imaging of periradicular lesion of each root of a multirooted tooth: a case report. J Endod 2006;32:583-87.
248. Nalçaci R, Erdemir EO, Baran I. Evaluation of the oral health status of the people aged 65 years and over living in near rural district of Middle Anatolia, Turkey. Arch Genrontol Geriat 2007;45:55-64.
249. Newman HN. Foccal infection. J Dent Res 1996;75:1912-19.
250. Nicopoulou-Karayianni K, Bragger U, Patrikiou A, Stassinakis A, Lang NP. Image processing for enhanced observer agreement in the evaluation of periapical bone changes. Int Endod J 2002;35:615-22.
251. Nielsen RB, Alyassin AM, Peters DD, Carnes DL, Lancaster J. Microcomputed tomography: an advanced system for detailed endodontic research. J Endod 1995;21:561-68.
252. Nisengard RJ, Newman MG. Oral Microbiology and Immunilogy. 2nd ed. Philadelphia: Sauders;1994. 477p.
253. Nori Y, Ehara A, Kawahara T, Takemura N, Ebisu S. Participation of bacterial biofilms in refractory and chronic periapical periodontitis. J Endod 2002;28:679-83.
254. Ödesjö B, Helldén L, Salonen L, Langeland K. Prevalence of previous endodontic treatment, technical standard and occurrence of periapical lesions in a randomly selected adult, general population. Endod Dent Traumatol 1990;6:265-72.
255. Oguntebi BR, DeSchepper EJ, Taylor TS, White CL, Pink FE. Postoperative pain incidence related to the type of emergency treatment of symptomatic pulpitis. Oral Surg Oral Med Oral Pathol 1992;73:479-83.
256. Oppenheim JJ. Forward. In: The cytokine handbook. Thomson AW. 2nd ed. London: Academic Press;1994.

257. Ørstavik D, Kerekes K, Eriksen HM. The periapical index: a scoring system for radiographic assessment of apical periodontitis. Endod Dent Traumatol 1986;2:20-24.
258. Ørstavik D, Pitt-Ford TR. Apical periodontitis: microbial infection and host response. In: Essential Endodontology. Oxford: Blackwell, 1998.
259. Osborn JW, Ten Cate AR. Histologia Dental Avançada. 4th ed. São Paulo: Quintessence Books;1988. p.81-95.
260. Patel S, Dawood A, Pitt Ford T, Whaites E. The potential applications of cone beam computed tomography in the management of endodontic problems. Int Endod J 2007;40:818-23.
261. Paterson SA, Curzon ME. The effect of amoxycillin versus penicillin V in the treatment of acutely abscessed primary teeth. Br Dent J 1993;174:443-49.
262. Paz EC, Dahlén G, Molander A, Möller A, Bergenholtz G. Bacteria recovered from teeth with apical periodontitis after antimicrobial endodontic treatment. I Endod J 2003;36:500-08.
263. Peciuliene V, Reynaud AH, Balciuniene I, Haapsalo M. Isolation of yeasts and enteric bacteria in root-filled teeth with chronic apical periodontitis. Int Endod J 2001;34:429-43.
264. Petersson K, Lewin B, Håkansson J, Olsson B, Wennberg A. Endodontic status and suggested treatment in a population requiring substantial dental care. Endod Dent Traumatol 1989;5:153-58.
265. Petersson K, Petersson A, Olsson B, Håkansson J, Wennberg A. Technical quality of root fillings in an adult Swedish population. Endod Dent Traumatol 1986;2:99-102.
266. Petersson K. Endodontic status of mandibular premolars and molars in an adult Swedish population. A longitudinalstudy1974-85. Endodontics and DentalTraumatology 1993;9:13-18.
267. Pickenpaugh L, Reader A, Beck M, Meyers W, Peterson L. Effect of prophylactic amoxicilin on endodontic flare-up in asymptomatic, necrotic teeth. J Endod 2001;27:53-56.
268. Pierce A. Pathophysiological and therapeutic aspects of dentoalveolar resorption. Austr Dent J 1989;34:437-48.
269. Pitt-Ford TR. The effects of the periapical tissues of bacterial contamination of the filled root canal. Int Endod J 1982;15:16-20.
270. Ranta H, Haapasalo M, Kontiainem S, Kerosuo E, Valtonem V. Bacteriology of odontogenic apical periodontitis and effect of penicillin treatment. Scan J Infect Dis 1988;20:187-92.
271. Ray HA, Trope M. Periapical status of endodontically treated teeth in relation to the technical quality of the root filling and the coronal restoration. Int Endod J 1995;28:12-18.
272. Reit C, Dahlén G. Decision making analysis of endodontic treatment strategies in teeth with apical periododontitis. Int Endod J 1988;16:207-10.
273. Reit C, Grøndahl HG. Application of statistical decision theory to radiographic diagnosis of endodontically treated teeth. Scand J Dent Res 1983;9:213-18.
274. Reit C. Decision strategies in endodontics: on the design of a recall program. Endod Dent Traumatol 1987;3:233-39.
275. Ribeiro FC, Consolaro A. Aspectos morfológicos dos biofilmes microbianos na osteomielite crônica supurativa e correlações endodôntica e parendodôntica. Rev Fac Odontol Bauru 1999;7:41-47.
276. Ribeiro FC. Distribuição das bactérias nas estruturas mineralizadas de dentes com necrose pulpar e granuloma apical. (Master´s Thesis). University of São Paulo, 1997.
277. Ribeiro-Sobrinho AP, Barros MHM, Nicoli JR, Carvalho MAR, Farias LM, Bambirra EA, Bahia MGA, Vieira EC. Experimental root canal infection in conventional and germ-free mice. J Endod 1998;24:405-08.
278. Rimmer A. The flare-up index: a quantitative method to describe the phenomenon. J Endod 1993. 19:255-56.
279. Rocha MJC. Estudo microscópico e imuno-histoquímico dos cistos periodontais apicais de dentes tratados ou não endodonticamente. Sua relação com a regressão não cirúrgica. (Doctoral Thesis). University of São Paulo, 1991. 149p.
280. Rohlin M, Kullendorff B, Ahlquist M, Henrikson CO, Hollender L, Stenstrom B. Comparison between panoramic and periapical radiography in the diagnosis of periapical bone lesions. DentoMax Facial Radiol 1989;18:151-55.
281. Rohlin M, Kullendorff B, Ahlqwist M, Stenstrom B. Observer performance in the assessment of periapical pathology: a comparison of panoramic with periapical radiography. DentoMax Facial Radiol 1991;20:127-31.
282. Rubin E, Farber JL. Patologia. 1st ed. Rio de Janeiro: Interlivros;1990.
283. Sacks HS, Berrier J, Reitman D, Ancona-Berk VA, Chalmers TC. Meta-analyses of randomized controlled trials. N Engl J Med 1987;316:450-51.
284. Safavi KE, Rossomando ER. Tumor necrosis factor identified in periapical tissue exsudates of teeth with apical periodontitis. J Endod 1991;17:12.
285. Saunders MB, Gulabivala K, Holt R, Kahan RS. Reliability of radiographic observation recorded on a proforma measured using inter- and intraobserver variation: a preliminary study. Int Endod J 2000;33:272-78.
286. Saunders WP, Saunders EM, Sadiq J, Cruickshank E. Technical standard of root canal treatment in an adult Scottish sub-population. Brit Dent J 1997;182:382-86.
287. Scarfe WC, Farman AG, Sukovic P. Clinical applications of cone-beam computed tomograghy in dental practice. J Can Dent Ass 2007;72:75-80.
288. Schaeffer MA, White RR, Walton RE. Determining the Optimal Obturation Length: A Meta-Analysis of Literature. J Endod 2005;31:271-4.
289. Segura-Egea JJ, Jiménez-Pinzón A, Poyato-Ferrera M, Velasco-Ortega E, Ríos-Santos JV. Periapical status and quality of root fillings and coronal restorations in an adult Spanish population. Int Endod J 2004;37:525-30.
290. Seltzer S, Bender ID, Turkenkopf S. Factors affecting successful repair after root canal treatment. J Am Dent Assoc 1963;67:651-62.
291. Seltzer S, Bender ID. Epithelial proliferation in periapical lesions. Oral Surg Oral Med Oral Pathol 1969;27:111-21.

292. Seltzer S, Farber PA. Microbiologic factors in endodontology. Oral Surg Oral Med Oral Pathol 1994;78:634-45.
293. Seltzer S, Naidorf IS. Flare-ups in Endodontics. I. Etiological factors. J Endod 1985;11:472-76.
294. Seltzer S, Naidorf IS. FLare-ups in Endodontics. II. Therapeutic measures. J Endod 1985;11:559-65.
295. Sen BH, Safavi KE, Spangberg LSW. Growth patterns of *Candida albicans* in relation to radicular dentin. Oral Surg Oral Med Oral Pathol 1997;84:68-73.
296. Shovelton DS. The presence and distribuition of microorganisms within non vital Teeth. British Dental J 1964;117:101-07.
297. Sidaravicius B, Aleksejuniene J, Eriksen HM. Endodontic treatment and prevalence of apical periodontitis in an adult population of Vilnius, Lithuania. Endod Dent Traumatol 1999;15:210-15.
298. Simon JHS, Enciso R, Malfaz JM, Rogers R, Bailey-Perry M, Patel A. Differential diagnosis of large periapical lesions using cone-beam computed tomography measurements and biopsy. J Endod 2006;32:833-37.
299. Simon JHS. Incidence of periapical cysts in relation to root canal. J Endod 1980;6:845-48.
300. Simon JHS. Patologia Periapical. In: Caminhos da Polpa. Cohen S, Burns RC. 6th ed. Guanabara Koogan: Rio de Janeiro;1997.
301. Siqueira JF Jr. Endodontic infections: concepts, paradigms, and perspectives. Oral Surg Oral Med Oral Pathol Oral Radiol Endod, 2002;94:281-93.
302. Siqueira JF, Rôças I N. Polymerase chain reaction-based analysis of microorganisms associated with failed endodontic treatment. Oral Surg. Oral Med. Oral Pathol Oral Radiol Endod 2004;97:85-94.
303. Siqueira JF, Rôças IN, Souto R, Uzeda M.;Colombo A.P. Checkerboard DNA-DNA hibridization analysis of endodontic infections. Oral Surg Oral Med Oral Pathol Oral Radiol Endod 2000;89:744-48.
304. Siqueira Jr JF, Rôças IN, Alves FRF, Campos LC. Periradicular status related to the quality of coronal restorations and root canal fillings in a Brazilian population. Oral Surg Oral Med Oral Pathol Oral Radiol Endod 2005;100:369-74.
305. Siqueira Jr JF, Rôças IN, Favieri, Machado AG, Gahyva, Oliveira JCM, Abad EC. Incidence of postoperative pain after intracanal procedures based on an antimicrobial strategy. J Endod 2002;28: 457-60.
306. Siqueira-Jr JF. Microbial causes of endodontic flare-ups. Int Endod J 2003;36:453-63.
307. Sirén EK, Haapasalo PP, Ranta K, Salmi P, Kerosuo ENJ. Microbiological findings and clinical treatment procedures in endodontic cases selected for microbiological investigation. Int Endod J 1997;30:91-95.
308. Siwek J, Gourlay ML, Slawson DC, Shaughnessy AF. How to write an evidencebased clinical review article. Am Fam Physician 2002;65:251-58.
309. Sjögren U, Fidgor D, Pearsson S, Sundqvist G. Influence of infection at the time of root filling on the outcome of endodontic treatment of teeth with apical periodontitis. Int Endod J 1997;30:297-306.
310. Sjögren U, Hägglund B, Sundqvist G, Wing K. Factors affecting the long-term results of endodontoc treatment. J Endod 1990;16:498-504.
311. Sjögren U, Hanstrom L, Happonen RP, Sundqvist G. Extensive bone loss associated with periapical infection with *Bacteroides gingivalis*: a case report. Int Endod J 1990;23:254-62.
312. Sjögren U, Happonen RP, Kahnberg KE, Sundqvist G. Survival of *Arachinia propionica* in periapical tissue. Inter Endod J 1988;21:277-82.
313. Sjögren U, Sundqvist G, Nair PNR. Tissue reaction to gutta-percha of various sizes when implanted subcutaneously in guinea pigs. Eur J Oral Sci 1995;103:313-18.
314. Skudutyte-Rysstad R, Eriksen HM. Endodontic status amongst 35-year-old Oslo citizens and changes over a 30-year period. Int Endod J 2006;39:637-42.
315. Slavikin HC. Emerging and re-emerging infectious diseases: a biological evolutionary drama. J Amer Dent Assoc 1997;128:108-12.
316. Slots J, Taubman MA. Contemporany Oral Microbiology and Immunology. Mosby;1992. 649p.
317. Socransky SS, Haffajee AD. Microbial mechanisms in the pathogenesis of destructive periodontal disease: a critical assesseement. J Periodont Res 1991;26:195-212.
318. Socransky SS, Haffajee AD. The bacterial etiology of destructive periodontal disease: current concepts. J Periodontol 1992;63:322-31.
319. Soikkonen KT. Endodontically treated teeth and periapical findings in the elderly. Int Endod J 1995;28:200-3.
320. Southard D, Rooney TP. Effective one-visit therapy for the acute periapical abscess. J Endod 1984;10:580-83.
321. Souza V, Bernabé PFE, Holland R, Nery MJ, Mello W, Otoboni-Filho JA. Tratamento não-cirúrgico de dentes lesões periapicais. Rev Bras Odontol 1989;46:39-46.
322. Stashenko P, Wang CY. Characterization of bone resorptive mediators in active periapical lesions. Proc Finn Dent Soc 1992;88:427-32.
323. Stashenko P. The role of imunne cytokines in the pathogenesis of periapical lesions. Endod Dent Traumatol 1990;6:86-96.
324. Stavropoulos A, Wenzel A. Accuracy of cone-beam dental CT, intraoral digital and conventional film radiography for the detection of periapical lesions. An ex-vivo study in pig jaws. Clin Oral Invest 2007;11:101-06.
325. Stheeman SE, Mileman PA, Van't Hof MA, Van Der Stelt PF. Diagnostic confidence and the accuracy of reatment decisions for radiopaque periapical lesions. Int Endod J 1995;28:121-28.
326. Strindberg LZ. The dependence of the results of pulp therapy on certain factors. An analytical study based on radiographic and clinical follow-up examinations. Acta Odontol Scand 1956;14:1-175.
327. Sunay H, Tanalp J, Dikbas I, Bayirli G. Crosssectional evaluation of the periapical status and quality of root canal treatment in a selected population of urban Turkish adults. Int Endod J 2007;40:139-45.
328. Sundqvist G, Eckerbom MI, Larsson AP, Sjögren UT. Capacity of anaerobic bacteria from necrotic dental pulps to induce purulent infections. Infec Immun 1979;25:685-93.
329. Sundqvist G, Figdor D, Persson S, Sjögren U. Microbiologic analysis of teeth with failed endodontic treatment and the outcome of conservative retreatment. Oral Surg Oral Med Oral Pathol 1998;85:86-93.

330. Sundqvist G, Figdor D. Life as an endodontic pathogen. Ecological differences between the untreated and root-filled root canals. Endodontic Topics. 2003;6:3–28.
331. Sundqvist G, Johansson E, Sjögren U. Prevalence of black-pigmented *Bacteroides* species in root canal infections. J Endod 1989;15:13-19.
332. Sundqvist G, Johansson E. Neutrophil chemotaxis induced by anaerobic bacteria isolated from necrotic dental pulps. Scand J Dent Res 1980;88:113-21.
333. Sundqvist G, Reuterving CO. Isolation of *Actinomyces israelli* from periapical lesions. J Endod 1980;6:602-6.
334. Sundqvist G. Associations between microbial species in dental root canal infections. Oral Microbiol Immunol 1992;7:257-62.
335. Sundqvist G. Bacteriological studies of necrotic dental pulps. (Master´s Thesis). Umea: University of Umea, Sweden;1976. 94p.
336. Sundqvist G. Ecology of the root canals flora. J Endod 1992;18:427-30.
337. Sundqvist G. Taxonomy, ecology and pathogenicity of the root canal flora. Oral Surg Oral Med Oral Pathol 1994;78:522-30.
338. Sutherland S, Matthews DC. Emergency management of acute apical periodontitis in the permanent dentition: a systematic review of the literature. J Can Dent Assoc 2003;69:160A-160I.
339. Swartz DB, Skidmore AE, Griffin JA. Twenty years of endodontic success and failure. J Endod 1983;9:198-202.
340. Sydney GB, Estrela C. The influence of root canal preparation on anaerobic bacteria in teeth with asymptomatic apical periodontitis. Braz Endod J 1996;1:12-15.
341. Tsesis I, Faivishevsky V, Fuss Z, Zukerman O. Flare-ups after endodontic treatment: a meta-anlysis of literature. J Endod 2008;34(doi.10.1016/j.joen.2008.07.016).
342. Ten Cate AR. The epithelial cells rests of Malassez and the genesis of the dental cysts. Oral Surg Oral Med Oral Pathol 1972;34:957-62.
343. Torabinejad M, Cymerman JJ, Frankson M, Lemon RR, Maggio JD, Schilder H. Effectiveness of various medications on postoperative pain following complete instrumentation. J Endod 1994;20:345-53.
344. Torabinejad M, Dorn SO, Eleazer PD, Frankson M, Jouhari B, Mullin RK, Soluti A. Effectiveness of various medications on post-operative pain following root canal obturation. J Endod 1994;20:427-31.
345. Torabinejad M, Eby WC, Naidorf IJ. Inflammatory and immunological aspects of the pathogenesis of human periapical lesions. J Endod 1985;11:479-88.
346. Torabinejad M, Kettering JD, McGraw JC, Cummings RR, Dwyer TG, Tobias TG, Tobias TS. Factors assocciated with endodontic interappointment emergencies of teeth with necrotic pulps. J Endod 1988;14:261-66.
347. Tronstad L, Asbjornsen K, Doving L, Pedersen I, Eriksen HM. Influence of coronal restorations on the periapical health of endodontically treated teeth. Endod Dent Traumatol 2000;16:218-21.
348. Tronstad L, Barnett F, Cervone F. Periapical bacterial plaque in teeth refratory to endodontic treatment. Endod Dent Traumatol 1990;6:73-77.
349. Tronstad L, Barnett F, Riso K, Slots J. Extra-radicular infections. Endod Dent Traumatol 1987;3:86-90.
350. Tronstad L, Kreshtool D, Barnett F. Microbiological monitoring and results of treatment of extraradicular endodontic infection. Endod Dent Traumatol 1990;6:129-36.
351. Trope M, Pettigrew J, Petras J, Barnett F, Tronstad L. Differentiation of radicular cyst and granulomas using computerized tomography. Endod Dent Traumatol 1989;5:69-72.
352. Trope M. Flare-up rate of single-visit endodontics. Int Endod J 1991;24:24-26.
353. Trope M. Relationship of intracanal medicaments to endodontic flare-ups. Endod Dent Traumatol 1990;6:226-29.
354. Trowbridge HO, Emling RC. Inflamation – A review of the process. 4th ed. Quintessence books: Illinois;1993. 172p.
355. Tsanova STs. Early clinical results from the use of 5% potassium nitrate in polycarboxylate cement for biological treatment of reversible pulpitis. Folia Med (Plovdiv) 2003;45:36-41.
356. Tsuneishi M, Yamamoto T, Yamanaka R, Tamaki N, Sakamoto T, Tsuji K, Watanabe T. Radiographic evaluation of periapical status and prevalence of endodontic treatment in an adult Japanese population. Oral Surg Oral Med Oral Pathol Oral Radiol Endod 2005;100:631-35.
357. Vaes G. Cellular biology and biochemical of bone resorption: a review of recent developments on the formation and mode of action of osteoclasts. Clin Ortp Related Res 1985;231:239-271.
358. Van der Stelt PF. Experimentally produced bone lesions. Oral Surg Oral Med Oral Pathol Oral Radiol Endod 1985;59:306-12.
359. Velvart P, Hecker H, Tillinger G. Detection of the apical lesion and the mandibular canal in conventional radiography and computed tomography. Oral Surg Oral Med Oral Pathol Oral Radiol Endod 2001;92:682-88.
360. Vigil GV, Wayman BE, Dazey SE, Fowler CB, Bradley-Jr DV. Identification and antibiotic sensitivity of bacteria isolated from periapical lesions. J Endod 1997;23:110-14.
361. von Stechow D, Balto K, Stashenko P, Müller R. Three-dimensional quantitation of periradicular bone destruction by micro-computed tomography. J Endod 2003;29:252-56.
362. Waltimo T, Trope M, Haapasalo M, Ørstavik D. Clinical efficacy of treatment procedures in endodontic infection control and one year followup of periapical healing. J Endod 2005;31:863-66.
363. Waltimo TMT, Siren EK, Ørstavik D, Haapasalo MPP. Susceptibility of oral *Candida* species to calcium hydroxide in vitro. Int Endod J 1999;32:94-98.
364. Waltimo TMT, Siren EK, Torkko HLK, Olsen I, Haapasalo MPP. Fungi in therapy-resistant apical periodontitis. Int Endod J 1997;30:96-101.

365. Walton RE, Chiappinelli J. Prophylactic penicillin: Effect on Post-treatment symptoms following root canal treatment of asymptomatic periapical pathosis. J Endod 1993;19:466-70.
366. Walton R, Fouad A. Endodontic interappointment flare-ups: a prospective study of incidence and related factors. J Endod;1992, 18:172-77.
367. Walton RE, Holton IF Jr, Michelich R. Calcium hydroxide as an intracanal medication: effect on post-treatment pain. J Endod 2003;29:627-29.
368. Walton RE, Torabinejad M. Principles and practice of Endodontics. 2nd ed. Saunders Company: Philadelphia;1996. 558p.
369. Wayman BE, Murata SM, Almeida RJ, Fowler CB. A bacteriological and histological evaluation of 58 periapical lesions. J Endod 1992;18:152-55.
370. Weiger R, Hitzler S, Hermle G, Löst C. Periapical status, quality of root canal fillings and estimated endodontic treatment needs in an urban German population. Endod Dent Traumatol 1997;13:69-74.
371. White SC, Atchison KA, Hewlett ER, Flack VF. Efficacy of FDA guidelines for prescribing radiographs to detect dental and intraosseous conditions. Oral Surg Oral Med Oral Pathol Oral Radiol Endod 1995;80:108-14.
372. Wittgow-Jr WC, Sabiston-Jr CB. Microorganisms from pulpal chambers of intact teeth with necrotic pulps. J Endod 1975;1:168-71.
373. World Health Organization. Application of the International Classification of Diseases to Dentistry and Stomatology. 3rd ed. Geneva: WHO;1995. p.66-67.
374. Yajima A, Otonari-Yamamoto M, Sano T, Hayakawa Y, Otonari T, Tanabe K, Wakoh M, Mizuta S, Yonezu H, Nakagawa K, Yajima Y. Cone beam CT (CB Throne) applied to dentomaxillofacial region. Bull Tokyo Dent Coll 2006;47:133-41.
375. Yamamoto K, Fukushima H, Tsuchiya H, Sagawa H. Antimicrobial susceptibilities of *Eubacterium, Peptostreptococcus*, and *Bacteroides* isolated from root canals of teeth with periapical pathosis. J Endod 1989;15:112-16.
376. Yared GM, Bou Dagher FE. Influence of apical enlargement of on bacterial infection during treatment of apical periodontitis. J Endod 1994;20:535-37.
377. Yingling NM, Byrne BE, Hartwell GR. Antibiotic use by members of the American Association of Endodontists in the year 2000: report of a national survey. J Endod 2002;28:396-404.
378. Yoldas O,Topuz A, Iscxi AS, Oztunc H. Postoperative pain after endodontic retreatment: Single- versus two-visit treatment. Oral Surg Oral Med Oral Pathol Oral Radiol Endod 2004;98: 483-87.
379. Yoshida M, Fukushima H, Yamamoto K, Ogawa K, Toda T, Sagawa H. Correlation between clinical symptoms and microorganisms isolated from canals of teeth with periapical pathosis. J Endod 1987;13:24-28.

# Differential Diagnosis of Apical Periodontitis

**M. R. Bueno**
*University of Cuiabá, Cuiabá, MT, Brazil*

**C. Estrela**
*Federal University of Goiás, Goiânia, GO, Brazil*

Chapter contents

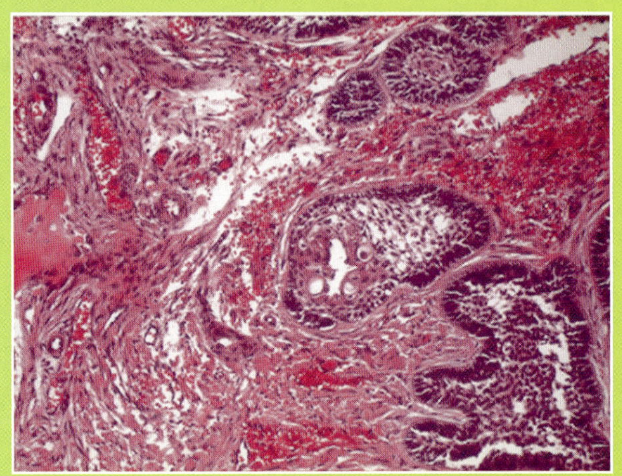

Microscopy of ameloblastoma. Parenchyma exhibit a basal layer, cuboidal cells with reverse polarity, resembling ameloblast-like cells; epithelial cells mimic the stellate reticulum of the enamel organ (H. & E., X40).

Chapter contents

## 11.1 Introduction

Radiographic images of periapical bone rarefactions similar to those of apical periodontitis can represent another entity that frequently does not require endodontic treatment. It can be an atypical anatomical repair, a developmental disturbance or pathology similar to a periapical lesion that does not have a direct relationship with pulp necrosis. Tooth loss due to fractures or hidden perforations, revealed in conventional radiographic exams and the tissue repair area deserve special care during diagnosis. In the absence of correct diagnosis a tooth can be endodontically treated unnecessarily and the dentist will await a repair that does not occur. Correct endodontic treatment is performed through correct diagnosis, which depends on a perfect anamnesis, a detailed anatomical recognition of the teeth, bone structures of the jaws and of the face, the dental development stages, and the pathologies that are part of the differential diagnosis in endodontics.

Before discussing the variations from normality, development disturbances, pathological processes and other conditions that are similar to apical periodontitis, it is appropriate to do a short review of the radiographic and clinical aspects of apical periodontitis.

### Apical foramen position and accessory foramen presence

In most cases, the radiographic aspect of apical periodontitis shows an enlargement of the apical periodontal space, with circumscribed or diffuse radiolucence. Depending on the anatomical variations of the root curvature or of the position of the apical foramen opening, (mesial or distal, buccal or palatine) the image of a lesion of endodontic origin could suggest that its origin is not associated with the tooth (Fig. 11.1, 11.2) and can initially raise doubts in the diagnosis. A tooth can present other foramen (lateral, secondary, accessory, apical delta) in addition to the apical root foramen. Some of these root canals can have a considerable caliber and in the case of pulp necrosis can produce a lesion in a lateral position (atypical), which leads to doubts during diagnosis. A tooth can also present two roots radiographically superimposed, and only the shortest root with a lateral apical opening can show apical bone rarefaction projected in a lateral position of the longest root (Fig. 11.3). In this case, the pulp vitality test is an important aid in diagnosis.

### Symptomatic apical periodontitis and abscess without fistula

Alterations of inflammatory origin: symptomatic apical periodontitis (traumatic or infectious), periapical abscess without fistula (initial, developing or developed) are inflammatory processes established in the apexes of teeth. The radiographic aspects can be identical and the clinical aspects similar.

The acute clinical manifestations of great extent are not always associated with wide radiographic images of bone rarefaction. The radiographic results can be discreet or even null, because there may not have been enough time for visible bone alterations to occur - there has to be from 30% to 50% of bone loss before it begins to be perceptible in periapical radiography. In these cases, the radiographic aspects do not depend on the clinical aspects, but mainly on the length of time the injuries have been present.

The radiographic aspects of a lesion can be null, or only a thickened apical periodontal space established by local pressure due to the edema. If the injuries continue there can be an increase in thickness, and when they become established, reabsorption of the apical lamina dura and afterwards, a diffuse apical lesion can occur. After a longer time, if there is no treatment, the lesion tends to become more radiolucent, with more defined margins (asymptomatic lesion).

The abscesses can be formed from an initial apical alteration or exacerbation of a chronic inflammatory process. Granulomas and infected cysts can develop and behave as typical abscesses.

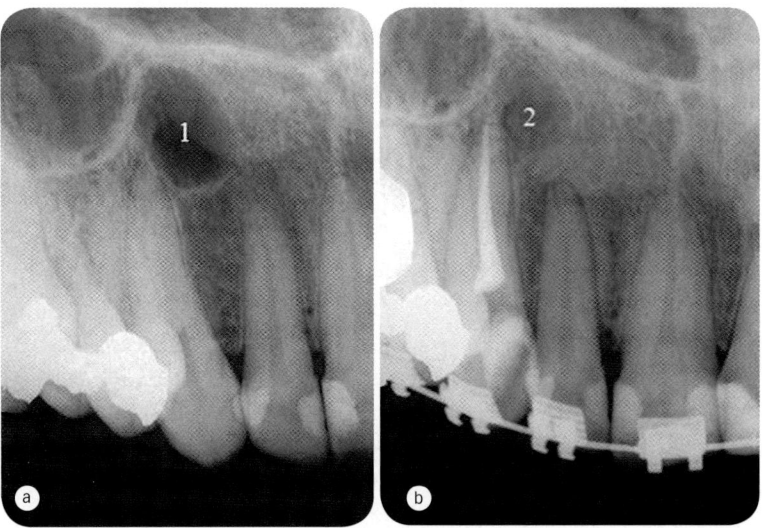


**Figure 11.1** - (**A**) Circumscribed radiolucent area (1) above and in front of the apex of tooth #13, with radiographic appearance of not being in direct contact with the apex, preserved apical periodontal space and nevertheless, it was a lesion of endodontic origin. (**B**) Bone repair (2) 11 months after the endodontic treatment.

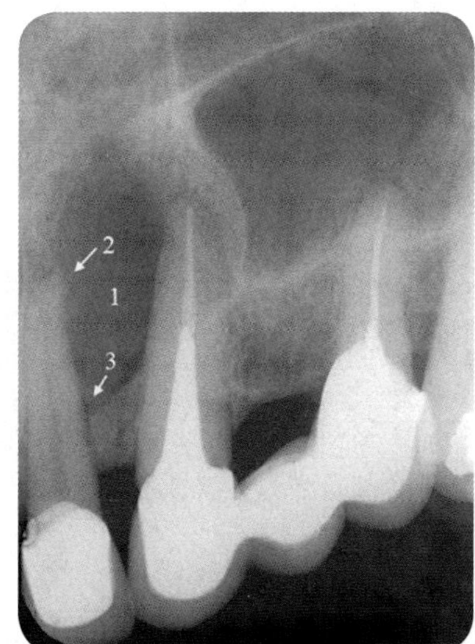


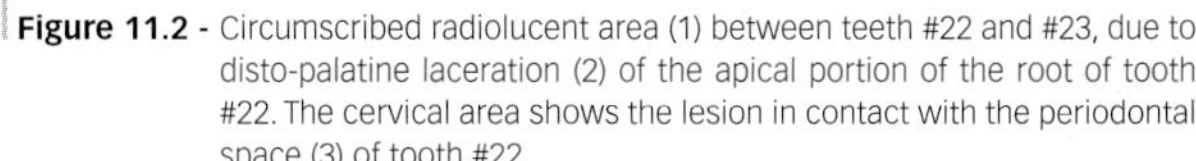

**Figure 11.2** - Circumscribed radiolucent area (1) between teeth #22 and #23, due to disto-palatine laceration (2) of the apical portion of the root of tooth #22. The cervical area shows the lesion in contact with the periodontal space (3) of tooth #22.

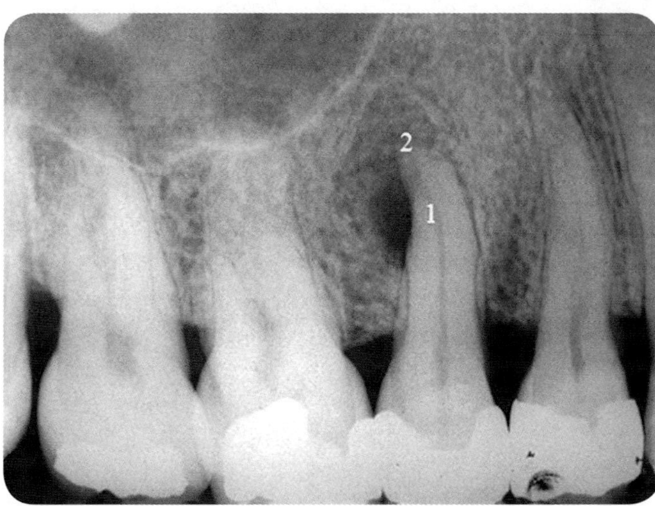


**Figure 11.3** - Tooth #15 is bi-radicular, with lateral root bone lesion due to apical periodontitis of the buccal root (1) with apical foramen moved in the distal direction, superimposed on the longer palatine root (2).

In addition to the apical region, apical periodontitis and periapical abscesses can also grow on the side of the root of a tooth, due to conditions, such as lateral foramens, fractures and root perforations.

The periapical abscess can develop into acute osteomyelitis, which can later become chronic, although it is uncommon in developed societies nowadays. Immunologically debilitated individuals, and decrease in the local bone blood supply in the cases of some pathologies that lead to a primary or secondary form are factors that contribute to the establishment of osteomyelitis.

Occasionally, aggressive cases of symptomatic abscesses with the manifestation of cellulite in the submandibular region can lead to a serious type of pathology called Ludwig's Angina. In about 70% of the cases of this pathology, it develops in the mandibular molars. Initially, the edema is unilateral, but characteristically it extends to the opposite side, pressing the floor of the mouth upward, and causing the tongue to protrude. There can be pain and regional hyperemia, fever, weakness of the organism, among many other signs and symptoms.

The formation of another serious and uncommon type of cellulite, called cavernous sinus thrombosis, can occur in different teeth through several approaches. Usually, tumefaction develops in the periorbital region, which later extends to the cavernous sinus.

In the cases of Ludwig's Angina and cavernous sinus thrombosis of odontogenic origin, the possible radiographic characteristics of the apical areas of the teeth are the same as those of symptomatic abscesses. The patients have to be treated in a hospital environment, because these are serious pathologies that can lead to the death.

Figures 11.4 to 11.6 show radiographic aspects associated with the periapical inflammatory alterations previously described.

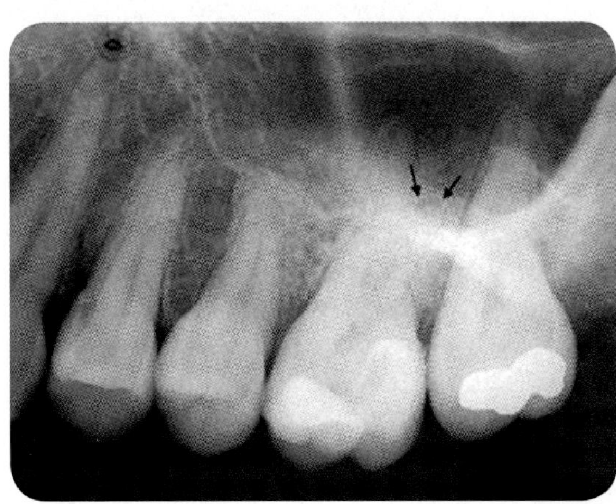

**Figure 11.4 -** Radiographic image associated with symptomatic apical periodontitis with intense and diffuse pain, on the whole left side of the maxilla, diffusing to the mandible on the same side. The patient did not define which tooth the pain originated from or whether it was a maxillary or mandibular tooth, for four days. The periapical exam showed a deep plastic restoration and a discreet periodontal thickness in the distobuccal root of tooth #26. Although it was discreet, this thickness was a result of the injuries. The crown opening led to the immediate relief of pain.

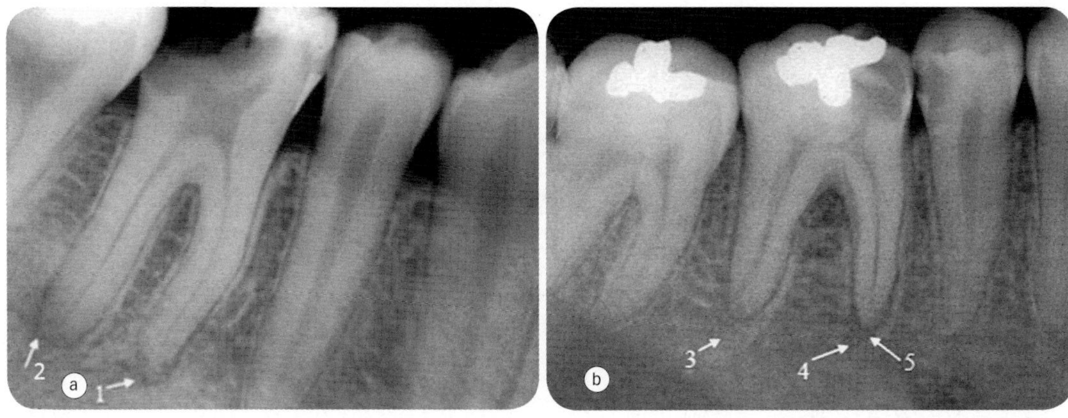


Figure 11.5 - (A) Radiographic image associated with periapical abscess without fistula. Tooth #46, origin of the injuries, presented thickening of the apical periodontal space in the mesial root (1) and in the distal root, thickness in which the lamina dura is already breaking (2). (B) Tooth #46, origin of the injuries, with loss of the trabecular pattern in the distal root (3) and diffuse bone rarefaction (4), with complete reabsorption of the apical lamina dura (5).

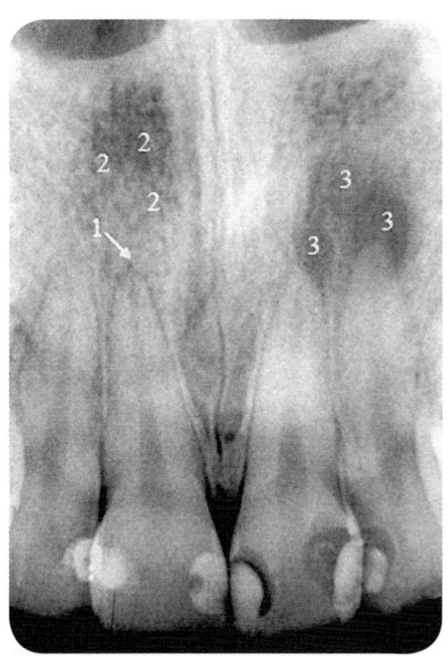


Figure 11.6 - Radiographic image associated with periapical abscess without fistula. Tooth #11 presented a discreet and irregular thickness of the periodontal space, with the onset of reabsorption of the lamina dura (1) and a wide, diffuse lesion (2) with discreet visibility and indefinite margins, in the region of projection of the nasal opening. Tooth #11 with negative pulp vitality test. Teeth #21 and #22, also with negative pulp vitality test, and clinically with an abscess with fistula, with more intense rarefaction (3) than tooth #11. The lesion has partially defined margins.

## Periapical abscess with fistula

Periapical abscess with fistula, is an inflammatory process that leads to the continuous extravasation of purulent content, and in some cases it can be intermittent. The long time duration leads to bone destruction that it is usually well visible in periapical radiographic exams, with the margins of the diffuse area of radiolucence reasonably well delimited. In some cases, the existent bone rarefaction can present discreetly or even be hidden in conventional radiographic exams. Periapical abscess with fistula can develop into an acute situation or chronic osteomyelitis when the local defense or nutriment is decreased (Fig. 11.7, 11.8).

Considering that the gold standard in the diagnosis of apical periodontitis, at the moment, indicates that the histopathological exam of the granuloma and the cyst it will be represented by asymptomatic apical periodontitis.

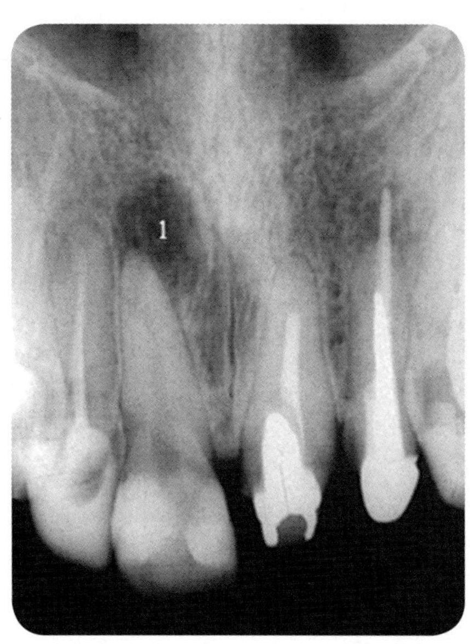


**Figure 11.7** - Radiographic image of tooth #11 with negative pulp vitality test, clinical aspects of abscess with fistula, with intense rarefaction and margins with partial definition, mainly in the mesial region (1). Tooth #22 with reabsorption and overfilling.

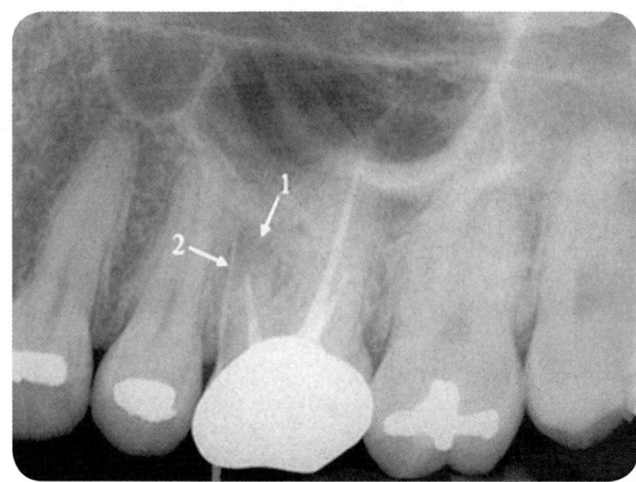


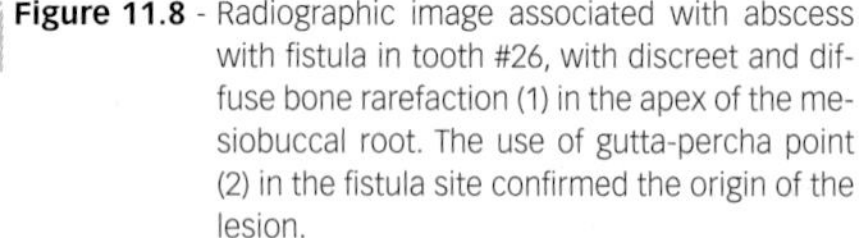

**Figure 11.8** - Radiographic image associated with abscess with fistula in tooth #26, with discreet and diffuse bone rarefaction (1) in the apex of the mesiobuccal root. The use of gutta-percha point (2) in the fistula site confirmed the origin of the lesion.

## Asymptomatic apical periodontitis (Periapical granuloma)

Asymptomatic apical periodontitis (periapical granuloma) can originate from a developed abscess or directly as an initial process. It can become a radicular cyst or still exacerbate into an abscess without fistula or with fistula. The granuloma does not grow as markedly as some cysts.

Radiographically the asymptomatic apical periodontitis can show an image that varies from discreet, imprecise limits, to a radiolucent image with well defined margins, similar, or even identical to the apical radicular cyst (Fig. 11.9). Another possibility is hidden apical granuloma in the periapical radiographic exams, even with variations of angulations, but that can be visualized in cone beam computed tomography (CBCT). The pulp vitality test is negative and the appropriate endodontic treatment provides a favorable prognosis.

The safer way to differentiate the granuloma from periapical cyst is by histopathological analysis.

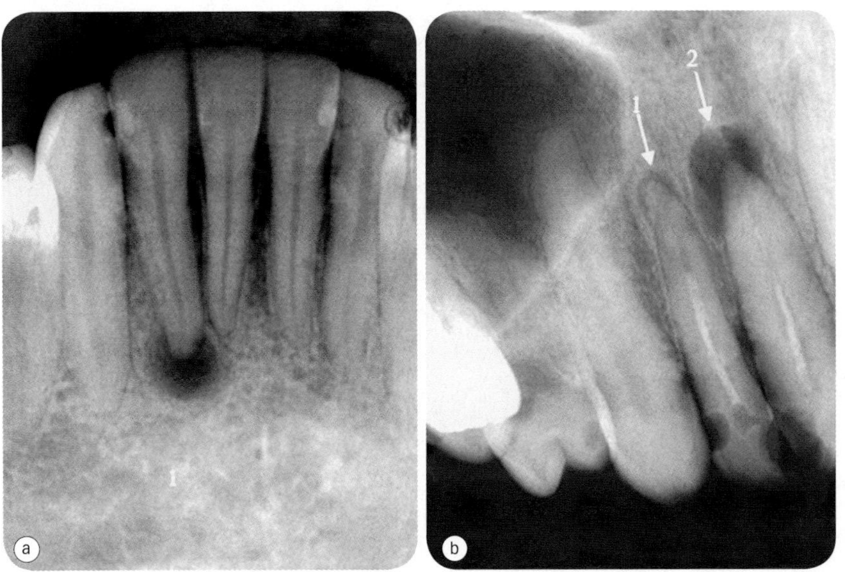


Figure 11.9 - (A,B) Asymptomatic apical periodontitis images varying from partially radiolucent areas with defined (1) or clear (2) margins.

## Asymptomatic apical periodontitis (Periapical cyst)

The periapical cyst has asymptomatic slow growth. It can be small or even reach large dimensions. Radiographically it can present indefinite margins, but it usually shows clear margins and may or may not have a radiopaque halo. When a cyst is infected, or is decompressed by drainage, the margins can lose their typical clarity. Infected cysts can develop and behave as typical abscesses (Fig. 11.10).

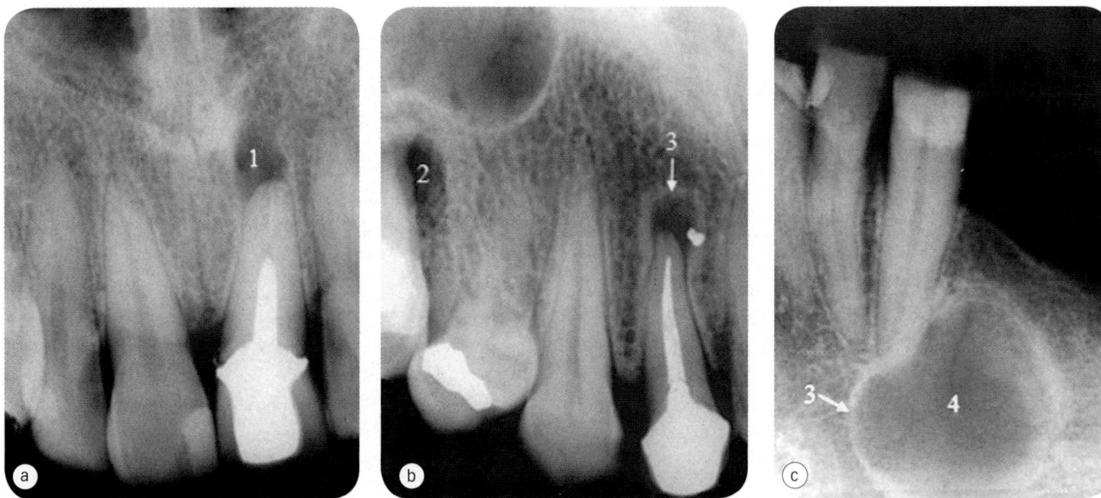


Figure 11.10 - (A-C) Radiographic images of asymptomatic apical periodontitis (1 and 2) that can have radiopaque haloes (3), mainly when they are bulky (4).

## Asymptomatic apical periodontitis (Lateral radicular cyst)

An inflammatory cyst that originated from a necrosed tooth, cannot grow in the apical area, but grows laterally. The injuries that lead to the proliferation of epithelial cells present in the periodontal spaces can be caused by microorganisms or toxins through either the lateral canal or secondary canal, by perforation, fissure or root fracture. The lateral periodontal space is shown to be affected by an image of bone rarefaction (Fig. 11.11, 11.12).

A Globulemaxillary cyst can occur between the lateral incisor and the maxillary canine, which radiographically appears pear shaped, as it is of cleft origin. This subtype of cyst does not exist, and the cases found have been established as being lateral radicular cysts, lateral periodontal cysts or odontogenic keratocysts.

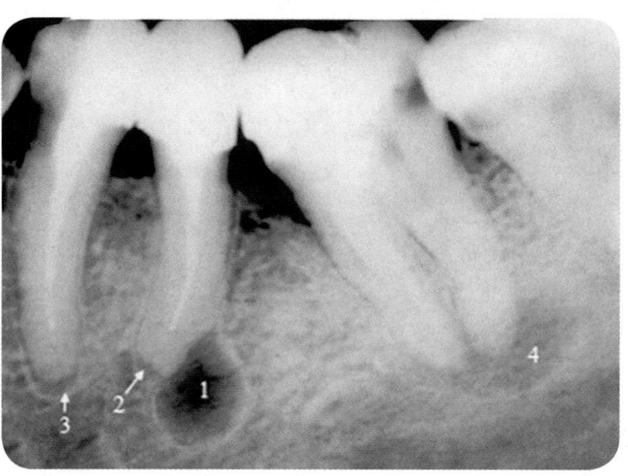


**Figure 11.11** - Radiographic image of asymptomatic apical periodontitis (1) in the distal position of the apical third of tooth #35, with discreet apical bone rarefaction (2), which is and a little more intense in tooth 34 (3). Tooth #37 with AP leading to diffuse bone rarefaction.

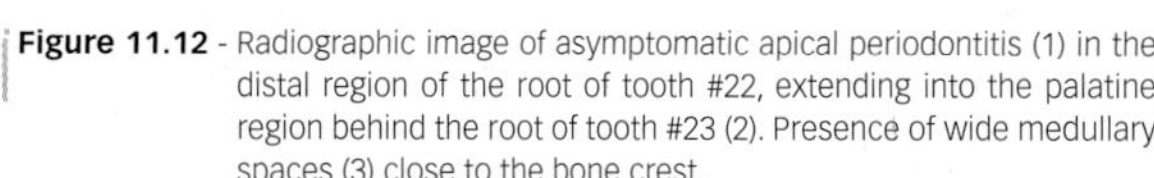

**Figure 11.12** - Radiographic image of asymptomatic apical periodontitis (1) in the distal region of the root of tooth #22, extending into the palatine region behind the root of tooth #23 (2). Presence of wide medullary spaces (3) close to the bone crest.

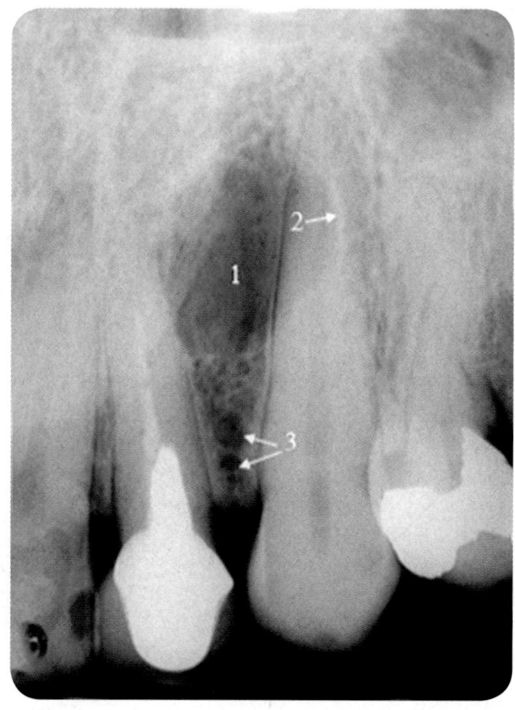

### Asymptomatic apical periodontitis (Residual cyst)

As a radicular cyst cannot be removed during extraction, it can become residual, could regress or continue developing without the presence of the progenitor tooth. When it is close to one of its neighbors, it can be confused with apical periodontitis, and this subject will be discussed later on the differential diagnoses.

### Differential Diagnoses

The differential diagnoses were divided into two groups, although they are frequently ascribed to:

1 - Anatomical variations and conditions that do not require treatment
2 - Variations due to pathological processes

Anatomical variations and conditions that do not require treatment

| Anatomical variations: Maxilla and Mandible |
|---|
| • Open apical foramen (incomplete rhizogenesis) |
| • Large medullary spaces |
| • Focal osteoporotic marrow defect |
| • Radiolucence due to reduced bone thickness |
| • Ghost image of the vertebral column - panoramic radiography |

| Anatomical variations: Maxilla |
|---|
| • Wide nasopalatine foramen |
| • Nasopalatine canal |
| • Upper opening of nasopalatine canals |
| • Nasal opening |
| • Incisive fossa |
| • Myrtiform fossette |
| • Pneumatization of maxillary sinus-alveolar |
| • Pneumatization of maxillary sinus-recess |
| • Greater palatine foramen |
| • Nasolacrimal canal |

| Anatomical variations: Mandible |
|---|
| • Mental foramen |
| • Mandibular para-radicular third molar radiolucencies |
| • Radiographic proximity of the mandibular third molar to the inferior alveolar canal |
| • Submandibular fossa |
| • Latent bone cavity |
| • Sublingual fossa |
| • Mental fovea |

| Other conditions that do not require treatment |
|---|
| • Surgical cavities |
| • Bone healing |
| • Fibrous healing defect |
| • Orthodontic movement |
| • Stains in conventional radiographic exams |

## Variations due to pathological processes

**Conditions that result from or lead to inflammatory processes**

- Residual cysts
- Lesions due to root fractures
- Lesions due to root perforations
- Marginal periodontitis
- Radicular grooves
- Furcation lesion
- Extra-radicular infections

**Lesions originated from development alterations, tumors and systemic disturbances**

- Supernumerary bone crypt
- Gingival cysts of the adults
- Dentigerous cyst
- Root bifurcation cyst
- Primordial cyst
- Cyst of the incisive papilla
- Solitary bone cyst
- Focal cemento-osseous dysplasia
- Familial gigantiform cementoma
- Central giant cell granuloma
- Central hemangioma
- Falciform anemia
- Intraosseous cancer
- Periodontal lateral cyst
- Botryoid odontogenic cyst
- Paradental cyst
- Odontogenic keratocyst
- Nasopalatine cyst
- Median palatal cyst
- Periapical cemento-osseous dysplasia
- Florid cemento-osseous dysplasia
- Ameloblastoma
- Hyperparathyroidism
- Hematological disturbances
- Thalassemia
- Metastasis

**Other conditions**

- Other pathologies

## 11.2 Anatomical Variations: Maxilla and Mandibula

*Incomplete rhizogenesis*

Teeth with incomplete rhizogenesis present areas of low tissue density at their apical ends, showing radiolucent images that can be similar to apical periodontitis in the initial stages. Anamnesis, verifying the signs and symptoms, image of the characteristic format of the apical opening, associated with dental age are helpful steps in diagnosis (Fig.11.13).

### Wide medullary space

The bone trabeculae of the jaw must be well known by the professional (shape, number, disposition and texture, variations in agreement with their anatomical locations, and as well as variations from one person to another). Local and systemic pathologies can alter the pattern of the bone trabeculae. The trabeculae present a pattern with small trabeculae in the maxilla, and more spaced trabeculae in the mandible, mainly in the posterior area, and this could also occur in the anterior area (Fig.11.14).

In some cases the formation of trabeculae can occur with wide medullary spaces, close to the apexes of teeth, similar to circumscribed bone lesions. One should observe whether the cortical bone of the lamina dura close to root of the teeth is integral. It may also be necessary to verify the integrity of tooth and perform a pulp vitality test. In some more doubtful cases it may be necessary perform a cone beam computed tomography, because the integrity of the apical lamina dura observed in the periapical radiograph is not a guarantee of continuity.

### Focal osteoporotic marrow defect

The focal osteoporotic marrow defect is usually more extensive than the wide medullary space, which is a localized presence of bulky hematopoietic bone marrow that produces either discreet or accentuated radiolucence. In many cases, it has the particularity of fine partially regular lines within the rarefaction. It can be similar to a residual or tumoral bone lesion, or apical periodontitis with lateral involvement.

The reason for the presence of this medullary tissue is still obscure, but there are three more accepted theories: aberrant bone regeneration, persistence of the fetal mar-

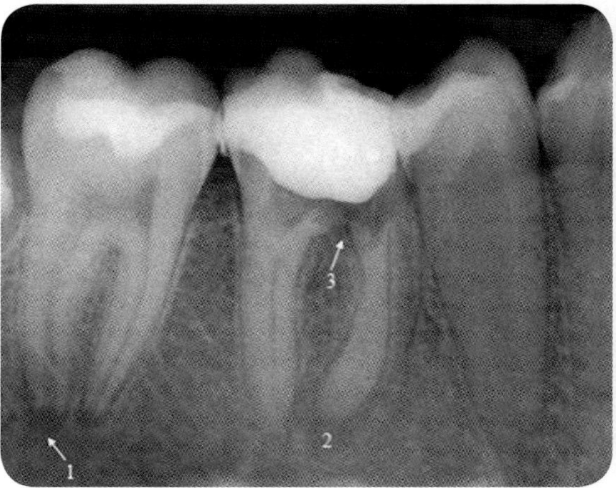


**Figure 11.13** - Tooth #47 with radiolucent area in the apical region due to incomplete rhizogenesis (1) and tooth #46 due to an apical periodontitis (2). Perforation in the furcation area (3).

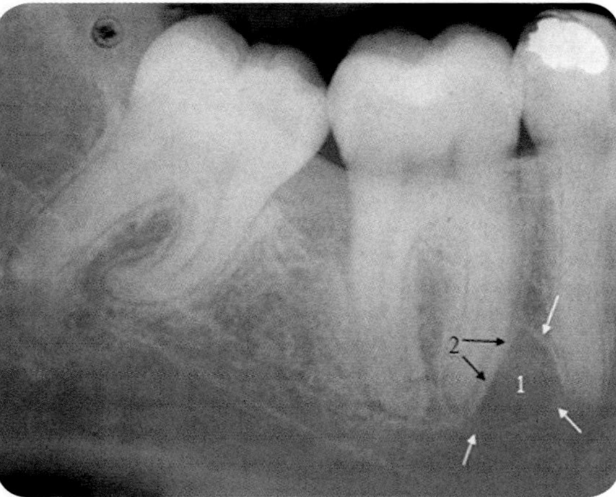


**Figure 11.14** - Large medullary gap with wide trabeculae (1) in the mesial area of the apical third of tooth #47 similar to apical periodontitis, but only a variation of normality. Adjacent lamina dura preserved (2).

row and medullary hyperplasia. In 75% of the cases, it involves adult women, and 70% of the posterior area of the mandible (a previous extraction site), ranging from millimeters to centimeters in size. It is asymptomatic and it does not produce bone expansion.

Signs, symptoms and images with the presence of fine, partially regular lines inside, associated with unchanged size as shown in successive radiographic controls are the means used for diagnosis. In extreme situations a histopathological exam may be required (Fig.11.15, 11.16).

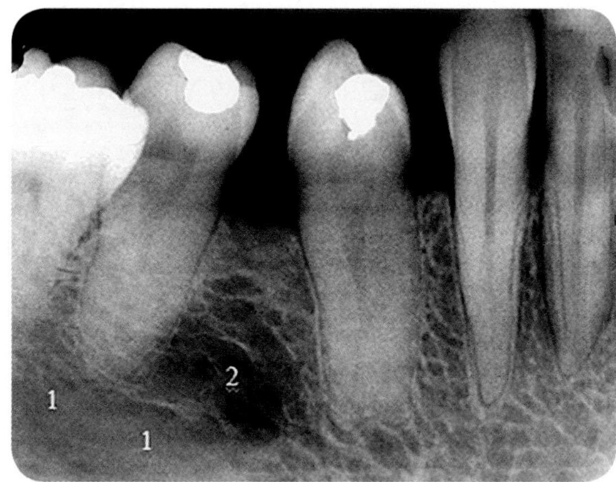


**Figure 11.15** - Focal osteoporotic marrow defect manifesting as a radiolucent area below the apex of tooth #45 (1), extending to the mesial region, where it shows an even lower image density (2). Imprecise margins, with spaced trabeculae and fine lines inside. Periodontal space of tooth #45 preserved.

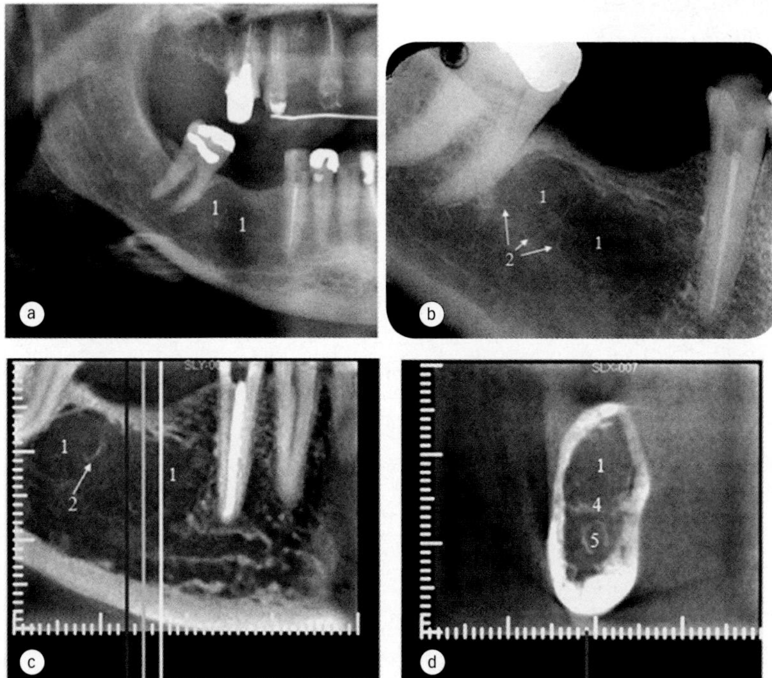


**Figure 11.16** - (**A**) Focal osteoporotic marrow defect with the presence of discreet wide radiolucent area (1), in the region of tooth #46 (absent). (**B**) The same image as the one in the panoramic radiograph, now observed in the periapical radiograph, with slightly more defined margins, although imprecise, with fine lines inside. (**C** and **D**) In slices of cone beam computed tomography, show the radiolucence (1) with the lack of trabeculae, fine lines inside (2) and inferior delimitation (4). The mandibular canal can be observed lower down (5).

### Radiolucence because of reduced bone thickness

A thin alveolar ridge with reduced bone thickness, can occur, mainly when it has not functioning for several years (process of atrophy). In some cases it can show an image of a well defined, delimited radiolucent area, similar to that of a residual lesion, and if it is close to the root of a tooth, it can be similar to a lateral root lesion. A cone beam computed tomography image shows that it is not a very thick area, but one without local bone lesion (Fig.11.17).

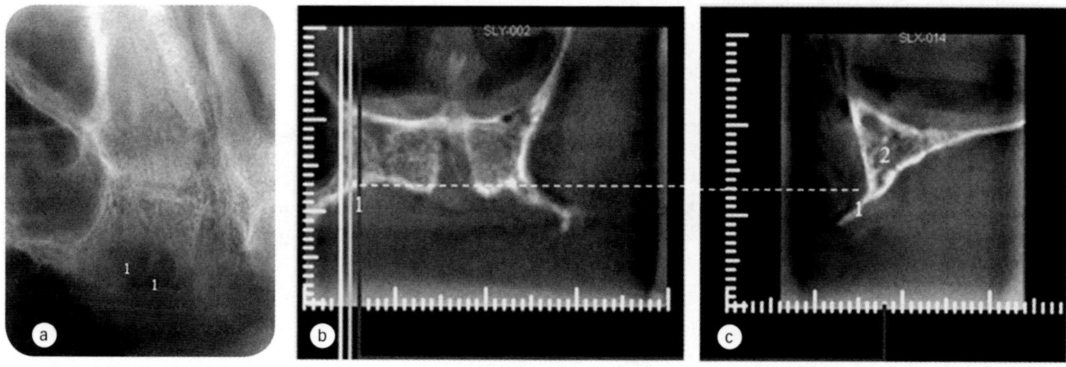


**Figure 11.17** - (**A**) Region with absence of teeth, formation of a partially delimited area (1) that can be a residual lesion of apical periodontitis, or another bone pathology. (**B**) longitudinal coronal slice of the cone beam computed tomography exam shows the origin of the cross sections. The thinner area (1) is out of this slice plane. (**C**) Transversal slice of cone beam computed tomography shows an area with extremely reduced bone thickness (1), leaving a thin area that facilitates penetration of the x-rays, adjacent to another much thicker area (2) leading to density contrast that induces an image, similar to that of the bone lesion.

### Ghost images of vertebral column (Panoramic radiography)

Radiolucent images of intervertebral spaces of the atlanto-occipital joint can be projected close to the apexes of the maxillary incisors in panoramic radiography. They are two independent radiotransparent images, delimited by a radiopaque area, without focus lines, positioned diagonally, and with lateral portions lower than the medial region.

Radiolucent ghost images of intervertebral spaces can also be projected in the mentum area - among the canine teeth, but in this case with a rounded aspect. In this area there are also similar images, such as the one of the digastric fossa - bilateral and low - and of the mental fossa - central and tall.

The panoramic radiograph is not an exam that shows details, especially in the anterior tooth area, because this area is not as clear as the posterior tooth area and these areas are subject to ghost images.

The radiographic aspects of the intervertebral spaces can be similar to apical periodontitis, but as it can appear only in panoramic radiography, a periapical radiographic exam that aids in the diagnosis and that reduces the doubts, is indicated (Fig.11.18 to 11.20).

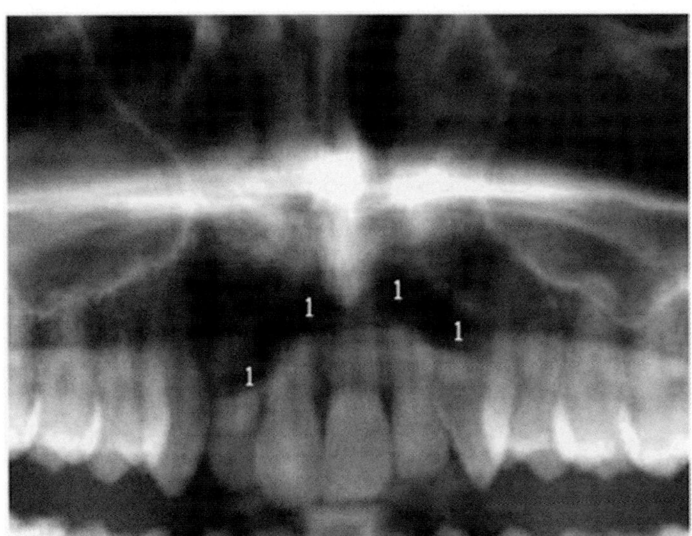


**Figure 11.18** - Radiolucent images of intervertebral spaces of the atlanto-occipital joint (1) projected close to the apexes of the maxillary incisors - without apical lesion – in a panoramic radiograph.

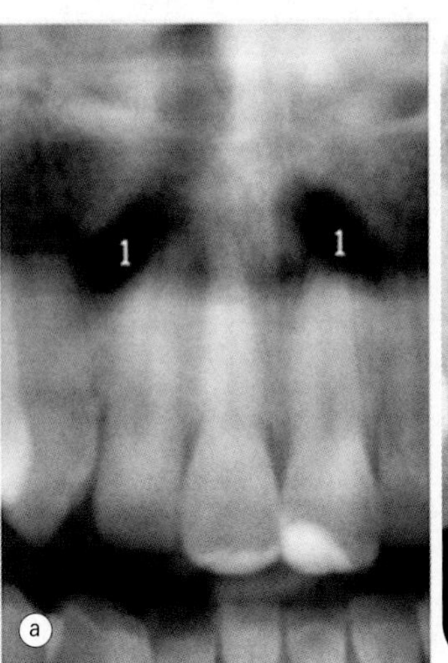


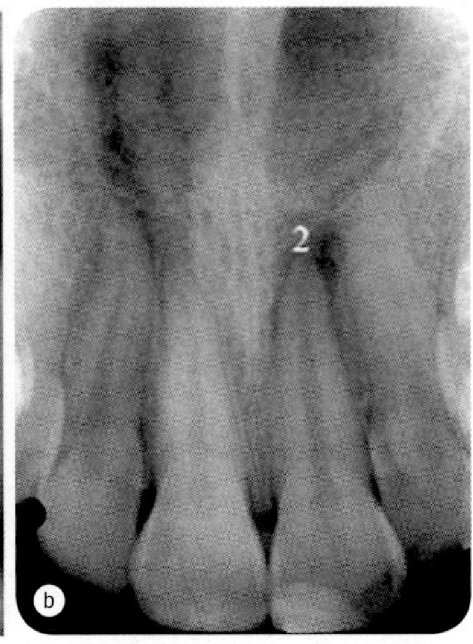


**Figure 11.19** - (**A**) Intervertebral spaces (1) projected close to the apexes of the maxillary incisors in a cut of a panoramic radiograph. (**B**) In the same patient only tooth #21 presents apical lesion (2) in the image of the periapical radiograph.

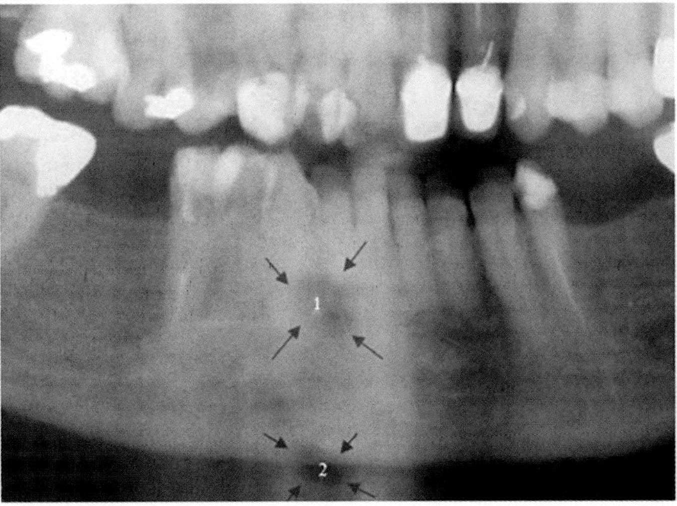


**Figure 11.20** - Intervertebral spaces, in the panoramic radiograph, projected in the anterior area of the mandible in high (1) and low (2), positions in a case of cervical vertebrae with displacement to the right side.

## 11.2.1 Anatomical Variations in the Maxilla

### Wide nasopalatine foramen

The nasopalatine foramen, present between the maxillary central incisors in the palatine region is one of the anatomical structures that most varies radiographically in the maxillae. It can be discreet, almost imperceptible or very visible, low, close to the cervical third, or higher up, close to the root apexes. It can be narrow or wide, up to 6 mm in diameter, considered as the maximum limit for this foramen, because of a larger load, if suggests a nasopalatine duct cyst. When the incisor foramen is projected onto the apex of a central incisor, depending on the X-rays angulation towards the distal region, it can be confused with the image of apical periodontitis. For this reason, the apical area of a maxillary central incisor should not be evaluated to diagnose an apical lesion, with a radiograph positioned for a lateral incisor or canine. The correct procedure is to perform only orthoradial periapical radiography (Fig.11.21 and 11.22).



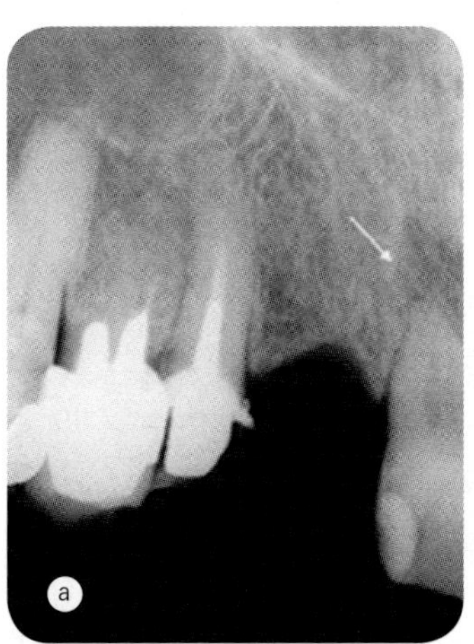


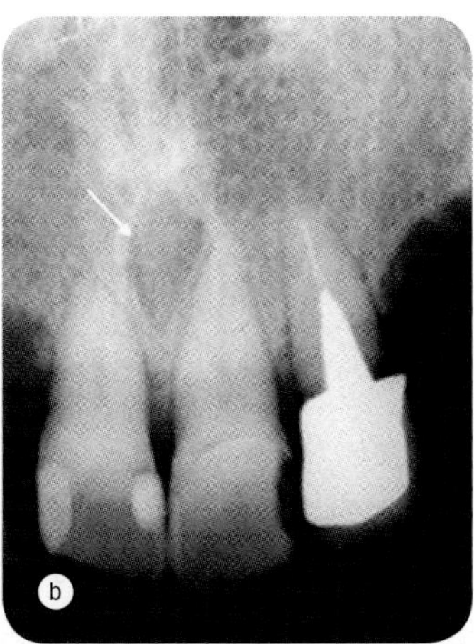


**Figure 11.21** - (**A**) Incisor foramen projected onto the apex of tooth #11 in a radiographic exam with the X-rays appliance moved along the patient's right side. (**B**) Image of the same case shows the foramen in a normal position, but wide, with diameter of 6 mm, at the limit of the normality, with the suspicion of a nasopalatine duct cyst, however without increase in volume, with radiographic control over a medium period.

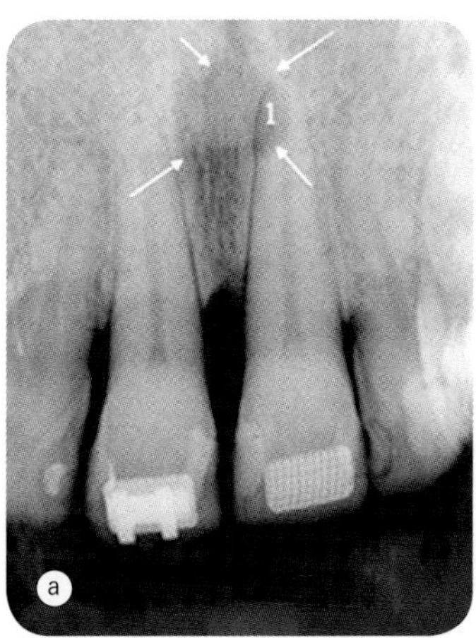


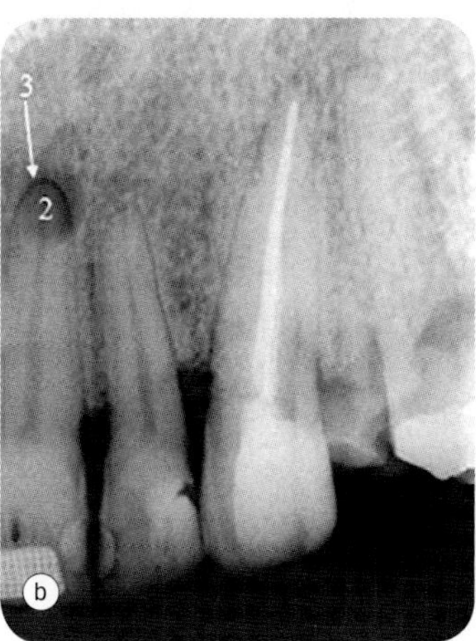


**Figure 11.22** - (**A**) Incisor foramen moderately displaced to the left and partially superimposed by (1) the mesial apical portion of the root of tooth #21. (**B**) Incisor foramen more intensely overlapping (2) the apical area of tooth #21, similar to apical periodontitis. Apical periodontal space of tooth #21 preserved (3). Due to the width, at the limit of normality, radiographic control is indicated, because it could be a nasopalatine duct cyst.

## Nasopalatine canal (Incisive canal)

The incisive canals come out of the floor of the nasal fossa and go towards the incisor foramen. In radiographs positioned for lateral incisors or canines this can lead to doubts in the diagnosis of apical periodontitis of maxillary central incisors.

The higher openings of the incisive canals present two foramens that can occasionally be projected onto the apexes of the central incisors in radiographs, with an exaggerated vertical angulation associated with the presence of low nasal fossa.

With the observation of the format of long and parallel lines of the margins of the incisive canals, an aspect not present in apical lesions, it is important to evaluate the apical area of the central incisors in orthoradial radiographic exams for these teeth. This way the doubt will be removed. When one observes the format of long and parallel lines of the incisive canal margins, an aspect not present in apical lesions, it is important to evaluate the apical area of the central incisors in orthoradial radiographic exams of these teeth (Fig. 11.23).

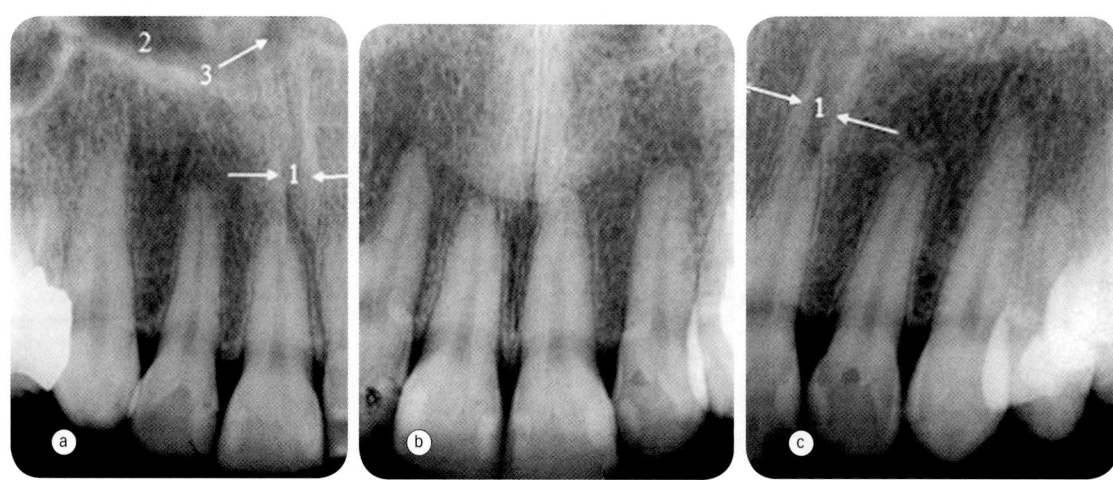


**Figure 11.23** - (**A**) Partial projection of the incisive canal in the apex of tooth #11. Nasal fossa (2) and discreet oval radiolucent image of the maxillary foramen (nasal) of the incisive canal on the right side, high in this patient, but it can be lower in others. (**B**) Image of absence of overlapping in teeth #11 and 21 in the orthoradial periapical exam. (**C**) Projection of the left incisive canal in the apex of tooth #21. In images **A** and **B**, observe the parallelism of the lateral cortical of the incisive canal that discards the possibility of an apical periodontitis.

## Nasal opening

The nasal openings in soft tissues can be projected onto the areas of the maxillary incisors apexes and cause doubts in the diagnosis, because the apical area can be more radiolucent, with discreet diffused aspect, similar to that of a residual lesion or bone lesion caused by apical periodontitis in the initial stages or in the repair phase. The images of the nasal openings can be visible bilaterally in some patients, above and next to the tip of the nose.

The outlines of the soft tissues of the nose, observation of the periodontal space preserved in maxillary incisors, and when necessary, change in angulation of the X-ray can help in the diagnosis (Fig. 11.24).

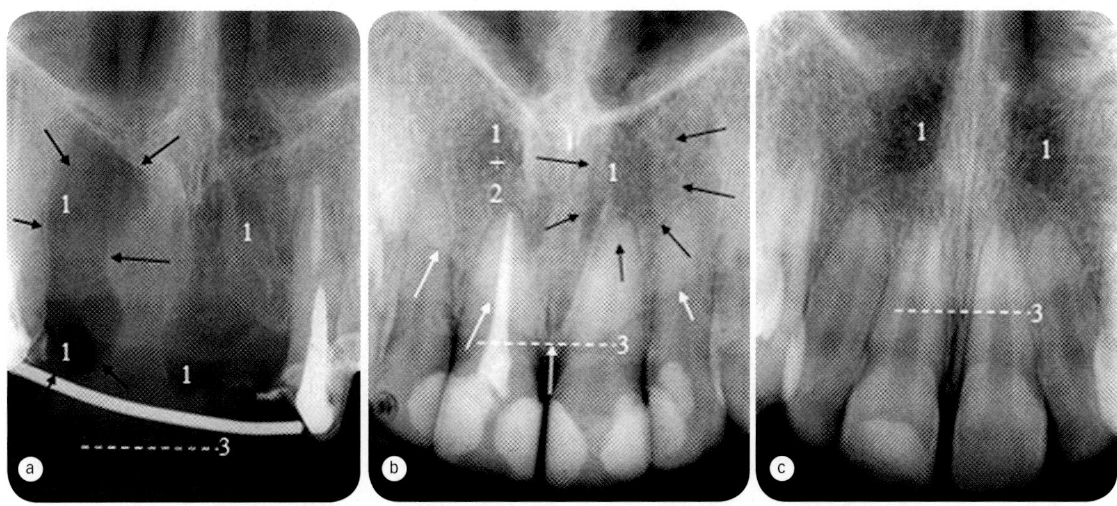


**Figure 11.24AC** - Images of the nasal opening (1) right and left (with arrows only in the area of tooth #11 in image **A** and of tooth #21 in **B** to reduce the pollution of the image), projected onto the alveolar ridge in the maxillary central incisor area, leaving it more radiolucent. (1) In the three images (**A-C**), note the change in the height of the nasal apex (3) accompanied by the height of the nasal openings (1) - superior displacement. (**B**) Tooth #11 with bone repair (2) in progress and overlapping the nasal opening (1). Tooth #21 with radiolucent area in the apical region similar to that of diffuse apical periodontitis with change in the trabecular pattern and preserved periodontal space, but in relation to the overlapping of the nasal opening. (1) In **C**, due to the high projection of the nose (3) the openings (1) also become higher, and are further from the apexes of the incisors.

### *Incisor fossa*

The incisor fossa is a smooth depression in the anterior portion of the maxilla, close to the apical region of the maxillary lateral incisor. Radiographically, there is no defined delimitation of the margins. In some cases, this depression can be more accentuated than normal, showing an exacerbated radiolucence, approaching the aspect of a diffused and discreet apical lesion.

A process of necrosis frequently begins in the maxillary lateral incisors. Signs and symptoms, pulp vitality test, apical periodontal space preserved in the periapical radiographic exam, are essential resources of diagnoses (Fig. 11.25).

## Myrtiform fossette

The myrtiform fossette is a depression that occurs at the insert of the homonymous muscle, (called the depressor of the septum). Situated between the central and lateral incisor, it is usually prolonged and discreet, well-marked in some patients, and in certain cases it can also lead to the impression of causing divergences of the tooth roots. In these cases, it can become similar to a bone lesion of lateral root origin, or apical periodontitis with lateral extension (Fig. 11.25 and 11.26).

## Nasal fossa

The nasal fossa does not usually present difficulties with diagnosis, but it could be confused with some other lesion, close to the apexes of incisors, although it is not in contact with them. This confusion can happen when the periapical radiographic technique was not well performed, or in the case of low nasal fossae and particularly in patients with incomplete, or surgically treated palatine fissure. Anamnesis, clinical exam and occlusal radiographs of the maxilla are solutions to the doubts (Fig. 11.27 and 11.28).

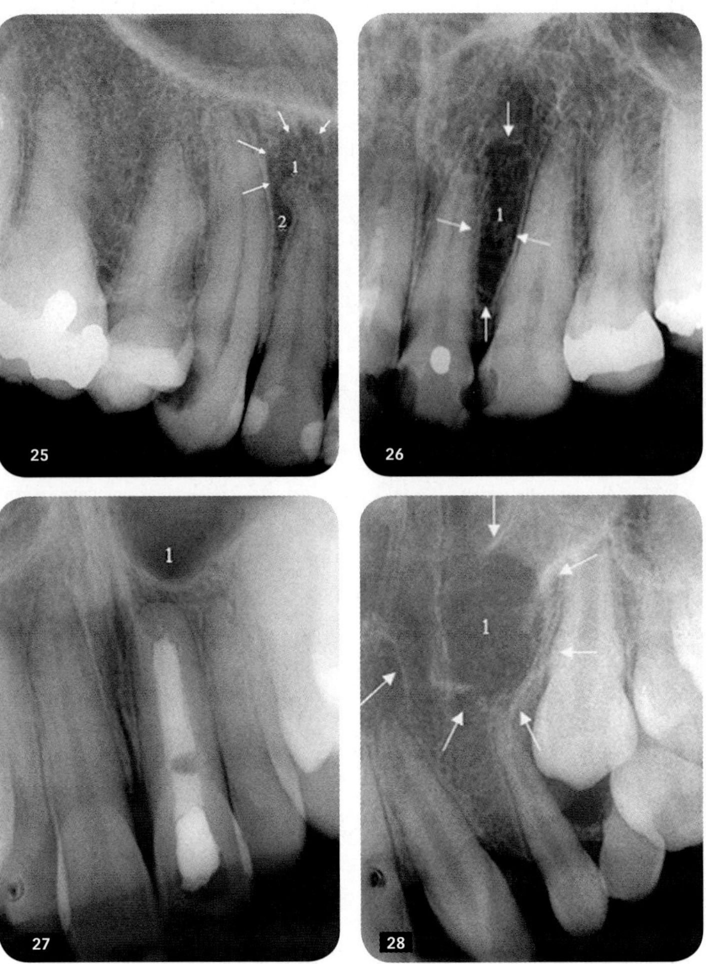


**Figure 11.25** - Smooth depression close to the apical region of the maxillary lateral incisor #12 in relation to the incisor fossa (1). A little below, between teeth #12 and 13, the moderate appearance of the myrtiform fossette (2).

**Figure 11.26** - The myrtiform fossette (1) between teeth #22 and #23 can be similar to a lateral root lesion or an apical lesion with lateral extension.

**Figure 11.27** - Nasal fossae (1) projected close to, but not in contact with tooth #21 in an asymmetrical radiograph in a patient with low nasal fossae.

**Figure 11.28** - Incomplete palatine fissure with involvement of the left nasal fossae (1), projected close to the apex of tooth #22, complete and with normal vitality.

Pneumatization of maxillary sinus - alveolar

The sinus of the face can present extensions due to pneumatization, this process intensifies with increasing age, although it can be present even in adolescents, varying from one person to another. There is a trend towards pneumatization of the maxillary sinus – in an alveolar direction to areas of dental loss, and due to the migration of neighboring teeth, it can have the appearance of dental divergences that occur in some lesions. It can also appear as though the root is positioned inside the sinus, although it is usually separated by a lamina dura. In some cases it can really be in direct contact with the soft tissues of the maxillary sinus.

The maxillary sinus, as well as the other paranasal sinuses, can present extensions with septa, and with recesses forming true chambers. These septa form images of radiopaque halos, which can also be found in cystic lesions and in some benign tumors. The proximity to dental apexes can show the appearance of apical periodontitis or, depending on the position, be similar to lateral or residual lesions. Panoramic radiography can partially help in the diagnostic process, because one can visualize the continuity of the maxillary sinus with the suspect recess, but not in all cases; there may still be doubts.

In addition to observation of the periodontal space, it is fundamental to seek continuous lines in the periapical radiograph. Frequently there are sinuous vascular canals of varied calibers present in the walls of normal maxillary sinuses. In the case of the presence of local bone lesion, loss of this vascular pattern occurs. In darker radiographies the image should be cleared by hyper- illumination when film is used, or by software in the case of digital radiography, in order to identify the presence of these vascularizations (Fig. 11.29 to 11.33).

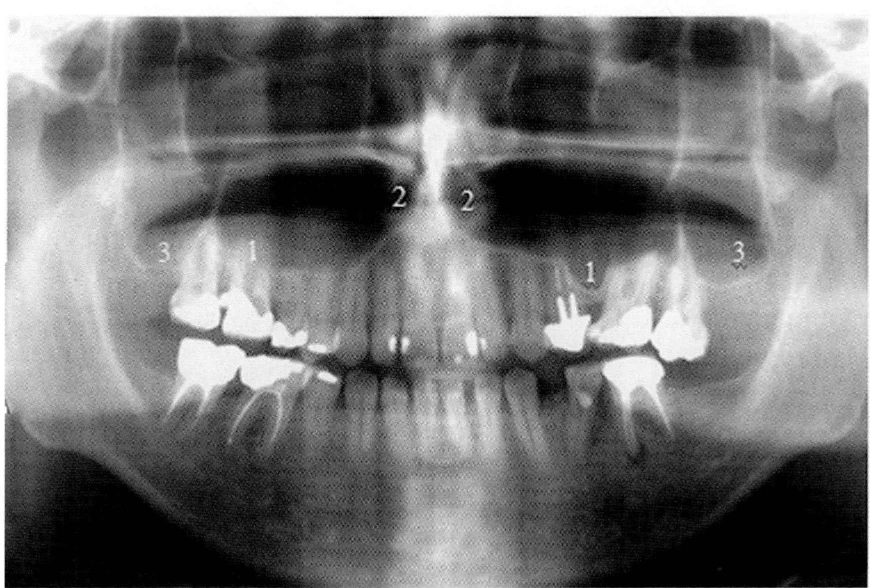


**Figure 11.29** - Extensions of the maxillary sinus: alveolar extension (1), anterior extension (2) and extension to the tuber (3).

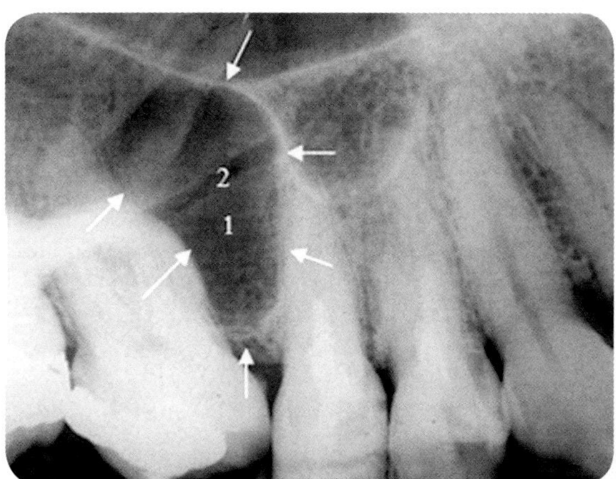


**Figure 11.30** - Alveolar extension of the right maxillary sinus in the extraction site of tooth #16, in the area delimited with the arrows (1), with a wide radiolucent line in relation to the canal of the posterior superior alveolar artery (2).

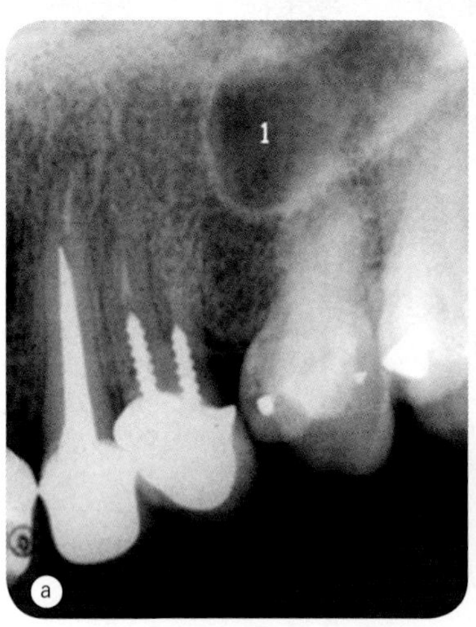


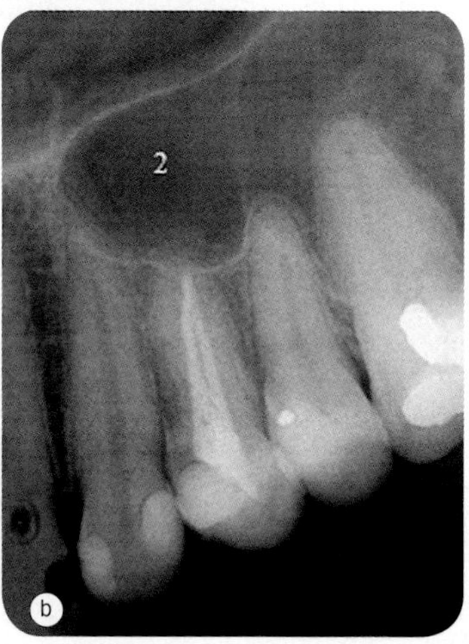


**Figure 11.31** - (**A**,**B**) Alveolar extensions of the left maxillary sinuses (1 and 2) forming recesses (chambers) similar to those in apical periodontitis. The chamber of the extension can present walls with concavities in the anterior direction (2) which indicates that it is not an expandable lesion.

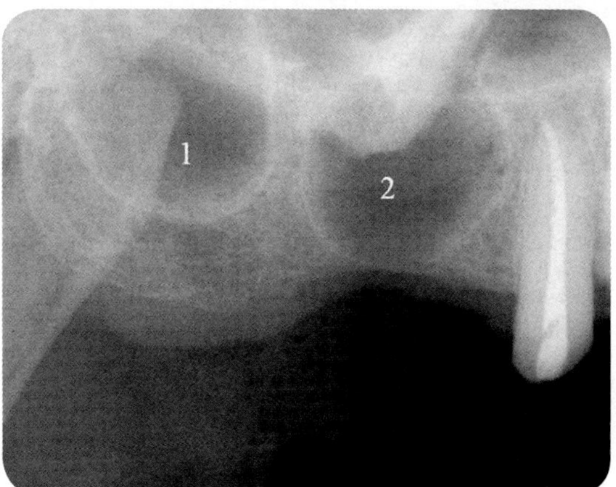


**Figure 11.32** - Alveolar extensions of the maxillary right sinus forming cavities (1 and 2) in the area of molars. Radiographic aspect similar to that of circumscribed bone lesions, such as residual cysts, but they are only variations of normality.

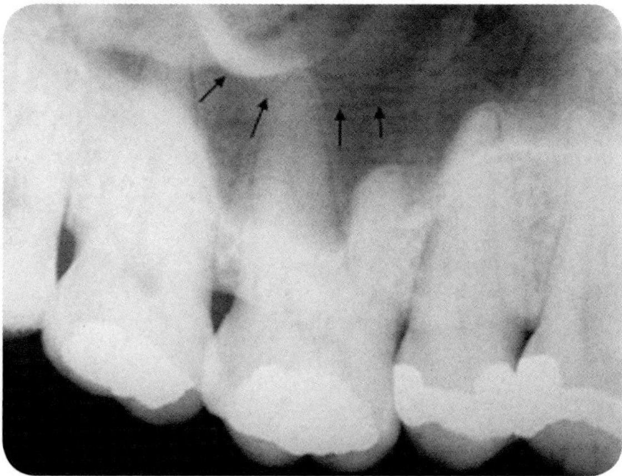

**Figure 11.33** - Alveolar extension of the maxillary sinus between the roots of the molars #17 and #16, extending towards the anterior direction. Observe the radiolucent lines in relation to the vascular canals (particularly), and of innervations observed in radiographs with hyper-illumination; lines that define the presence of the sinus and do not have the appearance of local lesion. In this image it is only a line demarcated with arrows, but there are dozens of others in several directions.

## Pneumatization of maxillary sinus – recess

In addition to the alveolar extension, there are other extensions of the maxillaries sinus: extension of the tuber, palatine, zygomatic and anterior extension, and the latter can lead to doubts in the diagnosis in the anterior area of the maxilla. In some patients the maxillary sinus can project even into the proximities of the midline of the incisors (Fig. 11.34 and 11.35).

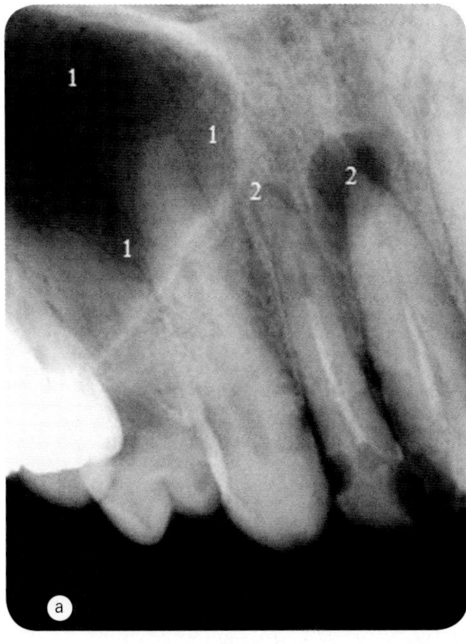


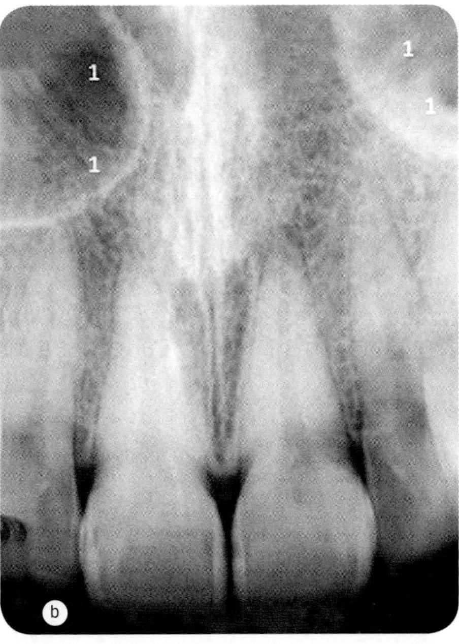


**Figure 11.34** - (**A**,**B**) Anterior extension of the maxillary sinus (1). Teeth #12 and #11 with root canals partially filled and with apical lesions (2).

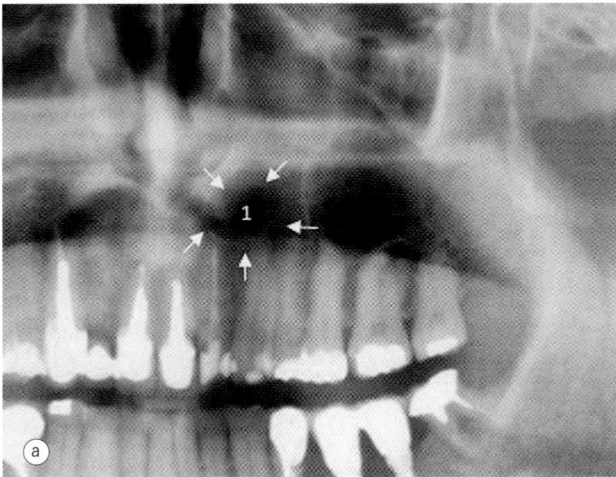


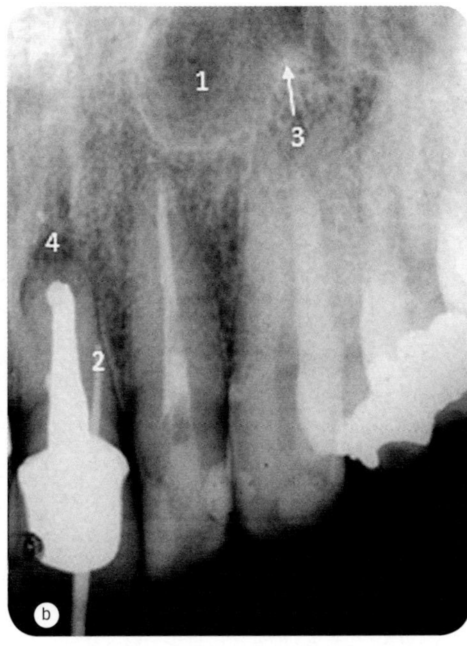


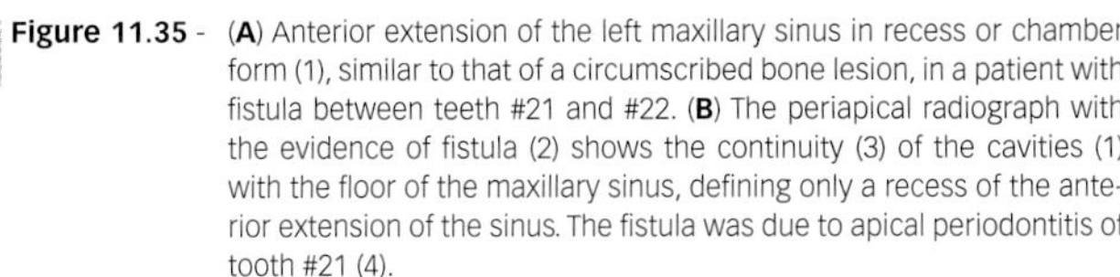

**Figure 11.35** - (**A**) Anterior extension of the left maxillary sinus in recess or chamber form (1), similar to that of a circumscribed bone lesion, in a patient with fistula between teeth #21 and #22. (**B**) The periapical radiograph with the evidence of fistula (2) shows the continuity (3) of the cavities (1) with the floor of the maxillary sinus, defining only a recess of the anterior extension of the sinus. The fistula was due to apical periodontitis of tooth #21 (4).

## Greater palatine foramen

The greater palatine foramen is situated in the third maxillary molar area, between the alveolar ridge and the hard palate. Usually this foramen is not apparent in conventional radiographic exams, because of its anatomical outline in drop form, and its inclination. Although it is very uncommon, depending on the anatomical variation and the angulation of the periapical radiograph, the greater palatine foramen can be projected close to the apex of a third or second molar, with the appearance of apical periodontitis in periapical radiography. The pulp vitality test may be necessary, and a cone beam computed tomography exam could be indicated (Fig. 11.36).

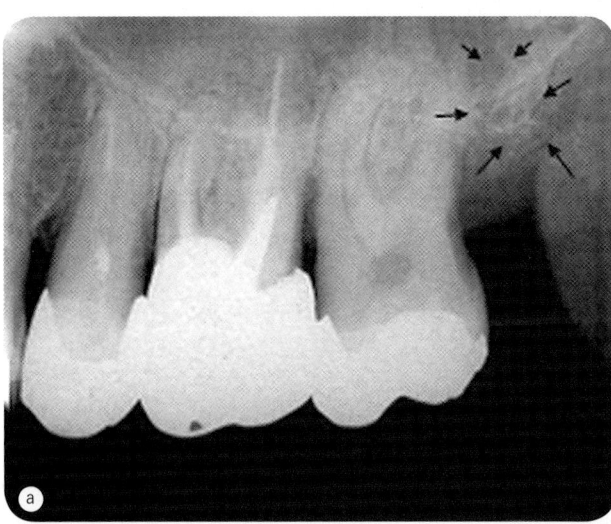

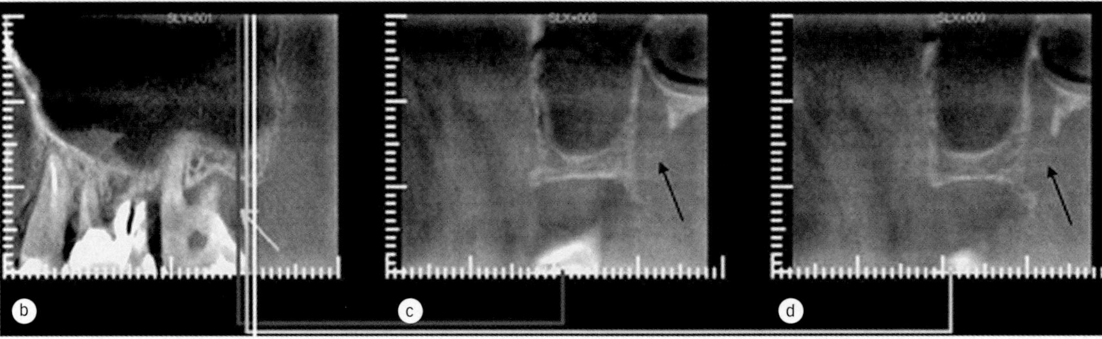

**Figure 11.36** - (**A**) Discreet image projected with an oval format in the periapical radiograph, close to the distal root portion of tooth #27, showing an uncommon case of the greater palatine foramen apparent in a periapical. (**B**) Longitudinal slice guide of cone beam computed tomography, showing a much larger bone loss than apparent in the periapical radiograph. (**C**, **D**) Fissure of the greater palatine foramen.

### Nasolacrimal canal

The nasolacrimal canal is not usually visible in periapical radiography, but it can be apparent and well-evident in occlusal radiography, projected into the molar area, in the palatine direction. For the diagnosis it is important to observe its wide, bilateral presence, and its oval, almost round shape. In cases of facial asymmetry or the patient's asymmetrical positioning in relation to the X-ray beam, the two nasolacrimal canals can be projected at different heights, capable of being more visible on one side than the other. In the occlusal radiographs it is also important to identify the maxillary sinus with and without palatine extension, because the two forms can show images similar to those of bone lesions (Fig. 11.37).

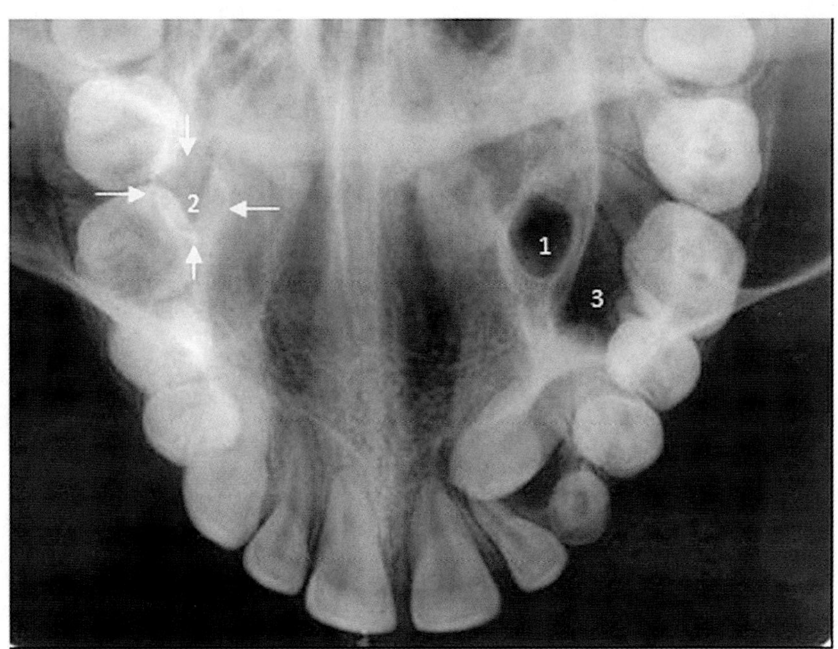


**Figure 11.37** - Well-visible nasolacrimal canal on the left side (1) and with low visibility, due to the overlapping, on the right side (2). Maxillary sinus projected towards the palatine region on the left side (3).

## 11.2.2 Anatomical Variations in Mandibula

### Mental foramen

The mental foramen opens close to the mandibular premolars, varying in height, and can be further ahead of the first premolar area or behind it, in the second premolar area. Sometimes it can extend further towards the canine tooth area or to the first molar. When it is projected onto the apex of a tooth, it can be similar to apical periodontitis. The presence of preserved apical periodontal space is a good indication of normality. When necessary, the angulation of the X-ray can be changed in a new radiographic exam. If the image leaves out the mental foramen, it changes position, usually with discreet movement, in the opposite direction to the change of the X-ray angulation. If the image leaves out a lesion, and this is centralized in the buccal-lingual direction, it stays in the same position as in the previous radiograph (Fig. 11.38 and 11.39).

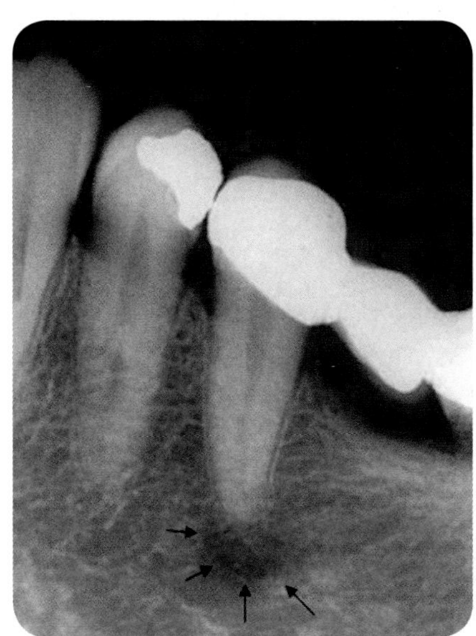

**Figure 11.38** - Mental foramen close to the apex of tooth #35, similar to apical periodontitis. Apical periodontal space preserved.

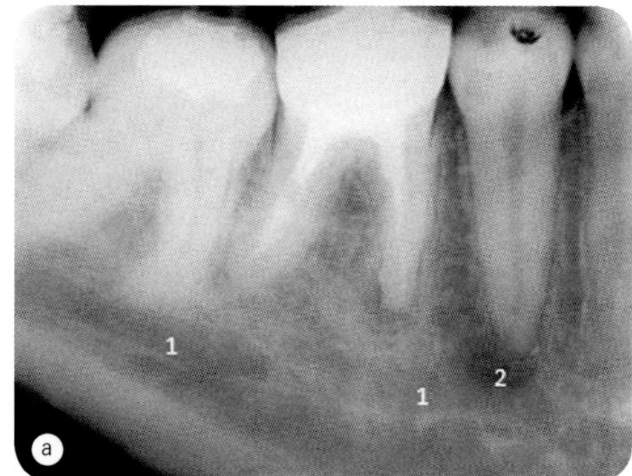


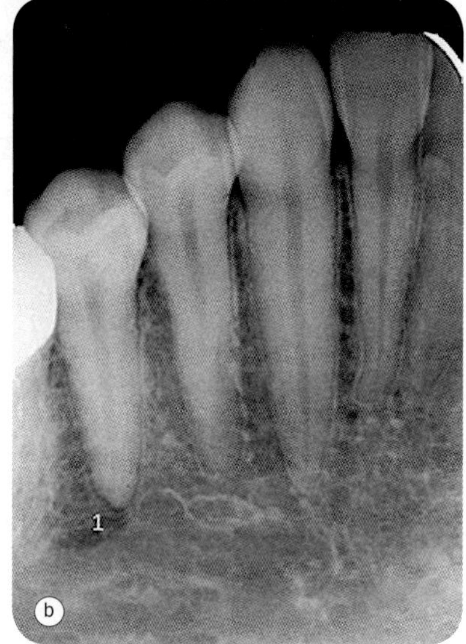


**Figure 11.39** - (**A**) Continuity of the mandibular canal; (1) it leads to the mental foramen (2) projected close to the apex of tooth #45, similar to apical periodontitis. (**B**) Same case with a change in x-ray angulation towards the mesial direction, with a discreet variation of the position of the mental foramen (1) in the opposite direction, distinguishing the bone lesion. Periodontal space of tooth #45 preserved.

### Mandibular third molar para-radicular radiolucency

Oval shaped radiolucencies surrounded by a discreet radiopaque line can be found adjacent to the posterior and inferior portion of the distal root of the mandibular third molar - only in the distal portion of this tooth - in almost 8% of the patients, more frequently in women. Usually unilateral, it can occasionally present on both sides. The origin is uncertain, but it is probably an anatomical variation with a decrease in the local bone density. The lamina dura and the periodontal space of the third molar are preserved. The formation is not connected with cases of chronic pericoronitis or with paradental cyst, since the position of para-radicular radiolucencies is lower, approaching the third molar apex distally, which could lead to confusing it with apical periodontitis. The absence of signs and symptoms, associated with the characteristic anatomical position, together with radiographic control, if indicated, are usually sufficient as diagnostic methods (Fig. 11.40).

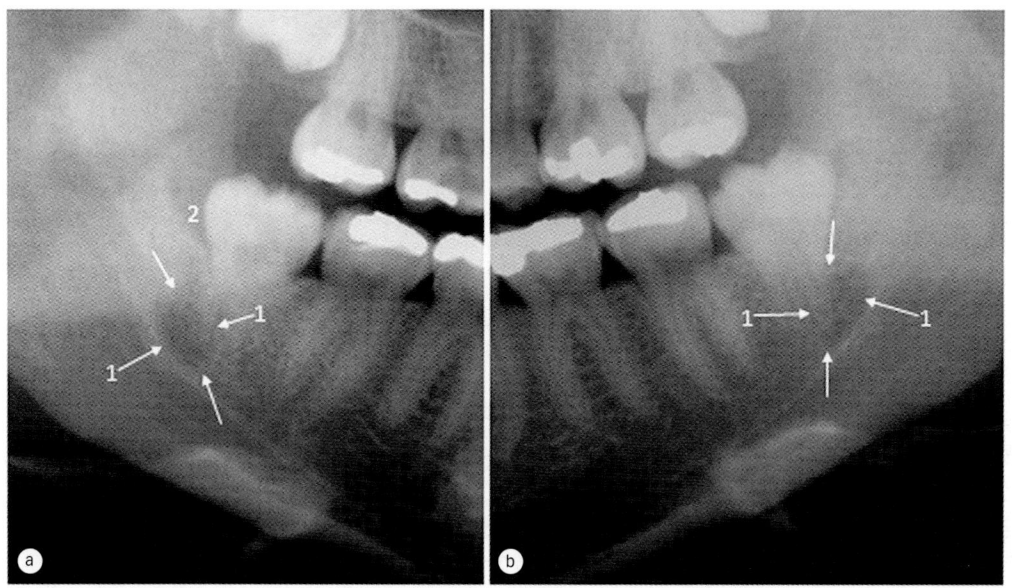


Figure 11.40 - (A,B) Patient with bilateral para-radicular radiolucencies of the mandibular third molar (1). Oval format, adjacent to the distal root portion, close to the apical area. Tooth #48 with chronic pericoronitis (2).

## Radiographic proximity of the mandibular third molar to the inferior alveolar canal

The overlapping of root apexes with the mandibular canal can give the apical area of the mandibular third molars a more radiolucent, more evident appearance than usually presented, although the difference may be discreet. Even when it is discreet it can lead to doubts in the diagnosis in the case of thickening of the periodontal space, with or without symptoms, compatible with apical periodontitis in the initial stages (Fig. 11.41).

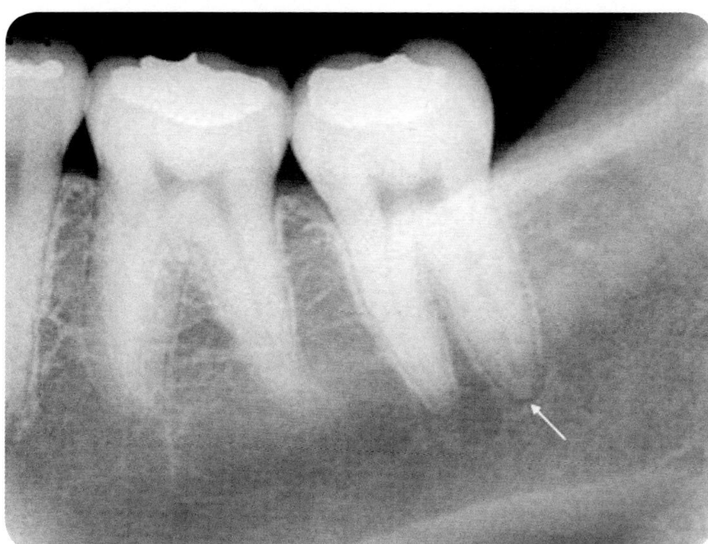

Figure 11.41 - Overlapping of the distal root of tooth #37 with the mandibular canal leaving the apical periodontal space more evident.

## Submandibular fossa

The submandibular fossa is a depression in the lingual portion of the mandibular body, to accommodate the salivary submandibular gland. In some patients it can be very pronounced, causing the mandibular body to be thinner. In this case, X-ray penetration is facilitated, marking the film or the digital sensor a great deal. The area is radiographically darker, radiolucent, and similar to a bone lesion. In some cases, the submandibular fossa can be much more evident on one side of the mandible than on the other. In a panoramic radiograph, in case of doubt between the presence of a pronounced submandibular fossa or lesion, a periapical radiograph should be taken of the area, and if it is really a submandibular fossa, this new exam would show that the area is more radiolucent, with spaced but normal trabeculae. In more accentuated cases, if the doubt remains even after having taken the periapical radiograph, a cone beam computed exam should be performed. In this exam the lingual depression of the submandibular fossa is evident, with the fine lingual cortical curve, preserved with features of morphologic variation, without the need for any treatment (Fig. 11.42 to 11.45).

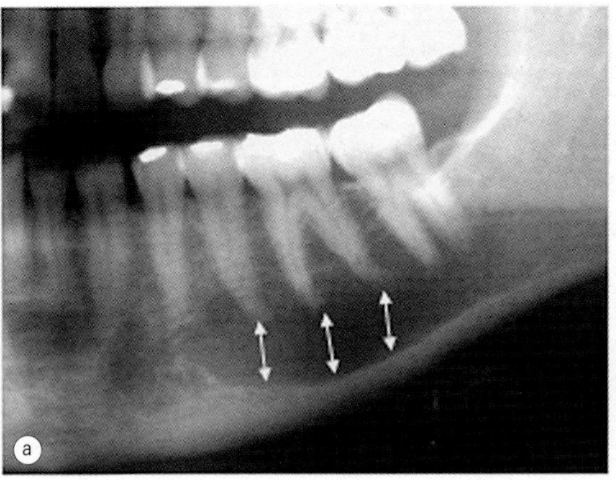


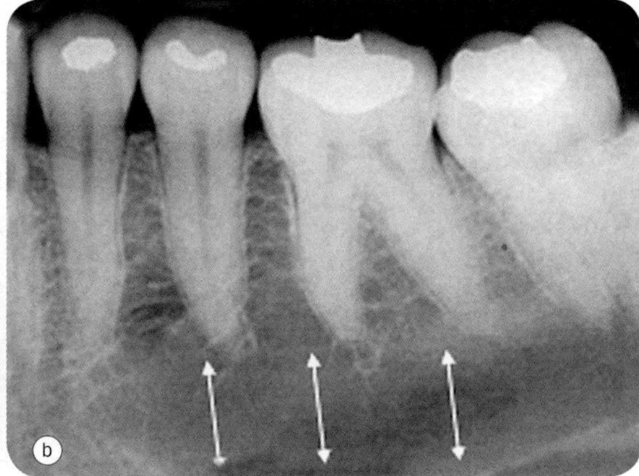


**Figure 11.42** - (**A**) Pronounced submandibular fossa (1) below the apexes of teeth #36, #35 and neighboring region, similar to a bone lesion. (**B**) In the same patient's periapical radiograph, the margins indicate that there is no lesion, although this exam does not show this distinction.

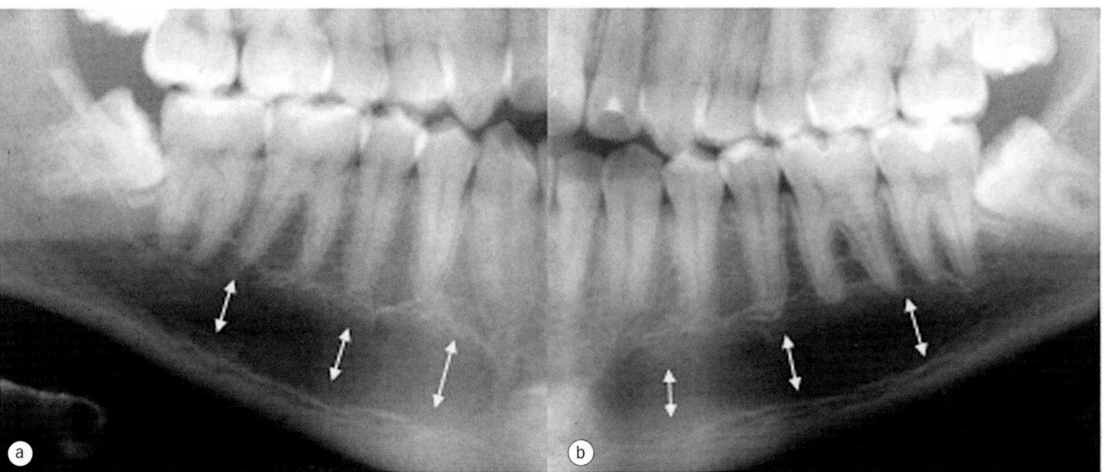


**Figure 11.43** - (**A**,**B**) Images of the right and left submandibular fossa of the same patient, pronounced and extending up to the area of canine teeth, similar to a pathological process, but identified as anatomical variation in cone beam computed tomography exam.

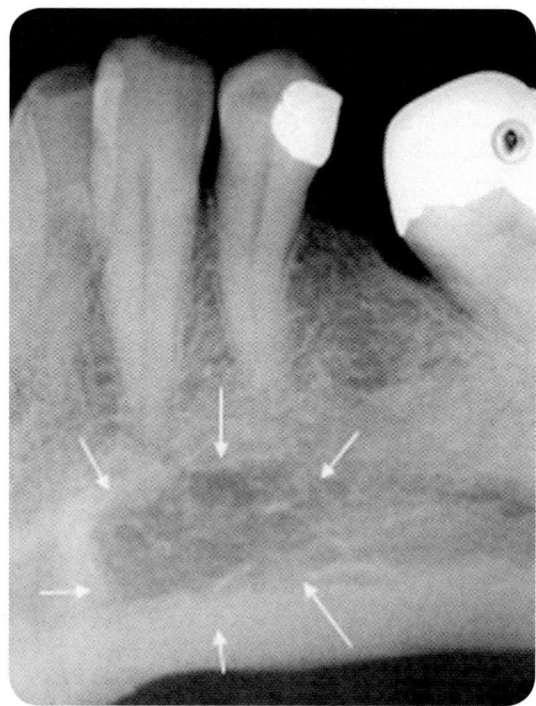

**Figure 11.44** - Anterior portion of the pronounced submandibular fossa, below the apexes of teeth #34 and #33. Position below the mylohyoid line distinguishes it from the sublingual fossa.

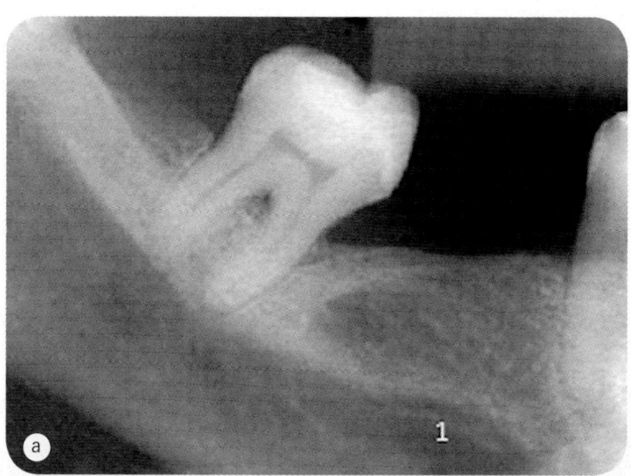


**Figure 11.45** - (**A**) Pronounced submandibular fossa (1) in a periapical radiograph. (**B**) In a longitudinal slice of cone beam computed tomography, in transversal slice, showing the accentuated depression, with a thin lingual cortical preserved. Presence of the mandibular canal (2).

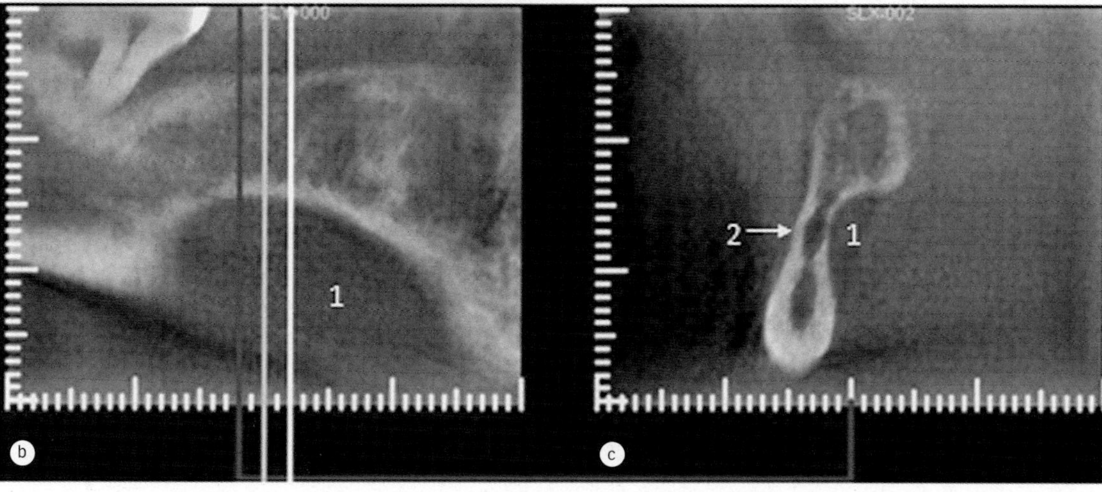

## Latent bone cavity

It is known by several names, such as: static bone cavity, Stafne's cyst, Stafne's defect, depression of the lingual mandibular cortical, among others.

It is a developmental alteration, either congenital or not, present in 0.1% to 1.8% of the population. It is a depression that accommodates the tissues of normal salivary glands, and in most cases, other types of tissues could also be present, or it could be empty. It has a characteristic appearance, usually unilateral, in the posterior area of the mandibular body, just ahead of the mandibular angle, below the mandibular canal. These alterations can also be found less frequently, in the anatomical areas corresponding to the sublingual and parotid salivary glands. The developmental bone defect of the mandible, when present in a higher position than the normal, or in a lower mandibular body, can approach the root apex and lead to suspicion of apical periodontitis or a residual lesion close to an apex.

As it is not a pathological process, only a morphologic variation, no treatment is necessary (Fig. 11.46 to 11.48).

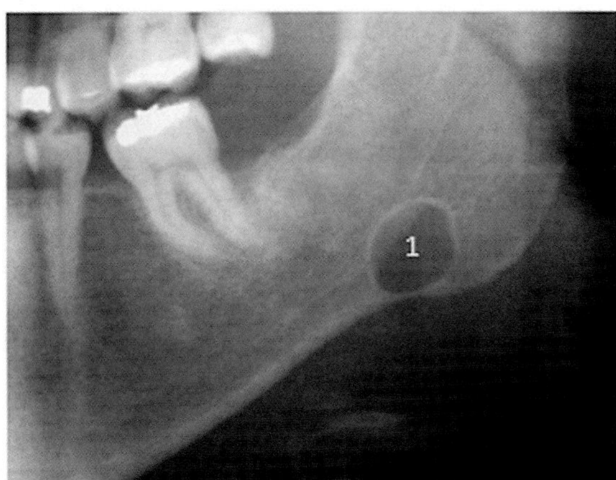


**Figure 11.46** - Developmental defect of the mandible (Stafne's defect) (1).

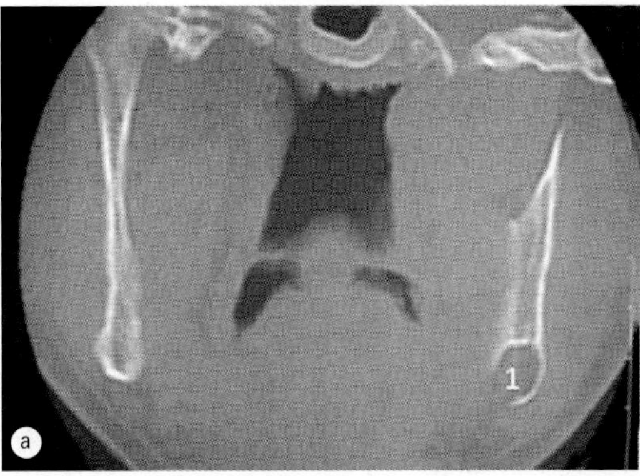


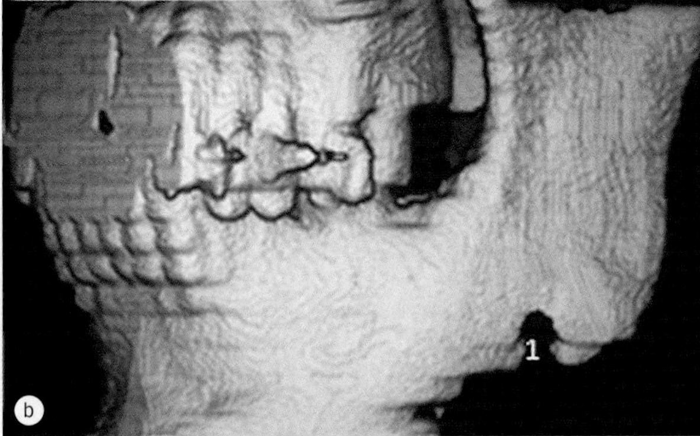


**Figure 11.47** - (**A**) Developmental defect of the mandible (1) in coronal slice in cone beam computed tomography. (**B**) Three-dimensional reconstruction, showing transfixation of the mandible.

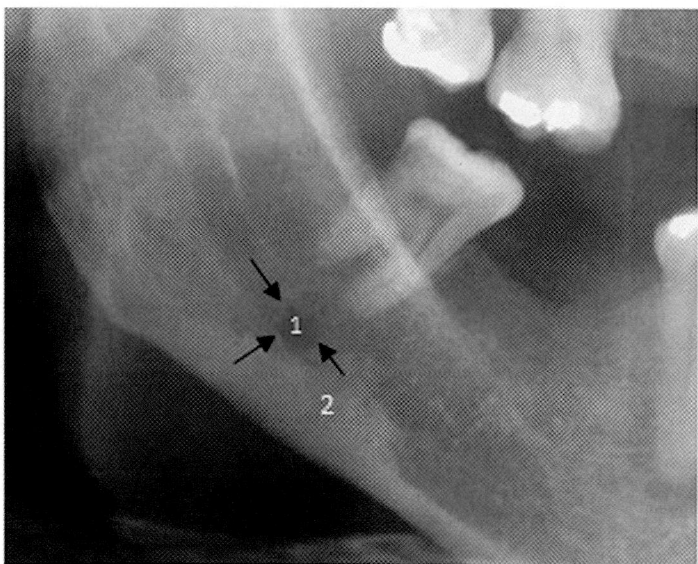


**Figure 11.48** - Developmental defect of the mandible in panoramic radiograph in an atypical location, overlapping the mandibular canal, nearing the apex of tooth #48.



## Sublingual fossa

The sublingual fossa is a bilateral, usually flat, triangular shaped depression, located on the internal surface of the mandible body, anterior to the submandibular fossa, however, above the mylohyoid line, and it accommodates the sublingual salivary gland. This fossa can sometimes be more pronounced than normal, showing a radiolucent image that can raise doubts in the diagnosis. There is usually a bilateral similarity, although one side can be much more evident than the other. Although uncommon, or even rare, a locally developed bone defect can occur, and make the depression still more accentuated, with clear delimitation, similar to apical periodontitis.

Observation of the triangular format of the fossa, presence of internal trabeculae and signs and symptoms, are usually sufficient to enable diagnosis (Fig. 11.49).

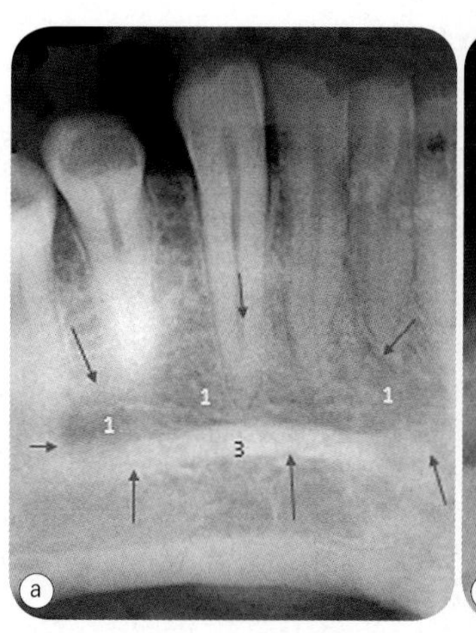


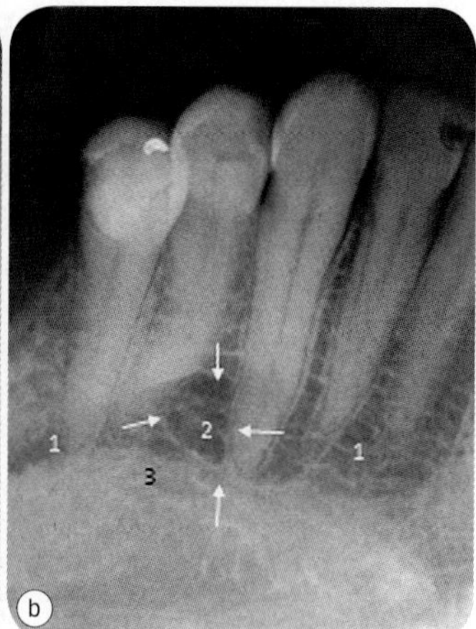


**Figure 11.49** - (**A**) Sublingual fossa determined by depression with triangular format below the apexes of tooth #42 up to #45, above the mylohyoid line. (**B**) Sublingual fossa, with larger penetration in the mandible, forming a loculus, similar to that of apical periodontitis in tooth #44. It is an overlapping case caused by a developmental defect in the mandible.

## Mental fovea

The mental fovea is an anatomical repair characterized by a depression located in the area of the mandibular incisors, and on the outside in the buccal area. It can be accentuated in some patients, causing the alveolar ridge area to become thinner. Thus, X-ray penetration is easier than in the neighboring bone tissues, showing a radiolucent image in the radiographic exams, similar to that of a bone lesion and leading to it being confused with wide apical periodontitis. One of the important lines for diagnosing pronounced mental fovea, is the presence of the vertically guided and very evident nutritive canals. These lines are not usually present in bone lesions. As it is not a pathological process, but only a morphologic variation, no treatment is necessary (Fig. 11.50 and 11.51).

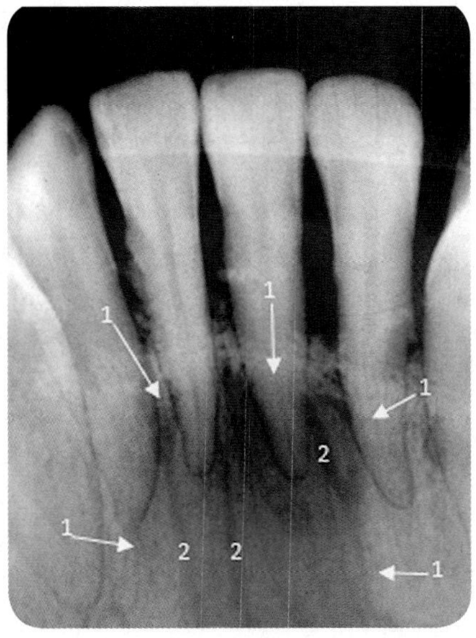

**Figure 11.50** - Pronounced mental fovea (1), similar to a bone lesion below the apex of the central incisors. Presence of nutritive canals in the vertical direction (2).

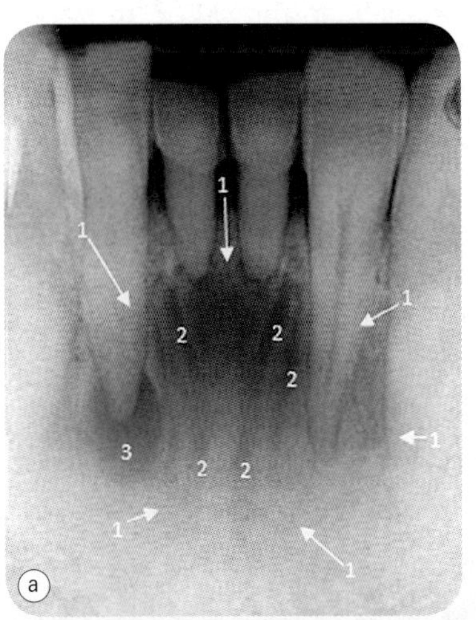

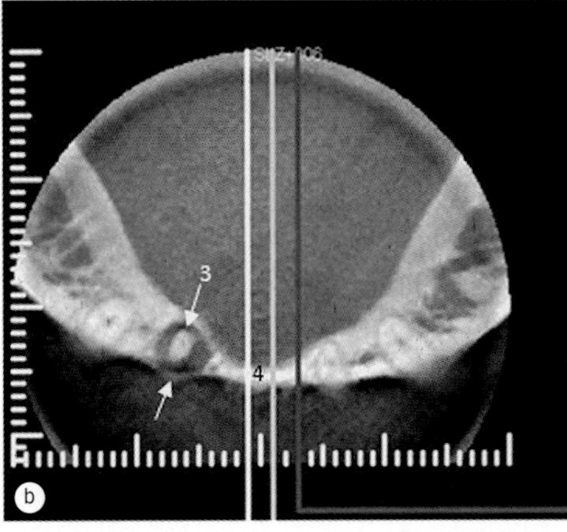

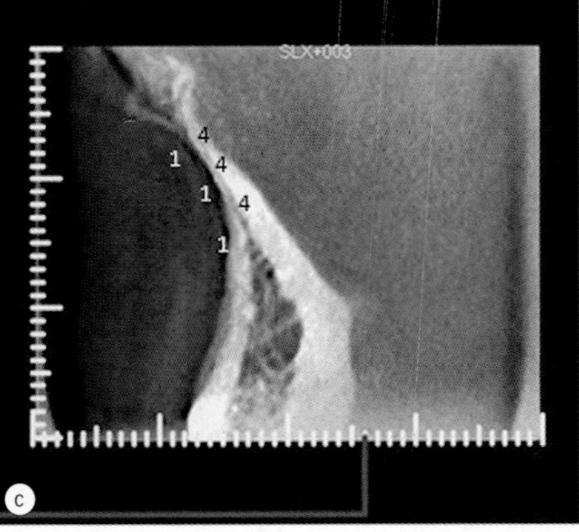

**Figure 11.51** - (**A**) Pronounced mental fovea (1), similar to bone lesion in periapical radiography. Presence of nutritive canals (2) in the vertical direction and apical lesion (3) in tooth #43. Patient with agenesis of the permanent mandibular central incisors. (**B**) In the same case, in an axial slice of cone beam computed tomography, showing the thinness of the area (4) and apical lesion (3) in tooth #43. (**C**) Transversal sagittal slice, showing the depression of the pronounced mental fovea and the thinness (4) of the area, facilitating X-ray penetration.

## 11.3 Other Conditions that do not Require Treatment

### Surgical cavities

Surgery that involves bone tissues, takes on the formation of a cavity, and if no graft is used, the immediate radiographic result shows a radiolucent area that can be similar to that of apical periodontitis, depending on the position. This doubt can occur when the image is observed in isolation, a few weeks after the surgery, before the beginning of bone repair, by a professional that ignores the previous intervention (Fig. 11.52).

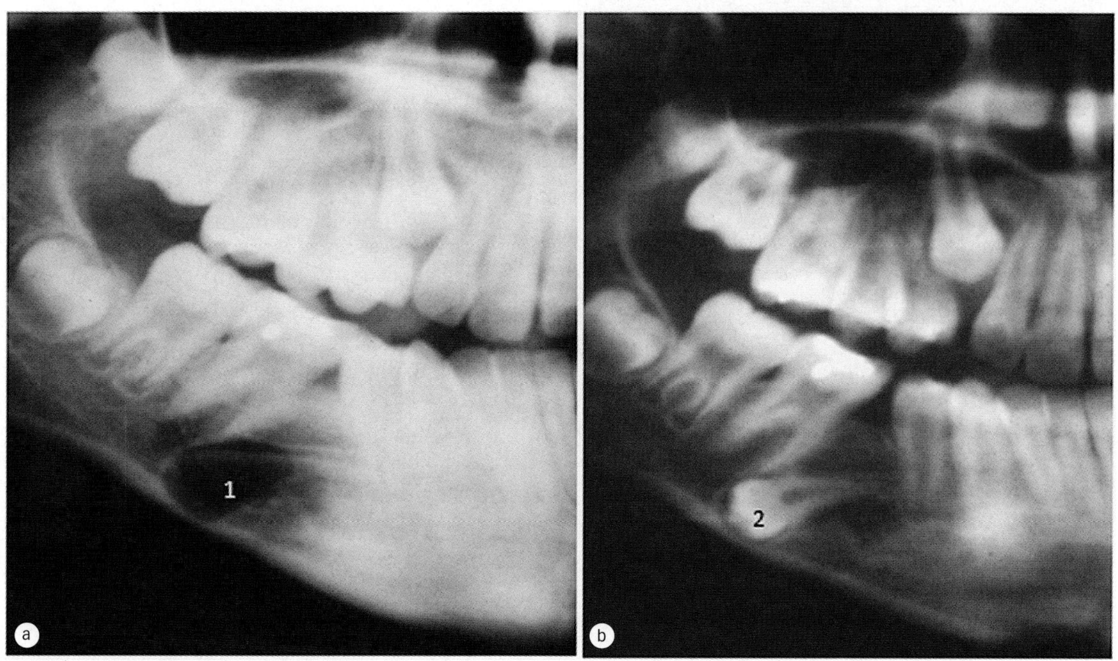


**Figure 11.52** - (**A**) Extraction of tooth #45, performed a month earlier, can form surgical cavities (1) close to the apical area of tooth #45, similar to a lesion resulting from apical periodontitis. (**B**) To evoke the previous exam, the submerged tooth was observed in position (2).

### Bone healing

At first sight, a radiolucent area can indicate a lesion in an endodontically treated tooth. In reality, it can be an area in which bone repair is occurring, a case that was treated by other professional few weeks before, for example. The initial bone repair in progress can have an appearance identical to that of apical periodontitis. Signs and symptoms, time elapsed and radiographic control, are necessary for this evaluation. In the beginning, it is not possible to distinguish the repair radiographically from a lesion, but after some months the lesion begins to decrease and discreet lines can be present in its margins, tending to be concentric towards the "opening" of the lesion (Fig. 11.53).

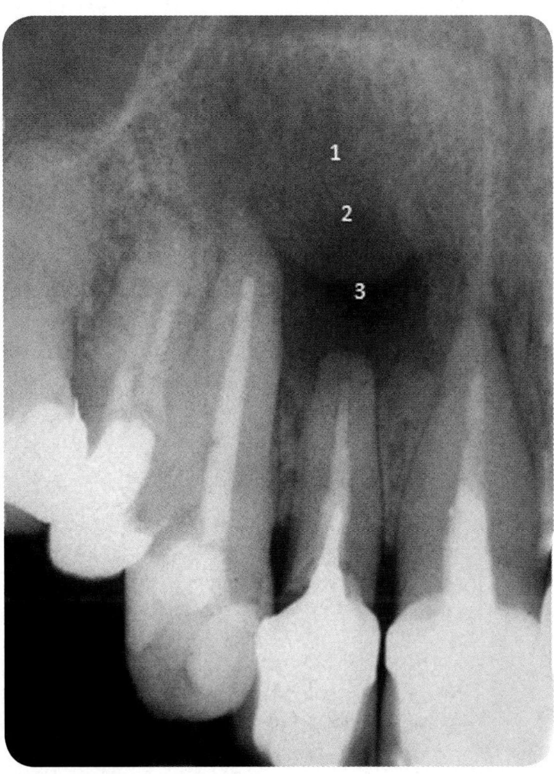


**Figure 11.53** - Area of a wide apical lesion in tooth #12 with bone repair in progress, post-treatment, with bone areas already formed at the periphery, but still having a different trabecular pattern (1) with normal bone in the neighboring area. Presence of the margins of the more radiolucent central area (3), of discreet lines in area in which there was no bone formation, with concentric tendencies (2) towards the "opening" (3) of the lesion.

## Fibrous healing defect

A bone lesion in a tooth that received appropriate endodontic treatment usually develops bone repair, but repair can also develop with fibrous conjunctive tissue, and be considered a successful repair as well. A mixed condition can occur in peripheral bone repair, and in the center, a fibrous repair remainder that could disappear completely with time, or leave signs for a short while, or for the rest of the patient's life. As the fibrous area has a lower density than the neighboring bone tissue, it shows a radiolucent image, radiographically similar or even identical to apical periodontitis.

The observation of the signs and symptoms, associated with the periapical radiographic controls, with radiographic exams in the same position, indicates a stabilized radiolucent area, or one slowly decreasing, but never increasing in size.

Simple fibrous repair occurs when there was no surgical intervention locally, and it becomes dominated by surgical fibrous repair (surgical scar), much more frequently than what usually occurs with the loss of the periosteum and buccal or palatine cortical, particularly when the loss of both occurs, thus forming a "tunnel". In the surgical case, the radiographic aspect is very suggestive of a radiolucent area, usually overlapped by a halo of medium density, followed by the neighboring bone tissue of greater density. The margins are clear, with or without visible cortical limits. The surgical fibrous repair could be confused with apical periodontitis, but anamnesis indicates local surgery and the highly suggestive radiographic aspects facilitate the diagnosis. In case of doubt persisting, radiographic control is indicated, as mentioned above (Fig. 11.54 and 11.55).

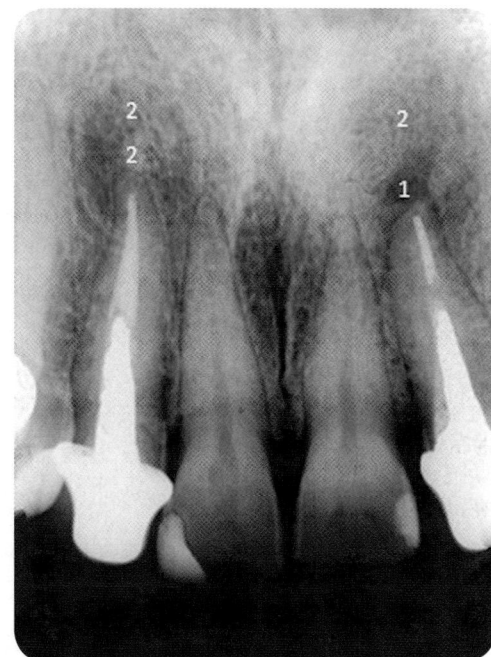


**Figure 11.54** - Area of fibrous healing defect (1) in the apical area of tooth #22, submitted to an apicetomy (discreet radiographically), with the presence of outlying bone repair (2). On the opposite side tooth #12 developed with a conventional bone repair (2) of variable density, after endodontic treatment.

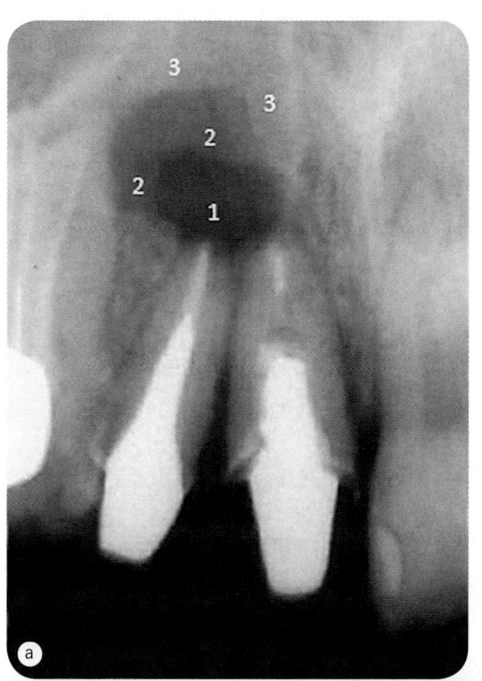


**Figure 11.55** - (**A**) Fibrous healing defect (1) in the apical area of tooth #12, submitted to an apicetomy in a case of wide lesion. Central area extremely radiolucent (1), overlapped by a halo of medium density (2), followed by the neighboring bone tissue of greater density (3). (**B**) A longitudinal slice of cone beam computed tomography shows the width of the area of fibrous repair. (**C**, **D**) Transversal slices in cone beam computed tomography show the buccal-palatine communication in a tunnel form.

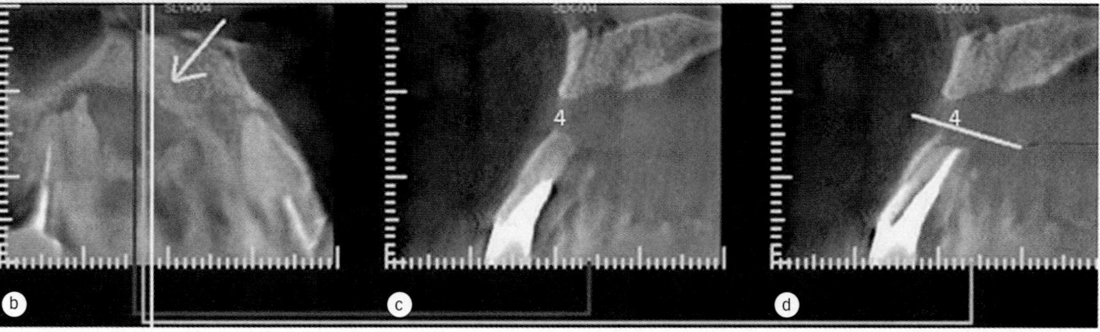

## Orthodontic movement

Active orthodontic movement leads to an increase in the apical and lateral periodontal space, and radiographically, neighboring teeth can present a greater increase than others. This increase should be taken into account when the differential diagnoses of apical periodontitis is being established.

When the movement is fast, the image of the alveolus can be apparent, with an aspect similar to that of apical periodontitis that leads to bone destruction in the periapical area. Anamnesis and careful clinical exams are important in the diagnosis. The vitality test is indicated, because this type of movement can, in some cases, lead to pulp necrosis (Fig. 11.56).

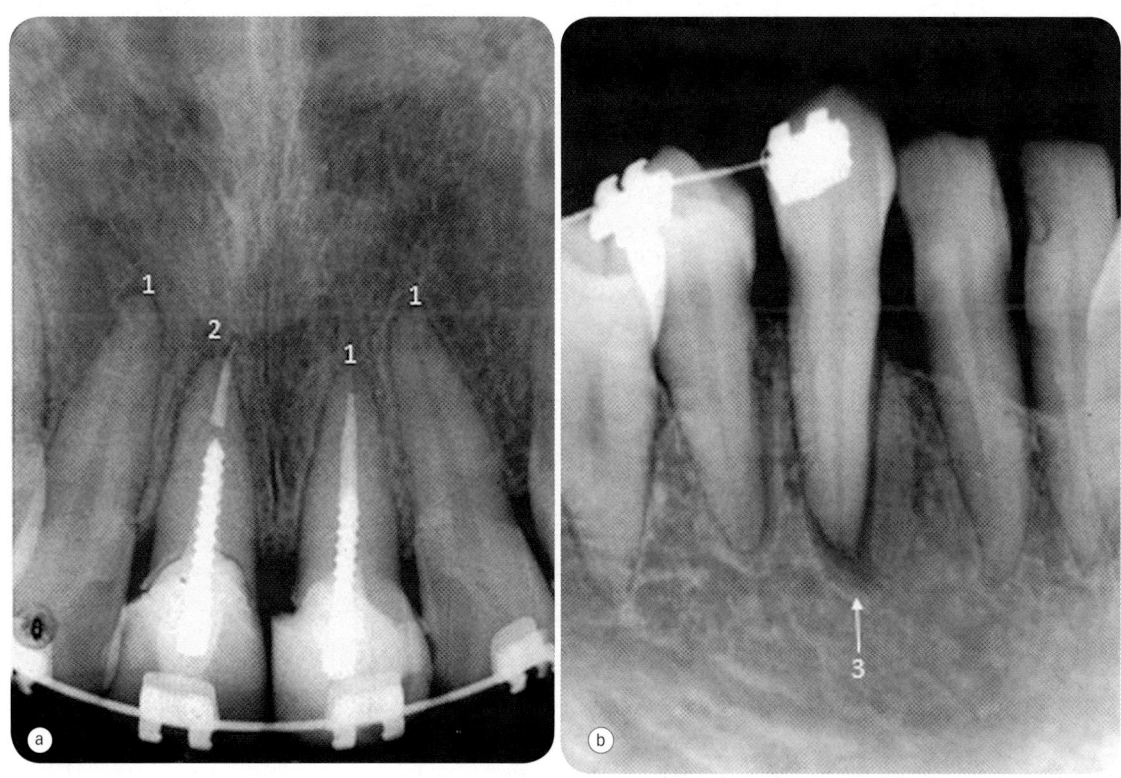


**Figure 11.56** - (**A**) Orthodontic movement can induce thickness of the periodontal space (1). Tooth #11 with overfilling, root fractures in the apical third and discreet diffuse bone apical rarefaction (2). (**B**) Orthodontic device, only part of the arch inducing the extrusion of tooth #43, extreme mesial region, establishing a radiolucent apical area (3) similar to that of AP.

## Stains in conventional radiographic exams

Stains can occur in radiographic films for several reasons, such as an area of the film that was pressed against body before the radiographic exam, or during processing and drying of the films. It could also be a stain of an X-ray mount that was not noticed and overlapped the radiograph. Depending on the position, the stain can be similar to a fracture or apical periodontitis. If the suspicion persists, a new radiographic exam will be the solution (Fig. 11.57 and 11.58).

One of the great advantages of digital radiology is that it is free from processing and editing stains.

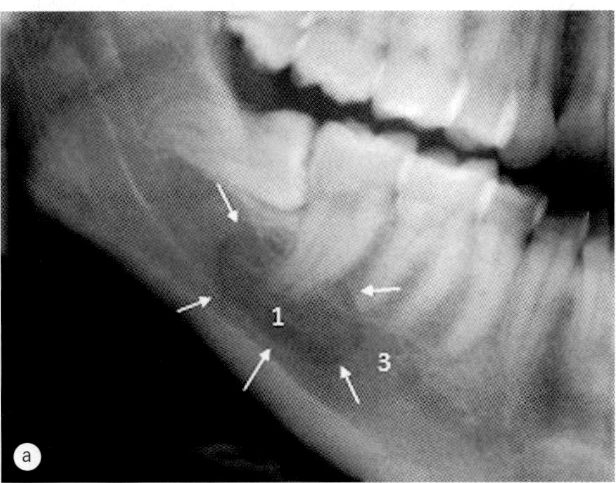


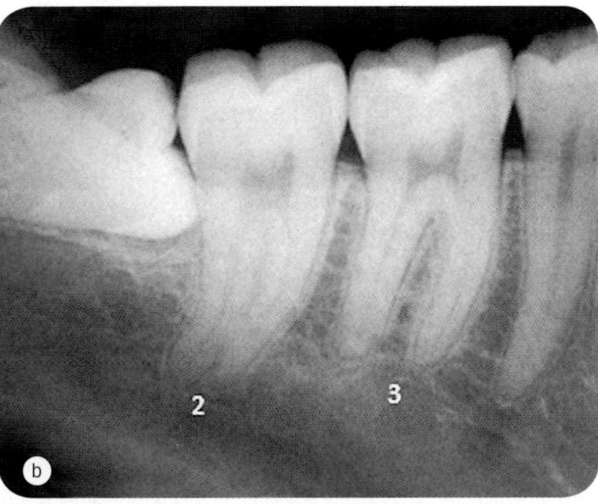


**Figure 11.57** - (**A**) Processing stains (1) in a panoramic segment, overlapping the apex of tooth #47, similar to apical lesion. (**B**) Periapical radiograph of the same area shows lack of treatment of rarefaction area (2). Wide medullary space (3) close to the apical area of tooth #46.

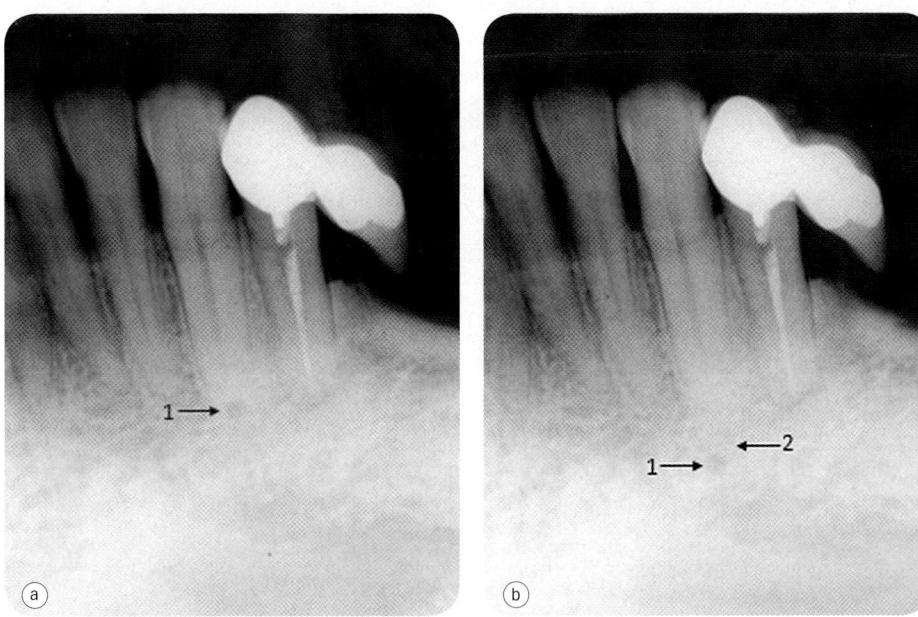


**Figure 11.58** - (**A**) Stains (1) in the transparent plastic X-ray mount overlapped the apex of tooth #33. (**B**) The same anterior radiograph as before, when moving the film a little higher, the stain (1) of the X-ray mount was left behind, moving away from the apex (2).

## 11.4 Results of Pathological Processes

### Conditions that result from or lead to inflammatory processes

#### Residual cyst

Depending on the position, shape and size of a residual cyst, it can cause confusion with a lateral or apical lesion originating in a neighboring tooth. In many cases the absence of a tooth in the area and image of extraction repair indicate this lesion, pointing to the diagnosis (Fig. 11.59).

#### Lesions due to root fractures

Root fractures produce clefts that frequently develop into an aggressive process in the neighboring bone tissues. The inflammatory reaction established at the site, can develop into an abscess without or with a fistula, granuloma, or a cyst.

Root fractures are only visible in conventional radiographic exams, when the angulation of the fracture line is favorable to the X-ray angulation. Most of the root fractures are hidden in conventional radiographic exams. Even if the fracture line is not seen, after a while, an inflammatory reaction with enlargement of the periodontal space in the form of a half moon, can be observed. However, this image cannot be present (Fig. 11.60 to 11.62).

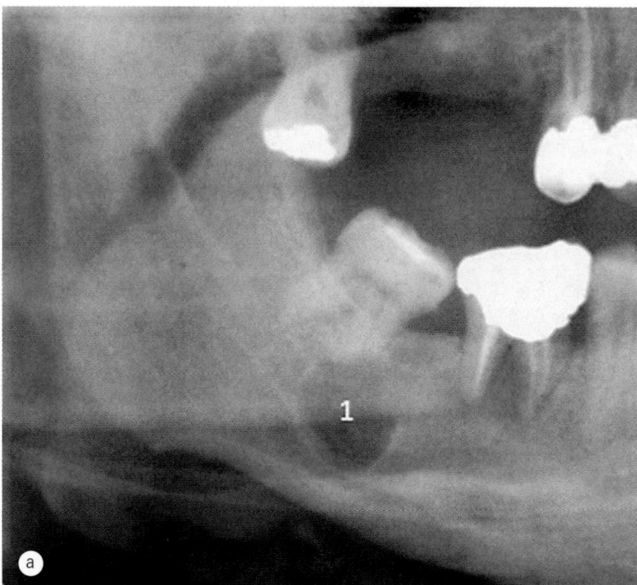


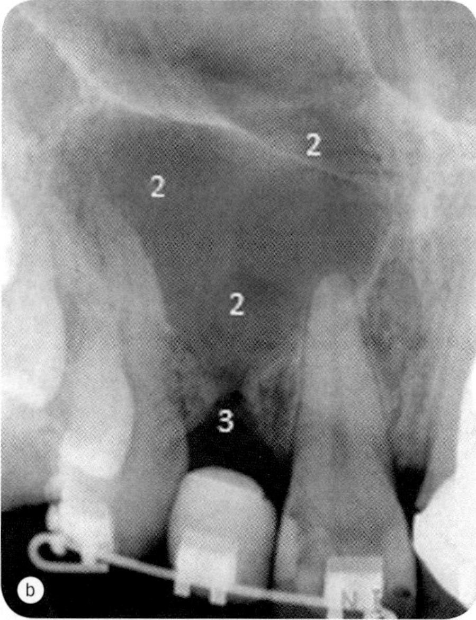


**Figure 11.59** - (**A**) Residual cyst (1) of tooth #47 (absent) close and similar to a lesion originating from tooth #48 that had perfect vitality. (**B**) Wide residual cyst (2) of tooth 12 with signs (3) of extraction.

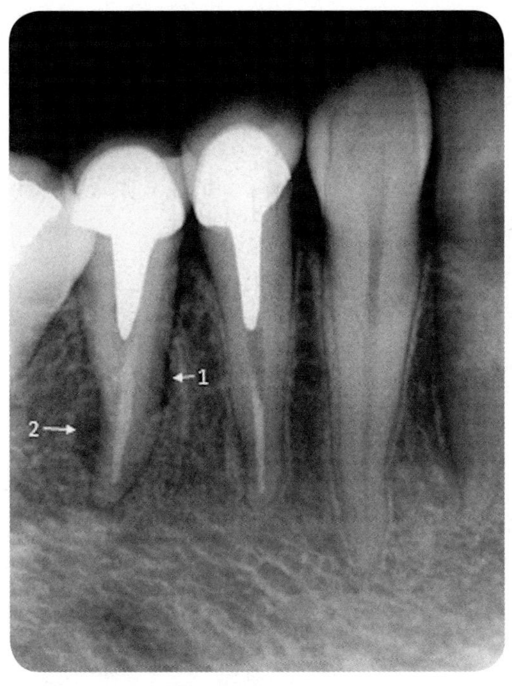


**Figure 11.60** - Tooth #45 with root fracture without precise visualization of the dental structure, presence of thickened lateral periodontal space in form of a "half moon" (1) in the mesial region and diffuse bone rarefaction (2) in the distal region, indicating the presence of fracture.



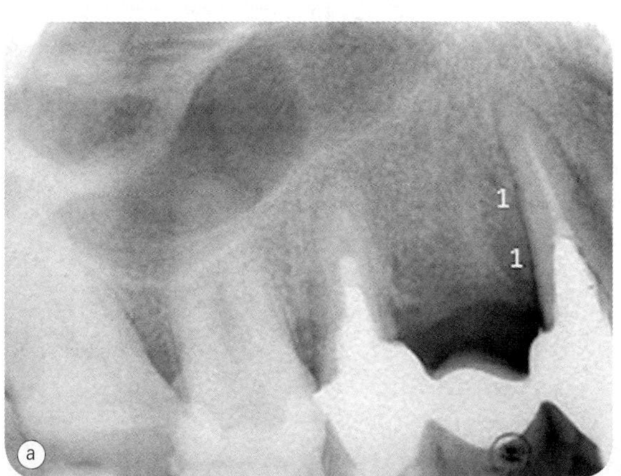


**Figure 11.61** - (**A**) Tooth #13 with hidden root fracture in the periapical exam, with diffuse bone rarefaction in the distal region (1), indicating the presence of fracture, perforation, and periodontitis observed in lateral canal or periodontal lesion (most probable lesions). (**B**) Referential longitudinal slice of cone beam computed tomography shows that the bone rarefaction is intense (1). (**C**, **D**). Transversal slices of cone beam computed tomography show the presence of fracture line (2), hidden in the periapical radiograph.

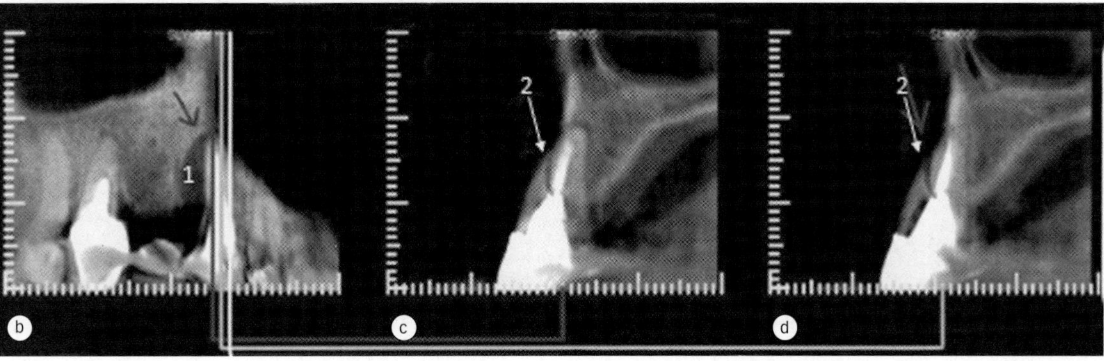

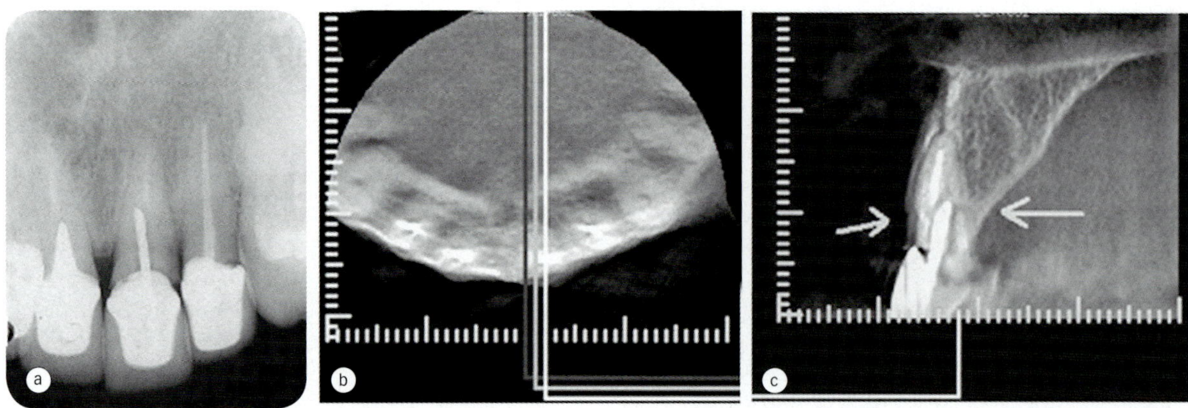

**Figure 11.62** - (**A**) Tooth #21 with filled root canal and intracanal post moved distally, with root fracture hidden in the periapical exam, also not presenting bone rarefaction. (**B**) Referential longitudinal slice of cone beam computed tomography. (**C**) Transversal slice of cone beam computed tomography shows the post in the distal position and presence of fracture line, hidden in the periapical radiograph.

## Lesions due to root perforations

After some time, root perforation usually presents lateral bone lesion with patterns similar to those described in root fractures (in some cases identical), therefore, fractures and root perforation are very close in the diagnosis with images. When located adjacent to the apical area, it can be confused with apical periodontitis, or could be the very cause of it (Fig. 11.63).

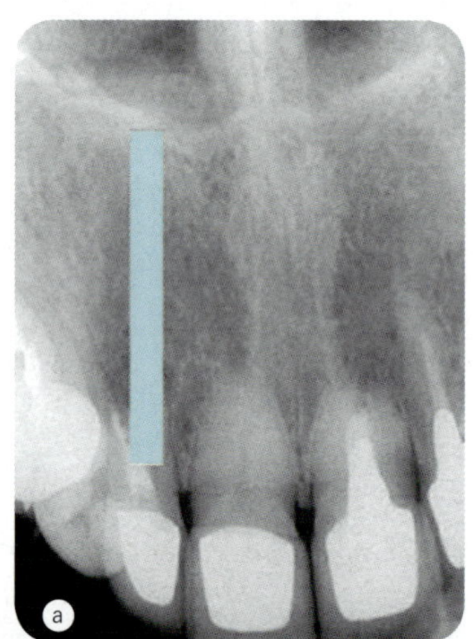

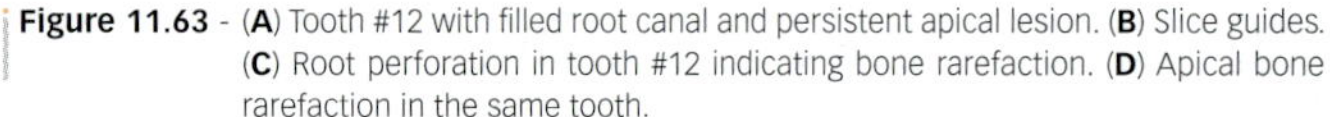

**Figure 11.63** - (**A**) Tooth #12 with filled root canal and persistent apical lesion. (**B**) Slice guides. (**C**) Root perforation in tooth #12 indicating bone rarefaction. (**D**) Apical bone rarefaction in the same tooth.

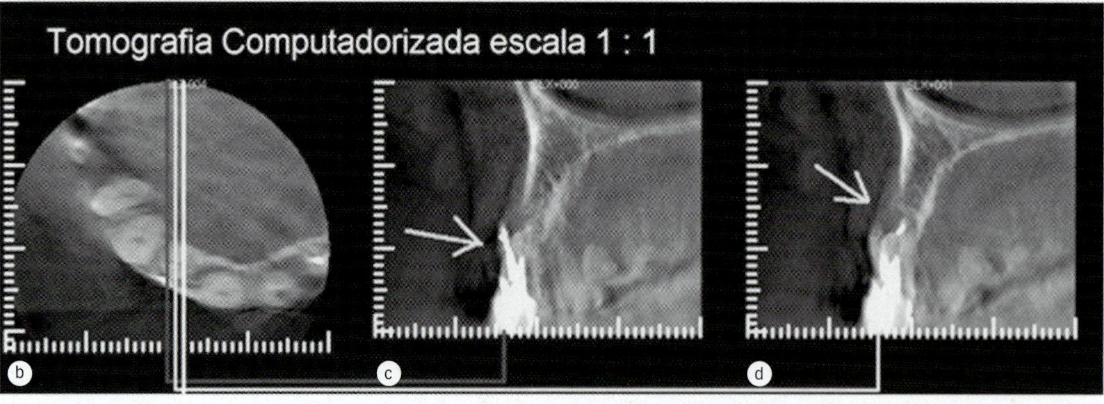

## Marginal periodontitis

Atypical cases of marginal periodontitis can eventually reach a tooth from the buccal or lingual side, giving the appearance of bone integrity in the proximal areas (mesial and distal) close to the crown. In these cases, as there is no visible, radiographically continuous bone loss starting from the cervical third, the existent rarefaction could lead to the suspicion of reaction to a hidden fracture line, perforation, or other lateral lesion that involves the periodontal space. In some cases the marginal periodontitis go as far as the apical area without presenting radiographically visible bone loss in the area of the cervical third of the root, capable of being similar to apical periodontitis with lateral involvement.

Marginal periodontitis can eventually become established, which leads to the deposition of salivary calculus towards the apex, starting with a pronounced radicular groove and progressing towards a developmental defect (Fig. 11.64 and 11.65).

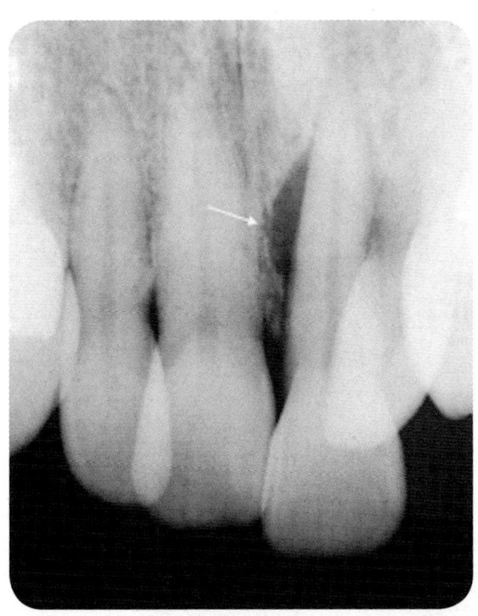

**Figure 11.64** - Marginal periodontitis in tooth #21 leading to mesial bone loss, with the cervical area atypically preserved.

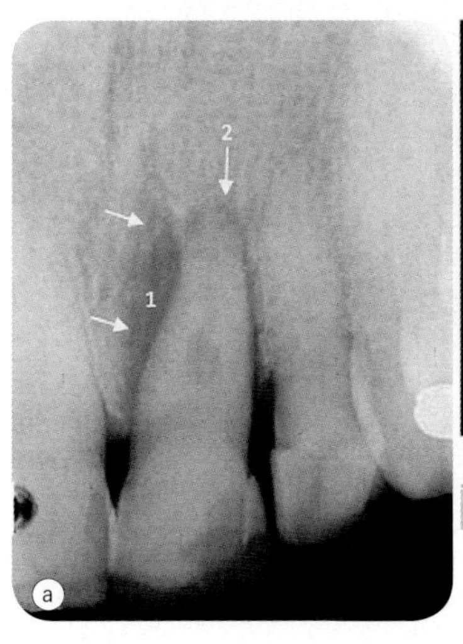


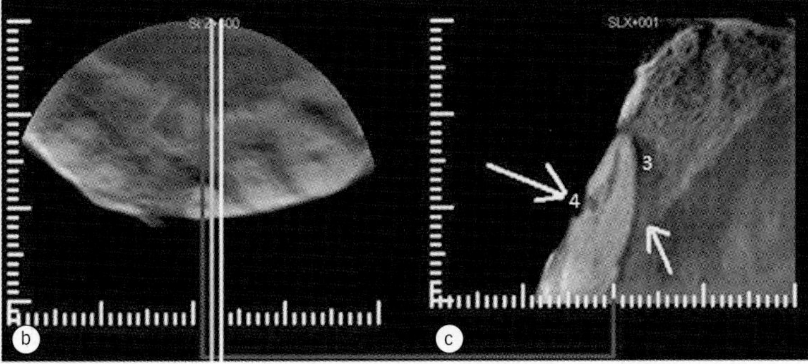


**Figure 11.65** - (**A**) Marginal periodontitis in tooth #21 leading to mesial and apical bone loss (1) (2) observed in the periapical radiograph, similar to apical periodontitis with lateral involvement. (**B**) Axial guide slices. (**C**) The cone beam computed tomography exam shows the inclusion of the palatine face (3) in the periodontitis (not observed in the periapical radiograph) leading to an endoperiodontal lesion. Root reabsorption (4) on the buccal face of tooth #21.

## Furcation lesion

A furcation lesion can show an atypical image, only bone rarefaction on the side of a tooth root, leading to the suspicion of a fracture, root perforation or another lateral lesion.

Furcation lesion may not be seen on a radiographic image, but it can develop to an abscess with or without fistula, leading to clinical suspicion of a hidden apical periodontitis. An endodontist should be well-prepared to perform delicate periodontal probes in the event of clinical indication (Fig. 11.66 and 11.67).

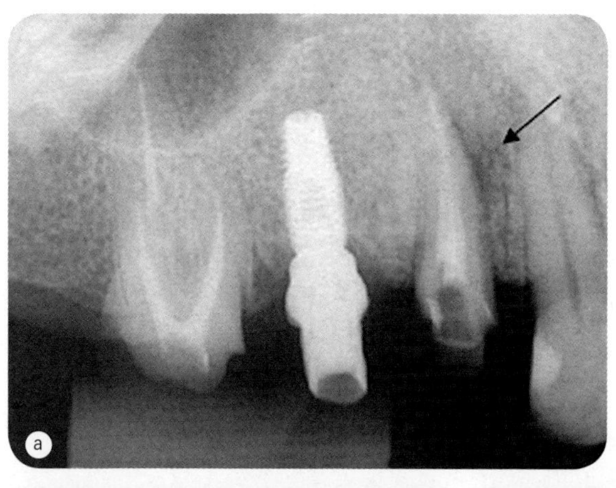


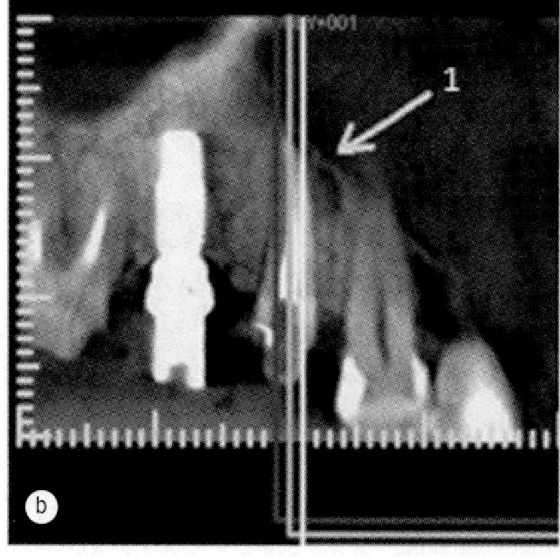


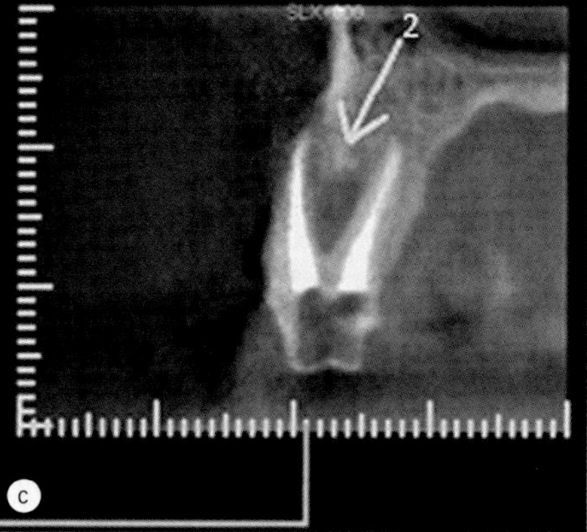


**Figure 11.66** - (**A**) Bone rarefaction (arrow) in relation to furcation lesion in tooth #14, hidden in the periapical radiograph, similar to a lateral root lesion. (**B**) Longitudinal slice of cone beam computed tomography confirms bone rarefaction (1). (**C**) Transversal slice of cone beam computed tomography shows the presence of furcation lesion (2).

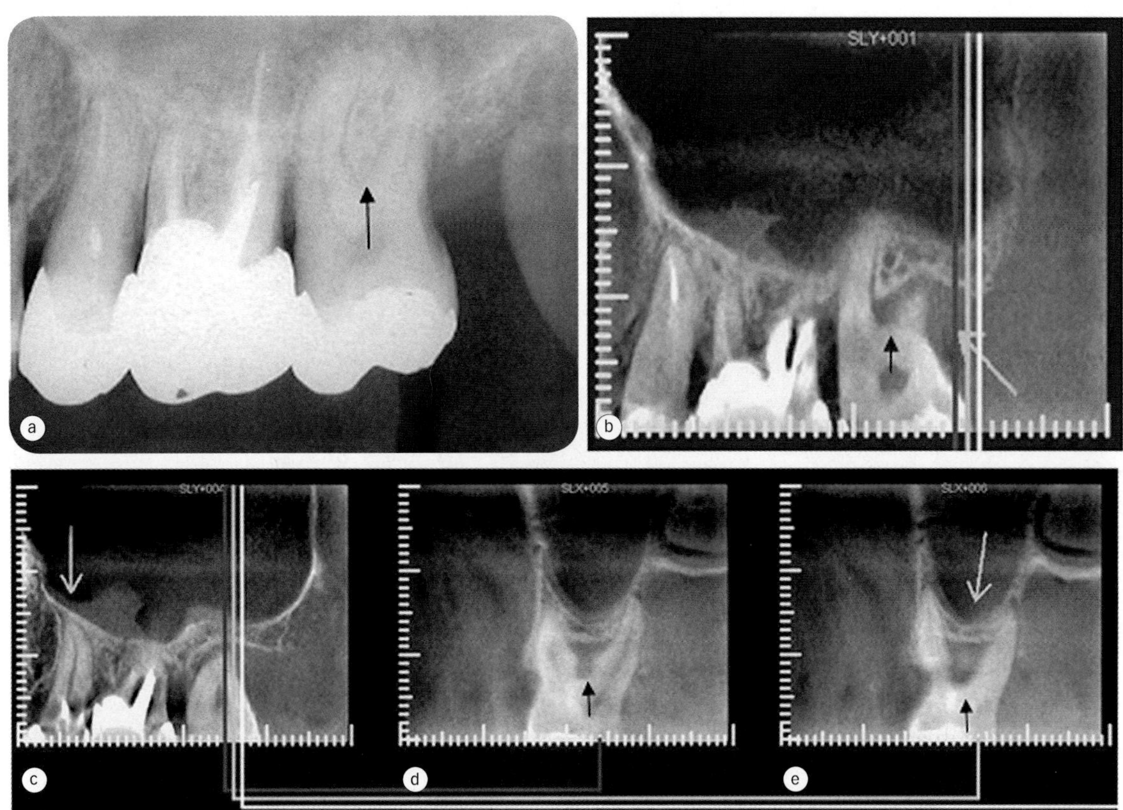


**Figure 11.67** - (**A**) Hidden furcation lesion in tooth #27 hidden in the periapical radiograph, with symptoms similar to apical periodontitis. (**B**) Longitudinal slice of cone beam computed tomography shows the presence of furcation lesion. (**C**) Slice guides. (**D**, **E**) Transversal slice shows the presence of furcation lesion.

## Extra-radicular infections

A tooth with apical periodontitis can lead to the formation of a periapical abscess with intra-oral fistula. If these abscesses are present for a prolonged period, and the root is close to the external middle with fistula, there is increased chance of salivary calculus deposition on the root surface near the affected area. With the presence of calculus adhered to the root, the formation of bone lesion occurs at the site of the aggression, because these calculus are infected (Fig. 11.68).

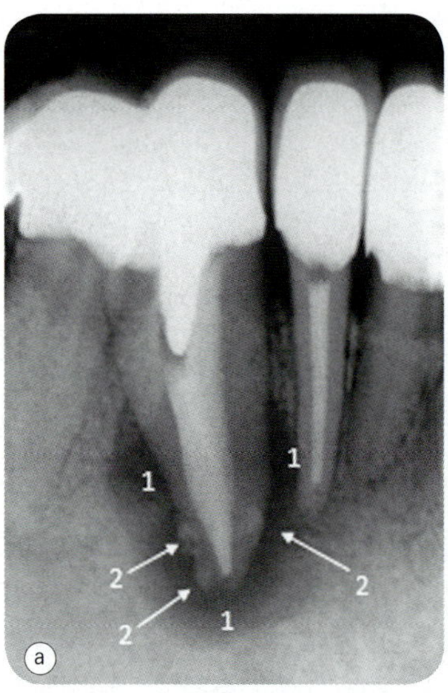


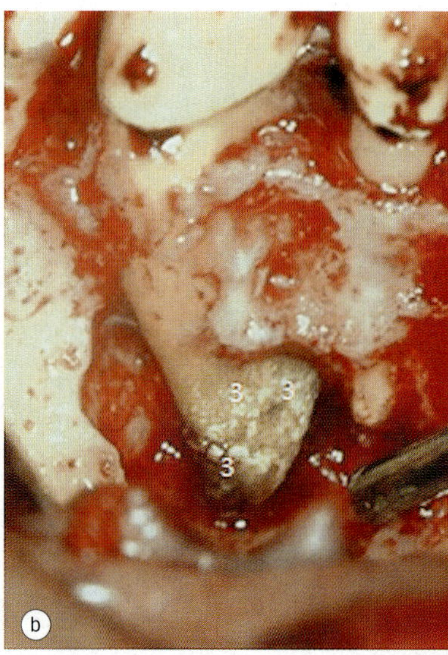


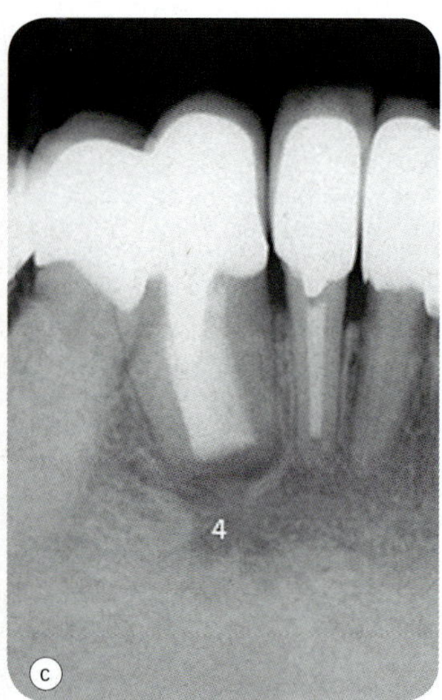


**Figure 11.68** - (**A**) There was presence of a fistula in Tooth #43 for a long time, later it was endodontically treated. The expected bone repair did not take place after the treatment, as the fistula remained, without decrease in the apical bone rarefaction (1), and presence of radiopaque areas in the apical third of the root (2). (**B**) The radiopaque areas observed in the image of Figure **A** (1) were salivary calculus (3), visualized by performing a surgical flap. (**C**) The treatment option was apicetomy, due to the presence of calculus in the lingual area of the root. Bone repair (4) 3 years after the radiograph shown in Figure A.

## 11.5 Lesions that Originated from Developmental Alterations, Tumors and Systemic Disturbances

### Supernumerary bone crypt

A bone crypt of a tooth in the initial stage of formation is a radiolucent area, delimited by a radiopaque halo. When this crypt occurs in its normal place, at the normal dental age, it is not difficult to diagnose. A crypt of a supernumerary, not in the natural period of germ formation, which can occur at the end of adolescence and in young adults, depending on its position, can be confused with a lateral root lesion, or even with apical periodontitis.

The next stage after the crypt formation, is the beginning of calcification. In case of doubt, radiographic control will show the stages of calcification (Fig. 11.69).

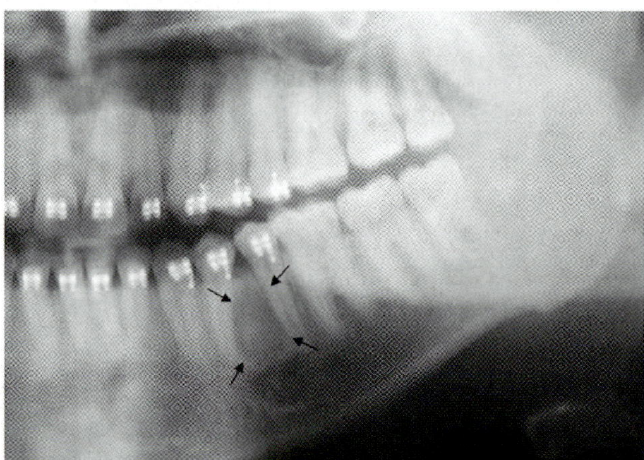

**Figure 11.69** - Bone crypt of a supernumerary in the beginning of calcification. Similar to cemento-osseous dysplasia in the beginning of the osteocementum formation phase.

## Lateral periodontal cyst

The lateral periodontal cyst is a developmental cyst that occurs due to multiplication of lateral epithelial tissue without pulp induction. This cyst does not have direct relationship with pulp necrosis, as does the lateral root cyst.

Radiographically, it is an image such as that of other cysts, with a radiolucent central area and clear margins, varying from hardly any, to well-defined limits, with or without a radiopaque halo. The position can be lateral towards the buccal or lingual regions, which appear to be more discreet in the radiograph. In the case of being more centralized, it can lengthen with growth, due to pressure from the neighboring teeth, frequently leading to root divergences.

Radiographically, the image of the lateral periodontal cyst, lateral root cyst (inflammatory) and of odontogenic keratocyst can be identical, however these three entities have different clinical and microscopic characteristics. This cyst can occur at any height of the lateral periodontal space. If the position is close to the cervical and middle third of the root, it is similar to other circumscribed lateral lesions. If it occurs close to the apical area, it can be confused with apical periodontitis.

When a lateral periodontal cyst occurs in soft tissues, it is called Adult's gingival cyst. Volumetric increase in gingival tissues can occur, in the form of tense tumefaction that can lead to adjacent bone absorption by pressure, which in this case, usually presents moderately imprecise limits. Depending on the position of this bone loss, the result can be similar to that of a lateral root lesion.

The lateral periodontal cyst may eventually become only a cavity, but a polycystic variant with the appearance of a bunch of grapes", with a multilocular radiographic aspect, and in these occurrences it is called a botryoid odontogenic cyst, and is of a slightly more aggressive nature (Fig. 11.70 to 11.72).



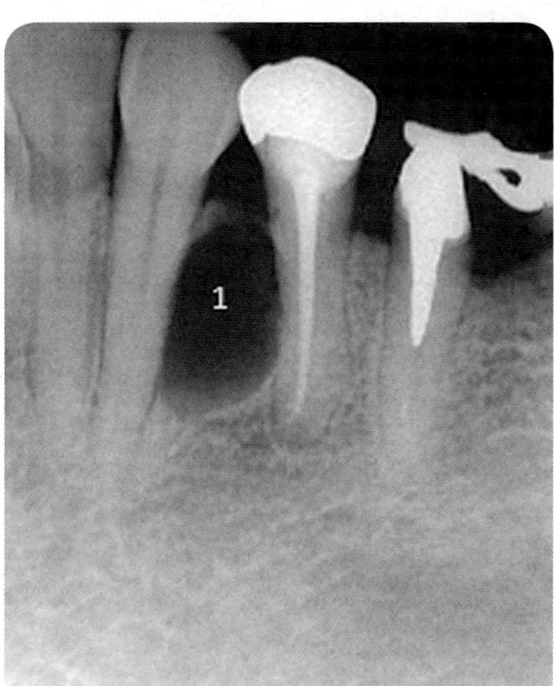


**Figure 11.70** - Lateral periodontal cyst (1) in tooth #33 extending until tooth #34.

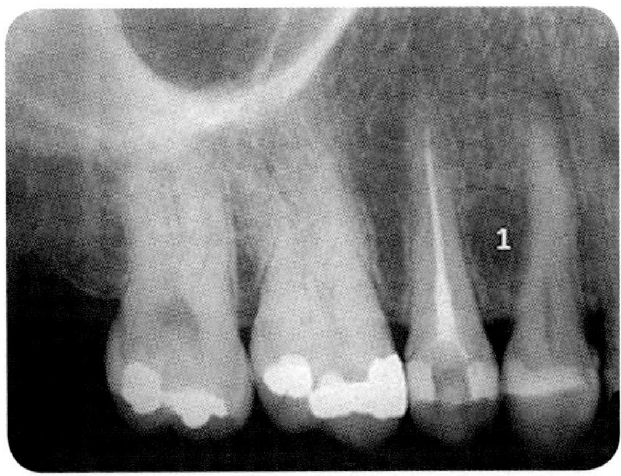


**Figure 11.71** - Adult's gingival cyst between teeth #15 and #14 with local volumetric increase in the gingival tissue and adjacent bone resorption by pressure, with moderately imprecise limits.

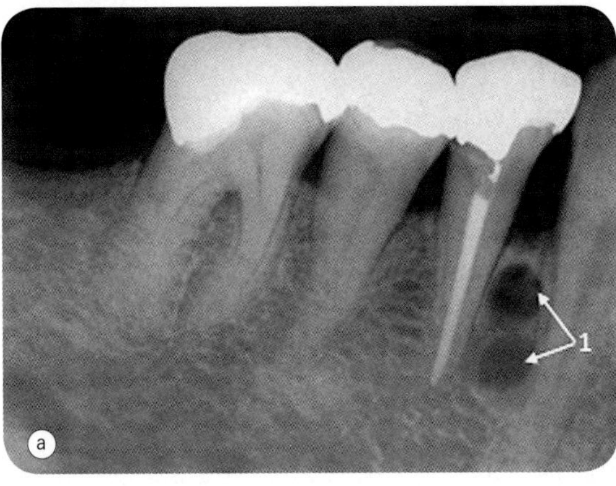


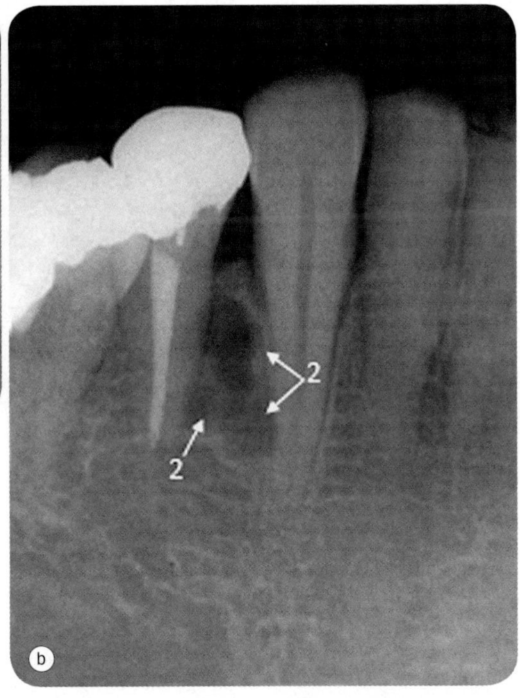


**Figure 11.72** - (**A**) Botryoid odontogenic cyst between teeth #43 and #44 in polycystic form. (**B**) The same case with change of the x-ray angulation shows the polycystic form with the appearance of "bunch of grapes."

## Dentigerous cyst

Dentigerous cyst is a developmental cyst that can occur in any retained tooth. Radiographically, there is an accentuated increase in the pericoronal space, place of origin, in a circumscribed form, with radiopaque halo defined by reagent bone cortical. The location can be restricted to the crown, in a centralized position or even lateral. It can also involve the root, starting from the crown.

The dentigerous cyst radiolucent area overlapping the lateral root region of a neighboring tooth can lead to doubts in the diagnosis of a lateral lesion. The possibility of overlapping exists in the apical area and it can be confused with apical periodontitis in a neighboring tooth. A more careful observation shows the pericoronal involvement (Fig. 11.73 to 11.75).

Another pathological entity called paradental cyst, of an inflammatory origin, is similar to a dentigerous cyst that occurs laterally, but it respects the pericementum space and the adjacent lamina dura. When it occurs the paradental cyst is more common in the distal region of the partially erupted mandibular third molars, but it can even be located in the buccal region of a permanent mandibular molar (particularly first molars) due to an uncommon defect of enamel development, that overlaps the cementum, called root bifurcation cyst, which is also inflammatory.

During the eruption of a tooth with a dentigerous cyst, the cyst can be left behind" and depending on its position, now outside the crown, it is capable of being close to the root apex, leading to doubts about the diagnosis.

Another condition is a result from endodontic treatment, or apical periodontitis, which can communicate with a dentigerous cyst of a neighboring tooth and infect it. In these cases the bone cortical of the cyst can be reabsorbed, masking the diagnosis.

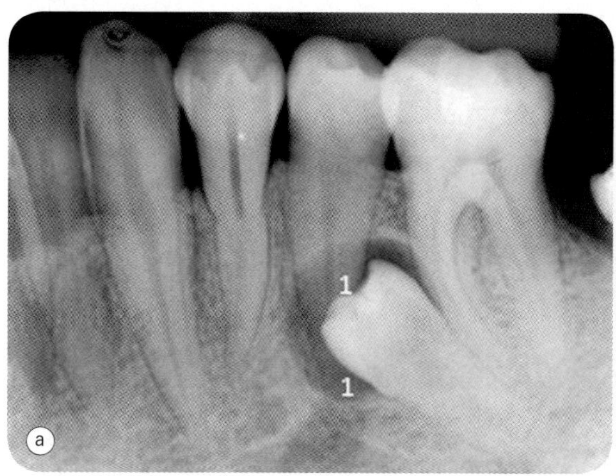


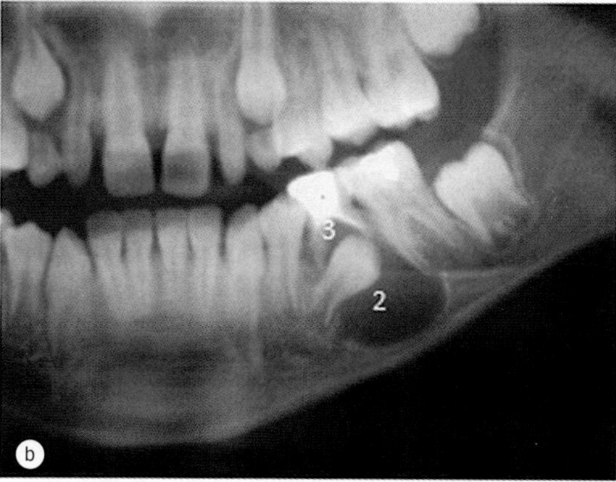


**Figure 11.73** - (**A**) Dentigerous cyst (1) of a supernumerary tooth close to the middle and apical third of the root of tooth #75. (**B**) Wide dentigerous cyst (2) in tooth #35 retained, below the apex of tooth #75 with endodontic treatment and rarefaction in the furcation area (3).

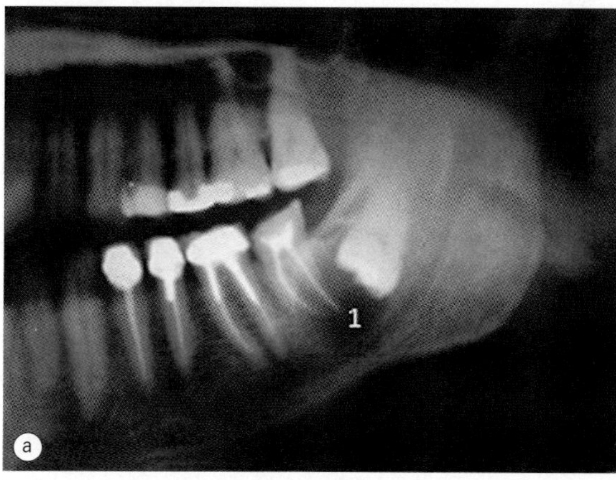


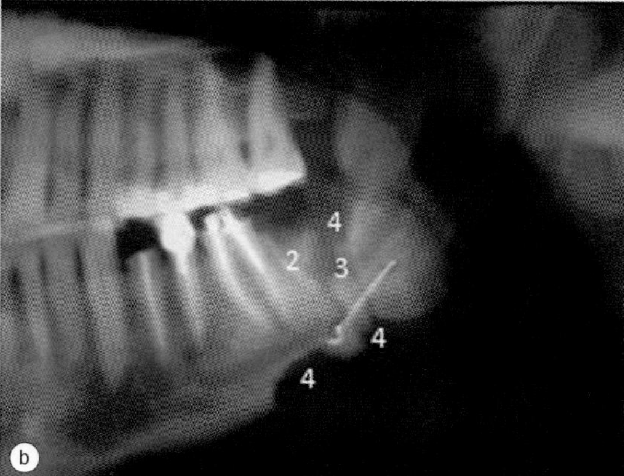


**Figure 11.74** - (**A**) Retained dentigerous cyst (1) in the crown of tooth #38. Loss of typical clearness at the margins of the cystic lesion due to partial decompression with endodontic treatment, and process of infection, similar to persistent apical periodontitis in tooth #37. Presence of local bone fragility. (**B**) During extraction of tooth #38, a mandibular fracture occurred (3) also with loss of tooth #37 (2), followed by pseudoarthrosis with severe detriment of local bone structures (4).

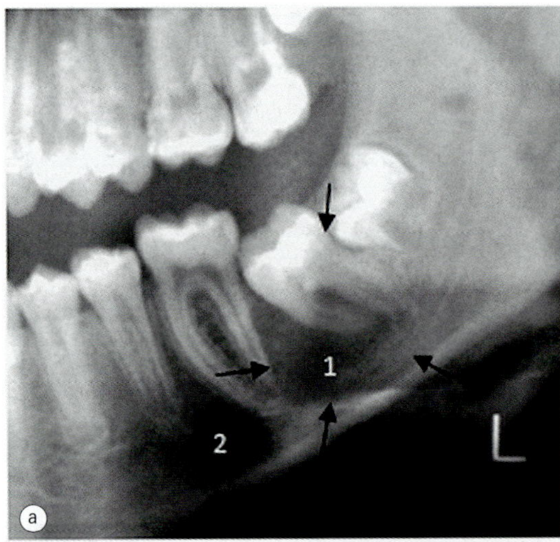


Figure 11.75 - (**A**) Retained dentigerous cyst (1) at the side of the crown of tooth #37, which led to a discreet and indefinite radiolucent area between tooth #37 and #36. (**B**) The longitudinal slice in the cone beam computed tomography shows the wide lesion, in contact (4) with the root of tooth #36. (**C-D**) The transversal slices of the cone beam computed tomography indicate connection of the cyst with the periodontal buccal space (3) of the crown of tooth #37. Submandibular fossa characterized in the panoramic radiograph and CBCT images (2).

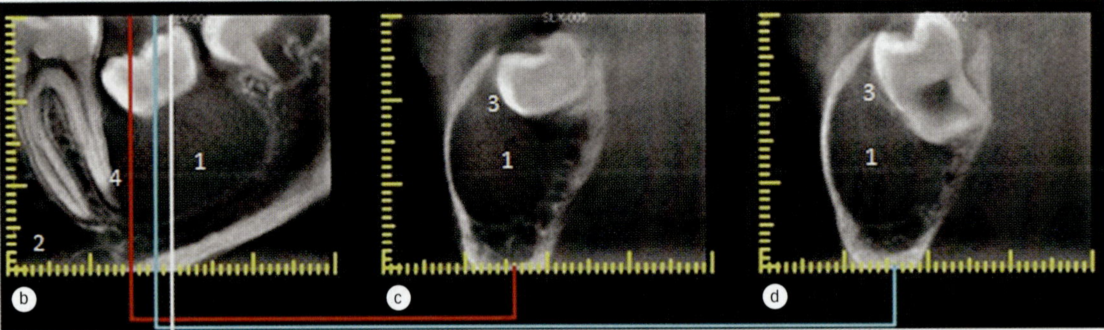


## Odontogenic keratocyst

The odontogenic keratocyst is an uncommon lesion that develops through cystic degeneration and liquefaction of the enamel organ, before calcification of the enamel or dentin of a dental germ occurs. It can be multilocular, similar to the ameloblastoma or unilocular.

When it is circumscribed, depending on its location, it has a well-defined aspect, usually with sclerotic limits. It can be similar to a lateral periodontal cyst, lateral root cyst, residual cyst or dentigerous cyst. The keratocyst can appear close to the apex of a tooth or it can be large enough to approach this area, and in these cases, it can be confused with apical periodontitis (Fig. 11.76).

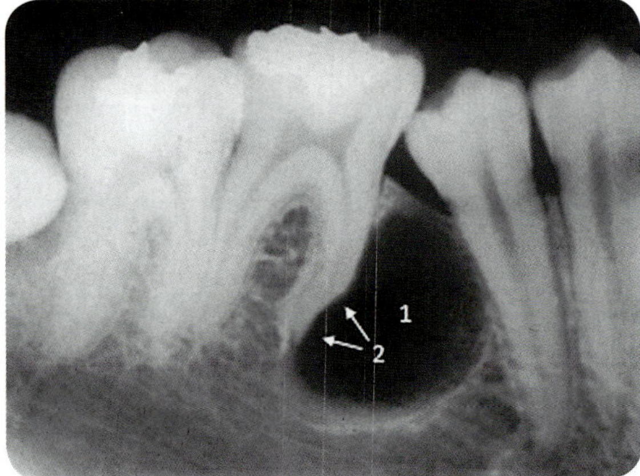


Figure 11.76 - Odontogenic keratocyst (1) between teeth #45 and #46, causing partial reabsorption (2) of the apical third of the root of tooth #46. Aspect similar to apical periodontitis of tooth #46 which, however, had positive pulp vitality.

## Nasopalatine cyst

The nasopalatine cyst is the most frequent of the non-odontogenic cysts, happening in about 1% of the population (an occurrence considered high) with three times higher incidence in men. It is believed to originate from embryonic tissue of the nasopalatine duct. The size of this cyst can vary from 6 mm in small lesions up to 6 cm or more in large ones, 1 to 2.5 cm being more common. When extensive, it can cause palatine, and in some cases also buccal crowning. It can occur in a high position, adjacent to the nasal fossa, or even low, close to the opening of the incisor foramen. It occurs in the median area of the maxilla, and in radiographs appears with a round, oval, or inverted pear shape when pressed by the roots of the maxillary central incisors. When its location is high and radiographically overlapping the area of the anterior nasal spine or the nasal septum, it can be heart-shaped. This shape can also occur, less frequently in the case of the formation of two independent cysts, one in each incisive canal. In reality, the duct system of the incisive canals consists of 4 ducts, two smaller (Scarpa) medium and two larger (Stenson) lateral ducts, that can go down separately or they can fuse before arriving at the incisor foramen.

This cyst can occur inside, or next to only one incisive canal, being moved sideways, increasing initial doubts about the diagnosis. It is a type of pathology that can be similar to apical periodontitis and lead to mistakes in diagnosis. Although it is usually asymptomatic, it can cause discreet symptoms. The bone cavity of this cyst is not closed, but communicates directly with the oral and nasal cavity. It could eventually drain into the oral cavity by a fistulous pathway caused by previous surgical intervention or by embryonic remains of the nasopalatine duct. The drainage can be constant or intermittent, discreet to the point of not being easily detected, and a fine probe is indicated to confirm it. The occurrence of drainage limits the size, stabilizing the growth of the nasopalatine duct cyst.

In the case of doubt between the presentation of a bulky incisor foramen or the presence of the nasopalatine duct cyst, a diameter larger than 6 mm tends to indicate the presence of the pathological process. The lateral margins are usually clear, with apparent cortical in the cyst and in some foramens. The superior and inferior margins are usually clearer in the cysts. Oval or irregular radiolucencies with diffuse margins are more likely to be a wide incisor foramen. Round radiolucencies with all margins defined have a greater possibility of being a cyst.

The pulp vitality test is important in the diagnosis because this pathology does not originate from pulp necrosis. A cone beam computed tomography exam show that the cystic area do not have direct connection with the teeth in the area.

When the cystic formation occurs in the area of the incisor foramen opening, it presents either no radiographic lines, or discreet lines establishing the crowning of soft tissue in the palatine area corresponding to the blooming of the foramen, and is called an incisor papilla cyst; one that occurs rarely (Fig. 11.77 to 11.80).

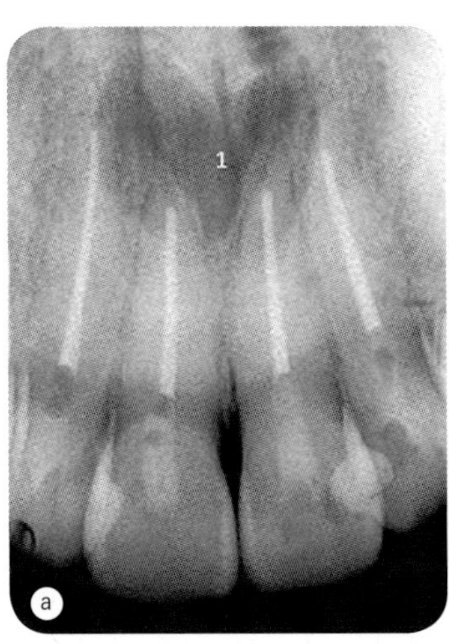


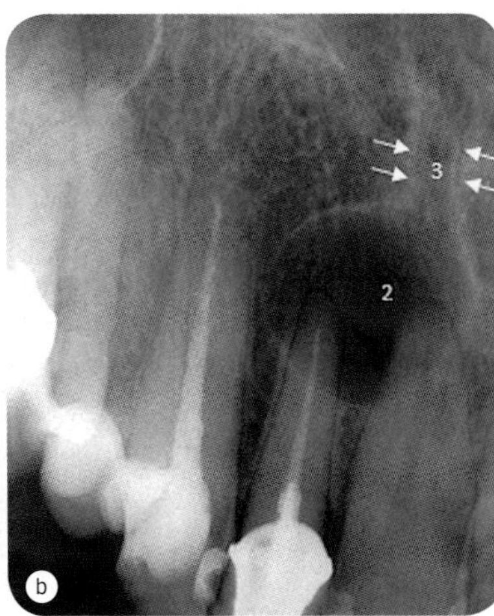


**Figure 11.77** - (**A**) A heart-shaped nasopalatine cyst above the apexes of the maxillary incisors, and for this reason, no endodontic treatment was necessary. (**B**) Nasopalatine cyst projected into the apical area of teeth #12 and #11.

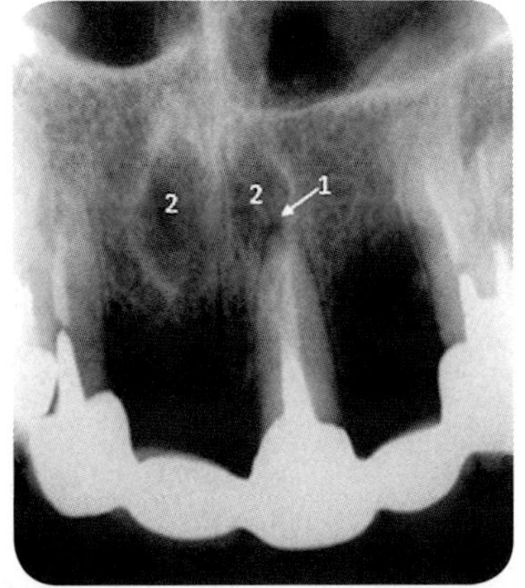


**Figure 11.78** - Double nasopalatine cyst (2) – in independent canals, with the larger heart-shaped cyst on the right side. On the left side the duct cyst overlaps a discreet apical lesion in the apex of tooth #21.

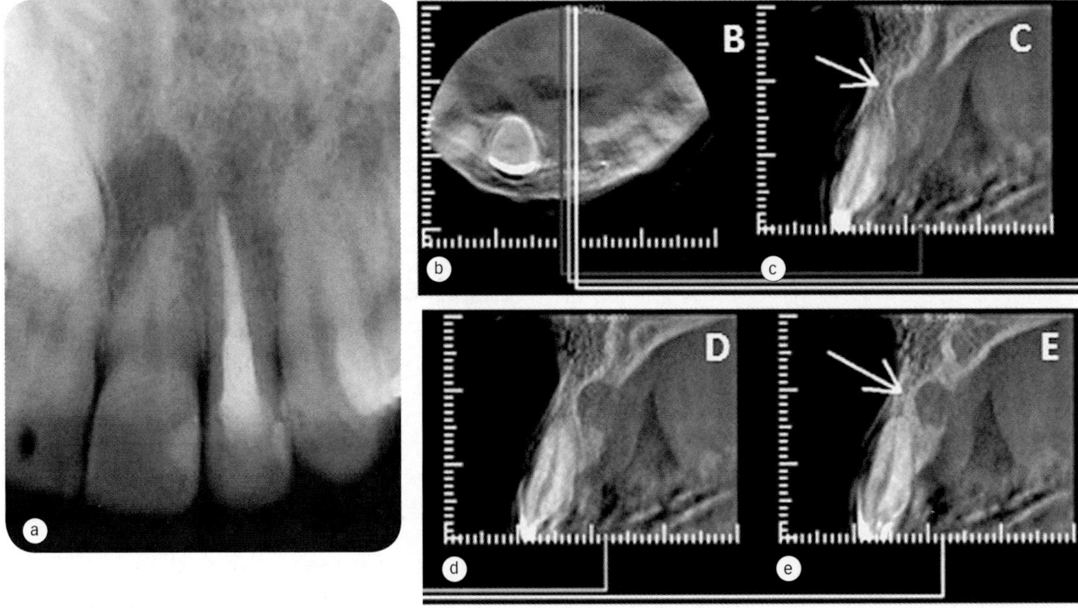


**Figure 11.79** - (**A**) Nasopalatine cyst above the apex of tooth #21, moved to the left side in the periapical radiograph, similar to apical periodontitis. (**B**) the axial slice of cone beam computed tomography confirms the displacement of the lesion to the left. (**C**) Transversal slice in cone beam computed tomography shows involvement of the left incisive canal with the cyst. (**D**, **E**) Cyst without contact with the root of tooth #21.

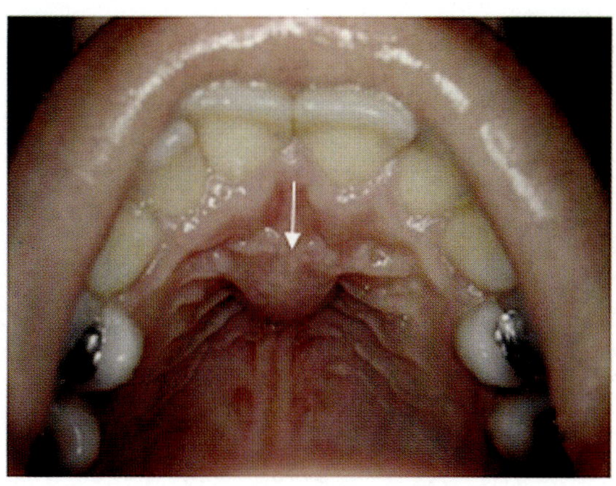

Figure 11.80 - Incisor papilla cyst with palatine crowning in the central area of the palate, corresponding to the opening of the incisor foramen. In this patient it presented in a high position. There was no radiographic evidence of volumetric increase of the incisor foramen.

### Median palatal cyst

This developmental cyst is rare and occurs, as the name suggests, in the median area of the palate, in a posterior position to the incisive canal, and in the conventional radiograph, higher than the nasopalatine cyst. Due to this high position, in some situations it may not appear in a periapical radiograph, but sometimes it does appear in an occlusal radiograph.

In a case of a patient with a low nasal fossa and formation of the cyst in the anterior position of the palate, an increased vertical angulation, enables this cyst to be radiographically projected onto the dental apexes. It can be confused with the nasopalatine cyst, if the anatomical position is not well-observed. Palatine crowning is usually present (Fig. 11.81).

### Solitary bone cyst

This type of cyst can also be called a traumatic bone cyst or hemorrhagic cyst, among other designations. In reality, in spite of the name, it is not a true cyst, because it does not have the typical epithelial covering that characterizes cysts. Although of uncertain origin, one of the theories is that it is caused by some type of trauma type that leads to hemorrhage into the bone trabeculae, with a clot forming an internal hematoma that is not organized, so it dissolves, forming an empty or blood-filled cavity. There are few reports of this lesion in the maxilla, but a significant prevalence is shown in the mandible, in patients between 10 and 20 years of age. This lesion rarely appears in children under the age of 5, and individuals over 35 years of age.

It is found during a routine radiographic exam, presenting an image of a well-delimited lesion with high and low density margins, sometimes located in a cavity, in which case it is imprecise. Usually the margins are a little irregular, with some flat walls or inverted concavities, showing no growth by hydric pressure, which is typical of the true cysts, although these characteristics can occur in other lesions. When it involves roots, it seldom requires removal, or causes reabsorption, but preserves the roots. It is common for the lamina dura to be saved, establishing an interdigitation image with the appearance of "glove fingers", as if it were hugging the tooth, without causing pulp necrosis. The radiographic aspect is highly suggestive but not conclusive. Depending on the amount of reabsorbed buccal-lingual trabecular bone, this lesion can be radiolucent in a very intense or discreet way, in some cases even similar to a large trabecula.

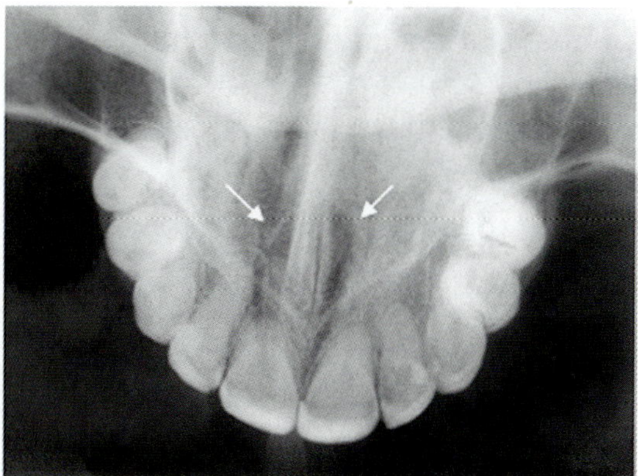

Figure 11.81 - Median palatine cyst similar to the nasopalatine cyst, but higher and in a posterior position.

In most cases, there are no signs and symptoms. In 20% of cases, a moderate painless, local volumetric increase occurs. Although not common, pain and paresthesia can eventually be present.

The indicated treatment is aspiration followed by biopsy in the same section, although it is difficult to collect material. If the cavity is empty, which occurs in 1/3 of cases, or filled with liquid in 2/3 of the occurrences, the chances of it being a solitary bone cyst increase. The treatment is usually the same as procedure initially followed for diagnosis; in other words, opening for surgical exploration, liquid aspiration, if there is any, followed by curettage to obtain material (scarce) for the histopathological exam, trying not to cause bleeding inside the cavity, and finally, suturing. After this, radiographic control should be done in order to verify bone repair, which it is usually fast and could occur in 6 months, even in large lesions.

Solitary bone cysts can be large or small and close to a tooth, in which case they are similar to apical periodontitis, and without doubt, they are much commoner than the literature relates. This is due to the difficulty of obtaining of appropriate material for histopathological exams (Fig. 11.82 to 11.85).

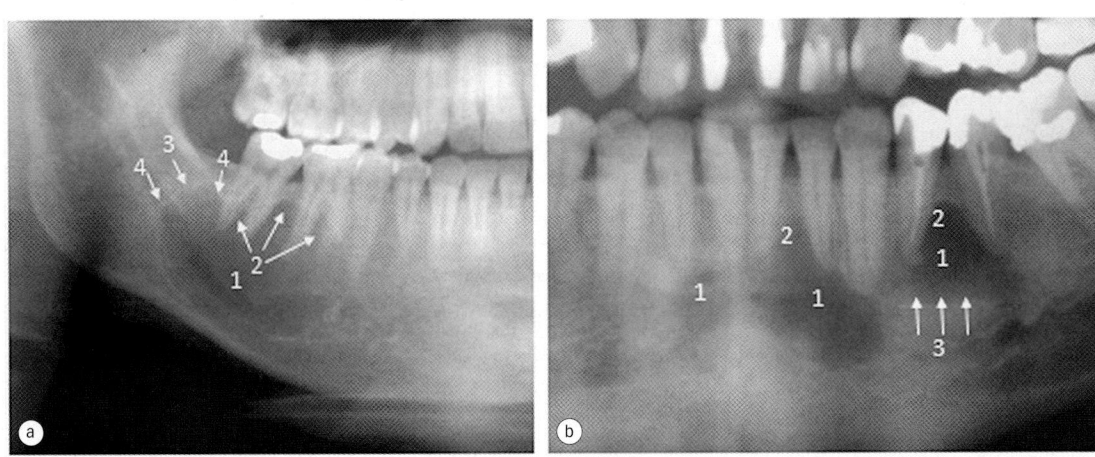


**Figure 11.82** - (**A**) solitary bone cyst (1) close to the apexes of teeth #45, 46 and 47, following the root outlines (2), with small continuation of the flat distal wall (3) and others with discreet reverse concavities, towards the interior (4). (**B**) Solitary bone cyst (1) with double image, extending into the complete area from tooth #35 to tooth 42, also with a flat wall (3).

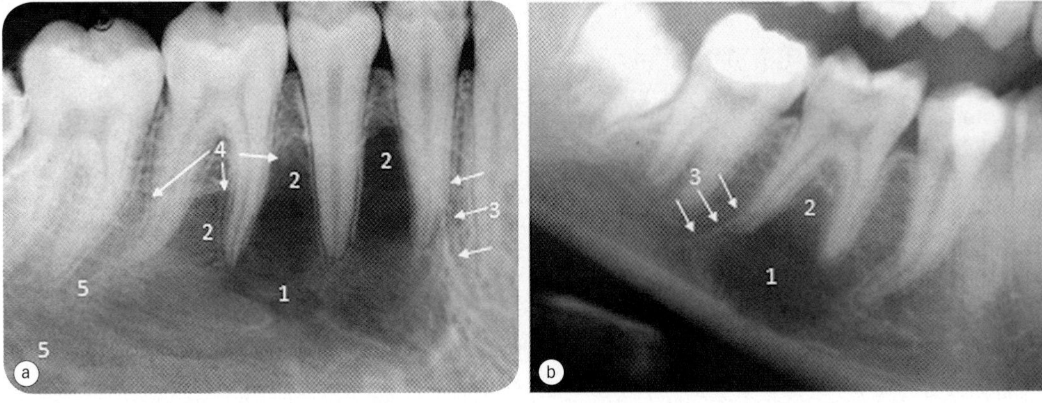


**Figure 11.83** - (**A**) Solitary bone cyst (1) close to the apexes of teeth #44, #45, #46 and #47, following the root outlines (2), with some clear margins and others indefinite (5), with a flat mesial (3) and superior wall, in the area of tooth #46, with discreet reverse concavity, towards the interior (4). (**B**) Solitary bone cyst (1) between the roots (2) of tooth #46, similar to apical periodontitis, with a flat distal wall (3) and partially defined and discrete irregular margins.

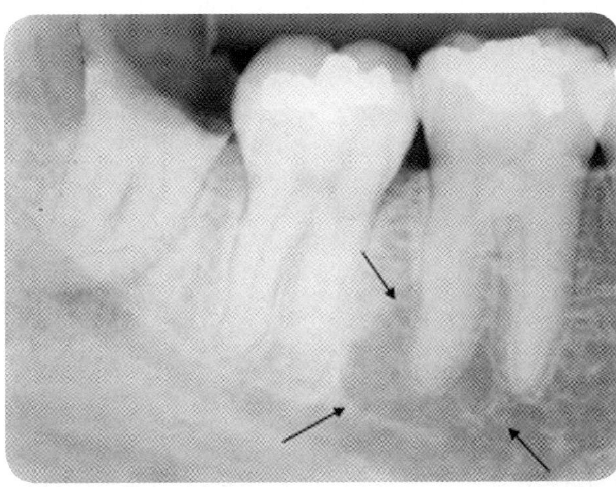

**Figure 11.84** - Solitary bone cyst involving the distal root of tooth #46, with an atypical, round aspect, similar to that of a wide medullary space or to apical periodontitis. Cortical of the apical lamina dura preserved.



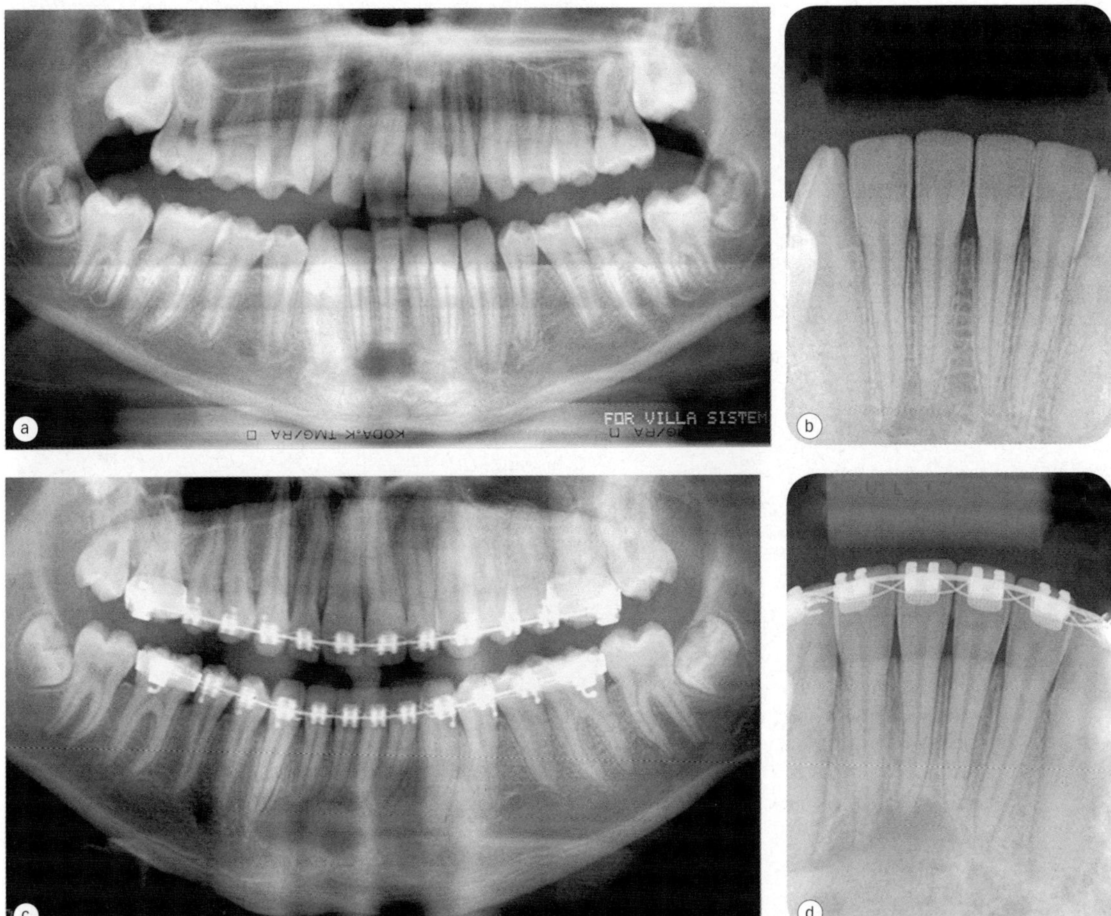


**Figure 11.85** - (**A**) Panoramic radiography showing radiolucent area on the periapex of teeth #41-42, that was considered as radiographic device (December/2004). (**B**) Periapical radiography of tooth # 42 showed small radiolucent area below of the apexes that seemed to be normal (December/2004). (**C**) Panoramic radiography showing on periapical region of teeth # 31-42 large well circumscribed radiolucent image (April, 2007). (**D**) Periapical radiography with large well circumscribed radiolucent area on teeth # 31-42 (April, 2007).

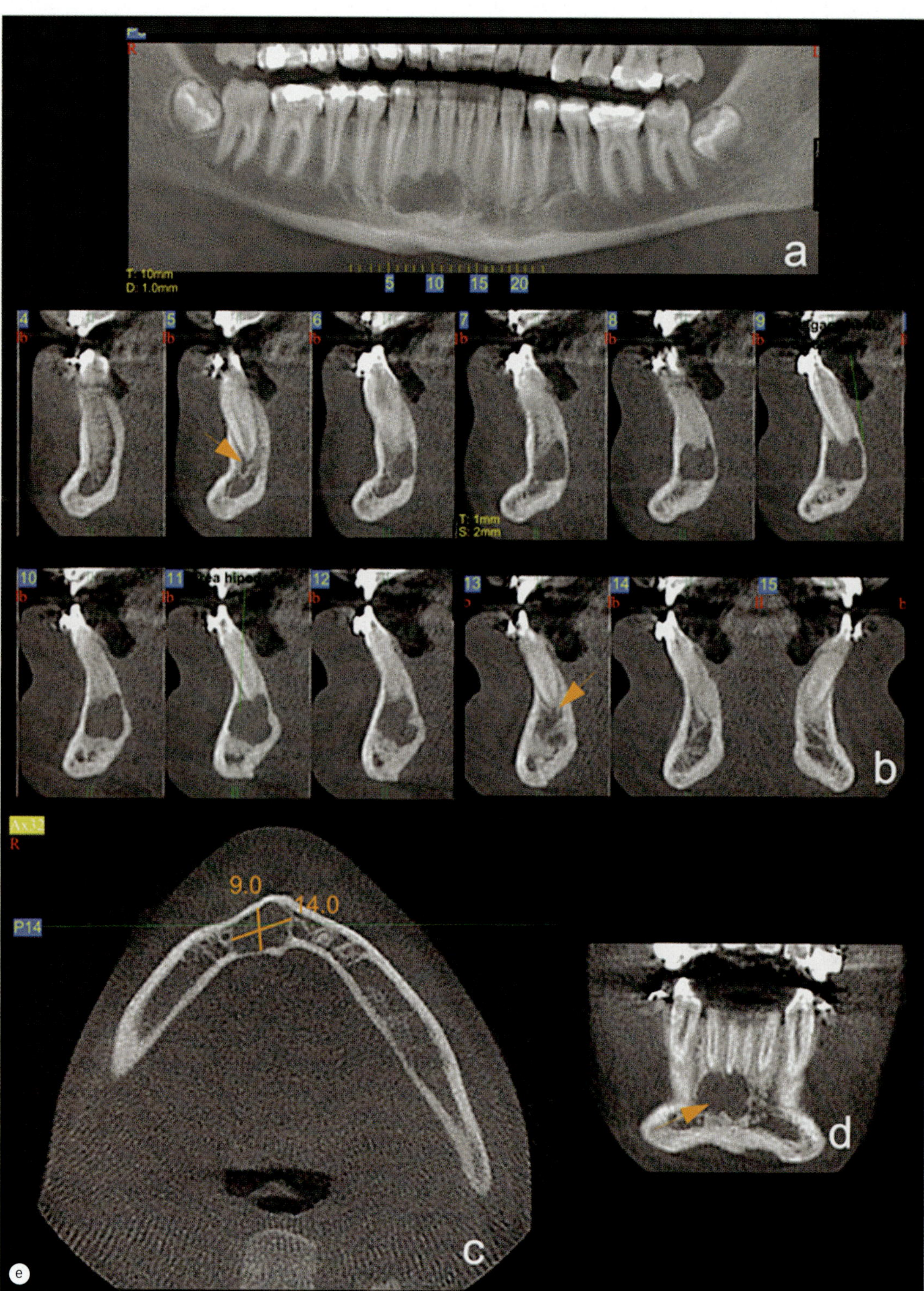


Figure 11.85 - (E) Cone beam computed tomography, A. Panoramic image, B. Transaxiais; C. Axial; D. Coronal.

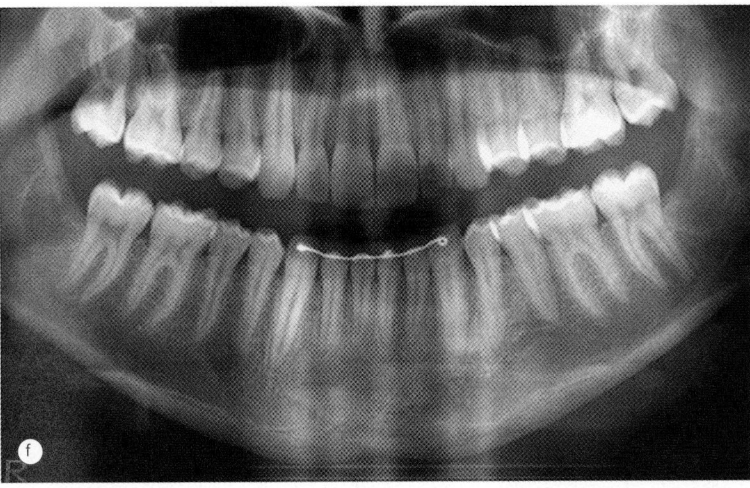

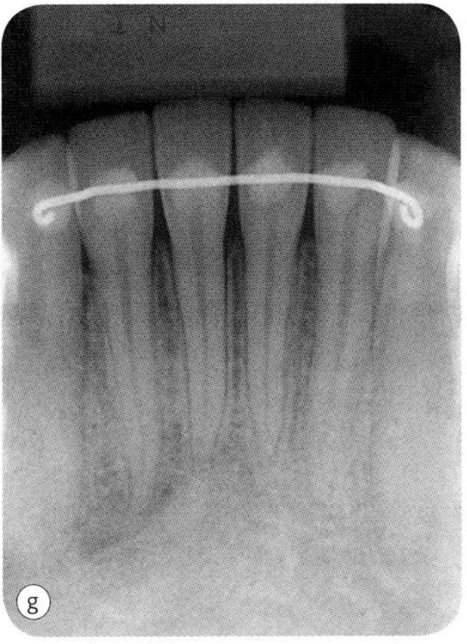

**Figure 11.85** - (**F**) Panoramic image showing normal aspect on periapical area of teeth # 31-42, 6 months after surgery. (**G**) Periapical radiography presenting normal aspect on periapical area of teeth #31-42, remaining only small radiolucid adjacent area to the apex of tooth #41, 6 months after surgery.

## Cemento-osseous dysplasia

Cemento-osseous dysplasia now denominated bone dysplasia by the World Health Organization (WHO) are fibro-bone lesions that usually present cementoid tissue close to the bone. These dysplasias are limited to the gnathic bones leading to the belief that they originated in the periodontal ligament. The etiopathology of this lesion is still obscure, however it is possibly of reactive or dysplastic origin. Some of these lesions can rupture and expand the cortical.

It concerns a group of 4 entities:

1. Periapical cemento-osseous dysplasia (Periapical bone dysplasia)
2. Localized cemento-osseous dysplasia (Focal bone dysplasia)
3. Florid cemento-osseous dysplasia (Florid bone dysplasia)
4. Familial gigantiform cementoma

These lesions occur in three phases:

1. Phase 1: bone destruction with radiolucent image of different widths
2. Phase 2: radiolucent image of bone destruction together with radiopaque image of osteocementum formation starting from the center
3. Phase 3: radiopaque image of more intense formation of osteocementum, but still with a radiolucent line at the margins that tend to decrease with the passage of time.

## Periapical cemento-osseous dysplasia

Periapical cementum-osseous dysplasia occurs mainly in the apical area of the mandibular incisors and less frequently in other teeth. It usually affects a group of teeth, or only one. It has a high predilection for women (14:1) black persons between the ages of 30 to 50, it is asymptomatic (when it does not come in contact with the external environment) and is usually discovered in routine radiographic exams, or because of other symptoms.

This lesion goes through the three phases previously described. When it is in the initial stage (phase 1) it can be identical to apical periodontitis, and lead to mistakes in diagnosis and unnecessary endodontic treatment. The pulp vitality test is fundamental. In addition to this, radiographic control is necessary as a complement to diagnosis, which will characterize the lesion when it enters the mixed phase (phase 2), with mineralization starting from the center, and an appearance similar to that of "cotton clots". In the final phase, (phase 3) the mineralization is more intense, but there continues to be a radiolucent line at the margins, which decreases with time. The maximum size of this lesion is usually limited to 1 cm. The diagnosis is clinical and radiographic. Biopsy is not usually indicated, because it exposes the mineralized bone tissues with low vascularization, which can become necrosed, isolated and enter a chronic state of osteomyelitis, with acute outbreaks. The low local vascularization leads to a poor response to antibiotic therapy. Endodontic treatment itself can infect the apical area with dysplasia and lead to a condition of osteomyelitis of varying degrees of intensity, with all its signs and symptoms. In this case the apical area can be exposed to the outside environment, which is difficult to repair (Fig. 11.86 to 11.88).

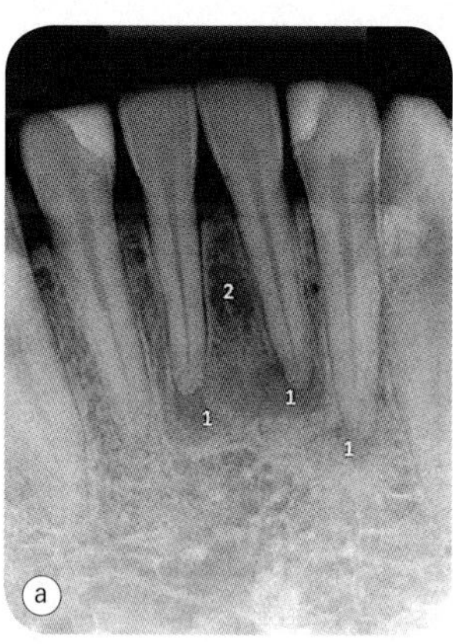


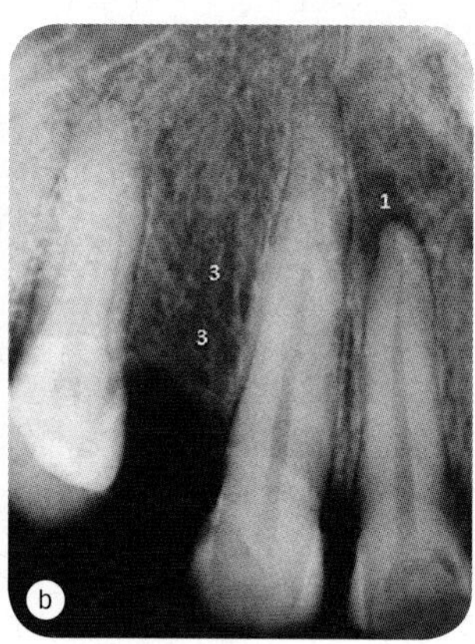


**Figure 11.86** - (**A**) Periapical cemento-osseous dysplasia (1) in phase 1 in the apical area of teeth #32 (discreet), #31 and #41. It could be confused with apical periodontitis due to the apical rarefactions and presence of local trauma, because teeth #32 and #42 suffered crown fractures. Thin anatomical area (2), with variation of normality. (**B**) Periapical cemento-osseous dysplasia in the apical area of tooth #12, uncommon location, identical to apical periodontitis. Additional radiographic exams also revealed the presence of this dysplasia in the apical area of the mandibular incisors. Area of bone repair (3) in the extraction area of tooth #14.

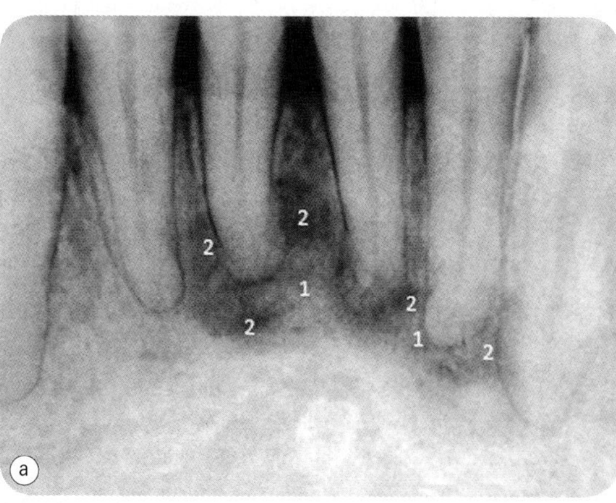


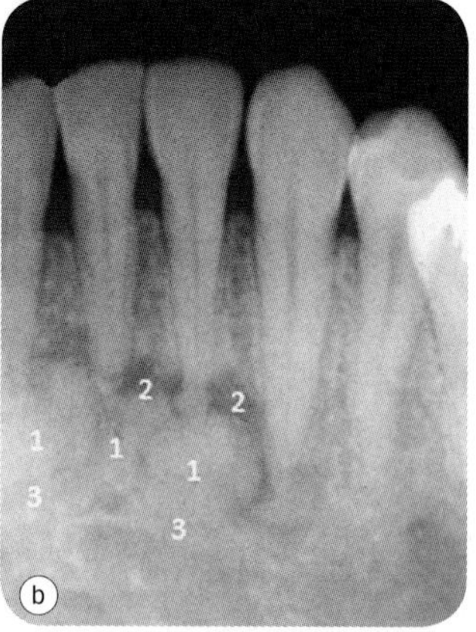


**Figure 11.87** - (**A**) Periapical cemento-osseous dysplasia in phase 2 in the apical area of incisors #32, #31, #41, with osteocalcification, starting from the center, with an appearance similar to that of "cotton clots" (1) with diffuse margins and with wide strip of bone rarefaction delimited by an indefinite outline (2). (**B**) Periapical cemento-osseous dysplasia in phase 2, close to phase 3, in the apical area of teeth #33, #32, #31, #41, with osteocalcification starting from the center, and an appearance similar to that of "cotton clots" (1), now with a more intense band of radiopacity and rarefaction (2) than in the previous case, mainly at the inferior margin (3), almost obliterated.

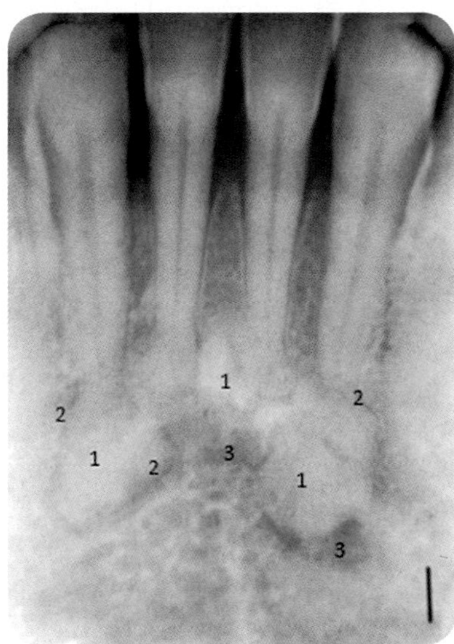

**Figure 11.88** - Periapical cemento-osseous dysplasia in phase 3 in the apical area of the mandibular incisors, with osteocalcification starting from the center, with an appearance similar to that of "cotton clots" (1), with more intense radiopacity than the neighboring bone tissue. Fine external line of delimitation (2), denser and thicker in some areas. (3)

## Focal cemento-osseous dysplasia

The name "Focal" indicates a single affected area. Similar to periapical cemento-osseous dysplasia, it goes through three phases, and is more prevalent in the age group between 40 and 50 years. But, differently from the previous dysplasia, it more frequently occurs in men, with only a slight predilection for the black race.

When it is in phase 1, or at the beginning of phase 2, it can be confused with apical periodontitis. The diagnosis and the care required are the same as for periapical cemento-osseous dysplasia. The maximum size of this lesion is usually limited to 1.5 cm.

A panoramic radiograph is indicated to verify whether there is incidence of it in other areas, and is so, to treat it in the same way as for florid or periapical dysplasia (Fig. 11.89 and 11.90).



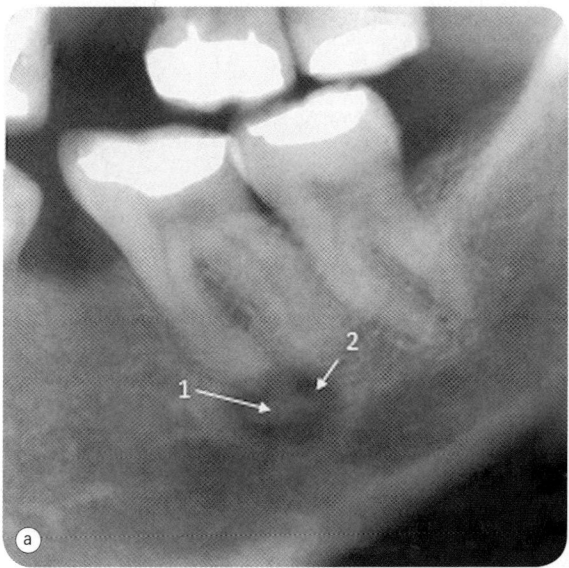

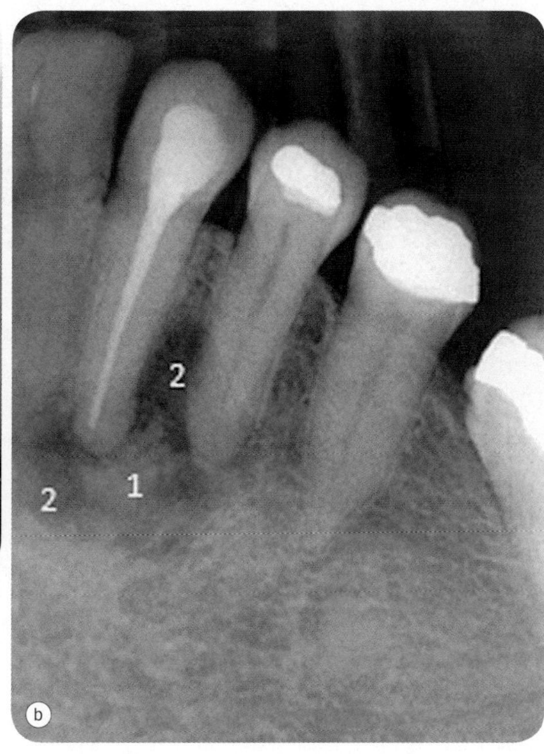

**Figure 11.89** - (**A**) Focal cemento-osseous dysplasia in the beginning of phase 2, in the apical area of the mesial root of tooth #46, similar to apical periodontitis, particularly when it was in phase 1. Mineralization starting from the center (1), with radiolucent margin (2). (**B**) Focal cemento-osseous dysplasia in phase 2, in the apical area of tooth #43. Due to being similar to apical periodontitis, the tooth was inadvertently submitted to endodontic treatment. Presence of mineralization starting from the center (1), with wide radiolucent margin (2).

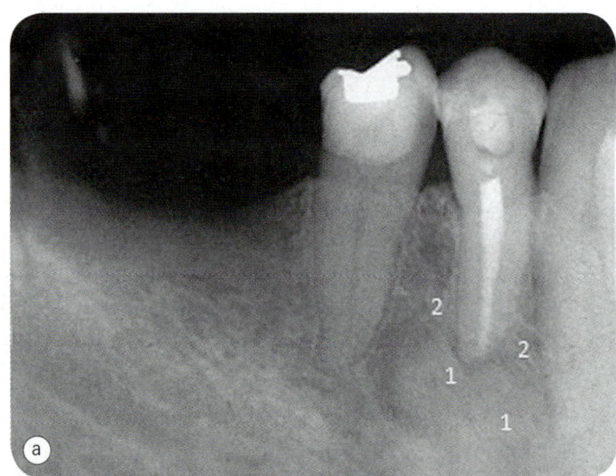


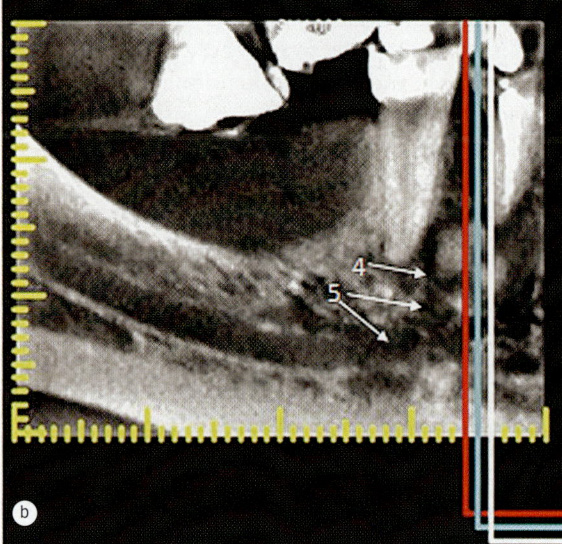


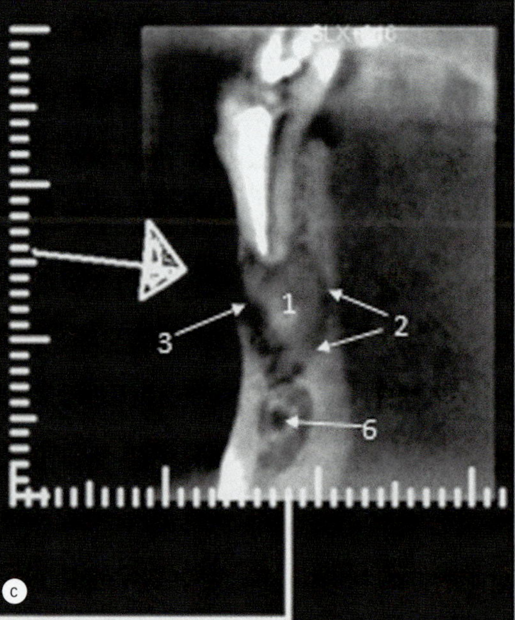


**Figure 11.90** - (**A**) Focal cemento-osseous dysplasia in phase 3 in the apical area of tooth #44, with mineralization (1) starting from the center, with more intense radiopacity than the neighboring bone tissue and with a fine external line of delimitation (2). (**B-C**) Slices of the cone beam computed tomography of the same patient as shown in the previous periapical radiograph, revealing mineralization (1) starting from the center, with a thicker delimitation line than the line visible in the periapical radiograph, rupturing the buccal cortical (3), this image is not the mental foramen (4), subsequently out of the cut area, following the continuity of the mandibular canal (5). Presence of the mandibular incisive canal (6).

## Florid cemento-osseous dysplasia (florid bone dysplasia)

Similar to the previous cases of cemento-osseous dysplasia, it goes through three phases, but it is wider. The name "Florid" was given with the intention of indicating extensive lesions dispersed throughout several places, often symmetrical in opposed quadrants of the dental arches. As in the case of periapical cemento-osseous dysplasia, there is a high predilection for women of the black race between the ages of 30 and 50 years.

When it is in phase 1 or right at the beginning of phase 2, it can be confused with apical periodontitis. The pulp vitality test, radiographic control and the necessary care are auxiliary diagnostic resources. In florid dysplasia, there is a greater chance of the lesion communicating with the outside environment, infection and osteomyelitis setting in with various degrees of aggressiveness. A panoramic radiograph is also indicated as an additional diagnostic resource, because it reveals its width in several places of the dental arch (Fig. 11.91 and 11.92).

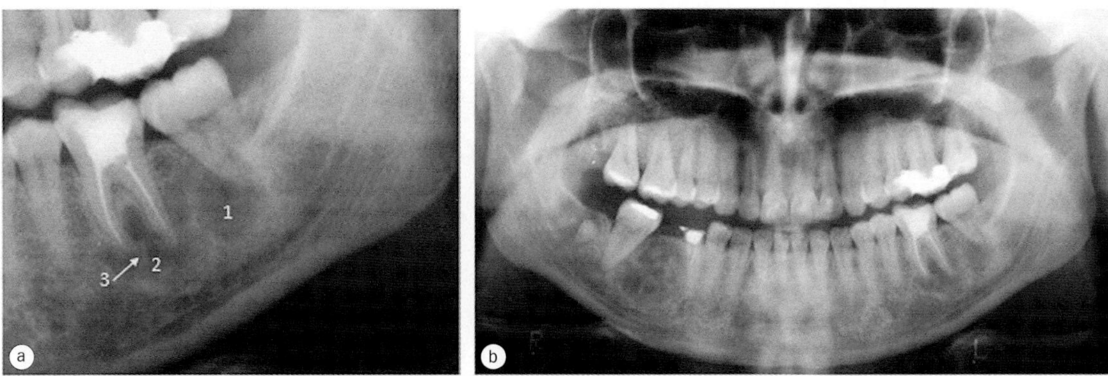


**Figure 11.91** - (**A**) Florid cemento-osseous dysplasia in phase 1 (1) in the apical area of teeth #36 and in the beginning of phase 2 (2) in the area of tooth #36, with mineralization starting from the center (3), close to the apex and with radiolucent margins. (**B**) The same as the previous case of florid cemento-osseous dysplasia, showing the bilateral involvement in other areas of the dental arch.

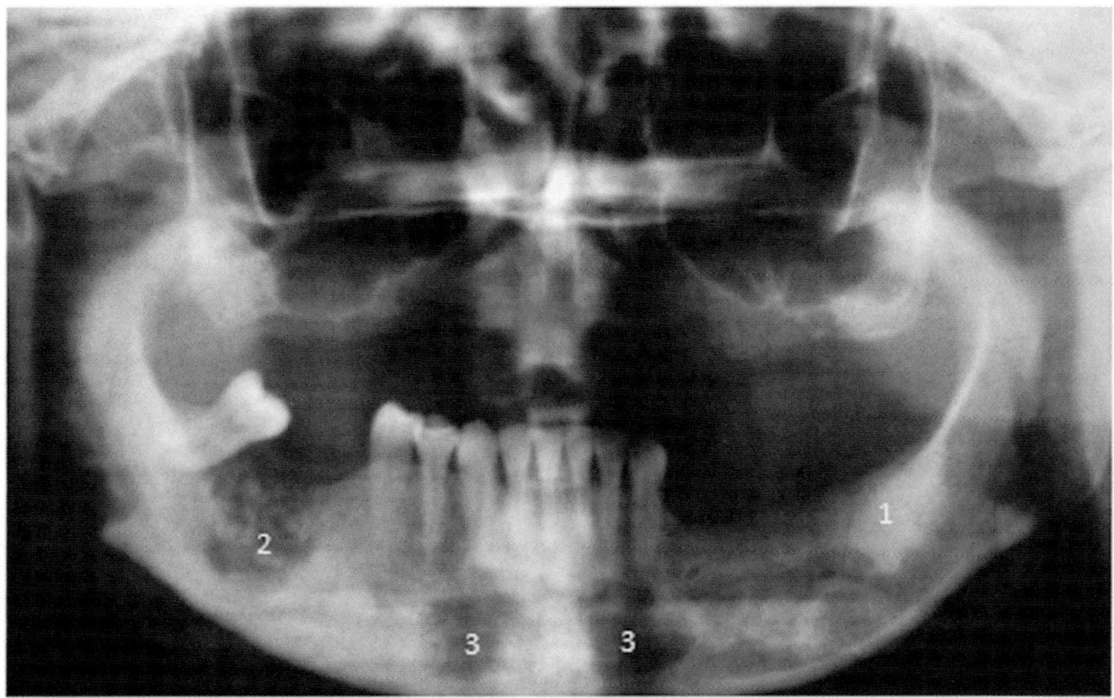


**Figure 11.92** - Florid cemento-osseous dysplasia in phase 3, with an area of high radiopacity in the area of the third molar #38, confirmed by a periapical radiograph. Image visualized in the area of teeth #46 and #47 are not mixed areas of the florid dysplasia but of the triturated bone gráft (2) inserted surgically in the place, and the mental area (3) as donor area bilaterally, observed in the postoperative radiographs. Previously to the tissue removal from the area of teeth #46 and #47, a great area of dysplasia, a yellowed osteocementum block in an isolated form, infected and in contact with the buccal environment, with the presence of fistula, resistant to antibiotic therapy. A typical case of chronic osteomyelitis due to the infection of the areas of osteocementum dysplasia that came into contact with the buccal environment.

## Familial gigantiform cementoma

The familial gigantiform cementoma has been described as the florid cemento-osseous dysplasia, but later it was considered a different entity, because it presents some particular clinical characteristics. There is no predilection for sex, it almost always affects caucasians and it seems to be a hereditary syndrome, usually with autossomal dominant inheritance. It goes through the three phases of maturation of the cemento-osseous dysplasia already described. In some cases, it can be wide and exuberant, leading to asymmetry of the dental arches and accentuated facial asymmetry.

Analyzing a periapical radiograph in isolation can lead to it being confused with apical periodontitis. The panoramic radiograph is indicated as an auxiliary diagnostic resource, because it reveals its width and distribution (Fig. 11.93 and 11.94).

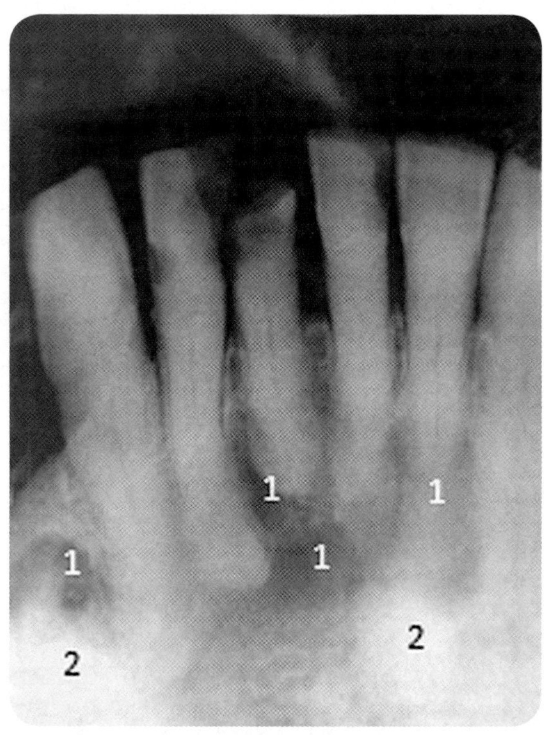


**Figure 11.93** - The area below the mandibular incisors, with an extensive bone rarefaction (1) below the mandibular incisors, up to the distal region of tooth #43, with sclerotic formations (2) higher density than the adjacent bone in a case of familial gigantiform cementoma.

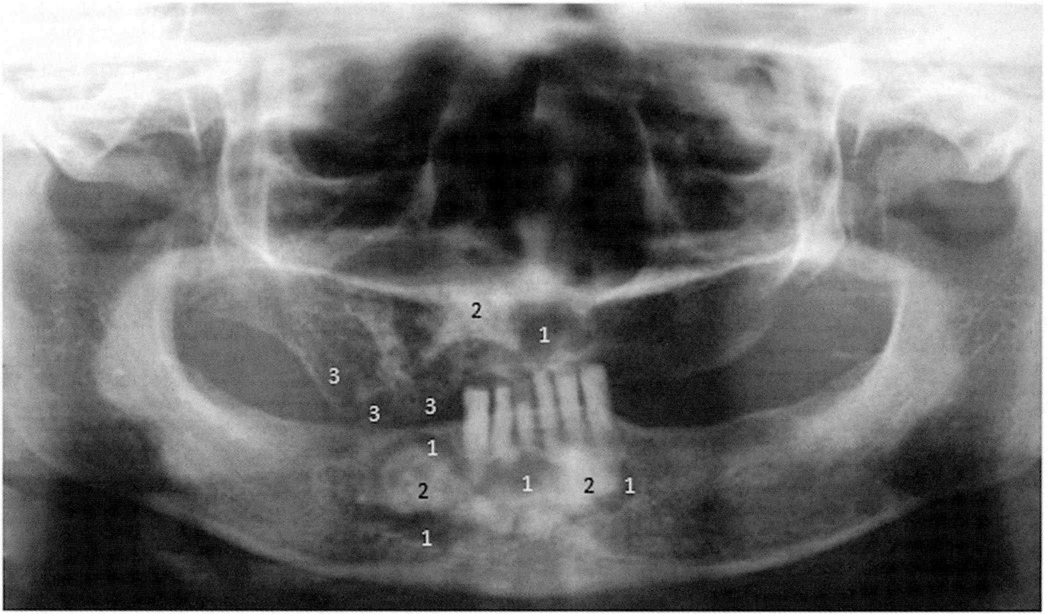


**Figure 11.94** - The same as the previous case of familial gigantiform cementoma, in addition to the areas of bone rarefactions (1) and sclerotic formations (2), an accentuated expansion is observed in the area to the right of the maxilla (3).

## Ameloblastoma

Ameloblastoma is one of the many types of odontogenic tumors that affect the maxilla. When they begin to form, and are of reduced size and close to dental apexes, they can be confused with apical periodontitis.

It is an aggressive lesion, with radiolucent image with margins varying from imprecise to clear ones, capable either of forming sclerotic radiopaque halos, or not. It can be multilocular and unilocular, and the latter causes more doubt at the initial phase of diagnosis. This lesion has slow or fast growth; it frequently causes divergence of the dental roots, and is capable of leading to resorption. It causes lateral expansion, which can initially pass unnoticed. Teeth respond positively to the pulp vitality test. Surgical intervention is indicated and the definitive diagnosis is performed through the histopathological exam. In lesions considered small, excisional biopsy should be performed to enable evaluation based on microscopic analysis, without the need for a further intervention, thus increasing the safety margin, if the first surgical intervention was sufficient for diagnosing the case (Fig. 11.95 and 11.96).



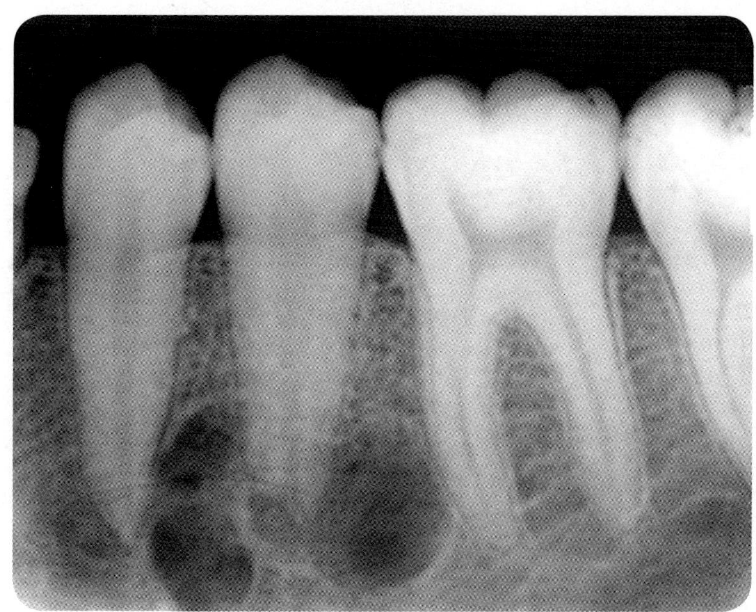

**Figure 11.95** - Ameloblastoma with multilocular radiolucent images of "soap bubbles" below and beside the apex of tooth #35, extending to the mesial region of teeth #36 and #34.

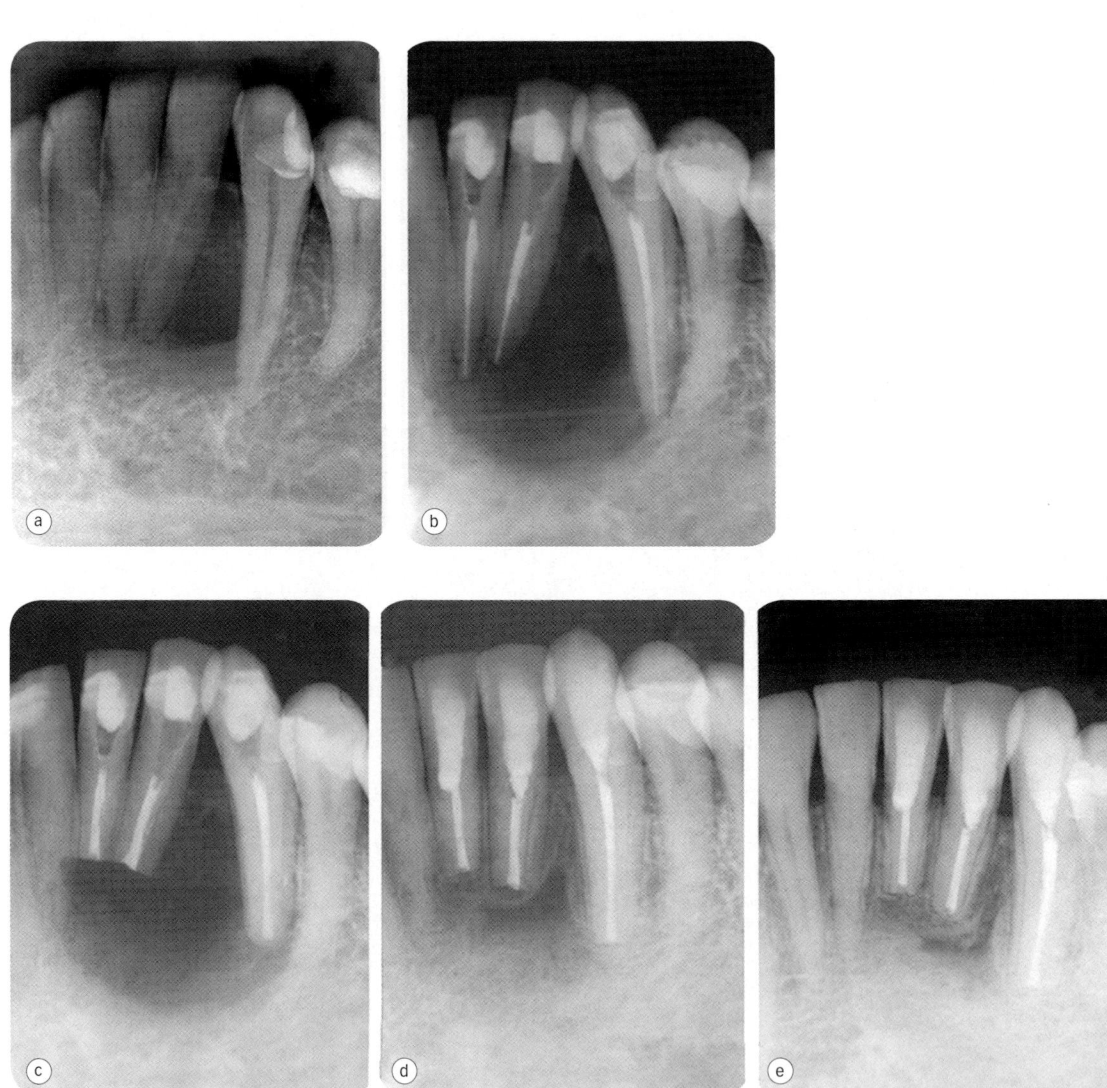


**Figure 11.96** - (**A**, **B**) Periapical radiograph showing radiolucent area well-defined among periapical area of teeth #31-33. (**B**) Endodontic treatment of teeth #31-33.(**C**) Periapical radiograph after periapical surgery (enucleation of lesion and apicectomy of #31 and #32 teeth). (**D**, **E**) Radiographs showing follow-up of 3 and 4 years, respectively[45].

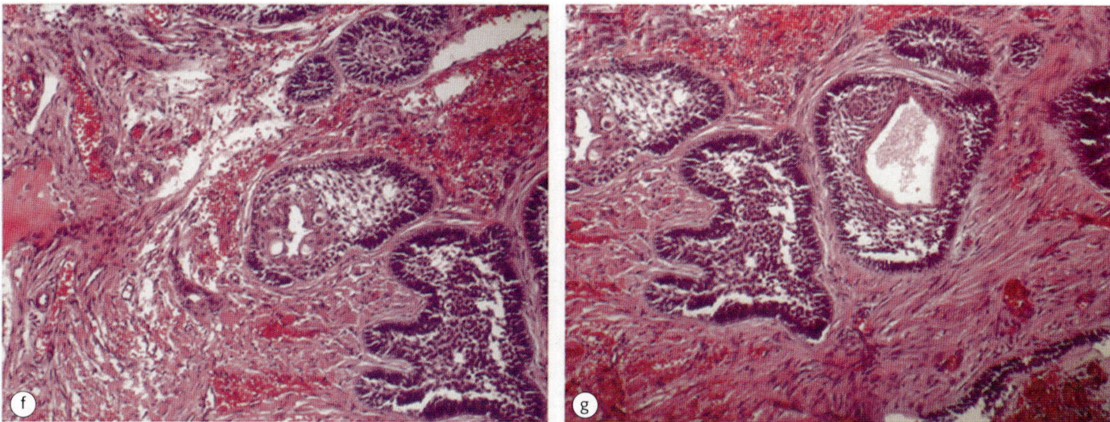

**Figure 11.96** - Microscopy of ameloblastoma. (**F**) Parenchyma exhibit a basal layer, cuboidal cells with reverse polarity, resembling ameloblast-like cells; epithelial cells mimic the stellate reticulum of the enamel organ (H & E, X40). (**G**) It is observed squamous metaplasia and formation of cysts spaces (H & E, X40)[45].



## Central giant cell granuloma

The central giant cell granuloma is one of the many types of non-odontogenic tumors that affects the maxilla and when close to dental apexes, it can be confused with apical periodontitis.

It is a highly vascularized lesion with a radiolucent aspect, imprecisely defined, irregular margins, and could contain lines inside it that indicate an infiltrative characteristic. This lesion frequently causes divergence of the dental roots. The definitive diagnosis is made through the histopathological exam (Fig. 11.97).

## Hyperparathyroidism

Some systemic diseases can lead to the condition of bone loss or can hinder bone repair. It is very important, to perform a perfect anamnesis and clinical exam, to verify the correlations between the general and local conditions.

Hyperparathyroidism is a pathology that causes a series of systemic alterations, such as the loss of calcium in the bones of the body, including the face, leading to structural fragility. Radiographically, it can reveal reduced bone density leading to change in the trabecular pattern orientation, with approximation of the trabecula, creating a dysplastic appearance. In more advanced cases general bone loss occurs, with obliteration of the cortical bones, and as the teeth continue to have normal density because they do not lose calcium, radiographs show contrast between the radiopaque teeth (light), and the radiolucent bone (dark). In some areas, in a focal form, the bone loss can be even more intense and it could be confused with apical periodontitis, when located close to dental apex.

Patients with hyperparathyroidism frequently present a brown tumor; a lesion that is radiographically and microscopically identical to the central giant cell granuloma. It could be solitary, or more usually, multiple, presenting in the body, face and gnathic bones, and in the initial stage, can also be confused with apical periodontitis (Fig. 11.98).

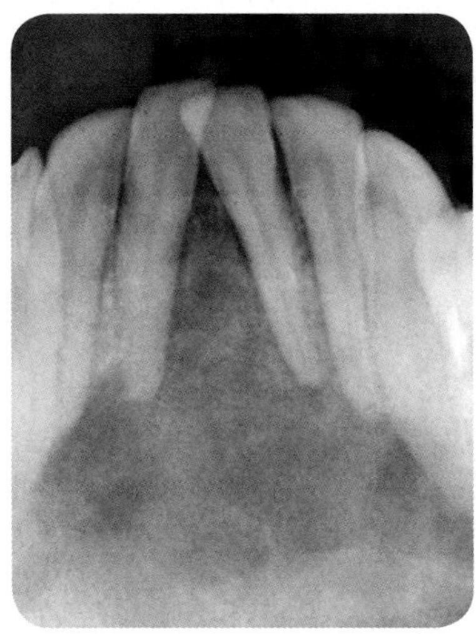

**Figure 11.97** - Central giant cell granuloma, below the mandibular incisors, causing divergence of the roots. Radiolucent area of medium density, radiograph shows dysplastic area with irregular margins and fine, irregular bone lines in the lesion.

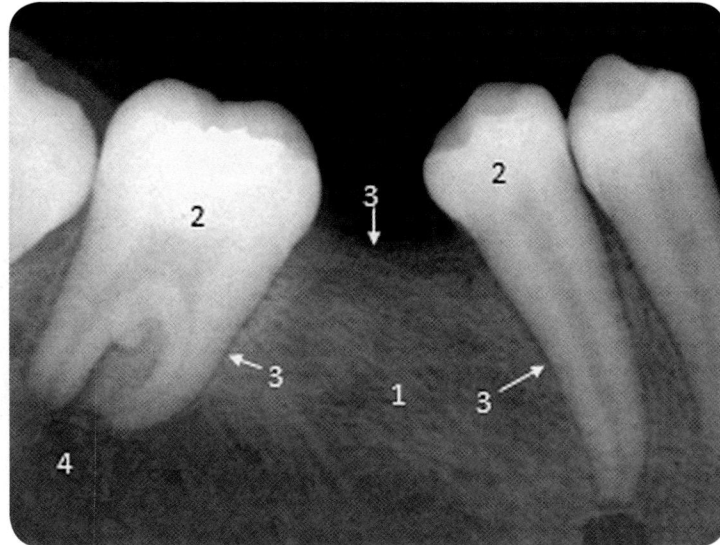


**Figure 11.98** - A case of hyperparathyroidism with general reduced bone density, accentuated approximation of the trabecula, guided in a pattern that has a dysplastic aspect, similar to that of unpolished glass (1) associated with radiopaque teeth (2). Deletion by reabsorption of the cortical bone (3) of the lamina dura and the alveolar ridge. More intense rarefaction (4), close to the apex of tooth #47 that lead to the suspicion of apical periodontitis, but it is an effect of hyperparathyroidism itself.

## Central hemangioma

The intra-osseous central hemangioma is a non-odontogenic tumor that requires special care, because in the event of an imprudent intervention, it puts the patient's life at risk.

Radiographically it presents radiolucence with undefined, irregular margins, and it could have lines inside it that indicate infiltrative characteristics. These lines are found in the central giant cell granuloma and in several other types of aggressive pathologies. In some cases it presents relatively clear margins and can be multilocular or unilocular. The lines, which are characteristic of low or moderately aggressive lesions, could be radiographically similar to an ameloblastoma, another similar tumor, or even to a cyst. As the central hemangioma can be radiographically similar to many other benign or invasive lesions, fine-needle aspiration is indicated before surgical intervention in any lesion. In the case of very easy aspiration, add the collected blood to coagulate, usually on a glass plate. This indicates hemangioma and surgery would be not indicated, or special preparation would be required together with specialist professionals. A small central hemangioma close to dental apexes is easily confused with apical periodontitis.

## Hematological disturbances

Some hematological disturbances such as falciforme anemia and thalassemia can change the trabecular pattern, especially of the mandible, with reduction in the number of trabeculae, due to their wider spacing as a result of increase in hematopoiesis in the medullary spaces, although these aspects are not exclusive to these disturbances. The aspect of loss of lacunar density of bone in the radiograph can be confused with apical periodontitis, in the case of wide medullary space, delimited close to the apex of a tooth, enabling selective visualization of the image of this site only. If the neighboring areas of tooth were observed, one would see that this pathology also affects other areas, even on the opposite side.

Hematological disturbances can also be apparent in radiographies of the patient's skull in falciforme anemia and particularly in thalassemia, showing images with aspects of "strands of hair " in the outlying cranial periphery (Fig. 11.99).

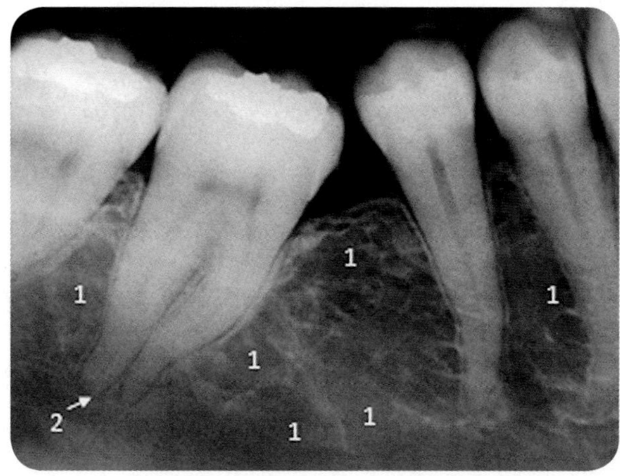


Figure 11.99 - Patient with falciforme anemia leading to bone loss with increase in spaces the trabecula (1) and generally reduced bone density. Presents cortical of the lamina dura, discrete in some places, with preserved periodontal spaces (2).



## Intraosseous cancer

In the great majority of cases of mouth cancer, the origin is in soft tissues, and if it is not treated it can invade bone tissues. Adequate anamnesis and careful clinical exam are indicated. For malignant neoplasia, the bone invasion radiographically reveals a highly aggressive and infiltrative radiolucent image, with completely irregular margins and unpreserved cortical. A malign neoplasia rarely arises centrally in the bone tissue of the maxilla.

Metastases can affect the gnathic bones centrally. Although remote, there is the chance of a supposed apical periodontitis being confused with a primary central bone cancer or metastases in the same position (Fig. 11.100 to 11.108).

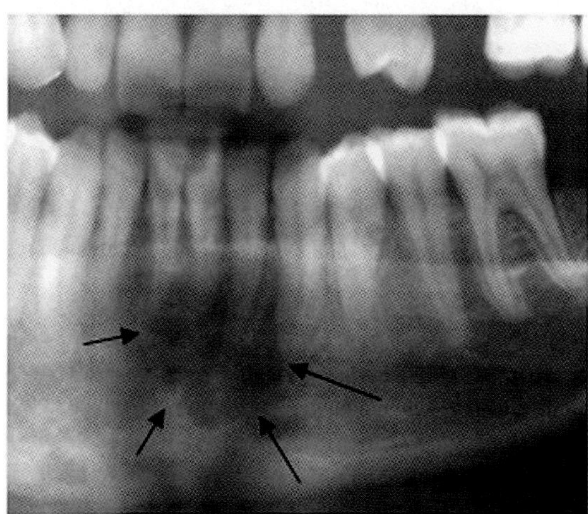

Figure 11.100 - Metastases of breast cancer in the apical area of teeth #33/32/31 and #41, radiographically similar to apical periodontitis. There was also invasion in the area of the mandibular molars on the opposite side.

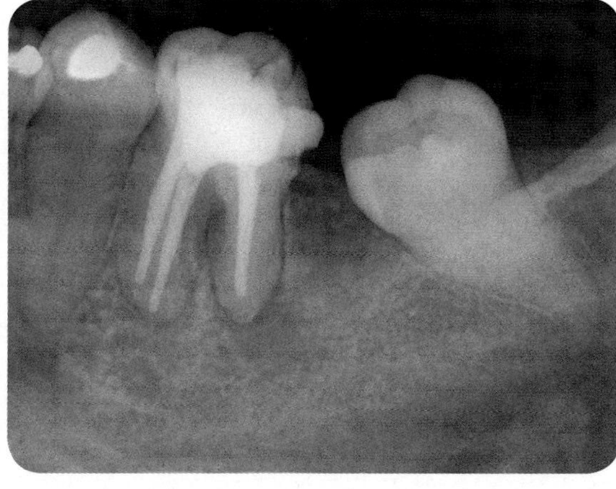

Figure 11.101 - Periapical radiograph of tooth #37 shows root canal filling and apical periodontitis. Radiolucency in furcation area is suggestive of a lesion[15].

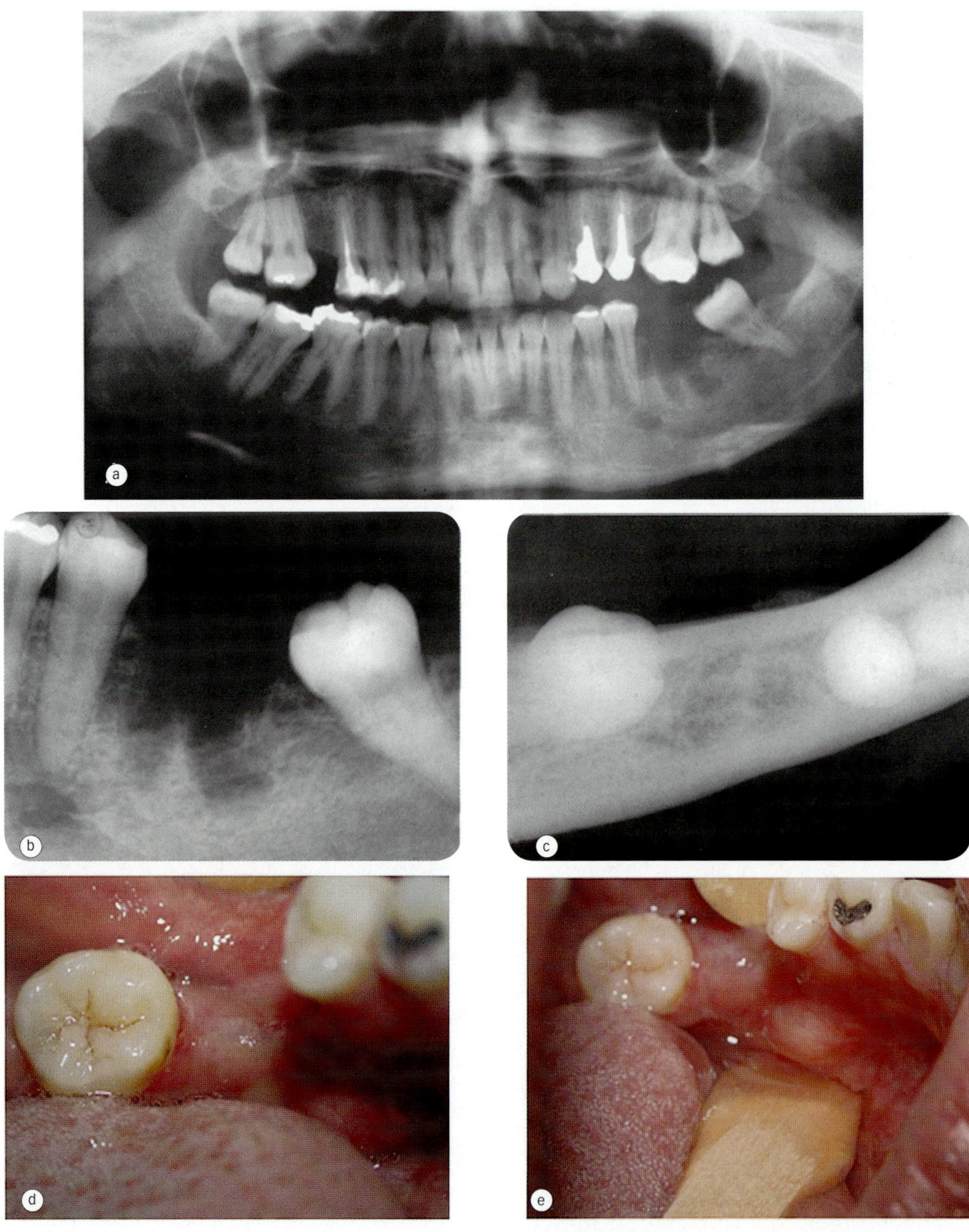

**Figure 11.102** - (**A-B**) Panoramic and periapical radiographs show absence of tooth #37, recently extracted. (**C**) Occlusal image of tooth #37 area shows increased lingual bone structure. (**D-E**) Clinical image shows swelling caused by lesion and compromised bite[15].

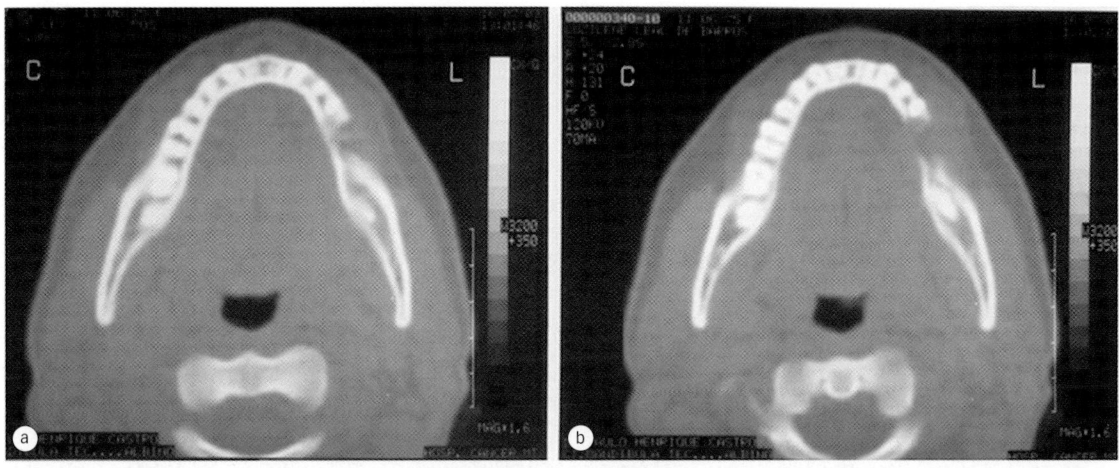

Figure 11.103 - (A-B) Axial CT scan shows destructive radiolucent area in left posterior mandible.

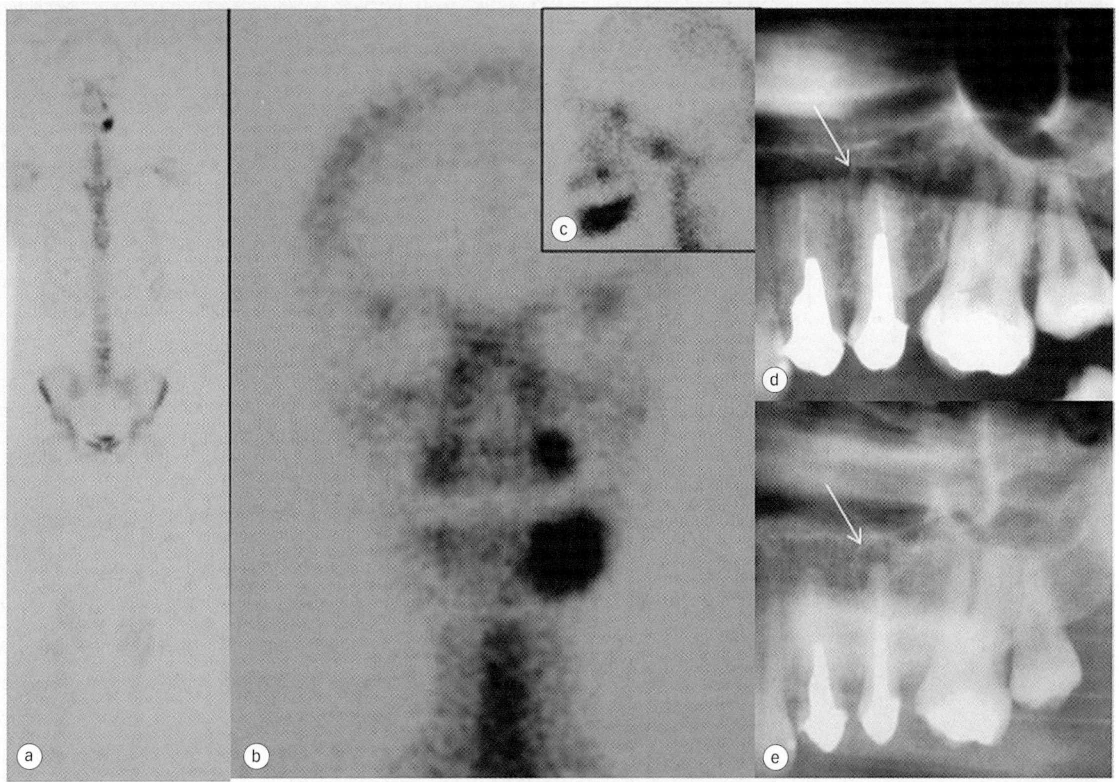

Figure 11.104 - (A-C) Bone cintilography image shows radiolucent area in left posterior mandible, as well as in tooth #25 region; apical periodontitis before and after endodontic treatment (D-E)[15].

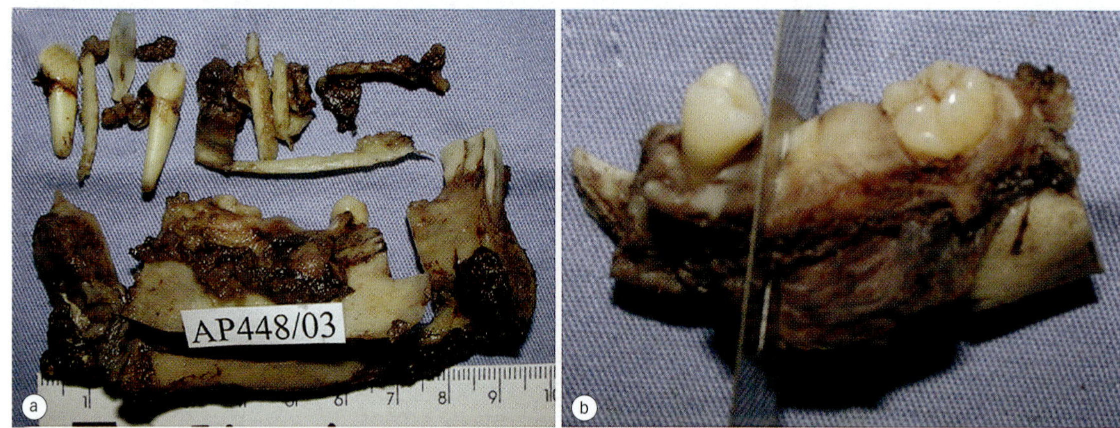


**Figure 11.105** - (**A**) Surgical specimen sent to pathology laboratory with longer axis measuring 9.5 cm. Central block (also shown in Fig. 105B) was surgically removed for transoperative evaluation of margins in an attempt to have a more conservative intervention. Macroscopic and histopathological examinations of central block revealed involvement of the surgical margin, and surgical excision was extended. Macroscopic and histopathological examination of surgical specimen of partial hemimandibulectomy revealed free surgical margins. (**B**) Central block of surgical specimen at macroscopic examination. A blade, used to remove representative fragments of lesion, cut specimen easily, which confirmed destruction of cortical and spongy bone[15].

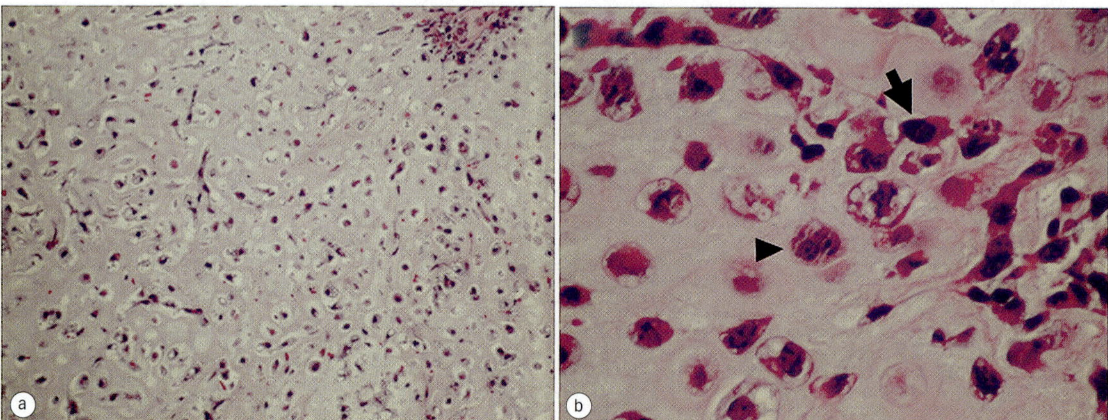


**Figure 11.106** - (**A**) Neoplastic tissue mimics hyaline cartilage and is composed of cells with intense pleomorphism; several hyperchromatic cells with two or multiple nucleus and loss of nucleus/nucleolus and nucleus/cytoplasm ratios (X100 magnification, Hematoxylin &Eosin). (**B**) Neoplastic binucleate cell (arrowhead) and undifferentiated cells with intense cellular hyperchromatism; details of remarkable cellular pleomorphism at greater magnification (X400 magnification, Hematoxylin & Eosin) (Diagnosis – Mesenchymal chondrosarcoma)[15].

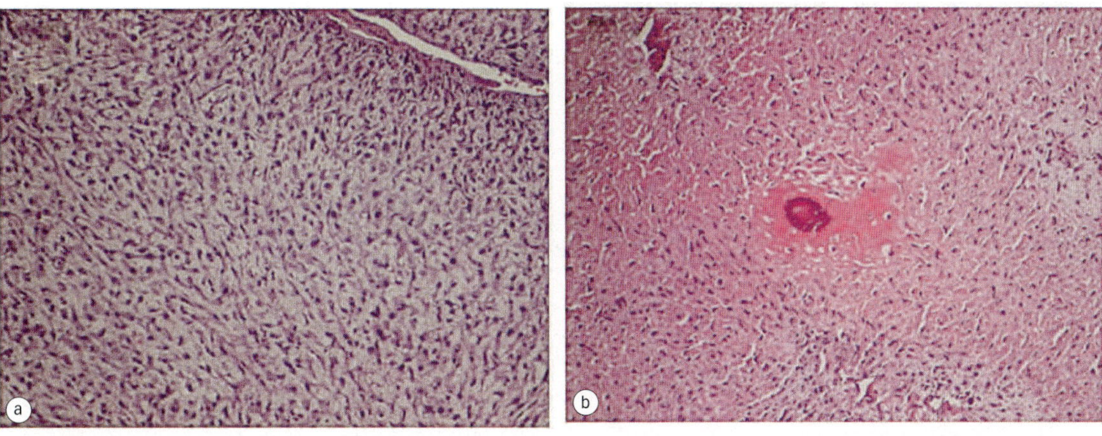

**Figure 11.107** - (**A**) Richly neoplastic mass composed of anaplastic cells indicates poor differentiation and high malignancy (X100 magnification, Hematoxylin & Eosin). (**B**) Extensive areas of necrosis suggest high mitotic activity (X100 magnification, Hematoxylin & Eosin) (Diagnosis – Mesenchymal chondrosarcoma)[15].

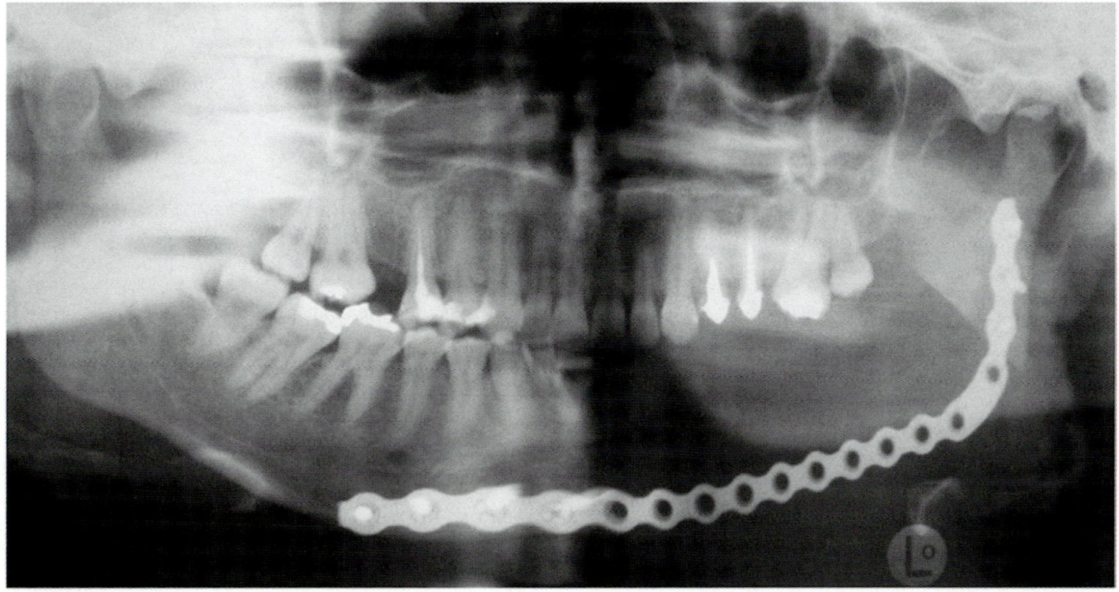

**Figure 11.108** - Panoramic radiograph shows hemimandibulectomy with wide surgical margins.

## 11.6 Other Pathologies Similar to Apical Periodontitis

In addition to the previously reported pathologies, there are others that could be similar to apical periodontitis. Correct anamnesis and careful clinical exam are always fundamental.

Cone beam computed tomography is an exam that has come to revolutionize Dentistry, and when suitable for the case and well interpreted, it can be an excellent diagnostic aid. It is very important to consider that in some situations, for instance, radiographic and clinical control themselves become means of diagnosis. When indicated, the histopathological exam will provide a definitive diagnosis of the surgically removed tissues.

## References and further reading




1. Allan BP, Egbert MA, Myall RWT. Orbital abscess of odontogenic origin: case report and review of the literature, J Oral Maxillofac Surg 1991;20:268-70.
2. Allard RHB, van der Kwast WAM, van der Waal I: Nasopalatine duct cyst: review of the literature and report of 22 cases. Int J Oral Surg 1981;10:447-61.
3. Altini M, Shear M. The lateral periodontal cyst: an update, J Oral Pathol Med 1992;21:245-250.
4. Aziz SR, Miremadi AR, McCabe JC: Mesenchymal chondrosarcoma of the maxilla with diffuse metastasis: Case report and literature review. J Oral Maxillofac Surg 2002;60:931-5.
5. Azma NEA, Razzak MYA, Saaid HY. Correlation between histological and radiographic appearance of periapical radiolucencies. Egypt Dent J 1990;36:245-259.
6. Baqain ZH, Jayakrishnan A, Farthing PM, Hardee P. Recurrence of a solitary bone cyst of the mandible: case report. Br J Oral Maxillofac Surg 2005;43:333–5.
7. Barker BF, Jensen JL, Howell FV. Focal osteoporotic marrow defects of the jaws. Oral Surg Oral Med Oral Pathol 1974;38:404-13.
8. Bender IB, Seltzer S. Roentgenographic and direct observation of experimental lesions in bone I. J Am Dent Ass 1961;62:152–60.
9. Bender IB, Seltzer S. Roentgenographic and direct observation of experimental lesions in bone II. J Am Dent Ass 1961;62:708–16.
10. Bhaskar SN. Periapical lesions-types, incidence, and clinical features. Oral Surg Oral Med Oral Pathol Oral Radiol Endod 1966;21:657–71.
11. Borax S. Diagnóstico bucal. 2nd ed. São Paulo: Artes Médicas, 1999.
12. Brannon RB: The odontogenic keratocyst- a clinicopathologic study of 312 cases. Part I: Clinical features, Oral Surg Oral Med Oral Pathol 1976;42:54-72.
13. Brown FH, Houston GD, Lubow RM, Sagan MA. Cyst of the incisive (palatine) papilla: report of a case. J Periodontol 1987;58:274-5.
14. Browne RM, Edmondson HD, Rout PGJ. Atlas of dental and maxillofacial radiology and imaging. Barcelona: Mosby-Wolfe, 1995. 281p.
15. Bueno MR, Carvalhosa AAC, Castro PHS, Pereira KC, Borges FT, Estrela C. Mesenchymal chondrosarcoma mimicking apical periodontitis. J Endod 2008; 34:1415-19.
16. Bueno MR, Estrela C. Prevalência de tratamento endodôntico e periodontite apical em várias populações do mundo, detectados por radiografias panorâmicas, periapicais e tomografias computadorizadas cone beam. Rev Bras Odontol Brasil Central 2008;17:79-90.
17. Bueno MR, Estrela C, Azevedo BC, Brugnera-Jr. A, Azevedo JR. Tomografia computadorizada Cone Beam: Revolução na odontologia. Rev Ass Paul Cir Dent 2007;61:325-8.
18. Carvalhosa AA, Junior DSP, Cavalcanti MGP, Nunes FD, Jorge WA. Calcifying epithelial odontogenic cyst (Gorlin cyst): reporto f a case. Histopathological and radiological correlation. Rev Pos Grad USP 2004;11:257-63.
19. Casati Alvares L, Tavano O. Curso de radiologia em odontologia. 4th ed. São Paulo: Ed. Santos, 2000.
20. Cavézian R, Pasquet G. Diagnóstico por la imagen en odonto-estomatología. Barcelona: Masson, 1993. 249p.
21. Chiba I, The BG, Iizuka T, Fukuda H. Conversion of a traumatic bone cyst into central giant cell granuloma: implications for pathogenesis—a case report. J Oral Maxillofac Surg 2002;60:222–5.
22. Christensen RE. Mesenchymal chondrosarcoma of the jaws. J Oral Surg 1982;54:197-206.
23. Coleman GC, Nelson JF. Princípios de diagnóstico bucal. Rio de Janeiro: Guanabara Koogan, 1996.
24. Cotti E, Campisi G. Advanced radiographic techniques for the detection of lesions in bone. Endodontic Topics 2004;7:52–72.
25. Cotton TP, Geisler TM, Holden DT, Schwartz SA, Schindler WG. Endodontic applications of cone-beam volumetric tomography. J Endod 2007;33:1121–32.
26. Craig GT. The paradental cyst. A specific inflammatory odontogenic cyst, Brit Dent J 1976;141:9-14.
27. Crawford BE, Weather DR. Osteoporotic marrow defects of the jaws, J Oral Surg 1970;28:600-3.
28. Cunha EM, Fernandes AV, Versiani MA, Loyola AM. Unicystic ameloblastoma: a possible pitfall in periapical diagnosis. Int Endod J 2005;38:334-40.
29. Curi MM, Dib LL, Pinto DS. Management of solid ameloblastoma of the jaws with liquid nitrogen spray cryosurgery. Oral Surg Oral Med Oral Pathol Oral Radiol Endod 1997;84:339-44.
30. Daley TD, Wysocki GP. The small dentigerous cyst. A diagnostic dilemma. Oral Surg Oral Med Oral Pathol Oral Radiol Endod 1995;79:77-81.
31. Diago MP, Bielsa JMS, Bonet-Marco J, Sanz JMM. Surgical treatment and follow-up of solitary bone cyst of the mandible: a report of seven cases. Br J Oral Maxillofac Surg 2001;39:221-3.
32. Donizete CR, Estrela C. Traumatic bone cyst suggestive of large apical periodontitis. J Endod 2008;34:484-9.
33. Douglas CR. Patofisiologia Oral. São Paulo: Pancast, 1998. v. 2.
34. Erasmus JH, Thompson IO, van Rensburg LJ, van der Westhuijzen AJ. Central calcifying odontogenic cyst. A review of the literature and role of advanced imaging techniques. Dentomaxillofac Radiol 1998;27:30-5.
35. Erikisson L, Hansson GL, Åkesson L, Ståhlberg F. Simple bone cyst: a discrepancy between magnetic resonance imaging and surgical observations. Oral Surg Oral Med Oral Pathol Oral Radiol Endod 2001;92:694–8.

36. Eriksen HM, Kirkevang L-L, Petersson K. Endodontic epidemiology and treatment outcome: general considerations. Endodontic Topics 2002;2:1–9.
37. Estrela C. Ciência Endodôntica. 1st ed. Artes Médicas: São Paulo, 2004. 1010p.
38. Estrela C, Bueno MR, Azevedo B, Azevedo JR, Pécora JD. A New Periapical Index Based on Cone Beam Computed Tomography. J Endod 2008; 34:1325-31.
39. Estrela C, Bueno MR, Leles CR, Azevedo B, Azevedo JR. Accuracy of cone beam computed tomography and panoramic and periapical radiography for detection of apical periodontitis. J Endod 2008;34:273–9.
40. Estrela C, Leles CR, Hollanda ACB, Moura MS, Pécora JD. Prevalence and risk factors of apical periodontitis in endodontically treated teeth in a selected population of Brazilian adults. Braz Dent J 2008;19: 34-39
41. Estrela C, Lopes HP, Pécora JD. Radicular grooves in maxillary lateral incisor: case report. Braz Dent J 1995;6:143-6.
42. Estrela C, Decúrcio DA, Silva JA, Mendonça EF, Estrela CRA. Persistent apical periodontitis associated with calcifying odontogenic. Int Endod J 2009 (in press).
43. Eversole LR, Leider AS, Hansen LS. Ameloblastomas with pronounced desmoplasia. J Oral Maxillofac Surg 1984;42:735– 40.
44. Eyrich, G. Is primary chronic osteomyelitis a uniform disease? Proposal of a classification based on a retrospective analysis of patients treated in the past 30 years. J Craniomaxillofac Surg 2004;32:43-50.
45. Faitaroni LA, Bueno MR, Carvalhosa AA, Ale KAB, Estrela C. Ameloblastoma suggesting large apical periodontitis. J Endod 2008;34:216-9.
46. Farman, AG, Nortjé CJ, Wood RE. Oral and maxillofacial diagnostic imaging. St. Louis: Mosby, 1993. 448p.
47. Figueiredo MAZ, Figueiredo JAP, Porter S. Root resoption associated with mandibular bone erosion in a patient with scleroderma. J Endod 2008;34:102-3.
48. Finical SJ, Kane WJ, Clay RP, Bite U. Familial gigantiform cementoma. Plast Reconstr Surg 1999;103:949-54.
49. Gardner AF. The odontogenic cyst as a potencial carcinoma: a clinicopathologic appraisal. J Am Dent Assoc 1969;78:746-55.
50. Gardner DG, Corio RL. The relationship of plexiform unicystic ameloblastoma to conventional ameloblastoma. Oral Surg Oral Med Oral Pathol Oral Radiol Endod 1983;56:54–60.
51. Garlock JA, Pringle GA, Hicks ML. The odontogenic keratocyst. A potential endodontic misdiagnosis. Oral Surg Oral Med Oral Pathol Oral Radiol Endod 1988;85:452-6.
52. Gibilisco JA. Diagnóstico radiográfico bucal de Stafne. 5th ed. Rio de Janeiro: Discos CBS, 1986. 493p.
53. Goaz PW, White SC. Oral radiology: principles and interpretation. 3rd ed. St. Louis: Mosby, 1994.
54. Gordon NC, Swann NP, Hansen LS. Median palatine cyst and maxillary antral osteoma: report of an unusual case. J Oral Surg 1980;38:361-5.
55. Gorlin RJ, Pinborg JJ, Clausen FP, Vickers RA. The calcifying odontogenic cyst – a possible analogue of the cutaneous calcifying epithelioma of Malherbe. Oral Surg Oral Med Oral Pathol 1962;15:1235-43.
56. Groot RH, van Merkesteyn JPR, Bras J. Diffuse sclerosing osteomyelitis and florid osseous dysplasia. Oral Surg Oral Med Oral Pathol Oral Radiol Endod 1996;81:333-42.
57. Gurol M, Burkes EJ Jr, Jacoway J. Botryoid odontogenic cyst: analysis of 33 cases. J Periodontol 1995;66:1069-73.
58. Halse A, Molven O, Fristad I. Diagnosing periapical lesions: disagreement and borderline cases. Int Endod J 2002;35:703–9.
59. Hansen LS, Sapone J, Sproat RC. Traumatic bone cysts jaws. Oral Surg Oral Med. Oral Pathol 1974;37:899–910.
60. Harris SJ, O'Carroll MK, Gordy FM. Idiopathic bone cavity (traumatic bone cyst) with the radiographic appearance of a fibro-osseous lesion. Oral Surg Oral Med Oral Pathol 1992;74:118–23.
61. Haug RH, Hauer CA, Smith B, Indresano AT. Reviewing the unicystic ameloblastoma: report of two cases. J Am Dent Assoc 1990;121:703–5.
62. Higashi T, Shiba, JKC, Ikuta H. Atlas de diagnóstico oral por imagens. 2nd ed. São Paulo: Ed. Santos, 1999. 269p.
63. Hirshberg A, Buchner A. Metastatic tumours to the oral region. An overview. Eur J Cancer B Oral Oncol 1995;31:355-60.
64. Howe GI. Haemorrhagic cysts of the mandible. Br J Oral Surg 1965;3:55–91.
65. Hülsmann M. Dens invaginatus: aetiology, classification, prevalence, diagnosis, and treatment considerations. Int Endod J 1997;30:79.
66. Huumonen S, Ørstavik D. Radiological aspects of apical periodontitis. Endodontic Topics 2002;1:3–25.
67. Kaffe I, Ardekian L, Taicher S, Littner MM, Buchner A. Radiologic features of central giant cell granuloma of the jaws. Oral Surg Oral Med Oral Pathol Oral Radiol Endod 1996;81:720-6.
68. Kaugars GE Cale AE. Traumatic bone cyst. Oral Surg Oral Med Oral Pathol 1987;63:318-24.
69. Kerr DA, Ash MM, Millard HD. Oral diagnosis. St. Louis: Mosby; 1978:13–77.
70. Khan A, Bilezikian J. Primary hyperparathyroidism: pathophysiology and impact on bone. CMAJ 2000;163:173-5.
71. Kim SG, Jang HS. Ameloblastoma: a clinical, radiographic, and histopathologic analysis of 71 cases. Oral Surg Oral Med Oral Pathol Oral Radiol Endod 2001;91:649 –53.
72. Kirkevang L-L, Ørstavik D, Hörsted-Bindslev P, Wenzel A. Periapical status and quality of root fillings and coronal restorations in a Danish population. Int Endod J 2000;33:509–15.
73. Koorbsch GF, Fotos P, Terhark K. Retrospective assessment of osteomyelitis: etiology, demographics, risk factors, and management in 35 cases. Oral Surg Oral Med Oral Pathol 1992;74:149-54.
74. Kusukawa J, Irie K, Morimatsu M, Koyanagi S, Kameyama T. Dentigerous cyst associated with a deciduous tooth: a case report. Oral Surg Oral Med Oral Pathol 1992;73:415-8.
75. Langlais RP, Langland OE, Nortjé CJ. Diagnostic imaging of the jaws. Philadelphia, USA: Willians & Wilkins – A lea & lebiger Book, 1995.
76. Langland OE et al. Panoramic radiology. 2nd ed. Philadelphia: Lea & Febiger, 1989.

77. Langland OE, Langlais RP. Princípios do diagnóstico por imagem em odontologia. São Paulo: Ed. Santos, 2002. 463p.
78. Lascala CA et al. Fundamentos de odontologia: radiologia odontológica e imaginologia. Rio de Janeiro: Guanabra Koogan, 2006. 358p.
79. Laskaris G. Color atlas of oral diasease. 2nd ed. New York: Thieme, 1994.
80. Laux M, Abbott PV, Pajarola G, Nair PNR. Apical inflammatory root resorption: a correlative radiographic and histological assessment. Int Endod J 2000;33:483–93.
81. LeCorn DW, Bhattacharyya I, Vertucci FJ. Peripheral ameloblastoma: a case report and review of the literature. J Endod 2006;32:152– 4.
82. Lee JJ, heng SJ, in SK, chiang CP, Yu CH, Kok SH. Gingival squamous cell carcinoma mimicking a dentoalveolar abscess: report of a case. J Endod 2007;33:177-80.
83. Li T-J, Kitano M, Arimura K, Sugihara K. Recurrence of unicystic ameloblastoma. A case report and review of the literature. Arch Pathol Lab Med 1998;122:371-4.
84. Li TJ, Wu YT, Yu SH, Yu GY. Unicystic ameloblastoma: a clinic pathologic study of 33 Chinese patients. Am J Surg Pathol 2000;24:1385–92.
85. Lichtenstein L, Bernstein D: Unusual benign and malignant chondroid tumors of bones: A survey of some mesenchymal cartilage tumors and malignant chondroblastic tumors including a few multicentric ones as well as many atypical benign chondroblastomas and chondromyxoid fibroma. Cancer 1959;12:1142.
86. Lofthag-Hansen S, Hummonen S, Gröndahl K, Gröndahl H-G. Limited cone-beam CT and intraoral radiography for the diagnosis of periapical pathology. Oral Surg Oral Med Oral Pathol Oral Radiol Endod 2007;103:114 –9.
87. Marx RE, Stern D. Oral and maxiloffacial pathology: A rationale for diagnosis and treatment. Carol Stream: Quintessence, 2003. 908p.
88. Matsumura S, Murakami S, Kakimoto N, Furukawa S, Kishino M, Ishida T, Fuchihata H. Histopathologic and radiographic findings of the simple bone cyst. Oral Surg Oral Med Oral Pathol Oral Radiol Endod 1998;85:619-25.
89. Matsuzaki H, Asaumi JI, Yanagi Y, et al. MR imaging in the assessment of a solitary bone cyst. Eur J Radiol Extra 2003;45:37– 42.
90. McMinn RMH, Hutchings RT, Logan BM. Atlas colorido de anatomia da cabeça e do pescoço. São Paulo: Artes Médicas, 1983. 240p.
91. Meltzer JA. Lateral periodontal cyst: report of a case with 1-year reentry. Int Periodontics Restorative Dent 1999;19:299-303.
92. Miyashita K. Contemporany cephalometric radiography. Tokyo: Quintessence, 1996. 291p.
93. Molven O, Halse A, Fristad I. Long-term reliability and observer comparisons in the radiographic diagnosis of periapical disease. Int Endod J 2002;35:142–7.
94. Moreland LW, Corey J, Mckenzie R. Ludwig's angina: report of a case and review of the literature, Arch Intern Med 1988;148:461-6.
95. Mourshed F, Tuckson C. A study of radiographic features of the jaws in sickle-cell anemia. Oral Surg Oral Med Oral Pathol 1974;37:812-9.
96. Nair MK, Nair UP. Digital and advanced imaging in endodontics: a review. J Endod 2007;33:1– 6.
97. Nair PNR, Pajarola G, Schroeder HE. Types and incidence of human periapical lesions obtained with extracted teeth. Oral Surg Oral Med Oral Pathol Oral Radiol Endod 1996;81:93–102.
98. Nair PNR, Sjögren U, Figdor D, Sundqvist G. Persistent periapical radiolucencies of root-filled human teeth, failed endodontic treatments, and periapical scars. Oral Surg Oral Med Oral Pathol Oral Radiol Endod 1999;87:617–27.
99. Nair PNR, Sjögren U, Schumacher E, Sundqvist G. Radicular cyst affecting a rootfilled human tooth: a long-term post-treatment follow-up. Int Endod J 1993;26:225-33.
100. Nair PNR. New perspectives on radicular cysts: do they heal? Int Endod J 1998;31:155-60.
101. Nair PNR. Pathogenesis of apical periodontitis and the causes of endodontic failures. Crit Rev Oral Biol Med 2004;15:348-81.
102. Nakamura N, Higuchi Y, Mitsuyasu T, Sandra F, Ohoshi M. Comparison of long-term results between different approaches to ameloblastoma. Oral Surg Oral Med Oral Pathol Oral Radiol Endod 2002;93:13–20.
103. Nakashima Y, Krishnan K, Shives T. Mesenchymal chondrosarcoma of bone and soft tissue: A review of 111 cases. Cancer 1986;57:2444-53.
104. Nakata K, Naitoh M, Izumi M, Inamoto K, Ariji E, Nakamura H. Effectiveness of dental computed tomography in diagnostic imaging of periradicular lesion of each root of a multirooted tooth: a case report. J Endod 2006;32:583–7.
105. Neville BW, Damm DA, Allen CM, Bouquot JE. Oral maxillofacial pathology. 2nd ed.Philadelphia: WB Saunders Company, 2002.
106. Nielsen RB, Alyassin AM, Peters DD, Carnes DL, Lancaster J. Microcomputed tomography: an advanced system for detailed endodontic research. J Endod 1995;21:561– 8.
107. Oda Y, Kagami H, Tohnai I, Ueda M. Asynchronously occurring bilateral mandibular hemorrhagic bone cysts in patient with idiopathic thrombocytopenic purpura. J Oral Maxillofac Surg 2002;60:95–9.
108. Okada H, Davies JE, Yamamoto H. Brown tumor of the maxilla in a patient with secondary hyperparathyroidism: a case study involving immunohistochemistry and electron microscopy. J Oral Maxillofoc Surg 2000;58:233-8.
109. Olaitan AA, Adekeye EO. Clinical features and management of ameloblastoma of the mandible in children and adolescents. Br J Oral Maxillofac Surg 1996;34:248.
110. Pasler F, Visser H. Radiologia odontológica: procedimentos ilustrados. 2nd Ed. Porto Alegre: Artmed, 2001. 331p.
111. Pasler FA. Color atlas of dental medicine. New York: Thieme, 1993. 266p.
112. Philipsen HP, Reichart PA. Unicystic ameloblastoma: a review of 193 cases from the literature. Oral Oncol 1998;34:317–25.
113. Pileggi R, Dumsha TC, Myslinksi NR. The reliability of electric pulp test after concussion injury. Endod Dent Traumatol 1996;12:16 –9.

114. PittFord TR, Patel S. Technical equipment for assessment of dental pulp status. Endod Topics 2004;7:2–13.
115. Pompura JR, Sàndor GKB, Stoneman DW. The buccal bifurcation cyst. A prospective study of treatment outcomes in 44 sites. Oral Surg Oral Med Oral Pathol Oral Radiol Endod 1997;83:215-21.
116. Poyton HG, Davey KW. Thalassemia: changes visible in radiographs used in dentistry, Oral Med Oral Pathol 1968;25:564-76.
117. Praetorius F, Ledesma-Montes C. Calcyfing cystic odontogenic tumor. In: Barnes L, Evenson JW, Reichart P, Sidransky D. WHO classification of tumors. Pathology and genetics. Head and neck tumors. Chapter 6. Lyon: IACR; 2005. p.
118. Puricelli E, Chaves KDB, Ligocki AF, et al. Cisto ósseo traumático em área de rizogênese: relato de um caso. Rev Fac Odontol Porto Alegre 1997;38:19–25.
119. Regezi JA, Kerr DA, Courtney RM. Odontogenic tumors: analysis of 706 cases. J Oral Surg 1978;36:771.
120. Regezi JA, Sciubba JJ, Pogrel MA. Atlas de patologia oral e maxilofacial. Rio de Janeiro: Guanabra Koogan, 2002.
121. Regezi JA, Sciubba JJ. Oral pathology – clinical pathologic correlations. 3rd ed. Philadelphia, W.B. Saunders Comp., 1999.
122. Reichart PA, Philipsen HP. Atlas colorido de odontologia: patologia bucal. Porto Alegre: Artmed, 2000. 283p.
123. Reyes D, Villanueva J, Espinosa S, Cornejo M. Odontogenic Calcificant cystic tumor: a report of two clinical cases. Med Oral Patol Oral Cir Bucal 2007;12:26-9.
124. Robinson L, Martinez MG. Unicystic ameloblastoma: a prognostically distinct entity. Cancer 1977;40:2278–85.
125. Rohlin M, Kullendorff B, Ahlquist M, Henrikson CO, Hollender L, Stenstrom B. Comparison between panoramic and periapical radiography in the diagnosis of periapical bone lesions. Dentomax Radiol 1989;18:151–5.
126. Rohlin M, Kullendorff B, Ahlqwist M, Stenstrom B. Observer performance in the assessment of periapical pathology: a comparison of panoramic with periapical radiography. DentoMax Facial Radiol 1991;20:127–31.
127. Rushton VE, Horner K. Calcifying odontogenic cyst – a characteristic CT finding. Br J Oral Maxillofac Surg 1997;35:196-9.
128. Rushtton MA. Solitary bone cysts in the mandible. Br Dent J 1946;81:37– 49.
129. Saddy MS, Chilvarquer I, Dib LL, Sandoval RL. Aspectos clínicos, radiográficos e terapêuticos do Ameloblastoma. RPG Rev Pós Grad 2005;12:460 –5.
130. Sahno NAM, Shukur ST, Abulkhail A: Mesenchymaf chondrosarcoma of the maxilla: Report of a case. J Oral Maxillofac Surg 1988;46:887-9.
131. Salvador AH, BeaboutJW, Dahlin DC. Mesenchymaf chondrosarcoma: Observations on 30 new cases. Cancer 1971;26:605-15.
132. Sapp JP, Eversole LR, Wysocki GP. Contemporary oral and maxillofacial pathology. 2nd ed. St. Louis: Mosby; 2004:123–33.
133. Saunders MB, Gulabivala K, Holt R, Kahan RS. Reliability of radiographic observation recorded on a proforma measured using inter- and intraobserver variation: a preliminary study. Int Endod J 2000;33:272– 8.
134. Scarfe WC, Farman AG, Sukovic P. Clinical applications of cone-beam computed tomograghy in dental practice. J Can Dent Ass 2007;72:75– 80.
135. Scully C, Flint SR, Porter SR. Oral diseases. 2nd ed. Saint Louis: Mosby, 1996.
136. Selden HS, Manhoff DT, Hatges NA, Michel C. Metastatic carcinoma to the mandible that mimicked pulpal/periodontal disease. J Endod 1998;24:267-70.
137. Seltzer S. Endodontology – biologic considerations in endodontic procedures. 2nd ed. Philadelphia: Lea & Febiger; 1988:140–4.
138. Shafer WA. Tratado de patologia bucal. 4th ed. Rio de Janeiro: Interamericana, 1985.
139. Shear M, Speight P. Cysts of the oral and maxillofacial regions. 4th ed. London: Blackwell; 2007.
140. Shear M. Cysts of the oral regions. 3rd ed. Oxford: Wright, 1992.
141. Silva TA, Batista AC, Camarini ET, Lara VS, Consolaro A. Paradental cyst mimicking radicular cyst on the adjacent tooth: case report and review of terminology. J Endod 2003;29:73.
142. Silverman S Jr, Eversole LR, Truelove EL. Essentials of oral medicine. Ontário: BC Decker, 2001.
143. Silverman S Jr, Ware WH, Gillooly C. Dental aspects of hyperparathyroidism. Oral Surg Oral Med Oral Pathol 1968;184-9.
144. Simon JHS, Enciso R, Malfaz JM, Rogers R, Bailey-Perry M, Patel A. Differential diagnosis of large periapical lesions using cone beam computed tomography measurements and biopsy. J Endod 2006;32:833–7.
145. Slutzky-Goldberg I, Heling I. Healing of a fibrous dysplastic lesion in a permanent molar after endodontic therapy. J Endod 2007;33:314-7.
146. Sobotta, J. Atlas de anatomia humana. 22nd ed. Rio de Janeiro: Guanabara Koogan, 2006. v1.
147. Stanley HR Jr, Krogh HW. Peripheral ameloblastoma: report of a case. Oral Surg Oral Med Oral Pathol Oral Radiol Endod 1959;12:760–5.
148. Stavropoulos A, Wenzel A. Accuracy of conebeam dental CT, intraoral digital and conventional film radiography for the detection of periapical lesions: an ex-vivo study in pig jaws. Clin Oral Invest 2007;11:101– 6.
149. Steiner DR. A lesion of endodontic origin misdiagnosed as a globulomaxillary cyst. J Endod 1999;25:277-81.
150. Swanson KS, Kaugars GE, Gunsolley JC. Nasopalatine duct cyst: an analysis of 334 cases. J Oral Maxillofac Surg 1991;49:268-71.
151. Tien N, Chaisuparat R, Fernandes R, Sarlani E, Papadimitriou JC, Ord RA, Nikitakis NG. Mesenchymal Chondrosarcoma of the Maxilla: Case Report and Literature Review. J Oral Maxillofac Surg 2007;65:1260-6.
152. Tomasi D, Hann JR. Traumatic bone cyst: report of case. J Am Dent Assoc 1985;111:56–7.
153. Tommasi, AF. Diagnóstico em patologia bucal. 3rd ed. São Paulo: Pancast, 2002.
154. Tronstad L, Barnett F, Riso K, Slots, J. Extra-radicular infections. Endod Dent Traumatol 1987;3:86-90.

155. Trope M, Pettigrew J, Petras J, Barnett F, Tronstad L. Differentiation of radicular cyst and granulomas using computerized tomography. Endod Dent Traumatol 1989;5:69 –72.
156. Van der Stelt PF. Experimentally produced bone lesions. Oral Surg Oral Med Oral Pathol Oral Radiol Endod 1985;59:306 –12.
157. Velvart P, Hecker H, Tillinger G. Detection of the apical lesion and the mandibular canal in conventional radiography and computed tomography. Oral Surg Oral Med Oral Pathol Oral Radiol Endod 2001;92:682– 8.
158. Vencio EF, Reeve CM, Unni KK, Nascimento AG. Mesenchymal chondrosarcoma of the jaw bones: clinicopathologic study of 19 cases. Cancer 1998;82:2350-5.
159. von Stechow D, Balto K, Stashenko P, Müller R. Three-dimensional quantitation of periradicular bone destruction by micro-computed tomography. J Endod 2003;29:252– 6.
160. Waldron CA. Odontogenic cysts and tumors. In: Neville BW, Damm DD, Allen CM, Bouquot JE. Oral maxillofacial pathology. 2nd ed. Phladelphia, USA: WB Saunders Company, 2002. p:506-9.
161. Weiger R, Hitzler S, Hermle G, Löst C. Periapical status, quality of root canal fillings and estimated endodontic treatment needs in an urban German population. Endod Dent Traumatol 1997;13:69 –74.
162. Whaites, E. Princípios de radiologia odontológica. 3rd ed. Porto Alegre: Artmed, 2003.
163. White SC, Atchison KA, Hewlett ER, Flack VF. Efficacy of FDA guidelines for prescribing radiographs to detect dental and intraosseous conditions. Oral Surg Oral Med Oral Pathol Oral Radiol Endod 1995;80:108–14.
164. White SC, Pharoah MJ. Oral radiology: principles and interpretation. 5th ed. St. Louis: Mosby, 2004.
165. Wood NK, Goaz PW. Differential diagnosis of oral and maxillofacial lesions. 3rd ed. St Louis, MO: Mosby, 1985.
166. Wysocki GP, Brannon RB, Gardner DG, Sapp P. Histogenesis of the lateral periodontal cyst and the gingival cyst of the adult. Oral Surg Oral Med Oral Pathol 1980;50:327-34.
167. Wysocki GP, Goldblatt LI. The so-called "globulomaxilliary cyst" is extinct. Oral Surg Oral Med Oral Pathol 1993;76:185-6.
168. Xanthinaki AA, Choupis KI, Tosios K, Pagkalos VA, Papanikolau SI. Traumatic bone cyst of the mandible of possible iatrogenic origin: a case report and brief review of the literature. Head Face Med 2006;2:40–5.
169. Yamaguchi S, Nagasawa H, Susuki T, Fujii E, Iwaki H, Takagi M, Amagasa T. Sarcomas of the oral and maxillofacial region: a review of 32 cases in 25 years. Clin Oral Investig 2004;8:52-5.
170. Young SK, Markowistz NR, Sullivan S, Seale TW, Hirschi R. Familial gigantiform cementoma: classification and presentation of a large pedigree. Oral Surg Oral Med Oral Pathol 1989;68:740-7.

# Endodontic Infection Control

**C.R.A. Estrela**
*Brazilian Dentistry Research and Learning Center, CEPOBRAS, Goiânia, GO, Brazil*

**C. Estrela**
*Federal University of Goiás, Goiânia, GO, Brazil*

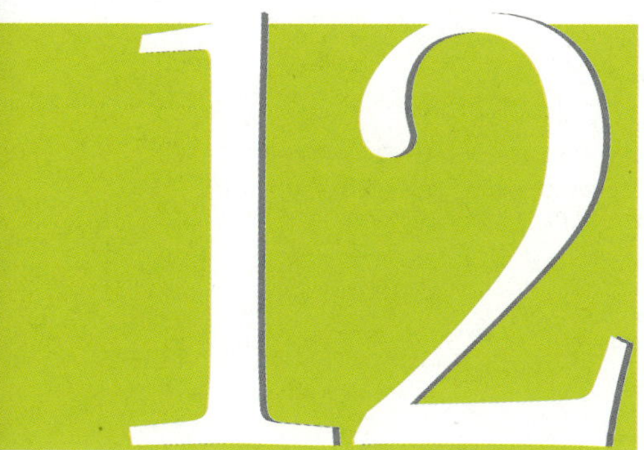

Chapter contents

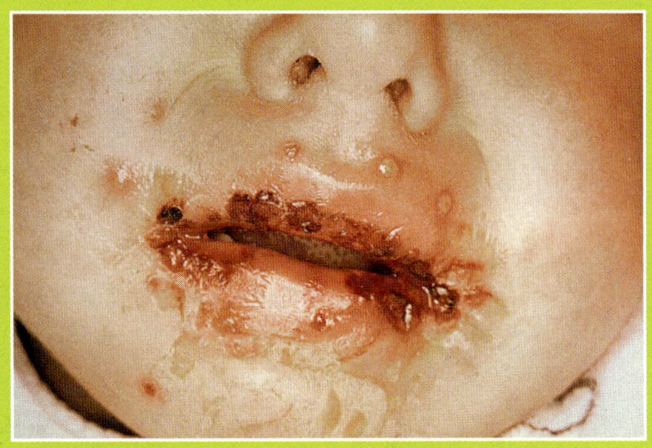

Primary Herpes infection
(Stomatology Service of São Lucas Hospital of PUC-RS/
Prof. Dr. Maria Antônia Zancanaro Figueiredo).

## 12.1 Introduction

The importance of infection control in health areas, especially after the first reports about the Acquired Immunodeficiency Syndrome (AIDS), set off the adoption of a series of measures to avoid cross-contamination. Distrust of contamination by the human immunodeficiency virus (HIV) has led to many studies with the aim of better clarifying the pathogenicity mechanisms and the most efficient alternatives for the control of microorganisms.

Concern with infection control must integrate the protocols of clinical attendance of all areas of health, without giving preference to any particular one.

Among health professionals, the dentist runs the greatest risk of contamination by the B hepatitis virus (HBV). This can be explained by some of the peculiarities of the work environment. The oral cavity is one of the most septic environments of the organism and can lodge from 400 to 1000 microbial species. Therefore, from a quantitative and qualitative point of view, it can be affirmed that the oral cavity presents a complex microbiota, (Gram-positive bacteria, Gram-negative bacteria, viruses, fungi and protozoa), and these microorganisms are distributed into 4 main oral ecosystems: oral epithelium, dorsum of the tongue, supragingival tooth surfaces and dental and epithelial subgingival surfaces, in addition to saliva, which does not present its own specific microbiota, and presents partially, microorganisms that are to be found in other oral sites[21]. In addition to these characteristics of the oral cavity, other areas should be stand out, as shown in Table 12.1. Figure 12.1 shows the sources of contamination during endodontic treatment. Figures 12.2 to 12.8 show some of the diseases caused by microorganisms that can be disseminated in the dental office.

**Table 12.1** - Peculiarities of the dentist's work environment

| |
|---|
| Great proximity to the patient (focus of infection) |
| Working environment that is difficult to access, visualize, and is rich in resident and transient pathogenic microorganisms |
| Manipulation of sharp material / instruments |
| Use of material / instruments that generate aerosol |

(Pimenta et al.[181], 1999)

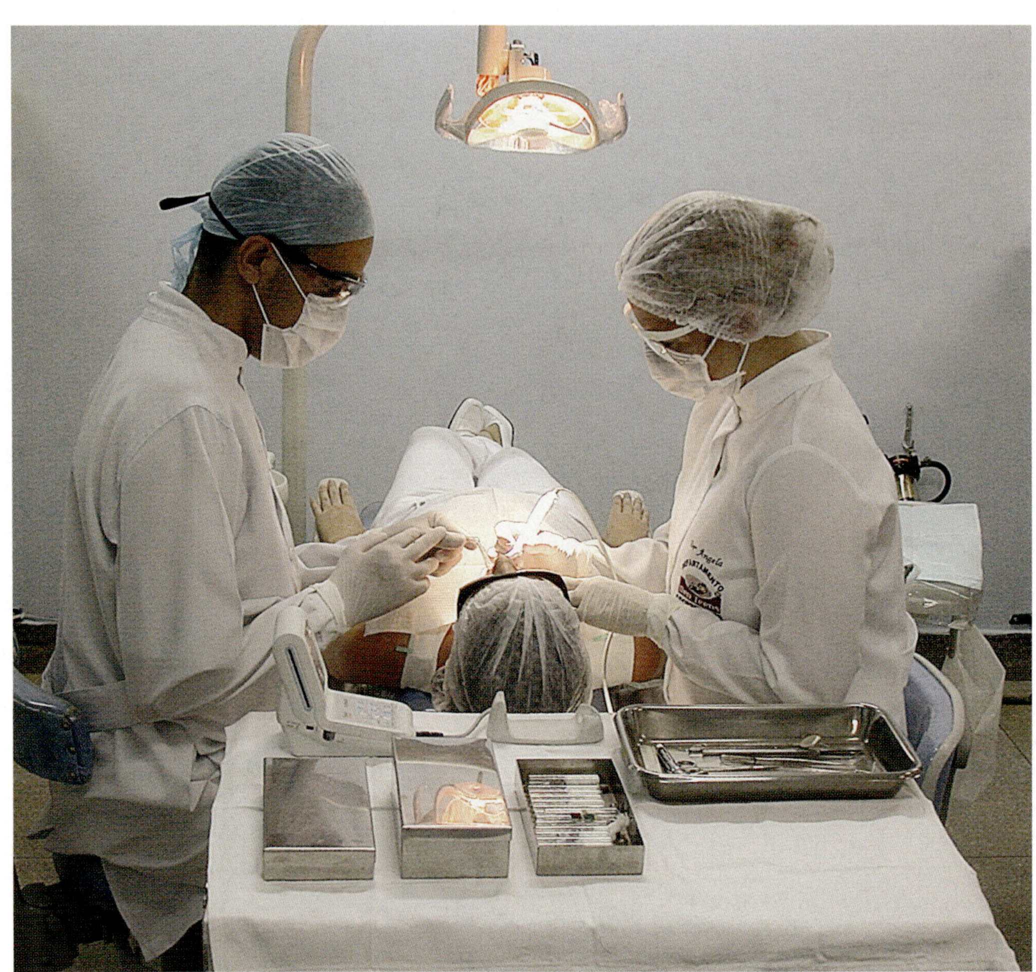

Figure 12.1 - Sources of contamination during the endodontic treatment.

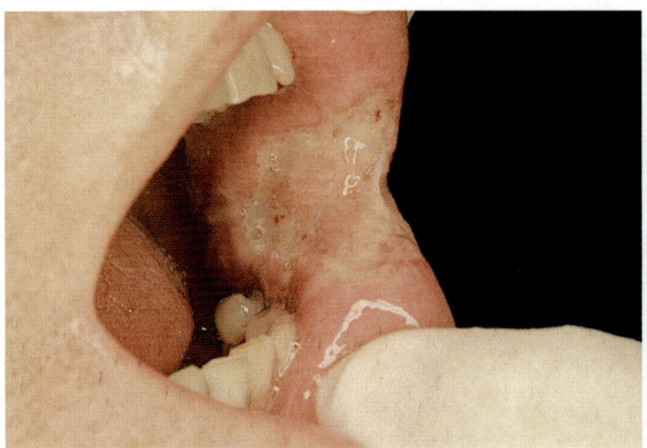

Figure 12.2 - Oral lesion of tuberculosis (Stomatology Service of São Lucas Hospital of PUC-RS/ Prof. Dr. Maria Antônia Zancanaro Figueiredo).

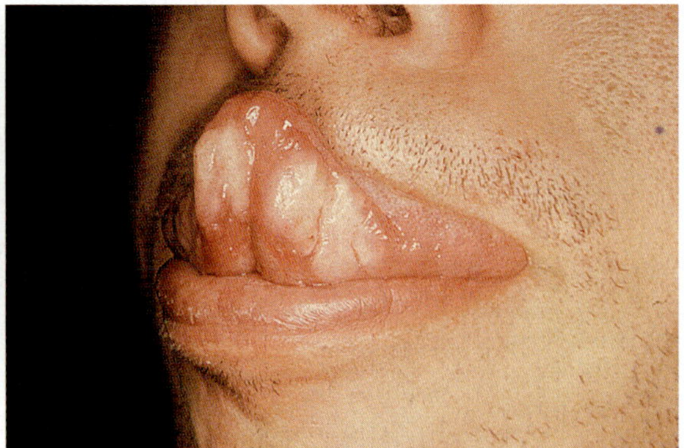

Figure 12.3 - Secondary syphilis (Stomatology Service of São Lucas Hospital of PUC-RS/ Prof. Dr. Maria Antônia Zancanaro Figueiredo).

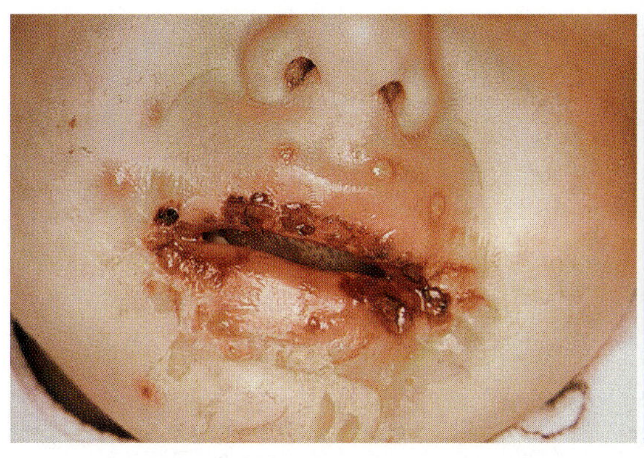

**Figure 12.4** - Primary herpes infection (Stomatology Service of São Lucas Hospital of PUC-RS/ Prof. Dr. Maria Antônia Zancanaro Figueiredo).

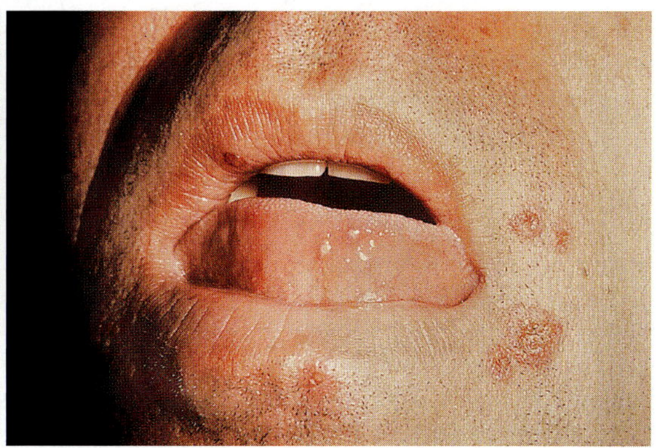

**Figure 12.5** - Recurrent herpes in HIV positive patient (Stomatology Service of São Lucas Hospital of PUC-RS/ Prof. Dr. Maria Antônia Zancanaro Figueiredo).

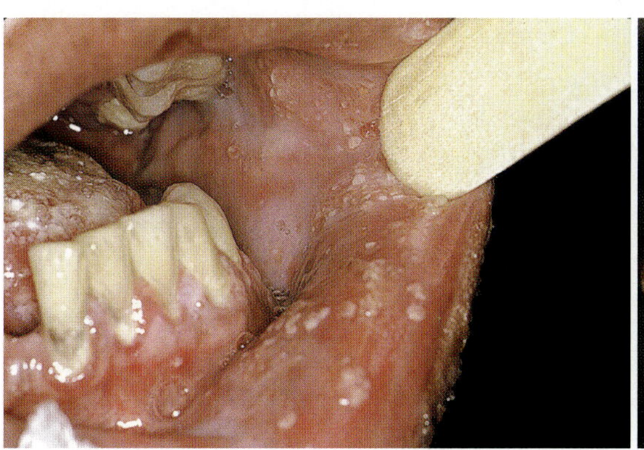

**Figure 12.6** - Herpes zoster in HIV positive patient (Stomatology Service of São Lucas Hospital of PUC-RS/ Prof. Dr. Maria Antônia Zancanaro Figueiredo).

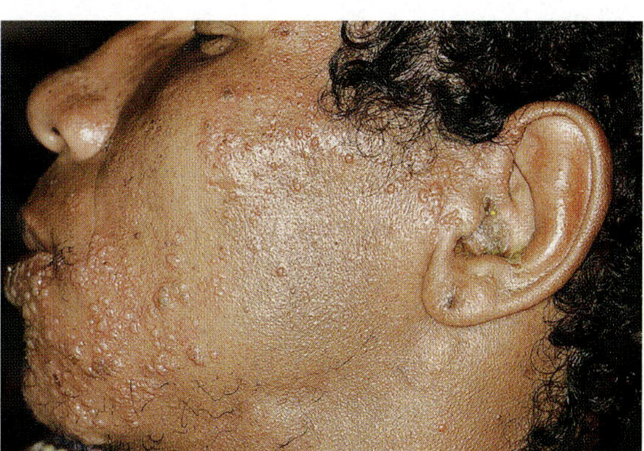

**Figure 12.7** - Herpes zoster in HIV positive patient (Stomatology Service of São Lucas Hospital of PUC-RS/ Prof. Dr. Maria Antônia Zancanaro Figueiredo).

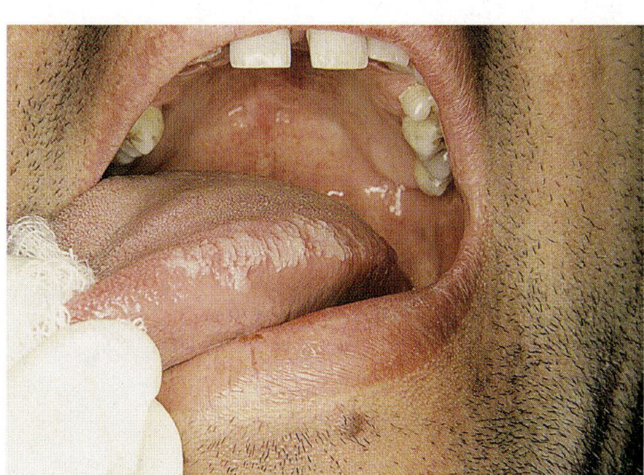

**Figure 12.8** - Hairy leukoplakia in HIV positive patient (Stomatology Service of São Lucas Hospital of PUC-RS/ Prof. Dr. Maria Antônia Zancanaro Figueiredo).

The Endodontist is a specialist that works directly with the focus of infection and particularly with the blood system; thus he/she may act as a disseminator of different diseases, as can be seen in Tables 12.2 to 12.5. It must be emphasized that health professionals, more specifically of the dental team, must use all the Individual Protection Equipment – IPE (long sleeved gown, protective headgear, mask, protective eyewear and gloves), which are essential for the control and prevention of cross-infection and other possible contaminations.

**Table 12.2** - Main bacterial diseases of importance to the dental team

| | Tuberculosis | Syphilis | Diphtheria |
|---|---|---|---|
| **Etiological agent** | *Mycobacterium tuberculosis* | *Treponema pallidum* | *Corynebacterium diphtheriae* |
| **Transmission** | Aerosol, contaminated droplets | Sexual, direct contact with lesions, blood transfusions, vertical | Aerosol, contaminated droplets |
| **Diagnosis** | Clinical, laboratorial | Clinical, laboratorial | Clinical, laboratorial |
| **Treatment** | Chemotherapeutics | Antibiotics / Chemotherapeutics | Diphtheria antitoxin |
| **Prevention** | Immunization (BCG) | Safe sex | Immunization DPT or Dt |

**Table 12.3** - Main viral diseases of importance to the dental team

| | Herpes labialis | Varicella | Herpes zoster | Measles | Mumps | Rubeola |
|---|---|---|---|---|---|---|
| **Etiologic agent** | Herpes simplex virus type 1 | Varicella zoster virus | Varicella zoster virus | Measles virus | Mumps virus | Rubeola virus |
| **Transmission** | Direct contact with lesions, contaminated objects, droplets of spittle, aerosol | Aerosol | Aerosol | Respiratory secretions | Droplets of spittle | Respiratory secretions, aerosol |
| **Diagnosis** | Clinical, laboratorial | Clinical | Clinical | Clinical | Clinical | Clinical, laboratorial |
| **Treatment** | Antivirals | Antivirals, Interferon | Antivirals, Interferon | Nonexistent | Symptomatic | Nonexistent |
| **Prevention** | Barriers, IPE | Barriers, IPE | Barriers, IPE | Immunization (MMR) | Immunization (MMR) | Immunization (MMR) |

**Table 12.4** - Viral hepatitis of importance to the dental team

| | Hepatitis A | Hepatitis B | Hepatitis C |
|---|---|---|---|
| **Etiological agent** | HAV | HBV | HCV |
| **Transmission** | Fecal oral (enteric) | Parenteral | Parenteral |
| **Diagnosis** | Clinical, laboratorial | Clinical, laboratorial | Clinical, laboratorial |
| **Treatment** | Ingestion of liquids, rest, controlled feeding Interferon (chronic infections) | Ingestion of liquids, rest, controlled feeding Interferon (chronic infections) | Ingestion of liquids, rest, controlled feeding Interferon (chronic infections) |
| **Prevention** | Educational programs, basic sanitation, personal hygiene, immunization | Care of blood and hemoderivatives, sterilized and disposable materials, immunization | Care of blood and hemoderivatives, sterilized and disposable materials, immunization |

(Adopted from Santos et al.[201], 2002)

**Table 12.5** - Acquired immunodeficiency syndrome (AIDS)

| | |
|---|---|
| **Etiological agent** | Human immunodeficiency virus (HIV) |
| **Transmission** | Sexual, blood, vertical (congenital, perinatal or post-natal), occupational |
| **Diagnosis** | Clinical - laboratorial |
| **Treatment** | Antiretrovirals |
| **Prevention** | Educational programs, blood and hemoderivatives control, adoption of infection control norms |

Endodontists must adopt several procedures to ensure infection control and avoid cross-infection. The basic, easily performed procedure, essential for infection control is hand washing. Other procedures that must be included in the clinical attendance routine in order to avoid the dissemination of microorganisms, are as follows: accurate clinical examination, following the dental handbook correctly, personal and equipment protection; surgical scrubbing; processing and sterilization of instruments; workbench organization; cleanliness and disinfection of the dental office; dental waste disposal and management[71].

## 12.2 Clinical Examination

The foundation of good endodontic treatment is diagnosis. Different factors are involved, and are essential for the recognition of a certain illness. The challenge to find the agent responsible for the alteration in the oral structures, emphasizes the need to perform a refined clinical examination, and shows the stage of diagnosis to be basic and of supreme importance in the search for the cure. It is essential for the investigator to verify the etiological factor of a certain pathology by analysis, collection, tabulation identification, and interpretation of data, signs and characteristic symptoms of the possible abnormality of the tissue structure.

The oral health professional needs an adequate dental treatment plan, not only to know the factors responsible for the illness, but also to verify the general health status of the individual; former and current illnesses, and the biophysiological aspects of all the organs of his/her organism.

Therefore, when the relevance of prevention of cross-infection in the dental office is considered, it becomes opportune and necessary to maintain a frequent and up-dated inquiry into the patient's medical health.

Valuable information as regards the possible transmissibility of important illnesses such as hepatitis, AIDS and several others can be obtained from the case history. The care taken at the time of clinical attendance must always favor the "Universal Precautions" (all individuals must receive the same attendance, backed by all the special care taken to control infection and potential contaminant agents). In the data investigated through the medical history, important details about the individual general state of health, from birth until the present moment must be sought, which involves former illnesses, infections, immunization, allergies, hospitalizations, and the current health status. All the factors involved, including profession (occupation), habits, daily activities, emotional state must be well analyzed. It is opportune to evaluate the possible alterations in various organic systems.

Thus, to investigate and obtain information about oral health requires knowledge and study of the normality status (health) of organic tissues, and adequate mastery of the semiologic technique for structuring the diagnosis, so that the hypothesis about the identity of the pathology can be reached in a controlled manner. Systematic recording of the collected and tabulated data can lead in the right direction to interpret and identify the alteration.

Some pathologies can present pre-clinical signs and symptoms, or even typical and evident aspects that allow them to be differentiated (pathognomonic characteristics). In other situations, however, antagonistic signs and symptoms can be evidenced, or inconsistent responses to the semiotechnical resources used, which makes it difficult to recognize them. Differential diagnosis allows comparison of the similar signs and symptoms among certain pathologies, and exclusion analysis often leads to diagnosis by elimination of signs and symptoms that are similar.

Successful treatment depends on determining the diagnosis correctly, and this is only complete when it is performed in a rational and intelligent manner, directed towards resolution of the patient's problem, and not exclusively and essentially that of the tooth.

When considering all the important requirements for achieving diagnosis, it is commonly observed that while the case history is being recorded and the clinical examination performed, we frequently see our patient with a problem, but we do not perceive; we hear, but do not listen". Chapter 4 presents the necessary steps to accurate diagnosis - essential to the success of endodontic treatment - in greater detail, as well as details concerning inquiry into the patient's general health, which must be contained in the dentistry handbook.

## 12.3 Personal and Equipment Protection

The aim of a personal protection system (patient, professional, assistant) in a clinical environment is to ensure the prevention of microbial contamination and cross-infection during dental appointments. The dental team's exposure to infectious/contagious illnesses on a day-by-day bases is significant.

Contagion can occur when the infectious agent comes into contact with the uncontaminated receiver or remains exposed to the environment. The sources of contagion in the clinical environment are composed of the professional, patient, assistant, equipment (instruments) and the environment itself (Fig. 12.1).

The precautions taken with the personal protection and equipment that comes into direct or indirect contact with the patient must be strictly implemented in order to diminish the possibility of cross-infection.

The set of factors that involve the infection process, denominated the "infection chain", by Molinari[156], is made up of the etiological agent, transmissibility, and the susceptible host. Among the etiological agents are bacteria, fungi and viruses. The ability to cause illness depends on the microbial virulence (attack armamentarium), number of colony forming units, and number of inoculations that occurred. The transmissibility from the source to the susceptible host can occur by direct and/or indirect contagion.

Direct contagion can take place through contact with flügge, a droplet of particles bigger than 50 μm, easily decanted or sedimented, or aerosol particles, smaller than 50 μm, capable of floating in the air for a long time)[181].

The significant increase in infectious-contagious illnesses makes it necessary for the dental surgeon to know the biological risks, and adopt methods to control infection during professional practice, such as prevention of contact with the contaminant agent and microbial propagation; and the use of protective equipment and safe manipulation of dental equipment.

Infection control in the dental office demands protocols to prevent and reduce the dissemination of infectious agents that can occur between:

1. Patient and the dental team;
2. Dental team and the patient;
3. Patient to patient;
4. Dental office to the community, including relatives of the dental team;
5. Community to the patient.

It is basic to establish a protocol for clinical attendance, with the goal of preventing cross-infection, and admit that all patients must be considered as infective agents, and in the same way as the dental team, infectant vectors of cross-infection.

Cross-infection can be prevented by the adoption of different behavior patterns, and using protocol barriers.

## 12.4 Personal Protection (Individual Protection Equipment – IPE)

The aim of concern about microbial contamination in the dental office is to prevent the transmission and the dissemination of microorganisms (infectant agents) during dental attendance. Among the different agents of transmission the microorganisms present in the oral cavity, skin injuries and in contaminated equipment are outstanding. Infectant droplets (exhaled during the act of coughing, sneezing), the aerosols (produced by high speed hand pieces, air/water syringe handling, ultrasound apparatus), instruments (that can induce perforating-cutting wounds) constitute potential agents responsible for causing infectious processes.

With the intention of minimizing the contamination process and reducing the biological risks during clinical attendance of the patient, protective barriers have been used, which represent physical resources responsible for blocking infectant agents. To protect the dental team, routine use of individual protection equipment has been indicated, such as long-sleeved gowns, protective clothing for the head, masks, protective eyewear, protective footwear and gloves.

To control microbial dissemination, different resources have been added to the equipment and routine during the dental attendance. Among the ways of protecting the equipment the following have been indicated: the use of a surgical drape; using of protective sheets of aluminum foil and/or plastic; modern dental chairs that have foot controls; a line with an aseptic disinfection system; hand pieces with air reflux; cleanliness of the environment; devices capable of cleaning the air in the clinical environment.

### 12.4.1 Gown

The gown is a means of protecting the dental team's clothing and hindering the transport and dissemination of microorganisms to other places and people. Its use is indispensable. The objective of using it is to protect the professional, therefore it must be long, have a high collar, long sleeves with adequate cuffs, and minimum porosity.

The use of a gown must be restricted to the clinical attendance environment. The gown can be disposable or reusable, provided that it is closed in front when used in semicritical procedures. Moreover, the gown for use in critical procedures (surgical cloak), closes at the back and must always be sterilized.

After clinical attendance, the gown must receive special treatment during transport and laundering (when using an non-disposable gown). After use, the contaminated gown must be placed in a plastic bag and sealed. Ideally it should be laundered in a laundry with a special decontamination process, for example, the use of appropriate disinfectants and hot water, or ozone water treatment. When it is washed at home, it must be handled separately, using enzymatic substances and sodium hypochlorite (sanitary water). Surgical cloaks or gowns must be treated carefully (autoclaving before the surgical procedure and special laundering after use).

### 12.4.2 Cap, mask, protective eyewear and protective footwear

It is mandatory for the dental team to use individual protection equipment. The cap protects the hair against saliva droplets, contaminated blood and other infectant microparticles. The women in the dental team must take special care of their hair. It must be tied up and protected with the cap, which must be changed before each critical procedure, and discarded after each period of attendance. If the cap is not disposable, the same care must be taken with the laundering and processing, as for the gown.

The masks, which must be changed after each patient, protect the dental team's upper airways (the mucous membranes of the nose and mouth) from contact with aerosol particles (*spray*) or oral fluids coming from the patient, rich in transmissible microorganisms via the airways. *Mycobacterium tuberculosis* found in aerosols, can cause respiratory infections. Therefore, it is necessary to use special masks in cases where there is a history or suspicion of tuberculosis. The mask chosen by the professional, must come with information about previous analysis of its filtration potential. It should provide triple protection, with an internal barrier capable of filtering particles released by aerosols. It must also fit well and be comfortable, antiallergic and allow normal breathing. The choice should be masks that do not fog up the eyewear. After clinical attendance, the mask must be discarded. It is opportune to point out that the use of a rubber sheet is a valuable resource in diminishing the aerosol of saliva and contaminated blood.

Protective eyewear is an important barrier that prevents contamination of the eyes with microorganisms, blood droplets or secretion (fluid), and must be decontaminated after each attendance.

Furthermore, it provides protection against operational accidents, and it is important to point out that both the dental team and the patient must wear protective eyewear during the clinical attendance. The risk of accidents is very high and everyone is susceptible to operational accidents capable of involving the eyes, as procedures involving cutting and grinding, produced by the high-speed handpiece are capable of causing microparticles and metal fragments, enamel and dentine to fly out of the patient's mouth.

Protective footwear constitutes barriers with the goal of avoiding the transmission of microorganisms to other areas of the dental office. The shoes worn during clinical attendance must be restricted to and used exclusively in this environment, with care about decontamination and cleanliness that have to be strictly followed. In critical procedures, protective footwear must be worn, in order to reduce contamination of the clinical environment.

### 12.4.3 Gloves

Wearing gloves in dental procedures is considered a routine protocol. Gloves are the best physical protection for the dental team's hands against contact with the saliva, blood, mucous fluids (tissues), and prevents the possible transmission and dissemination of infectant agents. The professional wears this type of mechanical barrier exclusively for each patient, and it is discarded immediately at the end of the attendance.

While the professional is wearing gloves, manipulation of any object out of the area of clinical attendance must be prevented. In surgical procedures with extreme bleeding, two pairs of gloves must be worn. Every time the gloves are removed, the hands must immediately be well washed.

Different types of gloves are found on the dental market: unsterilized latex gloves (indicated for semicritical procedures: dentistry, radiology, orthodontics and dental prosthesis); sterilized latex gloves (indicated for critical procedures: surgery, periodontology and endodontics); vinyl gloves (worn as "overgloves" to prevent the contamination of latex gloves, for example, while taking x-rays). Rubber gloves (thick latex) are still available for use in instrument cleaning and disinfection procedures, handling contaminated material and equipment, or for manipulating chemical substances. After the procedures, these rubber gloves must be disinfected, washed with soap and water and be air dried inside out.

### 12.4.4 Immunization

In addition to all the means of personal protection of the dental team against cross-infections, immunization against some preventable diseases is not only opportune but essential.

Immunization is a procedure that prevents the transmission of illnesses, by blocking the dissemination of the microorganisms. It presents a lower cost and is better than treating illnesses. Immunization can block the dissemination of a virus, bacterium or bacterial toxin, which favors reduction in the number of susceptible hosts in a population. However, there is a great deal of disinformation and even resistance, on the part of health professionals. Therefore, to be effective, the vaccination project must be mandatory, but the health professionals must also be made aware of its importance, considering that while many do not place value on immunization, others are unaware of the risk of acquiring infectious diseases, or think they are excluded from the group considered at risk of contamination. The use of individual protection equipment associated with immunization, reduces the risk of contamination of the dental team. Sterilization and disinfection procedures, together with IPEs and immunization constitute efficient ways of reducing the risk of cross-infection among the dental team, patients and their relatives.

### 12.4.5 Hand washing with antiseptic cleaner

Hand and arm washing with an antiseptic cleaning agent is one of the most essential measures of cross-infection control by the dental team at the dental clinic. The hands are capable of sheltering microorganisms that could be responsible for infections when they come into contact with exposed tissues.

The use of antimicrobial substances for degerming and antisepsis of the hands, and use of sterilized gloves, constitute a routine protocol recommended for all clinical procedures. These precautions prevent resident and transitory microbiota of the hands from being introduced into the depths of tissues during an invasive operative procedure.

The adoption of an aseptic technique during any clinical operative procedure, requires efficient hand washing with antiseptic cleaners that have a strong antimicrobial effect (immediate and residual), making it possible to reduce the microbial population considerably.

Within the scope of microbiology, degerming can be considered a process by which the microorganisms on tissue surfaces are mechanically removed (for example hand washing); antisepsis means the control of potential pathogenic "unsporulated" microorganisms present on the skin and mucosa, by the "cid" or "static" effect obtained with the use of chemical substances, called antiseptics.

Degerming and antisepsis are phases of procedures carried out by the surgical team, and should not be considered separately, but as a set with the aim of controlling infection properly. The majority of cutaneous microorganisms live and multiply in the corneous extract and on the surfaces of the pillous follicles, easily removed by degerming. Approximately 20% of these microbiota, however, are located deeply and escape the action of the normal processes of decontamination and antisepsis.

The object of antisepsis of the hands is to eliminate pathogenic microorganisms that have become deposited on the hands and constitute transitory microbiota. The preparations used for this antisepsis must act quickly, in a short period of time, and preferably maintain a residual effect on the amphibiotic microorganisms. Transitory microbiota are constituted of microorganisms with varied pathogenicity (mainly Gram-negative bacteria – responsible for part of hospital infections), whereas, the resident microbiota are considered pathogenic, and thought of as part of the colonized microbiota (constituted mainly of Gram-positive bacteria). These microbiota are difficult to remove with simple scrubbing, and require the use of antiseptic solutions. It must be considered that these microbiota hardly ever cause serious problems in normal patients, however, in immunodepressed patients it can induce complications. It is always important and essential to degerm the dental team's hands to reduce contamination by the amphibiotic microbiota, and also as a result of possible micro-perforations in the gloves, which can only be verified later after the clinical attendance. It is mandatory to wash the hands well before putting on and after removing the gloves in the clinical attendance of any patient. Another resource to reduce the cross-contamination is to reduce the microbiota of the mouth through the use of oral antiseptic solutions, like mouth washing with chlorhexidine solutions before clinical procedures, as it presents an immediate and residual effect.

In attempts to control the microorganisms present in the hand microbiota, different substances have been proposed for hand antisepsis. Amongst these, are:

1. 2% chlorhexidine digluconate;
2. Preparations with polyvinylpyrrolidone-iodine (PVP-I, alcohol solution, degerming solution, all of them 10%, with 1% of active iodine);
3. 1% iodized alcohol solution;
4. 1% tryclosan;
5. 70% isopropyl alcohol.

Caldart et al.[37] analyzed the antimicrobial effect of two pre-surgical hand degerming techniques (with and without scrubbing, associated with the use of 4% chlorhexidine digluconate). The samples had been collected from the hands of 20 students, with and without experience in pre-surgical procedures. The results showed that the two evaluated techniques of degerming, associated with the use of 4% chlorhexidine digluconate, in the time considered, presented a potential to reduce the amphibiotic microbiota of the hands.

Some precautions must, however, be adopted before degerming and antisepsis of the hands, such as: removing rings, earrings, watches and bracelets; tie up long hair, put on a cap and mask, put on and adjust protective eyewear; the tap for hand washing must be turned on by foot, elbow or photosensitive device, and the sink must not be touched. Hand washing must be performed to enable clean work; considering the presence of dirt on the hands after using the toilet, coughing, sneezing or blowing the nose, before and after caring for the patient; at the end of the day's work; before meals and after using the telephone

After the hands have been scrubbed, the gown must be put on with the help of the assistant. After hand scrubbing and putting on all the protective clothing, no surface or object may be touched.

Tables 12.6 to 12.8 describe in sequence, the stages of simple hand washing, hand degerming for clinical procedures and the degerming and antisepsis for surgical procedures.

**Table 12.6** - Sequence of the simple hand washing

| | |
|---|---|
| **1** | Open the tap with foot or elbow, or by a photosensitive device, wet the hands, without touching the sink; |
| **2** | Apply the appropriate antiseptic associated with a detergent; |
| **3** | Soap the hands, rubbing them for approximately 30 seconds, the palm and the back of hands, interdigital spaces, thumbs, joints, nails and extremities of the fingers; |
| **4** | Rinse the hands under running water, completely removing all residues of detergent, then with hands upright, proceed with drying; |
| **5** | Dry well with paper towels. |

**Table 12.7** - Sequence of hand degerming for clinical procedures (without scrubbing)

| | |
|---|---|
| **1** | Open the tap and wet the hands; |
| **2** | Apply detergent into the cup of the hand; |
| **3** | Rub the palms of the hands backwards and forwards; |
| **4** | Rub palm to palm with fingers entwined; |
| **5** | Rub the back of left hand with right palm, back of right hand with the left palm; |
| **6** | Rub interdigital spaces; |
| **7** | Rub the left thumb, the right one, the joints; |
| **8** | Rub the nails; |
| **9** | Rub the left wrist, the right one; |
| **10** | Rinse the hands under running water, completely removing all residues of detergent, keep hands upright, while drying well with sterilized compresses. |

**Table 12.8** - Sequence of hand degerming and antisepsis for surgical procedures (with scrubbing)

| | |
|---|---|
| **1** | Open the tap and wet the hands and arms; |
| **2** | Apply an antiseptic detergent into a cupped hand, soap the hands and the arms, ensuring the application of detergent and antiseptic; |
| **3** | Clean the nails with a plastic or wooden stylet and brush the nails; |
| **4** | Brush the back of fingers, interdigital spaces and fingers; |
| **5** | Brush the palm and the back of hands; |
| **6** | Brush the back of the arm; brush forearms; |
| **7** | Rinse the hands and arms well under running water, completely removing all residues of detergent; hold hands upright while drying well with sterilized compresses. |

In the case of wounds, impermeable dressings should be applied before washing, and it is necessary to work with two pairs of gloves; a separate sterilized compress must be used with each patient.

## 12.5 Organization of the Instruments

For efficient and systematic endodontic treatment, it is essential to have organized work benches. A good professional is easily recognized by the preparation of the operating table. Thus, for good clinical performance, the table must be prepared in accordance with the clinical procedure to be performed. The minimum of instruments required and strict control of aseptic technique favor the calm development of the treatment.

Taking into consideration the aim, the instruments must be in a suitable condition to ensure performance of the sterilization process. Thus, the instruments can be laid out in stainless steel boxes, composed of the instruments necessary for each stage of the operation:

1. Clinical instruments;
2. Endodontic instruments;
3. Instruments and material for absolute isolation;
4. Instruments for coronal opening;
5. Complementary instruments;
6. Endodontic material.

## 12.6 Instrument Cleaning

Correct cleaning of the instruments used in the dental office represents an essential stage in microbial control. The removal of adhered blood, saliva, remains of organic and inorganic material, residual dental materials, favors elimination of the microorganisms present on the instruments before the sterilization process. The goal of this decontamination using physical and/or chemical means is to inactivate the pathogenic agents in order to keep the manipulation and disposal safe.

The clinical instrument decontamination procedures before sterilization, increase the dental team's safety, to protect them from exposure to pathogenic agents, as these agents can be isolated by the presence of organic material. Subsequent to the clinical procedures, it is mandatory for the instruments to be submitted to the decontamination process, from precleaning using enzymatic detergents that favor the effectiveness of the process. Amongst the resources routinely used for instrument precleaning are: manual scrubbing and ultrasonic cleaning.

The enzymatic substance selected for cleaning with ultrasound must be in accordance with the type of contamination (presence of organic material or dental material – cements). The enzymatic substances contain different enzymes that act on the remainders of dirt adhered to the instruments (for instance: protease, amylase, lipase, carbohydrase).

Manual cleaning consists of decontaminating the clinical instruments before washing and scrubbing (brushing). After the use of the clinical instrument, it is conditioned by using a system containing two plastic cuvettes (one internal, with perforations and one external, without perforations containing an enzymatic substance for decrusting, for a period of 5 to 20 minutes, depending on the type of substance used, and on the clinical origin of the instruments. After the necessary time for decontamination has elapsed, the instruments are carefully removed with the perforated cuvette, rinsing abundantly under running water, and after this are removed with Collins 2S forceps and scrubbed with water and detergent. After these procedures, the plastic cuvettes also have to be appropriately washed.

The precleaning performed in the ultrasound unit is done by piezo-electric oscillators that raise the pressure fluctuation in the liquid, created by the sound effect on the water. The different amplitudes create microscopic vacuum bubbles (high frequency sound waves); when these bubbles implode, they create small areas of vacuum that facilitate detachment of the dirt or the adhered material (scrubbing action). This process reaches these small and difficult spaces better than manual scrubbing does. Basically, it should be explained and remembered that this precleaning process does not dispense the need of the sterilization process. Nevertheless, it is an excellent opportunity to decontaminate the instruments first, in order to favor the complete elimination of microbes by sterilization.

The ultrasonic cleaning process has several advantages over manual cleaning, amongst them following are emphasized; reduced risk of accidents with perforating-cutting instruments, reduced working time, and a more efficient cleaning process.

The effective precleaning process time with the ultrasonic system ranges from 5 to 10 minutes, depending on the type of instrument, contaminated material, enzymatic solution and the device manufacturer's specifications. The tray, containing the instruments must not be crowded, and instruments that are connected, must be disconnected. The solution must cover all the surfaces of the instruments, not less than 3 cm from the bottom of the cuvette, and not more than 1 cm from the top edge. In some ultrasonic cuvettes, these divisions are already demarcated (Figs. 12.9 and 12.10). After the cleaning process, the tray containing the liquid and instruments is removed, well rinsed preferably in warm water, then the precleaned instruments are scrubbed with water and detergent.

## 12.7 Drying and Packaging

It is mandatory to comply with all the procedures necessary to control infection in the dental office. Thus, none of the stages involved in this decontamination process must be omitted. Drying and the packaging are also important phases and must be observed. Drying the instruments with a clean and dry cloth, or in a kiln at 60°C are procedures in accordance with basic decontamination protocols.

The packaging of the clinical instruments in packets, metal boxes or bottles with cloth or paper lids, plastic perforated envelopes or crepe paper, follows the clinical recommendations. Plastic envelopes make it easy to see the contents, as one of the sides is transparent.

When packaging for autoclaving, it is recommended that the packs are made of raw cotton, double, with an adjustable textile closing device; surgical paper; Kraft paper, polyamide film and plastic envelopes. It is important for the instruments to be adequately packed for sterilization.

There are commercial sealers on the market that help the packaging of instruments in plastic envelopes (Figs. 12.11 and 12.12).

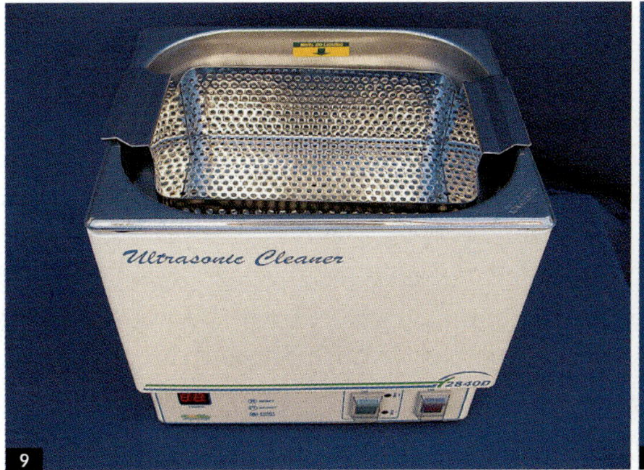


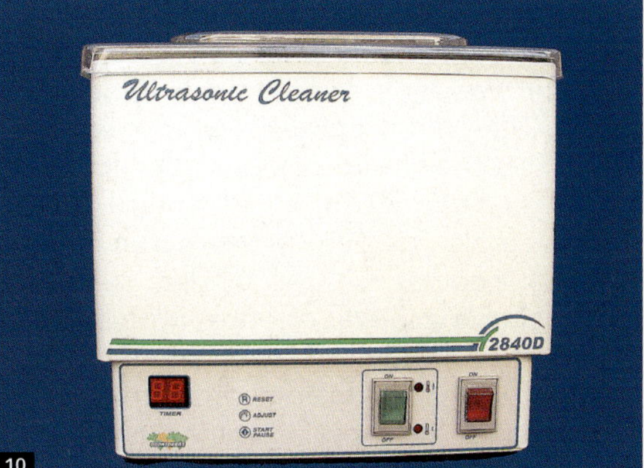


**Figures 12.9 and 12.10** - Ultrasonic system.

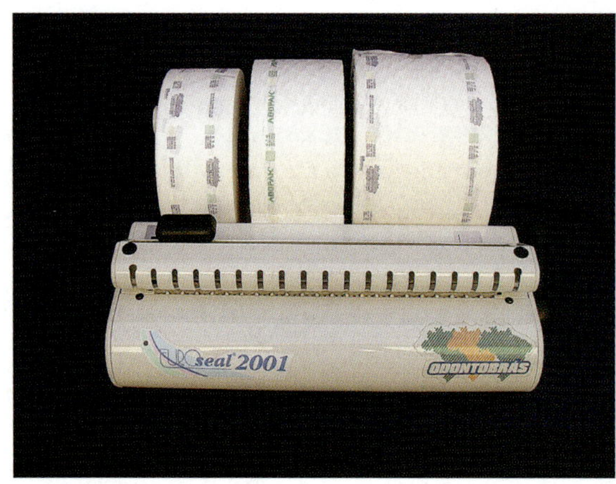


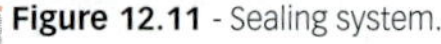

Figure 12.11 - Sealing system.

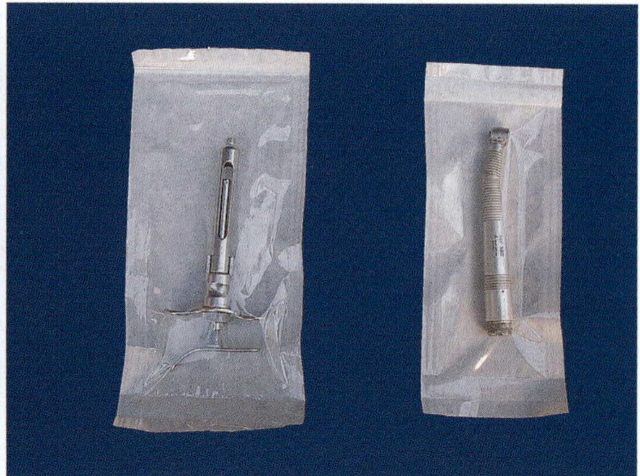

Figure 12.12 - Packaging of instruments and dental material.

## 12.8 Sterilization Processes

The decontamination process consists of cleanliness, disinfection and sterilization. The preparation of contaminated instruments for reuse in clinical procedures is considered a basic factor in cross-infection control. The processing of contaminated instruments involves different stages, such as: pre-cleaning, quality control of the instruments (corrosion, lubrication, damage etc.), drying, wrapping up, sterilization, monitoring of sterilization and handling of sterilized instruments.

With the aim of assuring a suitable process for decontaminating inanimate objects (articles, equipment, instruments), Spauding[218] classified them into three levels according to infection risks: non critical, semicritical and critical. The critical articles require sterilization. These items are composed of instruments that penetrate the mucous membrane, incomplete skin, tissues, vascular system – for example: needles, scalpel blades, surgical instruments, explorers, curettes, probes etc. The semiciritcal articles need sterilization, however, when they do not tolerate this, they must receive "high-level" disinfection. They are composed of items that come into contact with complete mucosa – for example, the amalgam condenser etc. The non-critical articles must be cleaned and disinfected, because they are items that are in contact with the complete skin and do not come into contact with the patient – for example, the switch, the reflector, the door handle, the chair, the worktable etc.

Cottone et al.[57,58] emphasized that the basic protocol for infection control recommends that "you must not disinfect when you can sterilize". One could add though, that sterilization certainly represents an essential stage in the program of cross-infection control.

Sterilization is a procedure that is responsible for the complete destruction of every microbial form of life (resistant forms, like bacterial spores, mycobacteria, unwrapped viruses – without lipid – and fungi). This process can be developed in physical ways (humid heat – steam under pressure, autoclave; dry heat – Pasteur oven, kiln; ultraviolet radiation, ionizing radiation) by gases, steam (ethylene oxide, formaldehyde, hydrogen peroxide, plasma) and chemical processes (glutaraldehyde).

The sterilization methods that involve physical processes, particularly, humid heat (performed by autoclave) and dry heat (developed by kiln), represent the most frequent sterilization methods used in dental offices. These methods are recommended for most instruments, except those sensitive to heat or those that present toxic or volatile chemical substances.

Other methods have also been used, such as ultraviolet and ionizing radiation (gamma rays). Ultraviolet radiation is used to disinfect the laminar flow chamber, the dental offices (surgical rooms). To disinfect the surrounding air, it is important for the lights to be at the top part of the room. Nowadays, there are ultraviolet devices on the market, for the purpose of disinfecting the surrounding air present by ultraviolet radiation. It is important to emphasize that to obtain the desired effect, it is necessary to expose the microorganism directly to the light. The effectiveness of the ultraviolet radiation is associated with lethal mutation (chemical alterations in DNA, intervening in its later replication).

The ethylene oxide is another important system for sterilization, operated by gas heat. Nevertheless, there are regulations limiting its use, particularly as a result of its toxicity. It has a wider application in hospitals and some clinics. In dental offices, generally, this method is less used. The exposure time for the process to be effective is relatively long.

Another resource used for microbial control is formaldehyde gas. Currently its use is reduced, because of its limitations, in addition to being considered a carcinogenic substance.

Plasma is a mixture of electrons and ions produced by the discharge of electromagnetic forces, at low gas pressure. Reactive free reagents with the frequency of a microwave oven or radio frequency are produced, constituting a new method capable of effective sterilization. This method does not produce toxic derivatives. In addition to eliminating bacteria, fungi, viruses and spores, it is also able to remove microorganisms from the instrument surface, which emphasizes its importance as a significant sterilization resource even more. It is believed that this process will eventually substitute the applications of ethylene oxide.

Among the substances considered as chemical sterilizers, glutaraldehyde is an effective alternative (considered as high level disinfecting), for the purpose of sterilizing instruments sensitive to heat and to replace deodorants with chlorine (due to possibility of damaging instruments and surfaces. However, when manipulating this chemical substance, care must be taken, because of the possibility of irritating the eyes, and the respiratory mucosa. 2% Glutaraldehyde alkaline is effective on spores, bacilli (such as *Mycobacterium tuberculosis*), fungi and a large variety of viruses. The instruments must remain immersed in the solution for ten hours.

Other chemical sterilizer used for instruments sensitive to heat is peracetic acid. It is a highly biocidal oxider with rapid action – 30 minutes under 50 to 56°C (122°F to 133°F). It must be remembered that when manipulating chemical substances the dental team must use all the individual protection equipament.

### 12.8.1 Sterilization with humid heat (vapor under pressure, autoclave)

Sterilization performed by water vapor under pressure (done by autoclave) is the fastest and the most efficient method. The high temperature produces denaturation of microbial proteins, since there is greater heat penetration under pressure, therefore, the humidity (water) catalyzes the protein coagulation. Microorganisms are quickly destroyed during autoclaving, but this is influenced by temperature, time, volume of the autoclave, vapor flow speed, density and size of the material placed in the chamber.

The autoclave sterilization process is generally carried out over a period of 20 minutes at a temperature of 250°F (121°C) and under a pressure of 15 pounds. A great deal of care is required not to create air pockets, as they can interfere with the steam penetration. As the material is wet at the end of the sterilization, an additional period of time is needed for drying it. In this process there is the problem of corrosion on metal instruments because of the high amount of oxygen present. As way to minimize and prevent corrosion, the addition of a chemical substance (1% sodium nitrite), which evaporates during the sterilization process, has been considered[57,58].

There are different models of autoclaves (as for example, vacuum autoclaves) with a shorter sterilization time (from 3 to 6 minutes), and higher temperature and pressure (273°F/134°C/30 pounds). The variation in the period of time of the vacuum autoclaves depends on the time required to exclude the residual air, create a vacuum and saturate the chamber with water vapor (Figs. 12.13 and 12.14).

The autoclave sterilization procedures must be carefully and strictly obeyed, always following the manufacturer's instructions. The sterilization cycle must be guided by the type of instrument that must be presented clean, dry and duly conditioned. The volume of loading that fills the autoclave must not exceed two thirds of the chamber capacity, so that the instruments must be accommodated in a way that does not interfere with the steam circulation (the folds of the packages must be placed upside down to facilitate steam penetration). The packages must not touch the lateral or posterior surfaces of the device, and must be correctly packed (amount and thickness adjusted in the packages). It is important to maintain space between the packages to ensure steam circulation, and concave objects must be placed upside down. After the instruments are removed from the autoclave, they must be kept in a clean place until use. The evidence of extreme humidity in the packages, and the presence of perforations, are indications of the possibility that the process has failed. Table 12.9 describes some characteristics of autoclave and kiln sterilization.

### 12.8.2 Sterilization with dry heat (Pasteur furnace, kiln)

The sterilization by dry heat (operated by kiln) is the resource dentists most frequently use. The unit, known as the kiln and sold under this name, consists of a metal container with double walls; coated with asbestos on the outside and on the inside it has electric filaments regulated by a thermostat, normally enabling it to maintain a maximum temperature of 300°C (572°F).

Dry heat needs long periods and high temperatures for the sterilization process, when compared with the humid heat or the plasma system, because the diffusion and heat penetration are slow. To perform the sterilization process effectively, one hour at the temperature of 170°C (338°F), or two hours at 160°C (320°F) are required. The microorganism destruction mechanism is developed by microbial protein oxidation. This method preserves the instrument from corrosion, but damages plastic materials (rubber), polymers, cellulose, and fabrics. For sterilization in the kiln, it must be heat when the instruments are introduced into the kiln (160-170°C/320-338°F – the time of one or two hours is counted according to this temperature) and removed only at the end of this time, to accomplish complete sterilization. Currently, there is a kiln with door constraint that only allows the door to open after the complete performance of the programmed sterilization process. The cycle to be completed by the kiln must not be interrupted at any moment. It is important to take care with exposure to an exaggerated temperature, because this could cause problems with some instruments. The instrument is placed in the kiln (packed adequately) using metal boxes or aluminum foil, kept closed and identified (date and type of material) (Fig. 12.15).

**Table 12.9** - Sterilization by humid heat (autoclave) and dry heat (kiln)

| Autoclaves | Conventional | Automatic |
|---|---|---|
| Temperature<br>Pressure<br>Cycle (time) | 121ºC (250ºF)<br>15 pounds (psi)<br>15 to 20 minutes | 132ºC (270ºF)<br>30 pounds (psi)<br>3 to 6 minutes |
| **Kiln** | | |
| Temperature<br>Cycle (time) | 160ºC (320ºF)<br>2 hours | 170ºC (338ºF)<br>1 hour |

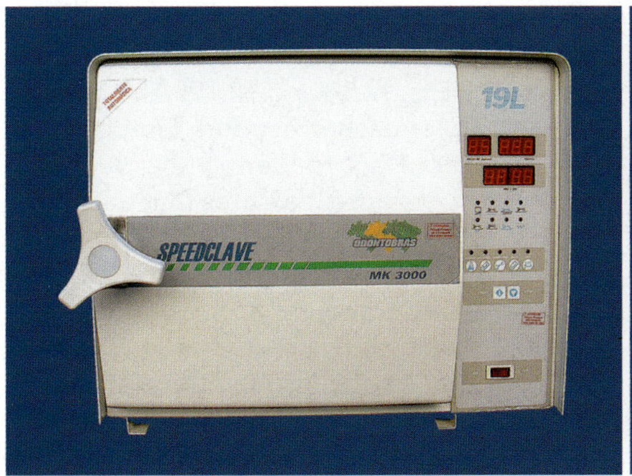


**Figure 12.13** - Conventional Autoclave.

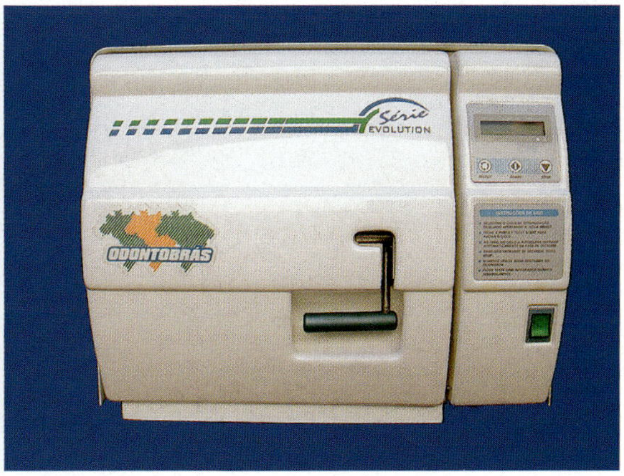

**Figure 12.14** - Vacuum Autoclave.

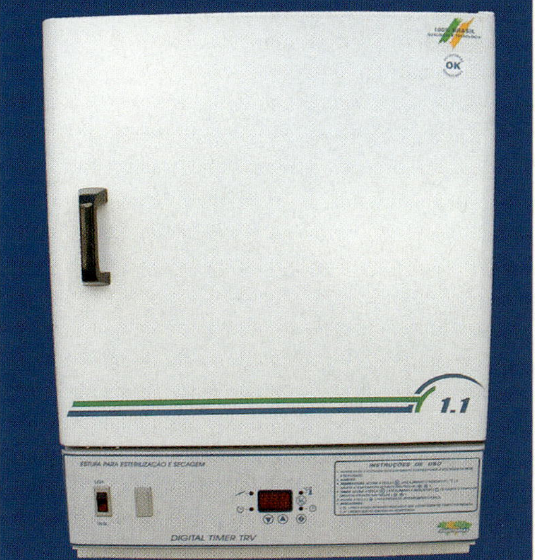


**Figure 12.15** - Kiln.

### 12.8.3 Monitoring the Sterilization Process

The procedures that involve sterilization must be carefully and regularly analyzed to be certain of successful decontamination and therefore prevent possible imperfections. For example, in some situations it can be evident that temperatures recorded by the thermometer are not real (true).Therefore, monitoring is important, and the three markers can be used: biological, chemical and physical. To guarantee effective sterilization, also imposes control of the markers themselves.

Biological markers consist of bacterial spores. For the autoclave the spores indicated are *Bacillus stearothermophilus* and for the kiln *Bacillus subtilis*. These spores can be found in different forms, impregnated in strips of filter paper or in small bottles (blisters). The spores presented in bottles are practical, made up of a blister with a double chamber, with the presence of spores on the inner surface, and a culture medium on the outer. After the autoclaving process, the blisters are removed and squeezed or twisted slightly, allowing the spores to come into contact with the culture medium and subsequently incubated for 7 days at 56°C (133°F) (for *Bacillus stearothermophilus*) or at 37°C (99°F) (for *Bacillus subtilis*). Imperfection in the process is indicated by the presence of blurring in the culture medium, whereas the absence of blurring is indicative of successful sterilization (Figs. 12.16 and 12.17).

Another type of biological marker consists of traps, impregnated with spores that can be sent to the laboratory for culture, soon after being exposed, or up to 7 days after exposure.

Two aspects must be verified when monitoring sterilization: human error in performance of the procedures, and mechanical failures.

The chemical markers consist of chemical substances (chemical reagents), present on traps, labels, envelopes and in small bottles, whose color changes (either on paper, or in the liquid) when submitted to the sterilization process. There are markers that evaluate only the temperature aspects and the presence of steam and those that evaluate time, presence of steam and temperature. For autoclaves and kilns there are adhesive ribbons, resistant to high temperatures that change color after completing the sterilization cycle (Figs. 12.18 and 12.19). The ribbons are specific for each procedure (autoclave or kiln). It is important to identify the packages with ribbon, because it assures that they were submitted to heat.

The physical markers consist of thermometers and manometers (temperature and pressure markers). In some situations, the effectiveness of the sterilization process cannot be guaranteed. For this reason, it is necessary to constantly gauge the exact functioning of the devices (by thermometer, manometer and thermostat).

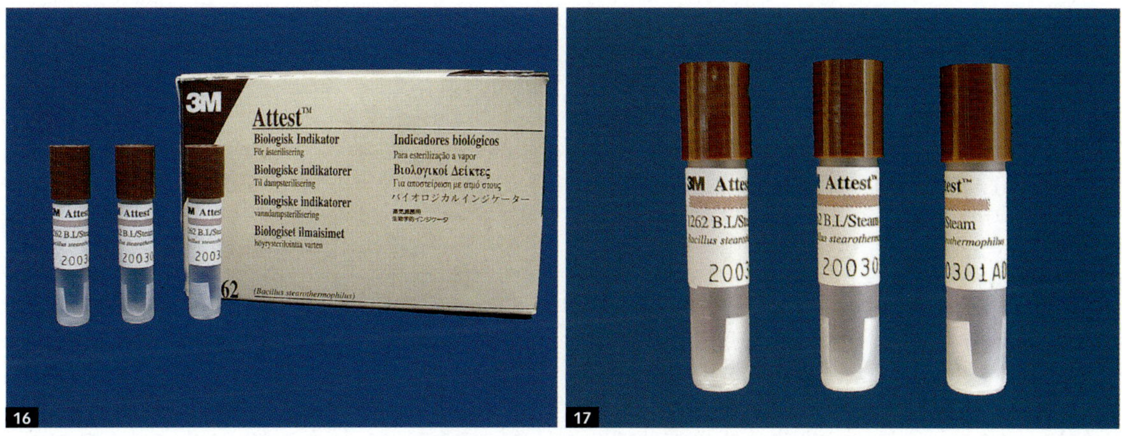


Figures 12.16 and 12.17 - Biological marker.

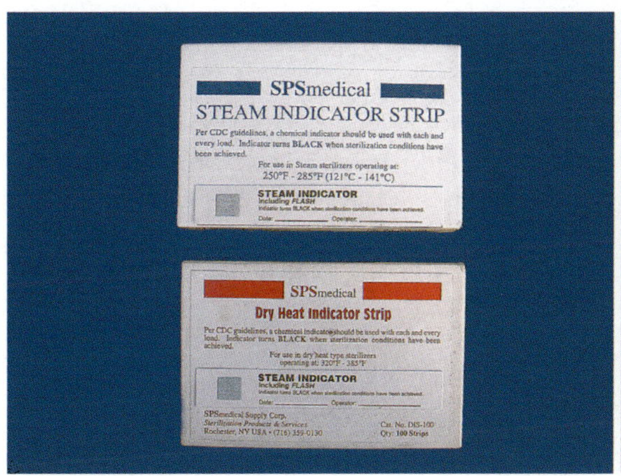


Figure 12.18 - Chemical marker.

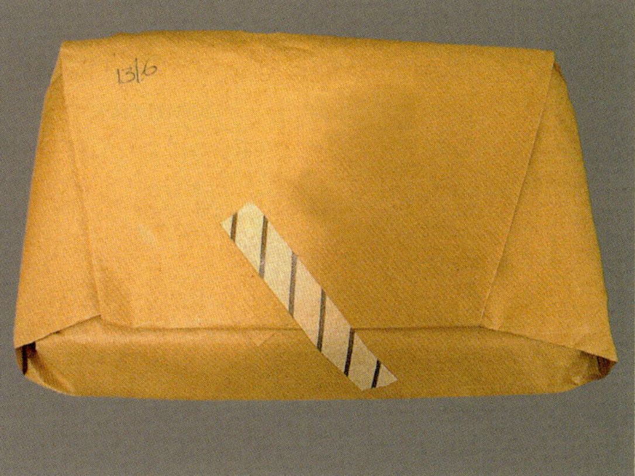

Figure 12.19 - Ribbons marker.

## 12.9 Disinfection

Disinfection consists of procedures that endeavor to destroy pathogenic microorganisms in the vegetative form (not affecting spores), through chemical agents (disinfectant substances) on inanimate surfaces. It is important to emphasize that sterilization is the process that really promotes complete and effective microbial destruction, which should not be confused with disinfection.

Disinfection processes can be classified into three levels of effectiveness: high, intermediate (medium) and low. High level disinfection is designated to objects involved in critical procedures (invasive) that would not tolerate sterilization (for example, surgical instruments with plastic components that can not be autoclaved). In these cases, disinfection needs to be preceded by adequate cleaning (precleaning to remove the organic material). Among the high level disinfectants, are 2% glutaraldehyde. Intermediate level disinfection (medium) is indicated for cleaning in semicritical conditions (little possibility of contamination by bacterial spores and resistant microorganisms). The agents most recommended as disinfectants are iodized-alcohol, iodine composites, chlorine composites, and phenolic composites. Low level disinfection is used for non-critical situations. The most recommended agents are the ammonium quaternary composites.

Thus, the level of the disinfectants for surfaces is determined by the risk of constituting a reservoir of pathogenic microorganisms. It is important to consider the contact time necessary for the disinfection agent to exert its real effectiveness, and also, whether its action occurs only by friction, or whether the instrument needs to be immersed in the chemical substance. Among the factors that modify the activity of the disinfectants the degree of contamination (number and resistance of microorganisms), concentration of the disinfectant, and exposure time must be considered.

### 12.9.1 Antisepsis

Antisepsis comprises the attempt to destroy pathogenic microorganisms in animate beings (for example: the oral cavity, skin), by antiseptic substances. Antisepsis can involve extra-oral and intra-oral procedures. According to the Brazilian Health Ministry (2000)[153] norms for infection control, the indications for extra-oral antiseptics include the 10,0% PVPI-based solutions (with 1.0% of available iodine) and 2.0 and 4.0% chlorhexidine. For the intra-oral antisepsis iodine composites (PVPI), chlorhexidine and ammonium quaternary composites can be used.

### 12.9.2 Disinfecting Substances

#### Aldehydes

Aldehydes are represented by formaldehyde and glutaraldehyde (high level disinfectants). These substances exert their effects by the alkylation of sulphydril radicals, hydroxyl, carboxylic and amine group of proteins and nucleic acids of the microorganisms, with DNA, RNA and protein synthesis alterations.

Glutaraldehyde is constituted of two units of aldehyde (di-aldehyde), being more active at an alkaline pH, however, less steady. At the concentration of 2%, it was shown to be effective on bacteria in the vegetative form (*M. tuberculosis*), fungi and viruses, presenting the ability of destroying spores, after 10 hours of immersion. This substance was shown to be a tissue irritant, being able to cause burns on the skin or mucosa. Glutaraldehyde is also inactivated by organic material, which requires the precleaning of the material to be sterilized.

#### Halogen composites

Halogen composites are widely used as deodorants, represented by composites that contain iodine or chlorine.

The composites that contain iodine are also efficient for disinfection. The action mechanism of iodine provides high reactivity, precipitating proteins and oxidizing essential proteins. With the presence of organic and inorganic substances, iodine activity can be reduced. The iodine can be dissolved in water, potassium iodide, alcohol, or complexed with a transporter (known as iodophore). The iodophores are iodized composites (prepared with a surface tension reducer substance and stabilizer), classified as medium level disinfectants (these composites are also used as antiseptics). An iodized product widely used as preoperative antiseptic solution, is PVPI (10% polyvinylpyrrolidone-iodine in alcoholic solution with 1% active iodine).

The hypochlorites are known as halogen composites and their use began in 1792, when they were produced for the first time and received the name Javele Water. In 1820, Labarraque, a French chemist obtained sodium hypochlorite with 2.5% active chlorine, began to be used as a wound disinfectant. In 1915, Dakin, an American chemist, during the First World War, proposed a new solution of sodium hypochlorite with 0.5% active chlorine, neutralized by boric acid. The solution of sodium hypochlorite with high pH (around 11 to 12) is stabler, and chlorine release is slower. As soon as the pH of the solution is reduced, either with boric acid, or with sodium bicarbonate (Dausfrene Solution), the solution is stabler and the loss of chlorine is faster. This means that useful life of the solution is short. Sun light and high temperature cause the chlorine release, leaving the solution inefficient. The verification of the active chlorine content is important, as the professional must not use the modified product, therefore, the expected efficiency as disinfectant is compromised. The effectiveness of sodium hypochlorite is due to the antimicrobial properties and the ability to dissolve tissue. This solution is presented as an intermediate level disinfectant (medium).

The action mechanism of sodium hypochlorite has been discussed because of its physical-chemical and antimicrobial properties. Sodium hypochlorite is elected as an efficient disinfectant solution at higher concentrations. This is because of the action mechanism of this solution, able to promote biosynthetic cellular alterations; alterations in cell metabolism and destruction of phospholipids; formation of chloramines that intervene in the cell metabolism; oxidant action, with irreversible enzymatic inhibition in bacteria; degradation of fatty acids and lipids. Sodium hypochlorite can be found in the following concentrations of active chlorine: 5% (chlorinated soda), 2.5% (Labaraque solution), 1% (Milton solution) and 0.5% (Dakin solution).

Sodium hypochlorite solution presents fast antimicrobial action, and a significant ability to dissolve organic material. The antimicrobial effect and the ability of tissue dissolution are directly proportional to the concentration of the solution.

Following the guidelines on infection control recommended by the Brazilian Health Ministry (2000)[153], there are indications for the disinfection of instruments, when it is impossible to submit the articles to the sterilization process, by immersion in 1% sodium hypochlorite solution, or 2% glutaraldehyde water solution for 30 minutes. For metal disinfection, glutaraldehyde solution (with time cycle in accordance with the manufacturer's specifications) is more suitable, as sodium hypochlorite presents a corrosive action with a cumulative effect. After using sodium hypochlorite on metal surfaces, they must be rinsed and dried immediately.

### Alcohols

The antimicrobial action of alcohols occurs on vegetative bacteria, mycobacteria, some fungi and viruses that contain lipids. Alcohols present poor activity on bacterial spores and on some fungi and viruses that do not contain lipids, and its effectiveness rises with the increase in the length of the chain. Alcohols are considered intermediate level bactericides, being inefficient on the hydrophilic viruses (such as Hepatitis B).

The most frequently used alcohols are ethyl and isopropanol alcohol. The 70% alcohol is more active than 95% alcohol, therefore its highest activity occurs in the presence of water. Alcohol is a surface disinfectant, and in association with iodofors it was shown to be efficient for antisepsis of the skin.

Since 1996, the ADA and CDC do not recommend 70% alcohol to disinfect the surfaces and the materials. The 70% alcohol does not present tuberculocide action[57, 147].

### Phenolic composites

The phenolic composites are considered intermediate level disinfectants. They present bactericide, fungicide and virucide actions, but the bacterial spores, and the hydrophilic viruses show resistance, whereas the lipophil virus are shown to be susceptible. These composites have been associated with detergents with the purpose of facilitating cleaning, and are recommended for surface disinfection, and for use in hospitals. They have been prepared for use by diluting them in water in a ratio of 1 to 50. The phenolic composites present toxic and irritant effects on the skin and eyes.

## 12.10 Cleaning and Disinfection of the Dental Office

The decontamination process of the dental office must be effective and able to prevent cross-infections. It is therefore essential to implement a routine, standard and rational cleaning and disinfection protocol that strives for the performance of an excellent aseptic treatment technique, capable of reducing the potential to transmit infectious diseases.

The aim of dental office cleaning disinfection is the complete, or partial elimination of microorganisms, and must be performed after the patient has been attended. The use of barriers (surface covers) on dental equipment constitutes an important procedure. It is opportune to stress that decontamination of the dental office must prioritize care to avoid infections, which imposes on all those involved, the mandatory use of individual protection equipment (rubber gloves, mask, protective eyewear, gown).

Mouth rinsing with antiseptic substances (such as chlorexidine digluconate) before the beginning of treatment, and the use of absolute isolation with a rubber dam, help reduction of the number of microorganisms that are spread during clinical attendance. Chlorexidine used as an antiseptic solution has shown to be efficient against oral cavity microbiota. The rubber dam acts as an effective barrier, capable of reducing the action of microorganism-rich aerosols from the oral cavity, hurled into the external environment by the high-speed or slow-speed hand pieces.

The environment of the dental office presents different areas of contamination, which have to be specially treated during the performance of the decontamination process. Thus, considering the level of contamination of each area, they can be divided into: critical area (treatment place, with a higher possibility of contamination, comprising the chair, equipment and auxiliary unit, which demand a high level of decontamination); semicritical area (limited to the treatment, – composed of the operating light, radiographic device, chair control switch); and the non-critical area (peripheral area that does not come into contact with the patient or the contaminating agent, or that involves areas distant from the treatment).

The adoption of an aseptic technique for clinical attendance is essential for preventing cross-infection. The dental team's work environment requires special treatment, supported by a strict decontamination protocol during office cleaning. Therefore, the dental appliances, room and closets also have to receive an suitable disinfection. It must be remembered that all instruments must be perfectly sterilized and correctly stored. When analyzing the conduct involved in cross-infection control in the dental office, the standard rule must be remembered: "do not disinfect what can be sterilized".

## 12.11 Dental Equipment

Perfect cleaning constantly requires washing with water and soap, before disinfection. The procedures involved in cleaning and disinfection will be presented, with emphasis on the standardized (universal) safety measures for infection control.

Modern equipment facilitates infection control, as it has been developed with the appropriate design to implement an aseptic technique. The dental equipment used in the cleaning and disinfection processes will be presented separately. The decontamination process will have a parameter that considers the infection risks from inanimate objects and the criteria adopted by Spauding, such as those shown in Table 12.10. The chemical substances used in this process will be considered as regards their effectiveness of disinfection, as shown in Table 12.11. It is convenient to point out that disinfectants can be used in different ways: by immersion of the articles (e.g., in 2% glutaraldehyde for longer than 6 hours); or by friction (disinfectants are applied on external surfaces, e.g., sodium hypochlorite). Adequate cleaning with soap and water is essential before the disinfection process. In some circumstances, the washing procedure is also recommended. For example, after cleaning an auxiliary unit with water and soap, and rubbing it with disinfectant (2.5% sodium hypochlorite), it can be washed with the same disinfectant substance. When choosing a substance to use as a deodorant, it must be analyzed with regard to its antimicrobial qualities and the risks inherent to its toxicity.

The parts of the dental equipment that need disinfection constitute all those that can be contaminated during dental procedures (by the dental team's hands, droplets with infectant agents and aerosols). The dental equipment involved in the decontamination process comprises the chair, equipment (support table, combination syringe, hand pieces (high and slow-speed), auxiliary unit (suction system), clinical table, radiography device, operating light and switches).



**Table 12.10** - Infection risks

| Articles | Infection risks by inanimate objects |
|---|---|
| **Critical** | Items that require sterilization. They comprise instruments that penetrate mucosa, incomplete and complete skin, tissues, vascular system – for example: needles, scalpels, surgical instruments, explorers, curettes, probes. |
| **Semicritical** | Items that need sterilization, but when they do not tolerate it, they must receive a "high level" disinfection. They comprise items that are in contact with complete mucosa. |
| **Non-critical** | Items that must be cleaned and disinfected, therefore, they comprise items that come into contact with the complete skin and do not come into contact with the patient – for example: switch, reflector, door handle, chair, bench. |

(Spauding[218], 1972)

**Table 12.11** - Levels of disinfectant effectiveness

| Level | Application |
|---|---|
| **High** | They comprise objects involved in critical procedures (invasive), which do not tolerate sterilization. Disinfection must be preceded by adequate cleaning (precleaning to remove the organic material). High level deodorants are composed of: glutaraldehyde 2%, peracetic acid. |
| **Medium** | Indicated for cleaning surfaces or instruments in semicritical situations (small probability of contamination by bacterial spores and resistant microorganisms). The most recommended agents are iodized-alcohol, iodophore compounds, chlorine compounds and phenolic composites. |
| **Low** | Used for non-critical situations, such as for surface disinfection. The most recommended agents are ammonium quaternary compounds, detergents. |

### 12.11.1 Chair

The dental chair is the place the patient is in direct contact with for a certain length of time, and where he/she is exposed to indirect contamination by aerosols, saliva droplets, blood and other infectant agents, produced during the clinical attendance. Therefore, barriers such as protector drapes for the chair, arms and head back-rest have been used. Disposable drapes must be replaced after each patient. On modern chairs the controls are foot operated to avoid direct contact with the professional. With chairs that have hand controls, it is safer to use plastic covers. Nevertheless, the chair must be cleaned with soap and water, followed by disinfection with 1% sodium hypochlorite (by friction with an absorbent sponge).

### 12.11.2 Control unit

The control unit can be the cart type, or associated with the chair-reflector set. Whatever the model, it must be protected with a drape or another type of protective barrier. Generally, some boxes with instruments for the clinical exam (complete isolation instruments, burs, tray are placed on the control unit surface. The control unit must undergo a disinfection procedure identical to that of the chair, (cleaning with soap and water, followed by disinfection with 1% sodium hypochlorite by rubbing the surface with an absorbent sponge).

On the control unit, there are the instrument tray and connectors for air/water syringe handle, high and slow-speed hand pieces. The hoses of the hand pieces must be smooth and must be protected with plastic barriers. The air/water syringe handle must be disinfected by friction with 1% sodium hypochlorite. After the hand pieces have been used, the asepsis system must be applied to the water supply line.

After the cleaning procedure, the high and slow-speed hand pieces must be sterilized by vacuum autoclave. In the course of time, sterilization can be responsible for damaging hand pieces structurally or mechanically, nevertheless, it is the safest resource for cross-infection control. After sterilization, the hand pieces must also be covered with protective barriers.

### 12.11.3 Auxiliary unit

The auxiliary unit requires particularly careful cleaning and disinfection procedures, as this equipment comes into direct contact with the organic fluids of the patient. The chosen disinfectant must present high antimicrobial effectiveness. The auxiliary unit (cuspidor) must be made of ceramic and be easy to remove, in order to avoid oxidation and corrosion, minimize the damage suffered during disinfection, as well as facilitate cleaning. This equipment is mobile, which allows it to be horizontally displaced in relation to the chair, in order to enable two pairs of hands to work. The auxiliary unit must be cleaned with the appropriate brush, soap and water, and be disinfected by friction with 2.5% sodium hypochlorite. The dental team professional that performs this procedure must wear thick rubber gloves.

The saliva ejector connector must preferably be a high power vacuum pump that diminishes the possibility of reflux. The saliva ejector must also be disposable, however, in surgical interventions metal units are indicated because they can be sterilized by autoclaving.

### 12.11.4 Reflector, X-ray machine, chair command switches

On these items of equipment, adhesive plastic barriers avoid direct contact with the professional's hands (or feet). This area is considered semicritical. Disinfection by friction with 1% sodium hypochlorite, must always be preceded by cleaning with soap and water).

## 12.12 Room (floor, wall, ceiling)

Every place that the professional and the dental team come into contact with can be contaminated, and must therefore undergo some type of decontamination process. The surfaces to be cleaned and disinfected could present dust and microorganisms. Therefore it must be possible to perform these decontamination and maintenance processes easily in all the places, which is easier if the surfaces are smooth.

The disinfection process for the walls, floor and ceiling is carried out by friction with 1% sodium hypochlorite, or a phenolic compound, preceded by washing with soap and water.

## 12.13 Material and Instruments for Clinical Use

The disinfection and sterilization procedure of material and instruments used in each specialty must follow the general infection control protocol, previously presented. It must be remembered at all times that disinfection is carried out in cases where sterilization is not possible, and that cross-infection is not something peculiar to one specialty, but must be prevented by all those related to the chain of infection.

In some clinical specialties (Operative Dentistry, Endodontics, Periodontics, Pedodontics, Prosthetics, Surgery), the set of instruments is basically composed of clinical instruments, specific instruments, instruments and materials for isolation, instruments for coronal opening and complementary instruments. Thus, all the necessary care must be taken with the goal of preventing cross-infection during dental attendance.

As regards the use of critical articles, such as anesthetic needles and scalpel blades, it is important to warn about the risks of occupational accidents. Before being discarded in the appropriate special packing for perforating-cutting articles, anesthetic needles and scalpel blades must be predisinfected by immersion in 2.5% sodium hypochlorite for 30 minutes in a rigid container.

## 12.14 Occupational Accidents (during the attendance or cleaning of the office)

An infectious contagious diseases is not always identified during the anamnesis and/or clinical exam, because at this time, it is difficult to recognize whether the patient is a carrier of a disease, and thus a potential infectant agent. Therefore, it is considered mandatory to implement universal standard precautions in all clinical attendances, which enable the prevention of possible infections. It is considered that the chain of infection (comprising the etiologic agent, transmissibility (material volume, type of exposure) and the susceptible host) makes the dental team vulnerable during any clinical attendance.

The Brazilian Health Ministry[153] (2000) guidelines for health services on handling occupational exposure by professionals, establishes that they must always have at their disposal, a system that includes:

- written protocols to report the fact;
- accident evaluation;
- notification;
- treatment and accompaniment of the health professional at risk of acquiring any infection.

Therefore, it is essential that the health professional informs the occurrence of the incident as quickly as possible, because when prophylactic measures are recommended, they must be implemented immediately after the accident. The procedures include local care of the exposed area, specific recommendations for immunization against tetanus, chemoprophylactic measures and serum follow-up for hepatitis B, C and AIDS. Among other local care for skin exposure to biological material, thorough cleaning with soap and water is recommended, and application of a degerming antiseptic solution (PVPI or chlorhexidine). When the mucosae have been exposed, exhaustive cleaning with water and physiological solution is recommended. Furthermore, in accordance with the Brazilian Health Ministry[153] (2000) recommendations, the professional will have to be followed-up for a period of 6 months after the accident with biological material contaminated by HIV, and in accidents with unknown patient-sources. In exposure to a patient-source non-reactive to HIV, the follow-up of the professional is indicated, in case there is the possibility of the patient-source's having been exposed to HIV in the last 3 to 6 months (immunological window).

## 12.15 Dental Garbage Monitoring

The dental team must take special care with every type of garbage produced in the dental offices (discarding material from clinical and surgical procedures), particularly with the purpose of avoiding a possible cross-infection. Many infectant agents can be present and can constitute contaminant vectors.

The education and the awareness of the dental team with regard to the measures established for taking care of residues produced by the health services (biological, chemical, physical), place value on management and reflects on the prevention of risks to public health.

The risks are associated with biological, chemical and physical agents. The biological risks are constituted of potentially pathogenic agents that can cause serious infections (viruses, bacteria, yeasts, protozoons, genetically modified organisms). The chemical risks are constituted of chemical products responsible for serious lesions and intoxications (corrosive, irritating, toxic, cancerigenous, explosive, inflammable products). The physical risks are constituted of physical aggressors (ionizing, non-ionizing radiations, noises, vibrations, ultrasound, extreme temperatures and others).

The biological risks are of concern to the dental team professionals because, according to the Brazilian Health Ministry[153] (2000), these professionals fit into the group that present a 3 to 6 times bigger risk of acquiring the hepatitis B virus, than the population in general. The possibility of serum conversion after the accident involving biological material is around 40%. The risk of acquiring AIDS is around 0.3% after a skin accident and 0.09% after exposure of the mucosa.

The inhalation of aerosols is pointed out as being among the main sources of clinical environment contamination, which needs to receive different treatment. Air can be decontaminated by ultraviolet machines.

A good health program must be based on the awareness and education of the entire community involved in the problem, as it is of collective interest, and constitutes a fundamental aspect of structuring a successful preventive program.

Disposal of garbage contaminated with infectious residues maintains the viability of pathogens with varying degrees of virulence, which can represent etiologic agents of contagious diseases. Thus, there are protocols that describe the transport and destination of products responsible for biological risks. All biological material must be sterilized before being discarded (or reused). For this purpose, incineration, sterilization or even disinfection procedures are more indicated.

The Brazilian Health Ministry[153] (2000) warns that perforating-cutting objects, such as anesthetic and suture needles, scalpel blades, files and similar items must be discarded immediately after use, in appropriate, rigid containers, with lids. There are special packagings on the market for discarding perforating-cutting materials, with a device for the disconnecting the needle from the anesthetic syringe (for example Descartex) (Figs. 12.20 and 12.21). At no time the collector should be filled with material above the dotted line. These containers have to be identified with the symbol "infectant" and "perforating-cutting material". After closing the material container, it must be placed into a milky white plastic bag, standardized in accordance with the Brazilian Association of Technical Norms[18,19] (NBR 9190/9191, 1993). Garbage containing perforating-cutting materials must have the words "perforating-cutting" recorded on the disposal containers, in addition to indicating the type of contamination present in it. Solid garbage, such as gauze, cotton, aspirators, and drapes, must be placed into milky white plastic bags, as described above, and they must only be filled up to 2/3 of their volume. The trash container must have foot operated pedals and covers.

The Brazilian National Environment Council (CONAMA, Number 5, 1993) recommends that all infectious disposals must be sterilized and incinerated. It is important to identify the type of residue. It is necessary to take care with amalgams, avoiding contact with the hands. Amalgam and mercuric residues must be put into containers with water, which minimizes mercurial contamination of the environment.

Incineration is a method indicated for the final treatment of contaminated garbage (organic material, of human or animal origin). This material must first be autoclaved, to assure previous sterilization. Contaminated material incineration is subject to approval by public health authorities, because of the possibility of air pollution.

The World Health Organization has adopted the following color code system to identify garbage: Green – common, non-recyclable objects; Red – residues with biological risk; Black – anatomic-pathological tissues (organic); White – plastic; Gray – paper, cardboard and similar materials.

It is important to use the color codes, symbols and signs that are representative of many conditions involved in the process of infection control. Nowadays, the "infectant" symbol is recognized by Health specialists all over the world (Fig. 12.22).



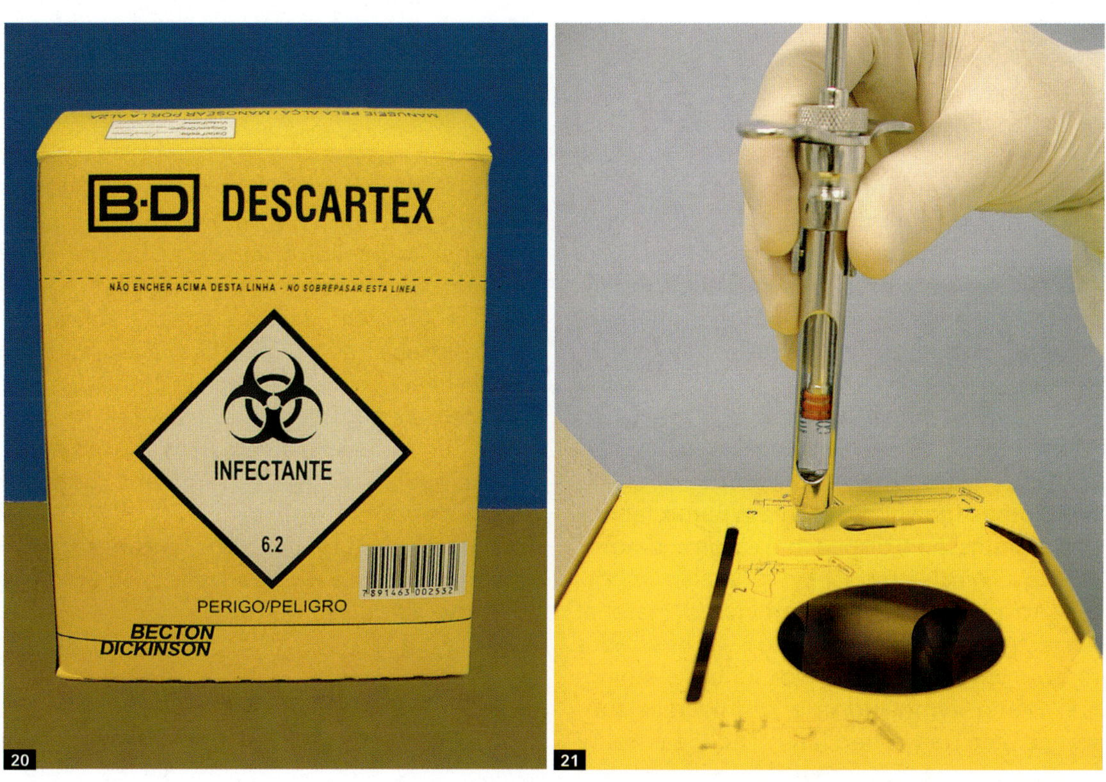


**Figures 12.20 and 12.21** - Special packagings on the market for discarding perforating-cutting materials (Descartex).

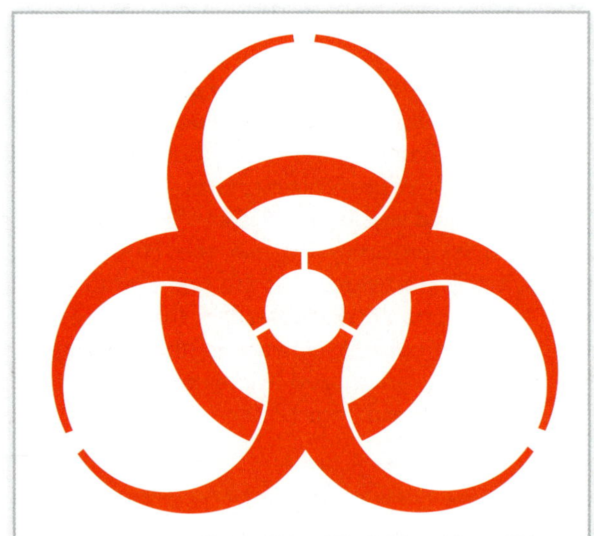

**Figure 12.22** - Symbol of infectious article.

It should be remembered that after an instrument has gone through a suitably severe sterilization process, in monitored machines in a perfect state, it is presumed that the instrument is free of microorganisms, that it is sterilized, which justifies the use of "sterilized" symbol.

Treatment of all the garbage produced in the dental office must receive special attention. Thus, it is necessary to take care with the clothes (gown) and contaminated fabrics (table cloths, non-disposable surgical drapes) during clinical attendance. It is also important to process this contaminated material correctly. Dirty clothes must be washed separately from the common household clothing, first being immersed in a disinfectant substance, and be washed later. The ideal would be to have them laundered in a specialized laundry (for example, one that has ozonified water processing and specialized treatment). After attendance, all the dirty clothing must be packed into plastic bags capable of preventing leakage, for transport from the place where they were used to the place where they will be washed.

It is prudent to warn that the recommendations described above need to be applied in order to minimize the risks of contamination through biological material.

The problem is not perfectly solved by professionals, authorities or the community, which needs to be made aware of the dangers for the benefit of personal and public health.

A fundamental question is the effective participation of the Government (Federal, State and City) with serious, well directed programs, divulged to the entire community, with the goal of garbage management in general.

1. Agolini G, Russo A, Clementi M. Effect of phenolic and chlorine disinfectants on hepatitis C virus binding and infectivity. Am J Infect Control 1999;27:236-39.
2. Aguiar CM, Pinheiro JT. Avaliação bacteriológica da qualidade da água utilizada nos equipos odontológicos. Rev Ass Paul Cir Dent 1999; 53.
3. Agut H. Prevention and control of viral hospital infections. Am J Infect Control 2001;29:244-46.
4. Alfa MJ, Jackson M. A new hydrogen peroxidebased medical-device detergent with germicidal properties: Comparison with enzymatic cleaners. Am J Infect Control 2001;29:168-77.
5. Allegra L, Blasi F, Tarsia P, Arosio C, Fagetti L, Gazzano M. A novel device for the prevention of airborne infections. J Clin Microbiol 1997;35:1918- 19.
6. Alves AC, Borges AC, Silva CCP, Pordeus IA, Paixão HH. O manuseio do lixo hospitalar pela equipe auxiliar odontológica: conhecimento de risco e comportamento. Rev CRO-MG 1996;2:87-93.
7. Alves-Rezende MCR, Lorenzato F. Avaliação dos procedimentos de prevenção dos riscos biológicos por cirurgiões-dentistas. Rev Ass Paul Cir Dent 2000; 54:446-54.
8. American Dental Association. Biological indicators for verifying sterilization. J Am Dent Assoc 1988;117:653-54.
9. American Dental Association. Council on Dental Materials and Devices, Council on Therapeutics: Infection control in the dental office. J Am Dent Assoc 1978; 97:673-77.
10. American Dental Association. Council on Dental Materials, Instruments and Equipament. Council on dental practice and council on dental therapeutics. Infection control recommendations for the dental office and the dental laboratory. J Amer Dent Ass 1988;116:241-48.
11. American Dental Association. Infection control recommendations for dental office and the dental laboratory. J Amer Dent Assoc 1996;127:672-80.
12. American Dental Association. Council on Scientific affairs. American Dental Association statement on dental unit waterlines. Texas Dent J 1996;113:23-24.
13. Andremont A. The future control of bacterial resistance to antimicrobial agents. Am J Infect Control 2001;29:256-58.
14. Andrés MT, Tejerina JM, Fierro JF. Reliability of biologic indicators in a mail return sterilizationmonitoring service: a review of 3 years. Quint Int 1995; 26:865-70.
15. Araújo LMA, Fernandes AL, Schwantes NA. O uso de barreiras de proteção no consultório odontológico na visão do paciente. Rev Fac Odontol UFPel 1994;5:3-9.
16. Associação Paulista de Estudos e Controle de Infecção Hospitalar. Limpeza, desinfecção de artigos e áreas hospitalares e anti-sepsia. São Paulo: APECIH; 1999. 74p.
17. Associação Paulista de Estudos e Controle de Infecção Hospitalar. Esterilização de artigos em unidades de saúde. São Paulo: APECIH; 1999. 74p.
18. Associação Brasileira de Normas Técnicas. Riscos de origem de serviços de saúde. NBR 10004; 1987.
19. Associação Brasileira de Normas Técnicas. Resíduos de serviços de saúde. NBR 12808; 1997.
20. Ayllffe GAJ, Babb JR, Quoraishi AH. A test for 'higienic' hand disinfection. J Clin Pathol 1978;31:923-8
21. Bammann LL, Estrela C. Aspectos microbiológicos em Endodontia. In: Endodontia: princípios biológicos e mecânicos. Estrela C, Figueredo JAP. São Paulo: Artes Médicas; 1999. p.167-189.
22. Barbieri DSV, Duarte DA, Higuti IH, Vicente VA. Isolamento e identificação de microrganismos em brinquedos utilizados em consultórios. Rev Ass Paul Cir Dent 1999;53:243-48.
23. Bastos GK, Souza IPR, Tura LFR, Vianna RBC. AIDS e controle de infecção, conhecimentos e atitudes dos pacientes. Rev Assoc Bras Odontol Nac 1997;4:39-41.
24. Bednarsh HS, Eklund KJ. Universal precautions reconsidered. Dent Assist 1997;62:13-35.
25. Belkin NL. Home laundering of soiled surgical scrubs: surgical site infections and the home environment. Am J Infect Control 2001;29:58-64.
26. Bentley CD, Burkhart NW, Crawford JJ. Evaluating spatter and aerosol contamination during dental procedures. J Am Dent Assoc 1994;125:579-84.
27. Berkelman RL, Anderson RL, Davis BJ. Lntrinsecbacterial contamination of a commercial iodophor solution investigation of the implicated manufacturing plant. Appl Environ Microbiol 1984;47:752-6.
28. Bernstein D, Schiff G, Echler G, Prince A, Feller M, Briner W. In vitro virucidal effectiveness of a 0.12% - chlorhexidine gluconate mouthrinse. J Dental Res 1990;69:874-76.
29. Bettner MD, Beiswanger MA, Miller CH, Palenik CJ. Effect of ultrasonic cleaning on microorganisms. Am J Dent 1998;11:185-88.
30. Bier O. Microbiologia e imunologia. 24th ed. São Paulo: Melhoramentos; 1990. 1234p.
31. Block SS. Disinfection, sterilization, and preservation. 4th ed. Philadelphia: Lea & Febiger; 1991. p.167-81.
32. Brattmall D, Köhler B. *Streptococcus mutans* serotypes: some aspects of their identification, distribuition, antigenic strifts and relationship to caries. J Dent Res 1976; 55:C15-C21.
33. Brooks GF, Butel SS, Morse SA. Microbiologia Médica. 21st ed. Rio de Janeiro: Guanabara Koogan; 2000. 611p.
34. Bulgarelli AF, Torquato TM, Costa LSS, Ferreira ZA. Avaliação das medidas de biossegurança no controle de infecção cruzada durante tratamento periodontal básico. Rev Bras Odontol 2001;58:188-190.
35. Cabrera RH, Caballero JG, Moreno JMM, Regadera MAGP, Rodrigues JP. Clinical assay of n-duopropenide alcohol solution on hand application in newborn and pediatric intensive care units: control of an outbreak of multiresistant *Klebsiella pneumonia* in a newborn intensive care unit with this measure. Am J Infect Control 2001;29:162-67.

36. Caldart LFM. Efeito antimicrobiano de técnicas précirúrgicas de degermação das mãos. (Master's Thesis) Federal University of Pelotas-RS-Brazil.
37. Caldart LFM, Zambrano CB, Mollnari JA, Bammann LL. Comparison of pre-surgical hand degermation procedures. J Dent Res 1997;76:435.
38. Compte DV, Roldan R, Sandoval S, Corominas R, Rosa M, Gordilho P, Volkow P. Surgical site infections in ambulatory surgery: a 5-year experience. Am J Infect Control 2001;29:99-103.
39. Cardo DM, Soule BM. Hospital infection prevention and control: a global perspective. Am J Infect Control 1999;27:233-35.
40. Cardoso CL, Pereira HH, Zequim JC, Guilhermetti M. Effectiveness of hand-cleansing agents for removing *Acinetobacter baumannii* strain from contaminated hands. Am J Infect Control 1999; 27:327-31.
41. Carmo CMR, Costa AMDD. Procedimentos de biossegurança em odontologia. J Bras Clín Estética Odontol 2001;5:116-19.
42. Carvalho A, Santos-Pinto MC, Pardini LC, Alonso Verri R, Ito IY. Efeitos do paraformaldeído e da temperatura em filmes radiográficos odontológicos durante sua esterilização. Estudo densitométrico. Odontol Mod 1989;16:22-6.
43. Carvalho PL, Papaiz EG. Controle de infecção em radiologia odontológica. Rev Ass Paul Cir Dent 1999;53:202-204.
44. Ceisel RJ, Osetek EM, Turner DW, Spear PG. Evaluating chemical inactivation of viral agents in handpiece splatter. J Am Dent Assoc 1995; 126:197-202.
45. Centers for Disease Control and Prevention. Recommended Infection Control Pratices for Dentistry. MMWR 1993; 42.
46. Chau TT, Kao KC, Blank G, Madrid F. Microwave plasmas for low-temperature dry sterilization. Biomaterials 1996;17:1273-77.
47. Checchi L, Matarasso S, Pirro P, D'Achile C. Topographical analysis of the facial areas most susceptible to infection with transmissible diseases in dentists. Inter J Periodontol Rest Dent 1991;11:165-172.
48. Chinellato LEM, Marques ALV. Hepatites virais: contágio e prevenção para o cirugião-dentista. Odont Mod 1993; 20.
49. Chinellato LEM, Santana E. Avaliação da efetividade de soluções desinfetantes utilizadas para o controle de infecção cruzada em filmes radiográficos intrabucais. Rev Fac Odontol Bauru 1997;5:37-44.
50. Chinellato LEM, Scheidt A. Estudo e avaliação dos meios de biossegurança para o cirurgião-dentista e auxiliares contra doenças infecto-contagiosas no consultório odontológico. Rev Fac Odontol Bauru 1993;1.
51. Chu NS, Chan-Myers H, Ghazanfari N, Antonoplos P. Levels of naturally occurring microorganisms on surgical instruments after clinical use and after washing. Am J Infect Control 1999;27:315-19.
52. Ciola BA. Readily adaptable cost-effective method of infection control for dental radiography. J Am Dent Assoc 1988; 117:349.
53. Clappison RA. Cross contamination control and the dental handpiece. J Prosthet Dent 1995;73:492-4.
54. Cleveland JL, Gooch BF, Lockwood AS. Occupational blood exposures in dentistry: a decade in review. Infect Control Hosp Epidemiol 1997;18:717-21.
55. Conceição OJG, Focaccia R. Hepatite A. In: Hepatites virais. Focaccia R. São Paulo: Atheneu;1997. p.23-26.
56. Cottone JA, Miller CH. The basic principies of infectious diseases as related to dental pratice. Topics in Oral Diagnoses II 1993; 37.
57. Cottone JA, Terezhalmy GT, Molinari JA. Practical infection control in dentistry. Philadelphia: Lea & Febiger;1991. 286p.
58. Cottone JA, Molinari JA. Infection control in Dentistry. J Amer Dent Ass 1991;123:33-41.
59. Cottone JA, Puttaiah R. Hepatitis B virus infection: current status in dentistry. Dental Clin N Amer 1996;40:293-307.
60. Couto JL, Cuto RS, Giorgi SM. Controle da contaminação nos consultórios odontológicos. Rev Gaúcha Odontol 1994;42:347-355.
61. Crawford JJ, Favero MS, Miller RL, Petersen NJ, Sabiston CB. Infection control in the dental office. J Amer Dent Assoc 1978;97:673-77.
62. Crawford JJ. Sterilization, disinfection, and aseps in dentistry. In: Disinfection, sterilization and preservation. Block SS. 3rd ed. Philadephia: Lea & Febiger; 1983. p.505-23.
63. Davies A. The mode of action of chlorhexidine. J Periodontol Res 1973; 8:68-75.
64. Dery S, Giard BJR, Valois M, Landry RG. Effectiveness of salt sterilizers for sterilising dental instruments. Int Dent J 1997;47:334-9.
65. Diangelis AJ, Martens LV, Little JW, Hastreiter RJJ. Infection control practices of Minnesota dentists: changes during 1 year. J Am Dent Assoc 1989;118:299-303.
66. Discacciati JAC, Neves AD, Pordeus IA. AIDS e controle de infecção cruzada na prática odontológica: percepção e atitudes nos pacientes. Rev Odontol Univ São Paulo 1999;13:75-82.
67. EN CY, Pereira AC, Daruge E. Avaliação das condições sanitárias em estabelecimento de assistência odontológica, consultório odontológico tipo I. Rev Paul Odontol 2001;23:4-10.
68. Engelhardt JP, Grun L, Dahl HJ. Factors affecting sterilization in glass bead sterilizers. J Endod 1984;10:465-70.
69. Ernest R, Loesche W. Measuring harmful levels of bacteria in dental aerosols. J Amer Dent Ass 1991; 122.
70. Estrela C. Dor odontogênica. São Paulo: Artes Médicas; 2001. 312p.
71. Estrela C, Estrela CRA. Controle de infecção em odontologia. São Paulo: Artes Médicas; 2003. 188p.
72. Estrela C, Figueredo JAP. Endodontia: princípios biológicos e mecânicos. São Paulo: Artes Médicas; 1999. 819p.
73. Exner M, Hartemann P, Kistemann T. Higiene and health - the need for a holistic approach. Am J Infect Control 2001;29:228-231.
74. Faecher RS. Tuberculosis: a growing concern for dentistry? J Am Dent Assoc 1993;94-104.
75. Faizibaioff R, Kignel S. Princípios de biossegurança em implantodontia. Rev Ass Paul Cir Dent 2000;54:329-34.
76. Faoagali JL, George N, Fong J, Davy J, Dowser M. Comparison of the antibacterial efficacy of 4% chlorhexidine gluconate and 1% triclosan handwash products in an acute clinical ward. Am J Infect Control 1999; 27:320-26.

77. Faraco FN, Moura APF. Controle de risco de transmissão de doenças infectocontagiosas no consultório odontológico. Parte 1. Rev Paul Odontol 1992;14:14-8.
78. Faraco FN, Moura APF. Controle de risco de transmissão de doenças infectocontagiosas no consultório odontológico. Parte 2. Rev Paul Odontol 1993;15:2836.
79. Fatinato V, Shimizu MT, Almeida NQ, Jorge AOC. Esterilização e desinfecção em odontologia: AIDS e hepatite. Rev Bras Odontol 1992;49:31-6.
80. Favero MS. Chemical disinfection of medical and surgical materiais. In: Disinfection, Sterilization and preservation. Block SS. 3rd ed. Philadelphia: Lea & Febiger; 1983. p.469-92.
81. Ferreira EL, Ferraz GA, Padilha JC, Ruthes S. Avaliação do efeito dos processos de esterilização e desinfecção em brocas de aço carbono e aço carbide associados ou não ao uso de lubrificantes. Rev Assoc Bras Odontol Nac 2001;8:375-81.
82. Ferreira RA. Barrando o invisível. Rev Ass Paul Cir Dent 1995; 49:417-27.
83. Fidgor D, Sjögren U, Sörlin S, Sundqvist G, Nair PNR. Pathogenicity of *Actinomyces israelli* and *Arachnia propionica*: experimental infection in guinea pigs and phagocytosis and intracellular killing by human polymorphonuclear leukocytes in vitro. Oral Microbial Immunol 1992;7:129-36.
84. Fine DH, Mendieta C, Barnett ML, Furgan D, Meyers R, Olshan A, Vincent J. Efficacy of preprocedural rinsing with an antiseptic in reducing viable bacteria in dental aerosols. J Periodontol 1992;63:821-42.
85. Fine DH, Rorik I, Furgan D, Myers R, Olshan A, Barnett ML, Vicent J. Assessing pre-procedural subgingival irrigation and rinsing with antiseptic mouthrinse to reduce bacteremia. J Am Dent Assoc 1996;127:641-6.
86. Focaccia R. Hepatites virais. São Paulo: Atheneu; 1997. 192p.
87. Focaccia R, Souza FV, Conceição OJG, Santos EB. Hepatite C. In: Hepatites virais. Focaccia R. São Paulo: Atheneu; 1997. p.51-65.
88. Fonseca JCF. Hepatite D. In: Hepatites virais. Focaccia R. São Paulo: Atheneu; 1997. p.67-80.
89. Fors UGH, Berg JO, Sandberg H. Microbiological investigation of saliva leakage between the rubber dam and tooth during endodontic treatment. J Endod 1986; 12:396-9.
90. Francls RD, Long WK. Hepatitis and tumor viruses. In: Dental microbiology. McGhee JR, Michalek SM, Cassel GH. Philadelphia: Harper & Row Publishers; 1982. p.628-39.
91. Gaetti-Jardim-Jr E, Pedrini D. Contaminação microbiana do sistema de água do equipo odontológico. Rev Fac Odontol Lins 1997;10:32-35.
92. Gaetti-Jardim-Jr E, Pedrini D. Avaliação dos níveis de contaminação microbiana em luvas cirúrgicas utilizadas por docentes e graduandos da Faculdade de Odontologia de Araçatuba-UNESP. Rev Fac Odontol Lins 1997;10:51-55
93. Garner JS. Guideline for Isolation precautions in Hospitais. Infect Control Hosp Epidem 1996;17:54-80.
94. Gerberding JL, Schecter WP. Surgery and AIDS: reducing the risk. J Am Med Assoc 1991; 265:1572-73.
95. Gilbert P, Das J, Foley I. Biofilm susceptibility to antimicrobials. Adv Dent Res 1997;11:160-7.
96. Gilbert P, Mcbain AJ. Biofilms: their impact on health and their recalcitrance toward biocides. Am J Infect Control 2001; 29:252-55.
97. Girouard S, Levine G, Goodrich K, Jones S, Keyserling H, Rathore M, Rubens C, Willlams E, Jarvis W. Infection control programs at children's hospitais: A description of structures and processes. Am J Infect Control 2001;29:145-151.
98. Glick M, Trope M, Bagasra O, Pliskin ME. Human immunodeficiency vírus infection of fibroblasts of dental pulp in soropositive patients. Oral Surg Oral Med Oral Pathol 1991;71:33-6.
99. Glass BJ. Infection Control in Dental Radiology. Current and future. NY St Dent J 1994;60:42-5.
100. Gonçalves-Jr FL. Hepatite por vírus B. In: Hepatites virais. Focaccia R. São Paulo: Atheneu; 1997. p.27-49.
101. Gonçalves PMJ. Controle da infecção cruzada na prática odontológica. Rev CRO-MG 1997;3:17-22.
102. Grenier D. Quantitative analysis of bacterial aerosols in two different dental clinic environments. Applied Enviroment Microbiol 1995;61:3165-68.
103. Gristina AG, Hobgood CD, Webb LX, Myrvik QN. Adhesive colonization of biomaterials and antibiotic resistance. Biomaterials 1987;8:423-6.
104. Gross KBW, Overman PR, Cobb C, Brockmann S. Aerosol generation by two ultrasonic scalers. J Dent Hyg 1992;66:314-8.
105. Guandalini SL, Melo NSFO, Santos ECP. Biossegurança em Odontologia. 1st ed. Curitiba: Odontex; 1998. 150p.
106. Guandalini SL, Santos ECP, Melo NSFO. Como controlar infecção na Odontologia. Paraná: Gnatus. 88p.
107. Guimarães-Jr J. Biossegurança e controle de Infecção Cruzada em consultórios odontológicos. 1st ed. 2001. 517p.
108. Guimarães-Jr J. Controle de infecção cruzada no consultório odontológico. Rev Assoc Paul Cir Dent 1992;46:711-6.
109. Haddad AJ, Girard JRB, Bouclin R, Valois M, Landry RG. Effectiveness of salt versus glass bead sterilizers. J Cand Dent Assoc 1997;63:448-53.
110. Harrel SK, Barnes JB, Hidalgo FR. Reduction of aerosols produced by ultrasonic scalers. J Periodontol 1996;67:28-32.
111. Harsfst SA. Personal barrier protection. Dent Clin North Am 1991;35:357-66.
112. Held-Filho A, Alcantara A. O cirurgião-dentista frente à AIDS. 1.ed. São Paulo: Pancast; 1996. 159p.
113. Hirata MH, Mancini-Filho J. Manual de Biossegurança. 1st ed. São Paulo: Manole; 2002. 496p.
114. Hobson DW, Seal LA. Evaluation of a novel, rapidacting, sterilizing solution at roam temperature. Am J Infect Control 2000;28:370-5.
115. Joklik WK, Willet HP, AMOS DB, Wilfert CM. Microbiología. 20ty ed. Panamericana: Buenos Aires; 1994. 1696p.
116. Jones RD. Bacterial resistance and topical antimicrobial wash products. Am J Infect Control 1999;27:351-63.
117. Jones RD, Jampani HB, Newman JL, Lee AS. Triclosan: A review of effectiveness and safety in health care settings. Am J Infect Control 2000;28:184-96.

118. King TC, Muzzin KB, Berry CW, Anders LM. The effectiveness of an aerosol reduction device for ultrasonic scalers. J Periodontol 1997; 68:45-9.
119. Larson EL, Ailled AE. Hygiene and health: an epidemiologic link? Am J Infect Control 2001;29:232-8.
120. Liberto MIM, Oliveira BCEPD, Cabral MC. Hepatites Virais. In: Introdução à virologia humana. Santos NSO, Romanos MTV, Wigg MD. Rio de Janeiro: Guanabara Koogan; 2002. p.135-156.
121. Lima SNM, Ito IY. Infecções odontogênicas - O controle de infecção no consultório odontológico. Sistema BEDA de controle - Parte I. Rev Paul Odontol 1993;25:46-47.
122. Lima SNM, Ito, IY. Infecções odontogênicas. O controle de infecção no consultório odontológico. Sistema BEDA de controle - Parte 3. Rev Paul Odontol 1994;26:44-6.
123. Lima SNM, Ito IY, Maia Campos G, Alonso Verri R, Ribas JP. Efeitos da raspagem ultra-sônica na alteração do número de *estreptococos* na área cervical do dente. Rev Paul Odontol 1990;13:18-28.
124. Loesche WJ. Oxygen sensitivity of various anaerobic bactéria. Appl Microbiol 1969; 18:723-7.
125. Loesche WJ. Cárie dental: uma infecção tratável. Rio de janeiro: Cultura Médica; 1993. 349p.
126. Logothetis DD, Martinez-Welles JM. Reducing bacterial aerosol contamination with a chlorhexidine gluconate pre-rinse. J Am Dent Assoc 1995; 126:1634-9.
127. Lopes-Neto EPA, Sette-Jr H. Hepatite E. In: Hepatites virais. Focaccia R. São Paulo: Atheneu; 1997. p.81-8.
128. Lotufo RFM, Giorgi SM. Infecção Cruzada: existe no seu consultório? Rev Assoc Paul Cir Dent 1990; 45:105-7.
129. Luby S. The role of handwashing in improving hygiene and health in low-income countries. Am J Infect Control 2001; 29:239-40.
130. Lucas RB, Kramer IRH. Bacteriologia. 1st ed. Rio de Janeiro: Científica; 1957. 267p.
131. Lynch P, Jackson M, Saint S. Research priorites project, year 2000: Establishing a direction for infection control and hospital epidemiology. Am J Infect Control 2001;29:73-8.
132. MacDonald G. Can the thermal disinfector outperform the ultrasonic cleaner? J Am Dent Assoc 1996;127:1787-8.
133. Magro-Filho O, Carvalho ACP. Aids. Esclarecimentos para o cirurgião-dentista. Odonto Moder 1988;15:28-35.
134. Magro-Filho O, Garcia-Jr IR, Souza AMM, D'Antônio GM, Moimaz SAS, Érnica NM. Lavagem das mãos com soluções de PVP-I, clorexidina e sabão líquido: estudo microbiológico. Rev Ass Paul Cir Dent 2000; 54.
135. Magro-Filho O, Melo MS, Martin SC. Métodos de esterilização, desinfecção e paramentação utilizados pelo cirurgião dentista e auxiliar no consultório odontológico. Levantamento entre profissionais. Rev Assoc Paul Cir Dent 1991; 45.
136. Mamizuka EM, Hirata MH. Manuseio, controle e descarte de produtos biológicos. In: Hepatites virais. Hirata MH, Mancini-Filho J. 1st ed. São Paulo: Manole; 2002. p.87-120.
137. Mandell ID. Occupation risks in dentistry: confort and concerns. J Amer Dent Ass 1993;124:419.
138. Mantecca MAM. Responsabilidade profissional frente à esterilização e higiene. Rev Odontol Univ Santo Amaro 1996;1:41-4.
139. Mathias SA, Mathias AL, Guadalini SL. Recomendações para o controle de infecção em laboratório de prótese odontológica. Rev Bras Prótese Clin & Laboratorial 2002;1:21-7.
140. McErlane B, Rosebush WJ, Waterfield JD. Assessment of the effectiveness of dental sterilizers using biological monitors. J Canad Dent Assoc 1992;58:481-3.
141. McGhee JR, Michalek SM. Host protetion from viruses: inactivation, chemotherapy, Interferon production and vaccination. In: Dental microbiology. McGhee JR, Michalek SM, Cassel GH. Philadelphia: Harper & Row Publishers; 1982. p.628-39.
142. McGuckin M, Waterman R, Porten L, Bello S, Caruso M, Juzaitis B, Krug E, Mazer S, Ostrawski S. Patient education model for increasing handwashing compliance. Am J Infect Control 1999;27:309-14.
143. McKinley IB, Ludlow MO. Hazards of laser smoke during endodontic therapy. J Endod 1994;20:558-9.
144. Medeiros UV, Cardoso AS, Ferreira SMS. Uso das normas de controle de infecção na prática odontológica. Rev Bras Odontol 1998;55:209-15.
145. Melo AMR, Carvalho RL, Araújo IC. Hepatite B: prevenção e tratamento em Odontologia. Uma revisão da literatura. Rev Paraense de Odontologia 1999;4:41-6.
146. Merchant VA. An update on infection control in the dental laboratory. Quint Dent Techol 1997;20:157-69.
147. Miller CH. Infection control. Dent Clin North Am 1996;40:437-56.
148. Miller CH, Cottone JA. The basic principles of infectious diseases as related to dental practice. Dent Clin North Am 1993; 37:1-20.
149. Miller CH, Palenik CJ. Infection Control and management of hazardous materials for the dental team. St Louis: Mosby; 1998. 362p.
150. Miller CH, Sheldrake MA. The ability of biological indicators to detect sterilization failures. Am J Dent 1994;7:95-7.
151. Miller RL, Micik RF, Able C, Ryge G. Studies on dental aerobiology. Microbial platters discharged from the oral cavity of dental patient. J Dent Res 1971;50:621-5.
152. Mills SE, Lauderdale PW, Mayhew RB. Reduction of microbial contamination in dental units with povidone-iodine 10%. J Am Dent Assoc 1986;113:280-4.
153. Ministério da Saúde. Controle de infecções e a prática odontológica em tempos de AIDS. Brasília: Manual de Condutas; 2000. 118p.
154. Ministério da Saúde. Secretaria de Assistência à Saúde. Processamento de artigos e superfícies em estabelecimentos de saúde. 2nd ed. Brasília; 1994. 50p.
155. Miranda MMFS. Propriedades gerais dos vírus. In: Introdução à virologia humana. Santos NSO, Romanos MTV, Wigg MD. Rio de Janeiro: Guanabara Koogan; 2002. p.1-10.

156. Molinari JA. Dental Infection control at the year 2000. J Am Dent Assoc 1990; 130.
157. Molinari JA. Practical infection control for the 1990s: Applying science to government regulations. J Am Dent Assoc 1994;125:1189-97.
158. Molinari JA, Runnells RR. Role of disinfection in infection control. Dent Clin North Am 1991;35:323-7.
159. Monfrin RCP, Ribeiro MC. Avaliação *in vitro* de anti-sépticos bucais sobre a microbiota da saliva. Rev Ass Paul Cir Dent 2000;54:400-8.
160. Moore RL, Brantley SW. Frequency of glove perforations. J Clin Orthod 1990;24:294-5.
161. Moriya TM, Cologna MHYT, Solé-Vernin C, Machado MH. Anti-sépticos e/ou desinfetantes: deterioração e contaminação. Rev Bras Enf 1982; 35:238-44.
162. Muenchinger FS. Evaluation of an electrosonic denture cleaner. J Prosthet Dent 1975;33:610-4.
163. Murphy CL, Mclaws ML. Variation in administrators 'and clinicians' atitudes toward critical elements of an infection control program and the role of the infection control practitioner in New South Wales, Australia. Am J Infect Control 2001;29:262-70.
164. Murray PR, Rosenthal KS, Kobayashi GS, Pfaller MA. Microbiologia Médica. 3rd ed. Rio de Janeiro: Guanabara Koogan; 1992. 513p.
165. Nair PNR. Apical periodontitis: a dinamic encounter between root canal infection and host response. Periodontology 2000 1997;13:121-48.
166. Nascimento WF, Borges ALS, Uemura ES, Moraes JV. Desinfecção de moldes: como, quando e por quê. Rev Ass Paul Cir Dent 1999;53:21-4.
167. Neaverth EJ, Pantera-Jr EA, Ga A. Chairside disinfection of radiographs. Oral Surg Oral Med Oral Pathol 1991;71:116-9.
168. Neely AN, Maley MP. Dealing with contaminated computer keyboards and microbial survival. Am J Infect Control 2001;29:131-2.
169. Nisengard RJ, Newman MG. Microbiologia Oral e Imunologia. 2nd ed. Rio de Janeiro: Guanabara Koogan; 1997. 395p.
170. Nunes MF, Freire MCM. AIDS e odontologia: conhecimentos e atitudes dos cirurgiões-dentistas. Rev Odontol Bras Central 1999;8:7-10.
171. Okamoto T, Gaetti-Jardim-Jr E, Ghaname ES. Efeitos da anti-sepsia com PVP-I sobre o crescimento bacteriano em suturas com fio de seda. Estudo microbiológico e histomorfológico em ratos. Rev Fac Odontol Lins 1997;11:36-41.
172. Oliveira BH, Moliterno LF, Marçal S. Medidas de precaução universal: o que são e para que servem? Rev Bras Odontol 1996;53:18-22.
173. Ollveira TC, Branchini MLM. Infection control in a Brazilian regional multihospital system. Am J Infect Control 1999;27:262-9.
174. Otis LL, Cottone JA. Prevalence of perforations in disposable latex gloves during routine dental treatment. J Am Dent Assoc 1989;118:321-4.
175. Panelick CJ, King TN, Newton CW, Miller CH, Koerber LG. A survey of sterilization practices in selected endodontic offices. J Endod 1986; 12:206-9.
176. Papaiz EG, Carvalho PL. Controle de infecção em radiologia Odontológica. Rev Ass Paul Cir Dent 1999; 53.
177. Pauson DS, Fendler EJ, Dolan MJ, Willians RA. A close look at alcohol gel as an antimicrobial sanitizing agent. Am J Infect Control 1999;27:332-8.
178. Pelczar-Jr MJ, Chan ECS, Krieg NR. Microbiology: concepts and applications. New York: McGraw-Hill; 1993.
179. Pelczar-Jr MJ, Chan ECS, Krieg NR. Microbiologia: conceitos e aplicações. 2nd ed. São Paulo: Makrom Books; 1996. 524p. 1.v.
180. Pelczar-Jr MJ, Chan ECS, Krieg NR. Microbiologia: conceitos e aplicações. 2nd ed. São Paulo: Makrom Books, 1996. 517p. 2.v.
181. Pimenta FC, Ito IY, Lima SNM. Biossegurança em Endodontia. In: Endodontia: princípios biológicos e mecânicos. Estrela C, Figueredo JAP. São Paulo: Artes Médicas; 1999. p.385-438.
182. Pinho JRR. Hepatite não A – E. In: Hepatites virais. Focaccia R. São Paulo: Atheneu; 1997. p.89-98.
183. Pinheiro JJV, Tucci R. Doenças infecciosas da cavidade bucal, emergentes e endêmicas no Brasil. Ver Paraense Odontol 2000;5:25-31.
184. Rabello SB, Godoy CVC, Santos FRW. Presença de bactérias em Instrumentais e superfícies do ambiente clínico odontológico. Rev Bras Odontol 2001;58:184-190.
185. Ramos INC, Markus C, Maia RAR. Riscos da endocardite infecciosa nos procedimentos odontológicos. J Brasil Clín Odontol Integr 2001;5:208-11.
186. Ranali J. Eficiência de máscaras cirúrgicas frente a aspersões produzidas por alta rotação. Rev Gaúcha de Odontol 1992; 16.
187. Reams GJ, Baumgartner JC, Kulild JC. Practical application of infection control in endodontics. J Endod 1995;21:281-4.
188. Rego A, Roley L. In use barrier integrity of gloves: latex and nitrile superior to vinil. Am J Infect Control 1999;27:405-10.
189. Rezende MCRA, Lorenzato F. Avaliação dos procedimentos de prevenção dos riscos biológicos por cirurgiões-dentistas. Rev Ass Paul Cir Dent 2000; 54:446-54.
190. Ribeiro EL, Andre AR, Maggi PS, Paiva EMM, Naves PLF, Pimenta FC. Avaliação da microbiota fúngica do ar da clínica de Periodontia - FO/UFG. In: II CUGO, Goiânia, Goiás, Brasil, 7/10 a 11/10, 1997.
191. Rimland D, Parkin WE, Miller GB, Schrack WD. Hepatitis B outbreak traced to oral surgeon. The New England J of Medicine 1997;296:953-8.
192. Rodrigues CF, Corrêa GM, Figueira CMM. Esterilização: uma necessidade na odontologia moderna. Rev Fac Odontol Lins 1995;8:23-8.
193. Roruquayrol MZ, Almeida-Filho N. Epidemiologia & Saúde. 5.ed. Rio de Janeiro: Medsi; 1999. 570p.
194. Rosebury T. Microorganisms Indigenous to man. New York: McGraw-Hill Book Company; 1962.
195. Rubino JR. Infection control practices in institutional settings. Am J Infect Control 2001; 29:241-3.
196. Russel AD. Mechanisms of bacterial insusceptibility to biocides. Am J Infect Control 2001;29:259-61.
197. Russo EMA, Carvalho RCR, Lorenzo JL, Garone-Neto N, Cardoso MV, Grossi E. Avaliação da intensidade de contaminação de pontas de seringa tríplice. Pesq Odontol Bras 2000;14:243-7.
198. Sabattini VB, Rosaia E, Franco M. Sterilizzazione e desinfezione. Dental Cadmos 1993;2:54-63.
199. Samaranayake LP, Scheutz F, Cottone JA. Controle de infecção para a equipe odontológica. 2.ed. São Paulo: Santos; 1995. 146p.

200. Sanchez S, MacDonald G. Decontaminating dental instruments: testing the effectiveness of selected methods. J Am Dent Assoc 1995;126:359-68.
201. Santos NSO. Patogenia das infecções virais. In: Introdução à virologia humana. Santos NSO, Romanos MTV, Wigg MD. Rio de Janeiro: Guanabara Koogan; 2002. p.11-18.
202. Santos NSO, Romanos MTV, Wigg MD. Introdução à virologia humana. Rio de Janeiro: Guanabara Koogan; 2002. 254p.
203. Sattar SA, Tetro J, Springthorpe VS, Giulivi A. Preventing the spread of hepatitis B and C viruses: where are germicides relevant? Amer J Infect Control 2001;29:187-197.
204. Slots J, Rams TE. Microbiology of periodontal disease. In: Contemporary oral microbiology and immunology. Slots J, Taubman MA. St Louis: Mosby; 1992. p.425-43.
205. Slots J, Rams TE, Schonfeld SE. In Vitro activity of chlorhexidine against enteric rods, pseudomonas and acinetobacter from human periodontitis. Oral Microbiol Immunol 1991;6:62-4.
206. Slots J, Taubman MA. Contemporary oral microbiology and immunology. St Louis: Mosby; 1992. 649p.
207. Stach DJ, Poline GNC, Newman SM, Tilliss TSI. Effect of repeated sterilization and ultrasonic cleaning on curet blades. J Dent Hyg 1995;69:31-9.
208. Savage NW, Walsh LJ. The use of autoclaves in the dental surgery. Aust Dent J 1995;40:197-200.
209. Scott E. The potential benefits of infection control measures in the home. Am J Infect Control 2001;29:247-9.
210. Scott HML, Bass C. Biofilm formation: attachment, growth, and detachment of microbes from surfaces. Am J Infect Control 2001;29:250-1.
211. Shearer BG. Biofilm and the dental office. J Am Dent Assoc 1996;127:181-9.
212. Shechmeister IL. Sterilization by ultraviolet irradiation. In: Disinfection, sterilization and preservation. Block SS. 4th ed. Philadephia: Lea & Febiger; 1991. p.553-65.
213. Souza ACS. Descontaminação prévia de materiais médico-cirúrgico: estudo comparativo entre desinfetantes químicos e água e sabão. (Dissertação de Mestrado em Microbiologia). Goiânia: Instituto de Patologia Tropical e Saúde Pública, Universidade Federal de Goiás; 1996.
214. Souza ACS, Bento DA, Pimenta FC. Rotina de procedimentos de descontaminação das clínicas da ABO-Goiás: Sistema BEDAC de controle. Goiânia. ABO-GO; 1997. (manual).
215. Souza AMM, Garcia-Jr IR, Magro-Filho O, *et al.* Lavagem das mãos com soluções de PVP-I, clorexidina e sabão líquido: estudo microbiológico. Rev Ass Paul Cir Dent 2000;54:25-8.
216. Souza HMMR. AIDS e o profissional de Odontologia. Rev Ass Bras Odontol Nac 1997;5:256-9.
217. Spach DH, Silverstein FE, Stamm WE. Transmission of infection by gastrointestinal endoscopy and bronchoscopy. Ann Int Med 1993;118:117-28.
218. Spauding EH. Chemical disinfection and antisepsis in the hospital. J Hosp Res 1972;9:5-31.
219. Sundqvist GK, Reuterving CO. Isolation of *Actinomyces israelli* from periapical lesion. J Endod 1980;6:602-6.
220. Tinsley D, Chadwick RG. The permeability of dental gloves folowing exposure to certain dental materiais. J Dent 1997;25:65-70.
221. Tripple AFV. As interfaces do controle de infecção em uma instituição de ensino odontológico. (Tese de Doutorado). Ribeirão Preto: Universidade de São Paulo; 2000. 177p.
222. Trabulsi LR, Toledo MRF. Microbiologia. 2nd ed. São Paulo: Atheneu; 1996. 386p.
223. Tortora GJ, Funke BR, Case CL. Microbiologia. 6th ed. Porto Alegre: Artes Médicas; 2000. 827p.
224. Ureña JL. Microbiología oral. México: Interamericana - McGraw-Hill; 1996. 565p.
225. Uzeda M. Microbiologia oral. Rio de janeiro: Medsi; 2002. 104p.
226. Vilar-Compte D, Roldán R, Sandoval S, Corominas R, De La Rosa M, Gordillo P, Volkow P. Surgical site infections in ambulatory surgery: A 5-year experience. Am J Infect Control 2001;29:99-103.
227. Voltz PA. Transmission of fungal spores in space and their conditions for survival: a review. Microbios 1997;91:145-51.
228. Watkins BJ. Sterilizer monitoring: An essential component of sterilization procedures. Compend Contin Educ Dent 1987;8:476-8.
229. White DO, Fenner F. Medical virology. 4th ed. New York: Academic; 1994.
230. Wigg MD. Vírus da Imunodeficiência Humana. In: Introdução à virologia humana. Santos NSO, Romanos MTV, Wigg MD. Rio de Janeiro: Guanabara Koogan; 2002. p.183-199.
231. Williams HN, Johnson A, Kelley JI, Baer ML, King TS, Mitchell B, Hasler JF. Bacterial contamination of the water supply in newly installed dental units. Quint Int 1995;26:331-7.
232. Williams HN, Kelley JI, Folineo D, Willians GC, Hawley CL, Sibiski J. Assessing microbial contamination in clean water dental - units and compliance with disinfection protocol. J Amer Dent Ass 1994;125:1205-1211.
233. Winchcombe J. Competency standards in the context of infection control. Am J Infect Control 2000;28:228-32.
234. Youg JM. Keys to sucessful hand piece maintenance. Texas Dent J 1997;114:15-9.
235. Young JM, Cottone JA. Dental handpieces: maintenance and sterilization. In: Practical infection control in dentistry. Cottone JA, Terezhalmy GT, Molinari JA. 2nd ed. Baltimore: Williams & Wilkins;1996. p.176-89.
236. Zancanaro-Jr O. Manuseio de produtos químicos e descarte de seus resíduos. In: Manual de Biossegurança. Hirata MH, Mancini-Filho J. 1st ed. São Paulo: Manole; 2002. p.121-183.
237. Zanon U. Infectantes ou desinfetantes hospitalares. Rev Div Nac Tuberc 1975;19:105-17.
238. Zaragoza M, Sallés M, Gomez J, Bayas JM, Trilla A. Handwashing with soap or alcoholic solutions? A randomized clinical trial of its effectiveness. Am J Infect Control 1999;27:258-61.
239. Zebral AA, Ether SS. Quimioprofilaxia na prevenção de endocardite bacteriana de origem dentária. Odonto Modern 1988;15:26-39.

# Internal Anatomy and Coronal Preparation


**C. Estrela**
*Federal University of Goiás, Goiânia, GO, Brazil*

**J. D. Pécora**
*University of São Paulo, Ribeirão Preto, SP, Brazil*

**D. A. Decurcio**
*Federal University of Goiás, Goiânia, GO, Brazil*

**A. M. Toledo**
*Brazilian Dentistry Research and Learning Center, CEPOBRAS, Goiânia, GO, Brazil*


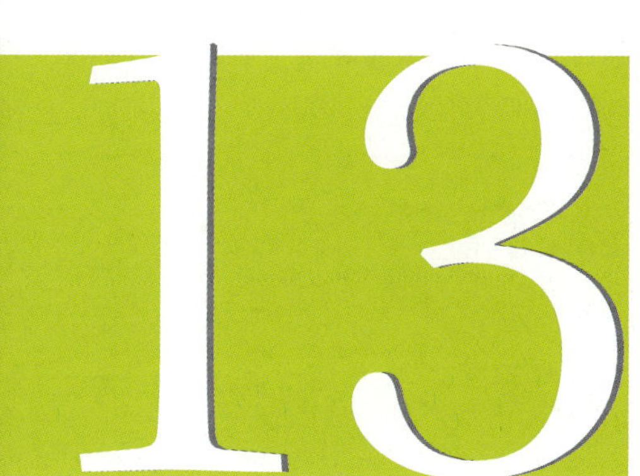


Chapter contents

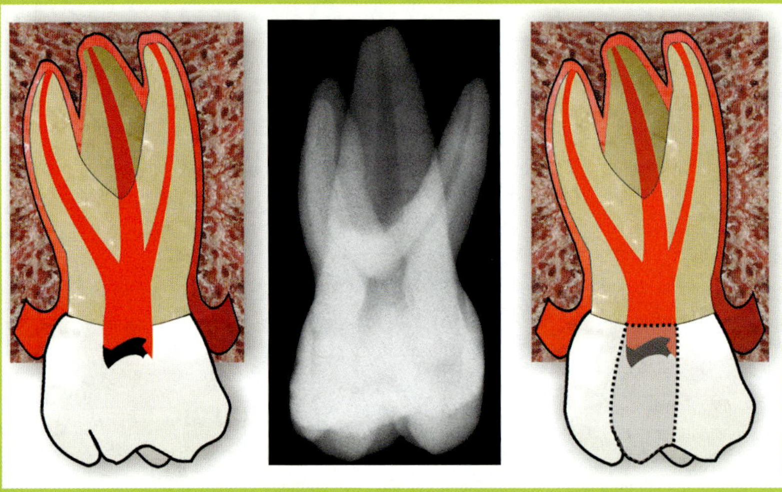

Pulp cavity and access cavity of maxillary molar.

## 13.1 Introduction

Knowledge of internal dental anatomy is fundamental for performing the sanitization process and root canal preparation perfectly, as the anatomic structure of the pulp cavity is considered very complex.

Once again, it can be illusory to verify the macroconfiguration of the pulp cavity illustrated by drawings, photographs, decalcification, moldings, serial cortex, scanning analysis, because they give a close up and projected idea of the internal micromorphology.

Endodontic treatment involves different operative steps. One of the great challenges is to strive against the internal shapes located in the different dental groups, which must never be underestimated, when the option is to seek successful endodontic treatment.

Several studies[1-177] of the pulp cavity morphology have been described in the literature. Many anatomic variations can be found, such as: dental ramifications, developmental disturbances, C shaped canals, dilacerated root canals (gradual and ungradual curvatures), calcification resorptions, flattened root canals, etc.

Burns & Buchanam[12] reported that it is discouraging to be conscious of the complexity of the spaces that are expected to be cleaned and filled. Now, however, it is known that present methods of endodontic treatment yield a high range of success. De Deus[23], in a study of 1140 human teeth from adult individuals, analyzed the distribution and frequency of accessory, secondary and lateral canals, and observed their presence in 27.4%; and also found 37.2% of apical deltas in 1166 teeth studied.

Taking into account the complexity of the pulp cavity and the difficulties encountered in achieving endodontic success, all the available resources must be used for the complete cleaning, preparation and filling of the root canal system. Considering the limitations imposed by the internal dental morphology on ideal endodontic treatment, it is necessary to respect the value of the radiograph examination. With the aim of associating knowledge of the internal morphology and the beginning preparation of the access cavity, a systematized analysis will be developed with a view of normality, which will reflect the high prevalence of anatomic characteristics. The most relevant aspects of the pulp cavity anatomy in each group will be associated with the required details for the access cavity, shown in summarized tables, followed by the schematic representation of each tooth, and shape of the access cavity.

## 13.2 Pulp Cavity

The pulp cavity, the space that accommodates the dental pulp is divided into two sites: one related to the crown named the pulp chamber, and the radicular part, called the root canal. Usually located in the central region of the tooth, the crown walls are denominated the buccal, lingual, mesial, distal, occlusal and cervical faces. The occlusal face is also called the pulp chamber roof, while the cervical face (present in the premolars and molars) corresponds to the floor of the pulp chamber.

The purpose of access cavity preparation is allow endodontic instruments to enter the root canal system.

Krasner & Rankow[75], analyzing 500 pulp chambers, verified that the cemento-enamel junction was an essential anatomic marker for the location of pulp chambers and root canal orifices. The associations presented in these laws are important help with locating calcified canal orifices. Based on the relationships of the pulp chamber with the clinical crown, and the pulp-chamber floor (Chart 13.1) some laws were established: "*1. law of symmetry 1: except for maxillary molars, the orifices of the canals are equidistant from a line drawn in a mesiodistal direction through the pulp chamber floor. 2. law of symmetry 2: except for maxillary molars, the orifices of the canals lie on a line perpendicular to a line drawn in a mesiodistal direction across the center of the floor of the pulp chamber. 3. law of color change: The color of the pulp chamber floor is always darker than the walls. 4. law of orifice location 1: the orifices of the root canals are always located at the junction of the walls and the floor. 5. law of orifice location 2: the orifices of the root canals are located at the angles in the floor – wall junction. 6. law of orifice location 3: the orifices of the root canals are located at the terminus of the root developmental fusion lines."*

Vertucci[164] studying root canal morphology and its relationship with endodontic procedures, concluded that the outcomes of non-surgical and surgical endodontic procedures are influenced by highly variable anatomic structures. Therefore clinicians ought to be aware of complex root canal structures, of cross-sectional dimensions and of iatrogenic alterations of canal anatomy. Careful interpretation of angled radiographs, proper access preparation and a detailed exploration of the interior of the tooth, ideally under magnification, are essential prerequisites for a successful treatment outcome.

The importance and limitations of images obtained by periapical radiography for identifying anatomical structures of root canals should be pointed it. The radiographic image corresponds to a two-dimensional aspect of a three-dimensional structure. There have been several advances in radiographic techniques for use in dentistry, as follows: digital radiography, densitometry methods, cone beam computed tomography, magnetic resonance imaging, ultrasound, nuclear techniques. Cone beam computed tomography has been used in endodontics for several purposes, such as: anatomic study of root canals, external and internal macromorphology in 3D-reconstruction of the teeth, evaluation of root canal preparation and obturation, re-treatment, coronal microleakage, detection of lesions in bone and in applications in experimental endodontology. These new images have enabled several anatomic aspects to be verified, which could previously not be seen with periapical radiography[31].

Estrela et al.[31] determined the accuracy of cone beam computed tomography, panoramic and periapical radiography for the detection of apical periodontitis. The findings of this investigation demonstrated that cone beam computed tomography images presented high accuracy for the recognition of apical periodontitis. Cone beam computed tomography images tend to offer higher scores than periapical and panoramic radiographs, suggesting that diagnosis of the degree of Apical periodondotitis, using conventional images, is underrated in a large number of cases. Apical periodondotitis was correctly identified in 54.5% using periapical radiographs, and in 27.8% using panoramic radiographs. Accuracy of periapical radiographs was significantly higher than that of panoramic radiographs. Apical periodontitis was correctly identified by conventional methods when a severe condition is observed.

In the apical region of the pulp cavity, the cemento-dentinal junction (CDJ) divides the cavity into two regions: the dentin canal and cement canal. Close to this region, in cases of vital pulp, is the apical extension that determines the preparation of the root canal. For situations of necrotic pulp, with or without periapical lesion, due to possible resorptions, the apical limit of choice must be aproximately 1-2 mm from the radiographic apex. Kutler[77] reports that the dentin canal narrows in the apical direction, and the cement canal opens up in the apical direction. The average distance observed from the foramen to the smaller diameter of the canal is 0.507 in young people, and 0.784 mm in adults. The root canal is divided into a long

**Chart 13.1** - Anatomy of the pulp-chamber floor (Krasner & Rankow[75])

**Relationships between the Pulp Chamber and the Clinical Crown**

*"1. The pulp chamber is always in the center of the tooth at the level of the Cemento-Enamel Junction (CEJ);*

*2. The walls of the pulp chamber are always concentric to the external surface of the crown at the level of the CEJ;*

*3. The distance from the external surface of the clinical crown to the wall of the pulp chamber is the same throughout the circumference of the tooth at the level of the CEJ."*

**Relationships on the Pulp-chamber Floor**

*"1. The floor of pulp chamber is always a darker color than the surrounding dentinal walls;*

*2. This color difference creates a distinct junction where the walls and the floor of the pulp chamber meet;*

*3. The orifices of the root canals are always located at the junction of the walls and floor;*

*4. The orifices of the root canals are located at the angles in the floor wall junction;*

*5. The orifices lie at the terminus of developmental root fusion lines, if present;*

*6. The developmental root fusion lines are darker than the floor color;*

*7. Reparative dentin or calcifications are lighter than the pulp chamber floor, and often obscure it and the orifices".*

conical dentinal portion and a short funnel-shaped cemental portion. The cemental portion is usually in the form of an inverted cone with the narrowest diameter at or near the cementodentinal junction, and its base at the apical foramen. Seltzer[144] related that occasionally the cementum abuts directly on the dentin at the apex; at times, the cementum extends for a considerable distance into the root canal, lining the dentin in an irregular manner. Burch & Hullen[11], analysing the relationship of the apical foramen with the root canal in 877 teeth, emphasized that in 92.3% of the teeth, the apical foramen opened up before the apical limit, however, the average distance from the radiographic limit to the apical foramen was 0.59 mm. The center of the apical root never coincides with the apical foramen. Pineda & Kuttler[127], studying the relationship between the apical root and apical foramen, verified that they had the same location in only 17% out of 7275 teeth analysed; thus, in 83% the foramen was about 2 to 3 mm away from the apical root.

Hess[58], studying the pulp cavity reported that this was a reflection of the external shape of teeth, which progressively reduces the light as the teeth age, featuring different apical and lateral ramifications. The process of aging modifies the anatomic aspect, by virtue of the continuous deposition of secondary dentin, or formation of reparative dentin, in response to the process of aggression, mainly represented by the dental caries process.

As regards the cement-dentin junction, Ricucci[135] based on a literature review, discussed the importance of the apical limit of instrumentation and obturation, which is one of the major controversial issues in root canal therapy. The results of longitudinal prognostic studies, basic on anatomical knowledge of the apical third of the root canal, and the histological pulp reaction to caries progression, demonstrated the presence of a vital pulp remnant, even in the presence of a periapical lesion. The location of the apical foramen in root canal treatment, most frequently ends short of the apex, often by several millimeters.

Ponce & Fernandez[132] histologically evaluated the location of the cement dentin canal junction, the diameters of the apical foramen and root canal at the cement dentin canal junction in anterior maxillary teeth. The results showed that: a. the cement dentin canal junction is simply the point at which two histological tissues converge inside the root canal, susceptible to modification depending on each particular clinical situation, and on the varying extensions of the cementum into the root canal; b. the apical constriction and the apical foramen are not reliable anatomic references to use to set the apical limit in preparations. Their use as a reference or apical stopping point can result in the production of lesions in the apical and periapical tissues.

Kojima et al.[73] by cumulative meta-analysis, analyzed the success rate of root canal filling, as well as the effect on the outcome of under extension, over extension, and flush filling. The cumulative success rate for treatment of teeth with vital pulp was higher than that of teeth with nonvital pulp. This result may be related to the pulp space of nonvital teeth often being infected. The results indicate that the success rates were the highest with flush filling, as confirmed by radiography of teeth with both vital and nonvital pulp. The main aspects of the results were as follows: a. a cumulative success rate of 82.8 ± 1.19% was obtained for teeth with vital pulp, and 78.9 ± 1.05% for those with nonvital pulp; b. the cumulative success rates with over extension, flush, and under extension for vital pulp and nonvital pulp were 70.8 ± 1.44, 86.5 ± 0.88, and 85.5 ± 0.98%, respectively; c. the cumulative success rates without and with periradicular lesion, were 82.0 ± 1.24 and 71.5 ± 1.60% respectively; d. in the analysis of success rate according to age group, the cumulative success rates for patients under 30 years of age, and those over 50 years of age were 78.4 ± 1.44% and 77.3 ± 2.58% respectively. Based on the use of cumulative meta-analysis, they proposed that the root canal should be filled to within 2 mm of the radiographic apex.

With regard to apical ramifications and lateral canals, it is important to report that they occur more frequently than one imagines.

## 13.3 Root Canal Ramifications

The ramifications found in the region of the dental root which, according to Pucci & Reig[133], deserve emphasis are:

1. **Main canal** – Present in the longitudinal axis of the teeth, passing from the roof of the pulp chamber to the apical foramen.
2. **Collateral canal** – Located parallel to the main canal, either capable of being reached or not by isolating the apical foramen, and shown to be smaller in volume than the main canal.
3. **Lateral canal** – shown to be in the cervical third and beginning of the middle third, going in the direction of the periodontium, either perpendicularly or not.
4. **Secondary canal** – shown to be in the apical third, being either perpendicular to the main canal or not, going in the direction of the periodontium.
5. **Acessory canal** – is a ramification of the secondary canal, which goes in the direction of the periodontium.
6. **Intercanal** – is the ramification between the main and collateral or secondary canal, and does not reach the periodontium.
7. **Recurring canal** – is part of the main canal going through a discreet passage, and returning to the main canal, not coming close to the apical region.
8. **Reticular canal** – represents the mixture of three or more canals, which run parallel, as ramifications of the intercanal, featuring a reticular aspect.
9. **Apical delta** – consists of several inset derivations in the region of the dental apices, which goes from the main canal in the direction of the apical periodontium.

Figures 13.1 and 13.2 show schematic representations of ramifications of the pulp cavity and area of the cemento-dentinal junction.

The value of knowing the internal morphology of the pulp cavity provides the opportunity to point out some of the factors that could complicate access to the root canals, either from the access cavity or the empty canal, such as the presence of nodules in the pulp chamber, calcification, dislocated tooth or a single denture covering the crown. However, before starting the access cavity, it is prudent to verify the radiographic image for the size and shape of the pulp chamber, inclination of the tooth in the arch. Minute analysis of the internal morphology by means of an initial radiograph is of significant value for the proper planning of the endodontic treatment.

Compatibility between the size of the pulp chamber and selection of the drill size to use is fundamental to the correct procedure of access cavity penetration, to allow the endodontic instrument the most direct and independent access to the root canal.

Some operative factors previous to the access cavity preparation are the removal of all caries tissue, restoration of defects and weakened dentin structure, which could change the coronal references. Some situations even demand a coronal reconstruction before the dental access.

The perfect access cavity can be prepared by meeting the following objectives: direct access to the root canal, complete elimination of the entire roof of the pulp chamber, respect for the pulp chamber floor, making no steps on the proximal walls of the pulp chamber and the proper selection of drills.

Coronal preparation in teeth with complete crowns has to be carefully performed, as a change in position could predispose to or be responsible for accidents. Before the endodontic treatment even of a left maxillary central incisor, considering the clinically favorable location of the tooth and its ideal morphology for endodontic treatment, no clinical procedure being instituted in any tooth must ever be underestimated.

The general characteristics of the pulp cavity of each dental group will be shown as being representative references to Endodontic procedures. Tables 13.1 to 13.28 show synthetic anatomical data, whose values represent results and averages obtained in different studies; such as those of Hess[57-59], Ingle & Taintor[68], Pucci & Reig[133], Pineda[127,128], Aprile & Figun[4], De Deus[23,24], Pécora[103-122], and important considerations with respect to the access cavity[1-177]. The estimate of percentage may involve other factors in addition to those introduced. Above all, the technical considerations of the access cavity are present. Figures 13.3 to 13.14 show schematic representations of the general considerations concerning the access cavity.

## Ramifications of the Pulp Cavity

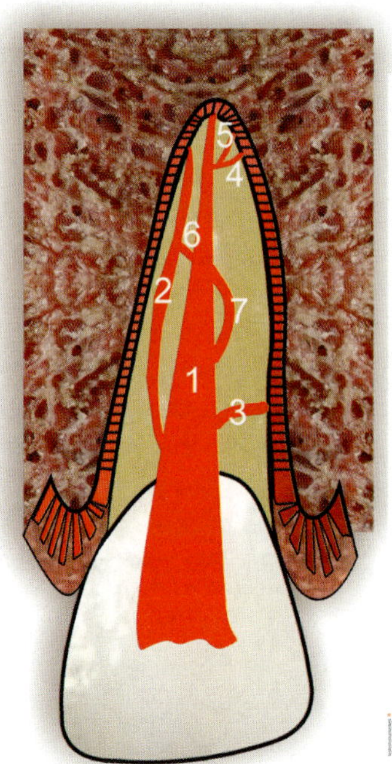


1. Main Canal
2. Collateral Canal
3. Lateral Canal
4. Secondary
5. Acessory Canal
6. Intercanal
7. Recurring Canal

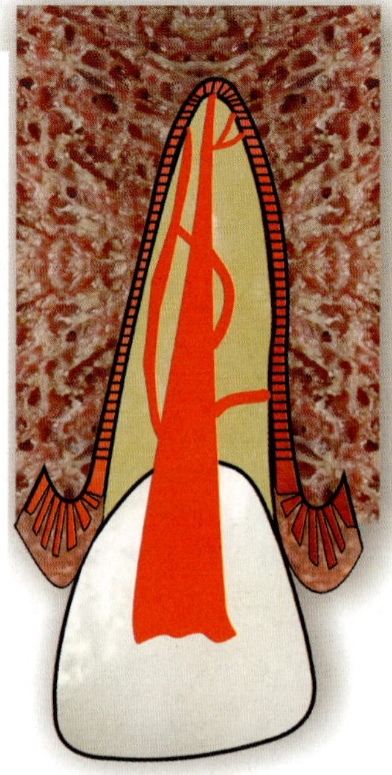

**Figure 13.1** - Root canal ramifications.

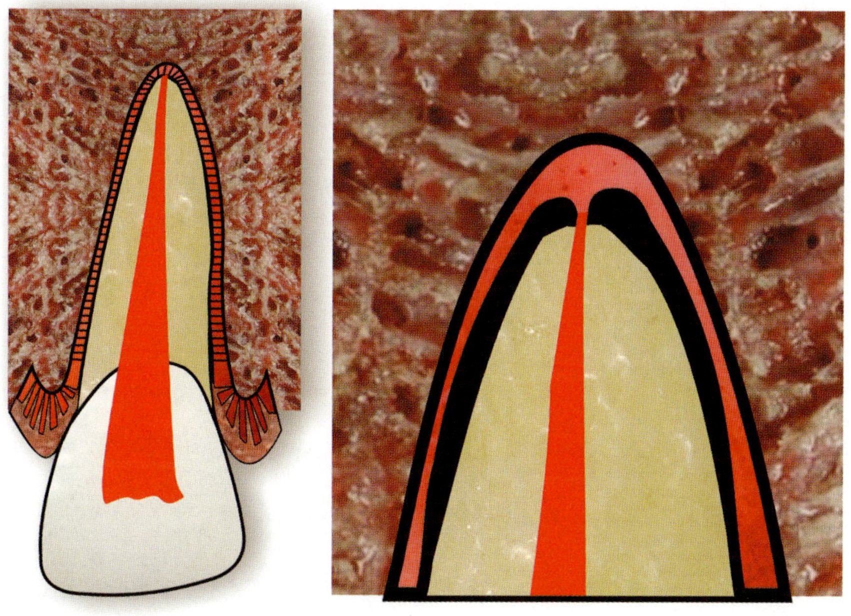

Figure 13.2 - Cemento-dentinal junction.

## Maxillary Central Incisor

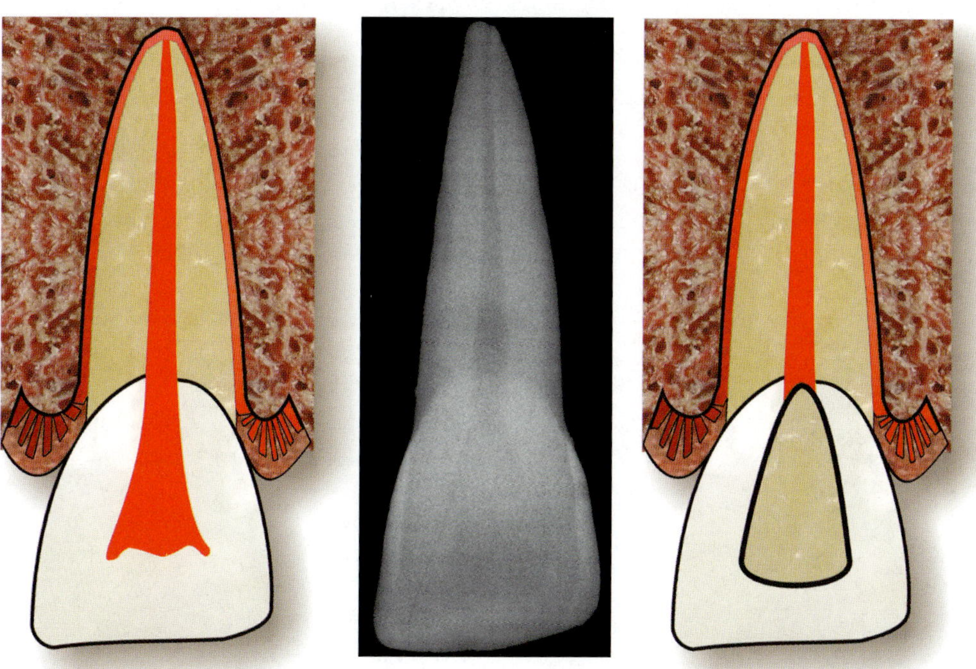

Figure 13.3 -Pulp cavity and access cavity of maxillary central Incisors.

**Table 13.1** - General characteristics of the pulp cavity of maxillary central Incisors

| **Maxillary Central Incisor Pulp Cavity** | |
|---|---|
| • Medium length | 23 mm |
| • Inclination to distal | 3° |
| • Inclination to palatine (apices closer to the buccal surface than to the palatine) | 15° |
| • Quantity of roots | 1 (100%) |
| • Quantity of canals | 1 (100%) |
| • Shape of canal | Conical pyramid |
| • Direction of the root | 75.0 % straight line<br>9.3 % buccal<br>7.8 % distal |
| • Period of eruption | 7 - 8 years |
| • Complete rhizogenesis | 10 years |

**Table 13.2** - Access cavity of maxillary central Incisor

| **Access Cavity** | |
|---|---|
| • Access preparation | Palatine face, close to the cingulum |
| • Type of drill | Diamond spherical #1012, 1013 |
| • Direction for access | Drill perpendicular in relation to the palatine face; after, the drill is inclined to the long axis of the tooth; the access is made by removal of the entire roof |
| • Shape of outline | Reflects the external shape of the tooth (triangular with base to the face of incision); proximal walls lightly expulsive |
| • Type of drill | Diamond conical # 3195 / 2200, mounted on micromotor |
| • Compensatory wearing | Removal of the palatine projection |
| • Type of drill | Orifice opening |

## Maxillary Lateral Incisor

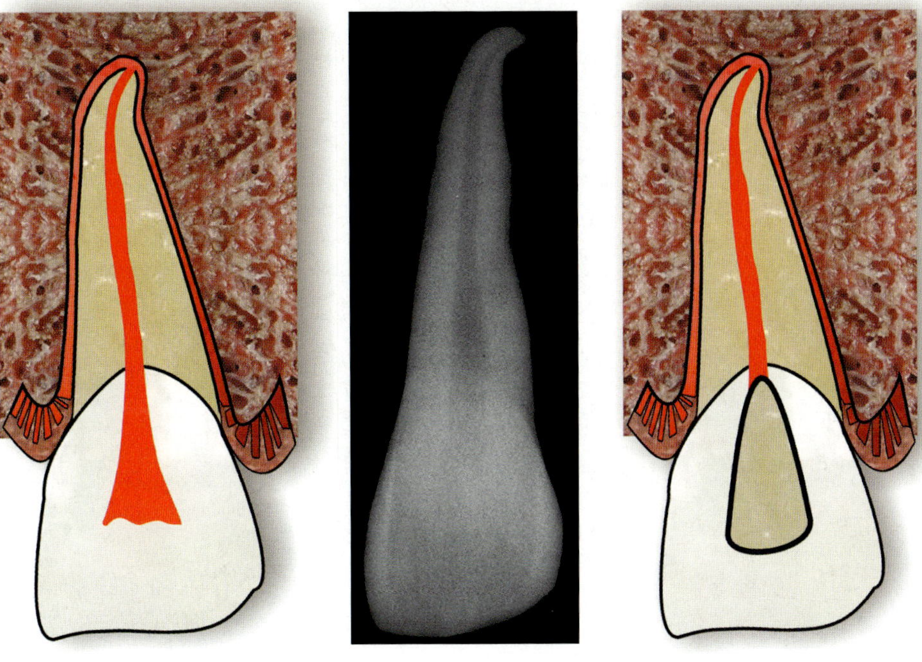

Figure 13.4 - Pulp cavity and access cavity of maxillary lateral Incisor.

**Table 13.3** - General characteristics of the pulp cavity of maxillary lateral Incisors

| Maxillary Lateral Incisor<br>Pulp Cavity | |
|---|---|
| • Medium length | 23 mm |
| • Inclination to distal | 5º |
| • Inclination to palatine (apices closer to the buccal surface than to the palatine) | 20º |
| • Quantity of roots | 1 (97%); 2 (3%) |
| • Quantity of canals | 1 (97%); 2 (3%) |
| • Shape of canal | Conical pyramid (oval section in mesio-distal direction) |
| • Direction of the root | 29.0 % straight line<br>49.2 % distal<br>3.9 % palatine |
| • Period of eruption | 8 - 9 years |
| • Complete rhizogenesis | 11 years |

**Table 13.4** - Considerations of access cavity of maxillary lateral Incisors

| Access Cavity | |
|---|---|
| • Access preparation | Palatine face, close to the cingulum |
| • Type of drill | Diamond spherical #1011, 1012 |
| • Direction to access | Drill perpendicular in relation to the palatine face; after, the drill is inclined to the long axis of the tooth; the access is conducted with removal of the entire roof |
| • Shape of outline | Reflects the external shape of the tooth (triangular with base to the face of incision); proximal walls lightly expulsive |
| • Type of drill | Diamond conical #2200, mounted on micromotor |
| • Compensatory wearing | Removal of the palatine projection |
| • Type of drill | Orifice opening |

## Maxillary Canine

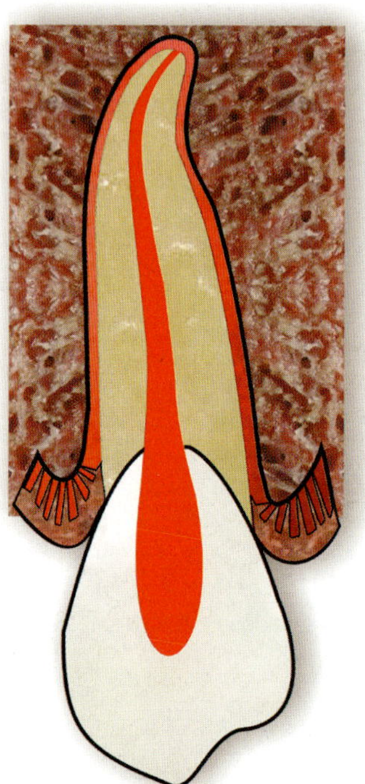

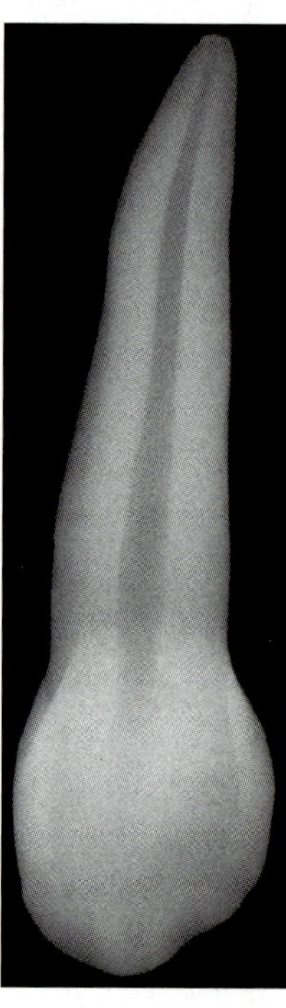

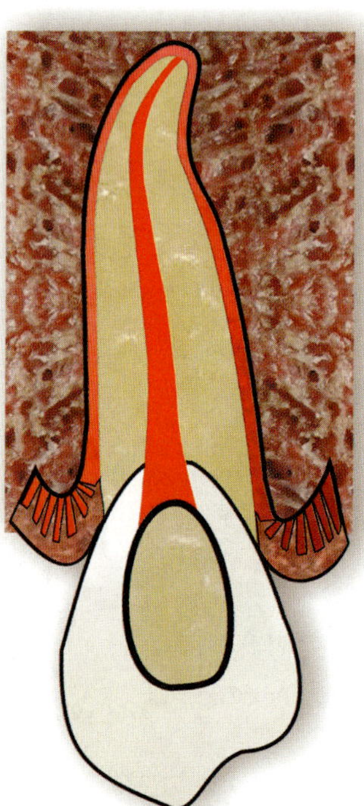

**Figure 13.5** - Pulp cavity and access cavity of maxillary canine.

**Table 13.5** - General characteristics of the pulp cavity of maxillary Canines

| Maxillary Canine<br>Pulp Cavity | |
|---|---|
| • Medium length | 25 mm |
| • Inclination to distal | 6° |
| • Inclination to palatine (apices closer to the buccal surface than to the palatine) | 17° |
| • Quantity of roots | 1 (100%) |
| • Quantity of canals | 1 (100%) |
| • Shape of canal | Conical pyramid (triangular section) |
| • Direction of the root | 38.5 % straight line<br>31.5 % distal<br>12.8 % buccal |
| • Period of eruption | 11 -12 years |
| • Complete rhizogenesis | 13 -15 years |

**Table 13.6** - Considerations of access cavity of maxillary canines

| Access Cavity | |
|---|---|
| • Access preparation | Palatine face, close to the cingulum |
| • Type of drill | Diamond spherical #1012, 1013 or 1014 |
| • Direction to access | Drill perpendicular in relation to the palatine face; after, the drill is inclined to the long axis of the tooth; the access is conducted, with removal of the entire roof |
| • Shape of outline | Reflects the external shape of the tooth (oval); proximal walls lightly expulsive |
| • Type of drill | Diamond conical #3195 / 2200, mounted on micromotor |
| • Compensatory wearing | Removal of the palatine projection |
| • Type of drill | Orifice opening |

**Table 13.7** - General characteristics of the pulp cavity of maxillary first premolars (BR – buccal root; PR – palatine root)

| **Maxillary First Premolar Pulp Cavity** | | |
|---|---|---|
| • Medium length | 21 mm | |
| • Inclination to distal | 7° | |
| • Inclination to palatine (apices closer to the buccal surface than to the palatine) | 11° | |
| • Quantity of roots | 1 (35.5%); 2 (42%) | |
| • Quantity of canals | 1 (8.3%); 2 (84.2%); 3 (7.5%) | |
| • Shape of canal | BR pyramidal<br>PR conical | |
| • Direction of the root | BR 27.8 % straight<br>14.0 % distal<br>36.2 % palatine<br>14.0 % buccal | PR 44.4% straight<br>14.0 % distal<br>8.0% palatine<br>27.8% buccal |
| • Period of eruption | 10 -11 years | |
| • Complete rhizogenesis | 12 -13 years | |

**Table 13.8** - Considerations of access cavity of maxillary first premolars

| **Access Cavity** | |
|---|---|
| • Access preparation | Oclusal face, center of mesiodistal track |
| • Type of drill | Diamond spherical #1012, 1013, 1014 |
| • Direction to access | Drill in relation to the long axis of the tooth until up to the pulp chamber, after, in the palatine direction; the access is conduct with removal of the entire roof |
| • Shape of outline | Reflects the external shape of the tooth (oval); proximal walls, lightly expulsive |
| • Type of drill | Diamond conical #3195 / 2200, mounted on micromotor |
| • Compensatory wearing | Proximal walls lightly expulsive |
| • Type of drill | Orifice opening |

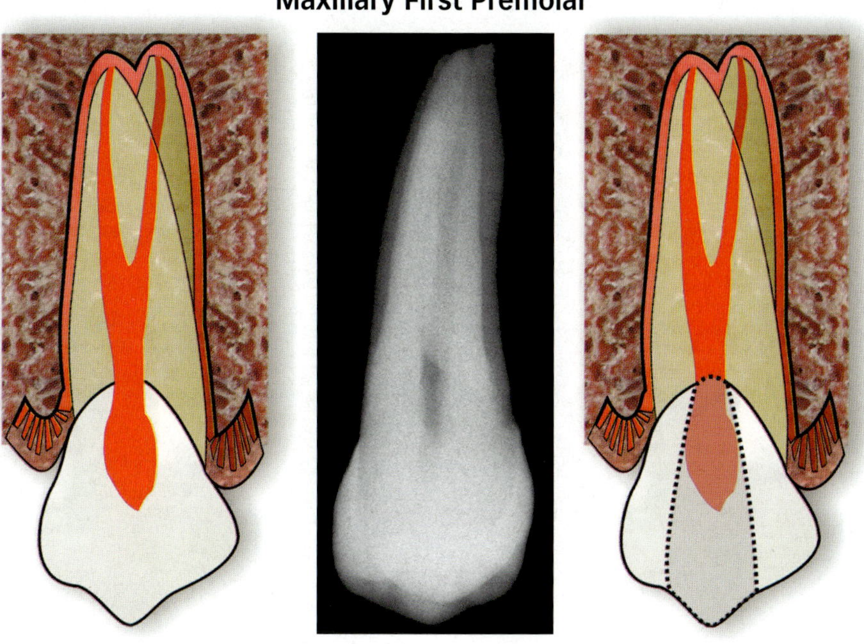


Figure 13.6 - Pulp cavity and access cavity of maxillary first premolar.



**Table 13.9** - General characteristics of the pulp cavity of maxillary second premolar

| Maxillary Second Premolar<br>Pulp Cavity | |
|---|---|
| • Medium length | 21 mm |
| • Inclination to distal | 7º |
| • Inclination to palatine (apices closer to the buccal surface than to the palatine) | 7º |
| • Quantity of roots | 1 (90.3%); 2 dif. (2%); 2 fus. (7.7%) |
| • Quantity of canals | 1 (53.7%); 2 (46.3%) |
| • Shape of canal | flattened mesiodistal (oval) |
| • Direction of the root | 37.4 % straight line<br>33.9 % distal<br>15.7 % buccal<br>13.0 % bayonet |
| • Period of eruption | 10 -12 years |

**Table 13.10** - Considerations of access cavity of maxillary second premolars

| Access Cavity | |
|---|---|
| • Access preparation | Oclusal face, center of mesiodistal track |
| • Type of drill | Spherical Diamond #1012, 1013, 1014 |
| • Direction to access | Drill in relation to the long axis of the tooth until up to the pulp chamber, after, in the palatine direction; the access is conducted with removal of the entire roof |
| • Shape of outline | Reflects the external shape of the tooth (oval); proximal walls lightly expulsive |
| • Type of drill | Diamond conical #3195 / 2200, mounted on micromotor |
| • Compensatory wearing | Proximal walls lightly expulsive |
| • Type of drill | Orifice opening |

**Maxillary Second Premolar**

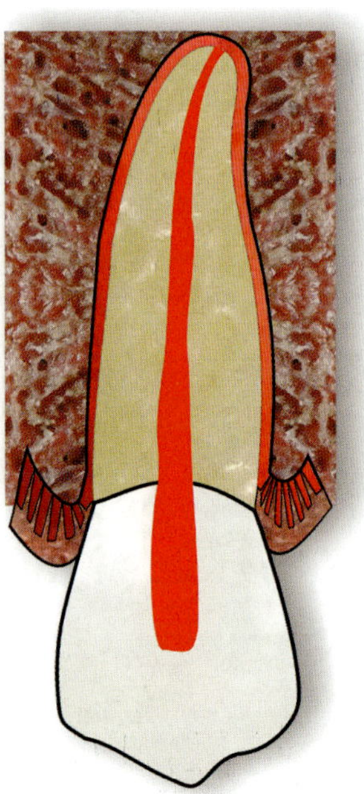

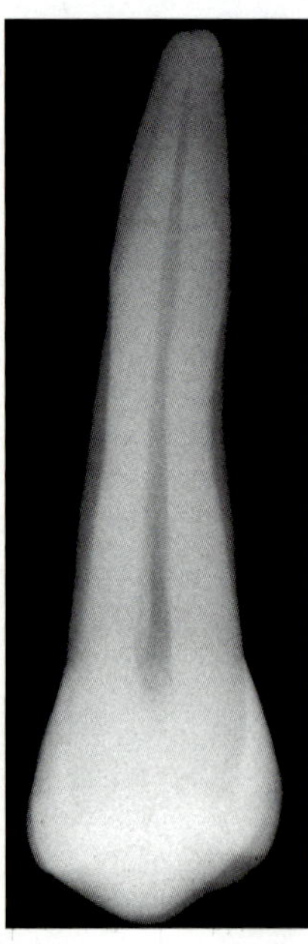

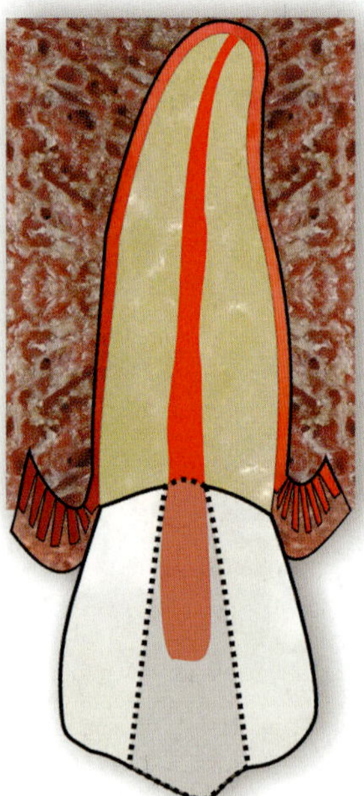

**Figure 13.7** - Pulp cavity and access of maxillary second premolars.

**Table 13.11** - General characteristics of the pulp cavity of maxillary first molars (PR – palatine root; MBR – mesio-buccal root; DBR – disto-buccal root)

| Maxillary First Molar<br>Pulp Cavity | |
|---|---|
| • Medium length | PR 21 mm; MBR and DBR 19mm |
| • Inclination to distal | 0° |
| • Inclination to palatine (apices closer to the buccal surface than to the palatine) | 15° |
| • Quantity of roots | 3 dif. (95%); 3 fus. (5%) |
| • Quantity of canals | 3 (60%); 4 (40%) |
| • Shape of canal | PR pyramidal (oval VP direction)<br>MBR flattened MD direction<br>DBR conical (circular) |
| • Direction of the root | PR 40% straight 55% buccal<br>MBR 21% straight 78% distal<br>DBR 54% straight 17% distal 19% mesial |
| • Period of eruption | 6 -7 years |
| • Complete rhizogenesis | 9 -10 years |

**Table 13.12** - Considerations of access cavity of maxillary first molars

| Access Cavity | |
|---|---|
| • Access preparation | Oclusal face in central pit |
| • Type of drill | Diamond spherical #1013, 1014 |
| • Direction to access | Drill parallel in relation to the long axis of the tooth, inclined to palatine |
| • Shape of outline | Reflects the external shape of the tooth (trapezoidal); proximal walls lightly expulsive (mesial) |
| • Type of drill | Diamond conical #3195FF / 2200, mounted on micromotor |
| • Compensatory wearing | Buccal face (mesio-buccal angle) |
| • Type of drill | Orifice opening |

## Maxillary Molar

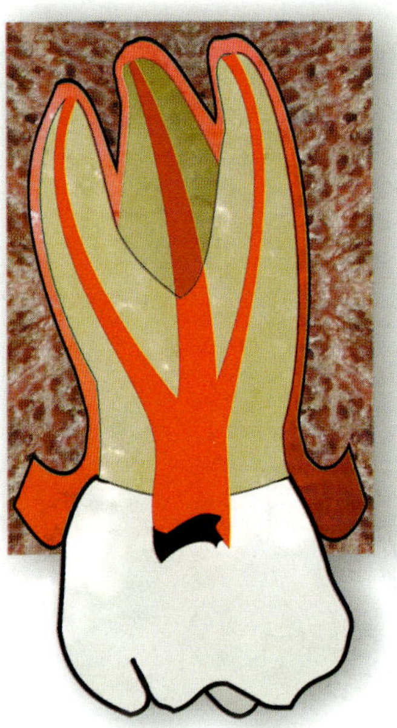

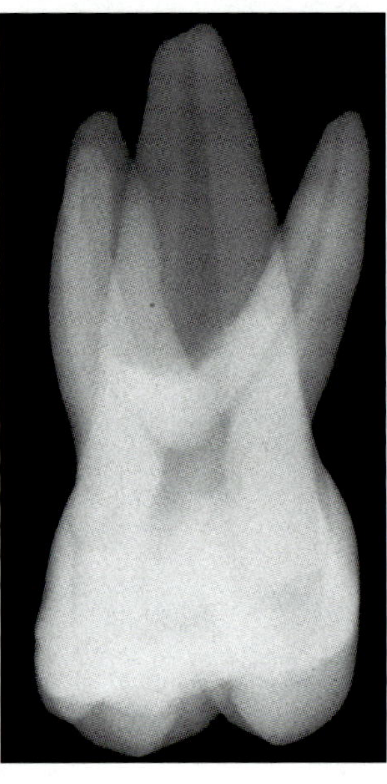

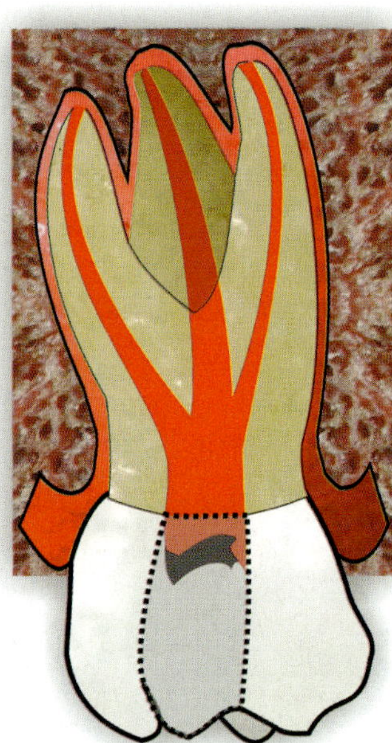

**Figure 13.8** - Pulp cavity and access cavity of maxillary molar.

**Table 13.13** - General characteristics of the pulp cavity of maxillary second molars (PR – palatine root; MBR – mesio-buccal root; DBR – disto-buccal root)

| Maxillary Second Molar<br>Pulp Cavity | |
|---|---|
| • Medium length | PR 21 mm; MBR and DBR 19mm |
| • Inclination to distal | 5° |
| • Inclination to palatine (apices closer to the buccal surface than to the palatine) | 11° |
| • Quantity of roots | 3 dif. (55%); 3 fus. (45%) |
| • Quantity of canals | 3 (70%); 4 (30%) |
| • Shape of canal | PR pyramidal (oval BP direction)<br>MBR flattened MD direction<br>DBR conical (circular) |
| • Direction of the root | PR 63% straight 37% buccal<br>MBR 22% straight 54% distal<br>DBR 54% straight 17% mesial |
| • Period of eruption | 12 -13 years |
| • Complete rhizogenesis | 14 -16 years |

**Table 13.14** - Considerations of access cavity of maxillary second molars

| Access Cavity | |
|---|---|
| • Access preparation | Oclusal face in central pit |
| • Type of drill | Spherical Diamond #1013, 1014 |
| • Direction to access | Drill parallel in relation to the long axis of the tooth, inclined to palatine |
| • Shape of outline | Reflects the external shape of the tooth (trapezoidal); proximal walls lightly expulsive (mesial) |
| • Type of drill | Conical Diamond #3195FF / 2200, mounted on micromotor |
| • Compensatory wearing | Buccal face (MB angle) |
| • Type of drill | Orifice opening |

**Table 13.15** - General characteristics of the pulp cavity of mandibular central Incisors

| Mandibular Central Incisor<br>Pulp Cavity | |
|---|---|
| • Medium length | 21 mm |
| • Inclination to distal | 0º |
| • Inclination to lingual (apices closer to the buccal surface than to the palatine) | 15º |
| • Quantity of roots | 1 (100%) |
| • Quantity of canals | 1 (73.4%); 2 (26.6%) |
| • Shape of canal | oval in buccal-lingual direction and flattened in mesio-distal direction |
| • Direction of the root | 66.7 % straight line<br>12.5 % distal<br>18.8 % buccal |
| • Period of eruption | 6 -7 years |
| • Complete rhizogenesis | 9 years |

**Table 13.16** - Considerations of access cavity of mandibular central Incisors

| Access Cavity | |
|---|---|
| • Access preparation | Palatine face, close to the cingulum |
| • Type of drill | Spherical Diamond #1011 |
| • Direction to access | Drill perpendicular in relation to the palatine face; after, the drill is inclined to the long axis of the tooth; the access is conducted with removal of the entire roof |
| • Shape of outline | Reflects the external shape of the tooth (triangular with base to the face of incision); proximal walls lightly expulsive |
| • Type of drill | Conical Diamond #2200, mounted on micromotor |
| • Compensatory wearing | Removal of the palatine projection |
| • Type of drill | Orifice opening |

## Mandibular Central Incisor

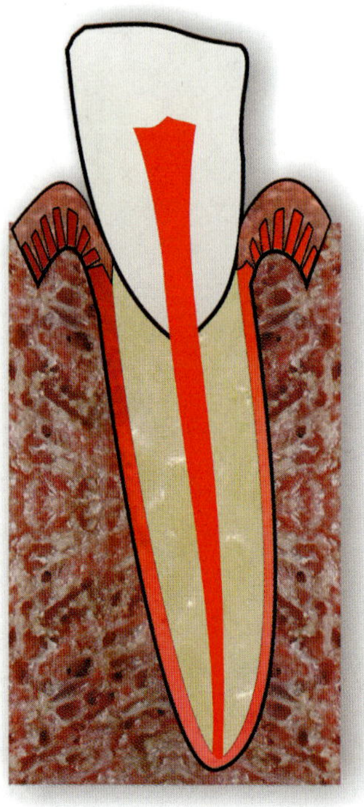

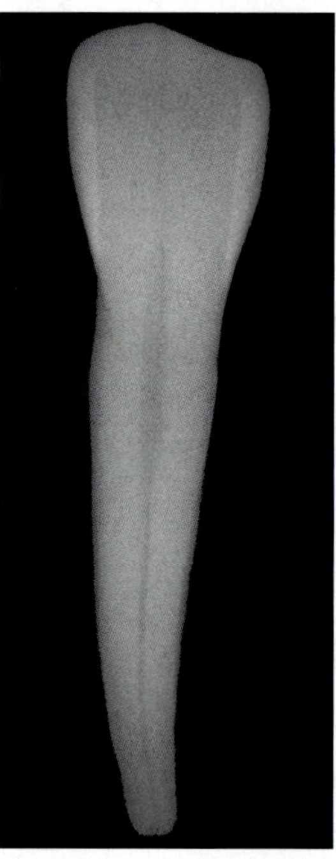

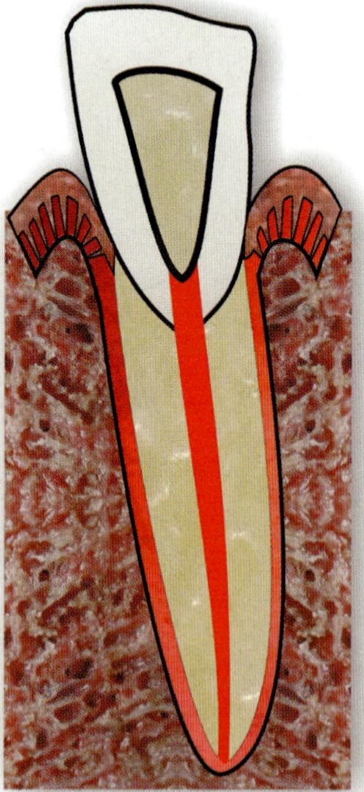

**Figure 13.9** - Pulp cavity and access cavity of mandibular central Incisor.

**Table 13.17** - General characteristics of the pulp cavity of mandibular lateral Incisors

| Mandibular Lateral Incisor Pulp Cavity | |
|---|---|
| • Medium length | 21 mm |
| • Inclination to distal | 0° |
| • Inclination to lingual (apices closer to the buccal surface than to the palatine) | 10° |
| • Quantity of roots | 1 (100%) |
| • Quantity of canals | 1 (84.6%); 2 (15.4%) |
| • Shape of canal | oval in buccal-lingual direction and flattened in mesio-distal direction |
| • Direction of the root | 54.0 % straight line<br>33.3 % distal<br>10.7 % buccal |
| • Period of eruption | 7 - 8 years |
| • Complete rhizogenesis | 10 years |

**Table 13.18** - Considerations of access cavity of mandibular lateral Incisors

| Access Cavity | |
|---|---|
| • Access preparation | Palatine face, close to the cingulum |
| • Type of drill | Spherical Diamond #1011 |
| • Direction to access | Drill perpendicular in relation to the palatine face; after the drill is inclined to the long axis of the tooth; the access is conducted with removal of the entire roof |
| • Shape of outline | Reflects the external shape of the tooth (triangular with base to the face of incision); proximal walls lightly expulsive |
| • Type of drill | Diamond conical #2200, mounted on micromotor |
| • Compensatory wearing | Removal of the palatine projection |
| • Type of drill | Orifice opening |

## Mandibular Lateral Incisor

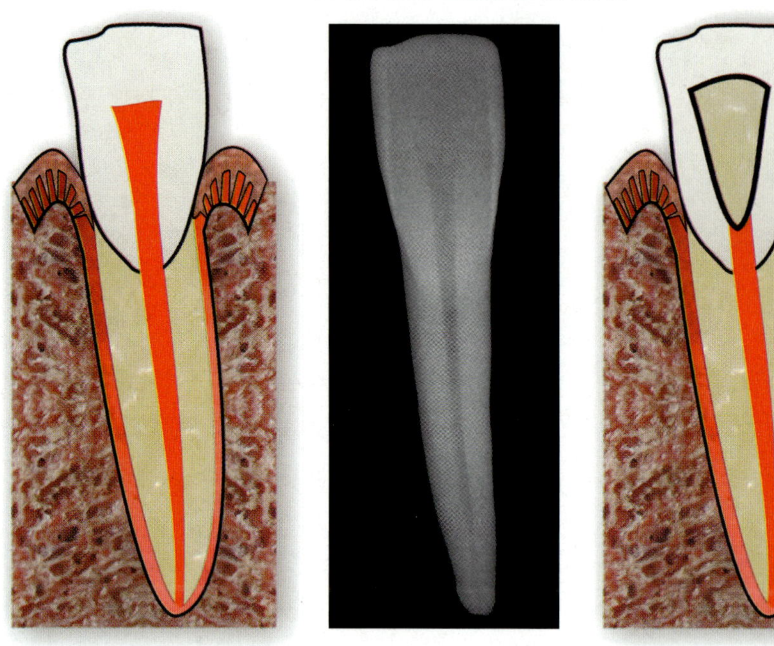

**Figure 13.10** - Pulp cavity and access cavity cavity of mandibular lateral Incisor.

**Table 13.19** - General characteristics of the pulp cavity of mandibular canines

| Mandibular Canine<br>Pulp Cavity | |
|---|---|
| • Medium length | 25 mm |
| • Inclination to distal | 3° |
| • Inclination to lingual (apices closer to the buccal surface than to the palatine) | 2° |
| • Quantity of roots | 1 (94%); 2 fus. (6%) |
| • Quantity of canals | 1 (88.2%); 2 (11.8%) |
| • Shape of canal | flattened in mesio-distal direction (oval); apice rounded |
| • Direction of the root | 68.2 % straight line<br>19.6 % distal<br>6.8 % buccal |
| • Period of eruption | 9 -10 years |
| • Complete rhizogenesis | 12 -14 years |

**Table 13.20** - Considerations of access cavity of mandibular canines

| Access Cavity | |
|---|---|
| • Access preparation | Palatine face, close to the cingulum |
| • Type of drill | Spherical Diamond #1012, 1013 |
| • Direction to access | Drill perpendicular in relation to the palatine face; after the drill is inclined to the long axis of the tooth; the access is conducted with removal of the entire roof |
| • Shape of outline | Reflects the external shape of the tooth (oval); proximal walls lightly expulsive |
| • Type of drill | Conical Diamond #3195 / 2200, mounted on micromotor |
| • Compensatory wearing | Removal of the palatine projection |
| • Type of drill | Orifice opening |



**Mandibular Canine**

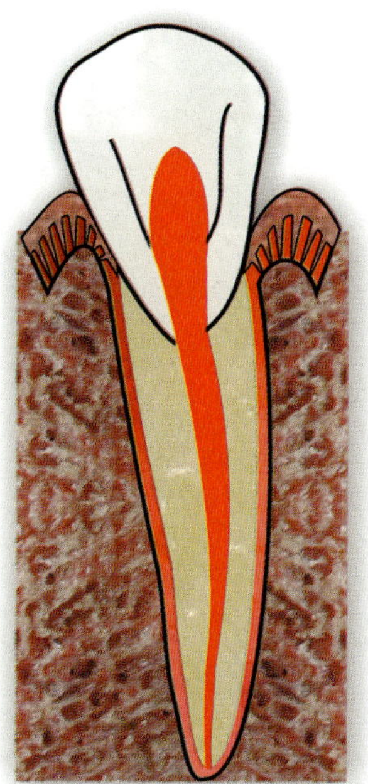
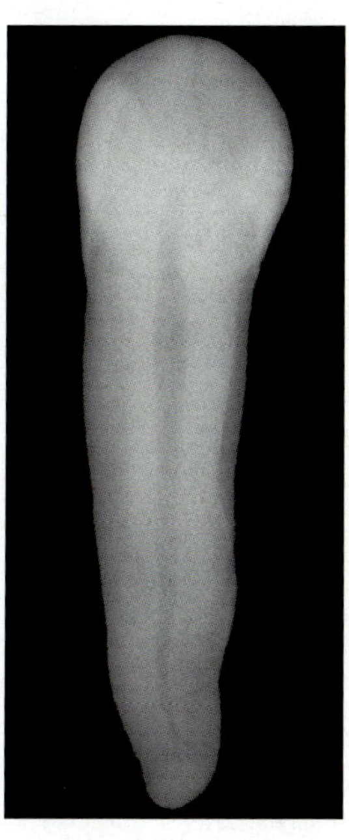
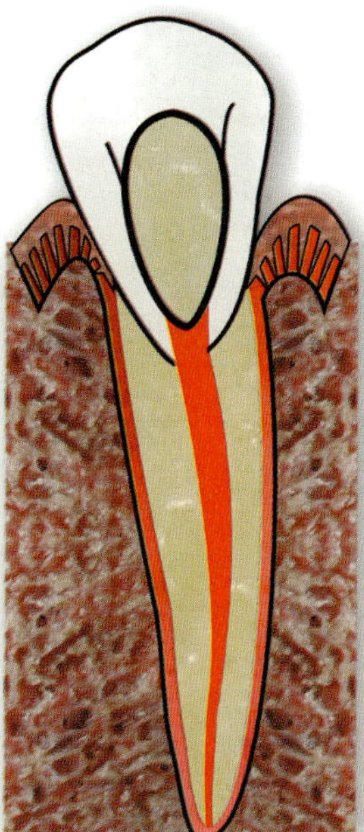

**Figure 13.11** - Pulp cavity and access cavity of mandibular canine.

**Table 13.21** - General characteristics of the pulp cavity of mandibular first premolars

| Mandibular First Premolar Pulp Cavity | |
|---|---|
| • Medium length | 21 mm |
| • Inclination to distal | 5º |
| • Inclination to lingual (apices closer to the buccal surface than to the lingual) | 3º |
| • Quantity of roots | 1 (82%); 2 fus. (18%) |
| • Quantity of canals | 1 (66.6%); 2 (31.3%); 3 (2.1%) |
| • Shape of canal | flattened in mesio-distal direction (oval); apice rounded |
| • Direction of the root | 47.5 % straight line<br>34.8 % distal<br>7.1 % lingual |
| • Period of eruption | 10 -12 years |
| • Complete rhizogenesis | 12 -13 years |

**Table 13.22** - Considerations of access cavity of mandibular first premolars

| Access Cavity | |
|---|---|
| • Access preparation | Oclusal face, center of mesiodistal track |
| • Type of drill | Spherical Diamond #1011 |
| • Direction to access | Drill in relation to the long axis of the tooth until up to the pulp chamber; the access is conducted with removal of the entire roof |
| • Shape of outline | Circular (oval in BL direction, near to mesial) |
| • Type of drill | Conical Diamond #3195 / 2200, mounted on micromotor |
| • Compensatory wearing | Proximal walls lightly expulsive |
| • Type of drill | Orifice opening |

## Mandibular First Premolar

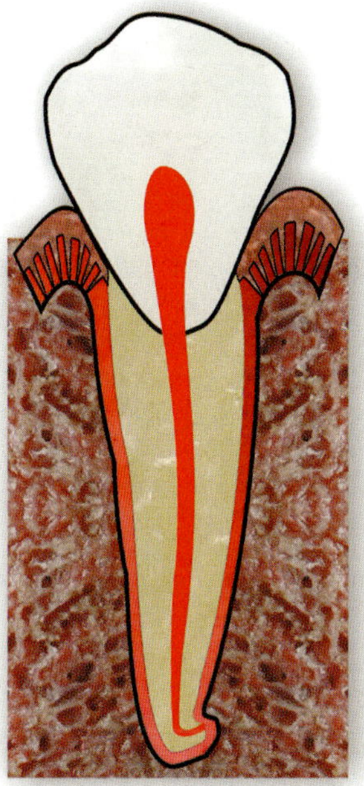

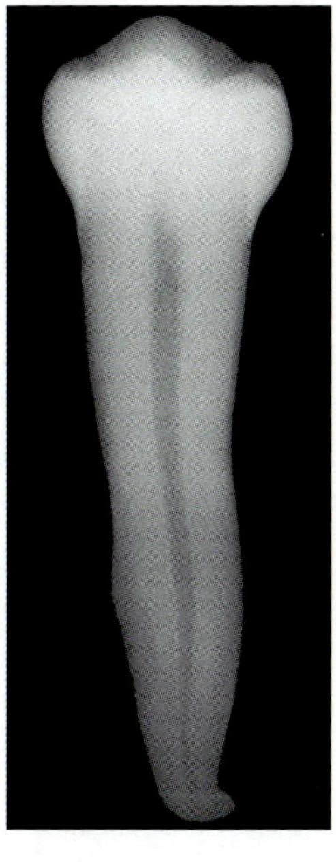

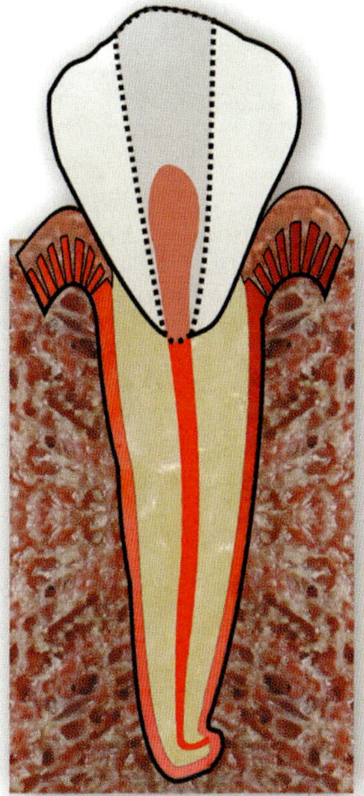

**Figure 13.12** - Pulp cavity and access cavity of mandibular first premolar.

**Table 13.23** - General characteristics of the pulp cavity of mandibular second premolars

| **Mandibular Second Premolar Pulp Cavity** | |
|---|---|
| • Medium length | 21 mm |
| • Inclination to distal | 5º |
| • Inclination to lingual (apices closer to the buccal surface than to the lingual) | 9º |
| • Quantity of roots | 1 (92%); 2 fus. (8%) |
| • Quantity of canals | 1 (89.3%); 2 (10.7%) |
| • Shape of canal | flattened in mesio-distal direction (oval); apice rounded |
| • Direction of the root | 38.5 % straight line<br>39.8 % distal<br>10.1 % buccal |
| • Period of eruption | 11 -12 years |
| • Complete rhizogenesis | 13 -14 years |

**Table 13.24** - Considerations of access cavity of mandibular second premolars

| Access Cavity | |
|---|---|
| • Access preparation | Oclusal face, center of mesiodistal track |
| • Type of drill | Spherical Diamond #1011 |
| • Direction to access | Drill in relation to the long axis of the tooth until up to the pulp chamber; the access is conducted with removal of the entire roof |
| • Shape of outline | Circular (oval in BL direction, near to mesial) |
| • Type of drill | Conical Diamond #3195 / 2200, mounted on micromotor |
| • Compensatory wearing | Proximal walls lightly expulsive |
| • Type of drill | Orifice opening |

## Mandibular Second Premolar

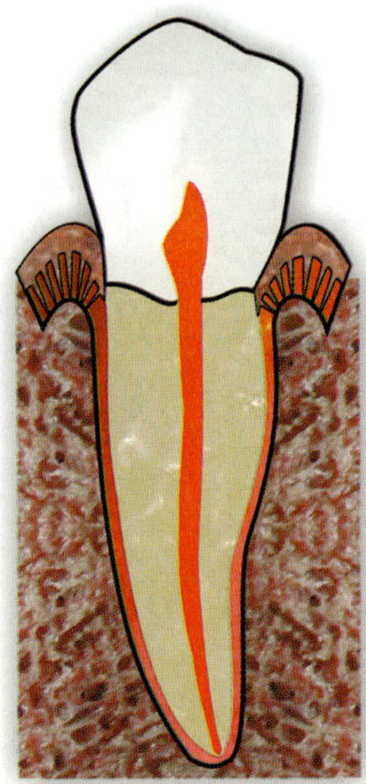

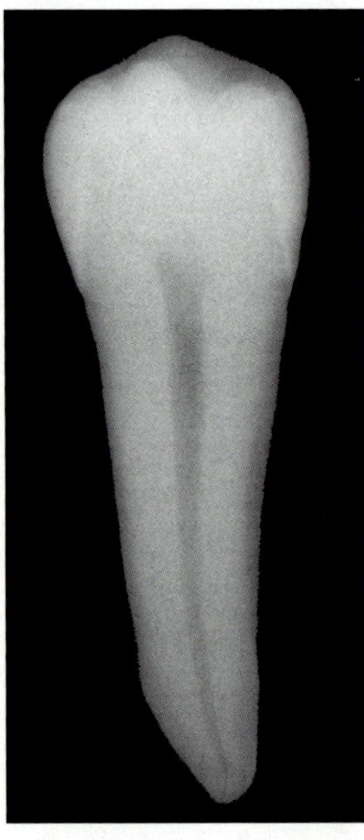

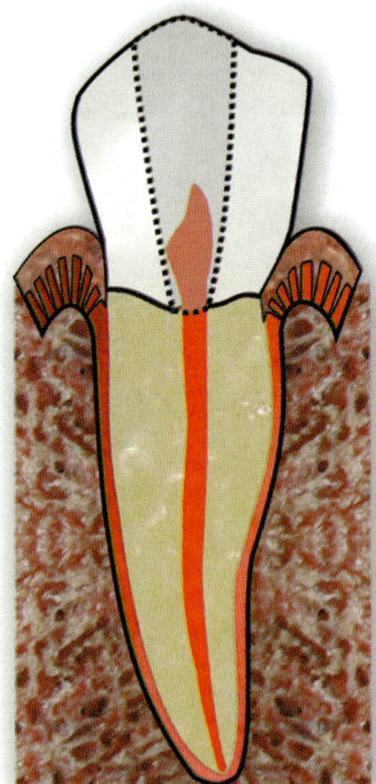

**Figure 13.13** - Pulp cavity and access cavity of mandibular second premolar.

**Table 13.25** - General characteristics of the pulp cavity of mandibular first molars (MR – mesio root; DR – distal root)

| Mandibular First Molar Pulp Cavity | | |
|---|---|---|
| • Medium length | 21 mm | |
| • Inclination to distal | 10º | |
| • Inclination to lingual (apices closer to the buccal surface than to the lingual) | 13º | |
| • Quantity of roots | 2 dif. (92.2%); 3 dif. (2.5%)<br>2 fus. (5.3%) | |
| • Quantity of canals | 2 (8%); 3 (56%); 4 (36%) | |
| • Shape of canal | Roots flattened in mesio-distal direction with longitudinal tracks and oval canals | |
| • Direction of the root | MR 16.5 % straight<br>84.0 % distal<br>8.5 % mesial | DR 73.5 % straight<br>18.0 % distal |
| • Period of eruption | 6 - 7 years | |
| • Complete rhizogenesis | 9 -10 years | |

**Table 13.26** - Considerations of access cavity of mandibular first molars

| Access Cavity | |
|---|---|
| • Access preparation | Oclusal face, central pit, union of MD and BL track |
| • Type of drill | Spherical Diamond #1012, 1013 |
| • Direction to access | Drill in relation to the long axis of the tooth until up to the pulp chamber; the access is conducted with removal of the entire roof |
| • Shape of outline | Almost rectangular with smaller side to distal |
| • Type of drill | Conical Diamond 2200, mounted on micromotor |
| • Compensatory wearing | Expulsive walls (especially the mesial) |
| • Type of drill | Orifice opening |

## Mandibular Molar

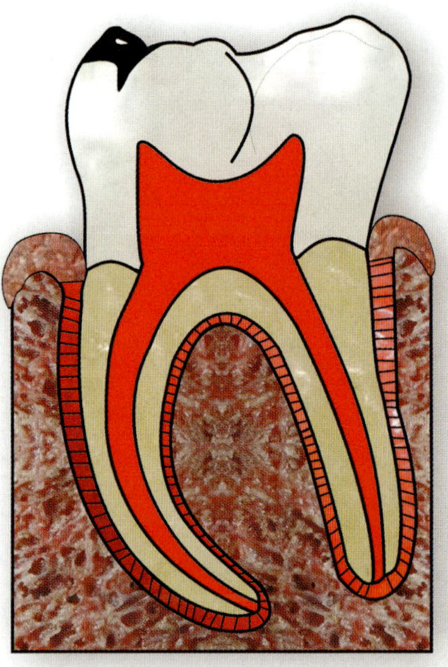
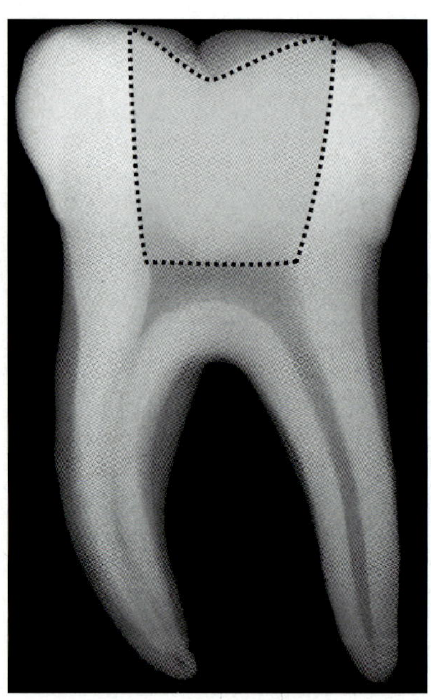

**Figure 13.14** - Pulp cavity and access cavity of mandibular first molar.

**Table 13.27** - General characteristics of the pulp cavity of mandibular second molars (MR – mesio root; DR – distal root)

| Mandibular Second Molar<br>Pulp Cavity | | |
|---|---|---|
| • Medium length | 21 mm | |
| • Inclination to distal | 15° | |
| • Inclination to lingual (apices closer to the buccal surface than to the lingual) | 12° | |
| • Quantity of roots | 2 dif. (68%); 2 fus. (30.5%); 3 (1.5%) | |
| • Quantity of canals | 2 (16.2%); 3 (72.5%); 4 (11.3%) | |
| • Shape of canal | Roots flattened in mesio-distal direction with longitudinal tracks and oval canals | |
| • Direction of the root | MR 27.2 % straight<br>60.8 % distal<br>4.0 % buccal | DR 57.6 % straight<br>18.4 % distal<br>13.6 % mesial |
| • Period of eruption | 11 -13 years | |
| • Complete rhizogenesis | 14 -15 years | |

**Table 13.28** - Considerations of access cavity of mandibular second molars.

| Access Cavity | |
|---|---|
| • Access preparation | Oclusal face, central pit, union of MD and BL track |
| • Type of drill | Spherical Diamond #1012, 1013 |
| • Direction to access | Drill in relation to the long axis of the tooth up to the pulp chamber; the access is conducted with removal of the entire roof |
| • Shape of outline | Almost rectangular with smaller side to distal |
| • Type of drill | Conical Diamond 2200, mounted on micromotor |
| • Compensatory wearing | Expulsive walls (especially the mesial) |
| • Type of drill | Orifice opening |

Taking into account all the knowledge of the pulp cavity anatomy, the commonest accidents observed during access cavity preparation deserve special reference, as they may lead to the failure of the endodontic treatment. Among them, the following are emphasized: 1. Caries tissue remaining in the pulp chamber; 2. Incorrect choice of the point for preparing the access cavity; 3. Incorrect selection of the drill (excessively large drill in relation to the size of the pulp chamber); 4. Error on the climbing of teeth with wrong position; 5. Incomplete access; 6. Not removing the coronal roof; 7. Buccal perforation in anterior teeth; 8. Perforation of the floor in molars; 9: Inadequate compensatory wearing; 10. Steps on the proximal walls.

Figures 13.15 and 13.16 show a maxillary lateral incisor with two roots, in which the endodontic treatment was performed in only one of them. Another procedure is required, which would probably indicate endodontic surgery. Figures 13.17 to 13.18 evidence radiographic aspects of mandibular and maxillary premolar with three root canals. Figures 13.19 to 13.23 show accidents that occurred while preparing the access cavity, causing perforations.

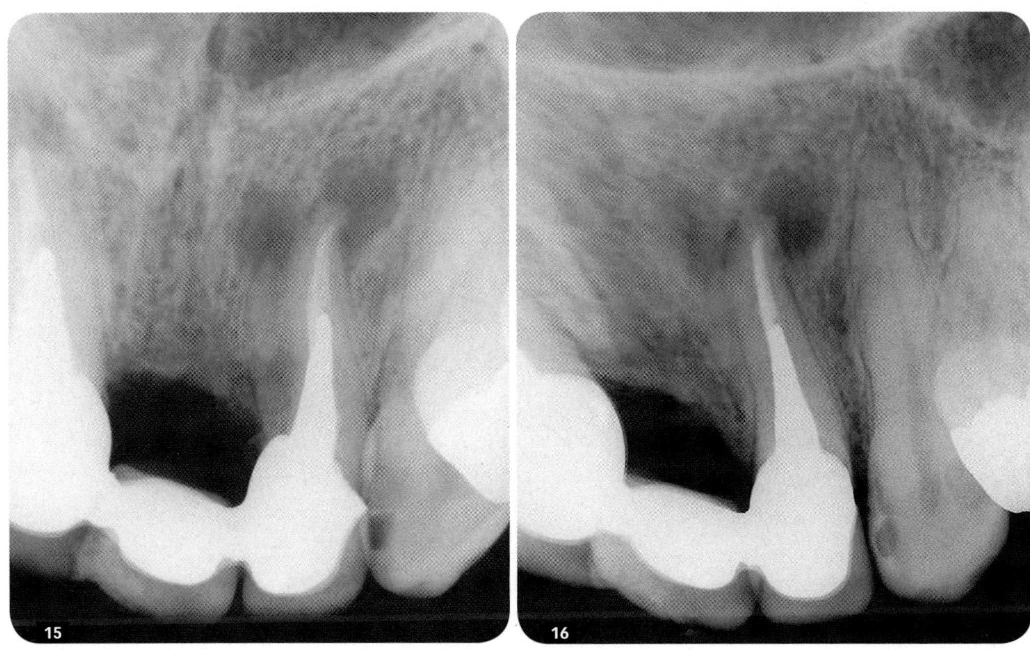


**Figures 13.15 and 13.16** - Maxillary lateral Incisor with two roots.

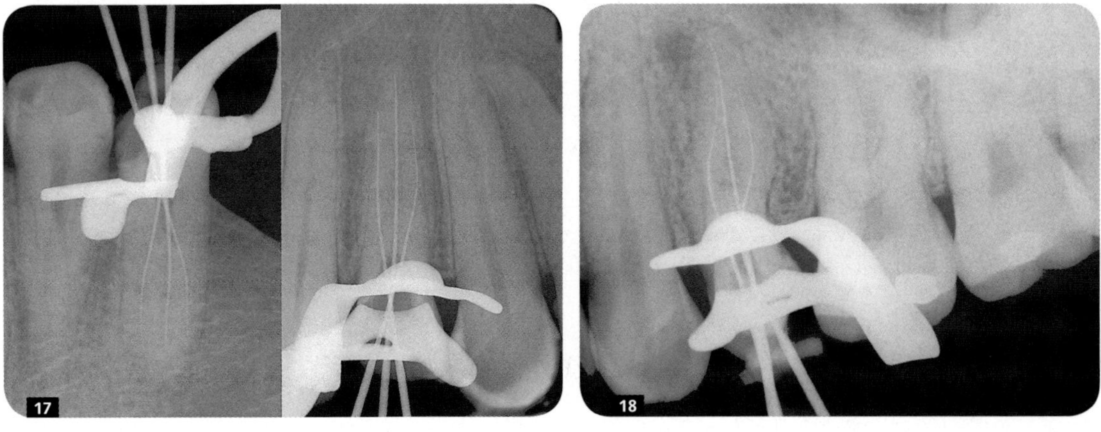


**Figures 13.17 and 13.18** - Mandibular and maxillary premolars with 3 root canals.

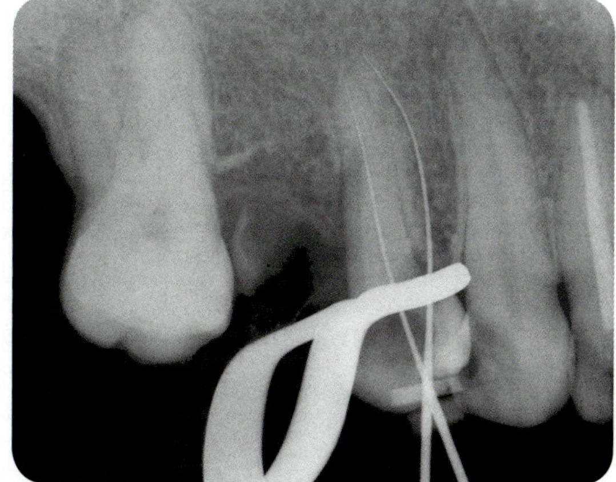

Figure 13.19 - Coronal perforations during the access cavity preparation.

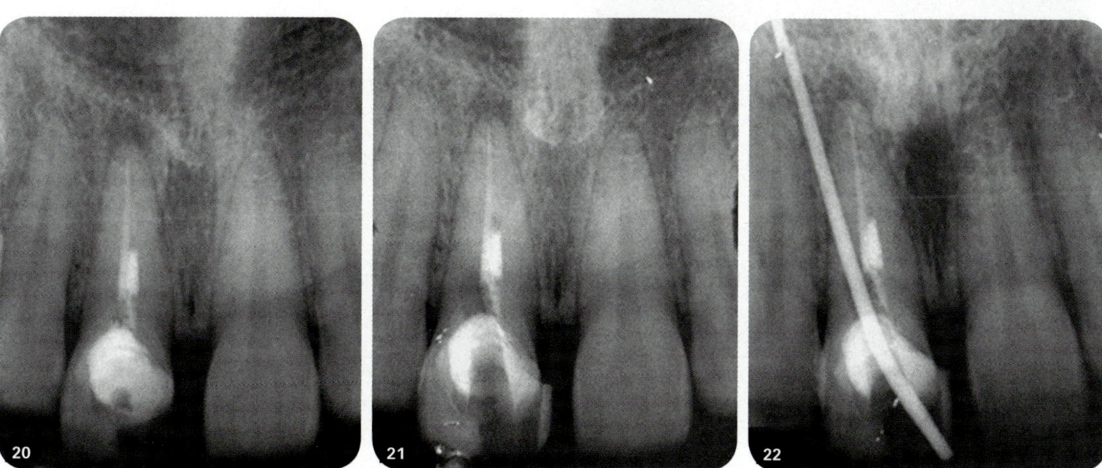


**Figures 13.20 to 13.22** - Coronal perforations during the access cavity preparation.

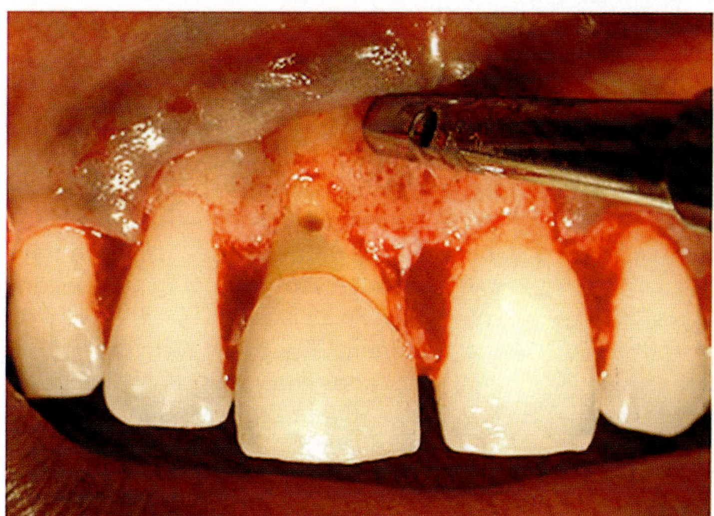

**Figure 13.23** - Coronal perforations during the access cavity preparation.

## 13.4 Disturbance of Dental Development

The disturbance of dental development shows deviations normally produced by local conditions through hereditary processes or by manifestations of systemic disturbances. These dental anomalies may involve the shape (germination, fusion, concrescence, laceration, radicular grooves, dens invaginatus, dens evaginatus), the size (microdontia and macrodontia), the number (anadontia, supernumerary teeth), the period of development (premature dentition, belated eruption) and its histological structure (imperfect odontogenesis – imperfect amelogenesis, hypercementosis)[5,44]. Among the anomalies important to endodontic treatment, those that involve the shape deserve special attention. Some alterations are only observed through a good radiographic exam.

### Germination

Germination is an attempted division of a dental germ resulting in the incomplete formation of two teeth. It normally appears with a bifid crown (larger than normal) with only one root[5] (Fig. 13.24 to 13.27).

### Fusion

Fusion is the union of two or more teeth during development, in which the dentin and other dental tissues are united. This union may occur in a stranger way, to compose a large tooth, or the union of the crowns, or the union of the roots[44].

### Concrescence

Concrescence corresponds to the union of two or more teeth, only by the cement, representing a type of fusion[5,44].

### Dens Invaginatus

Dens (Dens Invaginatus) represents an anomaly in the development of a tooth, with disorganization occurring in the enamel organ, featured by an invagination inside the dental body which is covered with enamel. Dens in dens may occur in any tooth, although its major prevalence is in the maxillary lateral incisors. Frequently, these are shown to be cuneiform. There are three types of dens in dens, based on the classification published by Ohlers in 1957[100]:

**Type I** - the invagination of the enamel circumscribes the area of the dental crown.

**Type II** - the invagination of the enamel extends up to the middle third of the root, finishing in a blind pouch (Fig. 13.28 and 13.29).

**Type III** - the invagination of the enamel extends up to the apical region of the tooth, so that it may compose several apical foramens (Fig. 13.30 and 13.31).

Type I Dens in dens does not make endodontic treatment difficult, as the invagination is small and is situated in the dental crown. Type 2 causes a certain difficulty in endodontic treatment, as it becomes necessary to remove it from the enamel invagination inside the root canal. Type 3 is the one that may create major difficulty in performing endodontic treatment. It is never possible to save a tooth with this type of anomaly.

### Dens Evaginatus (Talon Cusp)

Other anomaly that may occur in the central as well as in the maxillary lateral incisor, is Dens Evaginatus or Talon Cusp.

This anomaly consists of the evagination of the area of the cingulum of these teeth, producing an extra cusp. The presence of the extra cusp on the maxillary incisors may cause esthetic problems, caries because of the difficulty with hygiene, occlusion trauma, and also traumatized irritation of the tongue when chewing. Despite Dens Invaginatus, the treatment of a tooth with Talon Cusp is very simple, as the removal of the evagination is a procedure similar to that performed in a normal tooth.

### Radicular Grooves

The maxillary lateral incisor may show an anomaly that is difficult to diagnose - the presence of radicular depression (radicular groove). This depression is normally present on the lingual face of the lateral Incisors, in the area of the cingulum and extends to the root, capable of occurring at different points in the radicular region. The presence of the radicular depression provides a pathway for the penetration of microorganisms, which may definitively lead to a periodontal problem. Early diagnosis of this anomaly is important because the patient must be instructed to perform oral hygiene in order to avoid the onset of periodontal pockets. The Figures 13.32 to 13.36 demonstrate radicular grooves in a maxillary lateral incisor, featuring an area of communication between the root canal and the external surface (periodontium)[32].

### Consumptive Premolar (Evaginated Odontoma)

This anomaly features the presence of a protuberance on the occlusal surface of the premolars. This protuberance may vary in shape (rising from the center of occlusal surface and close the central furrow), or may rise from the lingual rim of the buccal cusp. It consists of an external coat of enamel covering the dentin, which has a pulp horn of varying size. The second premolars are frequently the most affected teeth and the anomaly is usually bilateral[44].

### Taurodontia

The characteristic of taurodontia is the large volume of the pulp chamber, which may reach the radicular portion. One of the consequences of this alteration is the presence of short root canals.

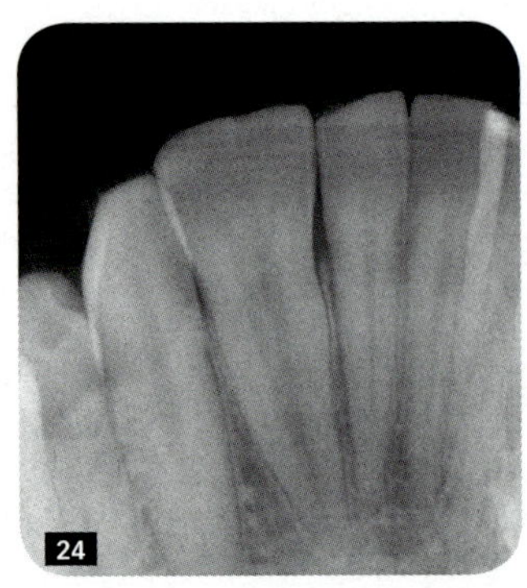


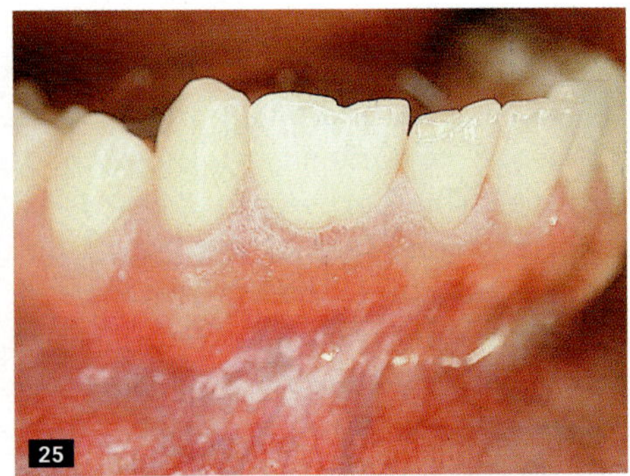


**Figures 13.24 and 13.25** - Germination.

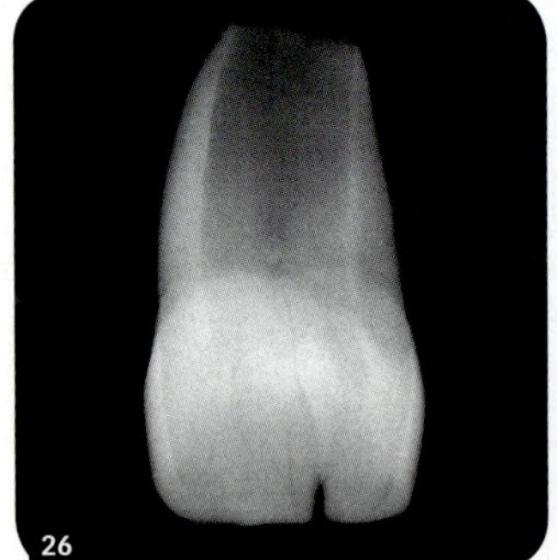


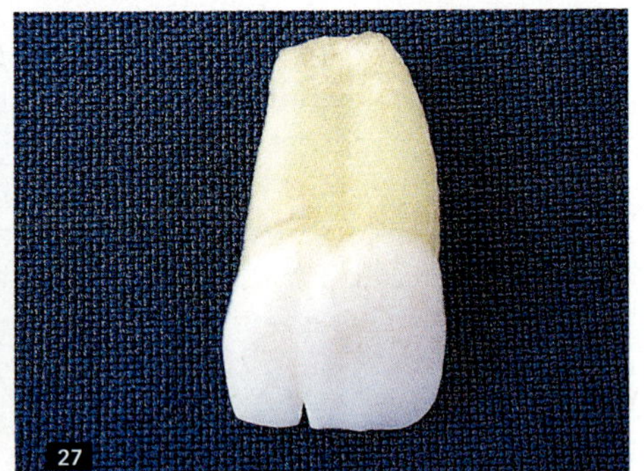


**Figures 13.26 and 13.27** - Germination.

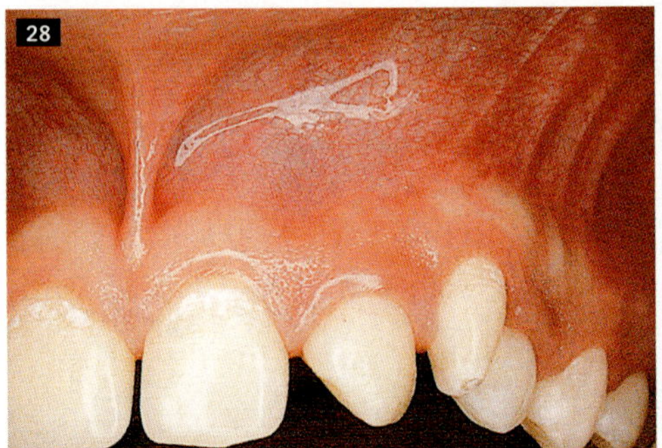


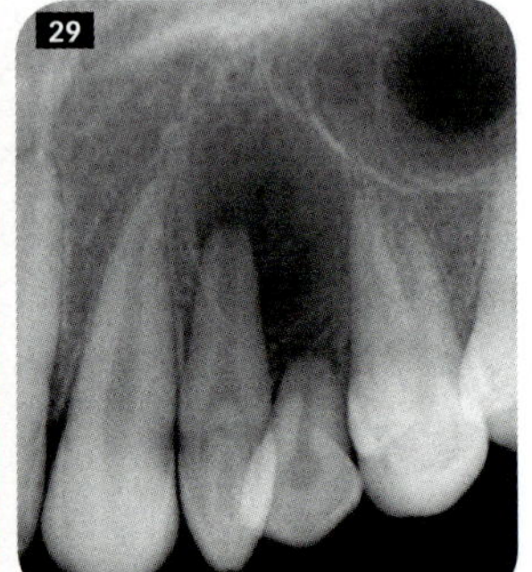


**Figures 13.28 and 13.29** - Dens invaginatus.

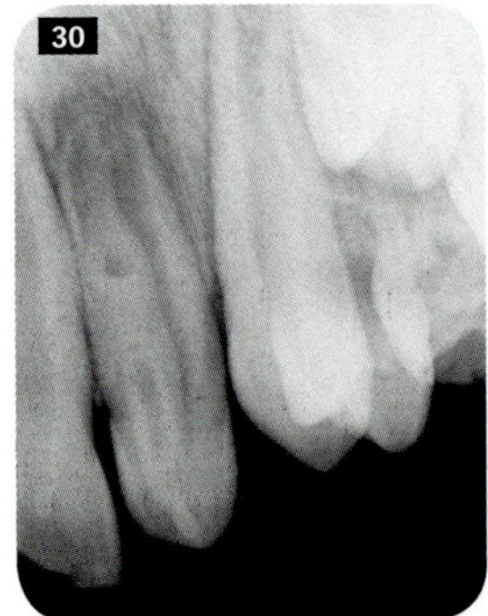


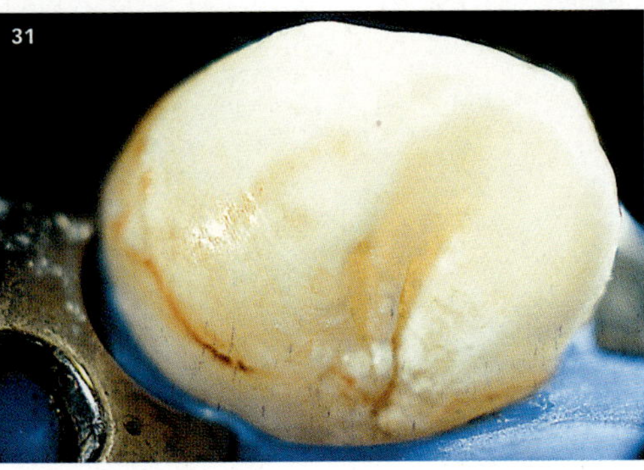


**Figures 13.30 and 13.31** - Dens invaginatus.

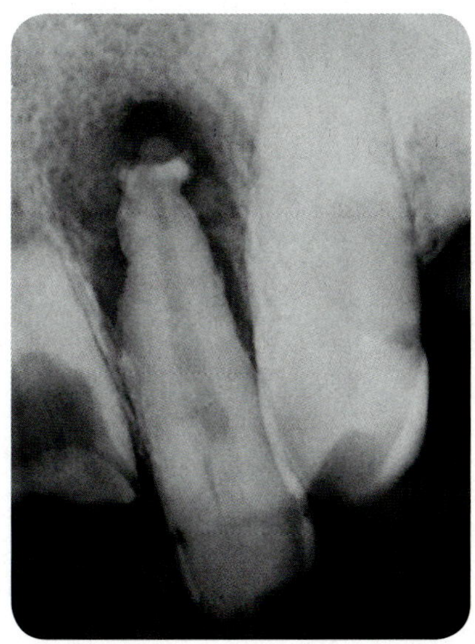

**Figure 13.32** - Radicular groove in maxillary lateral incisor.

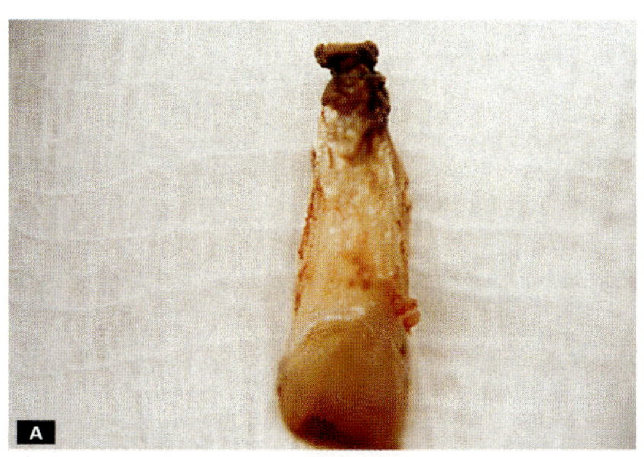

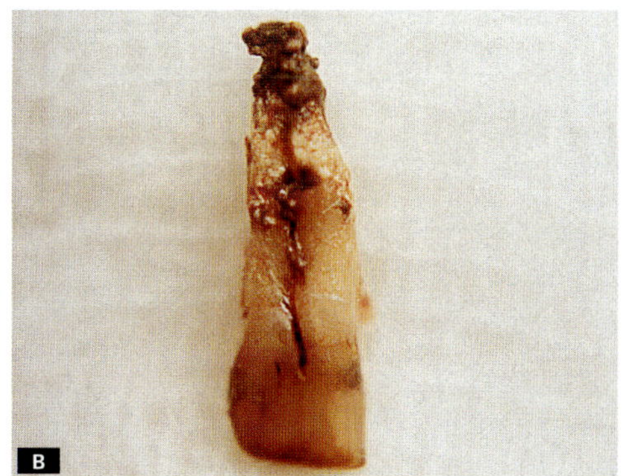

**Figure 13.33** - (**A-B**) Radicular Groove in maxillary lateral incisor.

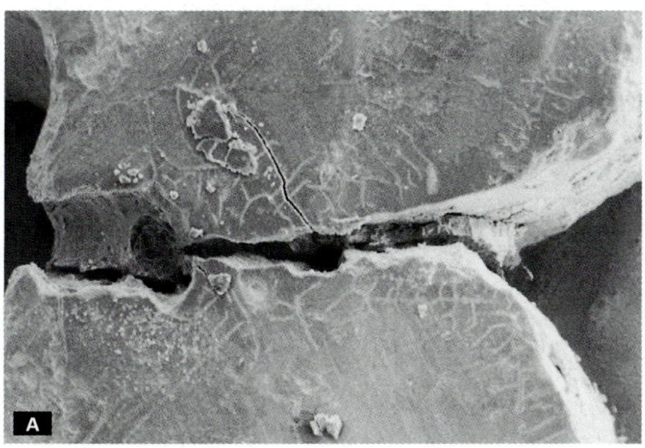

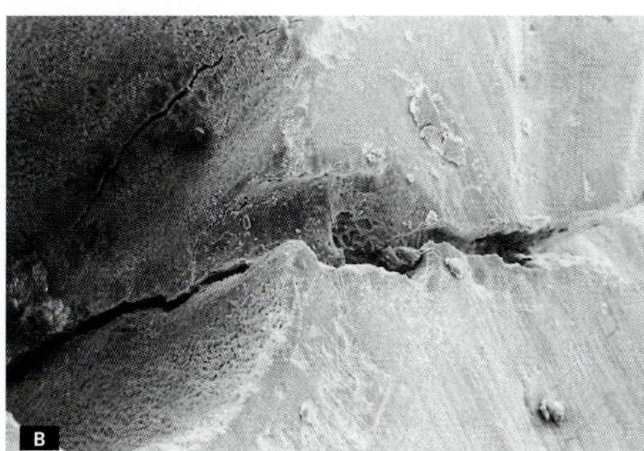

**Figure 13.34** - (**A-B**) Radicular Groove in maxillary lateral incisor.

## References and Further Reading


1. Album MM. Taurodontia in Deciduous First Molars. J Amer Dent Assoc 1958;56:562.
2. Allison ML, Wallace WR, Von Wyl H. Coronoid Abnormalities Causing Limitation of Mandibular Movement. Oral Surg Oral Med Oral Pathol 1969;27:229-33.
3. Amaral WJ, Jacobs DS. Aberrant Salivary Gland Defect in the Mandible: Report of a Case. Oral Surg Oral Med Oral Pathol 1961;14:748-52.
4. Aprile EC, Figun S. Anatomia odontológica. Bueno Aires: El Ateneo;1954.
5. Araújo NS, Araújo VC. Distúrbios de desenvolvimento. In: ______. Patologia Bucal. São Paulo: Artes Médicas 1984:11-37.
6. Benenati FW. Complex treatment of a maxillary lateral incisor with dens invaginatus and associated aberrant morphology. J Endod 1994;20:180-7.
7. Bergman G, Lysell L, Pindborg JJ. Unilateral Dental Malformation: Report of two cases. Oral Surg Oral Med Oral Pathol 1963;16:48-60.
8. Bolanos OR, Martell B, Morse DR. A unique approach to the treatment of a tooth with dens invaginatus. J Endod 1988;14:315-8.
9. Boyne P. Dens in dente: report of three cases. J Amer Dent Assoc 1952;45:208.
10. Bruce KW. Dental Anomaly: Early Exfoliatiom of Deciduous and Permanent Teeth. J Am Dent Ass 1954;48:414-21.
11. Burch RC, Hullen S. The relationship of the apical foramen to the anatomic apex of the tooth. Oral Surg Oral Med Oral Pathol 1972;34:262-8.
12. Burns RC, Buchanan SL. Tooth morphology and access openings. In: Pathways of the Pulp. Cohen S, Burns RC. 5th ed. St. Louis: Mosby;1991.
13. Caliskan MK, Pehlivan Y, Sepetçioglu F, Türkün M, Tuncer SS. Root Canal morphology of human permanent teeth in a Turkish population. J Endod 1995;21:200-4.
14. Callahan JR. Multiple apical foramina of tooth roots. J Nat A Ass 1916;3:85.
15. Carsen O. Root complex and root canal system: a correlation analysis using one-rooted mandibular second molars. Scand J Dent Res 1990;98:273-85.
16. Chen R, Yang J, Chao T. Invaginated tooth associated with periodontal abscess. Oral Surg Oral Med Oral Pathol 1990;69:659.
17. Chen RJ, Chen HS. Talon Cusp in primary dentition. Oral Surg Oral Med Oral Pathol 1986;62:67-72.
18. Christie WH, Peikoff MD, Acheson DW. Endodontic treatment of a maxillary lateral incisor with anomalous root formations. J Endod 1981;7:528-34.
19. Cooke HG, Cox FL. C-shaped canal configurations in mandibular molars. J Amer Dent Assoc 1979;99:836-40.
20. Costa WF, Sousa-Neto MD, Pécora JD. Upper molar dens in dente. Case report. Braz Dent J 1990;1:45-9.
21. Cunha ES. Diafanização de dentes pelo processo okumura-aprile. Rev Paul Cirurg Dent 1948;1:1-5.
22. Davis SR, Brayton SM, Goldman M. The morphology of the prepared root canal: a study utilizing injectable silicone. Oral Surg Oral Med Oral Pathol 1972;34:642-8.
23. De Deus QD. Frequency, location, and direction of the lateral, secondary, and accessory canals. J Endod 1975;1:361-6.
24. De Deus QD. Endodontia. 5th ed. Rio de Janeiro: Medsi;1992. 695p.
25. De Smith A, Demaut L. Nonsurgical endodontic treatment of invaginatus teeth. J Endod 1982;8:506-11.
26. De Grood ME, Cunningham CJ. Mandibular Molar with 5 Canals: Report of a Case. J Endod 1997;23:60-62.
27. Deveaux E. Maxillary second molar with two palatal roots. J Endod 1999;25:571-3.
28. Dummer PMM, Mc Ginn JH, Rees DG. The position and topography of the apical foramen. Int Endod J 1984;17:192-8.
29. Esberard RM, Consolaro A, Esberard RR. Considerações clínicas e morfológicas dos dens invaginatus. J Bras Endo Perio 2002;2:21-7.
30. Eskoz N, Weine FS. Canal configuration of the mesiobuccal root of the maxillary second molar. J Endod 1995;21:38-42.
31. Estrela C, Bueno MR, Leles CR, Azevedo B, Azevedo JR. Accuracy of cone beam computed tomography and panoramic and periapical radiography for detection of apical periodontitis. J Endod 2008;34:273-9.
32. Estrela C, Lopes HP, Pécora JD. Radicular grooves in maxillary lateral incisor: case report. Braz Dent J 1995;6:143-6.
33. Everett FG, Kramer GM. The dento-lingual groove in the maxillary lateral incisor. A periodontal hazard. J Periodontol 1972;42:352-61.
34. Fabra-Campos H. Failure of Endodontic Treatment due to a palatal Gingival Groove in a Maxillary Lateral Incisor with Talon Cusp and Two Root Canals. J Endod 1990;16:342-5.
35. Fabra-Campos H. Three canals in the mesial root of mandibular first permanent molars: a clinical study. Int Endod J 1989;22:39-43.
36. Fabra-Campos H. Unusual root anatomy of mandibular first molars. J Endod 1985;11:568-72.
37. Favieri RA, Rothier A, Fidel R. Estudo da anatomia interna dos molares inferiores, submetidos ao processo de injeção por resina plástica. Rev Bras Odontol 1986;43:42-5.
38. Ferguson F, Friedman S, Frazetto V. Sucessful Apexification technique in an immature tooth with dens in dente. Oral Surg Oral Med Oral Pathol 1980;49:356-9.
39. Ferraz JAB, Carvalho-Júnior JR, Saquy PC, Pécora JD, Sousa-Neto MD. Dental anomaly: dens evaginatus (Talon Cusp). Braz Dent J 2001;12:132-4.
40. Ferraz JAB, Pécora JD. Three-rooted mandibular molars in patients of mongolian, caucasian and negro origin. Braz Dent J 1992;3:113-7.
41. Ferreira CM, Moraes IG, Bernardineli N. Three rooted maxillary second premolar. J Endod 2000;26:105-6.
42. Fogel HM, Peikoff MD, Christie WH. Canal configuration in the mesiobuccal root of the maxillary first molar: a clinical study. J Endod 1994;20:135-40.
43. Gani O, Visvisian C. Apical canal diameter in the first upper molar at various ages. J Endod 1999;25:689-91.
44. Gibilisco JA. Diagnóstico radiográfico bucal de Stafne. Rio de Janeiro: Interamericana, 1986.p.17-24.
45. Goswami M, Chandra S, Chandra S, Singh S. Mandibular Premolar with Two Roots. J Endod 1997;23:187.
46. Green D. A stereo-binocular microscopic study of the root apices and surrounding areas of 100 man-

dibular molars. Oral Surg Oral Med Oral Pathol 1955;8:1298-1304.
47. Green D. A stereomicroscopic study of the root apices of 400 maxillary and mandibular anterior teeth. Oral Surg Oral Med Oral Pathol 1956;9:1224-32.
48. Green D. Double canals in single roots. Oral Surg Oral Med Oral Pathol 1973;35:689-96.
49. Green D. Morphology of the pulp cavity of the permanent teeth. Oral Surg Oral Med Oral Pathol 1955;7:743-59.
50. Green D. Stereomicroscopic study of 700 root apices of maxillary and mandibular posterior teeth. Oral Surg Oral Med Oral Pathol 1960;13:728-33.
51. Grossman LI. Endodontia Prática. 8th ed. Rio de Janeiro:Guanabara Koogan;1976.
52. Guerisoli DMZ, Souza RA, Sousa-Neto MD, Silva RG, Pécora JD. External and internal anatomy of third molars. Braz Dent J 1998;9:91-4.
53. Gutmann JL. Prevalence, location, and patency of accessory canals in the furcation region of permanent molars. J Periodontol 1978;49:21-6.
54. Haddad GY, Nehme WB, Ounsi HF. Diagnosis, classification, and frequency of C-shaped canals in mandibular second molars in the labanese population. J Endod 1999;25, 268-71.
55. Hasselgreen G, Tronstad L. The use of transparent teeth in the teaching of preclinical endodontics. J Endod 1975;8:25-34.
56. Hayashi Y. Endodontic treatment in taurodontism. J Endod 1994;20:357-8.
57. Hess W, Zurcher E. The anatomy of the root canals of the teeth of the permanent dentition. 1st ed. New York: Williams Wood Co;1925. 200 p.
58. Hess W. Formation of root canals in human teeth. J Am Dent Ass 1921;3:704-90.
59. Hess W. Zur anatomie der wurzelkanale des menschlichen gebisses mit berucksichtigung der feinern verzweigungen am foramen apicale, schweiz. Vierteljahrsschr. F Zahnheilk 1917;27:256-60.
60. Hession RW. Endodontic morphology. I. An alternative method of study. Oral Surg Oral Med Oral Pathol 1977;44:456-62.
61. Hession RW. Endodontic morphology. III. Canal preparation. Oral Surg Oral Med Oral Pathol 1977;44:775-85.
62. Hetem C, Madeira MC, Bernabé JM. Contribuição ao estudo dos caninos inferiores birradiculados. Rev Fac Odontol Araçatuba 1965;1:83-92.
63. Hill FJ, Bellis WJ. Dens Invaginatus and its management. British Dental J 1984;156:400-2.
64. Holtzman L. Endodontic treatment of maxillary canine with dens invaginatus and immature root. Oral Surg Oral Med Oral Pathol 1996;82:452-5.
65. Hovland EJ, Block RM. Nonrecognition and subsequent endodontic treatment of dens invaginatus. J Endod 1977;13:546-9.
66. Hülsmann M. A Maxillary First Molar with Two Distobuccal Root Canals. J Endod 1997;23:707-8.
67. Ida RD, Gutmann JL. Importance of anatomic variables in endodontic treatment outcomes: case report. Endod Dent Traumatol 1995;11:199-203.
68. Ingle IJ, Taintor JI. Endodontics. 3rd ed. Philadelphia: Lea & Febiger;1985. 881 p.
69. Jacobsen EL, Dick K, Bodell R. Mandibular first molars with multiple mesial canals. J Endod 1994;20:610-3.
70. Kerekes K, Tronstad L. Morphometric observations on root canals of human anterior teeth. J Endod 1977;3:24-9.
71. Kerekes K, Tronstad L. Morphometric observations on root canals of human molars. J Endod 1977;3:114-9.
72. Kim E, Jou YT. A supernumerary tooth fused to the facial surface of a maxillary permanent central incisor: case report. J Endod 2000;26:45-8.
73. Kojima K, Inamoto K, Nagamatsu K, Hara A, Nakata K, Morita I, Nakagaki H, Nakamura H. Success rate of endodontic treatment of teeth with vital and nonvital pulps. A meta-analysis. Oral Surg Oral Med Oral Pathol Oral Radiol Endod 2004;97:95-9.
74. Korzen BH, Pulver WH. Endodontic access cavities - the first step to success. Ontario Dentist 1978;55:19-22.
75. Krasner P, Rankow HJ. Anatomy of pulp chamber floor. J Endod 2004;30:5-16.
76. Kulild JC, Weller RN. Treatment considerations in Dens Invaginatus. J Endod 1989;15:381-4.
77. Kuttler Y. Microscopic investigation of root apexes. J Amer Dent Assoc 1955;50:544-52.
78. Lara VS, Consolaro A, Bruce RS. Macroscopic and Microscopic Analyses of the Palato-Gingival Groove. J Endod 2000;26:345-50.
79. LaTurno SAL, Zillich RM. Straight-line endodontic access to anterior teeth. Oral Surg Oral Med Oral Pathol 1985;59:418-9.
80. Lavagnoli G. La cavità d'accesso. Dental Cadmos 1984;52:17-22.
81. Leite APP, Silva RG, Cruz-Filho AM, Pécora JD. In vitro study of cervical enamel projection in human molars. Braz Dent J 1995;6:25-8.
82. Libfeld H, Rotstein I. Incidence of four-rooted Maxillary Second Molars: Literature Review and Radiographic Survey of 1,200 teeth. J Endod 1989;15:129-131.
83. Lonçali G, Hazar S, Altinbulak H. Talon Cusp: Report of five cases. Quintessence Int 1994;25:431-3.
84. Lowman JV, Burke RS, Pelleu GB. Patent accessory canals: incidence in molar furcation region. Oral Surg Oral Med Oral Pathol 1973;36:580-4.
85. Macri E, Zmener O. Five Canals in a Mandibular Second Premolar. J Endod 2000;26:304-5.
86. Madeira MC, Hetem S, Tagliavani O, Matheus MTG, Bernabé JM, Marchi F. Canal radicular bifurcado em dente canino inferior: ocorrência e significância clínica. Rev Fac Odontol Araçatuba 1973;2:27-30.
87. Madeira MC, Hetem S. Incidence of bifurcation in mandibular incisor. Oral Surg Oral Med Oral Pathol 1973;36:589-91.
88. Madeira MC. Anatomia da Face. 1st ed. São Paulo: Sarvier;1995. 174p.
89. Madeira MC. Raízes bifurcadas em incisivos superiores. Rev Fac Odont Araçatuba 1973;2:249-50.
90. Mader CL, Kellog SL. Primary Talon Cusp. J Dent Child 1985;52:223-6.
91. Mader CL. Talon Cusp. J Am Dent Ass 1981;103:244-6.
92. Malagnino V, Gallottini G, Passariello P. Some unusual clinical cases on root anatomy of permanent maxillary molars. J Endod 1997;23:127-8.
93. Mangani F, Ruddle CJ. Endodontic treatment of a "very particular" maxillary central incisor. J Endod 1994;20:560-4.

94. Matzer JAC. Anatomia interna e externa dos dentes de indígenas descendentes de maias da República da Guatemala. (Master's Thesis). Ribeirão Preto: University of São Paulo;1993. 178p.
95. Miyashita M, Kasahara E, Yasuda E, Yamamoto A, Sekizawa T. Root canal system of the mandibular incisor. J Endod 1997;23:479-84.
96. Moreinis AS. Avoiding perforation during endodontic access. J Amer Dent Assoc 1979;98:707-12.
97. Morfis A, Lentzari A. Dens Invaginatus with an open apex: a case report. Int Endod J 1989;22:190-2.
98. Nik-Hussein N. Dens invaginatus: complications and treatment of nonvital infected tooth. J Clin Pediatr Dent 1994;18:303-6.
99. Nunes E, Moraes IG, Novaes PMO, Sousa SMG. Bilateral fusion of mandibular second molars with supernumerary teeth: case report. Braz Dent J 2002;13:137-41.
100. Ohlers FAC. Dens Invaginatus (dilated composite odontoma). I - Variations of the invaginatus process and associated anterior crown form. Oral Surg Oral Med Oral Pathol 1957;10:1204-8.
101. Ohlers FAC. Dens Invaginatus (dilated composite odontoma). II - Associated posterior crown forms and pathogenesis. Oral Surg Oral Med Oral Pathol 1957;10:1302.
102. Okumura T. Anatomy of the root canals. J Amer Dent Assoc 1927;14:632-6.
103. Pécora JD, Conrado C, Zucolotto W, Souza N, Saquy PC. Root canal therapy of an anomalous Maxillary central incisor. Endod Dent Traumatol 1993;9:260-2.
104. Pécora JD, Cruz-Filho AM. Study of the incidence of radicular grooves in maxillary incisor. Braz Dent J 1992;3:11-6.
105. Pécora JD, Macchetti DD, Costa WF. Caso clínico Dens in Dente. Rev Odontol USP 1987;1:46-9.
106. Pécora JD, Santana SVS. Maxillary lateral incisors with two roots. Case report. Braz Dent J 1991;2:151-153.
107. Pécora JD, Saquy PC, Sousa-Neto MD, Cruz-Filho AM. Morfologia dos dentes humanos anteriores superiores - dimensões, direções das raízes e sistema de canais radiculares. Rev Inst Cienc Saúde 1991;9:5-8.
108. Pécora JD, Saquy PC, Sousa-Neto MD, Woefel JB. Root form and canal anatomy of maxillary first premolars. Braz Dent J 1991;2:87-94.
109. Pécora JD, Saquy PC, Sousa-Neto MD. Endodontic treatment of a maxillary lateral incisor presenting Dens Invaginatus and transposition to the region of the canine. A case report. Braz Dent J 1991;2:5-8.
110. Pécora JD, Savioli RN, Costa WF, Cruz-Filho AM, Fidel RS. Estudo da anatomia e do comprimento dos pré-molares inferiores humanos. Rev Bras Odontol 1991;48:31-6.
111. Pécora JD, Savioli RN, Murgel CAF. Estudo da incidência de dois canais nos incisivos inferiores humanos. Rev Bras Odontol 1990;47:44-7.
112. Pécora JD, Savioli RN, Vansan R, Silva RG, Costa WE. Novo método de diafanizar dentes. Rev Fac Odontol Ribeirão Preto 1986;23:1-5.
113. Pécora JD, Silva RS, Sousa-Neto MD. Apresentação de uma técnica simplificada de diafanização de dentes e sua inclusão em blocos transparentes. Odonto 1993;2:384-5.
114. Pécora JD, Sousa-Neto MD, Costa WF. Dens invaginatus in a maxillary canine: an anatomic, macroscopic and radiographic study. Aust Endod Newsletter 1992;18:12-3.
115. Pécora JD, Sousa-Neto MD, Santos TC, Saquy PC. In vitro study of the incidence of radicular grooves in maxillary incisors. Braz Dent J 1991;2:69-73.
116. Pécora JD, Sousa-Neto MD, Saquy PC, Leite APP. Endodontic treatment of a maxillary lateral incisors with a Talon cusp: a case report. Braz Dent J 1993;4:127-30.
117. Pécora JD, Sousa-Neto MD, Saquy PC, Woefel JB. In vitro study of root canal anatomy of maxillary second premolars. Braz Dent J 1992;3:81-5.
118. Pécora JD, Sousa-Neto MD, Saquy PC. Internal anatomy, direction and number of roots and size of human mandibular canines. Braz Dent J 1993;4:53-7.
119. Pécora JD, Vansan LP, Silva RG, Aiello JSS. Dens Invaginatus: Tratamento endodôntico em uma sessão. Rev Assoc Paul Cirurg Dent 1990;44:20-21.
120. Pécora JD, Vansan LP, Sousa-Neto MD, Saquy PC. Tratamento endodôntico de um dens evaginatus. Rev Ass Paul Cirurg Dent 1991;45:535-6.
121. Pécora JD, Woefel JB, Sousa-Neto MD, Issa EP. Morphology study of the maxillary molars. Part II: Internal anatomy. Braz Dent J 1992;3:53-7.
122. Pécora JD, Woelfel JB, Sousa-Neto MD. Morphologic study of the maxillary molars part I: external anatomy. Braz Dent J 1991;2:45-50.
123. Pereira AJA, Fidel RAS, Fidel SR. Maxillary lateral incisor with two root canals: fusion, germination or dens invaginatus? Braz Dent J 2000;11:141-6.
124. Peyrano A, Zmener O. Endodontic management of mandibular lateral incisor fused with supernumerary tooth. Endod Dent Traumatol 1995;11:196-8.
125. Philippas GG. Influence of occlusal wear and age on formation of dentin and size of pulp chamber. J Dent Research 1961;40:1186-98.
126. Picosse M. Anatomia Dental. 3. ed. São Paulo: Sarvier;1979. 57p.
127. Pineda F, Kuttler Y. Mesiodistal and buccolingual roentgenographic investigation of 7,275 root canals. Oral Surg Oral Med Oral Pathol 1972;33:101-10.
128. Pineda F. Roentgenographic investigation of the mesiobuccal root of the maxillary first molar. Oral Surg Oral Med Oral Pathol 1973;36:253-60.
129. Pinheiro-Júnior EC, Leite APP, Silva RG, Pécora JD. Relação entre sulcos radiculares e número de canais em pré-molares inferiores. Estudo in vitro. Rev Ass Bras Odontol Nac 1994;2:265-9.
130. Pomeranz HH, Eidelman DL, Goldberg MG. Treatment considerations of the middle mesial canal of mandibular first and second molars. J Endod 1981;7:565-8.
131. Pomeranz HH, Fishelberg G. The secondary mesiobuccal canal of maxillary molars. J Am Dent Ass 1974;88:119-24.
132. Ponce EH, Fernández JAV. The cemento-dentino-canal junction, the apical foramen, and the apical constriction: evaluation by optical microscopy. J Endod 2003;29:214-9.
133. Pucci EM, Reig R. Conductos radiculares. Anatomia, patologia y terapia. Montevideo: A. Barreiro y Ramos;1945.

134. Ricucci D, Pascon EA, Langeland K. Long-term follow-up on C-shaped mandibular molars. J Endod 1996;22:185-7.
135. Ricucci D. Apical limit of root canal instrumentation and obturation, part 1. Literature review. Int Endod J 1998;31:384-93.
136. Robertson D, Leeb J. The evaluation of a transparent tooth model system for the evaluation of endodontically filled teeth. J Endod 1982;8:317-20.
137. Rocha LFC, Sousa-Neto MD, Fidel SR, Costa WF, Pécora JD. External and internal anatomy of mandibular molars. Braz Dent J 1996;7:33-40.
138. Rotstein I, Stabholz A, Heling I, Friedman S. Clinical considerations in the treatment of dens invaginatus. Endod Dent Traumatol 1987;3:249-54.
139. Rushton MA. A New Form of Dentinal Displasia: Shell Teeth. Oral Surg Oral Med Oral Pathol 1954;7:543-9.
140. Sabala CL, Benenati FW, Neas BR. Bilateral root or root canal aberrations in a dental school patient population. J Endod 1994;20:38-42.
141. Santa-Cecília M, Lara VS, Moraes IG. The palatogingival groove. A cause of failure in root canal treatment. Oral Surg Oral Med Oral Pathol 1998;85:94-8.
142. Schulze C, Brand E. Über Den Dens Invaginatus. Zahnarztl Welt/Reform 1972;81:653-60.
143. Seidberg BH, Altman M, Guttuso J, Suson M. Frequency of two mesiobuccal root canals in maxillary permanent first molars. J Amer Dent Assoc 1973;87:852-6.
144. Seltzer S. Endodontology: biologic considerations in endodontic procedures. 2nd ed. Philadelphia, Lea & Febiger, 1988.
145. Sempira HN, Hartwell GR. Frequency of Second Mesiobuccal Canals in Maxillary Molars as Determined by Use of an Operating Microscope: A Clinical Study. J Endod 2000;26:673-4.
146. Serota KS, Watson ID, Lenkinski L. Endodontic access cavities. Oral Health 1985;75:45-9.
147. Shifman A, Tamir A. Dens Invaginatus with concrescent supernumerary tooth. Oral Surg Oral Med Oral Pathol 1979;47:391.
148. Shuler SE, Howell BT, Green DB. Unusual pattern of pulp canal obliteration following luxation injury. J Endod 1994;20:460-2.
149. Sidow SJ, West LA, Liewehr FR, Loushine RJ. Root Canal Morphology of Human Maxillary and Mandibular Third Molars. J Endod 2000;26:675-8.
150. Silva RG, Sousa-Neto MD, Carvalho-Júnior JR, Saquy PC, Pécora JD. Periapical cemental dysplasia: case report. Braz Dent J 1999;10:55-7.
151. Simon JHS, Dogan H, Ceresa LM, Silver GK. The Radicular Groove: Its Potential Clinical Significance. J Endod 2000;26:295-8.
152. Simon JHS, Glick DH, Frank AL. Predictable endodontic and periodontic failures as a result of radicular anomalies. Oral Surg Oral Med Oral Pathol 1971;31:823-6.
153. Siqueira EL, Silva YTC, Leite AMP, Pécora JD. Incidência de incisivos laterais coniformes. Rev Odonto 1994;2:416-8.
154. Skidmore AE, Bjorndal AM. Root canal morphology of the human mandibular first molar. Oral Surg Oral Med Oral Pathol 1971;32:778-84.
155. Sousa-Neto MD, Zuccolotto WG, Saquy PC, Grandini SA, Pécora JD. Treatment of dens invaginatus in a maxillary canine: case report. Braz Dent J 1991;2:147-50.
156. Stafne EC, Szabo SE. The Significance of Pulp Nodules. Dent Cosmos 1933;75:160-4.
157. Stambaugh RV, Wittrock JW. The relationship of the pulp chamber to the external surface of the tooth. J Prosthet Dent 1977;37:537-46.
158. Stropko JJ. Canal morphology of an maxillary molars: clinical observations of canal configurations. J Endod 1999;25:446-50.
159. Tamse A, Katz A, Pilo R. Furcation Groove of a Buccal Root of a Maxillary First Premolars - A Morphometric Study. J Endod 2000;26:359-63.
160. Tidmarsh BG. Micromorphology of pulp chambers in human molar teeth. Int Endod J 1980;13:69-75.
161. Trope M, Elfenbein L, Tronstad L. Mandibular premolars with more than one root canal in different race groups. J Endod 1986;11:343-5.
162. Vertucci FJ, Williams RG. Furcation canals in the human mandibular first molar. Oral Surg Oral Med Oral Pathol 1974;38:308-14.
163. Vertucci FJ. Root canal anatomy of the human permanent teeth. Oral Surg Oral Med Oral Pathol 1984;58:589-99.
164. Vertucci FJ. Root canal morphology and its relationship to endodontic procedures. Endod Topics 2005;10:3-29.
165. Vertucci FJ. Root canal morphology of mandibular pre-molars. J Am Dent Ass 1978;97:47.
166. Vincent-Townrend J. Dens Invaginatus. J Dent 1974;2:234-8.
167. Walvekar SV, Behbehani JM. Three Root Canals and Dens Formation in a Maxillary Lateral Incisor: A Case Report. J Endod 1997;23:185-6.
168. Weine FS, Healey HJ, Gerstein H, Evasnton L. Canal configuration in the mesiobuccal root of the maxillary first molars and its endodontic significance. Oral Surg Oral Med Oral Pathol 1969;28:419-25.
169. Weine FS, Pasiewicz RA, Rice RT. Canal configuration of the mandibular second molar using a clinically oriented in vitro method. J Endod 1988;14:207-13.
170. Weine FS. Case report: three canals in the mesial root of mandibular first molar. J Endod 1982;18:517-20.
171. Weine FS. O enigma do canal lateral. Clin Odontol Amer Norte 1987:209-228.
172. Weine FS. The C-shaped mandibular second molar: incidence and others considerations. J Endod 1998;24:372.
173. Weller RN, Niemczyk SP, Kim S. Incidence and position of the canal isthmus. Part I. Mesiobuccal root of the maxillary first molar. J Endod 1995;21:380-3.
174. Witkop-Júnior CJ. Manifestations of Genetic Diseases in the Human Pulp. Oral Surg Oral Med Oral Pathol 1971;32:278-316.
175. Wong M. Four root canals in a mandibular second premolar. J Endod 1991;17:125-6.
176. Wong M. Maxillary first molar with three palatal canals. J Endod 1991;17:298-9.
177. Yesilsoy C, Gordon W, Porras O, Hoch B. Observation of Depth and Incidence of the Mesial Groove Between the Mesiobuccal and Mesiolingual Orifices in Mandibular Molars. J Endod 2002;28:507-9.

# Challenges of Root Canal Preparation

**J. D. Pécora**
*University of São Paulo, Ribeirão Preto, SP, Brazil*

**C. Estrela**
*Federal University of Goiás, Goiânia, GO, Brazil*

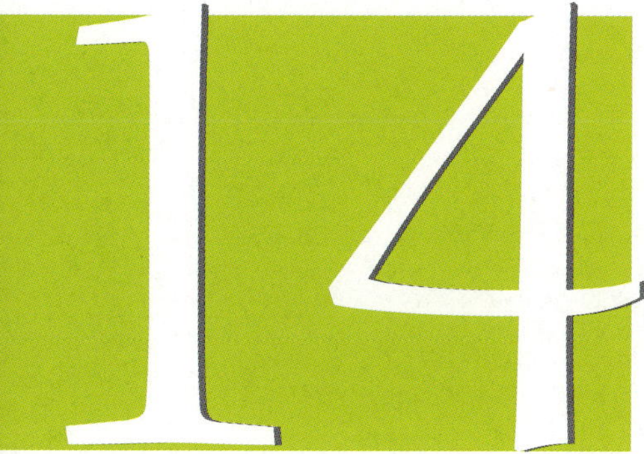

Chapter contents

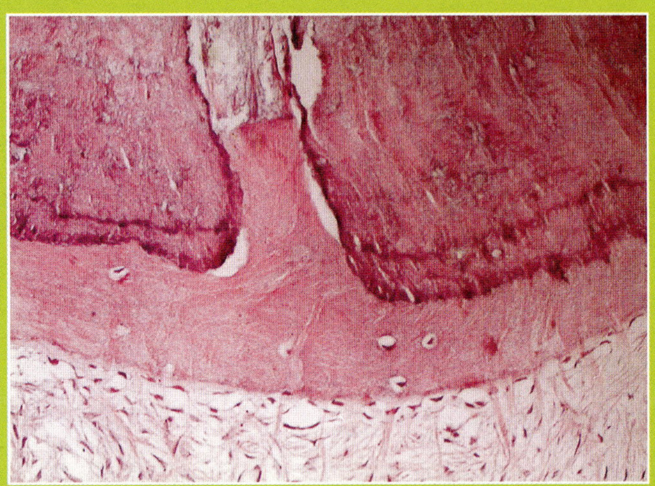

Sealer Plus without patency. Note total closure of the main root canal and an organized periodontal tissue (H&E., original magnification X100) (Courtesy Prof. Dr. Roberto Holland[20]).

## 14.1 Introduction

During endodontic treatment, several challenges may be encountered, such as a good understanding of internal morphology, victory over endodontic microbiota, and the immunological response. These aspects are associated with the professional's ability and scientific knowledge (Fig. 14.1). Specifically during the curved root canal preparation, some factors require greater attention. In this book, the subject of root canal preparation has been divided into several segments, so that each topic can be discussed at length.

For adequate root canal sanitization, sufficient knowledge of internal morphology is essential. The anatomical structure of the pulp cavity is considered very complex. Determination of the macro configuration of the pulp cavity requires specific attention. Drawings, photographs, decalcification, moldings, serial cortex, scanning analysis, once again, can be illusory, because they provide a close up and projected idea of the internal micromorphology. One of the greatest challenges is overcome the internal shapes located in different dental groups, which should never be underestimated. Many anatomical variations can be found, such as: dental ramifications, developmental anomalies, C shaped canals, dilacerated root canals (gradual and abrupt curvatures), isthmus areas, calcifications, resorptions, flattened root canals, etc.

Therefore, special attention should be paid at all times, given the limitations of internal morphology analysis. The first phase of structuring endodontic treatment is the accurate planning, in which a systematic exam of patient and tooth is required. Considering the root canal preparation phase, some aspects will be discussed in the order of their importance, but it is not within the scope of this chapter to finish the discussion on the challenges of root canal preparation. Knowledge of root canal curvature, determination of anatomical diameter and the influence of apical sanitization on the healing process are major factors in the present discussion about root canal preparation (Fig. 14.2).

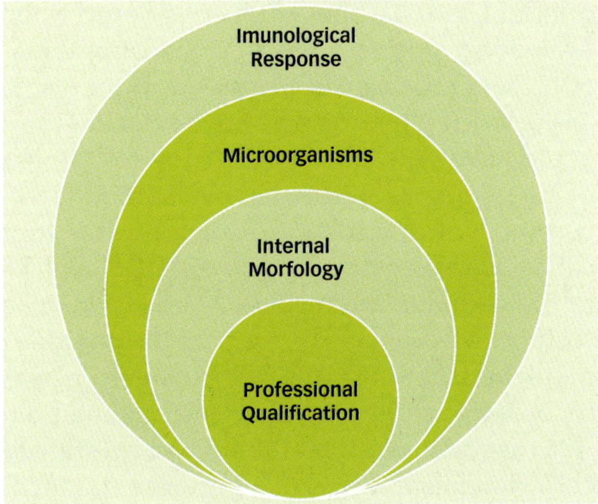


**Figure 14.1** - The challenges of endodontic treatment: understanding internal morphology, achieving victory over endodontic microbiota, understanding and obtainment of acceptable immunological responses, in conjunction with the professionalís ability and scientific knowledge.

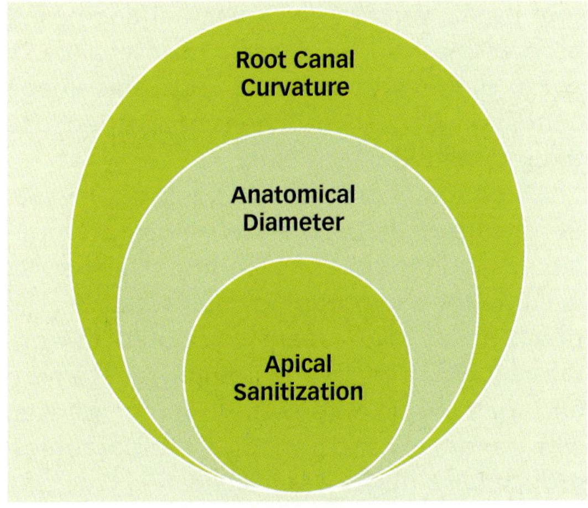


**Figure 14.2** - Root canal preparation challenges: understanding root canal curvature, determination of anatomical diameter and development of apical sanitization.

## 14.2 Root Canal Curvature

Standard root canal treatment is based on the processes of emptying, widening, sanitizing and filling the root canal. The eradication of healthy, inflamed or infected pulp tissue favors the root canal shape, and the sanitization process, allowing better action of the intracanal medications and free space for root canal filling.

Schilder[38] emphasized the need for a root canal to present a flared shape from the apical to coronal level, maintaining the apical foramen and not altering the original canal curvature. Many different techniques have been proposed to prepare the root canal system easily and more effectively[8,10-13,23,25-27,29,32,33,36,39], such as those using nickel-titanium instruments.

However, transportation of the apical foramen, creation of ledges, elbows, zips, perforations, fracture of instruments, as well as loss of working length can occur during curved root canal preparation[10,25-27,29,32,33].

Careful analysis of the anatomical complexity is prudent, and accurate endodontic treatment planning is an essential step in reducing the high failure rate.

Furthermore, periapical radiography is an indispensable alternative aid to endodontic diagnosis. All endodontic planning is associated with identifying the different aspects observed in the radiographic images, including anatomical complexity, the presence of material in the root canal, dental developmental anomalies, progression, regression and maintenance of apical periodontitis. The radiographic image corresponds to a two-dimensional aspect of a three-dimensional structure.

Depending on the morphological variations, surrounding bone density, x-ray angulations and radiographic contrast, failure can occur in the radiographic interpretation. The precision of cone beam computed tomography (CBCT) images to identify anatomical and pathologic alterations, in comparison with panoramic and periapical radiographies, reduce false-negative results[13].

Different anatomical configurations of root canals can lead to disastrous consequences during root canal preparation, such as dilacerated curves, which require careful choice of the endodontic instrument and technique. Several studies have determined the curvature of root canals by the angle and the radius methods, using periapical radiographic images[10,11,13,22,27,29,32,36].

Schneider[39] proposed a method to determine curvature based on angle, which is obtained by two straight lines, one parallel to the axis of the root canal, and the second being the line passes through the apical foramen up to its intersection with the first line, where the curvature starts to occur. The angle formed ($\alpha$) was named as the degree of root canal curvature (degrees of curvature: straight = 5° or less; moderate = 10-20 °; severe = 25-70°). Dobó-Nagy et al.[12] described root canal curvatures mathematically, and suggested a standard model, with help of differentiation geometrical pattern analysis, and computer graphics. Measured points of the same radiographs were approximated, using fourth degree polynomial functions, describing the imaginary axis of canals. This type of root canal classification is suitable for standardizing test specimens, including natural human teeth used for testing root forms: I (straight), J (apical curve), C (entirely curved), or S (multicurved). Pruett et al.[32] reported that the effect of the radius of curvature as an independent variable should be considered when evaluating studies of root canal instrumentation. Two root canals measured at the same angle in degrees by the Schneider method could have very different radii, or abruptness of curvatures. Lopes et al.[25] evaluated the occurrence of apical transportation after root canal instrumentation, using only K-Flexofiles or K-Flexofiles intercalated with K-Flexofile Golden Mediums. The degree (Schneider's method) and the radius of the curvature, was recorded before and after instrumentation. The results showed that there was no statistically significant difference between the techniques. The correlation between the degree and the radius of curvature of the root canal was not consistent, nor was there any relationship between the original radius of curvature and the apical transportation. Nevertheless, determination of curvature by use of its radius has proved to be an effective method. Sonntag et al.[40] presented a new method based on numerical calculus, to provide data on any type of root canal curvature, at any point of the long axis of the canal. Twenty severely curved, simulated root canals were prepared with rotary FlexMaster and Profile instruments in the crown-down technique, and manually in the step-back technique. The inner and outer curvatures were recorded in a system of coordinates before and after preparation, in increments of 0.5 mm. Using an equalizing function, the curvatures were first represented in graphic and algebraic form. The maximum and the mean curvature, as well as the length of the arc from the apical foramen to the point of maximum curvature were determined mathematically. An increase in maximum curvature was recorded for all four shaping systems investigated. The radius of the inner curvature decreased by 0.5–1.2 mm in the manual systems, as a result of the preparation. The Profile system displayed the smallest changes in radius (-0.9 mm), even with the outer curvature, and manual preparation with stainless steel files, showed the most pronounced change (-1.8 mm). The point of maximum curvature at the inner curvature was displaced by 1.6 mm to the apical foramen, through manual preparation with nickel-titanium instruments. At the outer curvature, the maximum displacement (1.8 mm) recorded was also the result of preparation with nickel-titanium instruments, while a displacement of only 0.3 mm to the apical foramen was recorded with the other systems. The method offers a means of determining curvatures precisely, without random specification of reference points. The method is also capable of registering only minor changes in curvature in the two-dimensional long axis of the canal.

Estrela et al.[14] suggested a method to determine the curvature radius of a curved root canal. This method uses two 6mm semi-straight lines superimposed on the root canal, the primary (red) line being the one to represent the longer continuity of the apical region, and the secondary (blue) line representing the middle and cervical thirds. Irrespective of the length of the secondary line, only the 6mm closest to the primary line are used to measure. The midpoint of each semi-straight line is recorded, and from there, two lines perpendicular to the semi- straight lines are made, until they meet at a central point. This point is called the circumcenter. The distance between the circumcenter and the center of each semi-straight line is the radius of the circumference[8] which determines the magnitude of the curve (Fig. 14.3A-C). These semi-straight lines can present a smaller measure. In images of high resolution quality, the measurement of radicular curvature radius can be obtained through circumcenter. Based on three mathematical points using the the software work tool named Planimp®, the curvature radius in both the for apical, and coronal both directions can be calculated. This method aided by CBCT images can favor the planning and curved root canal preparation. The values of the radicular curvature radius, considering the two 6 mm semi-straight lines, which can present a smaller measurement, were classified as: small radius $r \leq 4$ mm; severe curve, intermediary radius $r > 4$ and $< 8$ mm – moderate curve; major radius $r > 8$ mm – gentle curve.

The methodology suggested[14] for obtaining the radicular curvature radius is easy, reproducible and efficient, particularly when using CBCT images. The knowledge of the radicular curvature radius allows better planning of instrumentation, with a lower impact on the anatomical difficulties, and the limit of endodontic instruments. It is capable of maintaining the curves associated with the continuously tapered shape, and the instrument without undergoing structural deformations. Thus, a single aspect can reduce disastrous consequences such as loss of working length, transportation of the apical foramen, creation of ledges, elbows, zips, perforations, fracture of instruments.

In root canal curvature classifications, several root forms can be observed, such as: apical curve, gradual curve, sickle-shape curve, severe-moderate-straight curve, bayonet curve, dilacerated curve[26,39]. One hardly ever observes a standard sample of root canal morphology with a precise visual appearance. By the method suggested[14] for determining the curvature radius, it is possible to analyze a specific length of root canal, and not necessarily the total length of the root canal. This is important, because in the same root canal more than one curve can be found (such as in coronal and/or apical portion), which will not allow the radius throughout the entire root length to be correctly calculated.

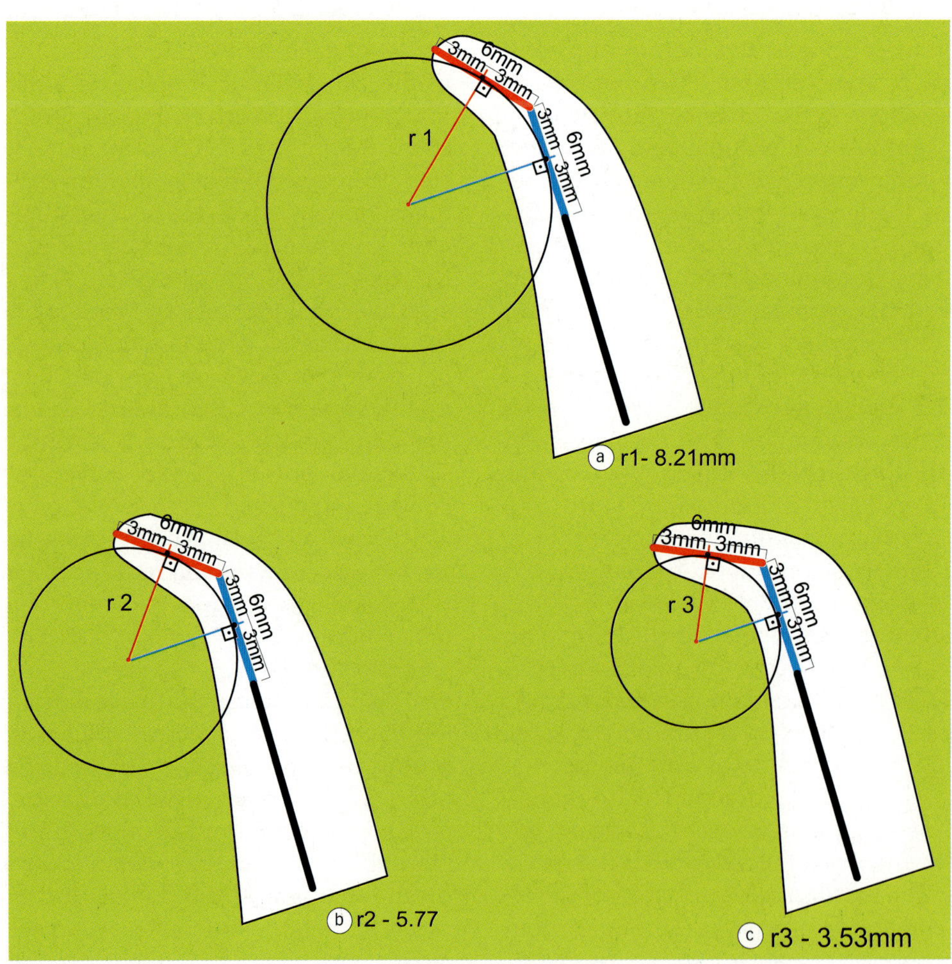


**Figure 14.3** - (**A-C**) The root curvature radius based on 3 mathematical points can be determined in both apical and coronal directions. Curvature radius considering the two 6-mm semistraight lines are classified as small radius (r≤4 mm): severe curvature; intermediary radius (r>4 and r≤8 mm): moderate curvature; and large radius (r>8 mm): mild curvature (From Estrela et al.[14]).

This aspect is in agreement with Lopes et al.[25] who reported that in a curved canal with the same radius, it is possible for there to be arcs (curved segments) with different lengths (angles with different degrees). These differences may influence the intensity of the tensile and compressive stresses induced in the helical shaft of an endodontic instrument, therefore altering its resistance to cyclic fatigue. Cunningham & Senia[11] studied the degree and configuration of canal curvature present in the mesial roots of 100 mandibular first and second molars. The teeth were radiographed in buccolingual (clinical) and mesiodistal (proximal) directions with #8 K files in place. One hundred percent of the specimens demonstrated curvature in both views. It was found that there was no correlation in degree of curvature between the clinical and proximal views. Secondary curvature, in a direction opposite to that of the principle curve was seen more frequently in the proximal view. In the proximal view, canals exhibited greater mean curvature than in the clinical view 38% of the time.

The values of radicular curvature radius[14], considering the two 6 mm semi-straight lines, was classified as follows: small radius $r \leq 4$ mm – severe curve; intermediary radius $r > 4$ and $< 8$ mm – moderate curve; major radius $r > 8$ mm – gentle curve (Fig. 14.3). The smaller radius of radicular curvature is associated with a severe curve. This aspect was observed in a previous study[26,36]. Root canals with small radius can be associated with a negative impact on instruments or instrumentation technique. Lopes et al.[26] related that the number of cycles necessary to induce cyclic fatigue fracture in ProTaper F3 instruments used in rotating-bending in canals with the same curvature radius, decreases as the lengths of the arcs increase.

Other aspect that cannot be overlooked before root canal preparation is to determine the anatomical diameter[33,41]. Pécora et al.[29] reported that the instrument binding technique for determining anatomical diameter at working length is not precise.

The visual appearance of root canal morphology, considering images obtained by CBCT, or periapical radiographs had more differences, mainly considering the high resolution quality offered by CBCT images. Estrela et al.[13] verified the accuracy of CBCT imaging and panoramic and periapical radiographs for the detection of apical periodontitis. The use of conventional radiographic images for detection of apical periodontitis should be done with care, because of the high possibility of false-negative diagnosis. A great advantage of using CBCT in endodontics refers to its usefulness in aiding the identification of essential anatomical structures and periapical lesions, and in a differential diagnosis with a highly accurate noninvasive technique. Apical periodontitis was correctly identified in 54.5% of the cases with periapical radiographs and in 27.8% of the cases with panoramic radiographs. Minor changes in sensitivity were found for the different tooth groups, except for incisors in panoramic radiographs. CBCT was proved to be an accurate diagnostic method.

Thus, incontestably, the determination of the root canal curvature is essential to endodontic treatment planning.

### 14.3 Root Canal Anatomical Diameter

Apical instrumentation is one of the most critical aspects of endodontic treatment, mainly in curved root canals. In Endodontics, a paradigm has been created[31]. Theories and techniques for instrumentation of curved root canals state that the use of a #25 file in the apical portion fulfills all the requisites for cleaning and shaping the root canal system. The theories emphasize that beyond this numbering (#25), failures such as deviations, perforations, zip, etc, could frequently occur[1,2,4,22].

Therefore, one created the paradigm of the instrumentation of curved root canals, stating that the apical portion must be instrumented up to a #25 file. As regards manual instrumentation, this approach is partly correct, considering that root canal instrumentation used to be performed with stainless steel instruments that did not present flexibility beyond #25. Nevertheless, during the course of the twentieth century, the findings of optical and scanning electron microscopic studies showed that the cleaning of curved root canals was indeed defective. To date, none of the techniques available have been capable of yielding thorough cleaning of the apical portion of curved root canals[4,6,16-18,21, 30,35,41-46].

Despite the evidence provided by the outcome of scientific investigations, the paradigm remained emphatic as regards the method for preparation of curved root canals, that is, instrumentation of the apical portion, up to the #25 file.

Nevertheless, anatomical studies have revealed that the anatomical diameter of the apical portion of the mesio-buccal/oral canals of maxillary molars correspond to the diameters of#25 or #30[41] files. Thus, it may be assumed that when a #25 file is the last one used for instrumentation, root canal cleaning has not been efficient. Although there is strong evidence of a lack of cleaning and preparation of the apical portion, the paradigm persists, even in spite of the outstanding technological advances, because all the development that has taken place has been adapted to the existing paradigm[31].

This paradigm[31] remained successful throughout the whole of the 20th century; however, it began to be modified in the 21$^{th}$ century, by the following approaches:

1. The existence of extremely flexible manual and rotary instruments made of nickel-titanium (NiTi) alloys, mainly those of .02 taper. If the operator is familiar with the instrumentation technique and has the skills to perform it, the apical portion of curved root canals may safely be prepared, using NiTi #40, #45 or #50 files (.02 taper), with no risk of causing deviations, perforations or zipping;

2. The real determination of the apical anatomical diameter or the real determination of the first initial instrument (Fig. 14.4A-B). For this purpose, the canals must be previously enlarged in the middle and cervical thirds with modern instruments (Orifice Shaper, Flare, Endo-Flare, Coronal Shaper, LA Axxess).

Pécora et al.[29] investigated the influence of cervical preflaring with different instruments (Gates-Glidden drills, Quantec Flare series instruments and LA Axxess burs) on the first file that binds at working length (WL) in maxillary central incisors. The instrument binding technique for determining anatomical diameter at WL is not precise. Preflaring of the cervical and middle thirds of the root canal improved anatomical diameter determination; the instrument used for preflaring played a major role in determining the anatomical diameter at the WL. Canals preflared with LA Axxess burs created a more accurate relationship between file size and anatomical diameter (Fig. 14.5A-F).

Barroso et al.[5] investigated the influence of cervical preflaring on the determination of the first file that binds at working length (WL) in buccal roots of maxillary premolars. Five groups (n=10) were formed at random and, after standard access cavities, the WL was determined 1 mm short from the apex. In group 1, the initial apical file was inserted without preflaring of cervical and middle thirds of the root canals. In groups 2 to 5, the cervical and middle thirds were enlarged with sizes 90 and 110 Gates-Glidden drills, K3 Orifice Opener instruments, ProTaper instruments and LA Axxess burs, respectively. Canals were sized manually with K-files, starting with #08 K-files inserted passively up to the WL. File sizes were increased until a binding sensation was felt at the WL and the size of the instrument was recorded. Transversal sections of the WL regions were examined under scanning electron microscopy and the discrepancies between the canal diameter and first file to bind at the WL were assessed. Significant differences were found between the groups. The major discrepancy was found without

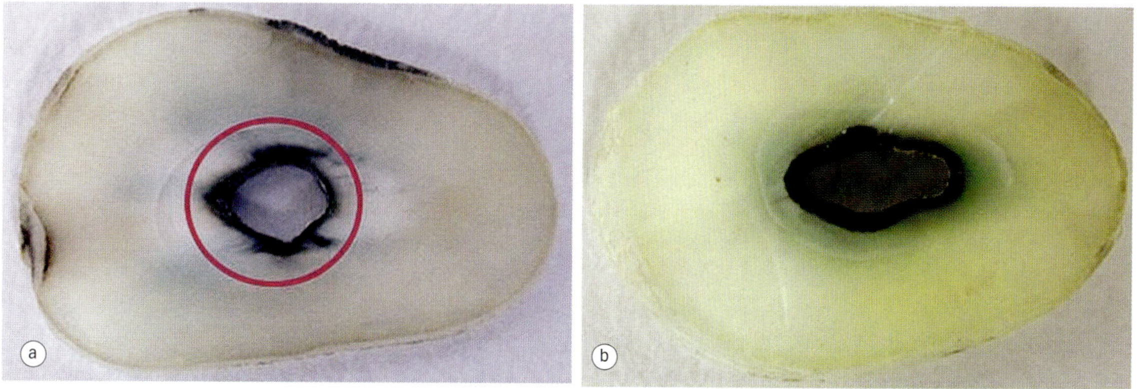

Figure 14.4 - (**A-B**) Anatomical diameter.

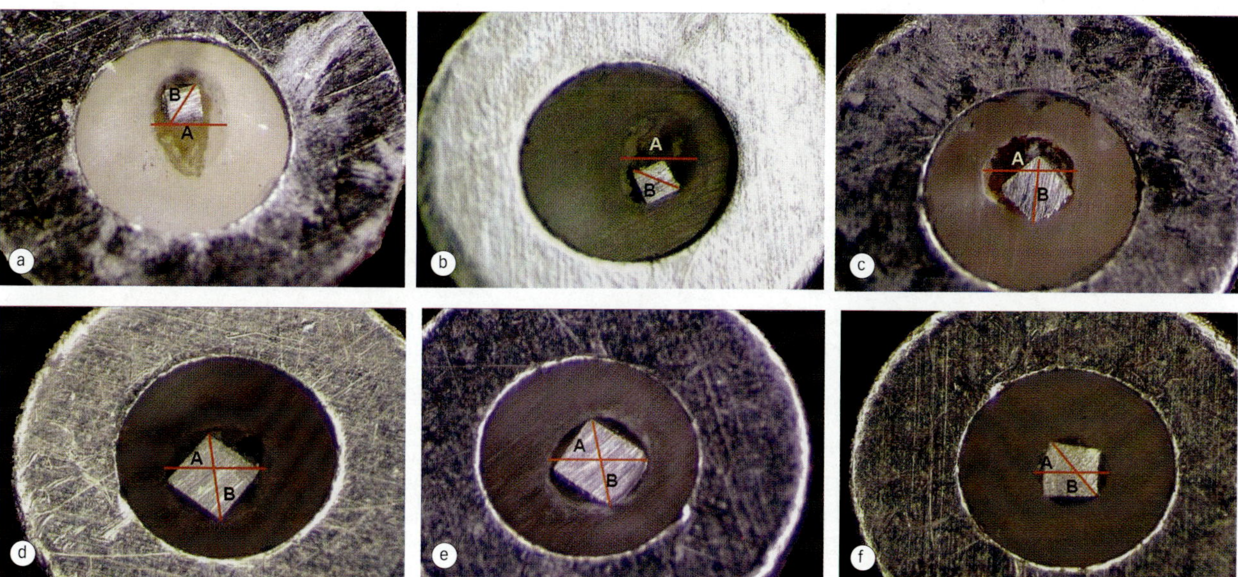

Figure 14.5 - (**A**) No cervical and middle preflaring. Transverse section at working length. A: instrument diameter; B: canal diameter. (**B**) Cervical and middle preflaring with Gates-Glidden drills. Transverse section at working length. A: Instrument diameter; B: canal diameter. (**C**) Cervical and middle preflaring with Quantec Flare series instruments. Transverse section at working length. A: Instrument diameter; B: canal diameter. (**D-F**)Cervical and middle preflaring with LA Axxess burs. Transverse section at working length. A:Instrument diameter; B: canal diameter (From Pécora et al.[29]).

preflaring (mean 157.8 µm). LA Axxess burs produced the smallest discrepancy (mean 0.8 µm). Gates-Glidden drills and K3 Orifice Opener instruments showed no significant differences between their results (83.2 µm and 73.6 µm, respectively). The discrepancy for ProTaper instruments was 35.4 µm on average. In conclusion, the instrument binding technique for determination of the anatomical diameter at the WL was not precise. Preflaring of the cervical and middle thirds improved the determination of the anatomical diameter at the WL, and the type of instrument played a major role. Canals preflared with LA Axxess burs showed a more accurate binding of the files to anatomical diameter (Fig.14.6A-J).

Schmitz et al.[41] studied the influence of cervical preflaring with different rotary instruments on determination of the initial apical file in mesiobuccal roots of mandibular molars. Fifty human mandibular molars whose mesial roots presented two clearly separated apical foramens (mesiobuccal and mesiolingual) were used. After standard access opening and removal of pulp tissue, the working length (WL) was determined at 1 mm short of the root apex. Five groups (n=10) were formed at random, according to the type of instrument used for cervical preflaring. In group 1, the size of the initial apical file was determined without preflaring of the cervical and middle root canal thirds. In groups 2 to 5, preflaring was performed with Gates-Glidden drills, ProTaper instruments, EndoFlare instruments and LA Axxes burs, respectively. Canals were sized manually with K-files, starting with size 08 K-files, inserted passively up to the WL. File sizes were increased until a binding sensation was felt at the WL and the size of the file was recorded. The instrument corresponding to the initial apical file was fixed into the canal at the WL with methylcyanoacrylate. The teeth were then sectioned transversally 1 mm short of the apex, with the IAF in position. Cross-sections of the WL region were examined under scanning electron microscopy and the discrepancies between canal diameter and the diameter of initial apical file were calculated using the tool "rule" (FEG) of the microscope's proprietary software. There were statistically significant differences among the groups ($p<0.05$). The non-flared group had the greatest discrepancy (125.30 ± 51.54) and differed significantly from all flared groups ($p<0.05$). Cervical preflaring with LA Axxess burs produced the least discrepancies (55.10 ± 48.31), followed by EndoFlare instruments (68.20 ± 42.44), Gattes Glidden drills (68.90 ± 42.46) and ProTaper files (77.40 ± 73.19). However, no significant differences ($p>0.05$) were found among the rotary instruments. In conclusion, Cervical preflaring improved the fitting of the IAF to the canals at the WL in mesiobuccal roots of maxillary first molars; 2. The non-flared group had the greatest discrepancy between the initial apical file diameter and canal diameter at the WL and differed significantly from all flared groups, regardless of the type of instrument; 3. The rotary instruments evaluated in this study (Gates-Glidden drills, EndoFlare instruments, ProTaper and LA Axxess burs) had similar performance to each other (Fig.14.7A-J).

3. Achievement of optimal shaping and cleaning of the apical portion, obtained by effective microsurgery of the root canals, using three or four instruments, above the one that determined the real anatomical diameter. Therefore, in this region, dentin will be removed at approximately 150 to 200 microns.

This change of attitude, based on the aforementioned features, led to these new hypotheses to create other theories and a new paradigm on the instrumentation of curved root canals. Therefore, this new insight will gradually modify the mentality of researchers and clinicians, but will still be open to further investigation.

The introduction of a new paradigm may face extraordinary difficulties because it creates a clash of paradigms. Whenever there is a clash of paradigms, antagonism and faulty communication are commonly observed among researchers[31].

There are those who remain locked in the past, to the ancient paradigm of instrumentation of curved root canals, not taking into account that it was based on the use of non-flexible stainless steel files.

Moreover, the corporations that produce rotary instruments have not become aware of the new paradigm that allows the instrumentation of curved root canals to be carried out with nickel-titanium instruments. They insist on divulging these new technologies, indicating their use according to the principles of the old paradigm. Such corporations insist on advising the use of these instruments, based on the crown-down technique, transposed from manual instrumentation. This is an error to be avoided, because the proposed instrumentation causes the tip of the instrument to engage during the preparation, thereby leading to instrument breakage as a result of torsional load. In order to overcome the problem of rotary instrument fracture, it is necessary to change the idea of the crown-down instrumentation adapted from manual instrumentation. A new concept of rotary instrumentation has been proposed (*Free Tip preparation*[30,31]), according to which, the tip of the instrument works freely inside the canal most of the time, acting as a guide to the instrument, thereby significantly minimizing the possibility of fracture by torsion[37].

Another mistake the manufacturers make is to manufacture instruments in which the taper of the #25 files is increased, but the tip of the file is maintained. Therefore, although the canals instrumented with the use of #25 taper. 04 or .06 files are well shaped, the apical portion is under prepared, and thus it is not clean, because the contaminated dentin is not properly removed. In addition, it is known that the greater the taper of a NiTi instrument, the less its flexibility. Therefore, in curved root canals, it is important for the apical third to be prepared with .02 taper files, thus preventing failures, and providing a more thorough cleaning. A NiTi #45 taper .02 file is flexible enough to be used in curved areas. Greater flexibility would be achieved, if parallel instruments (taper 00) were developed in the future.

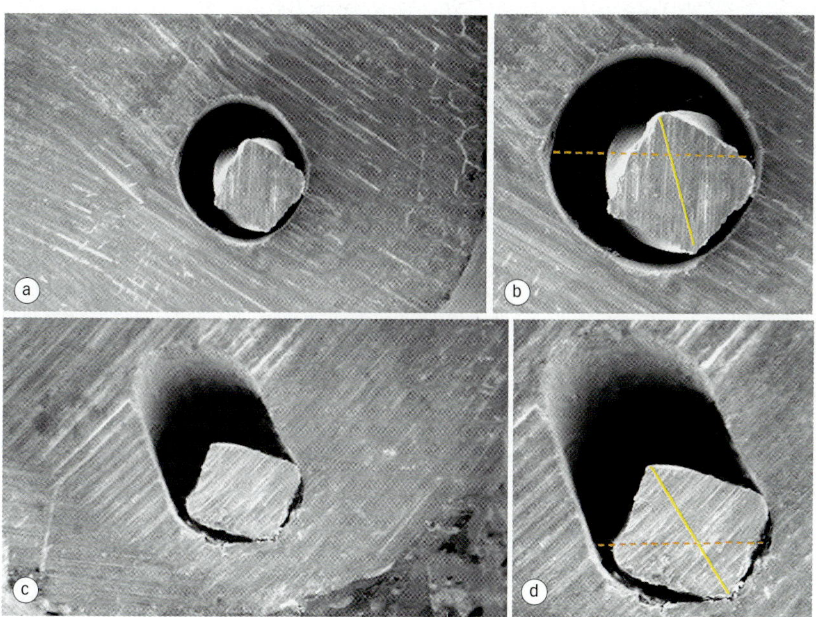


**Figure 14.6** - (**A-B**) SEM micrograph of Group 1 (no cervical and middle preflaring). Transverse section at the working length. (**C-D**) SEM micrograph of Group 2 (cervical and middle preflaring with Gates-Glidden drills). Transverse section at the working length (From Barroso et al.[5]).

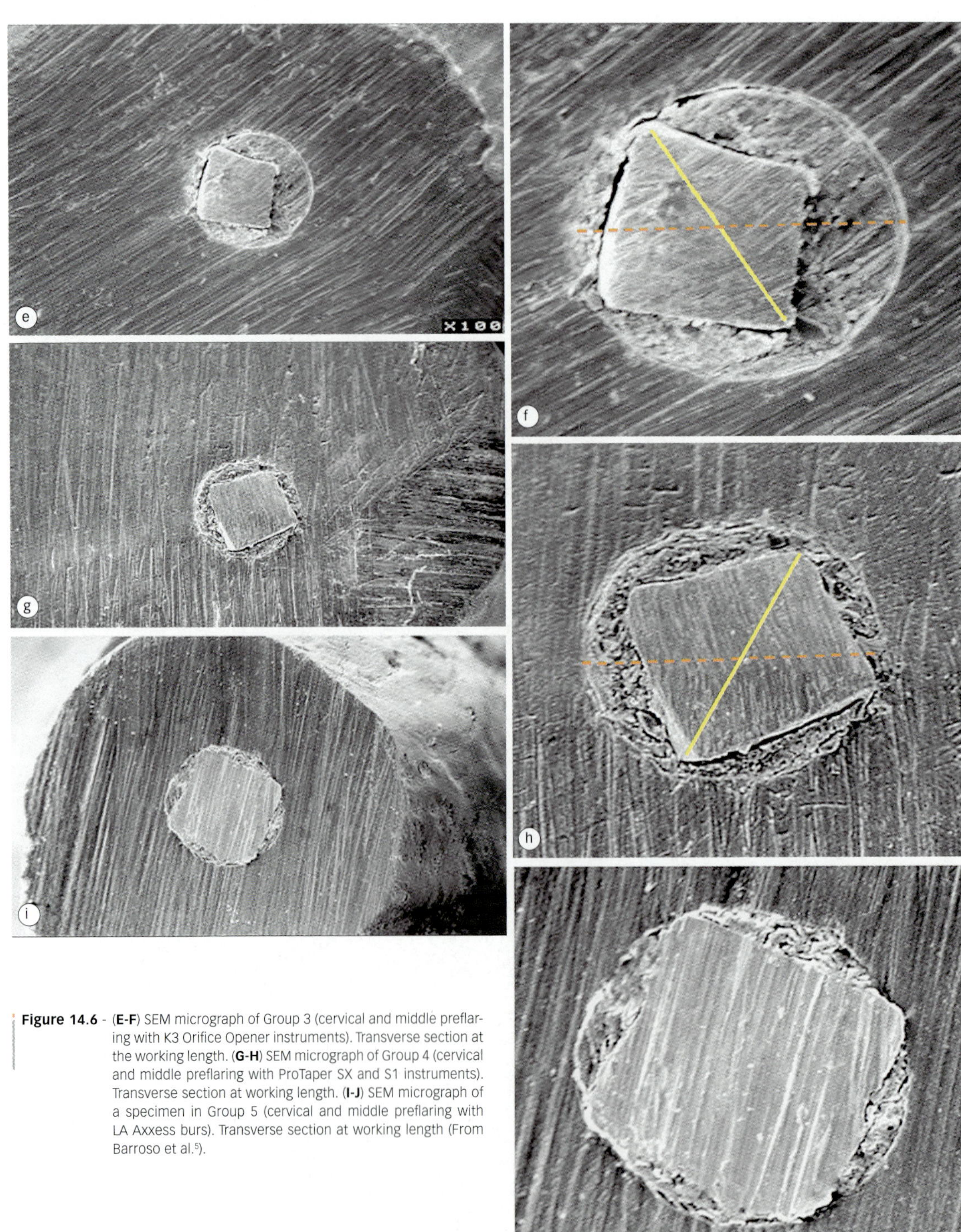


**Figure 14.6** - (**E-F**) SEM micrograph of Group 3 (cervical and middle preflaring with K3 Orifice Opener instruments). Transverse section at the working length. (**G-H**) SEM micrograph of Group 4 (cervical and middle preflaring with ProTaper SX and S1 instruments). Transverse section at working length. (**I-J**) SEM micrograph of a specimen in Group 5 (cervical and middle preflaring with LA Axxess burs). Transverse section at working length (From Barroso et al.[5]).

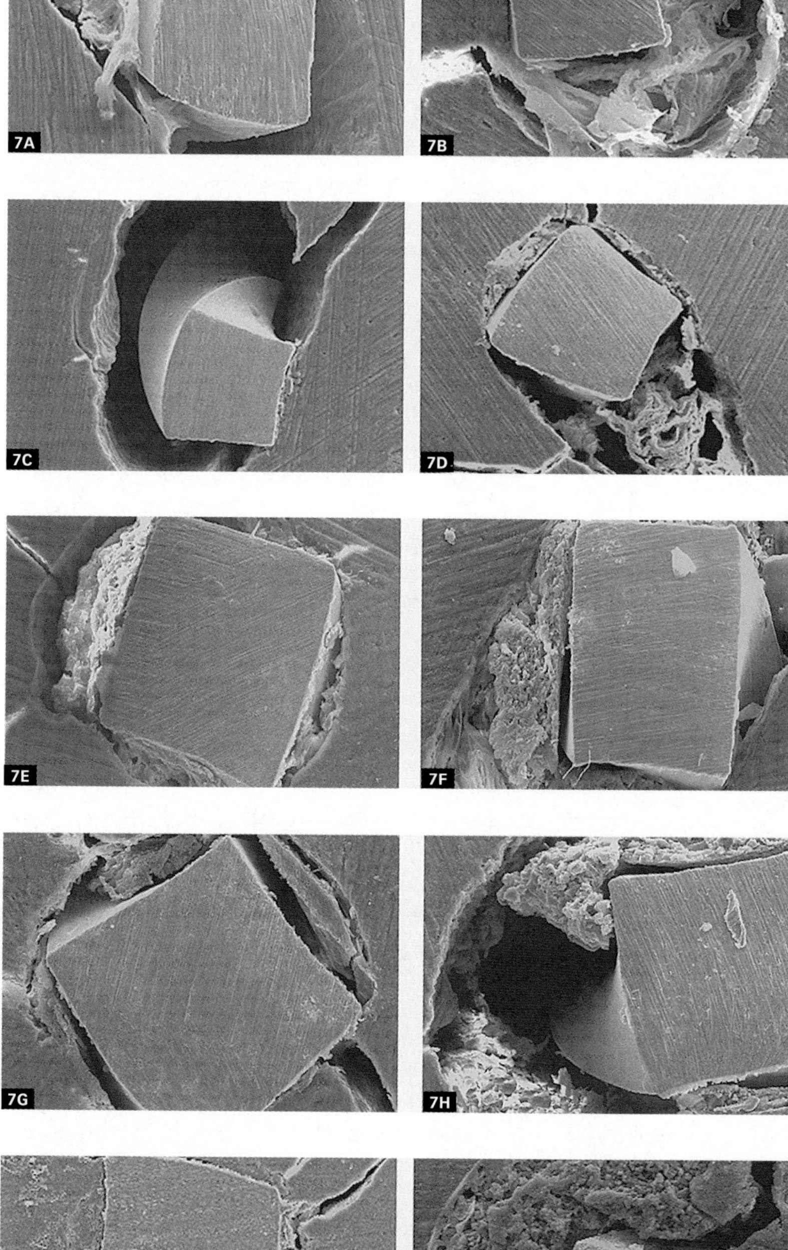


**Figure 14.7** - (**A-B**) SEM micrograph of Group 1 (no preflaring). Cross-section at the working length (X200). (From Schmitz et al.[41]).

**Figure 14.7** - (**C-D**) SEM micrograph of Group 2 (preflaring with Gates Glidden drills). Cross-section at the working length (X200). (From Schmitz et al.[41]).

**Figure 14.7** - (**E-F**) SEM micrograph of Group 3 (preflaring with ProTaper SX and S1 files). Cross-section at the working length (X200). (From Schmitz et al.[41]).

**Figure 14.7** - (**G-H**) SEM micrograph of Group 4 (preflaring with EndoFlare and Hero 25 .06 instruments). Cross-section at the working length (X200). (From Schmitz et al.[41]).

**Figure 14.7** - (**I-J**) SEM micrograph of Group 5 (preflaring with LA Axxes burs). Cross-section at the working length (X200). (From Schmitz et al.[41]).

In view of this, instrumentation of the apical portion of curved root canals must be performed with.02 taper files, because this region may be prepared with three, four or five instruments, beyond the real anatomical diameter. Nevertheless, the real anatomical diameter must be determined first.

According this reasoning, Estrela et al.[15] critically discussed the antibacterial efficacy of intracanal medications on bacterial biofilm. Longitudinal studies were evaluated by systematic review including articles from MEDLINE using various keywords involving root canal biofilm, from 1966 until August 1st 2007, and fom the Cochrane Library, during the same period. The selected articles were identified from titles, abstracts and complete articles by two independent reviews, considering the tabulated inclusion and exclusion criteria. The search of information found 91 related articles, and of these, 8.8% articles involved in vivo studies that demonstrated the lack of efficacy of endodontic therapy against bacterial biofilm.

The biofilm in the root canal system is a challenge to the outcome of root canal treatment. For all these reasons, considering the heterogeneity of guidelines to study antimicrobial strategies for endodontic infections, the higher estimate of clinical success, adequate sanitization process, assisted by the intracanal medications, reduce the bacterial population and favor the prognosis.

The antimicrobial efficacy of intracanal medications against bacterial biofilm still needs to be confirmed. In order to satisfy regulatory guidelines, to disrupt bacterial biofilm, the active participation of mechanical action of endodontic instruments, associated with antimicrobial medicaments is essential. Further studies are indispensable to offer new guidelines for the treatment protocol of endodontic biofilm.

The progress of endodontics is now leaving the artisanal (handicraft) stage behind, and entering the technological stage, in which the general practitioner will be able to perform the treatment of curved canals successfully, provided that he/she is familiar with the instrumentation technique.

## 14.4 Apical Sanitization

The relationship between endodontic infection and consequential host response has led to several therapeutic trends. The goal of endodontic therapy is to perform the sanitization process of an infected root canal by chemical and mechanical cleaning and shaping, thereby significantly reducing the number of microorganisms.

Root canal filling is the third of the significant steps in endodontic treatment (coronal access, sanitization-shaping and endodontic obturation-sealing). Thus, it reinforces the concept of eliminating empty spaces inside the tooth, which can harbor microorganisms. In this context, it allows tissue repair, because the periapical tissues are able to rest from the previous irritation, and to favor osteogenesis and cementogenesis (with formation of osteocement to substitute resorbed dentin), followed by reorganization of the periodontal ligament and reintegration of the lamina dura.

Schilder[38] reported several criteria that constitute the mechanical goal of root canal preparation: 1. A continuously tapering funnel going from the coronal access cavity to the root apex; 2. Confine instrumentation to the root canal and dentinal tissue; 3. Root canal preparation should flow with the shape of the original canal; 4. The apical foramen should remain in its original spatial relationship with both the bone and root surface. These factors must be taken into consideration because of the direct relationship between the root canal and the endodontic file, influencing this complete and intimate relationship.

One approach to control accumulation of debris in the apical region is the concept of apical patency. Apical patency has been recommended to prevent occlusion of the apical foramen and maintain control of the working length. Buchanan[9] analyzing the management of the curved root canal, reported that the patency file must passively move through the apical constricture, without widening it.

The apical limit of exploration can differ in two clinical situations: vital pulp and pulp necrosis. In vital pulp, exploration is restricted to the proximities of the cementum-dentin-canal junction, while in situations of pulp necrosis, the exploration should advance up to the radiographic apical vertex, allowing the cementum canal to be emptied. Sanitization of this area, considered critical, favors microorganism control.

It is impossible to obtain direct access to the lateral canal and ramifications with an endodontic instrument. Thus, cleaning and shaping in this region is restricted to the main canal. Ricucci & Langeland[34] report that one of the major controversies in endodontic therapy concerns the apical limit of instrumentation and obturation. The results of longitudinal studies, basic anatomical knowledge of the apical third of the root canal, and the histological pulp reaction to caries progression, demonstrated the presence of a vital apical pulp remnant, even in the presence of a periapical lesion.

As regards the apical limit of obturation, Kojima et al.[24] based on meta-analysis, determined the influence of factors such as apical limit (short vs. over extension), status of the pulp (vital vs. non vital), and periapical status (presence or absence of radiolucency) on endodontic prognosis. The study-list was obtained by using a MEDLINE search and Japana Centra Revuo Medicina search. Only articles in which the criteria for success or failure were exactly described, were accepted. A cumulative success rate of 82.8 ± 1.19% was obtained for teeth with vital pulp, and 78.9 ± 1.05% for those with a non vital pulp. There was a significant difference between the 2 groups (cumulative odds ratio, 1.18; 95% confidence intervals, 1.06 - 1.32). The cumulative success rates with over extension, flush, and under extension for vital pulp and non vital pulp were 70.8 ± 1.44, 86.5 ± 0.88, and 85.5 ± 0.98%, respectively. There was a significant difference between flush and over extension (cumulative odds ratio, 2.32; 95% confidence intervals, 2.07 ± 2.60) and between flush and under extension (cumulative odds ratio, 1.12; 95% confidence intervals, 1.00-1.27). The cumulative success rates, without a periapical lesion, and with one were 82.0 ± 1.24 and 71.5 ± 1.60%, respectively; and the difference between the 2 groups was significant (cumulative odds ratio, 2.79; 95% confidence intervals, 2.44 - 3.20). In the analysis of success rate by age group, the cumulative success rates for patients under 30 years of age and those over 50 years of age were 78.4 ± 1.44% and 77.3% ± 2.58, respectively. Nevertheless, there was no significant difference between these age groups (cumulative odds ratio, 0.97; 95% confidence intervals, 0.80-1.18). A significant difference in success rates was found when teeth with perirapical lesion were compared with those without lesion. Based on the use of cumulative meta-analysis, the authors proposed that the root canal should be filled to within 2 mm of the radiographic apex.

Holland et al.[19] evaluated the influence of the type of vehicle (distilled water or propyleneglycol) on the response of apical tissues of dog's teeth after root canal filling with Mineral Trioxide Aggregate (MTA) at two different limits. Forty roots of incisors and premolars of two adult dogs were used. After pulpectomy, the root canals were prepared biomechanically, and the apical cemented barrier of the roots was penetrated with a #15 K-file and widened to a #25 K-file. The root canals were assigned to four groups according to the vehicle used for MTA preparation, and the limit of root canal filling: group 1, filling with MTA/distilled water to the limit of the cemental canal; group 2, overfilling with MTA/distilled water; group 3, filling with MTA/propyleneglycol to the limit of the cemental canal; and group 4, overfilling with MTA/propyleneglycol. After 90 days, the results showed that MTA pastes prepared with either distilled water or propyleneglycol as vehicles, had similar biological behavior; root fillings placed at the cemental canal limit showed better results than the over fillings, and MTA/propyleneglycol paste was more easily put into the root canals than MTA/distilled water paste.

Holland et al.[20] investigated the periapical healing process of dog's teeth with or without apical patency, and after root canal filling with two types of sealers. Forty premolar and incisor roots were used. The root canals were over instrumented and dressed with a corticosteroid-antibiotic solution for 7 days to obtain an ingrowth of periapical connective tissue, into the canals. After this period, the tissue was removed in half of the specimens (groups with patency) and preserved in the other half (groups without patency). Canals were filled by lateral condensation technique with gutta-percha points, and either a calcium hydroxide-based sealer (Sealer Plus) or Grossmanís cement (Fill Canal). After histophatological analysis, it could be observed that both apical patency (presence or absence), and the type of root canal filling material, influenced the periapical healing process in dog's teeth with vital pulp, after root canal treatment. The use of a calcium hydroxide-based sealer in teeth without apical patency yielded the best results among the experimental conditions proposed (Fig. 14.8A-D).

Anjos-Neto[3] evaluated the apical patency in the repair of chronic periapical lesions induced in dog's teeth after intracanal medication with calcium hydroxide, and obturation with Sealapex or AH Plus sealers. Forty root canals (from 2 dogs) were exposed to the oral environment for 180 days, to induce the periapical lesions. After this period, the root canals were prepared up to the K-file # 55, under constant irrigation with 2.5% sodium hypochlorite. When root canal preparation on 20 specimens was concluded, perforation and amplification of the apical cement barrier was performed. Next, the 40 root canals were filled with a paste composed of calcium hydroxide, and the cavities were sealed with zinc

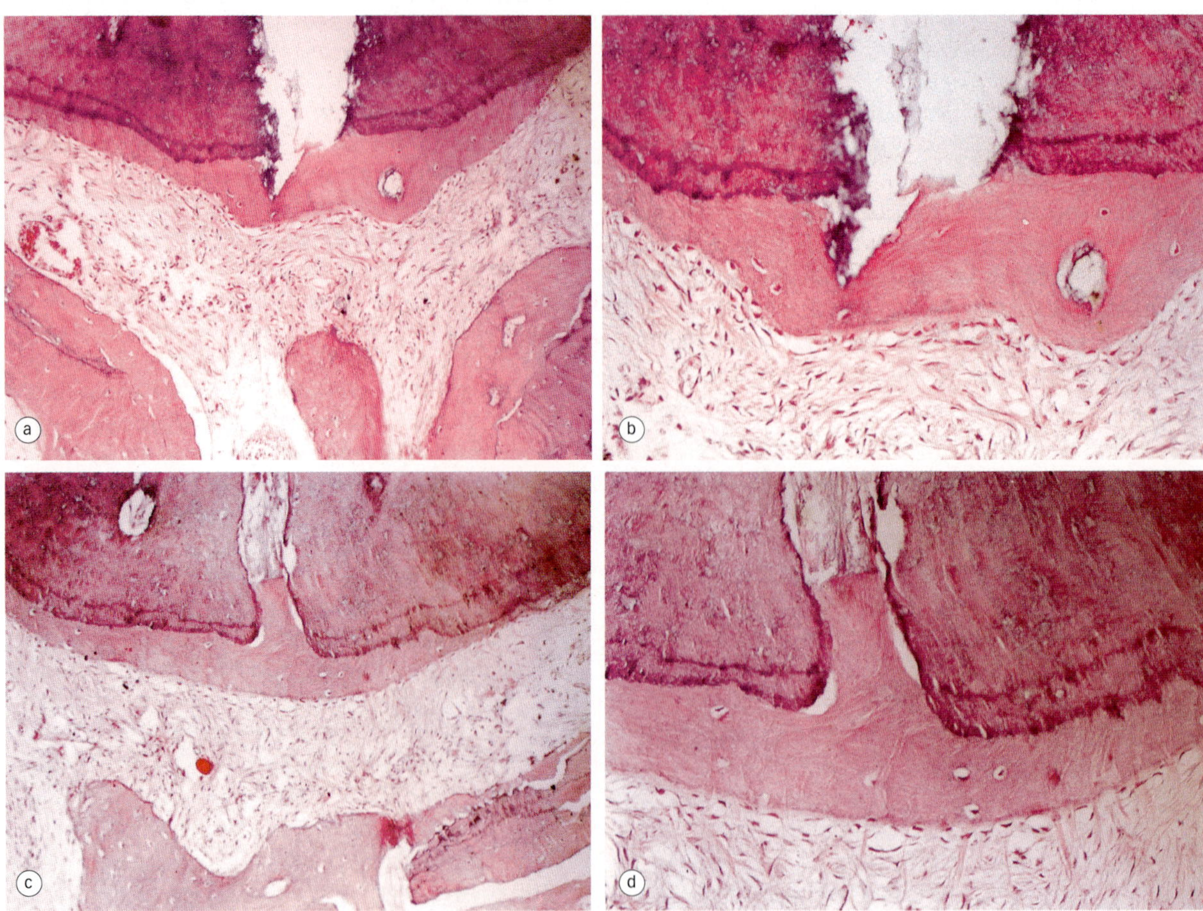


**Figure 14.8** - (**A-B**) Sealer Plus without patency. Biological closure by neoformed cementum deposition. H&E. (original magnification X100). (**C-D**) Sealer Plus without patency. Note total closure of the main root canal and an organized periodontal tissue (PT). H&E. (original magnification X100) (Courtesy Prof. Dr. Roberto Holland[19,20]).

oxide and eugenol. After a period of 21 days, the dressing was removed and obturation of the root canals began, being performed in 10 roots with apical patency using with AH Plus sealers, and in 10 without apical patency using Sealapex, under equal conditions. Thus, four experimental groups were defined with 10 in each group. After the postoperative period of 180 days, the animals were euthanized and the tissures obtained were prepared for histomorphologic and histomicrobiologic analysis. The 16 events analyzed were quantified with scores from 1 to 4, where 1 represented the best result and 4 the worst, with 2 and 3 in intermediate positions. Statistical analysis of the results showed that in general, the use of apical patency favored the treatment, irrespective of the sealer, and the Sealapex group was significantly better than the AH Plus group, irrespective of the apical patency.

Borlina[7] analyzed the influence of patency, with enlargement of the apical foramen, in the repair of chronic inflammatory periapical lesions induced in dog's teeth, after dressing with calcium hydroxide paste, and filling the root canals with Sealer 26 and Endomethasone sealers. Two dogs were selected to obtain a sample of 40 root canals which, after pulpectomy, were exposed to the oral environment for 180 days for the induction of periapical lesions. After this period, the biomechanical preparation of root canals was performed. Then, in twenty specimens, the apical cementum barrier was perforated and the foramen was enlarged, up to K-file # 25 (with apical patency), while in another twenty, the barrier was preserved (without apical patency). Throughout the preparation, the root canals were irrigated with 2.5% sodium hypochlorite. After this, all canals were dried and filled with EDTA for 3 minutes, after which, they were again irrigated with the same solution, and dried to receive the calcium hydroxide paste dressing with saline and iodoform. This was followed by coronal sealing with gutta percha and zinc oxide-eugenol cement. After 21 days the calcium hydroxide paste was removed from the root canals, using K-file # 15 and irrigation with saline. Finally, the canals were dried and filled with the cements according to the experimental group tested: Group I – Sealer 26 with patency; Group II – Sealer 26 without patency; Group III – Endomethasone with patency; Group IV - Endomethasone without patency. After 180 days of the treatments and histopathological analyses, it could be concluded that: 1) use of apical patency favored the treatment, irrespective of the cement used; 2) Sealer 26, was better than Endomethasone, irrespective of the apical patency, 3) the cement Sealer 26 group with patency, provided the best results.

The principle to reach favorable outcome on endodontic infection treatment requires to recognize and to remove aetiological factors. Nair et al.[28] reported the importance and necessity of stringently applying nonantibiotic chemomechanical measures in order to disrupt the biofilm and reduce the intraradicular microbial load to the lowest possible level to ensure the most favorable long-term prognosis for treatment of infected root canals.

The microenvironment of root canal presents excellent conditions to establish microbial growth. The endodontic microbiota reduction has been made by antimicrobial strategies like root canal preparation, irrigants solutions, intracanal dressing and root canal filling. The antimicrobial efficacy of intracanal medicaments on bacterial biofilm still did not confirmed[15]. In order to satisfy regulatory guidelines to disrupt bacterial biofilm is essential the active participation of mechanical action of endodontic instruments associated to antimicrobial medicaments.

## References


1. Abou-Rass M, Frank AL, Glick DH. The anticurvature filing method to prepare the curve root canal. J Am Dent Assoc 1980;101:792-4.
2. Al-Omari MAO, Dummer PMH. Canal blockage and debris extrusion with eight preparation techniques. J Endod 1995;21: 57-61.
3. Anjos-Neto DA. Influência da patência apical e dos cimentos Sealapex e AH Plus no reparo de lesões periapicais inflamatórias crônicas induzidas em dentes de cães, após curativo com hidróxido de cálcio (Master's Thesis), University of Marília, 2008; 222f.
4. Barbizam JV, Fariniuk LF, Marchesan MA, Pécora JD, Sousa-Neto MD. Efectiveness of manual and rotary instrumentation techniques for cleaning flattened root canals. J Endod 2002;28:365-6.
5. Barroso JM, Guerisoli DMZ, Capelli A, Saquy PC, Pécora JD. Influence of cervical preflaring on determination of apical file size in maxillary premolars: SEM analysis. Braz Dent J 2005;16:30-4.
6. Bolanos OR, Jensen JR. Scanning electron microscope comparison of the efficacy of various methods or root canal preparation. J Endod 1980;6:815-22.
7. Borlina SC. Influence of apical patency in induced chronic periapical lesions, after calcium hydroxide dressing and filling of the root canals of dogs´teeth with Sealer 26 and Endométhasone sealers. Dissertação (Master's Thesis), University of Marília, 2008; 215f.
8. Boyer CB. A History of Mathematics. 2nd ed. Revised by Merzbach UC. New York: Wiley; 1989.
9. Buchanan LS. Management of the curved root canal. J Calif Dent Assoc 1989;17:18-27.
10. Cimis GM, Boyler TF, Pelleu-Jr GR. Effect of three files studies of canal curvatures in the mesial roots of mandibular molars. J Endod 1988;14:441-4.
11. Cunningham CJ, Senia ES. A three dimensional studies of canal curvatures in the mesial roots of mandibular molars. J Endod 1992;18:294-300.
12. Dobó-Nagy C, Szabó J, Szabó J. A mathematically based classification of root canal curvatres on natural human teeth. J Endod 1995;11:567-60.
13. Estrela C, Bueno MR, Leles CR, Azevedo BC, Azevedo JR. Accuracy of computed tomography, panoramic and periapical radiographic for the detection of apical periodontitis. J Endod 2008;34:273-9.
14. Estrela C, Bueno MR, Sousa-Neto MD, Pécora JD. Method for determination of root curvature radius using cone-beam computed tomography images. Braz Dent J 2008;19:114-8.
15. Estrela C, Sydney GB, Figueiredo JAP, Estrela CRA. Antibacterial efficacy of intracanal medicaments on bacterial biofilm – a critical review. J Applied Oral Science, 2009; 17(1) (in press).
16. Gambarini G, Laszkiewicz J. A scanning electron microscopic study of debris and smear layer remaining following use of GT rotary instruments. Int Endod J 2002;35:422-7.
17. Grandini S, Balleri P, Ferrari M. Evaluation of Glyde File Prep in combination with sodium hypochlorite as a root canal irrigant. J Endod 2002;28:300-3.
18. Guerisoli DMZ, Marchesan MA, Walmsley AD, Pécora JD. Evaluation of smear layer removal by EDTAC and sodium hypochlorite with ultrasonic agitation. Int Endod J 2002;35:418-21.
19. Holland R, Mazuqueli L, Souza V, Murata SS, Dezan-Jr E, Suzuki P. Influence of the type of vehicle and limit of obturation on apical and periapical tissue response in dog's teeth after root canal filling with mineral trioxide aggregate. J Endod 2007;33:693–7.
20. Holland R, Sant'anna-Jr A, Souza V, Dezan-Jr E, Otoboni-Filho JA, Bernabé PFE, Nery MJ, Murata SS. Influence of Apical patency and filling material on healing process of dog's teeth with vital pulp after root canal therapy. Braz Dent J 2005;16:9-16.
21. Hülsmann M, Gressmann G, Schäfers F. A comparative study of root canal preparation using FlexMaster and HERO 642 rotary Ni-Ti instruments. Int Endod J 2003;36:358-66.
22. Hülsmann M, Schade M, Schäfers F. A comparative study of root canal preparation with HERO 642 and Quanted SC rotary Ni-Ti instruments. Int Endod J 2001;34:538-46.
23. Ingle JI, Taintor JF. Endodontics. 3rd ed. Philadelphia: Lea & Febiger; 1985.
24. Kojima K, Inamoto K, Nagamatsu K, Hara A, Nakata K, Morita I, Nakagaki H, Nakamura H. Success rate of endodontic treatment of teeth with vital and nonvital pulps. A meta-analysis. Oral Surg Oral Med Oral Pathol Oral Radiol Endod 2004;97:95-9.
25. Lopes HP, Elias CN, Estrela C, Siqueira JF Jr. Assessment of the apical transportation of root canals using the method of the curvature radius. Braz Dent J 1998;9:39-45.
26. Lopes HP, Moreira EJL, Elias CN, Almeida RA, Neves MS. Cyclic Fatigue of Protaper Instruments. J Endod 2008;33:55-7.
27. Moreira EJL, Lopes HP, Elias CN, Fidel RAS. Fratura por flexão em rotação de instrumentos endodônticos de NiTi. Rev. Bras. Odontol 2002;59:412–14.
28. Nair PNR, Henry S, Cano V, Vera J. Microbial status of apical root canal system of human mandibular first molars with primary apical periodontitis after one-visit-endodontic treatment. Oral Surg Oral Med Oral Pathol Oral Radiol Endod 2005;99:231–52.
29. Pécora JD, Capelli A, Guerisoli DMZ, Spanó JCE, Estrela C. Influence of cervical preflaring on apical file size determination. Int Endod J 38;430-35, 2005.
30. Pécora JD, Capelli A, Seixas FH, Maechesan MA, Guerisoli DMZ. Rotary Biomechanics: Reality or Future? http://www.forp.usp.br/restauradora/rotatorios/free/rotary_biomechanics.html.
31. Pécora JD, Capelli A. Shock of paradigms on the instrumentation of curved root canals. Braz Dent J 2006;17:3-5.

32. Pruett JP, Clement DJ, Carnes DL. Cyclic fatigue testing of nickel-titanium endodontic instruments. J Endod 1997;23:77-85.
33. Pucci FM, Reig R. Conductos radiculares. Buenos Aires: Médico-Quirurgica, 1944.
34. Ricucci D, Langeland K. Apical limit of root canal instrumentation and obturation, part. 2. A histological study. Int Endod J 1998;31:394-409.
35. Rödig T, Hülsmann M, Mühge M, Schäfers F. Quality of preparation of oval distal root canals in mandibular molars using nickel-titanium instruments. Int Endod J 2002;35:919-28.
36. Schäfer E, Florek H. Efficiency of rotary nickel–titanium K3 instruments compared with stainless steel hand K-Flexo-file. Part 1. Shaping ability in simulated curved canals. Int Endod J 2003:36:199–207.
37. Schäfers F, Schlingemann R. Efficiency of rotary nickel-titanium K3 instruments compared with stainless steel hand K-Flexofile. Part. 2. Cleaning effectiveness and shaping ability in severely curved canals of extracted teeth. Int Endod J 2003;36:208-17.
38. Schilder H. Cleaning and shaping the root canal. Dent Clin North Amer 1974;8:269–96.
39. Schneider SW. A comparison of canal preparations in straight and curved root canals. Oral Surg Oral med Oral Pathol 1971;32:271-5.
40. Sonntag D, Stachniss-Carp S, Stachniss C, Stachniss V. Determination of root canal curvatures before and after canal preparation (part II): A method based on numeric calculus. Aust Endod J 2006; 32:16–25
41. Schmitz MS, Santos R, Capelli A, Jacobovitz M, Spanó JCA, Pécora JD. influence of cervical preflaring on determination of apical file size in mandibular molars: SEM analysis. Braz Dent J 2008; 19:245-51.
42. Vanni JR, R Santos, Limongi O, Guerisoli DMZ, Capelli A, Pecora JD. Influence of cervical preflaring on determination of apical file size in maxillary molars: SEM analysis. Braz Dent J 2005;16:181-6.
43. West JD, Roane JB, Goerig AC. Cleaning and shaping the root canal system. In: Pathways of the Pulps. Cohen S, Burns RC (Editors). 6th ed. St. Louis: Mosby Year Book; 1994. p.179-218.
44. Wu MK, Kastakova A, Wesselink PR. Quality of cold and warm gutta-percha fillings in oval canals in mandibular pre-molars. Int Endod J 2001;34:485-91.
45. Wu MK, Roris A, Barkis D, Wesselink PR. Prevalence and extent of long oval shape of canals in the apical third. Oral Surg, Oral Med, Oral Pathol, Oral Radiol Endod 2000;89:739-43.
46. Wu MK, Wesselink PR. A primary observation on the preparation and obturation of oval canals. Int Endod J 2001;34:137-141.
47. Wu MK, Wesselink PR. Efficacy of three techniques in cleaning the apical portion of curved root canals. Oral Surg Oral Med Oral Pathol Oral Radiol Endod 1995;79:492-496.

# Development of Root Canal Preparation

**J. A. P. Figueiredo**
*Pontifical Catholic University of Rio Grande do Sul, Porto Alegre, RS, Brazil*

**P. M.H. Dummer**
*Cardiff University, Cardiff, United Kingdom*

**C. Estrela**
*Federal University of Goiás, Goiânia, GO, Brazil*

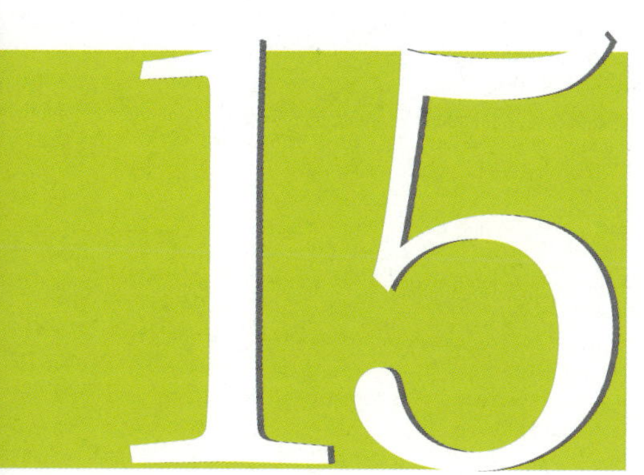


Chapter contents

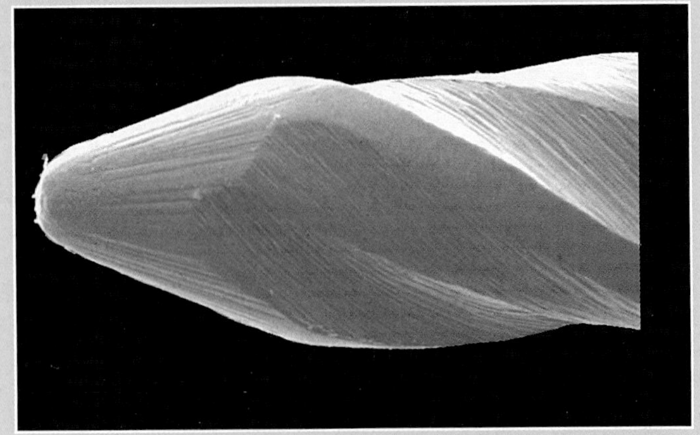

K3 instrument tip.

## 15.1 Introduction

The methods endodontists use to prepare root canals have changed substantially in recent years. The use of rotary, reciprocal, ultrasonic and other devices has enhanced the efficiency and effectiveness of canal shaping. These innovations in turn have encouraged more general practitioners to undertake root canal treatment, particularly in posterior teeth that are more often associated with a greater degree of difficulty. It is interesting to appreciate that although mechanical approaches are adopted, most techniques in use at present continue to make use of manual instruments to some degree. The standardized .02 taper stainless steel instruments have certain advantages that instruments manufactured from nickel-titanium alone are not able to reproduce.

Although there are no longitudinal studies showing that mechanical means of root canal preparation achieve better outcomes than manual techniques, the popularization of their use is a reality and an irreversible trend. In this context, it is important for clinicians and specialists to be capable of understanding the principles behind mechanical preparation, in order to provide the best possible canal shape with minimal risk.

The greatest problem associated with root canal preparation is a lack of understanding of the rationale behind instrument design, the inherent advantages and limitations of procedures and techniques, and the lack of precise indications for use of the various systems available. It is rather simplistic to believe that a given technique can be applied regardless of the tooth type and its anatomical variations and complexities. Furthermore, manufacturers fail to describe the way their instruments should be used, in sufficient detail to maximize their performance; at the same time clinical scientists take too long to provide adequate information, through research, of the outcome expected with a certain technique, or when analyzing a specific detail or design feature of an instrument.

This chapter endeavors to cover the development of root canal preparation, considering the properties of instruments, their techniques of use and limitations. It does not intend to describe clinical techniques in detail, but to point out important aspects of root canal preparation that should ultimately contribute to an understanding of the state of the art of what is probably the most time-consuming stage of the root canal treatment.

## 15.2 Development of Stainless Steel Instruments

The advent of nickel-titanium instruments could create a false assumption that this was the greatest development in root canal instrumentation. Indeed, when introduced many years ago, stainless steel instruments constituted a very effective move towards a systematic approach to root canal treatment. Until the 1950s, endodontic instruments were produced without specific design criteria or to defined standards. The father of modern Dentistry, Pierre Fauchard[24] (1745) used instruments in the root canal to cauterize the pulps; the role of bacteria in the cause and perpetuation of apical periodontitis was not understood. Thus, at that time, the purpose of using endodontic instruments was to physically create a space for obturation; it was not linked to the removal of microorganisms. Historical data[7] attribute to Maynard the first endodontic instruments consisting of notched round wires. Files were used by Arthur in 1852[7,33].

With the discovery of stainless steel, in 1912, by Henry Brearley[40], the chromium content in the steel provided the metal with protection. The principle being that the contact of chromium with air creates a pellicle of chromium oxide that adheres to the surface avoiding the action of aggressive agents. This pellicle rapidly regenerates but can be minimized or destroyed by chloride.[40] Stainless steel can be classified as austenitic, ferritic or martensitic, according to the type of microstructure and the additional alloys added. Endodontic instruments are generally austenitic, in which their crystal lattice configuration is described as a body centered cubic structure[36].

The K-file was introduced in 1915[33], but instrument manufacture was not standardized in terms of shape, length or diameter. Standardization of instruments was proposed in 1929 by Trebitsch and again by Ingle[34] in 1955 and Ingle and Levine[35] (in 1958). But, it was not until 1962 that the American Association of Endodontists (AAE) created a team to work with the manufacturers on standardization, which later resulted in the ISO specifications for endodontic instruments, published in 1974[33].

Ingle's contribution to Endodontology was substantial, as his concepts on instruments for root canal preparation systematically led to new concepts and techniques. Following the 'standard' preparation technique of Ingle, a large number of other techniques were proposed in the 1970s and 1980s. Clem[17] in 1969 introduced the 'step' preparation that recognized that canal preparation could be directed towards specific areas of the root canal, which resulted in greater emphasis on anatomical aspects of the root canal and the delivery of techniques and/or instrument maneuvers to overcome specific problems. This fundamental principle later contributed to the methods recommended for using different rotary techniques, as the engagement of the instrument in not more than one point is pivotal to preventing breakage.

The manipulation of hand instruments is a sensitive yet poorly explored issue in the dental literature. The push-pull motion is possibly used by most operators in the world, but there are no data to support its apparent superiority. Although it is claimed to provide effective cutting, it is more difficult to maintain a curvature using this motion alone. The stem-winding (or watch-winding) motion requires gentle pressure to maintain the file to length, has reduced cutting efficiency, but does provide control around canal curves even with stainless steel instruments[57]. It may take longer to prepare the canal using this method of manipulation, but it has the advantage of maintaining the original canal anatomy. Some authors prefer to combine different motions, using stem-winding to prepare the area of the curve, and push-pull in the straight area of the root canal. Others adopt a hybrid approach, stem-winding whilst push-pulling at the same time.

Allison et al.[4] histologically compared the effectiveness of canal wall planing when filing, reaming or step-back filing. They found that while reaming and filing planed the walls in a similar manner, step-back filing planed a greater percentage of walls in both straight and curved canals. Reaming resulted in fewer planed walls than filing or step-back filing. Reaming and filing produced more uniform preparations, but step-back produced a more thoroughly prepared, but more irregularly shaped preparation. According to the authors, filing tended to be the least effective technique.

The balanced force technique[50] consists of rotating the instrument ¼ clockwise, and with apical pressure, ¾ counter-clockwise. Such a movement tends to enlarge the apical area effectively, but produces a cylindrical preparation shape, as the instruments are effectively boring/drilling out the canal.

Emphasis has been laid on the anti-curvature approach, promoted by Abou-Rass et al.[1], which describes the inner portion of the curve as the danger zone for excessive dentin removal and perforation at the furca. To prevent this happening, the anti-curvature technique requires the file to be targeted preferentially away from the danger zone[23] (Fig. 15.1).

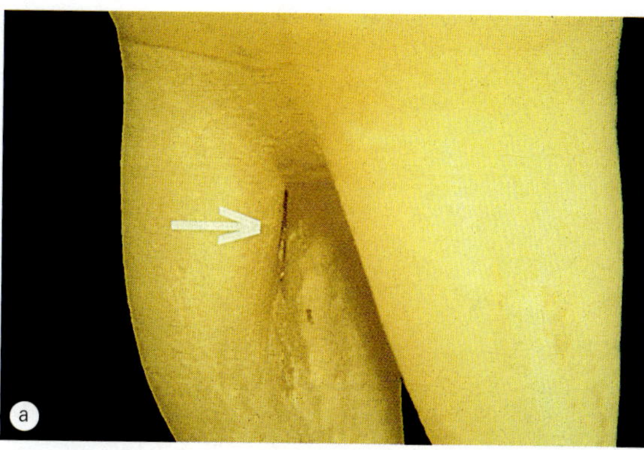

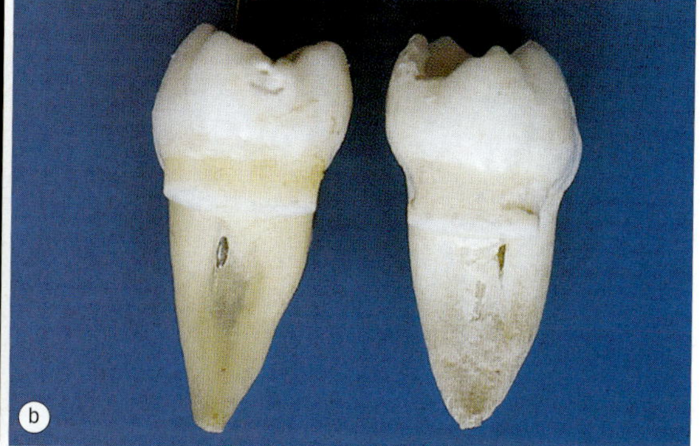

**Figure 15.1** - (**A-B**) The distal aspect of the mesiobuccal canal of the mandibular first molar may have thin dentin walls 2-3mm apically from the birfucation (danger zone); preparing this area may lead to perforation[23].

Weine et al.[71] suggested the use of modified instruments, in which the cutting flutes of a K-file were removed along the internal aspect of the curve coronally and along the external aspect of the curve apically, in an endeavor to avoid the formation of zips and danger zones. The Canal Finder system follows a similar concept using a handpiece that provides a push-pull motion and modified Hedströem files that have reduced flute depths along the inner portion of the curve, with greater depths on the outer aspect of the curve.

**Tip**

The design of an instrument tip can influence its ability to shape root canals. Miserendino et al.[41] found that specific design features of the tip, such as tip angle, length, cross-section, and geometry, significantly affected the cutting efficiency of endodontic instruments. According to Del Bello et al.[21], a pyramidal tip design has ridges on the face that enable it to cut in a forward (insertion) direction; these ridges intersect with the cutting edges, forming sharp points at the transition angle, which tend to remove excessive dentin at the curvature, leading to the file straightening the canal. This sharp transition angle can be useful for path finding in a straight canal, but dangerous when negotiating a curve. A conical-shaped tip has no ridges on its face, but the intersection of the face and the cutting edges can form sharp transition angles that can also cut dentin aggressively with the potential to straighten the canal. This can be reduced if a secondary cone is produced, removing the sharpness at the transition angle to provide a smooth surface that guides the tip through a curve (Fig. 15.2).

**Body**

The body of the instrument consists of an area that connects to the tip (inactive) and an active part, subdivided into the core or shank, and the flute or cutting edge. The active part is the one that varies most amongst instruments. Hand stainless steel instruments do not vary in taper (mostly .02), nor length (generally 16mm) but the manufacturing process is variable (Fig. 15.3).

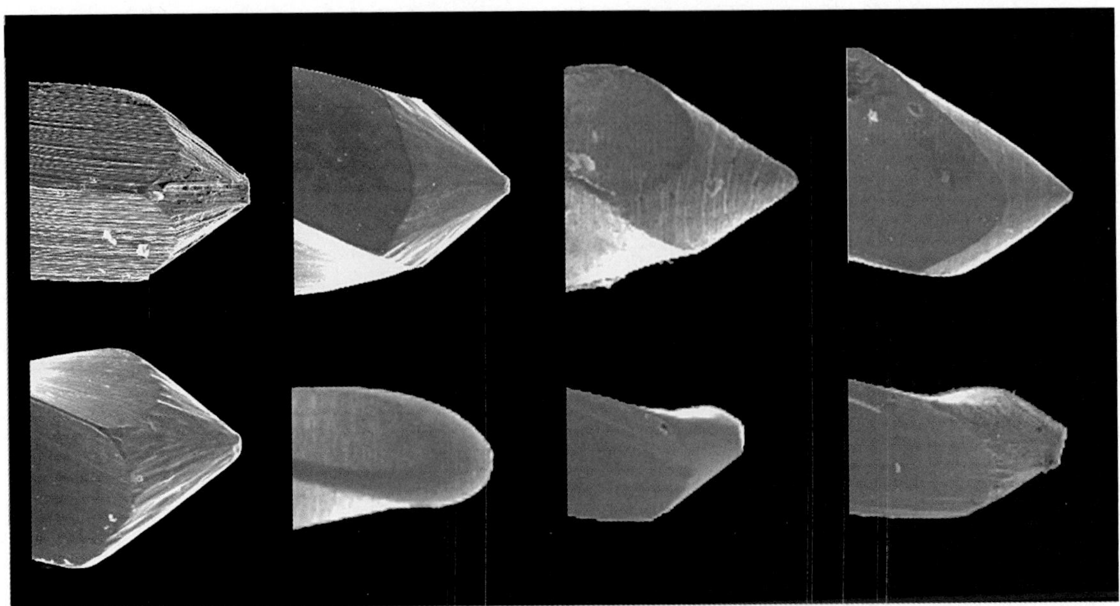

**Figure 15.2** - Designs of an instrument tip.

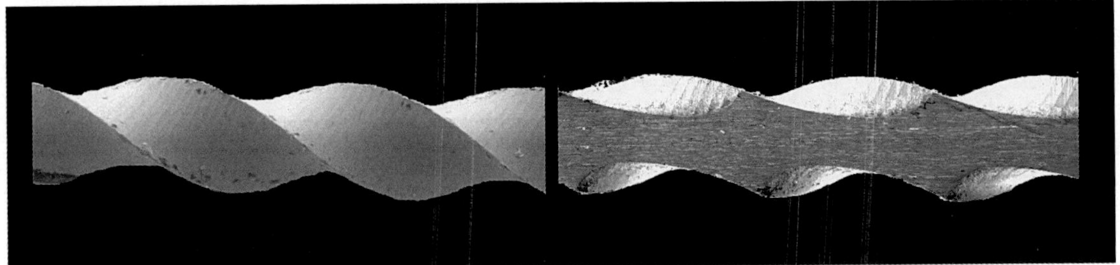

**Figure 15.3** - Several body designs that can influence the root canal shaping.

## Handle

The handle is important as it is the only part of the instrument that the operator can control directly. It varies in size, diameter, shape and texture depending on the manufacturer. For conventional stainless steel instruments color coding has facilitated standardization and recognition of the instrument to be used; more recent NiTi instruments have various, often non-standardized, color coding systems.

According to Grant et al.[30], grip strength is maximized by smaller handles with a consequent reduction in effort required. According to Osawa et al.[45] the handle size has an effect on reaming time and muscle activity and can therefore influence operator performance during instrumentation.

Chandler & Bloxham[14] found differences in operating time according to the handle design, with a barrel-shaped handle allowing more preparation both with and without gloves.

Handles are available in metal or plastic, whilst recently soft-texture silicone has been introduced with the aim of increasing tactile sensation from the instrument. However, to date no studies have been published to confirm such claims.

One important development in the use of stainless steel instruments is related to pathfinding that generally requires small files[3]. Unfortunately, regular files lack the rigidity to traverse constricted spaces and often buckle when vertical watch-winding forces are directed apically. Larger or more tapered files would have the necessary rigidity but are too bulky to pass through a constricted space. One method of overcoming the limitations of regular files is to grind a size # 08 or 10 K-file at the tip with a diamond disc, so as to obtain more rigidity as a result of the slightly larger diameters created further back from the tip[38]. More recently, however, manufacturers have started producing files specifically for pathfinding. In these instruments the tip is active, and stainless steel instruments are heat tempered to increase stiffness. Carbon steel is also useful to enhance sharpness[6]. Variations in shape, design, pitch, and taper have also been considered to maximize the necessary balance between small size, increased rigidity, and minimal deformation[12,13,19,20,39]. Allen et al.[3] compared several pathfinding instruments and reported a number of features that can influence the efficiency of these instruments. The pitch of an instrument may be important, because the more flutes an instrument has, the less flexible it becomes, and the more points of contact it creates for contributing to tactile sensation. An instrument with reduced pitched will be inherently more effective for filing, less effective for reaming. Other aspects include tip design, degree of spiraling, taper, cross-sectional design, heat tempering, metal type, operator skills, and clinical conditions.

### 15.3 Nickel-titanium Instruments

The use of nickel-titanium (NiTi) instruments can be considered a recent innovation. Their use in Dentistry was first described by Civjan et al.[16], using *Nitinol* (Ni – nickel; Ti – titanium; Nol – Naval ordnance Laboratory) in orthodontic wires. The satisfactory results obtained in their study made them suggest the use of NiTi alloys for cutting instruments, such as endodontic files. NiTi is composed of 55% nickel and 45% titanium, approximately (Fig. 15.4).

Miura et al.[42] tested the elastic modulus of NiTi in comparison with that of stainless steel. The low elasticity modulus of (5-6 x $10^3$ Kg/mm$^2$), contrasted with that of stainless steel (17-20 x $10^3$ Kg/mm$^2$), and this property of NiTi alloy was named superelasticity.

Walia et al.[69] were the first to study the use of #15 NiTi endodontic instruments, comparing them with stainless steel instruments of the same caliber. In addition to being more flexible, NiTi files had more resistance to torsion.

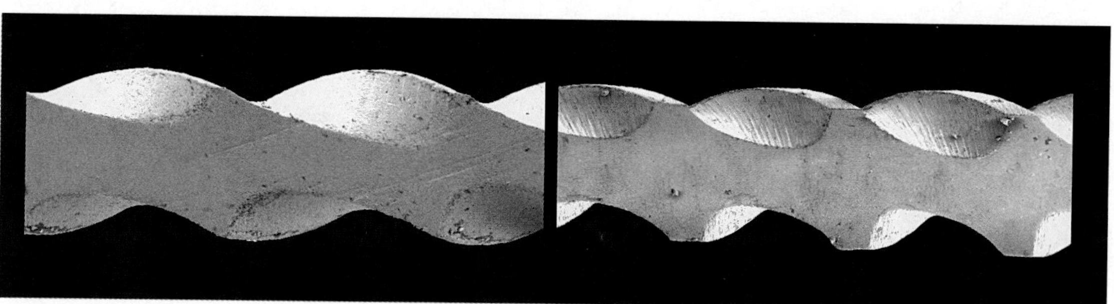

**Figure 15.4** - The body of a Niti instrument. The upper right image is a longitudinal section showing the shank and flutes[25].

Thompson[58] described the process of manufacturing nickel-titanium endodontic instruments, which requires the metal alloy to be cast under vacuum into an ingot. The instrument shape is ground from blanks produced from the cast; thus, it is important to understand that NiTi instruments differ from most stainless steel instruments that are twisted to create the cutting flutes.

According to Hülsmann et al.[33], NiTi is a 'shape memory alloy', existing in two different crystalline forms: austenite and martensite. The austenitic phase transforms into the martensitic phase on stressing at a constant temperature and in this form needs only light force for bending. After stress is released, the metal transforms back into the austenitic phase and the instrument regains its original shape. This means these instruments have the capability of retaining their original shape after mechanical deformation by temperature elevation.

Several studies on NiTi endodontic instruments followed the studies by Walia et al.[69], and considerable changes in instrument design and mode of use occurred. The curved canal became easier to negotiate, and lower stresses were exerted on dentin walls, allowing the creation of instruments with greater and more variable tapers, variable helical angles, rake angles and cross-sections. Nickel-titanium can reduce the incidence of transportation (Fig. 15.5) when compared with stainless steel instruments[18,27-29,48,58-64]. However, some reports show no difference in the incidence of transportation; particularly when stainless steel instrumentation was performed with either a balanced force technique or a turn-pull technique[32,51]. Less time is required for root canal preparation, and less extrusion of debris occurs when using rotary nickel-titanium instruments, compared with root canal preparation using stainless steel instruments[28,29].

The possibility of effectively increasing the taper within root canals is one of the most important advantages of NiTi instrumentation, as it can have a major influence on the ability of irrigants to penetrate deeply into the canal, as well as provide a better shape to fill it. The conventional step-back technique using .02 taper stainless steel instruments can provide canal tapers of .05 (1 mm step-back) or .10 (0.5 mm step-back); however, this requires a large series of instruments. On the other hand, a rotary .06 taper instrument will provide a taper of .06, with a single instrument if it goes to the length (Fig. 15.6).

Use of instruments of greater taper powered by an electric motor at low speeds and controlled torque has become popular and information on their safe use has emerged over the last few years.

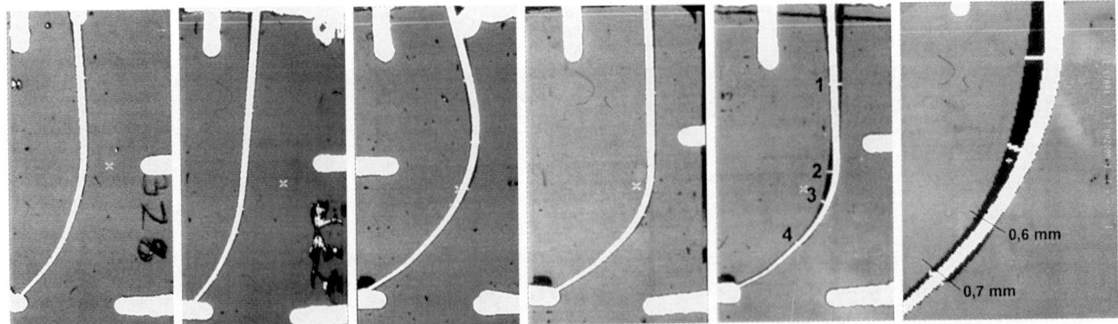


**Figure 15.5** - Simulated canals in resin blocks showing centered canals when NiTi (Pow-R) instruments were used (left and center images), and zip formation when stainless steel instrument (Flex-R) was used (image at the right) (Dummer, Bryant, Figueiredo et al – study performed in 1998 – 80 simulated canals were used to compare Pow-R rotary vs Flex-R stainless steel hand instrument – not published).

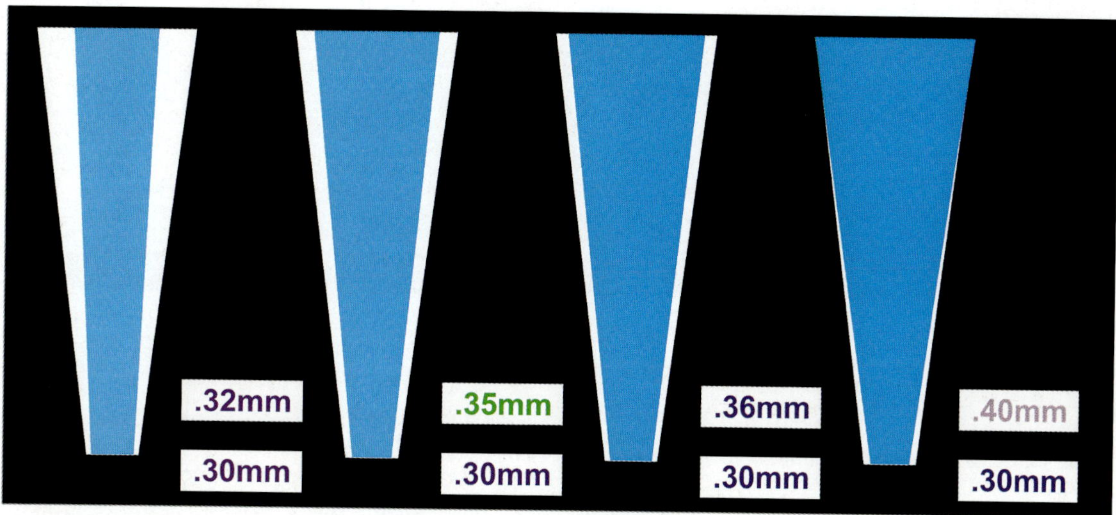


**Figure 15.6** - Representation of the effect of preparation on root canal taper. A conventional step-back technique can provide tapers of .05 or .10. However, it requires a large number of instruments stepping back every mm (.05 taper) or ½ mm (.10 taper). With one rotary NiTi instrument, similar tapers can be achieved (e.g .06 taper) using a tapered instrument (e.g. .06) (Adapted from Y-L Ng – UCL Eastman Dental Institute).

One design feature that remains controversial is the radial land and is it not known for certain whether this feature is beneficial or not for shaping canals (Fig. 15.7).

It can be hypothesized that the radial land reduces cutting efficiency and tends to allow the instruments to remain centered in the canal, thus increasing safety. Instruments without radial land would tend to be more aggressive, can be filed against the canal in a circumferential manner to plane more of the canal wall and are perceived to be more efficient. Modifying design features such as cutting angle, number of blades, tip design, taper and cross-section, further influences the flexibility, cutting efficacy, and strength of NiTi instruments[58] (Table 15.1).

Some of the rotary instrument designs are available in manual form. Such hand instruments can create space (glide path) for the rotary instruments that follow and allow them to function with less stress. Alternatively, they can be used to overcome sharp curves in a hybrid technique with rotary instruments or simply used alone. The manipulation of NiTi hand instruments with greater tapers can vary and include stem-winding, with balanced force, or a rotational movement.

The ADA identified a number of clinically relevant laboratory tests for nickel-titanium rotary instruments for comparing eight brands to provide the dental practitioner with appropriate comparative scientific information to assist in the purchase of these instruments (ADA Professional Product Review, 2006). The tests included the following: Dimensions (accuracy of the dimensions of the instrument specified by the manufacturer); Corrosion (ability of instruments to withstand repeated steam and heat sterilizations without exhibiting signs of corrosion); Stiffness (tests the flexibility of the instrument); Resistance to Fracture by twisting; Resistance to fatigue (the ability of an instrument to resist fracture when rotated in a flexed state at the manufacturer's recommended rotational speeds)[36].

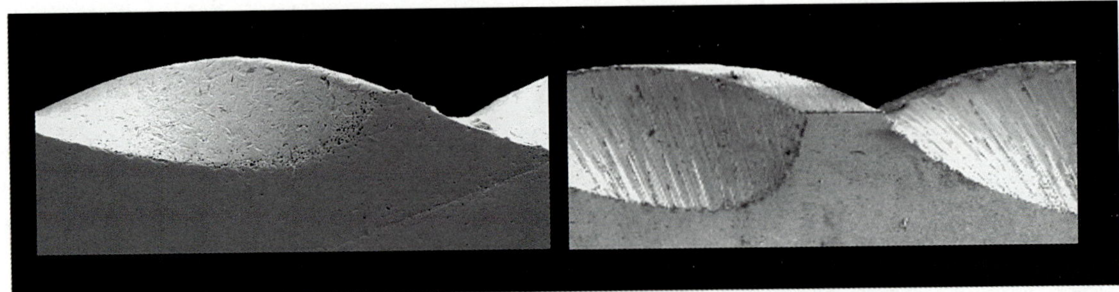

Figure 15.7 - A Rotary NiTi without radial land (left) compared with one containing.

**Table 15.1** - Summarizes the features of most of the rotary instruments available at present

| | Section | Tip | Radial Land | Rake Angle | Helical Angle | Taper & System |
|---|---|---|---|---|---|---|
| **Hero** | | Inactive | No | + | Variable | Variable .02 .04 .06 |
| **LightSpeed** | | Inactive | Complete | Neutral | - | - Sizes 20-100 |
| **Profile** | | Inactive | Complete | Neutral | Constant | Constant .04. 06 |
| **GT** | | Inactive | Complete | Neutral | Variable | Variable .06 .08 .10 .12 |
| **Quantec** | | Both | Hollow | + | Variable | Variable .02 .03 .04 .05 .06 |
| **K3** | | Inactive | Hollow | + | Variable | Variable .02 .04 .06 .08 .10 |
| **RaCe** | | Active | No | - | Alternating Helix | Variable |
| **ProTaper** | | Active | No | - | Variable | Progressive multitaper |
| **Pow-R** | | Active | No | - | Constant | Variable .02 .04 .06 |
| **FlexMaster** | | Active | No | - | Constant | Variable .02 .04 .06 |
| **ProTaper Universal** | | Inactive | No | + | Variable | Progressive multitaper |
| **Mtwo** | | Inactive | Hollow | + | Variable | Variable .02 .04 .05 .06 .07 |

Instrument fracture remains a problem with NiTi instruments. The main difficulty is that most practitioners prepare root canals with a NiTi rotary instrument as they would with a stainless steel hand instrument. Placing excess pressure on instruments, not moving them constantly within the canal, and using the step-back approach, are typical procedures that users of stainless-steel instruments undertake; however, such approaches with NiTi instruments can be catastrophic. Other risk factors include poor access cavity preparation, the use of high or variable rotational speeds, the use of deformed instruments, and not cleaning the instruments so that debris becomes packed along the flutes.

There are two main modes of instrument fracture. *Flexural fracture* consists of repeated compression and tension along the length of an instrument as it rotates in a curved canal when not moving in and out. This generally occurs with larger instruments, fracturing at the curvature and leaving a longer fragment within the canal. *Torsional fracture* is the shear fracture of the instrument when its tip becomes wedged and slows down in relation to the speed of the motor or does not rotate further. This occurs with smaller instruments, fracturing at the tip and leaving smaller fragments in the canal. Parashos et al.[47] found that about 70% of fractures were attributable to flexural fatigue. This is understandable as most root canals are curved.

Clearly, an instrument will cut only where it touches the canal wall. However, a large contact area increases the stress within the instrument, and breakage can occur. Reducing the contact area reduces the risk of breakage. Using a crown-down approach, with instruments of greater taper in a coronal direction, and of smaller taper apically (varied taper sequence), or larger sizes coronally and smaller sizes apically (varied tip sequence), or by varying both size and taper whilst allowing the instrument to go further down the canal (varied taper, varied tip sequence), promotes contact of small portions of the instrument against the dentin wall, reducing the risk of fracture. Alternatively, some instruments (e.g. ProTaper) have a variable taper and this automatically reduces the contact with the canal walls without the need to adopt a special technique.

All the available NiTi systems require straight line access to the coronal portion of the canal to reduce tension coronally that ultimately could lead to breakage.

The crown-down-pressureless technique[43] was adapted to the use of rotary instruments by using decreasing sizes of .04 or .06 instruments.

Calas & Vulcain[11] suggested a crown-down approach, in which the .06 instruments prepare the coronal third, the .04 taper prepares the middle third and the .02 taper prepares the apical third. It is claimed that this procedure facilitates the management of curved canals.

The VTVT (Varied Taper Varied Tip) sequence was proposed by Serota et al.[53] in 2004 and consists of a gentle "engage-disengage" pecking motion, with approximately 1-2mm depth per engagement; 5 gentle pecks to resistance with #25/.10 then #25/.08, working length determination, then 5 gentle pecks of #35/.06, #30/.04, #25/.06, #20/.04 in sequence, repeating the series until working length is reached. The apical portion can be increased with .02 hand rotary NiTi instruments. The aim of this sequence is to respect the apical anatomy and reach the length with a small set of instruments.

The only rotary NiTi technique that uses apical preparation to length initially is Lightspeed (LS), which consists of preparation to length beginning with the smallest LS instrument that binds and continues with sequentially larger sizes. The final apical preparation size is determined using the "12 pecks" rule, which ensures the canal is instrumented to a size large enough to ensure optimal canal debridement[52]. The cutting blade of LS instrument is small (0.25-2 mm in length), which permits large apical preparation with minimal risk of breakage.

Serota et al.[53] advocate the 'Apical Control Zone', which they describe as a matrix-like region created in the apical third of the root canal space. The zone demonstrates an exaggerated taper from the apical constriction defined spatially by the clinician as either a linear or point determination, which is claimed to provide resistance to the condensation pressures of obturation and acts to prevent the extrusion of the filling material.

Estrela & Figueiredo[22] suggest a hybrid technique that uses gauging, preparation of the orifice and cervical third of the root canal (with Gates-Glidden or LAAxxess burs followed by NiTi tapered orifice shapers), followed by length determination and preparation of the apical third using both NiTi and stainless steel instruments.

Wolcott & Himel[72] compared the torsional properties of NiTi and stainless steel files, and observed that fracture caused by torsion increased with increase in size. Camps & Pertot[12,13] showed that the opposite is observed for stainless steel files, i.e. an increase in size results in a decrease in fractures caused by torsion.

Cheung & Darwell[15] verified that the fatigue behavior of NiTi rotary instrument is typical of most metals, provided that the analysis is based on the surface strain amplitude, and showed a high-cycle and a low cycle fatigue (LCF) region. The LCF life is adversely affected by water.

A more robust flute in relation to the core of the instrument is also an important aspect of resistance. Biz & Figueiredo[8] assessed the shank-to-flute ratio in rotary nickel-titanium instruments and verified that the linear measurements of the instruments tested was similar amongst them; the area of the flute, however, tended to be greater in the more resistant instruments (Fig. 15.8).

Pre-flaring the root canal removes the curvature positioned along the coronal third of the canal, allowing free entrance of the instrument. This is not a new approach, since as early as 1885 the Gates Glidden drills, which are rotary stainless steel instruments, were used. Maintaining a glide path, particularly in the apical third facilitates control of the instrument, and cutting of strategic portions of dentin to avoid pressure. The pressure must be light and gentle, always respecting the anatomical variations of the canal system.

The number of uses negatively affects the resistance to fracture of rotary NiTi instruments (Fig. 15.9). Troian et al.[65] demonstrated that distortion of spirals and wear increased with progressive use of RaCe instruments, whereas K3 instruments remained relatively undamaged after their fifth use. Simulated canals with smaller radii of curvature were positively associated with fracture of RaCe instruments.

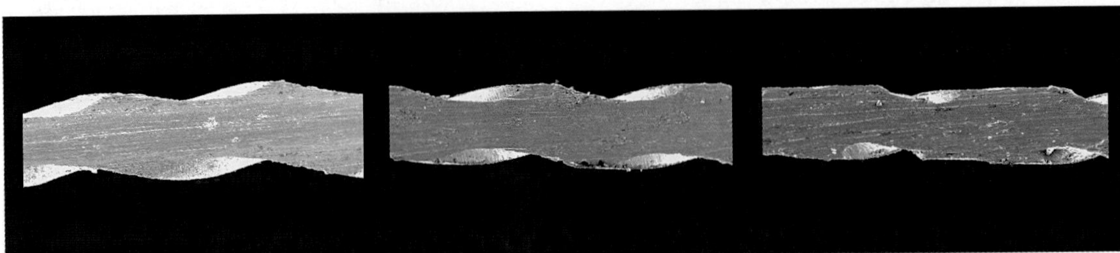

**Figure 15.8** - The increased amount of flute area influences the resistance to breakage of the instruments. The more robust the flute, the more resistant the instrument is. (SEM Images – Biz & Figueiredo[8]).

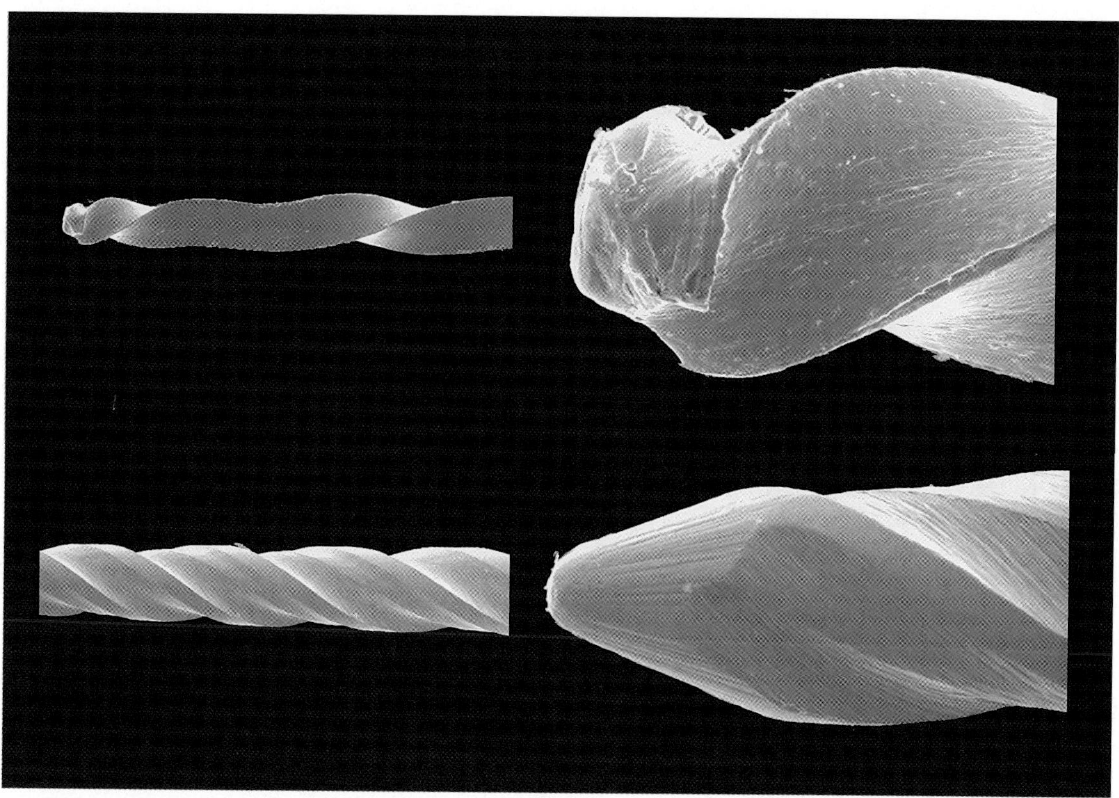

**Figure 15.9** - RaCe instruments (above) were affected by the repetitive use in simulated canals; K3 (below) was not affected. It is possible to speculate that the robust flute area of K3 contributed to the results (Troian et al.[9]).

All new instruments contain small cracks that propagate with repeated use. Electropolishing has been suggested as a method of overcoming this problem, as it has the potential to enhance the resistance of the instruments. According to Anderson et al.[5], electropolished instruments performed significantly better than non-electropolished instruments in cyclic fatigue testing, and to a lesser extent, under static torsional loading. When viewing electropolished instruments by SEM, milling grooves, cracks, pits, and areas of metal rollover were observed, although they were more evident in the non-electropolished instruments. Electropolishing may have beneficial effects on prolonging the fatigue life of rotary NiTi endodontic instruments, probably by a reduction in surface irregularities that serve as points for stress concentration and crack initiation.

Keeping NiTi rotary instruments moving within the canal reduces crack propagation. In addition, periodic cleaning of dentin and pulp debris from the flutes reduces friction against canal walls (Fig. 15.10). The flutes must be checked after every use, and instrument discarded if any alteration in shape is noted; some manufacturers advise a single use for their NiTi rotary instruments, and the dental authorities in some countries, e.g. the UK., have made single use of endodontic instruments compulsory.

Canal anatomy is a major challenge for successful root canal preparation. Root canal systems vary in terms of the number of canals in each root, their length, curvature and diameter.[33] The apical anatomy with accessory canals and ramifications adds to the challenge. Communications between the canal space and the lateral periodontium and

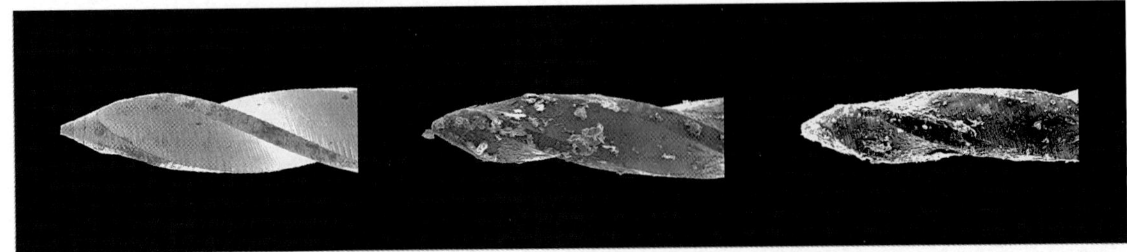

**Figure 15.10** - Instruments considered ready for use may not be clean. Only the first instrument is properly decontaminated.

the furcation area, the dentinal tubular system and the effect of microorganisms living in an anaerobic environment with sufficient nutrients for the biofilm to sustain bacterial growth, or survival under stringent conditions, are some of the factors that influence the effect of shaping as an adjunct to the cleaning procedures[31] (Fig. 15.11).

## 15.4 Reciprocating Devices

Canal preparation using reciprocating handpieces is an alternative to hand and rotary instrumentation for primary root canal treatment, as well as for endodontic retreatment. The handpiece provides 30° to 90° reciprocal (back and forth) movement and the attached instruments remove dentin more rapidly and more aggressively. M4, Endo-Gripper, Endo-Eze, Intra-Endo, amongst others, were all developed from the Giromatic handpiece, originally designed and marketed in the 1950s. The Giromatic technique did not become popular world-wide because the instruments had poor design features, did not shape canals effectively, and were associated with inappropriate filling techniques and materials.

The use of a reciprocating handpiece helps the development of tactile control differing from that obtained by hand instrumentation, and may allow a transitional stage for the operator to eventually move towards mechanical rotary instrumentation. Another advantageous feature of reciprocating devices is that they have the potential for allowing the operator to better prepare oval and mesiodistally flattened root canals[73].

The disadvantage of reciprocating instrumentation is that it tends to fail to negotiate curves[46]. Because of this, the Endo-Eze system recommends this mechanical approach be used in a crown-down mode only until approximately 3 mm short of the canal length. The apical files with the system are hand files with shortened cutting flutes to cut only in the apical region of the canal and are used in a clockwise turn and pull motion. Studies with this system have shown good cutting efficiency, especially in canals with oval cross-section, but not as good a performance along the curve.

## 15.5 Endosonics

Ultrasonics can be defined as the science of sound waves above the limits of human audibility (20-100 KHz). The sound transmits vibration through an elastic medium which may be a solid, liquid, or a gas. This produces shock events that are sources of a single compression wave that radiates from the source, either through magnetostriction or through a piezoelectric effect. Magnetostriction converts electromagnetic energy into mechanical energy. The piezoelectric principle consists of a crystal that changes dimension when an electrical charge is applied, converting the energy into mechanical oscillation without producing heat[56]. Piezoelectric units are extensively used in endodontics, as they are more powerful and generate less heat[56].

Endosonics is the use of ultrasonics for endodontic purposes, bringing together the separate procedures of canal debridement, cleansing, irrigation, disinfection and shaping. They produce two effects: cavitation, which is the stable or transient formation of gas or vapor filled bubbles growing under negative pressure until they collapse under compression to gen-

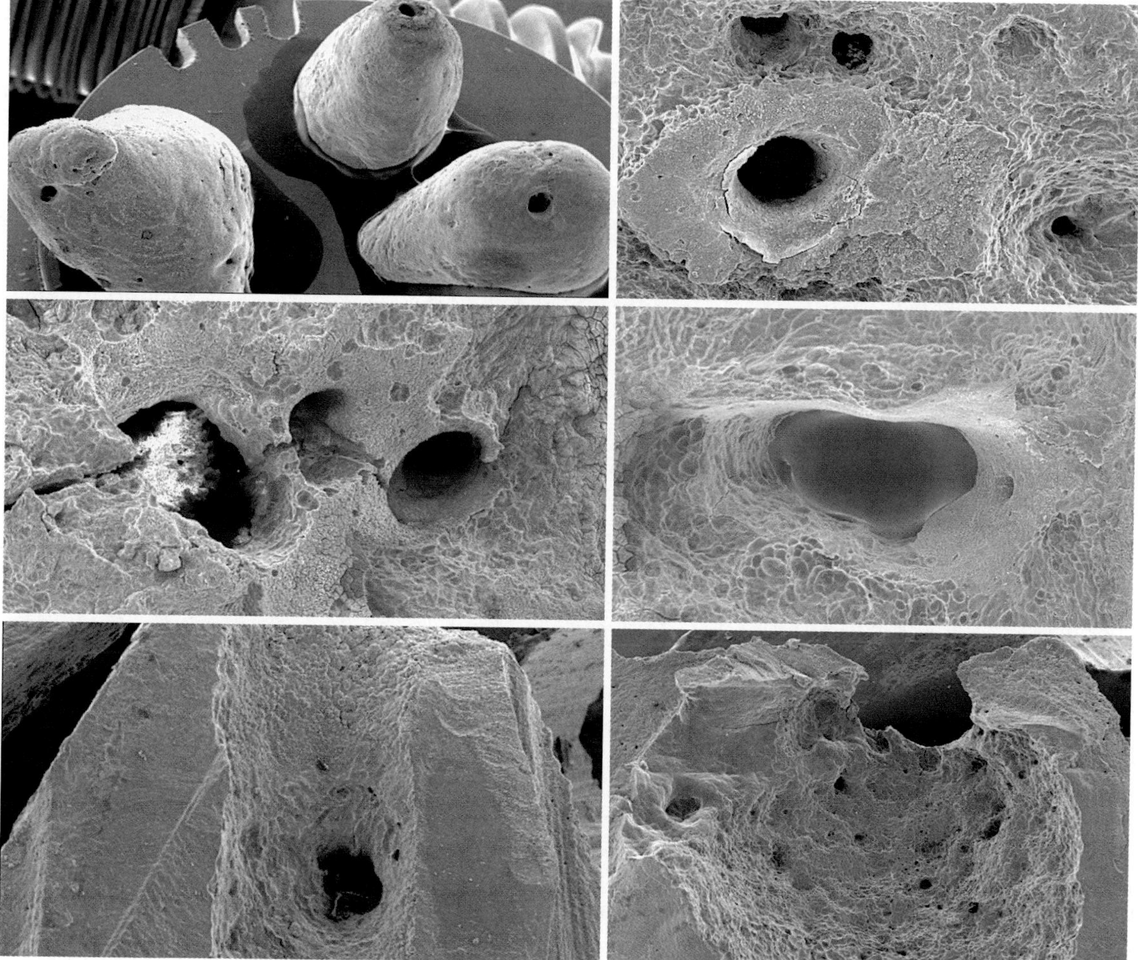

**Figure 15.11** - Apices of root canals showing diverse aspects of the foraminal anatomy, and the influence of apical infection that results in root resorption, which contributes to the difficulties during root canal treatment (Vier & Figueiredo[67,68]).

erate a new cycle of bubble growth; acoustic micro-streaming is the creation of intense circular fluid movements or flow patterns around vibrating files, which enhance the cleaning effect of the irrigating solution in the pulp space through hydrodynamic shear stress.

Although the potential uses for ultrasonics suggest a highly effective and efficient system, the literature is conflicting on the efficacy of ultrasonic devices, particularly for shaping canals. Reasons for the lack of consistent research results can be explained by the variation in the endosonic systems tested, the different instrument designs used with the systems, as well as variations with the methodology. Other factors influence their shaping ability include, power output, interfacial force, and direction of file oscillation[9,10,49].

It is widely accepted that endosonics is a useful and effective method for cleaning canals. In association with NaOCl and EDTA, the technique removes the smear layer and exposes dentinal tubules and canalicules, facilitating disinfection and filling of the root canal system (Fig. 15.12).

Controversy surrounds the use of endosonic devices in terms of whether they should be used with active or passive manipulation within the canal system. Passive activation implies that no attempt is made to instrument, plane, or contact the canal walls with the vibrating file, to allow its free oscillation.

When a file touches the dentin wall the amplitude of oscillation will diminish[70]. With the vibrating file oscillating freely in a prepared canal with larger dimensions after instrumentation, reports have indicated they have been cleaner than when the file contacted the canal wall[2]. To maximize the effects of acoustic streaming, smaller files should be used within the canal space.

The presence of flutes along the endosonic files is another matter of debate. Van der Sluis et al.[66] suggested that a smooth wire is able to clean canal walls sufficiently well to improve the sealing ability of canal fillings. However, Munley & Goodel[44] demonstrated that a standard fluted file used for 3 minutes with passive ultrasonic irrigation was superior for debris removal when considering the entire canal space. When used with ultrasonics, non-fluted finger spreaders did not improve debris removal.

To improve shaping ability of endosonics it is advisable to use a small, precurved flexible file (e.g. #15), applying a high power setting coronally and lower power setting apically, in an attempt to avoid apical transportation.

## 15.6 Laser

The word Laser is an acronym for Light Amplification by Stimulated Emission of Radiation. According to Kimura et al.[37] a laser is a device that transforms light of various frequencies into a chromatic radiation in the visible, infrared, and ultraviolet regions with all the waves in phase capable of mobilizing immense heat and power when focused at close range.

Lasers have been suggested in endodontics for several uses:

- *Low intensity*: Diagnosis of pulp blood flow (Laser Doppler flowmetry); treatment of dentinal sensitivity; pulpotomies (biostimulation); post-surgical endodontics (pain reduction + healing acceleration).
- *High intensity*: Treatment of dentin sensitivity; pulpotomies; endodontic surgery (apicectomy); root canal cleaning (removal of smear layer); root canal sterilization (dentin melting); root canal shaping; root canal obturation.

Sydney et al.[55] studied the effect of irrigation on endodontic shaping with Nd-YAG laser. The absence of irrigation resulted in various levels of dentin melting, whilst the use of a water delivery system along the fiber optic tip resulted in different patterns of smear layer removal. The influence of the laser was dependent on the action of the fiber optic tip, as well as the angle at which the beam touched the canal walls. In one case, a ledge appeared to have been created. These unclear benefits, together with the high costs, and the safety implications, mean that lasers in endodontic treatment require further development in order to be considered for daily use in a dental practice.

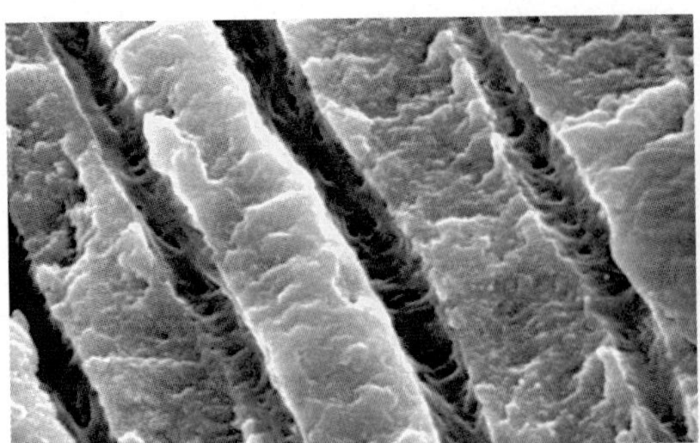
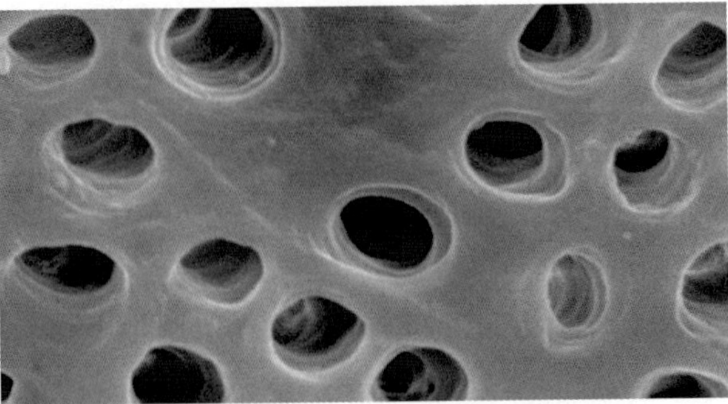

**Figure 15.12** - SEM of root canals cleaned with endosonics in combination with NaOCl and EDTA. Note that the longitudinal sections as well as the tubule openings show clean tubules exposing canalicules.

## References



1. Abou-Rass M, Frank AL, Glick DH. The anticurvature filing method to prepare the curved root canal. J Amer Dent Assoc 1980;101:792-4.
2. Ahmad M, Pitt Ford TJ, Crum LA. Ultrasonic debridement of root canals: acoustic streaming and its possible role. J Endod 1987;13:490–9.
3. Allen MJ, Glickman GN, Griggs JA. Comparative analysis of endodontic pathfinders. J Endod 2007;33:723-6.
4. Allison DA, Weber CR, Walton RE. The influence of the method of canal preparation on the quality of apical and coronal obturation. J Endod 1979;5:298-304.
5. Anderson ME, Price JWH, Parashos P. Fracture resistance of electropolished rotary nickel–titanium endodontic instruments. J Endod 2007;33:1112-6.
6. Ashby M, Jones D. Engineering Materials 2. Oxford: Pergamon Press; 1992. p.11. Chapter 12.
7. Bellizzi R, Cruse WP. A historic review of endodontics, 1689–1963. Part III. J Endod 1980;6:576–80.
8. Biz MT, Figueiredo JAP. Morphometric analysis of shank-to-flute ratio in rotary nickel-titanium files. Int Endod J 2004;37:353-8.
9. Briggs P, Gulabivala K, Stock CJR, Setchell DJ. The dentine-removing characteristics of an ultrasonically energised K-File. Int Endod J 1989;22:259–68.
10. Briggs P, Gulabivala K, Setchell DJ. Dentine-removing characteristics of K-files energised by the PiezonEndo. Int Endod J 1992;25:6–14.
11. Calas P, Vulcain JM. Le concept du HERO 642. Rev Odont-Stom 1999;28:1–10.
12. Camps J, Pertot W. Relationship between file size and stiffness of stainless steel instruments. Endod Dent Traumatol 1994;10:260–3.
13. Camps JJ, Pertot WJ. Torsional and stiffness properties of nickel-titanium K files. Int Endod J 1995;28:239–43.
14. Chandler N, Bloxham G. The influence of two handle designs and gloves on the performance of a simulated endodontic task. J Endod 1990;16:541-2.
15. Cheung GSP, Darvell BW. Fatigue testing of a NiTi rotary instrument. Part 1: strain-life relationship. Int Endod J 2007;40:612-8.
16. Civjan S, Huget EF, DeSimon LB. Potential applications of certain nickel-titanium (nitinol) alloys. J Dent Res 1975;54:89-96.
17. Clem WH. Endodontics: the adolescent patient. Dent Clin North Amer 1969; 13:483-93.
18. Coleman CL, Svec TA, Rieger MR, Suchina JA, Wang MM, Glickman GN. Analysis of nickel–titanium versus stainless steel instrumentation by means of direct digital imaging. J Endod 1996;22:603–7.
19. Cormier CJ, von Fraunhofer JA, Chamberlain JH. A comparison of endodontic file quality and file dimensions. J Endod 1988;14:138–42.
20. Dearing GJ, Kazemi RB, Stevens RH. An objective evaluation comparing the physical properties of two brands of stainless steel endodontic hand files. J Endod 2005;31:827–30.
21. Del Bello TPL, Wang N, Roane JB. Crown-Down tip design and shaping. J Endod 2003;29:513-18.
22. Estrela C. Estudo comparativo do desgaste dentinário da parede distal do canal mesiovestibular do 1° molar inferior, produzido por três técnicas de instrumentação. (Master's Dissertation), Federal University of Pelotas, 1990.
23. Estrela C, Figueiredo JAP. Técnica híbrida para preparo de canais curvos. Rev Odontol Brasil Central 2001;10:14-21.
24. Fauchard P. Le chirurgien-dentiste – traite des dents. 2 nd ed. Paris: Chez Pierre Jean Marriete; 1745. 182p.
25. Filippini HF, Figueiredo JAP. Evaluation of endodontic file surface on EDX and SEM. J Dent Res 2002;81:B42-B42.
26. Freund J, Toivonen R, Takala E-P. Grip forces of the fingertips. Clin Biomech 2002;17:515-20.
27. Gambill JM, Alder M, del Rio CE. Comparison of nickel–titanium and stainless steel hand-file instrumentation using computed tomography. J Endod 1996;22:369–75.
28. Glosson CR, Haller RH, Dove SB, del Rio CE. A comparison of root canal preparations using Ni–Ti hand, Ni–Ti engine-driven and K-Flex endodontic instruments. J Endod 1995;21:146–151.
29. Gluskin AH, Brown DC, Buchanan LS. A reconstructed computerized tomographic comparison of Ni–Ti rotary GT™ files versus traditional instruments in canals shaped by novice operators. Int Endod J 2001;34:476–84.
30. Grant KA, Habes DJ, Steward LL. An analysis of handle designs for reducing manual effort: The influence of grip diameter. Int J Ind Ergon 1992;10:199-206.
31. Gulabivala K, Patel B, Evans G, Ng Y-L. Effects of mechanical and chemical procedures on root canal surfaces. Endod Topics 2005;10:103-22.
32. Harlan AL, Nicholls JI, Steiner JC. A comparison of curved canal instrumentation using nickel–titanium or stainless steel files with the balanced-force technique. J Endod 1996;22:410–3.
33. Hulssmann M, Peters OA, Dummer PMH. Mechanical preparation of root canals: shaping goals, techniques and means. Endod Topics 2005;10:30-76.
34. Ingle JI. Standardized endodontic technique utilizing newly designed instruments and filling materials. Oral Surg Oral Med Oral Pathol 1961;14:83-91.
35. Ingle JI, Levine M. The need for uniformity of endodontic instrument, equipments and filling materials. 2nd International Conference on Endodontics; 1958.
36. Jambi S. Fatigue life of Profile nickel-titanium rotary instrument under pure bending stresses. MClinDent thesis, UCL Estman Dental Institute; 2007.
37. Kimura Y, Wilder-Smith P, Matsumoto K. Lasers in endodontics: a review. Int Endod J 1999;33:173-85.
38. Kobaiashi C. Penetration of constricted canals with modified K files. J Endod 2007; 23:391–3.
39. Krup JD, Brantley WA, Gerstein H. An investigation of the torsional and bending properties of seven brands of endodontic files. J Endod 1984; 10:372– 80.
40. Lopes HP, Elias CN, Siqueira Jr JF. Instrumentos endodonticos. In: Lopes HP, Siqueira Jr JF. Endodontia: biologia e tecnica. 2nd ed. Rio de Janeiro: Guanabara Koogan; 2004. pp.323-417.

41. Miserendino LJ, Moser JB, Heuer MA, Osetek EM. Cutting efficiency of endodontic instruments. Part II: Analysis of tip design. J Endod 1986;12:8-12.
42. Miura F, Mogi M, Ohura Y, Hamanaka H. The super-elastic property of the japanese NiTi alloy wire for use in orthodontics. Am J Orthod Dentofacial Orthop 1986;90:1-10.
43. Morgan LA, Montgomery S. An evaluation of the crown-down pressureless technique. J Endod 1984;10:491-8.
44. Munley PJ, Goodell GG. Comparison of passive ultrasonic debridement between fluted and nonfluted instruments in root canals. J Endod 2007;33:578-80.
45. Ozawa T, Nakano M, Sugimura H, Tahata K, Nakamura J, Shiozawa K. Effects of endodontic instrument handle diameter on electromyographic activity of forearm and hand muscles. Int Endod J 2001;34:100-6.
46. Paque F, Barbakow F, Peters OA. Root canal preparation with Endo-Eze AET: changes in root canal shape assessed by micro-computed tomography. Int Endod J 2005;38:456–64.
47. Parashos P, Gordon I, Messer HH. Factors influencing defects of rotary nickel-titanium endodontic instruments after clinical use. J Endod 2004;30:722-5.
48. Pettiette MT, Metzger Z, Phillips C, Trope M. Endodontic complications of root-canal therapy performed by dental students with stainless-steel K-files and nickel–titanium hand files. J Endod 1999;25:230–4.
49. Regan JD, Sherriff M, Meredith N, Gulabivala K. A survey of interfacial forces used during endosonic instrumentation of root canals. Int Endod J 2001;34:54–62.
50. Roane JB, Sabala CL, Duncanson MG. The balanced force concept for instrumentation of curved canals. J Endod 1985;11:203-11.
51. Schäfer E. Effects of various sterilization procedures on the cutting efficiency of root-canal instruments. Deutsche Zahn Zeitschrift 1995;50:150–3.
52. Senia ES, Wildey WL. The LightSpeed root canal instrumentation system. Endod Topics 2005;10:148-50.
53. Serota KS, Nahmias Y, Barnett F, Brock M, Senia ES. Predeictable endodontic success: the apical control zone. Oral Health 2003;3:75-89.
54. Serota KS, Vera J, Barnett F, Nahmias Y. The new era of foramenal location. Oral Health 2004;4:48-54.
55. Sydney GB, Figueiredo JAP, Melo LL. SEM analysis of cleaning and shaping canals with Nd: YAG laser. J Dent Res 1999;78:1028.
56. Stock CJR. Current status of the use of ultrasound in endodontics. Int Dent J 1991;41:175– 82.
57. Stock C, Walker R, Gulabivala K. Endodontics. 3rd ed. London: Elsevier Mosby; 2004. 324p.
58. Thompson SA. An overview of nickel–titanium alloys used in dentistry. Int Endod J 1980;33:297-310.
59. Thompson SA, Dummer PMH. Shaping ability of Lightspeed rotary nickel-titanium instruments in simulated root canals. Part 2. J Endod 1997;23:742-7.
60. Thompson SA, Dummer PMH. Shaping ability of ProFile.04 Taper Series 29 rotary nickel–titanium instruments in simulated root canals. Part 2. Int Endod J 1997;30:8-15.
61. Thompson SA, Dummer PMH. Shaping ability of NT Engine and McXim rotary nickel–titanium instruments in simulated root canals. Part 2. Int Endod J 1997; 30:270-8.
62. Thompson SA, Dummer PMH. Shaping ability of Mity Roto 360 and Naviflex rotary nickel–titanium instruments in simulated root canals. Part 2. J Endod 1998;24:135-42.
63. Thompson SA, Dummer PMH. Shaping ability of Quantec Series 2000 rotary nickel–titanium instruments in simulated root canals. Part 2. Int Endod J 1998;31:268-74.
64. Thompson SA, Dummer PMH. Shaping ability of Hero 642 rotary nickel–titanium instruments with ISO sized tips in simulated root canals. Part 1. Int Endod J 2000;33:248-54.
65. Troian CH, So MVR, Figueiredo JAP, Oliveira EPM. Deformation and fracture of RaCe and K3 endodontic instruments according to the number of uses. Int Endod J 2006;39: 616–625.
66. van der Sluis LWM, Shemesh H, Wu MK, Wesselink PR. An evaluation of the influence of passive ultrasonic irrigation on the seal of root canal fillings. Int Endod J 2007;40:356–61.
67. Vier FV, Figueiredo JAP. Prevalence of different periapical lesions associated with human teeth and their correlation with the presence and extension of apical external root resorption. Int Endod J 2002;35:710-9.
68. Vier FV, Figueiredo JAP. Internal apical resorption and its correlation with the type of apical lesion. Int Endod J 2004;37:730–7.
69. Walia H, Brantley WA, Gerstein H. An initial investigation of the bending and torsional properties of nitinol root canal files. J Endod 1988;14:346–51.
70. Walmsley AD. Ultrasound and root canal treatment: the need for scientific evaluation. Int Endod J 1987;20:105–11.
71. Weine FS, Kelly RF, Lio PJ. The effect of preparation procedures on original canal shape and on apical foramen. J Endod 1975; 1: 255-262.
72. Wolcott J, Himel VT. Torsional properties of nickel-titanium versus stainless steel endodontic files. J Endod 1997;23:217-20.
73. Zmener O, Pameijer CH, Banegas G. Retreatment efficacy of hand versus automated instrumentation in oval-shaped root canals: an ex vivo study. Int Endod J 2006;39:521-6.

Carlos Estrela

# Endodontic Science

Volume 2

# Endodontic Science

**Carlos Estrela, DDS, MSc, PhD**
Chairman and Professor of Endodontics,
Department of Stomatologic Sciences
Federal University of Goiás, Goiânia, GO, Brazil

Volume 2

**2009**

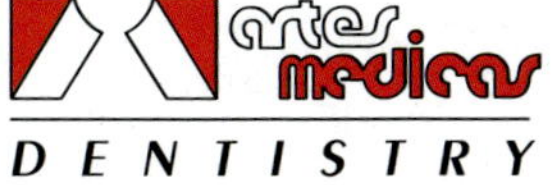

Endodontic Science

ISBN 978-85-367-0083-0



**Publishing Director**

Milton Hecht

**Production Manager**

Fernanda Matajs

**Editorial Production/Cover**

Júnior Bianchi

**Translation Reviewing**

Margery Galbraith

**Printing**

RR Donnelley

Dados Internacionais de Catalogação na Publicação (CIP)
(Câmara Brasileira do Livro, SP, Brasil)

Estrela, Carlos
Endodontic science / Carlos Estrela ; [translation reviewing Margery Galbraith]. - - São Paulo : Artes Médicas, 2009.

Título original: Ciência endodôntica.
Vários colaboradores.
Obra em 2 v.
Bibliografia.
ISBN 978-85-367-0083-0

1. Endodontia I. Título.

08-10697 CDD-617.6342

Índices para catálogo sistemático:

1. Endodontia 617.6342

**Editora Artes Médicas Ltda.**

R. Dr. Cesário Motta Jr, 63 - Vila Buarque - 01221-020 - São Paulo - SP - Brazil

www.artesmedicas.com.br - artesmedicas@artesmedicas.com.br

Tel.: 55 11 3221-9033 - Fax: 55 11 3223-6635

# About the Author

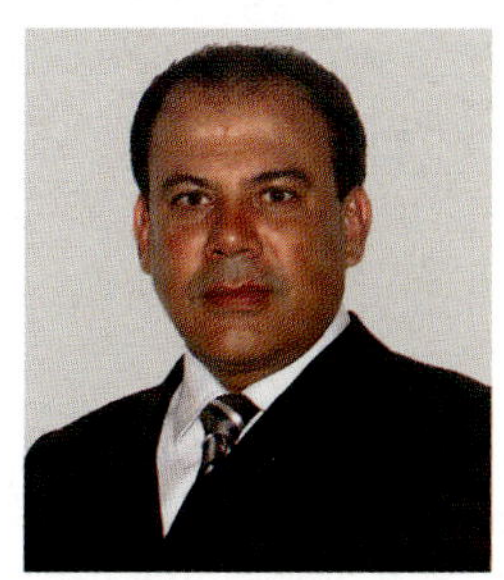


**CARLOS ESTRELA, DDS, MSc, PhD**

Chairman and Professor of Endodontics,
Department of Stomatologic Sciences
Federal University of Goiás, Goiânia, GO, Brazil


Carlos Estrela graduated from Dental School in 1983, in Anápolis, GO, Brazil, and specialized in Endodontics in 1988 from the Brazilian Dental Association in Goiania, GO, Brazil. He completed the MSc Course in Endodontology at the Federal University of Pelotas in 1990. He obtained his PhD in 1994, at the University of São Paulo, Brazil. In 1997 he obtained the position of Free Lecturer from the University of Sao Paulo, in Ribeirao Preto, SP, Brazil. Since 1993 he has taught at the Dental School of the Federal University of Goias, where he has served as Professor and Chairman of Endodontology since 1995. Dr Estrela has been published in the field of Endodontics and Dentistry, having authored 8 books in Dentistry in Portuguese, with 2 translated into Spanish and 1 currently being translated into English. He has published 130 papers in refereed journals and 130 chapters in books. He has lectured extensively in Brazil and Latin America, with more than 300 courses in Endodontics in different countries. He is the Coordinator of the Specialty Course in Endodontology of the Brazilian Dental Association of Goias, Brazil, since 1993. He participates in the Post-graduate Programs in Dentistry at the Masters and PhD levels of the Federal University of Goias and the Federal University of Uberlandia, in Brazil. He is a member of the Editorial Board of several journals in Dentistry, including the prestigious International Endodontic Journal. His areas of interest in research are Oral Microbiology, Endodontic irrigation and medication, Endodontic techniques and imaging related to the root canal system.

# Dedication

To Master Jesus, who showed us the importance of love, the need for faith, hope, charity, essential ingredients for excellence in life.

To all spiritual protectors and friends, for the affection, security, harmony and peace, factors that strengthened our emotions.

To my angels, and loves, gifts from Heaven – Cyntia, Lucas, Matheus, Maria Cristina and Pedro; my parents, Odilon and Maria, indispensable to my life.

To the eternal friend Hildeberto Francisco Pesce, for believing in the possibility of the invisible, coherence of the complex, to see the color of wind and time without space. Here it is my Master, thank you for existing, for walking with me and keeping our commitments.

To all estimated researchers, clinicians and friends who share the same scientific emotions, essential in building this book, my admiration, respect and great affection.

**Roberto Holland, DDS, MSc, PhD**
*Professor of Endodontics, São Paulo State University, Araçatuba, SP, Brazil*

**P. N. Ramachamdran Nair, BVSc, DVM, PhD, Senior Scientist**
*Institute of Oral Biology, Center of Dental and Oral Medicine,University of Zurich, Zurich, Switzerland*

**Carlos Alberto Souza Costa, DDS, MSc, PhD**
*Professor of Oral Pathology, São Paulo State University, Araraquara, SP, Brazil*

**José Antônio Poli de Figueiredo, DDS, MSc, PhD**
*Professor of Endodontics, Pontifical Catholic University of Rio Grande do Sul, Porto Alegre,RS, Brazil*

**Josimery Hebling, DDS, MSc, PhD**
*Professor of Pediatric Dentistry, São Paulo State University, Araraquara, SP, Brazil*

**Ana Helena G. Alencar, DDS, MSc, PhD**
*Professor of Endodontics, Federal University of Goiás, Goiânia, GO, Brazil*

**Sueli Satomi Murata, DDS, MSc, PhD**
*São Paulo State University, Araçatuba, SP, Brazil*

**Cyntia R.A. Estrela, DDS, MSc, PhD**
*Brazilian Dentistry Research and Learning Center, CEPOBRAS, Goiânia, GO, Brazil*

**Mike Reis Bueno, DDS, MSc, PhD**
*Professor of Diagnosis and Radiology, University of Cuiabá, Cuiabá, MT, Brazil*

**Lili Luesche Bammann, DDS, MSc, PhD**
*Professor of Microbiology, Federal University of Pelotas, Pelotas, RS, Brazil*

**Jesus Djalma Pécora, DDS, MSc, PhD**
*Professor of Endodontics, University of São Paulo, Ribeirão Preto, SP, Brazil*

**Paul M.H. Dummer, DDS, MSc, PhD**
*Department of Adult Dental Health, Dental School, Wales College of Medicine, Cardiff University, Cardiff, UK*

**Gilson Blitzkow Sydney, DDS, MSc, PhD**
*Professor of Endodontics, Federal University of Paraná, Curitiba, PR, Brazil*

**Hélio Pereira Lopes, DDS, MSc, PhD**
*Professor of Endodontics, Brazilian Endodontic Association, Rio de Janeiro, RJ, Brazil*

**Carlos Nelson Elias, DDS, MSc, PhD**
*Engeneering Military Institute, Rio de Janeiro, RJ, Brazil*

**Manoel Damião Sousa Neto DDS, MSc, PhD**
*University of São Paulo, Ribeirão Preto, SP, Brazil*

# Collaborators

**Lourdes Esponda, DDS, MSc**
*Professor of Endodontics, University of Mexico, MX, Mexico*

**Álvaro Gonzalez Cruz, DDS, MSc**
*Professor of Endodontics, University of Guadalajara, Jal, Mexico*

**João Carlos Gabrielli Biffi, DDS, MSc, PhD**
*Federal University of Uberlândia, Uberlândia, MG, Brazil*

**Marcelo Sampaio Moura, DDS, MSc, PhD**
*Brazilian Dentistry Research and Learning Center, CEPOBRAS, Goiânia, GO, Brazil*

**Maria Ilma de Souza Côrtes, DDS, MSc, PhD**
*Pontifical Catholic Uniersity of Minas Gerais, Belo Horizonte, MG, Brazil*

**Juliana Vilela Bastos, DDS, MSc, PhD**
*Federal University of Minas Gerais, Belo Horizonte, MG, Brazil*

**Pedro Felício Estrada Bernabé, DDS, MSc, PhD**
*São Paulo State University, Araçatuba, SP, Brazil*

**Elismauro Francisco de Mendonça, DDS, MSc, PhD**
*Professor of Oral Pathology, Federal University of Goiás, Goiânia, GO, Brazil*

**Daniel Almeida Decurcio, DDS, MSc**
*Professor of Endodontics, Federal University of Goiás, Goiânia, GO, Brazil*

**Aleimar Moraes Toledo, DDS, Fellow**
*Postgraduate Student, Federal University of Goiás, Goiânia, GO, Brazil*

**Cláudio Rodrigues Leles, DDS, MSc, PhD**
*Professor of Prosthesis, Federal University of Goiás, Goiânia, GO, Brazil*

**Júlio Almeida Silva, DDS, MSc**
*Professor of Endodontics, Federal University of Goiás, Goiânia, GO, Brazil*

**Luiz Augusto Faitaroni, DDS, Fellow**
*Brazilian Dentistry Research and Learning Center, CEPOBRAS, Goiânia, GO, Brazil*

**Orlando Aguirre Guedes, DDS, MSc**
*Professor of Endodontics, Federal University of Goiás, Goiânia, GO, Brazil*

**Welington Pereira Júnior, DDS, MSc**
*Brazilian Dentistry Research and Learning Center, CEPOBRAS, Goiânia, GO, Brazil*

**Sicknan S. Rocha, DDS, MSc, PhD**
*Professor of Prosthesis, Federal University of Goiás, Goiânia, GO, Brazil*

**João Batista de Souza, DDS, MSc, PhD**
*Professor of Oral Pathology, Federal University of Goiás, Goiânia, GO, Brazil*

**Adair Luiz Stefanello Busato, DDS, MSc, PhD**
*Professor of Operative Dentistry, Luteran University of Canoas, Canoas, RS, Brazil*

# Preface

It is with great satisfaction that we receive the publication of the book Endodontic Science, by Professor Carlos Estrela. His previous books were written either in Portuguese or in Spanish, with enormous impact in Latin America, particularly in Brazil. The book, now in English, makes his valuable knowledge reachable to a much wider readership. For a long time we have been following the scientific evolution of Professor Carlos Estrela. His original research contributions to endodontics and related areas have been extensive as can be judged through the numerous scientific publications appearing in a regular and sustained manner. This book not only draws heavily from his own reserves but also enriches itself through the support and participation of several reputed scientists and clinicians. The given guidelines of endodontic treatment are based on sound scientific works with clinical and histopathological confirmations that confers great strength and validity to the referred procedures. The Endodontic Science organizes the current knowledge on the principles and practice of endodontic treatment in a very didactic mode with the highest available level of evidence. Therefore, we feel very comfortable and confidant to recommend this valuable work in endodontology to students and colleagues who strive for excellence in research, teaching and patient-care.

**Roberto Holland**

*Department of Endodontics, School of Dentistry*
*São Paulo State University São Paulo, Brazil*

**P. N. Ramachandran Nair**

*Institute of Oral Biology School of Dental & Oral*
*Medicine University of Zurich, Switzerland*

Endodontic Science was built from knowledge based on scientific evidences, analyzed from the perspective of reflection, scientific evidence, and a hard work of researchers, clinicians and idealists.

The primary focus of the study was to bring scientific knowledge for the best use of endodontic materials and techniques in different clinical conditions. The magnum regent, the host, was extremely valuable, not only from the perspective of the application of a material or technique for the treatment of the injured tooth, but the context was based on the scientific process of the real state of healing.

The study and understanding of the knowledge of endodontic science transcends the particular knowledge of the material principle, which, in particular, requires the knowledge of the vital principle. Understanding mechanisms of action and reaction is essential to the knowledge of the factors involved in the processes of disease and healing. The biological mechanisms related to the aggression factors and defense of the host, identify the existence of the vital principle, which is the major impetus to the study of endodontic natural structures and their characteristics.

Several challenges have been met with levels of complexity proportional to their sizes. The first dimension (the empirism), involving all new procedures, lack a standard of basic science. The second dimension consisted of images of oral structures in two dimensions. In the third dimension, we move in depth, we began to imagine all the best in several senses. With the fourth dimension we valued even more microscopic structures, allowing more secure procedures. The fifth dimension favored the mysteries of pain, essential to the healing procedures. Well, the sixth dimension is still the challenge, as it rules all the events and the balance of the essential human phenomenon.

The scientific learning should overcome the practical operational limits, besides requiring the privilege of clinical manifestations, the biological aspects that govern them. Clinically we cannot see the microscopic beings (cells, microorganisms) that monitor the organic responses, but it is necessary to understand them for the best treatment.

# Challenges of Endodontic Science

Endodontic Science aims to offer endodontic expressive essence of the knowledge of biological events related to the phenomena of aggression and healing. Therefore, it reflects the incessant search of the most appropriate treatment options for the moment, using biological bases from significant scientific evidences.

Thus, if we knew all the answers of life, the work would make no sense. If we knew fully the science of health, the disease would make no sense. If we knew how to heal the wound, pain would not be felt. The work, the disease and the pain, are strong reasons to struggle for evolution and indicates our limitations in science.

I thank all researchers and teachers who worked in this book, the editor of Artes Medicas, Mr. Milton Hecht, the entire support staff in the person of Renata Bertaco, and their confidence and professionalism in the conduct of this book, which content sought to reflect science.

**Carlos Estrela**

# Contents

# Root Canal Preparation


## C. Estrela

*Federal University of Goiás, Goiânia, GO, Brazil*

## G. B. Sydney

*Federal University of Paraná, Curitiba, PR, Brazil*

## J. A. P. Figueiredo

*Pontifical Catholic University of Rio Grande do Sul, PUCRS, Porto Alegre, RS, Brazil*


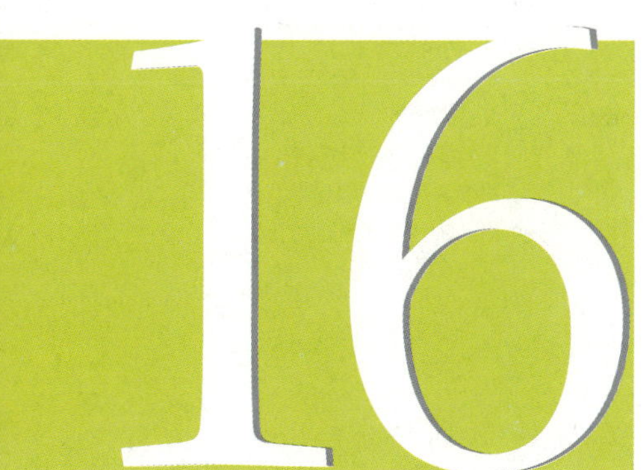

Chapter contents

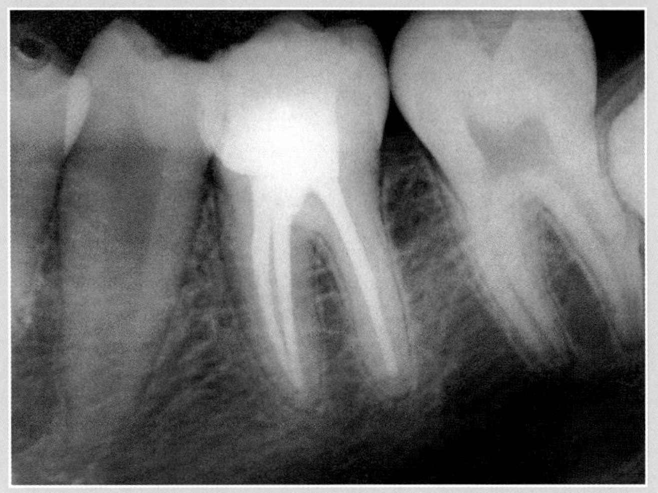

Endodontic therapy.

## 16.1 Introduction

The actual concept of root canal preparation is intimately related to the process of sanitizing the dentinal tubule system. There are important associations among the process required during root canal preparation, such as, emptying and enlarging the root canal, the endodontic instrument and instrumentation technique used, and the operator's experience.

Significant changes, sophisticated technological resources and materials with excellent biological, physical-chemical and mechanical properties have been presented and discussed in contemporary endodontics[1-310]. Flexible instruments and effective techniques have appeared, and have reduced the working time and professional stress, thereby simplifying the operative steps. The challenge of altering the norms already established as correct remains, as does the challenge to overcome the complex internal anatomy, microorganisms and host response. Therefore, the search for an intelligent instrument continues. The advances attained with flexible instruments and the development of rotary systems favor the predictability of success or failure in shaping.

Several studies have presented different instruments, rotary systems, instrumentation techniques, and their influence on the sanitization process[1-310].

Different terms have been used to denominate root canal preparation, each defining the concerns of the different historical phases of endodontics. Among others, this stage has been denominated mechanical preparation, instrumentation, biomechanical preparation, chemical-mechanical preparation, cleaning and shaping and root canal preparation[2,19,50,60-64,68,81,87,105,109,116,118,119,125,158,174,181,196,285]. Schilder[217] used the term cleaning and shaping. Not only the technical-mechanical nature of the procedure is pointed out, but also the influence it has on the tissues and consequently, the biological principles. Cleaning involves emptying of the root canal, irrespective of the prevailing clinical situation (vital pulp, pulp necrosis or filled root canal content). It is the first step of enlargement and is a determinant of success. The sanitization process consists of the combined use of endodontic instruments with irrigant solutions, in addition to the effect of the intracanal dressing. Shaping is responsible for regularizing and planing the root canal walls, with the aim of better seating of the filling material, as well as favoring the perfect sealing of the dentinal tubules. This reasoning indicates the use of a preparation technique with a progressive advance from the cervical to apical third. A significant improvement has been observed in the quality of shape preparation after the advent of the new era of nickel-titanium instruments with recognized flexibility, either hand held or driven by continuous rotary electric motors[9-11,16,32,119-122,143,146-151,183,184,187,209-215,222,223-225,244-246,251-264,299].

It seems, however, opportune to emphasize the need for correct canal cleaning, which requires effective emptying followed by appropriate enlargement, including the apical root third. Thus, the selection of an ideal instrument depends on: the knowledge of internal anatomy, command of the operative technique, and analysis of the instrument characteristics. When selecting instruments for root canal preparation, perfect balance must be attained, in order to avoid irreversible accidents and mistakes.

The major problem is to make the instrument enlarge the canal and adapt to its shape, without deforming it. For several years, the step back techniques were used with the goal of overcoming these difficulties. They reduced the deformities in the shape of the curved root canal, during preparation with stainless steel files. Nowadays, the prevailing thought is the crown down preparation, with progressive advance. Nevertheless, it is important to obey the biologic and mechanical parameters that should monitor the entire the operative technique (Fig.1 A-D).

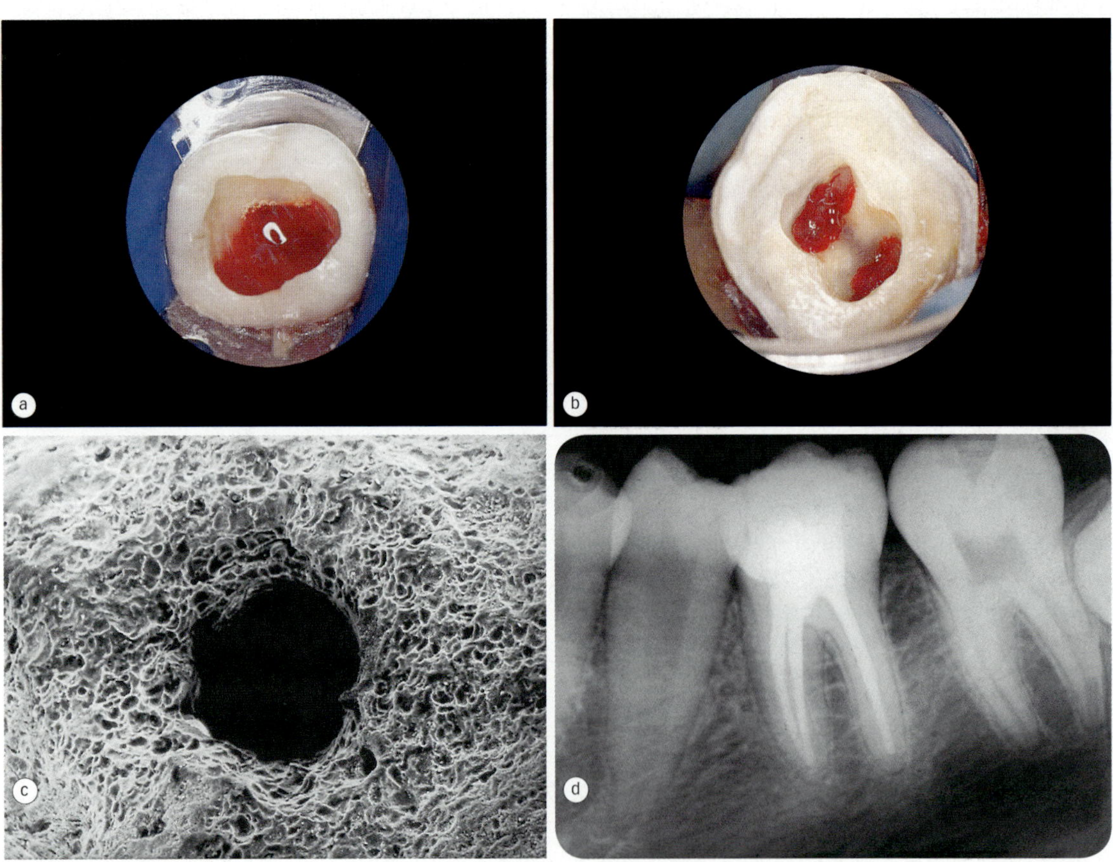


**Figure 16.1** - **(A-D)** Endodontic therapy involves several stages. Therefore, they are all associated with biological principles.

## 16.2 Biological and Mechanical Parameters

In this book, the subject of root canal preparation has been divided into several segments, in order to favor better discussion of each of them. Several challenges can be encountered in endodontic treatment, but specifically during curved root canal preparation, some of these require major attention.

Accurate endodontic treatment planning involves the systematic exam of the patient. Considering the root canal preparation stage, some essential aspects have been discussed in separate topics, such as root canal curvature, the determination of anatomic diameter, and the influence of apical patency on the healing process of teeth with vital and infected pulp.

The sanitization process of the dentinal tubule system, obtained by emptying the contents, requires direct and free access to the entire root canal system. Provided that the principles considered mechanical are complied with, they interact with the biological principles, particularly as regards periapical tissues.

Schilder[217] emphasized some of the criteria that are the mechanical purposes of root canal preparation: 1. prepare with *continuously tapering funnel from the access cavity to apical foramen*; 2. preparation *should maintain the path of the original root canal*; 3. *the apical foramen should remain in its original position*; 4. *the apical opening should be kept as small as is practically possible.*

These criteria should be considered, as the endodontic instrument and the root canal establish a direct relationship of complete and intimate association.

Selection of the ideal instrument depends on the knowledge of internal anatomy, operative technique, and analysis of the characteristics of the instrument. The outstanding problem is to make the instrument enlarge the canal, and to adapt to its shape without deformities. With the aim of overcoming these difficulties, for some time, the step back techniques were used, as they reduced the deformities in the shape of curved root canals. Nowadays the prevailing thought is the crown down preparation, with progressive advance. Nevertheless, it is necessary to comply with the biologic and mechanical parameters which should monitor all the operative techniques.

The anatomic variations that occur in root canals were responsible for the appearance of several shaping techniques which, for a long time, were not shown to have a global pattern. It is emphasized that root canal shaping is based on clear and specific purposes: to regularize and plane the root canal walls without altering their original shape.

The sanitization process requires free access to the entire pulp cavity. During the shaping process, the direct relationship between the root canal walls and the endodontic instruments imposes patterns that should be well guided, particularly with respect to individuality of the root canal.

Considering Schilder's[217] observations on root canal cleaning and shaping, the following biologic and mechanical parameters governing this stage must be emphasized: complete removal of the root canal content, and longitudinal and transversal shaping.

### 16.2.1 Complete Emptying of the Root Canal Content

Complete cleanliness of the root canal, under any of the different therapeutic conditions, such as pulpitis or pulp necrosis, represents an essential point for performing the sanitization process in the endodontic space. This is achieved by removing the tissue or material present by means of pulpectomy, a sanitization process, or the removal of filling material that was placed during retreatment, and enlargement of the root canal.

The current concept heads is to perform complete root canal sanitization, preferably in the same section. Microbial control is increased by intracanal dressing, such as calcium hydroxide paste (Chapter 20).

The natural and logical entry access to the pulp cavity is via the cervico-apical pathway, and must lead to the removal of the root canal content and enlargement.

There are several benefits to previous preparation of the cervical third. The removal of the root canal content in the cervico-apical direction should maintain the conical funnel shape, capable of completely sanitizing the root canal.

### 16.2.2 Longitudinal Shaping

After complete removal of the root canal content, there is the longitudinal coronal-apical shaping, which consists of the regularizing and planing the root canal walls throughout the determined length, from the cervical third to 1-2 mm below the radiographical apex, in the surroundings of the cementum dentinal canal junction. Careful sanitization of the apical third is very important, particularly in cases of endodontic infections. Nevertheless, the preparation should maintain the filling material inside the dentinal canal, with an apical limit capable of providing complete support for the filling material, and avoiding material extrusion.

Furthermore, the enlargement must be gradual and conical in shape. Perfect instrument kinematics should be developed in accordance with the technical standards and the type of file selected. For root canal exploration, when the file is initially introduced, it must first be rotated ¼ of a turn clockwise, then anti-clockwise, and after that it must be extracted without any rotation.

During instrumentation with stainless steel files, the action of each instrument should be constant, following short longitudinal movements (0.5 to 2 mm), oblique to the occlusal direction, traversing the entire canal perimeter, until the instrument is free. For other techniques and continuous or alternate systems, each instrument maintains its own inherent particularities[53].

### 16.2.3 Transversal Shaping

Transversal and longitudinal shaping must be guided by strict planning and discipline, and be based on the anatomic structures. The lateral limit of cervical and apical enlargement should be appropriate, as the radiographic aspect does not represent a precise reference to the real dentinal thickness, and the illusion of the radiographic image can be responsible for insufficient or excessive wear. During endodontic exploration, it is possible to plan the transversal enlargement.

The degree of enlargement becomes important, as it positively influences the sanitization process. On the other hand, excessive wear does not mechanically favor the root canal filling, and it can cause several difficulties during curved or dilacerated root canal fillings. Canals that deviate, present more complications to overcome, particularly as the original root canal shape is enlarged to receive the filling material.

Planning, good sense and anatomic knowledge are significant at this stage of the operation. Determination of the lateral enlargement limit should take into account the anatomic and pathological condition, intensity of the root canal bend, transversal section and the flexibility of the endodontic instrument.

Preparation of the cervical third makes it possible to remove the dentinal prominences (constriction areas) and favors determination of the anatomic diameter of the root canal.

Nevertheless, this recommended enlargement limit merits questioning, because the more contamination removed during the sanitization processes of infected root canals, the more effective they will be. This removal imposes the need for root canal enlargement, which favors the effectiveness of the medications used during irrigation, or the intracanal dressing. Certainly, a great enlargement will favor the root canal filling. These factors emphasize the importance of enlargement, as long as it is compatible with the internal anatomy.

Sydney & Estrela[241] studied the influence of root canal enlargement to eliminate anaerobic bacteria in teeth with asymptomatic apical periodontitis. When preparing the root canal using saline solution and 1% sodium hypochlorite, it was shown that the concept of enlarging the root canal three or four sizes larger than the initial file, is not enough to eliminate bacteria from infected root canals.

Before root canal exploration, it is impossible to exactly define the lateral limit of enlargement. It must be considered that maintenance of the original position of the foramen is as important as the primitive position of the root canal. During root canal instrumentation, transport of the foramen and/or the main canal deviation (with consequent loss of the working length), can be controlled when the endodontic instruments are known, manipulated, and used cautiously and rationally in a good shaping technique.

Stainless steel instruments are manufactured from quadrangular or triangular stems, twisted to the left of their long axes, and when they are pre-bent for curved root canal enlargement, they tend to return to their original position (unfolding capacity). Furthermore, when the amplitude of the movement is high, the pre-bending can be undone. With the highly flexible nickel titanium instruments development occurs during the maintenance of the original shape of the root canal. It should be emphasized that for curved root canal situations, in which the professional selects manual preparation, the K-Flexofile files must be preferred.

Cervical enlargement must be carefully observed, particularly after the introduction of instruments with high taper, which can be responsible for excessive attrition in thin root canal regions, such as the distal wall of the mesial root of mandibular molars. These aspects must be analyzed and considered, since there is a direct and intimate relationship between endodontic instruments and root canals.

## 16.3 Root Canal Instrumentation

Several researches have studied ways to improve the preparation of curved root canals, and to inspect biological and mechanical principles. The innovations and investigations studied and developed flexible endodontic instruments[1-310]. An important step was to suggest a standardized system for instruments, as proposed by Ingle[124,125] (Table 16.1). Manufacturers have introduced a diversity of models in dentistry, such as the cross-section with square or triangular configurations (Fig. 16.2-16.3A-C).

A revolutionary development in endodontics, was the introduction of nickel-titanium instruments[119-122,143-158,252-264] (Fig. 16.2-16.4). Made from a precious alloy, their properties offer a significant dimension to clinical endodontics. The property of superelasticity that nickel-titanium has allows it to return to its original shape after significant deformation, and differentiates it from other metals, such as stainless steel that sustains deformation and retains a permanent shape change. These properties make nickel-titanium instruments more flexible and capable of conforming better to canal curvature, and wear less than stainless steel instruments[126].

The next chapter critically discusses the efficacy of nickel-titanium instruments on shaping curved root canals.

**Table 16.1** - Diameter of endodontic instruments (ADA Specification #28, Tolerance ± 0.02 mm)

| Number | Series | *D 1* - Diameter (mm) | *D16* - Diameter (mm) | Color |
|---|---|---|---|---|
| 06 | | 0.06 | 0.38 | Lilac |
| 08 | | 0.08 | 0.40 | Gray |
| 10 | **Special** | 0.10 | 0.42 | Purple |
| 15 | | 0.15 | 0.47 | White |
| 20 | | 0.20 | 0.52 | Yellow |
| 25 | | 0.25 | 0.57 | Red |
| 30 | | 0.30 | 0.62 | Blue |
| 35 | **1ª** | 0.35 | 0.67 | Green |
| 40 | | 0.40 | 0.72 | Black |
| 45 | | 0.45 | 0.77 | White |
| 50 | | 0.50 | 0.82 | Yellow |
| 55 | | 0.55 | 0.87 | Red |
| 60 | | 0.60 | 0.92 | Blue |
| 70 | **2ª** | 0.70 | 1.02 | Green |
| 80 | | 0.80 | 1.12 | Black |
| 90 | | 0.90 | 1.22 | White |
| 100 | | 1.00 | 1.32 | Yellow |
| 110 | | 1.10 | 1.42 | Red |
| 120 | | 1.20 | 1.52 | Blue |
| 130 | **3ª** | 1.30 | 1.62 | Green |
| 140 | | 1.40 | 1.72 | Black |

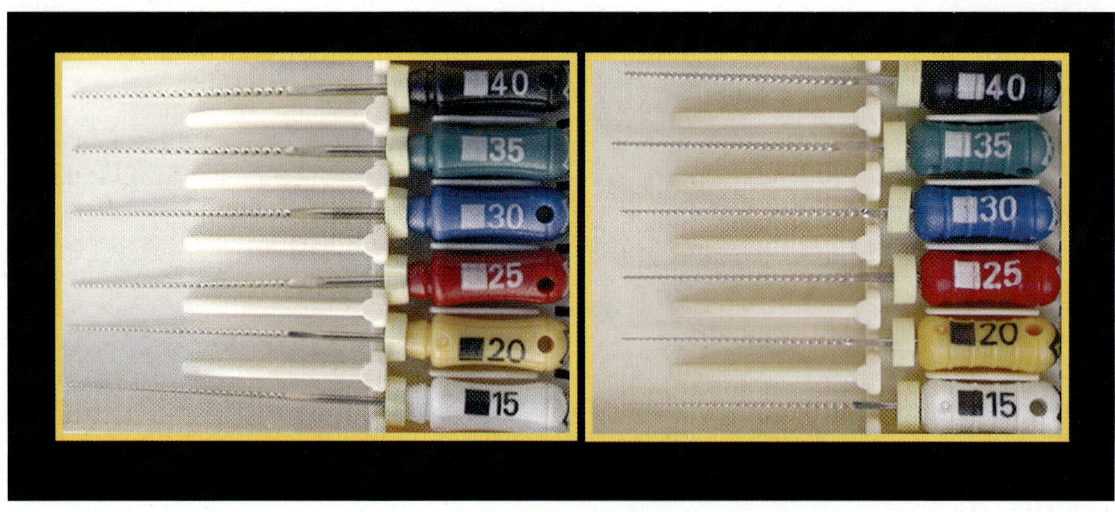


**Figure 16.2** - Endodontic instruments of stainless steel (K-File, K-Flexofile).

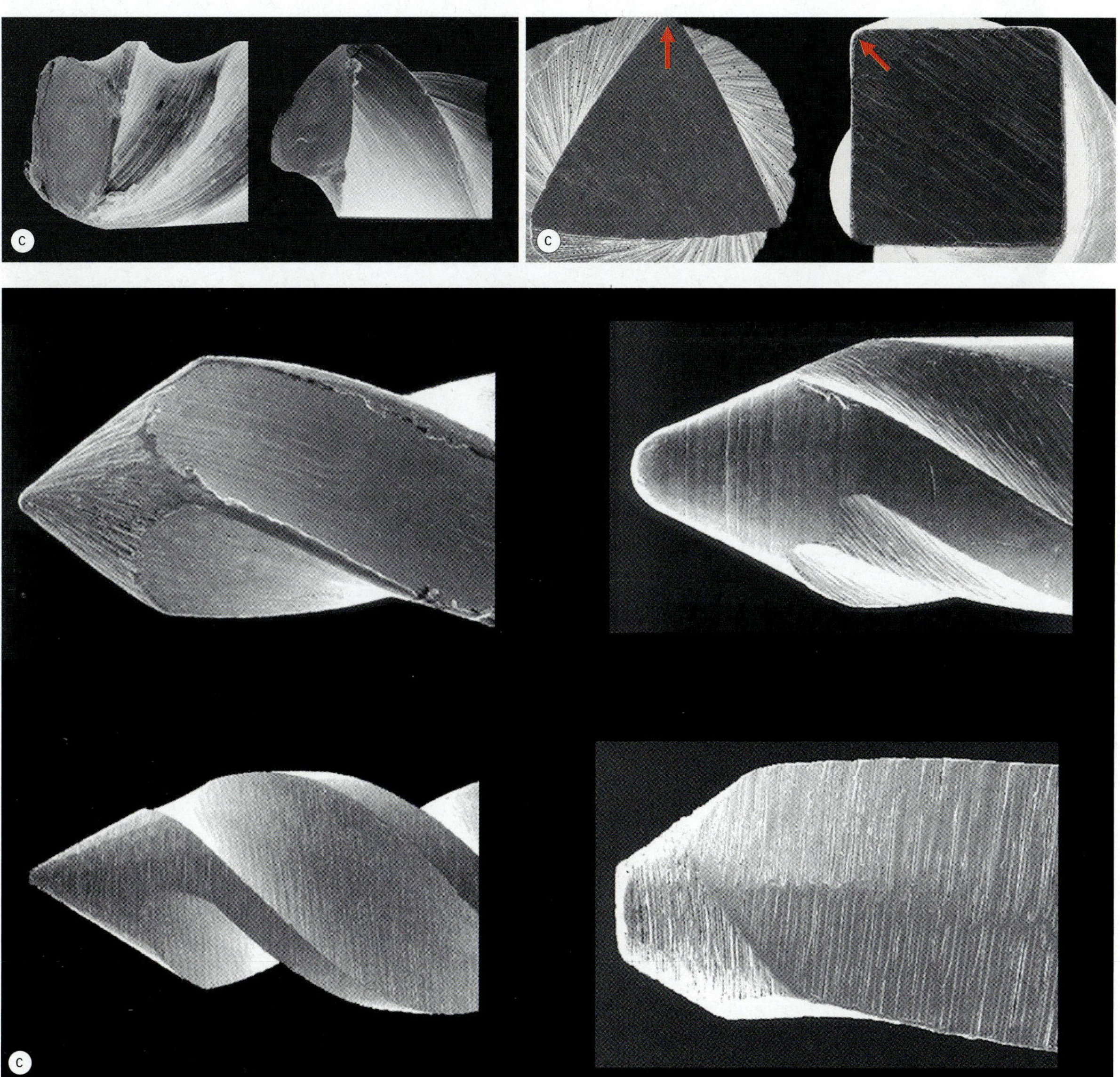


**Figure 16.3** - (**A-B**) Cross-section with square or triangular configurations. (**C**) Design of several tips of endodontic instruments (Courtesy Prof. Dr. Hélio P. Lopes).

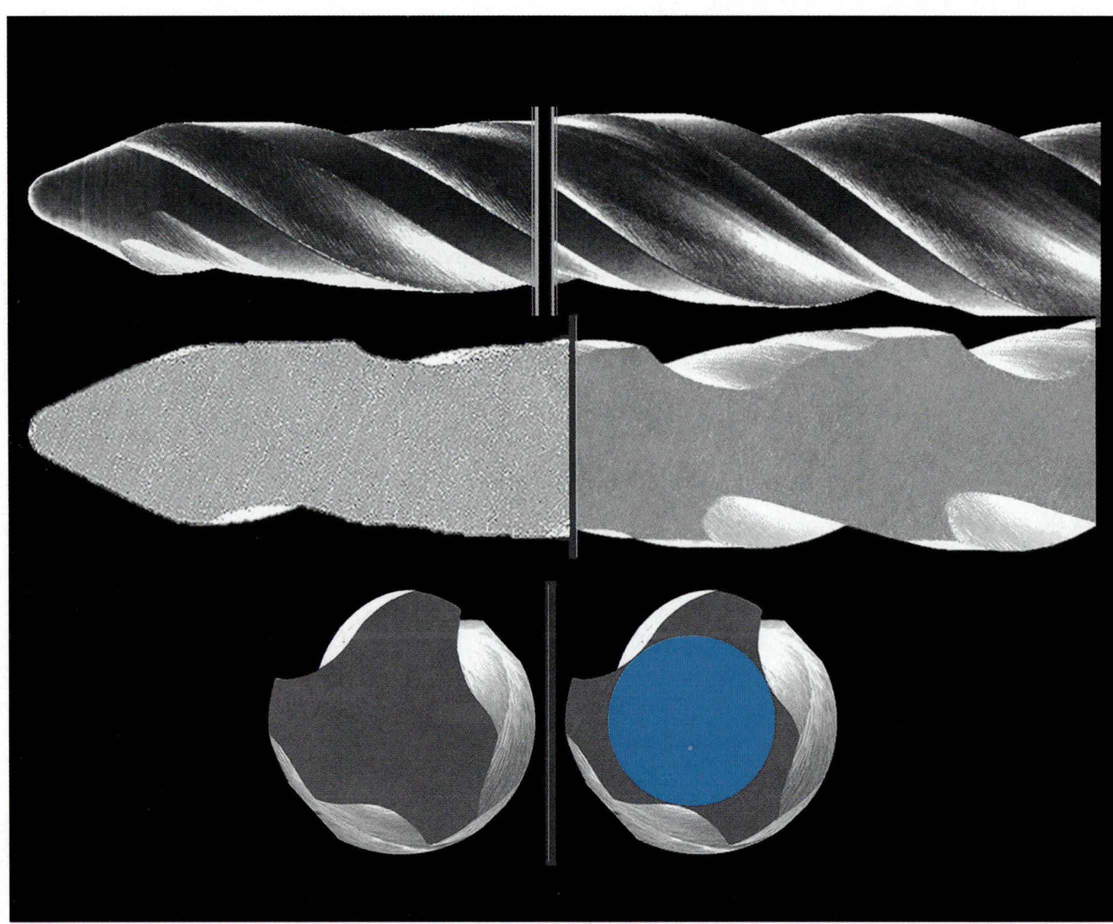

**Figure 16.4** - NiTi instruments, cross-section, K 3 (Courtesy Prof. Dr. Hélio P. Lopes).

## 16.4 A general clinical protocol

Definition of the final configuration, obtained after root canal preparation has been completed, represents a very special objective. The absence of a reliable and applicable methodology for evaluating the quality of the preparation, and for qualifying and defining a well prepared root canal, constitutes a difficult and challenging task, and is also a very personal matter. When the influence of the apical curvature has been overcome by preparation of the cervical third, the final shape is better and the preparation becomes more efficient. The principles and the surgical steps in the preparation of curved root canals, serve as support for the preparation of straight root canals.

The large number of root canal preparation techniques[1-310] was sustained by justifications involving the complex anatomy and endodontic instruments available, which did not lead to general consensus. The new treatment alternatives and arrival of nickel-titanium instruments for use in continuous rotation represent a good alternative to obtain the final quality of the preparation.

With respect to standardization, the need is emphasized for obtaining a well defined conical preparation in multiple planes, with a decreasing diameter in the apical direction, so that the surgical canal obtained by shaping the anatomical canal, allows the perfect adaptation and accommodation of the filling material, and favors its complete sealing.

The alternative to definition of the final shape to be obtained in curved root canals represents a differential. Nevertheless, it is of significant importance to observe the biologic and mechanical parameters previously discussed: complete emptying of the root canal, longitudinal and transversal shaping. This definition of the ideal final shape can be achieved by the cervical and apical preparation, thus qualifying not only the sanitization and shaping process, but also making the physical and biological qualities of filling the dentinal tubule system more efficient.

Shovelton[227], analyzing the presence and distribution of microorganisms in teeth with pulp necrosis, observed that the largest volume of microorganisms is in the cervical third, decreasing in the apical direction. This can be explained by the larger pulp volume, number and volume of dentinal tubules that are larger in the cervical than in the middle and apical thirds.

The present technique discussed and suggested in this chapter consists of a preparation with reverse enlargement and progressive advance from the cervical to apical third. Based on clear and specific principles, one of the alternatives for overcoming the influence of the apical curvature is in the capacity of stabilizing it, from the compensation offered, through the preparation of the entrance and the cervical third of the root canal. It should be emphasized that in molars there is a progressive increase in dentinal thickness on the floor of the chamber, with age. Thus, this concrescence of dentin on the mesial wall of the mesial root of mandibular molars, and in the mesial region of the mesial-buccal canal of maxillary molars, gives the apical curvature an obscure characteristic. The elimination of this interference decreases the initial pressure (that can constitute a fulcrum point on the distal wall of the mesial-buccal canals of mandibular molars), which allows greater freedom for working in the apical third.

Leeb[140] believes it is difficult to determine the diameter of the canal using a locked instrument, since this impediment can occur in the cervical third (near the entrance of the orifice of the root canal). Wu et al.[296] verified the relationship between the anatomic instrument and the diameter of the canal in the apical region. To do this, two groups of mandibular curved premolars were selected. After the coronal opening and pulpectomy, the anatomic instrument was determined. In one group, the K-Flex, and in the other, the Lightspeed file was used. After fixing the instruments in position, the apices were cut until the working length, and the diameters of the instruments were analyzed. In 75 % of the root canals, the instrument locked on only one wall; in 25%, the instrument did not touch any wall. In 90% of the canals, the diameter of the instrument was smaller than the diameter of the canals. This difference was bigger than 0.19 mm. No difference was observed between the instruments. Therefore, observations showed that neither of the instruments that locked at the working length, reflected the anatomic apical diameter of the curved mandibular premolars. Thus, removal of dentin on the entire circumference of the canal, by preparing it with only 3 instruments above the anatomic diameter is uncertain. Pécora et al.[186] investigated the influence of the cervical preparation with different instruments (Gates-Glidden burs, Flare files, LA Axxess burs) on the first file that adjusts to the working length, in maxillary central incisors. The results showed that determining the anatomic diameter by the working length is not accurate, and cannot be used as parameter; cervical preparation favors establishment of the anatomic diameter; the canals prepared with LA Axxess, presented lower values of difference between the size of the file and the anatomic diameter.

The method of preparation proposed is based on rational and deductive observations, in an endeavor to promote better definition of the final shape, obtained in curved root canals. It is imperative to emphasize that the technique should make the instrument adapt to the root canal, and not the root canal to the instrument. Moreover, progressive cervical-apical advance, in addition to acting in areas with more organic material (larger amount of microorganisms), favors the irrigation system, action of the endodontic instrument, releases it apically, and finally, provides better conditions for root canal filling[83].

### 16.4.1 Sequence of the Technique

#### Exploration of the Root Canal (initial emptying)

When preparing the root canal, the first step is to clinically identify its entrance orifice and explore it, allowing the canal to be mapped and to determine its anatomic diameter, direction of the curvature and obstacles, frequently not visualized in the radiograph, to create a first pathway for the following instruments. This exploring instrument is essential to successful root canal preparation, and it is necessary for it to have a small diameter and a curved tip. Thus, it can overcome the obstacles more easily[83].

The parameter for the initial measurement of the exploring instrument should be the mean of the length of the tooth and its length as shown on the initial radiograph minus 2 mm. This stage allows initial planning of the difficulties to be faced next. Moreover, it is a first parameter for determining the lateral limit of instrumentation. One of the objectives of exploration is known to be removal of the remaining material in the root canal.

When faced with curved molar canals, initial exploration using a #8 or #10 file, and partial emptying performed with a file up to #15 is recommended, thus favoring conditions for the penetration of subsequent instruments. The exploration in narrow (constricted) root canals favors the preparation of the canal entrance and cervical third. The kinematics developed by the exploratory penetration occur with the initial introduction of the file, by moving it a ¼ of a turn clockwise, then anticlockwise, followed by removing it without rotation. Intensive irrigation and aspiration should be performed constantly, parallel to the action of each instrument. This exploration should be done in steps, from the cervical to apical region, advancing progressively, and when resistance is encountered, the instrument should not be forced. It should be retrieved and the initial maneuvers of penetration, short clockwise rotation, and retraction should be repeated.

The apical limit of exploration differs in two clinical situations: that of vital pulp and of pulp necrosis. In vital pulp, exploration is restricted to the proximities of the cementum-dentin-canal junction, while in situations of pulp infection, the exploration should advance as far as the radiographic apex, allowing the cementum canal to be emptied. The sanitization of this area, considered critical, is significant for the control of microorganisms and removal of debris. Exploration is the first step, and is essentially important to the success of emptying and sanitizing the root canal.

In situations of vital pulp, exploration is performed before pulpectomy. In cases of pulp necrosis, exploration allows partial emptying. Consequently, this initial emptying and sanitization process, which is really developed simultaneously, needs special care to avoid extrusion of necrotic remainders, dentinal chips and microorganisms to the periapex. The sequences of pulpectomy and sanitization techniques that involve this operation are given below (Fig. 16.5-16.7).

**Pulpectomy Technique** (Emptying in Vital Pulp)

1 Anaesthesia, absolute isolation and antisepsis of the operative field;
2 Coronary opening, complete removal of the roof of the pulp chamber;
3 Removal of the coronary pulp with curettes of intermediate length and well sharpened;
4 Intensive irrigation-aspiration of the coronal chamber with 1% sodium hypochlorite;
5 Observe the complete removal of the entire roof of the coronal chamber with an explorer and, if necessary, complement the coronal opening;
6 Find the entrance of the root canals by using an endodontic explorer;
7 For the wide root canals, the radicular pulp is excised with a Hedströem file, while in the narrow (constricted) root canals, this is removed during the root canal preparation, by fragmentation (crushing). For this, introduce a small diameter K-file (#10/#15), between the root canal wall and the dental pulp, with the objective opening a space and releasing the tissue. This instrument is used to explore and release the canal automatically, until the probable limits of its length are determined;
8 Once the apical limit for the pulpectomy is established, penetrate with a Hedströem file, following the pathway created by the K-file, pressing the pulp tissue against the buccal wall, and withdraw the instrument. The dental pulp is not always removed the first time, which means the procedure must be repeated until it is completely removed;
9 In situations in which the tissue is condensed in the apical third, one should take care not to push it into the periapical region. Using thin instruments, try to displace it with a K-file, for later removal;
10 In narrow (constricted) canals, after the length has been determined, the pulp tissue is removed by fragmentation (crushing) during root canal enlargement;
11 Copious irrigation-aspiration with 1% sodium hypochlorite should be done immediately after the pulpectomy, to remove all pulp remains and coagulated blood, which helps to avoid coronal darkening;
12 After the pulpectomy, root canal preparation and filling are performed in the same appointment, when possible, or an intracanal dressing can be used, and the filling done in a second appointment (Fig. 16.5).

**Sanitization Technique** (Emptying in Pulp Necrosis)

1 Anaesthesia, absolute isolation and antisepsis of the operative field;
2 Coronal opening with complete removal of the roof of the pulp chamber;
3 Copious irrigation-aspiration with 1-2.5% sodium hypochlorite, followed by the eventual removal of the contents of the pulp cavity with curettes of intermediate length;
4 Filling of the coronal chamber with 1-2.5% sodium hypochlorite;
5 Introduction of an instrument of small diameter (#08 to #15), depending on the diameter of the root canal, with progressive movement of penetration and withdrawal (forwards and backwards), dislocating the organic remains, followed by neutralization with sodium hypochlorite. The coronary chamber roof is completely removed using an explorer, and if necessary, the coronary opening is complemented;
6 The neutralization of the septic content is neutralized in steps, working in small longitudinal amplitudes that allow the chemical substance to act on the necrotic residues released from the walls of the root canals by the mechanical action of the files;
7 In exploration, the working length adopted is based on the length determined only from an initial radiograph, and the average length of the tooth. Complete emptying and disinfectant penetration are performed after the entrance orifice and cervical third have been prepared and the length determined;
8 After performing these operative steps, disinfectant penetration and emptying are completed up to the radiographic apical vertex. Copious irrigation-aspiration with sodium hypochlorite should be done frequently to ensure the complete removal of possible necrotic remainders and / or automatically neutralize them;
9 After the sanitization process, prepare the root canal apply the intracanal dressing (calcium hydroxide paste) (Fig. 16.6).

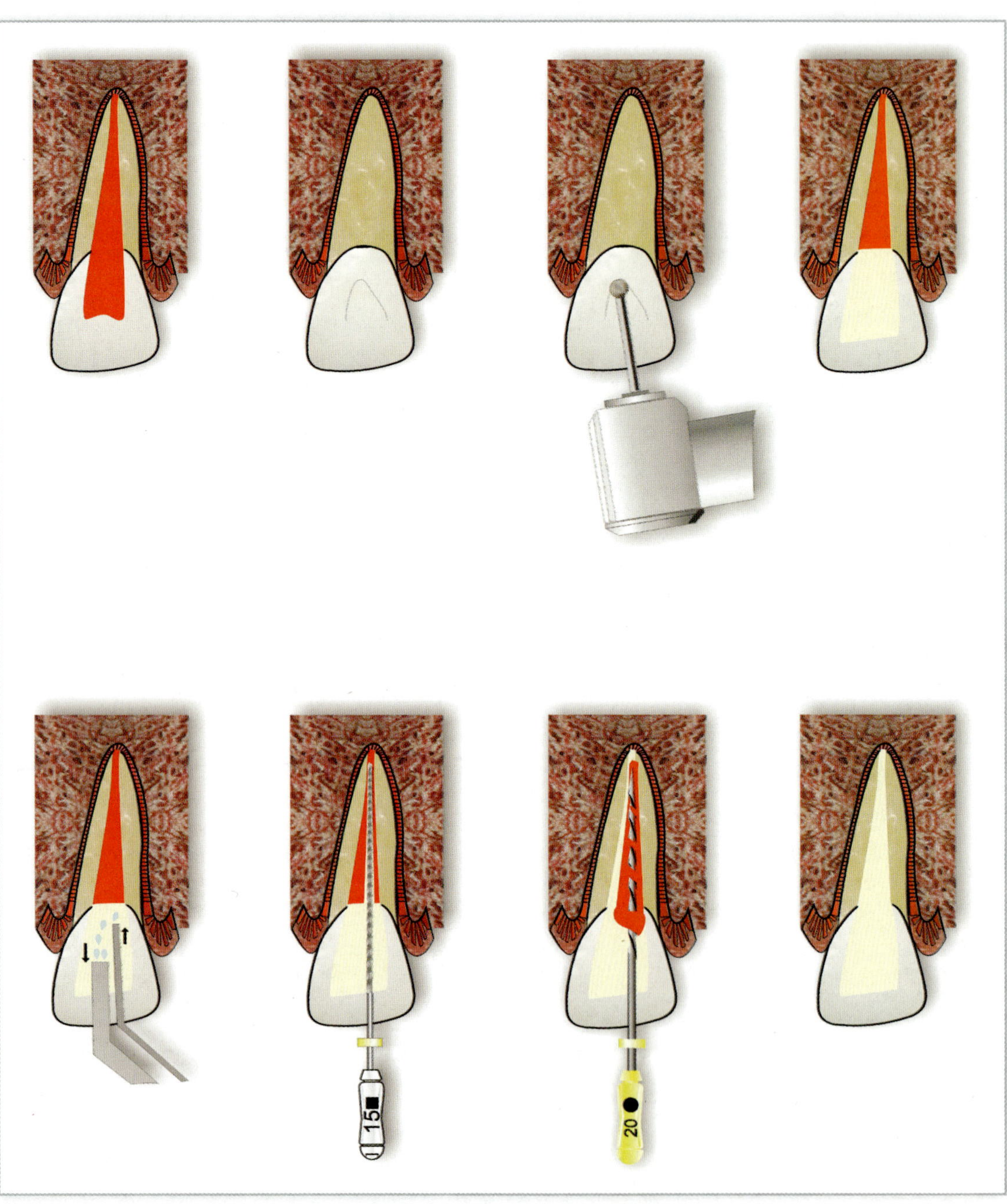


Figure 16.5A - Schematic representation of pulpectomy.

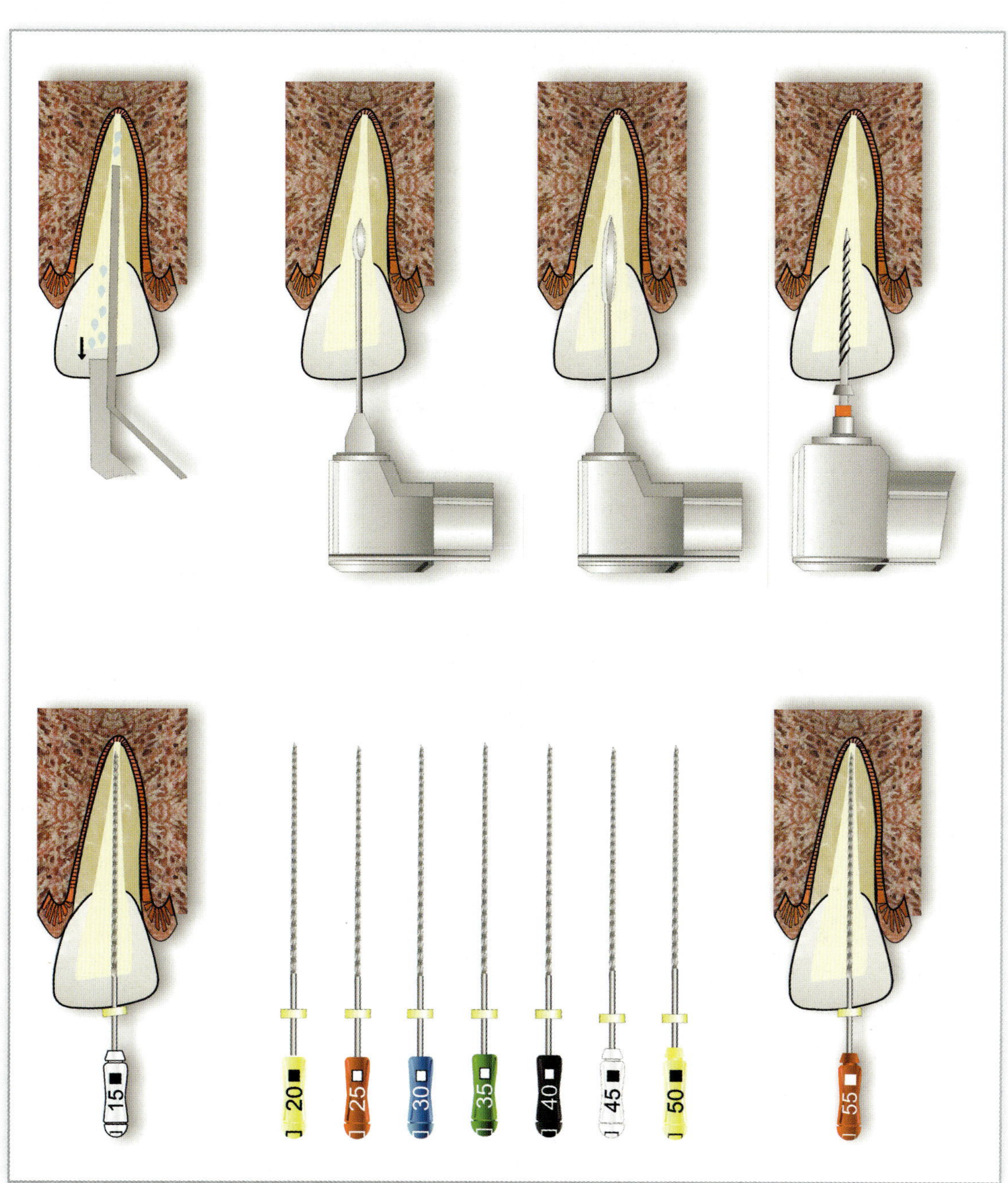


**Figure 16.5B** - Schematic representation of root canal preparation.

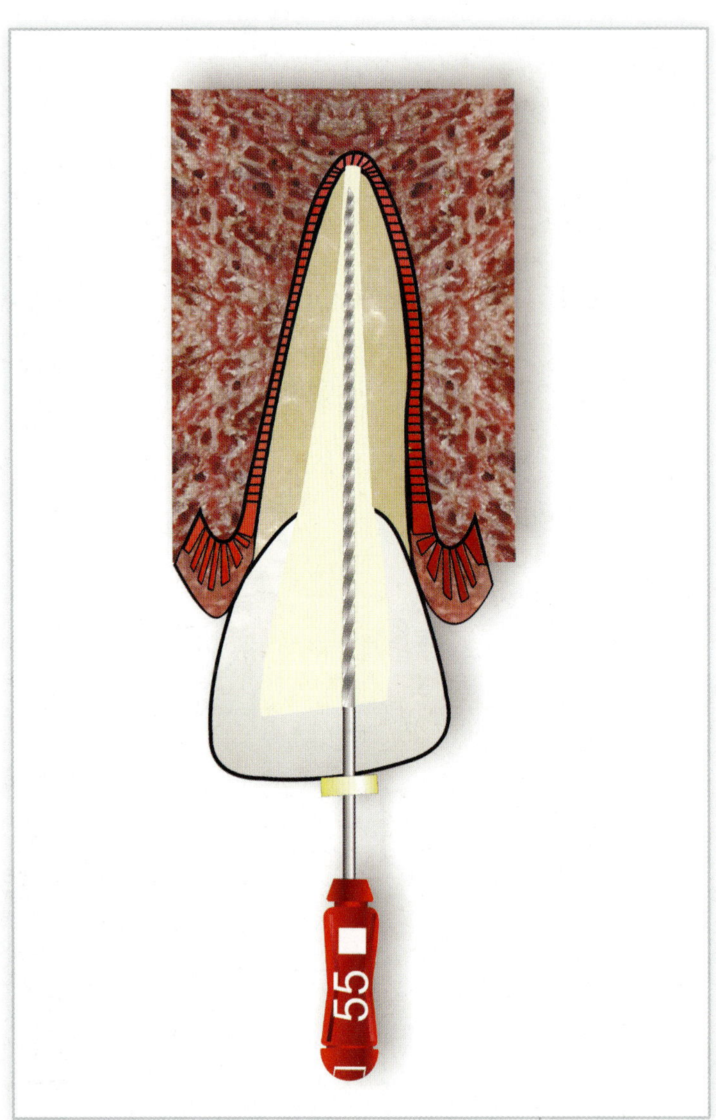


**Figure 16.5C** - Schematic representation of root canal preparation.

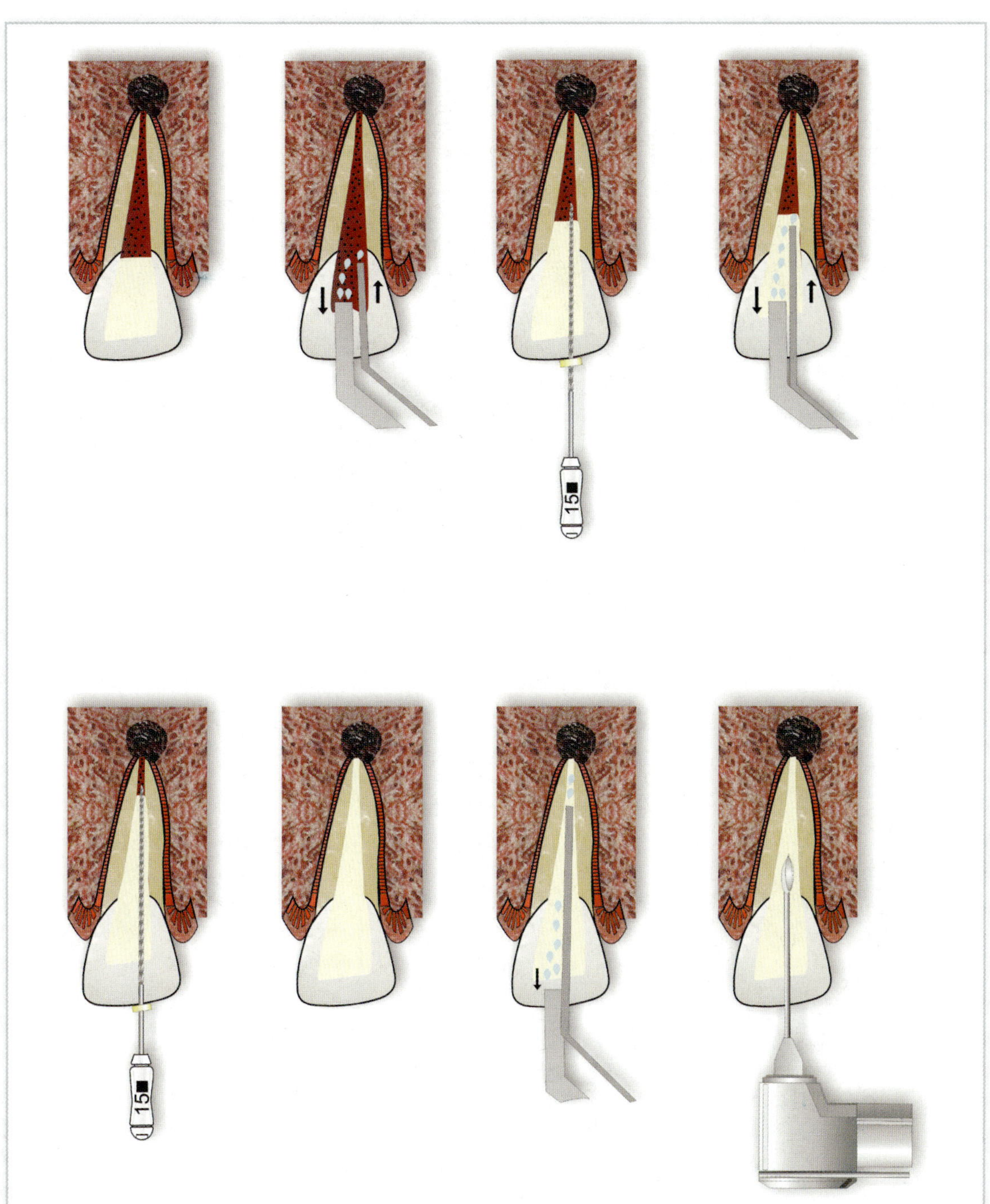


**Figure 16.6A** - Schematic representation of the sanitization process.

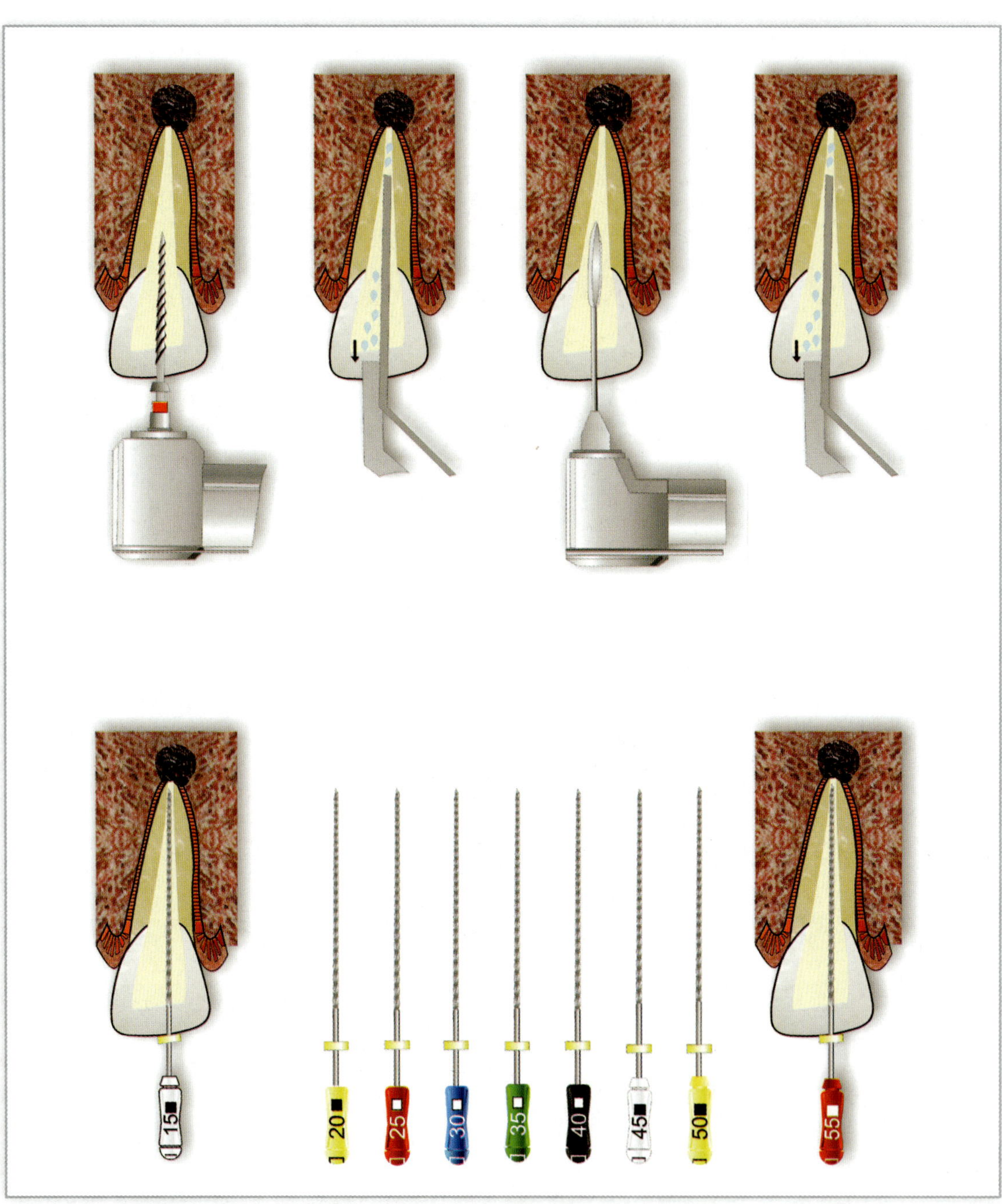


**Figure 16.6B** - Schematic representation of the sanitization process.

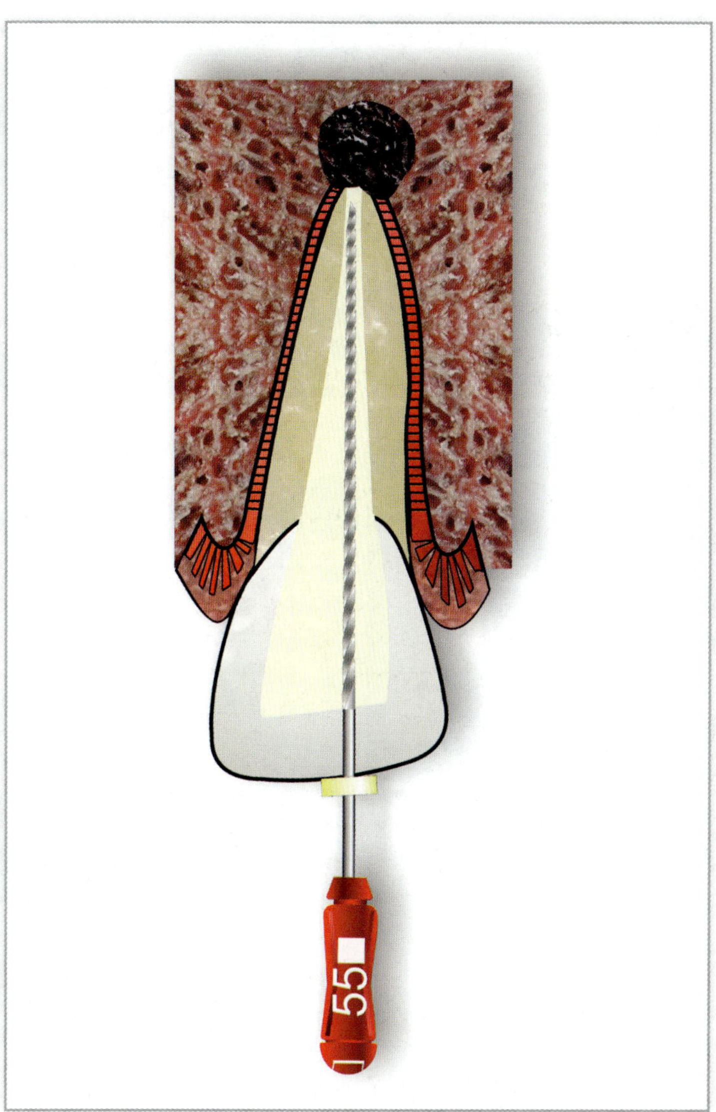


Figure 16.6C - Schematic representation of root canal preparation.

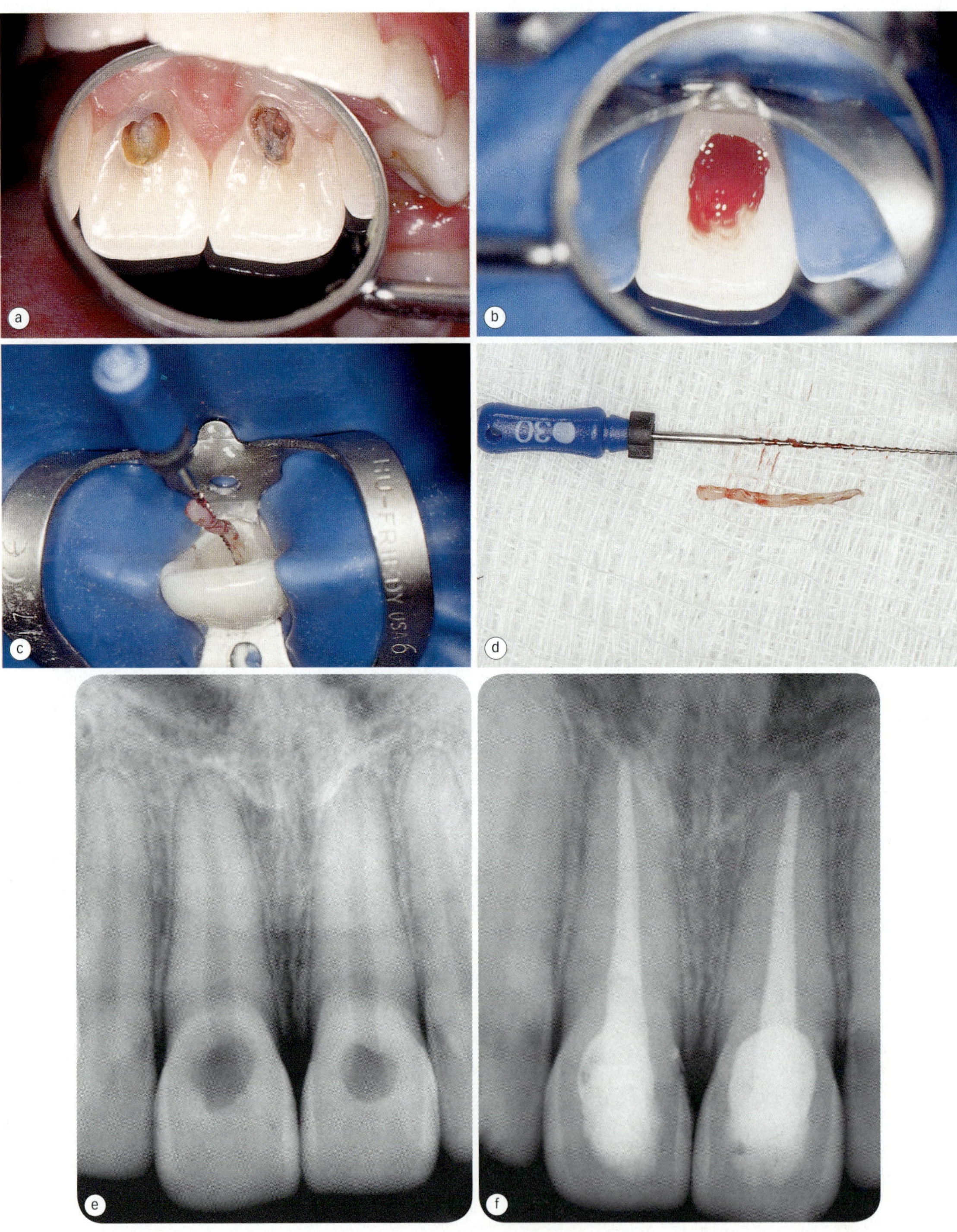


**Figure 16.7** - (**A-F**) Clinical case, showing pulpectomy.

## Preparation of the Entrance Orifice and Cervical Third

One of the most important concepts that resulted in one of the great advances of modern endodontic therapy, was the cervical-apical preparation. In reality, the adoption by Goerig et al.[99] of the procedure of root access before preparation of the apical area was the most significant because, irrespective of the technique used, it brought innumerable benefits such as: minimal occurrence of defects in the apical area, the possibility of more extensive enlargement of this area, less risk of debris extrusion, and consequently enabling the instruments to touch the walls better, thereby providing more efficient irrigation and better cleaning.

This operative step is no more than an extension of the coronal access cavity to the interior of the root canal, consisting of two different stages accomplished almost simultaneously: preparation of the entrance to the root canal, and preparation of the cervical third.

Recently, instruments with different tapers have been introduced with the purpose of providing a more extensive enlargement of the middle and cervical thirds, gaining in taper and in regularity of the walls.

Because of the need for a defined, conical preparation tapering towards the apex, which allows more contact of the instrument along the root canal wall after the mapping done during the exploration, the entrance orifice and the cervical third must be prepared. In anterior teeth, observe the dentinal projections in the palatine or lingual regions, and in the molars, in the cervical region. Furthermore, observe that one of the causes of iatrogenic procedures during endodontic preparation is the absence of control over the active part of the instrument which, in a huge number of cases, precludes the perfect regularization and planing of the root canal walls. However, it is pointed out that the zone of smaller canal diameter is located in the region of the entrance orifice of the cervical third, and not in the more apical area, in agreement with Leeb[84], who analyzed maxillary and mandibular molars. Thus, the choice of the initial instrument for preparation and measurement lacks accuracy, due to the possible adjustment in the cervical third, and more freedom in the apical third of the root canal.

Indeed, in order to achieve the above-mentioned objectives, the use of manual orifice openers is recommended (Auerback Opener) (Fig. 16.8A-C), to enable enlargement of this region. Thus, the dentinal concrescence on the mesial walls of mandibular and maxillary molars, which interferes in correct preparation, is removed. It is emphasized that care must be taken as regards dentin projections, especially in mandibular molars, because if the instrument is directed towards the anti furcation, there is a risk of perforation, as it has a fulcrum point on a thin wall, with a higher tendency to wear out.

The entrance orifice in anterior teeth is prepared during the compensatory maneuvers, shared with coronal opening.

Initially, to analyze quality of the preparation, take the shape of the entrance orifice of the root canal, which is an excellent reference, as a basis.

From the above discussion it is clear that the adoption of simple and practical solutions can reduce operating time and provide a gain in quality.

Therefore, it is pointed out that the influence of apical curvature can be overcome by preparation of the cervical third. For this purpose, merely planning the cervical access on the opposite side of the curvature will allow the instrument to work in a straighter pathway up to the apical curvature, as well as enable greater control over the instrument, decreasing tension during the operation. Unquestionably the cervical preparation assumes a strategic and important role, since it facilitates emptying of the root canal, creates an evasion pathway, and decreases the pressure during irrigation.

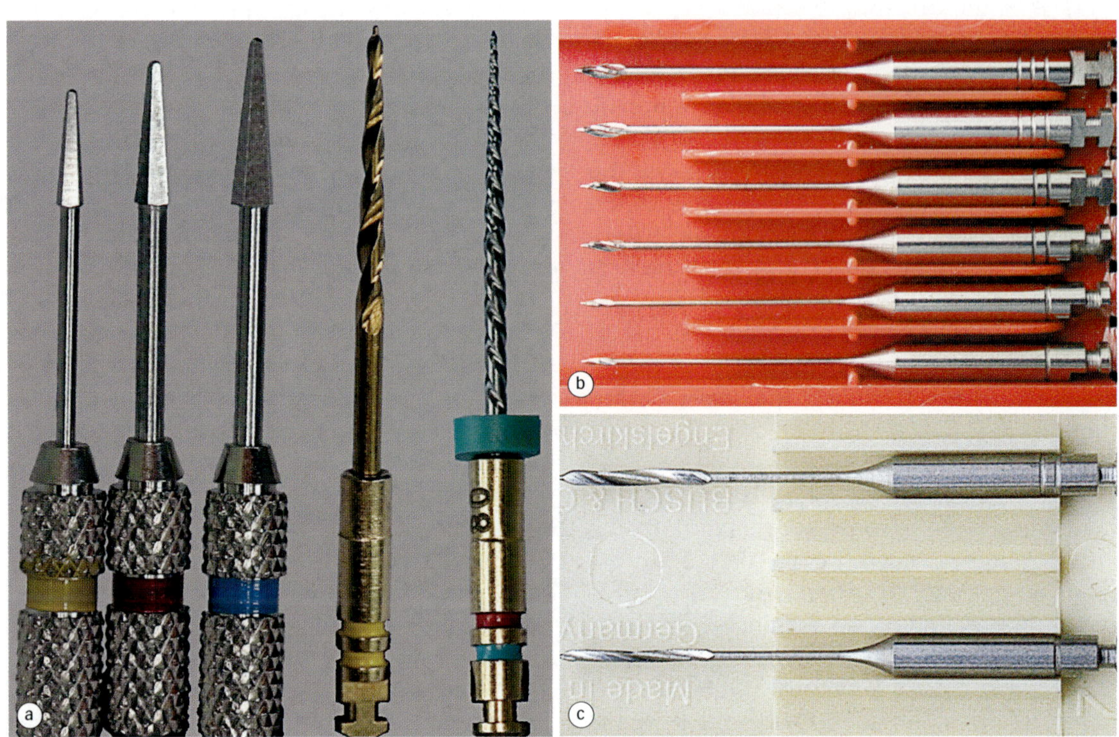

**Figure 16.8** - (**A-C**) Instruments used for preparation of cervical third (Auerback Opener; LA Axxess; K 3 orifice oppener). (**B**) Gates-Glidden and (**C**) Largo burs.

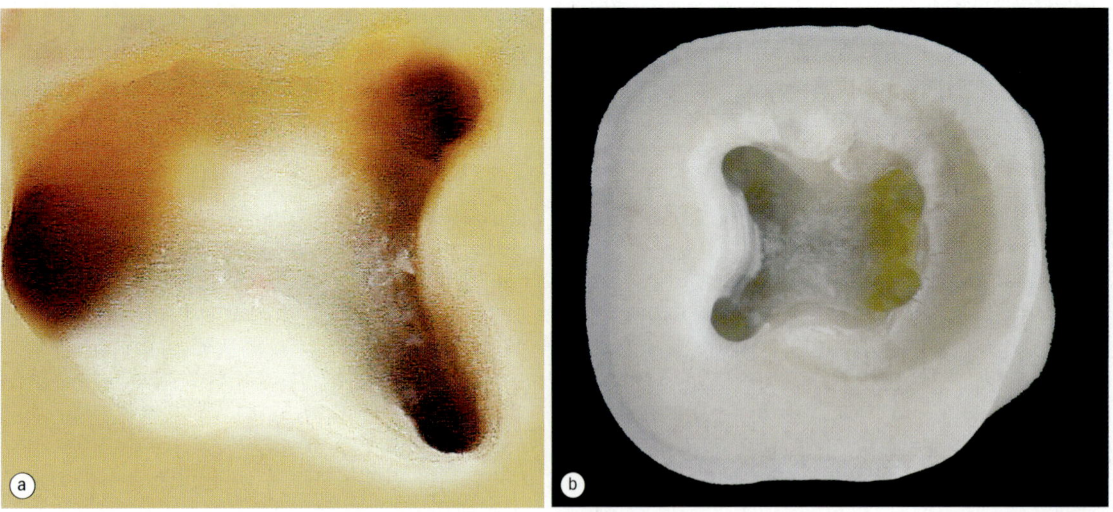

**Figure 16.9** - (**A-B**) Preparation of the entrance orifice and cervical third.

The advantages of preparing the cervical third beforehand emphasize the straighter access to the apical third, allowing more freedom of action of the instrument in the apical region and decreasing a possible change in the longitudinal limit of work. It has been observed that when using manual preparation, more of the content and contamination in the cervical third is removed; the irrigating solution penetrates more efficiently, and there is less possibility of the formation of steps, perforation and fracture of the endodontic instrument; it is easier to place the intracanal dressing and filling; and there is less prevalence of post-operative pain due the lower extrusion of necrotic remainders and microorganisms (Fig. 16.9A-B).

## Gates-Glidden burs

The Gates-Glidden drills have been the instruments indicated for preparation of cervical third (Fig. 16.8B). Nevertheless, their unique diameter and restricted area of cut, result in compaction of the dentine, which requires the professional's skill to obtain regularity of the walls.

The options for the preparation of this entrance region of the root canal have been widely discussed in a large number of models[1-310]. For many years, the most used resources were the Gates-Glidden and Largo burs. The use of the Gates-Glidden burs, to facilitate the opening of root canals, is not recent. Otollengui[179] in 1892 and Callahan[39] in 1894 presented considerations about the risks and benefits of their use.

In the same way as any other instruments, the Gates-Glidden burs should be manipulated with care. When incorrectly used, fractures and perforations are among the most frequent inconveniences. In teeth with thin walls, perforation of a wall due to an oversize bur causes unnecessary wear during instrumentation, particularly on the distal wall of the mesial root of mandibular molars. This same incident can also occur during instrumentation with nickel-titanium instruments of .04 and .06 taper, if the diameter of the file is not suited to the dentinal volume of the root canal walls. Estrela[76] conducted a comparative study of the dental wear on the distal wall of the mesial-buccal canal of the mandibular first molar, produced by three instrumentation techniques with different standards of enlargement. The objective was to evaluate the risk of perforating and creating very thin walls in the distal region of the mesiobuccal canal of the mandibular first molar during instrumentation. The average dentinal thickness at levels 2, 3, 4 and 5 mm from the radicular furcation, for Group 1 (Control), for Group 2 (anti-curvature enlargement, corresponding up to file #35), for Group 3 (enlargement corresponding up to file #35, with step-back up to file #60), for Group 4 (enlargement corresponding up to file #35, associated with the use of Gates-Glidden burs # 2 and 3), were of 0.819 mm, 0.648 mm, 0.492 mm and 0.351 mm, respectively. When comparing level 2 with 3, and 4 with 5, there was no significant difference. However, when levels 2 and 3, were associated with levels 4 and 5, there was significant difference. Nevertheless, when analyzing levels 2 and 3, in the canals instrumented with Technique 3, an average dentinal thickness of 0.285 mm and 0.291 mm, respectively was obtained. Lower indexes of thickness were observed in the walls of the canals prepared using the Gates-Glidden bur #3 (corresponding to file #90). There was a case of perforation at the levels of 2 and 3 mm of the furcation. The canals instrumented by the conventional technique with the aid of Gates-Glidden burs #2 and #3, were the ones that had thinner walls and presented lower thickness. This technique presented a higher possibility of perforation (Fig. 16.10A-F). Figure 16.11 show radiographic aspects with lateral perforations, due to excessive wear in thin walls.

The Gates-Glidden burs act better in circular canals, such as the mesial canals of mandibular molars, buccal canals of maxillary molars, premolars and incisors. For flattened canals, the difficulty with using Gates-Glidden burs lies in its cutting power being directed towards the equator of the helical guide of the bur, which causes circular wear. For root canals with a flattened shape, rotary instruments, such as the orifice openers (Orifice Shaper or Line-Angle Axxess) have showed interesting results.

**CP DRILL (INJECTA)**

The rotary CP Drill instruments are made of stainless steel, have a long shaft and small active part, designed for removing dental deposits at the entrance of root canals, and for preparing the cervical third. They are composed of three instruments with the following characteristics:

- CP Drill #1 - Identified by a black ring on its shaft, it has a diameter of 0.40 at its tip and a taper of 0.22. It active part measures 7.0 mm.
- CP Drill #2 - Identified by a blue ring on its shaft, it has a diameter of 0.30 at its tip and a taper of 0.18. Its active part measures 5.0 mm.
- CP Drill #3 - Identified by a red ring on its shaft, it has a diameter of 0.25 at its tip and a taper of 0.14. Its active part measures 5.0 mm.

One notes that the taper variations among the burs are small, in comparison with the reduced active part. This allows to the instrument to penetrate the cervical third smoothly way and to achieve the goal regularizing the walls.

**PRE - RACE (FKG)**

Another option that seems very effective is the use of the Pre-Race instruments. Although these instruments are designed for automated preparation in continuous rotation, they are also available in stainless steel, which allows them to be used in normal handpieces, and because of their characteristics, they are excellent for performing root access.

The lateral cutting edge is 60° and the vertex of the lateral cutting edge angle is acute, which contributes to its great cutting capacity. Its rank angle is negative.

Pre-Race instruments are available in two models:

- #40/0.10 – tip diameter is 0.40 and taper 0.10.
- #35 / 0.08 – tip diameter is 0.35 and taper 0.08.

They have an active part measuring only 9 mm and a length of 19 mm. One of the characteristics of these instruments with different tapers is taking the best direction in anti-curvature. It is important to remember that the instruments do not know where to act. The professional has to direct it. Thus, when working with the instrument, kinematics involves conducting it to the anti-curvature and guiding it to touch all the walls, which involves oblique traction.

### LA AXXESS (Sybron Endo)

The Line-Angle Axxess instruments were introduced by Sybron Endo for the preparation of the cervical third. They are stainless steel instruments, composed of shaft, intermediate and active blade.

The series is composed of 3 instruments, all with a taper of 0.06, with lengths of 19 mm, 12 mm having active blades and 7 mm with an intermediate blade. LASS #1 has a diameter of 0.20 mm at the tip, LASS #2 0.35 mm and LASS #3 0.45 mm. According to Lopes et al.[150] its helical shaft has a straight traversal section, with two lateral cutting edges formed by the intersection of the radial land and the attack surface of the helical flute. The lateral cutting edges are diametrically opposite (180°) and its internal angle is approximately 90°. The rank angle is positive and the angle of inclination of the helix is approximately 15°. They have a parabolic-shaped tip, actually, more cylindrical with a round extremity.

LASS instruments have been good for the removal of dental deposits of teeth with wide root canals. Their use in root canals of smaller diameter, such as the buccal canals of maxillary molars and the mesial canals of mandibular molars is more critical, because of their large diameter. The manufacturer's information indicates diameters of 0.20 mm, 0.35 mm and 0.45 mm and taper of 0.06. This is true, but this diameter really corresponds to its parabolic tip, so that it only acts as a guide. One millimeter beyond the tip, the diameter increases considerably. The LASS instrument tip measurements were recorded by a digital pachymeter at 1 and 2 mm. The data obtained for LASS instruments were as follows: LASS 1 (#20), 0.28 mm diameter; 1 mm beyond the tip, the diameter verified was 0.53, and for 2 mm it was 0.79 mm; at the end of its active part, the corresponding value was 1.20 mm. For LASS 2 (#35) the measurements obtained were: at the tip it was 0.35 for 1 mm; and 0.76 mm for 2 mm; 0.90 and 1.20 at the end of the active part. LASS 3 (#45) presented the following diameters: it was 0.46 at the tip for 1 mm; for 2 mm it was 0.90; and 1.06 and 1.20 mm at the end of the active part (Fig. 16.8A).

Table 16.2 shows the advantages of preparing the entrance orifice and cervical third.

**Table 16.2** - Advantages of preparation of the entrance orifice and cervical third

| |
|---|
| Removal of coronal contamination; |
| Reduction of disastrous consequences such as the loss of working length, transportation of apical foramen, creation of ledges, elbows, zips, perforations, fracture of instruments; |
| Preparation allows greater control of the active part of the endodontic instrument; |
| Produces the greatest possible penetration of irrigant; |
| Supports the exit of irrigant solution and a better sanitization process; |
| Allows better action of the instrument in curved root canals; |
| Allows the adequate introduction of intracanal dressing (such as calcium hydroxide paste), the management of filling material, development of the gutta-percha lateral condensation technique; |
| Favors the preparation for intracanal post, removal of incomplete obturation during endodontic retreatment. |

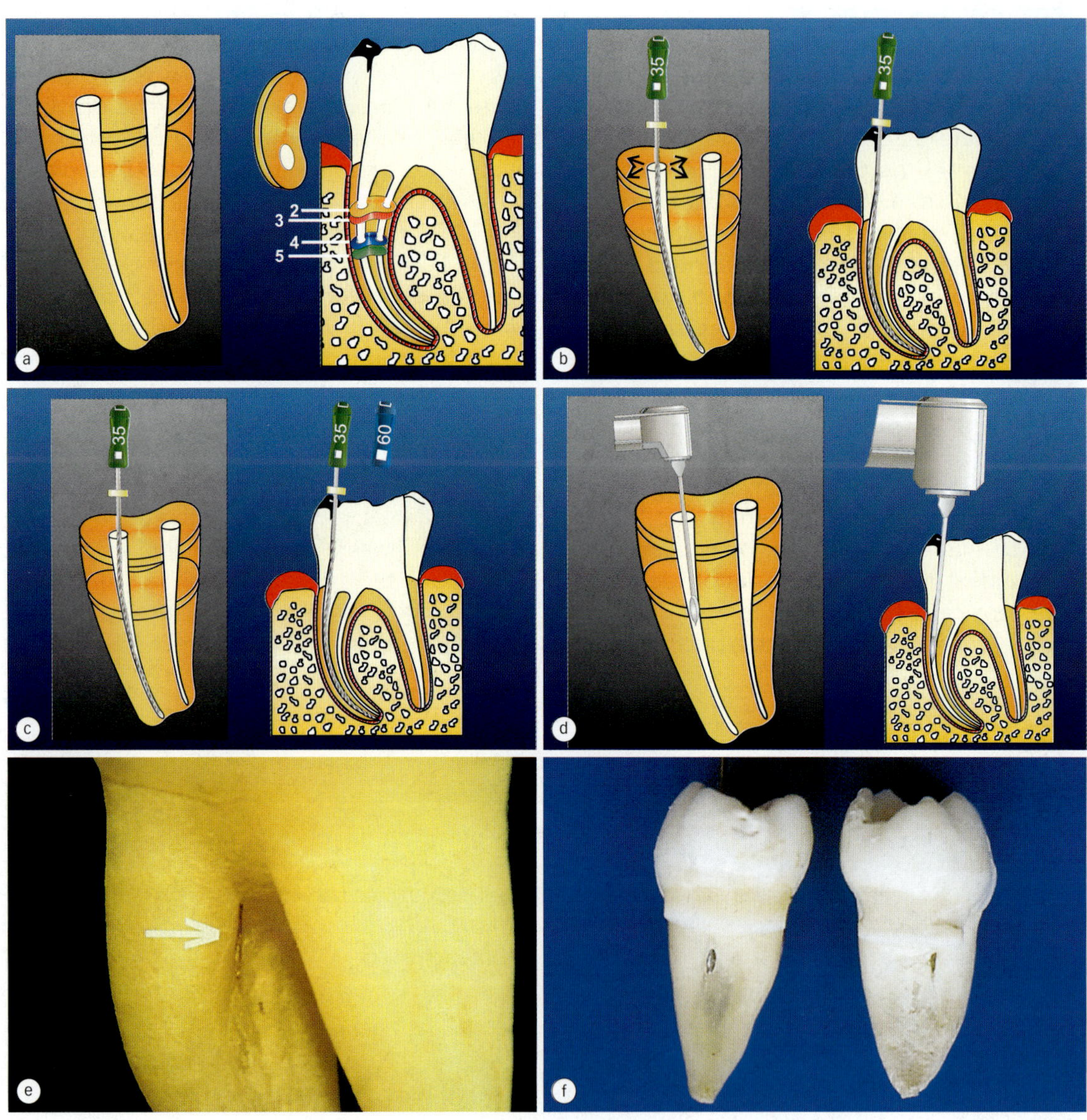


**Figure 16.10** - (**A-F**) Experimental study design, with risk of perforating thin walls in first mandibular molars[76].

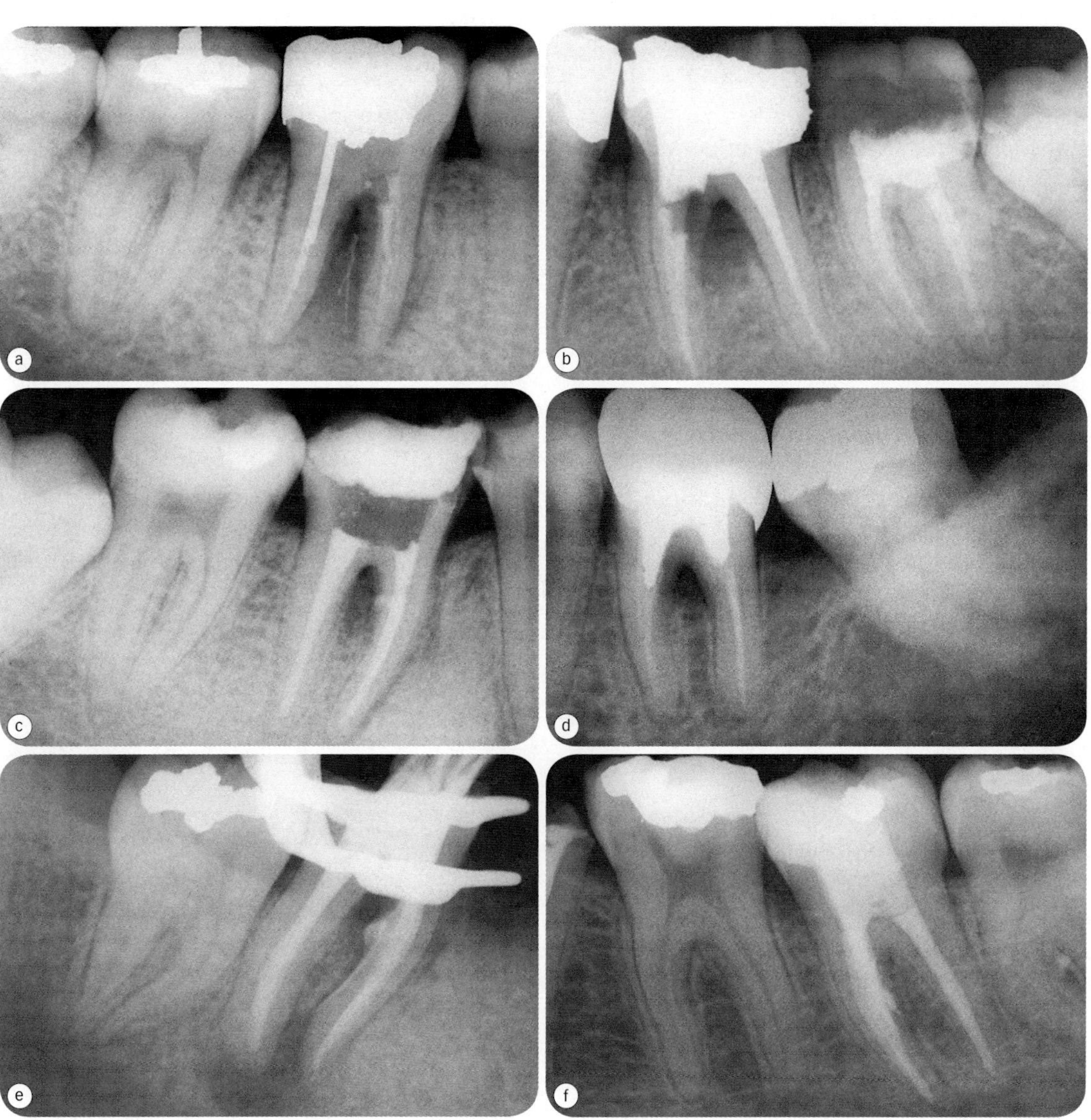


**Figure 16.11** - (**A-F**) Radiographic aspects with lateral perforations, due to excessive wear in thin walls[81].

### Determination of the Working Length

At this moment, establishment of the apical working limit allows greater control over possible variations in the working length that exist during preparation, and once the entrance orifice and the cervical third of the root canal have been prepared, smaller changes in length are seen, due to the rectification already done in this cervical region. Moreover, it allows greater control of the changes in the diameters of the endodontic instruments.

Pesce et al.[190] evaluated the variations of the working length in the coronal third of curved root canals. It was demonstrated that before and after the preparation of the cervical third, an average difference occurred for the mesial-buccal and mesial-lingual canals of mandibular first molars, ranging from 0.308 mm to 0.261 mm, respectively.

Determination of the longitudinal extent of work is based on the method proposed by Ingle & Taintor[126] as follows:

1. Obtain the average between the mean length of the tooth and the length of the tooth on the initial radiograph;
2. Subtract 2 mm from this measurement (due to possible distortions) and introduce a file into the root canal to measure this length and take a radiograph;
3. In the radiograph, verify the distance between the end of the endodontic instrument and the tooth radiographic apex. To maintain the preparation limit in the proximities of the cementum dentinal canal junction, retrieve approximately 1 mm, increasing or decreasing the length of the file, visualized in the radiograph;

When the difference is greater than 1 mm, repeat the radiograph to confirm. This maneuver should be repeated until one is certain of the adequate limit for the preparation of the root canal (Fig. 16.12A-B).

Different systems for determining the working length of the root canal have been suggested (Fig. 16.13).The association of electronic apex locators with an inspection radiograph length, is more frequently recommended.

According Serota et al.[223-225], there are several basic conditions that ensure accuracy during use of all generations of foramen locators; 1. Preliminary debridement should remove most tissue or debris obstructions; 2. Cervical leakage must be eliminated and excess fluid removed from the chamber, as this may cause inaccurate readings; 3. Extremely dry canals may result in low readings (long working length); 4. Long canals can produce high readings (short working lengths); 4) Lateral canals may give a false foramen reading, and 5) With open apices their use is contraindicated. The residual fluid in the canal should have a low conductivity value.

Wu et al.[299], based on biologic and clinical principles, reported that the after pulpectomy, the best success rate has been decrypted when the procedures terminated 2 to 3 mm short of the radiographic apex. With pulpal necrosis, bacteria and their byproducts, as well as infected dentinal debris may remain in the most apical portion of the canal; these irritants may jeopardize apical healing. In these cases, better success was achieved when the procedures terminated at or within 2 mm of the radiographic apex (0 to 2 mm). When the therapeutic procedures were shorter than 2 mm from or past the radiographic apex, the success rate for infected canals was approximately 20% lower than that when the procedures terminated at 0 to 2 mm. Clinical determination of apical canal anatomy is difficult. An apical constriction is often absent. Based on biologic and clinical principles, instrumentation and obturation should not extend beyond the apical foramen.

Considering the actual importance of evidence-based dentistry, and the role of meta-analysis to search outcome for clinical decisions, it is essential to examine studies based on meta-analysis. [18,28] As regards the apical limit of obturation, Kojima et al.[134] based on meta-analysis, determined the influence of factors such as apical limit (short vs. over extension), status of the pulp (vital vs. non vital), and periapical status (presence or absence of radiolucency) on endodontic prognosis. The study-list was obtained by using a MEDLINE search and Japan Centra Revuo Medicina search. Only articles in which the criteria for success or failure were exactly described, were accepted. A significant difference in success rates was found when teeth with perirapical lesion were compared with those without lesion. Based on the use of cumulative meta-analysis, the authors proposed that the root canal should be filled to within 2 mm of the radiographic apex. In another meta-analysis, Schaeffer et al.[216] determined the termination of instrumentation and obturation. Correlations were made as to success/failure as related to length of obturation from the apex. When comparing group A (obturated 0–1 mm from apex) versus group C (obturated past apex) using the DerSimonian and Laird estimates, group A showed a marginally better success rate than group C by 28.8%. Group A had better success than group B (obturated 1 mm short); the difference was insignificant. The results were similar after controlling for study quality using a single random effects regression model. In conclusion, the meta-analysis indicated that a better success rate is achieved when treatment includes obturation short of the apex.



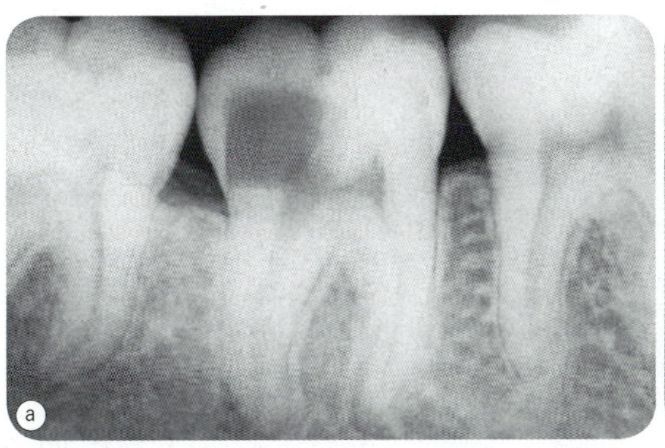


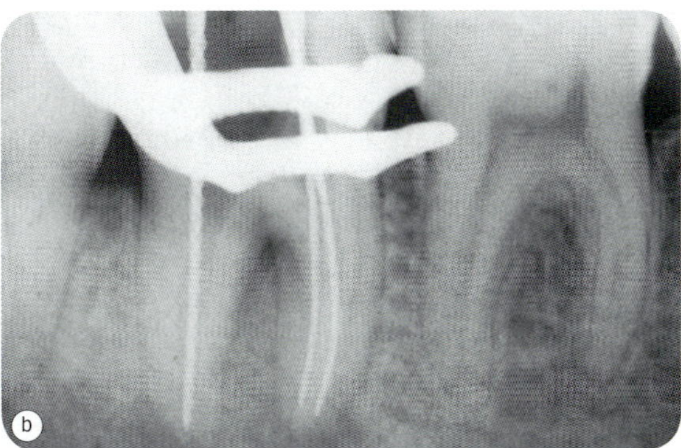


**Figure 16.12** - (**A-B**) Radiographic aspect visualizing determination of the working length.

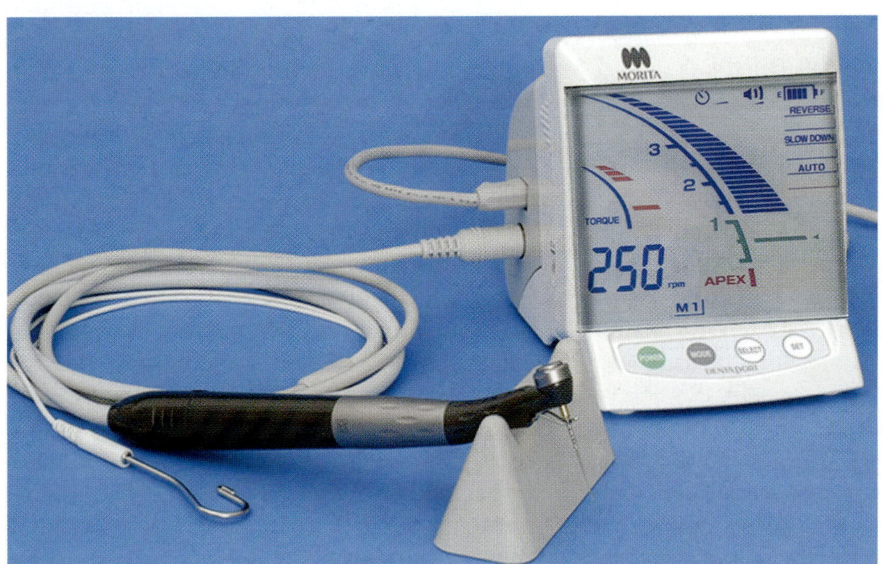


**Figure 16.13** - Apex locators (Courtesy of J. Morita).

Moura et al.[173] determined the influence of length of root canal obturation on apical periodontitis detected using periapical radiography and cone beam computed tomography. A total of 503 root canal obturations were evaluated using periapical radiography and cone beam computed tomography (CBCT). Distances from the radiographic apex to the tip of filling material were measured and classified as close to 2 mm, 1 mm short or beyond apex, and at the apex. Obturations at the apex were associated with apical periodontitis (AP). Periapical radiographs showed that root canal obturations were 1 to 2 mm short of the apex in 88%, 89.3% and 95% of the anterior teeth, premolars and molars. CBCT images showed obturations had the same length in 70%, 73.7% and 79% of anterior teeth, premolars and molars. The frequency of AP was significantly greater in molars than in the other tooth groups, regardless of diagnostic method. AP was detected more frequently when CBCT was used. AP was detected at all lengths of root canal obturation, and length was not associated with AP when root canals were not cleaned, shaped and three-dimensionally filled with good coronal restorations. The analyses of diagnostic methods showed that AP was detected more frequently when CBCT was used.

## Preparation of the Apical Third

Finally, the apical third still has to be prepared. Once again, through progressive advance, enlargement will be made easier.

Once the working length has been established, return to the exploring instrument (#8, #10, #15), empty the rest of the apical root canal and start the apical shaping. This instrument with a small diameter is more flexible and adapts better to the curvatures of the canal. It must be emphasized that the first instrument that reaches the ideal working limit is the one that should be called the identifier, because it allows the individuality of the canal to be recognized. Up until now, the canal has been seen only as a radiographic image, which has frequently been inconclusive and undefined. By means of this instrument, however, it is possible to establish the "identity" of the root canal, favor the plan of cleaning and shaping, select the most suitable anatomic instrument (the one that penetrates the root canal tightly), and favors the predictability of determining the lateral limit of enlargement.

For curved root canals the instrument should be preceded by a pre-curvature compatible with the root canal. One should be aware that the curved instrument can undergo unfolding in the straight region of the canal; therefore, the amplitude of the longitudinal movement should be small, not exceeding 2 mm. Endodontic instruments are capable of unfolding, and have a natural tendency of returning to the original position.

With instrument #10, start the rasping movement that consists of negative pressure on penetration and positive pressure against all the walls during traction, because the highest control over the tip of the instrument occurs during its removal and not at the time when it penetrates. Add movements of small amplitude, between 0.5 mm and 2.0 mm, until the freedom of the file in the root canal is noted. If resistance is noted when changing from one instrument to another, preferably return to the one first used, and proceed with instrumentation until it is free again. After the preparation with instrument #10, proceed to the next, #15, and make the same movements as described for the earlier instrument. Thus, the root canal is shaped. Frequently, difficulty is found in curved root canals when using stainless steel instruments #25 and #30, which in many cases, make it necessary to revert to files with smaller diameters, and preferably the instrument first used. Furthermore, it is accepted that the choice of the first instrument is as important as the choice of the last, and it is the intensity of the curvature, diameter of the root canal, thickness of the walls and the flexibility of the instrument itself that dictate the limits of enlargement.

For straight root canals, the kinematics of the instrumentation adopted during conventional instrumentation with stainless steel files is practically the same. When working in a rotary, oscillatory movement during its traction, the instrument should obey a movement of bias traction, in an oblique direction to the occlusal region, and follow the course of all the root canal walls.

Furthermore, if resistance is encountered when following the gradual increase in instrument size, return to the latter one, which can serve as the memory that will act throughout the entire working length. There is no predetermined rule to establish the memory instrument, because, it is the curvature and the anatomic diameter of the canal that do so. Thus, the memory can be the #30, #35, #40 or #45. The other instruments that follow obey anatomic recoil, where first resistance is the point that limits the working length. It is pointed out that once the anatomy is compatible, a higher degree of enlargement favors the sanitization process, placement of the intracanal dressing, and consequently, the filling.

The appearance of more flexible instruments with good cutting capacity have reduced the number of defects in the final shape of the root canal. When concluding the root canal preparation, before placing the intracanal dressing in pulp necrosis situations, it is important to repeat the foramen cleaning with low caliber files (#10 or #15), to unblock the cementum canal by removing the dentinal scraps that were extruded and compacted.

Pesce et al.[189,190] emphasized that, once the instrument is used, its cutting capacity decreases, because of deformation and / or dulling of its blades; from the first to the second use, there is a cutting loss of around 30%. Thus, it should not be mixed with others of that have been in use for a longer time, given the difficulty of maintaining the rhythm of work and serialization.

At this time, it is emphasized that preparation of the apical matrix (shoulder, backstop) in curved root canals is achieved with the gradual increase in the size of the instruments. This does not differ much from the procedure in straight canals, apart from the increase in dentinal wear, yet could spin (rotation movement) by additional rotary movement of the last instrument, with the objective of better defining the apical matrix, responsible for allowing a base to the main cone and serve as support for the filling material during the lateral condensation.

This preparation technique was compared with different instrumentation techniques and showed significant results in maintaining a tapering conical shape, retaining the original shape of the canal and of the apical foramen, regularity of the walls, and being easy to perform.

It is important to remember that the root canal, should be full of irrigant solution throughout the shaping procedure, and be renewed after every file change. After this, the root canal must be dried and completely filled with EDTA, pH 7.2 (close to neutral), and agitated for 3 minutes. Then, irrigation with sodium hypochlorite should be repeated, not with the objective of neutralizing the EDTA, but to potentiate its effect, because now it will probably penetrate more effectively, liberating more nascent chloride and hypochlorous acid, and recognized antimicrobial agents.

Thus, irrigation with EDTA after the root canal preparation has been concluded is performed for the purpose of removing the organic and inorganic dentinal magma.

Considering the actual state of Endodontics, with the advent of several facilitating resources, it is not exaggerated care to think of defining the final shape of the prepared curved canals better. Although aware of the absence of a reliable and applicable methodology to evaluate the quality of the preparation, it is a challenging and difficult task to qualify and conceive a well prepared canal, and it also bears a very personal stamp.

The canal preparation technique described presents an alternative to better define the shape of the curved root canals, especially present in the molars. It starts with logical and deductive observations, such as the shortest distance between two points is a straight line. Thus, when the influence of the apical curvature has been overcome, and beginning with an adequate cervical preparation, the better the final shape will be standardized and the more efficient will be the root canal preparation.

More important than the euphoria of the discovery of magic formulas and modern equipment that solve all the problems, it is the esteem and respect for the biologic principles that govern their indications and declare their efficiency. Thus, by the survival of these new systems it is observed that research and time are impartial judges. Evaluations with different methodologies and longitudinal studies are necessary to confirm the results recorded up to now. It is, however admitted that a new generation of nickel-titanium instruments will occupy a special place in the shaping of curved root canals.

Some considerations should be adopted during the instrumentation of root canals to avoid fractures of endodontic instruments, since this uncomfortable accident places the success of endodontic treatment at risk. Attitudes that should be taken, to prevent fracture of endodontic instrument can be grouped as follows (Table 16.3).

Figures 16.14A-D illustrate a schematic representation of a sequence of the preparation technique using stainless steel and NiTi instruments. Figures 16.15A-T exhibit radiographic aspects of root canals prepared using this root canal technique.

**Table 16.3** - Considerations to prevent accidents during root canal preparation

| |
|---|
| Use of a smooth instrument and with small caliber (special series # 06, 08, 10) for the initial exploration of the root canals (emptying and planning the root canal preparation); |
| Keep the sequence of gradual increase during the lateral enlargement (transversal preparation); |
| Always work with the root canal full of chemical substance, renewing it after every endodontic file change; |
| Any stainless steel instrument that becomes stuck on the root canal walls should be removed without rotary movement, only with a simple traction movement; |
| Always start the root canal preparation with manual files, for later preparation with nickel-titanium instruments, driven by electric motors; |
| Do not abuse nickel-titanium instruments in root canals with severe curvature; |
| Continuous renewal of endodontic instruments. Although it is difficult to determine the number of times that the instrument is really capable of working, it should be examined with a magnifier and adequate light after every use, not underestimating the time of action for the preparation, Irrespective of the number of times it has been used. For the files # 06, 08, 10 and 15, change after every use; |
| Always develop the previous preparation of the cervical third, which allows an action with more freedom for the endodontic instrument in the apical third; this facilitates a higher penetration and action of the chemical substance in depth, thus favoring the maneuvers of root canal filling; |
| Never underestimate the true macro-configuration of the pulp cavity judged simply by the radiographic aspect; |
| The quality of preparation is more significant than the speed of preparation. |

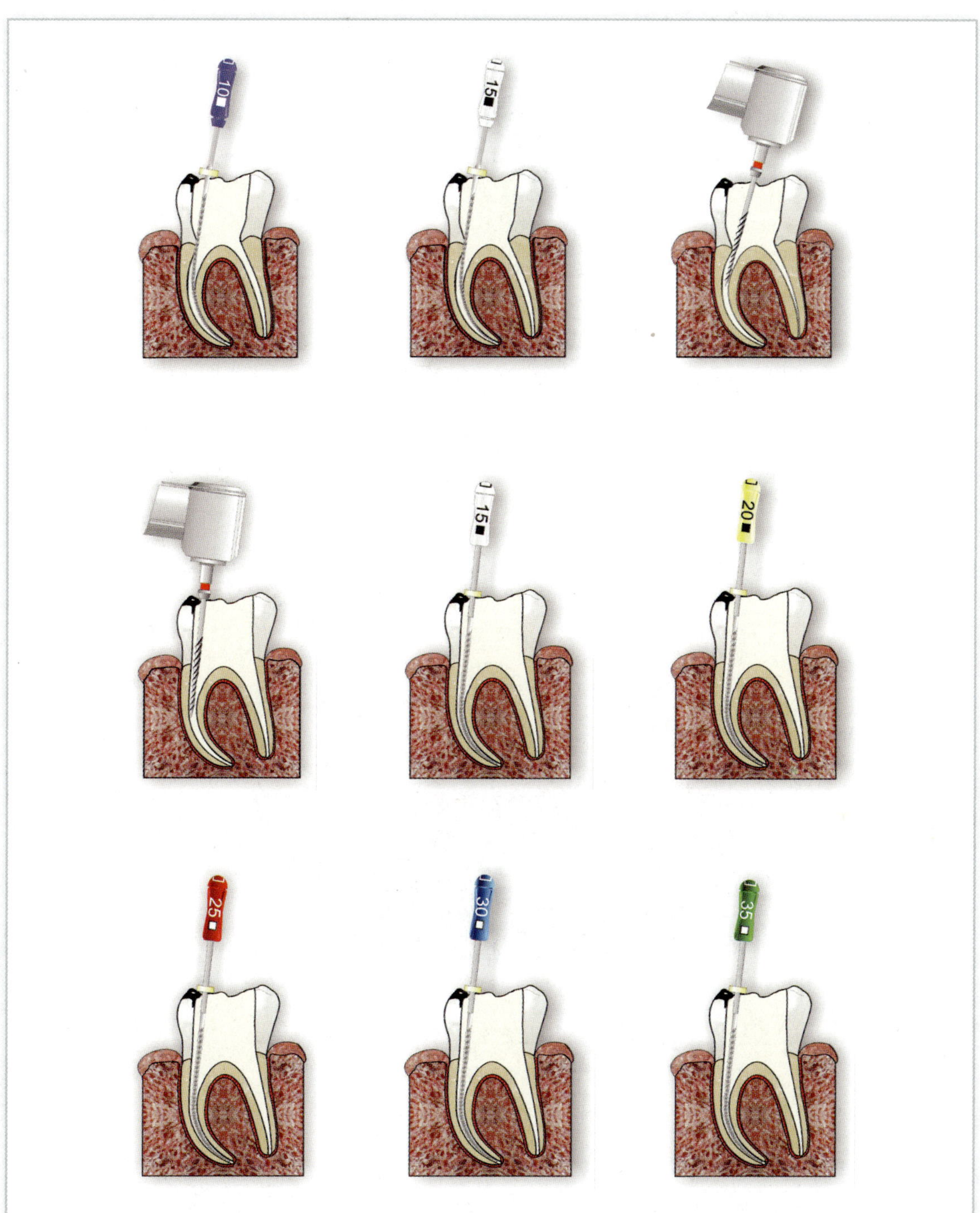


**Figure 16.14A** - Schematic representation of a sequence of the preparation technique using stainless steel instruments (Chapter 17).

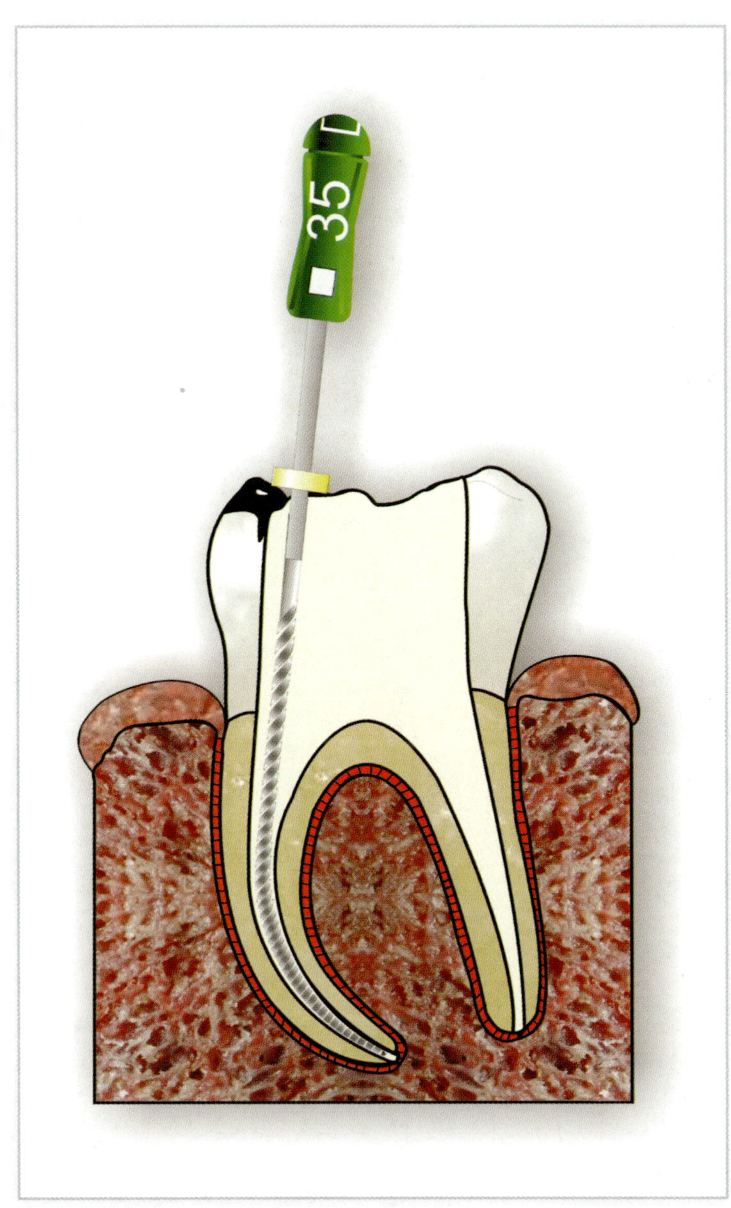


**Figure 16.14B** - Schematic representation using stainless steel instruments.

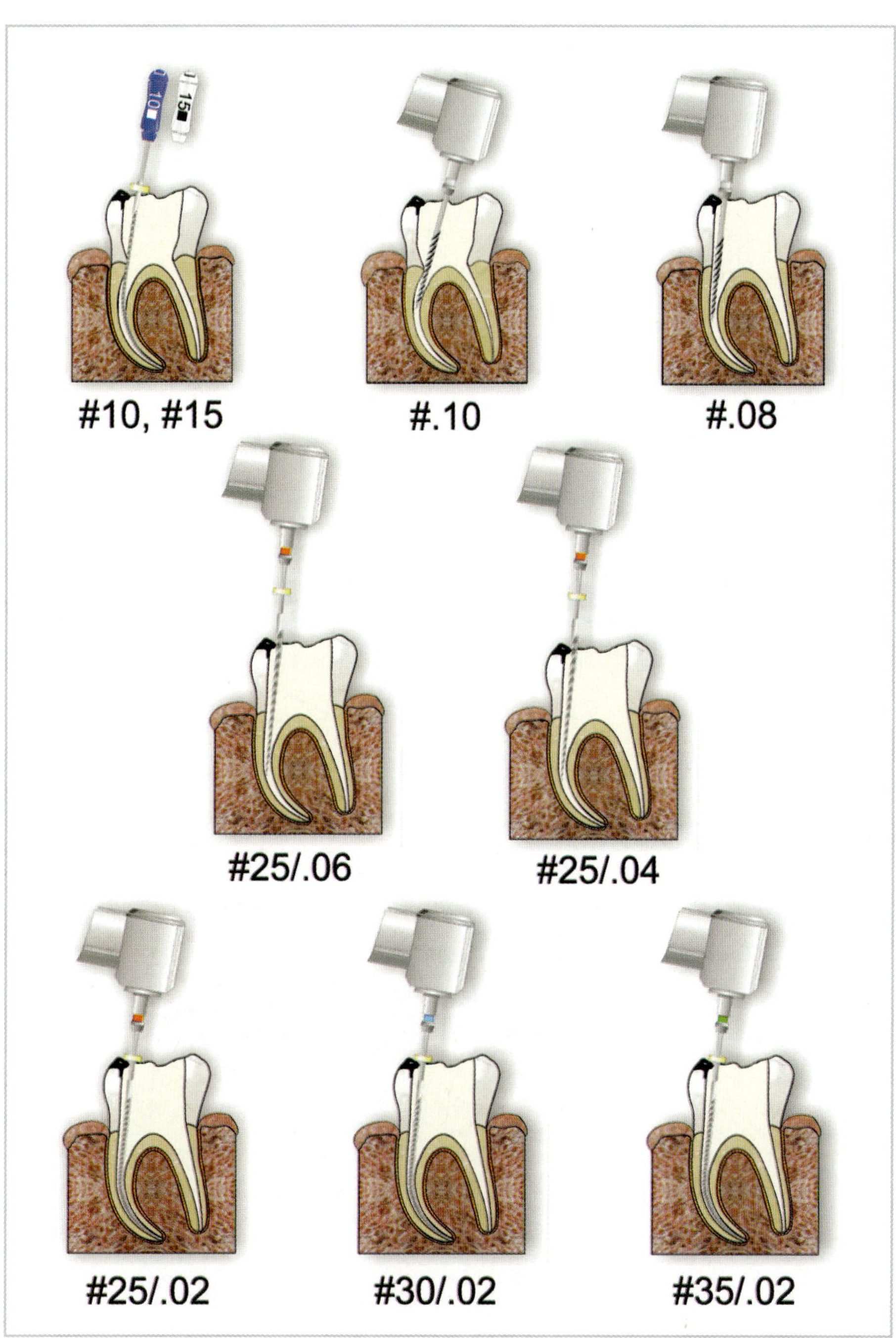


**Figure 16.14C** - Schematic representation of a sequence of the preparation technique using NiTi instruments (Chapter 17).

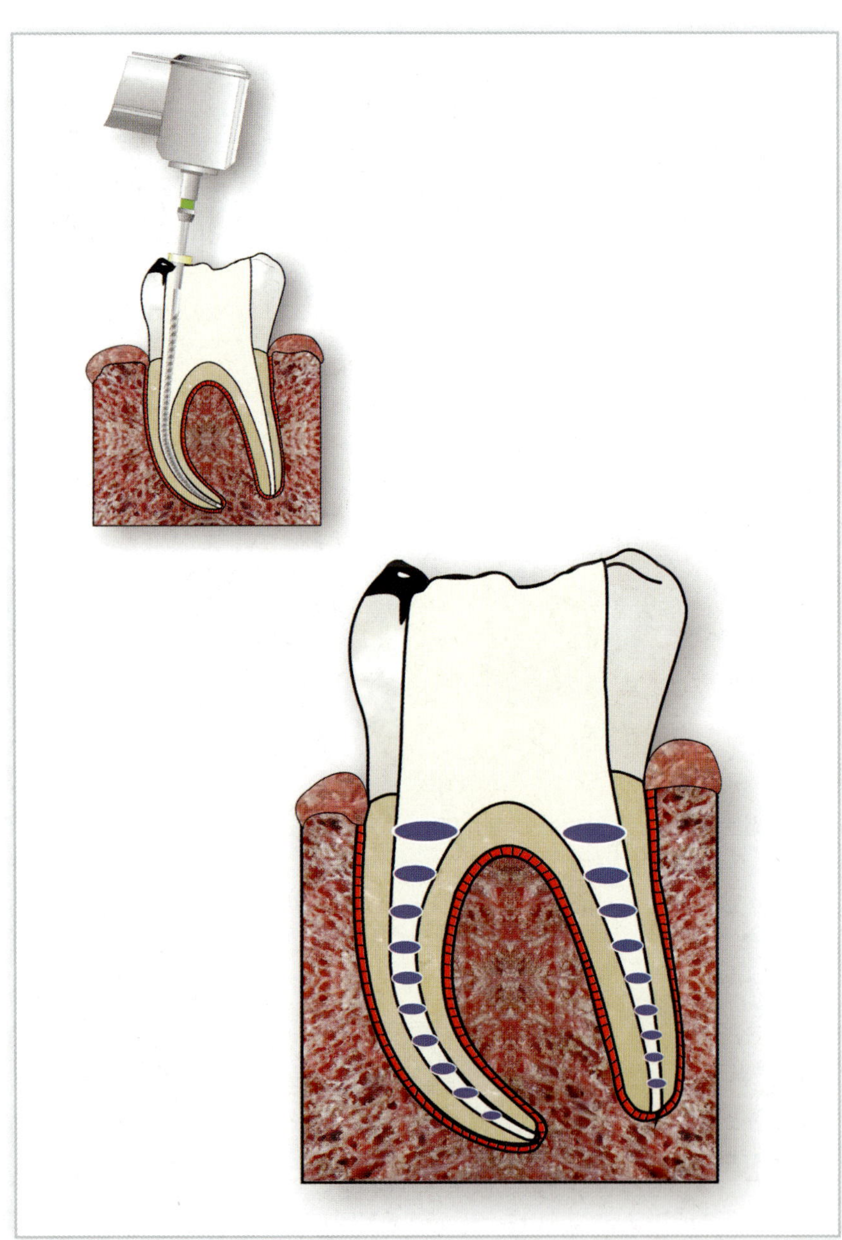

**Figure 16.14D** - Schematic representation using NiTi instruments.

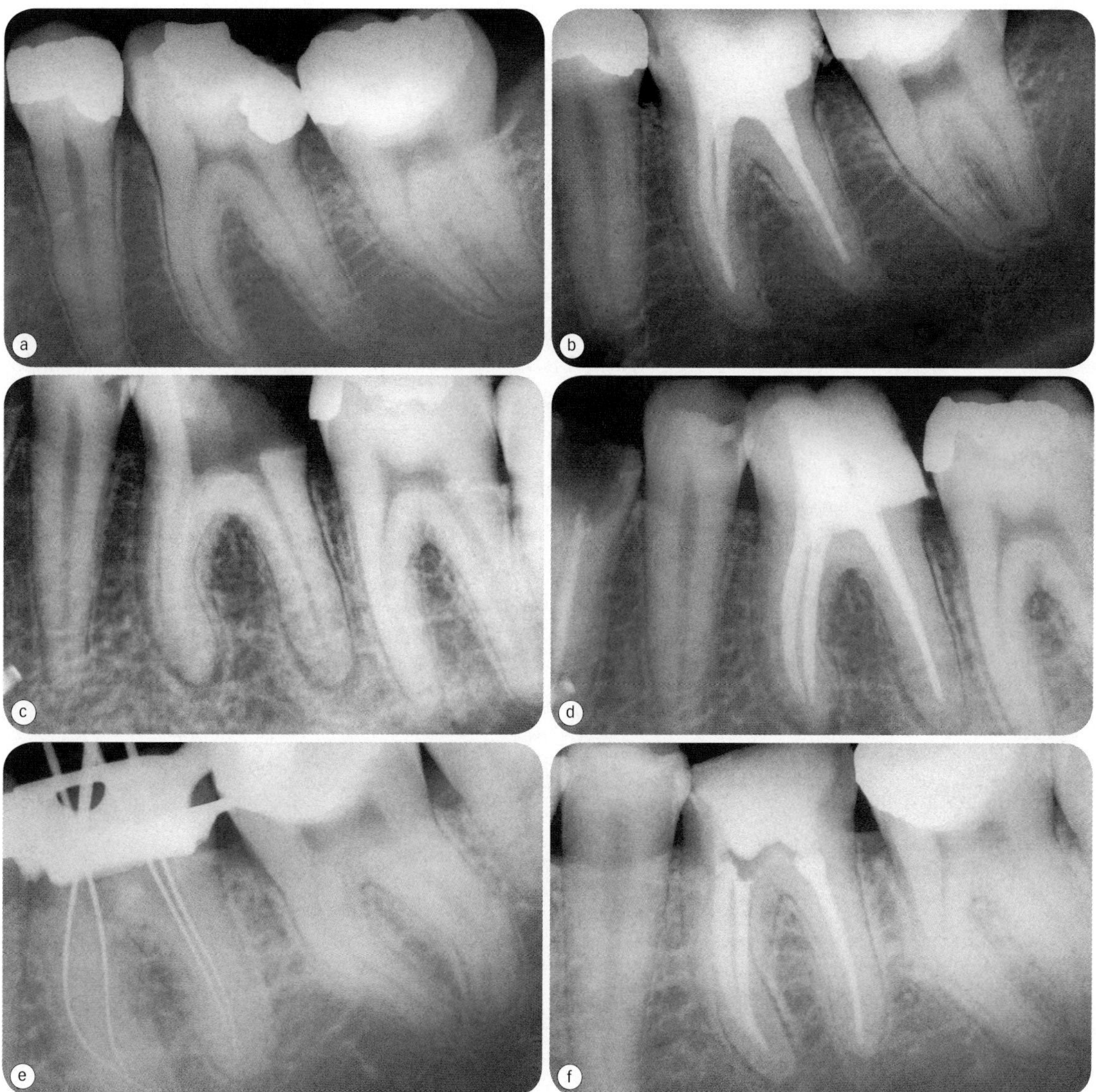


**Figure 16.15** - (**A-F**) Radiographic aspects of root canals prepared using this root canal technique.

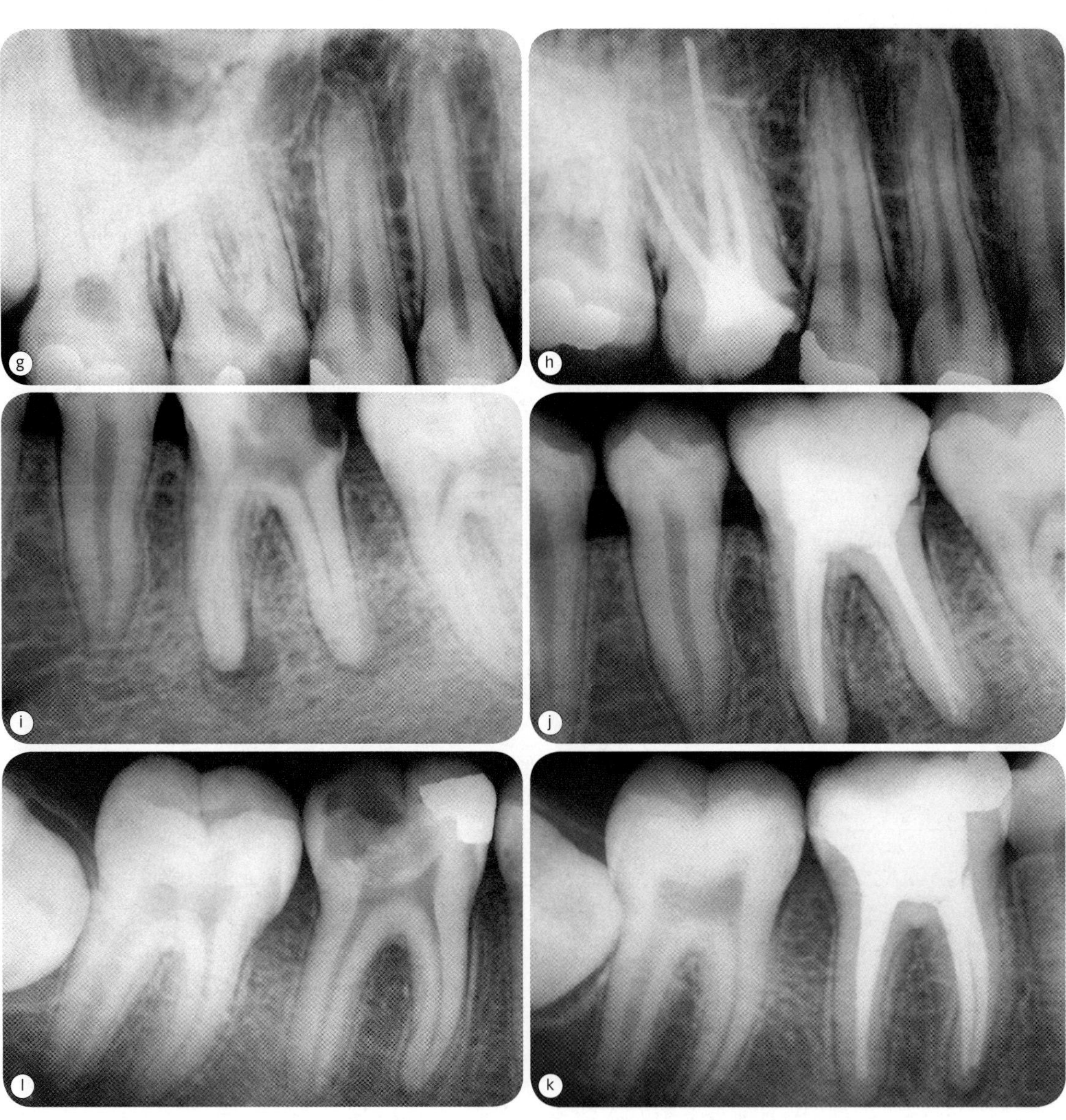

**Figure 16.15** - (**G-K**) Radiographic aspects of root canals prepared using this root canal technique.

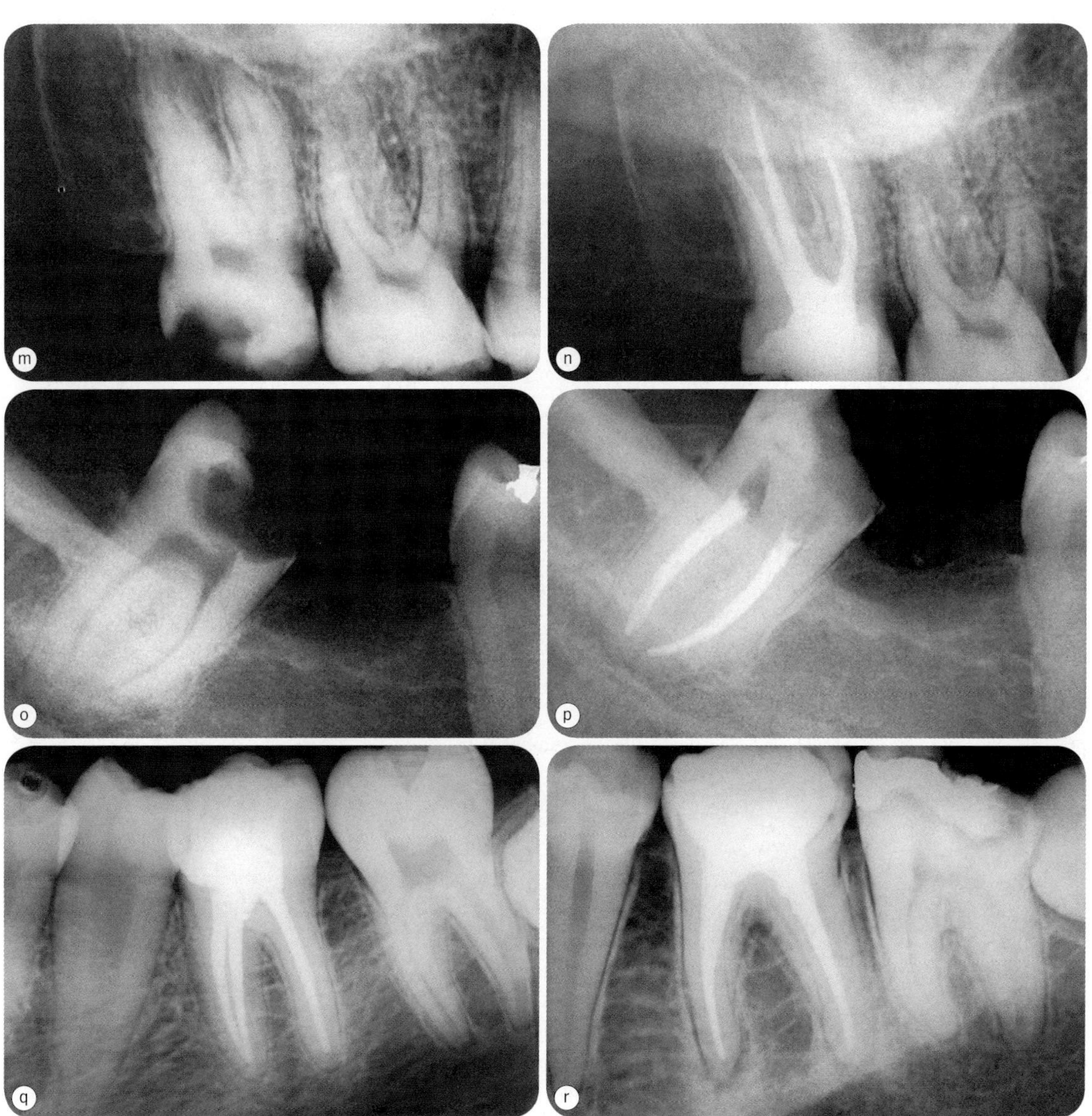


**Figure 16.15** - (**M-R**) Radiographic aspects of root canals prepared using this root canal technique.

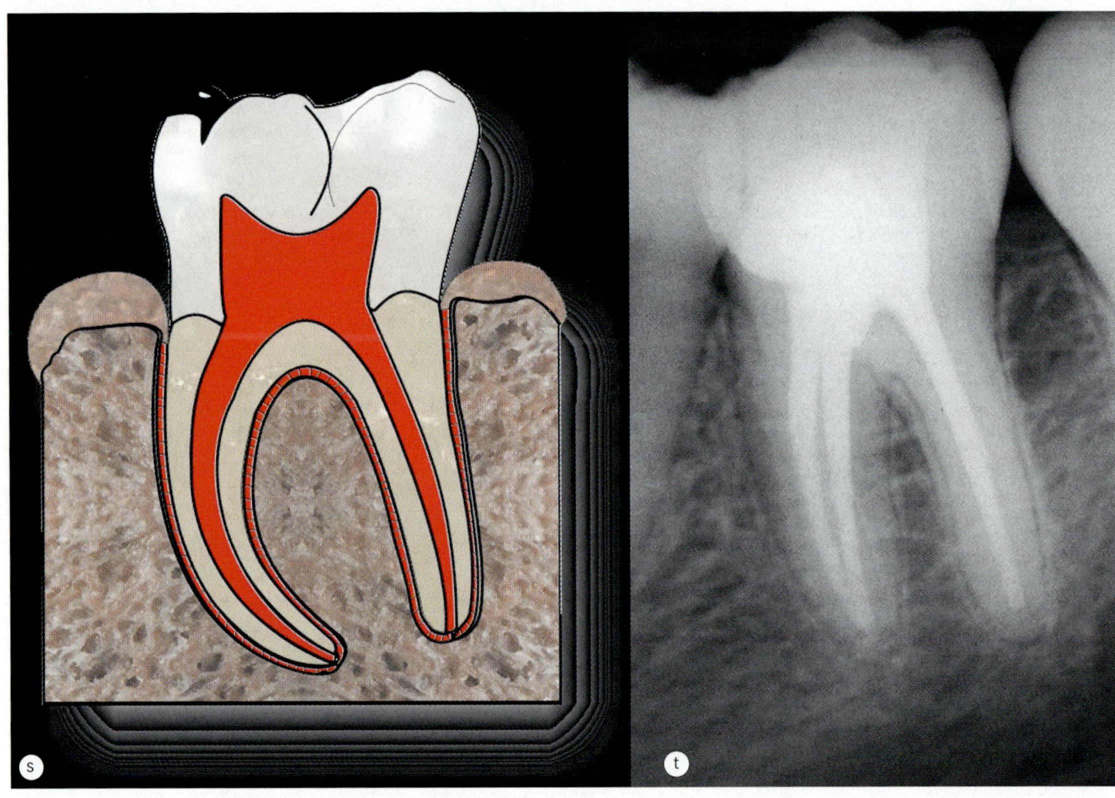

**Figure 16.15** - (**S-T**) Radiographic aspects of root canals prepared using this root canal technique.

1. Abou-Rass M, Ellis MA. Comparison of three methods of hand and automated instrumentation using the CFS and M4 for preparations of curved and narrow simulated root canals. Braz Endod J 1996;1:25-33.
2. Abou-Rass M, Frank AL, Glick DH. The anticurvature filing method to prepare the curve root canal. J Am Dent Ass 1980;101:792-4.
3. Abou-Rass M, Jastrab RJ. The use of rotary instruments as auxiliary aids to root canal preparation of molars. J Endod 1982;8:78-82.
4. Ahmad M, Pitt Ford TJ, Crum LA. Ultrasonic debridement of root canals: acoustic streaming and its possible role. J Endod 1987;13:490-9.
5. Allen MJ, Glickman GN, Griggs JA. Comparative analysis of endodontic pathfinders. J Endod 2007;33:723-6.
6. Allison DA, Weber CR, Walton RE. The influence of the method of canal preparation on the quality of apical and coronal obturation. J Endod 1979;5:298-304.
7. Alodeh MHA, Doller R, Dummer PMH. Shaping of simulated root canals in resin blocks using the step-back technique with K-files manipulated in a simple in/out motion. Int Endod J 1989;22:107-17.
8. Alodeh MHA, Dummer PMH. A comparison of the ability of K-files to shape simulated root canals in resin blocks. Int Endod J 1989;22:226-35.
9. Al-Omari MAO, Dummer PMH, Newcombe RG, Doller R. Comparison of six files to prepare simulated root canals. Part 1. Int Endod J 1992;25:57-66.
10. Al-Omari MAO, Dummer PMH, Newcombe RG. Comparison of six files to prepare simulated root canals. Part 2. Int Endod J 1992;25:67-81.
11. Al-Omari MAO, Dummer PMH. Canal blockage and debris extrusion with eight preparation techniques. J Endod 1995;21:57-61.
12. Anderson ME, Price JWH, Parashos P. Fracture resistance of electropolished rotary nickel–titanium endodontic instruments. J Endod 2007;33:1112-6.
13. Andrade MS. Características estruturais e termomecânicas de uma liga NiTi aproximadamente equiatômica na faixa de temperatura 20-100°C. (Master's Thesis). Federal University of Minas Gerais; 1978. 114p.
14. Anjos-Neto DA. Influência da patência apical e dos cimentos Sealapex e AH Plus no reparo de lesões periapicais inflamatórias crônicas induzidas em dentes de cães, após curativo com hidróxido de cálcio. (Master's Thesis). Univesity of Marília, 2008.
15. Ashby M, Jones D. Engineering Materials 2. Oxford: Pergamon Press; 1992. p.11. Chapter 12.
16. Bahia MGA. Resistência à fadiga e comportamento em torção de instrumentos endodônticos de NiTi. (Doctoral Thesis). Federal University of Minas Gerais, 2006. 213p.
17. Barbizam JV, Fariniuk LF, Marchesan MA, Pécora JD, Sousa-Neto MD. Efectiveness of manual and rotary instrumentation techniques for cleaning flattened root canals. J Endod 2002;28:365-6.
18. Barroso JM, Guerisoli DMZ, Capelli A, Saquy PC, Pécora JD. Influence of cervical preflaring on determination of apical file size in maxillary premolars: SEM analysis. Braz Dent J 2005;16:30-4.
19. Batista A, Sydney GB. Preparo do canal radicular curvo. J Bras Endo/Perio 2000;1:43-51.
20. Baugh D, Wallance J. The role of apical instrumentation in root canal treatment: a review of the literature. J Endod 2005;31:333-40.
21. Bellizzi R, Cruse WP. A historic review of endodontics, 1689–1963, Part III. J Endod 1980;6:576–80.
22. Bishop K, Dummer PMH. A comparison of stainless steel Flexofiles and nickel-titanium NiTi Files during the shaping of simulated canals. Int Endod J 1997;30:25-34.
23. Biz MT, Figueiredo JAP. Morphometric analysis of shank-to-flute ratio in rotary nickel-titanium files. Int Endod J 2004;37:353-8.
24. Blum JY, Machtou P, Micallef JP. Location of contact areas on rotary ProFile instruments in relationship to the forces developed during mechanical preparation on extracted teeth. Int Endod J 1999;32:108-114.
25. Bolanos OR, Jensen JR. Scanning electron microscope comparison of the efficacy of various methods of root canal preparation. J Endod 1980;6:815-22.
26. Bombana AC. Análise química-quantitativa das ligas de aço inoxidável de alguns instrumentos endodônticos de diferentes tipos e procedências. Contribuição ao estudo. (Doctoral Thesis). University of São Paulo, 1986.
27. Borlina SC. Influence of apical patency in induced chronic periapical lesions, after calcium hydroxide dressing and filling of the root canals of dog's teeth with Sealer 26 and Endomethasone sealers. (Master's Thesis). Univesity of Marília, 2008; 215p.
28. Bower RC. Furcation morphology relative to periodontal treatment. J Endod 1979;50:366-74.
29. Boyer CB. A History of Mathematics. 2nd ed. Revised by Merzbach UC. New York: Wiley; 1989.
30. Briggs P, Gulabivala K, Setchell DJ. Dentine-removing characteristics of K-files energised by the Piezo-Endo. Int Endod J 1992;25:6–14.
31. Briggs P, Gulabivala K, Stock CJR, Setchell DJ. The dentine-removing characteristics of an ultrasonically energised K-File. Int Endod J 1989;22:259–68.
32. Bryant ST, Dummer PMH, Pitoni C, Bourba M, Moghal S. Shaping ability of .04 and .06 taper ProFile rotary nickel-titanium instruments in simulated root canals. Int Endod J 1999;32:155-64.
33. Bryant ST, Thompson SA, Al-Omari MAO, Dummer PMH. The shaping ability of ProFile rotary nickel-titanium instruments with ISO sized tips in simulated root canals: Part 1. Int Endod J 1998;31:275-81.
34. Buchanan LS. Management of the curved root canal. J Calif Dent Assoc 1989;17:18-27.
35. Buehler WJ, Cross WB. 55-Nitinol uniques wire alloy with a memory. Wire J 1969;2:41-49.
36. Burch JE, Hulen S. The relationship of the apical foramen to the anatomic apex of the tooth root. Oral Surg Oral Med Oral Pathol 1974;34:262-8.

37. Byström A, Sundqvist G. Bacteriologic evaluation of the efficacy of mechanical root canal instrumentation in endodontic therapy. Scand J Dent Res 1981;89:321-8.
38. Calas P, Vulcain JM. Le concept du HERO 642. Rev Odont-Stom 1999;28:1–10.
39. Callahan JR. Periscope. Dent Cosmos 1894;36: 329-31.
40. Camps J, Pertot W. Relationship between file size and stiffness of stainless steel instruments. Endod Dent Traumatol 1994;10:260–3.
41. Camps JJ, Perlot WJ. Torsional and stiffness properties of nickel-titanium K files. Int Endod J 1995;28:239-43.
42. Canalda-Sahli C, Brau-Aguade E, Berastegui-Jimeno E. Torsional and bending properties of stainless steel and nickel-titanium Canal Master U and Flexogate instruments. Endod Dent Traumatol 1996;12:141-5.
43. Card SJ, Sigurdsson A, Orstavik D, Trope M. The effectiveness of increased apical enlargement in reducing intracanal bacteria. J Endod 2002;28:779-83.
44. Carrascoza A. Análise morfológica comparativa, em dentes humanos extraídos, de duas técnicas propostas para o emprego de canais radiculares curvos. (Master's Thesis). University of São Paulo; 1994.
45. Carvalho LAP, Bonetti I, Borges MAG. A comparison of molar root canal preparation using stainless steal and nickel titanium instruments. J Endod 1999;25:807-10.
46. Chan AWK, Cheung GSP. A comparison of stainless steel and nickel-titanium k-files in curved canals. Int Endod J 1996; 29:370-5.
47. Chandler N, Bloxham G. The influence of two handle designs and gloves on the performance of a simulated endodontic task. J Endod 1990;16:541-2.
48. Chapman CE. A microscopic study of the apical region of human anterior teeth. J Brit Endod Soc 1969;3:52-61.
49. Cheung GSP, Darvell BW. Fatigue testing of a NiTi rotary instrument. Part 1: strain-life relationship. Int Endod J 2007;40:612-8.
50. Cimis GM, Boyler TF, Pelleu-Jr GR. Effect of three files studies of canal curvatures in the mesial roots of mandibular molars. J Endod 1988;14:441-4.
51. Civjan S, Huget EF, Simon LB. Potential applications of certain nickel-titanium (nitinol) alloys. J Dent Res 1975;54:89-96.
52. Clem WH. Endodontics: the adolescent patient. Dent Clin N Amer 1969; 13:483-93.
53. Coffae KP, Briliant JD. The effect of serial preparation on tissue removal in the root canal of extracted mandibular human molars. J Endod 1975;1:211-4.
54. Coleman CL, Svec TA, Rieger MR, Suchina JA, Wang MM, Glickman GN. Analysis of nickel titanium versus stainless steel instrumentation by means of direct digital imaging. J Endod 1996; 22:603-7.
55. Contreras MAL, Zinman EH, Kaplan SK. Comparison of the first file that fits at the apex, before and after early flaring. J Endod 2001;27:113-6.
56. Cormier CJ, von Fraunhofer JA, Chamberlain JH. A comparison of endodontic file quality and file dimensions. J Endod 1988;14:138–42.
57. Courtney TH. Mechanical behavior of materials. USA: Mc Grow Hill, 1990.
58. Cunningham CJ, Senia ES. A three dimensional studies of canal curvatures in the mesial roots of mandibular molars. J Endod 1992;18:294-300.
59. Dalton BC, Orstavik D, Phillips C, Pettiette M, Trope M. Bacterial reduction with nickel-titanium rotary instrumentation. J Endod 1998;24:763-7.
60. Davis SR, Brayton SM, Goldman M. The morphology of the prepared root canal a study utilizing injectable silicone. Oral Surg Oral Med Oral Pathol 1972;34:642-8.
61. De Deus QD. Endodontia. 5th ed. Medsi: Rio de Janeiro; 1992. 695p.
62. Dearing GJ, Kazemi RB, Stevens RH. An objective evaluation comparing the physical properties of two brands of stainless steel endodontic hand files. J Endod 2005;31:827–30.
63. Debelian G, Trope M. BioRace: efficient, safe and biological based sequence files. Roots 2008;1:20-26.
64. Del Bello TPL, Wang N, Roane JB. Crown-Down tip design and shaping. J Endod 2003;29:513-8.
65. Deplases P, Peters O, Barbakow F. Comparing apical preparations of root canals shaped by nickel-titanium rotatory instruments and nickel-titanium hand instruments. J Endod 2001;27:196-202.
66. Dietz DB, Di Fiore PM, Bahcall JK, Launtenschlager EP. Effect of rotational speed on the breakage of nickel-titanium rotary files. J Endod 2000;26: 68-71.
67. Dobó-Nagy C, Szabó J, Szabó J. A mathematically based classification of root canal curvatres on natural human teeth. J Endod 1995;11:557-60.
68. Dummer PMH, Alodeh MHA, Al-Omari MAO. A method for the construction of simulated canals in clear resin blocks. Int Endod J 1991;24:63-6.
69. Dummer PMH, Alodeh MHA, Doller R. Shaping of simulated root canals in resin blocks using files activated by a sonic handpiece. Int Endod J 1989;24:211-25.
70. Dummer PMH, Al-Omari J. Shaping of simulated root canals in resin blocks using files activated by sonic handpiece. Int Endod J 1989; 22:211-5.
71. Dummer PMH, Hutchings R, Hartles FR. Comparison of two sonic handpieces during the preparation of simulated root canals. Int Endod J 1993;26:159-68.
72. Eggeler G, Hornbogen E, Yawny A, Heckmann A, Wagner M. Strutural and functional fatigue of NiTi shape memory alloys. Materials Science and Engineering A 2004;378:24-33.
73. ElDeeb ME, Boraas JC. The effect of different files on the preparation shape of severely curved canals. Int Endod J 1985;18:1-7.
74. Elias CN, Lopes HP. Materiais dentários. Ensaios Mecânicos. São Paulo: Santos, 2007.
75. Esposito PT, Cunninghan CJ. A comparation of canal preparation with nickel-titanium and stainless steel instruments. J Endod 1995;21:173-6.
76. Estrela C. Estudo comparativo do desgaste dentinário na parede distal do canal mésiovestibular do 1° molar inferior, produzido por três técnicas de instrumentação. (Master's Thesis). Federal University of Pelotas; 1990.
77. Estrela C. Preparo do Canal Radicular. In: Estrela C. Ciência Endodontia. São Paulo: Artes Médicas, 2004.

78. Estrela C, Bueno MR, Leles CR, Azevedo BC, Azevedo JR. Accuracy of computed tomography, panoramic and periapical radiographic for the detection of apical periodontitis. J Endod 2008;34:273-9.
79. Estrela C, Bueno MR, Sousa-Neto MD, Pécora JD. Method for determination of root curvature radius using cone-beam computed tomography images. Braz Dent J 2008;19:114-8.
80. Estrela C, Figueiredo JAP, Pesce HF. Avaliação da ocorrência do desvio apical, tendo como fonte de variação o instrumento memória, quando do emprego da técnica escalonada. Rev Bras Odontol 1993;50:3-6.
81. Estrela C, Figueiredo JAP. Endodontia: princípios biológicos e mecânicos. São Paulo: Artes Médicas, 1999. 819 p.
82. Estrela C, Figueiredo JAP. Técnica hídrida para preparo de canais radiculares curvos. Rev Odontol Brasil Central 2001;10:14-21.
83. Estrela C, Pesce HF, Stephan IW. Proposição de uma técnica de preparo cervical para canais radiculares curvos. Rev Odontol Brasil Central 1992;2:21-5.
84. Estrela C, Santos M, Bombana AC, Pesce HF. Análise da composição química de aços inoxidáveis de brocas Gates-Glidden de diferentes procedências. Rev Odontol USP 1993;7:251-5.
85. Estrela C, Sydney GB, Figueiredo JAP, Estrela CRA. Antibacterial efficacy of intracanal medicaments on bacterial biofilm – a critical review. J Applied Oral Science, 2009; 19(1) (in press).
86. Fauchard P. Le chirurgien-dentiste – traite des dents. 2nd ed. Paris: Chez Pierre Jean Marriete. 1745, 182p.
87. Fava LRG. Ampliação Reversa: Instrumental e técnicas. Contraste: São Paulo; 1996. 80p.
88. Fava LRG. Uma variação do preparo biomecânico escalonado: preparo biomecânico biescalonado. Rev Ass Paul Cirur Dent 1983;37:100-6.
89. Figueiredo JAP, Milano NF, Dummer PMH. Análise comparativa da formação do Zip apical em canais curvos e atresiados produzido *in vitro* por duas técnicas de instrumentação. Rev Fac Odontol URGS 1991;32:2-5.
90. Filippini HF, Figueiredo JAP. Evaluation of endodontic file surface on EDX and SEM. J Dent Res 2002;81:B42-B42.
91. Freund J, Toivonen R, Takala E-P. Grip forces of the fingertips. Clin Biomech 2002;17:515-20.
92. Gabel WP, Hoen M, Sterman HR, Pink FE, Dietz R. Effect of rotational speed on nickel-titanium file distortion. J Endod 1999;25:752-4.
93. Gambarini G, Laszkiewicz J. A scanning electron microscopic study of debris and smear layer remaining following use of GT rotary instruments. Int Endod J 2002;35:422-7.
94. Gambarini G. Rationale for the use of low-torque endodontic motors in root canal instrumentation. Endod Dent Traumatol 2000;16:95-100.
95. Gambill JM, Alder M, Del Rio CE. Comparison of nickel–titanium and stainless steel hand-file instrumentation using computed tomography. J Endod 1996;22:369–75.
96. Gavini G, Estrela C, Santos M, Fellipe-Jr O. In Vitro analysis of the desmineralizing effect of some endodontic irrigants. J Dent Res 1995;74:796.
97. Glosson CR, Haller RH, Dove SB, Del Rio CE. A comparison of root canal preparations using Ni-Ti hand, Ni-Ti engine-driven and K-flex endodontic instruments. J Endod 1995;21:146-51.
98. Gluskin AH, Brown DC, Buchanan LS. A reconstructed computerized tomographic comparison of Ni–Ti rotary GT™ files versus traditional instruments in canals shaped by novice operators. Int Endod J 2001;34:476-84.
99. Goerig AC, Michelich RJ, Schultz HH. Instrumentation of root canals in molar using the step-down technique. J Endod 1982;8:550-4.
100. Goldberg F; Massone EJ. Patency file and apical transportation: An in vitro study. J Endod 2002;28:7:510-1.
101. Grandini S, Balleri P, Ferrari M. Evaluation of Glyde File Prep in combination with sodium hypochlorite as a root canal irrigant. J Endod 2002;28:300-3.
102. Grant KA, Habes DJ, Steward LL. An analysis of handle designs for reducing manual effort: The influence of grip diameter. Int J Ind Ergon 1992;10:199-206.
103. Green DA. Stereomicroscopic study of 700 the root apices of maxillary and mandibular posterior teeth. Oral Surg Oral Med Oral Pathol 1956;13:728-733.
104. Green DA. Stereomicroscopic study of the root apices of 400 maxillary and mandibular anterior teeth. Oral Surg Oral Med Oral Pathol 1956; 9:1224-32.
105. Grossman LI. Endodontic Practice. 2nd ed. Lea & Febiger: Philadelphia; 1988.
106. Gu LS, Ling Q, Wei X, Huang Y. Efficacy of Protaper universal rotary retreatment system for gutta-percha removal from root canals. Int Endod J 2008;41:229-95.
107. Guerisoli DMZ, Marchesan MA, Walmsley AD, Pécora JD. Evaluation of smear layer removal by EDTAC and sodium hypochlorite with ultrasonic agitation. Int Endod J 2002;35:418-21.
108. Guilford WL, Lemons BS, Eleager PD. A comparison of torque required to fracture rotary files with tips bound in simulated curved canal. J Endod 2005;31:468-70.
109. Gulabivala K, Patel B, Evans G, Ng Y-L. Effects of mechanical and chemical procedures on root canal surfaces. Endod Topics 2005;10:103-22.
110. Gutiérrez JH, Garcia J. Microscopic and macroscopic investigation on results of mechanical preparation of root canals. Oral Surg Oral Med Oral Pathol 1968;25:108-16.
111. Haga WE. Microscope measurements on root canal preparations following instrumentation. J Brit Endod Soc 1968;2:41-6.
112. Haikel Y, Serfaty R, Batenan G, Senger B, Allemann. Dynamic and cyclic fatigue of engine-driven rotator nickel-titanium endodontic. J Endod 1999;25:434-40.
113. Harlan AL, Nicholls JI, Steiner JC. A comparison of curved canal instrumentation using nickel–titanium or stainless steel files with the balanced-force technique. J Endod 1996;22:410–3.
114. Hession RW. Endodontic morphology. III. Canal preparation. Oral Surg Oral Med Oral Pathol 1977;44:775-85.
115. Himel VT, Ahmed KM, Wood DM, Alhadainy HA. An evaluation of Nitinol and stainless steel files used by dental students dureing a laboratory proficiency exam. Oral Surg Oral Med Oral Pathol 1995;79:232-7.

116. Holland R, Mazuqueli L, Souza V, Murata SS, Dezan-Jr E, Suzuki P. Influence of the type of vehicle and limit of obturation on apical and periapical tissue response in dogs' teeth after root canal filling with mineral trioxide aggregate. J Endod 2007;33:693–7.
117. Holland R, Sant'anna-Jr A, Souza V, Dezan-Jr E, Otoboni-Filho JA, Bernabé PFE, Nery MJ, Murata SS. Influence of Apical patency and filling material on healing process of dogs' teeth with vital pulp after root canal therapy. Braz Dent J 2005;16:9-16.
118. Holland R, Souza V, Otoboni-Filho JA, Nery MJ, Bernabé PFE, Mello W. Técnicas mistas de preparo do canal radicular. Rev Paul Cirur Dent 1991;13:17-23.
119. Hülsmann M, Gressmann G, Schäfers F. A comparative study of root canal preparation using FlexMaster and HERO 642 rotary Ni-Ti instruments. Int Endod J 2003;36:358-66.
120. Hülsmann M, Schade M, Schäfers F. A comparative study of root canal preparation with HERO 642 and Quanted SC rotary Ni-Ti instruments. Int Endod J 2001;34:538-46.
121. Hülsmann M, Stryga F. Comparison of root canal preparation using different automated devices and hand instrumentation. J Endod 1993, 19:141-5.
122. Hülssmann M, Peters OA, Dummer PMH. Mechanical preparation of root canals: shaping goals, techniques and means. Endod Topics 2005;10:30-76.
123. Inan U, Aydin C, Tunca YM. Cyclic fatigue of ProTaper Rotary nickel-titanium instruments in artificial canals with 2 different radii of curvature. Oral Sur Oral Med Oral Pathol Oral Radiol Endod 2007;104:837-40.
124. Ingle JI, Levine M. The need for uniformity of endodontic instrument, equipaments and filling materials. Presented to the 2nd International Conference on Endodontics; 1958.
125. Ingle JI. Standardized endodontic technique utilizing newly designed instruments and filling materials. Oral Surg Oral Med Oral Pathol 1961; 14:83-91.
126. Ingle JI, Taintor JF. Endodontics. 3rd ed. Philadelphia: Lea & Febiger; 1985.
127. Kessler JR, Peters DD, Lorton L. Comparation of the relative risk of molar root perforation using various endodontic instrumentation techniques. J Endod 1983;9:439-47.
128. Kfir A, Rosenberg E, Zuckerman O, Tamse A, Fuss Z. Comparison of procedural errors resulting during root canal preparations completed by senior dental students in patients using an '8-step method' versus 'serial step-back technique'. Oral Surg Oral Med Oral Pathol Oral Radiol Endod 2004;97:745-8.
129. Kherlakian D, Ferreira MO, Zuolo ML. Quantec 2000: uma nova técnica para instrumentação de canais. Rev Ass Paul Cir Dent 1997;51:333-7.
130. Kimura Y, Wilder-Smith P, Matsumoto K. Lasers in endodontics: a review. Int Endod J 1999;33:173-85.
131. Kitchens Jr GG, Liewehr FR, Moon PC. The effect of operational speed on the fracture of nickel-titanium rotary instruments. J Endod 2007;33:52-4.
132. Kobaiashi C. Penetration of constricted canals with modified K files. J Endod 2007;23:391-3.
133. Koch K, Brave D. Real world endo: design features of rotary files and how they affect clinical performance. Oral Health 2002;39-49.
134. Kojima K, Inamoto K, Nagamatsu K, Hara A, Nakata K, Morita I, Nakagaki H, Nakamura H. Success rate of endodontic treatment of teeth with vital and nonvital pulps. A meta-analysis. Oral Surg Oral Med Oral Pathol Oral Radiol Endod 2004;97:95-9.
135. Kosa DA, Mershall G, Baungartner JG. An analysis of canal antering using mecanical instrumentation techniques. J Endod 1999;25:441-5.
136. Krup JD, Brantley WA, Gerstein H. An investigation of the torsional and bending properties of seven brands of endodontic files. J Endod 1984;10:372– 80.
137. Kuhn G, Tavernier B, Jordan L. Influence of structure on nickel-titanium endodontic instruments failure. J Endod 2001;27:516-20.
138. Kuttler Y. Microscopic investigation of root apexes. J Am Dent Ass 1955;50:544-52.
139. Lasala A. Endodoncia. Barcelona: Salvat, 1979.
140. Leeb J. Canal orifice enlargements related to biomechanical preparation. J Endod 1983;9:463-70.
141. Lim KC, Webber R. The validity of simulated root canal for the investigation for the prepared root canal shape. Int Endod J 1985;18:240-6.
142. Lim SS, Stock CJR. The risk of performance in the curved canal: anticurvature filing compared with the step-back technique. Int Endod J 1987;20:33-9.
143. Lopes HP, Elias CN, Estrela C, Fontes PP, Tuchman D. Emprego de limas acionadas a motor no preparo de canais radiculares. Rev Bras Odontol 1996;53:20-5.
144. Lopes HP, Elias CN, Estrela C, Pellegrinelli A, Leite HAS. Aquecimento na superfície radicular, durante a criação do espaço para pino. Estudo *in vitro*. Rev Ass Paul Cir Dent 1995;49:299-302.
145. Lopes HP, Elias CN, Estrela C, Siqueira JF Jr. Assessment of the apical transportation of root canals using the method of the curvature radius. Braz Dent J 1998;9:39-45.
146. Lopes HP, Elias CN, Estrela C, Siqueira-Jr JF, Fontes PP. Influência de limas endodônticas de NiTi de aço inoxidável, manuais e acionadas a motor, no deslocamento apical. Rev Bras Odontol 1997;54:67-70.
147. Lopes HP, Elias CN, Estrela C, Toniasso S. Mechanical stirring of smear layer removal: influence of the chelating agent (EDTA). Braz Endod J 1996;1:52-5.
148. Lopes HP, Elias CN, Mangelli M, Moreira EJL. Instrumentos endodônticos de NiTi de diferentes conicidades. Fratura por torção em flexão. Rev Bras Odontol 2006;63:113-6.
149. Lopes HP, Elias CN, Maria CR, Estrela C. Fratura, em rotação e flexão, de brocas Gates-Glidden e de Largo. Rev Bras Odontol 1995; 52:18-22.
150. Lopes HP, Elias CN, Siqueira Jr JF. Instrumentos endodônticos. In: Lopes HP, Siqueira Jr JF. Endodontia: biologia e técnica. 2nd ed. Rio de Janeiro: Guanabara Koogan, 2004;323-417.
151. Lopes HP, Elias CN, Siqueira-Jr JF, Estrela C. Considerações sobre a conicidade e o diâmetro das limas endodônticas. Rev Paul Odontol 1998;20:8-14.
152. Lopes HP, Elias CN, Siqueira-Jr JF. Fratura por torção das limas endodônticas de aço inoxidável. Rev Bras Odontol 2000;57:142-6.
153. Lopes HP, Elias CN, Siqueira-Jr JF. Mecanismo de fratura dos instrumentos endodônticos. Rev Paul Odontol 2000;22:4-9.

154. Lopes HP, Elias CN, Viana CSC, Estrela C. Estudo da fratura de limas endodônticas. Rev Bras Odontol 1995; 52:7-11.
155. Lopes HP, Elias CN. Fratura das limas endodônticas tipo K. Fundamentos teóricos e práticos. Rev Bras Odontol 2001;58:406-10.
156. Lopes HP, Elias CN. Fratura dos instrumentos endodônticos de níquel-titânio acionados a motor. Fundamentos teóricos e práticos. Rev Bras Odontol 2001;58:207-10.
157. Lopes HP, Moreira EJL, Elias CN, Almeida RA, Neves MS. Cyclic Fatigue of Protaper Instruments. J Endod 2008;33:55-7.
158. Lopes HP, Siqueira-Jr JF. Endodontia: biologia e técnica. Rio de Janeiro: Medsi, 1999. 650 p.
159. Marshall FJ, Papin J. A crown-down presureless preparation root canal enlargement technique. Technique Manual. Oregon Health Sciences University. Oregon: Portland; 1980.
160. Martin H. A telescope technique for endodontics. J Dent Can Dent Soc 1974;49:12-9.
161. Martin H. Ultrasonic disinfection of the root canal. Oral Surg Oral Med Oral Pathol 1976;42:92-9.
162. McSpadden JT. Advanced geometrics in endodontic micro files: the rationale. Chattanooga: TN:N.T. Company; 1996.
163. Melo LL, Pesce HF, Sydney GB. Estudo comparativo *in vitro* da flexibilidade e resistência à torção das limas K-Flex e Flexo-File. Rev Paul Odontol 1988;34-42.
164. Melo LL, Sydney GB, Pesce HF. Estudo comparativo *in vitro* da flexibilidade das limas Flexo-File, Tri- File e K-Flex. Rev Paul Odontol 1992;14:10-6.
165. Melo LL, Sydney GB. Novas técnicas de instrumentação endodôntica. In: Atualização na clínica odontológica. Gonçalves EAN, Feller C. Artes Médicas: São Paulo; 1998. p.167-199.
166. Melo MCC. Avaliação da resistência à fadiga de instrumentos de níquel-titânio acionados a motor. (Master´s Thesis). Federal University of Minas Gerais; 1999. 153p.
167. Miserendino LJ, Moser JB, Heuer MA, Osetek EM. Cutting efficiency of endodontic instruments. Part 1: a quantitative comparison of the tip and fluted regions. J Endod 1985;11:435-41.
168. Miserendino LJ, Moser JB, Heuer MA, Osetek EM. Cutting efficiency of endodontic instruments. Part 2: analysis of tip design. J Endod 1986;12:8-12.
169. Miura F, Mogi M, Ohura Y, Hamanaka H. The superelastic property of the japanese NiTi alloy wire for use in orthodontics. Am J Orthod Dentofacial Orthop 1986;90:1-10.
170. Montgomery S. Root canal wall thickness of mandibular molars after biomechanical preparation. J Endod 1985;11:257-63.
171. Moreira EJL, Lopes HP, Elias CN, Fidel RAS. Fratura por flexão em rotação de instrumentos endodônticos de NiTi. Rev Bras Odontol 2002;59:412–14.
172. Morgan LF, Montgomery S. An evaluation of the crown-down pressureless technique. J Endod 1984;10:491-8.
173. Moura MS, Guedes OA, Alencar AHG, Azevedo BC, Estrela C. Influence of apical limit of root canal obturation on apical periodontitis detected by periapical radiography and cone beam computed tomography. 2008; (submitted).
174. Mullaney TP. Instrumentation of finely curved canals. Dent Clin North Amer 1979;23:575-92.
175. Munley PJ, Goodell GG. Comparison of passive ultrasonic debridement between fluted and nonfluted instruments in root canals. J Endod 2007;33:578-80.
176. Nagy CD, Bartha K, Bernaf M, Verdes E, Szabó J. The effect of root canal morphologic on canal shape following instrumentation using different techniques. Int Endod J 1997;30:133-40.
177. Nasser SN, Guo WG. Superelastic and cyclic response of NiTi SMA at various strain rates and temperatures. Mechanics of Materials 2006;38:463-74.
178. O'Connell DT, Bryton SM. Evaluation of root canal preparation with two automated endodontic hand pieces. Oral Surg Oral Med Oral Pathol 1975;39:298-303.
179. Ottolengui R. Methods of filling teeth. Dent Cosmos 1892;34:807-23.
180. Ozawa T, Nakano M, Sugimura H, Tahata K, Nakamura J, Shiozawa K. Effects of endodontic instrument handle diameter on electromyographic activity of forearm and hand muscles. Int Endod J 2001;34:100-6.
181. Paiva JG, Antoniazzi JH. Endodontia - Bases para a prática clínica. 2nd ed. Artes Médicas: São Paulo; 1988. p.531-88.
182. Paque F, Barbakow F, Peters OA. Root canal preparation with Endo-Eze AET: changes in root canal shape assessed by micro-computed tomography. Int Endod J 2005;38:456–64.
183. Parashos P, Gordon I, Messer HH. Factors influencing defects of rotary nickel-titanium endodontic instruments after clinical use. J Endod 2004;30:722-25.
184. Parashos P, Messer HH. Rotary NiTi instrument fracture and its consequences. J Endod 2006;32:1031-43.
185. Parashos P, Messer HH. The diffusion of innovation in dentistry: a review using rotary nickel-titanium technology as an example. Oral Surg Oral Med Oral Pathol Oral Radiol Endod 2006;101:395-401.
186. Pécora JD, Capelli A, Guerisoli DMZ, Spano JCE, Estrela C. Influence of cervical preparation on apical file size determination. Int Endod J 2005;38:430-5.
187. Pécora JD, Capelli A, Seixas FH, Marchesan MA, Guerisoli DMZ. Biomecânica Rotatória: Realidade ou futuro? Rev Assoc Paul Cir Dent 2002;56:4-6.
188. Pécora JD, Capelli A. Shock of paradigms on the instrumentation of curved root canals. Braz Dent J 2006;17:3-5.
189. Pesce HF, Carrascoza A, Medeiros JMF, Estrela C. An *in vitro* evaluation of the effects of golden medium files on the preparation of curved canals. Rev Odont UNICID 1996;8:25-9.
190. Pesce HF, Estrela C, César OVS. Évaluation des variations de la longueur de travail aprés préparation du tiers coronaire des canaux radiculaires courbes. Rev Française d'Endodontie 1994;13:9-12.
191. Pessoa OF, Estrela C, Pesce HF. Estudo morfológico de canais radiculares preparados com duas técnicas manuais de instrumentação. Rev Odontol UNICID 1993; 5:21-26.
192. Peters OA, Barbakow F, Peters CI. An analysis of endodontic treatment with three nickel-titanium rotary root canal preparation techniques. Int Endod J. 2004;37:849-59.

193. Pettiette MT, Metzger Z, Phillips C, Trope M. Endodontic complications of root canal therapy performed by students with stainless-steal K-files and nickel titanium hand files. J Endod 1999;25:230-34.
194. Philipas GG. Influence of oclusal wear and age on formation of dentin and size of pulp chamber. J Dent Reasch 1961;40:1186-98.
195. Pruet JP, Clement DJ, Carnes-Jr DL. Cyclic fatigue testing of Nickel-Titanium endodontic instruments. J Endod 1997;23:77-85.
196. Pucci FM, Reig R. Conductos radiculares. Buenos Aires: Médico-Quirurgica, 1944.
197. Regan JD, Sherriff M, Meredith N, Gulabivala K. A survey of interfacial forces used during endosonic instrumentation of root canals. Int Endod J 2001;34:54–62.
198. Reis WP, Elias CL. Ligas de Ni-Ti com superelasticidade e memória de forma. Rev Bras Odontol 2001;58:300-4.
199. Ricucci D, Langeland K. Apical limit of root canal instrumentation and obturation, part. 2. A histological study. Int Endod J 1998;31:394-409.
200. Roane JB, Sabala CL, Duncanson MG. The balanced force concept for instrumentation of curved canals. J Endod 1985;11:203-11.
201. Roane JB, Sabala CL. Clockwise or counterclockwise. J Endod 1984; 10:349-53.
202. Rödig T, Hülsmann M, Mühge M, Schäfers F. Quality of preparation of oval distal root canals in mandibular molars using nickel-titanium instruments. Int Endod J 2002;35:919-28.
203. Rogers EM. Diffusion of innovations. 5th ed. New York: Free Press, 2003.
204. Rowan MB, Nicholls JI, Steiner JC. Torsional properties of stainless steal and nickel titanium endodontic files. J Endod 1996;22:341-5.
205. Royal JR, Donnelly JC. A comparison of maintenance of curvature using Balanced Force instrumentation with three different file types. J Endod 1995;21:300-4.
206. Sabala CL, Roane JB, Southard LZ. Instrumentation of curved canals a modified tipped instrument: a comparison study. J Endod 1988;14:59-64.
207. Samyn JA, Nicholls JI, Steiner JC. Comparison of stainless steal and nickel titanium instruments in molar root canal preparation. J Endod 1996;22:177-81.
208. Sattapan B, Nervo GJ, Palamara JEA, Messer HH. Defects in rotatory nickel-titanium files after clinical use. J Endod 2000;25:161-5.
209. Schäfer E, Florek H. Efficiency of rotary nickel-titanium K3 instruments compared with stainless steel hand K-Flexofile. Part 1: Shaping ability in simulated curved canals. Int Endod J 2003;36:199-207.
210. Schäfer E, Schlingemann R. Efficiency of rotary nickel-titanium K3 instruments compared with stainless steel hand K-Flexofile. Part.2. Cleaning effectiveness and shaping ability in severely curved canals of extracted teeth. Int Endod J 2003;36:208-17.
211. Schäfer E, Schulz-Bongert U, Tulus G. Comparison of hand stainless steel and nickel titanium rotary instrumentation: a clinical study. J Endod 2004;30:432-5.
212. Schäfer E, Tepel J, Hoppe W. Properties of endodontic hand instruments used in rotary motion. Part 2. Instrumentation of curved canals. J Endod 1995;21:493-7.
213. Schäfer E. Effects of four instrumentations techniques on curved canals: a comparison study. J Endod 1996;22:685-9.
214. Schäfer E. Effects of various sterilization procedures on the cutting efficiency of root-canal instruments. Deutsche Zahn Zeitschrift 1995;50:150–3.
215. Schäfers F, Schlingemann R. Efficiency of rotary nickel-titanium K3 instruments compared with stainless steel hand K-Flexofile. Part. 2. Cleaning effectiveness and shaping ability in severely curved canals of extracted teeth. Int Endod J 2003;36:208-17.
216. Schaeffer MA, White RR, Walton RE. Determining the Optimal Obturation Length: A Meta-Analysis of Literature. J Endod 2005;31: 271-4.
217. Schilder H. Cleaning and shaping the root canal. Dent Clin N Amer 1974;18:269-96.
218. Schilder H, Yee FS. Canal debridement and disinfection. In: Pathways of the Pulp. Cohen S, Burns RC. 3rd ed. St Louis, MO, USA: The CV Mosby Company; 1984. p.175.
219. Schineider SW. A comparison of canal preparations in straight and curved root canals. Oral Surg Oral med Oral Pathol 1971;31:96-193.
220. Schineider SW. A comparison of canal preparations in straight and curved root canals. Oral Surg Oral Med Oral Pathol 1971;32:271-5.
221. Senia ES, Wildey WL. The LightSpeed root canal instrumentation system. Endod Topics 2005;10:148-50.
222. Serene TP, Adams JD, Saxena A. Nickel-Titanium instruments: applications in Endodontics. Ihiyama Euro America Inc: St Louis; 1995. 112p.
223. Serota KS, Nahmias Y, Barnett F, Brock M, Senia ES. Predictable endodontic success: the apical control zone. Oral Health 2003;3:75-89.
224. Serota KS, Vera J, Barnett F, Nahmias Y. The new era of foramenal location. Oral Health 2004;4:48-54.
225. Serota KS. Nahmias Y. Predictable Endodontic Success: The hybrid approach – Part 1. Oral Health 2003:41-48.
226. Seto BG, Nicholls JI, Harrington GW. Torsional properties with twisted and machined endodontic files. J Endod 1990;16:355-60.
227. Shovelton DS. The presence and distribution of microorganisms with non-vital teeth. Brit Dent J 1964;3:101-7.
228. Shuping G, Orstavick D, Sigurdsson A, Trope M. Reduction of intracanal bacteria using nickel-titanium rotary instrumentation and various medications. J Endod 2000;26:751-5.
229. Sonntag D, Stachniss-Carp S, Stachniss C, Stachniss V. Determination of root canal curvatures before and after canal preparation (part II): A method based on numeric calculus. Aust Endod J 2006;32:16–25
230. Southard DW, Oswald RJ, Natkin E. Instrumentation of curved molar canals with the Roane Technique. J Endod 1987;13:479-89.
231. Souza RA. Endodontia clínica. São Paulo: Santos, 2003. 319p.
232. Souza RA. Limpeza do forame – uma análise crítica. J Bras Endo/Perio 2000;1:72-78.
233. Souza V, Otoboni-Filho JA, Holland R, Nery MJ, Bernabé PFE, Dezan-Jr E. Avaliação de alguns aspectos relacionados ao preparo manual e automatizado do canal radicular. Rev Paul Odont 2001;23:22-24.

234. Stock C, Walker R, Gulabivala K. Endodontics. 3rd ed. London: Elsevier Mosby. 2004, 324p.
235. Stock CJR. Current status of the use of ultrasound in endodontics. Int Dent J 1991;41:175-82.
236. Svec TA, Powers JM. Effects of simulated clinical conditions on nickel-titanium rotatory files. J Endod 1999;25:759-60.
237. Sydney GB, Batista A, Deonizio MD. Acesso Radicular. Rev Odontol Brasil Central 2008;17:1-12.
238. Sydney GB, Batista A, Estrela C, Pesce HF, Melo LL. SEM analysis of smear layer removal after root canal preparation by hand and with an automated handpiece. Braz Dent J 1996;7:19-26.
239. Sydney GB, Batista A, Melo LL. Alargadores para contra-ângulo: uma opção como auxiliar no preparo do canal radicular. Rev Bras Odontol 1994;51:41-4.
240. Sydney GB, Batista A. Diagnóstico e viabilização do retratamento endodôntico. p.5113-144, In: Dib LL; Saddy MS Atualização Clínica em Odontologia, Artes Médicas, São Paulo, 2006, 577p.
241. Sydney GB, Estrela C. The Influence of root canal preparation on anaerobic bacteria in teeth with asymptomatic apical periodontitis. Braz Endod J 1996;1:7-10.
242. Sydney GB, Estrela C, Carrascoza A, Pesce HF. Avaliação morfológica de canais radiculares curvos após o preparo com a técnica cervical auxiliada por brocas Gates-Glidden e com o Canal Finder System. Rev Ass Bras Odontol Nac 1995;2:427-30.
243. Sydney GB, Ferreira JL, Berger CR, Pellissari CA. Estudo comparativo do preparo do canal radicular realizado manualmente e acionado a motor com rotação alternada. Rev Bras Odontol 2000;57:91-5.
244. Sydney GB, Figueiredo JAP, Melo LL. SEM analysis of cleaning and shaping canals with Nd : YAG laser. J Dent Res 1999;78:1028.
245. Sydney GB. K3 – A nova geração de instrumentos de níquel-titânio. J Bras Endod 2002; 3:33-38.
246. Sydney GB. Preparo automatizado. In: Atualização na clínica odontológica. Feller C, Gorab R. São Paulo: Artes Médicas, 2000. p 250-293.
247. Taintor JF. Use of the Gates-Glidden bur in endodontics. J Neb Dent Ass 1978;10-2.
248. Tan BT, Messer H. The effect of instrument type and preflaring on apical file size determination. Int Endod J 2002;35:752-8.
249. Tepel J, Schäffer E, Hoppe W. Properties of endodontic hand instruments used in rotatory motion. Part 1: Cutting efficiency. J Endod 1995;21:418-21.
250. Tepel J, Schäffer E, Hoppe W. Properties of endodontic hand instruments used in rotatory motion. Part 3: Resistance to bending and fracture. J Endod 1997;23:141-5.
251. Tepel J, Schäffer E, Hoppe W. Root canal instruments for manual use: cutting efficiency and instrumentation of curved canals. Int Endod J 2000;28:68-76.
252. Thompson AS. An overview of nickel-titanium alloys used in dentistry. Int Endod J 2000;33:297-310.
253. Thompson SA, Dummer PMH. Shaping ability of Hero 642 rotary nickel-titanium instruments in simulated root canals. Part 1. Int Endod J 2000;33:248-54.
254. Thompson SA, Dummer PMH. Shaping ability of Hero 642 rotary nickel-titanium instruments in simulated root canals. Part 2. Int Endod J 2000;33:255-61.
255. Thompson SA, Dummer PMH. Shaping ability of Lightspeed rotary nickel-titanium instruments in simulated root canals. Part 1. J Endod 1997;23:698-702.
256. Thompson SA, Dummer PMH. Shaping ability of Lightspeed rotary nickel-titanium instruments in simulated root canals. Part 2. J Endod 1997;23:742-7.
257. Thompson SA, Dummer PMH. Shaping ability of Mity Roto 360° and Naviflex rotary nickel-titanium instruments in simulated root canals. Part 1. J Endod 1998;24:128-34.
258. Thompson SA, Dummer PMH. Shaping ability of Mity Roto 360° and Naviflex rotary nickel–titanium instruments in simulated root canals. Part 2. J Endod 1998;24:135-42.
259. Thompson SA, Dummer PMH. Shaping ability of NT Engine and McXim rotary nickel-titanium instruments in simulated root canals. Part 1. Int Endod J 1997;30:262-9.
260. Thompson SA, Dummer PMH. Shaping ability of NT Engine and McXim rotary nickel–titanium instruments in simulated root canals. Part 2. Int Endod J 1997;30:270-8.
261. Thompson SA, Dummer PMH. Shaping ability of Profile .04 Series 29 rotary nickel-titanium instruments in simulated root canals. Part 1. Int Endod J 1997;30:1-7.
262. Thompson SA, Dummer PMH. Shaping ability of Profile .04 Series 29 rotary nickel-titanium instruments in simulated root canals. Part 2. Int Endod J 1997;30:8-15.
263. Thompson SA, Dummer PMH. Shaping ability Quantec Series 2000 rotary nickel-titanium instruments in simulated root canals. Part 1. Int Endod J 1998;31:259-67.
264. Thompson SA, Dummer PMH. Shaping ability Quantec Series 2000 rotary nickel-titanium instruments in simulated root canals. Part 2. Int Endod J 1998;31:268-74.
265. Tidmarsh BG. Preparation of the root canal. Int Endod J 1982;15:53-61.
266. Troian CH, So MVR, Figueiredo JAP, Oliveira EPM. Deformation and fracture of RaCe and K3 endodontic instruments according to the number of uses. Int Endod J 2006;39:616–25.
267. Tronstad L, Niemczyk SP. Efficacy and safety tests of six automated devices for root canal instrumentation. Endod Dent Traumatol 1986;2:270-6.
268. Trope M, Debelian G. Endodontic treatment of apical periodontitis chapter 12, 347-380, In: Orstavik D, Pitt Ford T Essential Endodontology, Blackwell Munksgaard, 2nd ed., 2008. 477p.
269. Turek T, Langeland K. A light microscopic study of the efficacy of the telescopic and the Giromatic preparation of root canals. J Endod 1982;8:437-43.
270. Turpin Y, Chagneau F, Vulcain J. Impact of two theorical cross-sections on torsioal anda bending stresses of NiTi root canal instrument models. J Endod 2000;26:414-7.
271. Ullmann CJ, Peters OA. Effect of cyclic fatigue on static fracture loads in ProTaper nickel-titanium instruments. J Endod 2005;31:183-6.
272. van der Sluis LWM, Shemesh H, Wu MK, Wesselink PR. An evaluation of the influence of passive ultrasonic irrigation on the seal of root canal fillings. Int Endod J 2007;40:356–61.

273. Vanni JR, R Santos, Limongi O, Guerisoli DMZ, Capelli A, Pécora JD. Influence of cervical preflaring on determination of apical file size in maxillary molars: SEM analysis. Braz Dent J 2005;16:181-6.
274. Vargas FLH, Estrela C, Pesce HF. Estudio comparativo de la morfologia del conducto radicular producida después de la instrumentación ultrasónica y manual. Rev Espanhola d'Endodoncia 1997;15:26-30.
275. Vessey RA. The effect of felling versus reaming on the shape of the prepared root canal. Oral Surg Oral Med Oral Pathol 1969; 27:543-47.
276. Vier FV, Figueiredo JAP. Prevalence of different periapical lesions associated with human teeth and their correlation with the presence and extension of apical external root resorption. Int Endod J 2002;35:710-9.
277. Vier FV, Figueiredo JAP. Internal apical resorption and its correlation with the type of apical lesion. Int Endod J 2004;37:730–7.
278. Walia H, Brantley WA, Gerstein H. An initial investigation of the bending and torsional properties of Nitinol root canal files. J Endod 1988;14:346-57.
279. Walmsley AD. Ultrasound and root canal treatment: the need for scientific evaluation. Int Endod J 1987;20:105–11.
280. Walton RE, Rivera EM. Cleaning and Shaping. In: Principles and practice of endodontic. Walton RE, Torabinejad M. 2nd ed. Philadelphia: WB Saunders; 1996. 201-33.
281. Wei X, Ling J, Jiang J, Huang X, Liu L. Modes of failure of ProTaper nickel-titanium rotary instruments after clinical use. J Endod 2007;33:276-9.
282. Weiger R, Bartha T, Kalwitzki M, Lost C. A clinical method to determine the optimal apical preparation size – Part 1. Oral Surg Oral Med Oral Pathol Oral Radiol Endod 2006;102:686-91.
283. Weine FS, Kelly RF, Bray KE. Effect of preparation with endodontic handpieces on original canal shape. J Endod 1976;2:298-301.
284. Weine FS, Kelly RF, Lio PJ. The effect of preparation procedures on original canal shape and on apical foramen shape. J Endod 1975;1:255-62.
285. Weine FS. Intracanal treatment Procedures, basic and advanced topics. In: Endodontic Therapy. 4th ed. Mosby: St Louis; 1989. p.277-369.
286. Weine FS. Tratamento endodôntico. 5th ed. São Paulo: Editora Santos, 1998. 862p.
287. Weisy G. A clinical study using automated instrumentation in root canal therapy. Inter Endod J 1985; 18:203-09.
288. West JD, Roane JB, Goerig AC. Cleaning and shaping the root canal system. In: Pathways of the Pulps. Cohen S, Burns RC. 6th ed. St. Louis, USA: Mosby Year Book, 1994. p179-218.
289. Wilcox LR, Swift ML. Endodontic retreatment in small and large curved canals. J Endod 1991;17:313-5.
290. Wildey WL, Senia S, Montgomery S. Another look at root canal instrumentation. Oral Surg Oral Med Oral Pathol 1992;74:499-507.
291. Wildey WL, Senia S. A new root canal instrument and instrumentation technique: a preliminary report. Oral Surg Oral Med Oral Pathol 1989;67:198-207.
292. Wolcott J, Himel VT. Torsional properties of niquel titanium versus stainless steel endodontic files. J Endod 1997;23:217-20.
293. Wu MK, Barkis D, Roris A, Wesselink PR. Does the first file to bind correspond to the diameter of the canal in the apical region? Int Endod J 2002;35:264-7.
294. Wu MK, Fan B, Wesselink PR. Leakage along apical root filling in curved root canals. Part 1. Effects of apical transportation on seal of root fillings. J Endod 2000;26:210-6.
295. Wu MK, Kastakova A, Wesselink PR. Quality of cold and warm gutta-percha fillings in oval canals in mandibular pre-molars. Int Endod J 2001;34:485-91.
296. Wu MK, R'oris A, Barkis D, Wesselink PR. Prevalence and extend of long oval canals in the apical third. Oral Surg Oral Med Oral Pathol Oral Radiol Endod 2000;89:739-43.
297. Wu MK, Wesselink PR. A primary observation on the preparation and obturation of oval canals. Int Endod J 2001;34:137-41.
298. Wu MK, Wesselink PR. Efficacy of three techniques in cleaning the apical portion of curved root canals. Oral Surg Oral Med Oral Pathol Oral Radiol Endod 1995;79:492-6.
299. Wu M-K, Wesselink P, Walton R. Apical terminus location of root canal treatment procedures. Oral Surg Oral Med Oral Pathol Oral Radiol Endod 2000;89: 99-103.
300. Yang SF, Pai SF. An accident with Gates-Glidden drill an endodontic practice. J Endod 2000;26:49-50.
301. Yao JH, Schwartz SA, Beeson TJ. Cyclic fatigue of three types of rotary nickel-titanium files in a dynamic model. J Endod 2006;32:55-7.
302. Yared GM, Bou Dagher FE, Machtou P. Influence of rotational speed, torque and operator's proficiency on Profile failures. Int Endod J 2001;34:47-53.
303. Yared GM, Bou Daugher FE, Machtou P, Kulkarni GK. Influence of rotational speed, torque and operator's proeficiency on failure of Greater Tapper files. Int Endod J 2002;35:7-12.
304. Yared GM, Bou Daugher FE, Machtou P. Cyclic fatigue of Profile rotary instruments after simulated clinical use. Int Endod J 1999;32:115-9.
305. Yared GM, Bou Daugher FE. Influence of apical enlargement on bacterial infection treatment of apical periodontitis. J Endod 1994;20:535-7.
306. Yoshida T, Shibata T, Shinohara T, Gomyo S, Sekine I. Clinical evaluation of efficacy of EDTA solution as an endodontic irrigant. J Endod 1995;21:592-3.
307. Young GR, Parashos P, Messer HH. The principles of techniques for cleaning root canals. Aust Endod J 2007;52:522-63.
308. Zelada G, Varela P, Martín B, Bahílio JG, Magan F, Ahn S. The effect of rotational speed and the curvature of root canals on the breakage of rotary endodontic instruments. J Endod 2002;28:540-2.
309. Zmener O, Balbachan L. Effectiveness of niquel titanium files for preparing curved root canals. Endod Dent Traumatol 1995;11:121-3.
310. Zmener O, Pameijer CH, Banegas G. Retreatment efficacy of hand versus automated instrumentation in oval-shaped root canals: an ex vivo study. Int Endod J 2006;39:521–6.

# A Critical Review of Efficacy of Nickel-Titanium Instruments in Shaping Curved Root Canals

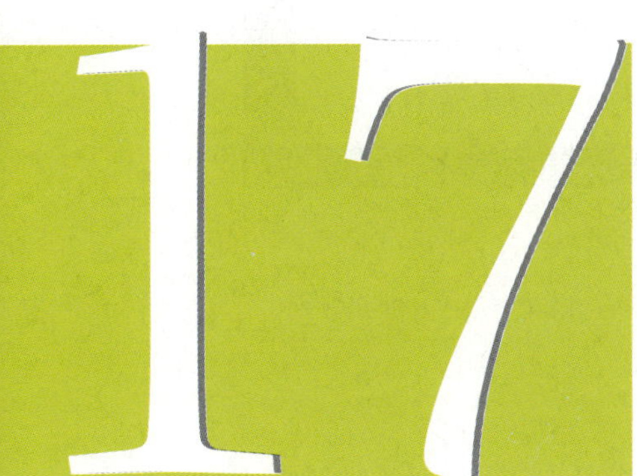

**G. B. Sydney**
*Federal University of Paraná, Curitiba, PR, Brazil*

**C. Estrela**
*Federal University of Goiás, Goiânia, GO, Brazil*

Chapter contents

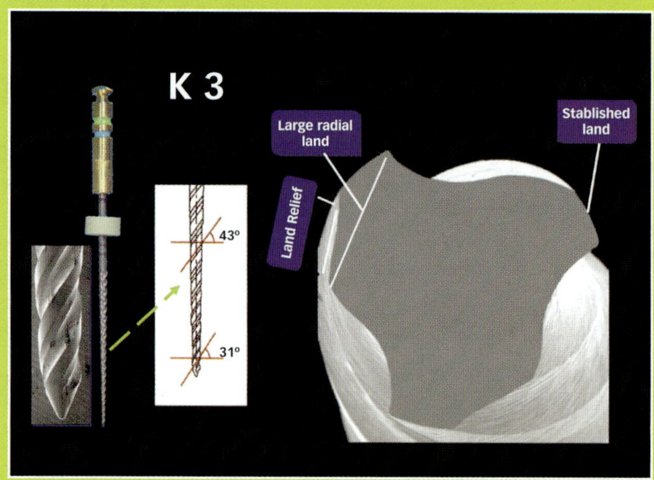


Characteristics of K3 instrument.

## 17.1 Introduction

Recent advances in the field of root canal preparation have led to the use of nickel-titanium instruments. The NiTi alloy used to manufacture endodontic instruments is composed of approximately 56% (wt) nickel and 44% (wt) of titanium, known as 55- Nitinol. The improved flexibility and unique properties of NiTi alloy provide advantages and the instrument can be used in a rotary movement inside the root canal at a controlled speed. It was possible to engineer instruments with greater tapers (4 to 12 per cent) allowing better control of the root canal shape, a more tapered preparation improving cleaning and shaping and eliminating some of the shortcomings of traditional preparation.

A large number of new rotary instruments have come onto the market with their own particular characteristics. Engineering philosophies have created different systems and the clinician is dependent on the findings of in vitro studies and clinical trials for information and guidance, as there is no specific rule for the outcome of their use[9,23].

The systems differ based on their sectional areas, cutting angles, helicoidal angles, grooves and radial land. The choice of a system is depends on different thoughts as regards instrument taper. Thus, it is fundamental to understand what each available taper means and when it may be used (Fig. 17.1).

## 17.2 The Taper

Series with taper # 0.12, # 0.10 and # 0.08 are indicated for radicular access. They remove dentin from the entrance creating a straight line access to the root canal.

These instruments may be used from the large to the small taper when a large canal is going to be prepared. In atresic root canals the order may be reversed: a smaller taper first and then the largest taper. Important consideration must be given as regards the movement. First of all, the instrument is introduced into the root canal until it fits the canal wall. It is tried again to free the tip and then turned on. Secondly: it must be used in an anticurvature movement. This is classical. Direct the instrument to the safety zone. Thirdly, the instrument must be directed to all the canal walls with an anticurvature movement, by pulling it out in an oblique movement (oblique pull out), mainly in the cervical and middle third where an ovoid form may be present. It is important to remember that the instrument does not know where to work. It is necessary to tell it where it must work. So, two orders have to be given: 1. work in an anticurvature movement and 2. Touch all the dentin walls. Thus we can define the movement as an anticurvature filling and oblique pull out[19,21].

Only two instruments are really necessary: *# 0.12 and # 0.10* or a *# 0.10 and # 0.08* may be selected. These three instruments are available in most of the systems and some of them will make two of them available.

### Series with taper # 0.06

These files will start the crown-down technique. After the cervical third preparation they will start the crown-down preparation until the beginning of the curvature; this means the straight part of the root canal. But pay attention!!! The files must not go into the curvature area. The movement requires the same care described for the instruments used for radicular access.

All series are available with taper # 0.06 but bearing in mind that the clinical anatomical diameter of a mesial root canal of a mandibular molar, 1 mm from the apex, corresponds to a file *# 25*, it is sensible to select only one file: *# 25/0.06*.

**Series with taper # 0.04**

These instruments will continue the crown-down preparation, but differently from series 0.06, they advance into the curvature but do not complete it. With the same concept determined for the 0.06 series, we need only one instrument: *# 25/0.04*.

**Series with taper # 0.02**

Instruments with taper 0.02 are responsible for enlarging the apical area, which is why you need # 25/0.02, # 30/0.02; # 35/0.02 and # 40/0.02.

Until some years ago, taper 0.04 was more common because of the sectional area of the instruments. When comparing the sectional area of the early instruments, such as Profile with the new concept on this topic, it becomes easy to understand why it is now called the new generation of rotary root canal instruments.

Turpin et al.[25] presented a study comparing the torsional and bending properties of NiTi alloys with different sectional areas: triple U and triple helix models. The two models showed very different stresses in terms of intensity and distribution. For identical working diameters, the area of the triple helix cross-section is 30% greater than that of the triple U, thus generating more massive structures. A triple helix cross-section thus has more than double the torsional inertia of a triple U cross-section. Thus, triple helix instruments should be able to resist higher moments because of lower and more evenly distributed stresses. On the other hand, triple U instruments would require much lower moments, especially because the highest stresses are concentrated in the flutes, thus increasing the risk of breakage. Triple helix models are thus less flexible than triple U models. However, in endodontic procedures, bending is not caused by operator pressure but by canal curvature.

The authors showed that a bending moment for triple helix model almost double that of the triple U would be required to obtain the same bend radius in the two models. This is extremely important in endodontic treatment, in order to avoid straightening curved canals. Triple U instruments are extremely flexible but have little torsional strength, and should preferably be used for canals where there is little risk of instrument blockage. A hand file is required to prepare the pathway of the root canal before the use of a rotary triple U instrument. These instruments are more flexible but have little torsional strength. Thus, a large number of instruments are necessary to reduce the risk of instrument blockage and breakage. The risk of exceeding the limit of elasticity is high, that is why a low-speed and highly stable motor must be used. Little operating pressure is required to avoid embedding the file in the canal wall.

The stresses are more spread out and better distributed in the triple helix model thus it is possible to use higher, less stable speeds and nonspecific motors. That is why angles have been used for these instruments. Figure 17.2 shows the differences between this new concept in cross-sectional area.

The new generation of rotary nickel-titanium instruments is represented here by: Protaper, K3, Hero, NiTi Tee, Race and BioRace.

## 17.3 K 3 (Sybron, Kerr)

The K3 series was developed with this new concept of cross-sectional area. Its strength comes from the mass of the material encompassed in the core area of the instrument (Fig.17.3.). It is the key to resisting torsional and rotary stresses. The amount of material supporting the cutting blades of the instrument, called the radial land, is critical to the instrument. The less the amount of metal behind the cutting edge (blade support), the less resistant the instrument is. The reduction in the size of the radial land, equals the decrease in the strength of the instrument.

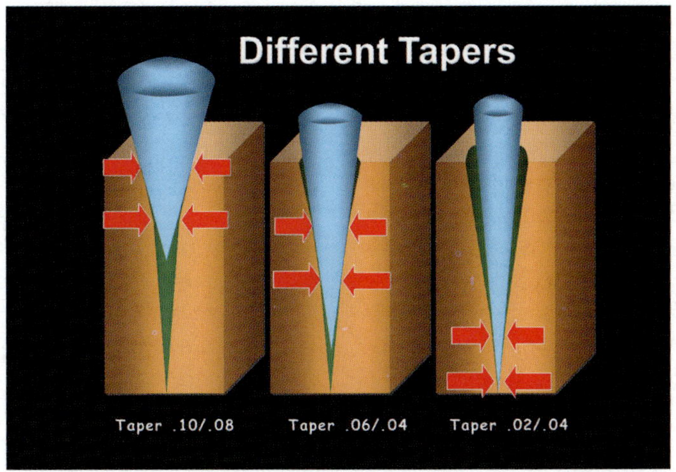


**Figure 17.1A** - Each taper is designed to be used in different thirds of the root canal.

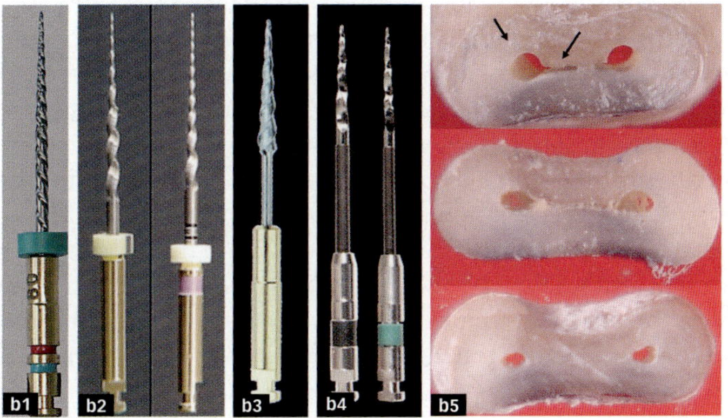


**Figure 17.1B** - Different instruments for the radicular access: (**b1**)K3. (**b2**) Protaper. (**b3**) Endo Flare and (**b4**) Pré-Race. If you don't say the instrument to work in an anti-curvature and an oblique pull out movement it will work in the danger zone and will not touch all the canal walls.

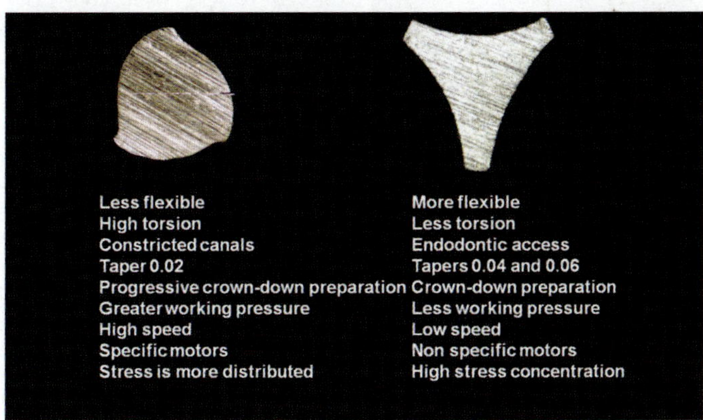


**Figure 17.2** - Main differences between cross-section area.

K3 instruments have two blades with a relief area giving the blade more efficiency. The K3 blade relief area reduces frictional resistance and controls the depth at which the flutes engage the dentin. Increased radial land increases peripheral strength behind the cutting blade. The third one has no relief and is called the established blade. Therefore, the peripheral mass prevents the propagation of cracks and reduces the chances of separation and deformation due to torsional stresses. Clinically this is extremely important.

Another important innovation is the variable helical flute angle. This enables the instrument not to engage the dentin walls and allows more debris to be carried out via the variable flute design of the file (Fig. 17.3).

The proportion of the core diameter to the outside diameter is greatest at the tip, where strength is most important. This proportion decreases uniformly as the fluting moves up the taper, resulting in greater flute depth and increased flexibility while maintaining strength. This characteristic allows the debris to be removed more efficiently.

K3 access handle is shorter making it easier for the operator to have a view of the cavity access. The instrument has a safe-ended non-cutting tip that avoids transportation, and follows the root canal safely.

Three tapers are now available: 0.06, 0.04 and 0.02. The first is Orange, 0.04 is green and 0.02 is purple. There are two color bands on the handle: the top band signifies the taper, and the bottom band conforms to standard ISO sizing (Fig. 17.4).

K3 has a positive rake angle. The cutting efficiency of an instrument depends on the overall rake angle of the cutting blades. An instrument with a negative rake angle results in a scraping rather than a cutting action, a difficult and inefficient condition. That is why the new generation of NiTi rotary instruments tends to have positive rake angles.

## Clinical considerations

The cross sectional area has made the instrument safe and efficient. It works smoothly on the canal walls and presents good flexibility, low rate of fracture and good cutting efficiency. Although it has a tactile sense of rigidity or "stiffness" in hand because of the variable core diameter, the smallest tip sizes are excellent as an aid to helping create or specially accentuate the glide path. After establishing a glyde path with # 10 and/or # 15 manual K-file, the 0.02 or 0.04 taper (according to the canal diameter) slide close to the working length and accentuate the initial shape. This flow creates efficiencies to insertion of subsequent files making root canal preparation easier (Fig 17.5).

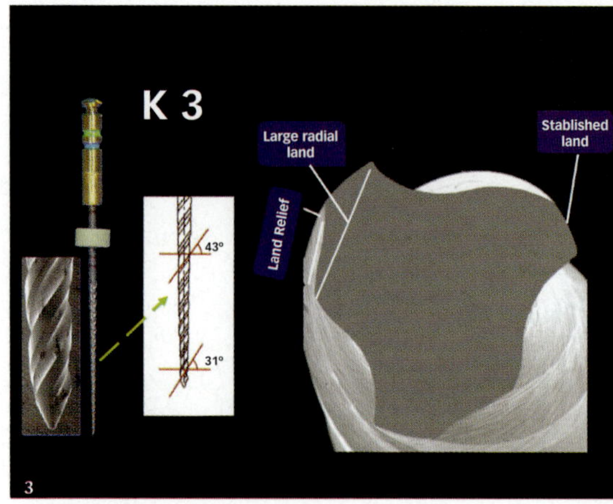


**Figure 17.3** - Figure 17.3. Characteristics of K3 instrument.

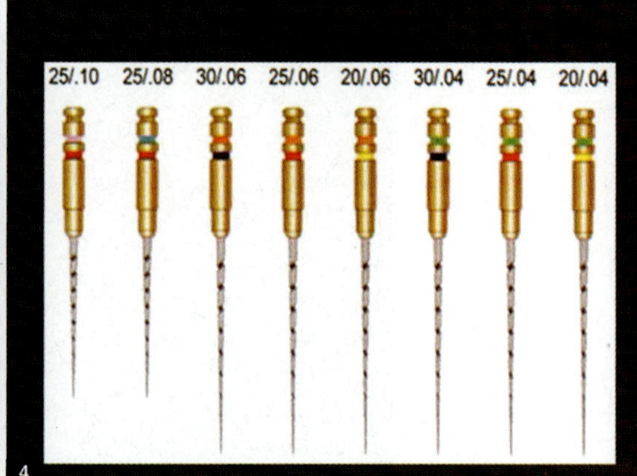


**Figure 17.4** - The K3 serie.

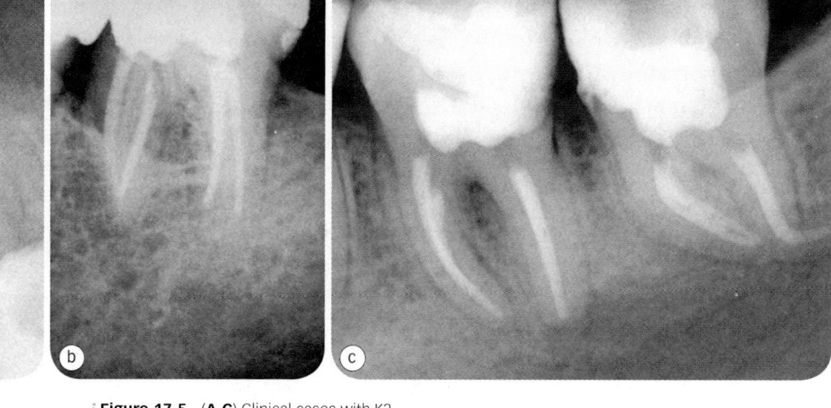

**Figure 17.5** - (**A-C**) Clinical cases with K3.



## 17.4 Hero 642 ( Micro-Mega)

Hero is the rotary instrument from Micro-Mega (France) and is the acronym of High Elasticity in Rotation. As described by Spangberg, the instrument has a trihelical Hedström design with rather sharp flutes. Due to a progressively increasing distance between the flutes, there is a reduced risk of binding when used in the root canal (Fig. 17.6).

The number 642 represents the three tapers available: 0.06, 0.04 and 0.02. Taper 0.06, 21mmm long and taper 0.04, 25mmm long are available for instruments # 20, # 25 and # 30. Taper 0.02 is available for instruments from # 20 to # 45, 25mm long.

Hero, like others of the new generation, has the cross-sectional area of a triple helix with a positive cutting, leading edge and a large central core that provides extra strength. It has a progressive and variable helical angle that reduces engagement in the canal walls and a non-cutting tip, similar to other NiTi rotary instruments. It results in excellent resistance, greatly reducing the chances of breakages.

For radicular access, an instrument with exactly the same morphological characteristics as Hero 642, named Endoflare is available (Fig. 17.7). The taper of this instrument is 0.12 and the tip is # 25, 15.0 mm long. The blade strength is only 10.0mm, which is the only difficulty with this series, since the pulp chambers of many molars require more than 10.0mm.

### Hero Shaper

The Hero Shaper series are NiTi instruments with taper 0.06 and 0.04., # 20, # 25 and # 30. The idea is to prepare the root canal with few instruments. Two files: # 30/0.06 for the crown-down and # 30/0.04 for the apical preparation in easy cases. Three files: # 25/0.06, # 25/0.04 and # 30/0.04 in the same concept. For teeth with severe curvature, four instruments are suggested: # 20/0.06, # 20/0.04, # 25/0.04 and # 30/0.04. The significant characteristic of the Hero Shaper is the adapted pitch that makes the instrument safe with no screwing effects, gives it more flexibility and perfect debris evacuation (Fig. 17.8).

## Hero Apical

Hero apicals are NiTi instruments designed for enlargement of the apical third after preparation with Hero 642 or Shaper, in order to eliminate contaminated dentin layers (Fig. 17.7). Two instruments are offered: 0.06 taper # 30 and 0.08 # 30, with 4mm active part. The non-active part of the instrument presents a reversed tapering to prevent bending of the active part. It is available with a length of 25mm, presents a very good flexibility and high resistance to breakage. The long pitch promotes excellent debris evacuation plus increased cutting power.

## Clinical considerations

Preparing the root canal with Hero 645 is easy and comfortable. The cutting area is efficient and the cross-section reduces breakage. Hero Shaper is a very good instrument for light and moderate curvatures but the suggested technique is not easy when severe curvatures are present.

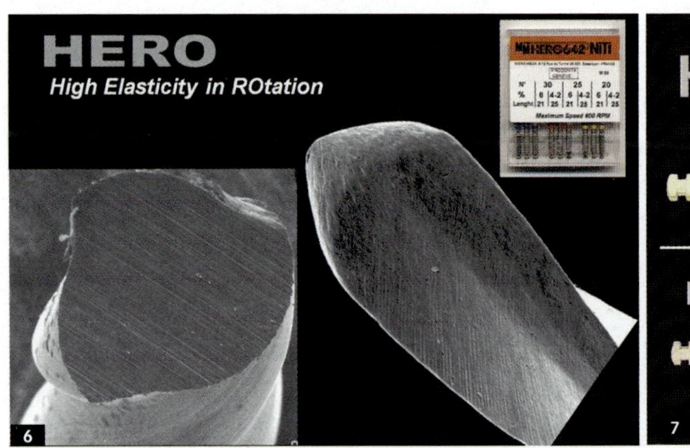


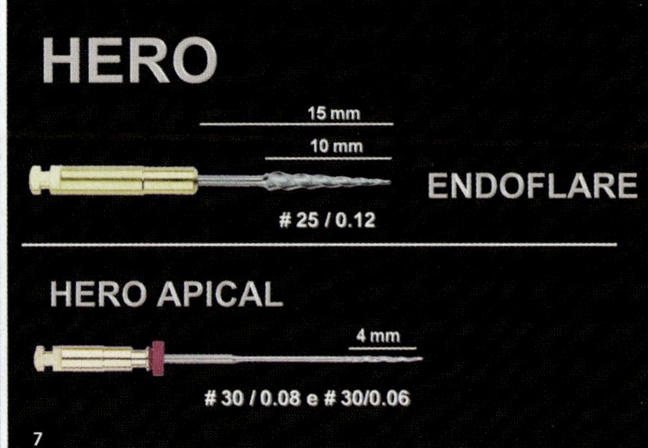


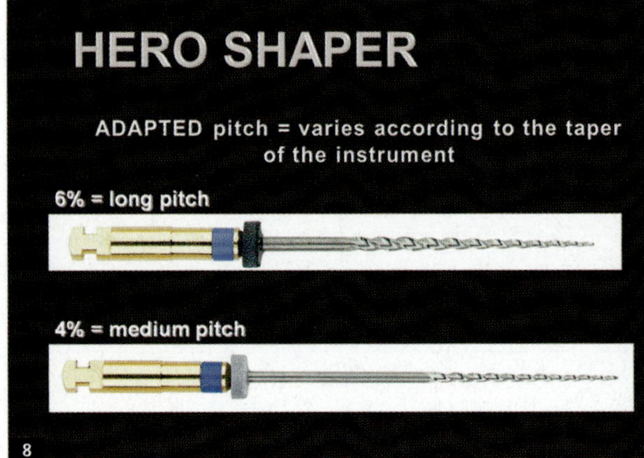


**Figure 17.6** - HERO from Micro Mega.
**Figure 17.7** - ENDOFLARE for Radicular access and HERO apical for enlargement of the apical area.
**Figure 17.8** - The HERO SHAPER series.

## 17.5 Protaper (Dentsply, Maillefer)

The Protaper system is based in a unique concept: a different taper in the same instrument. The aim is to reduce the number of instruments necessary for preparing the root canal. There are three instruments for shaping and three for finishing the root canal.

More recently, The ProTaper NiTi rotary system was upgraded to the ProTaper Universal system, which includes shaping, finishing and retreatment instruments.

Protaper has a convex triangular cross-section and progressive taper (Fig. 17.9). The convex area reduces the contact of the instrument with the canal walls and the cutting efficiency is related to the balance of the pitch of the spirals and the helicoidal angle.

The goal of a multiple taper with progressive conicity is to reduce the instrument fatigue and contact with the canal walls, thereby greatly diminishing the chances of fracture.

The shaping instruments are: SX, S1 and S2 (Fig. 17.10). The SX instrument is for radicular access. It is 19.0 mm long and the blade strength is 14.0mm. The taper is 3,5% from the tip and 19% to the end of the blade. It works in the cervical third but as mentioned before, care must be taken to make the instrument work in an anticurvature filling and oblique traction. The manufacturer's instruction to use the instrument in an up and down movement is not efficient. The tip of the instrument is always free.

The second instrument is S1. It is used for preparation of the middle third of the root canal. Its identification is a pink band on the handle. As the SX prepared the cervical third, the S1 that has a tip diameter of 0.17 with taper beginning at 2% and ending at 11%; it prepares the middle third maintaining the tip of the instrument free, obtaining the working length with minimal pressure.

The last instrument of the shaping series is S2, identified by a white band on the handle. This instrument has a 0.20 tip diameter and taper of 4% and 11.5%. Changes were made to this instrument in order to make the tip less aggressive and the transition to F1 more comfortable. For this purpose, the taper was reduced a little and the transition angle of the tip was eliminated.

To prepare the apical third three instruments complete the ProTaper Universal series: F1, F2 and F3, with color code yellow, red and blue respectively (Fig. 17.10). F1 has a tip diameter of # 20, F2, # 25 and F3 # 30. Taper of F1 is 7%, F2 is 8% and the taper at the end is 5.5%. Changes occurred in F3. The cross-section was modified in order to have more metal supporting the band giving the instrument more flexibility and reducing its rigidity (Fig. 17.11)

The new series presents two other instruments for larger root canals: F4 and F5 (Fig. 17.11). F4 is identified by two black bands on the handle; the tip diameter is # 40 and conicity in the first millimeters is 6%. F5 is identified by two yellow bands on the handle, the tip diameter is # 50 and conicity in the first millimeters is 5%.The cross-section presents the same alterations as those made in F3 (Fig. 17.11).

### Protaper for retreatment

ProTaper Universal retreatment files (D1, D2 and D3) are designed to remove filling material from the root canal when retreatment is indicated. There are three instruments: D1, D2 and D3 (Fig. 17.12).

The handles of these instruments are shorter (11 mm) for a better visualization of the pulp chamber. One, two or three white bands on the handle identify D1, D2 and D3, respectively. The taper of the tips are 9%, 8% and 7% and the tip diameter # 30, # 25 and # 20, respectively.

The tip of D1 was modified in order to remove the filling material from the cervical third. Its working tip is active, and facilitates its initial penetration into filling materials. Whereas, the tips of D2 and D3 are inactive, because these instruments act on the middle and apical thirds (Fig. 17.12).

Various instruments have been suggested for gutta-percha removal: hand files, Gates-Glidden burs, ultrasonic tips, ultrasonic tips and heat bearing instruments. Well condensed filling material is difficult and time consuming to removed with hand files. Since the new instruments for radicular access were introduced, they became a good option for removing the filling material from the cervical and middle thirds (the straight part of the root canal)[20]. Filling material is removed in a short time without the use of a solvent, and it is required only to help to remove the gutta-percha from the apical third.

Protaper for retreatment was developed with this aim. The three instruments have various tapers and diameters at the tip. Early studies on the efficiency of Protaper for retreatment in removing the filling material are controversial. Some point out better filling material removal than other techniques, but others do not.

It seems clear that a rotary NiTi instrument is capable of removing gutta-percha from the root canal because it tends to pull gutta-percha into the file flutes and direct it towards the orifice. Of course some frictional heat may be produced, plasticizing the gutta-percha, which then presents less resistance to removal. The cross sectional area of the instrument is important and efficient in Protaper. But it seems to be impossible to remove all traces of gutta-percha / sealers from root canals in any retreatment technique[28] (Fig. 17.13). Recently, Gu et al.[8], analyzing the efficacy of Protaper Universal for retreatment, demonstrated that although Protaper removed the filling material faster than other hybrid techniques tested, all of them left 10% - 17% of the canal area covered with gutta-percha sealer remnants.

## Technique for retreatment with a NiTi rotary instrument

1. A straight access to the root canal entrance is necessary.
2. Identify gutta-percha in the canal entrance and certify that it is gutta-percha. If it is not, a long neck round bur # 2 will remove it.
3. Establish a pilot hole using small sized stainless steel hand file (# 10, # 15 or # 20) associated with an orange solvent. These small stainless steel hand files can be prepared from used instruments by removing their destroyed parts to produce a small instrument (15/16mm). It is short and has good torsional properties.
4. Select a NiTi for radicular access (Pre-Race # 40/0.010 or Protaper Universal for retreatment D1). Apply a slight apical pressure advancing into the filling material not more than 3mm. Remember what you have to tell the instrument to do. Remove the instrument and inspect the blade for obturation material, and clean it from the flutes. Repeat this step three or four times.
5. Select Pre-Race # 35/0.08 or Protaper Universal for retreatment D2 and go to the middle third or the straight part of the root canal, taking care and repeating the same steps described before. Always advance a few millimeters. If the rotary file cannot go deeper, take a manual file Lu point # 10 or # 15 and overcome the resistance and confirm canal patency. Repeat the step.
6. If Protaper Universal for retreatment is the instrument of choice select D3 and go to the apical third to remove the filling material in this area. If not, a manual instrument associated with an orange solvent will remove the filling material from the apical third.
7. Bear in mind that these instruments provide very special help with removing the filling material, but this is not complete. Effective root canal re-preparation is the most important goal for thorough cleaning (Fig. 17.14 and 17.15)

## Clinical considerations

Preparing the root canal with Protaper is easy if a moderate curvature is present (Fig. 17.14). In spite of the recent changes, there is still too much taper In root canals with severe curvature, and frequently it is not possible to achieve the determined working length. If more pressure is applied to the instrument, it may fracture or the tip of the instrument will be active and not free, resulting in transportation.

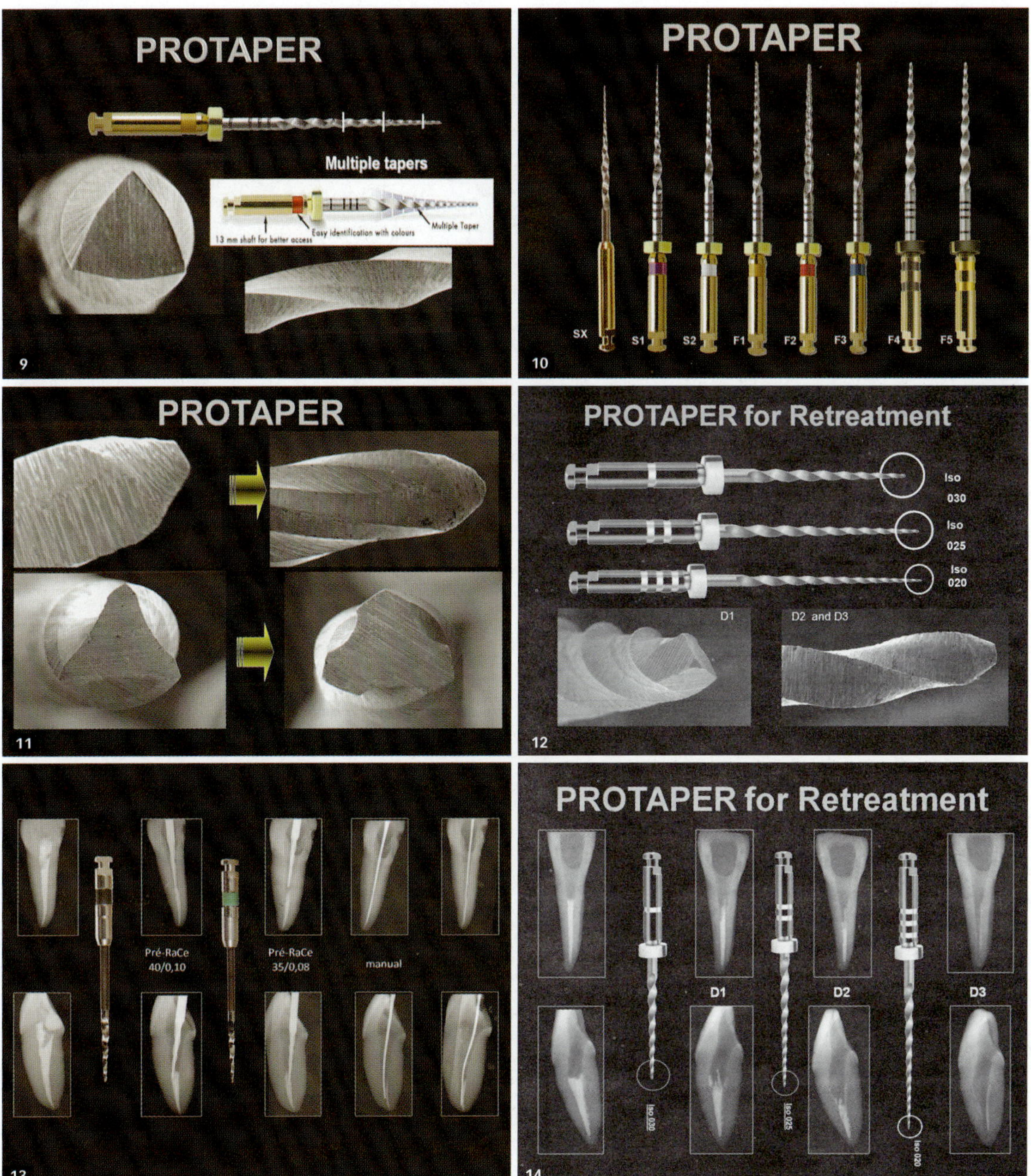


**Figure 17.9** - The Protaper characeristics: A convex triangular cross-section and multiple tapers in the same instrument.
**Figure 17.10** - The Protaper series instruments.
**Figure 17.11** - Changes in F serie tip: the transition angle was removed and a more rounded tip. F3, F4 and F5 have a new sectional area to reduce rigidity and to give the instrument more flexibility.
**Figure 17.12** - The Protater series for retreatment: D1, D2 and D3. The tip of D1 is more agressive and the tip of D2 and D3 are rounded.
**Figure 17.13** - The suggested technique using instruments for radicular access to help removing the filling material. Bear in mind that complete remotion is got only with complete repreparation of the radicular space.
**Figure 17.14** - Removing the filling material with Protaper for Retreatment.

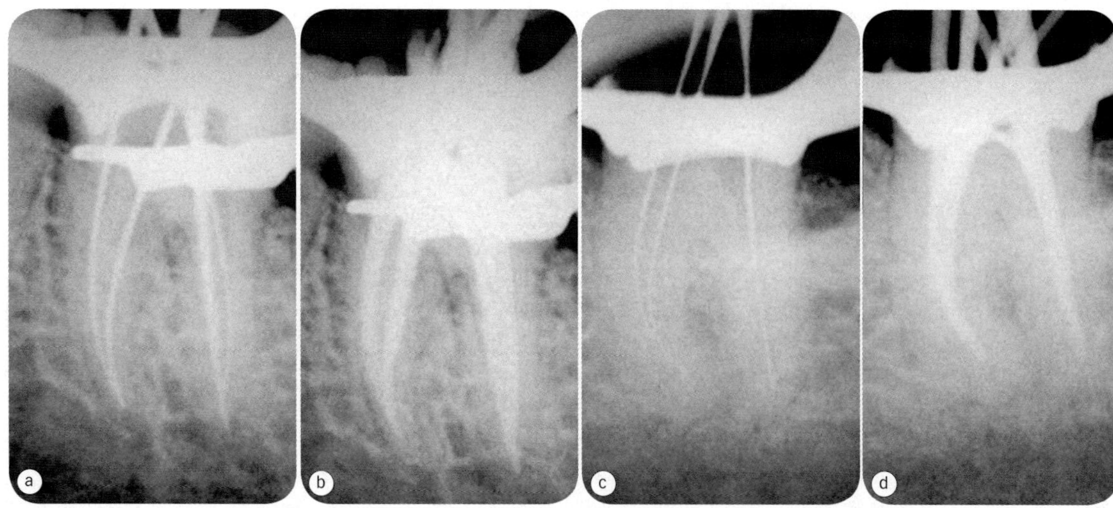

**Figure 17.15** - (**A-D**) Clinical cases with Protaper.

Protaper Universal for retreatment will help you remove the filling material faster, but not completely. Re-preparation is the most important step. Bear in mind that there is a tendency for the instrument to touch the same canal walls it touched in the first treatment, as shown by Wilcox et al 1987. So, try to make the instrument act in all areas (Fig. 17.15).

## 17.6 Race (FKG)

The FKG rotary Niti instrument is RACE, the acronym for Reaming with Alternating Cutting Edges and there are four technical innovations present. It has a sharp cutting edge resulting from its triangular cross-section. A triangular cross-section could be dangerous because of the tendency of engaging the canal walls with the risk of fracture. But Race has alternating cutting edges, only to avoid self-threading, which made it a very safe instrument. The tip is a non-cutting safety tip and the surface has been submitted to an electro-chemical surface polishing in order to reduce the stress on the instrument (Fig. 17.16 and 17.17).

A safety memory disc (SMD) was introduced to control the instrument stress. Each SMD has eight petals corresponding to a maximum of eight times of using the instrument. The SMDs remain in the instrument and are sterilizable. After each use of the instrument a petal is removed and the remaining petals indicate the possibility of further use. The SMD instructions are that if a simple root canal (25mm radius) is prepared, one petal is removed; if a medium complexity root canal is prepared (radius 25 until 11mm) two petals must be removed; and in a very complex root canal (radius 11mm until 8mm) three petals are removed.

There are different tapers available: 0.10. 0.08, 0.06 and 0.02. The instruments for radicular access are: #40/0.10 and # 35/0.08. Taper 0.06 is offered in sizes # 20, # 25 and # 30. Taper 0.04 is available in sizes # 25, # 30 and # 35. Taper 0.02 to prepare the apical third is available from size 15 to # 60 (Fig. 17.18).

### Clinical considerations

Race is one of the best NiTi rotary instruments and presents excellent cutting ability and flexibility. The file cuts dentin effectively, yet does not pull itself into the canal apically. It is able to prepare single and difficult cases safely and quickly (Fig. 17.19).

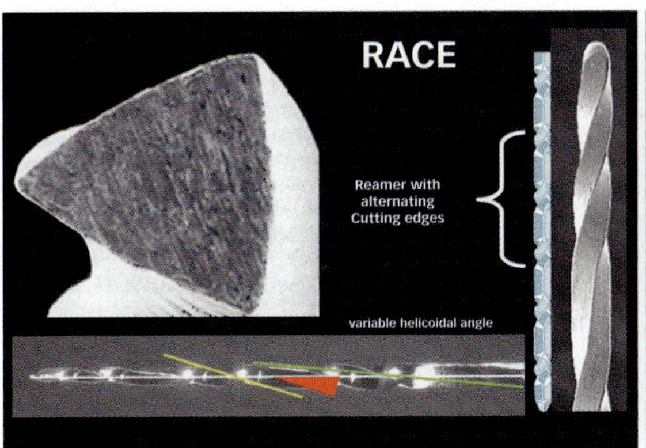


**Figure 17.16** - Characteristics of Race.

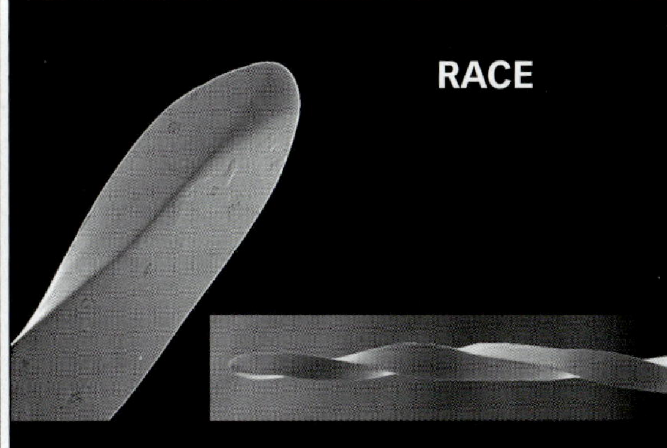


**Figure 17.17** - The surface has been submitted to an electro-chemical surface polishing in order to reduce the stress on the instrument.

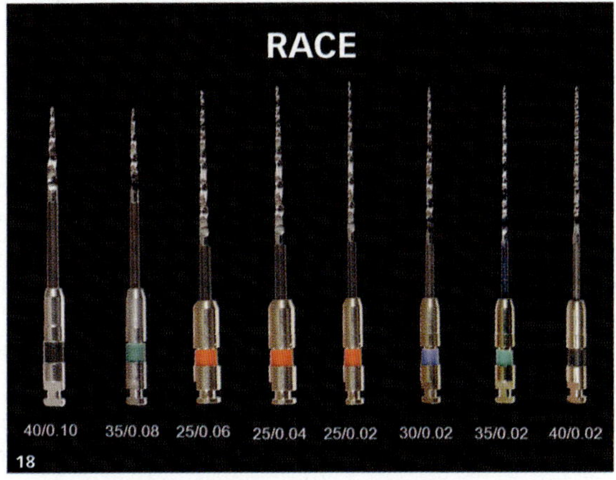


**Figure 17.18** - The Race series according to the text.

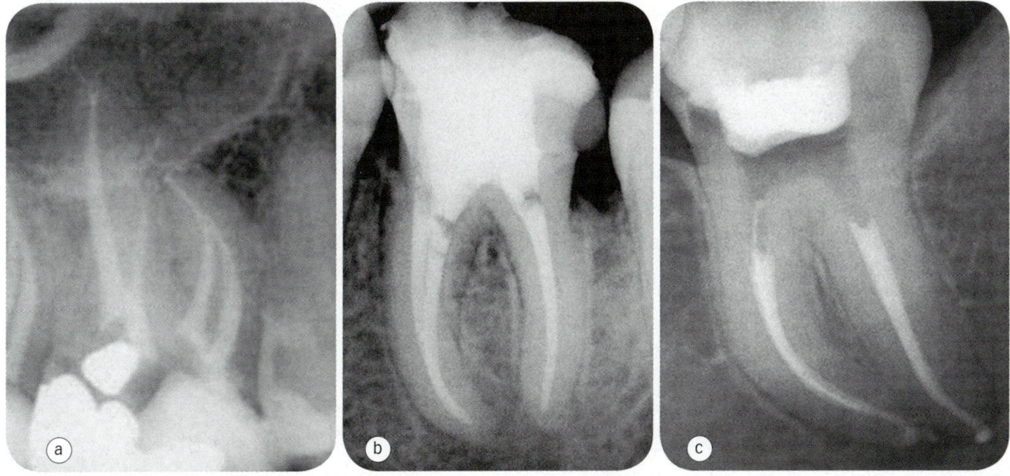


**Figure 17.19** - (**A-C**) Clinical cases with Race.

### 17.7 BioRace (FKG Dentaire)

BioRace is the upgrade of Race from FKG. It Differs from the RaCe instruments as regards instrument sizes, tapers and sequence. The physical characteristics are the same as RaCe. It has been designed to clean the root canal efficiently and safely with few instruments. The major goal of BioRace is to achieve apical preparation sizes that have been scientifically proved to effectively disinfect the root canal.

Since root canal infection is the cause of apical periodontitis, the biological aim of endodontic treatment is the prevention or elimination of root canal microbes. The apical seat preparation is not enough to eliminate microorganisms from the middle and apical third. Studies have shown that the apical third must be instrumented to certain minimum sizes (see apical seat x apical stop preparation) and then additional files are necessary, which takes time and becomes expensive for the practitioner.

With this concept in mind, the BioRace sequence was developed to achieve the required apical sizes without the need for additional steps and files. The order is to achieve the biologic aim of root canal treatment without compromising efficiency.

The BioRaCe coding system has changed, in an endeavor to simplify it for the practitioner, by using a single mark on the instrument handle. No tip number and taper defines the code. All instruments are BR, numbered from 0 to 5. BR0 is a #25/0.08, 19mm long and has no code on the handle; BR1 is a # 15/05 with 25mm and one single mark on the handle; BR2 is a # 25/04 with 25mm long and two marks on the handle; BR3 is a # 25/0.06, 25mmm long and three marks on the handle; BR4 is a # 35/04, 25mm with a large and a single mark on the handle; BR5 is a # 40/0.04, 25mm with a large and two single marks on the handle (Fig. 17.20). This is a BioRaCe Basic Set (Fig. 17.21). There is a BioRaCe extended Set for severe curvature and extra widening. The BioRaCe extended Set is composed of: BR4C that is a # 35/0.02, 25mm, an extra groove on the handle and a SMD; BR5C is a # 40/0.02, 25mm with an extra groove on the handle and two single marks. These instruments are used to prepare severely or atresic and curved canals. This kit also has BR6 a # 50/04, 25mm one large and three single grooves and BR7 a # 60/02, 25mm with two large and one single groove on the handle (Fig. 17.22).

Debelian & Trope[5] suggest a clinical protocol for BioRaCe:

First of all, the root canal must be reached to the working length with an instrument # 10 and # 15 with minimal pressure.

- The BR0 (#25/0.08/19mm) is then used in the coronal aspect of the canal with 4 steady strokes. As can be seen from Figure 8 about 4 mm of the file will be in contact with the canal in the most coronal part and the tip will work freely.
- The #15 K-file should then be used again to confirm that the pathway to the apical part of the canal could easily be achieved.
- BR1 (#15/0.05) follows and since a #15 file has already been used, the contact area for BR1 will be in the middle aspect of the file only.
- BR2 (#25/ 0.04 taper) contacts mostly the apical part of the canal since the previous file was a 0.05 taper file.
- BR3 (#25/0.06) has the same tip size as BR2 but a larger taper. Thus the contact area moved again to the coronal / middle aspect of the canal and the tip of this instrument will work freely.
- BR4 (#35/0.04) and BR5 (#40/ 0.04) are files with smaller tapers than BR3 and so they will cut only in the apical third thus getting to biological sizes safely. It is important to understand that apart from BR0 all instruments are used to working length. The entire protocol with the Bio RaCe basic set is shown in Figure 17.23.

For some difficult cases when severe curvatures are present, the instruments BR4C and BR5C, respectively # 35 and # 40 /0.02 are available in the BioRaCe extended kit. These files are used when BR3 (#25, 0.06) in the basic set has difficulty in getting to working length. The rule to know when it does not get to the working length is when no more than a double repetition of 4 steady insertions is performed. It is an indication that the 0.04 files would be unduly stressed to get to working length. The stress is based on anatomical considerations (Fig. 17.23). In these cases the files BR4C and BR5C are used since they get to working length with less stress (Fig. 17.24).

Instruments BR6 and BR7 (# 50/0.04 and # 60/0.02) are used in canals where BR5 (#40/0.04) is not large enough to reach biological sizes.

**Clinical considerations**

The alternating sequence of sizes and tapers of the BioRace system has allowed the required apical stop to be achieved without increasing the number of instruments. It is possible because the BioRace does not progress in a uniform sequential fashion. Thus unnecessary stress on the tip of the instruments is avoided even at full working length. However, because of the different tapers and tip sizes of the instruments, contact points (and thus stress) on the files is minimized thus maintaining the safety of this sequence. Since this sequence alternates between sizes and taper in a non sequential fashion, the coding system used for Bio RaCe is based on coding bars (Fig. 17.25).

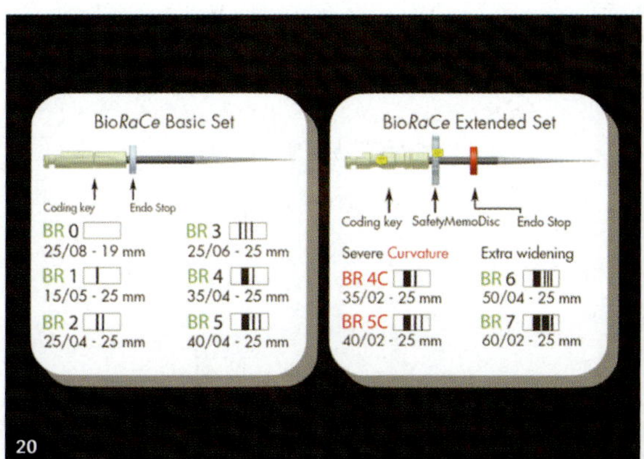


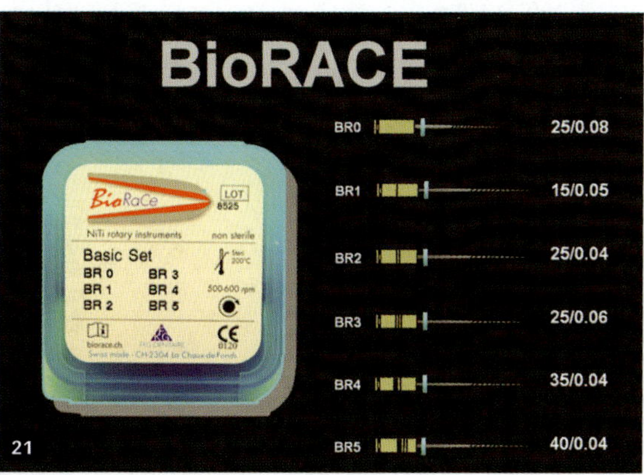


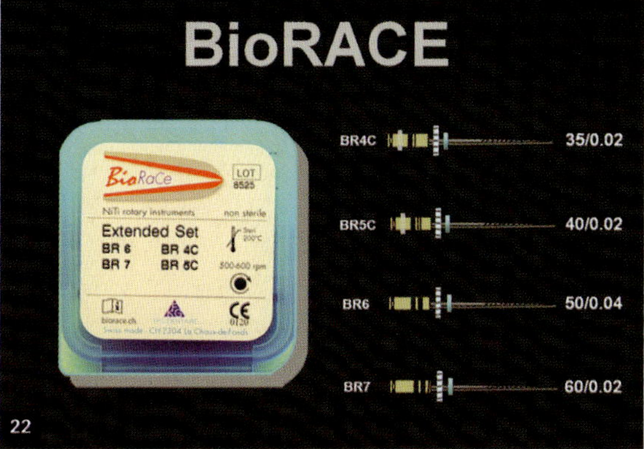


**Figure 17.20** - BioRaCe coding system.
**Figure 17.21** - BioRaCe basic set.
**Figure 17.22** - BioRaCe extended set.

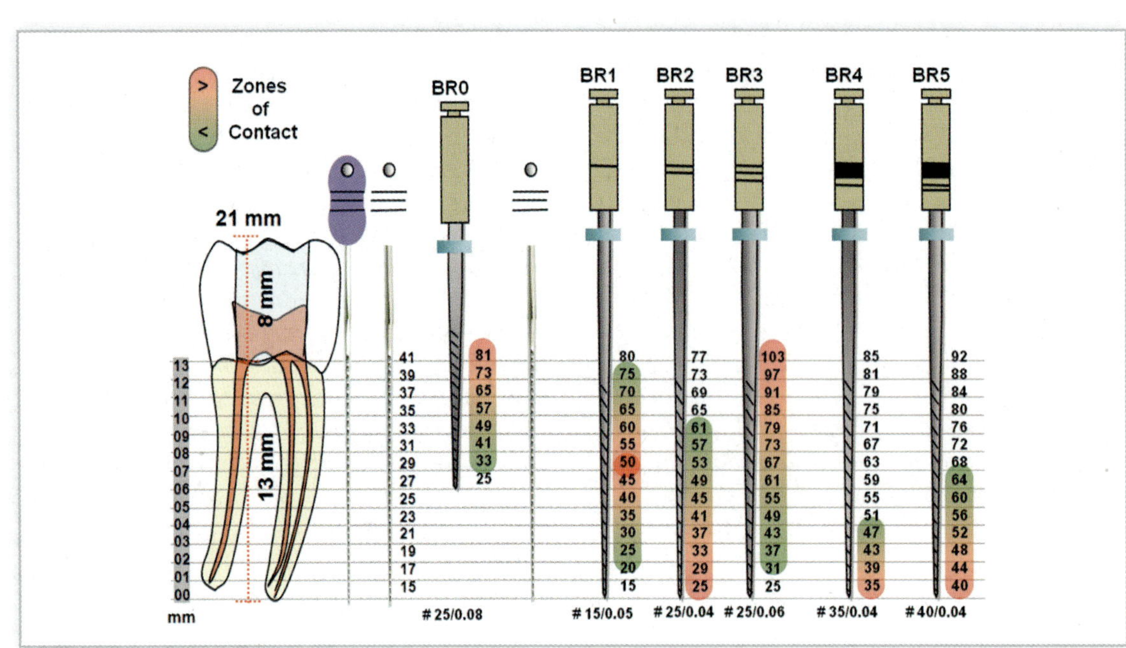


Figure 17.23 - BioRaCe basic set protocol.

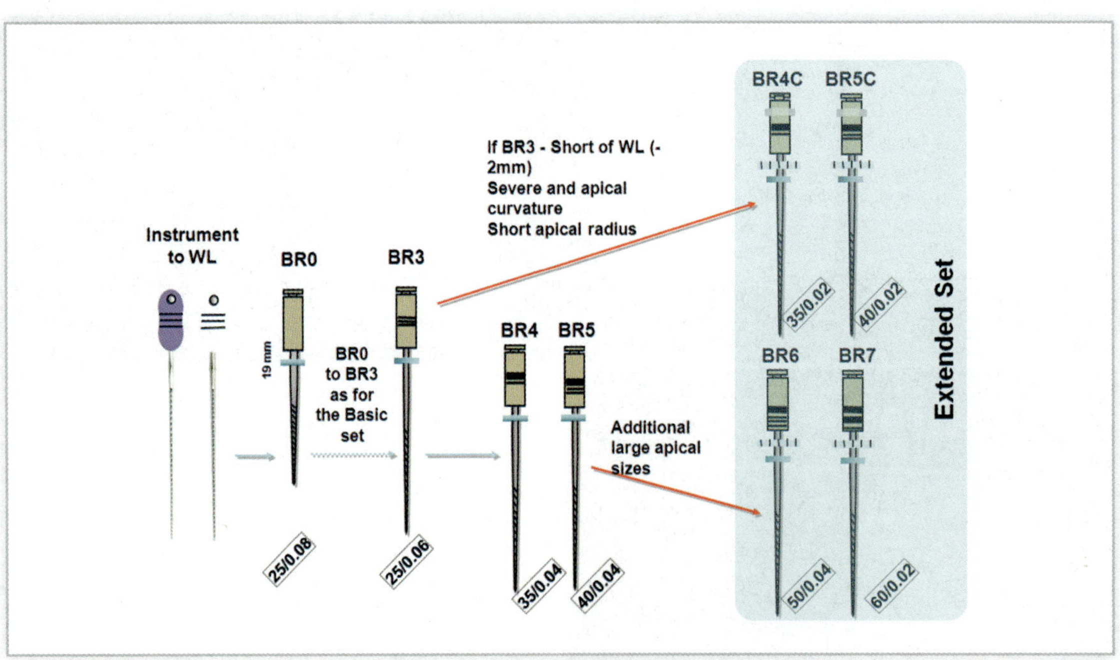


Figure 17.24 - The protocol for BioRaCe in difficult cases.

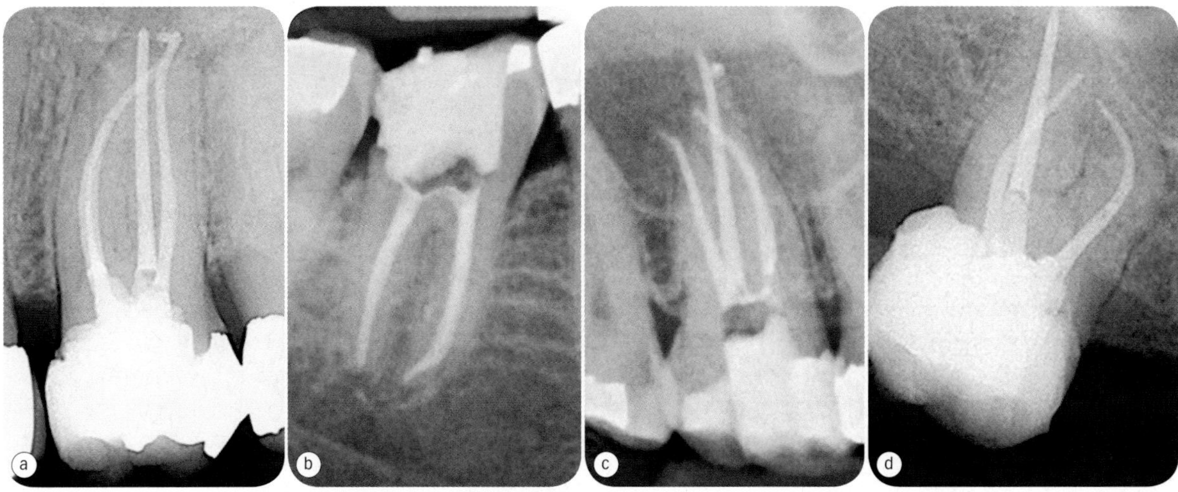

**Figure 17.25** - (**A-D**) Clinical cases with BioRaCe (Courtesy of Prof. Gilberto Debelian).

## 17.8 The Apical Seat versus the Apical Stop Preparation

If the aim of endodontic therapy is to prevent or cure apical periodontitis, then the most important step is root canal preparation. During mechanical instrumentation microorganisms are removed from the canal space with the help of antibacterial irrigants, and it becomes the critical stage in canal disinfection[22,24,26,27].

To what extent the root canal must be enlarged has been questioned for decades. Two concepts are available: the apical seat and apical stop preparation. Apical seat means not to enlarge the apical third too much, and obtaining disinfection by the use of irrigants at high concentrations (5.25% sodium hypochlorite). Apical stop means to enlarge the apical third with large instruments keeping this area 1mmm short of the apex. The irrigant concentration used is 1% sodium hypochlorite.

In the apical seat preparation concept the instrument acts up to the radiographic apex. The gutta-percha point is set 1mmm short. The problem is the apical limit: the vertices of the apex and the number of the instrument to do it: a # 25 file. When a # 25 file is reached the apical terminus it is not a patency, it is a foraminal cleanliness. Patency is what is done with a # 10 or # 15 file. The American Association of Endodontics glossary of terms defines patency as "a cabal preparation technique where the apical portion of the canal is maintained free of debris by recapitulation with a small file through the apical foramen".

The study by Goldberg & Massone[7] showed that the use of stainless steel or NiTi manual files # 10 to # 25 as patency files are capable of producing apical transportation. In 10 of the 30 specimens evaluated (33.3%), transportation started when a # 10 file size was used. As the foramen frequently emerges laterally from the apex, it means that the patency file acted on one wall of the apical foramen, irrespective of the file size or motion applied. The authors observed that when transportation started, it was increased with the increment in the file size. With these results in mind, it is difficult to understand how a # 25 file can safely be used in the vertices of the apex. That is why root canal filling shows cement in the periapical tissue. *So, confine yourself to the canal.*

The concept of apical stop preparation determines that instrumentation is kept inside the root canal, 1mm short. So it is possible to enlarge the apical third too much and make a stop at the master cone. Patency is performed with a # 10 or/and # 15 in all cases of necrotic pulp tissue, in order to help clean up, prevent occlusion of the apical foramen and maintain control of working length, only at the beginning after preliminary debridement, and after the use of the master file[13,21].

The apical constriction is the narrowest part of the root canal and the location where the pulp ends and the periodontium begins. It is generally ovoid or irregular shaped. Therefore an instrument size equal to the largest diameter of this area means the instrument of the anatomical diameter. Based on the anatomical diameter of the root canals from different studies, it becomes easier to understand why the evidences are conclusive that a step-back technique and an apical seat preparation are insufficient to clean most canals[1,3,4,18].

The study from Wu et al.[29] and Batista et al.[2] point to an anatomical clinical diameter of the root canals at different levels. The data pointed out a mean diameter corresponding to a #25 file to the mesio-buccal and bucco-lingual root canal Fig. 17.26 and 17.27). If it is an anatomical clinical diameter it means that a file #25 is not efficient in a preliminary debridement. The data for maxillary molars pointed out an anatomical diameter 1 mm from the apex of a diameter corresponding to a file # 20 or # 25. So, how can it achieve disinfection?

Kerekes & Tronstad[9], in a morphologic study on root canals in human molars pointed out that 95% of the molar mesial canals evaluated would have required at least a size #60 apical preparation to fully instrument the apical 1 mm.

Microbiological studies have shown that larger apical preparation sizes significantly reduced bacteria in the canal space when compared with smaller apical sizes. Card et al.[3] confirmed the Shuping et al.[18] study, that increasing instrumentation sizes of the apical area improved bacterial reduction. The root canals were instrumented with at least Profile # 45 and final enlargement performed with a Light Speed # 57.5 to # 60.

Debelian & Tope[5] affirmed that an additional problem of using minimal apical instrumentation sizes and irrigating solutions is that the effectiveness of these solutions is neutralized when the apical third of the canal is instrumented to smaller sizes. In the same way medications cannot reach the apical third.

It was really impossible when the technique was limited to a step-back preparation, because it was not possible to enlarge the apical third to a biological size with large tapered instruments, since the coronal half of the canal would be prepared correctly. So there are two important concepts: *the radicular access*[6] *and the biological root canal preparation*[5]. The first will allow one to gain straight access to the apex and to enlarge the apical third with larger instruments. The *biological preparation concept* is based on the anatomical diameter of the root canal in all areas.

## 17.9 A General Clinical Protocol

As described, each system has its own suggestion about how to prepare the root canal. But there is no specific rule for the outcome of its use. The following protocol for general rotary instrument use will enable everyone to safety and efficiently prepare the root canal (Fig. 17.28).

1. Coronal access
2. Clean the pulp chamber in order to remove all deposits on the pulp floor and locate all the root canal entrances.
3. Next step is to negotiate the root canal. This preliminary debridement and passive exploration of the canal is extremely important. It will map the root canal, identifying curvatures and anatomical challenges, obtaining a glide path to the apex preparing the pathway for the rotary instrument[19]. Hand files # 10 and # 15 are used in a watch winding motion: quarter turn clockwise followed by a quarter turn counterclockwise.

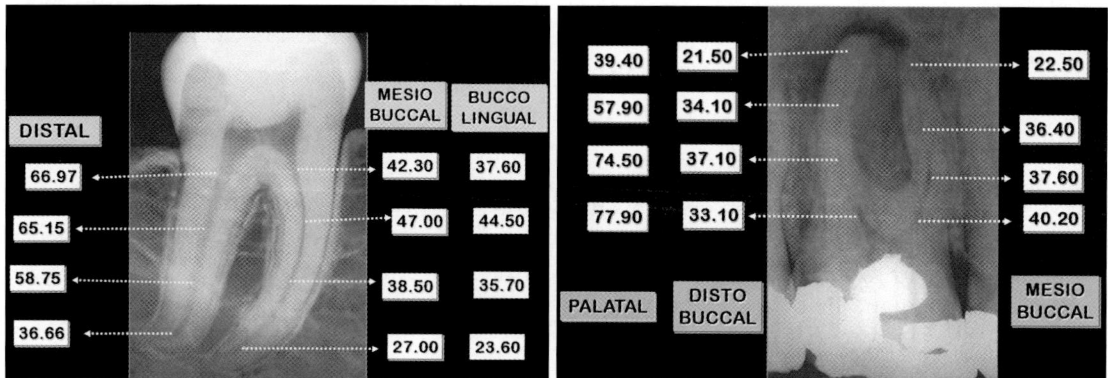


**Figure 17.26** - The clinical anatomic diameter in lower molars.

**Figure 17.27** - The clinical anatomic diameter in upper molars.

This feeds the file into the canal until it first binds. Once engaged the file is retrieved coronally, back no more than 2mm to ensure that the path of penetration is retained. It will continue until the apical terminus is reached. This step must be carefully performed. Clinical experience will dictate to what extent these instruments will be used in order to form a consistent glide path before any other step.

4. Use the radicular access instruments taper #0.10 and # 0.08 in order to get a straight line to the curvature. The depth of insertion is up to the anatomical aspects. Bear in mind that the aim of these instruments is to relocate the coronal aspects of the canal entrance away from external cavities. Remember: minimal pressure, insertion of 2 or 3 mm each time in order to allow a passive cut guiding the instrument to the anticurvature and telling it to touch all the external walls, which means with oblique pressure.
5. Start the crown-down preparation with a 0.06 taper instrument (#25). Introduce the instrument in the root canal until it binds the canal walls, withdraw until it is free in the canal and then move it. First of all, brush to the anticurvature cut with oblique pressure and then advance 2 or 3mm and pull away with the same combined movement. Repeat the procedure until completing the entire straight part of the root canal. Do not go into the curvature.
6. Continue the crown-down preparation, now with a 0.04 taper instrument (#25) following the same procedures described before. The 0.04 taper instrument advances into the curvature but does not complete it. Now it is important to understand that if we have a moderate curvature and a large canal, a # 25/0.04 instrument may complete the curvature and go to the working length, but with minimal pressure. In small canals and severe curvature the 0.04 instrument does not complete the curvature.
7. Now the # 25/0.02 instrument is inserted in the root canal and it will complete the curvature and get to the working length.
8. The next step is to prepare the apical third using # 30/02, #35/0.02 and depending on the canal diameter and the canal curvature an instrument #40/0.02 may prepare the apical third (Fig. 17.29).

When canal curvature and diameter allow the # 25/0.04 instrument to complete the curvature and reach the working length, the next step is to enlarge the root canal with file # 30/0.04 and # 35/0.04. Sometimes it will be safe to enlarge the apical third with # 30/0.02, # 35/0.02, # 40/0.02 and perhaps # 45/0.02.

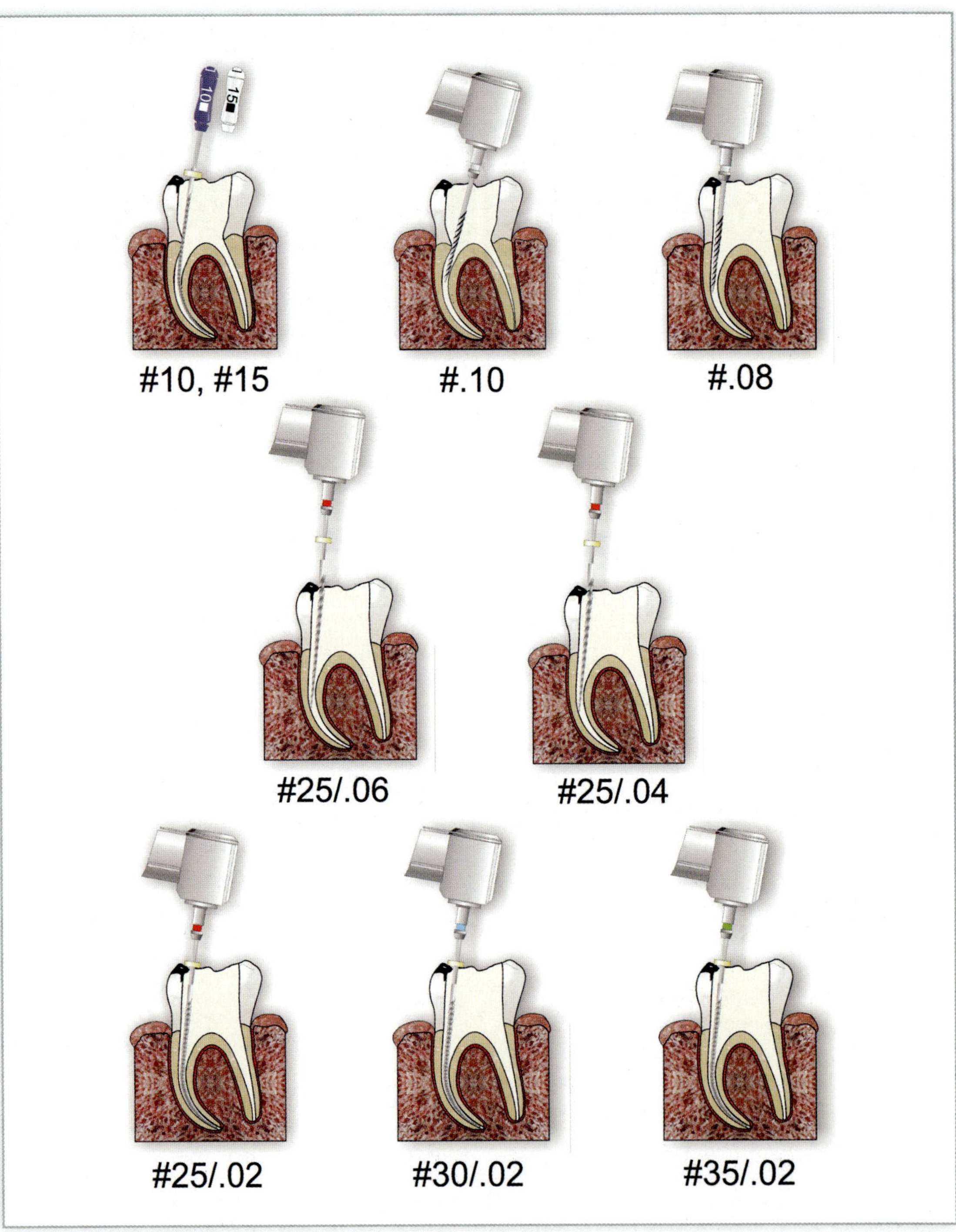


**Figure 17.28** - Schematic protocol for rotary instrument.

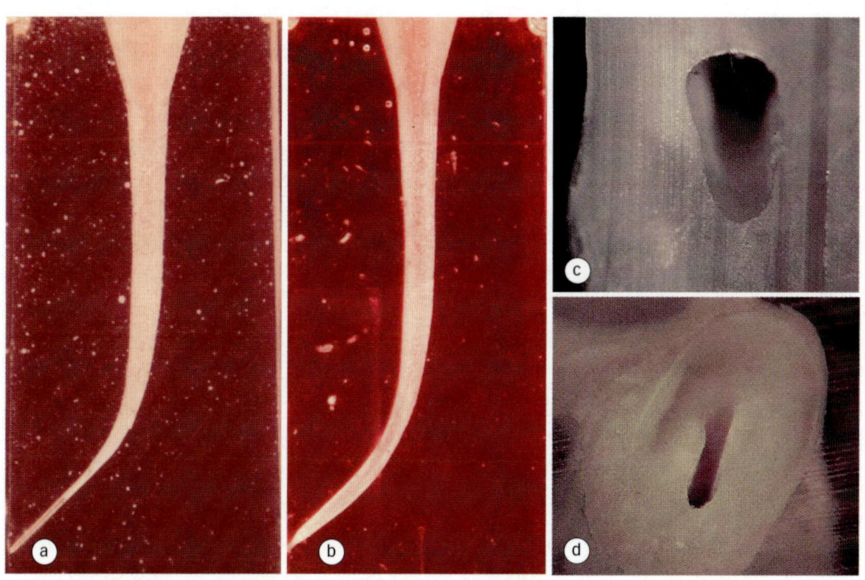


**Figure 17.29** - (**A**) Root canal preparation after the crown-down. (**B**) Final root canal aspects after enlarging the apical third. (**C-D**) Root canal anatomy must be maintained after enlargement independent of the curvature.

## 17.10 New Advances in NiTi Instruments

Niti instruments are manufactured by grounding the nickel titanium blanks. Through propriety process of heating and cooling, nickel titanium can be transitioned into a state known as *R-phase*. This crystalline structure state allows nickel titanium to be twisted. It is really a revolution in NiTi instruments because it opens up new possibilities for file design and optimizes its properties.

Grinding nickel-titanium is responsible for the creation of microcracks that can act as the precursor of fracture sites for the file if it is exposed to excessive torsion or cyclic fatigue. With the *r-phase* the crystalline structural modification maximises flexibility and resistance to breakage and the surface treatment increase hardness[11].

The new file based on this technology is the Twisted File (TF) from Sybron endo (Orange, California, USA).

### *Twisted File (Sybron Endo)*

The twisted file (TF) is the first instrument of nickel titanium manufactured by twisting the blank as described by Mounce[11] (Fig. 17.30). It has a triangular cross section and a surface deoxidant treatment thart respects underlying grain structure and is gentler than other methods, protects file integrity and improves file durability and cutting performance (Fig. 17.31).

Presents a variable pitch that minimizes "screw-in" effect, allows debris to be channeled effectively and greatly reduces torsional stress. As any other automated system has a safe-ended tip in order to minimizes canal transportation and becomes canal path easy to be followed.

It is available in 23mm and 27mm lenghths and in 5 tapers of: 0.12, 0.10, 0.08, 0.06 and 0.04. All of them have a # 25 size tip diameter. The TF file is color coded by two bands on the handle: the top band indicates the taper and the botton band the tip size. As all files are # 25 size tip the botton band is orange. The taper color codes are: 0.12 is purple, 0.10 is pink, 0.08 is aqua, 0.06 is orange and 0.04 is green (Fig. 17.30). Another important important characteristic of the TF is that the handle is not crimped on the nickel titanium shaft of the instrument.

The TF file is packaged in "large" pack assortments with 0.10, 0.08 and 0.06 tapers and "small" packs with 0.08, 0.06 and 0.04 tapers. The large pack is for typical cases like upper anteriors, cuspids, single root premolars and distal roots of lower molars and palatal roots of upper molars. The small pack is for mandibular incisors, multi-canal premolars, mesial roots of lower molars and buccal roots of upper molars.

### Clinical considerations

The twisted files make the crown-down technique easy and fast. The tapers available provide to be used in any canal anatomy. Cutting efficiency is significant and tracks smoothly. As the tip size is always # 25 and the actual biological preparation concept is to enlarge the apical area to greater sizes, it is possible to get it manually or using any other instrument with adequate tip size, taper 0.04 or 0.02.

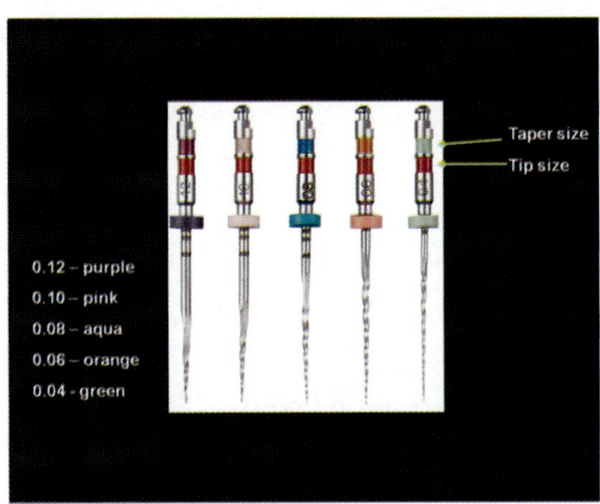


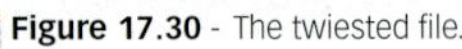

**Figure 17.30** - The twiested file.

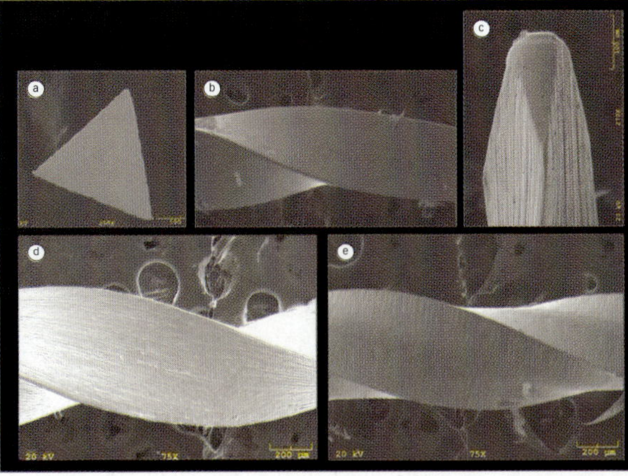


**Figure 17.31** - Twisted file design: in (**A**) Triangular cross-section; (**B**) Surface treatment; (**C**) Safe-ended tip; (**D**) File twisted mantain grain structure what does not happen in (**E**) Grounded file.

## 17.11 Clinical Analysis of the Efficacy of Nickel-Titanium Instruments

Several studies have investigated the main characteristics of NiTi instruments, especially the ability to maintain the shape in curved root canals. However, little information is observed on the discrepancy in clinical outcomes of teeth treated endodontically using the different NiTi rotary instruments. Thus, a systematic review was made to evaluate the clinical outcome obtained following root canal treatment performed when using different NiTi rotary instruments. The search strategies included electronic searches (MEDLINE, EMBASE, CENTRAL), since 1966 until December 18, 2007 and the Cochrane Library, in the same period. For the search strategy the following terms were used as keywords in several combinations: *Nickel Titanium and Endodontic Instruments*. The studies were selected by two independent reviewers that determined the inclusion and exclusion criteria (Table 17.1). The search presented 536 articles, of which 60 articles were literature reviews, 3 articles of case reports, 24 articles were in vivo (16 in humans, 8 clinical studies) and 364 were in vitro studies (human teeth - 190 articles; artificial canal - 89 articles; endodontic instruments - 25 articles; 50 articles without abstracts; and 25 other studies) (Fig. 17.32). From these studies 31 articles were associated with K3, 68 articles with Pro Taper, 29 with Hero, 154 articles with Profile, 33 articles with Quantec, 22 articles with Race, 43 with Greater Tapper and 156 with other systems. NiTi instruments showed good performance with favorable outcomes on shaping curved root canals. The combination of results was impossible because the studies presented different methodologies. There was absence of research that satisfied the inclusion criteria. Three interesting recently published studies contemplated the clinical aspects of the research on the efficacy of Nickel-Titanium instruments in shaping curved root canals.

**Table 17.1.** Inclusion and exclusion criteria

| **Inclusion Criteria** | |
|---|---|
| **1** | Studies in vivo, in humans |
| **2** | Prospective Studies |
| **3** | Randomized controlled trial studies (RCT) |
| **4** | Experimental and control group |
| **5** | Related to the quality of shape after the root canal preparation with Nickel-Titanium instruments |
| **6** | Studies published in English |
| **7** | Rub the left thumb, the right one, the joints; |
| **Exclusion Criteria** | |
| **1** | Studies in vitro |
| **2** | Studies developed in animals |
| **3** | Studies only with abstract or with absence of abstract |
| **4** | Studies of literature review |
| **5** | Studies involving case reports |
| **6** | Studies published in other languages |
| **7** | Studies that evaluated aspects other than the shape of the root canal |

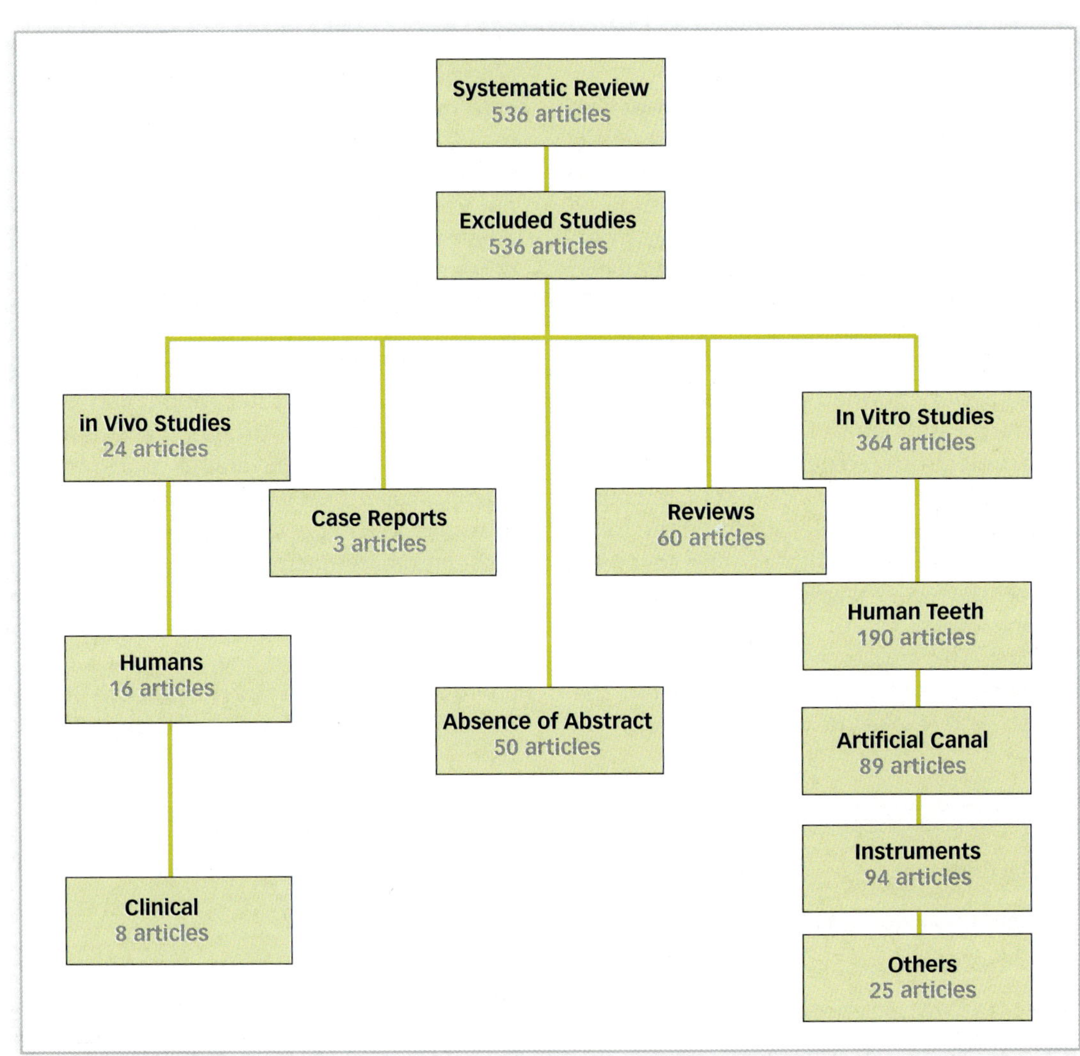


**Figure 17.32** - Distribution of articles for systematic review.

Kfir et al.[10] compared procedural errors that occur in patients during root canal preparation by senior dental students using a new - 8-step method - versus the traditional - serial step-back technique. Senior dental students treated 221 root canals of maxillary and mandibular teeth. Instrumentation included coronal flaring with Gates-Glidden reamers and standardized stainless steel K-files in all teeth. A new 8-step method was used to prepare 67 canals using standardized stainless steel hand instruments (8-step SS) and 69 canals using the rotary Nickel Titanium instruments (8-step NiTi). The traditional serial step-back technique (step-back) was used for 85 root canals. In the apical third, reaming or filing motions were used up to sizes 25 and only reaming motion in sizes larger than 25 with the new 8-step method. A filing motion was used in the step-back for all sizes.

Root canals of all groups were obturated with gutta-percha points and AH26 using a lateral condensation technique. Pre- and postoperative radiographs were taken of each tooth. Procedural errors were recorded and statistically analyzed using a bionomic test for comparison of proportion. The procedural errors detected consisted of 2 canals with transportation (3%) with the 8-step SS, and 3 canals (4%) with transportation with 8-step NiTi. There were no canal obstructions or instrument separations. With the step-back, 20 canals were transported (24%), 7 canals had obstructions (8%), and in 1 canal instrument was separated (1%). A reported complication when using rotary NiTi instruments is the tendency to separate in the root canal. In the present study none of the rotary NiTi instruments separated when used by inexperienced students. Adhering to the instructions for each rotary instrument, including proper motion in the root canal, avoiding overuse, and maintaining adequate speed of the motor could have minimized instrument breakage. The 8-step method is useful when used by senior dental students for preparing root canals in patients. It resulted in less procedural errors than the traditional serial step-back technique and allowed integration between traditional instruments and techniques with the modern rotary NiTi instruments and new techniques.

Peters et al.[14] investigated the clinical results of root canal treatment performed with the aid of nickel-titanium (NiTi) rotary instruments. A total of 179 patients underwent root canal treatment with either Lightspeed, or ProFile.04 or ProFile.04 and.06 or GT rotary instruments to create tapered preparations. In groups A and B, laterally condensed gutta-percha and AH Plus were used. Canals in group C were obturated with System B, Obtura II and Rothís 801 sealer. Initial and recall radiographs were assessed using the periapical index (PAI). Outcomes were analyzed using chi-square tests, event-time analyses and logistic regression models. Two hundred and thirty-three teeth were radiographically assessed after a mean interval of 25.4 ± 11.8 months. Favorable outcome of treatment, defined as PAI < 3 at recall was 86.7%. Logistic regression analysis and univariate analyses indicated that teeth with preoperative PAI scores >2 and retreated teeth had a significantly lower chance of healing compared with periapically healthy teeth and primary treatments, respectively. Preparation technique, length of fill and the type of sealer did not significantly affect healing rates. Two important key learning points included - the root canal treatment with NiTi root canal instrumentation systems renders favorable outcomes in more than 86% of the cases; outcome is significantly affected by preoperative diagnoses but not by the specific choice of instrumentation system.

Schäfer et al.[17] compared the effect of hand instruments and rotary nickel titanium Flex-Master files used by eight experienced dentists in private practice on the extent of straightening curved root canals. In patients, 110 canals were prepared by FlexMaster instruments, and 84 canals were enlarged using hand instruments. After instrumentation, all canals were obturated. Preoperative and postoperative radiographs were taken of each tooth using customized bite blocks. Straightening of the canal curvatures was determined with a computer image analysis program. Preparation time and size of the master apical file were also recorded. The use of FlexMaster instruments resulted in significantly less straightening and a shorter preparation time compared with hand instrumentation. Master apical file sizes were significantly greater for FlexMaster than for hand instruments. This clinical study indicated that the original curvature was significantly better maintained with automated FlexMaster files than with hand instruments. The hand instrumentation left the possibility of the canal space being inadequately debrided of vital or necrotic pulp tissue, which might result in an inadequate obturation of the root canal space. However, it must be borne in mind that this study investigated technical quality, which might not necessarily result in a higher prognosis for the teeth prepared with FlexMaster files. Certainly, follow-up examinations of the teeth treated in this study are necessary.

Nickel-titanium systems have been shown to allow preparation of root canals with fewer procedural errors and expressive performance with encouraging outcomes on shaping curved root canals.

There is no doubt that the NiTi rotary instrument has revolutionized the root canal technique. It is a very important innovation. As described by Parashos et al.[12], an innovation is an idea, practice, or object that is perceived as new. The problem is dissemination of the innovation. Dissemination refers to the process whereby an innovation spreads. Innovation is disruptive when it redefines a procedure and is sustaining when it is the better way of doing something. In the literature, innovation and technology seem to be used interchangeably.

Rogers[15] describes that there are 4 main elements in dissemination: the innovation itself, the communication channels, time and the social system. The members of a social system are classified into 5 adopter categories: innovators, early adopters, early majority, late majority and laggards. According to the author we are in the early majority of NiTi rotary instrument use. Late adopters probably will be more receptive to the innovation because of their characteristics of being less able to cope with uncertainty and risk. They are dependant not only on the accumulated experience of others but also on further improvements and understanding of the technology.

Change will occur only when people are shown how to change their old patterns and develop commitments to new ones. Change is inevitable but it is important to realize that dentists must perceive a need to change.

But an innovation in dentistry is related to research, education and credibility. The problem is the continuing education courses. Most of the professionals that attend these courses do not introduce the knowledge/know-how into their practices. An increased frequency of use of new technology and purchasing new technology does not necessarily lead to correct use and incorporation into practice[12].

Rotary systems are excellent auxiliary aid in root canal therapy. It is possible to make root canal preparation easy and fast but you must develop a clinical criterion to determine when hybridization is necessary in order to get the best with these systems. It is important to remember that "more important than the instrument or automated handpiece is the professional working with it. His guidelines for the particular aspects of each clinical case will result in a well conducted root canal preparation, leading to a succesful endodontic therapy".

1. Baugh D, Wallance J. The role of apical instrumentation in root canal treatment: a review of the literature. J Endod 2005;31:333-40.
2. Batista A, Sydney GB. An in vitro study of the clinical anatomic diameter in human molars. (in print – Aust Endod J).
3. Card SJ, Sigurdsson A, Ørstavik D, Trope M. The effectiveness of increased apical enlargement in reducing intracanal bacteria. Endod 2002;28:779-83.
4. Dalton BC, Orstavik D, Phillips C, Pettiette M, Trope M. Bacterial reduction with nickel-titanium rotary instrumentation. J Endod 1998;24:763-7.
5. Debelian G, Trope M. BioRace: efficient, safe and biological based sequence files. Roots 2008;1:20-26.
6. Goerig AC, Michelich RJ, Schultz HH. Instrumentation of root canals in molar using the step-down technique. J Endod 1982;8:550-4.
7. Goldberg F; Massone EJ. Patency file and apical transportation: An in vitro study. J Endod 2002;28:7:510-1.
8. Gu LS, Ling Q, Wei X, Huang Y. Efficacy of Protaper universal rotary retreatment system for gutta-percha removal from root canals. Int Endod J 2008;41:229-95.
9. Kerekes K, Tronstad L. Morphologic observations on root canals of human molars. J Endod 1977;3:114-8.
10. Kfir A, Rosenberg E, Zuckerman O, Tamse A, Fuss Z. Comparison of procedural errors resulting during root canal preparations completed by senior dental students in patients using an '8-step method' versus 'serial step-back technique'. Oral Surg Oral Med Oral Pathol Oral Radiol Endod 2004; 97:745-8.
11. Mounce RE. Rotary Nickel-Titanium instrumentation revolutionized: The twisted file. Oral Health 2008;6-9.
12. Parashos P, Messer HH. The diffusion of innovation in dentistry: a review using rotary nickel-titanium technology as an example. Oral Surg Oral Med Oral Pathol Oral Radiol Endod 2006;101:395-401.
13. Pécora JD, Capelli A, Guerisoli DMZ, Spano JCE, Estrela C. Influence of cervical preparation on apical file size determination. Int Endod J 2005;38:430-5.
14. Peters OA, Barbakow F, Peters CI. An analysis of endodontic treatment with three nickel-titanium rotary root canal preparation techniques. Int Endod J. 2004; 37:849-59.
15. Rogers EM. Diffusion of innovations. 5th ed. New York: Free Press, 2003.
16. Serota KS. Nahmias Y. Predictable Endodontic Success: The hybrid approach - Part 1. Oral Health 2003:41-48.
17. Schäfer E, Schulz-Bongert U, Tulus G. Comparison of hand stainless steel and nickel titanium rotary instrumentation: a clinical study. J Endod. 2004;30:432-5.
18. Shuping G, Ørstavick D, Sigurdsson A, Trope M. Reduction of intracanal bacteria using nickel-titanium rotary instrumentation and various medications. J Endod 2000;26:751-5.
19. Sydney GB. Como preparar o canal radicular com rapidez e eficiência, cap.10, p. 189-218, In: Cardoso,RJ; Gonçalves, EAG Odontologia: *Endodontia / Trauma*, Artes Médicas, São Paulo,2.002,476p.
20. Sydney GB, Batista A. Diagnóstico e viabilização do retratamento endodôntico, cap. 5113-144, In: Dib LL; Saddy MS Atualização Clínica em Odontologia, Artes Médicas, São Paulo, 2006, 577p.
21. Sydney GB, Batista A, Deonizio MD. Acesso Radicular. Rev Odontol Brasil Central 2008;17:1-12.
22. Sydney GB, Estrela C. Influence of root canal preparation on anaerobic bacteria in teeth with asymptomatic apical periodontitis. Braz Endod J 1996;1:7-10.
23. Thompson AS. An overview of nickel-titanium alloys used in dentistry. Int Endod J 2000;33:297-310.
24. Trope M, Debelian G. Endodontic treatment of apical periodontitis chapter 12, 347-380, In: Ørstavik D, Pitt Ford T Essential Endodontology, Blackwell Munksgaard, 2nd ed. 2008, 477p.
25. Turpin Y, Chagneau F, Vulcain J. Impact of two theorical cross-sections on torsioal anda bending stresses of NiTi root canal instrument models. J Endod 2000;26:414-7.
26. Young GR, Parashos P, Messer HH. The principles of techniques for cleaning root canals. Aust Endod J 52:522-63,2007.
27. Weiger R, Bartha T, Kalwitzki M, Lost C. A clinical method to determine the optimal apical preparation size - Part I. Oral Surg Oral Med Oral Pathol Oral Radiol Endod 2006;102:686-91.
28. Wilcox LR, Swift ML. Endodontic retreatment in small and large curved canals. J Endod 1991;17:313-5.
29. Wu MK, Ríoris A, Barkis D, Wesselink PR. Prevalence and extend of long oval canals in the apical third. Oral Surg Oral Med Oral Pathol Oral Radiol Endod 2000;89:739-43.

# Fractures of Motor-driven NiTi Endodontic Instruments: theoretical and practical concepts

**H. P. Lopes**
*Brazilian Endodontic Association, Rio de Janeiro, RJ, Brazil*

**C. N. Elias**
*Engeneering Military Institute, Rio de Janeiro, RJ, Brazil*

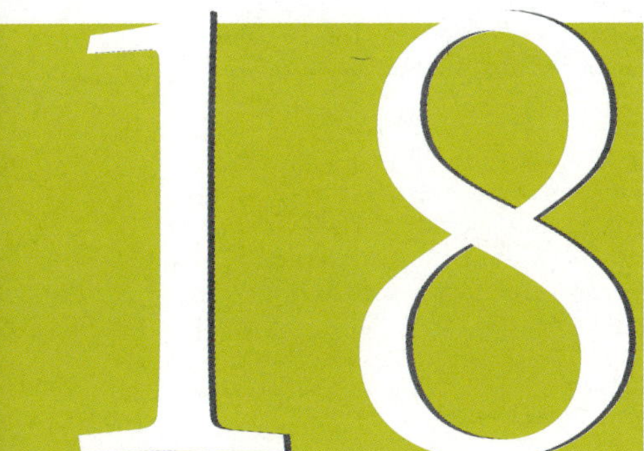

Chapter contents

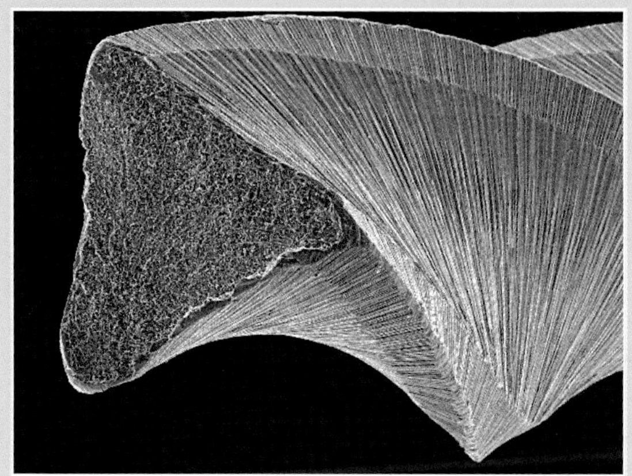

Cyclic fatigue fracture. Absence of plastic deformation in the cutting blade of the instrument. Plane fracture surface and perpendicular to the axis of the instrument (250X).

## 18.1 Introduction

The chemical-mechanical preparation of an atresic and curved root canal to enlargement and maintain its original form is a challenge to endodontics. Rotary nickel-titanium (NiTi) endodontic instruments have been indicated, particularly in the preparation of curved root canals, due to their greater elasticity when compared with stainless steel instruments. This greater elasticity has demonstrated little or no canal transportation in root canal preparation. However, the largest concern with rotary nickel-titanium (NiTi) endodontic instruments has been their fracture[5,8,11,17]. Rotary instruments can fracture due to torsion or cyclic fatigue force[16,17,23].

## 18.2 Torsion Fracture

For a torsion fracture to occur, it is necessary for the tip of the endodontic instrument to remain immobilized and torque (rotation force), to be greater than the fracture strength limit of the instrument to be applied at the other extremity (fixation and activation shaft)[16,17].

With immobilization of the tip of the endodontic instrument, the rotation force to the right passes the flow limit of the NiTi alloy causing a plastic deformation (distortion) located in the helical shaft of the instrument. This plastic deformation increases the mechanical hardening of the material. The continual increase in the rotation force (torque) can cross the limit of fracture resistance of the endodontic instrument, causing it to rupture into two parts close to the immobilization point[18].

The torsion fracture of an endodontic instrument can be evaluated and analyzed by mechanical testing or clinical use.

To perform mechanical testing it is necessary to use specific devices[10,18,22,25]. The instrument tip is usually immobilized with a bench vise that has a 3 mm deep backstop (step). The rotation force is obtained through specific devices coupled to an Instron testing machine[18,22,24,25]. By means of mechanical torsion testing one can quantify the rotation and the torque at failure that the endodontic instrument withstood under a determined loading condition. The rotation at failure determines the maximum number of turns that the endodontic instrument resists before the fracture. It can be quantified in number of turns or in degrees.

The torque at failure determines the maximum load that the endodontic instrument resists before the fracture. Torque can be defined as a rotary effect created by the application of a force (F) distant from the rotation axis (R) of an object. It is calculated by the equation: Torque = Forces x Radius.

With the results obtained in the mechanical torsion testing it is possible to anticipate the performance of an endodontic instrument during the clinical use.

In the torsion test many factors, such as the diameter in $D_0$, taper, instrument design, cross-sectional area of the straight section, core diameter, production technique, surface finish and the direction of rotation can influence the evaluated parameters (rotation and torque at failure).

For some authors, the rotation at failure decreases with the increase in diameter ($D_0$ or taper)[2,3,17]. For others, there is no direct relationship between the values of rotation at failure and diameter of the instruments[1,9]. Rotation at failure is a safety factor of the instrument, because the higher the rotation at failure, higher will be the possibility of the endodontic instrument not rupturing inside of a root canal.

As regards the torque at failure, the results shown in the literature demonstrated that the values increased with the increase in the diameter of the instrument ($D_0$ or taper)[10,15,23,26].

The mean values of rotation at failure and torque at failure withstood by the K3 rotary NiTi endodontic instruments are represented in Tables 18.1 and 18.2.

**Table 18.1** - Mean and standard deviation (SD) of rotation at failure of the instruments K3 #25 and tapers 0.02-0.04 and 0.06 mm

| Instrument K³ Number/Taper | Sample Size | Deformation in mm (DP) | Rotation at failure | |
|---|---|---|---|---|
| | | | Turns | Degree |
| 25/0.02 | 10 | 98.63 (10.92) | 3.93 | 1413.49 |
| 25/0.04 | 10 | 70.59 (14.79) | 2.81 | 1011.64 |
| 25/0.06 | 10 | 65.75 (7.68) | 2.62 | 942.28 |

The mean value of rotation at failure of the evaluated instruments was statistically higher for the endodontic instruments with smaller taper.

**Table 18.2** - Mean and standard deviation (SD) of the force (gf) and torque (gf.mm) at failure of the instruments K3 #25 and taper 0.02-0.04 and 0.06 mm

| Instrument K³ | | | |
|---|---|---|---|
| Number/Taper | Sample Size | Force at failure (SD) | Torque at failure |
| 25/0.02 | 10 | 154.8 (8.34) | 619.2 |
| 25/0.04 | 10 | 196.4 (15.99) | 785.6 |
| 25/0.06 | 10 | 337.3 (38.74) | 1349.2 |

The mean values of the force and torque at failure of the evaluated instruments was statistically higher for the instruments with larger taper.

For torsion fracture to occur during clinical use it is necessary for the tip of the endodontic instrument to be immobilized inside of a root canal, and for the torque of a hand piece connected to an electric motor to be applied at the other extremity[17].

If the professional can avoid immobilizing the tip of the instrument inside the root canal during clinical use, torsion fracture will not occur, irrespective of the torque applied. Torsion fracture can also be reduced by discarding instruments whose conical helical shaft have become distorted.

The study of the torsion fracture of endodontic instruments due to clinical use is of limited mechanical value. This is because, in clinical studies, the variables of the anatomical conditions of root canals (root canal length, radius of curvature of the root canal, length and location of the arch of the root canal and hardness of the dentin) and of the operators are not usually considered.

Thus, it is impossible or even imprudent to compare with safety the limits of resistance to torsion fracture of the endodontic instruments used in root canal instrumentation. Moreover, due the combinations of tensions that occur during root canal instrumentation, it is extremely difficult to classify and explain the fracture mechanism of endodontic instruments.

Clinical studies should endeavor to describe technical procedures capable of reducing the fracture of the endodontic instruments, and propose maneuvers for cases with endodontic instrument fragments retained inside the root canals.

Immobilization of an endodontic instrument inside a root canal can be controlled:

- Reducing the advance of the instrument in apical direction. The cutting action of rotary instruments is to enlarge the canal by continuous rotation, advancing from 1 to 2 mm in the apical direction of the root canal, interrupted at intervals with removal (pecking motion). Greater advances increase the cutting resistance of the dentinal wall, which can cause immobilization of the tip of the instrument and induce a loading that exceeds its limit of resistance to torsion fracture;
- Performing the root canal preparation in the crown-down direction. The previous enlargement of the cervical and middle segment of the root canal with instruments of larger diameter, allows instruments of smaller diameter used in the preparation of the apical segment of the root canal to be submitted to a smaller loading, which reduces the cutting effort and the possibility of the tip being immobilized.

Another resource to minimize the torsion fracture is to use the electric motor to interrupt the turn when the instrument becomes immobilized inside the root canal. The torque pre-established by the manufacturer or programmed by the operator should remain below the maximum limit of resistance to torsion fracture of the instrument used. It is difficult to reach this objective for several reasons:

- The operator should know the probable value of the torque that will induce the fracture of each endodontic instrument used. It is worth emphasizing that these values are not informed by the manufacturers;
- The torque is a measurement related to radius. With a conical geometric configuration of the helical shaft, the limit of resistance to torsion fracture of an endodontic instrument is variable. Consequently the torque is variable and it depends on the diameter of the conical helical shaft of the instrument near the point of its immobilization inside the root canal;
- The accentuated variations between the real diameters and the proposed nominal value, as well as, several surface finishing defects (grooves, burrs, and microcavities) existent in the endodontic instruments work as stress concentration points, and can lead to their premature fracture at torque levels below the predictable values.

It can not be denied that items of equipment with programmed torques to activate endodontic instruments are a technological advance. Nevertheless, the best resource for reducing torsion fracture of motor-driven endodontic instruments is to keep them from becoming immobilized during root canal preparation. This is achieved with the knowledge of the mechanical principles of instrumentation, with adequate technique, ability and professional experience. For Sattapan et al.[23] torsion fracture occurred in 55.7% of all the fractured NiTi instruments during the routine clinical use. They also affirmed that this fracture is caused by the increase in loading of the instrument in the apical direction during the root canal preparation.

In a recent study[28] of 100 fractured NiTi instruments, in 91% of the cases the fracture occurred as a result of cyclic fatigue, in 3% by torsion and in 6% by combination of these. According to Yared et al.[30], for experienced professionals the use of motors with torques smaller than the limit of resistance to torsion fracture of the instrument used is not important to reduce the plastic deformation or the incidence of instrument fracture.

Thus, it can be affirm that the biggest disadvantage of the use of rotary instruments is not torsion fracture, but fracture by cyclic fatigue (low-cycle fatigues).

## 18.3 Cyclic Fatigue Fracture

Cyclic fatigue fracture of a rotary endodontic instrument occurs when it rotates inside a curved root canal. In the cyclic fatigue area of the endodontic instrument, alternate tensile and compressive stresses are induced. The cyclic repetition of these stresses promotes cumulative micro-structural changes that induce the nucleation of cracks that increase, coalesce and spread until the fatigue fracture of the endodontic instrument.

Cyclic fatigue fractures can be evaluated and analyzed by mechanical testing or clinical use.

To perform mechanical testing it is necessary to use specific devices. The endodontic instrument rotates inside a curved artificial root canal with pre-determined curvature radius and length of the arch. The artificial root should present a larger diameter than that of the instrument to be evaluated. The endodontic instrument is activated at a pre-determined speed using a hand piece connected to an electric micro-motor. The artificial root canal, hand piece/electric micro-motor set is fixed in a supporting device with the main purpose of eliminating the interference of the operator in inducing tensions on the endodontic instruments during the cyclic fatigue test[11,18,21].

From the cyclic fatigue test we can quantify the number of cycles that an endodontic instrument is capable of resisting to fatigue fracture under a certain loading condition.

The number of cycles is obtained by multiplying the speed of rotation in the test by the time it takes for the endodontic instrument fracture to occur. It is cumulative and related to the intensity of the tensile and compressive stress imposed on the cyclic fatigue area of the endodontic instrument. The intensity of the stresses is a specific parameter and it is related to the radius of the curvature of the root canal, length of the arch and diameter and rigidity of the instrument used. The smaller the radius of curvature of the root canal, the greater will be the length of the arch, and the greater the diameter and rigidity of the instrument used, the lower will be the number of cycles until the fracture withstood by the evaluated endodontic instrument[12,18,21,27].

For cyclic fatigue testing performed under the same loading condition, the rotation speed does not have a significant influence on the number of cycles required to fracture the NiTi rotary endodontic instrument. This is because higher speeds reduce the time required to reach the number of cycles until the fracture occurs[4,13,21,31].

However, for other authors the increase in speed significantly reduces the number of cycles required to fracture NiTi rotary endodontic instruments[5,6,8,11,19].

The data relative to the cyclic fatigue test using the ProTaper F3 and F4 instruments are presented in the Table 18.3.

**Table 18.3** - Mean and standard deviation (SD) of the time and the number of cycles required for fatigue fracture to occur in ProTaper instruments

| Speed Rpm | Sample Size | ProTaper F3 | | ProTaper F4 | |
|---|---|---|---|---|---|
| | | Time (s) | NCF (DP) | Time (s) | NCF (DP) |
| 300 | 10 | 76 | 380 (42.10) | 56.2 | 281 (39.28) |
| 600 | 10 | 27 | 270 (46.43) | 21.8 | 218 (34.89) |

The comparison of the number of cycles for the fracture NCF between the two speeds evaluated with the ProTaper F3 and F4 instruments revealed that for the F3 and F4 instruments the NCF was statistically higher when the speed of 300rpm was used in the test.

For Eggeler et al.[6], the effect of the rotation speed on the fracture of a NiTi test specimen is related to the production of heat during the formation of the martensite induced by stress. To form the martensite, the austenite-martensite interface has to move and that movement dissipates energy and produces heat. Higher speeds produce more heat than lower speeds and thus increase the temperature of the test specimen faster, which leads to fast increase in the tension on the surface making the fatigue fracture occur sooner.

The fatigue fracture is unexpected and happens without any previous warning. This fracture does not depend on the torque applied to the rotary endodontic instrument.

For the cyclic fatigue fracture to occur during clinical use it is necessary for the endodontic instrument to rotate inside a curved root canal. Clinical use is of limited mechanical value for evaluating the fatigue fracture of endodontic instruments submitted to cyclic fatigue inside of curved root canals. This is due to great anatomical diversity of the root canals and the variables of the operators, which make it impossible to safely control the number of cycles and the intensity of the stresses in the cyclic fatigue region of the endodontic instrument used in root canal instrumentation.

Thus, to predict the number of root canals in which a rotary NiTi endodontic instrument can be used with safety in relation to fatigue fracture is at least an empirical and irresponsible conduct.

However, clinical study is important to describe technical procedures capable of increasing the useful life of an endodontic instrument when submitted to cyclic fatigue inside a root canal.

The following are clinical recommendations to reduce the incidence of cyclic fatigue fracture of an endodontic instrument:

- Keep the instrument rotating inside a curved root canal for the shortest possible time;
- Maintain the instrument inside a curved root canal in a constant forward and backward movement in the apical direction (pecking motion);
- Do not buckle the instrument inside a root canal;
- The smaller the radius of curvature of the root canals, the smaller should be the taper of the instrument used.

Another way to reduce to fatigue fracture is by prematurely discarding the instrument before it reaches the limit of useful life. However, this procedure elevates the cost of the endodontic treatment, and is considered a disadvantage.

## 18.4 Scanning Electronic Microscopy Evaluation

By scanning electronic microscopy (SEM) analysis it can be observed that the fracture surfaces of rotary NiTi endodontic instruments, when submitted to torsion loading, are plane and perpendicular to the axes of the instruments. On the torsion fracture to the right, plastic deformation occurs on the helical shaft of the instrument, represented by the reversal of the original direction of its helixes (Figs. 18.1A-B). On rupture by cyclic fatigue, the fracture surface can be plane, when originating from of the propagation of a single crack, or it can present several planes, when the rupture originates from of the propagation of more than one crack. Usually, in the second, case crack propagations occur in opposite directions and are separated by small distances. In cyclic fatigue fracture, no plastic deformation of the helical shaft of the instrument occurs (Figs. 18.2A-B). The morphology of the fracture surface of rotary NiTi endodontic instruments, by torsion or by cyclic fatigue, presents characteristics of a ductile type. In it, micro-cavities with varied shapes were identified (Figs.18.3A-B)[11,17,18,20].

Defects originating from the manufacture of endodontic instruments can act to concentrate stress. During the machining operations, small marks and undulations are introduced on the surface of the endodontic instruments by cutting tools. The presence of these surface finishing defects act by concentrating stress and induce fracture of the instrument during the clinical use under lower loading values than those expected and obtained in mechanical testing of only one cycle (torsion or cyclic fatigue) (Figs.18.4A-B). The larger the number and size of the defects on the helical shaft of an instrument, the lower will be the stress required for it to fracture (Figs.18.5 and 18.6A-B)[7,14,17,18,29].

Because of this, it can be affirmed that the problem of using rotary NiTi endodontic instruments in the preparation of curved root canals will not be solved by the production of sophisticated and highly expensive electric motors, but with:

- More precision in the dimensions of the endodontic instruments;
- Better surface finishing of the endodontic instruments;
- Incorporation of new chemical elements in the NiTi alloy;
- More knowledge about the mechanical properties of the endodontic instruments;
- The professional's better technical knowledge of the indications and use of the working tool (endodontic instruments).

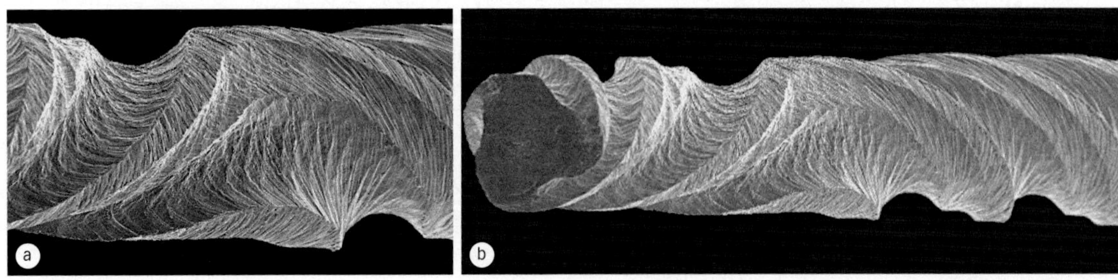


**Figure 18.1** - Torsion fracture (**A**) plastic deformation in the cutting blade of the instrument, with reversal of the original direction of the helixes (X100); (**B**) plane fracture surface and perpendicular to the axis of the instrument (X80).

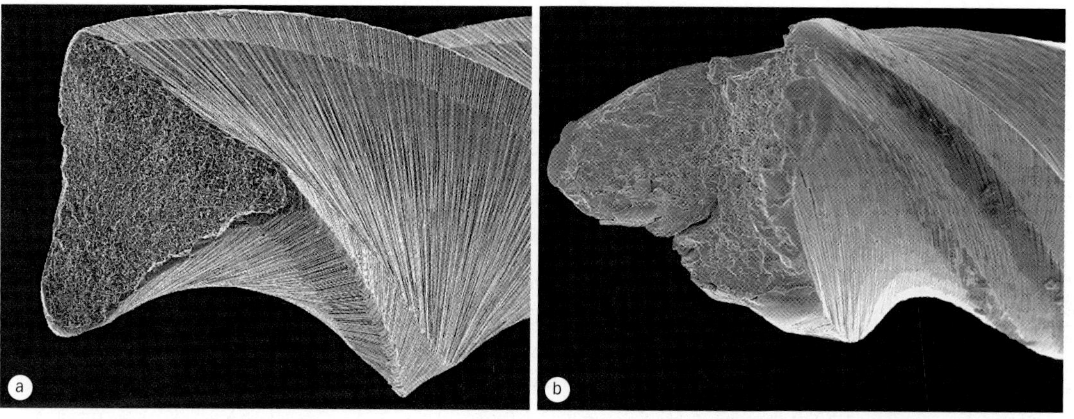

**Figure 18.2** - Cyclic fatigue fracture. Absence of plastic deformation in the cutting blade of the instrument. (**A**) Plane fracture surface and perpendicular to the axis of the instrument (X250); (**B**) fracture surface in two planes (degrees) (X300).

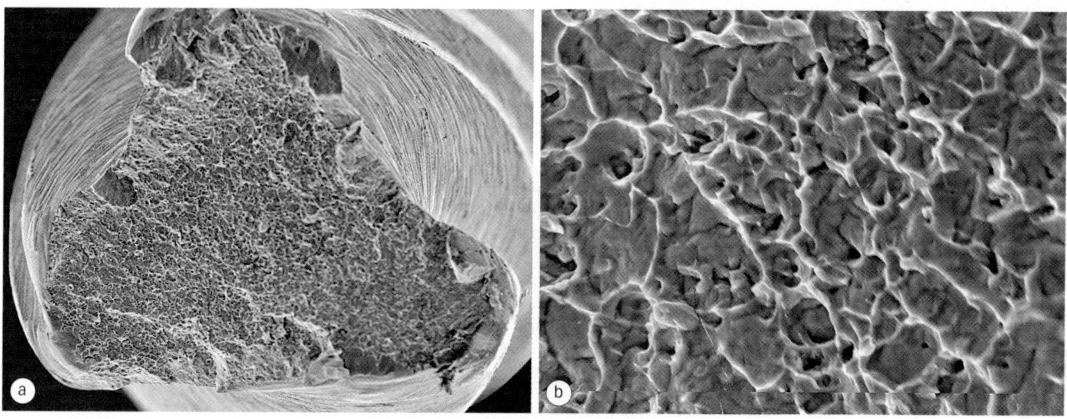

**Figure 18.3** - Torsion fracture. Morphology of the fracture surface. (**A**) Characteristic of ductile type of fracture (X200); (**B**) Magnification of the previous image (X2000).

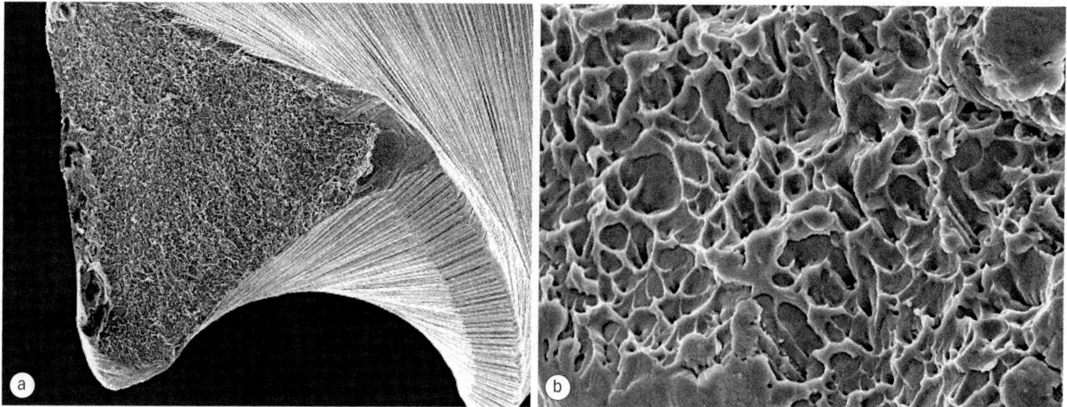

**Figure 18.4** - Cyclic fatigue fracture. Morphology of the fracture surface. (**A**) Characteristic of ductile type of fracture (X250); (**B**) Magnification of the previous image (X2000).

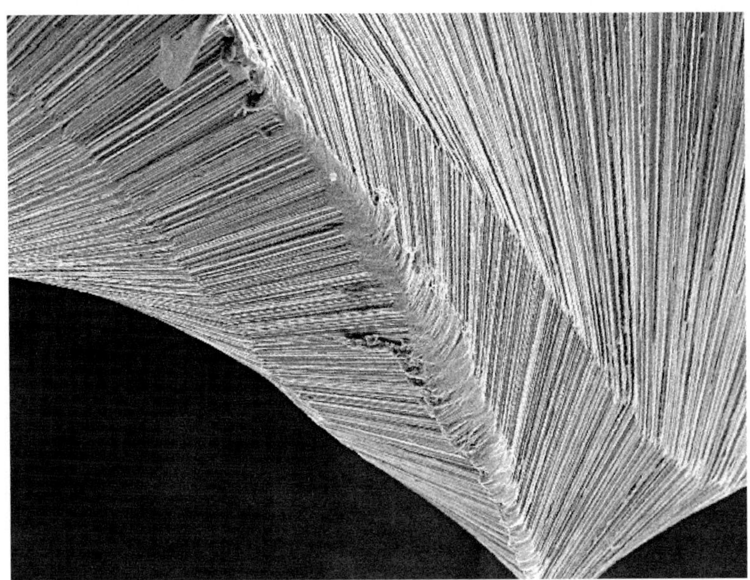

**Figure 18.5** - Surface finishing. Presence of groove (X800).

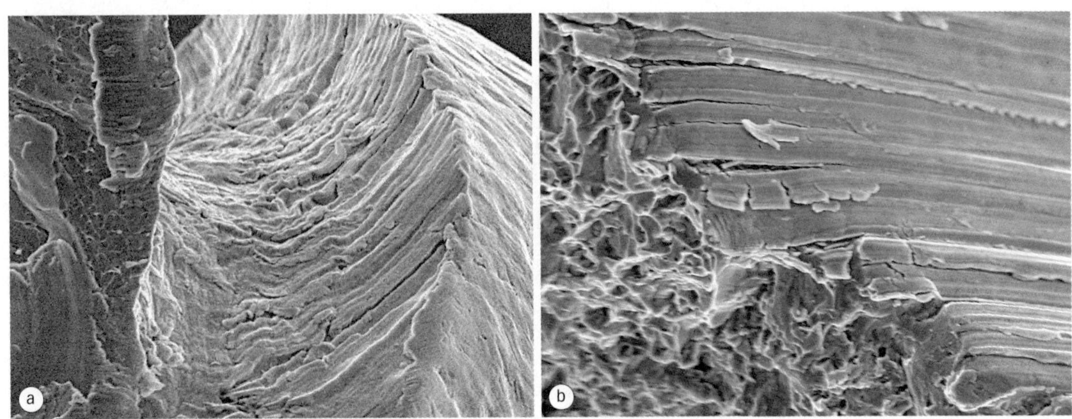


**Figure 18.6** - Presence of cracks in the groove areas. (**A**) Torsion fracture (X1000); (**B**) cyclic fatigue fracture (X1000).

1. Bahia MGA. Resistência à fadiga e comportamento em torção de instrumentos endodônticos de NiTi. (Doctoral Thesis). Federal University of Minas Gerais, 2006. 213p.
2. Camps JJ, Perlot WJ. Torsional and stiffness properties of nickel-titanium K files. Int Endod J 1995;28:239-43.
3. Canalda-Sahli C, Brau-Aguade E, Berastegui-Jimeno E. Torsional and bending properties of stainless steel and nickel-titanium Canal Master U and Flexogate instruments. Endod Dent Traumatol 1996;12:141-5.
4. Courtney TH. Mechanical behavior of materials. USA: Mc Grow Hill, 1990.
5. Dietz DB, Di Fiore PM, Bahcall JK, Launtenschlager EP. Effect of rotational speed on the breakage of nickel-titanium rotary files. J Endod 2000;26:68-71.
6. Eggeler G, Hornbogen E, Yawny A, Heckmann A Wagner M. Strutural and functional fatigue of NiTi shape memory alloys. Materials Science and Engineering A 2004;378:24-33.
7. Elias CN, Lopes HP. Materiais dentários. Ensaios Mecânicos. São Paulo: Santos, 2007.
8. Gabel WP, Hoen M, Sterman HR, Pink FE, Dietz R. Effect of rotational speed on nickel-titanium file distortion. J Endod 1999;25:752-4.
9. Gambarini G. Rationale for the use of low-torque endodontic motors in root canal instrumentation. Endod Dent Traumatol 2000;16:95-100.
10. Guilford WL, Lemons BS, Eleager PD. A comparison of torque required to fracture rotary files with tips bound in simulated curved canal. J Endod 2005;31:468-70.
11. Haikel Y, Serfaty R, Batenan G, Senger B, Allemann. Dynamic and cyclic fatigue of engine-driven rotator nickel-titanium endodontic. J Endod 1999;25:434-40.
12. Inan U, Aydin C, Tunca YM. Cyclic fatigue of ProTaper Rotary nickel-titanium instruments in artificial canals with 2 different radii of curvature. Oral Sur Oral Med Oral Pathol Oral Radiol Endod 2007;104:837-40.
13. Kitchens Jr GG, Liewehr FR, Moon PC. The effect of operational speed on the fracture of nickel-titanium rotary instruments. J Endod 2007;33:52-4.
14. Kuhn G, Tavernier B, Jordan L. Influence of structure on nickel-titanium endodontic instruments failure. J Endod 2001;27:516-20.
15. Lopes HP, Elias CN, Mangelli M, Moreira EJL. Instrumentos endodônticos de NiTi de diferentes conicidades. Fratura por torção em flexão. Rev Bras Odontol 2006;63:113-6.
16. Lopes HP, Elias CN, Siqueira-Jr JF. Mecanismo de fratura dos instrumentos endodônticos. Rev Paul Odontol 2000;22:4-9.
17. Lopes HP, Elias CN. Fratura dos instrumentos endodônticos de NiTi acionados a motor. Fundamentos teóricos e práticos. Rev Bras Odontol 2001;58:207-9.
18. Lopes HP, Moreira EJL, Elias CN, Almeida RA, Neves MS. Cyclic fatigue of ProTaper instruments. J Endod 2007;33:55-7.
19. Nasser SN, Guo WG. Superelastic and cyclic response of NiTi SMA at various strain rates and temperatures. Mechanics of Materials 2006; 38:463-74.
20. Parashos P, Messer HH. Rotary NiTi instrument fracture and its consequences. J Endod 2006;32:1031-43.
21. Pruett JP, Clement DJ, Carnes DL Jr. Cyclic fatigue testing of nickel-titanium endodontic instruments. J Endod 1997;23:77-85.
22. Rowan MB, Nichows JI, Steiner J. Propriedades torsionales de las limas endodónticas de acero inoxidável y de níquel-titanio. J Endod 1997;3:66-72. (ed. Español)
23. Sattapan B, Nervo GJ, Palamara JEA, Messer HH. Defects in rotatory nickel-titanium files after clinical use. J Endod 2000;25:161-5.
24. Serene TP Adams JD, Saxena A. Niquel-titanium instruments: applications in endodontics. St Louis: Ishiyaku Euro America 113, 1995.
25. Seto BG, Nicholls JI, Harrungton GW. Torsional properties of twisted and machined endodontic files. J Endod 1990;16:335-60.
26. Svec TA, Powers JM. Effects of simulated clinical conditions on nickel-titanium rotator files. J Endod 1999;25:759-60.
27. Ullmann CJ, Peters OA. Effect of cyclic fatigue on static fracture loads in ProTaper nickel-titanium instruments. J Endod 2005;31:183-6.
28. Wei X, Ling J, Jiang J, Huang X, Liu L. Modes of failure of ProTaper nickel-titanium rotary instruments after clinical use. J Endod 2007;33:276-9.
29. Yao JH, Schwartz SA, Beeson TJ. Cyclic fatigue of three types of rotary nickel-titanium files in a dynamic model. J Endod 2006;32:55-7.
30. Yared GM, Bou Dagher FE, Machtou P. Influence of rotational speed, torque and operator's proficiency on Profile failures. Int Endod J 2001;34:47-53.
31. Zelada G, Varela P, Martín B, Bahílio JG, Magan F, Ahn S. The effect of rotational speed and the curvature of root canals on the breakage of rotary endodontic instruments. J Endod 2002;28:540-2.

# Root Canal Irrigants

**C. Estrela**

*Federal University of Goiás, Goiânia, GO, Brazil*

**J. D. Pécora**

*University of São Paulo, Ribeirão Preto, SP, Brazil*

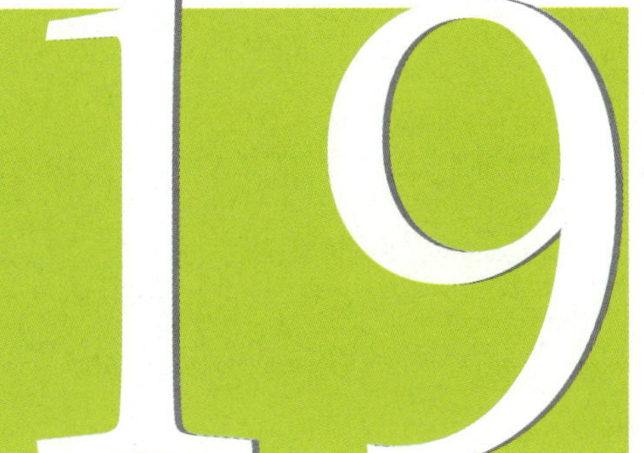

Chapter contents

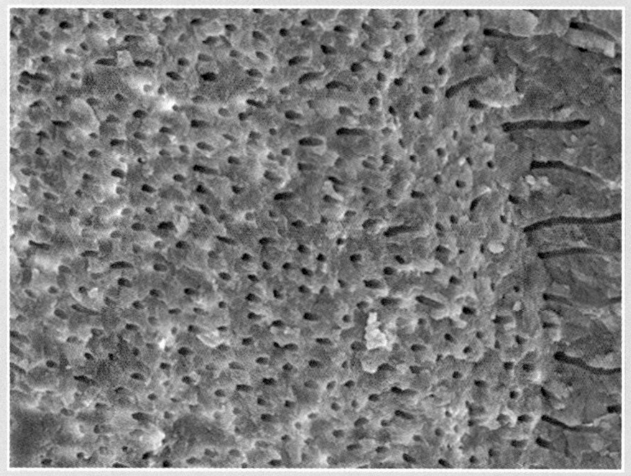

Root dentinal tubules opened after 5 min of apple vinegar (X500).

## 19.1 Introduction

The success of endodontic treatment is directly influenced by the elimination of microorganisms in infected root canals. Irrigant solutions are very important during root canal preparation because they help to clean the root canal, lubricate the files, flush out debris, and have an antimicrobial and tissue-dissolution effect, without damaging periapical tissues. The selection of an ideal irrigant depends on its action against microorganisms and on periapical tissues.

The importance of microorganisms in root canal therapy has been discussed for many years[1-434]. The sanitization process of infected root canals is the main purpose of endodontic therapy.

The process observed between endodontic infection and consequent host response has led to several therapeutic trends. Chemical and mechanical cleaning and shaping significantly reduce the number of microorganisms, but do not eliminate them[42,47-52,90,94-96,98,229,248,379]. Various irrigants have been indicated for the sanitization process in root canal infection. Although many of them have shown varied degrees of antimicrobial effectiveness [12,22,42-51,89-113,124,126,131,133-36,139,147-150,164-171,178,182-184,186-189,223,229,239,246,258,265,275,276,279,299,302,306,312,341,345-51,389,400,401], it is difficult to choose the ideal irrigant solution and its concentration.

The use of irrigant solutions has several objectives and properties (Table 19.1). These include antimicrobial efficacy, tissue dissolution capacity, and tissue tolerance, which must always be evaluated before choosing the ideal irrigant solution. There are two essential clinical conditions to consider: the presence or absence of microorganisms (pulp inflammation or pulp necrosis). Other characteristics, however, must also be analyzed such as; presence or absence of fistula, open or closed cavity, presence or absence of pain, complete or incomplete rhizogenesis, and traumatic dental injuries (such as an avulsed tooth).

A number of different irrigant solutions to reduce endodontic infection, and contribute to the sanitization process have been suggested, including: halogenated compounds (concentrations of 0.5%, 1.0%, 2.5% and 5.25% of sodium hypochlorite), chlorhexidine, detergent (anionic, cationic), chelating agents (EDTA, citric acid), (RC Prep, EDTAC, Gly-oxide, sodium hypochlorite + hydrogen peroxide) and others (MTAD, ozonated water, apple vinegar).

It is essential, however, to consider that as important as the irrigant solution are the penetration depth of the irrigating cannula, frequency of irrigation, abundance of irrigation and the concentration of irrigant solutions, in order for the sanitization process to be effective (Fig. 19.1). An irrigant can penetrate into the infected root canal, but this does not mean that the concentration was sufficiently high to kill the bacteria[97].

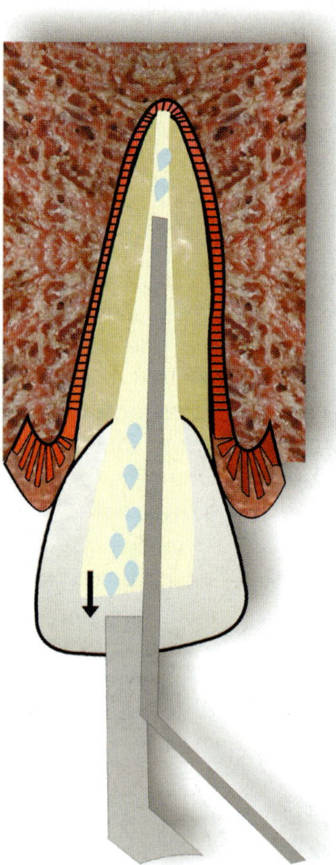

**Figure 19.1** - Irrigation process.

**Table 19.1** - Objectives and properties of irrigant solutions.

| | |
|---|---|
| **1** | Be highly efficacious against endodontic microbiota; |
| **2** | Neutralize the components of endodontic infection (to inactivate endotoxin); |
| **3** | Allow more direct and intense action against endodontic microbiota; |
| **4** | Facilitate the action of endodontic instrumentation (low coefficient of viscosity; low superficial tension; lubricant); |
| **5** | Alter the pH of the environment; |
| **6** | Remove blood in pulp cavity (to prevent alteration in the color of the coronal chamber); |
| **7** | Prevent the formation of a smear layer; favor the action of intracanal dressing or filling materials; |
| **8** | Remove organic matter (pulp rests) and inorganic (debris, dentin chips); to dissolve necrotic pulp tissue remnants (solubilize organic or inorganic matter); |
| **9** | Have good tissue tolerance (the irrigant solution cannot be irritant to periapical tissues; low toxicity and good tissue tolerance); |
| **10** | The irrigant solution must penetrate into the entire root canal (the irrigating cannula must penetrate up to 3 mm before the cement dentin canal junction). |

## 19.2 Irrigant Solutions

Sodium hypochlorite and chlorhexidine are antimicrobial agents frequently used in the treatment of endodontic and periodontal infections[1-143].

The use of sodium hypochlorite as an antimicrobial solution began at the end of the 18th century, with the `water of Javele (in 1792), a solution containing sodium and potassium hypochlorite[300]. Labaraque's liquor, a solution containing 2.5% sodium hypochlorite, appeared in 1820. A solution containing 0.5% of available chlorite with boric acid to reduce its pH was proposed by Dakin[79-80], in order to disinfect wounds during Word War I. Walker[404], introduced the use of 5% sodium hypochlorite in dentistry, and this was reinforced by Grossman & Maiman[142].

Sodium hypochlorite is the present day irrigant of choice, due to its antimicrobial effectiveness, tissue-dissolving effects and its tissue tolerance at adequate clinical concentrations. One of the problems with the use of sodium hypochlorite concerns its appropriate concentration, due to cellular damage caused by its extrusion into the periapical tissue.

Chlorhexidine is a cationic agent (biguanide group; 4-chlorophenyl radical) that has antibacterial activity. The cationic nature of the compound produces binding to the anionic compound at the bacterial surface (phosphate groups of teichoic acid in Gram-positive and lipopolysaccharide in Gram-negative bacteria) capable of altering their integrity. The potassium ion, being a small entity, is the first substance to appear when the cytoplasm membrane is damaged. Alteration of the cytoplasm membrane permeability promotes precipitation of cytoplasm proteins, alters cellular osmotic balance, interferes with metabolism, growth, cell division, inhibits the membrane ATPase and inhibits the anaerobic process[104,180,181,186,187,309].

Although sodium hypochlorite and chlorhexidine present antibacterial activity, the two substances have distinct characteristics. Various research results have shown disagreement when comparing the antimicrobial effect of these solutions[12,95-98,110,111,133-136,199,308,345,346]. Different experimental methods, biological indicators, concentrations, or the period of analysis may have caused these differences.

Several studies have evaluated the antimicrobial effectiveness of different irrigant solutions[1,3,7,12,16,17,23,26,42-45,47-52,55,56,85-112,114,117-124,126,131,133-136,147-150,153,156,157,164-171,186,210,213,219,220,229,246,257,258,260,265-268,275,276,299,302,305,306,311,337,345,346,351,364,379,389-391,397,400,401,423,429-431]. Vahdaty et al.[397] analyzed the efficacy of 2% chlorhexidine and 2% sodium hypochlorite in dentinal tubules infected with *E. faecalis*. Dentine was removed from the canal wall with sterile burs of increasing diameter to provide samples of 100, 100-300 and 300-500 µm deep. The results indicated that chlorhexidine and sodium hypochlorite were equally effective antibacterial agents at similar concentrations against the test microorganism. They significantly reduced the bacterial counts in the first 100 µm of dentinal tubules; however, up to 50% of dentine samples remained infected after the use of both agents. Jeansonne & White[186] compared 2% chlorhexidine and 5.25% sodium hypochlorite as antimicrobial endodontic irrigants in freshly extracted human teeth with pulp disease. The results showed that the number of post-irrigant positive cultures and the number of colony-forming units in positive cultures obtained from chlorhexidine-treated teeth, were lower than the numbers obtained from sodium hypochlorite-treated teeth, but the differences were not statistically significant. Heling & Chandler[164] investigated the antimicrobial effect of irrigant combinations within dentinal tubules, and concluded that 0.12% chlorhexidine and 1% sodium hypochlorite were similarly effective. Byström & Sundquist[51] examined the bacteriologic effect of 0.5% sodium hypochlorite solution in *in vivo* endodontic therapy. With 0.5% sodium hypochlorite, no bacteria could be recovered from 12 of 15 root canals at the fifth appointment. This was compared with 8 of 15 root canals, when saline solution was used as the irrigant. Ohara et al.[258] compared six irrigants against selected anaerobic bacteria. 0.2% chlorhexidine was the most effective; 3% hydrogen peroxide, 5.25% sodium hypochlorite and 17% REDTA were less effective, while the saturated solution of calcium hydroxide and saline proved to be completely ineffective. Ayhan et al.[12] reported the antimicrobial effects of various endodontic irrigants on selected microorganisms, and observed that 5.25% sodium hypochlorite was superior, and the reduced concentration of 0.5% resulted in significantly decreased antimicrobial effectiveness. Gomes et al.[135] investigated the in vitro antimicrobial activity of several concentrations of sodium hypochlorite and chlorhexidine in eliminating *E. faecalis*. Chlorhexidine (1% and 2%) and 5.25% sodium hypochlorite required significantly less time to eliminate *E. faecalis*. Silva[345] verified the in vivo antimicrobial action of 1% sodium hypochlorite and 2% chlorhexidine as endodontic irrigants. Using 1% sodium hypochlorite as irrigant, 16.7 and 83.3% of the canals appeared to be positive in the microbiological test, immediately, and after 7 days of therapy; with 2% chlorhexidine, the percentages of positive cultures were 8.3 and 41.7%, taking into account the immediate and residual effects, indicating that both irrigants have the same effect immediately after biochemical treatment. Nevertheless, irrigation with 2% chlorhexidine was shown to be more efficient than 1% sodium hypochlorite when 7-day residual effectiveness was considered.

Estrela et al.[99] evaluated the influence of irrigants on the antimicrobial potential of calcium hydroxide paste in dog teeth with apical periodontitis. Forty-eight premolar teeth of adult mongrel dogs had their root canals opened to the oral environment for 6 months. The root canals were prepared and treated with different irrigating solutions and intracanal medicaments, according to the following groups: 1. 2.5% sodium hypochlorite + calcium hydroxide paste (CHP); 2. 2% chlorhexidine gel + CHP; 3. vinegar + CHP; 4. vinegar + vinegar. In group 4, both the irrigating solution and intracanal medicament were vinegar, which was renewed every for 7 days. After 21 days, all experimental groups had microbial growth, however, in different percentages: group 1 - 30%; group 2 - 30%; group 3 - 40%; group 4 - 60% (Fig. 19.2). All materials tested had antimicrobial potential; however, the influence of calcium hydroxide paste on the control of microorganisms must be remembered.

Other properties, in addition to those of antimicrobial activity, must also be investigated before the final choice of an irrigant solution for clinical use is made, such as their physical-chemical properties, minimum inhibitory concentration, tissue dissolution capacity, detoxification of endotoxin (lipid A) and acceptable tissue tolerance.

Pécora et al.[280] studied the shelf-life of 5% sodium hypochlorite solutions. The effects of storage time and temperature on the stability of 5% sodium hypochlorite solutions were studied for 18 months. The samples were stored at ambient temperature, in the refrigerator (9°C) and in a place where they received direct sunlight. The available chloride was determined quantitatively each month by iodometric titration. All solutions showed degradation versus time, and no significant difference in the chorine loss was found among the three groups (Fig. 19.3).

Buck et al.[42] evaluated the detoxification of endotoxin by endodontic irrigants (chlorhexidine, sodium hypochlorite, chlorhexidine chloride, ethanol, EDTA, water) and calcium hydroxide. The results showed that the biologically active portion of endotoxin, lipid A, is hydrolyzed by highly alkaline chemicals, namely calcium hydroxide, or the mixture of chlorhexidine, sodium hypochlorite and ethanol. EDTA, sodium hypochlorite, chlorhexidine, chlorhexidine chloride, ethanol and water (control) showed little or no detoxifying ability for lipid A.

Some physical-chemical properties (density, surface tension, pH, viscosity, wetting capacity and conductivity) of sodium hypochlorite solutions at the concentrations of 0.5%, 1%, 2.5% and 5% were analyzed by Guerisoli et al.[143]. It was found that density, pH, viscosity, wetting capacity and conductivity of the solutions are directly proportional to their concentration of sodium hypochlorite. Surface tension values did not show significant differences among the solutions (Table 19.2).

Some of the physical-chemical characteristics of sodium hypochlorite are mentioned as follows. It has excellent tissue dissolving capability. Grossman & Meiman[142], observing pulp tissue dissolution capacity, reported that 5% sodium hypochlorite dissolves this tissue in 20 minutes to 2 hours.

Spanó et al.[361] studied the in vitro solvent effect of four concentrations of sodium hypochlorite solutions (0.1%, 1%, 2.5% and 5.0%) on bovine pulp tissue, and the level of residual chlorine pH and surface tension before and after tissue dissolution. Fragments of fresh bovine mandibular central incisor pulps were obtained and weighed. An apparatus was made and connected to a peristaltic pump that agitated the solution to evaluate dissolution. The peristaltic pump was turned on and a chronometer was activated when the pulp fragment was put into the apparatus. Time of dissolution was recorded as the time from placing the pulp fragment in the solution, until its total disappearance. Based on the time of pulp dissolution and its respective mass, the speed of dissolution was calculated. After dissolution, the remaining liquid was analyzed for pH, surface tension, ionic conductivity and remanent chlorine. The data were submitted to statistical analysis and in accordance with the methodology and the



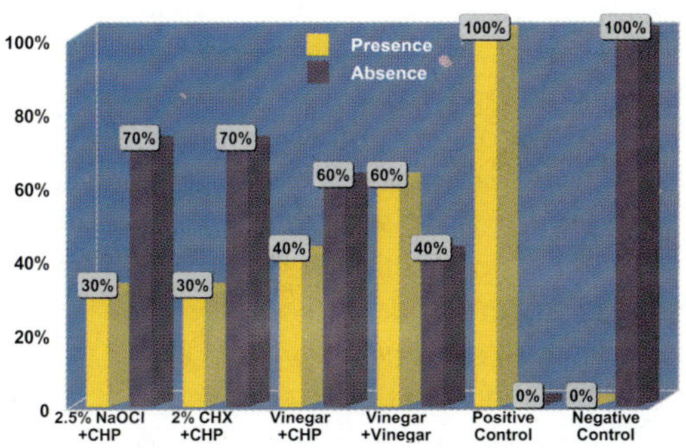


Figure 19.2 - Antimicrobial potential of the intracanal medicaments after 21 days in infected root canals of dog teeth.

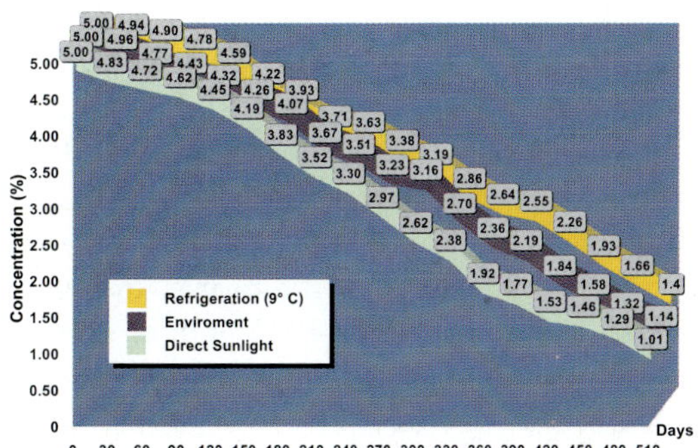


Figure 19.3 - Shelf-life of 5% sodium hypochlorite solutions.

**Table 19.2** - Mean values of the physical-chemical properties of NaOCl solutions

| | 0.5% NaOCl | 1% NaOCl | 2.5% NaOCl | 5%NaOCl |
|---|---|---|---|---|
| Density (g/cm³) | 1.00 | 1.04 | 1.06 | 1.09 |
| Surface Tension (dynes/cm) | 74.3 | 75.0 | 75.7 | 73.8 |
| pH | 11.98 | 12.60 | 12.65 | 12.89 |
| Viscosity (centiPoise) | 0.956 | 0.986 | 1.073 | 1.110 |
| Wetting capacity (time) | 2h 20 min. | 1h 27 min. | 1h 23min. | 18 min. |
| Conductivity (miliSiemens) | 26.0 | 65.5 | 88.0 | 127.5 |

(Guerisoli et al.[143])

results, it was concluded that: a) the bovine pulp fragment dissolution speed was directly proportional to the concentration of the sodium hypochlorite, or in other words, the higher the concentration, the faster the dissolution; b) the percent variation of pH of the sodium hypochlorite solutions, after dissolution, was inversely proportional to the initial concentration of the solution, or in other words, the higher the initial concentration of the sodium hypochlorite solutions, the smaller was the reduction in their pH; c) at the concentrations studied, the sodium hypochlorite solutions reduced the values of ionic conductivity after the process of bovine pulp tissue dissolution in a statistically similar manner; d) evaluation of the surface tension of these solutions, before and after tissue dissolution, showed that this property varied in a directly proportional manner to concentration, or in other words, the higher the initial concentration of the sodium hypochlorite solution, the greater was the reduction in surface tension; e) the level of remanent chorine in the sodium hypochlorite solutions after the pulp dissolution process, was directly proportional to concentration, or in other words, the higher the initial concentration of chlorine, the higher was the concentration of the remanent chlorine.

Estrela et al.[101] analyzed the tissue dissolution capacity and surface tension of the ESP substance (apple vinegar), solutions of 1% and 2.5% sodium hypochlorite and 2% chlorhexidine. The tissue dissolution test was performed with 50 bovine maxillary central incisor pulps. Initially, the pH of the experimental solutions was verified before use. To test the tissue dissolution speed a peristaltic pump was connected to the end of a urethane hose. The hose at the pump outlet was adapted to a plastic platform containing a nylon net on which the pulp remained suspended and in the same position during the experimental test, allowing full contact with a continuous flow of the test solutions. Five hundred milliliters of the irrigant solution were placed in the system, which allowed continuous circulation through the peristaltic pump in a closed circuit system. The observation period was 60 minutes. The surface tension was verified by means of a tensiometer. The results demonstrated that the capacity for dissolving bovine dental pulps was verified in the studied interval (60 minutes) in the 1% and 2.5% sodium hypochlorite solution, which was not observed in the substances ESP and 2% chlorhexidine (Fig. 19.4). The surface tension and pH of the solutions showed the following values: Substance ESP - 62.87 dynes/cm - pH 2.9; 1% sodium hypochlorite - 75.00 dynes/cm - pH 12.5; 2.5% sodium hypochlorite - 73.00 dynes/cm - pH 12.3; 2% chlorhexidine - 55.50 dynes/cm - pH 5.9.

The action of the irrigant solutions on the dentinal structure enhances the property of surface tension. This method consists of the application of force to separate a platinum ring immersed in the substances. Thus, torsion was applied to the screw until the platinum ring separated, while substances were being tested. Estrela et al.[98] evaluated the surface tension of 2% chlorhexidine digluconate, 3% sodium lauryl ether sulphate, sodium hypochlorite using tensiometer (Fig. 19.5-6). The association of chlorhexidine plus calcium hydroxide showed a high surface tension (58.00 dynes/cm) and pH values equal to 10.2; 3% sodium lauryl ether sulphate plus calcium hydroxide presents a low surface tension (31.60 dynes/cm) and high pH (12.5). Sodium hypochlorite presented a high surface tension (75.00 dynes/cm) and high pH (12.6).

The majority of dentists use and indicate of sodium hypochlorite, because this irrigant presents important properties, such as antimicrobial effect, tissue dissolution capacity and acceptable tissue tolerance at less concentrated solutions (0.5% - 1%). Pashley et al.[274] evaluated the cytotoxicity of various dilutions of sodium hypochlorite and reported that the use of 5% sodium hypochlorite for root canal preparation is a highly effective, and clinically accepted procedure. But it must be used judiciously, and with great caution, to prevent it from reaching the periapex, where it can cause severe inflammatory reactions.

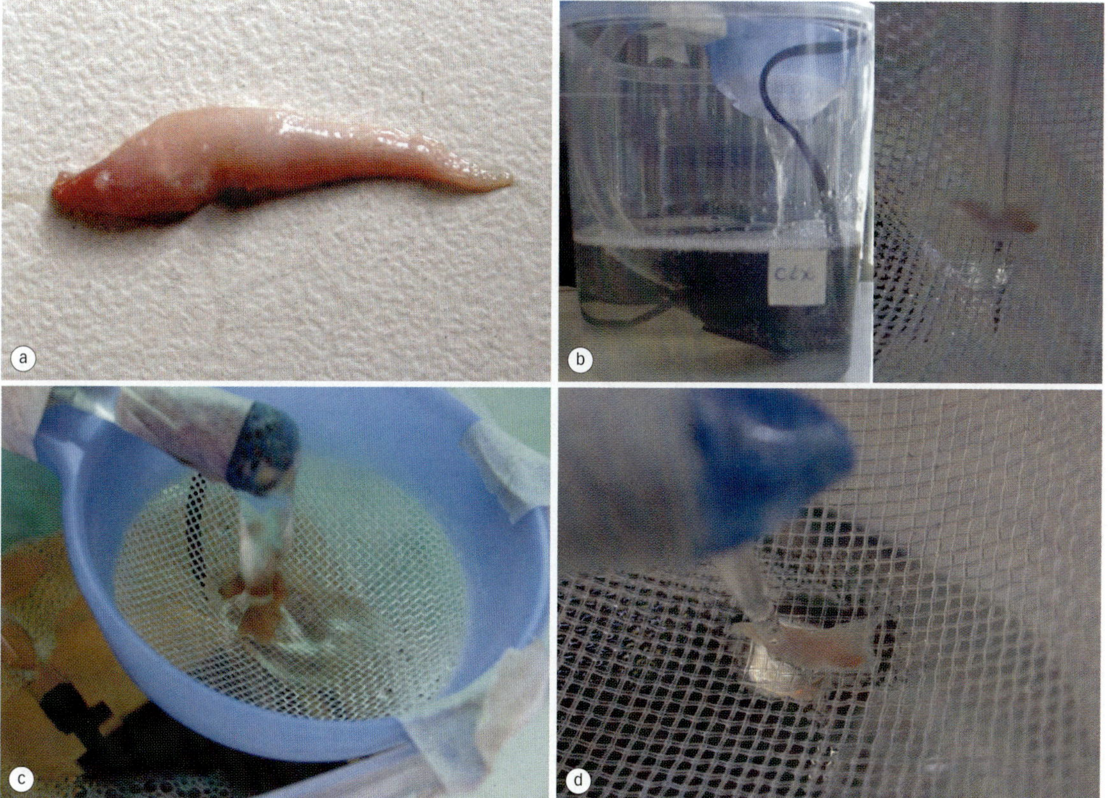


**Figure 19.4** - (**A-D**) Experimental survey of tissue dissolution of bovine pulp tissue[100].

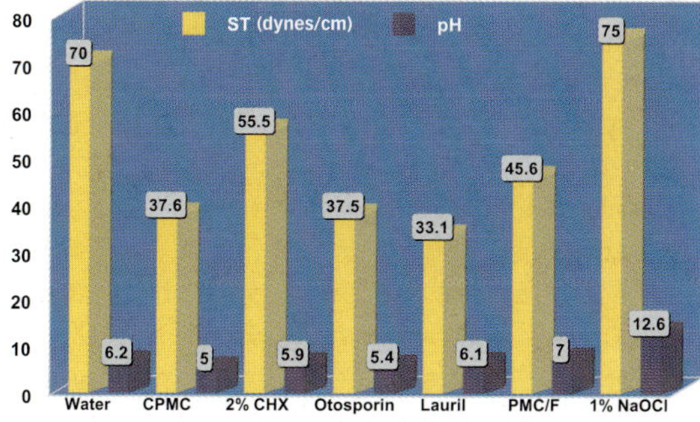


**Figure 19.5** - Surface tension and pH of various substances[100].

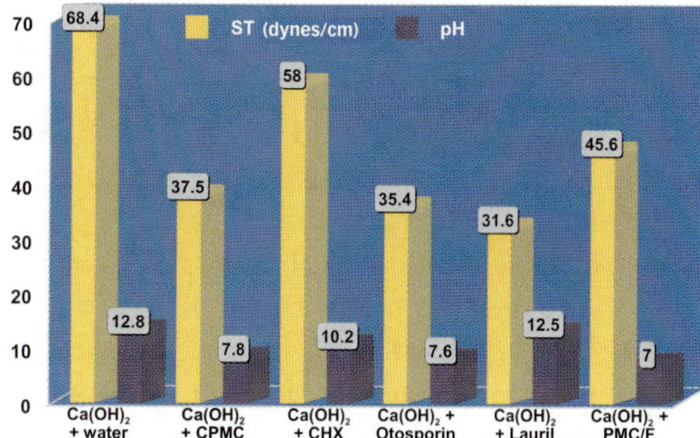


**Figure 19.6** - Surface tension and pH of calcium hydroxide solutions.

## 19.3 Mechanism of Action of Sodium Hypochlorite

The choice of an irrigating solution for use in infected root canals requires previous knowledge of the microorganisms responsible for the infectious process, as well as the properties of different irrigating solutions. Complex internal anatomy, host defenses and microorganism virulence are important factors in the treatment of teeth with asymptomatic apical periodontitis. Irrigating solutions must have significant antimicrobial action and tissue dissolution capacity. Sodium hypochlorite is the most used irrigating solution in endodontics, because its mechanism of action causes biosynthetic alterations in cellular metabolism and phospholipids destruction, formation of chloramines that interfere in cellular metabolism, oxidative action with irreversible enzymatic inactivation in bacteria, and lipid and fatty acid degradation[95].

The worldwide use of sodium hypochlorite as a root canal irrigating solution is due mainly to its efficacy for pulp dissolution and antimicrobial activity.

Pécora et al.[279] reported that sodium hypochlorite exhibits a dynamic balance as is shown by the reaction:

$NaOCl + H_2O$ « $NaOH + HOCl$ « $Na^+ + OH^- + H^+ + OCl^-$

The chemical reactions verified between organic tissue and sodium hypochlorite are shown in Figures 19.7-19-9.

When interpreting these chemical reactions, it can be observed that sodium hypochlorite acts as an organic and fat solvent degrading fatty acids, transforming them into fatty acid salts (soap) and glycerol (alcohol), that reduces the surface tension of the remaining solution (Fig. 19.7. saponification reaction). Sodium hypochlorite neutralizes amino acids forming water and salt (Fig. 19.8. neutralization reaction). With the exit of hydroxyl ions, there is a reduction in pH. Hypochlorous acid, a substance present in sodium hypochlorite solution, acts as solvent when in contact with organic tissue, and releases chlorine, which combined with the protein amino group, forms chloramines (Fig. 19.9. chloramination reaction). Hypochlorous acid ($HOCl^-$) and hypochlorite ions ($OCl^-$) lead to amino acid degradation and hydrolysis.

The chloramination reaction between chlorine and the amino group (NH) forms chloramines that interfere in cell metabolism. Chlorine (strong oxidant) presents antimicrobial action, inhibiting bacterial enzymes, leading to an irreversible oxidation of SH groups (sulphydryl group) of essential bacterial enzymes.

Sodium hypochlorite is a strong base ($pH>11$). At 1% concentration, sodium hypochlorite presents a surface tension equal to 75 dynes/cm, viscosity equal to 0.986 cP; conductivity of 65.5 mS; density of 1.04 $g/cm^3$, and moistening capacity equal to 1 hour and 27 minutes. Its antimicrobial mechanism of action can be observed by verifying its physical-chemical characteristics and its reaction with organic tissue.

Considering the available knowledge about pH processes and isolated activities in essential enzymatic sites, such as those in the membrane, it is enlightening to associate sodium hypochlorite (high pH, over 11), with harmful biological effects on bacterial cells, in order to explain part of its mechanism of action.

Estrela et al.[107] studied the biological effect of pH on the enzymatic activity of anaerobic bacteria. Because enzymatic sites are located in the cytoplasmic membrane, which is responsible for essential functions such as metabolism, cellular division and growth, and take part in the last stages of cellular wall formation, biosynthesis of lipids, transport of electrons and oxidative phosphorylation, the authors believe that hydroxyl ions from calcium hydroxide develop their mechanism of action in the cytoplasmic membrane. Extracellular enzymes act on nutrients, carbohydrates, proteins and lipids that favor digestion through hydrolysis. Intracellular enzymes located in the cell favor respiratory activity of the cell wall structure. The pH gradient of the

**1. Saponification reaction**

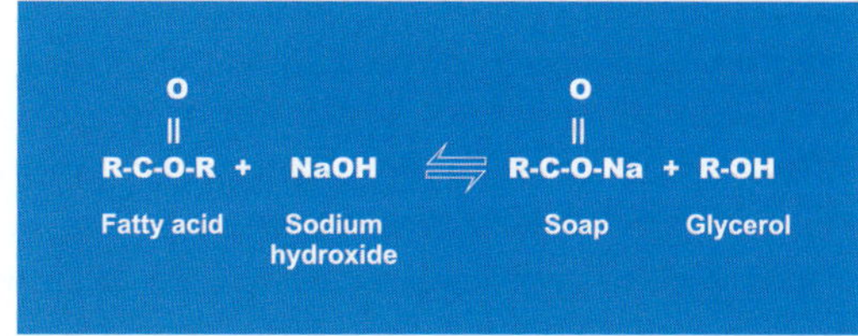


Sodium hydroxide reacts with grease acids (oils and lipids) present in the organic matter forming grease acid salts (soap) & glycerol (alcohol) [reaction 1]

7

**2. Amino acid neutralization reaction**

H O
| //
R-C-O-C + NaOH ⇋ R-C-O-C + $H_2O$
| \
$NH_2$ OH → $NH_2$ Na

Amino acid | Sodium hydroxide | Salt | Water

Sodium hydroxide reacts with protein amino acids forming salt + water [reaction 2]

8

**3. Chloramination reaction**

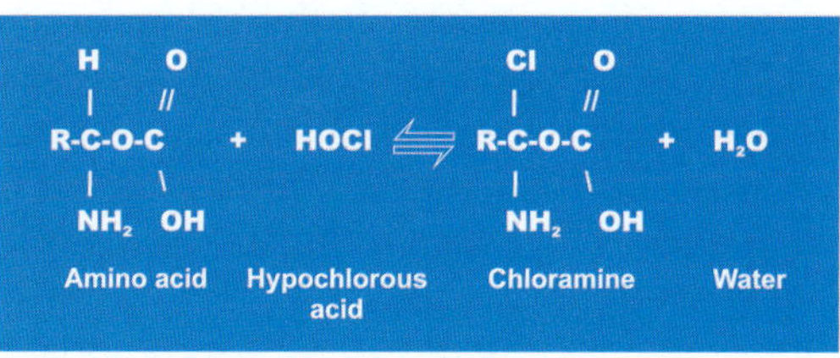


Hipochlorous acid reacts with amine group of amino acids forming chloramine + water [reaction 3]

9

**Figures 19.7 to 19.9** - Chemical reactions verified between organic tissue and sodium hypochlorite[95].

cytoplasmic membrane is altered by the high concentration of hydroxyl ions of calcium hydroxide acting on the proteins of the membrane (protein denaturation). The high pH (12.5), influenced by the release of hydroxyl ions, alters the integrity of the cytoplasmic membrane, by means of chemical injuries to organic components and nutrient transportation, or by means of degrading phospholipids or unsaturated fatty acids of the cytoplasmic membrane, observed in the peroxidation process, which is a saponification reaction[107].

The antimicrobial effectiveness of sodium hypochlorite, based on its high pH (hydroxyl ions action), is similar to the mechanism of action of calcium hydroxide. The high pH of sodium hypochlorite interferes in the cytoplasmic membrane integrity with irreversible enzymatic inhibition, biosynthetic alterations in cellular metabolism and phospholipid degradation observed in lipidic peroxidation. The amino acid chloramination reaction (reaction 3) forming chloramines interfere with cellular metabolism. Oxidation promotes irreversible bacterial enzymatic inhibition replacing hydrogen with chlorine. This enzyme inactivation can be observed in the reaction of chlorine with amino groups ($NH_2$) and irreversible oxidation of sulphydryl groups (SH) of bacterial enzymes (cysteine).

Thus, sodium hypochlorite presents antimicrobial activity with action on enzymatic sites essential for bacterial viability, promoting irreversible inactivation originated by hydroxyl ions and chloramination action. Dissolution of organic tissue can be verified in the saponification reaction, when sodium hypochlorite degrades fatty acids and lipids resulting in soap and glycerol.

The greatest concern in the selection of any irrigant solution or medication, is the knowledge of its mechanism of action against the predominant bacterial microflora. Knowledge about morphology, structure and physiology of microorganisms that are responsible for pain and destruction of periapical tissues led to several therapeutic trends. The first step of endodontic treatment is the knowledge of the interrelation between microorganisms and host, together with the chemical and biological dynamics of antimicrobial medications. Root canal preparation and the use of irrigant solutions, such as sodium hypochlorite are responsible for eliminating the majority of microorganisms in an infected root canal system.The use of intracanal dressings, however, is essential to eliminate surviving microorganisms.Calcium hydroxide has been the most studied and used intracanal dressing.

Sodium hypochlorite is recommended and used by the majority of dentists, because it presents several important properties: antimicrobial effect, tissue dissolution capacity and acceptable biological compatibility in less concentrated solutions. As regards its antimicrobial effect, studies have shown that sodium hypochlorite decreases the number of microorganisms during the treatment of teeth with apical periodontitis.

The efficacy of root canal irrigating solutions (1, 2 and 5% sodium hypochlorite, 2% chlorhexidine digluconate, 1% calcium hydroxide, and HCT20, a solution of calcium hydroxide associated with a detergent) against *S. aureus, E. faecalis, P. aeruginosa, B. subtilis, C. albicans* and a mixture of these microorganisms was studied by Estrela et al.[113]. The purpose was to determine the minimum inhibitory concentration of the tested solutions with a serial dilution in the proportion of 1:10, and antimicrobial activity with direct exposure for 5, 10, 15, 20 and 30 minutes. It was concluded that the minimum inhibitory concentration of sodium hypochlorite solutions required for inhibiting *S. aureus, E. faecalis, P. aeruginosa* and *C. albicans* was 0.1%, and for *B. subtilis* and the mixture it was 1%. All microorganisms were inactivated by these solutions in all experimental periods (5, 10, 15, 20 and 30 minutes). 2% chlorhexidine digluconate showed a minimum inhibitory concentration of 0.000002% for *S. aureus*, 0.002% for *P. aeruginosa*, 0.02% for *E. faecalis, B. subtilis, C. albicans* and the mixture. Antimicrobial effectiveness in the direct exposure test was observed in all experimental periods for *S. aureus, E. faecalis* and *C. albicans*, but it was ineffective against *P. aeruginosa, B. subtilis* and for the mixture in all periods. For 1% calcium hydroxide solution, a minimum inhibitory concentration equal to 1% was shown for *P. aeruginosa* but it was not effective against the other microorganisms. The antimicrobial activity by the direct exposure test was evident against *S. aureus, E. faecalis* and *P. aeruginosa* after 30 minutes, although it was not effective against *B. subtilis, C. albicans* and the mixture in all periods analyzed in this study. The solution of calcium hydroxide associated with a detergent (HCT20) showed the minimum concentration to be ineffective against *E. faecalis*. In the direct exposure test, the effectiveness was observed after 20 minutes for *S. aureus* and 30 minutes for *E. faecalis*. This solution was not effective against *P. aeruginosa, B. subtilis, C. albicans* and the mixture. Sodium hypochlorite presents high surface tension (75 dynes/cm) and a minimum inhibitory concentration lower than 1% for resistant microorganisms (*S. aureus, E. faecalis, P. aeruginosa, B. subtilis* and *C. albicans*). The rise in concentration is directly proportional to the antimicrobial effect and tissue dissolution capacity and inversely proportional to biological compatibility. Thus, considering the high surface tension, and that antimicrobial action can be achieved with the less concentrated solution, the better option is 1% sodium hypochlorite.

The comparison between the antimicrobial effect of 2% sodium hypochlorite and 2% chlorhexidine was analyzed by Estrela et al.[103] who observed that sodium hypochlorite showed the best performance of antimicrobial effectiveness when using the direct exposure test, and chlorhexidine, when using the agar diffusion test. The magnitude of antimicrobial effect was influenced by the experimental methods, biological indicators and exposure time.

Physical-chemical characteristics of sodium hypochlorite are important for explaining its mechanism of action. The saponification, amino acid neutralization and chloramination reactions that occur in the presence of microorganisms and organic tissue, lead to the antimicrobial and tissue dissolution process. The antimicrobial activity is related to enzymatic sites essential for bacteria, where hydroxyl ions and the chloramination reaction promote irreversible inactivation. The organic dissolution action can be observed in the saponification reaction when sodium hypochlorite degrades lipids and fatty acids, resulting in the formation soap and glycerol.

Sodium hypochlorite in higher concentrations is more aggressive, while in lower concentrations (0.5% to 1%) there is more tissue tolerance[318]. For a substance to be biocompatible, it must present little or no tissue reaction in all periods, and moderate to intense tissue reaction at 7 days, which decreases in intensity over the course of time until non-significant tissue reaction is reached[62].

## 19.4 Efficacy of Irrigant Solution in Endodontic Infections

The pathogenicity of endodontic microorganisms responsible for stimulating apical periodontitis has made it necessary to find efficient antimicrobial medicaments[98,246,247,374]. Sodium hypochlorite and chlorhexidine are the antimicrobial agents most frequently studied and used for the treatment of root canal infections[1-434]. When the two substances are compared, they present chemical characteristics responsible for different results. These variations probably occur as a result of methodology, biological indicators, concentrations or exposure times[104].

The contemporary literature contains numerous reports on their antimicrobial effectiveness in many experimental models, such as infected human teeth in vivo[48-51,246], infected human teeth ex-vivo[7,43,97,103,109,220], infected dog teeth in vivo[49,98,176,177], infected bovine teeth ex-vivo[136,148,265,293,316], biofilm model in membrane filters[131,346,364], direct contact and agar diffusion tests[493,103,135].

*E. faecalis* represents an extensively evaluated biological indicator[109,110,188,239,243,299,374,375] and several factors explain the concern this bacterium causes in endodontic infections. Its high prevalence in cases with post-treatment disease associated with virulence factors (aggregation substance, enterococcal surface proteins (Esp), gelatinase, cytolysin toxin, extracellular superoxide production, capsular polysaccharides, antibiotic resistance determinant) can facilitate its adherence to host cells and extracellular matrix, tissue invasions, immunomodulation effects and cause toxin mediated damage[188,243,299].

Present day thinking has recommended the implementation of Dentistry based on scientific evidences, which places a value on studies involving the systematic review or meta-analysis.

Previous studies conducted with experimental models in vitro have confirmed the significant antimicrobial effectiveness of sodium hypochlorite and chlorhexidine against *E. faecalis*[97,103,186,243], therefore, depending on the study design, this cannot occur[97,109]. Relevant clinical questions based on evidences, with regard to *E. faecalis* resistance to NaOCl or chlorhexidine requires further investigation.

Estrela et al.[105] verified the antibacterial efficacy of sodium hypochlorite or chlorhexidine against *E. faecalis* from endodontic infection, by means of a systematic review and meta-analysis. This work was planned, using an analysis of longitudinal studies from a quantitative systematic review. Prospective studies about the efficacy of sodium hypochlorite and chlorhexidine against *E. faecalis*, identified in endodontic infection before and after root canal preparation, were selected. Sources electronics of bibliographic catalogue were used. The following databases were searched on January 2nd of 2007: MEDLINE (without filter, from 1966 to January 2nd of 2007), EMBASE (without filter, from 1980 to January 2nd of 2007), Cochrane Oral Health Group Trials Register and Cochrane Central Register of Controlled Trials (CENTRAL). For the search strategy the following terms were used as keywords in several combinations: 1. *faecalis* and sodium hypochlorite OR, 2. *faecalis* and chlorhexidine OR, 3. *faecalis* and root canal infections OR, 4. *faecalis* and endodontics infections OR, 5. *faecalis* and root canal irrigants OR, 6. *faecalis* and irrigant solution OR, 7. *faecalis* and endodontics irrigants OR, 8. *faecalis* and intracanal irrigants.

The handsearching was conducted by the exam of the reference lists of the potentially eligible clinical trials and the review author's personal databases of trial reports in an attempt to identify any other relevant study.

The selected articles were identified from the titles and abstracts, considering the tabulated inclusion criteria, independently by two reviewers. The criteria of inclusion were studies in humans, studies related to the efficacy of the NaOCl or CHX on *E. faecalis*, nonsurgical root canal treatment was taken during the study, subjects had a noncontributory medical history, microbiological samples collected before and after the root canal preparation and studies published in English. For the criteria of exclusion, were studies in vitro, studies developed in animals, studies related to the efficacy of others medicaments (except NaOCl or CHX), studies without microbiological samples before or immediately after the root canal preparation, studies published in others languages, studies only with abstract or with absence of abstract, literature review studies, studies involving deciduous teeth, studies involving case reports, studies related just to the microorganisms identification or studies involving others microorganisms, except *E.faecalis*. Full copies of all relevant and potentially relevant studies, those appearing to meet the inclusion criteria, or for which there were insufficient data in the title and abstract to make a clear decision, were obtained[105].

The model to develop this meta-analysis was based on suggestions made by Cochrane Collaboration's and from preceding study made by Sathorn et al.[322]. Chi-square test was used to analyse the heterogeneity between studies. The essential analysis of antibacterial efficacy was risk difference (difference in the proportion of bacterial positive obtained by culture or PCR techniques between pre- and post-sanitization process). Risk differences of included studies were combined as generic inverse variance data type (Review Manager Version 5.0 - Cochrane Collaboration, http://www.cc-ims.net, accessed 15 May 2008), taking into account the separate tracking of positive and negative cultures/PCR. The level of statistical significance was $p<0.05$.

The success of endodontic treatment is closely associated with the control of endodontic microbiota. Thus, the ideal solution must be carefully selected, mainly in view of the innumerable articles with contradictory conclusions. Studies with similar results were reported when they compared sodium hypochlorite and chlorhexidine[135,186]. Other researches, however, have shown that sodium hypochlorite presents better antimicrobial activity than chlorhexidine[12,308,348], or, conversely, that chlorhexidine has better antimicrobial activity than sodium hypochlorite[135]. Recently, in a model with *E. faecalis* biofilm in human root canals, it was shown, that ozonated water, 2.5% sodium hypochlorite, 2% chlorhexidine and the application of gaseous ozone for 20 minutes were not sufficient to inactivate *E. faecalis*[97].

It is important to point out the study methods used in the present investigation. Studies based on scientific evidence have been well emphasized in dentistry[104,209,322]. There are several advantages to systematic reviews, such as explicit methods that limit bias in identifying and rejecting studies; hence, conclusions are more reliable and accurate; large amounts of information can be assimilated quickly by health care providers, researchers and policy makers; delay in research discoveries and implementation of effective diagnostic and therapeutic strategies is potentially reduced; results of different studies can be formally compared to establish generalization of findings and consistency (lack of heterogeneity) of results; reasons for heterogeneity (inconsistency in results across studies) can be identified and new hypothesis generated about particular subgroups; quantitative systematic reviews (meta-analysis) increase the precision of the overall result[132,352].

The investigation model adopted in the present evaluation[105] did not allow an ideal combination of results, making its correlation critical, because of the variability of the delineations used, which characterized the heterogeneity of the clinical protocols adopted. This limited the performance of the meta-analysis. Longitudinal studies that seek answers to clinical questions based on scientific evidences to confirm the efficacy of the sodium hypochlorite and chlorhexidine on *E. faecalis* showed only reduction of the biological indicator analyzed. Exactly the same problem occurred with calcium hydroxide, when tested on *E. faecalis*[92,103,209,322]. It can be verified that depending on the methodology - direct contact, agar diffusion or contaminated dentin test - these intracanal medicaments may or may not present effectiveness, but in human tests, this has not been confirmed[117,275,276,418,432]. The application and validation of the results of longitudinal studies, from an evidence-based point of view are essential aspects when analyzing the scientific value of the selected studies. This requires knowledge of the strategies to apply in order to select studies to be analyzed. Therefore, this study model requires notable prudence during its planning and development[132].

The first aspect to consider is the localization of the bacteria - if they are present only on the root canal surface, where the medicaments being discussed could show their true potential action, sodium hypochlorite and chlorhexidine could present efficacy against *E. faecalis*. However, if the bacteria are limited to inside the dentinal tubules or in the deep layer, this bacterium can show resistance, as these medicaments will not have their full antimicrobial effectiveness.

Five studies satisfied the inclusion criteria[117,275,276,418,432]. Peciuliene et al.[275] observed *E. faecalis* in twenty-five asymptomatic teeth with secondary infection. Taking care to avoid contamination, microbiological samples were taken from the canals before and after preparation and irrigation with sodium hypochlorite and EDTA. *E. faecalis* was isolated from 14 of the 20 culture positive teeth, usually in pure culture, or as a major component of the flora. Second samples taken after preparation, revealed growth in 7 of the 20 teeth. Five of the seven cases were *E. faecalis* in pure culture. Isolation of *E. faecalis* was not related to the use of any particular root filling material in the original root filling. In another study, Peciuliene et al.[276] determined the occurrence and role of yeasts, enteric Gram-negative rods and *Enterococcus* species in root-filled teeth with chronic apical periodontitis. After the first microbiological sample, the root canals were prepared to size 40 using 2.5% sodium hypochlorite and 17% EDTA as irrigating solutions. Microbes were isolated from 33 of 40 teeth in the initial sampling. Yeasts were isolated from 6 teeth, 3 of them together with *E. faecalis. E. faecalis* was isolated from 21 of the 33 culture positive teeth, 11 in pure culture. Growth was detected in 10 teeth of the second batch of samples. Six of the 10 cases were *E. faecalis*, with five being a pure culture. Ferrari et al.[117] detected enterococci, enteric bacteria and yeast species from 25 root canals with primary endodontic infections before and after canal preparation, and also tested the antibiotic susceptibility of enterococcal strains isolated. The canals were instrumented, using a simple stepback technique with Endo PTC cream associated with 0.5% sodium hypochlorite and EDTA. Microorganisms were isolated from 92% of the samples following intracoronal access, 22% were enterococci, enteric bacteria or yeast species. After biomechanical preparation, these species were no longer detected. After 7 days without intracanal dressing, 100% of the canals contained microorganisms, 52% of which were target species. *E. faecalis* and *E. faecium* were resistant to removal by root canal preparation followed by intracanal dressing. Zerella et al.[432] compared the effect of a slurry of calcium hydroxide mixed with aqueous 2% chlorhexidine versus aqueous calcium hydroxide slurry alone for disinfecting the pulp space of failed root-filled teeth during endodontic re-treatment in 40 teeth. The root canal was cleaned and shaped with endodontic files using a conventional endodontic technique. A copious amount of 1% sodium hypochlorite solution was used for irrigation. The results of this analysis have previously been reported. The teeth were nonsurgically retreated and medicated over 3 treatment visits at 7-10-day intervals with either calcium hydroxide in water or calcium hydroxide in 2% aqueous chlorhexidine. Of the total sample population, 12 of 40 teeth (30%) were positive for bacteria before root filling. The control medication disinfected 12 of 20 (60%) teeth including 2 of 4 teeth originally diagnosed with enterococci. The experimental medication resulted in disinfecting 16 of 20 (80%) teeth at the beginning of the third appointment. None of the teeth originally containing enterococci showed remaining growth. Canal dressing with a mixture of 2% chlorhexidine and calcium hydroxide slurry is as efficacious as aqueous calcium hydroxide for disinfecting failed root-filled teeth. Williams et al.[418] compared real-time quantitative PCR (qPCR) assay with cultivation for *E. faecalis* detection and quantification during endodontic treatment. Final shaping and mechanical debridement of the canal was achieved, using nickel-titanium files in a rotary crown-down technique. Teeth were irrigated with 1.05% sodium hypochlorite between files and after the final file. In primary infections, *E. faecalis* was found to be present in sample 1 in 7% (1/15) of the cases by cultivation, and in 13% (2/15) by qPCR. No tooth was positive for the bacterium, either in sample 2 or sample 3 by cultivation, indicating the removal of culturable *E. faecalis* by instrumentation - irrigation protocol. Using qPCR, 3 teeth (the two teeth identified at sample 1 and another tooth) harbored the bacterium in both sample 2 and sample 3. As observed with the primary infections, there was an insignificant trend towards increase to 57% (8/14) in the number of *E. faecalis* positive cases detected by qPCR in sample 2 and to 50% (7/14) in sample 3. In sample 1 up to three times more *E. faecalis* was detected by qPCR than by cultivation, but the difference was not statistically significant. At sample 2 and sample 3 collection times, more *E. faecalis* infections in refractory lesions were identified by qPCR than by cultivation (Table 19.3).

The search presented 229 related articles, with 6 of these as literature review articles, 39 articles were related with in vivo studies (27 in humans and 12 in animals), and 189 included in vitro studies. From the 39 in vivo studies, 5 studies satisfied the inclusion criteria. On the 5 studies included, from the total of 159 teeth with endodontic infections primary or secondary, the *E. faecalis* was detected initially in 16 (10%) teeth by PCR and 42 (26.4%) teeth by culture, and after the sanitization process (effect of root canal enlargement associated with action of irrigant solution) in 11 (6.9%) teeth by PCR and 12 (7.5%) teeth by culture. It was observed the absence of longitudinal studies in humans about the efficacy of NaOCl and CHX on *E. faecalis* from endodontic infection (Table 19.3).

The outcomes of five included studies are shown in Tables 19.4 and 19.5. The analysis was made between pre- and post-sanitization of the same root canals. The five studies were heterogeneous (Test of Homogeneity Chochran), considering samples evaluated by culture technique ($\chi^2$ =45.85, df=4, p<0.00001) and by PCR technique ($\chi^2$ =1.65, df=1, p=0.20). Thus, the NaOCl or CHX showed low ability to eliminate *E. faecalis* when evaluate by culture or PCR techniques. The complexity involved in comparing the included studies was due to differences in the strategies used, such as standardization of the limit of preparation, the choice of the preparation technique, standardization of tooth and size of the selected sample, time of the initial endodontic treatment in cases of secondary infection, quality control of the irrigant solution and variation in its concentration, periapical lesion detection criteria, and various hidden data important for complete evaluation[104].

As a result, the selection of endodontic irrigants containing the maximum number of ideal properties required attention. One precaution that was taken in this meta-analysis was to eliminate the risk of extrapolating in vitro results to the clinical situation, which is an unacceptable strategy for making clinical decisions as regards therapeutic protocols in humans. Therefore, this systematic review caused concern about the process for making clinical decisions about the control of microorganisms in endodontic infections.

In summary, the sanitization process consisting of emptying and enlarging the root canal, and the action of sodium hypochlorite, reduces the remaining endodontic microbiota, which certainly potentiates the action of the intracanal dressing and favors a higher level of success in endodontic treatment.

**Table 19.3.** Studies included related to the efficacy of the NaOCl and CHX on *E. faecalis*

| Studies (ref.) | N | IET | Baseline infection types | *E. faecalis* before RCP | | Irrigants | *E. faecalis* after RCP | |
|---|---|---|---|---|---|---|---|---|
| | | | | PCR | Culture | | PCR | Culture |
| Willian et al.[418] | 29 | >5 years | primary (n=15)<br>secondary (n=14) | 2 (13.3%)<br>6 (42.8%) | 1 (6.6%)<br>2 (14.2%) | 1% NaOCl | | 0 (0%)<br>1 (7.1%) |
| Zerella et al.[432] | 40 | - | secondary | 8 (20%) | - | 1% NaOCl | | 0 (0%) |
| Ferrari et al.[117] | 25 | - | primary | - | 4 (16%) | 0.5% NaOCl + Endo PTC | | 0 (immediately) (0%)<br>11 (after 7 days) (44%) |
| Peciuliene et al.[275] | 40 | 5-10 years | secondary | - | 21 (52.5%) | 2.5% NaOCl | | 6 (15%) |
| Peciuliene et al.[276] | 25 | - | secondary | - | 14 (56%) | 2.5% NaOCl | | 5 (20%) |
| **Total** | 159 | - | - | 16 (10%) | 42 (26.4%) | - | | 12 (7.5%) |

(n - number of samples, IET- initial endodontic treatment, RCP - root canal preparation)

**Table 19.4.** Forest Plot 1. Studies included related to the efficacy of the NaOCl and CHX on *E. faecalis* when evaluated by culture technique. Horizontal line shows 95% confidence interval. Negative and positive values of risk difference are used to indicate the differences in directions of the values[105].

| Study of Subgroup | Before RCP | | After RCP | | Weight | Risk Difference |
|---|---|---|---|---|---|---|
| | Events | Total | Events | Total | | M-H, Random, 95% CI |
| Ferrari et al.[117] | 4 | 25 | 11 | 25 | 18.0% | -0.28 [-0.52, -0.04] |
| Peciuliene et al.[275] | 14 | 25 | 5 | 25 | 17.8% | 0.36 [0.11, 0.61] |
| Peciuliene et al.[276] | 21 | 40 | 6 | 40 | 19.7% | 0.38 [0.18, 0.57] |
| Williams et al.[418] | 3 | 29 | 1 | 29 | 21.5% | 0.07 [-0.06, 0.20] |
| Zerella et al.[432] | 0 | 40 | 0 | 40 | 23.0% | 0.00 [-0.05, 0.05] |
| **Total (95% CI)** | | **159** | | **159** | **100%** | **0.10 [-0.11, 0.32]** |
| Total events | 42 | | 23 | | | |

Heterogeneity: $Tau^2$=0.05; $Chi^2$=45.85, df=4 (P < 0.00001); $I^2$=91%
Test for overall effect: Z=0.92 (P=0.36)



**Table 19.5.** Forest Plot 2. Studies included related to the efficacy of the NaOCl and CHX on *E. faecalis* when evaluated by PCR. Horizontal line shows 95% confidence interval. Negative and positive values of risk difference are used to indicate the differences in directions of the values[105].

| Study of Subgroup | Before RCP | | After RCP | | Weight | Risk Difference |
|---|---|---|---|---|---|---|
| | Events | Total | Events | Total | | M-H, Random, 95% CI |
| Williams et al.[418] | 8 | 29 | 3 | 29 | 46.5% | 0.17 [-0.02, 0.37] |
| Zerella et al.[432] | 8 | 40 | 8 | 40 | 53.5% | 0.00 [-0.18, 0.18] |
| **Total (95% CI)** | | **69** | | **69** | **100%** | **0.08 [-0.09, 0.25]** |
| Total events | 16 | | 11 | | | |

Heterogeneity: $Tau^2$=0.01; $Chi^2$=1.65, df=1 (P < 0.20); $I^2$=39%
Test for overall effect: Z=0.93 (P=0.35)

Chlorhexidine is an antimicrobial substance that has been indicated in several studies for the treatment of endodontic infection. Estrela et al.[111], using a systematic review, evaluated the efficacy of chlorhexidine in endodontic infections. The search strategies included electronic searches (MEDLINE, EMBASE, CENTRAL) and searches using various keywords concerning chlorhexidine and (endodontic* OR endodontic* infection* OR root canal infection*). The studies were selected by two independent reviewers, who determined the inclusion and exclusion criteria. The search presented 196 articles, of which, 19 were literature reviews, 1 meta-analysis, 48 were *in vivo* studies (humans or animals) and 132 were *in vitro* studies. (1.chlorhexidine and endodontic or (n = 98 articles); 2.chlorhexidine and endodontic or (n = 136 articles); 3.chlorhexidine and endodontic infections or (n = 10 articles); 4.chlorhexidine and endodontic infection or (n = 13 articles); 5.chlorhexidine and root canal infections or (n = 24 articles); 6.chlorhexidine and root canal infection or (n = 20 articles). Out of 48 *in vivo* studies, 7 articles[89,223,273,347,349,400,401] satisfied the inclusion criteria. In the included studies analyzed, there were 117 teeth with primary endodontic infection. These experiments detected microorganisms in all the teeth initially, and after treatment, by two identification methods. After root canal preparation microorganisms were detected in 16 teeth by PCR, and in 45 by culture. It was impossible to combine the results by meta-analysis, because the studies differed. When chlorhexidine was used as irrigants in the prepared infected root canals, residual endodontic microbiota decreased.

Various studies showed the need for more attention to the properties of chlorhexidine[20,26,426]. Yeung et al.[426] evaluated the antioxidant and pro-oxidant properties of chlorhexidine. The scavenging and generation of reactive oxygen species (ROS) by chlorhexidine, in the presence or absence of saturated calcium hydroxide solutions, was evaluated. The reaction emitted chemiluminescence in the presence of lucigenin thus, an illuminometer was used to evaluate the levels of ROS production. Changes in DNA conformation were analyzed by agarose gel electrophoresis. Chlorhexidine (0.00002-0.02%) effectively scavenged 56-88% of the superoxide radicals generated by the xanthine/xanthine oxidase reaction. Through analysis of PUC18 DNA conformation changes, chlorhexidine was shown to be a mild scavenger of hydroxyl radicals generated by $H_2O_2$ plus $FeCl_2$. Nevertheless, chlorhexidine (>0.083%) decreased the mobility of PUC18 plasmid DNA with potential production of DNA-DNA cross-link and severe DNA breaks (presence of DNA smear) at higher concentrations. Chlorhexidine induced ROS production including $H_2O_2$ and superoxide radicals in 0.1N NaOH (pH = 12.76) or calcium hydroxide (pH = 12.5) solutions. Chlorhexidine exhibited both antioxidant and pro-oxidant properties under different conditions. These events are possibly involved in the killing of root canal and periodontal microorganisms when chlorhexidine and calcium hydroxide were used in combination, or separately. Potential genotoxicity and tissue damage, when chlorhexidine is extruded into the periapical tissue, and also when used in higher concentrations, should be considered during periodontal and endodontic treatment.

Successful endodontic therapy depends upon root canal sanitization and hermetic obturation. Biomechanical preparation, however, does not always provide an adequate microbial reduction. Due to the inherent unreliability of the treatment, some cases are unsuccessful. Calcium hydroxide pastes have been used with the aim of improving the effectiveness of antisepsis in root canal treatments, in addition to stimulating the recovery of tissues affected by endodontic infection. Chlorhexidine digluconate has been used in endodontics due to its broad action spectrum, mainly against *E. faecalis* and *C. albicans*, and has been added to calcium hydroxide pastes so that the advantages of one would compensate for the deficiencies of the other. Yet the structure of the chlorhexidine molecule, in addition to the high pH values promoted by calcium hydroxide, pose a systemic risk when they are used, due to the likely decomposition of chlorhexidine into free radicals and *para*-chloroaniline, which the International Agency for Research on Cancer (IARC) has classified as a possible carcinogenic agent in humans. Barbin et al.[20] studied the chemical analysis of chlorhexidine digluconate at 0.2%, isolated or mixed with calcium hydroxide, using Mass Spectrometry and High-Efficiency Liquid Chromatography. The analyses were performed shortly after the samples were prepared, and after 7 and 14 days of storage at 36.5°C. It was found that the isolated chlorhexidine digluconate solution formed different byproducts, including *para*-chloroaniline, posing systemic risks. In contact with calcium hydroxide, chlorhexidine decomposes completely and forms different compounds. Though the study did not demonstrate the presence of *para*-chloroaniline in the medication paste, the high number of reactive species poses a high risk to the genetic material of the host cells, affected by intracanal medication. It is mandatory to establish a precise diagnostic-therapeutic relationship by developing clinical protocols that would restrict the use of these intracanal medications to clinical conditions with disseminated endodontic infection and persistent apical periodontitis. There is a need for more efficient strategies, that use more effective biomechanical processes and intracanal medications that do not offer any local or systemic risk, so that root canal treatment goals can be predictably and safely considered (Fig.19.10-19.18).

The association of chlorhexidine with calcium hydroxide has been shown not to influence the time required and efficacy for bacterial inactivation[113]. Thus, calcium hydroxide paste with aqueous vehicle reduces the endodontic microorganisms and favors the prognosis. Thus, the expressive role of sodium hypochlorite used as irrigant solution and calcium hydroxide as intracanal dressing must not be forgotten.

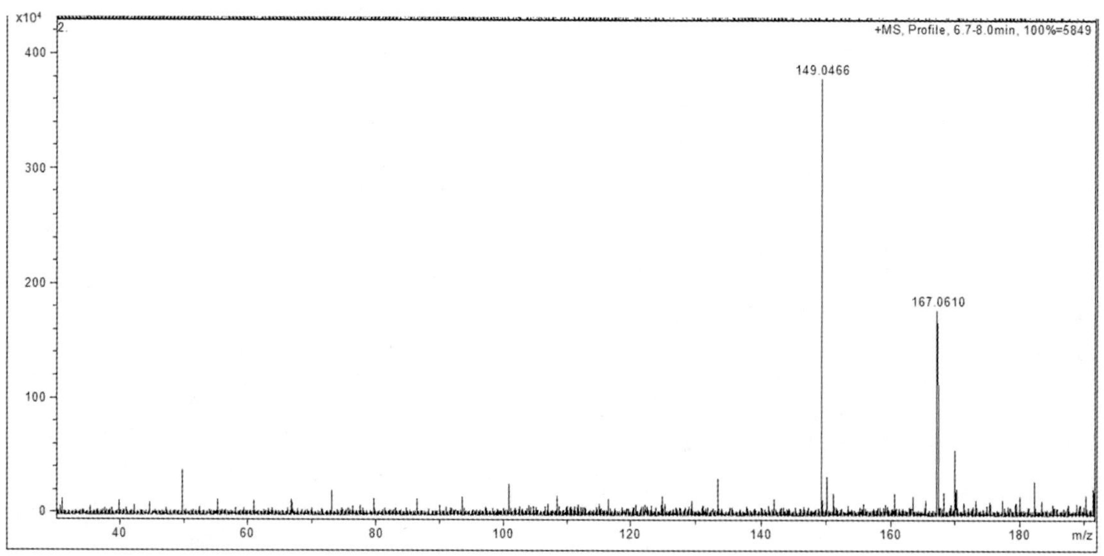


**Figure 19.10** - The mass spectrum shows a relation between mass and load (m/z) of ionized molecules in the sample with peaks at 149 m/z and 167 m/z immediately after preparation of PCA solution. These values indicate the presence of PCA. The difference might be due the presence of sodium.

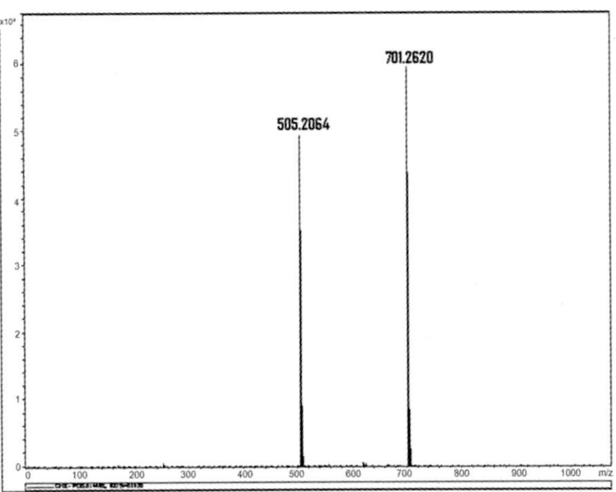


Figure 19.11 - Mass spectrometry analysis of 0.2% CHX immediately after its preparation presented peaks at 505 and 701 m/z, which confirms the high degree of purity of this sample. Presence of PCA was not verified.

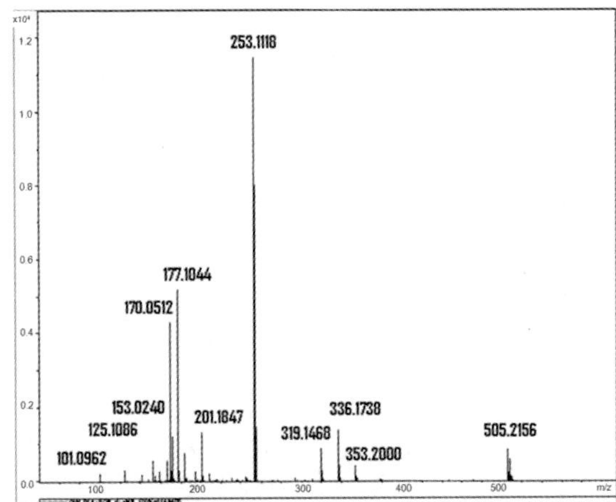


Figure 19.12 - Mass spectrometry analysis of a solution of 0.2% CHX after 7 days. The chromatographic analysis showed decomposition into several sub-products with different values (101, 125, 152, 170, 177, 201, 319, 336, 353 and 505 m/z).

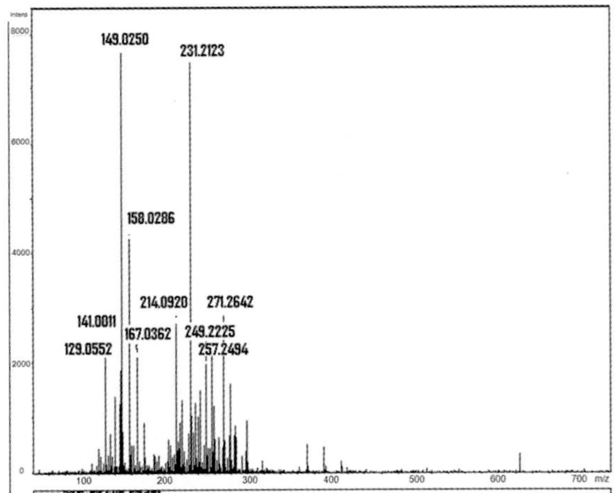


Figure 19.13 - Mass spectrometry analysis of a solution of 0.2% CHX after 14 days. It can be observed a total degradation of CHX. The initial peaks (505 and 701 m/z) are not observed. There are peaks of 129 m/z (literature-based indicator) and 149 and 167 m/z (experimental indicators), which suggest the presence of PCA after 14 days.

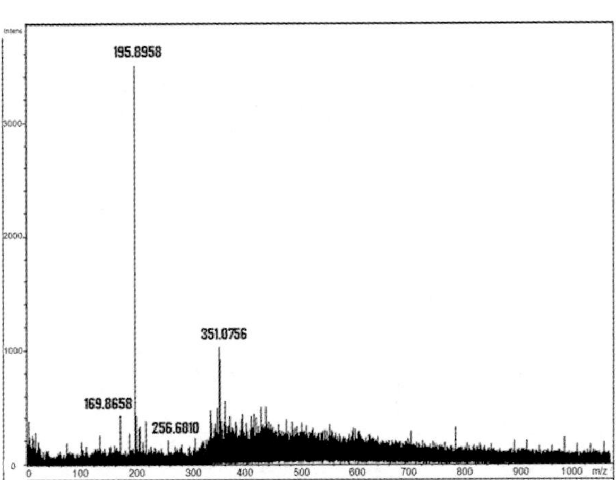


Figure 19.14 - Mass spectrometry analysis of a solution of CHP + 0.2% CHX. The chromatographic analysis of the CH + 0.2% CHX mixture immediately after its preparation showed peaks of 169, 195, 256 and 351 m/z. The peak of 169 m/z corresponds to chlorophenyl guanide. These results explain the ability of CH to separate the CHX molecule in positions containing groups $NH_n$. The peak of 195 m/z was probably originated by production of reactive compounds, due the high concentration of hydroxyl ions (alkaline environment) in the presence of CHX. Indicators for PCA were not found.

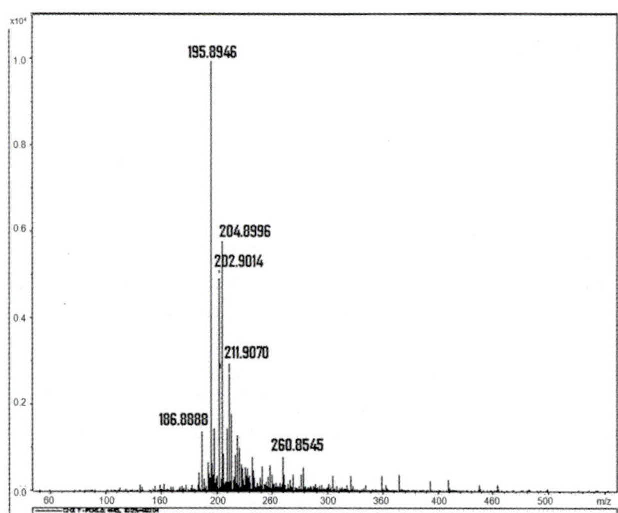


Figure 19.15 - Mass spectrometry analysis of a solution of CH mixed 0.2% CHX after 7 days. The chromatographic analysis shows absence of peaks at 505 and 701 m/z, which suggests a total degradation of CHX. ROS were observed, but indicators for PCA were not detected.

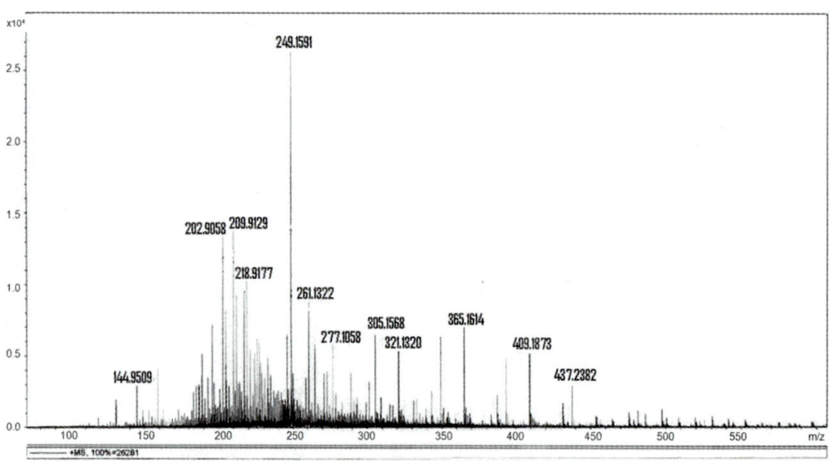


**Figure 19.16** - Mass spectrometry analysis of a solution of CH mixed 0.2% CHX after 14 days. The chromatographic analysis shows absence of peaks at 505 and 701 m/z, which suggests a total degradation of CHX. ROS were observed, but indicators for PCA were not detected.

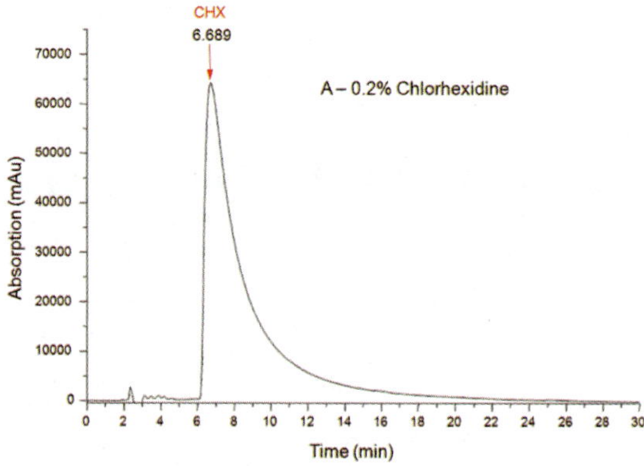


**Figure 19.17** - High-performance liquid chromatography (HPLC). Chromatogram of the analysis of compounds in the standard solution of CHX immediately after preparation showed that the time of retention of this substance was 6.7 min.

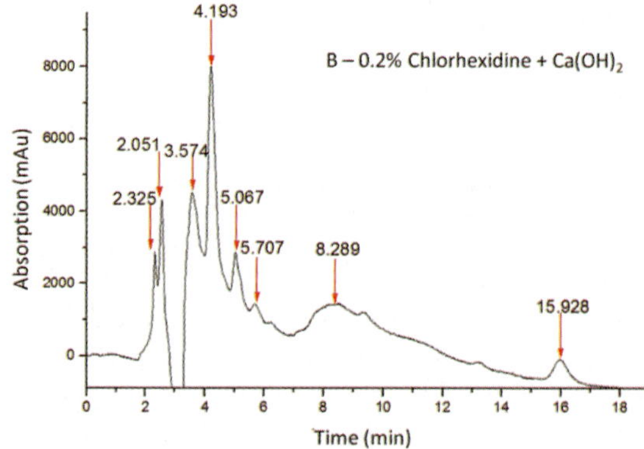


**Figure 19.18** - High-performance liquid chromatography (HPLC). Chromatogram of the analysis of the CH + 0.2% CHX mixture indicated that CHX was no longer present after 6.7 min. This result confirms the degradation of CHX after preparation of the mixture.

### 19.4.1 Antimicrobial efficacy of ozone against endodontic infection

The outcome of root canal treatment in the presence of apical periodontitis is directly influenced by the use of acceptable clinical procedures under strictly aseptic conditions, in addition to the host's immunological response. The patient's nutritional status and the selective pressures related to oxidation-reduction potential, nutrient supply and microbial interactions are related to the maintenance of endodontic infections.

*E. faecalis* has been the focus of attention as a recognized pathogen, isolated both in mixed microbiota and in monocultures. Several virulence factors (aggregation substance, enterococcal surface proteins (Esp), gelatinase, cytolysin toxin, extracellular superoxide production, capsular polysaccharides, antibiotic resistance determinant) can facilitate the adherence to host cells and extracellular matrix, tissue invasions, immunomodulation effect and cause toxin mediated damage[188,299,374]. Love[219] investigated a possible mechanism that would explain how *E. faecalis* could survive and grow within dentinal tubules and reinfect obturated canals. The author postulated that a virulence factor of *E. faecalis* in failed endodontically treated teeth may be related to *E. faecalis* cells maintaining the capability of invading dentinal tubules and adhering to collagen in the presence of human serum. Evans et al.[114] reported the mechanisms involved in *E. faecalis* resistance to calcium hydroxide. *E. faecalis* was resistant to calcium hydroxide at pH 11.1, but not at pH 11.5. Pre-treatment with calcium hydroxide (pH 10.3) induced no tolerance to further exposure at pH 11.5. Survival of *E. faecalis* in calcium hydroxide seemed to be unrelated to stress induced protein synthesis, but a functioning proton pump was critical for *E. faecalis* survival at high pH.

Spratt et al.[364] studied the bactericidal effect of 2.25% sodium hypochlorite, 0.2% chlorhexidine, 10% iodine or phosphate buffered saline on single-species of biofilms (*P. intermedia, P. micros, S. intermedius, F. nucleatum and E. faecalis*) derived from a range of root canal isolates. They concluded that the efficacy of a particular agent was dependent on the nature of the organism in the biofilm, and on the contact time. Sodium hypochlorite was generally the most effective agent tested, followed by iodine. The clinical effectiveness of these agents, however, must be regarded in the light of the complexity of root canal anatomy and polymicrobial nature of root canal infections. Abdullah et al.[3] evaluated and compared the efficacy of 3% sodium hypochlorite, 10% povidone iodine, 0.2% chlorhexidine, 17% EDTA and calcium hydroxide against a clinical isolate of *E. faecalis* grown as biofilm or planktonic suspension phenotype. The difference in gradients of bacterial killing among the biofilm, planktonic suspension or pellet presentation was significant, and dependent upon the agent, except for sodium hypochlorite and calcium hydroxide, in which no difference could be detected. Sodium hypochlorite was the most effective agent and achieved 100% kill for all presentations of *E. faecalis* after a 2-minutes contact time.

Ideally, an intracanal medicament should be able to neutralize the virulence of microorganisms and pathogenic factors (such as proteins, enzymes, toxins, aggregation substances) and induce a host response that favors periapical tissue healing.

Nevertheless, the continuous presence of positive microbial cultures after root canal shaping, disinfection and use of calcium hydroxide as inter-appointment intracanal dressing, justifies the investigation of other antimicrobial substances.

The use of ozonated water for treatment of endodontic infections has been suggested[97,170,245]. Ozone has also been used in the water industry to eliminate bacteria[214,215]. The properties of ozone could be useful in Dentistry[29]. Ozone is a blue gas containing three oxygen atoms; it is irritant, toxic and unstable; it is also very reactive. Studies have reported interesting results when ozone-treated water was used in the dental unit[24,120,214,215,242].

Nagayoshi et al.[245] examined the *in vitro* effect of ozonated water against *E. faecalis* and *S. mutans* infections in bovine dentin and compared the cytotoxicity against L-929 mouse fibroblasts between ozonated water and sodium hypochlorite. In conclusion, ozonated water had nearly the same antimicrobial activity as 2.5% sodium hypochlorite during irrigation, especially when combined with sonication (flow rate: 30 mL/min), and showed a low toxicity level against cultured cells. In this experiment, root canals were irrigated by flushing for 10 min (flow rate, 30 mL/min) with the following solutions: 4 mg/L of ozonated water ($O_3aq$), 4 mg/L of $O_3aq$ plus ultrasonication, distilled water (DW) and DW with plus ultrasonication. One specimen was not irrigated and acted as a positive control, while another specimen was flushed with 2.5% sodium hypochlorite for 2 minutes (flow rate, 30 mL/min) and acted as a negative control. Hems et al.[170], however, evaluating the ability of ozone to kill an *E. faecalis* strain, verified that its antibacterial efficacy was not comparable to that of sodium hypochlorite.

Modern concepts of microbial control have been directed towards the use of intracanal medications that acted effectively against different types of respiratory bacteria (aerobic, anaerobic and microaerophiles), which have the ability to affect cell wall synthesis, or alter the cytoplasmic membrane permeability and interfere with protein synthesis or chromosomal replication[106,107]. In primary endodontic infection, there is a predominance of Gram-negative anaerobic bacteria and it is conceivable that oxygen toxicity would be able to inactivate all anaerobic bacteria. It is not known, however, whether oxygen behaves in the same way, as in cases of secondary infection, in which facultative Gram-positive bacteria are predominantly found.

Several questions about the effects of ozone on endodontic microbiota remain unclear, for example, the ideal ozone concentration, its depth of action in dentinal tubules, and the ideal time for it to reach full antimicrobial efficacy.

Estrela et al.[97] determined the antimicrobial efficacy of ozonated water, gaseous ozone, sodium hypochlorite and chlorhexidine in human root canals infected by *E. faecalis* biofilm. Thirty human maxillary anterior teeth were prepared and inoculated with *E. faecalis* for 60 days. Eppendorf tubes were connected to the coronal portion of the teeth. Urethane hoses were attached to the tubes and to the inlet of a peristaltic pump. The outlet of the apparatus corresponded to the apical portion of the root canals. The test irrigant solutions were ozonated water, gaseous ozone, 2.5% sodium hypochlorite, 2% chlorhexidine, that circulated at a constant flow of 50 $mL.min^{-1}$ for 20 minutes (Fig.19.19). Samples from the root canals were collected and immersed in 7 mL Letheen Broth, followed by incubation at 37°C for 48 hours. Bacterial growth was analyzed by turbidity of the culture medium and subculture on a specific nutrient broth. The 0.1 mL inoculums obtained from Letheen Broth were transferred to 7 mL of Brain Heart Infusion and incubated at 37°C for 48 hours. Bacterial growth was checked by turbidity of the culture medium carried out in triplicate. The positive culture of microorganisms following the application of the irrigating solutions (ozonated water, gaseous ozone, 2.5% sodium hypochlorite, 2% chlorhexidine) that circulated at a constant 50 $mL.min^{-1}$ flow for 20 minutes, confirmed a lack of antimicrobial efficacy in infected human root canals. Thus, it appears that a 60-day period was enough for *E. faecalis* to invade root dentinal tubules and show resistance to ozonated water, ozone, 2.5% sodium hypochlorite, 2% chlorhexidine.

It is inferred that when a medication does not reach the target microorganism, its real efficacy to kill them cannot be expressed. Therefore, it cannot be stated whether the microbial strains were resistant to one or other medication or not. In this case, it is likely that the microorganisms were able to survive, adapt and tolerate the critical ecological conditions[97].

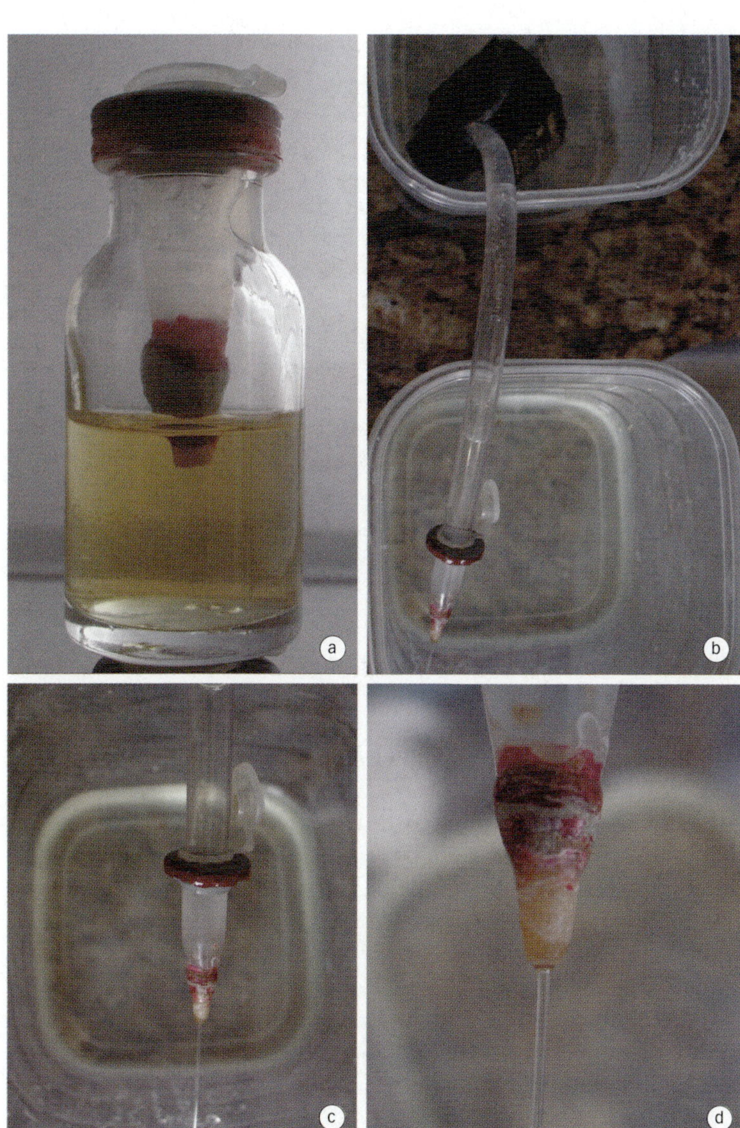

**Figure 19.19** - Overall view of the study model used to assess the antimicrobial efficacy of the irrigants in infected human root canals. (**A**) Platform used for inoculation with the biological indicator for 60 days; (**B**) irrigating system with peristaltic pump; (**C**) irrigants circulating at a constant flow of 50 mL/min)1; (**D**) closer view of the previous image.

The findings of this investigation[97] are consistent with those of previous studies that showed bacterial persistence after use of potent irrigants in endodontic infections. Therefore, it is important to take into consideration that root canal infection is not a random event, as observed by Sundqvist & Fidgor[374] in a study about the survival of endodontic pathogens. The types and combinations of microorganisms are developed in response to the surrounding environment. Factors that influence whether species shall die or survive include the particular ecological niche, nutrition, anaerobiosis, pH and competition with other microorganisms.

The use of ozone is justified as a new option of irrigant agent with antimicrobial action. The antimicrobial effect of ozone results from oxidation of microbial cellular components. Ozone is a highly reactive form of oxygen that is generated by passing oxygen through high-voltage[393].

Oxidation is the removal of electrons from an atom or molecule, a reaction that often produces energy. Several biological oxidations involve the loss of hydrogen atoms (dehydrogenation reactions). Oxygen is essential for the survival of cells that follow aerobic metabolism, although it has a dramatically toxic effect on microaerophiles and anaerobic bacteria[393]. Aerobic respiration involves ATP generation at specific sites in the electron transport chain via oxidative phosphorylation (the final electron acceptors include oxygen). Although aerobic bacteria contain a variety of enzymes that protect them from oxygen toxicity, microaerophilic and anaerobic bacteria are devoid of these protective mechanisms. The final electron acceptors in anaerobic respiration include inorganic substrate - sulfate ions, nitrate ions and carbonate ions. Oxygen is not used in the fermentation process; anaerobic bacteria use organic compounds as final oxygen acceptor during their energy metabolism[393].

Therefore, root canal preparation with careful sanitization and use of an intracanal medication that has good antimicrobial efficacy, tissue dissolution capacity, and acceptable biocompatibility, will definitely improve the prognosis of treatment of apical periodontitis. It should be kept in mind that the major factor contributing to the healing or maintenance of an infection involves the host immunological response. Studies should be carried out to investigate the applicability of ozone in different clinical situations.

## 19.5 Chelating Agents

The chelating solution (EDTA, ethylenediamine tetra acetic acid) was proposed by Nygaard-Østby in 1957[269] to aid during the root canal preparation, especially in calcified root canals. The EDTA at a neutral pH produces calcium chelation in dentin[183].

The smear layer is a material found on the canal walls during root canal instrumentation, composed of dentin, remnants of pulp tissue and odontoblastic processes (organic and inorganic components), and microorganisms.

The advantages and disadvantages of the presence of smear layer, and whether it should be removed or not from instrumented root canals, are still controversial[183]. The smear layer also acts as a physical barrier interfering with adhesion and penetration of sealers into dentinal tubules. It may affect the sealing efficiency of root canal obturation. When it is not removed, the durability of the apical and coronal seal should be evaluated over a long period. When the smear layer is removed, EDTA and sodium hypochlorite solutions have been shown to be more effective[279,285].

EDTA complements the action of sodium hypochlorite, by chelating calcium ions in dentin and making instrumentation of the root canal easier, especially in narrow canals. Because it is a chelating agent, EDTA is not dependent on a high hydrogen ion concentration to accomplish decalcification, and is effective at neutral pH[183,279]. McComb & Smith[232] related that smear layer is a factor that interferes in root canal sealing because of its weak adherence to the root canal walls hindering sealer adhesion, this being the reason for concern about removing it before obturation, to allow intimate contact of the sealer with the dentin surface. Byström & Sundquist[51] analyzed 0.5% and 5% sodium hypochlorite and observed that there was no difference between the effect of these solutions. The combined use of EDTA and 5% sodium hypochlorite solution was more efficient than the use of NaOCl alone. Abbott et al.[1] reported that sodium hypochlorite associated with EDTAC produced clean canal walls, but ultrasound did not enhance the cleansing action of these solutions. Pécora[289] studied the effect on root dentin permeability of Dakin's solution (0.5% sodium hypochlorite) and 15% EDTA, used separately, alternately, or mixed during instrumentation of root canals. Dakin's solution and EDTA produced statistically similar dentin permeability, however, greater than that of water. The use of Dakin's solution and EDTA, alternately or mixed, showed greater dentin permeability than the use of these solutions separately, however statistically similar. Dentin permeability of the cervical and middle thirds of the roots of human maxillary central incisors was statistically similar and greater than the permeability of the apical region.

Estrela et al.[102] compared the capacity of root canal surface cleaning produced by apple vinegar, 2.5% sodium hypochlorite, 2% chlorhexidine gel and EDTA in 24 extracted human maxillary incisor teeth. The samples were observed by scanning electronic microscopy, and evaluated for the quantity of smear layer. The statistical analysis was verified by non-parametric test for comparison of groups. The level of significance was 5%. The combination of EDTA with the irrigant solutions significantly increased the cleaning capability in all cases. In a complete comparison of irrigant solutions the best result was obtained by apple vinegar associated with EDTA (Fig. 19.20-19.23).

Spanó[362] evaluated the smear layer removal capacity of 15% EDTA, 10% citric acid, 10% sodium citrate, apple vinegar, 5% acetic acid and 1% sodium hypochlorite using scanning electronic microscopy, and flame atomic absorption spectrophotometry. Forty-two maxillary central incisors were used. Access surgery, removal of the cervical shoulder and compensatory wear were performed in these teeth. The working length was checked with a #10 K-type file that was introduced in the root canal of each tooth, until it was seen at the apex, then one millimeter was subtracted. The anatomical diameter of the canal along the working length was also determined, by introducing K-type instruments of the first series, with successively larger diameters. The anatomical diameter of the root canal was recorded, when one of the instruments showed resistance to being removed from the working length. All the teeth that presented a canal diameter of over 40 hundredths millimeters along the working length were discarded and replaced others. Thus, a standard wear of 20 hundredths millimeter in the apical third was obtained. The free tip preparation technique was used up to a #60- diameter instrument and.04 taper reached the entire working length. A 1.0% sodium hypochlorite solution was used during the biomechanical preparation. The teeth had their root canals washed with 20 milliliters of deionized water, using Milli-Q water purification system, for removal of possible dentin chips from inside the root canal. After the biomechanical preparation, the teeth were randomly divided into 7 groups of 6 teeth each: Group 1: teeth with final irrigation with 15% EDTA solution, Group 2: teeth with final irrigation with 10%citric acid solution, Group 3: final irrigation with 10% sodium citrate solution, Group 4: final irrigation with apple vinegar, Group 5: final irrigation with 5% acetic acid solution, Group 6: final irrigation with 5% maleic acid solution and Group 7: teeth only instrumented and irrigated with sodium hypochlorite, without final irrigation. Each solution remained in the root canal for 5 minutes. The teeth were sectioned in the buccal-palatine direction and then subjected to scanning electron microscopy and photographed at X1000 magnification. The solutions collected were submitted to chemical analysis through flame atomic absorption spectrophotometry. It was concluded that 15% EDTA and 10% citric acid, used for 5 minutes, are effective for removing the smear layer. The apple vinegar, 10% sodium citrate, 5% acetic and maleic acids and sodium hypochlorite were not effective for removing the smear layer from root canals. The 15% EDTA presented a higher concentration of calcium ions in solution, followed by 10% citric acid. Intermediary results were observed for apple vinegar, 5% acetic and maleic acids, and the lowest concentration of calcium ions was obtained with the 10% sodium citrate.

Thus, for clinical procedures sodium hypochlorite (0.5%-1% sodium hypochlorite for vital pulp and 2.5% sodium hypochlorite for necrotic pulp) has been indicated for irrigation during instrumentation, for each file used. Teeth were kept in 15%-17% EDTA (pH 7.2) for 3-5 minutes and then irrigated again with sodium hypochlorite. Figures 19.24-19.31 show various dentinal structures with and without smear layer.

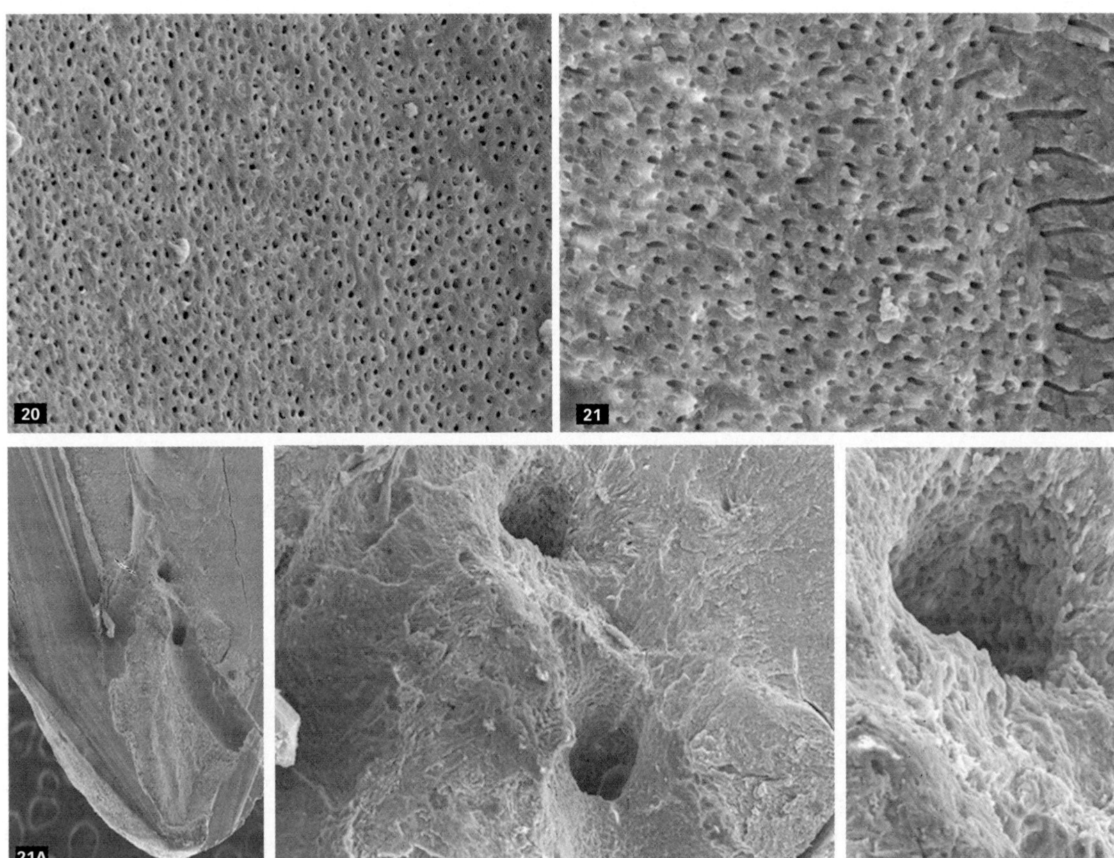


**Figure 19.20** - Root dentinal tubules opened after 5 min of apple vinegar plus 17% EDTA(X500).
**Figure 19.21** - Root dentinal tubules opened after 5 min of apple vinegar (X500).
**Figure 19.21** - (**A**) Root dentinal tubules opened after 5 min of apple vinegar plus 17% EDTA.

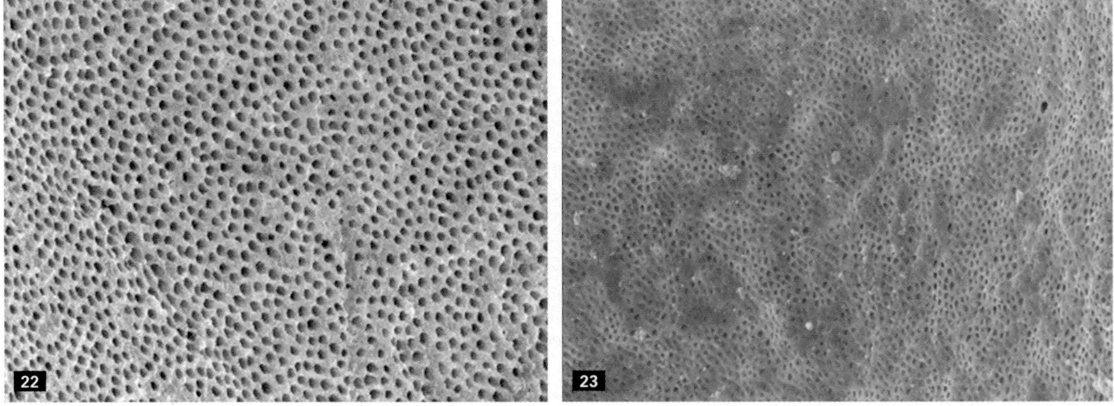


**Figure 19.22** - Root dentinal tubules opened after 5 min of 2.5% NaOCl plus 17% EDTA(X500).
**Figure 19.23** - Root dentinal tubules opened after 5 min of 2% chlorhexidine gel plus 17% EDTA(X500).

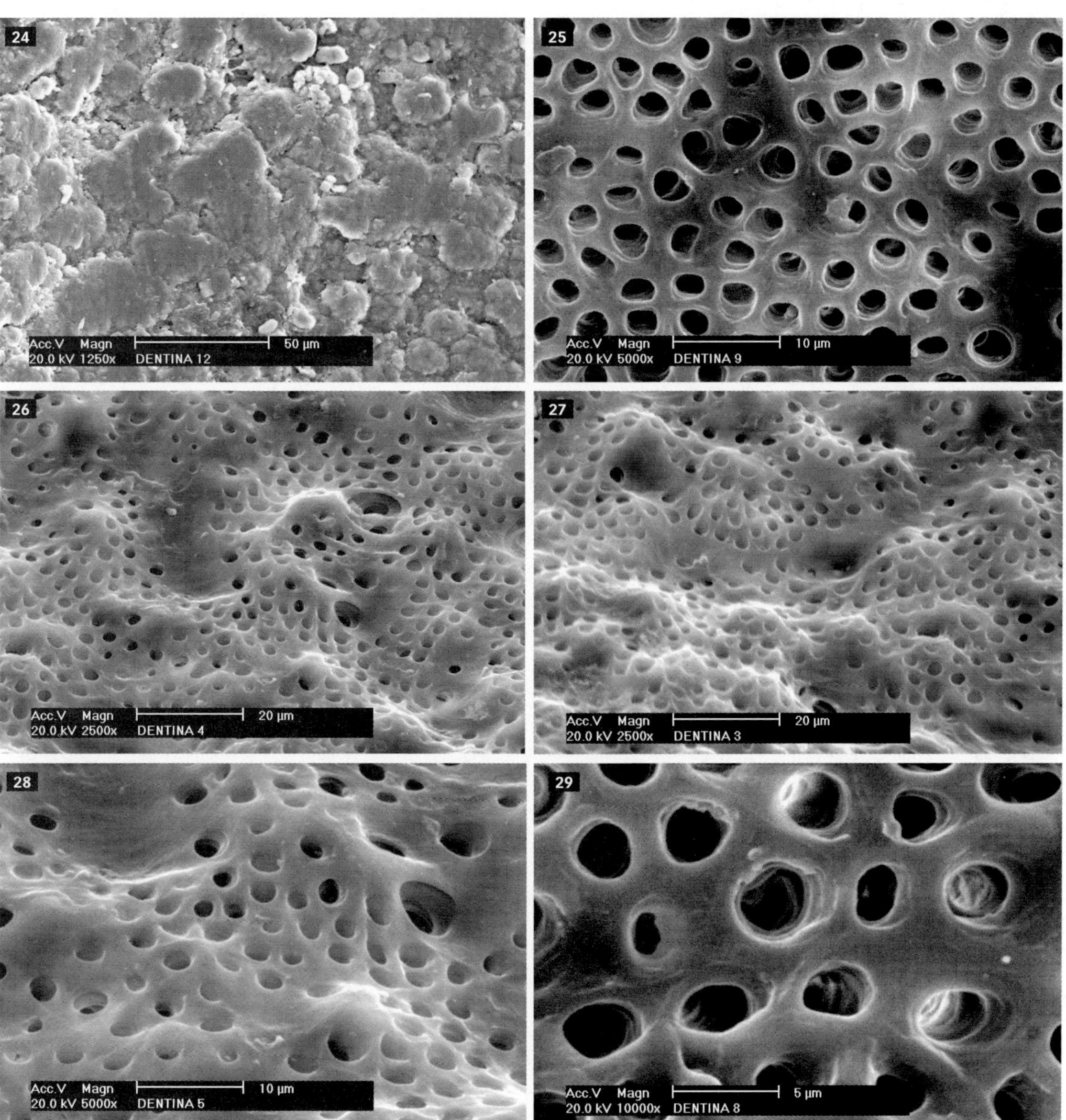


**Figure 19.24** - Root canal wall with smear layer (permission Prof. JAP Figueiredo).
**Figure 19.25** - Root canal wall without smear layer (permission Prof. JAP Figueiredo).
**Figures 19.26 to 19.28** - Root dentinal tubules (permission Prof. JAP Figueiredo).
**Figure 19.29** - Root dentinal tubules opened after 5 min of 17% EDTA (permission Prof. JAP Figueiredo).

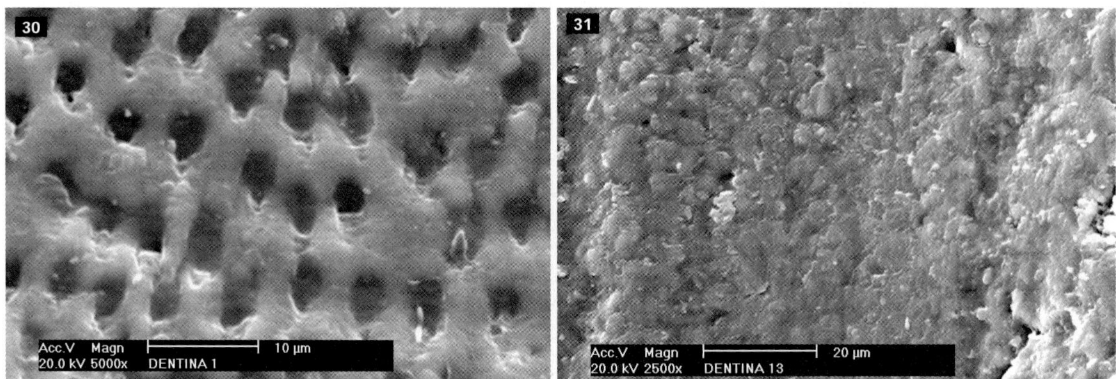


**Figure 19.30** - Root dentinal tubules with smear plug (permission Prof. JAP Figueiredo).
**Figure 19.31** - Root dentinal tubules with smear layer (permission Prof. JAP Figueiredo).

Torabinejad et al.[390] studied a new solution for smear layer removal. Various organic acids, ultrasonic instruments, and lasers have been used to remove the smear layer from the surface of instrumented root canals. The purpose of this study was to investigate the effect of a mixture of a tetracycline isomer, an acid, and a detergent (MTAD) as a final rinse for the surfaces of instrumented root canals. Forty-eight extracted maxillary and mandibular single-rooted human teeth were prepared by using a combination of passive step-back and rotary 0.04 taper nickel-titanium instruments. Sterile distilled water or 5.25% sodium hypochlorite was used as intracanal irrigant. The canals were then treated with 5 ml of one of the following solutions as a final rinse: sterile distilled water, 5.25% sodium hypochlorite, 17% EDTA, or a new solution, MTAD. The presence or absence of smear layer and the amount of erosion on the surface of the root canal walls at the coronal, middle, and apical portion of each canal were examined by scanning electronic microscopy. It seems that MTAD is an effective solution for the removal of the smear layer, when used as a final rinse. It does not significantly change the structure of the dentinal tubules when used in conjunction with NaOCl as a root canal irrigant. Studies are in progress to determine the efficacy of MTAD as a root canal irrigant, with and without NaOCl for removing the smear layer and completely disinfecting the root canal system.

## 19.6 A Model System to Study Antimicrobial Strategies Against Endodontic Biofilms

Root canal infection is an extraordinary microenvironment for several microorganism species to become attached to the dentinal surface and form a dense bacterial plaque[246]. These bacterial biofilms are prevalent on most surfaces of a damp nature, and can cause environmental problems, representing a common cause of persistent infections[65,378].

The stages of structural organization of biofilm, composition and activities of the colonizing microorganisms in various environments may differ, although the establishment of a micro-community on a surface seems to follow essentially the same series of developmental stages, including deposition of a conditioning film, adhesion and colonization of planktonic microorganisms in a polymeric matrix, co-adhesion of other organisms, and detachment of biofilm microorganisms into surroundings[378].

Successful infected root canal treatment is dependent on inactivation of the microorganisms present in the biofilm and planktonic environment. Root canal preparation with antimicrobial agents, such as irrigants and/or intracanal dressings, can contribute to the reduction of endodontic microbiota[83,97,246].

The microbiota of a necrotic root canal is dependent on the type of bacteria present in the oral cavity, especially in plaque, and on the ecological conditions in the root canal, such as infective microbiota, presence of oxygen (redox potential), availability of nutrients, and the host's defense[375]. Sundqvist & Fidgor[374] reported that infection of the root canal is not a random event. Species that establish a persistent root canal infection are selected by the phenotypic traits that they share in common and that are suited to the modified environment. Some of these shared characteristics include the capacity to penetrate and invade dentin, a growth pattern of chains or cohesive filaments, resistance to antimicrobial agents used in endodontic treatment, as well as an ability to grow in monoinfections, survive periods of starvation and evade the host response[374].

*E. faecalis* has been shown to be potentially important in colonization or overgrowth in endodontic infections, being the dominant microorganism in post-treatment apical periodontitis[125,374,375], and has often been isolated from the root canal in pure culture. It has, however, also found together with other bacteria and yeasts. In mixed infections, *E. faecalis* is typically the dominant isolate. The pathogenicity of *E. faecalis* in endodontic infections is well documented[93,125,148,149,150,188,243,299,374,375].

Several studies were developed with different bacterial biofilm models to test the antimicrobial effectiveness of endodontic medicaments[97,83,148,170,179,188,203,204,208,216,219,224,265,364]. Investigations have shown either antimicrobial effectiveness or ineffectiveness of intracanal medicaments against bacterial biofilm. The planktonic or biofilm environment can influence the effectiveness of antimicrobial agents.

Bacteria growing on a surface display a novel phenotype[208]; consequently they have increased resistance to antimicrobial agents. This can result from restricted inhibitor penetration, slower bacterial growth rates, transfer of resistance genes, suboptimal environmental conditions for inhibitor activity, and the expression of a resistant phenotype[224].

The large number of researches published about biofilm certainly can bring contradictory positions on antimicrobial strategies into context, particularly as a result of the variability between the methodologies. Thus, the purpose of this work was to develop a model system, to study antimicrobial strategies against endodontic biofilm[224].

Haapasalo & Ørstavik[148] used bovine teeth in an in vitro model for dentinal tubule infection. The study evaluated the antimicrobial effect of camphorated paramonochlorophenol (CMCP) and a calcium hydroxide compound (Calasept®) against tubule infection by *E. faecalis* for up to 28 days. CMCP in liquid form proved highly effective inside the tubules while Calasept® was completely ineffective. Estrela et al.[97] determined the antimicrobial efficacy of ozonated water, gaseous ozone, sodium hypochlorite and chlorhexidine against endodontic biofilm developed on human teeth for 60 days. The antimicrobial medicaments were not sufficient to inactivate *E. faecalis*, biofilm.

Estrela et al.[109] proposed a model system to analyze antimicrobial strategies against endodontic biofilm. An *E. faecalis* suspension was colonized in 10 human root canals. Five milliliters of Brain Heart Infusion were mixed with 5 mL of the bacterial inoculums (*E. faecalis*), inoculated with sufficient volume to fill the root canal for 60 days. This procedure was repeated every 72 hours, always using 24-hour pure culture, prepared and adjusted to No. 1 MacFarland turbidity standard. The biofilm formation was analyzed by scanning electronic microscopy (SEM). *E. faecalis* consistently adhered to collagen structures, colonized the dentinal surface, progressed towards the dentinal tubules and formed a biofilm. The model seems to be feasible for studies on antimicrobial strategies. The proposed biofilm model allows satisfactory colonization time of selected bacteria with virulence and adherence properties. Based on several investigations and analyzing various biofilm models, the purpose of this essay[109] was to review biofilm models and to develop a model system, to study antimicrobial strategies (Fig. 19.32A-D, 19.33A-D).

Bacteria produce a variety of different surface structure appendages that are involved in colonization of the host. They mediate bacterial adhesion to host surfaces, promote invasion of host cells, allow bacterial cell-cell contact and communication, or protect bacteria from host immune defenses[248].

The biofilm study model that reflects the real environment is the human root canal itself with variations and anatomic complexity[7,97,103,148,220,263,265,291-294,315,336,344,397]. Shovelton[344] observing bacteria diffusion in human root dentinal tubules, verified by histological methods that the number of bacteria-containing tubules was highly variable from tooth to tooth. The invasion of root dentinal tubules by root canal bacteria is a multifactorial event, and a limited number of oral bacterial species have the necessary properties to participate in it[220]. The penetration of microorganisms into infected root dentin has shown variations with respect to the experimental model, biological indicator and incubation time used in the studies[125,148,315]. The development and modification of *E. faecalis* biofilm in root canals and its penetration into the dentinal tubules have been associated with the prevailing environmental conditions[125]. The bacterial colonization structure on dentinal collagen constitutes a natural biological representation. Dentinal tubules contain a considerable quantity of unmineralized collagen[78], and Type I collagen serves as an adhesion substrate for oral streptococci[216]. The differences in behavior have been demonstrated between planktonic bacteria and bacteria in biofilm in laboratory tests of antimicrobial substances. Certainly, there are differences between artificial surfaces and natural oral hard tissues as regards bacterial adhesion and plaque formation.

Biofilm produced by membrane filter was used in some investigations[131,348,364]. This model may not provide an accurate representation of the antimicrobial efficacy of the substance tested, but this model has its merits, which include no need for extracted teeth and their time-consuming preparation[364].

The bacterial species that was observed in the largest number of studies was *E. faecalis,* and its importance in endodontics is well documented[3,77,97,103,104,114,117,125,131,134,136,170,188,194,212,219,263,275,276,299,306,316,330,351,371,375,418]. *E. faecalis* is a Gram-positive coccus, facultative anaerobe, present in normal human gastrointestinal infection and common in secondary apical periodontitis. Enterococci are variably classified as the second to third most common organisms found in hospital-acquired infections, and 85-95% of these isolates are *E. faecalis*[188,243]. The virulence of enterococci involves the need for adherence to host tissues encounter a vastly different environment during the process of tissue invasion, with higher redox potentials and limited essential nutrients. Infecting enterococci probably express genes favoring growth under these alternate environmental conditions and express factors that permit adherence to host cells and extracellular matrix, facilitate tissue invasion, interfere in immunomodulation, and cause toxin-mediated damage[188].

Adhesion to the dentin surface is an essential step that determines the pathogenic potential of *E. faecalis*. The influence of *E. faecalis* proteases and the collagen-binding protein have been studied[179,188,203,204,248,310]. Collagen-binding protein, serine protein, Ace and possibly gelatinase are potential virulence factors that give *E. faecalis* the ability to bind to dentin[179]. Kristich et al.[203] used independent experimental approaches to characterize biofilm formation by *E. faecalis*, which forms robust biofilms and its development is modulated by the prevailing environmental conditions. Neither the esp gene product, nor the remainder of the genes encoded by the known *E. faecalis* pathogenicity island, are required for the development of biofilms with complex architecture. A secreted metalloprotease, GelE, enhances biofilm formation of *E. faecalis* but otherwise, the genetic determinants controlling biofilm development remain unknown. Enterococcal lipoteicoic acid may serve as a virulence factor by modulating inflammatory responses, and by facilitating plasmid transfer[188]. The prevalence, virulence, phenotype and genotype of oral and endodontic enterococci was recently studied[328-330]. Phenotypic and genotypic evidence of potential virulence factors were identified in endodontic *Enterococcus spp.*, specifically production of gelatinase and response to pherormones.

It has been postulated that *E. faecalis* cells maintain the capability of invading dentinal tubules and adhering to collagen in the presence of human serum[219]. This bacterium persists, resistant even in critical environments where nutrients are reduced and in the presence of antimicrobial agents like calcium hydroxide, sodium hypochlorite, chlorhexidine, ozone[97,98,104,108]. Thus, the selection of *E. faecalis* as a biological indicator in several studies is well documented. Bacterial colonization and invasion of surface and root dentinal tubules include significant factors such as nutrient supply and time for colonization.

The ability of *E. faecalis* to invade dentinal tubule has been reported[148,265,315]. To establish the ideal time taken to contaminate the dentinal surface and deep layers of root canal to form the bacterial biofilm, is uncertain. Unquestionably, over a longer time, the structural organization of biofilm in an adequate microenvironment will be better. The time taken for the biofilm to form in various studies showed significant variations (15 minutes to 60 days)[97,110]. *E. faecalis* has shown its important role in endodontic infections, with particular strategies to form biofilm, substantial virulence factors[179,188,203,204,243,248,310,328-330,375], adherence capability on dentin collagen[179,188,203,204], survival in critical environment[78,219], and resistance to endodontic therapy[97,246,375].

Haapasalo et al.[149] analyzed a literature review on the effects of dentin on the antimicrobial properties of endodontic medicaments. Successful treatment of apical periodontitis is dependent on the elimination of infective microflora from the necrotic root canal system. Antimicrobial irrigating solutions and other locally used disinfecting agents and medicaments play a key role in the eradication of the microbes. While most, if not all presently used disinfecting agents rapidly kill even the resistant microbes when tested in vitro, in a test tube, the effectiveness of these same agents is clearly weaker than it is under the in vivo conditions. Recent studies have provided valuable information about the interaction of endodontic disinfecting agents with dentin and other compounds present in the necrotic root canal. As a result of these interactions, the antimicrobial effectiveness of several of our key disinfectants may be weakened, or even eliminated under certain circumstances. Different disinfectants show different sensitivity to the action by the various potential inactivators, such as dentin, serum proteins, hydroxyapatite, collagen derived from different sources, and microbial biomass.

The problem of solving endodontic biofilm, involves the need for a standard model to compare the antimicrobial endodontic materials under several conditions. A model of mature *E. faecalis* biofilm on human root dentin is suggested, with 60 days to develop under low oxygen and a nutrient-rich environment (Fig. 19.32A-D, 19.33A-D).

Estrela et al.[110] conducted a critical discussion on the antibacterial efficacy of intracanal medicaments against bacterial biofilm. Longitudinal studies were evaluated by systematic review (SR) including articles searched in electronic basis (MEDLINE, EMBASE, CENTRAL) and manual searches, using various keywords involving root canal biofilm, from 1966 through to August 1, 2007. The selected articles were identified from titles, abstracts and complete articles independently by two reviewers, considering the tabulated inclusion and exclusion criteria. Disagreements were resolved by consensus. The search of information of the present study found 91 related articles, so that from of these, 17 (18.7%) articles were literature reviews, 8 (8.8%) articles involved studies in vivo (7 in humans and 1 in animals), 19 (20.1%) included studies in vitro 7 (7.7%) articles about a biofilm model on membrane filter, 12 (13.1%) articles with biofilm model on root dentin, 9 (10%) studies associated with non- endodontic biofilm and 33 (36.2%) articles related to others studies. Of the 8 in vivo articles, no study satisfied the inclusion criteria. The analysis demonstrated lack of efficacy of endodontic therapy against bacterial biofilm. The biofilm in the root canal system is a challenge to the outcome of root canal treatment.

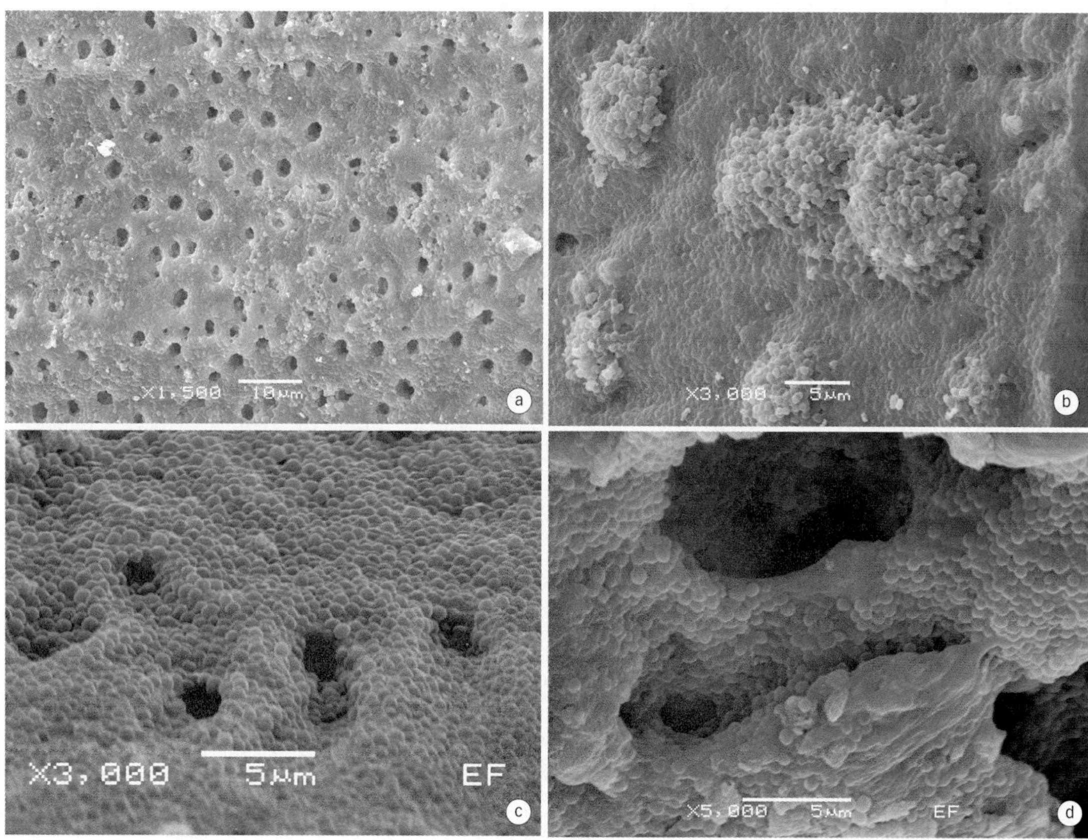


**Figure 19.32** - SEM of (**A**) Various areas covered by *E. faecalis* biofilm on root dentinal surface (X1,500). (**B**) Root dentinal surface completely covered by *E. faecalis* biofilm, and no dentinal tubule openings (X3,000). (**C**) Evidence of root dentinal surface completely covered by *E. faecalis* biofilm (X3,000). (**D**) Bacterial penetration into dentinal tubules (X5,000) (Estrela, Sydney, Figueiredo, Estrela, J Applied Oral Sci 2009[109]).

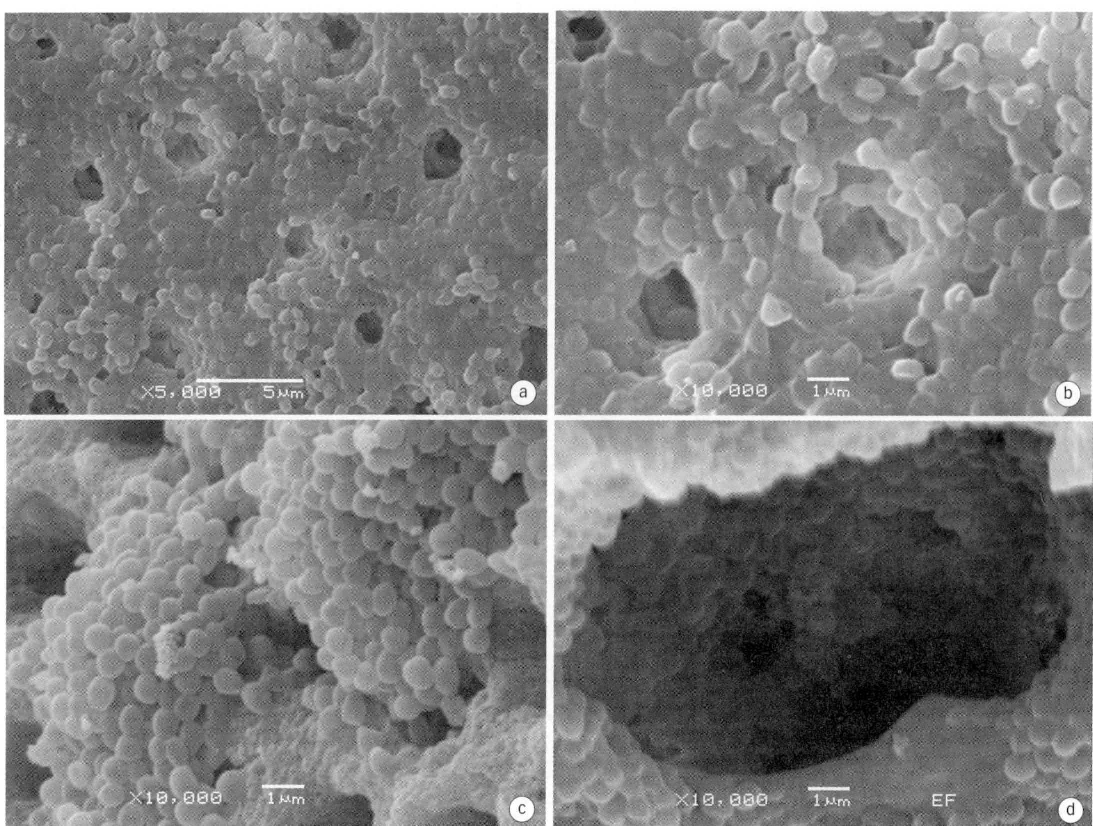


**Figure 19.33** - SEM of (**A**) Root dentinal surface covered by *E. faecalis* biofilm (X5,000). (**B**) Magnification area of previous picture (X10,000). (**C,D**) Aggregated bacterial cells on and in dentinal tubules (X10,000) )(Estrela, Sydney, Figueiredo, Estrela, J Applied Oral Sci 2009[109]).

## References


1. Abbott PV, Heijkoop PS, Cardaci SC, Hume WR. An SEM study of the effects of different irrigation sequences and ultrasonics. Int Endod J 1991;24:308-16.
2. Abbott PV, Heithersay GS, HumeWR. Release and diffusion through human tooth roots in vitro of corticosteroid and tetracycline trace molecules from Ledermix paste. Endod Dent Traumatol 1988;4:55-62.
3. Abdullah M, Ng Y-L, Gulabivala K, Moles D, Spratt DA. Susceptibilities of two *Enterococcus faecalis* phenotypes to root canal medications. J Endod 2005;31:30-6.
4. Abou-Rass M, Oglesby SW. The effects of temperature, concentration, and tissue type on ability of sodium hypochlorite. J Endod 1981;7:376-7.
5. Abou-Rass M, Piccinino MV. The effectiveness of four clinical irrigation methods on the removal of root canal debris. Oral Surg Oral Med Oral Pathol 1982;54:323-8.
6. Agarwal S, Piesco NP, Peterson De, Charon J, Suzuki JB, Godowski K, Southard GL. Effects of sanguinarium, chlorhexidine and tetracycline on neutrophil viability and functions in vitro. J Period Res 1997;32:335-44.
7. Akpata ES, Blechman H. Bacterial invasion on pulpal dentin wall in vitro. J Dent Res 1982;61:435-8.
8. Albergaria S. Substâncias químicas auxiliares da instrumentação dos canais radiculares utilizadas nas universidades brasileiras. Rev Fac Odont Univ Fed Bahia 1988-9;8/9:1-13.
9. Al-Nazhan S, Spångberg L. Morphological cell changes due to chemical toxicity of a dental material: an electron microscopic study on human periodontal ligament fibroblasts and L929 cells. J Endod 1990;16:129-34.
10. Andersen M, Andreasen JO, Andreasen FM. In vitro solubility of human pulp tissue in calcium hydroxide and sodium hypochlorite. Endod Dent Traumatol 1992;8:104-8.

11. Auerbach MB. Antibiotics vs instrumentation in endodontic. NY St Dent J 1953;19:225-8.
12. Ayhan H, Sultan N, Cirak M, Ruhi MZ, Bodur H. Antimicrobial effects of various endodontic irrigants on selected microorganisms. Int Endod J 1999;32:99-102.
13. Babich H,Wurzburger BJ, RubinYL, SinenskyMC, Blau L. An in vitro study on the cytotoxicity of chlorhexidine digluconate to human gingival cells. Cell Biol Toxicol 1995;11:79-88.
14. Badan M. Oxigenoargentoterapia. São Paulo, Mogi-Mirim:Pacini;Piccolomini;1949.
15. Baker NA, Eleazer PD, Auerbach RE, Seltzer S. Scanning electron microscopic study of the efficacy of various irrigating solutions. J Endod 1975;1:127-35.
16. Bammann LL, Estrela C. Aspectos microbiológicos em Endodontia. In: Estrela C, Figueiredo JAP. Endodontia: princípios biológicos e mecânicos. São Paulo: Artes Médicas;1999. p.168-89.
17. Barbeyrac B, Perro G, Quentin C, Cutillas M, Bebear C, Sanchez R. Influence of chlorhexidine on the flora of burns. Pathol Biol 1985;33:635-8.
18. Barbin EL, Spanó JCE, Silva RS, Pécora JD. Análise in vitro da variação térmica durante a utilização do hipoclorito de sódio, em diferentes concentrações, com peróxido de hidrogênio a 3%. Rev Odont USP 1995;9: 189-92.
19. Barbin EL. Estudo in vitro do efeito da adição de lauril dietileno glicol éter sulfato de sódio nas soluções hipoclorito de sódio sobre suas propriedades físico-químicas anteriores e posteriores à dissolução do tecido pulpar bovino. (Master's thesis). Ribeirão Preto, University of São Paulo;1999. 108p.
20. Barbin LE, Saquy PC, Guedes DFC, Sousa-Neto MD, Estrela C, Pécora JD. Determination of para-chloraline and reactive oxygen species in chlorhexidine and chlorhexidine associated with calcium hydroxide. J Endod 2008; 34:1508-14.
21. Barbosa SV, Almeida D. HCT 20 - Uma solução irrigadora para canais radiculares humanos. Análise in vitro. Rev Bras Odontol 1987;44:21-8.
22. Barbosa SV, Spångberg LSW, Almeida D. Low surface tension of calcium hydroxide solutions in an effective antiseptic. Int Endod J 1994;27:6-10
23. Barker BC, Lockett BC. Experiments using a glucocorticosteroid/antibiotic paste in infected root canals of a dog. J British Endod Society 1971;5:60-8.
24. Barker BC, Lockett BC. Reaction of dog pulp and periapical tissue to two glucocorticosteroid preparations. Oral Sur Oral Med Oral Pathol 1972;33: 249-62.
25. Barret MT. The Dakin-carrel antiseptic solution. Dent Cosmos 1917;59:446-8.
26. Basrani BR, Manek S, Sodhi RNS, Fillery E, Manzur A. Interaction between sodium hypochlorite and chlorhexidine gluconate. J Endod 2007; 33:966 -9.
27. Baumgartner JC, Cuenin PR. Efficacy of several concentrations of sodium hypochlorite for root canal irrigation. J Endod 1992;18:605-12.
28. Baumgartner JC, Ibay AC. The chemical of irrigants used for root canal debridement. J Endod 1987;13:47-51.
29. Baysan A, Lynch E. The use of ozone in dentistry and medicine. Prim Dent Care 2005;12:47-52.
30. Becking AG. Complications in the use of sodium hypochlorite during endodontic treatment. Oral Sur Oral Med Oral Pathol 1991;71:346-8.
31. Beltes P,Koulaouzidou E, KotoualaV, Kortsaris AH. In vitro evaluation of the cytotoxicity of calcium hydroxide-based root canal sealers. Endod Dent Traumatol 1995;11:245-9.
32. Berbert A, Bramante C, Bernadineli N. Irrigações em Endodontia. In: Endodontia Prática. São Paulo: Sarvier;1980.
33. Berbert A. Hidráulica das irrigações e aspirações dos canais radículo-dentários. Parte I. Ensaios preliminares. Rev Bras Odontol 1969;26:181-94.
34. Berbert A. Influência dos ductos de cânulas, dos seus aproveitamentos nos canais radiculares e da velocidade de irrigação, sobre a pressão apical nas irrigações simples. (Doctoral Thesis). Bauru, University of São Paulo;1971.
35. Bergqvist-Karlsson A. Delayedandimmediate-type-hypersensitivity to chlorhexidine. Contact Dermatitis 1988;18:84-8.
36. Berutti E, Marini R, Angeretti A. Penetration ability of different irrigants into dentinal tubules. J Endod 1997;23:725-7.
37. Blechman H, Cohen M. Use of aqueous urea solution in the field of Endodontia: Preliminary report. J Dent Res 1951;30:503-4.
38. Bowden JR, Brennan PA. Life-threatening airway obstruction secondary to hypochlorite extrusion during root canal treatment. Oral Surg Oral Med Oral Pathol Oral Radiol Endod 2006;101:402-4.
39. Braguetto CA, Souza-Neto MD, Cruz-Filho AM, Silva RG, Saquy PC, Pécora JD. Ação da solução de EDTA e da solução de Dakin, utilizadas isoladamente, misturadas ou alternadas na limpeza do canal radicular. Rev Odontol USP 1997;11:67-70.
40. Brise-o BM, Wirth R, Hamm G, Standhartinger W. Efficacy of different methods and concentrations of root canal irrigations on bacteria in the root canal. Endod Dent Traumatol 1992;8:6-11.
41. Brown DC, Moore BK, Brown CE Jr, Newton CW. An in vitro study of apical extrusion of sodium hypochlorite during endodontic canal preparation. J Endod 1995;21:587-91.
42. Buck RA, Cai J, Eleaser PD, Staat RH, Hurst HE. Detoxification of endotoxin by endodontic irrigants and calcium hydroxide. J Endod 2001;27:325-7.
43. Buck RA, Eleaser PD, Staat RH. In vitro disinfection of dentinal tubules by various endodontics irrigants. J Endod 1999;25:786-8.
44. Buck RA, Eleazer PD, Staat RH, Scheetz JP. Effectiveness of three endodontic irrigants at various tubular depths in human dentin. J Endod 2001;27:206-8.
45. Bui TB, Baumgartner JC, Mitchell JC. Evaluation of the interaction between sodium hypochlorite and chlorhexidine gluconate and its effect on root dentin. J Endod 2008; 34:181-5.
46. Buttler TK, Crawford JJ. The detoxifying effect of varying concentrations of sodium hypochlorite on endotoxins. J Endod 1982;8:59-66.
47. Byström A, Claesson R, Sundqvist G. The antibacterial effect of camphorated paramonochlorophenol, camphorated phenol and calcium hydroxide in the treatment of infected root canals. Endod Dent Traumatol 1985;1:170-5.

48. Byström A, Happonen RP, Sjögren U, Sundqvist G. Healing of periapical lesions of pulpless teeth after endodontic treatment with controlled asepsis. Endod Dent Traumatol 1987;3:58-63.
49. Byström A, Sundqvist G. Bacteriologic evaluation of the efficacy of mechanical root canal instrumentation in endodontic therapy. Scand J Dent Res 1981;89:321-8.
50. Byström A, Sundqvist G. The antibacterial action of sodium hypochlorite and EDTA in 60 cases of endodontic therapy. Int Endod J 1985;18:35-40.
51. Byströn A, Sundqvist G. Bacteriologic evaluation of the effects of 0.5% sodium hypochlorite in endodontic therapy. Oral Surg Oral Med Oral Pathol 1983;55:307-12.
52. Calas P, Rochd T, Druilhet P, Azais J. In vitro adhesion of two strains of *Prevotella nigrescens* to the dentin of the root canal: the part played by different irrigation solutions. J Endod 1998;24:112-5.
53. Caliskan MK, Turkun M, Alper S. Allergy to sodium hypochlorite during root canal therapy: a case report. Int Endod J 1994;27:163-7.
54. Callahan JR. Sulfuric acid for opening root canals. Dent Cosmos 1894;36:957-9.
55. Cervone F, Tronstad L, Hammond B. Antimicrobial effect of chlorhexidine in a controlled release delivery system. Endod Dent Traumatol 1990;6:33-6.
56. Chow TW. Mechanical effectiveness of root canal irrigation. J Endod 1983;9:675-9.
57. Ciancio SG. Antimicrobianos e Antibióticos. In: Nisengard RJ, Newman MG. Microbiologia oral e imunologia. 2nd ed. Rio de Janeiro: Guanabara Koogan;1994. p.364-372.
58. Cobe S. Investigations of a new dental chemotherapeutic agent in presence of blood. Oral Surg Oral Med O Pathol 1960;13:678-85.
59. Cohen S, Stewart GG, Laster LL. The effects of acids, alkalies, and chelating agents on dentine permeability. Oral Surg Oral Med Oral Pathol 1970;29:631-4.
60. Coolidge ED. Studies of germicides for the treatment of root canals. J Am Dent Assoc 1929;16:698-712.
61. Coolidge ED. The diagnosis and treatment of conditions from diseased dental pulps. J Am Dent Assoc 1919;6:337-49.
62. Costa CAS. Teste de biocompatibilidade dos materiais odontológicos. In: Estrela C. Metodologia Científica: Ciência, Ensino, Pesquisa. 2nd ed. São Paulo: Artes Médicas; 2005.
63. Costa ED, Souza-Filho FJ, Barbosa SV. Tissue reactions to a component of root canal system bacteria: lipoteichoic acid. Braz Dent J. 2003;14:95-8.
64. Costa WF, Antoniazzi JH, Campos MNM, Pécora JD, Robazza CRC. Avaliação comparativa sob microscopia ótica, da capacidade de limpeza da irrigação manual convencional versus ultrasônica dos canais radiculares. Rev Paul Odontol 1986;8:50-60.
65. Costerton JW, Cheng KJ, Geesey GG, Ladd TI, Nickel C, Dasgupta M, Marrie TJ. Bacterial biofilms in nature and disease. Annual Reviews of Microbiol. 1987;41:435-64.
66. Crabb HSM. The cleaning of root canals. Int Endod J 1982;15:62-6.
67. Cruz-Filho AM, Sousa-Neto MD, Saquy PC, Pécora JD. Evaluation of the effect of EDTAC, CDTA, and EGTA on radicular dentin microhardness. J Endod 2001;27:183-4.
68. Cunninghan WT, Balekjian AY. Effect of temperature on collagen-dissolving ability of sodiun hypochlorite endodontic irrigant. Oral Surg Oral Med Oral Pathol 1980;49:175-7.
69. Cunninghan WT, Joseph SW. Effect of temperature on the bactericidal action of sodium hypochlorite endodontic irrigant. Oral Surg Oral Med Oral Pathol 1980;50:569-71.
70. Cunninghan WT, Martin H, Forrest W. Evaluation of root canal debridament by the Endosonic Ultrasonic Synergistic System. Oral Surg Oral Med Oral Pathol 1982;53:401-4.
71. Cunninghan WT, Martin H, Pelleu GB, Stoops DE. A comparison of antimicrobial effectiveness of Endosonic and Hand root canal therapy. Oral Surg Oral Med Oral Pathol 1982;54:238-41.
72. Cunninghan WT, Martin H. A scanning electron microscopic evaluation of root canal debridament with the Endosonic Ultrasonic Synergistic System. Oral Surg Oral Med Oral Pathol 1982;53:527-31.
73. Cvek M. Treatment of non-vital permanent incisors with calcium hydroxide I. Follow-up of periapical repair and apical closure of immature roots. Odontol Rev 1972;23:27-44
74. Cvek M, Hollender L, Nord CE. Treatment of non-vital permanent incisors with calcium hydroxide VI. A clinical, microbiological and radiological evaluation of treatment in one sitting of teeth with mature or immature root. Odont Rev 1976;27:93-108.
75. Cvek M, Nord CE, Hollender L. Antimicrobial effect of root canal debridement in teeth with immature root. A clinical and microbiologic study. Odontol Rev 1976;27:1-10.
76. D'Arcangelo C, Varvara G, DeFazio P. An evaluation of the action of different root canal irrigants on facultative aerobic-anaerobic, obligate anaerobic and microaerophilic bacteria. J Endod 1999;25:351-3.
77. Dahlén G, Samuelsson W, Molander A, Reit C. Identification and antimicrobial susceptibility of enterococci isolated from the root canal. Oral Microbiol Immunol. 2000;15:309-12.
78. Dai X-F, Ten Cate AR, Limeback H. The extent and distribution of intratubular collagen fibrils in human dentine. Arch Oral Biol. 1991;36:775-8.
79. Dakin HD. On the use of certain antiseptic substances in the treatment of infected wounds. Br Med J 1915;2:318-20.
80. Dakin HD. The antiseptic action of hypochlorites: the ancient history of the new antiseptic. Br Med 1915;2:809-10.
81. Delany GM, Patterson SS, Miller CH, Newton CW. The effect of chlorhexidine gluconate irrigation on the root canal flora of freshly extracted necrotic teeth. Oral Sur Oral Med Oral Pathol 1982;53:518-23.
82. Denton GW. Chlorhexidine. In: Block SS. Disinfection, sterilization and preservation. 4th ed. Philadelphia: Lea & Febiger;1991. p 274-289.
83. Duggan JM, Sedgley CM. Biofilm formation of oral and endodontic *Enterococcus faecalis*. J Endod. 2007;33:815-8.
84. Ehrich DG, Brian JD Jr, Walker WA. Sodium hypochlorite accident: inadvertent injection into the maxillary sinus. J Endod 1993;19:180-2.

85. Emilson CG. Potential efficacy of chlorhexidine against mutans streptococci and human dental caries. J Dent Res 1994;73:682-91.
86. Emilson CG. Susceptibility of various microorganisms to chlorhexidine. J Dent Res 1977;85:255-65.
87. Engström B, Spångberg L. Toxic and antimicrobial effects of antiseptics in vitro. Svensk Tandläkare Tidskrift 1969;543-9.
88. Engstron B, Spångberg L. Studies on root canal medicaments. 1- Cytotoxic effect of root canal antiseptics. Acta Odontol Scand 1967;25:77-84.
89. Ercan E, Ozekinci T, Atakul F, Gul K. Antibacterial activity of 2% chlorhexidine gluconate and 5.25% sodium hypochlorite in infected root canal: in vivo study. J Endod 2004;30:84-7.
90. Estrela C. Ciência Endodôntica. 1st ed. São Paulo: Artes Médicas;2004.
91. Estrela C. Metodologia Científica: ensino e pesquisa em odontologia. 1st ed. São Paulo: Artes Médicas;2001.
92. Estrela C, Bammann LL, Pimenta FC, Pécora JD. Control of microorganisms in vitro by calcium hydroxide pastes. Int Endod J 2001;34:341-5.
93. Estrela C, César OVS, Leles CR, Pimenta FC, Alencar AHG. Avaliação em estudos longitudinais da eficácia do hidróxido de cálcio sobre o *Enterococcus faecalis* em infecções endodônticas - Revisão Sistemática. Rev Bras Odontol 2007;64:117-128.
94. Estrela C, Estrela CRA, Bammann LL, Pécora JD. Two methods to evaluate the antimicrobial action of calcium hydroxide paste. J Endod 2001;27:5-7.
95. Estrela C, Estrela CRA, Barbin EL, Spanó JC, Marchesan MA, Pécora JD. Mechanism of action of sodium hypochlorite. Braz Dent J 2002;13:113-7.
96. Estrela C, Estrela CRA, Cruz-Filho AM, Pécora JD. Substância ESP: opção na terapêutica endodôntica. J Bras Endod 2005;5:273-9.
97. Estrela C, Estrela CRA, Decurcio DA, Hollanda ACB, Silva JA. Antimicrobial efficacy of ozonated water, gaseous ozone, sodium hypochlorite and chlorhexidine in infected human root canals. Int Endod J 2007;40:85-93.
98. Estrela C, Estrela CRA, Guimarães FL, Silva RS, Pécora JD. Surface tension of calcium hydroxide associated with different substances. J Appl Oral Sci 2005;13:152-6.
99. Estrela C, Holland R, Bernabé PFE, Souza V, Estrela CRA. Antimicrobial potential of medicaments used in healing process in dog's teeth with apical periodontitis. Braz Dent J 2004;15:181-5.
100. Estrela C, Holland R. Calcium hydroxide: study based on scientific evidences. J Appl Oral Sci 2003;11:269-282.
101. Estrela C, Hollanda ACB, Decurcio DA, Guedes OA, Pécora JD. Substância ESP: análise da dissolução tecidual e tensão superficial - parte 1. Rev Odontol Bras Central 2005;14:11-8.
102. Estrela C, Lopes HP, Elias CN, Leles CR, Pécora JD. Limpeza da superfície do canal radicular pelo vinagre de maçã, hipoclorito de sódio, clorexidina e EDTA. Rev Ass Paul Cir Dent 2007;61:117-22.
103. Estrela C, Pimenta FC, Ito IY, Bammann LL. Antimicrobial evaluation of calcium hydroxide in infected dentinal tubules. J Endod 1999;25:416-418.
104. Estrela C, Ribeiro RG, Estrela CRA, Pécora JD, Sousa-Neto MD. Antimicrobial effect of 2% sodium hypochlorite and 2% chlorhexidine tested by different methods. Braz Dent J 2003;14:58-62.
105. Estrela C, Silva JA, Decurcio DA, Alencar AHG, Leles CR. Efficacy of sodium hypochlorite and chlorhexidine on *Enterococcus faecalis* - a systematic review and meta-analysis. J Appl Oral Sci 2008;16:364-8.
106. Estrela C, Siqueira RMG, Resende EV, Silva AS, Silva FA. Influência da substância química, do cimento obturador e do número de sessões na incidência de pericementite traumática. Rev Odontol Brasil Central 1996;6:9-13.
107. Estrela C, Sydney GB, Bammann LL, Felippe-Júnior O. Estudo do efeito biológico do pH na atividade enzimática de bactérias anaeróbias. Rev Fac Odontol Bauru 1994;2:31-38.
108. Estrela C, Sydney GB, Bammann LL, Felippe-Júnior O. Mechanism of action of calcium and hydroxyl ions of calcium hydroxide on tissue and bacteria. Braz Dent J 1995:6:85-90.
109. Estrela C, Sydney GB, Figueiredo JAP, Estrela C. A model system to study antimicrobial strategies on endodontic biofilms. J Appl Oral Sci 2009;17(2) (in press).
110. Estrela C, Sydney GB, Figueiredo JAP, Estrela C. Antibacterial efficacy of intracanal medicaments on bacterial biofilm - A Critical Review. J Appl Oral Sci 2009;17(1) (in press).
111. Estrela CRA, Ávila GEG, Decurcio DA, Silva JA, Estrela C. Efficacy of chlorhexidine in endodontic infection - Systematic Review. Rev Bras Odontol 2008;65: (in press).
112. Estrela CRA, Estrela C, Carvalho AL, Gonella ANPF, Pécora JD. Controle microbiano e químico de diferentes soluções de hipoclorito de sódio. Rev Odontol Bras Central 2002;11:16-21.
113. Estrela CRA, Estrela C, Reis C, Bammann LL, Pécora JD. Control of microorganisms in vitro by endodontic irrigants. Braz Dent J 2003;14:187-92
114. Evans M, Davies JK, Sundqvist G, Figdor D. Mechanisms involved in the resistance of *Enterococcus faecalis* to calcium hydroxide. Int Endod J 2002;35:221-8.
115. Farber PA, Seltzer S. Endodontic Microbiology I. Etiology. J Endod 1988;14:363-71.
116. Feirer WA, Leonard V. Hexylresorcinol in oral antisepsis with special reference to solution 37. Dent Cosmos 1927;69:882-92.
117. Ferrari PH, Cai S, Bombana AC. Effect of endodontic procedures on enterococci, enteric bacteria and yeasts in primary endodontic infections. Int Endod J. 2005;38:372-80.
118. Ferraz CCR, Gomes BPFA, Zaia AA, Teixeira FB, Souza-Filho FJ. In vitro assessment of the antimicrobial action and the mechanical ability of chlorhexidine gel as an Endodontic irrigant. J Endod 2001;27:452-55.
119. Ferreira CM, Bonifácio KC, Fronner IC, Ito IY. Evaluation of the antimicrobial activity of three irrigants solutions in teeth with pulpal necrosis. Braz Dent J 1999;10:15-21.
120. Filippi A. Water disinfection of dental units using ozone - microbiological results after 11 years

and technical problems. Ozon Sci & Engineering 2002;24:479-83.
121. Foley DB, Weine FS, Hagen JC, Deobarrio JJ. Effectiveness of selected irrigants in the elimination of *Bacteroides melaninogenicus* from the root canal system: an in vitro study. J Endod 1983;9:236-41.
122. Foschi F, Cavrini F, Montebugnoli L, Stashenko P, Sambri V, Prati C. Detection of bacteria in endodontic samples by polymerase chain reaction assays and association with defined clinical signs in Italian patients. Oral Microbiol Immunol. 2005;20:289-95.
123. Fouad AF, Zerella J, Barry J, Spångberg LS. Molecular detection of *Enterococcus species* in root canals of therapy-resistant endodontic infections. Oral Surg Oral Med Oral Pathol Oral Radiol Endod. 2005;99:112-8.
124. Gambarini G, DeLuca M, Gerosa R. Chemical stability of heated sodium hypochlorite endodontic irrigants. J Endod 1998;24:432-4.
125. George S, Kishen A, Song KP. The role of environmental changes on monospecies biofilm formation on root canal wall by *Enterococcus faecalis*. J Endod. 2005;31:867-72.
126. Georgopoulou M, Kontakiotis E, Nakou M. Evaluation of the antimicrobial effectiveness of critic acid and sodium hypochlorite on the anaerobic flora of the infected root canal. Int Endod J 1994;27:139-43.
127. Gerhardt DE, Williams HN. Factors affecting the stability of sodium hypochlorite solutions used to disinfect dental impressions. Quintessence Int 1991;22:587-91.
128. Gernhardt CR, Eppendorf K, Kozlowski A, Brandt M. Toxicity of concentrated sodium hypochlorite used as an endodontic irrigant. Int Endod J 2004;37:272-80.
129. Geurtsen W. Biocompatibility of root canal filling materials. Aust Endod J 2001;27:2-21.
130. Geurtsen W, LeyhausenG. Biological aspects of root canal filling materials - Histocompatibility, cytotoxicity, and mutagenicity. Clin Oral Invest 1997;1:5-11.
131. Giardino L, Ambu E, Savoldi E, Rimondini R, Cassanelli C, Debbia EA. Comparative evaluation of antimicrobial efficacy of sodium hypochlorite, MTAD, and Tetraclean against *Enterococcus faecalis* biofilm. J Endod 2007;33:852-5.
132. Glenny AM, Esposito M, Coulthard P, Worthington HV. The assessment of systematic reviews in dentistry. Eur J Oral Sci 2003;111:85-92.
133. Gomes BP, Pinheiro ET, Gade-Neto CR, Sousa EL, Ferraz CC, Zaia AA, Teixeira FB, Souza-Filho FJ. Microbiological examination of infected dental root canals. Oral Microbiol Immunol 2004;19:71-6.
134. Gomes BP, Pinheiro ET, Sousa EL, Jacinto RC, Zaia AA, Ferraz CC, de Souza-Filho FJ. *Enterococcus faecalis* in dental root canals detected by culture and by polymerase chain reaction analysis. Oral Surg Oral Med Oral Pathol Oral Radiol Endod 2006;102:247-53.
135. Gomes BPFA, Ferraz CCR, Vianna ME, Berber VB, Teixeira FB, Souza-Filho FJ. In vitro antimicrobial activity of several concentrations of sodium hypochlorite and chlorhexidine gluconate in the elimination of *Enterococcus faecalis*. Int Endod J 2001;34:424-28.
136. Gomes BPFA, Souza SFC, Ferraz CCR, Teixeira FB, Zaia AA, Valdrigui L, Souza-Filho FJ. Effectiveness of 2% chlorhexidine gel and calcium hydroxide against *Enterococcus faecalis* in bovine root dentine in vitro. Int Endod J 2003;36:67-75.
137. Gordon TM, Damato D, Christine P. Solvent of various dilutions of sodium hypochlorite on vital and necrotic tissue. J Endod 1981;7: 466-69.
138. Gordon TM, Ranly DM, Boyan BD. The effects of calcium hydroxide on bovine pulp tissue: variations in pH and calcium concentration. J Endod 1985;11:156-60.
139. Gray JH, Henry DA, Forbes M, Germann E, Roberts FJ, Snelling CF. Comparison of silver sulphadiazine 1%, silver sulphadiazine 1% plus chlorhexidine digluconate 0.2 % and mafenide acetate 8.5% for topical antibacterial effect in infected full skin thickness rat burn wounds. Burns. 1991;17:37-40.
140. Greenhalgh T. How to read a paper: the basics of evidence based medicine. 2nd ed. London: BMJ Books;2001.
141. Grossman LI. Irrigation of root canals. J Am Dent Assoc 1943;30:1915-7.
142. Grossman LI, Meiman BW. Solution of pulp tissue by chemical agent. J Amer Dent Ass 1941;28:223-5.
143. Guerisoli DMZ, Silva RS, Pécora JD. Evaluation of some physico-chemical properties of different concentrations of sodium hypochlorite solutions. Braz Endod J 1998;3:21-3.
144. Guerisoli DMZ, Souza-Neto MD, Pécora JD. Ação do hipoclorito de sódio em diversas concentrações sobre a estrutura dentinária. Rev Odont UNAERP 1998;1:7-11.
145. Gultz J, Do L, Boylan R, Kaim J, Scherer W. Antimicrobial activity of cavity disinfectants. Gen Dent 1999;47:187-90.
146. Gutierrez JH, Jofre A, Villena F. Scanning electron microscope study on the action of endodontic irrigants on bacteria invading the dentinal tubules. Oral Surg Oral Med Oral Pathol 1990;69:491-501.
147. Haapasalo HK, Sirén EK, Waltimo TMT, Ørstavik D, Haapasalo MPP. Inactivation of local root canal medicaments by dentine; an in vitro study. Int Endod J 2000;33:126-31.
148. Haapasalo M, Ørstavik D. In vitro infection and disinfection of dentinal tubules. J Dent Res 1987;66:1375-9.
149. Haapasalo M, Qian W, Portenier I, Waltimo T. Effects of dentin on the antimicrobial properties of endodontic medicaments. J Endod 2007;33:917-25.
150. Haapasalo M, Udnes T, Endal U. Persistent, recurrent, and acquired infection of the root canal system post-treatment. Endod Topics 203;6:29-56.
151. Hales JJ, Jackson CR, Everett AP, Moore SH. Treatment protocol for the management of a sodium hypochlorite accident during endodontic therapy. Gen Dent 2001;49:278-81.
152. Hammarström L, Blomlöf L, Feiglin B, Andersson L, Lindskog S. Replantation of teeth and antibiotic treatment. Endod Dent Traumatol 1986;2:51-7.
153. Hand RE, Smith ML, Harrison JW. Analysis of the effect of dilution on the necrotic tissue dissolution property of sodium hypochlorite. J Endod 1978;4:60-4.

154. Hanks CT, Diehl ML, Craig RG, Makinen PL, Pashley DH. Characterisation of the 'in vitro pulp chamber' using the cytotoxicity of phenol. J Oral Pathol Med 1989;18:97-107.
155. Hannan M, Juste RN, Umasanker S, Glendenning A, Nightingale C, Azadian B, Soni N. Antiseptic-bonded central venous catheters and bacterial colonization. Anaesthesia. 1999;54:868-72.
156. Harrison JW, Hand RE. The effect of dilution and organic matter on the antibacterial property of 5.25% sodium hypochlorite. J Endod 1981;7:128-32.
157. Harrison JW, Wagner GW, Henry CA. Comparison of the antimicrobiol effectiveness of regular and fresh scent clorox. J Endod 1990;16:328-30.
158. Hasselgren G, Olsson B, Cvek M. Effect of calcium hydroxide and sodium hypochlorite on the dissolution of necrotic porcine muscle tissue. J Endod 1988;14:125-7.
159. Hauman CHJ, Love RM. Biocompatibility of dental materials used in contemporary endodontic therapy: a review. Part 2. Root-canal filling materials. Int Endod J 2003;36:147-60.
160. Hauman CHJ, Love RM. Biocompatibility of dental materials used in contemporary endodontic therapy: a review. Part 1. Intracanal drugs and substances. Int Endod J 2003;36:75-85.
161. Heggers JP, Sazy JA, Stenberg BD, Strock LL, McCauley RL, Herndon DN, Robson MC. Bactericidal and woundhealing properties of sodium hypochlorite solutions: the 1991 Lindberg Award. J Burn Care Rehabilit 1991;12:420-4.
162. Heil J, Reiterscheid G, Waldmann P, Leyhausen G, Geurtsen W. Genotoxicity of dental materials. Mutation Res 1996;368:181-94.
163. Helgeland K, Heyden G, Rolla G. Effect of chlorhexidine on animal's cells in vitro. Scand J Dent Res 1971;79:209-15.
164. Heling I, Chandler NP. Antimicrobial effect of irrigant combinations within dentinal tubules. Int Endod J 1998;31:8-14.
165. Heling I, Irani E, Karni S, Steinberg D. In vitro antimicrobial effect of RC-Prep within dentinal tubules. J Endod 1999;25:782-5.
166. Heling I, Pecht M. Eficacy of Ledermix paste in eliminating *Staphylococcus aureus* from infected dentinal tubules in vitro. Endod Dent Traumatol 1991;7:251-4.
167. Heling I, Rotstein I, Dinur T, Szwec-Levine Y, Steinberg D. Bactericidal and cytotoxic effects of sodium hypochlorite and sodium dichloroisocyanurate solutions in vitro. J Endod 2001;27:278-80.
168. Heling I, Sommer M, Steinberg D, Friedman M, Sela MN. Microbiological evaluation of the efficacy of chlorhexidine in a sustained-release devise for dentine sterilization. Int Endod J 1992;25:15-19.
169. Heling I, Steinberg D, Kenig S, Gavrilovich I, Sela MN, Friedman. Efficacy of a sustained-release devise containing chlorhexidine and calcium hydroxide in preventing secondary infection of dentinal tubules. Int Endod J 1992;25:20-4.
170. Hems RS, Gulabivala K, Ng Y-L, Ready D, Spratt DA. An in vitro evaluation of the ability of ozone to kill a strain of *Enterococcus faecalis*. Int Endod J 2005;38:22-9.
171. Hennessey TD. Some antibacterial properties of chlorhexidine. J Periodontol Res 1973;12:61-7.
172. Hermann BW. Calciumhydroxid Als Mittel Zum Behandel and Füllungen Von Zahnwurzelkanälen. (Doctoral Thesis), Würzburg;1920.
173. Hoffmann PN, Death JE, Coates D. The stability of sodium hypochlorite solutions. In: Collins CH et al. Disinfectants: their use and evaluation of effectiveness. London: Academic Press;1981.
174. Holland R, Ingle JI, Valle GF, Taintor JF. Influence of bony resorption on endodontic treatment. Oral Surg Oral Med Oral Pathol 1983;55:191-203.
175. Holland R, Otoboni Filho JA, Bernabe PF, de SouzaV, Nery MJ, Dezan-Júnior E. Effect of root canal filling material and level of surgical injury on periodontal healing in dogs. Endod Dent Traumatol 1998;14:199-205.
176. Holland R, Otoboni-Filho JA, Souza V, Nery MJ, Bernabé PFE, Dezan-Júnior E. A comparison of one versus two appointment endodontic therapy in dogs' teeth with apical periodontitis. J Endod 2003;29: 121-5.
177. Holland R, Otoboni-Filho JA, Souza V, Nery MJ, Bernabé PFE, Dezan-Júnior E. Tratamiento endodontico en una o en dos visitas. Estudio histológico en dientes de perros con lesión periapical. Endodoncia 2003;21:20-7.
178. Holland R, Soares IJ, Soares IM. Influence of irrigation and intracanal dressing on the healing process of dog's teeth with apical periodontitis. Endod Dent Traumatol 1992;8:223-9.
179. Hubble TS, Hatton JF, Nallapareddy SR, Murray BE, Gillespie MJ. Influence of *Enterococcus faecalis* proteases and the collagen-binding protein, Ace, on adhesion to dentin. Oral Microbiol Immunol 2003;18:121-6.
180. Hugo WB, Longworth AR. Some aspects of the mode of action of chlorhexidine. J Pharmacol 1964;16:655-62.
181. Hugo WB, Russel AD. Pharmaceutical Microbiology. 5th ed. Oxford: Blackwell;1992. p 245-99.
182. Hülsmann M, Hahn W. Complications during root canal irrigation - literature review and case reports. Int Endod J 2000;33:186-93.
183. Hülsmann M, Heckendorff M, Lennon Á. Chelanting agents in root canal treatment: mode of action and indications for their use - a review. Inter Endod J 2003;36:810-30.
184. Ingle JI, Zeldow BJ. An evaluation of mechanical instrumentation and the negative culture in endodontic therapy. J Amer Dent Ass 1958;50:471.
185. ISO. Biological evaluation of dental materials. International Organization for Standardization. Technical Report 7405;1984.
186. Jeansonne MJ, White RR. A comparison of 2% chlorhexidine gluconate and 5.25% sodium hypochlorite as antimicrobial endodontic irrigant. J Endod 1994;20:276-8.
187. Jenkins S, Addy M, Wade W. The mechanism of action of chlorhexidine. J Clin Periodontol 1988;15:415-24.
188. Jett BD, Huycke MM, Gilmore MS. Virulence of *Enterococci*. Clin Microbiol Rev 1994;7:462-78.

189. Johnson BR, Remeikis NA. Effective shelf-life of prepared sodium hypochlorite solution. J Endod 1993;19:40-3.
190. Kamburis JJ, Barker TH, Barfield RD, Eleazer PD. Removal of Organic Debris from Bovine Dentin Shavings. J Endod 2003;29:559-61.
191. Kaufman AY, Keila S. Hypersensitivity to sodium hypochlorite. J Endod 1989;15:224-6.
192. Keresztesi K, Kellner G. The biological effect of root filling materials. Inter Dent J 1966;16:222-3.
193. King SR, McWhorterAG, Seale NS. Concentration of formocresol used by pediatric dentists in primary tooth pulpotomy. Pediat Dent 2002;24:157-9.
194. Kishen, A., C. P. Sum, S. Mathew and C. T. Lim. Influence of irrigation regimens on the adherence of *Enterococcus faecalis* to root canal dentin.J Endod 2008;34:850-4.
195. Kjolen H, Andersen BM. Handwashing and disinfection of heavily contaminated hands--effective or ineffective? J Hosp Infect. 1992;21:61-71.
196. Klotz MD, Gerstein H, Bahn AN. Bacteremia after topical use of prednisolone in infected pulps. J Am Dent Assoc 1965;71:871-5.
197. Kojima K, Inamoto K, Nagamatsu K, Hara A, Nakata K, Morita I, Nakagaki H, Nakamura H. Sucess rate of endodontic treatment of teeth with vital and nonvital pulps. A meta-analysis. Oral Surg Oral Med Oral Pathol Oral Radiol Endod 2004;97:95-9.
198. Kolokuris I, Economides N, Beltes P, Vlemmas I. In vivo comparison of the biocompatibility of two root canal sealers implanted into the subcutaneous connective tissue of rats. J Endod 1998;24:82-5.
199. Komorowski R, Grad H, Wu XY, Friedman S. Antibacterial substantivity of chlorhexidine-treated bovine root dentin. J Endod 2000;26:315-7.
200. Kontakiotis, E. G., I. N. Tsatsoulis, S. I. Papanakou and G. N. Tzanetakis. Effect of 2% chlorhexidine gel mixed with calcium hydroxide as an intracanal medication on sealing ability of permanent root canal filling: a 6-month follow-up. J Endod 2008;34: 866-70.
201. Koskinen KP, Meurman JH, Stenvall H. Dissolution of bovine pulp by endodontic solutions. Scand J Dent Res 1980;88:397-405.
202. Koulaouzidou EA, Margelos J, Beltes P, Kortsaris AH. Cytotoxic effects of different concentrations of neutral and alkaline EDTA solutions used as root canal irrigants. J Endod 1999;25:21-3.
203. Kristich CJ, Li Y-H, Cvitkovitch DG, Dunny GM. Esp-Independent biofilm formation by *Enterococcus faecalis*. J Bacteriol. 2004;186:154-163.
204. Kowalski WJ, Kasper EL, Hatton JF, Murray BE, Nallapareddy SR, Gillespie MJ. *Enterococcus faecalis* adhesion, ace, mediates attachment to particulate dentin. J Endod. 2006;32:634-7.
205. Kunert IR, Bertschinger B. Uso de uma solução de Dehyquart-A na irrigação de canais radiculares. Rev Bras Odontol 1976;33:381-2.
206. Kuruvilla JR, Kamath P. Antimicrobial activity of 2.5% sodium hypochlorite and 0.2% chlorexidine gluconate separately and combined, endodontic irrigants. J Endod 1998;24:472-6.
207. Lamers AC, Vanmullen PJ, Simon M. Tissue reactions to sodium hypochlorite and iodine potassium iodine under clinical conditions in monkey teeth. J Endod 1980;6:788-92.
208. Lamont RS, Jenkinson HF. Adhesion as an ecological determinant in the oral cavity. In: Kuramitsu HK, Ellen RP. Oral bacterial ecology - the molecular basis. Horizon Scientific Press, England, 2000.
209. Law A, Messer H. An evidence-based analysis of the antibacterial effectiveness of intracanal medicaments. J Endod. 2004;30:689-94.
210. Lawrence CA. Antimicrobial activity in vitro of chlorhexidine. J Amer Pharmaceut Ass 1960;49:731-4.
211. Lehman J, Bell WA, Gerstein H. Sodium lauryl sulfate as an endodontic irrigant. J Endod 1981;7:381-4.
212. Lee Y, Han SH, Hong SH, Lee JK, Ji H, Kum KY. Antimicrobial efficacy of a polymeric chlorhexidine release device using in vitro model of *Enterococcus faecalis* dentinal tubule infection. J Endod 2008;34: 855-8.
213. Leonardo MR, Tanomaru Filho M, Silva LAB, Nelson Filho P, Bonifácio KC, Ito IY. In vivo antimicrobial activity of 2% chlorhexidine used as a root canal irrigation solution. J Endod 1999;25:167-71.
214. Lezcano I, Rey RP, Gutiérrez MS, Baluja C, Sánchez E. Ozone inactivation of *Pseudomonas aeruginosa*, *Escherichia coli*, *Shigella sonnei* and *Salmonella typhimurium* in water. Ozon Sci & Engineering 1999;21:293-300.
215. Lezcano I, Rey RP, Gutiérrez MS, Baluja C, Sánchez E. Ozone inactivation of microorganisms in water. Gram positive Bacteria and yeast. Ozon Sci & Engineering 2001;23:183-7.
216. Liu T, Gibbons RJ. Binding of streptococci of the mutans group to type 1 collagen associated with apatitic surfaces. Oral Microbiol Immunol 1990;5:131-6.
217. Lopes HP, Elias CN, Estrela C, Toniasso S. Mechanical stirring of smear layer removal: influence of the chelating agent (EDTA). Braz Endod J 1996;1:52-5.
218. Lopes HP, Siqueira JFJr. Endodontia. Rio de Janeiro: Guanabara Koogan;2004. p.964
219. Love RM. *Enterococcus faecalis* - a mechanism for its role in endodontic failure. Int Endod J 2001;34:399-405.
220. Love RM. Invasion of dentinal tubules by root canal bacteria. Endod Topics 2004;9:52-65.
221. Machtou PP, Yana Y. L'Irrigation en endodontie. Chir Dent France 1990;60:25-30.
222. Maiden MFJ, Lai CH, Tanner A. Characteristics of oral Gram-positive bacteria. In: Slots J, Taubman MA, eds. Contemporary Oral Microbiology and Immunology. St Louis, MO: Mosby 1992, pp. 342-72.
223. Manzur A, Gonzales AM, Pozos A, Silva-Herzog D, Friedman S. Bacterial quantification in teeth with apical periodontitis related to instrumentation and different intracanal medications: a randomized clinical trial. J Endod 2007;33:114-8.
224. Marsh PD. Plaque as a biofilm: pharmacological principles of drug delivery and action in the sub- and supragingival environment. Oral Diseases. 2003;9:16-22.
225. Martin DM, Crabb HS. Calcium hydroxide in root canal therapy. A review. Br Dent J 1977;142:277-83.
226. Martin H, Cunningham WT. An evaluation of postoperative pain incidence following Endosonic and conventional root canal therapy. Oral Surg Oral Med Oral Pathol 1982;54:74-6.
227. Martin H, Cunningham WT. Endosonic endodontics: the Ultrasonic Synergistic System. Int Endod J 1984;34:198-203.

228. Martin H, Spring S. Quantitative bactericidal effectiveness of an old and new endodontic irrigant. J Endod 1975;1:164-7.
229. Martinho FC, Gomes BPFA. Quantification of endotoxins and cultivable bacteria in root canal infection before and after chemo-mechanical preparation with 2.5% sodium hypochlorite. J Endod 2008;34:268-72.
230. Matsumoto K, Inoue K, Matsumoto A. The effect of newly developed root canal sealers on rat dental pulp cells in primary culture. J Endod 1989;15:60-7.
231. McComb D, Smith DC, Beagrie GS. The results of in vivo endodontic chemo-mechanical instrumentation - a SEM study. J Brit Endod Soc 1976;9:11-7.
232. McComb D, Smith DC. A preliminary scanning electron microscopic study of root canal after endodontic procedures. J Endod 1975;1:238-42.
233. McIntosh HM, Woolacoot NF, Bagnall AM. Assessing harmful effects in systematic Reviews. BMC Med Res Method 2004;4:1-6.
234. McNamara JR, Heithersay GS, Wiebkin OW. Cell responses to Hydron by a new in vitro method. Int Endod J 1992;25:205-12.
235. Mehra P, Clancy C, Wu J. Formation of a facial hematoma during endodontic therapy. J Am Dent Assoc 2000;131:67-71.
236. Mentz TCF. The use of sodium hypochlorite as a general endodontic medicament. Int Endod J 1982;15:132-6.
237. Meryon SD, Brook AM. In vitro comparison of the cytotoxicity of twelve endodontic materials using a new technique. Int Endod J 1990;23:203-10.
238. Meryon SD, Tobias RS, Jakeman KJ. Smear removal agent: a quantitative study in vivo and in vitro. J Prosth Dent 1987;57:174-9.
239. Molander A, Reit C, Dahlén G. The antimicrobial effect of calcium hydroxide in root canals pretreated with 5% iodine potassium iodide. Endod Dent Traumatol. 1999;15:205-9.
240. Moodnik RM, Dorn SO, Feldman MJ, Levey M, Borden BG. Efficacy of biomechanical instrumentation: a scanning electron microscopic study. J Endod 1976;2:261-6.
241. Morgan RW, Canes DL, Montgomery S. The solvent effects of calcium hydroxide irrigating solution on bovine pulp tissue. J Endod 1991;17:165-8.
242. Murakami H, Mizuguchi M, Hattori M, Ito Y, Kawai T, Hasegawa J. Effect of denture cleaner using ozone against methicillin-resistant *Staphylococcus aureus* and *E. coli* T1 phage. Dent Materials 2002;21:53-60.
243. Murray BE. The life and times of the *Enterococcus*. Clin Microbiol Rev. 1990;3:46-65.
244. Naenni N, Thoma K, Zehnder M. Soft Tissue Dissolution Capacity of Currently Used and Potential Endodontic Irrigants. J Endod 2004;30:785-7.
245. Nagayoshi M, Kitamura C, Fukuizumi T, Nishihara T, Terashita M. Antimicrobial effect of ozonated water on bacteria invading dentinal tubules. J Endod 2004;30:778-81.
246. Nair PNR, Henry S, Cano V, Vera J. Microbial status of apical root canal system of human mandibular first molars with primary apical periodontitis after 'one-visit' endodontic treatment. Oral Surg Oral Med Oral Pathol Oral Radiol Endod 2005;99:231-52.
247. Nair PNR, Sjögren U, Krey G, Kahnberg KE, Sundqvist G. Intraradicular bacteria and fungi in root filled, asymptomatic human teeth with therapy-resistant periapical lesions: a long-term light and electron microscopic follow-up study. J Endod 1990;16:580-8.
248. Nallapareddy SR, Qin X, Weinstock GM, Höök M, Murray BE. *Enterococcus faecalis* adhesion, ace, mediates attachment to extracellular matrix proteins collagen type IV and laminin as well as collagen type I. Infec Immun. 2000;68:5218-24.
249. Naumovich DR. Surface tension and pH of drugs in root canal therapy. Oral Surg Oral Med Oral Pathol 1963;16:965-8.
250. Nery MJ. Reação do coto pulpar e tecidos periapicais de cães a algumas substâncias empregadas no preparo biomecânico dos canais radiculares. (Doctoral Thesis). Araçatuba: São Paulo State University;1973.
251. Netuschil L, Reich E, Brecx M. Direct measurement of the bactericidal effect of chlorhexidine on dental plaque. J Clin Periodontol 1998;16:484-8.
252. Nicholls E. The efficacy of cleansing of the root canal. Br Dent J 1962;112:167-70.
253. Nikolaus BE, Wayman BE, Encinas E. The bactericidal effect of citric acid and sodium hypochlorite on anaerobic bacteria. J Endod 1988;14:31-4.
254. Nisengard RJ, Newman MG. Microbiologia oral e imunologia. 2nd ed. Rio de Janeiro: Guanabara Koogan;1994.
255. Nyborg H. Healing processes in the pulp on capping: a morphological study. Experiments on surgical lesions in the pulp in dog and man. Acta Odont Scand 1955;13:1-130.
256. Oda Y, Nakamura S, Oki I, Kato T, Shinagawa H. Evaluation of the new system (umu-test) for the detection of environmental mutagens and carcinogens. Mutation Res 1985;147:219-29.
257. Oguntebi BR. Dentine tubule infection and endodontic therapy implications. Int Endod J 1994;27:218-22.
258. Ohara PK, Torabinejad M, Kettering JD. Antibacterial effect of various endodontic irrigants on selected anaerobic bacteria. Endod Dent Traumatol 1993;9:95-100.
259. Okino LA, Siqueira EL, Santos M, Bombana AC, Figueiredo JAP. Dissolution of pulp tissue by aqueous solution of chlorhexidine digluconate and chlorhexidine digluconate gel. Int Endod J 2004;37:38-41.
260. Olgart L, Brannstron M, Johnson G. Invasion of bacteria into dentinal tubules. Acta Odontol Scand 1974;32:61-70.
261. Olsson B, Siwkowski A, Langeland K. Intraosseus implantation for biological evaluation of endodontic materials. J Endod 1981;7:253-65.
262. Olsson B, Siwkowski A, Langeland K. Subcutaneous implantation inthe biological evaluation of endodontic material. J Endod 1981;7:355-8.
263. Oncaag O, Gogulu D, Uzel A. Efficacy of various intracanal medicaments against *Enterococcus faecalis* in primary teeth: an in vivo study. J Clin Pediatr Dent 2006;30:233-7.
264. Oncag O, Hosgor M, Hilmioglu S, Zekioglu O, Eronat C, Burhanoglu D. Comparison of antibacterial and toxic effects of various root canal irrigants. Int Endod J 2003;36:423-32.

265. Ørstavik D, Haapasalo M. Disinfection by endodontic irrigants and dressing of experimentally infected dentinal tubules. Endod Dent Traumatol 1990;6:142-9.
266. Ørstavik D, Hongslo JK. Mutagenicity of endodontic sealers. Biomaterials 1985;6:129-32.
267. Ørstavik D, Mjör IA. Histocompatibility and X-ray microanalysis of the subcutaneous tissue response to endodontic sealers. J Endod 1988;14:13-23.
268. Ørstavik D. Antibacterial properties of endodontic materials. Int Endod J 1988;21:161-9.
269. Østby NB. Chelation in root canal therapy. Ethylenediamine tetracetic acid for cleasing and widening of root canals. Odontol Tidskrift 1957;65:3-11.
270. Pader M. Cosmetic science and technology series. Products components: therapeutic agents. New York Marcell Dekker Incorporat 1988;6:313-81.
271. Painter RB. Rapid test to detect agents that damage human DNA. Nature 1977;265:650-1.
272. Paiva JG, Antoniazzi JH. Endodontia - bases para a prática clínica. 1st ed. São Paulo: Artes Médicas;1984.
273. Paquete L, Legner M, Fillery ED, Friedman S. Antibacterial efficacy of chlorhexidine gluconato intracanal medication in vivo. J Endod 2007;33:788-95.
274. Pashley EL, Birdsong NL, Bowman K, Pashley DH. Cytotoxic effects of NaOCl on vital tissue. J Endod 1985;11:525-8.
275. Peciuliene V, Balciuniene I, Eriksen HM, Haapasalo M. Isolation of *Enterococcus faecalis* in previously root-filled canals in a Lithuanian population. J Endod. 2000;26:593-5.
276. Peciuliene V, Reynaud AH, Balciuniene I, Haapasalo M. Isolation of yeasts and enteric bacteria in root-filled teeth with chronic apical periodontitis. Int Endod J. 2001;34:429-34.
277. Pécora JD. Contribuição ao estudo da permeabilidade dentinária radicular. Apresentação de um método histoquímico e análise morfométrica. (Master's Dissertation). Ribeirão Preto, University of São Paulo;1985. 110p.
278. Pécora JD. Efeito das soluções de Dakin e de EDTA, isoladas, alternadas e misturadas, sobre a permeabilidade da dentina radicular. (Livre-Docência Thesis). Ribeirão Preto, University of São Paulo;1993. 148p.
279. Pécora JD. Estudo da permeabilidade dentinária do assoalho da câmara pulpar dos molares inferiores humanos, com raízes separadas. (Doctoral Thesis). Ribeirão Preto, University of São Paulo;1990. 117p.
280. Pécora JD, Barbin EL, Spanó JC, Silva RS. In vitro analysis of gas released using different concentrations of sodium hypochlorite with 3% hydrogen peroxide. Braz Endod J 1997;2:16-18.
281. Pécora JD, Costa WF, Campos GM, Roselino RB. Presentation of a histochemical method for the study of root dentine permeability. Rev Odont USP. Bauru 1987;1:3-9.
282. Pécora JD, Estrela C. Hipoclorito de sódio. In: Estrela C. Ciência Endodôntica. São Paulo: Artes Médicas;2004. p.415-55.
283. Pécora JD, Guerisoli DMZ, Silva RS, Vansan SP. Shelf-life of 5% sodium hypochlorite solutions. Braz Endod J 1997;2:43-5.
284. Pécora JD, Guimarães LF, Savioli RN. Surface tension of several drugs used in Endodontics. Braz Dent J 1991;2:123-7.
285. Pécora JD, Murgel CAF, Guimarães LFL, Costa WF. Verificação do teor de cloro ativo de diferentes marcas de líquido de Dakin encontrados no mercado. Rev Odont Univ São Paulo 1988;2:10-3.
286. Pécora JD, Murgel, CAF, Savioli RN, Costa WF, Vansan LP. Estudo sobre o *shelf life* da solução de Dakin. Rev Odont Univ São Paulo 1987;1:3-7.
287. Pécora JD, Sousa-Neto MD, Saquy PC, Silva RG, Cruz Filho AM. Effect of Dakin's and EDTA solutions on dentin permeability of root canals. Braz Dent J 1993;4:79-84.
288. Pécora JD, Sousa-Neto MD, Estrela C. Soluções irrigadoras auxiliares do preparo do canal radicular. In: Estrela C, Figueiredo JAP. Endodontia - Princípios biológicos e mecânicos. São Paulo: Artes Médicas;1999. p 552-569.
289. Pécora JD, Sousa-Neto MD, Saquy PC, Silva RG, Cruz-Filho AM. Effect of Dakin's and EDTA solutions on dentin permeability of root canals. Braz Dent J 1993;4:79-84.
290. Pécora JD, Sousa-Neto MD, Guerisoli DMZ, Marchesan MA. Effect of reduction of the surface tension of different concentrations of sodium hypochlorite solutions on radicular dentine permeability. Braz Endod J 1998;3:38-40.
291. Perez F, Rochdt T, Lodter JP, Calas P, Michel G. In vitro study of the penetration of three bacterial strains into root dentine. Oral Surg Oral Med Oral Pathol Oral Radiol Endod 1993;76:97-103.
292. Peters LB, Wesselink PR, Buijs JF, van Winkelhoff AJ. Viable bacteria in root dentinal tubules of teeth with apical periodontitis. J Endod 2001;27:76-81.
293. Peters LB, Wesselink PR, Moorer WR. Penetration of bacteria in bovine root dentine in vitro. Int Endod J 2000;33:28-36.
294. Peters LB, Wesselink PR, Moorer WR. The fate and role of bacteria left in root dentinal tubules. Int Endod J 1995;28:95-9.
295. Phillips I, Lobo AZ, Fernandes R, Gundara NS. Acetic acid in the treatment of superficial wounds infected by *Pseudomonas aeruginosa*. Lancet 1968;6:11-2.
296. Pierce AN, Heithersay G, Lindskog S. Evidence for direct inhibition of dentinoclasts by a corticosteroid/antibiotic endodontic paste. Endod Dent Traumatol 1988;4:44-5.
297. Pierce AN, Lindskog S. The effect of an antibiotic/corticosteroid paste on inflammatory root resorption in vivo. Oral Surg Oral Med Oral Pathol 1987;64:216-20.
298. Piskin B, Turkun M. Stability of various sodium hypochlorite solutions. J Endod 1995;21:253-5.
299. Portenier I, Waltimo TMT, Haapasalo M. *Enterococcus faecalis* - the root canal survivor and 'star' in post-treatment disease. Endod Topics 2003;6:135-59.
300. Pucci EM, Reig R. Conductos radiculares. Anatomia, patologia y terapia. Montevideo: A. Barreiro y Ramos; 1945.
301. Ram Z. Effectiveness of root canal irrigation. Oral Surg Oral Med Oral Pathol 1977;44:306-12.
302. Ranta K, Haapasalo M, Renta H. Monoinfection of root canal with *Pseudomonas aeruginosa*. Endod Dent Traumatol 1988;4:269-72.

303. Raphael D, Wong TA, Moodnik R, Borden BG. The effect of temperature on the bactericidal efficiency of sodium hypochlorite. J Endod 1981;7:330-4.
304. Rappaport HM, Lilliy GE, Kapsimalis P. Toxicity of endodontic filling materials. Oral Surg Oral Med Oral Pathol 1964;18:785-802.
305. Reeh ES, Messer HH. Long-term paresthesia following inadvertent forcing of sodium hypochlorite through perforation in maxillary incisor. Endod Dent Traumatol 1989;5:200-3.
306. Reynaud Af Geijersstam AH, Ellington MJ, Warner M, Woodford N, Haapasalo M. Antimicrobial susceptibility and molecular analysis of *Enterococcus faecalis* originating from endodontic infections in Finland and Lithuania. Oral Microbiol Immunol 2006;21:164-8.
307. Ribeiro RG. Estudo da permeabilidade dentinária das paredes dos canais radiculares instrumentados com diferentes soluções irrigantes, associados ou não à irradiação de laser. (Master's Dissertation). Ribeirão Preto, University of São Paulo;2001.100p
308. Ringel AM, Patterson SS, Newton CW, Miller CH, Mulhern JM. In vivo evaluation of chlorhexidine gluconate solution and sodium hypochlorite solution as root canal irrigants. J Endod 1992;8:200-04.
309. Rolla G, Melsen B. On the mechanism of the plaque inhibition by chlorhexidine. J Dent Res 1975;54:57-62.
310. Rozdzinski E, Marre R, Susa M, Wirth R, Muscholl-Silberhorn A. Aggregation substance-mediated adherence of *Enterococcus faecalis* to immobilized extracellular matrix proteins. Microb Pathol. 2001;30:211-20.
311. Safavi KE, Dowden WE, Introcaso JH, Langeland K. A comparison of antimicrobial effects of calcium hydroxide and iodine-potassium iodine. J Endod 1985;11:454-6.
312. Safavi KE, Nichols FC. Effect of calcium hydroxide on bacterial lipopolysaccharide. J Endod 1993;19:76-8.
313. Safavi KE, Nichols FC. Alteration of biological properties of bacterial lipopolysaccharide by calcium hydroxide treatment. J Endod 1994;20:127-9.
314. Safavi KE, Pascon EA, Langeland K. Evaluation of tissue reaction to endodontic materials. J Endod 1983;9:421-9.
315. Safavi KE, Spångberg LSW, Langeland K. Root canal dentinal tubule disinfection. J Endod 1990;16:207-10.
316. Saleh IM, Ryuter IE, Haapasalo MPP, Ørstavik D. Survival of *Enterococcus faecalis* in infected dentinal tubules after root canal filling with different root canal sealer in vitro. Int Endod J 2004;37:193-8.
317. Sanchez IR, Nusbaum KE, Swaim SF, Hale AS, Henderson RA, McGuire JA. Chlorhexidine diacetate and povidone-iodine cutotoxicity to canine embryonic fibroblasts and *Staphylococcus aureus*. Veter Surg 1988;17:182-5.
318. Sant'anna-Jr A. Influência da preservação ou não do coto pulpar e do tipo de cimento obturador no preparo de dentes de cães após biopulpectomia e tratamento endodôntico. (Master's Dissertation). Marília: University of Marília;2001. 205p.
319. Santa-Cecília M. Avaliação de algumas propriedades fisico-químicas e biológicas de um solução clorada experimental, para a irrigação de canais radiculares. (Doctoral Thesis). Bauru, University of São Paulo;1999. 164 p.
320. Santos TC. Estudo ìin vitroî do efeito do aumento da temperatura nas soluções de hipoclorito de sódio sobre suas propriedades físico-químicas anteriores e posteriores à dissolução do tecido pulpar bovino. (Master's thesis). Ribeirão Preto, University of São Paulo;1999. 108p.
321. Saquy PC, Maia-Campos GM, Souza-Neto MD, Guimarães LF, Pécora JD. Evaluation of chelating action of EDTA in association with Dakin's solutions. Braz Dent J 1994;5:65-70.
322. Sathorn C, Parashos P, Messer H. Antibacterial efficacy of calcium hydroxide intracanal dressing: a systematic review and meta-analysis. Int Endod J. 2007;40:2-10.
323. Savioli RN, Costa WF, Saquy PC, Antoniazzi JR, Pécora JD. Estudo comparativo entre o hipoclorito de sódio e o ácido cítrico na capacidade de limpeza do canal radicular. Rev Odontol USP 1993;7:273-7.
324. Schilder H. Limpeza e desinfecção dos canais radiculares. In: Caminhos da Polpa. Cohen S, Burs RC. 2nd. ed. Rio de Janeiro: Guanabara Koogan;1980.
325. Schmalz G, Schweikl H. Characterization of an in vitro dentin barrier test using a standard toxicant. J Endod 1994;20:592-4.
326. Schmalz G, Schweikl H, Eibl M. Growth kinetics of fibroblasts on bovine dentin. J Endod 1994;20:453-6.
327. Schmalz G. Concepts in biocompatibility testing of dental restorative materials. Clin Oral Invest 1997;1:154-62.
328. Sedgley CM, lennan L, Clewell DB. Prevalence, phenotype and genotype of oral enterococci. Oral Microbiol Immunol. 2004;19:95-101.
329. Sedgley CM, Molander A, Flannagan SE, et al. Virulence, phenotype and genotype characteristics of endodontic *Enterococcus* spp. Oral Microbiol Immunol. 2005;20:10 -19.
330. Sedgley CM, Nagel AC, Shelburne CE, Clewell DB, Appelbe O, Molander A. Quantitative real-time PCR detection of oral *Enterococcus faecalis* in humans. Arch Oral Biol. 2005;50:575-83.
331. Segura JJ, Calvo JR, Guerrero JM, Jiménez-Planas A, Sampedro C, Llamas R. EDTA inhibits in vitro substrate adherence capacity of macrophages: Endodontic Implications. J Endod 1997;23:205-8.
332. Segura JJ, Calvo JR, Guerrero JM, Sampedro C, Jimenez A, Llamas R. The disodium salt of EDTA inhibits the binding of vasoactive intestinal peptide to macrophage membranes: endodontic implications. J Endod 1996;22:337-40.
333. Segura JJ, Jiménez-Rúbio A, Guerrero JM, Calvo JR. Comparative effects of two endodontic irrigants, chlorhexidine digluconate and sodium hypochlorite, on macrophage adhesion to plastic surfaces. J Endod 1999;25:243-6.
334. Seltzer S. Endodontology. 2nd edn. Philadelphia, USA: Lea & Febiger, 1988.
335. Seltzer S, Farber PA. Microbiologic factors in endodontology. Oral Surg Oral Med Oral Pathol 1994;78:634-45.
336. Sen BH, Piskin B, Demirci T. Observation of bacteria and fungi in infected root canals and dentinal tubules by SEM. Endod Dent Traumatol 1995;11:6-9.
337. Sen BH, Safavi KE, Spångberg LSW. Antifungal effects of sodium hypochlorite and chlorhexidine in root canals. J Endod 1999;25:235-8.

338. Sen BH, Safavi KE, Spångberg LSW. Colonization of *Candida albicans* on cleaned human dental hard tissues. Arch Oral Biol 1997;42:513-20.
339. Sen BH, Safavi KE, Spångberg LSW. Growth patterns of *Candida albicans* in relation to radicular dentin. Oral Surg Oral Med Oral Pathol 1997;84:68-73.
340. Sen BH, Wesselink PR, Türkün M. The smear layer: a phenomenon in root canal therapy. Inter Endod J 1995;28:141-8.
341. Senia ES, Marshall FJ, Rosen S. The solvent action of sodium hypochlorite on pulp tissue of extracted teeth. Oral Surg Oral Med Oral Pathol 1971;31:96-103.
342. Shih M, Marshall FJ, Rosen S. The bactericidal efficiency of sodium hypochlorite as an endodontic irrigant. Oral Surg Oral Med Oral Pathol 1970;29:613-9.
343. Shiozawa A. Characterization of reactive oxygen species generated from the mixture of NaOCl and H2O2 used as root canal irrigants. J Endod 2000;26:11-5.
344. Shovelton DS. The presence and distribution of microorganisms within Non-vital Teeth. British Dent J 1964;117:101-7.
345. Silva CAG. Efetividade antimicrobiana do hipoclorito de sódio e clorexidina como irrigantes endodônticos. (Master's thesis). Porto Alegre, Luteran University of Brasil, 1999.
346. Siqueira JF, Batista MD, Fraga RC, Uzeda M. Antimicrobial effects of endodontic irrigants on black-pigmented Gram-negative anaerobes and facultative bacteria. J Endodon 1998;24:414-6.
347. Siqueira JF, Paiva SSM, Rôças IN. Reduction in the cultivable bacterial populations in infected root canals by a chlorhexidine-based antimicrobial protocol. J Endod 2007;33:541-7.
348. Siqueira Jr JF, Rôças IN, Santos SRL, Lima KC, Magalhães FAC, Uzeda M. Efficacy of instrumentation techniques and irrigation regimens in reducing the bacterial population within root canals. J Endod 2002;28:181-184.
349. Siqueira JF, Rôças IN, Paiva SSM, Guimarães-Pinto T, Magalhães KM, Lima KC. Bacteriologic investigation of the effects of sodium hypochlorite and chlorhexidine during the endodontic treatment of teeth with apical periodontitis. Oral Surg Oral Med Oral Pathol Oral Radiol Endod 2007;104:122-30.
350. Siqueira JF, Uzeda M. Intracanal medications: evaluation of the antibacterial effects of chlorhexidine, metronidazole, and calcium hydroxide associated with three vehicles. J Endod 1997;23:167-9.
351. Sirén EK, Haapasalo MP, Waltimo TM, Orstavik D. In vitro antibacterial effect of calcium hydroxide combined with chlorhexidine or iodine potassium iodide on *Enterococcus faecalis*. Eur J Oral Sci 2004;112:326 -31.
352. Siwek J, Gourlay ML, Slawson DC, Shaughnessy AF. How to write an evidence-based clinical review article. Am Fam Physician 2002;65:251-8.
353. Sjögren V, Fidgor D, Spångberg L, Sundqvist G. The antimicrobial effect of calcium hydroxide as a short-term intracanal dressing. Int Endod J 1991;24:119-25.
354. Slots J, Taubman MA. Contemporany oral microbiology and immunology. Philadelphia: Mosby;1992. 649 p.
355. Snelling CF, Inman RJ, Germann E, Boyle JC, Foley B, Kester DA, Fitzpatrick DJ, Warren RJ, Courtemanche AD. Comparison of silver sulfadiazine 1% with chlorhexidine digluconate 0.2% to silver sulfadiazine 1% alone in the prophylactic topical antibacterial treatment of burns. J Burn Care Rehabil. 1991;12:13-8.
356. Snelling CF, Roberts FJ. Comparison of 1% silver sulfadiazine with and without 1% chlorhexidine digluconate for topical antibacterial effect in the burnt infected rat. J Burn Care Rehabil. 1988;9:35-40.
357. Sonat B, Dalat D, Günhan O. Periapical tissue reaction to root fillings with Sealapex. Int Endod J 1990;23:46-52.
358. Spångberg L, Engstrom B, Langeland K. Biological effect of dental materials: 3 - toxicity and antimicrobial effects of endodontic antiseptics in vitro. Oral Surg Oral Med Oral Pathol 1973;36:856-71.
359. Spångberg L, Rutberg M, Rydinge E. Biologic effects of endodontic antimicrobial agents. J Endod 1979;5:166-75.
360. Spångberg L. Biological effects of root canal filling materials. 7. Reaction of bony tissue to implanted root canal filling material in guinea pigs. Odontol Tidskrift 1969;77:133-59.
361. Spanó JCE, Barbin EL, Santos TC, Guimarães LF, Pécora JD. Solvent action of sodium hypochlorite on bovine pulp and physico-chemical properties of resulting liquid. Brazil Dent J 2001;12:154-7.
362. Spanó JCE. Limpeza das paredes dos canais radiculares promovida por agentes desmineralizantes e quelantes: estudo *in vitro* por microscopia eletrônica de varredura e espectrofotometria dos compostos. (Doctoral Thesis). Ribeirão Preto, University of São Paulo;2008. 93 p.
363. Spijkervet FK, van Saene HK, Panders AK, Vermey A, van Saene JJ, Mehta DM, Fidler V. Effect of chlorhexidine rinsing on the oropharyngeal ecology in patients with head and neck cancer who have irradiation mucositis. Oral Surg Oral Med Oral Pathol Oral Radiol Endod. 1989;67:154-61.
364. Spratt DA, Pratten J, Wilson M, Gulabivala K. An in vitro evaluation of the antimicrobial efficacy of irrigants on biofilms of root canal isolates. Int Endod J 2001;34:300-7.
365. Stanley H. Toxicity testing of dental materials. Boca Raton: CRC Press;1985.
366. Stea S, SavarinoL, Ciabett iG, Cenni E, Stea St,Trotta F,Morozzi G, Pizzoferrato A. Mutagenic potential of root canal sealers: evaluation through Ames testing. J Biom Material Res 1994;28:319-28.
367. Steinberg D, Abid-el-Raziq D, Heling I. In vitro antibacterial effect of RC-Prep components on *Streptococcus sobrinus*. Endod Dent Traumatol 1999;15:171-4.
368. Stewart GG, Cobe RM, Rappaport R. A study of a new medicament in chemomichanical preparation of infected root canals. J Amer Dent Ass 1961;63:33-7.
369. Stewart GG, Kapsimals P, Rappaport R. EDTA and urea peroxide for root canal preparation. J Am Dent Assoc 1969;78:335-8.
370. Stewart GG. The importance of chemo-mechanical preparation of root canal. Oral Surg Oral Med Oral Pathol 1955;8:993-7.
371. Strabelli TM, Cais DP, Zeigler R, Siciliano R, Rodrigues C, Carrara D, Neres S, Lessa S, Uip DE. Clustering of *Enterococcus faecalis* infections in a cardiolo-

gy hospital neonatal intensive care unit. Braz J Infect Dis. 2006;10:113-6.

372. Strindberg LZ. The dependence of the results of pulp therapy on certain factors. An analytic study based on radiographic and clinical follow-up examination. Acta Odontol Scand 1956;14:5-175.
373. Stuart KG, Miller CH, Brown CE, Newton CW. The comparative antimicrobial effect of calcium hydroxide. Oral Surg Oral Med Oral Pathol 1991;72:101-4.
374. Sundqvist G, Fidgor D. Life as an endodontic pathogen. Ecological differences between the untreated and the root-filled root canals. Endod Topics 2003;6:3-28.
375. Sundqvist G, Figdor D, Persson S, Sjögren U. Microbiologic analysis of teeth with failed endodontic treatment and the outcome of conservative re-treatment. Oral Surg Oral Med Oral Pathol Oral Radiol Endod 1998;85:86-93.
376. Sundqvist G. Taxonomy, ecology and pathogenicity of the root canal flora. Oral Surg Oral Med Oral Path 1994;78:522-30.
377. Suzuki S, Cox CF, Leinfelder KF, Snuggs HM, Powell CS. A new copolymerized composite resin system: a multiphased evaluation. Inter J Periodont Rest Dent 1995;15:482-95.
378. Svensäter G, Bergenholtz G. Biofilms in endodontic infections. Endod Topics. 2004;9:27-36.
379. Sydney GB, Estrela C. Influence of root canal preparation on anaerobic bacteria in teeth with asymptomatic apical periodontitis. Braz Endod J 1996;1:7-10.
380. Tassery H, Remusat M, Koubi G, Pertot WJ. Comparison of the intraosseus biocompatibility of Vitremer and superEBA by implantation into the mandible of rabbits. Oral Surg Oral Med Oral Radiol Endod 1997;83: 602-8.
381. Tatnall FM, Leigh IM, Gibson JR. Comparative study of antiseptic toxicity on basal keratinocytes, transformed human keratinocytes and fibroblasts. Skin Pharmacol 1990;3:157-63.
382. Taylor HD, Austin JH. The solvent action of antiseptics on necrotic tissue. J Exp Med 1918;2:155.
383. Taylor MA, Hume WR, Heithersay GS. Some effects of Ledermix paste and Pulpdent paste on mouse fibroblasts and on bacteria in vitro. Endod Dent Traumatol 1989;5:266-73.
384. Tepel J, Darwisch el Sawaf M, Hoppe W. Reaction of inflamed periapical tissue to intracanal medicaments and root canal sealers. Endod Dent Traumatol 1994;10:233-8.
385. Thacker E. O Vinagre. São Paulo: Pacific Post Com Ldta. 2000.
386. Thé SD, Maltha JC, Plaschart AJM. Reactions of guinea pig subcutaneous connective tissue following exposure to sodium hypochlorite. Oral Surg Oral Med Oral Pathol 1980;49:460-6.
387. Thé SD. The solvent action of sodium hypochlorite on fixed and unfixed necrotic tissue. Oral Surg Oral Med Oral Pathol 1979;47:558-61.
388. Thomas GP, Adrian JC, Banks KE, Robinson JA, Peagler FD. Biocompatibility evaluation of resins in hamsters. J Prosth Dent 1985;53:428-30.
389. Torabinejad M, Cho Y, Khademi AA, Bakland LK, Shabahang S. The effect of various concentrations of sodium hypochlorite on the ability of MTAD to remove the smear layer. J Endod 2003;29:233-9.
390. Torabinejad M, Khademi AA, Babagoli J, Cho Y, Johnson WB, Bozhilov K, Kim J, Shabahang S. A new solution for the removal of the smear layer. J Endod 2003;29:170-75.
391. Torabinejad M, Shabahang S, Aprecio RM, Kettering JD. The antimicrobial effect of MTAD: an in vitro investigation. J Endod. 2003;29:400-310.
392. Torneck CD. Reaction of hamster tissue to drugs used in the sterilization of the root canal. Oral Surg Oral Med Oral Pathol 1961;14:730-47.
393. Tortora GJ, Funke BR, Case CL. Microbiology - An Introduction, 6th ed. Menlo Park, CA: Benjamin/ Cummings Publ. Comp., 1998.
394. Trepagnier CM, Maden RM, Lazzari EP. Quantitative study of sodium hypochlorite as on in vitro endodontic irrigant. J Endod 1977;3:194-6.
395. Tucker JW, Mizrahi S, Seltzer S. Scanning electron microscopic study of efficacy of various irrigating solutions: urea, tubulicid red and tubulicid blue. J Endod 1976;2:71-7.
396. Türkün M, Cengiz T. The effects of sodium hypochlorite and calcium hydroxide on tissue dissolution and root canal cleanliness. Int Endod J 1997;30:335-42.
397. Vahdaty A, Pitt Ford TR, Wilson RF. Efficacy of chlorhexidine in disinfecting dentinal tubules in vitro. Endod Dental Traumatol 1993;9:243-8.
398. Valnet J. Aromathérapie. Paris: Librairie Maloine Éditeur. 1973.
399. Vande Visse JE, Brilliant JD. Effect of irrigation on the production of extrused material at the root apex during instrumentation. J Endod 1975;1:243-6.
400. Vianna ME, Horz HP, Conrads G, Zaia AA, Souza-Filho FJ, Gomes BPFA. Effect of root canal procedures on endotoxins and endodontic pathogens. Oral Microbiol Immunol 2002;22:411-8.
401. Vianna ME, Horz HP, Gomes BPFA, Conrads G. In vivo evaluation of microbial reduction after chemo-mechanical preparation of human root canals containing necrotic pulp tissue. Int Endod J 2006;39:484-92.
402. von der Fehr FR, Nygaard-Jstby B. Effect of EDTAC and sulphuric acid on root canal dentine. Oral Sur Oral Med Oral Pathol 1963;16:199-205.
403. Wadachi R, Araki K, Suda H. Effect of calcium hydroxide on the dissolution of soft tissue on the root canal wall. J Endod 1998;24:326-30.
404. Walker A. A definite and dependable therapy for pulpless teeth. J Am Dent Ass 1936;23:1418-25.
405. Walker C. Antimicrobial Agents and Chemoterapy I. In: Oral microbiology and immunology. Slots J, Taubman MA. St. Louis: Mosby Year Book;1992. p.5242-64.
406. Walker TL, del Rio CE. Histological evaluation of ultrasonic debridement comparing sodium hypochlorite and water. J Endod 1991;17:66-71.
407. Walters MJ, Baumgartner JC, Marshall JG. Efficacy of irrigation with rotatory instrumentation. J Endod 2002;28:837-9.
408. Waltimo TMT, Siren EK, Torkko HLK, Olsen I, Haapasalo MPP. Fungi in therapy-resistant apical periodontitis. Int Endod J 1997;30:96-101.
409. Walton RE, Torabinejad M. Principles and Practice of Endodontics, 2nd ed. Philadelphia:W.B. Saunders Co., 1996. p.214-5.
410. Washington BC, Villalba MR, Lauter CB, Colville J, Starnes R. Cefamandole-erythromycin-heparin

peritoneal irrigation: an adjunct to the surgical treatment of diffuse bacterial peritonitis. Surgery. 1983;94:576-81.

411. Wayman B, Kopp WM, Pinero GJ, Lazzari EP. Citric and latic acids as root canal irrigants in vitro. J Endod 1979;5:258-64.
412. Webb BC, Willcox MDP, Thomas CJ, Harty DWS, Knox KW. The effect of sodium hypochlorite on potential pathogenic traits of *Candida albicans* and other Candida species. Oral Microbiol Immunol 1995;10:334-41.
413. Weeks RS, Ravitch MM. The pathology of experimental injury to the cat esophagus by liquid chlorine bleach. Laryngoscope 1971;81:1532-41.
414. Weiss EI, Shalhav M, Fuss Z. Assesment of antibacterial activity of endodontic sealers by a direct contact test. Endod Dent Traumatol 1996;12:179-84.
415. Weller RN, Brady JM, Bernier WE. Efficacy of ultrasonic cleaning. J Endod 1980;6:740-3.
416. White RR, Hays GL, Janer LR. Residual antimicrobial activity after canal irrigation with chlorhexidine. J Endod 1997;23:229-31.
417. Williams DF. Definitions in Biomaterials. Oxford: Elsevier, 1987.
418. Williams JM, Trope M, Caplan DJ, Shugars DC. Detection and quantitation of *Enterococcus faecalis* by real-time PCR (qPCR), reverse transcription-PCR (RT-PCR), and cultivation during endodontic treatment. J Endod 2006;32:715-21.
419. Winkler KC. Bacteriologic results from 4000 root canal cultures. Oral Surg Oral Med Oral Pathol 1959;12:857-75.
420. Wittgow WC, Sabiston-Jr CB. Microorganisms from pulpal chambers of intact teeth with necrotic pulps. J Endod 1975;1:168-71.
421. Witton R, Henthorn K, Ethunandan M, Brennan PA. Neurological complications following extrusion of sodium hypochlorite solution during root canal treatment. Int Endod J 2005;38:843-8.
422. Yamada RS, Armas A, Goldman M, Lin SP. A scanning electron microscopic comparison of a high volume final flush with several irrigating solutions. J Endod 1983;9:137-42.
423. Yang SF, Rivera EM, Baugardner KR, Walton RE. Anaerobic tissue-dissolving abilities of calcium hydroxide and sodium hypochlorite. J Endod 1995;21:613-6.
424. Yang SF, Rivera EM, Walton RE, Baugardner KR. Canal debridement: Effectiveness of sodium hypochlorite and calcium hydroxide as medicaments. J Endod 1996;22:521-5.
425. Yesilsoy C,Whitaker E Cleveland D, Phillips E, Trope M. Antimicrobial and toxic effects of established and potential root canal irrigants. J Endod 1995;21:513-5.
426. Yeung SY, Huang CS, Chan CP, Lin CP, Lin HN, Lee PH, Jia HW, Huang SK, Jeng JH, Chang MC. Antioxidant and pro-oxidant properties of chlorhexidine and its interaction with calcium hydroxide solutions. Int Endod J 2007; 34:4-8.
427. Yoshida T, Shibata T, Shinohara T, Gomyo S, Sekine I. Clinical evaluation of the efficacy of EDTA solution as an endodontic irrigant. J Endod 1995;21:592-3.
428. Zamany A, Safavi K, Spångberg LS. The effect of chlorhexidine as an endodontic disinfectant. Oral Surg Oral Med Oral Pathol Oral Radiol Endod 2003;96:578-81.
429. Zehnder M, Grawehr M, Hasselgren G, Waltimo T. Tissue-dissolution capacity and dentin-disinfecting potential of calcium hydroxide mixed with irrigating solutions. Oral Surg Oral Med Oral Pathol Oral Radiol Endod 2003;96:608-13.
430. Zehnder M, Kosicki D, Luder H, Sener B, Waltimo T. Tissue-dissolving capacity and antibacterial effect of buffered and unbuffered hypochlorite solutions. Oral Surg Oral Med Oral Pathol Oral Radiol Endod 2002;94:756-62.
431. Zehnder M. Root canal irrigants. J Endod 2006;32:389-98.
432. Zerella JA, Fouad AF, Spångberg LS. Effectiveness of a calcium hydroxide and chlorhexidine digluconate mixture as disinfectant during retreatment of failed endodontic cases. Oral Surg Oral Med Oral Pathol Oral Radiol Endod 2005;100:756-61.
433. Zerlotti-Filho E. Contribuição à terapêutica dos condutos radiculares. (Docoral Thesis) Campinas, Universidade Católica de Campinas;1959.
434. Zuolo M, Murgel CAE, Pécora JD, Antoniazzi JH, Costa WF. Ação do EDTA e suas associações com tensoativos na permeabilidade da dentina radicular. Rev Odont USP 1987;1:18-23.

# Calcium Hydroxide

**C. Estrela**
*Federal University of Goiás, Goiânia, GO, Brazil*

**R. Holland**
*São Paulo State University, Araçatuba, SP, Brazil*

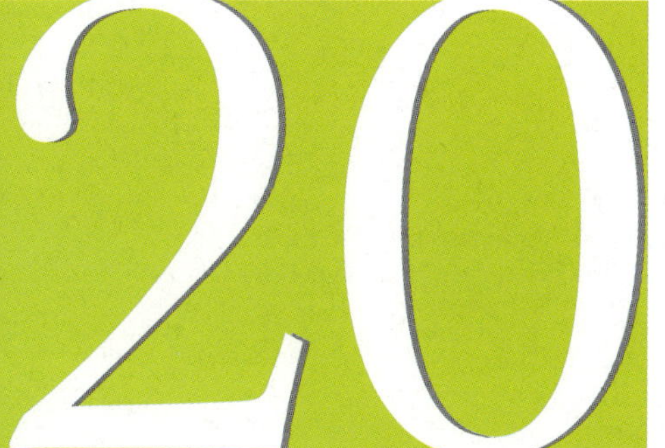

Chapter contents

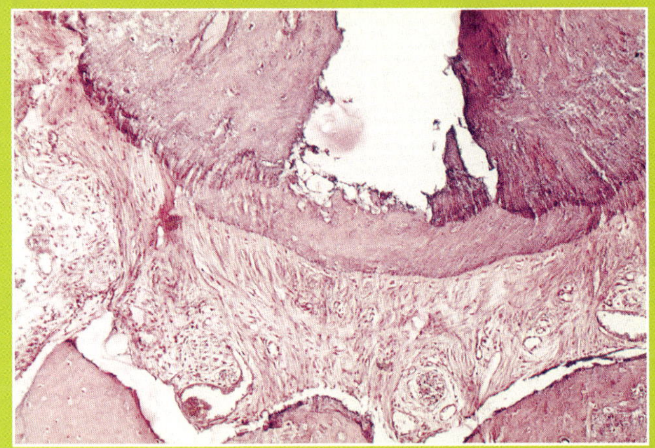

Calcium hydroxide used as an intracanal dressing. Complete closure of the main root canal by neoformed cementum (H.E. X100) (Holland et al.[265])

## 20.1 Introduction

Knowledge about the mechanisms of microbial aggression after pulp necrosis and therapeutic resources to neutralize them has motivated the study of intracanal medicaments. The importance of microorganisms in the root canal has been the object of discussion for many years. Microbial control in endodontic infections allows a high success rate in endodontic treatment[1-645].

The goal of endodontic treatment is to eliminate microorganisms from the root canal system by means of the association of procedures, i.e., biomechanical preparation, irrigation with different solutions, and the use of intracanal dressings. Nevertheless, root canal preparation under infected conditions does not allow complete microbial elimination.

Thus, it is necessary to consider that endodontic treatment performed in a single appointment is not the best therapeutic option, since several steps are required, which include: indicating an intracanal dressing – to maintain the sanitization process in difficult situations of vital pulp conditions; to reduce endodontic microbiota in primary and secondary infections; control persistent exudates; neutralize activity of the osteoclasts present in inflammatory dental resorption; treat large apical periodontitis; favor apical closure in apexification; and to treat root perforations.

Calcium hydroxide has been studied for many years[109-150,231-240,244-300]. The German, Bernhard W. Hermann (Würzberg, Germany, 1920) concluded his PhD in natural science with the pioneer research on calcium hydroxide[237] (Calxyl-Otto & CO; Frankfurt, Germany) and suggested it for dental pulp treatment. For Stanley[567] a new era had begun. Some years later, in 1966, in his PhD thesis, Holland[245,246] described the biologic mechanism of action of calcium hydroxide in the connective tissue of dogs, in his PhD thesis. In 1994 and 1995, Estrela et al.[146,147] discussed the probable antimicrobial mechanism of action of calcium hydroxide.

The selection of the intracanal dressing is based on important referential parameters – firstly, depending on its antimicrobial potential; secondly, histocompatibility and lastly, the capacity of favoring the tissue healing process. Thus, it is necessary to consider knowledge of the endodontic microbiota (primary or secondary infection); the mechanism of action of calcium hydroxide; antimicrobial efficacy of intracanal dressing - the time it takes to act in dentinal tubules, microbial resistance and tissue tolerance.

## 20.2 Chemical Characteristics of Calcium Hydroxide

Chemical analysis of the essential aspects of calcium hydroxide is important in order to use it correctly, i.e., the influence of the vehicle on the rate of ionic dissociation and diffusion into dentinal tubules, the influence on mineralization and antimicrobial effectiveness.

Calcium hydroxide is a strong base obtained by the calcination (heating) of calcium carbonate until it is transformed into calcium oxide. Calcium hydroxide is obtained through the hydration of calcium oxide, and the chemical reaction between calcium hydroxide and carbon dioxide forms calcium carbonate. It is a white powder with a high pH (12.6) and is slightly soluble in water (solubility of 1.2 g/L, at a temperature of 25°C) (Fig. 20.1)[109-111,130,587].

The properties of calcium hydroxide come from its dissociation into calcium and hydroxyl ions and the action of these ions on tissues and bacteria explains biological and antimicrobial properties of this substance. Changes in the biological properties can also be understood through the chemical reactions, since calcium hydroxide, in the presence of carbon dioxide, becomes calcium carbonate, and this product does not have the biological properties of calcium hydroxide, such as the mineralizing capability[146,147].

Estrela & Pesce[138] chemically analyzed the release of calcium and hydroxyl ions from calcium hydroxide pastes in the connective tissue of a dog, by means of conductimeter analysis. The vehicles had different acid-bases and hydrosolubility characteristics (saline, anesthetic and polyethylene glycol 400). The release of hydroxyl ions from the pastes can be demonstrated by the release of calcium ions and hydroxyl ions and the molecular weight of calcium hydroxide. Taking into account the molecular weight of calcium hydroxide, which is 74.08, using a rule of three, one can find the percentage of hydroxyl ions found in calcium hydroxide, which is 45.89%, while 54.11% corresponds to calcium ions. The percentage values of calcium and hydroxyl ions released by calcium hydroxide pastes over a period of 7, 30, 45 and 60 days, indicated greater ionic liberation for the pastes with hydrosoluble vehicles (Fig. 20.2-20.7).

The formation of calcium carbonate in the connective tissue of dogs showed that when a saline vehicle is used with calcium hydroxide, the formation rate of calcium carbonate is practically unaltered after 30 days, and up to 60 days (Fig. 20.8-9). The values in mass of calcium carbonate are small, with an increase up to 30 days and stabilizing at 30-60 days. After the initial reaction of calcium hydroxide with tissue, a reduction in the number of changes of the intracanal medication can be observed, especially after initial inflammatory alterations. Thus, with prudent clinical extrapolation, in extensive periapical lesions, dental trauma injuries, and apexification there can be a change of the calcium hydroxide paste after a long interval (i.e., 60 days). The characteristics of calcium hydroxide resulting from ionic release are directly influenced by carbon dioxide which, by forming a weak acid, could cause partial neutralization of the basic medication[137].

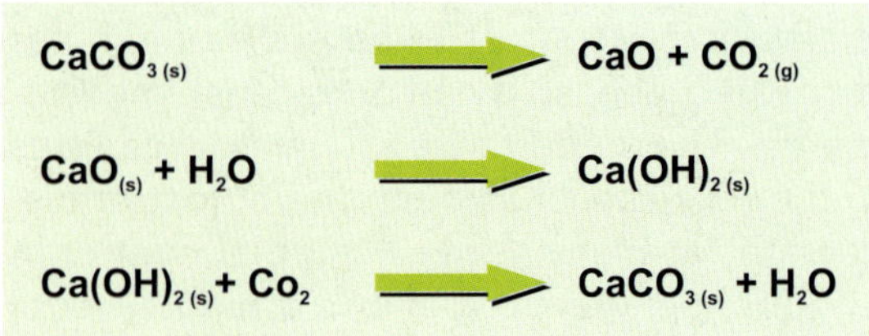


**Figure 20.1** - Calcium hydroxide production.

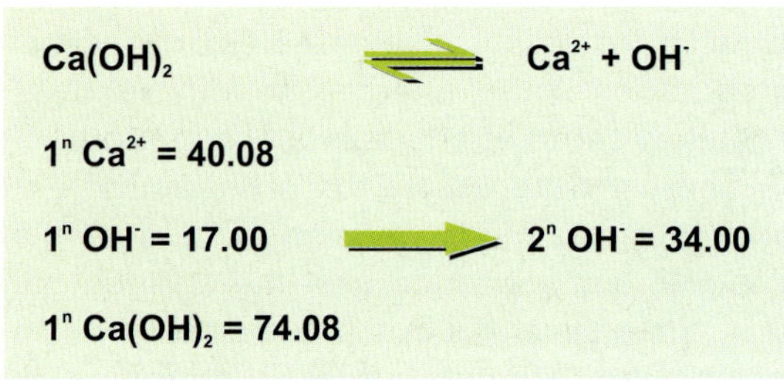


**Figure 20.2** - Ionic dissociation of calcium hydroxide.

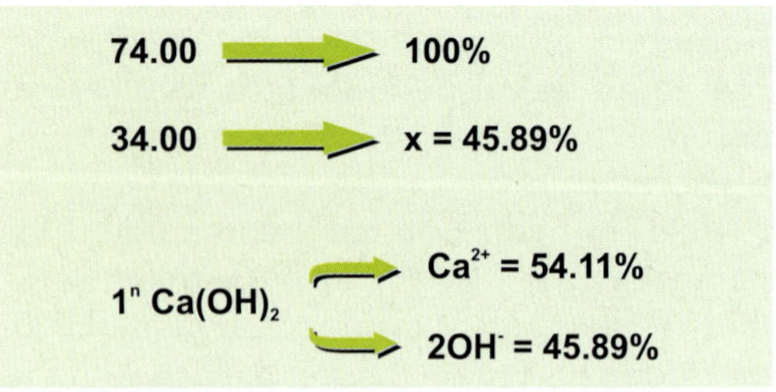


**Figure 20.3** - Ionic dissociation of calcium hydroxide

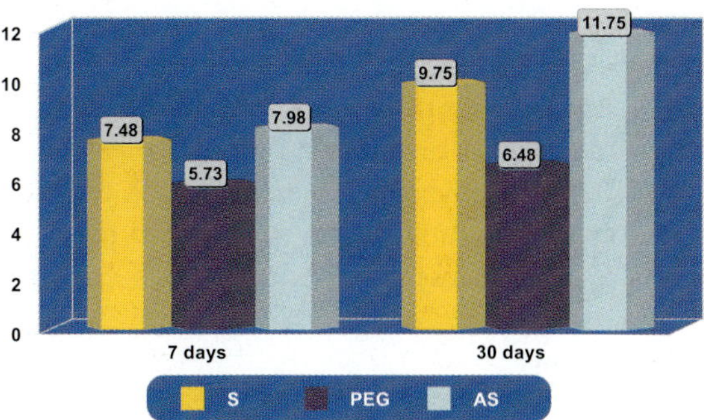


Figure 20.4 - Release of hydroxyl ions.

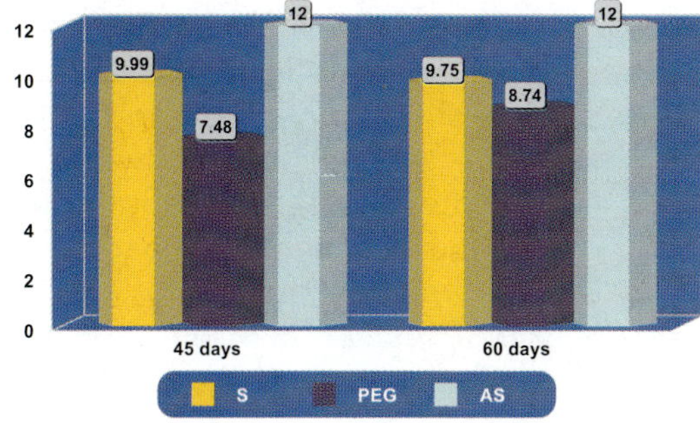


Figure 20.5 - Release of hydroxyl ions.

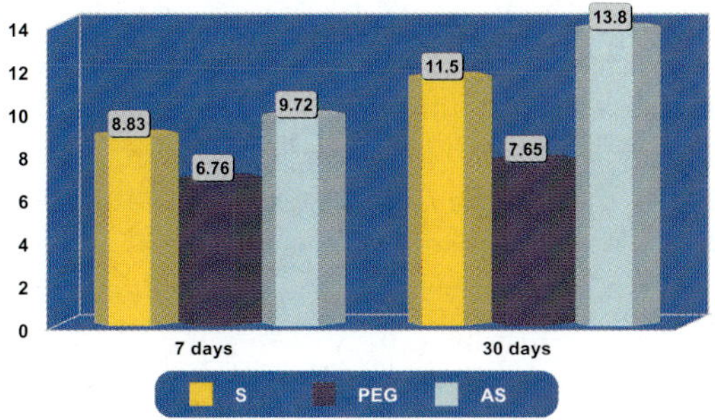


Figure 20.6 - Release of calcium ions.

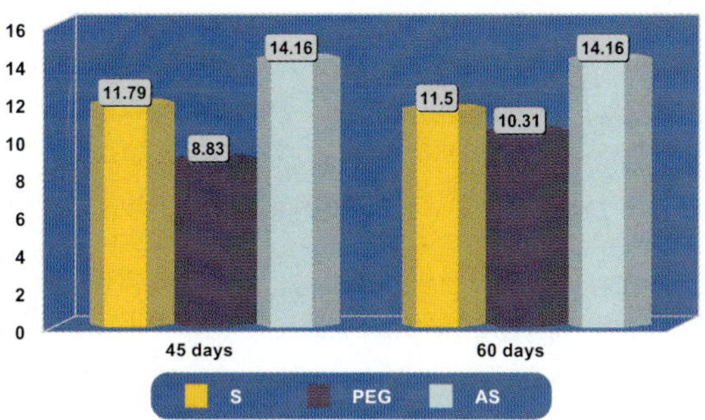


Figure 20.7 - Release of calcium ions.

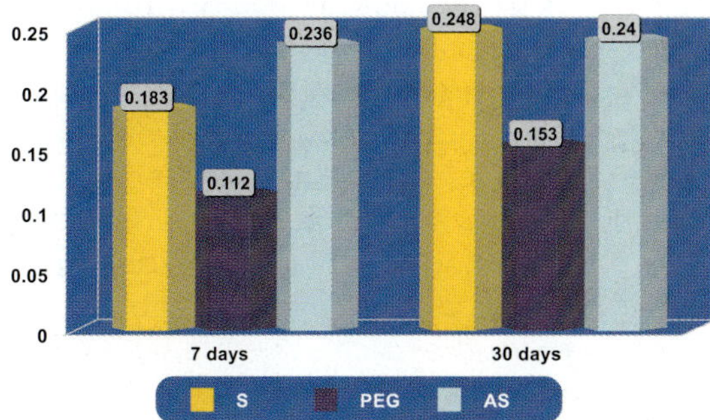


Figure 20.8 - Calcium carbonate formation.

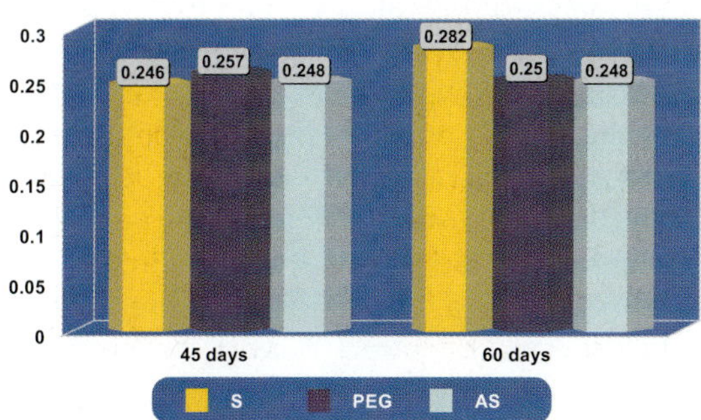


Figure 20.9 - Calcium carbonate formation.

Other chemical characteristics resulting from ionic dissociation of calcium hydroxide have been observed in various studies. Sciaky & Pisanti[509] and Pisanti & Sciaky[460] did not observe that any of the calcium ions in the mineralized barrier came from calcium hydroxide, used in the protection of the exposed pulps of dogs, and which contained radioactive calcium ($Ca^{45}$); or from the intravenous injection in dogs, with a solution containing radioactive calcium. This probably happened due to the methodology applied, since the authors used autoradiography.

Various studies showed the active participation of calcium ions from calcium hydroxide in mineralization (mineralization barrier on dental pulp, in apical biological sealing), in dentinal tubules, and in other areas involved in mineralization[244-301].

Through histochemical analysis, EDA[104] studied the mechanism of the formation of mineralized barriers after the application of direct pulp protection in dog teeth, through the action of calcium hydroxide, magnesium oxide, zinc fluorite and calcium fluorite pastes. After an observation period ranging from 30 minutes to 60 days, the author reported that during the initial stage of dentin formation, the mineralized barrier could be seen as extremely thin particles that reacted positively to von Kossa dye, and underlay the necrosed layer.

These small grains originated from the reaction of the capping material metal with the tissue carbon dioxide. Moreover, magnesium oxide and calcium hydroxide showed powerful effects on the new dentin formation. Nevertheless, Souza et al.[554], in a morphological study of the dental pulp behavior after pulpotomy, followed by protection, using magnesium oxide or calcium hydroxide, reported that the possibility of restoration using magnesium oxide was remote. Treatment in the pulp protected with calcium hydroxide was more effective, and eliminated the technical failure that occurred during the treatment with magnesium oxide.

A few minutes after the pulp tissue comes into contact with calcium hydroxide, necrotic areas begin to form. Right at the limit between the live and necrotic tissue there is deposition of calcium salts, and dentin is observed about 15 days after treatment[246]. Calcium hydroxide in direct contact with conjunctive tissue originates a zone of necrosis, altering the physical-chemical status of intercellular substance which, through rupture of glycoproteins, seems to determine protein denaturation[246].

Holland[245] analyzed the healing process in the dental pulp after pulpotomy and capping with calcium hydroxide, in a morphological and histochemical study carried out in dog teeth. The author reported that in the superficial grainy zone, interposed between the necrosed zone and the deep grainy zone, there was the presence of rough grains endowed with calcium salts, some of them composed of calcium carbonate, in the form of calcite and of calcium-protein compounds. These observations demonstrate the active participation of calcium ions from calcium hydroxide used as protective material, in the healing process. In this mineral fraction, there was positive reaction to chloranilic acid and the von Kossa method. Holland et al.[287], in another study in rat connective tissue after the implant of calcium hydroxide paste, verified the deposit of calcium salt (calcite) into dentinal tubules.

Seux et al.[521] obtained similar results to those of the Holland et al.[245] research. Seux et al.[521] studied odontoblast-like cytodifferentiation of human dental pulp cells in vitro in the presence of a calcium hydroxide-containing cement. The cement produced microcrystals of calcite by reaction with a culture medium supplemented with calf serum. Human dental pulp cells seeded on such a substrate adhered and aggregated preferentially around the microcrystals. Immunofluorescence and immunogold labeling revealed a high affinity of serum fibronectin molecules for the calcite crystals. At 4 weeks in the culture, the cells had various features of differentiated odontoblasts, notably nuclear polarization, typical appearance of the

Golgi apparatus, synthesis of type I collagen and absence of type III, and apical accumulation of actin and vimentin. These cells also elaborated a collagenous extracellular matrix that did not mineralize.

Holland et al.[286] analyzed the effect of calcium hydroxide on dentin. Dentin tubes filled with calcium hydroxide or zinc oxide-eugenol cement were implanted for 48 hours in rat subcutaneous connective tissue. Deep cavities, prepared in dog teeth, were protected with same materials, for 48 hours. The undecalcified specimens were prepared for histological analysis with polarized light. A highly birefringent structure, located in the interior of the dentin tubules was observed only in the dentin treated by calcium hydroxide. This result suggested that calcium hydroxide acts on dentin in the same way as it does on pulp tissue.

The behavior of periapical tissue filled with calcium hydroxide was observed in other studies[253] that demonstrated excellent results, particularly showing biological apical closure (Fig. 20.10–20.11).

Heithersay[231] admits that calcium ions may be of importance when calcium hydroxide is used in the treatment of pathologies associated with pulpless teeth. These ions can reduce capillary permeability in the mass of new capillaries in granulation tissue associated with these pulpless teeth. One particular enzyme involved in most productive energy-using processes, is pyrophosphatase, which is also calcium ion dependent. This enzyme is

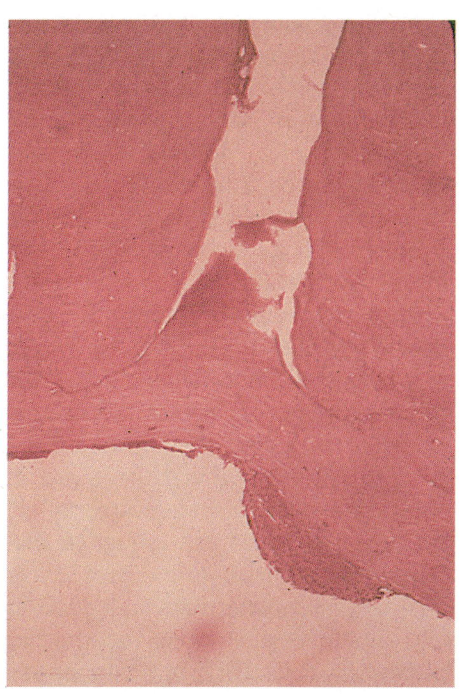

**Figure 20.10** - 180 days after calcium hydroxide filling in human tooth. Biological sealing (Holland et al.[253]).

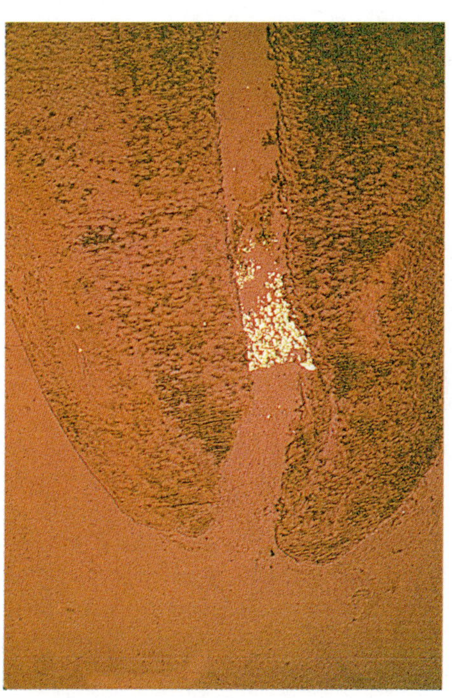

**Figure 20.11** - Undecalcified sections were examined under polarized light. Granulations of calcita (Holland et al.[253]).

a member of phosphatase enzymes, important in the mineralization process.

Other hydroxides were also evaluated regarding their effects on pulp tissue. Holland et al.[270] evaluated the effect of calcium hydroxide, barium hydroxide and strontium hydroxide after pulp capping, using histochemical analysis in the dental pulps of dogs. The results among the three hydroxides were similar, and showed deposits of strontium carbonate and barium carbonate grains, resembling the graining observed with calcium hydroxide. Since barium and strontium are not naturally present in the animal body, these grains originated from the capping material. They also reported that no presence of birefringent large grains was observed with the use of other hydroxides, such as magnesium hydroxide or sodium hydroxide, because the sedimentary reaction (sedimentation) only occurs with hydroxides that have solubility similar to that of calcium hydroxide. Magnesium hydroxide is insoluble and sodium hydroxide is highly soluble in pulp fluids. Barium hydroxide is slightly more soluble than strontium hydroxide, and this can be observed because barium hydroxide grains have been found deeper down than strontium hydroxide grains. Once again, this research confirms the active participation of calcium ions from the calcium hydroxide of the protective material in the healing process.

Pashley et al.[449], studied the effects of calcium hydroxide on dentin permeability. When the calcium hydroxide treated smear layer was exposed to 6% citric acid for two minutes, dentin permeability returned to the initial acid-etched value, demonstrating that calcium hydroxide offers little protection against acid challenge. Treatment of acid-etched dentin with calcium hydroxide produced a similar reduction in dentin permeability, which was restored to normal following acid challenge. Thus, calcium hydroxide is effective in vitro for reducing the permeability of both the smear layer and of acid-etched dentin. Wakabayashi et al.[619] evaluated the mechanism of dystrophic calcification, induced by calcium hydroxide in the connective tissue of a rabbit auricular chamber. The interactions between the microvessels and the calcium hydroxide were observed right after the application, and throughout the following 14 weeks. During the initial phases of tissue reaction, the results revealed the formation of a necrotic layer and calcifications seen as a fast sedimentation of crystals through neutralization, and immediately growing into a barrier (dystrophic calcification). They also observed that additional calcium and phosphorus was deposited right over the sedimentation particles. Furthermore, they found that in 24 hours, specimen sedimentation showed not only calcium peaks, but also weak peaks of phosphorus, sulphur and/or magnesium, in the melted portion among the crystals, and suggested that such sedimentation would have the potential to induce dystrophic calcification, which is in agreement with the findings of Holland et al.[245]

Tronstad et al.[598] verified pH changes in different areas of root dentin in monkey teeth after filling root canals with calcium hydroxide paste. Untreated teeth with pulp necrosis had a pH of 6.0 to 7.4 in the pulp, dentin, cementum, and periodontal ligament. Replanted and nonreplanted teeth with complete root formation and treated with calcium hydroxide showed pH values in the circumpulpal dentin of 8.0 to 11.1, and in the more peripheral dentin of 7.4 to 9.6. In teeth with incomplete root formation, the entire dentin showed a pH of 8 to 10. The pH of the cementum was not influenced by calcium hydroxide; however, in resorption areas, an alkaline pH was also observed on the exposed dentinal surfaces. Based on these results, it can be concluded that root canal filling with calcium hydroxide can influence the resorption areas (complicate the osteoclastic activities), and stimulate the repair process.

Holland et al.[287] observed the deposition of calcium salts in rat subcutaneous connective tissue reacting with implanted dentin tubes filled with mineral trioxide aggregate, Sealapex, Calciobiotic Root Canal Sealer (CRCS), Sealer 26, and the experimental material, Sealer Plus. The animals were sacrificed after 7 and 30 days, and the specimens were prepared for histological analysis after serial sections. The undecalcified sections were examined under polarized light after staining according to the Von Kossa technique for calcium. At the tube openings, there were Von Kossa-positive granules that were birefringent to polarized light. Next to these granulations, there was irregular bridge-like tissue that was Von Kossa positive. The dentin walls of the tubes exhibited a structure highly birefringent to polarized light, usually similar to a layer in the tubules. In conclusion, with the exception of CRCS, it is possible that the mechanism of action of the materials in encouraging hard tissue deposition is similar to the one described by Holland et al.[253] for calcium hydroxide.

Nerwich et al.[428] analyzed pH changes in root dentin over a 4-week period following root canal dressing with calcium hydroxide. Root canals in extracted human teeth were cleaned and shaped, and subsequently dressed with a calcium hydroxide root canal dressing. pH changes in the root dentin were measured over a 4-week period with microelectrodes in small cavities at apical and cervical levels in inner and outer dentin. The pH increased within hours in the inner dentin, peaking at pH 10.8 cervically and 9.7 apically. However, 1 to 7 days elapsed before the pH began to rise in the outer root dentin, reaching peak levels of pH 9.3 cervically and 9.0 apically after 2 to 3 weeks. Hydroxyl ions derived from a calcium hydroxide dressing do diffuse through root dentin faster and reach higher levels cervically than apically. Surface pH measurements showed that hydroxyl ions diffuse through the intact root surface only to an insignificant extent.

Estrela et al.[150] evaluated the dentinal diffusion of hydroxyl ions of calcium hydroxide pastes prepared with different acid-based vehicles, in a nitrogen inert atmosphere. Sixty maxillary central incisors with mature apexes were selected, and after access and root canal preparation, each root was filled with calcium hydroxide pastes prepared with different vehicles: saline solution, anesthetic and polyethylene glycol 400. The roots were then sectioned 2 mm from the apical vertex, and the teeth mounted in the center of a round platform, filled with saline solution up to 2 mm from the root tip. The platforms remained in a nitrogen inert atmosphere, completely sealed, in the absence of light and at a constant temperature of 36.5°C. Diffusion analysis of the hydroxyl ions was carried out by a colorimetric method on days 7, 15, 30, 45 and 60. Calcium hydroxide pastes prepared with saline solution and anesthetic showed a pH change of 6-7 to 7-8 after 30 days, and remained at this level at 60 days. In the polyethylene glycol 400 group, the same alteration occurred at 45 days, and continued at 60 days. Estrela & Sydney[145] determined in vitro, the influence of EDTA on root dentin pH during exchange of calcium hydroxide paste. Thirty maxillary central human incisors were selected, and after opening the pulp chamber, root canals were prepared using a stepback preparation technique. 1% sodium hypochlorite was used as the irrigant solution, and the root canals were the dried and filled with EDTA for 3 minutes. Root canals were then again irrigated with sodium hypochlorite, dried and completely filled with calcium hydroxide paste, using saline as the vehicle. Analysis of the diffusion of hydroxyl ions was carried out by a colorimetric method, using a universal indicating solution. This analysis was done at 7, 15, 30, 45, 60 and 90 days; after each analysis, the calcium hydroxide paste was exchanged in the root canals and EDTA was applied for 3 minutes. The results showed a pH change of 6-7 to 7-8 after 30 days, remaining at this level at 90 days in the apical and middle thirds; and in the cervical thirds there was a pH change of 6-7 to 7-8 after 30 days, and a change of pH to 8-9 at 60 days remaining at this level at 90 days. The Kruskal Wallis test showed no significant difference between the different thirds and the time.

Considering that the release of hydroxyl ions from calcium hydroxide is essential to the mineralization and microbial control processes, it is important to investigate the necessity of using vehicles that favor a quick ionic dissociation as well as maintaining a high pH during the entire period of activity.

The pH analyses of vehicles and pastes added to calcium hydroxide were performed over a period ranging from 0 to 160 days and the results were recorded in an electronic chart by Estrela et al.[135]. The pH of the following phenolic substances was studied: paramonochorophenol (5g) associated with Furacin® (28 ml) and camphorated paramonochorophenol, isolated and associated with 24 mg (0.12%) of calcium hydroxide P.A. The pH of the following non-phenolic substances was also studied: 0.1% sodium lauryl diethylene ether sulphate; 0.1%Tween 80; de-ionized distilled water; propylene glycol added to 24 mg (0.12%) of calcium hydroxide P.A., stored in plastic containers. Pastes with non-phenolic vehicles (de-ionized water, propylene glycol, sodium lauryl diethylene ether sulphate and Tween 80) showed high pH values (above 12). The paste, whose vehicle was camphorated paramonochorophenol, showed a pH around 7.8 during the entire period of observation and camphorated paramonochorophenol itself maintained a pH of 5. PMC-Furacin showed a pH of 7.0 and the paste containing this substance showed a pH of 10 during the period of observation.

The influence of vehicle on the rate of ionic dissociation of calcium hydroxide is a significant aspect related to its mechanism of action, and the importance of its role is emphasized when preparing the calcium hydroxide paste.

Safavi & Nakayama[490] evaluated the influence of the mixing vehicle on the dissociation of calcium hydroxide in solution. The antimicrobial effects of aqueous preparations of calcium hydroxide have been demonstrated in the past. Calcium hydroxide, when dissolved in water, dissociates into hydroxide and calcium ions. The presence of hydroxide ions in a solution makes it antimicrobial. Recently it was shown that the use of glycerin as a mixing vehicle facilitates placement of calcium hydroxide in the root canals. The influence of nonaqueous mixing vehicles on the dissociation of calcium hydroxide is not clearly understood. In this study the conductivity values for saturated solutions of calcium hydroxide in water was 7.3 $\pm$ 3 mS/cm. The conductivity of calcium hydroxide in pure glycerin or propylene glycol was essentially zero. It was concluded that the use of nonaqueous mixing vehicles might impede the effectiveness of calcium hydroxide as root canal dressing. Estrela et al.[128] studied the molar conductivity of different calcium hydroxide-based solutions. They investigated the molar conductivity of 120mg of calcium hydroxide combined with 0.1% sodium lauryl ether sulfate, 0.1% Tween 80, and deionized, distilled water (100 ml). The results for the solutions – 0.1%sodium lauryl ether sulfate, 0.1% Tween 80, and deionized water – combined with calcium hydroxide showed conductivity of 5057.74, 4976.87, and 4936.45 microsiemens, respectively. These differences were not significant.

Different substances (distilled water, saline solution, propylene glycol, camphorated paramonochorophenol(CMPC), chlorhexidine, glycerin, iodoform, barium sulfate, corticosteroid-antibiotic, antibiotics, anesthetic solution, methylcellulose, glycerin, detergent) have been associated with calcium hydroxide[130]. However, the change in dentinal pH caused by hydroxyl ions is slow and depends on several factors that can alter the rate of ionic dissociation and diffusion, such as the level of hydrosolubility of the vehicle used, difference in viscosity, acid-base characteristic, dentinal permeability, buffering capacity of dentin and level of existing calcification[130]. The viability of microorganisms is influenced by high pH values.

The pH of vehicles and calcium hydroxide pastes have presented interesting results, such as the low pH (5.0) of CMPC, the intermediate pH (7.8) resulting from the association of calcium hydroxide and CMPC and the high pH (12.6) of calcium hydroxide pastes associated with distilled water, sodium lauryl diethylene ether sulfate, Tween 80 and polyethylene glycol[135].

Knowledge of the influence of substances on ionic dissociation of calcium hydroxide and the capacity of hydroxyl ions to diffuse into the dentinal tubules is critical, because the result could affect its effectiveness.

Different properties of medications for endodontic use have been studied: antimicrobial effectiveness, biocompatibility, tissue solvency, pH, solubility, molar conductivity and surface tension, thus, their biological behavior is considered important. Nevertheless, for an endodontic substance to fully develop its action mechanism, it first needs to reach the target site. It is therefore essential to know the surface tension of the different substances for endodontic use, in order to select them based on their ability to penetrate dentin.

Özcelik et al.[445] compared the surface tension of calcium hydroxide alone, and its combinations with different vehicles (glycerin, Ringer's solution, anesthetic solution and saline. The results showed that the anesthetic solution is the most favorable vehicle, with the lowest surface tension values (44.00 and 51.00 dynes/cm).

Estrela et al.[125] evaluated the surface tension of calcium hydroxide, associated with different substances (deionized distilled water, CMPC, 2% chlorhexidine digluconate, Otosporin, 3% sodium lauryl ether sulphate; Furacin, PMC Furacin) using a tensiometer. The action of the substances studied on the dentinal structure enhanced the property of surface tension. This method consisted of the application of force to separate a platinum ring immersed in the substances. Thus, torsion was applied to the screw until the platinum ring separated during testing of the substances. Considering the methodology applied, it could be concluded that: distilled water alone or associated with calcium hydroxide presented a high surface tension (70.00 and 68.40 dynes/cm); calcium hydroxide in association with anionic detergent showed low surface tension (31.60 dynes/cm); camphorated paramonochorophenol plus calcium hydroxide presented low surface tension (37.50 dynes/cm); 2% chlorhexidine associated with calcium hydroxide showed high surface tension values (58.00 dynes/cm); Otosporin plus calcium hydroxide showed low surface tension (35.40 dynes/cm); paramonochorophenol Furacin mixed with calcium hydroxide presented surface tension equal to 45.50 dynes/cm; and sodium hypochlorite presented high surface tension (75.00 dynes/cm). The antimicrobial agents most indicated in endodontics, i.e. calcium hydroxide, chlorhexidine and hypochlorite, presented the highest surface tensions. The data obtained in this study[125] are shown in Figures 20.12 and 20.13. Although CMPC plus calcium hydroxide showed surface tension equal to 37.50 dynes/cm, the pH value was 7.8. Nevertheless, distilled water with calcium hydroxide presented high surface tension (68.40 dynes/cm), but the pH value was higher (12.80). Estrela et al.[136] determined the influence of vehicles (saline solution, CMPC, chlorhexidine, 3% sodium lauryl sulphate, Otosporin®) on the antimicrobial efficiency of calcium hydroxide paste. The various vehicles associated with calcium hydroxide pastes did not influence the time required for microbial inactivation, which suggests that they play a supportive role in the process by providing appropriate conditions for dissociation and diffusion, as well as enhancing complete filling of the root canal; these are important factors for antimicrobial potential and tissue healing capability[125].

The association of chlorhexidine plus calcium hydroxide showed a high surface tension (58.00 dynes/cm) and pH values equal to 10.2[125].

Nevertheless, the association of 3% sodium lauryl ether sulphate plus calcium hydroxide presented a low surface tension (31.60 dynes/cm) and high pH (12.5). Estrela et al.[128] observed no significant differences when comparing the molar conductivity of solutions containing sodium lauryl ether sulfate, Tween 80 and deionized water combined with calcium hydroxide. As irrigant solution, calcium hydroxide plus detergent (lauryl diethylene glycol ether sodium sulphate) did not show a stronger antimicrobial action, when compared with sodium hypochlorite or chlorhexidine[153].

Other chemical aspects are associated with the quality of calcium hydroxide, specifically in terms of the source of calcium carbonate present. Estrela et al.[132], using chemical analyses in their study, verified the formation of calcium carbonate in seven samples obtained from private Endodontic clinics, as follows: Quimis (Mallinckradt Inc., USA), PT Baker (USA), Calen (SS White, RJ, Brazil), Vigodent (RJ, Brazil), Merck (USA), Biodinâmica (PR, Brazil), Inodon (RS, Brazil). The presence of calcium carbonate in samples of calcium hydroxide stored for 2 years in containers under varying conditions was determined by means of volumetric analysis of neutralization, using hydrochloric acid, and visualization with methyl orange and phenolphthalein. The level of calcium hydroxide converted into calcium carbonate was not significant enough to interfere with its properties, ranging from 5 ± 1% to 11 ± 1%. Better results were obtained with samples of Quimis - 5%$CaCO_3$ and JT Baker - 6%$CaCO_3$.

The effectiveness of calcium hydroxide is as important as the correct filling of the radicular canal, as the lack of direct contact of this dressing interferes with its mechanism of action. Estrela et al.[133] investigated the density of calcium hydroxide pastes with different vehicles, without association with radiopaque substances and in comparison with dentin density using dog teeth. The results demonstrated that it is not necessary to add radiopaque substances to calcium hydroxide pastes, since pastes used without them showed densities similar to dentin, thus not justifying their use. Moreover, when any substance is added to calcium hydroxide, even an inert one, it represents one more factor to influence biological processes, also bringing the possibility of diminishing the amount of hydroxyl and calcium ions available, which is one of the reasons for using it.

## 20.3 Mechanism of action of Calcium hydroxide

Recent advances in cellular and molecular biology, biochemistry and microbiology have brought a better understanding and better definitions of certain mysteries still present in endodontics. Modern thinking has moved towards the use of an intracanal dressing, with a potentially effective action against dif-

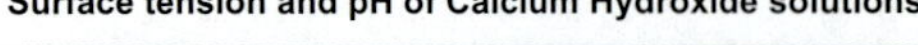


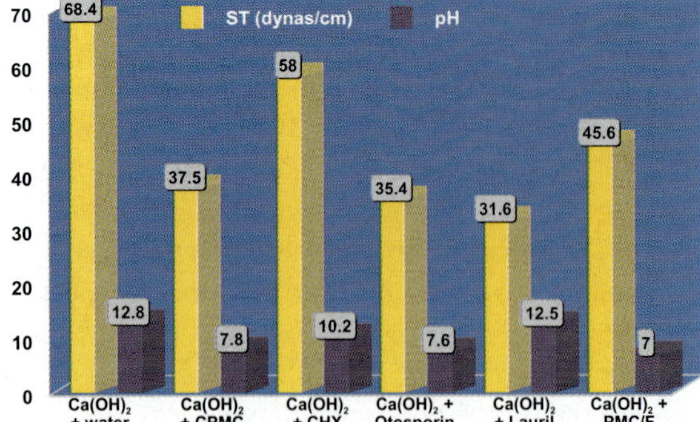


**Figure 20.12** - Surface tension of calcium hydroxide solutions.

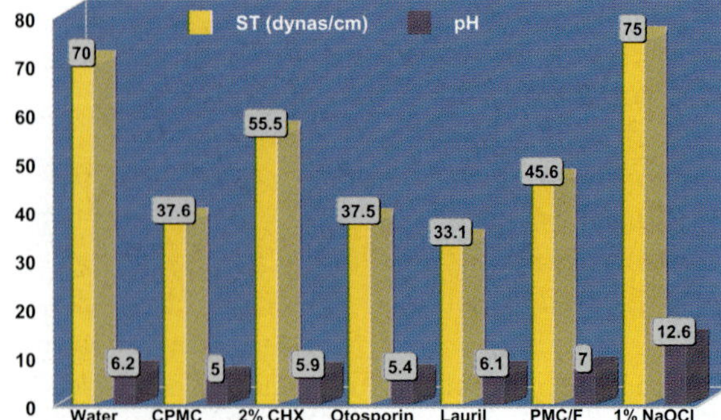


**Figure 20.13** - Surface tension of vehicles associated with calcium hydroxide.

ferent types of respiratory bacteria (aerobic, anaerobic and microaerophiles) which act by inhibiting the action of osteoclasts present in the area of dental resorption and favor the repair process of altered periapical tissue.

The destruction of bacterial life is dependent on the conditions related to their growth and multiplication, among which are physical-chemical factors such as: temperature, pH, osmotic pressure, concentrations of oxygen, carbon dioxide and substrate[46,597].

It has been noted that the response of the periapical tissues to endotoxins produced by Gram-negative bacteria, which are predominant in infected radicular canals, assures an opportunity for the repair of the destroyed tissue architecture. This can be observed by re-establishing the periodontal ligament, and reintegrating the alveolar bone, in conjunction with osteocement formation.

A primary root canal infection is associated with endodontic microbiota, generally composed of Gram-negative anaerobic bacteria. In secondary infection the microorganisms favor structured apical periodontitis. The microbiota present in this case (post-treatment disease) is largely composed of Gram-positive organisms, particularly *E. faecalis* (Fig. 20.14-20.17).

Ideally, an intracanal medicament should be able to neutralize the virulence of microorganisms and pathogenic factors (such as proteins, enzymes, toxins, aggregation substances), to alter growth and multiplication,



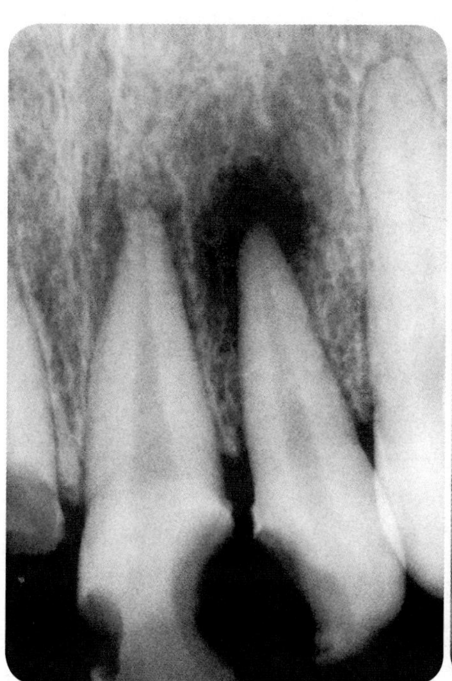

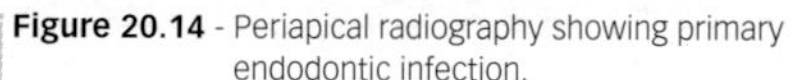

**Figure 20.14** - Periapical radiography showing primary endodontic infection.

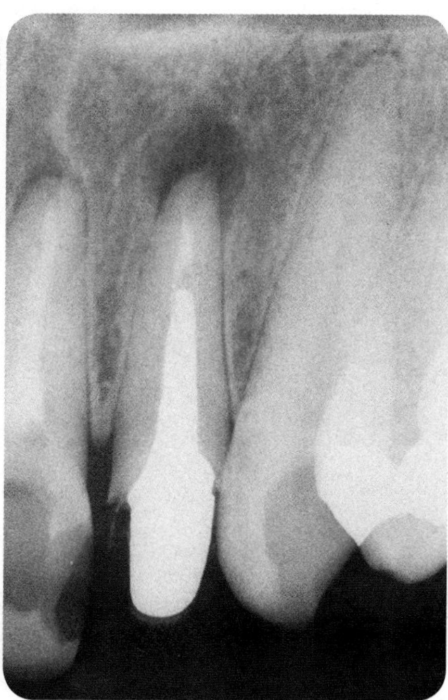

**Figure 20.15** - Periapical radiography showing secondary endodontic infection.

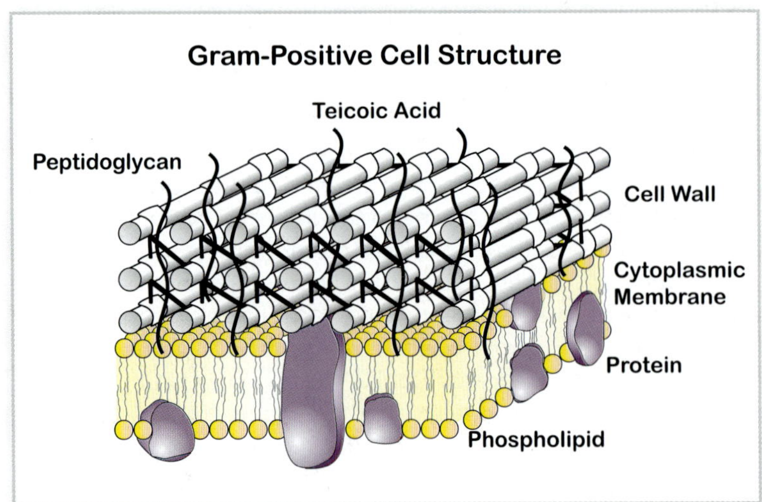


**Figure 20.16** - Diagram of the envelope of a Gram–positive cell (adjusted from Tortora et al.[597]).

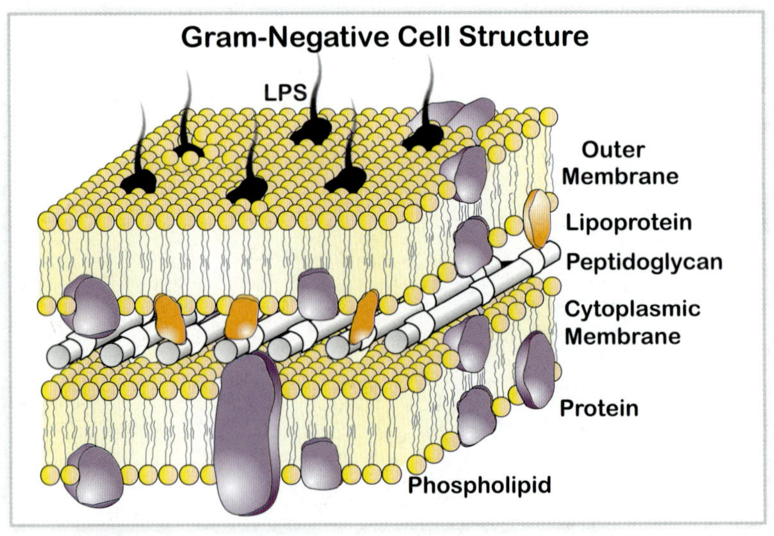


**Figure 20.17** - Diagram of the envelope of a Gram–negative cell (adjusted from Tortora et al.[597]).

and induce a host response that favors periapical tissue healing.

For this reason, the intracanal dressing must be effective against bacteria that may have escaped and survived after root canal preparation, the control of persistent exudates and the inactivation of the osteoclasts present in external dental resorption.

The success of calcium hydroxide as an intracanal dressing is due to its ionic effect observed by the chemical dissociation into calcium and hydroxyl ions and its action on tissue and bacteria[130,146,147].

Its capacity to stimulate tissue repair through the induction of mineralization, confirms the biological action of calcium hydroxide[246,247]. Its antibacterial action has also been shown to be superior when compared with other substances[146].

The greatest concern in the selection of any dressing, is the knowledge of its mechanism of action against the predominant microbiota in infected root canals. The mechanism of action of calcium hydroxide as an antimicrobial medication may be better understood, if one refers to knowledge about the microbiological and pharmacological properties of antibiotics/chemotherapeutics and their effects on microorganisms, and more specifically, their sites of action. Antimicrobial substances, such as antibiotics and/or chemotherapeutics have two types of effects on microorganisms: inhibit growth and reproduction, and induce cellular inactivation. These effects can be observed in cellular wall synthesis, altering the permeability of cytoplasmic membrane, chromosomal replication and intermediate metabolism[130,136,146,147].

From this line of reasoning, one can ask about the site of action of calcium hydroxide. Could its mechanism of action be considered similar to that of Penicillin or Cephalosporine, or identical to that of Nystatin or Polymyxin? The answer given by the literature at hand is that calcium hydroxide is an exceptional antibacterial agent due to its elevated pH.

Nevertheless, on adopting as a reference, the effects of antibiotics against bacteria, and more specifically the site of action, the phenomenon of the action of calcium hydroxide as an antibacterial agent will be better elucidated. For this reason it is important to analyze the isolated effect of pH on bacterial growth and metabolism, and cellular division[130,136,146,147].

The influence of pH on growth, metabolism and bacterial cell division is important to explain the mechanism of antimicrobial action of calcium hydroxide.

The locale of essential enzymatic systems of bacteria is the a cytoplasmic membrane where they involve themselves in the last stages of the formation of the cellular wall, participate in the bio-synthesis of lipids, and are responsible for the conveyance of electrons, as enzymes involved in the process of oxidative phosphorylation. Formed by a double phospholipoprotein layer, it acts as an osmotic barrier to ionized substances and to large molecules, being freely permeable to sodium ions and amino acids (selective permeability). When necessary, several bacteria produce proteinases that hydrolyze proteins and amino acids, since bacteria are generally incapable of using macro-molecules[111,335,358,427,468].

The enzymes located in the cytoplasmic membrane are related to the conveyance of substances to the interior and to the exterior of the cell, by structuring the cellular wall and respiratory activity. Extra-cellular enzymes act on the nutrients, carbohydrates, proteins and lipids which, by means of hydrolysis, favor digestion. To sum up, the enzymatic systems of the cytoplasmic membrane take on primordial functions for the bacteria, such as metabolism and cellular growth and division[335].

On the other hand, the catalytic activity of the enzymes can be regulated by variations in the pH of the medium. Each enzyme has an optimum pH at which its speed of reaction is maximum[29,335]. There is, however, a difference between the internal pH of the bacteria and that of the medium, possibly being responsible for the influence of pH on bacterial cellular activity, however, the mechanism that maintains the internal neutrality is unknown[335].

The enzymes present internally and externally in the cytoplasmic membrane influence their complex metabolic reactions, and the speed of the chemical reactions favored by these enzymes is influenced by the substrate. It is believed that control of the flow of nutrients alters chemical conveyance through the membrane, which is essential to bacterial life[335,358,427,468].

The energy necessary for the movement of organic nutrients and components into the cell, is obtained through a pH gradient, present in the cytoplasmic membrane, which can be altered by a change of pH in the medium. The effect of the pH on chemical movement can be direct or indirect. It is direct when the pH influences the specific activity of the proteins of the membrane, by combination with the specific chemical group. On the other hand, the indirect effect can lead to alterations in the ionization states of the organic components. The transfer through the membrane is easier for non-ionized than for ionized components. Depending on the pH, there will be an increase in nutrient availability, and an intense transfer can induce inhibition and toxic effects on the cell. Thus, the enzymatic activity of bacteria is inhibited under conditions of elevated pH (high concentration of hydroxyl ions)[335].

Adjustment of intracellular pH is influenced by different cellular processes such as: a) cellular metabolism, b) alterations in shape, mobility, adjustment of transporters and polymerization of cytoskeleton components, c) activation of cellular proliferation and growth, d) conductivity and transport through the membrane, and e) isosmotic cellular volume. Thus, many cellular functions can be affected by pH, including the enzymes that are essential to cellular metabolism[468].

The influence of the pH on the transfer and permeability of the cytoplasmic membrane probably explains the microbiological action of the hydroxyl ions of calcium hydroxide on the control of bacterial enzymatic activity. The conveyance of nutrients and the return of the catabolites through the cytoplasmic membrane must be carried out naturally.

Estrela et al.[147] in 1994 studied the biological effect of pH on the enzymatic activity of anaerobic bacteria. The authors believe that the hydroxyl ions from calcium hydroxide develop their mechanism of action in the cytoplasmic membrane, because enzymatic sites are located in the cytoplasmic membrane. This membrane is responsible for essential functions such as metabolism, cellular division and growth, and it takes part in the final stages of cellular wall formation, biosynthesis of lipids, transport of electrons and oxidative phosphorylation. Extracellular enzymes act on nutrients, carbohydrates, proteins, and lipids that favor digestion through hydrolysis. Intracellular enzymes located in the cell favor respiratory activity of the cellular wall structure. The pH gradient of the cytoplasmic membrane is altered by the high concentration of hydroxyl ions of calcium hydroxide acting on the proteins of the membrane (protein denaturation). The effect of the high pH of calcium hydroxide alters the integrity of the cytoplasmic membrane by means of chemical injury to organic components and transport of nutrients, or by means of the destruction of phospholipids or unsaturated fatty acids of the cytoplasmic membrane, observed in the peroxidation process, which is a saponification reaction.

During bacterial growth at a pH lower than the internal pH, the cytoplasm becomes more alkaline than the medium; when growth occurs at high pH, its cytoplasm becomes more acid[335,358,427,468]. Bacterial growth at high pH can induce more complex physiological complications.

Based on pH gradient, a few species of bacteria can grow at pH lower than 2 or higher than 10. Most of the pathogenic bacteria grow in neutral environments[434].

When exposed to a pH level above or below the ideal for its activity, reversible enzymatic inactivation could occur. At an ideal pH, the enzyme can recover its catalytic activity. Irreversible enzymatic inactivation can be observed under extreme conditions of pH over a long period of time, with complete loss of biological activity[109,358,427].

Extreme values of pH cause the development of most of the globular proteins, and the loss of their biological activities without breaking their covalent bonds in the polypeptidic skeleton. Therefore, it was demonstrated that as a result of pH, some denatured globular protein recovered its native structure and biological activities when the pH returned to normal values, this process being denominated renaturing[358].

For this reason, the elevated pH of calcium hydroxide, with values reaching 12.6, is due to the great release of hydroxyl ions which are capable of altering the integrity of the bacterial cytoplasmic membrane, either through the toxic effects generated during the transfer of nutrients, or through the destruction of the phospholipids of unsaturated fats[109,146,147].

Lehninger[358] relates that extreme pH values cause the uncoiling of many proteins, with loss of their biological activities. For many years the denaturation process was thought to be irreversible. If, however, pH returns to its normal value, the native structure of the lost biological activity is returned, that is to say, there is renaturation. Kodukula et al.[335] also consider that reactivation of catalytic activity is possible when the enzyme resumes operating in an ideal pH.

Understanding of the mechanism of action of the pH of calcium hydroxide in the control of bacterial enzymatic activity, allowed Estrela et al.[147] to propose the hypothesis of an irreversible bacterial enzymatic inactivation under extreme pH conditions for a long period of time, and also a temporary bacterial enzymatic inactivation with the restoration of normal activity when the pH returns to the ideal level for enzymatic activity. Irreversible enzymatic inactivation was demonstrated by Estrela et al.[141] who determined the direct antimicrobial effect of calcium hydroxide on different microorganisms (*M. luteus, S. aureus, P. aeruginosa, F. nucleatum, E. coli* and *Streptococcus sp.*) during periods of 0, 1, 2, 6, 12, 24, 48, and 72 hours and 7 days. The changes in the integrity of the cytoplasmic membrane of the microorganisms, which favored their destruction, occurred after 72 hours in both pure and mixed cultures. Reversible enzymatic inactivation could be observed in another study carried out by Estrela et al.[140] who assessed the antimicrobial effect of calcium hydroxide in dentinal tubules infected by different microorganisms, for periods of 0, 48, and 72 hours and 7 days. Calcium hydroxide was ineffective in action at a distance during a period of 7 days against *E. faecalis, S. aureus, P. aeruginosa* and *B. subtillis*. These biological activities of calcium hydroxide in tissues and against bacteria can be influenced by vehicles, making it necessary to know more about their importance and properties.

Rubin & Farber[483] reported that the action of hydroxyl ions on cellular membrane is produced by the chemical mechanism related to lipidic peroxidation. The loss of integrity of the membrane can be observed through the destruction of unsaturated fatty acids or phospholipids. When the hydroxyl ion removes a hydrogen atom from a fatty acid, a free lipidic radical is formed which, on reacting with the oxygen molecule, is transformed in a lipidic peroxide radical. The peroxide thus formed can act as a new inductor, drawing another hydrogen atom of a second unsaturated fatty acid, resulting in another lipidic peroxide and another new free lipidic radical, transforming itself into a chain reaction[483].

The neutralization of bacterial toxins is an essential aspect in the selection of an antimicrobial agent. Safavi & Nichols[492] studied the effect of calcium hydroxide on bacterial lipopolysaccharide (LPS). The calcium hydroxide treatment of LPS was shown to release elevated quantities of hydroxy fatty acids. It was concluded that calcium hydroxide hydrolyzed the lipid moiety of bacterial LPS, resulting in the release of free hydroxyl fatty acids. This result suggests that calcium hydroxide-mediated degradation of LPS may be an important reason for the beneficial effects obtained with calcium hydroxide use in clinical endodontics. In another study, Safavi & Nichols[491] investigated the alteration of biological properties of bacterial lipopolysaccharide by calcium hydroxide treatment. It was concluded that the treatment with calcium hydroxide may alter biological properties of bacterial LPS.

Buck et al.[44] analyzed the detoxification of endotoxin by endodontic irrigants (chlorhexidine, NaOCl, chlorhexidine chloride, ethanol, EDTA, water) and calcium hydroxide and reported that the biologically active portion of endotoxin, lipid A, is hydrolyzed by highly alkaline chemicals, namely calcium hydroxide or a mixture of chlorhexidine, sodium hypochlorite and ethanol. EDTA, NaOCl, chlorhexidine, chlorhexidine, chloride, ethanol and water (control) showed little or no detoxifying ability for lipid A.

Different studies[47,155,598] have shown that some bacteria can be resistant to calcium hydroxide when this medication has a pH of approximately 11. Evans et al.[155] studied the mechanisms involved in the resistance of *E. faecalis* to calcium hydroxide. *E. faecalis* was resistant to calcium hydroxide at a pH of 11.1 but not pH 11.5. No difference in cell survival was observed when protein synthesis was blocked during stress induction, however, addition of a proton pump inhibitor resulted in a dramatic reduction of cell viability of *E. faecalis* in calcium hydroxide. Survival of *E. faecalis* in calcium hydroxide appears to be unrelated to stress induced by protein synthesis, but a functioning proton pump is critical for the survival of *E. faecalis* at high pH.

Considering the previous discussion about the enzymatic characteristics of calcium hydroxide, irreversible enzymatic inactivation was demonstrated by the direct antimicrobial effect of calcium hydroxide on different microorganisms (*E. faecalis, S. aureus, P. aeruginosa* and *B. subtillis*). The changes in the integrity of the cytoplasmic membrane of the microorganisms favored their destruction, which occurred after 72 hours[141]. Reversible enzymatic inactivation could be observed in another study carried out by Estrela et al.[140] who assessed antimicrobial effect of calcium hydroxide in infected root canals by the same microorganisms, for periods of 0, 48, and 72 hours and 7 days. Calcium hydroxide was ineffective in action at a distance during a period of 7 days. Thus, the effectiveness by a direct contact of calcium hydroxide, such as intracanal dressing occurs immediately in all microorganisms of endodontic infection. However, for bacteria present in the dentinal tubules, the intracanal dressing requires time to dissociate and to diffuse dentin, and this depends on the time that the intracanal dressing is kept in the root canal. Thus, whenever possible, it is necessary to allow time for the calcium hydroxide paste to manifest its potential action on the microorganisms present in endodontic infections. The maintenance of a high concentration of hydroxyl ions can change enzymatic activity and promote its inactivation.

Based on these affirmatives, it is inferred that when a medication does not reach the target microorganisms, it cannot express its real efficacy to kill them. Therefore, one cannot say whether or not the microbial strains were resistant to one or other medication. In this case, it is likely that the microorganisms were able to survive, adapt and tolerate the critical ecological conditions[124].

On the other hand, it is also important to consider the biological mechanism of action on dental pulps, which was studied by Holland[246] (in 1966) and Holland et al.[244-301] in various investigations. The healing process of the dental pulp of dogs, after pulpotomy and protection with calcium hydroxide was characterized by the following zones[246]: 1. Necrotic zone – located under the calcium hydroxide and presenting both high reactivity to the histochemical stainings and resistance to the action of buffers and enzymes. 2. Outer granular zone - located immediately underneath the necrotic zone and characterized by birefringent granules that were formed by 2 fractions. A mineral fraction, positive to the calcium reaction, which contained glycoprotein complexes and metachromatic stainable material. 3. Inner granular zone - located under the outer granular zone and characterized by the presence of thin granulations that could be identified by von Kossa's method and by chloranilic acid. 4. Cellular proliferation zone - located under the inner granular zone and presenting connective cell proliferation; the cytoplasm of these cells had great amounts of RNA and glycoprotein complexes, and a small number of granulations containing glycogen. During the healing process some alterations could be seen, mainly in the granular and cellular proliferation zones. In the inner granular zone, there was a progressive increase in deposition of calcium compounds. In the cell proliferation zone, young odontoblasts determined dentin formation.

Researches about tissue repair induction in dental pulp and antimicrobial effectiveness in endodontic infections have shown calcium hydroxide as the best option[109-154,244-301] (Fig. 20.18-20.21). Two of the important enzyme properties of calcium hydroxide are the activation of tissue enzymes, such as alkaline phosphatase, causing a mineralizing effect, and the inhibition of bacterial enzymes causing an antimicrobial effect[130].



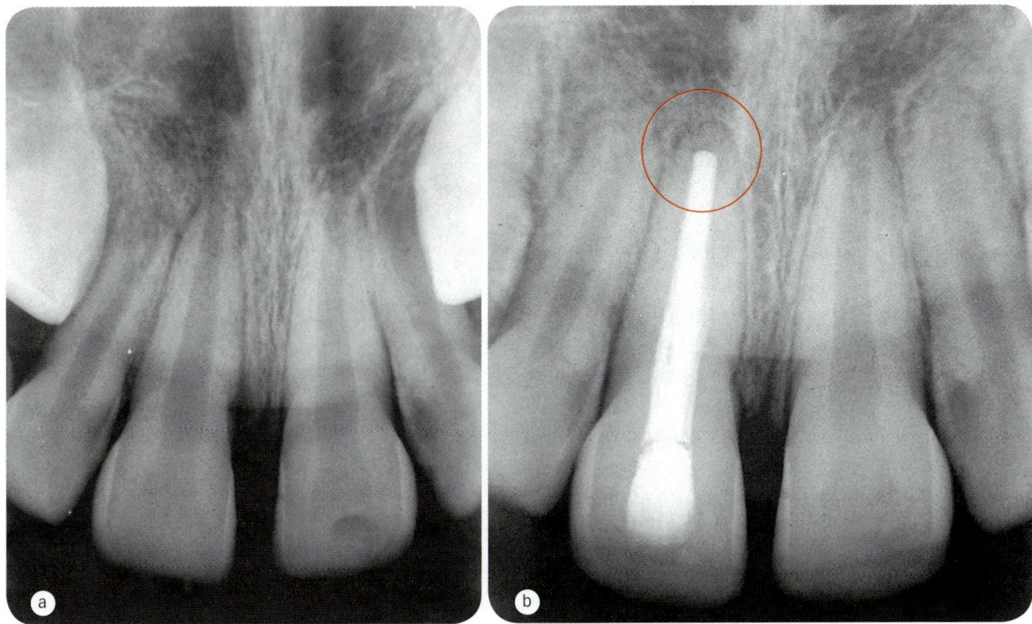


**Figure 20.18** - (**A-B**) Periapical radiograph shows complete mineralized barrier in the main root canal.

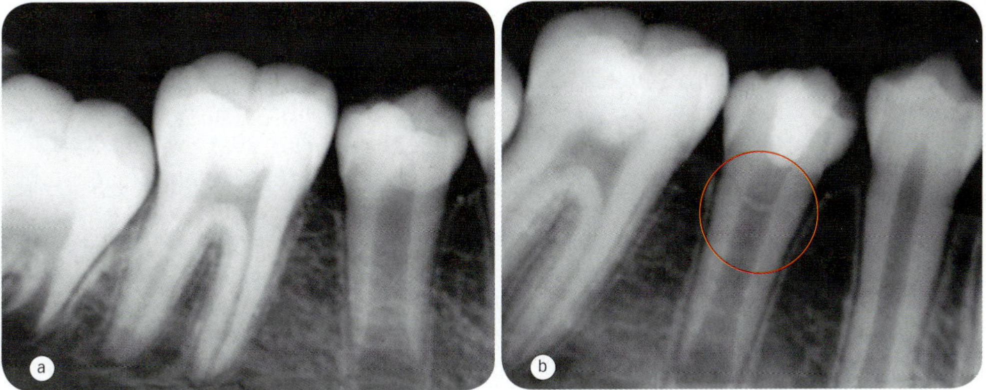


**Figure 20.19** - (**A-B**) Periapical radiograph shows complete mineralized barrier on the dental pulp.

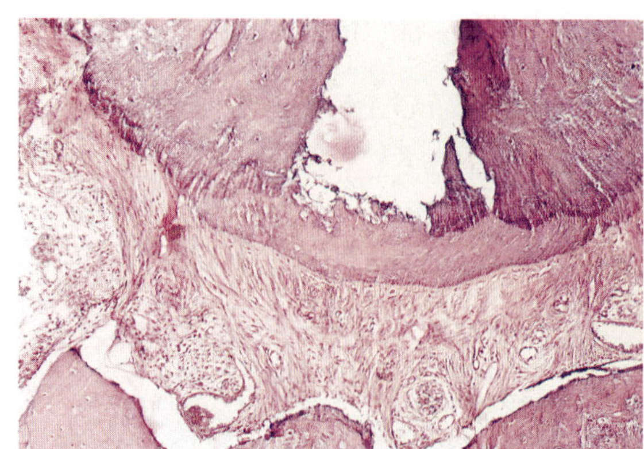

**Figure 20.20** - Calcium hydroxide used as an intracanal dressing. Complete closure of the main root canal by neoformed cementum (H.E. X100) (Holland et al.[265]).

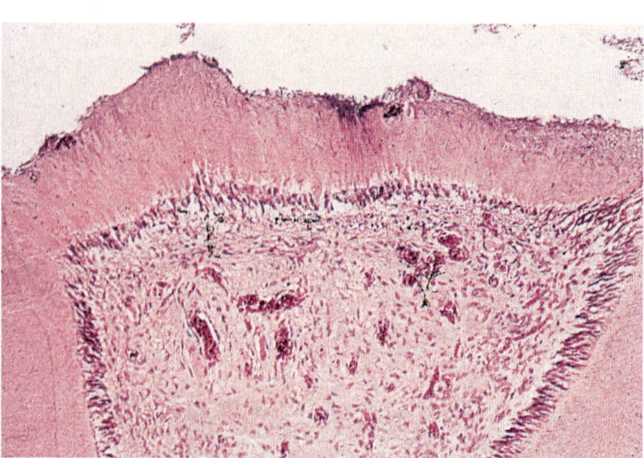

**Figure 20.21** - Calcium hydroxide - Complete hard tissue bridge on the dental pulp (H.E. X40) (Holland et al.[277]).

In addition to Calcium hydroxide being capable of bacterial enzymatic inhibition, which represents an important antibacterial property, it is capable of activating tissue enzymes, which favor tissue restoration through mineralization.

The elevated pH of calcium hydroxide activates alkaline phosphatase[211,231,232,404,587,595]; the best pH for the activation of this enzyme, which varies with the type and concentration of substratum, temperature and source of enzymes, ranges from 8.6 to 10.3[207,587].

Alkaline phosphatase is a hydrolytic enzyme that acts by means of the release of inorganic phosphate from the phosphate esters. It is believed to be intimately related to the process of mineralization[514]. This enzyme can separate the phosphoric esters, freeing phosphate ions which, once free, react with calcium ions in the blood stream to form a precipitate, calcium phosphate, in the organic matrix. This precipitate is the molecular unit of hydroxyapatite[514].

Mizuno & Banzai[406] investigated the effect of calcium ions on the dental pulp cells and the mechanism of dentine bridge formation by calcium hydroxide. Calcium ions release from calcium hydroxide stimulates fibronectin synthesis in dental pulp cells. Fibronectin might induce the differentiation of dental pulp cells to mineralized tissue forming cells that are the main cells to form dentine bridges, via direct contact.

Calcium hydroxide in direct contact with conjunctive tissue gives origin to a zone of necrosis, altering the physical-chemical state of intercellular substance which, through rupture of glycoproteins, seems to determine protein denaturation[245]. The formation of mineralized tissue after contact of calcium hydroxide with conjunctive tissue has been observed from about the 7th to the 10th day[245].

As regards the discussion about the mineralized barrier permeability, Holland et al.[277] observed the formation of a hard tissue bridge after pulpotomy with calcium hydroxide. They performed pulpotomy in 80 monkey teeth using calcium hydroxide. After 30 days, the dressings of 60 teeth were removed, allowing the hard tissue bridge to be seen. In order to evaluate permeability, the bridges were capped with silicate cement (20 teeth) or, zinc phosphate cement (20 teeth) and 20 teeth were exposed to the oral environment without any protection. The remaining 20 teeth were used as control. The pulp responses of the experimental groups resembled those of the control group. The complete bridges showed a high level of normal remnant pulp. Fragments of dentin were found in the incomplete bridges. The authors reported that these bridges were not permeable, and that porosity was not a contraindication to the procedures of direct pulp capping or pulpotomy.

Recently (in 1990) a new cement was developed at Loma Linda University. It has been accepted by the US Federal Drug Administration, and is commercially available as ProRoot MTA (Tulsa Dental Products, Tulsa, OK, USA) (Fig. 20.22A-B). Mineral trioxide aggregate (MTA) was shown to be capable of sealing communications between the tooth and the external surfaces[356,590-594]. This material was studied in a series of in vivo and in vitro investigations that reported good sealing ability[356,594] and tissue behavior[288-290,593]. Formation of new cementum over the material was reported in experimentally perforated furcation[269], in root end filling[590-594] and root canal filling of dog teeth[288,589-594]. Bridge-like dentin has been observed in cases of pulp capping and pulpotomy in monkey, and dog teeth[284].

There are some essential aspects to discuss with regard to the chemical and biological characteristics of mineral trioxide aggregate. Lee et al.[356] reported that the main components present in the MTA, would be the tricalcic silicate, the tricalcic aluminate, tricalcic oxide and silicate oxide. There were other mineral oxides that would be responsible for the chemical and physical properties of this aggregate. According to these authors, the MTA powder is constituted of thin, fine hydrophilic particles, that harden in the presence of water. Torabinejad et al.[590] analyzed the physical and chemical properties of MTA. MTA was divided into two specific phases, constituted of calcium oxide and calcium phosphate - calcium oxide presented discreet crystals and calcium phosphate an amorphous structure. Holland et al.[299] implanted tubes of dentin filled with calcium hydroxide or MTA in the subcutaneous tissue of rats. The tissues were removed after 7 or 30 days and processed without decalcification. Thus, cuts of hard tissue were analyzed with the aid of polarized light and Von Kossa coloration for calcium salts.



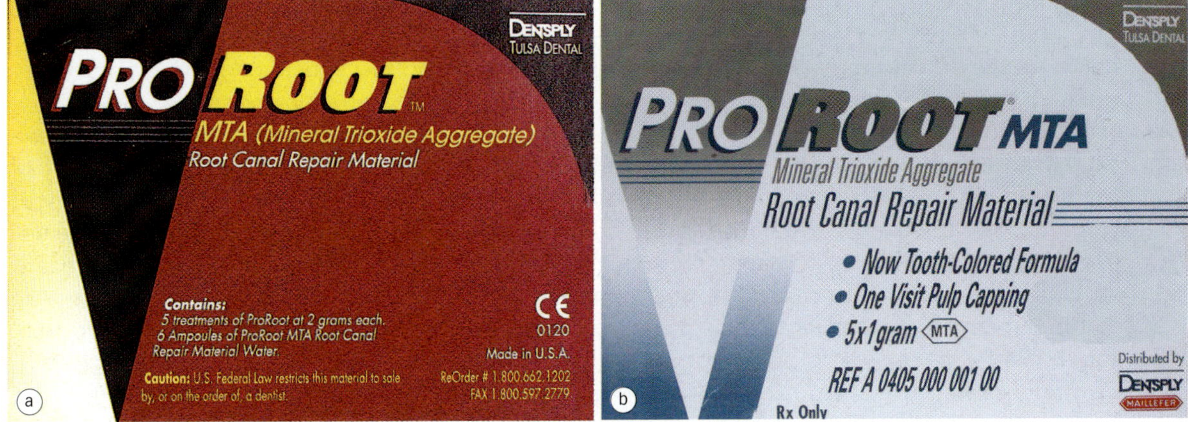


**Figure 20.22** - (**A-B**) Mineral trioxide aggregate (gray/white).

They observed that with calcium hydroxide, there was the formation of calcite granulations, birefringent to the polarized light, near the lumen of the tube. Under these granulations a von Kossa positive bridge of hard tissue was formed. Furthermore, the presence of calcite granulations, birefringent to the polarized light, was also observed inside the dentinal tubules. With MTA, the same situation was observed, but there was a slightly smaller number of calcite granulations than that observed with the calcium hydroxide, and that these granulations were in contact with the studied material, which did not occur with calcium hydroxide.

Wucherpfenning & Green[633] reported that both MTA and Portland cement seem almost identical macroscopically, microscopically, and by X-ray defraction analysis. They reported that both substances support matrix formation in a similar fashion in cultures of osteoblast-like cells, and also as apposition of reparative dentin, when used as direct pulp capping material in rat teeth.

Estrela et al.[112] studied the antimicrobial and chemical properties of some materials, including MTA and Portland cement. Analyses of the chemical elements present in MTA, and in two samples of Portland cement were performed with X-ray fluorescence spectrometry (XRF). They reported that Portland cement contained the same principle chemical elements as MTA, except that MTA also contains bismuth. Camilleri & Pitt Ford[60] reported that this study was the first research paper on the chemistry of Portland cement that had potential for dental use demonstrating the similarity of grey MTA to Portland cement.

Holland et al.[299] observed the reaction in the subcutaneous tissue of rats to dentin tubes filled with mineral trioxide aggregate, Portland cement or calcium hydroxide. The animals were sacrificed after 7 or 30 days and the undecalcified specimens were prepared for histological analysis with polarized light, and von Kossa technique for mineralized tissues. The results were similar for the studied materials. At the tube openings, there were von Kossa positive granules that were birefringent to polarized light. Next to these granulations, there was an irregular, bridge-like tissue that was von Kossa-positive. The dentin walls of the tubes exhibited a structure highly birefringent to polarized light in the tubules, usually layer-like and at different depths. Some similarity has been shown between the mechanisms of action of the studied materials. In another study, Holland et al.[284] considering several reports about the similarity between the chemical compositions of mineral trioxide aggregate and Portland cement, analyzed the behavior of dog dental pulp after pulpotomy and direct pulp protection with these materials. After pulpotomy, the pulp stumps of 26 roots of dog teeth were protected with MTA or Portland cement. Sixty days after treatment, the animal was sacrificed and the specimens removed and prepared for histomorphological analysis. There was a complete tubular hard tissue bridge in almost all specimens. In conclusion, MTA and Portland cement show similar comparative results when used in direct pulp protection after pulpotomy.

In various studies, Holland et al.[158,159,267,268,284,288,289,290,299,555] observed that calcium hydroxide showed the presence of calcite granulations in subcutaneous connective tissue, dental pulp[245,270] and periapical tissues[253,280]. These granulations are formed by the reaction of the calcium hydroxide with the carbonic gas of the tissue. The same granulations were described by Seux et al.[521] in an in vitro experiment. Moreover, these authors noticed an accumulation of fibronectin, a glycoprotein, in intimate contact with these calcite crystals, in a culture medium without cells. When pulp cells were placed in contact with this environment, there was formation of cells with the morphological aspect of odontoblasts. In the absence of calcite granulations there was only proliferation of fibroblasts. Seux et al.[521] concluded that these findings constituted strong evidence of the role of the calcite granulations and fibronectin as the beginning of the formation of a hard tissue barrier. Similarity was shown between the results of Calcium hydroxide and the MTA in subcutaneous tissue of rats[299]. Both materials determined the formation of calcite granulations and a subjacent hard tissue bridge.

The mechanism of action of the MTA would be the same as that of calcium hydroxide[299]. The calcium oxide in the MTA[112] powder is converted into calcium hydroxide, when the paste is prepared with water. This mixture in contact with the tissue fluids would dissociate into calcium and hydroxyl ions. The Calcium ions reacting with the carbonic gas of the tissues would originate the calcite granulations. Close to these granulations there is accumulation of fibronectin, which allows cellular adhesion and differentiation. After this there would be the formation of a hard tissue bridge.

A similar tissue reaction to that of the MTA can be observed with the filling sealer, Sealapex. This sealer contains calcium oxide in its formula. When Sealapex, also contained in the dentin tube, was implanted in the subcutaneous of rats, the same results were observed as with those found for MTA; in other words, there was calcite granulation and hard tissue bridge formation[299]. This observation with Sealapex reinforces the validity of the mechanism of action described for MTA. It could be highlighted that after the hydration of MTA, the solution is saturated with calcium ions ($Ca^{2+}$) and hydroxyl ions ($OH^-$) that will combine with ions of sulphate, silicate and aluminate, forming hydrated calcium silicates (50 to 60%), calcium hydroxide (20 to 25%) and calcium sulphoaluminates (15 to 20%), the main compounds of the hydrated paste[24].

Depending on the constant changes of ionic saturation, the calcium hydroxide formed can also solubilize and dissociate into calcium ($Ca^{2+}$) and hydroxyl ions ($OH^-$) that are mainly responsible for the mechanism of action of the material[245]. The carbon dioxide ($CO_2$) produced as result of the catabolism of our cells, solubilizes, diffusing to the interstitial liquids, and from these to the bloodstream, flowing to the lungs, from where it is exhaled in a gaseous state. The carbon dioxide ($CO_2$) in aqueous solution, such as the interstitial liquids or blood plasma, acts as a biological buffer, undergoing a series of reactions, including the participation of the enzyme carbonic anhydrate, with the purpose of regulating the pH of the environment where it is found in several forms: $CO_2$ (carbon dioxide), $H_2CO_3$ (carbonic acid), $HCO_3$ (bicarbonate ion), $CO_3$ (carbonate ion)[24,357,358,587]. The pH of the pulp and periapical tissues will be influenced by their inflammatory stages, or in other words, under normal conditions the pH is neutral or slightly alkaline (7.2 to 7.4). In acute inflammations, the pH decreases, becoming acid (6.5 or less) due to the lactic acid from the anaerobic glycolysis of the inflammatory cells and due to the accumulation of $CO_2$ in the location, derived from blood stasis. In chronic inflammations however, the pH returns to neutral (7.0 to 7.2) due to the increase of tissue vascularity[392]. Thus, when using a material of alkaline pH such as calcium hydroxide, MTA or Portland cement, over the pulp or in contact with the periapical tissues, the local tissue pH will be increased, due to the saturated solution of hydroxyl ions (OH). In order to balance the pH of the environment, the carbon dioxide ($CO_2$), carbonic acid ($H_2CO_3$) or bicarbonate ions ($HCO_3$-), present in the medium, will react with the hydroxyl ions, considerably increasing the concentration of carbonate ions ($CO_{3\ 2-}$). These will react with the calcium ions in solution ($Ca^{2+}$) forming calcium carbonate granulations, as a form of calcite ($CaCO_3$) in the tissue[245].

As mentioned before, Seux et al.[521] demonstrated in vitro that the fibronectin presents high affinity for calcium carbonate granulations, evidenced by the high concentration of fibronectin around the calcite crystals.

Fibronectin belongs to a group of substratum adhesion molecules responsible for cellular migration, adhesion and differentiation, being produced by fibroblasts, macrophages and endothelial cells[406,595].

Thus, fibronectin would be responsible for the migration and adhesion of pulp and periodontal cells that would synthesize and deposit collagen type I, forming the extracellular organic matrix. Moreover, the fibronectin would induce the differentiation of pulp cells into odontoblasts or of periodontium cells into cementoblasts, mainly responsible for the deposition of minerals[521].

The liquid phase saturated with hydroxyl ions also seems to be responsible for the slight layer of superficial pulp necrosis, situated between the mineralized tissue bridge and the material, and found in few specimens submitted to pulpotomy with MTA[546] or Portland cement[289]. These observations are a little different from those noted with several calcium hydroxide pastes submitted to the same conditions[255,546]. It is emphasized that this superficial necrosis is mostly absent, and when present, it is much thinner than that observed with chemically pure calcium hydroxide[255].

Holland et al.[299] found the same results between gray and white MTA, indicating that the mechanisms of action are similar. The reaction of rat subcutaneous connective tissue to the implantation of dentin tubes filled with white mineral trioxide aggregate, a material that will be marketed. The tubes were implanted into rat subcutaneous tissue and the animals were sacrificed after 7 and 30 days. The undecalcified tissues were prepared for histological analysis with polarized light and von Kossa technique for mineralized tissues. Granulations birefringent to polarized light and an irregular, bridge-like structure were observed next to the material; both were von Kossa positive. A layer of birefringent granulations was also observed in the dentin wall tubules.

Saidon et al.[496] studied the cell and tissue reactions to mineral trioxide aggregate and Portland cement. The authors observed that MTA and Portland cement showed comparative biocompatibility when evaluated in vitro and in vivo. The results suggest that Portland cement has the potential to be used as a less expensive root-end filling material.

In summary, Estrela & Holland[130] discussed the biological and antimicrobial role of calcium hydroxide, and reported that the characteristics of calcium hydroxide come from its dissociation into calcium and hydroxyl ions. The action of these ions on tissues and bacteria explains the biological and antimicrobial properties of this substance - 1. Dentin is considered the best pulp protective, and calcium hydroxide has proved, through numerous studies, to be capable of inducing the formation of a mineralized bridge over pulp tissue. 2. It is necessary, whenever possible, to allow time for the calcium hydroxide paste to manifest its potential of action against the microorganisms present in endodontic infections. The maintenance of a high concentration of hydroxyl ions can change bacteria enzymatic activity and promote its inactivation. 3. The site of action of hydroxyl ions of calcium hydroxide includes the enzymes in the cytoplasmic membrane. This medication has a broad scope of action, and therefore is effective against a wide range of microorganisms, regardless of their metabolic capability. In the microbial world, cytoplasmic membranes are similar, irrespective of the morphological, tinctorial and respiratory characteristics of microorganisms, which mean that this medication has a similar effect on aerobic, anaerobic, Gram-positive and Gram-negative bacteria. 4. Calcium hydroxide as a temporary dressing, used between appointments, promotes better results in the periapical healing process than the treatment performed in one appointment.

### 20.4.1 Inter-Appointment Medication (one versus two visits)

Establishing the strategies for microbial control of root canal requires knowledge of the relations between the bacteria, anatomy and host response. These are obstacles that the endodontist needs to overcome. Knowledge about microbiological phenomena and ultra-structural anatomy are important for achieving success in the treatment of endodontic infection. It is relevant and necessary to understand that it is the host that monitors the biological process to favor healing.

The choice of intracanal dressing correlates with two relevant aspects, namely: antimicrobial potential and tissue tolerance. In most clinical cases, these substances are in contact with only non vital tissue in the root canal and little contact with the periapical tissue. Their real function is to control microorganisms only in the root canal.

The main cause of apical periodontitis is endodontic infection (caused by bacteria and their by products). Thus, good therapeutic strategy is to solve the cause of the problem (microorganisms in the root canal) and naturally their consequences (pathological alterations) are better solved.

Identification and knowledge of the predominant microorganisms in infected root canals are decisive factors for effective microbial control.

The outcome of root canal treatment in the presence of apical periodontitis is directly influenced by the use of acceptable clinical procedures under strictly aseptic conditions, in addition to the host's immunological response. The patient's nutritional status and the selective pressures related to oxidation-reduction potential, nutrient supply and microbial interactions are important for the establishment and maintenance of polymicrobial infections in teeth with apical periodontitis.

Several reports have discussed factors related to the etiology of post-treatment disease in endodontics – 1. microbial etiologic factors (intraradicular and extraradicular infection – bacteria, fungi); 2. non-microbial etiologic factors (endogenous – true cysts; exogenous – foreign-body reaction)[419-424].

It is therefore important to consider the type of infection occurring. The primary root canal infection is associated with endodontic microbiota generally composed of Gram-negative anaerobic bacteria. In root-filled teeth, the microorganisms can persist and maintain the apical periodontitis. Microorganisms present in secondary root canal infection are those that were resistant to the first treatment or penetrated after the root canal filling and coronal sealing.

Sundqvist et al.[580] determined which microbial flora was present in teeth after failed root canal therapy, and established the outcomes of conservative re-treatment. The microbial flora was mainly composed of single species, mostly of Gram-positive organisms. The most commonly recovered isolates were bacteria of the species *E. faecalis*. The overall success rate of re-treatment was 74%. The microbial flora in canals after failed endodontic therapy differed markedly from the flora found in untreated teeth. The infection at the time of root filling and the size of the periapical lesion were factors that had a negative influence on the prognosis. Three out of four endodontic failures were successfully managed by re-treatment. Sundqvist & Figdor[581] in a discussion on the life of endodontic pathogens, related that root canal infection is not a random event. The type and the combination of the microbial flora developed in response to the surrounding environment. Factors that influence whether species shall die or survive are the particular ecological niche, nutrition, anaerobiosis, pH and competition with other microorganisms.

The chemical dynamics of calcium hydroxide, as demonstrated by ionic dissociation, characterizes its properties. The activation of tissue enzymes such as alkaline phosphatase, shows mineralizing effects and an inhibiting effect on bacterial enzymes, which leads to its antimicrobial property, illustrating the biological qualities of hydroxyl and calcium ions, in both tissue and microorganisms[130,146].

Modern concepts of microbial control have been directed towards the use of intracanal medicaments that act against different types of respiratory bacteria (aerobic, anaerobic and microaerophiles), have the ability to affect cell wall synthesis, or alter the cytoplasmic membrane permeability and interfere with protein synthesis or chromosomal replication[130,146].

Ideally, an intracanal medicament should be able to neutralize the virulence of microorganisms and pathogenic factors (such as proteins, enzymes, toxins, aggregation substances) and induce a host response that favors periapical tissue healing. The continuous presence, however, of positive microbial cultures after root canal shaping, sanitization and use of calcium hydroxide as interappointment, intracanal dressing justifies the investigations of antimicrobial substances.

It has been proposed to focus attention on solve all the endodontic problems immediately. The new direction of guidelines for universal endodontic treatment will be indicated, after scientific evidence has been found, and maintained by well-conducted research.

At this scientific moment it is prudent to discuss some of the questions concerning interappointment medication. Is there justification for indicating calcium hydroxide to control the endodontic infection? Do the vehicles influence the antimicrobial efficacy of calcium hydroxide pastes? Is calcium hydroxide paste effective against *E. faecalis* present in endodontic infection?

The dynamics observed between infection of the dentin-pulp complex and the development of apical periodontitis and consequent host response encouraged the search for greater knowledge about the structure of endodontic microbiota.

Knowledge about morphology, structure and physiology of microorganisms that are responsible for painful states and destruction of periapical tissues, motivated several therapeutic trends. The first step of endodontic treatment is knowledge of the interrelationship between microorganisms and host, and the chemical and biological dynamics of intracanal dressings.

Calcium hydroxide has been the most used, discussed and studied intracanal medication. Although this does not mean that this medication can cure all illnesses, calcium hydroxide has been the first choice as an intracanal dressing in different clinical situations.

Attempts have been made to establish appropriate criteria for use, including limits and implications, and at the same time, show the value of research to explain facts that are not yet clear or are mistakenly explained.

In endodontics, there are two clinical situations that require inter-appointment medication: in root canal infection, to prevent microbial growth and multiplication in dentinal tubules after cleaning and shaping; and occasionally in teeth with vital pulp. The goal of endodontic treatment is to eliminate microorganisms from the root canal system by means of the association of procedures, i.e., biomechanical preparation, irrigation with different solutions, and the use of intracanal dressings. The application of a new concept of root canal sanitization and shaping process has resulted in more successful endodontic treatment.

A long time ago, innumerous studies were conducted to determine the performance of calcium hydroxide in different clinical situations. The ability to stimulate mineralization, associated with its antimicrobial effectiveness has at present established its success as an endodontic medication.

Nevertheless, well-conducted research about the properties of calcium hydroxide, such as histocompatibility, antimicrobial potential, physical-chemical aspects, give credibility to the choice of this medication in several clinical situations.

Byström et al.[47] clinically evaluated the root canals of 65 single-rooted teeth with periapical lesions treated by calcium hydroxide, camphorated phenol and camphorated paramonoclorophenol. Bacteria were recovered from one out of 35 root canals treated by calcium hydroxide paste after 30 days. After the use of camphorated phenol and camphorated paramonoclorophenol as the dressing, bacteria were recovered from 10 out of 30 treated root canals. There was no indication that specific bacteria were resistant to the treatment. The results suggested that the endodontic treatment of infected root canals can be completed in two sessions when calcium hydroxide paste is used as an intracanal dressing.

Sjögren et al.[541] evaluated the antibacterial effectiveness of calcium hydroxide, when used as a short-term intracanal dressing in vivo. Thirty teeth were used, all of which had single roots containing necrotic pulps and radiographic evidence of periapical bone lesions. The teeth were enlarged to a size 40 Hedström or larger at the working length, and 0.5% sodium hypochlorite was used as irrigant. The teeth were divided into 2 groups: in 18 cases, calcium hydroxide was used as dressing for 7 days, and in 12 cases, for 10 minutes. Cultures were taken before and after the root canal preparation, and after the intracanal dressing period. The results showed that the 7-day dressing efficiently eliminated bacteria which survived biomechanical instrumentation of the canal, while the 10-minute application was ineffective.

Sydney[585] studied the endodontic microflora in teeth with asymptomatic apical periodontitis. Twenty maxillary single-rooted teeth were selected from patients between 20 to 40, and divided into two groups. Microbiologic samples were taken after the access cavity preparation. In group I, after instrumentation, the root canals were double sealed without intracanal medicament. In this group, microbiological samplings from the root canals were obtained 1 week and 6 weeks after the first visit. In group II, calcium hydroxide was used as intracanal medicament for a period of 1 week and 6 weeks, after the first visit. In this group, microbiological samplings were taken one week after the removal of calcium hydroxide, for both periods, which occurred 2 and 7 weeks afterwards. The results showed that anaerobic bacteria were the commonest microorganisms identified from the infected root canals. A combination of between 2 to 7 organisms was found in each root canal. After the use of calcium hydroxide as intracanal medicament for one week, the microflora was reduced to 77.8% and after 6 weeks, in only one instance, *E. faecalis* was isolated. Katebzadeh et al.[320], analyzing histological periapical repair after obturation of infected root canals in dogs, reported better results when root canal treatment was done in multiple sessions rather than in one session. Trope et al.[604] evaluated the radiographic healing of teeth with apical periodontitis treated in one or in two visits, and with or without calcium hydroxide paste as an intracanal dressing. The teeth that were left empty between appointments had clearly poorer healing results. The additional disinfecting action of calcium hydroxide paste before obturation resulted in a 10% increase in healing rates.

Holland et al.[268] observed the healing process in dog teeth with apical periodontitis after root canal treatment in one or two appointments. Premolars and anterior dog teeth had their root canals opened to the oral environment for 6 months before being treated. After root canal negotiation they were filled by the lateral condensation technique with gutta-percha points and Sealapex in one appointment or after a dressing with calcium hydroxide for 7 and 15 days. Six months after the treatment the animals were sacrificed and the tissues prepared for histomorphological analysis. Scores attributed to the different histomorphological events were submitted to statistical analysis, which resulted in ranking the experimental groups from the best to the worst in the following order: (a) calcium hydroxide 14 days; (b) calcium hydroxide 7 days; and (c) one appointment. It was concluded that the use of a calcium hydroxide dressing helps to achieve better results than the treatment in one appointment. The healing process observed in this experiment with the one appointment treatment was interesting. One believes that the results could partly be attributed to the Sealapex alkalinity. Some experiments in dog teeth with apical periodontitis showed better results in root canals filled with Sealapex than in root canals filled with zinc oxide-eugenol sealers. The groups with calcium hydroxide dressings exhibited the best results in this research. In another study Holland et al.[267] based their research on the same parameters to study Sealer 26. The results showed the better status of periapical tissue (with mineralized barrier) when the treatment performed in two appointments with use the intracanal dressing (calcium hydroxide paste) (Fig. 20.23 to 20.35).

Kvist et al.[346] evaluated the antimicrobial efficacy of endodontic procedures performed in one-visit (including a 10 minutes intra-appointment dressing with 5% iodine-potassium-iodide) was compared with a two-visit procedure (including an inter appoint-

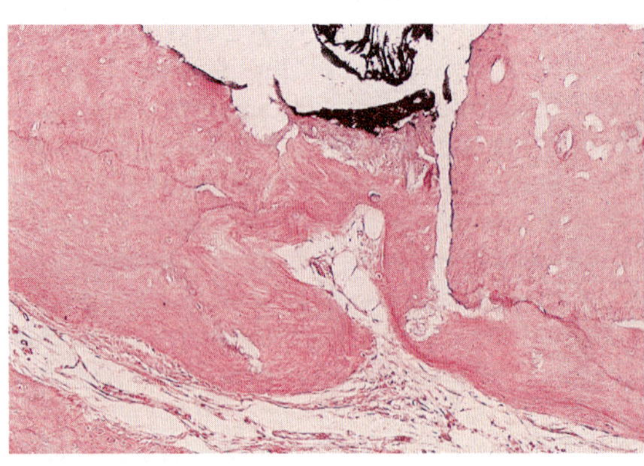

**Figure 20.23** - Calcium hydroxide 7 days. Complete closure of the main root canal by neoformed cementum (H.E. X100) (Holland et al.[267]).

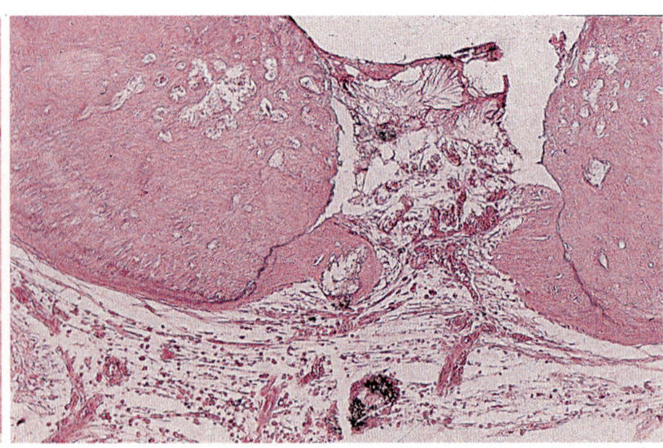

**Figure 20.24** - One visit. Neoformed cementum in the walls of the main root canal. There is a mild chronic inflammatory reaction (INF) in the periodontal ligament (H.E. X100) (Holland et al.[267]).

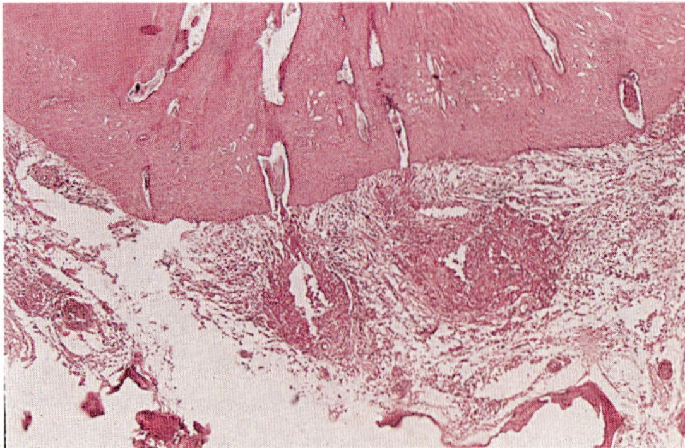

**Figure 20.25** - Control group. Areas of cementum resorptions (arrow), microabscess (M), and chronic inflammatory reaction (INF) in the apical periodontal space (H.E. X40) (Holland et al.[267]).

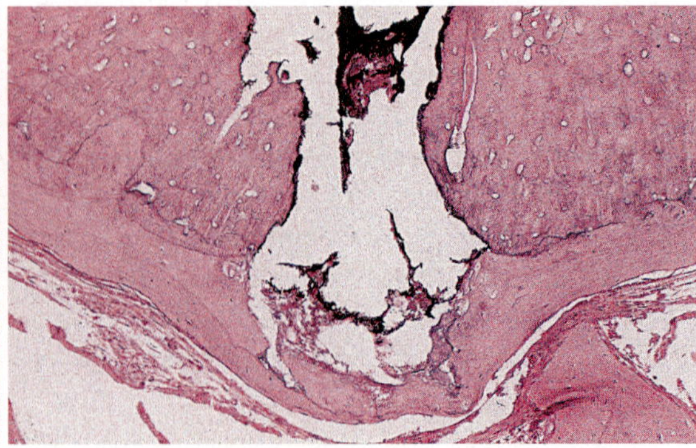

**Figure 20.26** - Calcium hydroxide 14 days. Complete closure of an accessory canal (arrow). There is a little overfilling (M) and closure (C) of the main root canal ( H.E. X100) (Holland et al.[267]).

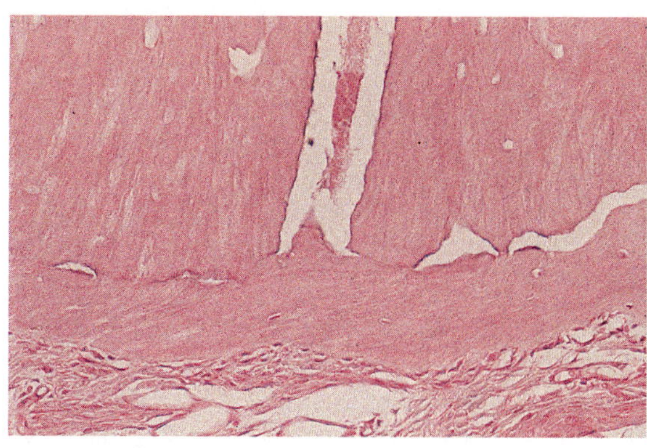

**Figure 20.27** - Calcium hydroxide 7 days. The neoformed cementum repaired resorption areas (arrow) and completely sealed (C) an apical accessory canal. Absence of inflammatory reaction (PL) in the periodontal ligament (hematoxylin and eosin; original magnification (H.E. X200) (Holland et al.[267]).

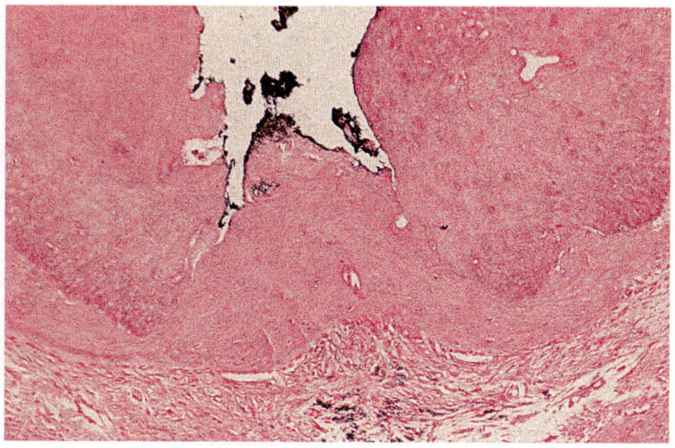

**Figure 20.28** - Calcium hydroxide 14 days. Complete closure of the main root canal (C). There are macrophages with black particles of the filling material (M) in the periodontal ligament (H.E. X100) (Holland et al.[267]).

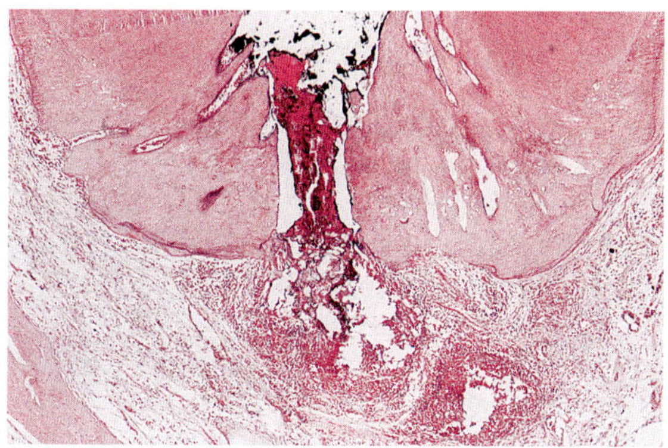

**Figure 20.29** - One visit. Intense chronic inflammatory reaction (INF) in the periodontal ligament (H.E. X40) (Holland et al.[267]).

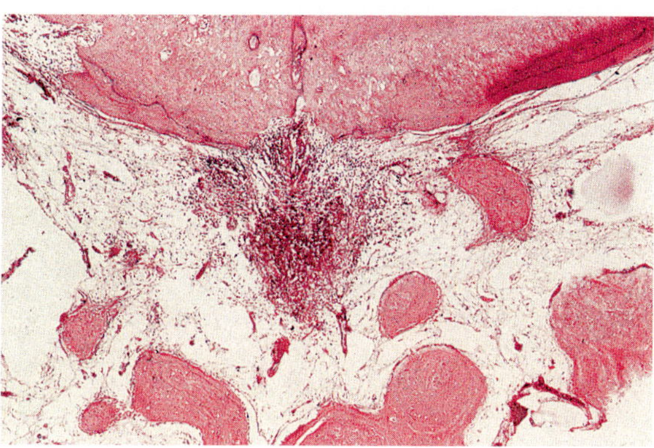

**Figure 20.30** - One visit. Intense chronic inflammatory reaction (INF) in the periodontal ligament (H.E. X40) (Holland et al.[267]).

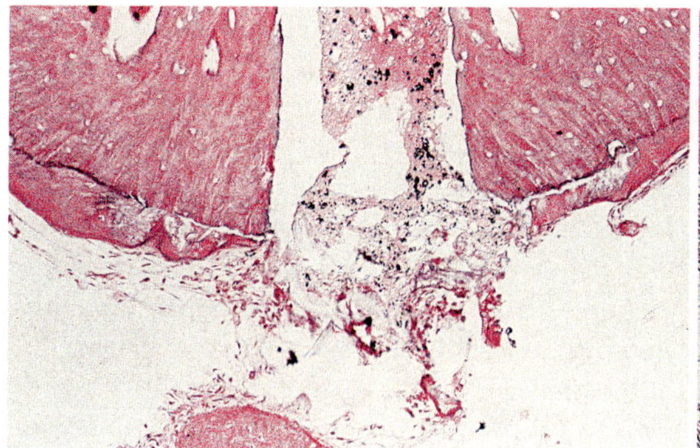

**Figure 20.31** - Calcium hydroxide 7 days. Few chronic inflammatory cells. (H.E. X100). (Holland et al.[268]).

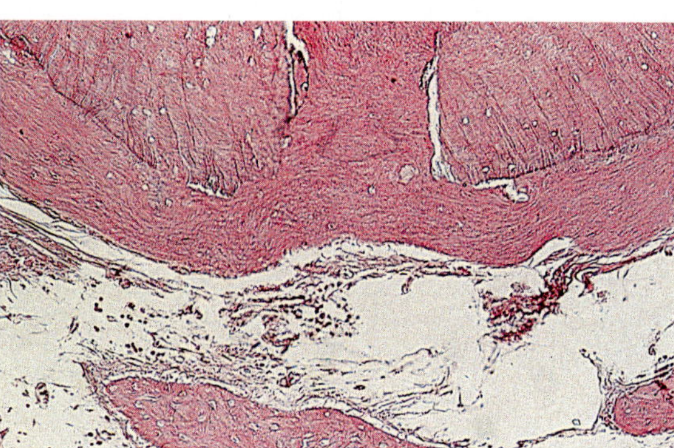

**Figure 20.32** - Calcium hydroxide 7 days. Complete biologic closure (H.E. X100) (Holland et al.[268]).

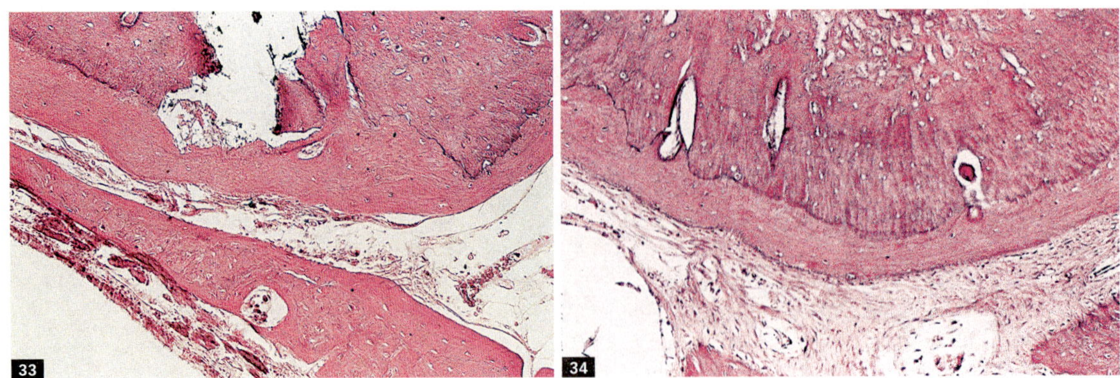

**Figures 20.33 and 20.34** - Calcium hydroxide 14 days. Complete biological closure. Absence of inflammatory cells. (H.E. 100X) (Holland et al.[268]).

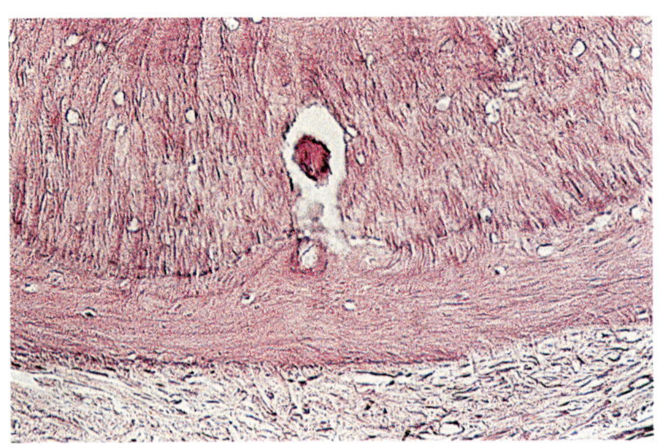

**Figure 20.35** - Higher magnification of Figure 20.34. Complete biological closure, Absence of inflammatory cells (H.E. 100X) (Holland et al.[268]).

ment dressing with calcium-hydroxide paste). Teeth with apical periodontitis were randomly assigned to either group. Root canal sampling and culturing were performed before and immediately after instrumentation, and after medication. Initial sampling demonstrated the presence of microorganisms in 98% of the teeth. Postinstrumentation sampling showed reduction of cultivable microbiota. Antibacterial dressing further reduced the number of teeth with surviving microbes. In the postmedication samples, residual microorganisms were recovered in 29% of the one-visit teeth and in 36% of the two-visit treated teeth. No statistically significant differences between the groups were discerned. It was concluded that from a microbiological point of view, treatment of teeth with apical periodontitis performed in two appointments was not more effective than the one-visit procedure investigated.

Estrela et al.[129] evaluated the influence of irrigants on the antimicrobial potential of calcium hydroxide paste in dog teeth with apical periodontitis. Forty-eight premolar teeth of adult mongrel dogs had their root canals opened to the oral environment for 6 months. The root canals were prepared and treated with different irrigating solutions and intracanal medicaments, according to the following groups: G1. 2.5% sodium hypochlorite + calcium hydroxide paste; G2. 2% chlorhexidine + calcium hydroxide paste; G3. vinegar + calcium hydroxide paste; G4. vinegar + vinegar. In group 4, both the irrigating solution and intracanal medicament were vinegar, which was renewed every 7 days. After 21 days, all experimental groups had microbial growth, however, in different percentages: group 1 - 30%; group 2 - 30%; group 3 - 40%; group 4 - 60%. All materials tested had antimicrobial potential; however, the influence of calcium hydroxide paste on the control of microorganisms must be remembered (Fig. 20.36).

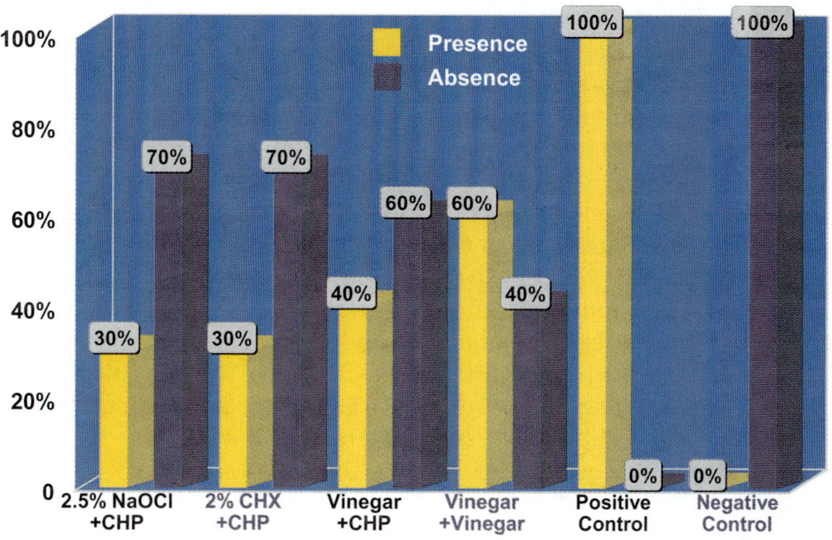


**Figure 20.36** - Antimicrobial potential of intracanal medicaments after 21 days in infected root canals of dog teeth.

Law & Messer[350] reviewed the literature evaluating the antibacterial effectiveness of intracanal medicaments used in the management of apical periodontitis. The total sample size in the studies included was 164 teeth. Microbiologic sampling was performed before endodontic treatment (S1), after instrumentation and irrigation (S2), and after intracanal medication (S3). At S2, 62% of canals were positive. After medication, 27% still showed detectable growth. Of cultures that were positive at S2, 45% were still positive at S3. Most studies did not address the issues of culture reversals or false positive and false negative cultures. The main component of antibacterial action appears to be associated with instrumentation and irrigation, although canals cannot be reliably rendered bacteria free. Calcium hydroxide remains the best medicament available to reduce residual microbial flora further. Sathorn et al.[503] determined to what extent calcium hydroxide intracanal medication eliminates bacteria from human root canals, compared with the same canals before medication, as measured by the number of positive cultures, in patients undergoing root canal treatment for apical periodontitis (teeth with an infected root canal system). The studies included were pre-/post-test clinical trials comparing the number of differences of included studies were combined, using the generic inverse variance and random effect method. Eight studies were identified and included in the review, covering 257 cases. Sample size varied from 18 to 60 cases; six studies demonstrated a statistically significant difference between pre- and post-medicated canals, whilst two did not. There was considerable heterogeneity among studies. The difference between pre- and post-medication was not statistically significant. Calcium hydroxide has limited effectiveness in eliminating bacteria from human root canal when assessed by culture techniques.

Nair et al.[422] assessed the in vivo intracanal microbial status of the apical root canal system of mesial roots of human mandibular first molars with primary apical periodontitis, immediately after one-visit endodontic treatment. The residual intracanal infection was confirmed by correlative light and transmission electron microscopy Study design. Sixteen diseased mesial roots of mandibular first molars were treated endodontically, each in one visit. Mesiobuccal canals were instrumented using stainless steel hand files and mesio-lingual canals with a nickel-titanium rotary system. The canals were irrigated with 5.25% sodium hypochlorite during the instrumentation procedures, rinsed with 10 mL of 17% EDTA, and obturated with gutta-percha and zinc oxide eugenol cement. Thereafter, the apical portion of the root of each tooth was removed by flap-surgery. The specimens were fixed, decalcified, subdivided in the horizontal plane, embedded in plastic, processed, and evaluated by correlative light and transmission electron microscopy. Fourteen of the 16 endodontically treated teeth revealed residual intracanal infection after instrumentation, antimicrobial irrigation, and obturation. The microbes were located in inaccessible recesses and diverticula of instrumented main canals, the intercanal isthmus, and accessory canals, mostly as biofilms. The results show (1) the anatomical complexity of the root canal system of mandibular first molar roots and (2) the organization of the flora as biofilms in inaccessible areas of the canal system that cannot be removed by contemporary instruments and irrigation alone in one-visit treatment. These findings demonstrate the importance of stringent application of all nonantibiotic chemo-mechanical measures to treat teeth with infected and necrotic root canals, so as to disrupt the biofilms and reduce the intraradicular microbial load to the lowest possible level so as to expect a highly favorable long-term prognosis of the root canal treatment.

*E. faecalis* has been the focus of attention as a recognized pathogen, isolated both in mixed microbiota and in monocultures. Several virulence factors (aggregation substance, enterococcal surface proteins (Esp), gelatinase, cytolysin toxin, extracellular superoxide production, capsular polysaccharides, antibiotic resistance determinant) can facilitate the adherence to host cells and the extracellular matrix, tissue invasions, immunomodulation effect and cause toxin mediated damage[465]. Sundqvist et al.[580] observed that the microbial flora of teeth with persistent apical periodontitis was mainly a simple species of predominantly Gram-positive organisms. *E. faecalis* (38%) was the species most commonly recovered, and the overall healing rate of re-treatment was 74%.

Love[373] investigated a possible mechanism that would explain how *E. faecalis* could survive and grow within dentinal tubules and reinfect obturated canals. The author postulated that a virulence factor of *E. faecalis* in failed endodontically treated teeth may be related to the fact that *E. faecalis* cells maintain the capability of invading dentinal tubules and adhere to collagen in the presence of human serum.

Evans et al.[155] reported the mechanisms involved in *E. faecalis* resistance to calcium hydroxide. *E. faecalis* was resistant to calcium hydroxide at pH 11.1, but not at pH 11.5. Pretreatment with calcium hydroxide (pH 10.3) induced no tolerance to further exposure at pH 11.5. Survival of *E. faecalis* in calcium hydroxide seemed to be unrelated to stress induced protein synthesis, but a functioning proton pump was critical for *E. faecalis* survival at high pH.

Based on an interesting review, Haapasalo et al.[217] discussed the mostly negative interactions between endodontic disinfecting agents and the various compounds present in the root canal environment. Successful treatment of apical periodontitis is dependent on the elimination of the infective microflora from the necrotic root canal system. Antimicrobial irrigating solutions and other locally used disinfecting agents and medicaments play a key role in eradicating the microbes. While most, if not all presently used disinfecting agents rapidly kill even the resistant microbes when tested in vitro in a test tube, the effectiveness of the same agents is clearly weaker under in vivo conditions. Recent studies have given valuable information about the interaction of endodontic disinfecting agents with dentin and other compounds present in the necrotic root canal. As a result of such interactions, the antimicrobial effectiveness of several of our key disinfectants may be weakened, or even eliminated under certain circumstances. Different disinfectants show different sensitivity to the action of the various potential inactivators, such as dentin, serum proteins, hydroxyapatite, collagen derived from different sources, and microbial biomass. There are several reasons for the lower in vivo performance, but clearly inactivation of the disinfectants by dentin and other substances present in the necrotic root canal is one of the contributory factors to the recognized difficulty of completely eradicating microorganisms from the root canal system.

Souza et al.[552] evaluated the predominant microbiota of infected necrotic pulps and the effects of calcium hydroxide therapy on these microorganisms by the checkerboard DNA-DNA hybridization technique. Conventional endodontic therapy associated with calcium hydroxide as intracanal dressing was performed in 12 single-rooted teeth with pulp necrosis and apical periodontitis. Samples were collected from the canal at baseline and 14 days after therapy, and the presence of 44 bacterial species was determined by the checkerboard method. Significant differences in the microbiota from baseline to post-therapy were sought by the paired-samples test. The most prevalent species included *F. nucleatum ss. vincentii, C. sputigena, C. ochracea, S. constellatus, V. parvula, P. gingivalis, P. melaninogenica*, and *S. sanguis*. Most of the microorganisms were reduced after treatment, particularly *A. gerencseriae, A. israelii, A. naeslundii, C. gingivalis, C. ochracea, P. gingivalis, S. noxia, S. sanguis*, and *S. oralis*. Conversely, *A. actinomycetemcomitans, C. sputigena*, and *E. corrodens* increased in numbers after therapy. These results indicate that conventional endodontic therapy with calcium hydroxide results in the reduction of pathogenic species associated with pulp necrosis.

Estrela et al.[119] evaluated longitudinal studies about the efficacy of calcium hydroxide on *E. faecalis* in endodontic infection, using a systematic review. A MEDLINE search strategy was developed to identify articles using the following uniterms: *Enterococcus faecalis* and Calcium hydroxide or, *Enterococcus faecalis* and Endodontic. The search included articles from the MEDLINE (http://www.ncbi.nlm.nih.gov/PubMed), from 1966 to 23 of November of 2006. The articles electronically identified by the search were selected by two independent reviewers. The selected articles were examined for inclusion or exclusion, based on several criteria. 178 articles were selected (5 articles of literature review, 35 articles about in vivo studies (human or animals) and 138 in vitro studies. Only 3 studies satisfied the inclusion and exclusion criteria. In these studies, 134 teeth had secondary endodontic infection. In 34 teeth *E. faecalis* was identified initially and after the intracanal dressing in 3, 6 and 2 samples of the included studies. The heterogeneity of the studies did not allow an adequate combination of results. Studies in vitro showed the effectiveness of the calcium hydroxide against *E. faecalis*. In the three studies in humans, which satisfied the inclusion criteria for analysis of scientific evidence, of a total of 94 teeth with secondary infections, *E. faecalis* was detected in 34 teeth at the beginning of the treatment and remained in 11 after the disinfections process and use of calcium hydroxide paste. Considering the exact estimative of clinical success of the analyzed studies, evidence of the reduction of *E. faecalis* after the sanitization process could be observed, including the use of calcium hydroxide (Table 20.1).

It is important to emphasize that several studies[47,124,140,155,465,580] showed that *E. faecalis* was more resistant to high pH.

**Table 20.1** - Included studies that allowed the efficacy of calcium hydroxide against *E. faecalis* to be analyzed

| Reference | n | ETi | Tooth | Tech. | *Ef* i | Inter. | Med | *Ef* f |
|---|---|---|---|---|---|---|---|---|
| Sundqvist et al.[580] (1998) | 54 G1 54 CH | 4-5 years | 49 (1r) 5 (2r) | culture | 9 | 0.5% SH + CH | 7-14 days | 3 |
| Peciuliene et al.[450] (2001) | 40 G1 20 CH G2 20 IKI | 5-10 years | 40 (1r) | culture | 21 | 2.5% SH + CH | 10-14 Days | 2 |
| Zerella et al.[643] (2005) | 40 G1 20 CH G2 20 CLX | - | 40 (1r) | culture/ PCR | 4 | 1.0% SH 1,.% + HC | 7-10 days | 2 |

Legend:
n - # of samples
ETi - Initial endodontic treatment
Tooth - 1(one) root; 2 (two) roots
Tech. - identification manner / culture or PCR
Ef initial - # initial samples of *E. faecalis*
Inter. - Intervention / sanitization process (SH - sodium hypochlorite / CH - calcium hydroxide)
Med - time of intracanal dressing
IKI- Iodine-Potassium Iodide solution
Ef final - number of final samples with *E. faecalis*

When the calcium hydroxide or any other medication used in intracanal dressing does not reach the target microorganism, its real efficacy to kill them cannot be expressed. Therefore, it cannot be stated whether or not the microbial strains were resistant to one or another medication. In this case, it is likely that the microorganisms were able to survive, adapt and tolerate the critical ecological conditions[124].

The lapse of time required for calcium hydroxide to express microbial inactivation is determined by several factors, i.e., quickness in dissociation and diffusion of hydroxyl ions, higher or lower dentinal permeability and buffering capacity of dentin.

Research currently indicates the need for an intracanal medication as an adjuvant in the microbial control and tissue healing process. The biological characteristics of calcium hydroxide, represented by its tissue healing and antimicrobial potential, make this material the best therapeutic choice as an intracanal dressing.

### 20.4.2 The role played by the vehicle associated with calcium hydroxide pastes

Several researches have studied the mixture of other substances with calcium hydroxide for the purpose of improving some of its properties. Among these additional substances are vehicles that can speed up or slow down ionic dissociation, and aid pulp cavity filling due to their consistency.

Thus, these different substances (distilled water, saline solution, propylene glycol, camphorated paramonochorophenol, chlorhexidine, glycerin, corticosteroid-antibiotic, antibiotics, anesthetic solution, methylcellulose, glycerin, detergent, iodoform, barium sulfate) have been added to calcium hydroxide in an attempt to enhance its antimicrobial activity, biocompatibility, ionic dissociation, and diffusion. A controversial factor when choosing a vehicle is the comparison of the antimicrobial effect of calcium hydroxide in association with hydrosoluble vehicles (distilled water, saline solution) and oily vehicles (camphorated paramonochorophenol). The experimental methods used to study the antimicrobial effects of substances with different dissociation and diffusion capabilities must be chosen carefully. Different tests to evaluate antimicrobial action of endodontic materials have been reported. Some studies have indicated calcium hydroxide plus camphorated paramonochorophenol as the best intracanal dressing for treatment of infected root canals. Other investigations have used histopathological analysis to demonstrate that calcium hydroxide plus a hydrosoluble vehicle provides favorable results for the treatment of teeth with apical periodontitis[130,136,].

The action of calcium hydroxide is directly influenced by the release of hydroxyl ions and by inactivation of enzymes of the cytoplasmic membrane of microorganisms, which chemically alters the organic components and transport of nutrients, causing toxic effects on the cells. The effectiveness of vehicles derives from their chemical characteristics (dissociation and diffusion). Chemically, hydrosoluble vehicles (distilled water, saline solution) induce a higher speed of ionic dissociation than viscous (polyethylene glycol) and oily vehicles (camphorated paramonochorophenol)[130,136,146,147].

Estrela et al.[136] determined the influence of vehicles on the antimicrobial efficiency of calcium hydroxide. Antimicrobial action was not sufficiently influenced by any of the vehicles to suggest that they play a supportive role in the process by providing appropriate conditions for dissociation and diffusion, and enhancing complete root canal filling; these are important factors for antimicrobial potential and tissue healing capability.

The methods used in research must also be considered. The Agar diffusion test (ADT), which evaluates microbial growth inhibition halos, may not offer equal conditions for comparing substances with different solubility and diffusibility and the correct performance of microbiological technique. Factors such as pre-incubation, dried culture medium, and maintenance for periods of time that exceed the ideal time for analysis, can yield doubtful results[114,130,136]. The ADT does not distinguish between bacteriostatic and bactericidal properties of dental materials, neither does it provide any information about the viability of the tested microorganism, or its limitation to measure the activity of soluble components. ADT requires careful standardization of inoculum density, medium content, agar viscosity, size, and number of specimens per plate[588]. The analysis of medications that have different dissociation and diffusion rates by means of an experimental model using liquid culture medium (broth) is more effective, than diffusion tests using agar as the culture medium. Agar is a semisolid medium that makes the diffusion of hydroxyl ions in calcium hydroxide pastes more difficult, requiring pre-incubation. Phenolic compounds, such as camphorated paramonochorophenol and calcium hydroxide plus camphorated paramonochorophenol, have shown satisfactory inhibition using ADT, but the size of the zone of microbial growth inhibition does not show their real antimicrobial effect[136]. Estrela et al.[130] reported that because the site of action of hydroxyl ions of calcium hydroxide includes the enzymes in the cytoplasmic membrane, this medication has a large scope of action, depending on its quantity, and therefore is effective on a wide range of microorganisms, regardless of their metabolic capability. Cytoplasmic membranes are similar regardless of their morphological, staining, and respiratory characteristics that mean that this medication has a similar effect on aerobic, anaerobic, Gram-positive, and Gram-negative bacteria. The choice of hydrossoluble vehicles can accelerate ionic dissociation and diffusion, and interfere with the bacterial enzyme and tissue systems[147]. Factors such as hydrosolubility of the vehicle (difference in viscosity), acid-based characteristics, higher or lower dentinal permeability, buffering capacity of dentin, and level of existing calcification can alter the rate of dissociation and diffusion of hydroxyl ions of calcium hydroxide and influence its properties, which lead to the choice of vehicles such as distilled water and saline solution.

Intracanal dressing represents a vast issue in Endodontics. For many years it was extensively valorized. Nowadays, controversial discussions are presented concerning its real function on teeth with apical periodontitis. It is known that the preparation of the root canal is potentially responsible for microbial control, particularly as regards the effective function of sanitization (emptying, enlargement, interaction of the irrigant agents).

The complete antimicrobial effectiveness of calcium hydroxide paste has been associated with availability, diffusiveness and velocity of the dissociation of ions, particularly the hydroxide ions[130,146,147].

Furthermore, the defense of study based on scientific evidence has been discussed. This aspect involves the realization of a systematic review or meta-analysis. The systematic review is a model of investigation focused on high-quality studies that intend to gather and examine evidences, in a systematic approach, taking care to avoid scientific distortions, which certainly influence decision making. The meta-analysis is a method of systematic review that involves the arrangement of results from several studies, in order to achieve a single point estimate (qualitative analysis, frequency, quantitative analysis). Not many systematic reviews and/or meta-analyses of studies have been conducted in Endodontics[119,120,143,350,503,589]. The main problem is to obtain support, based on evidence that indicates explanations that help with clinical decision making. Nevertheless, the question is to analyze the influence of the vehicle on the efficacy of calcium hydroxide in endodontic infections.

Effectiveness of the study begins with the analysis of investigations developed in human beings, which have provided answers to clinical questions, and goes through to the critical analysis of the longitudinal studies published.

Estrela et al.[120] selected prospective studies to investigate the influence of the vehicle on the efficacy of calcium hydroxide pastes in endodontic infections. To identify the studies, electronic searches and manual search strategies were used. The following databases were searched on January 2nd of 2007: MEDLINE (without filter, from 1966 to January 2nd of 2007), EMBASE (without filter, from 1980 to January 2nd of 2007), Cochrane Oral Health Group Trials Register and Cochrane Central Register of Controlled Trials (CENTRAL). The following descriptors were used as keywords in several combinations: 1. Calcium hydroxide and chlorhexidine OR, 2. Calcium hydroxide and root canal infection OR, 3. Calcium hydroxide and faecalis OR, 4. Calcium hydroxide and intracanal dressing OR, 5. Calcium hydroxide and endodontic infection OR, 6. Calcium hydroxide and intracanal medicament OR, 7. Calcium hydroxide and paramonochorophenol OR, 8. Calcium hydroxide and para monochlorophenol OR, 9. Calcium hydroxide and p-monochlorophenol. The manual search was conducted by the examining the reference lists of the potentially eligible clinical trials and the review author's personal databases of trial reports, in an endeavor to identify any other relevant studies.

The selected articles were identified from the titles and abstracts, considering the tabulated inclusion criteria, independently by two reviewers. Full copies of all relevant and potentially relevant studies, those that appeared to meet the inclusion criteria, or for which there were insufficient data in the title and abstract to enable one to make a clear decision, were obtained. The reviewers assessed the methodological quality of the studies using the same criteria. Next, for each selected study individually, the number of samples were calculated, the data were tabulated with regard to the type of infection (primary or secondary), the type of root canal involved in the research, the methods of identification of the bacteria, the presence of microorganisms in the initial samples, the vehicle associated with calcium hydroxide as intracanal dressing, medicament substances used during the sanitization process, the time the intracanal dressing was maintained before filling and the presence of microorganisms on the final samples. Evaluation of these combined factors brought a new group of associated data, which included all the selected samples.

At present, several questions remain with regard to intracanal dressing in the treatment of teeth with endodontic infections. The literature presents several investigations that were conducted to discuss the real indication of intracanal dressing. The proof of studies developed on the basis of scientific evidences has been considered an exclusion factor in the systematic investigations. The point of origin of a relevant clinical problem, which indicates a convincing and well founded solution, is part of the goal of a systematic review. Several decisions that guide the clinic ambit, have been upheld on controversial, and frequently inconclusive results.

It must be considered that the systematic review with meta-analysis is able to determine whether or not a clinical procedure (clinical decision) is applicable. Several precautions must be taken when a systematic review is undertaken, with or without meta-analysis, to start with the clinical relevance of the question, the aim of the study. Other fundamental aspects are connected with the criteria adopted in the search for the articles, selection of the inclusion and exclusion criteria, bias of publication, hierarchy of the studies and criteria of analysis. These factors can make a systematic review a study of extreme value for evaluating the clinical adoption of a conduct, as well as being an inquiry of particular value within the limits of this type of study. In general, care must be taken when extrapolating the results obtained in studies for adaptation to clinical conducts, considering that the results are frequently inconclusive, and do not allow a clinical decision applicable to therapeutic protocols in humans.

The quality of the systematic reviews published in connection with dentistry interventions were evaluated[193]. Only 19% demonstrated adequate care in identifying all the relevant studies.

In the present study[120], it was verified that most of the experiments were developed in vitro or in animals. Studies developed in humans must involve a strict methodology, guided entirely by present day bioethical parameters. Nevertheless, studies that are not essentially developed in humans cannot be disrespected, because some tests have been demanded for biologic evaluation of dental materials, which include the initial and secondary tests, until the stage of the application test is reached. It is natural to have a new view and scientific routine to verify the validation of studies, which seek to abate a discussion, and are frequently supported on the basis of evidence.

The search presented 303 related articles[120], and from these, 22 articles were literature reviews, 71 articles were related to in vivo studies (humans or animals), 34 studies were case reports, and 178 included in vitro studies. From the 71 in vivo studies, 5 studies satisfied the inclusion criteria, which enabled the data analysis (Table 20.2). The impossibility of combining the results, caused by differences in methodologies used in the studies did not allow a meta-analysis to be performed. In vitro studies showed that the vehicle influences the chemical characteristics of the calcium hydroxide paste with regard to the speed of diffusion an ionic dissociation, as occurs with aqueous hydrosoluble vehicles. This chemical characteristic reflects on the antimicrobial potential. In the five studies in humans, which satisfied the inclusion criteria for analysis of scientific evidence, out of a total of 110 teeth with endodontic infections subjected to the sanitization process with the use of calcium hydroxide paste as an intracanal dressing, microorganisms were detected in the final samples of 35 teeth.

Within the 5 studies included[72,444,457,552,643], interesting aspects were observed, but due to the absence of similarity in the experimental methods, it was not possible to make an ideal arrangement of the results. In these studies, primary and secondary endodontic infection were analyzed in 131 teeth. In the treated teeth with calcium hydroxide paste associated with the saline, 110 teeth were contaminated at the beginning of the endodontic treatment. After the sanitization process (root canal preparation, action of irrigant solutions - saline, 0.5 to 5.25% sodium hypochlorite), and application of the calcium hydroxide paste associated with the saline, in the period of 7 to 28 days, it was still possible to identify microorganisms in 35 of the teeth. Out of a total of 20 teeth treated with calcium hydroxide paste associated with chlorhexidine, after 14 to 21 days, 4 teeth still were contaminated.

In the data analysis of the studies included, it can be verified that some methodological data were hidden, which show a relative degree of significance, such as a radiographic admission after placement of the calcium hydroxide paste. Relevant aspects of the studies that met the inclusion criteria were considered, among them are: the presence of teeth involved in the research, method of identifying the bacterium, presence of microorganisms in the initial samples, vehicle associated with the calcium hydroxide paste, medication substances used during the sanitization process, period of maintaining the intracanal dressing before filling, and the presence of microorganisms in the final samples (Table 20.2).

The difficulty of comparing the studies included resulted from the differences in the experimental designs, such as: standardization of the limit of instrumentation after emptying the root canal, as well as the choice of the root canal preparation technique; standardization of the selected tooth and sample size; standardization of the test material, the technique of positioning the test material and verification of correct filling; quality control of the irrigating solution, as well as variation in its concentration; criteria for the detection of the periapical lesion, etc. The study model used did not allow perfect arrangement of the results, whose correlation was critical, particularly, characterizing heterogeneity of the clinic protocols adapted. This was one of the limitations to performing the meta-analysis.

The large number of investigations published can show a profile of context with con-

**Table 20.2** - Studies included that allowed the analysis of the influence of the vehicle on the efficacy of calcium hydroxide pastes in endodontic infections.

| Reference | n | Ti | Tooth | Technique | Vehicle | IS | Intervention | Med | Outcome |
|---|---|---|---|---|---|---|---|---|---|
| Ørstavik et al.[444] | 23 | 1ª | 23 uni | Culture | Saline | 22 | Saline | 7 d | 8 |
| Peters et al.[457] | 21 | 1ª | DNI | Culture | Saline | 21 | 2% SH + CH | 28 d | 2 |
| Souza et al.[552] | 12 | 1ª | 12 uni | Checkerboard DNA | Saline | 12 | 5.25% SH + CH | 14 d | 6 |
| Zerella et al.[643] | 20<br>20 | 2ª | 40 uni | Culture and PCR | Saline<br>2%CHX | 20<br>20 | 1% SH + CH | 14 to 21 d | 8<br>4 |
| Chu et al.[72] | 35 | 1ª | 18 uni<br>14 bi<br>3 tri | Culture | Saline | 35 | 0.5% SH + CH | 7d | 11 |

Legend:

n = number of samples, TI = Type of infection, Tooth = uniradicular / biradicular / triradicular, DNI = data not identified, Technique = kind of identification, IS = Initial microbiological sample, Med = time of maintenance of intracanal dressing; CHX = chlorhexidine; SH = sodium hypochlorite; CH = calcium hydroxide.

tradictory conclusions, as all the information of the experiments published and the actual nature of the trials indicate the critical involvement of this method of work.

The influence of the vehicles on the antimicrobial activities of calcium hydroxide was studied by Estrela et al.[114] using calcium hydroxide pastes in microbial suspensions (*S. mutans, E. faecalis, S. aureus, P. aeruginosa, B. subtilis, C. albicans* and a mixture of these microorganisms). The calcium hydroxide pastes studied were associated with the following vehicles: saline, camphor paramonochorophenol, solution of 1% chlorhexidine, 3% lauryl ether sodium sulfate, and Otosporin. After intervals of one minute, 48 and 72 hours, and 7 days, the microbial growth was evaluated by the turbidity of the culture medium. The antimicrobial effect of the paste, irrespective of the vehicle associated, occurred after 48 hours in all the microorganisms studied.

Safavi & Nakayama[490] evaluated the dissociation of calcium hydroxide added to two different non–aqueous vehicles. The authors prepared mixtures of glycerin or saturated propylenoglycol and calcium hydroxide, and separated the non soluble powder through a centrifuge. The values found for the association with water were of 7.3 $\pm$ mS/cm, while the behavior of the calcium hydroxide in glycerin or propylenoglycol was essentially zero. The association of calcium hydroxide with non – aqueous vehicles can obstruct its effectiveness as an intracanal dressing. Haenni et al.[218] evaluated the antimicrobial and chemical effects of calcium hydroxide pastes added to chlorhexidine, sodium hypochlorite or iodine potassium iodide. The authors studied the alterations of pH of the external surface of extracted teeth, and the antimicrobial action. The association of calcium hydroxide with the tested solution did not provide an increase in the antimicrobial efficacy, when compared with calcium hydroxide paste associated with saline.

In the endodontic context, analyzed on the basis of evidences, the vehicles do influence the association and ionic diffusion, which reflect the antimicrobial potential of calcium hydroxide paste. Hauman & Love[229] related that the arrangement of high-toxicity with limited clinical effectiveness, excludes the phenol compounds from the list of contemporary remedies for intracanal use.

Significant reduction of microorganisms has been found to occur in the sanitization process (emptying, irrigation, enlargement, intracanal medication), which has altered the procedures of modern Endodontology, based on evidence. The microorganisms prevalent in endodontic infections are determinant in the choice of the sanitization process. The attempt to solve a problem, after considering the possible inherent limitations, encourages new hypotheses, which will certainly influence new searches. There will probably be several future implications after this investigation, specially the valuation of studies in relation to scientific evidence. Considering the estimation of clinical success, an adequate sanitization process aided by the calcium hydroxide paste with aqueous vehicle, reduces the endodontic microorganisms, which favors the prognosis.

Calcium hydroxide encourages the deposition of a hard tissue bridge when in direct contact with the pulp tissue. Thus, the paste can be prepared in a pure form or by mixing it with distilled water. A controversial factor when choosing a vehicle, is the comparison of the antimicrobial effect of calcium hydroxide in association with hydrosoluble vehicles (distilled water, saline solution) and other vehicles, such as camphorated paramonochorophenol, chlorhexidine etc. The combination of a water-soluble vehicle (such as a saline solution) with calcium hydroxide pastes has shown better results when compared with camphorated paramonochorophenol.

Holland et al.[266] evaluated the healing of periapical tissues with different preparations of calcium hydroxide (Calen + polyethylene glycol 400; Calen + camphorated paramonochorophenol, and calcium hydroxide + anesthetic) in dog teeth. After a period of 6 months for the formation of periapical lesion, and another 6-month period for the histopathological evaluation following treatment, the results showed that the association between camphorated paramonochorophenol and Calen did not improve treatment results, and that the average total repair for the three groups was 50%. In another study, Holland et al.[248] studied the healing process in the roots of 60 teeth with periapical lesion, using calcium hydroxide in combination with saline solution, calcium hydroxide in combination with camphorated paramonochorophenol (CMPC), CMPC combined with furacin, and CMPC alone. The results were better with the use of calcium hydroxide associated with saline solution (approximately 60% of total repair and 40% of partial repair). In the case of calcium hydroxide associated with CMPC, results showed 20% of complete repair, 70% of partial repair, and 10% of unsuccessful repair. Treatment carried out in a single session showed 40% of unsuccessful repair, 40% of partial repair, and only 20% of complete repair (Fig. 20.37-20.41). It was observed that 6 months after obturation of root canals, the best rates of repair were obtained with an intracanal dressing with saline solution as the vehicle.

The association of chlorhexidine with calcium hydroxide has been shown not to influence the time required and efficacy for microbial inactivation[114].

The presence of para-chloroaniline (PCA) has already been detected in chlorhexidine (CHX) solutions[230,610]. The International Agency for Research on Cancer (IARC, 2006)[632] categorizes PCA in their 2B Group, which means that this agent is possibly carcinogenic to humans. The interaction of CHX with CH may generate reactive oxygen species (ROS), which play a critical role on the cellular wall and membrane structure of microorganisms[638].

Yeung et al.[638] evaluated the antioxidant and pro-oxidant properties of chlorhexidine. The scavenging and generation of reactive oxygen species (ROS) by chlorhexidine in the

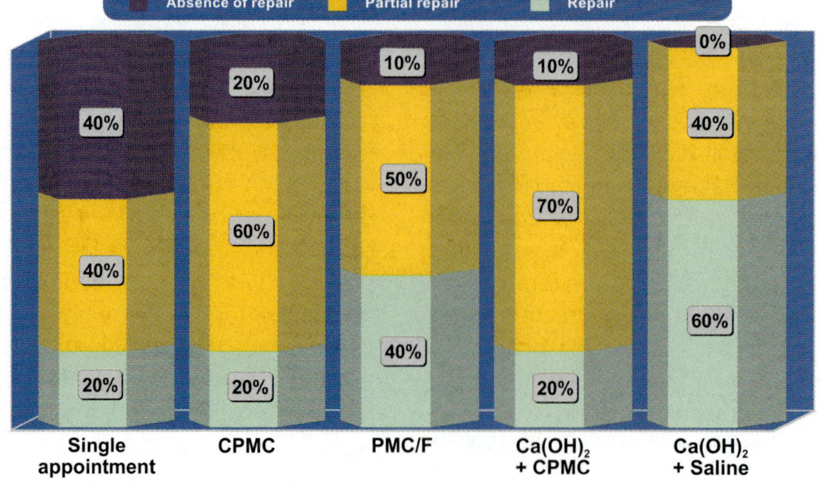


**Figure 20.37** - Effect of intracanal dressing on healing process in dog teeth with apical periodontitis (Holland et al.[248]).

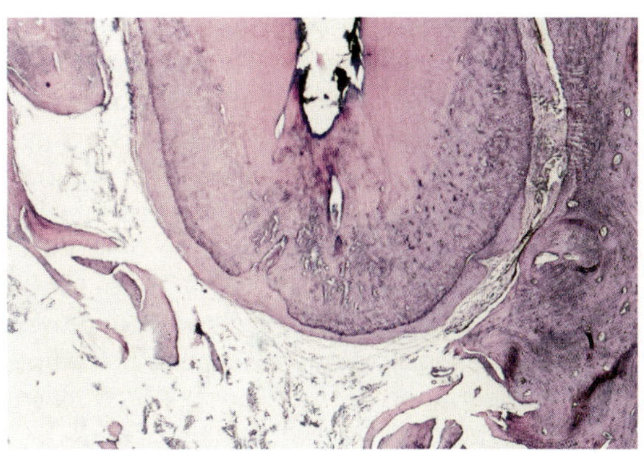

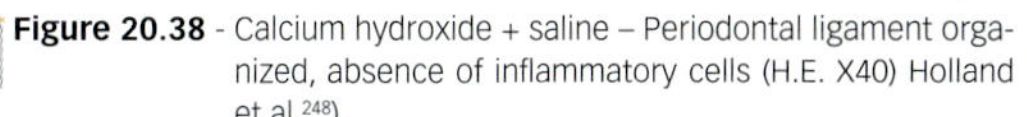

**Figure 20.38** - Calcium hydroxide + saline – Periodontal ligament organized, absence of inflammatory cells (H.E. X40) Holland et al.[248]).

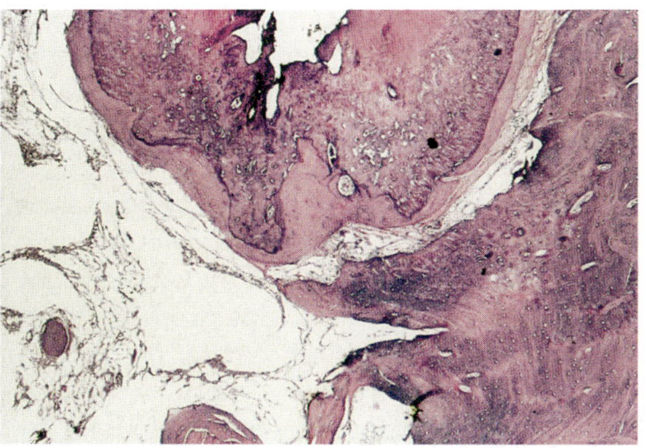

**Figure 20.39** - Calcium hydroxide + saline – Periodontal ligament organized, absence of inflammatory cells. Complete repair process (H.E. X40) Holland et al.[248]).

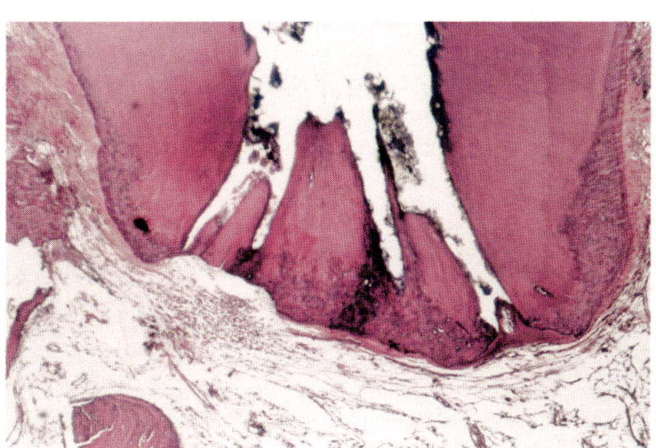

**Figure 20.40** - Calcium hydroxide + saline – Periodontal ligament organized, absence of inflammatory cells. Partial repair process (H.E. X40) Holland et al.[248]).

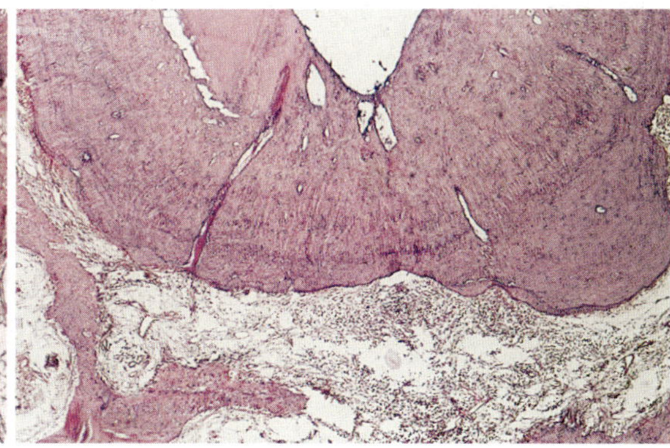

**Figure 20.41** - Calcium hydroxide + camphorated paramonochorophenol – Periodontal ligament with presence of inflammatory cells (H.E. X40)( Holland et al.[248]).

presence or absence of saturated calcium hydroxide solutions, was evaluated. The reaction emitted chemiluminescence in the presence of lucigenin, thus was determined by a luminometer to evaluate the levels of ROS production. Changes in DNA conformation were analyzed by agarose gel electrophoresis. Chlorhexidine (0.00002–0.02%) effectively scavenged 56–88% of the superoxide radicals generated by the xanthine/xanthine oxidase reaction. Through analysis of PUC18 DNA conformation changes, chlorhexidine was shown to be a mild scavenger of hydroxyl radicals generated by $H_2O_2$ plus $FeCl_2$. However, chlorhexidine (>0.083%) decreased the mobility of PUC18 plasmid DNA, with potential production of DNA–DNA cross-link and severe DNA breaks (presence of DNA smear) at further higher concentrations. Chlorhexidine induced ROS production including $H_2O_2$ and superoxide radicals in 0.1N NaOH (pH = 12.76) or calcium hydroxide (pH = 12.5) solutions. Chlorhexidine exhibited both antioxidant and pro-oxidant properties under different conditions. These events are possibly involved in the killing of root canal and periodontal microorganisms, when chlorhexidine and calcium hydroxide were used in combination or separately. Potential genotoxicity and tissue damage when extruded into the periradicular tissue and at higher concentrations should be considered during periodontal and endodontic practice.

Barbin et al.[19] studied the performance of a chemical analysis of 0.2% chlorhexidine digluconate, isolated or mixed with calcium hydroxide, using Mass Spectrometry and High-Efficiency Liquid Chromatography. The analyses were performed shortly after the samples were prepared, and after 7 and 14 days of storage at 36.5 °C. It was found that the isolated chlorhexidine digluconate solution formed different byproducts, including para-chloroaniline (PCA), posing systemic risks. In contact with calcium hydroxide, chlorhexidine decomposes completely and forms different compounds. Though the study did not demonstrate the presence of parachloroaniline in the medication paste, the high number of reactive species poses a high risk to the genetic material of the host cells affected by intracanal medication. It is mandatory to establish a precise diagnostic-therapeutic relation, by developing clinical protocols that would restrict the use of these intracanal medications to clinical conditions with disseminated endodontic infection and persistent apical periodontitis. There is a need for more efficient strategies that use more effective biomechanical processes and intracanal medications that do not offer any local or systemic risk, so that root canal treatment goals can predictability and safety be considered (Graphics 20.1-20.9).

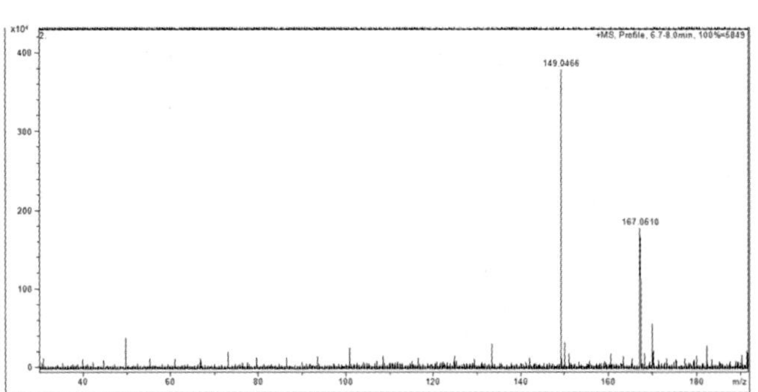


**Graphic 20.1** - The mass spectrum shows a relation between mass and load (m/z) of ionized molecules in the sample with peaks at 149 m/z and 167 m/z immediately after preparation of PCA solution. These values indicate the presence of PCA. The difference might be due the presence of sodium.

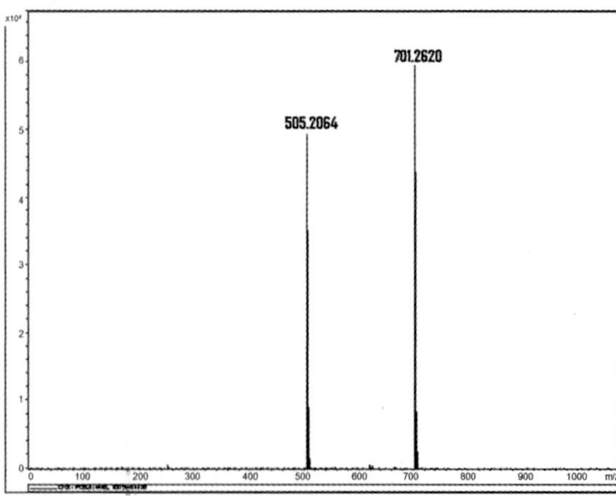


**Graphic 20.2** - Mass spectrometry analysis of 0.2% CHX immediately after its preparation presented peaks at 505 and 701 m/z, which confirms the high degree of purity of this sample. Presence of PCA was not verified.

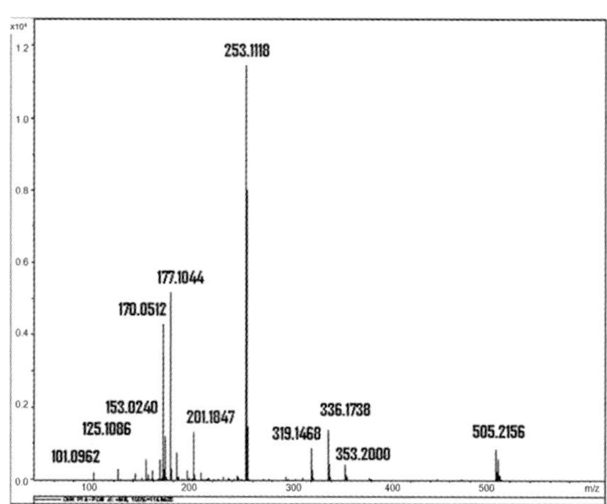


**Graphic 20.3** - Mass spectrometry analysis of a solution of 0.2% CHX after 7 days. The chromatographic analysis showed decomposition into several sub-products with different values (101, 125, 152, 170, 177, 201, 319, 336, 353 and 505 m/z).

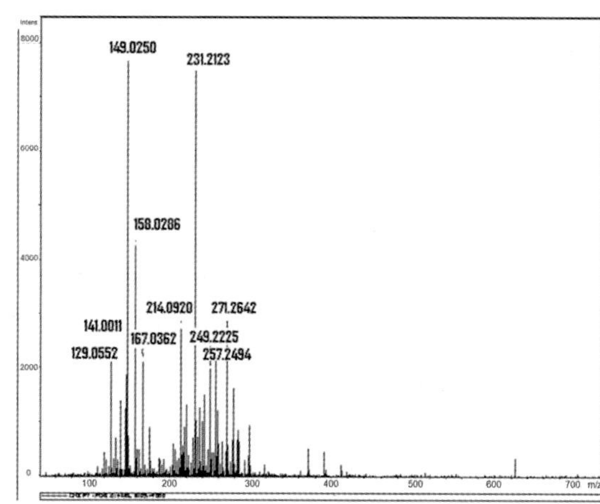


**Graphic 20.4** - Mass spectrometry analysis of a solution of 0.2% CHX after 14 days. It can be observed a total degradation of CHX. The initial peaks (505 and 701 m/z) are not observed. There are peaks of 129 m/z (literature-based indicator) and 149 and 167 m/z (experimental indicators), which suggest the presence of PCA after 14 days.

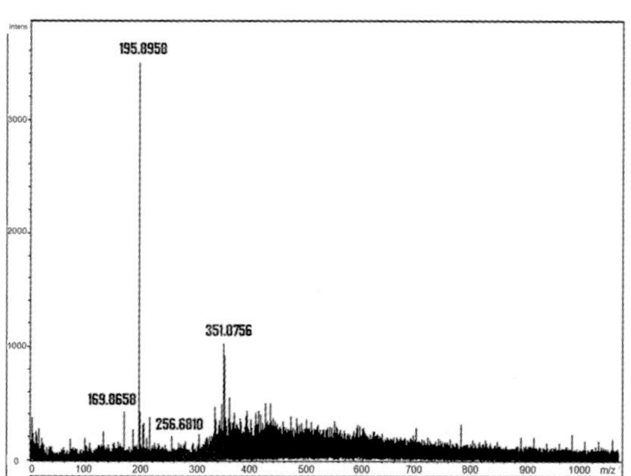


**Graphic 20.5** - Mass spectrometry analysis of a solution of CHP + 0.2% CHX. The chromatographic analysis of the CH + 0.2% CHX mixture immediately after its preparation showed peaks of 169, 195, 256 and 351 m/z. The peak of 169 m/z corresponds to chlorophenyl guanide. These results explain the ability of CH to separate the CHX molecule in positions containing groups $NH_n$. The peak of 195 m/z was probably originated by production of reactive compounds, due the high concentration of hydroxyl ions (alkaline environment) in the presence of CHX. Indicators for PCA were not found.

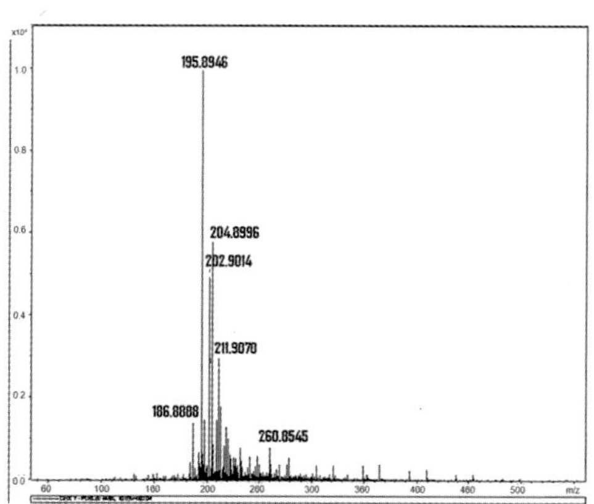


**Graphic 20.6** - Mass spectrometry analysis of a solution of CH mixed 0.2% CHX after 7 days. The chromatographic analysis shows absence of peaks at 505 and 701 m/z, which suggests a total degradation of CHX. ROS were observed, but indicators for PCA were not detected.

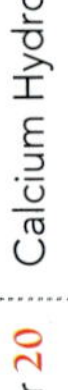


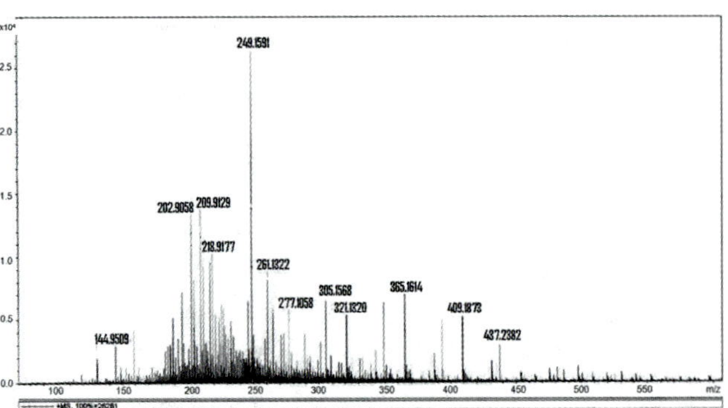


**Graphic 20.7** - Mass spectrometry analysis of a solution of CH mixed 0.2% CHX after 14 days. The chromatographic analysis shows absence of peaks at 505 and 701 m/z, which suggests a total degradation of CHX. ROS were observed, but indicators for PCA were not detected.

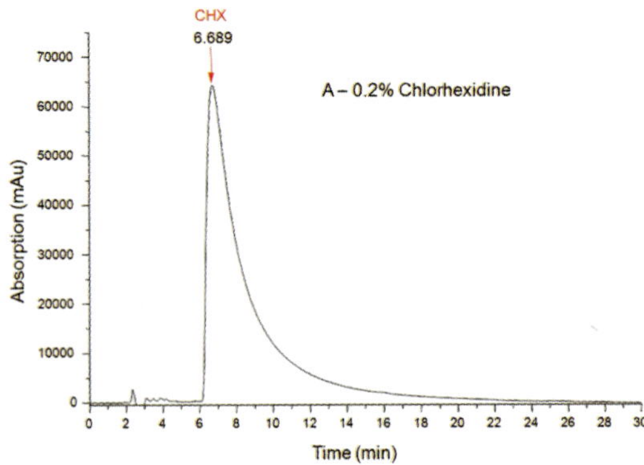


**Graphic 20.8** - High-performance liquid chromatography (HPLC). Chromatogram of the analysis of compounds in the standard solution of CHX immediately after preparation showed that the time of retention of this substance was 6.7 min.

B – 0.2% Chlorhexidine + $Ca(OH)_2$

Absorption (mAu)

Time (min)

**Graphic 20.9** - High-performance liquid chromatography (HPLC). Chromatogram of the analysis of the CH + 0.2% CHX mixture indicated that CHX was no longer present after 6.7 min. This result confirms the degradation of CHX after preparation of the mixture.

Other aspect that influenced the effectiveness of calcium hydroxide is the correct filling of radicular canal is as important as the effectiveness of calcium hydroxide, since the lack of direct contact of this dressing interferes with its mechanism of action. In order to better visualize the filling of pulp cavity, zinc oxide, iodoform and barium sulphate have been added to calcium hydroxide as radiopaque substances. Estrela et al.[133] observed that is not necessary to add radiopaque substances to calcium hydroxide pastes, because their density is similar that of dentin, provided the radicular canal had been properly filled. Moreover, when any substance is added to calcium hydroxide, even an inert one, it represents one more factor to influence biological processes also bringing the possibility of diminishing the amount of hydroxyl and calcium ions available, which is one of the reasons for its use.

Estrela et al.[126] verified the influence of iodoform on the antimicrobial potential of calcium hydroxide in several biological indicators (*E. faecalis, S. aureus, P. aeruginosa, B. subtillis, C. albicans* and a mix of these microbial samples). The substances tested were: calcium hydroxide + saline; calcium hydroxide + iodoform + saline; iodoform + saline. The calcium hydroxide associated with saline or iodoform plus saline, showed antimicrobial effectiveness in both experimental methods. The iodoform paste did not present antimicrobial effectiveness against all biological indicators tested.

### 20.4.3 Antibacterial Efficacy of Intracanal Medicaments on Bacterial Biofilm

This topic involves a critical analysis of published research that evaluated the antibacterial efficacy of intracanal medicaments against bacterial biofilm. The principle of treatment to reach a favorable outcome against endodontic infection, requires recognition of the problem and removal of the etiological factors. The micro-environment of root canal presents excellent conditions to establish microbial growth. The success of infected root canal treatment is influenced by discrepancy gradients of microorganism between the endodontic biofilm and planktonic suspension[124].

The phases for the microbial community to develop a biofilm and colonize the environment may be unusual, but basically occur with the same sequence of developmental steps - deposition of a conditioning film, adhesion and colonization of planktonic microorganisms in a polymeric matrix, co-adhesion of other organisms, and detachment of biofilm microorganisms into their surroundings[79,584].

The reduction in endodontic microbiota has been attained by antimicrobial strategies such as root canal preparation, irrigant solutions, intracanal dressing and root canal filling.

Several studies were developed with different bacterial biofilm models to test the antimicrobial effectiveness of endodontic medicaments[68,98,100,124,155,184,188,216,344,535,562]. Investigations have shown, either antimicrobial effectiveness[98,398], or ineffectiveness [3,68,98,124,155,216,332,422] of intracanal medicaments against bacterial biofilm, as well as the presence of biofilm, on all external root apex surfaces in teeth with pulp necrosis with radiographically visible periapical lesions[363]. The susceptibility of oral bacterial biofilm to antimicrobial agents indicates the necessity to think about in vivo conditions, where bacteria grow as biofilm on tooth surfaces[47].

Spratt et al.[562] verified the bactericidal effect of 2.25% NaOCl, 0.2% chlorhexidine, 10% iodine or phosphate buffered saline on single-species of biofilms (*P. intermedia, P. micros, S. intermedius, F. nucleatum* and *E. faecalis*) derived from a range of root canal isolates. The efficacy of a particular agent was dependent on the nature of the organism in the biofilm and on the contact time. NaOCl was generally the most effective agent tested, followed by iodine. Nevertheless, the clinical effectiveness of these agents must be regarded in the light of the complexity of root canal anatomy and the polymicrobial nature of root canal infections. Abdullah et al.[3] analyzed the efficacy of 3% NaOCl, 10% povidone iodine, 0.2% chlorhexidine, 17% EDTA and calcium hydroxide on a clinical isolate of *E. faecalis* grown as biofilm or planktonic suspension phenotype. The difference in gradients of bacterial killing amongst biofilm, planktonic suspension or pellet presentation was significant and dependent upon the agent, except for NaOCl and calcium hydroxide, in which no difference could be detected. NaOCl was the most effective agent and achieved 100% killing for all presentations of *E. faecalis* after a 2-min contact time. Estrela et al.[124] determined the antimicrobial efficacy of ozonated water, gaseous ozone, sodium hypochlorite and chlorhexidine in *E. faecalis* biofilm. The irrigation solutions tested for 20 minutes were not sufficient to inactivate *E. faecalis*. Nair et al.[422] suggested the need of non-antibiotic chemo-mechanical measures to treat teeth with infected and necrotic root canals so as to disrupt the biofilm.

On the other hand, evidence-based dentistry has been the ultimate goal, in which the observation of such evidences involves systematic review or meta-analysis. Within this context, based on systematic review, a critical analysis of therapeutic protocols for bacterial biofilm is essential. In order to develop this, studies in humans with definite clinical questions are required, using a critical longitudinal analysis of published articles. The focus on answering clinical questions can be structured by means of a problem, intervention, comparison and outcome (PICO).

An immense number of investigations about the antimicrobial potential of intracanal medicaments against bacterial biofilm have shown inconsistent results, but the clinical question on how to eliminate the endodontic bacterial biofilm remains unclear. Relevant clinical considerations are still not well elucidated, such as the efficacy of Intracanal medicament against bacterial biofilm, the time necessary for a mature endodontic biofilm to form, or the ideal biofilm model to assess antimicrobial endodontic substances.

Estrela et al.[149] based on the search strategy developed a quantitative systematic review using an analysis of longitudinal studies. Prospective studies were observed with regard to the efficacy of the intracanal medicaments against bacterial biofilm. Sources of a bibliographic catalogue were used, identified electronically as MEDLINE (http://www.ncbi.nlm.nih.gov/PubMed), from 1966, until 1st August of 2007, and Cochrane Library, during the same period. For the search strategy, the following terms were used as keywords in several combinations: 1. apical biofilm or, 2. apical biofilms or, 3. endodontic biofilm or, 4. endodontic biofilms or, 5. biofilm and root canal or, 6. biofilms and root canal or, 7. periapical biofilm or, 8. periapical biofilms or, 9. endodontic bacterial plaque or, 10. endodontic bacterial plaque or, 11. endodontic dental plaque or, 12. endodontic dental plaque or, 13. refractory endodontic plaque or, 14. biofilm and intracanal medicaments or, 15. biofilm and intracanal dressing.

The selected articles were identified from the titles, abstracts and complete articles independently, by two reviewers, considering the tabulated inclusion and exclusion criteria. Disagreements were resolved by consensus. Table 20.3 show the inclusion and exclusion criteria of selected studies.

The search of information for the present study[148] found 91 related articles, so that of these, 17 (18.7%) articles were literature reviews, 8 (8.8%) articles involved studies in vivo (7 in humans and 1 in animals), 19 (20.1%) included studies in vitro (7 (7.7%) articles of biofilm model on membrane filter, 12 (13.1%) articles with biofilm model on root dentin, 9 (10%) studies associated with nonendodontic biofilm and 33 (36.2%) articles related to others studies. Out of the 8 in vivo articles, no study satisfied the inclusion criteria (Table 20.4). Table 20.5 describes in vitro research articles showing several bacterial biofilm models, contamination time, process of cleaning and shaping and therapeutic efficacy. The analysis demonstrated lack of efficacy of endodontic therapy against bacterial biofilm

Systematic reviews, whether associated with the meta-analysis, or not, represent major positions on the evidence pyramid towards direct decision making, capable of indicating clinical procedures certificated by more trustable arguments. The biggest difficulty found was the large amount of information, and investigations with contradictory conclusions. The scientific evidence that confirms the efficacy of the intracanal medicaments against bacterial biofilm involve profound reflection and discussion, and despite the limits of the method[193,314,350,539], the longitudinal studies signaled that there is as yet no accurate solution to eliminate or disrupt the root canal bacterial biofilm. Moreover, the results of this critical review confirmed that root canal preparation, with careful sanitization process and using intracanal substances that provide good antimicrobial efficacy, tissue dissolution capacity, and acceptable biocompatibility, will definitely improve the prognosis of the treatment of apical periodontitis[350,422,503].

Out of 91 associated articles, 8.8% involved studies in vivo. There was absence of research that satisfied the inclusion criteria (Table 20.4)[17,330,363,432,433,602], particularly as a result of randomized controlled trial studies.

Interestingly, a recently published study contemplating the clinical aspects of bacterial biofilm, is the only one with a high level of evidence. Nair et al.[422] assessed intracanal microbial status of apical root canal system of mesial roots of human mandibular first molars with primary apical periodontitis immediately after one-visit endodontic treatment. The findings highlight the importance and necessity of stringently applying non antibiotic chemomechanical measures in order to disrupt the biofilm and reduce the intraradicular microbial load to the lowest possible level, to ensure the most favorable long-term prognosis for treatment of infected root canals.

In accordance with this study, other investigations also recovered microorganisms from teeth with endodontic infection, after antimicrobial endodontic therapy[47,69,129,155,410,580].

Considering in vitro essays[3,23,35,68,74,98,182,184,212,235,332,365,510,519,551,562] antimicrobial effectiveness of intracanal medicaments against bacterial biofilm can be observed[3,562], in a similar manner to that in vivo evaluations, involving the presence of biofilm on all external root apex surfaces in teeth with pulp necrosis with periapical lesions[363]. The majority of studies about endodontic biofilm are associated with in vitro experiments. Care should be taken to avoid inappropriate extrapolation of results, which does not allow a clinical decision for therapeutic protocols in humans. It is essential to consider the role and importance of biofilm in endodontology, as well as its definition. In many studies[3,17,23,35,68,74,98,182,185,212,235,330,332,365,432,430,50,510,551,562,602], considerable differences were observed in biofilm models, and in the time required for their development (Table 20.5). In the present study, it was not possible to obtain an ideal combination of results, considering the high heterogeneity of the clinical protocols adopted. This limited the performance of the meta-analysis.

The high number of papers published, can bring contradictory conclusions in its trail. The variability between the methodologies used, study selection, publication biases, absence of randomized controlled trials, access to all the information of the published experiments and the very nature of the essays, signals some of the critical implications of the equation of the problem.

A clinical question that supports the decision on the antibacterial efficacy of intracanal medicaments against bacterial biofilm, cannot be answered using a critical longitudinal analysis of published articles. Various obstacles to the analysis of the pertinent data of the included studies involved methodological data that were hidden, and that present a relative degree of importance. Relevant aspects of the studies that met the inclusion criteria were considered, such as the experimental model and sample size, the time lapsed from the initial endodontic treatment until the present moment, the method of identification of the bacteria, the presence of bacteria in the initial samples, the substances used during the sanitization process, the time of maintaining the intracanal dressing before filling and the efficacy of the medicaments against the bacteria studied. Yet, it was difficult to compare these studies, due to differences in their strategies, such as; standardization of the limit of amount of dentin removed after emptying the root canal, the choice of the preparation technique, tooth type and size of the selected sample, characteristics and technique of placement of the test material, and certification of its correct filling, the quality control of the irrigation solution, as well as the variation in its concentration, biofilm model, time for microbial colonization, criteria for the detection of the periapical lesion etc.

Despite the limitations, studies that were not essentially developed in humans must be considered. Before tests of application in humans, biologic evaluation of dental materials, initial and secondary test are required[566].

Other aspects that must be critically observed and judiciously analyzed are the biofilm model to test antimicrobial endodontic medicaments, the biological indicator; and the time necessary for biofilm formation.

Socransky & Haffajee[547] reported that the reason for the existence of a biofilm, is that it allows microorganisms to stick to, and multiply on surfaces. Thus, attached bacteria (sessile) growing in a biofilm, display a wide range of characteristics that provide a number of advantages over single-cell (planktonic) bacteria.

A major advantage is the protection the biofilm provides to colonizing species from competing microorganisms, environmental factors, such as host defense mechanisms, and from potentially toxic substances in the environment, such as lethal chemicals or antibiotics. Biofilms also can facilitate processing and the uptake of nutrients, cross-feeding (one species providing nutrients to another), removal of potentially harmful metabolic products (often used by other bacteria) as well as the development of an appropriate physicochemical environment (such as properly lowering the oxidation reduction potential).

Bacterial biofilm has an open architecture, with channels traversing from the biofilm surface. This structure affects the movement of molecules within plaque, and develops gradients in key determinants. Bacteria growing on a surface display a novel phenotype; one of the consequences is an increased resistance to antimicrobial agents. Resistance can result from restricted inhibitor penetration, slower bacterial growth rates, transfer of resistance genes, suboptimal environmental conditions for inhibitor activity, and the expression of a resistant phenotype[385]. Duggan & Sedgley[100] tested the hypothesis that the ability of *E. faecalis* to form biofilm, is related to the source of the strains. The variations observed in these clinical isolates suggested that biofilm formation might be a factor, when considering the virulence phenotype of endodontic strains in general.

Chávez de Paz[68] evaluated the possible role of biofilm communities. Changes in the environment, such as an increase in pH by calcium hydroxide or the effect of antimicrobials, are capable of triggering genetic cascades that modify the physiological characteristics of bacterial cells. Surface adherence by bacteria to form biofilms is a good example of bacterial adaptation. Increasing information is now available on the existence of polymicrobial biofilm communities on root canal walls, coupled with new data showing that the adaptive mechanisms of bacteria in these biofilms are significantly augmented for increased survival. This ecological view on the persisting infection problem in endodontics suggests that the action of individual species in persisting endodontic infections is secondary, when compared with the adaptive changes of a polymicrobial biofilm community undergoing physiological and genetic changes, in response to changes in the root canal environment.

The invasion of root dentinal tubules by root canal bacteria is a multi-factorial event, in which a limited number of oral bacterial species have the necessary properties to participate[374]. The penetration of microorganisms into infected root dentin have shown variations considering the experimental model, the biological indicator and the time of incubation used in the studies. Distel et al.[98] presented evidence of *E. faecalis* colonization and biofilm formation in root canals of human teeth. To develop new treatments to eradicate *E. faecalis* from persistent root canal infections, the mechanisms through which the bacterium maintains these infections, must be understood.

For all these reasons, considering the heterogeneity of guidelines to study antimicrobial strategies for endodontic infections, the higher estimate for clinical success, and adequate sanitization process assisted by intracanal medicaments reduces the bacterial population and favors prognosis.

The antimicrobial efficacy of intracanal medicaments against bacterial biofilm still needs to be confirmed. In order to satisfy regulatory guidelines to disrupt bacterial biofilm, the active participation of the mechanical action of endodontic instruments associated with antimicrobial medicaments is essential. Further studies are indispensable to offer new guidelines for the treatment protocol of endodontic biofilm.

**Table 20.3** - Inclusion and exclusion criteria

| **Inclusion Criteria** |
|---|
| 1. Studies in vivo, in humans<br>2. Related to the root canal biofilm<br>3. Randomized controlled trial (RCT) studies<br>4. Related to the efficacy of intracanal medicaments against biofilm<br>5. Studies published in English |
| **Exclusion Criteria** |
| 1. Studies in vitro<br>2. Studies developed in animals<br>3. Studies related only to the identification of microorganisms<br>4. Studies not related to the efficacy of intracanal medicaments against biofilm<br>5. Studies related to periapical biofilm<br>6. Studies related to non-endodontic biofilm<br>7. Studies with abstract only or with absence of abstract<br>8. Studies of literature reviews<br>9. Studies involving case reports |



**Table 20.4** - In vivo researches

| Author (ref.) | no. of samples | Criteria | Intervention | Appointment | Observation model | Outcome |
|---|---|---|---|---|---|---|
| Nair et al.[422] | 16 | 3 | Root canal preparation + 5.25% NaOCl + 17% EDTA | One-visit | LEM, TEM | Non efficacy |
| Araki et al.[17] | - | 3, 4, 5 | Er:Yag Laser | - | SEM | Efficacy |
| Khemaleelakul et al.[330] | 10 | 3, 4 | - | - | Visual, Fluorescent dye-staining | - |
| Noguchi et al.[432] | 27 | 3, 4, 5 | - | - | Immunohistochemical | - |
| Leonardo et al.[363] | 21 | 3, 4, 5 | - | - | SEM | - |
| Noiri et al.[433] | 6 | 3, 4, 5 | - | - | SEM | - |
| Tronstad et al.[602] | - | 3, 4, 5 | - | - | SEM | - |

(LEM = light emission microscopy, TEM = transmission electronic microscopy, SEM = scanning electronic microscopy).

**Table 20.5** - In vitro researches

| Author (ref.) | n | Biofilm model | Contamination time | Microorganims | Intervention | Observation model | Outcome |
|---|---|---|---|---|---|---|---|
| George & Kishen[184] | - | DC | - | *E. faecalis, A. actinomycetemcomitans* | - | - | Efficacy |
| Chavez de Paz et al.[68] | - | MF | - | *E. faecalis, L. paracasei, O. uli, S. anginosus, S. gordini, S. oralis, F. nucleatum* | - | Fluorescent staining | NE |
| Garcez et al.[182] | 10 | DC | 3 days | *P. mirabilis,P. aeruginosa* | Photodynamic therapy + laser light or root canal preparation | Bioluminescence imaging | Efficacy |
| Sena et al.[519] | - | MF | - | *E. faecalis, S. aureus, C. albicans, P. intermedia, P. gingivalis, P. endodontalys, F. nucleatum* | 2.5%, 5.25% NaOCl, 2% CHX gel and liquid | - | OD |
| Soukos et al. [551] | - | DC | 3 days | *E. faecalis* | Photodynamic therapy | - | NE |
| Bergmans et al.[35] | - | DC | 2 hours | *E. faecalis, A. naeslundii, S. anginosus* | Nd:YAG Laser | CSEM and ESEM | NE |
| Clegg et al.[74] | - | DC | 7 days | - | 6%, 3%, 1% NaOCl, 2% CHX + Biopure MTAD | SEM | Efficacy |
| Kishen et al.[332] | - | DC | 2, 4, 6 weeks intervals or 6 weeks | *E. faecalis* | - | x-ray diffraction, FTIR spectroscopy, SEM, LM and LCSM | OD |
| George et al.[185] | 45 | DC | 21 days | *E. faecalis* | - | SEM, LCSM and LM | OD |
| Abdullah et al.[3] | - | MF | - | *E. faecalis* | $Ca(OH)_2$, 0.2% CHX, 17% EDTA 10% povidone iodine and 3%NaOCl | - | Efficacy |
| Hems et al.[235] | - | MF | 48 hours | *E. faecalis* | Ozonated water and ozone gas | - | NE |
| Gulabivala et al.[212] | 198 | DC | 48 hours | *E. faecalis* | Neutral anolyte, acidic anolyte, catholyte and catholyte + neutral anolyte ultrasonicated or not | - | NE |
| Distel et al.[98] | 46 | DC | - | *E. faecalis* | $Ca(OH)_2$ paste or points | SEM and LCSM | NE |
| Seal et al.[510] | 35 | DC | 48 hours | *S. intermedius* | 3% NaOCl or TBO and 35-mW helium-neon low power laser | - | NE |
| Lima et al.[365] | - | MF | 1,3 days | *E. faecalis* | 2% CHX or antibiotics-based medications | - | Efficacy |
| Spratt et al.[562] | - | MF | 15 min or 1 hour | *P. intermedia, P. micros, S. intermedius, F. nucleatum, E. faecalis* | 2.25% NaOCl, 0.2% CHX, 10% iodine | - | Efficacy |
| Barrieshi et al. [23] | 40 | DC | - | *F. nucleatum, P. micros, C. rectus* | - | SEM | OD |

DC = dentinal contamination, MF = membrane filter, LM = light microscopy, LCSM = laser confocal scanning microscopy,
FTIR = Fourier transform infrared, CSEM = conventional scanning electron microscopy, ESEM = environmental scanning electron microscopy,
LEM = light electron microscopy, TEM = transmission electron microscopy, SEM = scanning electron microscopy, NE = Non efficacy

## 20.5 General Considerations

Intracanal dressing continues to be the target of discussions concerning several of its aspects. Considerations about the real necessity of its use in pulp necrosis and apical periodontitis, the selection of the substance to be used, the time it should remain in the radicular canal, its effect on different microorganisms found in endodontic infections, and its influence on tissue healing process are justifications for new researches structured within adequate critical analysis and well established methodologies.

Properties such as the hydrosolubility or not of the vehicle used (viscosity differences), acid-base characteristic, higher or lower dentinal permeability, buffering capacity of dentin, and level of calcification can influence the speed of diffusion of hydroxyl ions. For a medication to attain its complete antimicrobial and mineralizing effectiveness, the correct filling of the root canal is necessary.

Several different techniques for placing calcium hydroxide into root canals have been proposed. Cvek et al.[83] proposed the use of an injection syringe or Lentulo drill aided by effective lateral condensation. Webber et al.[627] highlighted the use of a plastic transporter that drives calcium hydroxide paste into the root canal followed by vertical compression, until its complete filling. Anthony & Senia[13] and Lopes et al.[370] suggested the use of a Lentulo drill. Krell & Madison[343] described the use of a Messing gun, stressing the simplicity and efficacy of this method. Estrela et al.[140] described root canal filling using files, absorbent paper points and vertical pluggers. Dunsha & Gutmann[101], evaluating different clinical methods for placing calcium hydroxide (amalgam carriers, Lentulo drill, injectable pastes, McSpadden compactors), pointed out that the clinician should know how to evaluate the situation and choose the most suitable method to promote the expected results. Sigurdsson et al.[529], comparing the Lentulo drill, endodontic file and syringe, reported that the best results were obtained with the Lentulo drill.

Estrela et al.[134] compared different techniques of root canal filling with calcium hydroxide pastes in dog teeth. The placement of calcium hydroxide with a file, absorbent paper points and vertical pluggers presented the lowest number of empty spaces in the three thirds of the root canal, followed by the Lentulo drill and the McSpadden compactor.

The apical third was the most difficult portion to fill completely. As regards the comparison between the use of these rotary instruments to fill root canals with calcium hydroxide paste, Lopes et al.[370] stressed that this difference may be related to the geometric shape of instruments. The McSpadden compactor has a larger straight section than the Lentulo drill, and when removed from the root canal, displaces the paste sideways, increasing the percentage of empty spaces. Another factor to consider is that calcium hydroxide paste does not contain a radiopaque substance, thus the paste should be very well condensed within the root canal to avoid empty spaces. Because the calcium hydroxide paste used in this study had a saline vehicle, it acquired a hydrossoluble nature, therefore its placement was more difficult and required the use of absorbent paper points and a vertical plugger to aid compression. Consistency is also an important aspect. A paste thicker than toothpaste that is put in place using a file provides a better filling. When this type of paste is placed with rotary instruments, a higher number of empty spaces can be observed. Width and curvature of the root canal can influence complete or incomplete filling. Sigurdsson et al.[529] compared placement techniques of calcium hydroxide paste, using Lentulo drill, endodontic file and syringe (Calasept paste system) in mesiobuccal canals of maxillary molars, prepared up to instrument #25 and concluded that the Lentulo drill presented the best results, filling the entire working length.

Another consideration is the possibility of root canal treatment in one sitting, in cases of vital pulp, which is not questioned. Nevertheless, it must be understood that it is not always possible to conclude treatment in only one session. In these cases, the integrity of the pulp stump and periapical tissues should be maintained, providing a repair close to the ideal, which is with apical closure by the deposition of hard tissue. The histological results of corticosteroid associated with an antibiotic, as a dressing in dog teeth, showed that these drugs were related to the preservation of pulp stump vitality and the integrity of the periapical tissues.

Holland et al.[265] studied the behavior of the periapical tissues of dog teeth after biopulpectomy and dressing with calcium hydroxide, or a corticosteroid-antibiotic association, before root canal filling with zinc oxide eugenol (ZOE) or Sealapex sealers. The teeth were overinstrumented and dressed for 7 days before the root canal filling. The animals were sacrificed 180 days after treatment and the specimens were prepared for morphological analysis. Specimens treated with Sealapex presented a higher number of cases with biological closure than ZOE. When the root canals were filled with ZOE, better results were observed with the use of the calcium hydroxide dressing. The authors concluded that: 1. Using Otosporin as the dressing, biological closure of the main foramen was observed in 73.35% of the cases when the filling material was Sealapex and 20% with the sealer ZOE; 2. Using calcium hydroxide as the dressing, biological closure of the main apical foramen was observed in 80% of root canals filled with Sealapex, and 40% with the sealer ZOE; 3. Using calcium hydroxide as the dressing, no difference was observed in relation to the small accessory root canals, with the two sealers; 4. When the dressing was Otosporin, the small accessory root canals showed a larger incidence of biological closure when the sealer was Sealapex; 5. When particles of Sealapex reach the periodontal ligament, they generally cause a mild inflammatory reaction, characterized mainly by macrophagic activity. In the absence of biological closure, and even without overfilling, ZOE frequently produced a mild chronic inflammatory reaction (Fig. 20.42-20.47).

Biological apical closure by deposit of neo-formed cementum after root canal filling with calcium hydroxide or calcium hydroxide-based sealers has been proved better when the filling material is placed in contact with an organized tissue rather than a blood clot[267,392]. Holland et al.[271] investigated the periapical healing process of dog teeth, with or without apical patency, and after root canal filling with two types of sealers. Forty roots of premolars and incisors were used. The root canals were overinstrumented and dressed with a corticosteroid-antibiotic solution for 7 days to obtain ingrowth of periapical connective tissue into the canals. After this period, the tissue was removed in half of the specimens (groups with patency) and preserved in the other half (groups without patency). Canals were filled by lateral condensation technique with gutta-percha points, and either a calcium hydroxide-based sealer (Sealer Plus) or a Grossman's cement (Fill Canal). The animals were killed 60 days after the endodontic treatment and anatomic pieces were obtained and prepared for histologic examination. Data were evaluated in a blind analysis, on the basis of several histomorphologic parameters. The groups without patency had better results than those in which the ingrown connective tissue was removed. When comparing the sealers, Sealer Plus had significantly better results than Fill Canal. In conclusion, both the apical patency (presence or absence) and the type of root canal filling material influenced the periapical healing process in dog teeth with vital pulp after root canal treatment. The use of a calcium hydroxide-based sealer in teeth without apical patency yielded the best results among the experimental conditions proposed.

Marion[382] analyzed the effect of using or not a corticosteroid-antibiotic (Otosporin) dressing on the healing process of dogs' teeth after pulpectomy and root canals filling with Sealapex or MTA with propylene glycol. Were used forty roots of incisives and pre-molars of two young adult mongrel dogs' from the same litter aging about 2 years old. The teeth were biomechanically prepared by reverse mixed technique. After that the cementary barrier was perforated and enlarged up to file K#25. Twenty canals received a dressing with Otosporin for 7 days aiming to allow the neo-formation of a pulp stump. Each root canal was then filled by the lateral condensation technique with gutta-percha points and one of the studied materials. The remaining 20 canals were filled in just one session using the same root canal filling technique and materials, but without the use of Otosporin dressing. After 90 days the animals were sacrificed and the jaws were removed the teeth were prepared for histomorphological and histomicrobiological analysis. The materials presented similar results independently of the use of the Otosporin. The Otosporin dressing favored the healing process with both studied filling material. In conclusion, the root canal filling with Sealapex or MTA with propylene glycol preceded by the Otosporin dressing improved the healing process (Fig.20.48-20.55).

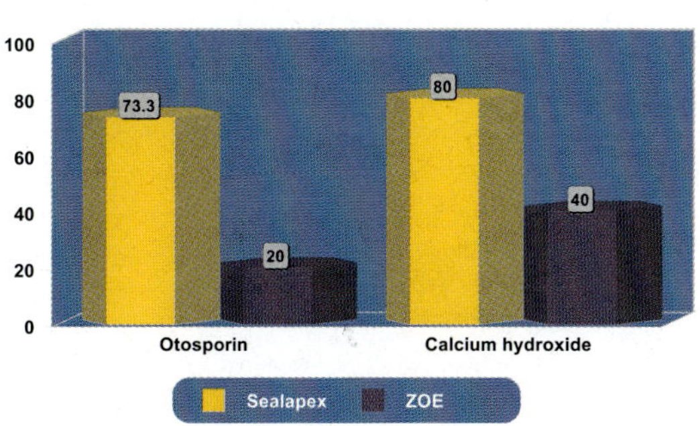


**Figure 20.42** - Biological closure observed in experimental groups (Holland et al.[265]).

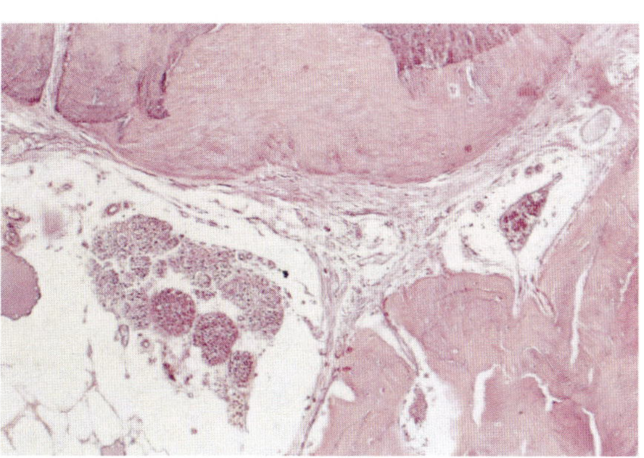

**Figure 20.43** - Otosporin-Sealapex - Complete closure of the main root canal (H.E. X100) (Holland et al.[265]).

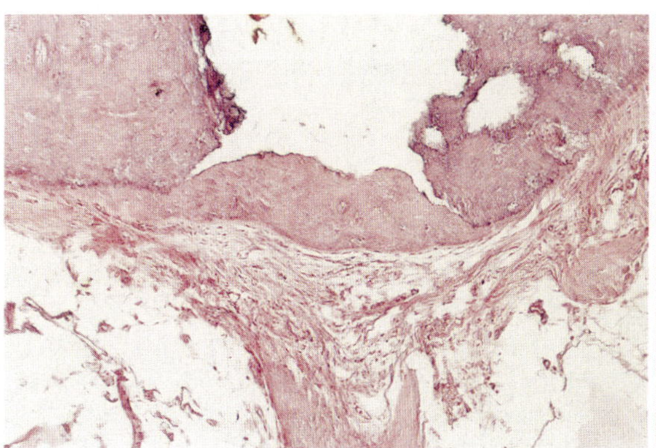

**Figure 20.44** - Calcium hydroxide-Sealapex - Complete closure of the main root canal (H.E. X100) (Holland et al.[265]).

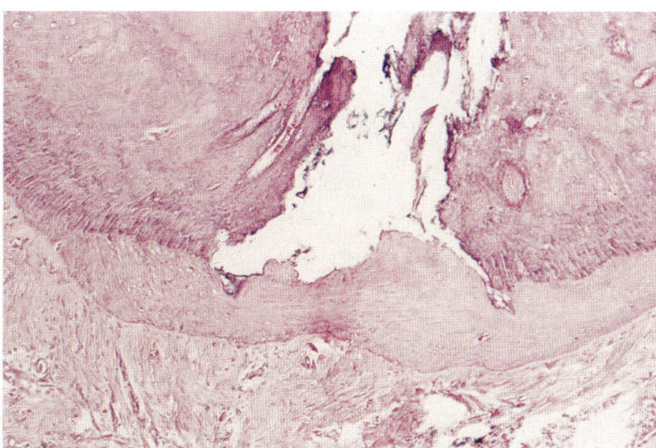

**Figure 20.45** - Calcium hydroxide-Sealapex - Closure biological of the main root canal (H.E. X100) (Holland et al.[265]).

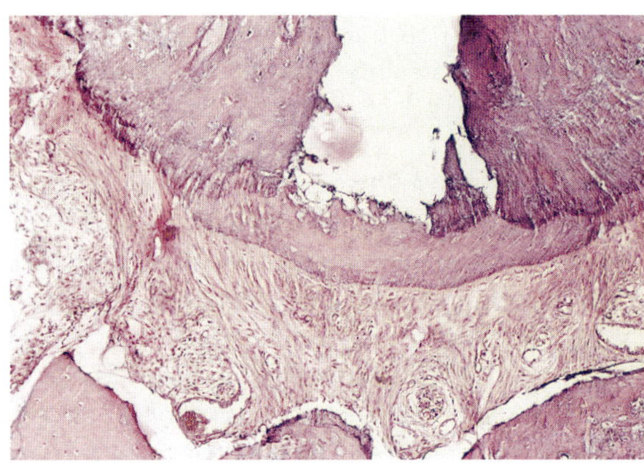

**Figure 20.46** - OZE-Sealapex - Closure biological of the main root canal (H.E. X100) (Holland et al.[265]).

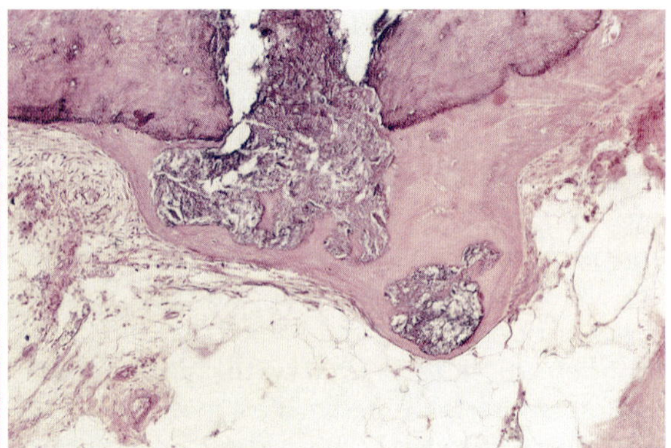

**Figure 20.47** - OZE-Sealapex – Presence of dentin chips - Closure biological of the main root canal (H.E. X100) (Holland et al.[265]).

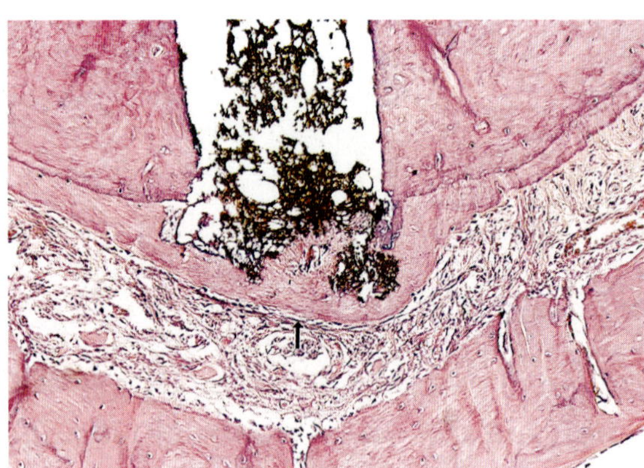

**Figure 20.48** - Sealapex without Otosporin. Biological closure. (Marion & Holland et al.[382]).

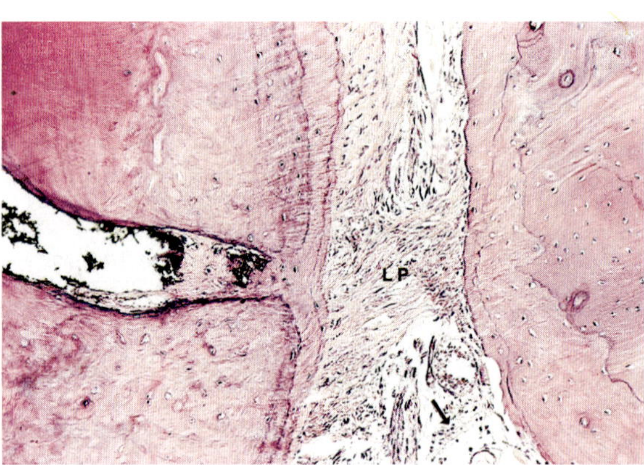


**Figure 20.49** - Complete closure of the Secondary canal (H.E. X100) (Marion & Holland et al.[382]).

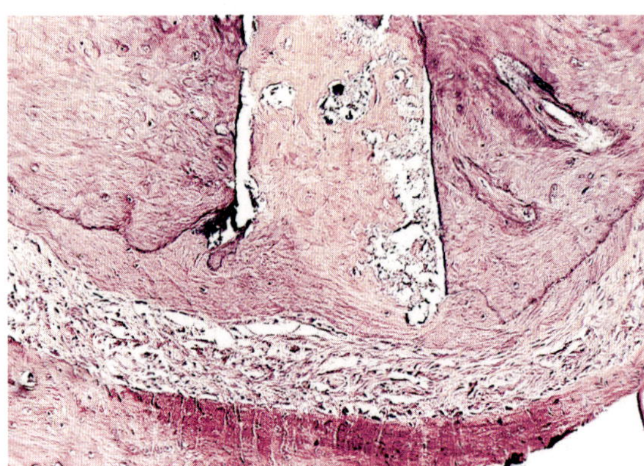

**Figure 20.50** - MTA without Otosporin - Complete closure of the main root canal (Marion & Holland et al.[382]).

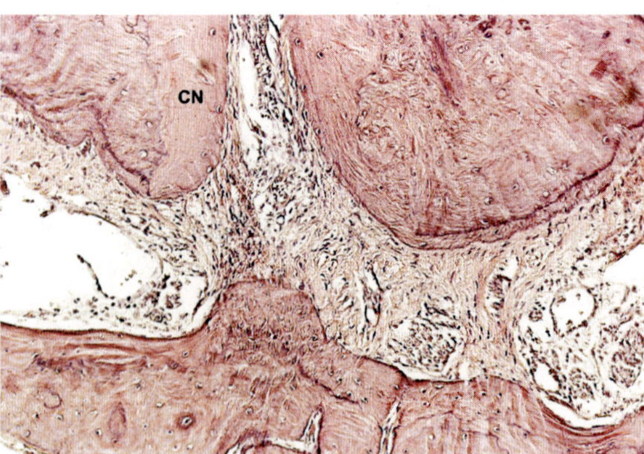


**Figure 20.51** - The neoformed cementum in main root canal (H.E. X100) (Marion & Holland et al.[382]).

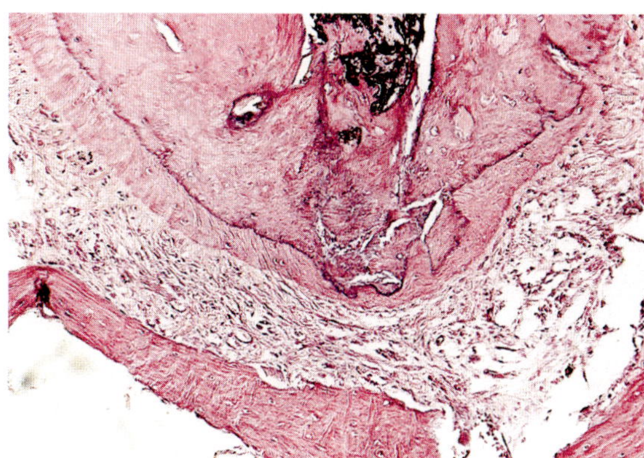

**Figure 20.52** - Sealapex with Otosporin. Closure biological of the main root canal (H.E. X100) (Marion & Holland et al.[382]).

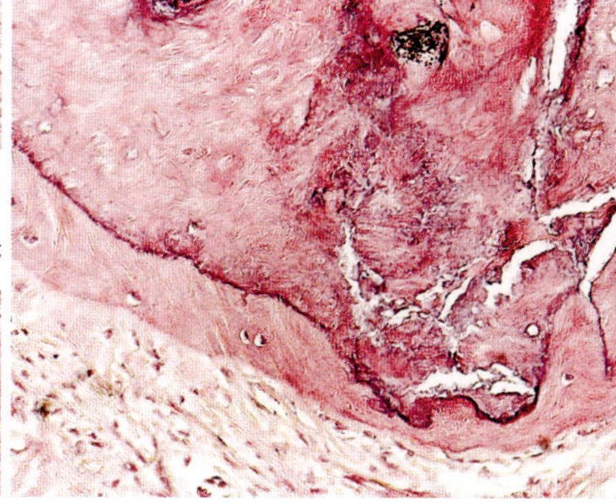

**Figure 20.53** - Closure biological of the main root canal (H.E. X200) (Marion & Holland et al.[382]).

Calcium hydroxide has been studied for many years, since Herman[237] in 1920 suggested calcium hydroxide for the treatment of dental pulp. A new era had begun. Calcium hydroxide encourages the deposition of a hard tissue bridge that usually protects the dental pulp. The ability to stimulate mineralization associated with the antimicrobial effectiveness, has conferred on it the current success as an endodontic medication.

Scientific research on the indication of calcium hydroxide in endodontics does not mean: habits of prescription, beliefs in beneficial effects or even the attempt to determine a drug able to heal all illnesses. It is only necessary to establish appropriate criteria for use, including limits and implications, and at the same time, show the value of research to explain facts that are not yet clear or have been mistakenly explained. Calcium hydroxide is an excellent therapeutic option when the clinical situation requires the use of a pulp capping agent and intracanal medication. Two effects of this medication need to be considered, its biological and antimicrobial effects.

It is necessary, whenever possible, to allow time for calcium hydroxide paste to manifest its potential action on the microorganisms present in endodontic infections. The maintenance of a high concentration of hydroxyl ions can change enzymatic activity and promote its inactivation. Obviously, the antimicrobial effect depends on the rate of release of hydroxyl ions, its availability, time of contact for direct or indirect action (diffusibility of hydroxyl ions within dentinal tubules) in order to show its real effectiveness. Thus, the reasoning should follow another direction. When the aim is to choose the intracanal dressing to use, it is necessary to consider the microbiota of the infected root canal, the host response, and the mechanism of action of the medication. Nevertheless, it is necessary for the medication to have enough time to be effective, able to act at a distance, and for neutralizing the residues of aggressor agents.

One must recognize that when a medication does not reach the target microorganisms, its real efficacy to kill them cannot be expressed. Therefore, it cannot be stated whether the microbial strains were resistant to one or another medication, or not. In this case, it is likely that the microorganisms were able to survive, adapt and tolerate the critical ecological conditions. The positive role of calcium hydroxide paste in the healing process must not be forgotten (Fig. 20.56-20.57).

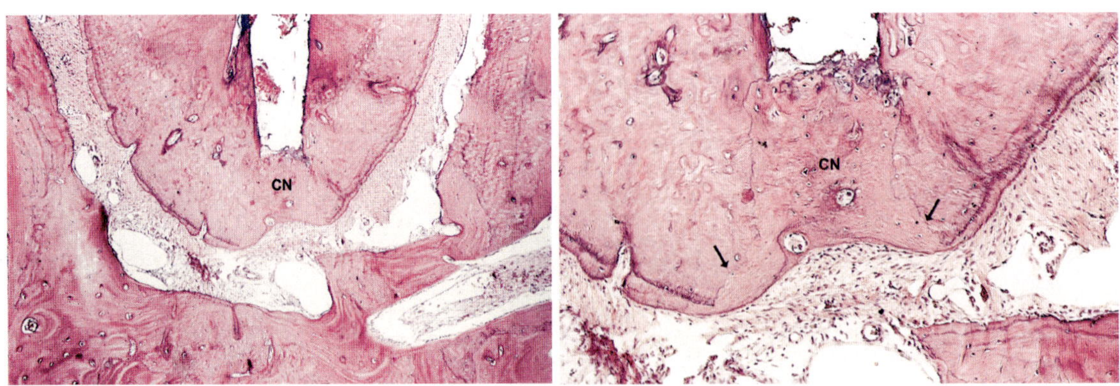


**Figure 20.54** - MTA with Otosporin. Closure biological of the main root canal (H.E. X40) (Marion & Holland et al.[382]).

**Figure 20.55** - Closure biological of the main root canal (H.E. X100) (Marion & Holland et al.[382]).

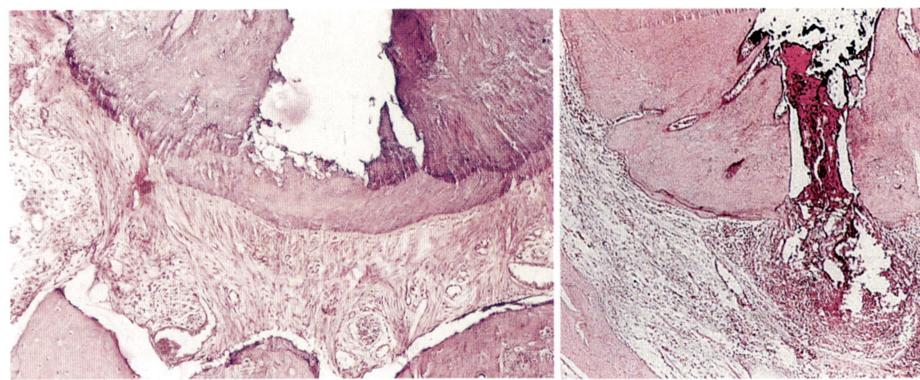

**Figure 20.56** - Biological closure. Complete closure of the main root canal by neoformed cementum (H.E. X100) (Holland et al.[267]).

**Figure 20.57** - Treatment in one visit – Chronic inflammatory reaction in the periodontal ligament (H.E. X100) (Holland et al.[267]).

The Figures 20.58 to 20.76 demonstrate clinical cases in which calcium hydroxide was used as intracanal dressing.

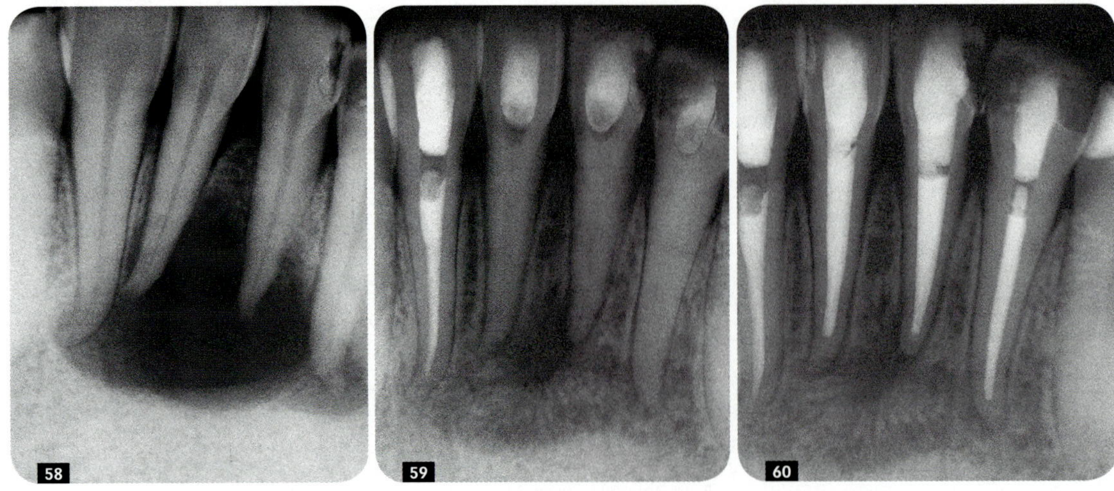


**Figures 20.58 to 20.60** - Asymptomatic apical periodontitis with a large bone radiolucence. Root canal treatment for 2 years, with changes of calcium hydroxide. Follow up for 2.5 years. Repair process of periapical lesion.

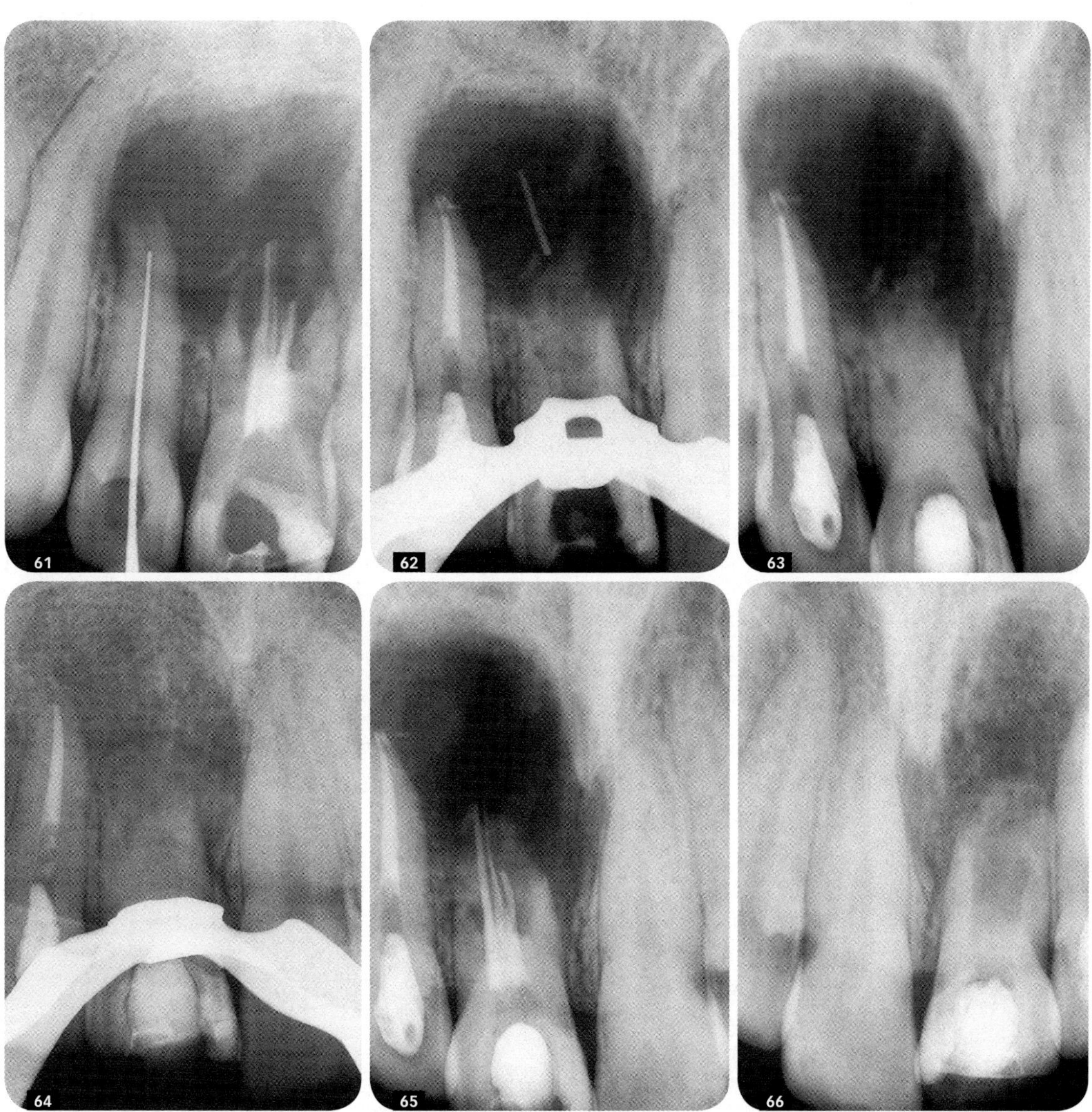


**Figures 20.61 to 20.66** - Asymptomatic apical periodontitis with a large bone radiolucence. Root canal treatment for 2 years, with changes of the calcium hydroxide. Follow up for 3 years. Repair process of periapical lesion.

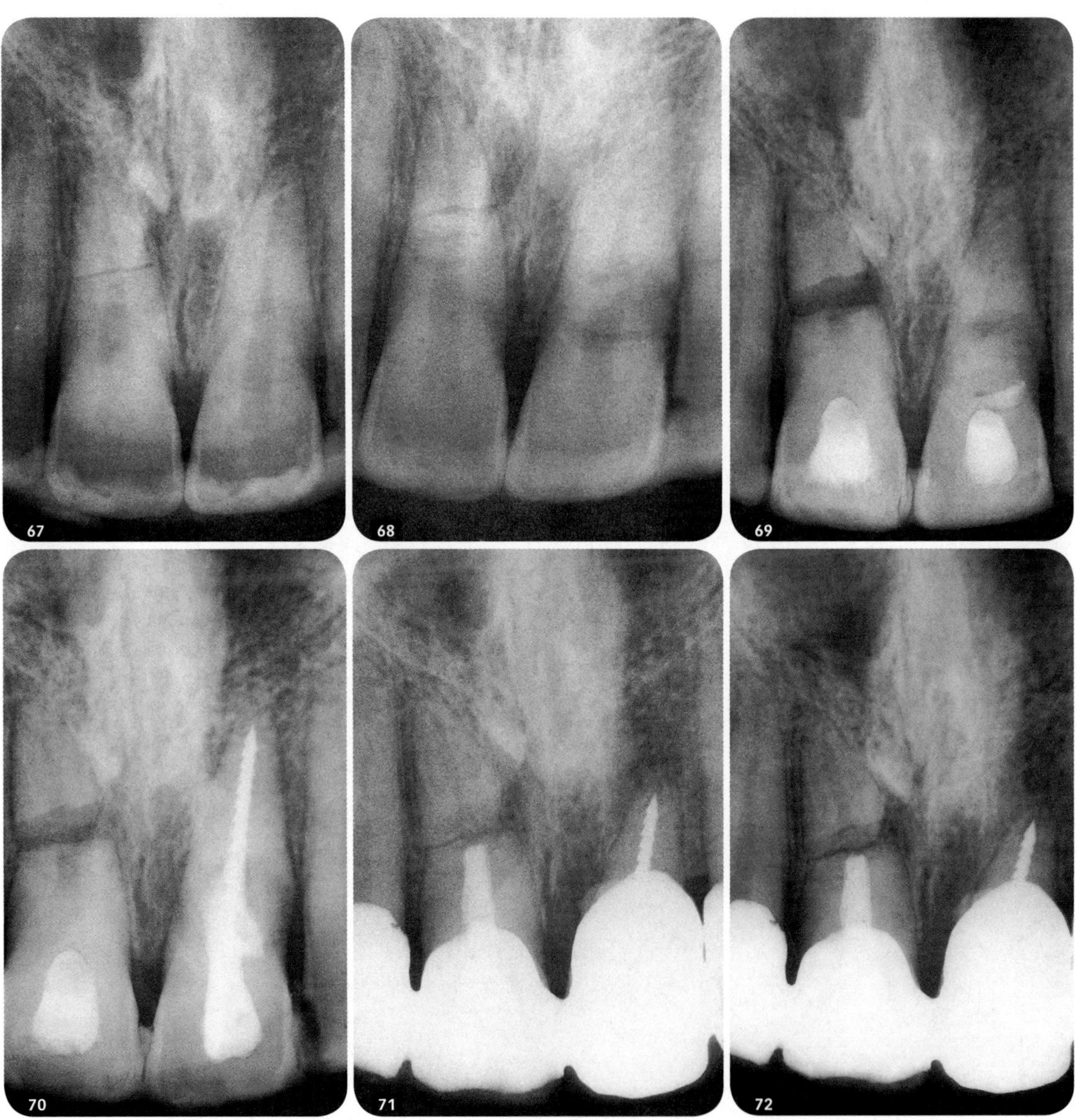


**Figures 20.67 to 20.72** - Root fracture. Root canal treatment using calcium hydroxide paste. Follow up for 10 years.

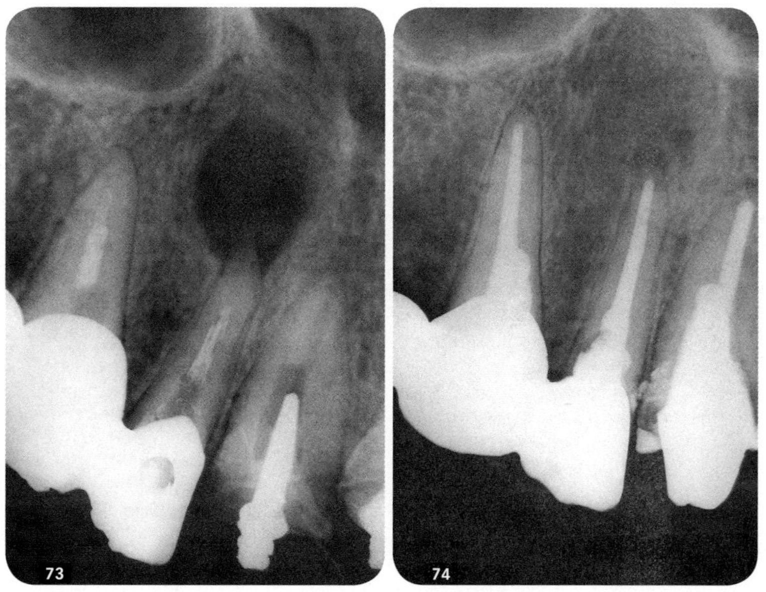


**Figures 20.73 and 20.74** - Asymptomatic apical periodontitis with a large bone radiolucence. Treatment for 2 years, with changes of calcium hydroxide. Follow-up for 3 years. Repair process of periapical lesion.

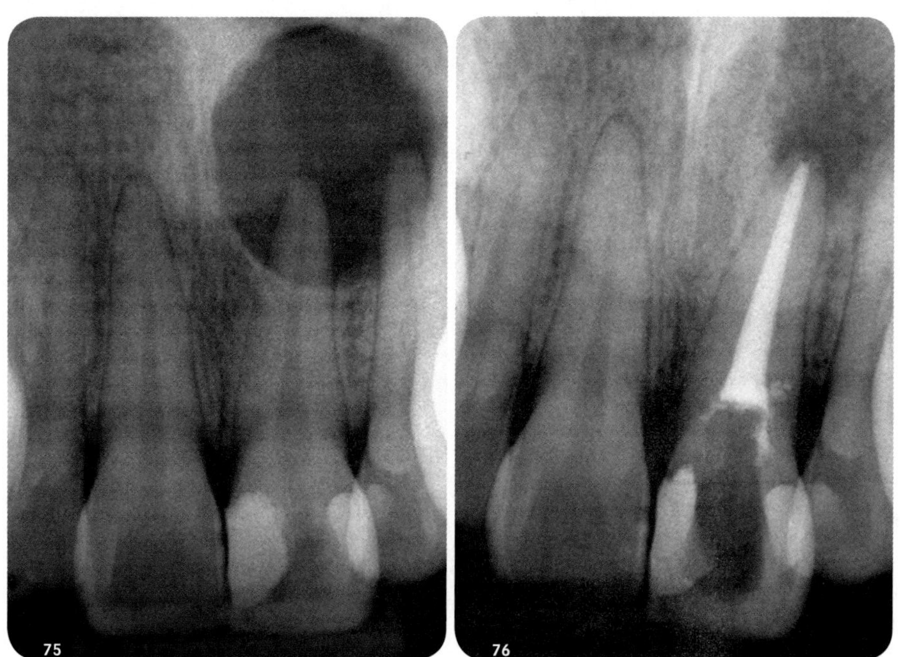


**Figures 20.75 and 20.76** - Asymptomatic apical periodontitis with a large bone radiolucence. Treatment using calcium hydroxide. Follow-up for 2 years. Repair process of periapical lesion.

## References


1. Abbott PV, Hume WR, Heithersay GS. Effects of combining Ledermix1 and calcium hydroxide pastes on the diffusion of corticosteroid and tetracycline through human roots in vitro. Endod Dent Traumatol 1989;5:188-92.
2. Abdullah D, Pitt Ford TR, Papaioannou S, Nicholson J, McDonald F. An evaluation of accelerated Portland cement as a restorative material. Biomaterials 2002;23:4001-10.
3. Abdullah M, Ng Y-L, Gulabivala K, Moles D, Spratt DA. Susceptibilties of two *Enterococcus faecalis* phenotypes to root canal medications. J Endod 2005;31:30-6.
4. Addy ML, Langeroudi M. Comparison of the immediate effects on the sub-gingival microflora of acrylic strips containing 40% chlorhexidine, metronidazole or tetracycline. J Clin Periodontol 1984;11:379-86.
5. Akpata ES, Blechman H. Bacterial invasion of pulpal dentin wall in vitro. J Dent Res 1982;61:435-8.
6. Alaçam T, Gorgul G, Omurlu H. Evaluation of diagnostic radiopaque contrast materials used with calcium hydroxide. J Endod 1990;16:365-8.
7. Alencar AH, Leonardo MR, Silva LA, Silva RS, Ito IY. Determination of the p-monochlorophenol residue in the calcium hydroxide + P-monochlorophenol combination used as an intracanal dressing in pulpless teeth of dogs with induced chronic periapical lesion. J Endod 1997;23:522-4.
8. Allard V, Stromberg V, Stromberg T. Endondontic treatment of experimentally induced apical periodontitis in dogs. Endod Dent Traumatol 1987;3:240-4.
9. Amabis JM, Martho GR, Mizuguchi Y. Biologia. São Paulo: Moderna;1976.
10. Andersen M, Lund A, Andreasen JO, Andreasen Al. In vitro solubility of human pulp tissue in calcium hydroxide and sodium hypochlorite. Endod Dent Traumatol 1992;8:104-8.
11. Ando N, Hoshino E. Predominant obligate anaerobes invading the deep layers of root canal dentine. Int Endod J 1990;23:20-7.
12. Anthony DR, Gordon TM, Del-Rio CE. The effect of three vehicles on the pH of calcium hydroxide. Oral Surg Oral Med Oral Pathol 1982;54:560-5.
13. Anthony DR, Senia ES. The use of calcium hydroxide as a temporary paste fill. Texas Dent J 1981;99:6-10.
14. Anwar H, Dasgupta MK, Costerton JW. Testing the susceptibility of bacteria in biofilms to antibacterial agentes. Amer Soc Microbiol 1990;34:2043-46.
15. Anwar H, Strap JL, Costerton JW. Establishment of aging biofilms: possible mechanism of bacterial resistance to antimicrobial therapy. Antimicrobial Agents Chemotherapy 1992;36:1347-51.
16. Apaydin ES, Shabahang S, Torabinejad M. Hard-tissue healing after application of fresh or set MTA as root-end-filling material. J Endod 2004;30:21-4.
17. Araki AT, Iraki Y, Kawakami T, Lage-Marques JL. Er:Yag laser irradiation of the microbiological apical biofilm. Braz Dent J 2006;17:296-9.
18. Balcow WN, Martindale W. The Extra Pharmacopeia, 26th edn. London: Pharmaceutical Press, 1972.
19. Barbin LE, Saquy PC, Guedes DFC, Souza-Neto MD, Pécora JD, Estrela C. Determination of para-chloraline and reactive oxygen species in chlorhexidine and chlorhexidine associated with calcium hydroxide. J Endod 2008;34:1508-14.
20. Barbosa CAM, Gonçalves RB, Siqueira JF Jr, Uzeda M. Evaluation of the antibacterial activities of calcium hydroxide, chlorhexidine and camphorated paramonochlorophenol as intracanal medicaments. A clinical and laboratory study. J Endod 1995;23:297-300.
21. Barbosa SV, Spångberg LSW, Almeida D. Low surface tension calcium hydroxide solution is an effective antiseptic. Int Endod J 1994; 27:6-10.
22. Barnett F, Trope M, Kreshtool D, Tronstad L. Suitability of controlled release delivery system for root canal disinfection. Endod Dent Traumatol 1986;2:71-4.
23. Barieshi KM, Walton RE, Jonhon WT, Drake DR. Coronal leakage of mixed anaerobic bacteria after obturation and post space preparation. Oral Surg Oral Pathol Oral med Oral radiol Endod 1991;84:310-4.
24. Bauer LAF. Materiais de Construção. 5th ed. Rio de Janeiro: LCT edit; 2007.
25. Baumgartner JC. Bacteria in the apical 5 mm of infected root canals. J Endod 1991;17:380-3.
26. Baumgartner JC. Serum IgG reative with oral anaerobic microorganisms associated with infections of endodontic origin. Oral Microbiol Imunol 1992;7:106-10.
27. Baumgartner JC, Watkins BJ, Bae K-S, Xia T. Association of black-pigmented bacteria with endodontic infections. J Endod 1999;25:413-5.
28. Baumgartner JC, Watts CM, Xia T. Occurrence of Candida albicans in infections of endodontic origin. J Endod 2000;26:695-8.
29. Bazin MJ, Prosser JI. Physiological models in microbiology. Flórida: CRC press;1988.
30. Behnen MJ, West LA, Liewehr FR, Buxton TB, McPherson JC. Antimicrobial activity of several calcium hydroxide preparations in root canal dentin. J Endod 2001;27:757-9.
31. Beltes P, Pissiotis E, Koulaouzidou E, Kortsaris AH. In vitro release of hydroxyl ions from six types of calcium hydroxide non-setting pastes. J Endod 1997;23:413-5.
32. Berbert A. Comportamento dos tecidos apicais e periapicais após biopulpectomia e obturação do canal com AH-26, hidróxido de calcio ou mistura de ambos. Estudo histológico em dentes de cães (Doctoral Thesis). Bauru, University of São Paulo, 1978.
33. Berck H. The effect of calcium hydroxidemethylcellulose paste on the dental pulp. J Dent Children 1950;17:65-8.
34. Bergenholtz G. Effects of bacterial produts on inflammatory reactions in the dental pulp. Scand J Dent Res 1977;85:122-9.
35. Bergmans L, Moisiadis P, Teughels W, Van Meerbeek B, Quirynen M, Lambrechts P. Bactericidal effect of Nd:YAG laser irradiation on some endodontic pathogens ex vivo. Inter Endod J 2006;39:547-7.
36. Bernabé PFE, Holland R, Souza V. Respostas dos tecidos periapicais ao tricresol formalina. Rev Fac Odontol Araçatuba 1972;1:45-51.

37. Bernabé PFE, Holland R. O emprego do hidróxido de cálcio nas cirurgias parendodônticas. Rev Ass Paul Cir Dent 1998;52:460-5.
38. Bhaskar SN, Cutright DE, Van Osdel V. Tissue response to cortisone containing and cortisone free calcium hydroxide. J Dent Children 1969;36:193-8.
39. Bhat KS, Walkevar S. Evaluation of bactericidal property of propylene glycol for its possible use in endodontics. J Health Sci 1975;1:54-9.
40. Binnie WH, Rowe AHR. A histological study of the periapical tissues of incompletely formed pulpless teeth filled with calcium hydroxide. J Dent Res 1973;52:1110-6.
41. Bramante CM, Benatti-Neto C, Lia RCC, Esberard RM. Tratamento das perfurações radiculares com pastas de hidróxido de cálcio e iodofórmio. Emprego de diferentes veículos - Estudo histológico em dentes de cães. Rev Bras Odontol 1986;43:22-30.
42. Brook I, Frazier EH, Gher ME. Aerobic and anaerobic microbiology of periapical abcess. Oral Microbiol Imunol 1991;6:123-5.
43. Brown LR, Rudolph-Jr CE. Isolation and identification of microorganisms from unexposed canals of pulp involved teeth. Oral Surg Oral Med Oral Pathol 1957;10:1094-9.
44. Buck RA, Cai J, Eleazer PD, Staat RH, Hurst HE. Detoxification of endotoxin by endodontic irrigants and calcium hydroxide. J Endod 2000;27:325-7.
45. Buclkey JPA. Rational treatment for putrescent pulps. Dent Rev 1906;18:1193-7.
46. Burnett GW, Schuster GS. Microbiologia Oral e Enfermidades infecciosas. Buenos Aires: Panamericana;1982.
47. Byström A, Claesson R, Sundqvist G. The antibacterial effect of camphorated paramonochlorophenol, comphorated phenol and calcium hydroxide in the treatment of infected root canals. Endod Dent Traumatol 1985;1:170-5.
48. Byström A, Happonen RP, Sjögren U, Sundqvist G. Healing of periapical lesions of pulpless teeth after endodontic treatment with controlled assepsis. Endod Dent Traumatol 1987;3:58-63.
49. Byström A, Sundqvist G. Bacteriologic evaluation of the effects of 0,5% sodium hypochlorite in endodontic therapy. Oral Surg Oral Med Oral Pathol 1983;55:307-12.
50. Byström A, Sundqvist G. Bacteriologic evaluation of the efficacy of mechanical root canal instrumentation in endodontic therapy. Scand J Dent Res 1981;89:321-8.
51. Çaliskan MK, Pehlivan Y. Prognosis of root-fractured permanent incisors. Endod Dent Traumatol1996;12:129-36.
52. Çaliskan MK, Sen BH, Ozinel BH. Treatment of extra oral sinus tracts from traumatized teeth with apical periodontitis. Endod Dent Traumatol 1994;10:115-20.
53. Çaliskan MK, Sen BH. Endodontic treatment of teeth with apical periodontitis using calcium hydroxide: a long term study. Endod Dent Traumatol 1996;12:215-21.
54. Çaliskan MK, Turkun M. Prognosis of permanent teeth with internal resorption: a clinical review. Endod Dent Traumatol 1997;13:75-81.
55. Çaliskan MK, Turkun M. Root canal treatment of a root-fractured incisor tooth with internal resorption: a case report. Int Endod J 1996;29:393-7.
56. Çalt S, Serper A, Özçelik B, Dalat MD. pH changes and calcium ion diffusion from calcium hydroxide dressing materials through root dentin. J Endod 1999;25:329-31.
57. Çalt S, Serper A. Dentinal tubule penetration of root canal sealers after root canal dressing with calcium hydroxide. J Endod 1999;25:431-3.
58. Camilleri J, Montesin FE, Brady K, Sweeney R, Curtis RV, Pitt Ford TR. The constitution of mineral trioxide aggregate. Dental Materials 2005;21:297-303.
59. Camilleri J, Montesin FE, Di Silvio L, Pitt Ford TR. The chemical constitution and biocompatibilility of accelerated Portland cement for endodontic use. Int Endod J 2005;38:834-42.
60. Camilleri J, Pitt Ford TR. Mineral trioxide aggregate: a review of the constituents and biological properties of the material. Int Endod J 2006:38:834-42.
61. Camp MA, Jeansonne BG, Lallier T. Adhesion of human fibroblasts to root-end-filling materials. J Endod 2003;29:602-7.
62. Castagnola L, Orlay HG. Treatment of grangene of the pulp by the Walkhoff method. Br Dent J. 1952;93:93-102.
63. Castagnola L. La Conservación de la Vitalidad de la Pulpa. Buenos Aires: Mundi, 1956.
64. Castagnola L. The use of iodoform paste (Walkhoff method) in modern endodontic therapy. Quintessence Int 1976;7:19-23.
65. Cervone F, Tronstad L, Hammond B. Antmicrobial effect of chlorhexidine in a controlled release delivery system. Endod Dent Traumatol 1990;6:33-6.
66. Chang YC, Huang FM, Cheng MH, Shen LSS, Chou MY. In Vitro evaluation of the cytotoxicity and genoxicity of root canal medicines on human pulp fibroblasts. J Endod 1998;24:604-6.
67. Chávez de Paz L. Redefining the persistent infection in root canals: possible role of biofilm communities. J Endod 2007;33:652-62.
68. Chávez de Paz LE, Bergenholtz G, Dahlén G, Svensäter G. Response to alkaline stress by root canal bacteria in biofilms. Int Endod J 2007;40:344-55.
69. Chávez de Paz LE, Dahlén G, Molander A, Möller A, Bergenholtz G. Bacteria recovered from teeth with apical periodontitis after antimicrobial endodontic treatment. Int Endod J 2003;36:500-8.
70. Chong BS, Pitt Ford TR. The role of intracanal medication in root canal treatment. Int Endod J 1992;25:97-106.
71. Chosak A, Sela J, Cleaton-Jones P. A histological and quantitative histomorphometric study of apexification of nonvital permanent incisors of vervet monkeys after repeated root filling with a calcium hydroxide paste. Endod Dent Traumatol 1997;13:211-7.
72. Chu FC, Leung WK, Tsang PC, Chow TW, Samaranayake LP. Identification of cultivable microorganisms from root canals with apical periodontitis following two-visit endodontic treatment with antibiotics/steroid or calcium hydroxide dressings. J Endod 2006;32:17-23.
73. Citrome GP, Kaminski EJ, Heuer MA. A comparative study of tooth apexification in the dog. J Endod 1979;5:290-7.

74. Clegg MS, Vertucci FJ, Walker C, Belanger M,Britto LR. The Effect of Exposure to irrigant solutions on apical dentin biofilms in vitro. J Endod 2006;32:434-7.
75. Codman WW. Ossification of the pulp of a tooth. Newsletter 1851;90. In: Malo PRT, Kessler Nieto F, Vadillo MVM. Hidroxido de calcio y picoformación. Rev Espan Endod 1987;5:41-61.
76. Cohen F, Lasfargues JJ. Quantitative chemical study of root canal preparations with calcium hydroxide. Endod Dent Traumatol 1988;4:108-13.
77. Costa CAS, Giro EMA, Nascimento ABL, Teixeira HM, Hebling J. Short-term evaluation of the pulpo-dentin complex response to a resin-modified glass-ionomer cement and a bonding agent applied in deep cavities. Dent Materials 2003;19:739-46.
78. Costa CAS. Teste de biocompatibilidade dos materiais odontológicos. In: Metodologia Científica: ensino e pesquisa em Odontologia. Estrela C. São Paulo: Artes Médicas; 2001.
79. Costerton JW, Cheng KJ, Geesey GG, Ladd TI, Nickel C, Dasgupta M, Marrie TJ. Bacterial biofilms in nature and disease. Annual Reviews of Microbiol 1987;41:435-64.
80. Cruz GA, Holland R, Alfaro JF. Efecto de la colocación de pastas de hidróxido de cálcio com diferentes vehiculos, como medicación intraconducto, sobre el sellado apical de la obturación endodóntica. Endodoncia 2001;19:284-92.
81. Cvek M, Hollender L, Nord CE. Treatment of nonvital permanent incisors with calcium hydroxide. VI. A clinical, microbiological and radiological evaluation of treatment in one sitting of teeth with mature or immature root. Odont Rev 1976;27:93-108.
82. Cvek M, Sundstrom B. Treatment of non-vital permanent incisors with calcium hydroxide. V - Histologic appearance of roentgenographically demonstrable apical closure of immature roots. Odontol Rev 1974;25:379-91.
83. Cvek M. Calcium Hydroxide in the Treatment of Traumatized Teeth. Stockholm: Eastman Institute, 1989.
84. Cvek M. Prognosis of luxated non-vital maxillary incisors treated with calcium hydroxide and filled with gutta-percha. A retrospective clinical study. Endod Dent Traumatol 1992;8:45-55.
85. Cvek M. Treatment of non-vital permanent incisors with calcium hydroxide. II - Effect on external root resorption in luxated teeth compared with effect of root filling with gutta-percha. A follow-up. Odontol Rev 1973;24:343-54.
86. Cvek M. Treatment of non-vital permanent incisors with calcium hydroxide. IV - Periodontal healing and closure of the root canal in the coronal fragment of teeth with intra-alveolar fracture and vital apical fragment. Odontol Rev 1974;25:239-46.
87. Cvek M. Treatment of non-vital permanent incisors with calcium hydroxide. I. Follow-up of periapical repair and apical closure of immature. Odontol Rev 1972;23:27-44.
88. Cwikla JR. The vaporization and capillarity effect of endodontic medicaments. Oral Surg Oral Med Oral Pathol 1972;34:117-21.
89. Dahlén G, Bergenholtz G. Endotoxic activity in teeth with necrotic pulps. J Dent Res 1980;59:1033-40.
90. Dahlén G, Hofstad T. Endotoxic activities of lipopolysaccharides of microorganisms isolated from an infected root canal in Macaca cynomolgus. Scand Dent Res 1977;85:272-8.
91. Dammaschke T, Gerth HU, Zuchner H, Schafer E. Chemical and physical surface and bulk material characterization of white ProRoot MTA and two Portland cements. Dent Materials 2005;21:731-8.
92. Danin J, Stromberg T, Forsgren H, Linder LE, Ramskold LO. Clinical management of nonhealing periradicular pathosis. Oral Surg Oral Med Oral Pathol 1996;82:213-7.
93. Deardorf KA, Swartz MI, Newton CW, Brown CE Jr. Effect of root canal treatments on dentin permeability. J Endod 1994;20:1-5.
94. Debelian GJ, Olsen I, Tronstad L. Bacteremia in conjuction with endodontic therapy. Endod Dent Traumatol 1995;11:142-9.
95. Denton GW. Chlorhexedine. In: Disinfection, sterilization and preservation. Block SS. 4th ed. Philadelphia: Lea & Febiger;1991. 274-89p.
96. Di Fiore PM, Peters DD, Setterstrom JA, Lorton L. The antibacterial effects of calcium hydroxide apexification pastes on *Streptococcus sanguis*. Oral Surg Oral Med Oral Pathol 1983;55:91-4.
97. Dilewski JJ. Apical closure of non-vital teeth. Oral Surg Oral Med Oral Pathol 1971;32:82-9.
98. Distel JW, Hatton JF, Gillespie J. Biofilm formation in medicated root canals. J Endod 2002;28:689-93.
99. Duarte MA, Demarchi AC, Yamashita JC, Kuga MC, Fraga SC. pH and calcium ion release of 2 root-end filling materials. Oral Surg Oral Med Oral Pathol Oral Radiol Endod 2003;95:345-7.
100. Duggan JM, Sedgley CM. Biofilm formation of oral and endodontic *Enterococcus faecalis*. J Endod 2007;33:815-8.
101. Dumsha TC, Gutmann M. Clinical techniques for the placement of calcium hydroxide. Compend Contin Educat Dent 1985;6:482-9.
102. Economides N, Pantelidou O, Kokkas A, Tziafas D. Short-term periradicular tissue response to mineral trioxide aggregate (MTA) as root-end filling material. Int Endod J 2003;36:44-8.
103. Eda S, Kawakami T, Hasegawa H, Watanabe I, Kato K. Clinico-pathological studies on the healing of periapical tissues in aged patients by root canal filling using pastes of calcium hydroxide added iodoforn. Gerodont 1985;1:98-104.
104. Eda S. Histochemical analysis on the mechanism of dentin formation in dog's pulp. Bull Tokyo Dent Coll 1961;2:59-88.
105. Eguren AEO. Vers la fermeture biologique du foramen apical en Endodontie. Rev Stomatol Chirurg Maxillo-Facialle 1971;72:310-3.
106. Engström B. The significance of enterococci in root canal treatment. Odontol Rev 1964;15:87-106.
107. Engström B, Spångberg L. Wound healing after partial pulpectomy. A histological study performed in contralateral pairs. Odontol Rev 1967;75:5-18.
108. Erdogan G. The treatment of non-vital immature teeth with calcium hydroxide-sterile water paste. Two case reports. Quint Int 1997;28:681-6.
109. Estrela C. Análise química de pastas de hidróxido de cálcio, frente à liberação de íons de cálcio, de íons hidroxila e ação do carbonato de cálcio na presença

de tecido conjuntivo de cão. (Doctoral Thesis). São Paulo: University of São Paulo - USP; 1994.
110. Estrela C. Ciência endodôntica. São Paulo: Artes Médicas; 2004.
111. Estrela C. Eficácia antimicrobiana de pastas de hidróxido de cálcio. (Livre Docência Thesis). Ribeirão Preto: University of São Paulo - USP; 1997.
112. Estrela C, Bammann LL, Estrela CRA, Silva RS, Pécora JD. Antmicrobial and chemical study of MTA, Portland cement, calcium hydroxide paste, Sealapex and Dycal. Braz Dent J 2000;11:3-9.
113. Estrela C, Bammann LL, Lopes HP, Moura J. Análise comparativa da ação antibacteriana de três cimentos obturadores contendo hidróxido de cálcio. Rev Ass Bras Odontol Nac 1995;3:185-7.
114. Estrela C, Bammann LL, Pimenta FC, Pécora JD. Control of microorganisms in vitro by calcium hydroxide pastes. Int Endod J 2001;34:341-5.
115. Estrela C, Bammann LL, Sydney GB, Moura J. Efeito antibacteriano de pastas de hidróxido de cálcio sobre bactérias aeróbias facultativas. Rev Fac Odontol Bauru 1995;3:109-14.
116. Estrela C, Bammann LL. Efeito enzimático do hidróxido de cálcio. Rev Ass Bras Odontol Nac 1999;7:32-42.
117. Estrela C, Bueno MR, Azevedo B, Azevedo JR, Pécora JD. A New Periapical Index Based on Cone Beam Computed Tomography. J Endod 2008;34:1325-31
118. Estrela C, Bueno MR, Leles CR, Azevedo B, Azevedo JR. Accuracy of cone beam computed tomography and panoramic and periapical radiography for detection of apical periodontitis. J Endod 2008;3: 273-9.
119. Estrela C, César OVS, Leles CR, Pimenta FC, Alencar AHG. Evaluation in longitudinal studies of efficacy of calcium hydroxide on ***Enterococcus faecalis*** in endodontic infection - systematic review. Rev Bras Odontol 2007;64: 117-28.
120. Estrela C, Decurcio DA, Alencar AHG, Sydney GS, Silva JA. Efficacy of calcim hydroxide dressing in endodontic infection treatment: a systematic review. Odonto Ciência 2008;23:82-6.
121. Estrela C, Decurcio DA, Silva JA, Mendonça EF, Estrela CRA. Persistent apical periodontitis associated with calcifying odontogenic cyst. Int Endod J 2009 (in press).
122. Estrela C, Estrela CRA, Bammann LL, Pécora JD. Two methods to evaluate the antimicrobial action of calcium hydroxide paste. J Endod 2001;27:720-3.
123. Estrela C, Estrela CRA, Barbin EL, Spanó JCE, Marchesan MA, Pécora JD. Mechanism of action of sodium hypochlorite. Braz Dent J 2002;13:113-7.
124. Estrela C, Estrela CRA, Decurcio DA, Hollanda ACB, Silva JA. Antimicrobial efficacy of ozonated water, gaseous ozone, sodium hypochlorite and chlorhexidine in infected human root canals. Int Endod J 2007;40:85-93.
125. Estrela C, Estrela CRA, Guimarães LF, Silva RS, Pécora JD. Surface tension of calcium hydroxide associated with different substances. J Appl Oral Sci 2005;13:152-6.
126. Estrela C, Estrela CRA, Hollanda ACB, Decurcio DA, Pécora JD. Iodoform effect on antimicrobial potential of intracanal medicament. J Appl Oral Sci 2006;14:33-7.
127. Estrela C, Estrela CRA, Pécora JD. A study of the time necessary for calcium hydroxide to eliminate microorganism in infected canals. J Appl Oral Sci 2003;12:133-7.
128. Estrela C, Estrela CRA, Silva RS, Pécora JD. Molar conductivity of calcium hydroxide solutions. Braz Endod J 2001;5:13-7.
129. Estrela C, Holland R, Bernabe PF, Souza V, Estrela CR. Antimicrobial potential of medicaments used in healing process in dogs' teeth with apical periodontitis. Braz Dent J 2004;15:181-5.
130. Estrela C, Holland R. Calcium Hydroxide: study based on scientific evidences. J Appl Oral Sci 2003;14:269-83.
131. Estrela C, Holland R, Bernabé PFE, Souza V, Estrela CRA. Antimicrobial potential of medicaments used in healing process in dogs teeth with apical periodontitis. Braz Dent J 2004;15: 181-5.
132. Estrela C, Lopes HP, Felippe-Jr O, Sydney GB. Chemical analysis of calcium carbonate present in various calcium hydroxide samples. Braz Endod J 1997;2:7-9.
133. Estrela C, Mamede-Neto I, Estrela CRA, Pécora JD. Evaluation of density of calcium hydroxide pastes in dog's mandible. Braz Endod J 1998;3:24-30.
134. Estrela C, Mamede-Neto I, Lopes HP, Estrela CRA, Pécora JD. Root canal filling with calcium hydroxide using different techniques. Braz Dent J 2002;13:53-6.
135. Estrela C, Pécora JD, Silva RS. pH analyse of vehicles and calcium hydroxide pastes. Braz Endod J 1998;3:41-7.
136. Estrela C, Pécora JD, Sousa-Neto MD, Estrela CRA, Bammann LL. Effect of vehicle on antimicrobial properties of calcium hydroxide paste. Braz Dent J 1999;10:63-72.
137. Estrela C, Pesce HF. Chemical analysis of the formation of calcium carbonate and its influence on calcium hydroxide pastes in the presence of connective tissue of the dog. Part II. Braz Dent J 1997;8:49-53.
138. Estrela C, Pesce HF. Chemical analysis of the liberation of calcium and hydroxyl ions of calcium hydroxide pastes in the presence of connective tissue of the dog. Part I. Braz Dent J 1996;7:41-6.
139. Estrela C, Pimenta FC, Estrela CRA. Testes microbiológicos aplicados à pesquisa odontológica. In: Estrela C. Metodologia Científica: Ensino e Pesquisa em Odontologia. São Paulo: Artes Médicas; 2001.
140. Estrela C, Pimenta FC, Ito IY, Bammann LL. Antimicrobial evaluation of calcium hydroxide in infected dentinal tubules. J Endod 1999;26:416-8.
141. Estrela C, Pimenta FC, Ito IY, Bammann LL. In vitro determination of direct antimicrobial effect of calcium hydroxide. J Endod 1998;24:15-7.
142. Estrela C, Ribeiro RG, Estrela CRA, Pécora JD, Souza-Neto MD. Antimicrobial effect of 2% sodium hypochlorite and 2% chlorhexidine tested by different methods. Braz Dent J 2003;14:58-62.
143. Estrela C, Silva JA, Alencar AHG, Decurcio DA, Leles CR. Efficacy of sodium hypochlorite and chlorhexidine on *Enterococcus faecalis* - systematic review and meta-analysis. J Appl Oral Sci 2008 (in press).

144. Estrela C, Siqueira RMG, Resende EV, Silva S, Silva FAC. Influência da substância química, do cimento obturador e do número de sessões na incidência de pericementite traumática. Rev Odontol Brasil Central 1996;6:9-13.
145. Estrela C, Sydney GB. EDTA effect on root dentin pH after exchange of calcium hydroxide paste. Braz Endod J 1997;2:20-3.
146. Estrela C, Sydney GB, Bammann LL, Felippe-Jr O. Mechanism of action of calcium and hydroxyl ions of calcium hydroxide on tissue and bacteria. Braz Dent J 1995;6:85-90.
147. Estrela C, Sydney GB, Bammann LL, Fellipe-Jr O. Estudo do efeito biológico do pH na atividade enzimática de bactérias anaeróbias. Rev Fac Odontol Bauru 1994;2:31-8.
148. Estrela C, Sydney GB, Figueiredo JAP, Estrela CRA. A model system to study antimicrobial strategies on endodontic biofilms. J Applied Oral Sci 2009;17(2) (in press).
149. Estrela C, Sydney GB, Figueiredo JAP, Estrela CRA. Antibacterial Efficacy of Intracanal Medicaments on Bacterial Biofilm - A Critical Review. J Applied Oral Sci 2009;17(1) (in press).
150. Estrela C, Sydney GB, Pesce HF, Felippe-Jr O. Dentinal diffusion of hydroxil ions of various calcium hydroxide pastes. Braz Dent J 1995;6:5-9.
151. Estrela CRA. Eficácia antimicrobiana de soluções irrigadoras de canais radiculares. (Master's Thesis) Goiânia: Instituto de Patologia Tropical e Saúde Pública, Federal University of Goiás; 2000.
152. Estrela CRA. Prevalência de *Streptococcus mutans, Enterococcus faecalis, Porphyromonas gingivalis* e *Prevotella intermadia* em diferentes sítios da boca detectados por reação em cadeia da polimerase. (Doctoral Thesis) Goiânia: Instituto de Ciências Biológicas, Federal University of Goiás; 2007.
153. Estrela CRA, Estrela C, Reis C, Bammann LL, Pécora JD. Control of microorganisms in vitro by endodontic irrigants. Braz Dent J 2003;11:133-7.
154. Estrela CRA, Ávila GEG, Decurcio DA, Silva JA, Estrela C. Eficácia da clorexidina em infecções endodônticas – Revisão sistemática. Rev Bras Odontol 2008. (in press)
155. Evans M, Davies JK, Sundqvist G, Fidgor D. Mechanism involved in the resistance of *Enterococcus faecalis* to calcium hydroxide. Int Endod J 2002;35:221-8.
156. Evans MD, Baumgartner JC, Khemaleelakul S, Xia T. Efficacy of Calcium Hydroxide: Chlorhexidine Paste as an Intracanal Medication in Bovine Dentin. J Endod 2003;29:338-9.
157. Fager FK, Messer HH. Systemic distribuition of camphorated monoclorophenol from cotton pellets sealed in pulp chambers. J Endod 1986;12:225-9.
158. Faraco IM, Holland R. Histomorphological response of dogs' dental pulp capped with white mineral trioxide aggregate. Braz Dent J 2004;15:104-8.
159. Faraco IM, Holland R. Response of the pulp of dogs to capping with mineral trioxide aggregate or a calcium hydroxide cement. Dent Traumatol 2001;17:163-6.
160. Farber PA, Seltzer S. Endodontic microbiology. I. Etiology. J Endod 1998;14:363-71.
161. Fava LRG. A clinical evaluation of one- and two-appointment root canal therapy using calcium hydroxide. Int Endod J 1994;27:47-51.
162. Fava LRG. Acute apical periodontitis: incidence of postoperative pain using two different root canal dressings. Int Endod J 1998;31:343-7.
163. Feirer WA, Leonard V. Hexylresorcinol in oral antisepsis with special reference to solution 37. Dent Cosmos 1927;69:882-92.
164. Feldman G, Solomon C, Notaro P, Moskowitz E. Endodontic treatment of vital and non-vital teeth with open apex. New York State Dent J 1973;39:277-80.
165. Felippe MCS. Estudo in vitro do transporte de íons hidroxila e cálcio através da dentina radicular. (Master's Thesis). Florianópolis: Federal University of Santa Catarina; 1998.
166. Fiore-Donno G, Baume LJ. Effects of capping compounds containing corticosteroids on the human dental pulp. Helvet Odontol Act 1962;6:23-32.
167. Flohr W. Die biologische Wurzelbehandlung. Zahnarzliche Rundschan 1936;31. In: Castagnola L.1956 La Conservación de la Vitalidad de la Pulpa. Buenos Aires: Mundi.
168. Foreman PC, Barnes IE. A review of calcium hydroxide. Int Endod J 1990;23:283-97.
169. Forsberg A, Hagglund G. Differential diagnosis of radicular cyst and granuloma. Use of X-ray contrast medium. Dent Radiog Photog 1960;33:84-8.
170. Foster KH, Kulild JC, Weller RN. Effect of smear layer removal on the diffusion of calcium hydroxide through radicular dentin. J Endod 1993;19:136-40.
171. Foster KH, Primack PD, Kulild JC. Odontogenic cutaneous sinus tract. J Endod 1992;18:304-6.
172. Frank AL. Endodontic endosseous implants and treatment of the wide open apex. Dent Clin North Am 1967;675-700.
173. Frank AL. Experimental efforts to effect a closing of the wide open pulpless tooth allowing conservative therapy rather than surgical intervention. Twenty-first Annual Meeting Am Assoc Endod. USA: Washington, DC; 1964.
174. Frank AL. Therapy for the divergent pulpess tooth by continued apical formation. J Amer Dent Assoc 1966;72:87-93.
175. Frank AL, Weine FS. Nonsurgical therapy for the perforative defect of internal resorption. J Am Dent Assoc 1973;87:863-8.
176. Freitas JF. Characterization and aqueous extraction of calcium hydroxide compounds. Aust Dent J 1982;2:352-6.
177. Fulghum RS, Wiggis CB, Mullaney TP. Pilot study of detecting obligate anaerobic bacteria in necrotic dental pulps. J Dent Res 1973;52:637.
178. Funteas UR, Wallace JA, Fochtman EW. A comparative analysis of Mineral Trioxide Aggregate and Portland cement. Aust Dent J 2003;29:43-4.
179. Fuss R, Rafaeloff R, Tagger M, Szajkis S. Intracanal pH changes of calcium hydroxide pastes exposed to carbon dioxide in vitro. J Endod 1996;22:362-4.
180. Fuss R, Szajkis S, Tagger M. Tubular permeability to calcium hydroxide and to bleaching agents. J Endod 1989;15:362-4.
181. Fuss R, Weiss EI, Shalhav M. Antibacterial activity of calcium hydroxide-containing endodontic sealers on *Enterococcus faecalis* in vitro. Int Endod J 1997;30:397-402.
182. Garcez AS, Riberio MS, Tegos GP, Nunez SC, Jorge AO, Hamblin MR. Antimicrobial photodynamic ther-

apy combined with conventional endodontic treatment to eliminate root canal biofilm infection. Lasers Surg Med 2007;39:59-66.

183. Genciglu N, Kulekçi G. Antibacterial efficacy of root canal medicaments. J Nihon Univ Sch Dent 1992;34:233-6.
184. George S, Kishen A. Photophysical, photochemical, and photobiological characterization of methylene blue formulations for light-activated root canal disinfection. J Biomed Opt 2007;12:034029.
185. George S, Kishen A, Song KP. The role of environmental changes on monospecies biofilm formation on root canal wall by *Enterococcus faecalis*. J Endod 2005;31:867-72.
186. Georgepoulou M, Kontakiotis E, Nakou M. In vitro evaluation of the effectiveness of calcium hydroxide and paramonoclorophenol on anaerobic bacteria form the root canal. Endod Dent Traumatol 1993;9:249-53.
187. Ghose U, Baghdady VS, Hykmat BYM. Apexification on immature apices of pulpless permanent anterior teeth with calcium hydroxide. J Endod 1987;13:285-90.
188. Giardino L, Ambu E, Savoldi E, Rimondini R, Cassanelli C, Debbia EA. Comparative evaluation of antimicrobial efficacy of sodium hypochlorite, MTAD, and Tetraclean against *Enterococcus faecalis* biofilm. J Endod 2007;33:852-5.
189. Gilbert B. Endodontic treatment of the open apex. Quint Int 1983;3:293-9.
190. Gimlin DR, Schindler WG. The management of postbleaching cervical resorption. J Endod 1990;16:292-7.
191. Girard C, Holz J. Short and long-term follow-up in the treatment of category IV pulp diseases with calcium hydroxide. Schweiz Monatsschr Zahnmed 1985;95:169-82.
192. Glass RL, Zander HA. Pulp healing. J Dent Res 1949;28:97- 107.
193. Glenny AM, Esposito M, Coulthard P, Worthington HV. The assessment of systematic reviews in dentistry. Eur J Oral Sci 2003;111:85-92.
194. Gloudeman EA. Endodontic management of the wide open apex. J Wiscon State Dent Soc 1968;44:49-53.
195. Goldman M. Root-end closure techniques including apexification. Dental Clinics of North America 1974;18:297-308.
196. Gomes BPFA, Ferraz CCR, Garrido FD, Rosalen PL, Zaia AA, Teixeira FB, Souza-Filho FJ. Susceptibility to calcium hydroxide pastes and their vehicles. J Endod 2002;28:758-61.
197. Gomes BPFA, Ferraz CCR, Vianna ME, Rosalen PL, Zaia AA, Teixeira FB, Souza-Filho FJ. In Vitro antimicrobial activity of calcium hydroxide pastes and their vehicles against selected microorganisms. Braz Dent J 2002;13:155-61.
198. Gomes BPFA, Ferraz FB, Teixeira FB, Souza-Filho FJ. In Vitro antibacterial activity of endodontic irrigants in the elimination of *Enterococcus faecalis*. J Endod 2000;26:555.
199. Gomes IC, Chevitaresse O, Almeida NS, Salles MR, Gomes GC. Diffusion of calcium through dentin. J Endod 1996;22:590-5.
200. Gordon DF, Sturman M, Loesche WJ. Improved isolation of anaerobic bacteria from gingival crevice area of man. Appl Microbiol 1971;21:1046-50.
201. Gordon TM, Alexandre JB. The effects of calcium hydroxide on bovine pulp tissue: variations on pH and calcium concentrations. J Endod 1985;11:156-60.
202. Granath L-E. Nagra synpukter pa behandlingen av traumatiserale incisiver pabarn. Odontol Rev 1959;10:272-86.
203. Granström G. Relationship of inorganic pyphosphatase and pnitrophenyl-phosphatase activities of alkaline phosphatase in the microsomal fraction of isolated odontoblasts. Scand J Dent Res 1982;90:271-7.
204. Granström G, Linde A. A biochemical study of alkaline phosphatase in isolated rat incisor odontoblast. Arch Oral Biol 1972;17:213-24.
205. Granström G, Linde A, Nygren H. Ultrastructural localization of alkaline phosphatase in rat incisor odontoblasts. J Histochem Cytochem 1978;26:359- 68.
206. Greenstein G, Berman C, Jaffin R. Chlorhexedine. An adjunct to periodontal therapy. J Periodontol 1986;57:370-6.
207. Greenwood NN, Earnshaw A. Cheminsty of the elements. New York: Pergamon Press;1984. p.117- 54.
208. Gregoriou AP, Jeansonne BG, Musselman W. Timing of calcium hydroxide therapy in the treatment of root resorption in replanted teeth of dogs. Endod Dent Traumatol 1994;10:268-75.
209. Guigand M, Vulcain J-M, Dantel-Morazin A, Bonnaure-Mallet M. In vitro study of intradentinal calcium diffusion induced by two endodontic biomaterials. J Endod 1997;23:387-90.
210. Guignes P, Burnel F, Maurette A. Elimination de deux présentations d'hydroxyde de calcium: etude au M.E.B. Rev Fran d'Endod 1991;10:29-35.
211. Guimarães SAC, Alle N. Estudo histoquímico da reação tecidual ao hidróxido de cálcio. Estomat Cult 1974;8:79-82.
212. Gulabivala K, Stock CJ, Lewsey JD, Ghori S, Ng YL, Spratt DA. Effectiveness of electrochemically activated water as an irrigant in an infected tooth model. Int Endod J 2004;37:624-31.
213. Gutmann JL, Fava LRG. Periradicular healing and apical closure of a non-vital tooth in the presence of apical contamination. Int Endod J 1992;251:307-11.
214. Haapasalo K, Sirén EK, Waltimo TMT, Ørstavik D, Haapasalo MPP. Inactivation of local root canal medicaments by dentine: an in vitro study. Int Endod J 2000;33:126-31.
215. Haapasalo M. The Bacteróides sp. in dental root canal infection. Endod Dent Traumatol 1989;5:1-10.
216. Haapasalo M, Ørstavik D. In vitro infection and desinfection of dentinal tubules. J Dent Res 1987;66:1375-79.
217. Haapasalo M, Qian W, Portenier I, Waltimo T. Effects of dentin on the antimicrobial properties of endodontic medicaments. J Endod 2007;33:917-25.
218. Haenni S, Schmidlin PR, Mueller B, Sener B, Zehnder M. Chemical and antimicrobial properties of calcium hydroxide mixed with irrigants solutions. Int Endod J 2003;36:100-5.
219. Haglund R, He J, Jarvis J, Safavi KE, Spångberg LS, Zhu Q. Effects of root-end filling materials on fibroblasts and macrophages in vitro. Oral Surg Oral Med Oral Pathol Oral Radiol Endod 2003;95:739-45.
220. Ham JW, Patterson SS, Mitchell DF. Induced apical closure of immature pulpless teeth in monkeys. Oral Surg Oral Med Oral Pathol 1972;33:438- 49.

221. Ham KA, Witherspoon DE, Gutmann JL, Ravindranath S, Gait TC, Opperman LA. Preliminary evaluation of BMP-2 expression and histological characteristics during apexification with calcium hydroxide and mineral trioxide aggregate. J Endod 2005;31:275-9.
222. Han GY, Park SH, Yoon TC. Antimicrobial activity of calcium hydroxide containing pastes with *Enterococcus faecalis* in vitro. J Endod 2001;27:328-32.
223. Hancock HH, Sigurdsson A, Trope M, Moiseiwitsch J. Bacteria isolated after unsuccessful endodontic treatment in a North American population. Oral Surg Oral Med Oral Pathol 2001;5:579-86.
224. Harrison JW. Continued apical formation in the immature non-vital teeth. J Amer Dent Assoc 1969;27:6-9.
225. Harrison JW, Madonia JV. The toxicity of paraclorophenol. Oral Surg Oral Med Oral Pathol 1971;32:90-99.
226. Harrison JW, Rakusin H. Intracanal cementosis following induced apical closure. Endod Dent Traumatol 1985;1:242-5.
227. Hasselgren G, Kerekes K, Nellestan P. pH changes in calcium hydroxide - covered dentin. J Endod 1982;8:502-11.
228. Hasselgren G, Olsson B, Cvek M. Effects of calcium hydroxide and sodium hypoclorite on the dissolution of necrotic porcine muscle tissue. J Endod 1988;14:125-7.
229. Hauman CHJ, Love RM. Biocompatibility of dental materials used in contemporary endodontic therapy: a review. Part 1. Intracanal drugs and substances. Int Endod J 2003;36:75-85.
230. Havlíyková L, Matysová L, Nováková L, Hájková R, Solich P. HPLC determination of chlorhexidine gluconate and p-chloroaniline in topical ointment. J Pharmaceutic Biomedic Anal 2007;43:1169-73.
231. Heithersay GS. Calcium hydroxide in the treatment of pulpless teeth with associated pathology. J Brit Endod Soc 1975;8:74-98.
232. Heithersay GS. Periapical repair following conservative endodontic therapy. Aust Dent J 1970;15:511-8.
233. Heithersay GS. Stimulation of root formation in incompletely developed pulpless teeth. Oral Surg Oral Med Oral Pathol 1970;29:620-30.
234. Heling I, Steinberg D, Kenig S, Gavrilovich I, Sela MN, Friedman M. Efficacy of a sustained-release devise containing chlorhexidine and calcium hydroxide in preventing secondary infection of dentinal tubules. Int Endod J 1992;25:20-4.
235. Hems RS, Gulabilavala K, Ng Y-L, Ready D, Spratt DA. An in vitro evaluation of the ability of ozone to kill a strain of *Enterococcus faecalis*. Int Endod J 2005;38:22-9.
236. Hermann BW. Biologische Wurzelbehandlung. Frankfurt arn Main: W. Kramer, 1936.
237. Hermann BW. Calciumhydroxyd als mittel zurn behandel und füllen vonxahnwurzelkanälen. (Doctoral Thesis) Würzburg;1920. 50p.
238. Hermann BW. Der desinfektorische Wert des Calxyl. Zahnarz Rundsch 1935;44:1929-34.
239. Hermann BW. Die biologische wurzelbehandlung. Zahnarz Rundsch 1935;44:1509-17.
240. Hermann BW. Die Kalziumkomponente in der Wurzelbehandlung. Deutsch Zahnarz Wochens 1935;38:461-5.
241. Hernandez EP, Botero TM, Mantellini MG, McDonald NJ, Nor JE. Effect of ProRoot MTA mixed with chlorhexidine on apoptosis and cell cycle of fibroblasts and macrophages in vitro. Int Endod J 2005;38:137-43.
242. Hess W. The treatment of teeth with exposed healthy pulps. Int Dent J 1950;1:10-35.
243. Holland GR. Periapical response to apical plugs of dentin and calcium hydroxide in ferret canines. J Endod 1984;10:71-74.
244. Holland R. Emprego tópico de medicamentos no interior de canais radiculares. Odonto Máster - Endodontia 1994;1:1-13.
245. Holland R. Histochemical response of amputed pulps to calcium hydroxide. Rev Bras Pesq Med e Biol 1971;4:83-95.
246. Holland R. Processo de reparo da polpa dental após pulpotomia e proteção com hidróxido de cálcio. (Doctoral Thesis). Araçatuba: São Paulo State University; 1966.
247. Holland R. Processo de reparo do coto pulpar e dos tecidos periapicais após biopulpectomias e obturação de canal com hidróxido de cálcio ou óxido de zinco e eugenol. Estudos histológicos em dentes de cães. (Livre Docência Thesis) Araçatuba: São Paulo State University; 1975.
248. Holland R, Cruz AG, Nery MJ, Souza V, Otoboni-Filho JA, Bernabé PFE. Efecto de los medicamentos colocados en el interior del conducto, hidrosolubles y no hidrosolubles en el proceso de reparación de dientes de perro con lesión periapical. Endodoncia 1999;17:90-100.
249. Holland R, Cruz AG, Souza V, Nery MJ, Bernabé PFE, Otoboni-Filho JA. Recambio del hidróxido de calcio después de la pulpotomia y su influencia en la reparación. Estudio histológico en dientes de monos. Endodoncia 1999;17:35-45.
250. Holland R, Delgado RJM, Souza V. Defeitos em forma de tunel em pontes de dentina são características exclusivas do emprego do hidróxido de cálcio? Rev Ciência Odontol 2001;4:51-6.
251. Holland R, Ingle JI, Valle GF, Taintor JF. Influence of bony resorption on Endodontic treatment. Oral Surg Oral Med Oral Pathol 1983;55:191-203.
252. Holland R, Maisto OA, Souza V, Maresca BM, Nery MJ. Acción y velocidad de reabsorción de distintos materiales de obturación de conductos radiculares em el tejido periapical. Rev Assoc Argentina 1981;69:7-17.
253. Holland R, Mello W, Nery MJ, Bernabé PFE, Souza V. Reaction of human periapical tissue to pulp extirpation and immediate root canal filling with calcium hydroxide. J Endod 1977;3:63-7.
254. Holland R, Mello W, Nery MJ, Souza V, Bernabé PFE, Otoboni-Filho JA. The influence of the sealing material in the healing process of inflamed pulps capped with calcium hydroxide or zinc oxide- eugenol cement. Acta Odontol Pediatr 1981;2:5-9.
255. Holland R, Mello W, Nery MJ, Souza V, Bernabé PFE, Otoboni-Filho JA. Healing process of Dog's dental pulp after pulpotomy and pulp covering with calcium hydroxide in powder or paste form. Acta Odontol Pediatr 1981;2:47-51.
256. Holland R, Mello W, Souza V, Nery MJ, Bernabé PFE, Otoboni-Filho JA. Reacción de la pulpa y tejidos

periapicales de dientes de perros, com forâmenes incompletamente formados, posteriormente a la pulpotomia y protección com hidróxido de cálcio o formocresol: estudo histologico a distância. Endodoncia 1983;1:33-8.
257. Holland R, Murata SS, Souza V, Lopes HP, Salia O. Análise do selamento marginal obtido com cimentos à base de hidróxido de cálcio. Rev Ass Paul Cir Dent 1996;50:61-4.
258. Holland R, Nery MJ, Mello W, Souza V, Bernabé PFE, Otoboni-Filho JA. Root canal treatment with calcium hydroxide I - Effect of overfilling and refilling. Oral Surg Oral Med Oral Pathol 1979;47:87-92.
259. Holland R, Nery MJ, Mello W, Souza V, Bernabé PFE, Otoboni-Filho JA. Root canal treatment with calcium hydroxide II - Effect of instrumentation beyond the apices. Oral Surg Oral Med Oral Pathol 1979;47:93-6.
260. Holland R, Nery MJ, Mello W, Souza V, Bernabé PFE, Otoboni-Filho JA. Root canal treatment with calcium hydroxide III - Effect of debris and pressure filling. Oral Surg Oral Med Oral Pathol 1979;47:185-8.
261. Holland R, Nery MJ, Souza V, Mello W, Bernabé PFE, Otoboni-Filho JA. The effect of corticosteroid-antibiotic dressing in the behaviour of the periapical tissue of dog's teeth after instrumentation. Rev Odontol UNESP 1981;10:21-5.
262. Holland R, Nery MJ, Souza V, Mello W, Bernabé PFE, Otoboni-Filho JA. The effect of the filling material in the tissue reactions following apical plugging of the root canal with dentin chips. A histologic study in monkey's teeth. Oral Surg Oral Med Oral Pathol 1983;55:398-401.
263. Holland R, Okabe JN, Souza V, Saliba O. Diffusion of corticosteroid-antibiotic solutinos through human dentine. Rev Odontol UNESP 1991;20:17-23.
264. Holland R, Otoboni-Filho JA, Bernabé PFE, Nery MJ, Souza V, Berbert A. Effect of root canal status on periodontal healing after surgical injury in dogs. Endod Dent Traumatol 1994;10:77-82.
265. Holland R, Otoboni-Filho JA, Souza V, Mello W, Nery MJ, Bernabé PFE, Dezan-Jr E. Calcium hydroxide and corticosteroid-antibiotic association as dressings in cases of biopulpectomy. A comparative study in dogs teeth. Braz Dent J 1998;9:67-76.
266. Holland R, Otoboni-Filho JA, Souza V, Nery MJ, Bernabé PFE, Dezan-Jr E. Reparação dos tecidos periapicais com diferentes formulações de Ca(OH)2 - Estudo em cães. Rev Ass Paul Cir Dent 1999;53:327-31.
267. Holland R, Otoboni-Filho JA, Souza V, Nery MJ, Bernabé PFE, Dezan-Jr E. A comparison of one versus two appointment endodontic therapy in dogs' teeth with apical periodontitis. J Endod 2003;29:121-5.
268. Holland R, Otoboni-Filho JA, Souza V, Nery MJ, Bernabé PFE, Dezan-Jr E.Tratamiento endodôntico em una o en dos visitas. Estudio histológico en dientes de perros con lesión periapical. Endodoncia 2003;21:20-7.
269. Holland R, Otoboni-Filho JA, Souza V, Nery MJ, Bernabé PFE, Dezan-Jr E. Mineral trioxide aggregate repair of root perforations. J Endod 2001;27:281-4.
270. Holland R, Pinheiro CE, Mello W, Nery MJ, Souza V. Histochemical analysis of the dog's dental pulp after pulp capping with calcium, barium and strontium hydroxides. J Endod 1982;8:444-7.
271. Holland R, Sant'anna-Jr A, Souza V, Dezan-Jr E, Otoboni-Filho PFE, Nery MJ, Murata SS. Influence of apical patency and filling material on healing process of dogs' teeth with vital pulp after root canal therapy. Braz Dent J 2005;16:9-16.
272. Holland R, Soares IJ, Soares TML, Dias NV. The effect of the dressing in the tissue reactions following apical plugging of the root canal of dogs' pulpless teeth with chips. Rev Odontol UNESP 1989;18:101-8.
273. Holland R, Souza V. Ability of a new calcium hydroxide root canal filling material to induce hard tissue formation. J Endod 1985;11:535-43.
274. Holland R, Souza V. Resposta da conjuntiva do olho de coelho a algumas substâncias empregadas na desinfecção dos canais radiculares. APUD: Souza V, Holland R, Nery MJ, Mello W. Emprego de medicamentos no interior dos canais radiculares. Ação tópica e a distância de algumas drogas. Ars Cvradi 1978;5:4-15.
275. Holland R, Souza V, Mello W, Nery MJ, Bernabé PFE, Mello W, Otoboni-Filho JA. Emprego da associação corticosteróide antibiótico durante o tratamento endodôntico. Rev Paul Endod 1980;1:4-7.
276. Holland R, Souza V, Mello W, Nery MJ, Bernabé PFE, Otoboni-Filho JA. Healing process of dog's dental pulp after pulptomy and protection with calcium hydroxide. Rev Odontol Unesp 1979/1980;8:67-73.
277. Holland R, Souza V, Mello W, Nery MJ, Bernabé PFE, Otoboni-Filho JA. Permeability of the hard tissue bridge formed after pulpotomy with calcium hydroxide: a histologic study. J Amer Dent Ass 1979: 99:472-5.
278. Holland R, Souza V, Mello W, Nery MJ, Bernabé PFE, Otoboni-Filho JA. Healing process of dog's dental pulp after pulpotomy and protection with calcium hydroxide or Dycal. Rev Odontol Unesp 1979;8:67-73.
279. Holland R, Souza V, Mello W, Russo MC. Healing process of the pulp stump and periapical tissues in dog teeth. II. Histological findings following root filling with zinc oxide-eugenol. Rev Fac Odontol Araçatuba 1977;6:59-67.
280. Holland R, Souza V, Mello W, Russo MC. Healing process of the pulp stump and periapical tissue in dog teeth. III - Histopathological findings following root filling with calcium hydroxide. Rev Fac Odontol Araçatuba 1978;7:25-30.
281. Holland R, Souza V, Milanezi LA. Behaviour of pulp stump and periapical tissues to some drugs used a root canal dressings. A morphological study. Rev Bras Pesq Med Biol 1969;2:13-23.
282. Holland R, Souza V, Milanezi LA. Estudo morfológico do coto pulpar e tecidos periapicais frente à alguns materiais empregados nas obturações dos canais radiculares. Ciência e Cultura 1968;20:355.
283. Holland R, Souza V, Milanezi LA. Resposta do coto pulpar e tecidos periapicais a algumas pastas empregadas na obturação dos canais radiculares. Arq Cent Est Fac Odontol 1971;8:189-97.
284. Holland R, Souza V, Murata SS, Nery MJ, Bernabé PFE, Otoboni-Filho JA, Dezan-Jr E. Healing process of dog dental pulp after pulpotomy and pulp covering with mineral trioxide aggregate or Portland cement. Braz Dent J 2001;12:109-13.

285. Holland R, Souza V, Murata SS. Técnica da pulpotomia com troca de hidróxido de cálcio. Rev Ciência Odontol 1999;2:7-12.
286. Holland R, Souza V, Nery MJ, Bernabé PFE, Mello W, Otoboni-Filho JA. The effect of calcium hydroxide in dentine. Rev Fac Odontol Araçatuba 1978;7:177-80.
287. Holland R, Souza V, Nery MJ, Bernabé PFE, Otoboni-Filho JA, Dezan-Jr E, Murata SS. Calcium salts deposition in rat connective tissue after the implantation of calcium hydroxide - containing sealers. J Endod 1979;28:173-6.
288. Holland R, Souza V, Nery MJ, Bernabé PFE, Otoboni-Filho JA, Dezan-Jr E. Agregado de trióxido mineral y cemento Portland en la obturación de conductos radiculares de perro. Endodoncia 2001;19:275-80.
289. Holland R, Souza V, Nery MJ, Faraco-Jr IM, Bernabé PFE, Otoboni-Filho JA, Dezan-Jr E. Reaction of Rat Connective Tissue to Implanted Dentin Tube Filled with Mineral Trioxide Aggregate, Portland Cement or Calcium Hydroxide. Braz Dent J 2001;12:3-8.
290. Holland R, Souza V, Nery MJ, Faraco-Jr IM, Bernabé PFE, Otoboni-Filho JA, Dezan-Jr E. Reaction of rat connective tissue to implanted dentin tubes filled with a white mineral trioxide aggregate. Braz Dent J 2002;13:23-6.
291. Holland R, Souza V, Nery MJ, Mello W, Bernabé PFE, Otoboni-Filho JA. Comportamento dos tecidos periapicais de dentes de cães com rizogênese incompleta após obturação dos canais radiculares com diferentes materiais obturadores. Rev Bras Odontol 1992;49: 49-53.
292. Holland R, Souza V, Nery MJ, Mello W, Bernabé PFE, Otoboni-Filho JA. Effect of the dressing in root canal treatment with calcium hydroxide. Rev Fac Odontol Araçatuba 1978;7:39-45.
293. Holland R, Souza V, Nery MJ, Mello W, Bernabé PFE, Otoboni-Filho JA. Root canal treatment of pulpless teeth with calvital or zinc oxide-eugenol, in one or two sittings. Histological study in dog. Rev Fac Odontol Araçatuba 1978;7:47-53.
294. Holland R, Souza V, Nery MJ, Mello W, Bernabé PFE, Otoboni-Filho JA. A histological study of the effect of calcium hydroxide in the treatment of pulpless teeth of dogs. J Brit Endod Soc 1979;12:15-23.
295. Holland R, Souza V, Nery MJ, Mello W, Bernabé PFE, Otoboni-Filho JA. Tissues reactions following apical plugging of the root canal with infected dentin chips. Oral Surg Oral Med Oral Pathol 1980;49:366-9.
296. Holland R, Souza V, Nery MJ, Mello, W, Bernabé PFE. Root canal treatment with calcium hydroxide. Effect of an oil water soluble vehicle. Rev Odontol Unesp 1983;12:1-6.
297. Holland R, Souza V, Nery MJ, Mello, W. Resposta ao tecido conjuntivo subcutâneo do rato ao implante de alguns materiais obturadores de canal. Rev Fac Odontol Araçatuba 1973;2:217-25.
298. Holland R, Souza V, Nery MJ, Otoboni Filho JA, Bernabé PFE, Dezan-Jr E. Reaction of dogs' teeth to root canal filling with mineral trioxide aggregate or a glass ionomer sealer. J Endod 1999;25:728-30.
299. Holland R, Souza V, Nery MJ, Otoboni-Filho JA, Bernabé PFE, Dezan-Jr E. Reaction of rat connective tissue to implanted dentin tubes filled with mineral trioxide aggregate or calcium hydroxide. J Endod 1999;25:161-6.
300. Holland R, Souza V, Russo MC. Healing process after root canal therapy in immature human teeth. Rev Fac Odontol Araçatuba 1973;2:269-73.
301. Holland R, Souza V, Tagliavini RL, Milanezi LA. Healing process of teeth with open apices: histological study. Bull Tokyo Dent Coll 1971;12:333-8.
302. Holt SC, Progulske A. General microbiology, metabolism, and genetics. In: Oral microbiology and Immunology. Nisengard RJ, Newman MG. 2nd ed. Philadelphia: Saunders; 1994. p.47-114.
303. Horiba N, Maekawa Y, Ito M, Matsumoto T, Nakamura H. Correlations between endotoxin and clinical symptoms or radiolucent areas in infected root canals. Oral Surg Oral Med Oral Pathol 1991;71:492-5.
304. Horsted P, Sendergaard B, Thylstrup A, El Attar K, Fejerskov O. A retrospective study of direct pulp capping with calcium hydroxide compounds. Endod Dent Traumatol 1985;1:29-34.
305. Hosoya N, Takahashi G, Arai T, Nakamura J. Calcium concentration and pH of the periapical environment after applying calcium hydroxide into root canals in vitro. J Endod 2001;27:343-6.
306. Huang TH, Ding SJ, Hsu TC, Kao CT. Effects of mineral trioxide aggregate (MTA) extracts on mitogen-activated protein kinase activity in human osteosarcoma cell line (U2OS). Biomaterials 2003;24:3909-13.
307. Huang TH, Yang CC, Ding SJ, Yeng M, Kao CT, Chou MY. Inflammatory cytokines reaction elicited by root-end filling materials. J Biomed Mat Res 2005;73:123-8.
308. Hugo WB, Russel AD. Pharmaceutical Microbiology. 5th ed. Oxford: Blackwell:1992. p.245-99.
309. Hume WR. In vitro studies on the local pharmacodynamics, pharmacology and toxicology of eugenol and zinc oxide-eugenol. Int Endod J 1988;21:130 - 134.
310. Hume WR. The pharmacologic and toxicological properties of zinc oxide-eugenol. J Amer Dent Ass 1986;113:789-91.
311. Hussey DL, Kennedy JG. Conservative treatment of a large radiolucent cyst-like apical lesion - a case report. Rest Dent 1990;6:12-3.
312. Ida K, Maseki T, Yamasaki M, Hirano S, Nakamura H. The pH values of pulp-capping agents. J Endod 1989;15:365-8.
313. Imanishi T. A clinico-pathological study of pulpotomy on deciduous teeth. J Tokyo Dent College Soc 1980;72:647-94.
314. Jadad AR, Cook DJ, Browman GP. A guide to interpreting discordant systematic reviews. Can Med Assoc J 1997;156:1411-6.
315. Jardim-Jr EG. Estudo da Microbiota anfibiôntica presente no interior de canais radiculares de dentes com polpa necrótica: susceptibilidade ao hidróxido de cálcio e fatores de virulência. (Livre Docência Thesis) Araçatuba, São Paulo State University;2001. 416p.
316. Jeansonne MJ, White RR. A comparison of 2% chlorhexidine gluconate and 5.25% sodium hypochlorite as antimicrobial endodontic irrigant. J Endod 1994;20:276-8.
317. Jenkins S, Addy M, Wade W. The mechanism of action of chlorhexidine. J Clin Periodontol 1988;15:415-24.
318. Juge H. Resorbable pastes for root filling. Int Dent J 1959;9:461-76.

319. Kakehashi S, Stanley HR, Fitzgerald RJ. The effects of surgical exposures of dental pulps in germ-free and conventional laboratory rats. Oral Surg Oral Med Oral Pathol 1965;20:340-9.
320. Katebzadeh N, Hupp J, Trope M. Histological periapical repair after obturation of infected root canals in dogs. J Endod 1999;25:364-8.
321. Kawakami T. An experimental study on tissue reaction to a paste made of calcium hydroxide and iodoform with an addition of silicone oil. J Tokyo Dent College Soc 1984;84:77-107.
322. Kawakami T, Nakamura C, Eda S. Effects of the penetration of a root canal filling material into the mandibular canal. 1 - Tissue reactions to the material. Endod Dent Traumatol 1991;7:36-41.
323. Kawakami T, Nakamura C, Hasegawa H, Akahane S, Eda S. Ultrastructural study of initial calcification in the rat subcutaneous tissues elicited by a root canal filling material. Oral Surg Oral Med Oral Pathol 1987;63:360-5.
324. Kawakami T, Nakamura C, Hasegawa H, Eda S. Fate of 14C-labeled dimethylpolysiloxane (silicone oil) in a root canal filling material embedded in rat subcutaneous tissues. Dent Materials 1987;3:256-60.
325. Kawakami T, Nakamura C, Hasegawa H, Eda S. Fate of 45Ca labeled calcium hydroxide in a root canal filling paste embedded in rat subcutaneous tissue. J Endod 1987;13:220-3.
326. Kawakami T, Nakamura C, Hayashi T, Eda S, Akahane S. Studies on the tissue reactions to the paste of calcium hydroxide added iodoform (root canal filling material: Vitapex1). First report: a histopathological study. Matsumoto Shigaku 1979;5:35-44.
327. Kawakami T, Nakamura C, Hayashi T, Eda S. Studies on tissue reactions to the paste of calcium hydroxide added iodoform (root canal filling material: Vitapex). Second report: an electron microscopic study. Matsumoto Shigaku 1979;5:161-70.
328. Keiser K, Johnson CC, Tipton DA. Cytotoxicity of mineral trioxide aggregate using human periodontal ligament fibroblasts. J Endod 2000;26:288-91.
329. Kennedy GDC, McLundy AC, Day RM. Calcium hydroxide. Its role in a simplified endodontic technique. Dent Manag Oral Topics 1967;84:51-7.
330. Khemaleelakul S, Baumgartner JC, Pruksakom S. Autoaggregation and coaggregation of bacteria associated with acute endodontic infections. J Endod 2006;32:312-8.
331. Kim M, Kim B, Yoon S. Effect on the healing of periapical perforations in dogs of the addition of growth factors to calcium hydroxide. J Endod 2001;27:426-9.
332. Kishen A, George S, Kumar R. *Enterococcus faecalis*-mediated biomineralized biofilm formation on root canal. J Biomed Mater Res 2006;77:406-15.
333. Kitagawa M. Clinico-pathological study on immediate root canal filling with improved Calvital after vital pulp extirpation. J Tokyo Dent College Soc 1969;69:2-5.
334. Kleier DJ, Averbach RE, Kawulok TC. Efficient calcium hydroxide placement within the root canal. J Prosth Dent 1985;53:509-510.
335. Kodukula PS, Prakasam TBS, Anthonisen AC. Role of pH in biological wastewater treatment process. In: Bazin MJ, Prosser JI. Physiological models in microbiology. Florida: CRC Press;1988. p.113-34.
336. Koh ET, McDonald F, Pitt Ford TR, Torabinejad M. Cellular response to Mineral Trioxide Aggregate. J Endod 1998;24:543-7.
337. Koh ET, Torabinejad M, Pitt Ford TR, Brady K, McDonald F. Mineral Trioxide Aggregate stimulates a biological response in human osteoblasts. J Biomed Materials Res 1997;37:432-9.
338. Kontakiotis M, Nakou M, Georgepoulou M. In vitro study of the indirect action of calcium hydroxide on the anaerobic flora of the root canal. Int Endod J 2001;28:285-9.
339. Koulaouzidou EA, Papazisis KT, Economides NA, Beltes P, Kortsaris AH. Antiproliferative effect of mineral trioxide aggregate, zinc oxide-eugenol cement, and glass- ionomer cement against three fibroblastic cell lines. J Endod 2005;31:44-6.
340. Krakow AA, Berck H, Gion P. Therapeutic induction of root formation in the exposed incompletely formed tooth with vital pulp. Oral Surg Oral Med Oral Pathol 1977;43:755-65.
341. Krakow AA, Berck H, Gion P. Tratamiento de la pulpa vital en la dentición permanente. In: Actas del Segundo Seminario de la Sociedad Argentina de Endodoncia. Buenos Aires: Argentina;1974.
342. Krasowska A, Chmielewska L, Adamski R, Luczynski J, Witek S, Sigler K. The sensitivity of yeast and yeast-like cells to new lysosomotropic agents. Cell Mol Biol Lett 2004;9:675- 83.
343. Krell FV, Madson S. The use of the Messing Gun in placing calcium hydroxide powder. J Endod 1989;11:233-4.
344. Kristich CJ, Li YH, Cvitkovitch DG, Dunny GM. Esp-Independent biofilm formation by *Enterococcus faecalis*. J Bacteriol 2004;186:154-63.
345. Kurimoto H. Experimental studies on the conservative treatment of experimental periapical lesion on the trial application of `Calsan B' as a root canal filling material. J Osaka Univ Dent Soc 1961;6:333-52.
346. Kvist T, Molander A, Dahlén G, Reit C. Microbiological evaluation of one- and two-visit endodontic treatment of teeth with apical periodontitis: a randomized, clinical trial. J Endod 2004;30:572-6.
347. Lana MA. Avaliação microbiológica de canais radiculares com necrose pulpar en três etapas do tratamento endodôntico. (Master's Thesis). Belo Horizonte: Federal University of Minas Gerais, 1999.
348. Larsen MJ, Hörsted-Bindslev P. A laboratory study evaluating the release of hydroxyl ions from various calcium hydroxide products in narrow root canal-like tubes. Int Endod J 2000;33:238-42.
349. Laurichesse JM. Le traitement endodontique des dents immatures par édification apicale (apexification). Actual Odontostomatolog 1980;131:459-76.
350. Law A, Messer H. An evidence-based analysis of the antibacterial effectiveness of intracanal medicaments. J Endod 2004;30:689-94.
351. Laws AJ. Calcium hydroxide as a possible root filling material. New Zealand Dent J 1962;58:199-215.
352. Laws AJ. Condensed calcium hydroxide root filling following partial pulpotomy. New Zealand Dent J 1971;67:161-8.
353. Lawson BF, Mitchell DF. Pharmacologic treatment of painful pulpitis. A preliminary, controlled double-blind study. Oral Surg Oral Med Oral Pathol 1964;17:47-61.

354. Lea FM. Lea's Chemistry of Cement and Concrete: 4th edn. London: Edward Arnold; 1998.
355. Lecazadieu M. Pharmacologic endodontique. In: Laurichesse J-M, Maestroni F, Breillat J, eds. Endodontie Clinique. Paris: Editions CDP; 1986.
356. Lee SJ, Monsef M, Torabinejad M. Sealing ability of a Mineral trioxide Agregate for repair of lateral root perforations. J Endod 1993;19:541-4.
357. Lee Y-L, Lee B-S, Lin F-H, Lin AY, Lan W-H, Lin C-P. Effects of physiological environments on the hydration behavior of mineral trioxide aggregate. Biomaterials 2004;25:787-93.
358. Lehninger AL. Princípios de bioquímica. 2nd ed. São Paulo: Sarvier; 1986.
359. Leksell E, Ridell K, Cvek M, Mejàre L. Pulp exposure after step-wise versus direct complete excavation of deep carious lesion in young posterior permanent teeth. Endod Dent Traumatol 1996;12:192-6.
360. Lengheden A, Blomlof L, Lindskog S. Effect of immediate calcium hydroxide treatment and permanent root-filling on periodontal healing in contaminated replanted teeth. Scandinavian J Dent Res 1991;99:139-46.
361. Leonardo MR, Almeida WA, Ito IY, Silva LAB. Radiographic and microbiologic evaluation of post-treatment apical and periapical repair of root canal of dogs' teeth with experimentally induced chronic lesion. Oral Surg Oral Med Oral Pathol 1994;78:232-8.
362. Leonardo MR, Almeida WA, Silva LAB, Utrilla S. Histopathological observations of periapical repair in teeth with radiolucent areas submitted to two different methods of root canal treatment. J Endod 1995;21:137-41.
363. Leonardo MR, Rossi MA, Silva LAB, Ito IY. EM evaluation of bacterial biofilm and microorganisms on the apical external root surface of human teeth. J Endod 2002;28:815-8.
364. Leonardo MR, Silva LAB, Utrilla LS, Leonardo RT, Consolaro A. Effect of intracanal dressings on repair and apical bridging of teeth with incomplete root formation. Endod Dent Traumatol 1993;9:25-30.
365. Lima KC, Fava LRG, Siqueira-Jr JF. Susceptibilities of *Enterococcus faecalis* biofilms to some antimicrobial medications. J Endod 2001;27:616-9.
366. Lindhe G. Antissépticos e antibióticos em Periodontia. In: Tratado de Periodontologia Clínica. Lindhe J. Rio de Janeiro: Guanabara Koogan;1995. p.270.
367. Lindskog S, Pierce AM, Blomlof L. Chlorhexedine as a root canal medicament for treating inflammatory lesions in the periodontal space. Endod Dent Traumatol 1998;14:186-90.
368. Lopes HP, Costa Filho AS. Tratamento endodôntico de dentes com rizogênese incompleta e necrose pulpar. Rev Bras Odontol 1984;41:2-12.
369. Lopes HP, Costa-Filho AS. O emprego do hidróxido de cálcio associado ao azeite de oliva. Rev Gaúcha Odontol 1986;34:306-13.
370. Lopes HP, Estrela C, Elias CN, Toniasso S. Smear layer: influence of the mechanical stirring of the chelting agent (EDTA): Braz Endod J 1996;1:52-55.
371. Lopes HP, Estrela C, Siqueira J, Fava LR. Considerações químicas, microbiológicas e biológicas do hidróxido de cálcio. Odonto Master 1996;1:1-17.
372. Lopes HP, Estrela C, Siqueira JF Jr. Tratamento endodôntico em dentes corn rizogênese incompleta. In: Berger CA. Endodontia. São Paulo: Pancast;1998.
373. Love RM. *Enterococcus faecalis* - mechanism for its role in endodontic failure. Int Endod J 2001;34:399-406.
374. Love RM. Invasion of dentinal tubules by root canal bacteria. Endodontic Topics 2004;9:52-65.
375. Ludlow MO. Apical closure after nonsurgical apical curetage. J Endod 1979;5:151-3.
376. Luvizotto AAV, Valdrighi L, Berbert CV, Murgel CAF. Apecificação. Formação de barreira apical em dentes imaturos com necrose pulpar. Rev Gaúcha Odontol 1996;44:287-91.
377. Lynne RE, Liewehr Fr, West LA, Patton WR, Buxton TB, McPherson JC. In vitro antimicrobial activity of various medications preparations on *Enterococcus faecalis* in root canal dentin. J Endod 2003;29:187-90.
378. MacDonald JB, Hare GC, Wood AWS. The bacteriologic status of the pulp chambers in intacts teeth found to be novital following trauma. Oral Surg Oral Med Oral Pathol 1957;10:318-22.
379. Maisto AO, Capurro MA. Obturación de conductos radiculares con hidróxido de cálcio-iodofórmio. Rev Assoc Odontol Argentina 1964;52:167-73.
380. Maisto OA, Erausquin J. Reacción de los tejidos periapicales del molar de la rata a las pastas de obturación, reabsorbibles. Rev Assoc Odontol Argentina. 1965;53:12-20.
381. Malo PRT, Kessler Nieto F, Vadillo MVM. Hidróxido, de calcio y apicoformación Rev Espan Endod 1987;5:41-61.
382. Marion JJC. Processo de reparo de dentes de cães após biopulpectomia e obturação dos canais radiculares com os cimentos Sealapex ou MTA manipulado com propilenoglicol, associados ao efeito do emprego ou não de um curativo de corticosteróide-antibiótico. (Master's Thesis), Marília, University of Marília; 2008.
383. Markowitz K, Moynihan M, Liu M, Kim S. Biologic properties of eugenol and zinc oxide-eugenol. Oral Surg Oral Med Oral Pathol 1992;73:729-37.
384. Marmasse A. Dentisterie Operatoire, vol. 1. Paris: JB Bailliere; 1953.
385. Marsh PD. Plaque as a biofilm: pharmacological principles of drug delivery and action in the sub- and supragingival environment. Oral Diseases 2003;9:16-22.
386. Martin DM, Crabb HSM. Calcium hydroxide in root canal therapy. Brit Dent J 1977;142:277-83.
387. Massler M, James E, Englander H. Histologic response of amputed pulps to calcium compounds and antibiotics. Oral Surg Oral Med Oral Pathol 1957;10:957-80.
388. Masterton JB. The healing of wounds of the dental pulp. An investigation of the nature of the scar tissue and of the phenomena leading to its formation. Dent Practitioner 1966;16:325-39.
389. Matsumiyas S, Kitamura M. Histopathological and histobacteriological studies of the relation between the condition of sterilization of the interior of the root canal and the healing process of periapical tissues in experimentally infected root canal treatment. Bull Tokyo Dent Coll 1950;1:1-19.

390. Matsumoto K, Inoue K, Matsumoto A. The effect of newly developed root canal sealers on rat dental pulp cells in primary culture. J Endod 1989;15:60-7.
391. Matsuzaki K, Fujii H, Machida Y. Experimental study of pulpotomy with calcium hydroxide-iodoform paste in dog's immature permanent teeth. Bull Tokyo Dent Coll 1990;31:9-15.
392. Mc Cormick JE. Tissue pH of developing periapical lesions in dogs. J Endod 1983;9:47-51.
393. Mejáre B. The incidence and significance of *Streptococcus sanguis*, *Streptococcus mutans* and *Streptococcus salivarius* in root canal cultures from human teeth. Odontol Rev 1974;25:359-77.
394. Mello W, Holland R, Souza V. Capeamento pulpar com hidróxido de cálcio ou pasta de óxido de zinco e eugenol. Rev Fac Odontol Araçatuba 1972;1:33-44.
395. Menezes R, Bramante CM, Letra A, Carvalho VG, Garcia RB. Histologic evaluation of pulpotomies in dog using two types of mineral trioxide aggregate and regular and white Portland cements as wound dressings. Oral Surg Oral Med Oral Pathol Oral Radiol Endod 2004;98:376-9.
396. Messer HH. Effect phosphate deficiency on pulp alkaline phosphatase and Ca2, Mg2 - ATPase activity in rats. J Dent Res 1982;61:1110-2.
397. Messer HH, Feigal RJ. A comparison of the antibacterial and citotoxic effects of parachlorophenol. J Dent Res 1985;64:18-821.
398. Metzler RS, Montgomery S. The effectiveness of ultrasonics and calcium hydroxide for the debridement of human mandibular molars. J Endod 1989;15:373-8.
399. Michanowicz J, Michanowcz A. A conservative approach and procedure to fill incompletely formed root using calcium hydroxide as an adjunct. J Dent Children 1967;32:42-7.
400. Milano NF, Kolling IG, Fachini EF. Tensão superficial de alguns auxiliares químicos em endodontia. Rev Gaúcha Odontol. 1983;31:37-8.
401. Miller WD. An introduction to the study of the bacteriopathology of the dental pulp. Dental Cosmos 1894;36:505-28.
402. Miller WD. The microorganisms of the human mounth. Philadelphia: S.S.White Dental Mfgo CO; 1890.
403. Miñana M, Carnes-Jr DL, Walker-III WA. pH changes at the surface of root dentin after intracanal dressing with calcium oxide and calcium hydroxide. J Endod 2001;27:43-5.
404. Mitchell OF, Shankawalker GB. Osteogenic potencial of calcium hydroxide and other materials in soft tissue and bone wounds. J Dent Res 1958;37:1157-63.
405. Mitchell PJC, Pitt Ford TR, Torabinejad M, McDonald F. Osteoblast biocompatibility of mineral trioxide aggregate. Biomaterials 1999;20:167-73.
406. Mizuno M, Banzai Y. Calcium ion release from calcium hydroxide stimulated fibronectin gene expression in dental pulp cells and the differentiation of dental pulp cells to mineralized tissue forming cells by fibronectin. Int Endod J 2008; 41:933-38.
407. Mjör IA, Furseth R. The inorganic phase of calcium hydroxide - and corticosteroid - covered dentine studied by electrom microscopy. Archs Oral Biol 1968;13:755-63.
408. Moghaddame-Jafari S, Mantellini MG, Botero TM, McDonald NJ, Nor JE. Effect of ProRoot MTA on pulp cell apoptosis and proliferation in vitro. J Endod 2005;31:387-91.
409. Molander A, Lundquist P, Papapanou PN, Dahlén G, Reit C. A protocol for polymerase chain reaction detection of *Enterococcus faecalis* and *Enterococcus faecium* from the root canal. Int Endod J 2002;35:1-6.
410. Molander A, Reit C, Dahlén G, Kvist T. Microbiological status of root-filled teeth with apical periodontitis. Int Endod J 1998;31:1-7.
411. Möller AJR. Microbiological examination of root canals and periapical tissues of human teeth. Odontol Tidskr 1966;74:1-38.
412. Möller AJR, Fabricus L, Dahlén G, Öhman AE, Heyden G. Influence on periapical tissues of indigeneous oral bacteria and necrotic pulp tissue in monkeys. Scand J Dental Res 1981;89:475-84.
413. Montgomery S. External cervical resorption after bleaching a pulpless tooth. Oral Surg Oral Med Oral Pathol 1984;57:203-6.
414. Morais JT. The use of calcium hydroxide as a dressing in root canal treatment. J Dent Assoc South Africa 1996;51:593-9.
415. Moretton TR, Brown CE, Legan JJ, Kafrawy AH. Tissue reactions after subcutaneous and intraosseous implantation of mineral trioxide aggregate and ethoxybenzoic acid cement. J Biomed Mater Res 2000;52:528-33.
416. Morgan RW, Carnes DL, Montgomery S. The solvent effects of calcium hydroxide irriganting solution on bovine pulp tissue. J Endod 1991;17:165-8.
417. Morse DR, O'Larnic J, Yesilsoy C. Apexification: review of the literature. Quint Int 1990;21:589-98.
418. Murata S. Experimental study on treatment of infected root canal of deciduous tooth with application of calcium hydroxide-eugenol. Japan J Conservat Dent 1959;3:163-5.
419. Nair PNR. Apical periodontitis: a dynamic encounter between root canal infection and host response. Periodontology 2000 1997;13:29-39.
420. Nair PNR. Light and electrom microscopic studies on root canal flora and periapical lesions. J Endod 1987;13:29-39.
421. Nair PNR. Pathobiology of the periapex. In: Pathways of the pulp. Cohen S, Burns RC. St. Louis: Mosby; 2001.
422. Nair PNR, Henry S, Cano V, Vera J. Microbial status of apical root canal system of human mandibular first molars with primary apical periodontitis after one-visit-endodontic treatment. Oral Surg Oral Med Oral Pathol Oral Radiol Endod 2005;99:231-52.
423. Nair PNR, Sjögren U, Kahnerg KE, Sundqvist G. Intraradicular bacteria and fungi in root - files, assymtomatic human teeth with therapy-resistant periapical lesions: A long-term light and electron microscopic follow-up study. J Endod 1990;16:580-8.
424. Nair PNR, Sjögren U, Schumacher E, Sundqvist G. Radicular cyst affecting a root-filled human tooth: a long-term post-treatment follow-up. Int Endod J 1993;26:225-33.
425. Naulin-Ifi C. Apexogenese apexification: données récentes. Rev Fran d'Endod 1986;5:75-83.
426. Naumovich DB. Surface tension and pH of drugs in root canal therapy. Oral Surg Oral Med Oral Pathol. 1963;16:965-8.

427. Neidhart FC. Physiology of the bacterial cell - a molecular approach. Massachussetts: Ed. Sinaver;1990.
428. Nerwich A, Figdor D, Messer HH. pH changes in root dentine over a 4 week period following root canal dressing with calcium hydroxide. J Endod 1993;19:302-6.
429. Nevins A, Finkelstein F, Laporta R, Borden B. Induction of hard tissues into pulpless open-apex teeth using collagen-calcium phosphate gel. J Endod 1978;4:76-81.
430. Nisengard RJ, Newman MG. Oral Microbiology and Immunology. 2nd ed. Philadelphia: Sauders;1994.
431. Noda M, Komatsu H, Inoue S, Sano H. Antibiotic susceptibility of bacteria detected from the root canal exudate of persistent apical periodontitis. J Endod 2000;26:221-4.
432. Noguchi N, Nori Y, Narimatsu M, Ebisu S. Identification and localization of extraradicular biofilm-forming bacteria associated with refractory endodontic pathogens. Appl Environ Microbiol 2005;71:8738-43.
433. Noiri Y, Ehara A, Kawahara T, Takemura N, Ebisu S. Participation of bacterial biofilms in refractory and chronic periapical periodontitis. J Endod 2002;28:679-83.
434. Nolte WA. Oral Microbiology. 4th ed. London: Mosby;1982. p.55-125.
435. Nosrat IV, Nosrat CA. Reparative hard tissue formation following calcium hydroxide application after partial pulpotomy in cariously exposed pulps of permanent teeth. Int Endod J 1998;31:221-6.
436. Nyborg H. Healing process in the pulp on capping. A morphologic study. Acta Odontol Scand 1955;13:1-129.
437. Nyborg H, Tullin B. Healing process after vital extirpation. An experimental study of 17 teeth. Odontol Tidskrift 1965;73:430-46.
438. Nygren J. Radgivare Angaende Basta Sattet Att Varda Ah Bevara Tandernas Fuskhet, Osv. Stockholm;1838.
439. Ogawa AT, Holland R, Souza V. Influência do selamento cavitário no processo de reparo da polpa dental após pulpotomia e proteção com hidróxido de calcio. Rev Fac Odontol Araçatuba 1974;3:51-9.
440. Ohara PK, Torabinejad M. Apical closure of an immature root subsequent to apical curettage. Endod Dent Traumatol 1992;8:134-7.
441. Olson A, Hoover JE. Remington's Pharmaceutical Sciences:15th ed. Easton: Mack Publishing Co; 1975.
442. O'Riordan M. Apexification of deciduous incisor. J Endod 1980;6:607-9.
443. Ørstavik D, Haapasalo M. Disinfection by endodontic irrigants and dressings of experimentally infected dentinal tubulares. Endod Dent Traumatol 1990;6:142-9.
444. Ørstavik D, Kerekes K, Molven O. Effects of extensive apical reaming and calcium hydroxide dressing on bacterial infection during treatment of apical periodontitis: a pilot study. Int Endod J 1991;24:1-7.
445. Özcelik B, Tasman F, Ogan C. A comparison of the surface tension of calcium hydroxide mixed with different vehicles. J Endod 2000;26:500-2.
446. Paiva JG, Antoniazzi JH. Endodontia - Bases para a prática clínica. 2nd ed. São Paulo: Artes Médicas;1988.
447. Panzarini SR, Souza V, Holland R, Dezan-Júnior E. Tratamento de dentes com lesão periapical crônica. Influência de diferentes tipos de curativo de devora e do material obturador de canal radicular. Rev Odontol UNESP 1998;27:509-26.
448. Parashos P. Apexification: case report. Aust Dent J 1997;42:43-6.
449. Pashley DH, Kalathoor S, Burnham D. The effects of calcium hydroxide on dentin permeability. J Dent Res 1986;65:417-20.
450. Peciuliene V, Reynaud AH, Balciuniene I, Haapasalo M. Isolation of yeasts and enteric bacteria in root-filled teeth with chronic apical periodontitis. Int Endod J 2001;34:429-34.
451. Pécora JD, Guimarães LF, Savioli RN. Surface tension of several drugs used in endodontics. Braz Dent J 1991;2:123-7.
452. Pécora JD, Souza-Neto MD, Saquy PC, Silva RG, Cruz-Filho AM. Effect of Dakin's and EDTA solutions on dentin permeability of root canals. Braz Dent J 1993;4:79-84.
453. Peniche CEC, Sampaio JMP, Collesi RR. Verificação do pH de diversas soluções à base de hidróxido de calcio. Rev Odontol Univ Santo Amaro 1996;1:58.
454. Pérez F, Franchi M, Péli JF. Effect of calcium hydroxide form and placement on root dentine pH. Int Endod J 2001;34:417-23.
455. Perez F, Rochdt T, Lodter JP, Calas P, Michel G. In vitro study of the penetration of three bacterial strains into root dentine. Oral Surg Oral Med Oral Pathol Oral Radiol Endod 1993;76:97-103.
456. Pertot WJ, Chemoul B, Camps J. Influence du mode de conservation et des solutions-vehicles sur le pH et la carbonatation de l'hydroxide de calcium. Rev Française Endod 1992;11:45-9.
457. Peters LB, Van Winkelhoff AJ, Buijs JF, Wesselink PR. Effects of instrumentation, irrigation and dressing with calcium hydroxide on infecton in pulpless teeth with periapical bone lesions. Int Endod J 2002;35:13-21.
458. Peters LB, Wesselink PR, Buijs JF, Van Winkelhoff AJ. Viable bacteria in root dentinal tubules of teeth with apical periodontitis. J Endod 2001;27:76-81.
459. Peters LB, Wesselink PR, Moorer WR. Penetration of bacteria in bovine root dentine in vitro. Int Endod J 2000;33:28-36.
460. Pisanti S, Sciaky I. Origin of calcium the repair wall after pulp exposure in the dog. J Dent Res 1964;43:641-4.
461. Pissiotis E, Spångberg LSW. Biological evaluation of collagen gels containing calcium hydroxide and hydroxyapatite. J Endod 1990;16:468-73.
462. Pitt Ford TR, Torabinejad M, Abedi HR, Bakland LK, Kariyawasan SP. Using mineral trioxide aggregate as a pulp-capping material. J Am Dent Assoc 1996;127:1491-6.
463. Pitt Ford TR, Torabinejad M, McKendry DJ, Hong CU, Kariyawasan SP. Use of mineral trioxide aggregate for repair of furcal perforations. Oral Surg Oral Med Oral Pathol 1995;79:756-62.
464. Porkaew P, Retief DH, Barfield RD, Lacefield WR, Soong S. Effects of calcium hydroxide paste as an intracanal medicament on apical seal. J Endod 1990;16:468-73.
465. Portenier I, Haapasalo H, Rye A, Waltimo T, Ørstavik D, Haapasalo M. Inactivation of root canal medicaments by dentine, hydroxiapatite and bovine serum albumin. Int Endod J 2001;34:184-8.
466. Pucci FM. Conductos radiculares. Vol. II. Montevideo: Casa A Barreiro y Ramos SA;1944/1945. p.344-77.

467. Pucci FM. Conductos radiculares: anatomia, patologia y terapia. Montevideo: Medico Quirurgica;1945.
468. Putnam RW. Intracellular pH regulation. In: Neid'hart FC. Cell physiology. San Diego: Academic Press;1995. p.212-29.
469. Quackenbush L. In vitro testing of three types of endodontic medicaments against anaerobic bacteria. J Endod 1986;12:132-6.
470. Quillin B, Dabirsiaghi CL, Krywolap GN, Dumsha TC. Antimicrobial effect of $Ca(OH)_2$ supplemented with metronidazole and chlorhexidine as intracanal medicaments. J Endod 1992;18:187.
471. Rabie G, Trope M, Trostad L. Treatment of a maxillary canine with external inflammatory root resorption. J Endod 1988;14:101-5.
472. Ranta K, Haapasalo M, Renta H. Monoinfection of root canal with *Pseudomonas aeruginosa*. Endod Dent Traumatol 1988;4:269-72.
473. Rantanen AV, Louhivuori A. The effect of calcium hydroxide upon human scrum proteins. Acta Odontol Scand 1959;17:103-11.
474. Rasmussen P, Mjor IA. Calcium hydroxide as ectopic bone inductor in rats. Scand J Dent Res 1971;79:24-30.
475. Ray HA, Trope M. Periapical status of endodontically treated teeth in relation to the technical quality of the root filling and the coronal restoration. Int Endod J 1995;28:12-8.
476. Rehman K, Saunders WP, Foye AH, Sharkey SW. Calcium ion diffusion from calcium hydroxide-containing materials in endodontically treated teeth. An in vitro study. Int Endod J 1996;29:271-9.
477. Reit C, Dahlén G. Decision making analysis of endodontic treatment strategies in teeth with apical periodontitis. Int Endod J 1988;21:291-9.
478. Ricci C, Travert V. L'hydroxyde de calcium em endodontie. Rev Fran d'Endod 1987;6:45-74.
479. Rohner W. Calxyl als wurzelfullings material nach pulpa extirpation. Schweizer Monatsschrift fur Zahnmedicin 1940;50:903-48.
480. Rolla G, Loe H, Schiott CR. Retention of chlorhexedine in the human oral cavity. Arch Oral Biol 1971;16:1109-16.
481. Rolla G, Melsen B. On the mechanism of the plaque inhibition by chlorhexedine. J Dent Res 1975;54:57-62.
482. Rotstein I, Friedman S, Katz J. Apical closure of mature molar roots with the use of calcium hydroxide. Oral Surg Oral Med Oral Pathol 1990;70:656-60.
483. Rubin E, Farber JL. Patologia. 1.ed. Rio de Janeiro: Interlivros;1990. p.2-30.
484. Russo MC, Holland R. Microscopical findings after protection with various dressings in pulpotomized deciduous teeth of dogs. Rev Fac Odontol Araçatuba 1974;3:113-23.
485. Russo MC, Souza V, Holland R. Effects of the dressing with calcium hydroxide under pressure on the pulpal healing of pulpotomized human teeth. Rev Fac Odontol Araçatuba 1974;3:303-11.
486. Rutherford RB, Spångberg L, Tucker M, Charette M. Transdentinal stimulation of reparative dentine formation by osteogenic protein-1 in monkeys. Arch Oral Biol 1995;40:681-83.
487. Rutherford RB, Wahle J, Tucker M, Rueger D, Charette M. Induction of reparative dentine formation in monkeys by recombinant human osteogenic protein-1. Archs Oral Biol 1993;38:571-576.
488. Sacks HS, Berrier J, Reitman D et al. Meta-analysis of randomized controlled trials. N Engl J Med 1987;316:450-51.
489. Safavi KE, Dowden WE, Introcaso JH, Langeland K. A comparison of antimicrobial effects of calcium hydroxide and iodine-potassium iodine. J Endod 1985;11:454-6.
490. Safavi KE, Nakayama TA. Influence of mixing vehicle on dissociation of calcium hydroxide in solution. J Endod 2000;26:649-51.
491. Safavi KE, Nichols FC. Alteration of biological properties of bacterial lipopolysaccharide by calcium hydroxide treatment. J Endod 1994;20:127-9.
492. Safavi KE, Nichols FC. Effect of calcium hydroxide on bacterial lipopolysaccharide. J Endod 1993;19:76-8.
493. Safavi KE, Spångberg LSW, Langeland K. Root canal dentinal tubule desinfection. J Endod 1990;16:207-10.
494. Sahli CC. L'hydroxyde de calcium dans le traitement endodontique des grandes lésions peariapicales. Rev Fran d'Endod 1988;7:45-51.
495. Sahli CC. Observación radiográfica y estudio histológico de un caso de apicoformación en un molar humano. Rev Espan Endod 1989;7:101-6.
496. Saidon J, He J, Zhu Q, Safavi K, Spångberg LSW. Cell and tissue reactions to mineral trioxide aggregate and Portland cement. Oral Surg Oral Med Oral Pathol 2003;95:483-9.
497. Saiijo Y. Clinico-pathological study on vital amputation with calcium hydroxide added to various kinds of antibacterial substances. J Tokyo Dent College Soc 1957;57:357-63.
498. Salamat K, Rezai RF. Nonsurgical treatment of extraoral lesions caused by necrotic nonvital teeth. Oral Surg Oral Med Oral Pathol 1986;61:618-23.
499. Santana-Jr A. Influência da preservação ou não do coto pulpar, e do tipo de cimento obturador, no processo de reparo de dentes de cães após biopulpectomia e tratamento endodôntico. (Master's Thesis). Marília: University of Marília; 2001. 205 p.
500. Santini AH. Intraoral comparison of calcium hydroxide (Calnex) alone and in combination with Ledermix in first permanent mandibular molars using two direct inspection criteria. J Dent 1985;13:52-9.
501. Santini AH. Long term clinical assessment of pulpotomy with calcium hydroxide containing Ledermix in human permanent premolars and molars. Acta Odontol Pediat 1986;7:45-50.
502. Santos KS. Hidróxido de calcio no tratamento das reabsorções cervicais extemas pós-clareamento em dente despolpado. Rev CRO Minas Gerais 1996;2:41-7.
503. Sathorn C, Parashos P, Messer H. Antibacterial efficacy of calcium hydroxide intracanal dressing: a systematic review and meta-analysis. Int Endod J 2007;40:2-10.
504. Sazak H, Gunday M, Alatti C. Effect of calcium hydroxide and combinations of Ledermix and calcium hydroxide on inflamed pulps in dog teeth. J Endod 1996;22:447-9.
505. Schäfer E, Behaissi AA. pH changes in root dentin after root canal dressing with gutta-percha points containing calcium hydroxide. J Endod 2000;26:665-7.

506. Schein B, Schilder H. Endotoxin content in endodontically involved teeth. J Endod 1975;1:19-21.
507. Schilder H, Amsterdam M. Inflammatory potential of root canal medicaments. Oral Surg Oral Med Oral Pathol 1959;12:211-21.
508. Schroeder A. Endodontics Science and Practice. Chicago: Quintessence;1981.
509. Sciaky I, Pisanti S. Localization of calcium placed over amputed pulps in dog's teeth. J Dent Res 1960;39:1128-32.
510. Seal GJ, Ng Y-L, Spratt D, Bhatti M, Gulabivala K. An in vitro comparison of the bactericidal efficacy of lethal photo - sensitization or sodium hyphochlorite irrigation on *Streptococcus intermedius* biofilms in root canals. Int Endod J 2002;35:268-274.
511. Sekine N, Asai Y, Nakamura Y, Tagami T, Nagakubo T. Clinico-pathological study of the effect of pulp capping with various calcium hydroxide pastes. Bull Tokyo Dent Coll 1971;4:149-73.
512. Sekine N, Machida V, Imanishi T. A clinico-pathological study on pulp extirpation and pulp amputation in the middle portion of the root canal. Bull Tokyo Dent Coll 1963;4:103-35.
513. Sekine N, Saiijo Y, Ishikawa T, Imanishi T, Asai Y, Narita M. Clinico-pathological study on vital pulpotomy with Calvital. J Tokyo Dent College Soc 1963;63:463-73.
514. Seltzer S, Bender IB. A polpa dental. 2nd ed. Rio de Janeiro: Labor;1979. 499p.
515. Seltzer S, Bender IB. Root canal dressings their usefulness in endodontic therapy reconsidered. Oral Surg Oral Med Oral Pathol 1961;14:603-10.
516. Seltzer S, Farber PA. Microbiologic factors in endodontology. Oral Surg Oral Med Oral Pathol 1994;78:634-45.
517. Semenoff TADV. Análise comparativa da reação do tecido submucoso de ratos ao implante de hidróxido de cálcio, de clorexidina e da mistura de ambos. (Master's Thesis). Porto Alegre: Luteran University of Brasil; 2003. 118 p.
518. Sen BH, Safavi KE, Spångberg LW. Antifungal effects of sodium hypochlorite and chlorhexedine in root canal. J Endod 1999;24:235-8.
519. Sena NT, Gomes BP, Vianna ME, Berber VB, Zaia AA, Ferraz CC, Souza-Filho FJ. In vitro antimicrobial activity of sodium hypochlorite and chlorhexidine against selected single-species biofilms. Int Endod J 2006;39:878-85.
520. Senzamici NP, Tesini DA. An approach to obturation using apical maturity as a consideration in endodontic treatment of young permanent teeth. J Pedodontics 1977;1:177-83.
521. Seux D, Couble ML, Hartman DJ, Gauthier JP, Magloire H. Odontoblast like cytodifferentation of human pulp cells in vitro in the presence of a calcium hydroxide contamining cement. Archs Oral Biol 1991;36:117-28.
522. Shabahang S, Torabinejad M, Boyne PP, Abedi H, McMillan P. A comparative study of root-end induction using osteogenic protein -1, calcium hydroxide, and mineral trioxide aggregate in dogs. J Endod 1999;25:1-5.
523. Shankle RJ, Brauer JS. Pulp capping. Oral Surg Oral Med Oral Pathol 1962;15:1121-7.
524. Shay DE, Sarubin LD, Spurrier HS, Sanders DJ. Pulp conservation with an antibiotic agent. J Dent Children 1960;36:5-12.
525. Sheehy EC, Roberts CJ. Use of calcium hydroxide for apical barrier formation and healing in non-vital immature permanent teeth: a review. Brit Dent J 1997;183:241-6.
526. Shibuya T. A histopathological study in dogs on the improvement of a paste for root canal filling. J Tokyo Dent College Soc 1980;80:417-46.
527. Shovelton DS. The presence and distribuition of microorganisms within Non-vital Teeth. British Dent J 1964;117:101-7.
528. Siwek J, Gourla ML, Slawson DC, Shanyhnessy AF. How to write an evidence-based clinical review article. Am Fam Physician 2002;65:251-8.
529. Sigurdson A, Stancill R, Madison S. Intracanal placement of calcium hydroxide: A comparison of techniques. J Endod 1992;18:367-70.
530. Silva CAG. Efetividade antimicrobiana do hipoclorito de sódio e clorexidina como irrigantes endodônticos. (Master's Thesis). Porto Alegre: Luteran University of Brasil;1999. 105p.
531. Silva FT, Pugliesi NS, Araújo VC. Resposta do tecido conjuntivo pulpar frente ao hidróxido de calcio PA associado à água destilada e ao hidróxido de cálcio associado ao soro fisiológico. Rev Pós-Grad FOUSP 1996;3:59-65.
532. Silveira FF. Efeito do tempo de ação do curativo de demora à base de hidróxido de cálcio, utilizado em canais radiculares de dentes de cães com lesão periapical crônica induzida. Análise histológica e microbiológica. (Master's Thesis). Araraquara: São Paulo State University; 1997. 218p.
533. Simon ST, Bhat KS, Francis R. Effect of four vehicles on the pH of calcium hydroxide and the release of calcium ion. Oral Surg Oral Med Oral Pathol 1995;80:459-64.
534. Simpson ST. Treatment of the open apex. Pulp involvement through trauma. Aust Dent J 1970;15:392-5.
535. Siqueira JFJr, Batista MMD, Fraga RC, Uzeda M. Antibacterial effects of endodontic irrigants on black-pigmented Gram-negative anaerobes and facultative bacteria. J Endod 1998;24:414-6.
536. Siqueira JFJr, Uzeda M. Disinfection by calcium hydroxide pastes of dentinal tubules infected with two obligate and one facultative anaerobic bacteria. J Endod 1996;22:674-6.
537. Siqueira JFJr, Uzeda M. Intracanal medicaments: evaluation of the antibacterial effects of chlorhexidine, metronidazole, and calcium hydroxide associated with three vehicles. J Endod 1997;23:167-9.
538. Sirén EK, Haapasalo MPP, Ranta K, Salmi P, Kerosuo ENJ. Microbiological findings and clinical treatment procedures in endodontic cases selected for microbiological investigation. Int Endod J 1997;30:91-5.
539. Siwek J, Gourlay ML, Slawson DC, Shaughnessy AF. How to write an evidence-based clinical review article. Am Fam Physician 2002;65:251-8.
540. Sjögren U, Figdor D, Persson S, Sundqvist G. Influence of infection at the time of root filling on the outcome of endodontic treatment of teeth with apical periodontitis. Int Endod J 1997;30:297-306.
541. Sjögren V, Figdor D, Spångberg L, Sundqvist G. The antimicrobial effects of calcium hydroxide as a short-term intra-canal dressing. Int Endod J 1991;24:119-25.

542. Slots J, Taubman MA. Contemporany Oral Microbiology and Immunology. Mosby;1992. 649 p.
543. Smith AJ, Cassidy N, Perry H, Begue-Kirn C, Ruch JV, Lesot H. Reactionary dentinogenesis. Int J Developm Biol 1995;39:273-80.
544. Smith AJ, Tobias RS, Cassidy N, Plant GC, Begue-Kirn C, Ruch JV, Lesot H. Odontoblast stimulation in ferrets by dentine matrix components. Arch Oral Biol 1994;39:13-22.
545. Smith JW, Leeb IJ, Torney DL. A comparison of calcium hydroxide and barium hydroxide as agent for inducing apical closure. J Endod 1984;10:64-70.
546. Soares IML. Resposta pulpar ao MTA - agregado de trióxido mineral _ comparado ao hidróxido de cálcio em pulpotomias. Histológico em dentes de cães. (Doctoral Thesis). Brazil: Federal University of Santa Catarina;1996.
547. Socransky SS, Haffajee AD. Dental biofilms: difficult therapeutic targets. Periodontol 2000;28:12-55.
548. Socransky SS, MacDonald JB, Sawyer S. The cultivation of Treponema microdentium as surfaces colonies. Arch Oral Biol 1959;1:171-2.
549. Soekanto A, Kasugai S, Mataki S, Ohaya K, Ogura H. Toxicity of camphorated phenol and camphorated parachlorophenol in dental pulp cell culture. J Endod 1996;22:284-6.
550. Sommer RF, Ostrander FD, Crowley MC. Endodoncia Clínica. Barcelona: Labor; 1975.
551. Soukos NS, Chen PS, Morris JT, Ruggiero K, Abernethy AD, Som S, Foschi F, Doucette S, Bammann LL, Fontana CR, Doukas AG, Stashenko PP. Photodynamic therapy for endodontic disinfection. J Endod 2006;32:979-84.
552. Souza CA, Teles RP, Souto R, Chaves MA, Colombo AP. Endodontic therapy associated with calcium hydroxide as an intracanal dressing: microbiologic evaluation by the checkerboard DNA-DNA hybridization technique. J Endod 2005;31:79-83.
553. Souza V, Bernabé PFE, Holland R, Nery MJ, Mello W, Otoboni-Filho JA. Tratamento não-cirúrgico de dentes com lesões periapicais. Rev Bras Odontol 1999;46:39-46.
554. Souza V, Holland R, Holland-Jr C, Nery MJ. Estudo morfológico do comportamento da polpa dentária após pulpotomia e proteção com óxido de magnésio ou hidróxido de cálcio. O Incisivo 1972;1:18-21.
555. Souza V, Holland R, Mello W, Nery MJ. Reaction of rat connective tissue to the implant of calcium hydroxide pastes. Rev Fac Odontol Araçatuba 1977;6:69-76.
556. Souza V, Holland R, Menezes MR. Comportamento biológico de cimento de óxido de zinco e eugenol após contato com o hidróxido de cálcio. Estudo histológico em tecido subcutâneo de ratos. Rev Bras Odontol 1991;48:2-10.
557. Souza V, Holland R, Nery MJ, Mello W. Emprego de medicamentos no interior dos canais radiculares. Ação tópica e à distância de algumas drogas. ARS Cvrandi 1978;5:4-15.
558. Souza V, Holland R, Souza RS. Tratamento endodôntico de dentes de cães com polpas vitais em uma ou duas sessões. Influência dos curativos de demora corticosteróide-antibiótico e hidróxido de cálcio. Rev Odontol UNESP 1995;24:47-59.
559. Spångberg L, Engström B, Langeland K. Biological effect of dental materials: 3 toxicity and antimicrobial effects of endodontic antiseptics in vitro. Oral Surg Oral Med Oral Pathol 1973;36:856-71.
560. Spångberg LSW. Intracanal medication. In: Ingle JI, Bakland LK, eds. Endodontics: 4th ed. Baltimore: Williams & Wilkins, 1994.
561. Spanó JCE, Barbin EL, Santos TC, Guimarães LF, Pécora JD. Solvent action of sodium hypochlorite on bovine pulp and physico-chemical properties of resulting liquid. Braz Dent J 2001;12:154-7.
562. Spratt DA, Pratten J, Wilson M, Gulabivala K. An in vitro of the antimicrobial efficacy of irrigants on biofilms of root canal isolates. Int Endod J 2001;34:300-7.
563. Staehle HJ, Thoma C, Möller HP. Comparative in vitro investigation of different methods for temporary root canal filling with aqueous suspensions of calcium hydroxide. Endod Dent Traumatol 1997;13:106-12.
564. Stamos DG, Haasch GC, Gerstein H. The pH of local anesthetic/calcium hydroxide solutions. J Endod 1985;11:264.
565. Stanley HR. Calcium hydroxide and vital pulp therapy. In: Hargreaves KM, Goodis HE. Seltzer and Bender's dental pulp. Quintessence books: Chicago;2002. p.309-24.
566. Stanley HR. Toxicity Testing of Dental Materials. Boca Raton, FL, CRC Press:1985.
567. Stanley HR, Pameijer CH. Dentistry's friend: calcium hydroxide. Operat Dent 1997;22:1-3.
568. Steiner JC, Dow PR, Cathey GM. Inducing root end closure of non-vital teeth. J Dent Children 1968;55:47-54.
569. Steiner JC, Van Hassel HJ. Experimental root apexification in primates. Oral Surg Oral Med Oral Pathol 1971;31:409-15.
570. Stevens RH, Grossman LI. Evaluation of the antimicrobial potential of calcium hydroxide as an intracanal medicament. J Endod 1983;9:372-4.
571. Stewart GG. Calcium hydroxide-induced root healing. J Am Dent Assoc 1975;90:793-800.
572. Stock CJR. Calcium hydroxide: root resorption and perio-endo lesions. Brit Dent J 1985;158:325-34.
573. Stromberg T. Wound healing after total pulpectomy in dogs. A comparative study between root fillings with calcium hydroxide, dibasic calcium phosphate and guttapercha. Odontol Rev 1969;20:147-63.
574. Stuart KG, Miller CH, Brown JR, Newton CW. The comparative antimicrobial effect of calcium hydroxide. Oral Surg Oral Med Oral Pathol 1991;72:101-4.
575. Sundqvist G. Associations between microbial species in dental root canal infections. Oral Microbiol Immunol 1992;7:257-62.
576. Sundqvist G. Bacteriological studies of necrotic dental pulps. (Dissertation Master). Umea: University of Umea, Sweden;1976. 94p.
577. Sundqvist G. Ecology of the root canals flora. J Endod 1992;18:427-30.
578. Sundqvist G. Taxonomy, ecology and pathogenicity of the root canal flora. Oral Surg Oral Med Oral Pathol 1994;78:522- 30.
579. Sundqvist G, Eckerbom MI, Larsson AP, Sjögren UT. Capacity of anaerobic bacteria from necrotic dental pulps to induce purulent infections. Infec Immun 1979;25:685-93.
580. Sundqvist G, Figdor D, Persson S, Sjögren U. Microbiologic analysis of teeth with failed endodontic treatment and the outcome of conservative retreatment. Oral Surg Oral Med Oral Pathol 1998;85:86-93.

581. Sundqvist G, Figdor D. Life as an endodontic pathogen. Ecological differences between the untreated and root-filled root canals. Endodontic Topics. 2003;6:3–28.
582. Sundqvist G, Johansson E. Neutrophil chemotaxis induced by anaerobic bacteria isolated from necrotic dental pulps. Scand J Dent Res 1980;88:113-21.
583. Suzuki K, Higuchi N, Horiba N, Matsumoto T, Nakamura H. Antimicrobial effect of calcium hydroxide in bacteria isolated from infected root canals. Dent Japan 1999;35:43-7.
584. Svensäter G, Bergenholtz G. Biofilms in endodontic infections. Endodontic Topics 2004;9:27-36.
585. Sydney GB. Identificação da microflora endodôntica após o preparo do canal radicular de dentes portadores de periodontite apical assintomática e o emprego de medicação de hidróxido de cálcio em diferentes tempos. (Doctoral Thesis). São Paulo, University of São Paulo;1996.
586. Sydney GB, Estrela C. The influence of root canal preparation on anaerobic bacteria in teeth with asymptomatic apical periodontitis. Braz Endod J 1996;1:12-5.
587. Thompson SW, Hunt RD. Selected histochemical and histopathological methods. Flórida: Charles C Thomas;1966. p.615-46.
588. Tobias RS. Antibacterial properties of Endodontic materials. Int Endod J 1988;21:155-60.
589. Torabinejad M, Bahjri K. Essential elements of evidence-based endodontics: steps involved in conducting clinical research. J Endod 2005:31563-9.
590. Torabinejad M, Hong CU, McDonald F, Pitt Ford TR. Physical and chemical properties of a new root-end filling material. J Endod 1995;21:349-53.
591. Torabinejad M, Hong CU, Lee SJ, Monsef M, Pitt Ford TR. Investigation of mineral trioxide aggregate for root-end filling in dogs. J Endod 1995;21:603-8.
592. Torabinejad M, Hong CU, Pitt-Ford TR, Kettering JD. Antibacterial effects of some root end filling materials. J Endod 1995; 21:403-06.
593. Torabinejad M, Pitt Ford TR. Root-endo filing materials: a review. Endod Dent Traumatol 1996;12:161-78.
594. Torabinejad M, Watson TF, Pitt Ford TR. Sealing ability of a Mineral trioxide Agregate when used as root end filling material. J Endod 1993;19:591-5.
595. Torneck CD, Howley TP. The effect of calcium hydroxide on porcine pulp fibroblasts in vitro. J Endod 1983;8:131-6.
596. Trowbridge HO, Emling RC. Inflamation. A review of the process. 4th ed. Chicago: Quintessence books, 1993.
597. Tortora GJ, Funke BR, Case CL. Microbiology. 6th.ed. Menho Park, Califórnia: Benjamin Cummings;1997.
598. Tronstad L, Andreassen JO, Hasselgren G, Kristerson L, Riis I. pH changes in dental tissues after root canal filling with calcium hydroxide. J Endod 1981;7:17-21.
599. Tronstad L, Asbjornsen K, Doving L, Pedersen I, Eriksen HM. Influence of coronal restorations on the periapical health of endodontically treated teeth. Endod Dent Traumatol 2000;16:218-21.
600. Tronstad L, Barnett F, Cervone F. Periapical bacterial plaque in teeth refratory to endodontic treatment. Endod Dent Traumatol 1990;6:73-7.
601. Tronstad L, Barnett F, Riso K, Slots J. Extra-radicular infections. Endod Dent Traumatol 1987;3:86-90.
602. Tronstad L, Kreshtool D, Barnett F. Microbiological monitoring and results of treatment of extraradicular endodontic infection. Endod Dent Traumatol 1990;6:129-36.
603. Tronstad L, Mjor IA. Pulp reactions to calcium hydroxide-containing materials. Oral Surg Oral Med Oral Pathol 1972;33:961-5.
604. Trope M, Delano O, Ørstavik D. Endodontic treatment of teeth with apical periodontitis: single vs. multivisit treatment. J Endod 1999;25:345-50.
605. Trope M, Moshonov J, Nissan R, Buxt P, Yesilsoy C. Short vs. long-term calcium hydroxide treatment of established inflammatory root resorption in replanted dog teeth. Endod Dent Traumatol 1995;11:124-8.
606. Trope M, Tronstad L. Long term calcium hydroxide treatment of a tooth with iatrogenic root perforation and lateral periodontitis. Endod Dent Traumatol 1985;1:35-8.
607. Trope M, Yesilsoy C, Koren L, Moshonov J, Friedman S. Effect of different endodontic treatment protocols on periodontal repair and root resorption of replanted dog teeth. J Endod 1992;18:492-6.
608. Tsuchima T. Clinico-pathological study of immediate root canal filling with paste, gutta-percha point and combination of the two after vital pulp extirpation. J Tokyo Dent College Soc 1970;70:1-4.
609. Türkün M, Cengiz T. The effects of sodium hypochlorite and calcium hydroxide on tissue dissolution and root canal cleanliness. Int Endod J 1997;30:335-42.
610. Usui K, Hishinuma T, Yamaguchi H, Tachiiri N, Goto J. Determination of chlorhexidine (CHD) and nonylphenolethoxylates (NPEOn) using LC-ESI-MS method and application to hemolyzed blood. J Chromatogr B 2006;831:105-9.
611. United States Pharmacopeia. 22nd revision. Rockville: The United States Pharmacopeial Convention, Inc;1989.
612. Van Hassel HJ, Natkin E. Induction of foraminal closure. J Can Dent Assoc 1969;35:606-8.
613. Van Hassel HJ, Natkin E. Induction of root end closure. J Dent Children 1970;37:57-9.
614. Vander Wall GL, Dowson J, Shipman C. Antibacterial efficacy and cytotoxicity of three endodontic drugs. Oral Surg Oral Med Oral Pathol 1972;33:230-41.
615. Vantuloki JC, Brown JI. An in vitro study of the diffusibility of camphorated parachlorophenol and metacresylacetate in the root canal. Oral Surg Oral Med Oral Pathol 1972;34:653-60.
616. Varella JAF, Paiva JG, Villa N. O uso de corticosteróides no tratamento conservador da polpa. Rev Fac Odontol USP 1966;4:153-64.
617. Vernieks AA. Calcium hydroxide induced healing of periapical lesions: a study of 78 non-vital teeth. J Brit Endod Soc 1978;11:61-9.
618. Vojinovic O, Srnié E. Induction of apical formation by the use of calcium hydroxide and iodoform - Chlumsky paste in the endodontic treatment of immature teeth. J Br Endod Soc 1975;8:16-22.
619. Wakabayashi H, Horikawa M, Funato A, Onodera A, Matsumoto K. Bio-microscopical observation of dystrophic calcification induced by calcium hydroxide. Endod Dent Traumatol 1993;9:165-70.

620. Wakabayashi H, Morita S, Koba K, Tachibana H, Matsumoto K. Effect of calcium hydroxide paste dressing on uninstrumented root canal wall. Endod Dent Traumatol 1993;9:165-70.
621. Wakai WT, Naito RM. Endodontic management of teeth with incompletely formed roots. J Hawaii Dent Assoc 1974;7:13-9.
622. Waltimo TMT, Ørstavik D, Sirén EK, Haapasalo MPP. In vitro susceptibility of Candida albicans to four disinfectants and their combinations. Int Endod J 1999;32:421-9.
623. Waltimo TMT, Sirén EK, Ørstavik D, Haapasalo MPP. Susceptibility of oral *Candida species* to calcium hydroxide in vitro. Int Endod J 1999;32:94-8.
624. Waltimo TMT, Sirén EK, Torkko LK, Olsen I, Haapasalo MPP. Fungi in therapy-resintant apical periodontitis. Int Endod J 1997;30:96-101.
625. Walton RE, Torabinejad M. Cleaning and shaping. In: Pedersen P, ed. Principles and Practice of Endodontics. Philadelphia: Saunders; 1989.
626. Wang JD, Hume WR. Difusion of hydrogen ion and hydroxil ion from various sources through dentine. Int Endod J 1988;21:17-26.
627. Webber RT, Schwiebert KA, Cathey GA. A technique for placement of calcium hydroxide in the root canal system. J Amer Dent Ass 1981;103:417-21.
628. Webber RT. Apexogenesis versus apexification. Dent Clinic North Am 1984;28:669-97.
629. Webber RT. Traumatic injuries and the expanded endodontic role of calcium hydroxide. In: Gerstein H, ed. Techniques in Clinical Endodontics. Philadelphia: Saunders; 1983.
630. Weinstein R, Goldman M. Apical hard-tissue deposition in adult teeth of monkeys with use of calcium hydroxide. Oral Surg Oral Med Oral Pathol 1977;43:627-30.
631. Wilson M. Susceptibility of oral bacterial biofilms to antimicrobial Agents. J Med Microbiol 1996;44:79-87.
632. World Health Organization. International Agency for Research on cance. IARC monography on the evaluation of carcinogenic risks to humans. Lyon-France, 2006;86:1-25.
633. Wucherpfening AL, Green DB. Mineral Trioxide Agregate vs Portland cement: two biocompatible filling materials. J Endod 1999;25:308 (Abstract).
634. Yang S-F, Rivera EM, Baungardner KR, Walton RE, Stanford C. Anaerobic tissue dissolving abilities of calcium hydroxide and sodium hypochlorite. J Endod 1995;21:613-6.
635. Yang S-F, Yang Z-P, Chang K-W. Continuing root formation following apexification treatment. Endod Dent Traumatol 1990;6:232-5.
636. Yates JA. Barrier formation time in non-vital teeth with open apices. Int Endod J 1988;21:313-9.
637. Yeung FJS, Newman HN, Addy M. Subgingival metronidazole in acrylic resin vs. chlorexidine irrigation in the control of cronic periodontitis. J Periodontol 1983;54:651-7.
638. Yeung SY, Huang CS, Chan CP, Lin CP, Lin HN, Lee PH, Jia HW, Huang SK, Jeng JH, Chang MC. Antioxidant and pro-oxidant properties of chlorhexidine and its interaction with calcium hydroxide solutions. Int Endod J 2007;40:837-44.
639. Yoshiba K, Yoshiba N, Iwaku M. Histological observations of hard tissue barrier formation in amputed dental pulp capped with a-tricalciumphosphate containing calcium hydroxide. Endod Dent Traumatol 1994;10:113-20.
640. Yoshida M, Fukushima H, Yamamoto K, Ogawa K, Toda T, Sagawa H. Correlation between clinical symptoms and microorganisms isolated from root canals of teeth periapical pathosis. J Endod 1987;13:24-8.
641. Zander HA. Reaction of the dental pulp to calcium hydroxide. J Dent Res 1939;181:373-9.
642. Zelante A, Oliveira MRB, Lia RCC, Benatti Neto C. Compatibilidade biológica em tecido conjuntivo subcutâneo do rato, de pastas à base de hidróxido de cálcio contidas em tubos de dentina humana. Rev Odontol UNESP 1992;21:37-46.
643. Zerella JA, Fouad AF, Spångberg LS. Effectiveness of a calcium hydroxide and chlorhexidine digluconate mixture as disinfectant during retreatment of failed endodontic cases. Oral Surg Oral Med Oral Pathol Oral Radiol Endod 2005;100:756-61.
644. Zerlotti E. Contribuição à terapêutica dos condutos radiculares. (Doctoral Thesis). Campinas: Faculdade de Odontologia de Campinas;1959. 87p.
645. Zielke DR, Heggers JP, Harrison JW. A statisical analysis of anaerobic versus aerobic culturing in endodontic. Oral Surg Oral Med Oral Pathol 1976;42:8-30.

# Root Canal Filling and Coronal Seal

**C. Estrela**
*Federal University of Goiás, Goiânia, GO, Brazil*

**J. A. P. Figueiredo**
*Pontifical Catholic University of Rio Grande do Sul, Porto Alegre, RS, Brazil*

**M. D. Sousa-Neto**
*University of São Paulo, Ribeirão Preto, SP, Brazil*

**L. A. Faitaroni**
*Brazilian Dentistry Research and Learning Center, CEPOBRAS, Goiânia, GO, Brazil*

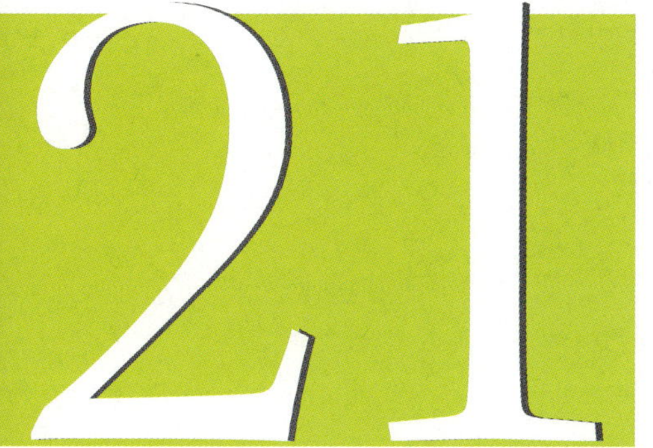


Chapter contents

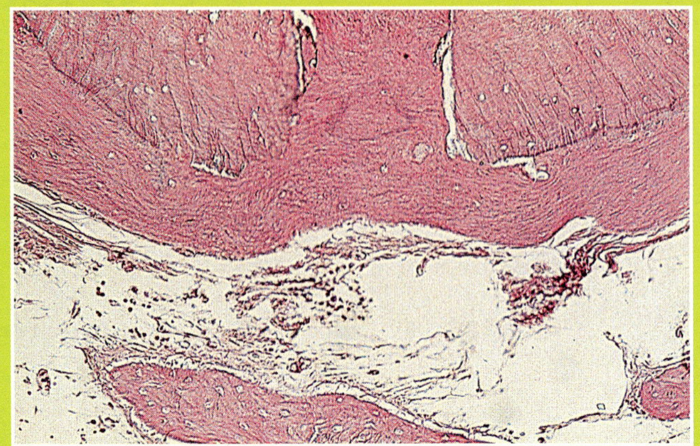

Complete biological sealing with formation of mineralized tissue (Cortesy Prof. Dr. Roberto Holland).

## 21.1 Introduction

Root canal filling is the third of the significant steps in endodontic treatment (coronal access, sanitization-shaping and endodontic filling-sealing). Thus, it reinforces the concept of eliminating empty spaces inside the tooth, which can harbor microorganisms.

In this context, it allows tissue repair, because the periapical tissues are able to rest from the previous irritation; it favors osteogenesis and cementogenesis, followed by the reorganization of the periodontal ligament and reintegration of the lamina dura. Biological filling is the sublime goal to achieve in modern endodontics (Fig.21.1).

The major objective of root canal system filling consists of complete three-dimensional filling. To reach this step of endodontic treatment there can be several challenges as regards the complex anatomy, specificity of microorganisms and the host response, in view of being limited to the two dimensions shown in radiographs[104,105] (Fig.21.2).

Nowadays a tridimensional image can be obtained by cone beam computed tomography, the new plane that has been added being the depth. In endodontics, in addition to evaluation the outcome of the endodontic treatment, it will be possible to solve various challenges and difficult situations with the aid of images obtained by cone beam computed tomography (apical periodontitis, differential diagnosis, fracture of endodontic instrument, perforation, overfilling)[53,54,104,105].

The principle of root canal filling places value on essential aspects, such as the performance capacity, microbial control and biological biocompatibility.

Likewise, this phase of the endodontic treatment involves many special details. However, after the well-oriented performance of each previous operating step, complete sealing of the dentine tubular system is the ultimate goal. Lack of a detailed view of this tubular system would jeopardize the operative procedure in such a way that this aim would not be reached. The high concept of endodontic sealing requires the operator to have special attributes. The radiographic view is only a clinical panorama of the quality of the treatment performed, and does not necessarily mirror the care taken to control of root canal infection, which should precede filling.

In many situations, the operating steps before filling are well conducted; however, defective points during this final stage can limit the achievement of a proper treatment.

Filling of dentinal tubule system should take into consideration the root formation (complete, incomplete), group of teeth (anterior, posterior, maxillary, mandibular), condition of infection (presence, absence), degree of difficulty (calcification; dilacerations; developmental disturbances; presence of degree, perforation, fractured instrument; retreatment in teeth with post or extensive prosthesis) and others.

Parallel to the scientific concerns as regards the endeavor to obtain perfect endodontic sealing, to avoid possible re-infection, several studies have verified the effectiveness of the coronal seal, seeking different factors which could influence the success of root canal filling, such as the real objectives of the root canal filling, the convenient moment to perform it, the filling materials, techniques used for filling, and the influence of the coronal sealing on the success of the endodontic treatment[1-549].

Some criteria for the radiographic analysis of endodontic success or failure were suggested by Strindberg[439] – "*success – a. the contours, width and structure of the periodontal margin are normal; b. the periodontal contours are widened mainly around the excess filling; failure – a. a decrease in the periapical rarefaction; b. unchanged periapical rarefaction; c. an appearance of new or an increase in the initial rarefaction; uncertain -a. there are ambiguous or technically unsatisfactory control radiographs, which for some reason, could not be repeated; b. the tooth is extracted before the 3-year follow-up owing to the unsuccessful treatment of another root of the tooth*".

## 21.2 Significance of Endodontic Sealing

Many professionals consider root canal filling the final phase of endodontic treatment, and express its quality as evaluated by the radiographic aspect, and although it has limitations, at present it is the only available complementary observation resource for use in a regular basis.

To completely fill the dentinal tubule system, once the sanitization process and endodontic molding have been concluded, it is necessary to eliminate the space previously occupied by the dental pulp, and prevent it from becoming an ideal shelter for microorganisms. In this connection, several studies were developed to evaluate different variables and factors that interfere in the efficacy of endodontic-coronal sealing[13,16,19-22,31-36,40-42,58,67-73,102,103,109,111-114,116,121,129,149,154,180-228,230,262,271,280-285,289-293,298,308,323-328,336-344,375,388-391,415-421,428-431,477,493,517,531,548].

All the spaces in the prepared canal must be well filled to avoid possible re-contamination. Holland et al.[204] verified intensive inflammatory reaction in dentinal tubes implanted in conjunctive tissue, when there were empty spaces measuring from 4 to 8 mm. These can be filled by microorganisms and tissue liquids and represent irritation to the periapical tissues[204,481,482].

The root canal filling stands out as being responsible for microbial control, which enhances its important participation as decisive contributor to the process of tissue repair. The root canal filling material, which must be contained only inside the root canal, must fill it completely, not to be an irritant, and possibly stimulate the healing process of the periapical tissues.

The endodontic sealing, in addition to being capable of controlling the microorganisms, if possible, must show antimicrobial activity. The role of the filling is to impede colonization by and invasion of microorganisms to the neighboring tissues and control their virulence potential. All the prepared space must be occupied by an inert material, which impedes the presence of tissue fluid and microorganisms. The sealer, in contact with this fluid, can become soluble and favor leakage. Degeneration of the tissue or fluid in the space created stimulates the inflammatory process and allows microorganisms to enter. It is universal consensus that every pulp cavity space which was submitted to the process of sanitization must be completely filled.

The process of tissue repair in the periapical region is jeopardized by the presence of spaces in the root canal filling, since they can serve to shelter microorganisms.

Ørstavik[324] emphasize that endodontic filling materials may be considered true implants, as they touch and are based on vital tissues of the body, and protrude to meet the external surface directly, or more appropriately, indirectly via another surface restoration seriously challenged by other synthetic materials in the production of root fillings.

## 21.3 Opportune Moment for the Root Canal Filling

The number of visits needed to conclude the endodontic treatment, as well as whether or not intracanal dressing is necessary, was discussed previously in the Chapter 20 (Calcium Hydroxide).

There is consensus about the idea that the canal must be cleaned and shaped before the filling. Shaping must allow the filling material to be accommodated throughout the full extent of the root canal. Moreover, so that the physical-chemical properties occur normally, the canal must be dried. In cases in which there is persistent exudate, the strategy involves the placement of an intracanal dressing, and/or application of a systemic medication. These aspects were exhaustively discussed in the chapter with reference to the diagnosis and treatment of the apical periodontitis (Chapter 10).

In teeth with vital pulps, independent on the inflammatory condition, it has been suggested, whenever possible, to prepare and fill the root canal in the same visit. The success rates in the case of vital pulp are not affected to the filling in one or two sessions. Under a histopathological point of view[194], it is admitted that the complete emptying, preparation and root canal filling can be achieved in the same session, not compromising tissue repair.

With regard to the influence of the root canal sealer and the number of sessions on the prevalence of symptomatic apical periodontitis in teeth with vital pulps, Estrela et al.[114] reported that Sealapex demonstrated lower percentage of post-operative pain (87.5% and 88.6% for the absence of pain, in 1 and 2 sessions), when compared with Fillcanal (Grossman sealer) (85.7% and 82.3% for the absence of pain, in 1 or 2 sessions), nevertheless, without statistically significant differences.

In the cases of pulp necrosis, the situation is completely changed. As discussed previously, in different studies conducted by Holland et al.[198,199], complete biological sealing by a barrier of mineralized tissue occurred after the application of the intracanal dressing with calcium hydroxide, and filling with Sealapex (Fig. 21.2).

To summarize, the ideal time for root canal filling is after the sanitization process, cleaning and shaping the root canal has been concluded. Furthermore, the root canal must be dry and asymptomatic.

As regards the apical limit of filling, Kojima et al.[262] based on meta-analysis, determined the influence of factors such as apical limit (short vs. overextension), pulp status (vital vs. nonvital), and periapical status (presence or absence of radiolucency) on endodontic prognosis. The study-list was obtained by using a MEDLINE search and Japana Centra Revuo Medicina search. A cumulative success rate of 82.8 ± 1.19% was obtained for teeth with a vital pulp, and 78.9 ± 1.05% for those with a nonvital pulp. There was a significant difference between the 2 groups. The cumulative success rates with overextension, flush, and under-extension for vital pulp and nonvital pulp were 70.8 ± 1.44, 86.5 ± 0.88, and 85.5 ± 0.98%, respectively. There was a significant difference between flush and overextension and between flush and under-extension. The cumulative success rates without a periapical lesion and with one were 82.0 ± 1.24 and 71.5 ± 1.60% respectively; and the difference between the 2 groups was significant. In the analysis of success rate by age group, the cumulative success rates for patients under 30 years of age and those over 50 years of age were 78.4 ± 1.44% and 77.3% ± 2.58 respectively. However, there was no significant difference between these age groups. A significant difference in success rates was found when teeth with a periapical lesion were compared with those without the lesion. These results agree with previous findings. Based on their use of cumulative meta-analysis, the authors proposed that the root canal should be filled to within 2 mm of the radiographic apex.

Moura et al.[315] determined the influence of length of root canal obturation on apical periodontitis using periapical radiography and cone beam computed tomography. A total of 503 root canal obturations were evaluated using periapical radiography and cone beam computed tomography (CBCT). Distances from the radiographic apex to the tip of filling material were measured and classified as close to 2 mm, 1 mm short or beyond apex, and at the apex. Obturations at the apex were associated with apical periodontitis (AP). Periapical radiographs showed that root canal obturations were 1 to 2 mm short of the apex in 88%, 89.3% and 95% of the anterior teeth, premolars and molars. CBCT images showed obturations had the same length in 70%, 73.7% and 79% of anterior teeth, premolars and molars (Tables 21.1 - 21.2). The frequency of AP was significantly greater in molars than in the other tooth groups, regardless of diagnostic method. AP was detected more frequently when CBCT was used. AP was detected at all lengths of root canal obturation, and length was not associated with AP when root canals were not cleaned, shaped and three-dimensionally filled with good coronal restorations. The analyses of diagnostic methods showed that AP was detected more frequently when CBCT was used.

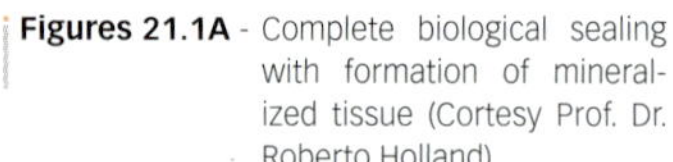

**Figures 21.1A** - Complete biological sealing with formation of mineralized tissue (Cortesy Prof. Dr. Roberto Holland).

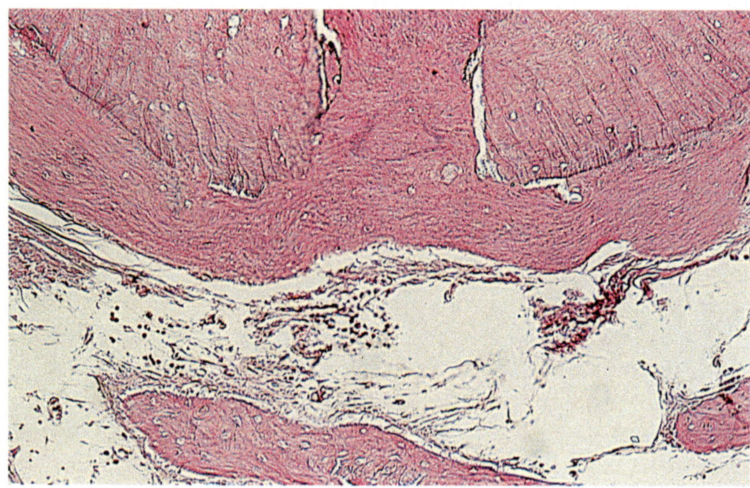

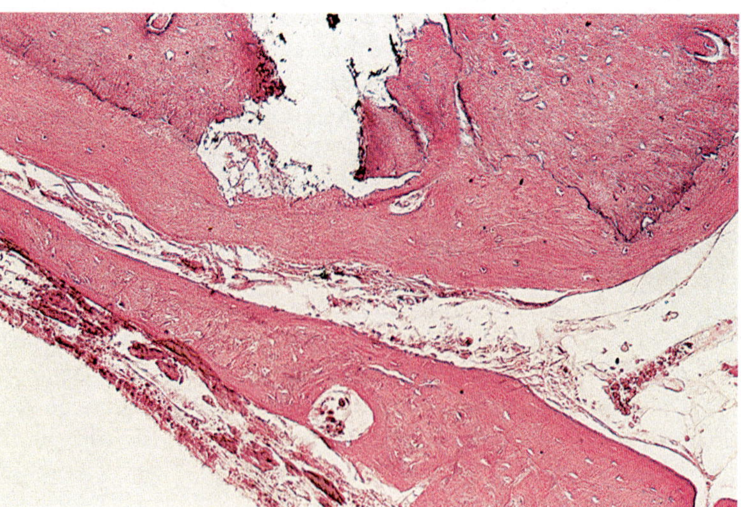

**Figures 21.1B** - Complete biological sealing with formation of mineralized tissue (Cortesy Prof. Dr. Roberto Holland).

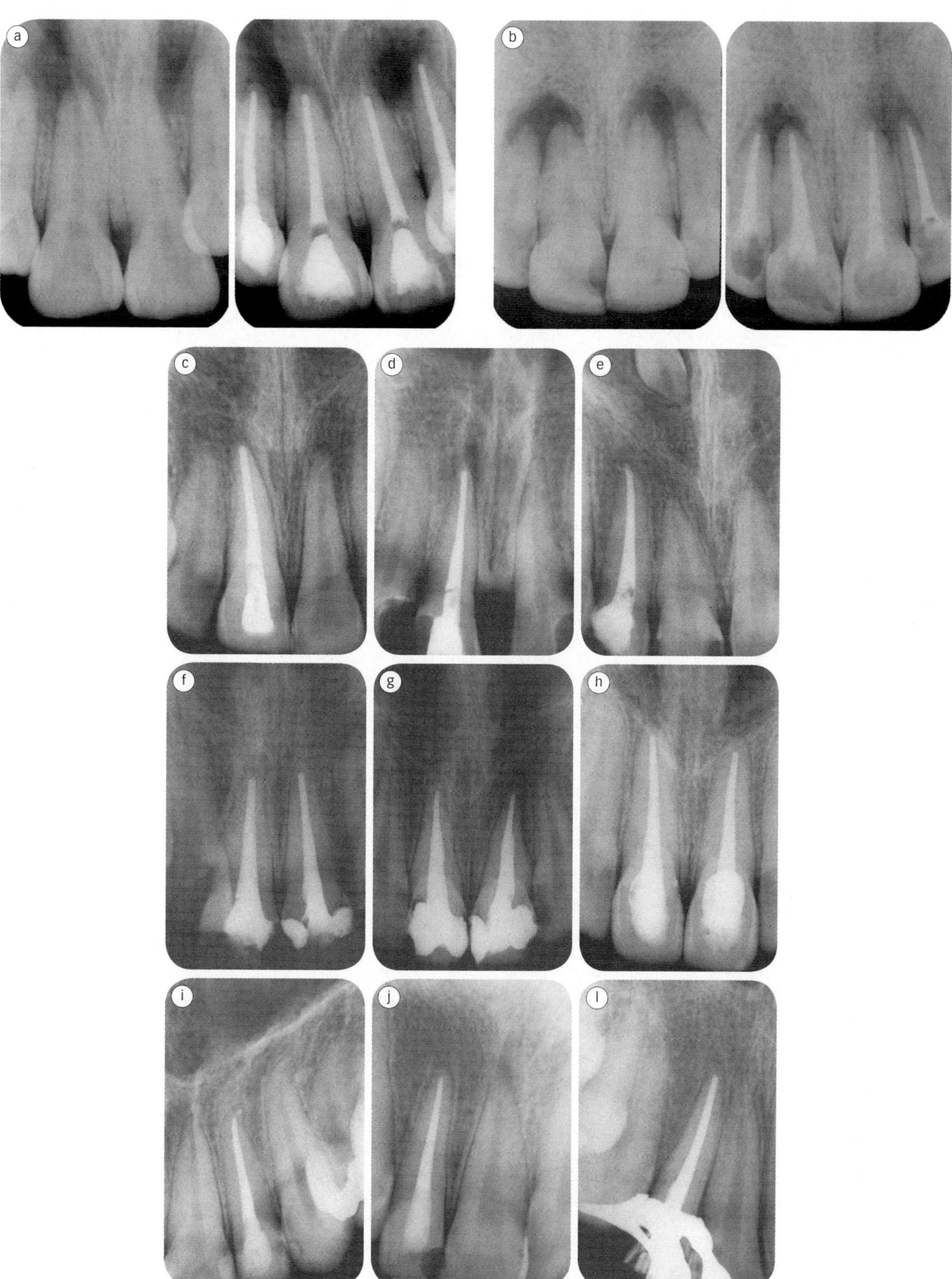


**Figure 21.2** - (A-L) Radiographic aspects of teeth adequately prepared and filled.

**Table 21.1** - Influence of length of root canal obturation on apical periodontitis detected by periapical radiographs[315].

| Length | Apical Periodontitis | Anterior n=100 | | OR | OR (CI 95%) | Premolar n=103 | | OR | OR (CI 95%) | Molar n=300 | | OR | OR (CI 95%) | p Chi-square test |
|---|---|---|---|---|---|---|---|---|---|---|---|---|---|---|
| | | | % | | | | % | | | | % | | | |
| -2 | Presence | 10 | 32.2 | 0.23 | 0.0782 - 0.6579 | 10 | 34.5 | 0.28 | 0.0938 - 0.8181 | 69 | 54.3 | 1.42 | 0.8638 - 2.319 | 0.027 |
| | Absence | 21 | 67.8 | | | 19 | 65.5 | | | 58 | 45.7 | | | |
| -1 | Presence | 18 | 31.6 | 0.21 | 0.0967 - 0.4692 | 10 | 15.9 | 0.04 | 0.0137 - 0.0926 | 85 | 53.8 | 1.36 | 0.8712 - 2.11 | 0.000 |
| | Absence | 39 | 68.4 | | | 53 | 84.1 | | | 73 | 46.2 | | | |
| 0 | Presence | 5 | 41.6 | 0.51 | 0.1007 - 2.5859 | 3 | 30 | 0.18 | 0.0271 - 1.244 | 10 | 66.6 | 4.00 | 0.8764 - 18.2562 | 0.167 |
| | Absence | 7 | 58.4 | | | 7 | 70 | | | 5 | 33.4 | | | |
| 1 | Presence | 0 | 0 | - | - | 0 | 0 | - | - | 0 | 0 | - | - | - |
| | Absence | 0 | 0 | | | 0 | 0 | | | 0 | 0 | | | |
| 2 | Presence | 0 | 0 | - | - | 1 | 100 | - | - | 0 | 0 | - | - | - |
| | Absence | 0 | 0 | | | 0 | 0 | | | 0 | 0 | | | |

(Anterior n=100; Premolar n=103; Molar=300)

OR< 1 indicates that absence of apical periodontitis is less probable than presence of this event.

OR> 1 indicates that absence of apical periodontitis is more probable than absence of this event.

OR=1 indicates events are equally probable

p<0.05 indicates statistically significant difference

**Table 21.2** - Influence of length of root canal obturation on apical periodontitis detected by CBCT images[315].

| Apical Limit | Apical Periodontitis | Anterior n=100 | | OR | OR (CI 95%) | Premolar n=103 | | OR | OR (CI 95%) | Molar n=300 | | OR | OR (CI 95%) | p Chi-square test |
|---|---|---|---|---|---|---|---|---|---|---|---|---|---|---|
| | | | % | | | | % | | | | % | | | |
| -2 | Presence | 12 | 63.1 | 2.93 | 0.7864 - 10.9823 | 9 | 40.9 | 0.479 | 0.1441 - 1.5945 | 72 | 75 | 9 | 4.6828-17.2974 | 0.008 |
| | Absence | 7 | 36.9 | | | 13 | 59.1 | | | 24 | 25 | | | |
| -1 | Presence | 22 | 43.1 | 0.57 | 0.2628 - 1.2601 | 12 | 22.2 | 0.082 | 0.0329 - 0.2022 | 104 | 73.7 | 7.9 | 4.6476-13.4307 | 0 |
| | Absence | 29 | 56.9 | | | 42 | 77.8 | | | 37 | 26.3 | | | |
| 0 | Presence | 11 | 55 | 1.49 | 0.4298 - 5.1923 | 7 | 30.4 | 0.191 | 0.0545 - 0.6721 | 34 | 60.7 | 3.2 | 1.4476-7.0836 | 0.025 |
| | Absence | 9 | 45 | | | 16 | 69.6 | | | 19 | 39.3 | | | |
| 1 | Presence | 3 | 37.5 | 0.36 | 0.0476 - 2.7254 | 1 | 33.3 | 0.25 | 0.0084 - 7.4523 | 8 | 80 | 16 | 1.7883-143.1561 | 0.129 |
| | Absence | 5 | 62.5 | | | 2 | 66.7 | | | 2 | 20 | | | |
| 2 | Presence | 1 | 50 | 1 | 0.0198 - 50.4004 | 1 | 100 | - | - | 0 | 0 | - | - | - |
| | Absence | 1 | 50 | | | 0 | | | | 0 | 0 | | | |

(Anterior n=100; Premolar n=103;Molar=300)

OR< 1 indicates that absence of apical periodontitis is less probable than presence of this event.

OR> 1 indicates that absence of apical periodontitis is more probable than absence of this event.

OR=1 indicates events are equally probable

p<0.05 indicates statistically significant difference

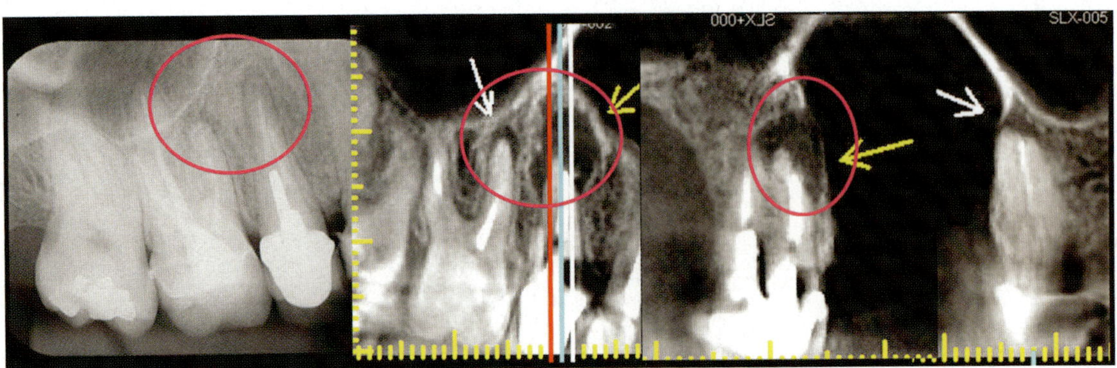


**Figure 21.3** - Length of root canal obturation observed by periapical radiographs and CBCT[315] (IORB, Brasília, DF, Brazil).

## 21.4 Root Canal Sealers

The literature is replete with studies evaluating the different properties (physical-chemical, biological and antimicrobial) of several materials recommended for root canal filling[1-549].

The use of sealer and gutta-percha is the most popular procedure as regards the materials indicated for filling the root canal. The differences lie in the selection of the root canal filling material and the filling technique.

Grossman[154] affirm that, irrespective of its type, the sealer should meet the following requirements:

1. It must be homogeneous, when manipulated, to promote good adherence between it and the root canal wall, when set;
2. It must promote a hermetic sealing;
3. It must be radiopaque, so that it can be visualized in the radiograph;
4. The particles of the powder must be very fine, so that they mix easily with the liquid;
5. It must not undergo contraction after hardening;
6. It must not spot the dental structure;
7. It must be bacteriostatic or, at least, not facilitate bacterial growth;
8. It must set slowly;
9. It must be insoluble in the oral fluids;
10. It must be tolerated by the tissues; that is, non-irritant to the periapical tissues;
11. It must be soluble in the common solvents, if it is necessary to remove the root canal filling.

Uniting different properties, especially adherence and biological compatibility, in the same material, continues to be an ideal to achieve. A material that is well tolerated by the tissues, but without good sealing capacity, or one that provides good sealing, but has an irritant action on the periapical tissues, must not be considered the best.

Wu et al.[519] based on a review of the literature about studies on leakage, observed that in studies published on endodontics, almost half would refer to this theme, with varied and contradictory results, and the methodology utilized. It is known that all the endodontic sealers allow some degree of dye leakage. The weight and size of the molecules of dyes, such as B rhodamine and methylene blue (indicators) are smaller than the bacterial cells present in the root canal.

Considering that the dye only leaks where there is space, and that all the sealers allow leakage, the hermetic sealing of the root canal system still is part of an objective to attain. Hovland & Dumsha[223] considered that leakage can occur at the interfaces of the sealer with the dentine, of the sealer with the gutta-percha, around the endodontic sealer or as a result of its dissolution. Therefore, it is understood that the endodontic sealer can be one of the critical points. Gutmann & Witherspoon[168] reported that to date, none of various materials and techniques used for root canal fillings have safely reached the highest biological and technical level. Ideally, future endeavors should focus on materials that *1. Penetrate the patent dentinal tubules; 2. Bind closely to both the organic and inorganic phases of dentin; 3. Neutralize or destroy microorganisms and their products; 4. Predictably induce a regenerative cement response on the apical foramen; and 5. Strengthen the root system. The delivery system of such materials requires it to be easy to place and set rapidly and thoroughly once in the canal system.*

With the objective of obtaining the ideal sealing different endodontic sealers have been manufactured. Some contain primarily zinc oxide and eugenol (Rickert sealer, N-Rickert, Grossman sealer, FillCanal, Endo-Fill, Tubliseal, Endomethasone), calcium oxide (Sealapex), calcium hydroxide (Sealer 26, Apexit), resin (AH 26, Diaket, Top Seal, AH Plus) or glass ionomer (Ketac-Endo).

In view of this varied quantity of endodontic sealers available, it is become necessary to analyze the relationship between their properties. It is fundamental to remember that the filling material must be confined only to the prepared root canal.

Grossman[155-159] idealized a sealer that became very popular amongst endodontists all over the world. By substituting eugenol for essential oils, eucalyptol and pepper leaf oil, the hardening period of the proposed sealer does not change.

Synthetic resins have been disseminated and used in endodontology[168,324]. The AH 26 sealer is a synthetic arrangement of macromolecules of the epoxy resin group. Other type of epoxy resin-based sealer introduced by Dentsply-Maillefer is AH Plus. Studies showed that AH 26 and AH Plus are toxic when freshly prepared[436] and toxicity decreases during setting, and after 24 hours[266].

Holland et al.[202] observed the good behavior of calcium hydroxide in connective tissue, especially as regards its capacity to stimulate biological apical sealing with mineralized tissue. Berbert[19] evaluated the behavior of the apical and periapical tissues in dog teeth after pulpectomy and filling with AH 26, calcium hydroxide or mixture of both, and showed that the mixture 20% of calcium hydroxide with AH 26 offered the best results. After this study[19], the Sealer 26 cement, which contains calcium hydroxide, bismuth oxide, hexamethylene tetramine and titanium dioxide agglutinated to epoxy bisphenol resin was introduced for use in endodontics. In the cytotoxicity analysis[12], Sealer 26 showed low cytotoxicity, when compared with other sealers, Fillcanal and N-Rickert.

It is universally accepted that sealers must be biologically compatible. In this sense, after the calcium hydroxide became available on the market, there were sealers with good biological compatibility. Sealapex demonstrated biocompatibility and capacity to induce apical closure by osteocement deposition[202].

Most of currently available sealers can be homogeneously mixed, provided they are correctly manipulated. However, the bonding to the dentinal tissue is more complex. The sealers containing glass ionomer have good bonding capacity to the dentinal surface. The best known of these sealers is Ketac-Endo.

The Figures 21.4 and 21.5 shows the some endodontic sealers used by endodontists all over the world.

**Table 21.3** - Sealapex™ (Approximate composition)

| | |
|---|---|
| Calcium oxide | 20.0% |
| Bismuth trioxide | 29.0% |
| Zinc oxide | 2.5% |
| Sub-micron silica | 3.0% |
| Titanium dioxide | 2.0% |
| Zinc stearate | 1.0% |
| Tricalcium phosphate | 3.0% |
| * Blend | 39% |
| * Ethyl toluene sulfonamide, poly (methylene methyl salicylate) resin, isobutyl salicylate and a pigment | |

(Sealapex™, Kerr SybronEndo, MI, USA)

**Table 21.4** - AH plus (Approximate composition)

| Paste A | Paste B |
|---|---|
| Epoxy resins | Amines |
| Calcium tungstate | Calcium tungstate |
| Zirconium oxide | Zirconium oxide |
| Silica | Silica |
| Iron oxide pigments | Silicone oil |

(AH-Plus, Dentsply Maillefer, Ballaigues, Switzerland)

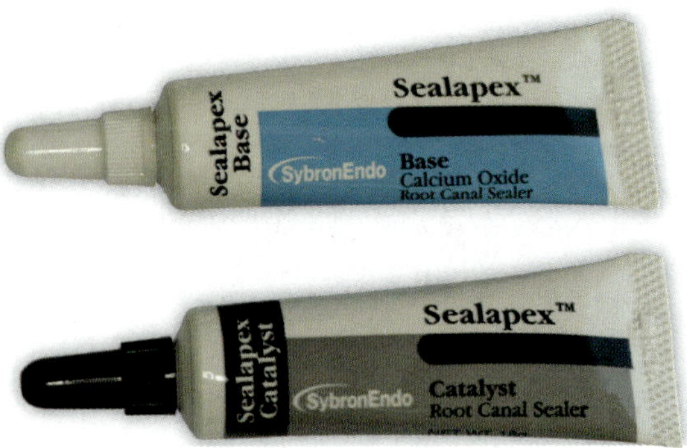


**Figures 21.4A** - Sealapex™ (Kerr SybronEndo, MI, USA).

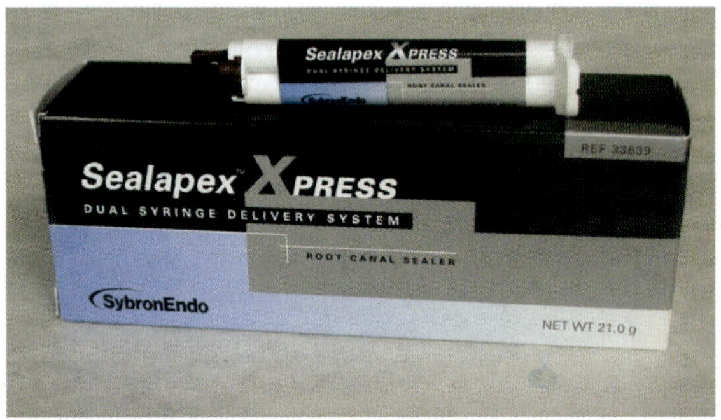


**Figures 21.4B** - Sealapex™.

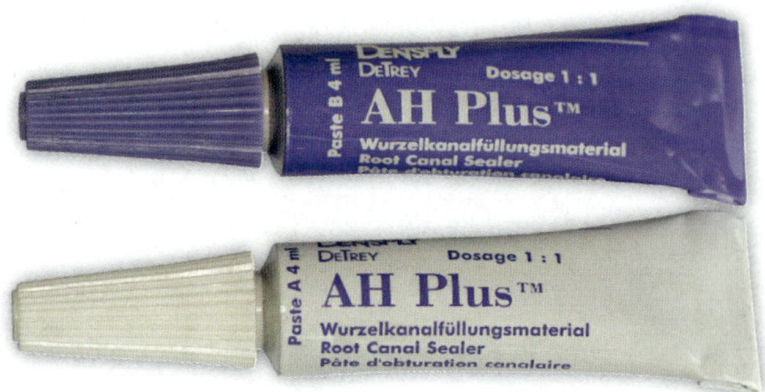


**Figures 21.5** - AH-Plus (Dentsply Maillefer, Ballaigues, Switzerland).

Present day thinking has recommended the implementation of dentistry based on scientific evidences, which places value on studies involving systematic review or meta-analysis. Studies based on scientific evidence have been emphasized in dentistry. Systematic review has several advantages, such as: explicit methods limit bias in identifying and rejecting studies; conclusions are hence more reliable and accurate; large amounts of information can be assimilated quickly by health care providers, researchers and policymakers; delay in divulging research discoveries, and implementation of effective diagnostic and therapeutic strategies is potentially reduced; results of different studies can be formally compared to establish generalization of findings and consistency (lack of heterogeneity) of results; reasons for heterogeneity (inconsistency in results across studies) can be identified and new hypothesis generated about particular subgroups; quantitative systematic reviews (meta-analyses) increase the precision of the overall result[96,97].

Estrela et al.[107] evaluated the biological sealing provided by endodontic sealer in longitudinal studies, through the systematic revision. Use was made of sources of bibliographic catalogation identified electronically by MEDLINE, EMBASE, CENTRAL (http://www.ncbi.nlm.nih.gov/PubMed) and hand-searches, from 1966 untill January 14, 2008. As search strategy the following terms were used – *Sealapex or AH Plus or Epiphany or Kerr Pulp Canal Sealer, or Grossman Sealer or Sealer 26* as keywords. The studies were selected by two independent reviewers, who also determined the inclusion and exclusion criteria. The search presented 456 related articles (Fig. 21.6), 132 articles being related to in vivo studies (humans or animals), 7 articles were case reports, 4 longitudinal studies, and 260 in vitro studies. Of the 132 in vivo studies, 1 satisfied the inclusion criteria (Table 21.5).

Taking values from the experimental design adopted in the included study (prospective analysis), it could be inferred that in the short term, the sealers containing calcium hydroxide or oxide showed better results, whereas, in the long term, there was no difference in the results when compared with the sealers containing zinc oxide and eugenol.

In the included study, Waltimo et al.[496] assessed three endodontics cements: Sealapex, CRCS and Procosol; 204 teeth were submitted to standardized endodontic treatment and then divided into 3 groups: PS Group (filled with gutta-percha and Procosol), CR Group (teeth filled with gutta-percha and CRCS) and SA Group (teeth filled with Sealapex and gutta-percha). The treatment was performed by graduates of the Dentistry Course at the University of Oslo - Norway, who used each cement at least 2 times each. The results were analyzed during the following 4 years, using the PAI - Periapical index. In the first years of analyses, it could be observed that the groups of filled teeth, in which cements containing oxide or hydroxide of calcium were used, showed higher clinical - radiographic success rates, when using the PAI index. Whereas in 3 and 4 years, this difference was not significant when the cements containing calcium hydroxide or oxide and the zinc oxide and eugenol-based cements were compared.

Considering the absence of studies in humans that involve biological sealing, investigations in dogs showed that Sealapex produced encouraging results as regards the biological sealing of the root canal system.

**Table 21.5** - Included study that it allowed the analysis of the biologic seal of the endodontics cement

| Reference | n | 1 year | 2 years | 3 years | 4 years | Exp. Oper. | Sanitization Process | Radiographic Follow-up | Clinical follow-up | Filling |
|---|---|---|---|---|---|---|---|---|---|---|
| Waltimo et al.[496] (2001) | 204 | 152 | 133 | 115 | 59 | Graduate | Stainless steel files | PAI score | Soft tissues, percussion and mobility tests, restorations, presence of contacts, marginal bony level | Lateral condensation |
| Sealapex | 56 | 48 | 41 | 37 | 16 | | | | | |
| Procosol | 95 | 68 | 60 | 45 | 25 | | | | | |
| CRCS | 52 | 34 | 31 | 28 | 14 | | | | | |

Legend:

n - Samples size

1 year, 2 years, 3 years, 4 years - number of samples in the clinical follow-up of 1 year, 2, 3 and 4 years

Exp. Oper. - Formation degree and experience of the operators of the study

Sanitization process - Prepare of the root canal

Filling - Filling technique accomplished by the operator in the study

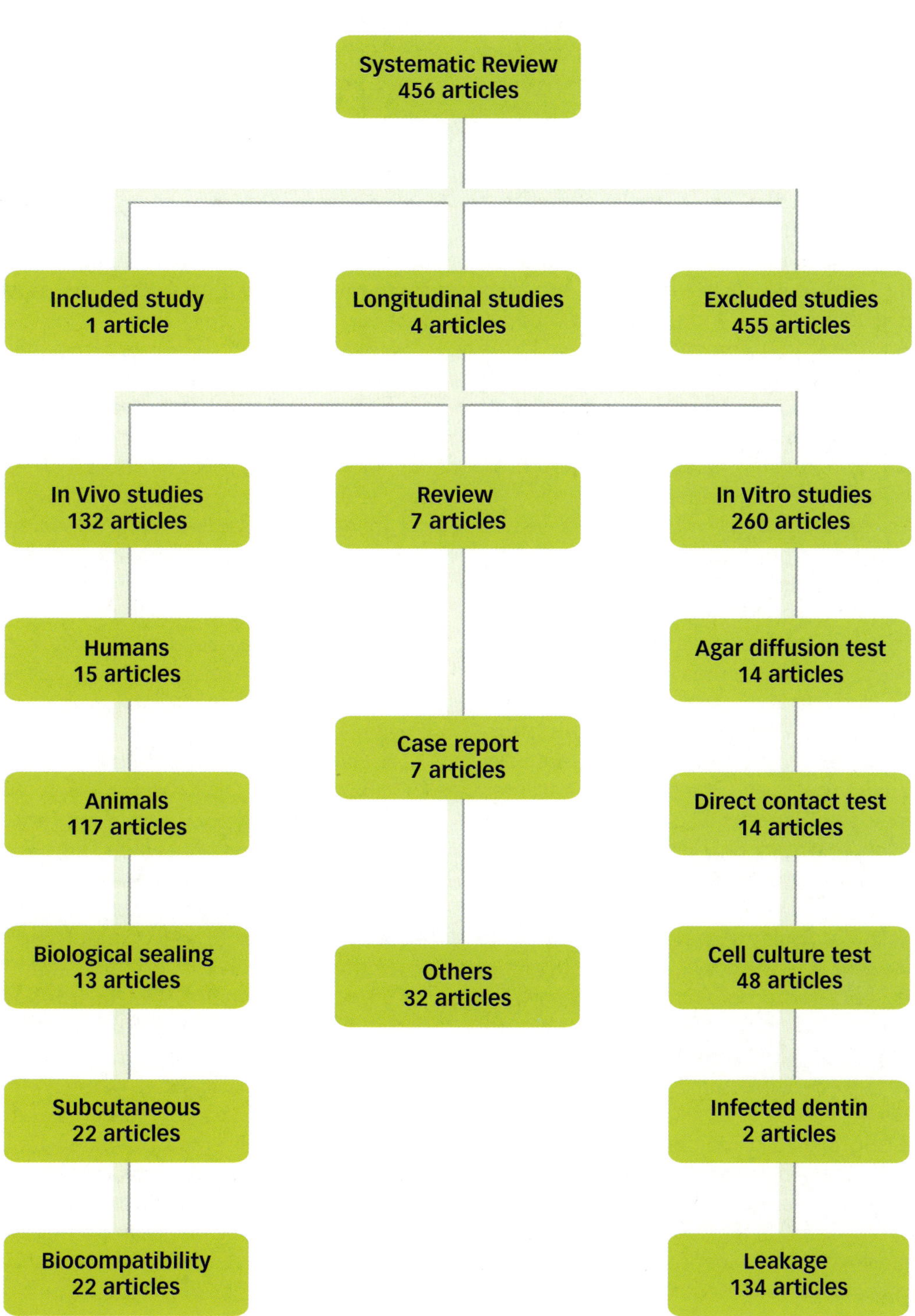


**Figure 21.6** - Distribution of the studies for the systematic review[107].

It is essential to consider various biological studies that are the basis of the biocompatibility of sealers containing oxide or hydroxide of calcium. Holland & Souza[202] evaluated the capacity of Sealapex to stimulate mineralized tissue deposition after the endodontic treatment in monkey's and dog's teeth. In the dog's experiment, 160 canals were used. The dental pulps were removed at two different levels: 1mm beneath the radiographic apex (partial pulpectomy) and at the radiographic apex (total pulpectomy). In Group 1, the pulp was removed with Hedström files, while in Group 2, the pulp was removed with Kerr type files, and filled by the lateral condensation technique with Sealapex and gutta-percha cones, Kerr Pulp Canal Sealer or calcium hydroxide associated with distilled water. The control group was not filled with any material. The chamber of all the groups was sealed with a zinc oxide and eugenol cement and restored with amalgam; each experimental group had 20 samples (root canals). After 180 days, the animals were sacrificed, and the segments of jaw were prepared for histological examination. In the study on monkeys, 80 canals were used. The teeth were treated similarly to those of the dogs, but the foramen was enlarged only up to file #25 in the experimental group (n=10), using the same previously described technique. The results suggest that Sealapex and calcium hydroxide induce apical closure by cement deposition. The cases of partial pulpectomy demonstrated the same percentage (70%) of apical closure for Sealapex and calcium hydroxide. In the cases of total pulpectomy, Sealapex demonstrated 33.3% of the cases with total closure, while calcium hydroxide demonstrated 10% of total closure. Apical closure was observed to less extent in the control group (5%), and the Kerr Pulp Canal Sealer group (10%), was associated with the presence of dentine chips. Both Sealapex and Kerr Pulp Canal Sealer, when overfilled, caused chronic inflammation in the periodontal ligament; however, Sealapex stimulated the deposition of mineralized tissue in this area, and was easily resorbed.

## 21.5 Root Canal Sealer Properties

Root canal filling materials have been analyzed from various aspects, in many studies, such as the tissue tolerance, physical-chemical, antimicrobial and clinical properties[1-549]. It is accepted that all these characteristics deserve to be valorized, however, it is essential to obtain an endodontic sealer capable of favoring more perfect sealing, and at the same time, being tolerated by the periapical tissues.

Holland et al.[191] evaluated the influence of the sealers Tubliseal, Maisto paste, Pulp Canal Sealer, Grossman sealer, AH 26, Endomethasone, zinc oxide and eugenol sealer, N2 and Diaket-A in the process of periapical repair in monkey's teeth, following apical filling with dentine chips. Most of the cases showed sealer deposition directly on the filling. In other cases, the dentine chips also deposited in the accessory canals. There was evidence of areas of sealer and resorbed dentine, which were completely repaired by cement on the root canal wall, with no inflammation.

Holland et al.[201] investigated the periapical healing process of dog's teeth with or without apical patency and after root canal filling with two types of sealers. Forty premolar and incisor roots were used. The root canals were overinstrumented and dressed with a corticosteroid-antibiotic solution for 7 days to obtain ingrowth of periapical connective tissue into the canals. After this period, the tissue was removed in half of the specimens (groups with patency) and preserved in the other half (groups without patency). Canals were filled by the lateral condensation technique with gutta-percha points and either a calcium hydroxide-based sealer (Sealer Plus) or a Grossman's cement (Fillcanal). Data were evaluated in a blind analysis on the basis of several histomorphologic parameters. The groups without patency had better results than those in which the ingrown connective tissue was removed. Comparing the sealers, Sealer Plus had significantly better results than Fillcanal. In conclusion, both the apical patency (presence or absence) and the type of root canal filling material influenced the periapical healing process in dog's teeth with vital pulp after root canal treatment. The use of a calcium hydroxide-based sealer in teeth without apical patency yielded the best results among the experimental conditions proposed (Fig 21.7).



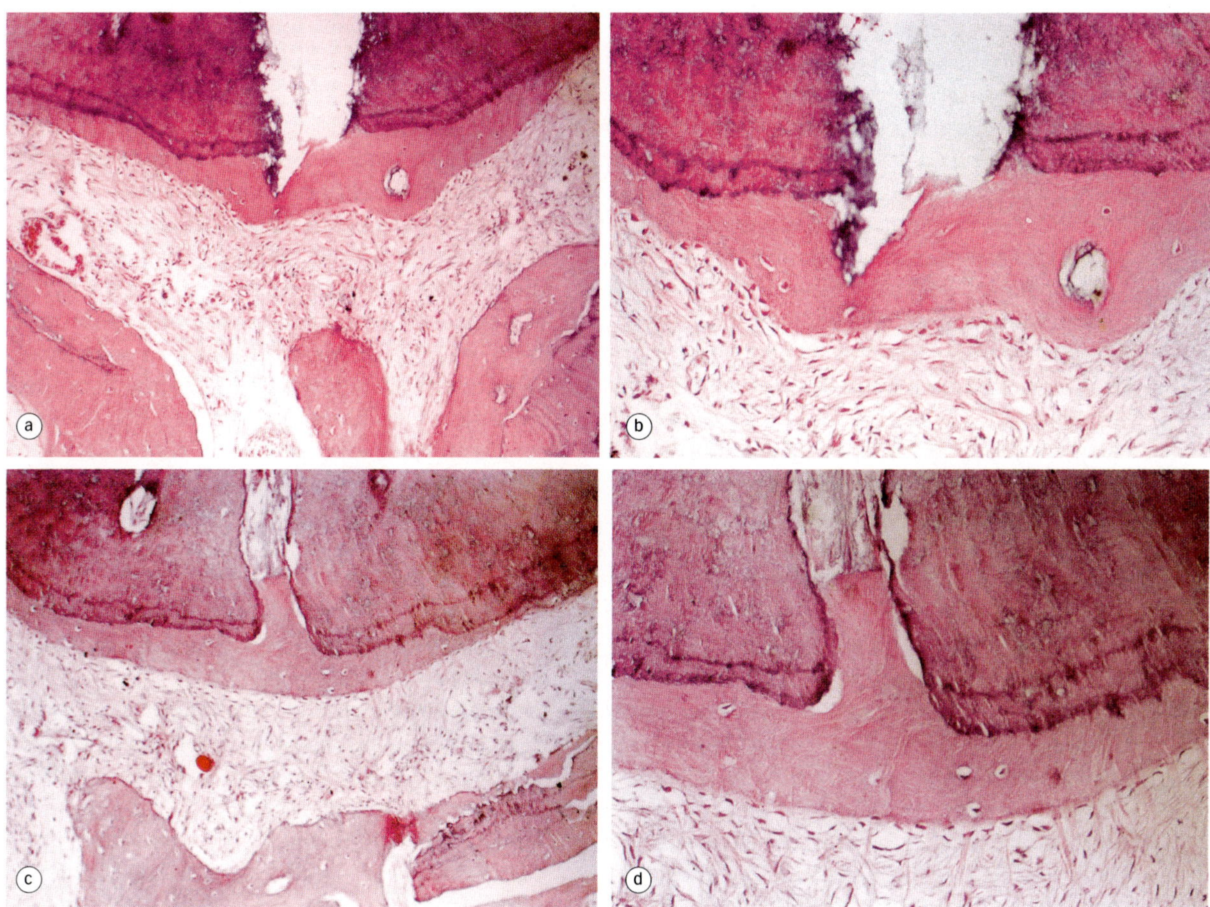


**Figure 21.7** - (A-B) Sealer Plus without patency. Biological closure of an accessory root canal by neoformed cementum deposition. H&E. (original magnification X100). (C-D) Sealer Plus without patency. Note total closure of the main root canal and an organized periodontal tissue, H&E. (original magnification X100)(Courtesy Holland et al.[202]).

Tagger et al.[446] studied the release of calcium and hydroxide ions from sealers containing calcium hydroxide (Sealapex, CRCS and Hermetic). Bases, analyzed for release of hydroxide ions were included for comparison, such as Life and Dycal. The materials were manipulated in accordance with manufacturers' instructions, and produced 2 samples for each material, approximately 7mm in diameter, and 3mm deep. After setting for a minimum period of 24 hours, the specimens were put into bi-distilled water (pH = 6.7) for 2 hours, changed every 15 minutes. The pH measurements were made after 15, 30, 45, 60, 75, 90, 105 and 120 minutes of sealer placement in distilled water. The release of calcium and pH exhibited by Sealapex was gradual and prolonged, as well as for Life and Dycal. After 60 and 45 minutes had elapsed, the Life and Dycal samples dissolved.

Leal et al.[272] compared the biocompatibility of the endodontic sealers Sealapex, CRCS, Fillcanal and N-Rickert in rat's subcutaneous connective tissues. After the periods of observation (4, 21 and 60 days), the implants were compared by microscopy analysis, with incisions in 6mm of thickness and staining with hematoxylin and eosin. All the tested materials showed irritation in the initial period. Sealapex and N-Rickert exhibited similar results, and minor tissue irritation, which was a little more accentuated than with the other sealers. Among the four tested sealers, Sealapex was the one that showed evidences of calcium salt deposition, similar to that observed with calcium hydroxide.

Barbosa et al.[23] verified the toxicity of the endodontic sealers (Fillcanal, N-Ricket, FS Paste and Sealer 26) in connective tissue cells, through the direct and indirect contact. The studied cells were fibroblasts L929 of rats, and periodontal joint cells, in cultures from 5 to 7 days. Spatulated sealers were analyzed (1, 7 and 14 days, after spatulation). The results showed that all the spatulated sealers caused significant cellular damages. The treatment was performed in two visits, and the canals were filled with gutta-percha points and zinc oxide and eugenol or Sealapex. In the second visit, the osseous tissue was exposed and two cavities were prepared in the bone, cementum and dentine. One cavity was prepared in the apical third and other cavity between the middle and cervical third. With Sealapex there was cementum deposition in the apical third with total closure in 8 cases, and in only 2 cases there was no deposition. Zinc oxide and eugenol showed total closure by deposition of cementum in the apical third in 5 specimens, and 3 specimens showed no cementum deposition. There was no inflammation in 8 cases, and other cases were similar to the previous group. In the cervical third, new cementum was absent in 6 specimens, there being only one case of total closure. Chronic moderate inflammation was present in 10 cases.

Fidel[121] studied the physical properties of the following root canal filling cements containing calcium hydroxide: Sealer 26, CRCS, Sealapex, Apexit and an experimental cement, PR-Sealer. Fillcanal cement was analyzed to compare it with other cements of the same type (CRCS and PR-Sealer). The American Dental Association (Specification 57)[14] for endodontic filling materials was used for the following tests: flow, work time, hardening time, film thickness, solubility and disintegration, dimensional stability and radiopacity. All of the cements studied showed flow compatible with the specification followed, with values varying from 28 to 47 mm. The cements could not be classified according to work time because the manufacturers did not provide this information. CRCS was the only cement that presented a hardening time in accordance with the time informed by the manufacturer. Sealapex and Sealer 26 had long hardening times, 45 hours and 34 minutes, and 41 hours and 22 minutes, respectively. Only Sealer 26 did not fill the requirements of film thickness of the specification followed. Fillcanal and Sealapex presented greater solubility and disintegration than that permitted values. Most of the cements presented expansion and complied with the standards of the specification. Sealapex was an exception and disintegrated, preventing testing. The radiopacity of all of the cements were acceptable, greater than 4 mm aluminum. Sealapex and Sealer 26 presented the lowest radiopacity. Bond to dentin of all the cements was measured. Fillcanal, Sealapex and Apexit showed lower bond strength. All the cements were alkaline, not only immediately after spreading, but also at the end of the experiment, 7 days after hardening.

Sacomani et al.[380] investigated the behavior of the periapical tissues of dog's teeth after preparation and filling with Sealer 26 cement and modified Sealer 26. After preparation, the canals were filled with Otosporin and 7 days later, they were dried and filled using the lateral condensation technique with gutta-percha and the root canal sealers. After 180 days had elapsed, the specimens were analyzed. When taken to the periapical tissues, the two sealers caused chronic inflammatory reaction observed 180 days after filling.

Holland et al.[209] observed the reaction of rat's subcutaneous connective tissues to the implant of dentine tubes filled with sealers containing calcium hydroxide. The tubes were filled with MTA, Sealapex, CRCS, Sealer 26 and an experimental sealer, Sealer Plus. The tubes were immediately implanted twice in the dorsal region of 60 rats, and the empty tubes were used as control in 10 additional animals. The animals were sacrificed after 7 and 30 days. The tube and adjacent tissue were removed and prepared for histological analysis. Some sections were also decalcified for 10 minutes in EDTA, before being stained. In the control groups, after 7 days, a surface of neutrophils covered the tubes, the presence of fibroblasts and chronic inflammatory cells being observed near this area; by 7 days, there were neutrophils present around the material, and by 30 days, there were fibroblasts and a chronic inflammatory reaction. All the other materials tested exhibited calcified structures by 7 and 30 days. The only difference was the quantity of these structures, which was more numerous in the MTA and Sealapex groups.

Pulgar et al.[365] determined whether the sealer AH 26 and AH Plus had osteogenic effects in vitro. Breast cancer cells MCF-F were put in 24-well plates at an initial concentration of 10,000 cells/well. The cells were left to jell for 24 hours; different concentrations of the materials being tested and added to the wells of the samples (AH 26 and AH Plus in dilutions of 1/100 up to 1/1,000,000). The experiment was observed after 144 hours. The authors observed that only the sealer AH 26 demonstrated osteogenic effect in vitro.

Holland et al.[208] observed the reaction of the apical tissues of dog's teeth after root canal filling with gutta-percha and mineral trioxide aggregate (MTA) or a glass ionomer (Ketac-Endo) as a sealer. The root canals were instrumented and filled by the lateral condensation technique with the studied sealers. Animals were killed 6 months later, and the specimens were removed and prepared for histological analysis. Results showed no inflammatory reaction of apical tissues and total closure of the apical foramen of all the teeth sealed with MTA. The teeth sealed with Ketac-Endo showed two cases of partial closure and different degrees of chronic inflammatory reaction. In conclusion, MTA exhibited better biological properties than Ketac-Endo.

Mileitic et al.[308] evaluated the penetration of *C. albicans* alone, and a combination of bacteria, through root canals filled with gutta-percha and one or two other root canal sealers, AH 26 and AH Plus. Eighty teeth were randomly divided into two groups of 40 teeth each and filled with gutta-percha using either AH26 or AH Plus sealer. A further 10 teeth served as negative controls and 10 as positive controls. The external surface of each root, except for the apical 2 mm, was covered with two layers of nail varnish. The teeth were inserted into Eppendorf plastic tubes and suspended in glass bottles containing sterile Schaedler broth. *S. mutans*, *S. mitis*, *P. melaninogenica* and *L. acidophilus* were placed in the access cavities of 20 teeth filled with AH 26 and 20 with AH Plus. *C. albicans* was placed in the access cavities of the other teeth. The culture medium with microorganisms was changed every 7 days. Every 72 h bacterial or fungal growth in the broth was tested for a period of up to 90 days. Leakage in the experimental teeth occurred between 14 and 87 days. Leakage was present in 47% of all samples. From the samples with AH26, 45% leaked bacteria and 60% leaked fungi; whilst from the samples with AH Plus, 50% leaked bacteria and 55% fungi. There was no statistically significant difference in penetration of bacteria and fungi between the sealers. In this in vitro study, gutta-percha and the sealers AH 26 and AH Plus allowed leakage of bacteria and fungi.

Estrela et al.[112] evaluated the apical sealing of teeth filled by the lateral condensation and Nguyen (lateral and vertical condensation) techniques by means of methylene blue, using N-Rickert and Sealapex. The Nguyen and lateral condensation techniques showed averages of leakage over 0.783mm and 0.935mm, when N-Rickert was applied, then 0.765 mm and 0.959mm, when Sealapex was applied, respectively. In another study, Estrela et al.[113], compared the apical leakage of different endodontic sealers (Fillcanal, N-Rickert, Sealapex and AH 26) and the technique of filling (active and passive lateral condensation), by means of with ethylene blue. All the sealers allowed apical leakage. There were no significant differences among the sealers when apical leakage was compared between active and passive lateral condensation. Fillcanal, Sealapex and AH26 demonstrated significant differences, with lower leakage values when active condensation was used. The sealer N-Rickert demonstrated no statistically significant differences between the techniques.

Holland & Murata[189] observed the effectiveness of filling the root canal system with Sealapex in 30 single rooted human teeth. After preparation, a lateral canal was simulated by a perforation with a size #15 instrument in the buccal-lingual direction and at right angles, from the cementum to the interior of the canal, followed by 3 minutes of irrigation with EDTA again. The canals were dried and filled by the lateral condensation technique, with cones of gutta-percha and the following sealers: N-Rickert, Sealapex and Apexit. The sealers were prepared in accordance with the manufacturers' instructions, and in the case of Sealapex, 1/3 of iodine was added. After the filling was concluded, mesio-distal and bucco-lingual periapical radiographs were taken to observe the extent of sealer penetrations through the perforations. Of the 10 specimen tested for each sealer, all the sealers were able to fill the lateral canals in all the specimen. As regards the apical ramifications, Sealapex filled 9 specimens, and Apexit and N-Rickert filled 8 specimens. The sealers were shown to have sufficient drainage for penetrating into the root canal system during filling by the lateral condensation technique.

Estrela et al.[111] used the agar diffusion test to compare the antibacterial action of 3 root canal sealers (Sealapex, Sealer 26 and Apexit), against the pure cultures of three optional aerobic bacteria: *E. coli, P. aeruginosa and S. faecalis*. The experimental root canal sealers showed no evidence of antibacterial potential when considering the above-mentioned bacteria.

Estrela et al.[102] investigated the antibacterial action of MTA, Portland Cement, calcium hydroxide paste, Sealapex and Dycal. The materials were tested against the following microorganisms: *S. aureus, E. faecalis, P. aeruginosa, B. subtilis and C. albicans*. For the agar diffusion test, the microorganisms were inoculated in 5 ml of agar BHI and incubated at 37°C for 24 hours. They were diluted in a saline suspension to obtain a mixture of the tested microorganisms. Then 0.1 ml of this suspension was inoculated in each one of 30 Petri plates containing 20 ml of agar BHI each. Three cavities, measuring 4mm of depth x 4mm of diameter, were concluded and filled with the tested materials. The plates were pre-incubated for 1 hour at room temperature, and then incubated at 37°C for 48 hours. Positive and negative controls were conducted, and the tests were performed in triplicate. Calcium hydroxide paste obtained the best results, showing inhibition zones varying from 6 to 9.5mm, and diffusion between 10 and 18mm. MTA, Portland cement and Sealapex demonstrated only diffusion zones; and amongst them, Sealapex obtained the largest zones (10 to 18 mm). Dycal demonstrated no inhibition and diffusion zones against the microorganisms tested.

## 21.6 Considerations Regarding Bond Strength of Endodontic Sealers to Root Canal Walls

The success of endodontic therapy is related to the appropriate execution of the different treatment phases. During biomechanical preparation, the removal of dentine tissue is necessary to promote cleaning and disinfection, as well as to prepare root canal system to receive the filling material. Complete root filling is achieved by the three-dimensional obturation of the root canal system with the association of a solid filling material[467,489]. Ideally, one of the key roles of the sealer is to aggregate the root filling material and maintain it as compact mass with no gaps that adheres to the canal walls and provides a single block configuration upon which the canal becomes hermetically sealed[406].

Adhesion of an endodontic sealer is defined as its capacity to adhere to the root canal walls and promote the union of the filling material to each other and to the dentine[430]. This property may be influenced by the treatment performed on the root canal walls as well as by the type of sealer used. The adhesion process involves mechanical forces that yields the intertwining of the material with the dentin structures[330] and may result in a greater sealing ability of the filling material, thus reducing the risk of root canal microleakage and maintaining cohesive filling mass[382]. This process is important in static and dynamic situations. In static circumstances, the adhesion eliminates spaces that allow the infiltration of fluids into the sealer/dentine interface. In dynamic situations, the adhesion is necessary to avoid the sealer dislodgment during operative procedures[330]. Therefore, the adhesion of the filling material to the intracanal walls has the additional benefit of reinforcing the roots of endodontically treated teeth[467].

Some variables may interfere with the outcome and understanding of sealer adhesion to root canal walls, namely the employed treatment of dentin surface, the type of material and methodology.

During biomechanical preparation of root canals, smear layer is formed on the dentin walls. According to Kennedy et al.[253], smear layer is a negative factor in root canal sealing because it forms an interface between the filling material and the root canal walls, hence reducing the adhesion of sealers. However, some studies have found higher bond strengths when the smear layer was not removed[383,447].

Different chemical solutions and their associations have been recommended for use with instrumentation of root canals to remove debris, smear layer and disinfect the root canal. Among the most commonly used irrigants, sodium hypochlorite presents capacity of dissolution of organic tissues, saponification of fats and neutralization of toxic products as well as antimicrobial and deodorizing action, while ethylenediaminetetraacetic acid disodium salt (EDTA) has a calcium ion chelating capacity and promotes dentine demineralization and smear layer removal. Nevertheless, the total cleaning of root internal surface is still a challenge[430].

In addition to the routinely used chemical substances, other technologies have been currently investigated for the treatment of root canal dentine, such as laser irradiation. In laser irradiated-surfaces, the absence of smear layer and exposure of dentine tubules[450] can facilitate the adaptation of the endodontic materials to root canal walls, thus improving the bond strength[429,430]. On the other hand, melting areas found in the laser irradiated-dentine can alter the surface permeability and decrease the bond strength of filling material.

Er:YAG, Nd:YAG and 980 nm diode lasers have been studied for applicability in Endodontics. Er:YAG lasers remove smear layer from the root canal walls, exposing dentinal tubules[52,428,451], while Nd:YAG lasers remove smear layer and melt and recrystallize dentinal tissue[386] and reduce apical leakage in teeth obturated with epoxy-based root canal sealers[335].

A new laser wavelength - 980-nm diode laser - has been recently launched to the market[377,403,497]. This laser transmits energy through thin flexible fibres that adapt perfectly to the tiny dimensions and curved shapes of the root canals[163]. Diode laser units have a low purchasing and maintenance cost as well as greater versatility due to their compact size[163,274,438] and Lee et al.[274] have observed a reduction of the microbial content in hard-to-reach areas, such as dentinal tubules, after diode laser irradiation. However, laser irradiation is applied inside the root canal and not perpendicular to a flat surface. According to Brugnera-Júnior et al.[52] and Alves et al.[19], smear layer removal depends on the angle of incidence of the fiberoptic tip and the dentinal surface.

Several studies have investigated the adhesion of different types of root canal sealers to root dentin and gutta-percha[178,382,430]. Regarding the composition of root canal sealers, they can be classified as calcium hydroxide-containing sealers, resin-based sealers, oxide de zinc eugenol-based sealers either containing or not medication, and glass ionomer sealers. While Trope & Ray[487] observed higher adhesion in tooth filled with glass ionomer-based sealers, Apicella et al.[18] did not find a difference between this sealer and the nonfilled teeth. Cobankara et al.[73] showed similar results between glass ionomer- and epoxy resin-based sealers, however, Lertchrakarn et al.[278] concluded that glass ionomer sealers were more effective in root reinforcement than the epoxy resin-based sealers.

Advances in adhesive technology have reinforced the search for means to minimize apical and coronal marginal leakage by improving sealer adhesion to the root canal walls[461] and thus reducing the susceptibility of endodontically treated teeth to fracture[467]. Among the resinous sealers, the epoxy resin-based cements have presented a good performance as root canal sealers [98,396]. AH Plus has been shown to have satisfactory physicochemical properties, low solubility and disintegration[63,396], good adhesion[98], antimicrobial action[249] and good biological properties[511].

Besides, a new generation of methacrylate resin-based sealers and self-etching primers increase the expectations of a better coronary and apical marginal sealing that could result in higher adhesion to tooth structure. Epiphany (Pentron Clinical Technologies, Wallingford, CT, USA) is a dual-cure methacrylate resin-based sealer used with a solid material named Resilon (Resilon Research LLC, Madison, CT, EUA), which contains a blend of synthetic thermoplastic polyester polymers. Obturation using the Epiphany/Resilon system is claimed to create a seal with the dentinal tubules within the root canal system[417,494]. In essence, it produces a "monoblock" effect, where the core material (Resilon), sealer (Epiphany) and dentinal tubules become a single solid structure. Shipper et al.[417] have suggested that this monoblock would be highly desirable to provide a thorough seal of the root canal system as it would be able to minimize cervical marginal infiltration in case of loss or fracture of the temporary coronal restoration. In vitro[417] and in vivo[416] studies have demonstrated a good resistance of the Epiphany/Resilon system monoblock to bacterial leakage.

However, the results obtained for Epiphany sealer were not higher than those obtained with AH Plus sealer[138]. On this concern, a recent investigation[371] reported that the Epiphany sealer presented the lowest bond strength values, which may be explained by the occurrence of physicochemical interferences during polymerization and primer interaction with the root canal walls submitted to different laser treatments. Composite resin polymerization is inhibited by the presence of oxygen and approximately 40 to 60% of the carbon bonds remain unsaturated[126,131]. It is likely that it inhibited the polymerization of Epiphany at sealer/dentine interface and inside the dentinal tubules. Failures at the sealer-dentine interface may also occur due to the polymerization of the methacrylate-based resin sealer immediately after its placement into the root canal[460]. In addition, the coronal photoactivation of the sealer, following the manufacturer's instructions, may reduce its flow and limit its contact with the primer and hence its penetration into the dentinal tubules. Another aspect that may interfere with the polymerization reaction of the sealer is the lack of photoactivation throughout the specimen extension, which contributes to its incomplete polymerization, leaving residual monomers in the sealer at the deepest regions of the specimen[371].

Although the American Dental Association (ANSI/ADA, 2000) has issued a series of regulations and tests for the study of the physical properties of root canal sealers, adhesion tests have not yet been standardized because no consensus regarding test parameters has been reached among researchers. Moreover, the divergent results obtained in the studies and the difficulties in testing materials with great plasticity, such as gutta-percha or Resilon, or materials with high modules of elasticity, such as radicular posts, have led to the development of different methodologies for determining the bond strength of endodontic sealers to the coronal or root dentin[150,178,430,447].

Bond strength of endodontic sealers to dentin and root canal filling material has been extensively investigated. These studies have attempted to establish a methodology that would provide a more standardized test model and overall investigated the adhesion of endodontic sealers to the coronal dentin rather to than root dentin[303, 318, 356, 428, 429]. Other studies tested coronal dentin discs cemented to gutta-percha discs[275,382].

Grossman[154] and Ørstavik[325] reported different experimental models designed to evaluate the adhesion of the root canal sealers. Grossman[154] proposed the use of an apparatus built from a "T" shaped shaft with two tackles and a string. One of the ends of the string is connected to the material to be tested and the other end receives additional load until the material separates from the dentine surface. The necessary mass for the rupture is related to the local gravity acceleration value, thus obtaining the traction force. The traction tension is calculated from the bonded area. Ørstavik[325] proposed the use of the universal testing machine. Various researchers[318,356,428,506] have performed the adhesion test with this method, which allows better precision of the applied forces i.e., intensity, velocity and direction and reproducibility of the experiment, and thus more reliable data. In addition, the values of tensile strength are expressed in MegaPascal (MPa), which allows the comparison of results with other studies.

Shear bond strength (SBS) test is a method in which the force is applied parallel to the interface between the material and the tested surface. This test has been developed to assess the adhesion of endodontic sealers to dentin and gutta-percha or Resilon® and has been proven to be effective and reproducible[98,172,173,178, 447]. A major problem of the shear testing is that it is difficult to align closely the shear-loading device with the bonded interface. The load is offset at some distance from the bonded interface, resulting in an unpredictable torque load on the specimen[498].

Another method that is largely used in Endodontic researches is push out test. Paterno et al.[345] proposed a method to evaluate resistance to traction of composites in cervical radicular dentine, in which the teeth were sectioned transversely to produce 4-mm thick cylindrical samples. Root canals were enlarged, adhesive was applied on the dentinal walls and resin was placed inside it for performing the push-out test. This experimental model could be adapted to the adhesion tests for root canal sealers. Sousa-Neto et al.[430] have pointed out the advantages of this method, including the possibility of placing the sealer in direct contact with the intracanal dentin walls, instead of a flat coronal dentin surface, which presents a different tubule arrangement pattern. Additionally, it provided homogenous results with considerably low variation of bond strength. Ungor et al.[489] used a push-out test with 1.13-mm root dentin cylinders to assess the bond strength of the Epiphany/Resilon resin-based root canal filling system in comparison to the bond strengths of different pairings of AH Plus, gutta-percha, Epiphany, Resilon. These authors observed that this method was effective and reproducible and allowed evaluating the adhesion of the endodontic materials even when bond strength was low.

The tensile bond strength test is more sensitive than the push-out test, in such a way that even small changes in the specimen or in stress distribution during load application affect significantly the results[492,489]. On the other hand, the micro-push-out test, for use in smaller areas, yields the development of a more uniform shear bond strength without the interference of the tensile component, thus producing a stress more reliably directed at the adhesive interface[150,350,489].

Another relevant aspect that should be considered is in adhesive tests, is the failure type obtained after debonding. The specimens should be to expose the internal portion of the canals to be analyzed at stereoscopic magnifying glass or scanning electron microscope to evaluate the presence/absence of sealer inside the dentinal tubules and to determine the failure modes. The fracture was considered adhesive – when occurred in the dentine/sealer or core material/sealer interface, cohesive – when the rupture happened in the filling material, and mixed - when combined both failure modes. In most cases, the sealer was almost completely dislodged from the specimen (dentin or solid material). In the SBS test to flat surface, the line located around the specimen favours an uniform distribution of the load applied during shearing rather than if the load would have been applied on a single point. Nevertheless, failure occurred on the sealer borders and sealer remnants are usually found on dentin surface in almost all debonded specimens. However, failure within the sealer is generally observed in the areas closer to the apex. Given that the debonding force exerted on the specimens in the push-out test is in the apex-cervical direction, it may be inferred that there is greater load distribution in the apical region, resulting in cohesive failure within the sealer in this area and part of the fractured sealer covering the dentin.

Although the test models cannot reproduce the exact clinical conditions, mainly because root dentin is not uniform and the surface of the canal walls prepared during the endodontic treatment may differ considerably[406], bonding laboratory tests can be used as a screening mechanism for predicting clinical performance.

It is important to emphasize that due to its resin nature, good flow and long setting time, adhesive sealer penetrates deeper into the surface microirregularities. These properties lead to greater intertwining of the sealer with dentin structure, which, together with the cohesion among the cement molecules[428], provides greater adhesiveness and resistance to dislodgment from dentin[430]. Nevertheless, these new resin based-filling materials have not had the same extensive evaluation that gutta-percha and conventional sealers have had.

Besides, because the adhesive capacity of internal radicular dentine is quite ambiguous and depends on the dentin tubule pattern, which differs significantly not only from one tooth to another but can also differ within the same tooth, there was a need to develop a method that would allow the evaluation of this adhesive capacity using internal radicular dentine as a sample, thus allowing the understanding of how adhesion occurs on dentine walls in a situation as close as possible of the root canal. Further studies with these promising adhesive materials should be conducted to search for an effective method to reduce the fracture susceptibility of root-filled teeth.

## 21.7 Gutta-percha Points

Gutta-percha is the core material in the cones for filling root canals. It consists of a vegetable substance from the genus Pallaquium, existent in Sumatra and Philippines, zinc oxide, calcium carbonate, barium sulfate and strontium sulfate, pulverized catgut, waxes, resins, tonic acids, dye and carnation oil. Gutta-percha has several advantages over other core materials, as follows: the possibility of condensation and adaptation to the irregularities of root canals, the capacity of being mollified by the heat or solvent, being inert, showing acceptable dimensional stability, being tolerated by the tissues, not altering the dental color, being radiopaque, and being easy to remove from the root canal.

Gutta-percha is insoluble in water, distinctly soluble in eucalyptol, soluble in ether, xylene, benzene, halothane, turpentine and chloroform. The chapter with regard to the retreatment techniques discusses the application of gutta-percha solvents.

The root canal must be hermetically filled in order to hinder communication between its interior and the periapical tissues. Many studies have been developed with the object of studying the factors that could influence the sealing property of root canal fillings. Thus, Holland et al.[183] determined whether gutta-percha points with calcium hydroxide improve the apical seal after root canal filling and whether the master point does it alone. Single, recently extracted human teeth were biomechanically prepared and the root canals filled by the lateral condensation technique with ZOE and gutta-percha points, with or without calcium hydroxide. The teeth were placed into a 2% methylene blue solution in a vacuum environment for 24 hours, after which they were processed for stereomicroscope evaluation. Better results were observed with the teeth filled with gutta-percha points with calcium hydroxide. These new points make a better apical seal and these results can also be obtained with the calcium hydroxide master point associated with regular ones. The real influence of apical leakage on the healing process after root canal treatment must be better analyzed.

## 21.8 Procedures Prior to Filling

Some procedures are carried out before filling, such as smear layer and intracanal dressing removal, when present. Removal of the smear layer, theme already discussed in the chapters about irrigant solutions and root canal preparation, must be done before placement of the intracanal medication. The remainder of the calcium hydroxide can reduce dentine permeability[207]. After removing the intracanal medication (calcium hydroxide paste), the main cone can be selected.

When considering smear layer removal before root canal filling, it is important to consider different investigations[37,284,468,469,513].

Some studies found that smear layer removal did not enhance the sealing ability[284,468,469,513]. On the other hand, the smear layer can undergo microbial leakage and provide a supportive substrate, interfering with the accurate adaptation of the material. Behrend et al.[37] observed that smear layer removal during canal filling enhanced sealability, as shown by increased resistance to bacterial penetration.

Shahravan et al.[413], based on a systematic review, determined whether smear layer removal reduces leakage of filled human teeth in vitro. PubMed was searched for articles published between 1975 and 2005, and results were categorized, based on the leakage test method. Among 26 eligible papers with 65 comparisons, 53.8% of the comparisons reported no significant difference, 41.5% reported a difference in favor of removing the smear layer, and 4.7% reported a difference in favor of keeping it; differences were significant. Of the 65 comparisons, 44 used the dye leakage test for evaluation. The combined effect in this group showed smear layer removal decreases dye leakage. According to a meta-regression, filling type, test site and duration, sealer and dye, and publication year had no effect on the results. In conclusion, considering the conditions of these in vitro leakage studies, smear layer removal improves the fluid-tight seal of the root canal system, whereas other factors, such as the filling technique or the sealer used, did not produce significant effects. The dye leakage test was the favorite means for evaluating the effects of smear layer removal, and the site of the test, type of dye, and year of publication did not significantly affect the final outcome.

### Main Cone Selection

The adequate adaptation of the main cone in the prepared pulp cavity must allow the minimum space for the filling sealer, as this material performs its unique and exclusive function of impermeableness and aggregation agent. The main cone should be manufactured in accordance with the size and shape of the last instrument that was used in the apical region. A gutta-percha conformer can be used to suit the main cone to the characteristics of the canal space.

The major problem of the main cones is the way it is produced. The type, and standard of the making depend on quality control.

The fit of the main cone to the walls of the root canal favors better endodontic sealing. The degree of enlargement and the instrumentation technique influence the adaptation of the main cone. The compatible diameter is chosen considering the diameter of the last instrument used in the root canal. The contraction and expansion limit of the main gutta-percha cone becomes critical, because, as these cones are more malleable, their diameters can be modified more easily.

The main cone must be selected by introducing it into the canal inundated by an irrigant. Adaptation means fitting it into the length must be done with apical pressure, and the cone should offer certain resistance to the removal.

## 21.9 Root Canal Filling Techniques

The literature shows that there are several techniques and systems of root canal filling (lateral condensation, vertical condensation, McSpadden, Schilder, Tagger techniques; Endotec, System B, Therma Fill, Obtura II, Ultra Fill systems, etc (Fig. 21.8). All these resources were developed with intention of overcoming the complex internal morphology, capable of being well sealed. Parallel to the filling techniques, root canal preparation techniques were developed in the search for a continuous taper, which favors root canal filling material insertion, and respects the anatomic particularities of the canals. A suitable process would be to use one technique for conventional situations, and when necessary, use non-conventional techniques.

## 21.10 Lateral Condensation Technique with Gutta-Percha

The lateral condensation technique with gutta-percha is the best known and most used root canal filling technique. After preparation of the root canal, which must have a conical shape, the main cone must be selected. Then, periapical radiography confirms its position in the length. The root canal is dried and the root canal sealer is prepared. The paper point must be sterilized. While the drying procedure is in progress, the main cone is kept in a plate with three divisions, immersed in sodium hypochlorite as a previous anti-sepsis.

Manipulation of the endodontic sealer varies according to the type of sealer chosen. It must comply with the proportion indicated by the manufacturer. For the paste/paste type sealers, the mixture must be homogeneous. For the sealers containing eugenol, care must be taken with the powder – liquid proportion as the higher the proportion of liquid in the sealer, the more irritant it becomes.

The sealer is taken to the root canal with the main cone, covering its entire extent, including its tip. The aim is to keep sealer in contact with all the walls of the root canal. Initially, two or three cones are introduced, stabilizing the main cone, and then the space among these and the lateral walls is opened with the accessory cone, which will penetrate to the same extent as the spreader. In some situations, the 2 or 3 first accessory cones are able reach the desired extent without the aid of the spreader. With the removal of the spreader an accessory cone of suitable diameter should immediately follow to occupy the space created. This procedure is repeated until the spreader does not find space to penetrate below the cervical third. It is convenient if the position of main cone is not changed with each insertion of new accessory cones; the ideal is that if it is kept in the buccal aspect of an anterior tooth, the same point of introduction of the spreader allows the placement of the following accessory cones.

The quality of the filling can be verified by periapical radiography, before the gutta-percha points are cut. If the apical third shows spaces, this can be still improved, or all the filling material can be removed and the operation repeated. The spaces in the cervical and middle thirds can be corrected with further lateral and vertical condensation. After the final quality of the filling has been verified, gutta-percha is cut in the opening of the canals with a heated condenser, to accommodate it inside the root canal. Figures 21.9AD to 21.11, by diagrammatic representations and radiographic aspects, show root canals filled by the lateral and vertical condensation techniques with gutta-percha.

Estrela et al.[109] determined the effectiveness of lateral condensation in the endodontic seal In longitudinal studies by means of a systematic review. A MEDLINE search strategy was developed to identify articles using the following uniterms: Root canal filling, condensation lateral, condensation vertical, McSpadden, Thermafil, System B, Thermal Compaction, Tagger, in different combinations. The search included articles from the bibliographic catalogue identified electronically (MEDLINE, EMBASE, CENTRAL) (http://www.ncbi.nlm.nih.gov/PubMed), from 1966 up to January 14$^{th}$ of 2008. The studies were selected by two independent reviewers, who had also determined the inclusion and exclusion criteria. The search presented 372 related articles (Fig. 21.12). Twenty nine articles were related to studies in vivo (human or animal), 267 in vitro studies and 92 were not related to root canal filling. Of the 29 in vivo studies, none satisfied the inclusion criteria, which disabled the analysis. The topic of the root canal filling generates few scientific conflicts, particularly because the lateral condensation technique with gutta-percha associated with filling cement became consensus between the majority of endodontists. Based on the method of study considered, it seems opportune to conclude that the articles that were analyzed did not satisfy the inclusion criteria. Considering the success of clinical behavior, the lateral condensation technique used by endodontists is the most studied and has the highest success rate.

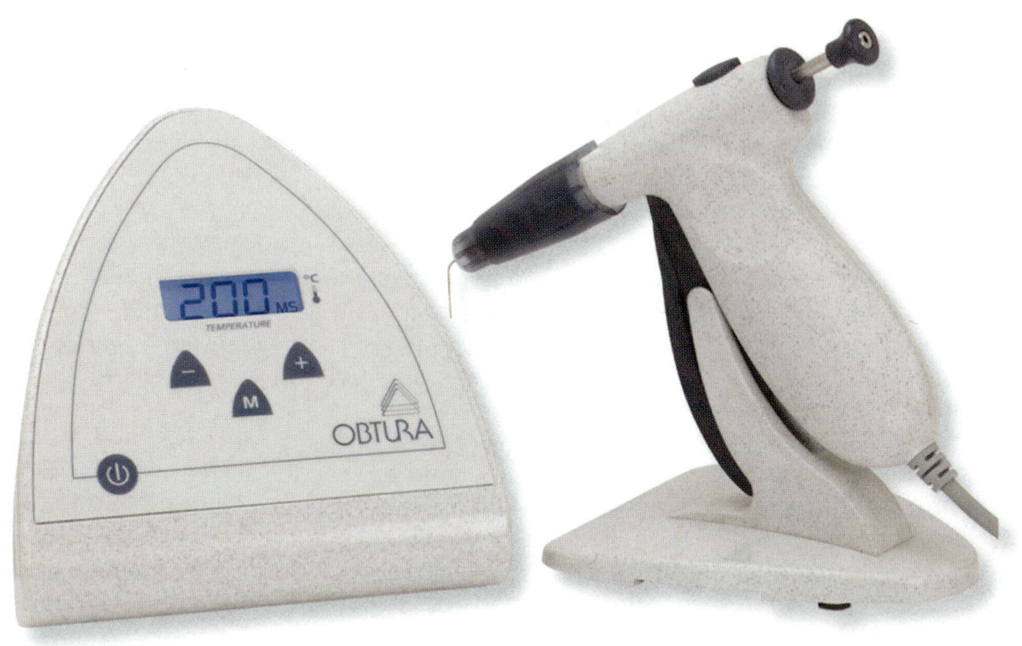


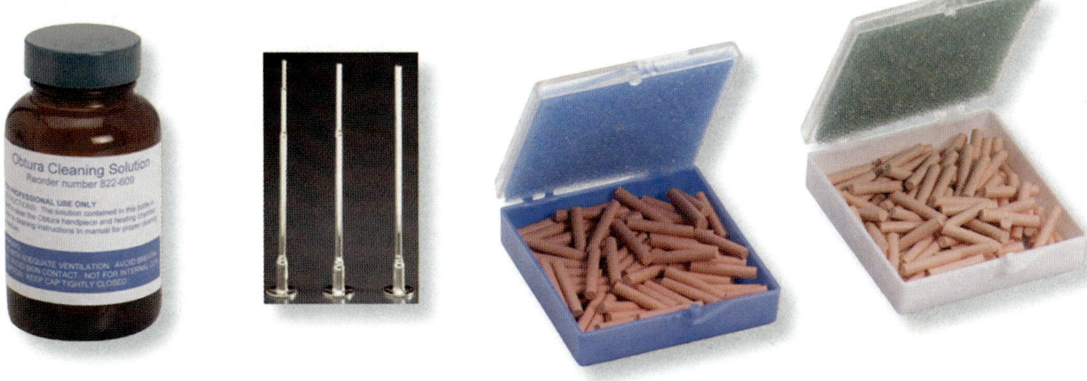


**Figure 21.8** - Obtura II System (Courtesy of J.Morita).

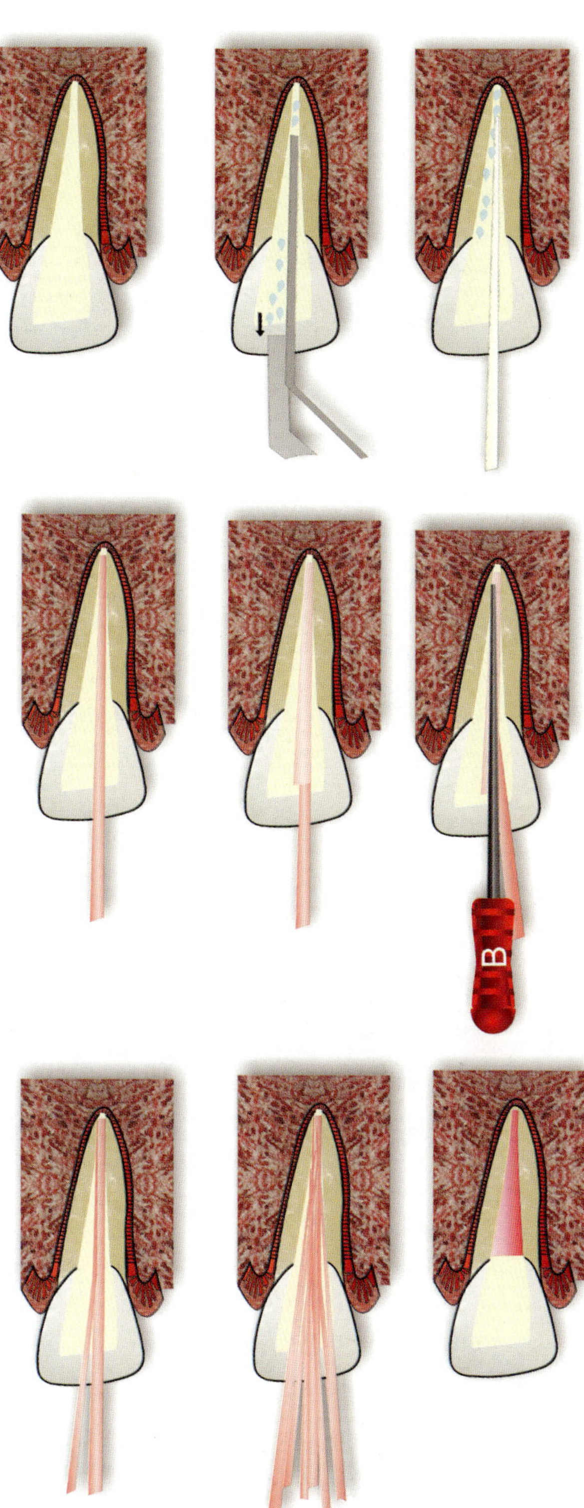


**Figure 21.9A** - Schematic representation of root canals filled by the lateral and vertical condensation techniques with gutta-percha.

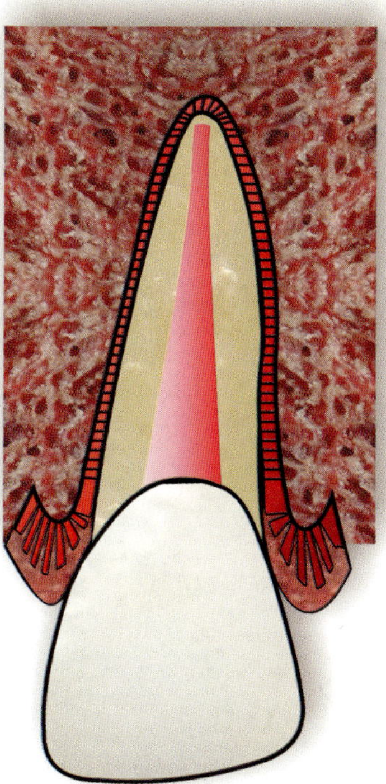

**Figure 21.9B** - Schematic representation of root canals filled by the lateral and vertical condensation techniques with gutta-percha.

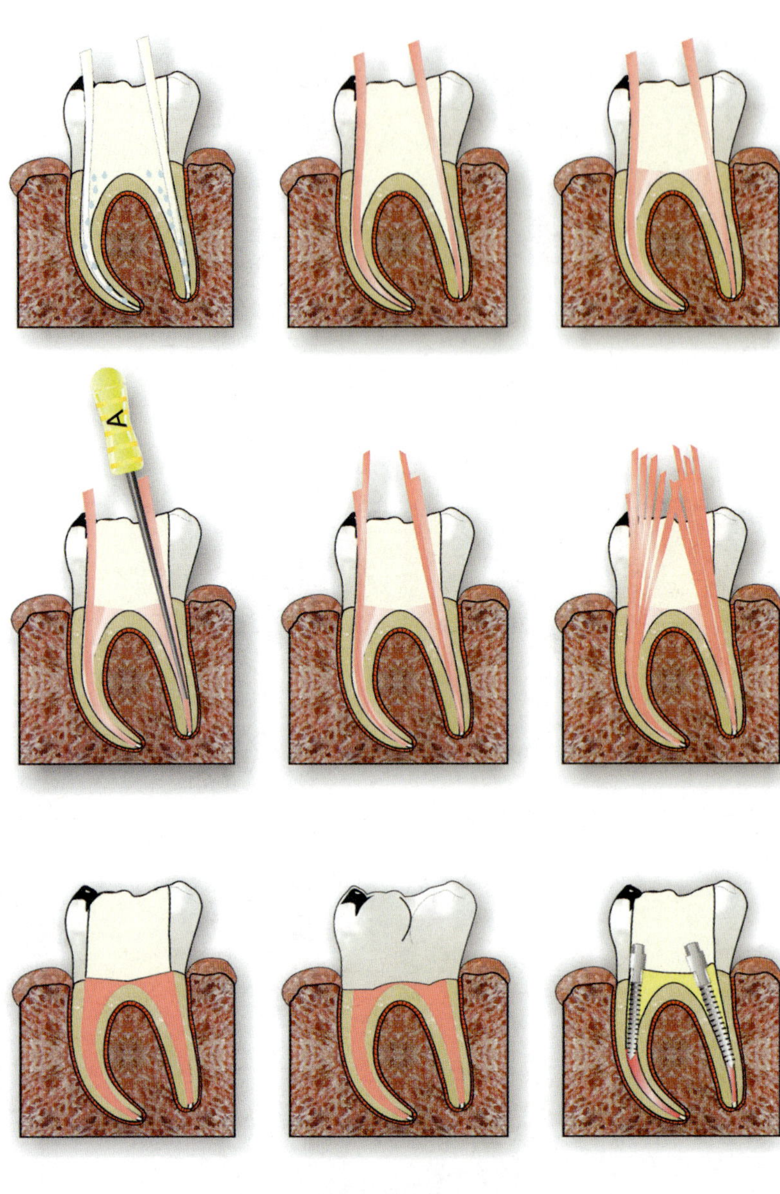


**Figure 21.9C** - Schematic representation of root canals filled by the lateral and vertical condensation techniques with gutta-percha.

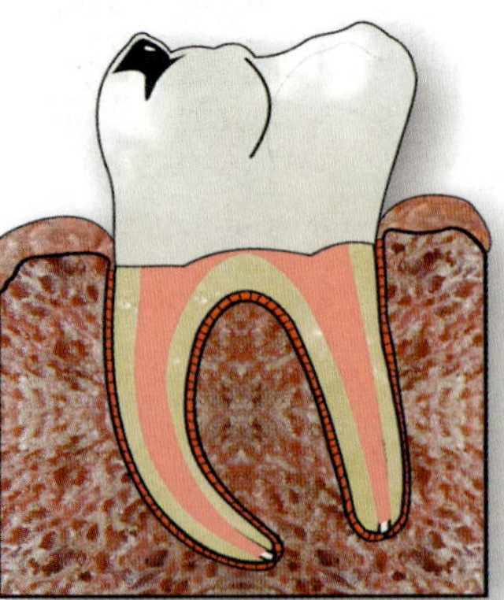

**Figure 21.9D** - Schematic representation of root canals filled by the lateral and vertical condensation techniques with gutta-percha.

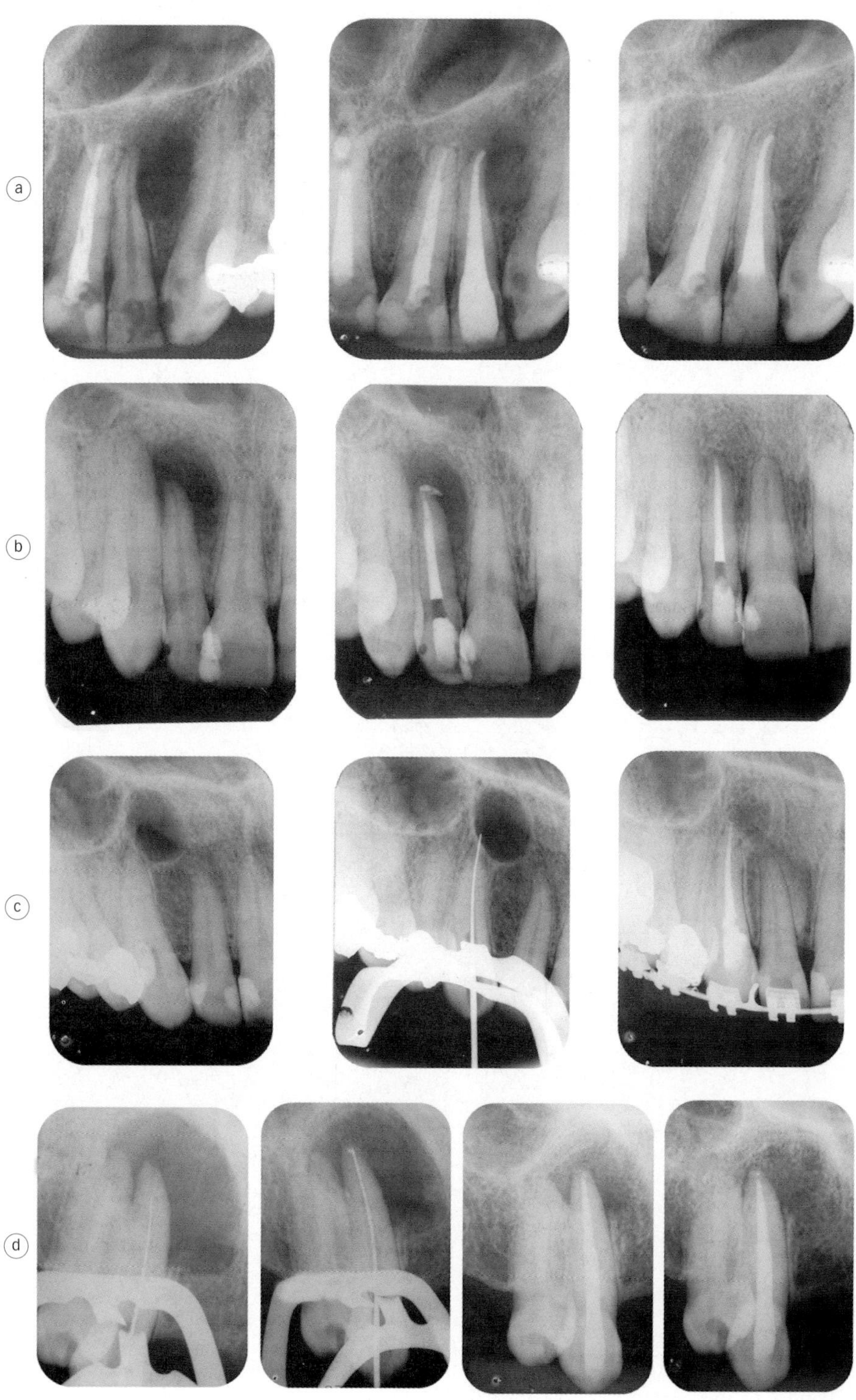


**Figure 21.10** - (A-D) Radiographic aspects show root canals filled by the lateral and vertical condensation techniques with gutta-percha.

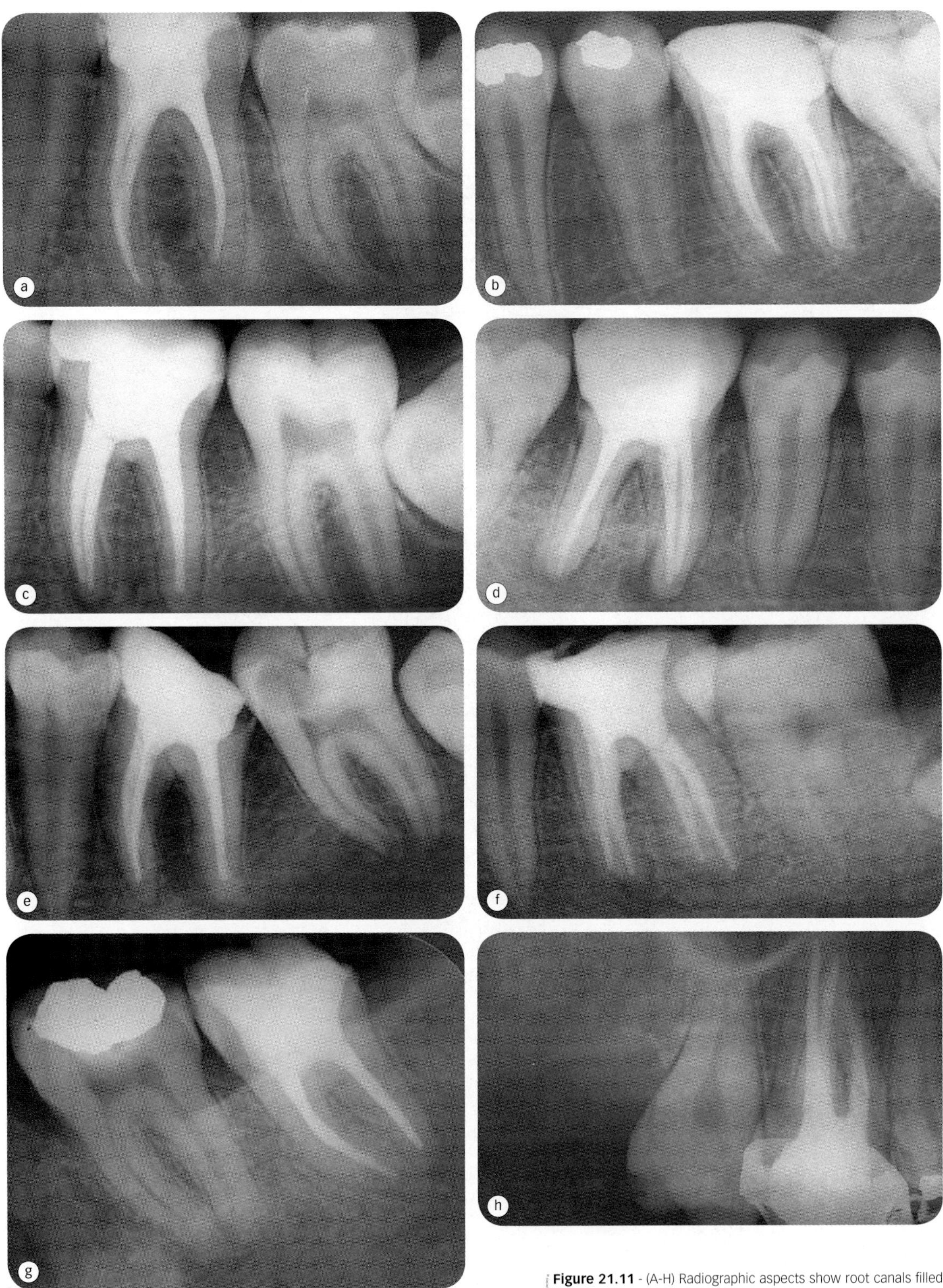


**Figure 21.11** - (A-H) Radiographic aspects show root canals filled by the lateral and vertical condensation techniques with gutta-percha.

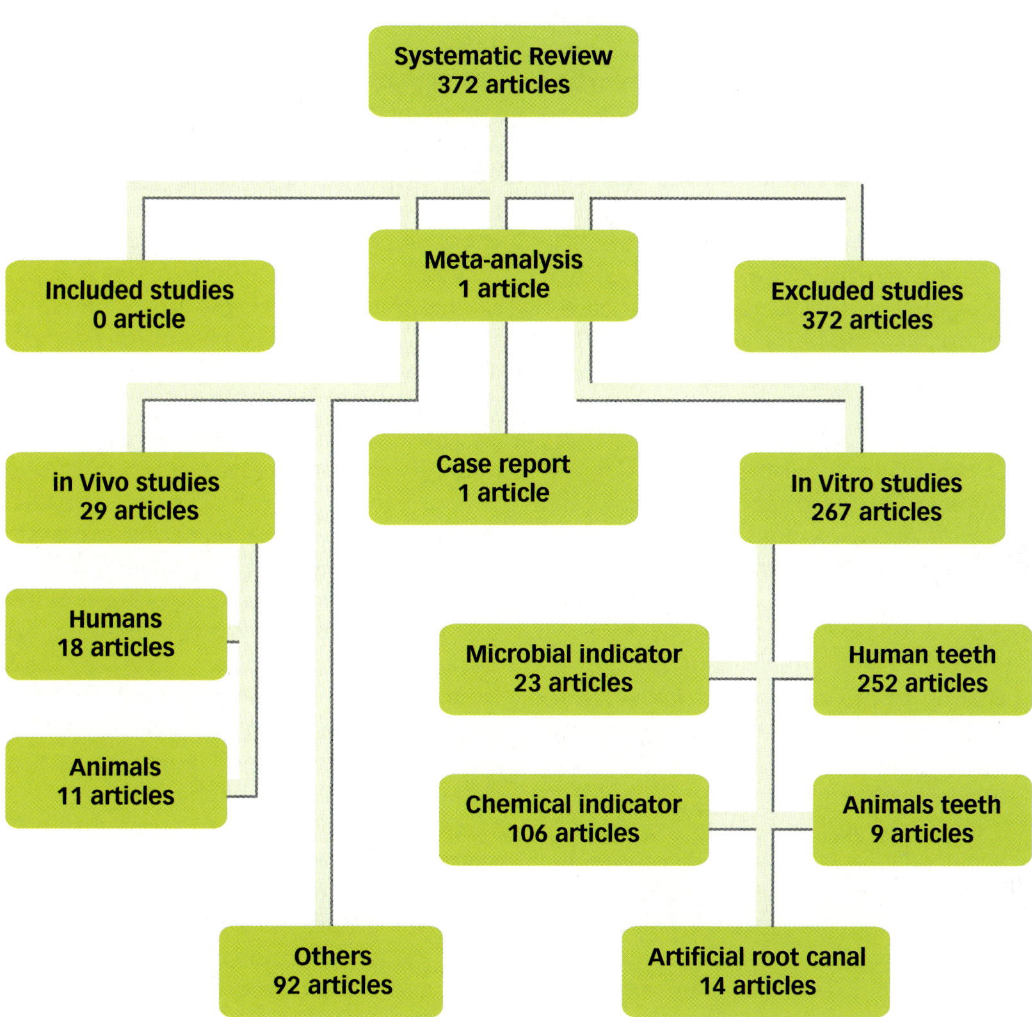


**Figure 21.12** - Distribution of the studies for the systematic review[109].

## 21.11 Contemporary Filling Alternatives

Some maneuvers complementary to the lateral condensation can be used in special situations. In extremely large canals, rolled points can be used. These cones are made utilizing 2 or 3 major core points. With two plates of glass, of which at least one has to be warmed, sliding on each other, the cones are interposed, until the heat plasticizes and then unites them. The plate which moves must be inclined to maintain the conic aspect of the newly prepared cone. By rubbing repeatedly, its diameter decreases. The cone, however, is made according to the need of the case, substituting the traditional main cone. The accessory cones supplement the customized cone by the lateral condensation technique. With the approach of cones with taper of 0.04 and 0.06mm, filling under these conditions is less complex. Another maneuver which can be used with lateral condensation is molding of the main cone. Using the heat resource, which can be the flame of a night lamp, the cone of more or less 2 cm is brought close to it, and then the cone is quickly put into to the root canal up to the working length. A mark is made on the cone (with a cotton tweezers) to determine the position in which it should be put back again.

The canal is dried, and lateral condensation is achieved as usual in the traditional technique. Several maneuvers can be developed for accommodating the material in the root canal, thus, part of the gutta-percha that fills the cervical and middle thirds can be removed, and reinforces the vertical condensation of the gutta-percha (described as the Nguyen[320] vertical and lateral condensation technique). A widely disseminated technique is the one proposed by Schilder[398-402]. However, the number of operating steps, need for skills and training on the operator's part are taken into account, because the technique has become more popular since it was published. This technique is only possible to perform in very well prepared and tapered canals. After the introduction of the endodontic sealer, the main cone is put into the length with more sealer. The cone is cut in the coronal portion with warmed instrument. With a vertical condenser, the cone is condensed in the apical direction. With heat carriers, 2 to 3mm of cone is cut, followed by vertical condensation with a cold instrument. This procedure must be repeated, with smaller instruments, until approximately 4mm of gutta-percha is left. These procedures are known as down-packing. The goal of this phase is to make the apical region susceptible to the action of the heat and pressure, which makes the gutta-percha flow to the ramifications, sometimes shown by radiography. The cervical and middle thirds, now empty, are filled by using small segments of warmed gutta-percha, put inside the root canal and compacted until all the space is filled.

The control of deviation of the filling material and the force exerted in the vertical condensation are imprecise. These critical aspects represent arguable points of the technique, as over-filling and vertical fracture can occur. To help to reduce the time taken to conclude filling by this technique, some devices were developed, such as Touch'n Heat (Analytic Technology, USA), the Endotec (Caulk-Dentsply) and the System B. These systems are automatic warmers with tips of different diameters and shapes.

McSpadden[301] showed a different way of warming and compacting gutta-percha. It consists of a rotary instrument, which looks like an inverted Hedströem file. The gutta-percha point is heated by rotating the instrument and is plasticized and compacted in the direction of the apices. The compaction leads the gutta-percha and the endodontic sealer into the lateral canals, and fills the ramifications, in similar way to Schilder's technique. The original technique recommended the use of a main cone of a larger diameter than the last apical instrument to be placed with endodontic sealer. The cone is plasticized and led to the apical region.

This technique underwent alterations. The most significant of them was the proposal of Tagger et al.[449] who associates lateral condensation with the use of the McSpadden compactor. The lateral condensation technique is carried out until the apical third is replete with secondary cones. The compactor is put into action slowly until 2mm of the working length, taking care to adjust the motor in the clockwise direction. With the gutta-percha plasticization and its pressure in the apical direction, the compactor is gradually pushed out of the canal. The result is generally a compact and homogeneous filling in the full extent of the canal, in a short time, and with small quantity of accessory cones. One must be reminded that the selected compactor must be two diameters bigger than the main gutta-percha cone.

The flutes of the McSpadden compactor had their angulations reduced, which made the compaction more controllable. The tip became inactive, which decreased the risk of fracture of the instrument and extrusion of the gutta-percha beyond the apical foramen.

Other items of equipment and techniques were proposed, in an attempt to valorize the advantages of gutta-percha thermo-plasticization, even considering the risks, especially of the absence of control over the plasticized material. Among the systems, some use pistols with thermo-plasticized gutta-percha, such as the Obtura System (Texaed-USA) and Ultrafill (Hygienic-USA).

Thermafil (Tulsa-USA) is another widely disseminated and developed technique after obtaining a solid nucleus around gutta-percha in the alpha phase. When put into a special oven for a short time, the gutta-percha becomes warmed and softened. It is then put inside the canal, after the sealer has been placed. The solid nucleus (made of plastic) is cut at the entrance of the root canal.

The lack of apical control is the major limitation of this system.

Peng et al.[348] related that a large number of in vitro studies were conducted to compare the outcome of root canal filling by warm gutta-percha with cold lateral condensation. The conclusions were inconsistent or contradictory, and less pertinent than those of clinical studies. In this study, based on meta-analysis, the authors evaluated the differences in the clinical outcome of root canal filling by warm gutta-percha (GP) or cold lateral condensation (CLC) through a systematic review and meta-analysis. There were 10 clinical studies evaluated. Postoperative pain, long-term outcomes, filling quality, and overextension were the characteristics investigated. The results suggest that the two filling techniques do not differ significantly, except as regards overextension. The relative risk (RR) value of warm GP versus CLC and 95% confidence interval (CI) of the first three criteria were 1.10 (0.71, 1.71), 0.78 (0.58, 1.05), and 1.31 (0.98,1.76), respectively. Overextension was more likely to occur in the warm GP filling group in comparison with the CLC group. The RR value and 95% CI were 1.98 (1.33, 2.93). The results of this meta-analysis demonstrated that a higher incidence of overextension was seen in the warm GP filling group than in the CLC group. The filling quality, long-term outcome, and prevalence of postoperative pain were similar between these two groups. A subgroup meta-analysis will be performed in the near future in new studies.

## 21.12 Coronal Seal

There is consensus at present that endodontic treatment ends with restoration of the tooth; that is, with the definitive coronal sealing. Thus, coronal sealing is as important as the sealing of the apical region (Fig. 21.13).

Wu & Wesselink[529] discussed the significance of coronal sealing as a determinant factor for the success of endodontic treatment. The basis of this investigation was the evaluation of semi-quantitative and quantitative methods. The studies used in this investigation evaluated the failure of endodontic treatments as a result of partially filled canals, or their inadequate instrumentation and sanitization. The results of most of the leakage in vitro's studies, have shown questionable clinical importance, since the lateral condensation technique used clinically, shows high success rates, but results of studies conducted in vitro reveal that over 1/3 of the canals filled with this technique show high levels of dye penetration. To try to reduce the variations among the methodologies applied, the length and anatomy of all the teeth should be similar and controlled, and pH of the known solutions used should preferably be neutral.

Ray & Trope[369] evaluated the relationship between the quality of the coronal restoration and the root canal filling, with the presence of periapical pathology. One thousand and ten radiographs of different teeth treated endodontically and restored with definitive restorations were selected. The results showed that 61.07% of the evaluated teeth did not present periapical inflammation. The good restoration resulted in significantly more cases of absence of periapical inflammation when compared with teeth with good endodontic treatment (80% versus 75.7%). The poor restorations resulted in significantly more cases of presence of periapical inflammation when compared with poor endodontics (30.2% versus 48.6%). The arrangement between good restoration and good endodontics resulted at 91.4% of cases of absence of periapical inflammation, while the arrangement of poor endodontics and poor restoration resulted at 18.1% of absence of periapical inflammation. Kirkevang et al.[259] evaluated the radiographs of 773 root-filled teeth to investigate the quality of endodontic treatments and coronal restorations as well as their association with periodontal status and reported a prevalence of 52.3% of AP. Inadequate root canal filling and coronal restoration were associated with an increased incidence of AP. Tronstad et al.[483] evaluated the possible relationship between the quality of the coronal restoration, the quality of the endodontic filling and the periapical health of 1001 endodontically treated teeth that had coronal restorations. Teeth with or without posts were considered during the radiographic analysis. The results showed 67.4% of endodontic success. Teeth with intra-radicular posts showed a success rate of 70.7%; while those without posts showed 63.6%. Good endodontics combined with good restorations showed 81% of success; good endodontics combined with poor restoration showed 71% of success; poor endodontics combined with good restoration showed 56% of success; poor endodontics combined with poor restoration showed 57% of success. Estrela et al.[110] assessed the prevalence and risk factors of apical periodontitis in endodontically treated teeth in a selected population of Brazilian adults. A total of 1,372 periapical radiographs of endodontically treated teeth were analyzed based on the quality of root filling, status of coronal restoration and presence of posts associated with apical periodontitis (AP). Data were analyzed statistically using Odds Ratio, Confidence Intervals and Chi-square test. The prevalence of AP with adequate endodontic treatment was low (16.5%). This number dropped to 12.1% in cases with adequate root filling and adequate coronal restoration. Teeth with adequate endodontic treatment and poor coronal restoration had a 27.9% prevalence of AP. AP increased to 71.7% in teeth with poor endodontic treatment associated with poor coronal restoration. When poor endodontic treatment was combined with adequate coronal restoration, the AP was 61.8%. The prevalence of AP was low when associated with high technical quality of root canal treatment. Poor coronal restoration increased the risk of AP even when endodontic treatment was adequate (OR=2.80; 95%CI=1.87-4.22). The presence of intracanal posts had no influence on the prevalence of AP (Table 21.6, Fig. 21.14).

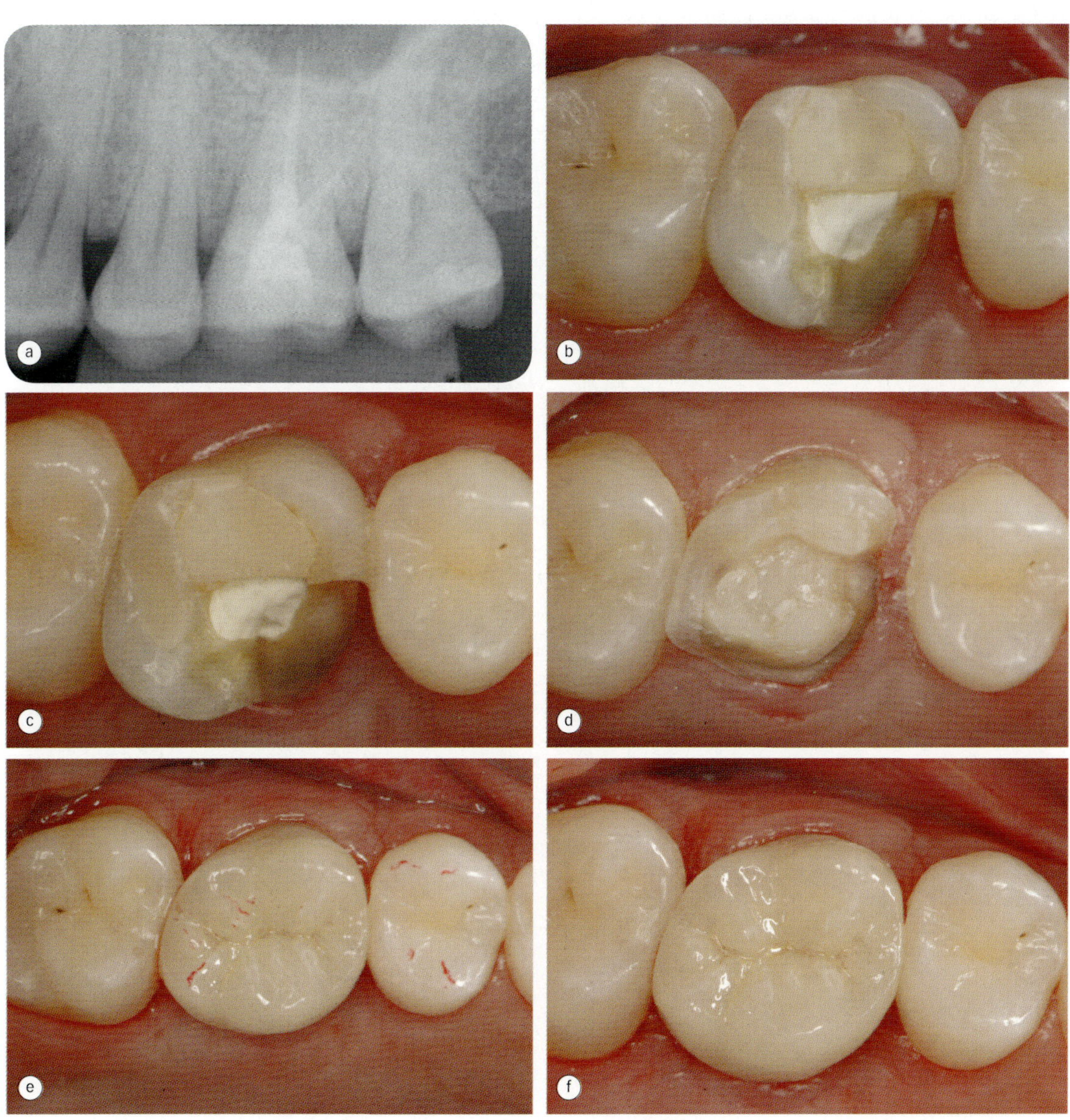


**Figure 21.13** - Coronal sealing (Courtesy of Prof. Lawrence Gonzaga Lopes).

**Table 21.6** - Prevalence of apical periodontitis as influenced by the quality of the endodontic treatment and coronal restoration, and the presence of intracanal post (n=1,372)

| Factor | n (%) | Prevalence of apical periodontitis n (%) | *p** | OR (CI 95%) |
|---|---|---|---|---|
| Endodontic treatment | | | | |
| Adequate | 781 (56.9) | 129 (16.5) | 0.000 | 9.96 (7.66 – 12.95) |
| Poor | 591 (43.1) | 392 (66.3) | | |
| Coronal Restoration | | | | |
| Adequate | 881 (64.2) | 265 (30.1) | 0.000 | 2.53 (2.00 – 3.20) |
| Poor | 491 (35.8) | 256 (52.1) | | |
| Intracanal Post | | | | |
| Absent | 768 (56.0) | 305 (39.7) | 0.134 | 0.85 (0.67 – 1.06) |
| Present | 604 (44.0) | 216 (35.8) | | |
| Combined endodontic treatment and coronal restoration | | | | |
| Adequate endodontic treatment (n=781) | | | | |
| Adequate coronal restoration | 562 (72.0) | 68 (12.1) | 0.000 | 2.80 (1.87 – 4.22) |
| Poor coronal restoration | 219 (28.0) | 61 (27.9) | | |
| Poor endodontic treatment (n=591) | | | | |
| Adequate coronal restoration | 319 (54.0) | 197 (61.8) | 0.011 | 1.57 (1.09 – 2.25) |
| Poor coronal restoration | 272 (46.0) | 195 (71.7) | | |

* Chi-square test

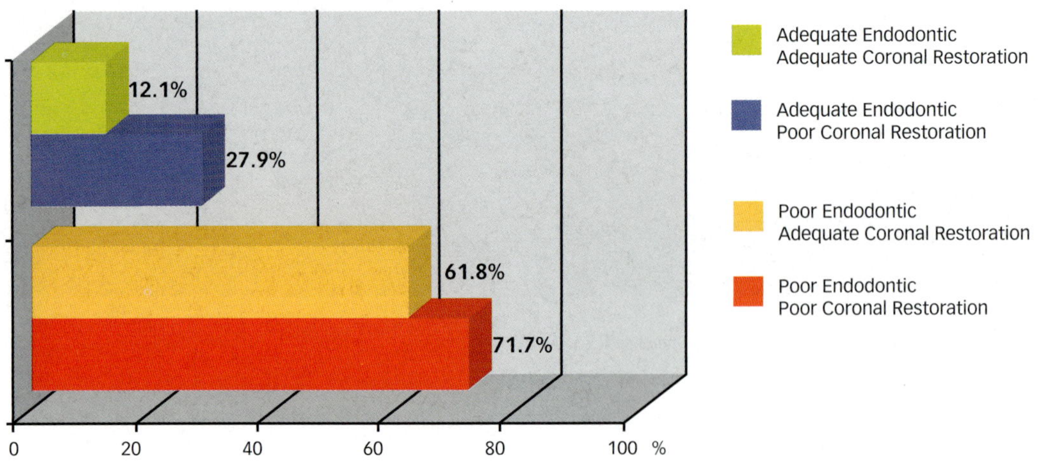


**Figure 21.14** - Prevalence of apical periodontitis as determined by the combination of endodontic treatment and coronal restoration

According to the final evaluation, it was postulated that from the radiographic point of view, the technical quality of the endodontic treatment is equally as important as the quality of the coronal restoration, when the analysis of the periapical region served as criterion of success.

Kersten et al.[254] investigated the capacity of filling to prevent the leakage of bacterial components and protein macromolecules; they also investigated whether the penetration of ethylene blue is comparable to the penetration of metabolic bacterial products of similar sizes. The endotoxin used was cytotoxic *E. coli* 055:B5. The bacterial particles and protein macromolecules cannot infiltrate with the use of sealer and pressure only at the time of the filling with gutta-percha. Leakage of small molecules, such as butyric acid, could not be prevented in this study, irrespective of the filling method used, the infiltration of butyric acid proved to be comparable with that of ethylene blue.

One of the serious problems that have been found in the endodontic clinic is the period in which the tooth remains with a temporary restoration until the definitive treatment. Considering all the inconveniences that occur due to coronal microbial infiltration, it is observed that the definitive restoration must be done immediately. The situation becomes a little more complex when the tooth receives preparation for an intraradicular retainer and remains with sealing on a temporary crown for a longer period. The internal sealing must as adequate as possible, in order to avoid possible re-infection. It is noticed that during the endodontic treatment, every care is taken to carry out an aseptic procedure. Similar care must be established as routine when the tooth is to receive an intraradicular retainer, irrespective of the operator's level of specialty. The ideal would be for the endodontist to prepare the root canal for the intraradicular retainer, and if necessary, to cement the post.

One of the materials that have been accepted as temporary restoration material is glass ionomer, in order to protect the fractured tooth and to prevent microbial leakage (Fig. 21.15).

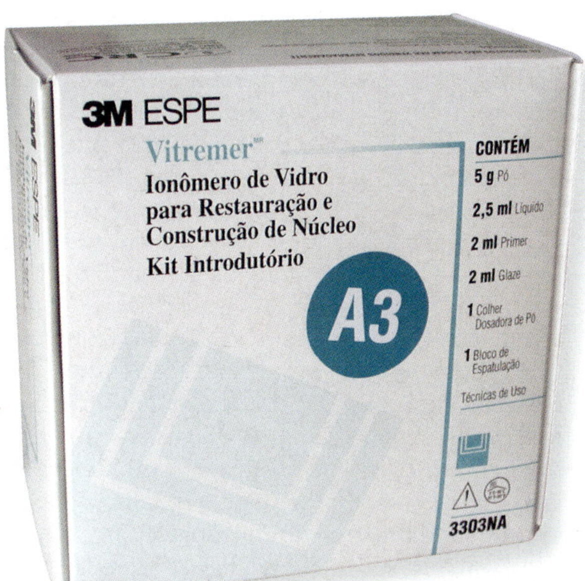


**Figure 21.15** - Glass ionomer.

Coronal and apical microbial leakage along with coronal restoration and apical root canal fillings have been considered strongly associated with endodontic failures. This fact shows the importance of guaranteeing endodontic infection control by perfect coronal-endodontic sealing. The factors, which are normally able to influence the prevalence of endodontic treatment success, emphasize the need for better knowledge about the performance of restoration materials after post space preparation in the presence of remaining apical root fillings. Lopes-Filho & Estrela[285] evaluated the sealing ability of root canal filling remnants when using Sealapex and EndoFill, by means of different microbial indicators. Thus, 40 single-rooted human teeth were used, which were shaped until the file #50 and assigned to 2 groups based on the endodontic sealers. For each group, there was a subdivision based on the length of the remaining apical filling (4, 5 and 6 mm). In the study model, a platform was used, which was split into two halves: an upper chamber – where the microbial suspension containing the biological indicators was introduced (*E. faecalis* + *S. aureus* + *P. aeruginosa* + *B. subtilis* + *C. albicans*); and a lower chamber containing the culture medium Brain Heart Infusion, in which 3 mm of the apical region of teeth were kept immersed. Interpretations of the time it took for microbial leakage to occur were made daily for 60 days, using the turbidity of the culture medium, which is indicative of microbial contamination, as a reference. The outcomes showed no significant difference between the sealers assessed, when the time it took for microbial leakage to occur was compared, and leakage was noted in all the comparative groups. When the results of the remaining filling level were compared, between 4 and 5 mm and 5 and 6 mm, no significant differences were found; however, when 4 and 6 mm levels were compared significant differences were noted. The Figures 21.16 show by schematic representation the endodontically treated tooth and the intraradicular retention associated with a coronal restoration.

Holland et al.[181] evaluated the influence of coronal leakage on the healing of dog's periapical tissues after root canal filling, post space preparation, and with or without protection with a temporary sealer plug. Forty root canals of dog teeth were instrumented and filled with gutta-percha points using the lateral condensation technique, and Endomethasone or CRCS sealers. After post space preparation, the remaining filling material was either protected or not, with a plug of temporary Coltosol sealer and exposed to the oral environment for 90 days. After this, the animals were sacrificed and the specimens were removed and prepared for histomorphological and histobacteriological analysis. The findings revealed 35% of microbial leakage in the groups without plugs and 15% of leakage in the groups with plugs. Statistical analysis showed that the use of a Coltosol plug significantly improved the histomorphological results, irrespective of the type of root canal sealer and that CRCS and Endomethasone sealers showed similar results.

Barbosa et al.[22] observed the influence of coronal leakage on the behavior of periapical tissues after root canal filling and post space preparation. Forty root canals of dog teeth were instrumented and filled with gutta percha points using the lateral condensation technique, and the cements Sealer 26 and Roth. After post space preparation, the remaining filling material was either protected or not with a plug of the temporary cement Lumicon. After root canal exposure to the oral environment for 90 days, the animals were killed and specimens were removed and prepared for histomorphological analysis. The Brown and Brenn technique showed 70% of cases with microorganism leakage for Roth cement, and 20% with Sealer 26. When a plug of Lumicon was used, there was 30% leakage for Roth cement and 0% for Sealer 26. A chronic inflammatory reaction was more frequently observed with Roth cement than with Sealer 26. It was concluded that a plug of Lumicon was efficient in controlling microorganism coronal leakage, and that Sealer 26 was more biocompatible and sealed root canals better than Roth sealer.

Holland et al.[182] evaluated the coronal leakage in vitro after root canal filling and post space preparation. One hundred single-rooted human teeth had their crowns removed and the canals prepared and filled with gutta-percha points using the lateral condensation technique and the sealers CRCS and Endofill (a Grossman sealer). After post space preparation, the remainder of the filling was either protected or not with 1mm of a plug of the following materials: Coltosol, Super Bonder (cyanoacrylate-ester), CRCS and Endofill. After 24 hours in saline solution, the specimens were immersed in a 2% methylene blue solution in a vacuum environment for 24 hours. The teeth were then sectioned longitudinally, leakage was evaluated linearly and the data obtained were submitted to the Kruskal-Wallis test. The results with the two studied sealers were similar between them and worse than the groups with a protector plug. The statistical analysis ranked the experimental groups from the best to the worst in the following order: a – Endofill-Super Bonder, CRCS-Super Bonder, CRCS-CRCS; b – Endofill-Endofill; c – Endofill-Coltosol, CRCS-Coltosol; d – Endofill, CRCS.



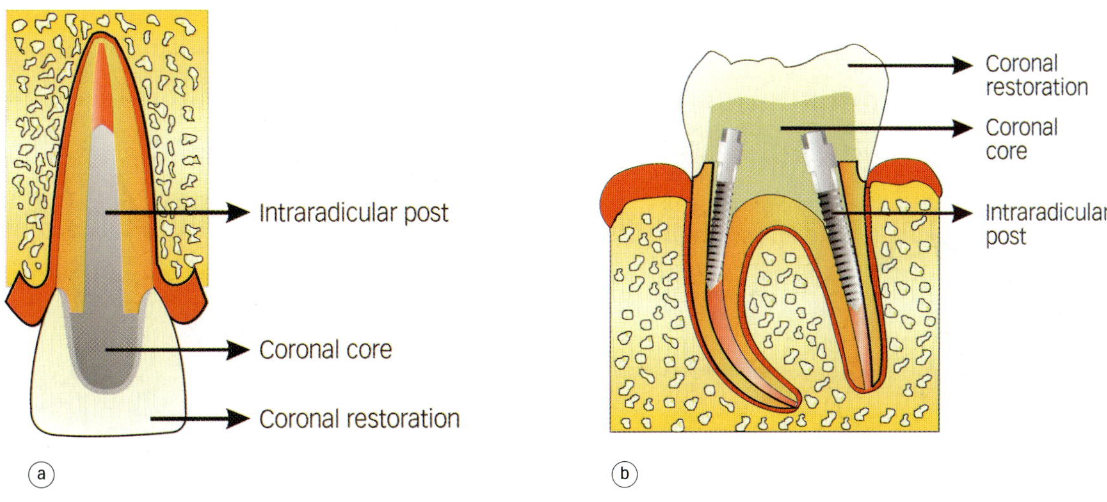


**Figure 21.16** - (A,B) Schematic representation of the endodontically treated tooth and the intraradicular retention associated with a coronal restoration.

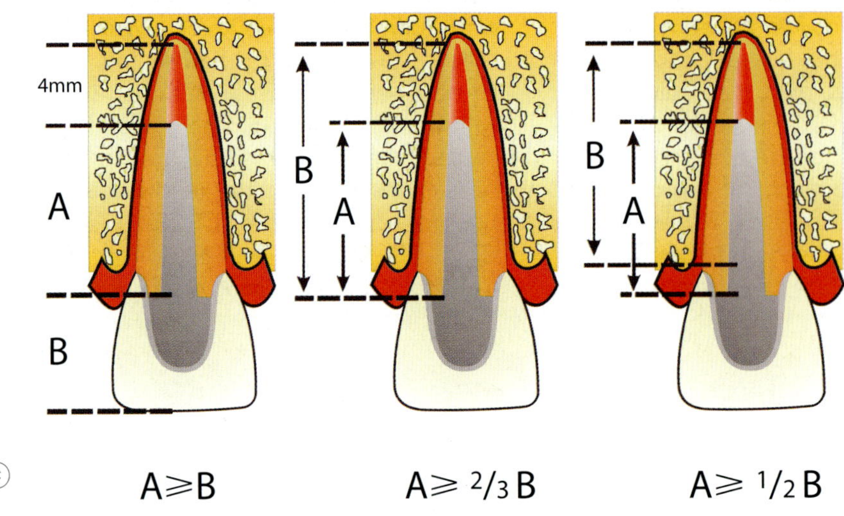


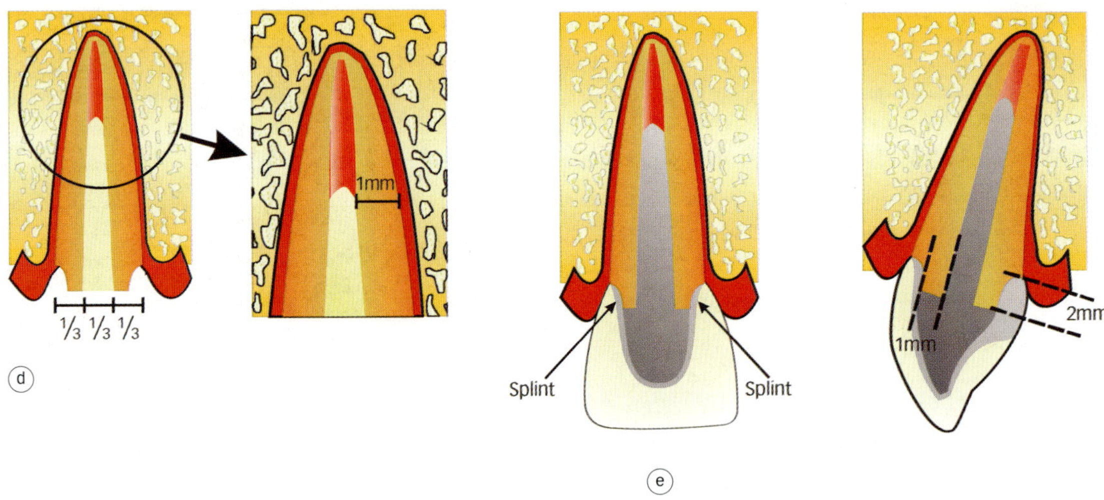


**Figure 21.16** - (C-E) Schematic representation of the endodontically treated tooth and the intraradicular retention associated with a coronal restoration.

Thus, a clinical condition that could be favorable to microbial leakage is responsible for a questionable prognosis and may be a critical factor in the future of endodontic treatment. Veloso et al.[493] investigated the microbial microleakage of temporary restorative materials after post space preparation. Forty-two maxillary anterior human teeth were distributed according to the temporary restorative materials used: Coltosol, IRM, Vidrion R. The teeth were prepared and filled with gutta-percha and Sealapex sealer using the lateral condensation technique, maintaining 4mm of remaining apical filling. Calcium hydroxide paste was used to fill the post space preparation, leaving 4mm in the cervical region to be filled by experimental materials. An in vitro microbial leakage test (MLT) with a split chamber was used in this assay. A mixture of polymicrobial marker (*S. aureus + E. faecalis + P. aeruginosa + B. subtilis + C. albicans*) was placed in the upper chamber and it could only reach the lower chamber containing Brain Heart Infusion broth by way of microleakage through the tested material. Microbial microleakage was verified daily for 90 days. The results showed that all the temporary restorative materials investigated (Coltosol, IRM, Vidrion R) allowed microbial microleakage during the 90 day period. The presence of calcium hydroxide paste in the post space did not interfere in the sealing ability. The quantity of microbial cells that promoted turbidity was not analyzed. The main focus was to evaluate the sealing potential of temporary restorations in teeth prepared for posts. Clinical considerations about the results of this study reinforces that in order to obtain an ideal performance of coronal restoration and a higher rate of endodontic treatment success, it is mandatory to provide an immediate and appropriate definitive coronal restoration as soon as possible after root canal treatment.

Therefore, it is important to consider that according Chailertvanitkul et al.[67], the number of microorganisms required to cause apical periodontitis is still unknown.

The current conception of a concluded endodontic treatment involves the perfect and definite coronal sealing. Some clinical conditions are necessary for preparing the post space, such as the maintenance of a small remaining apical root canal filling and the use of temporary restorative materials. In these cases, the teeth present a higher probability of microbial microleakage and this interferes in periapical health.

A new root filling material, claimed to have optimal sealing capacity has been introduced to Endodontics. Resilon Research LLC (Madison, CT, USA) proposed the use of Resilon filling cones associated with a resin-based sealer - Epiphany Root Canal Sealant (Pentron Clinical Technologies, Wallingford, CT, USA). According to the manufacturer, Resilon thermoplastic synthetic polymer-based cones have an optimal bond to both root dentin and resin-based endodontic sealers, such as Epiphany The so-called Resilon/Epiphany system creates a "monoblock" effect, in which Resilon cones, Epiphany sealer and dentin surface become a single structure[459-462,466,467,489].

Hollanda et al.[219] compared microorganism leakage through root canals filled with Sealer 26, AH Plus or Resilon/Epiphany. Forty maxillary anterior human teeth were randomly assigned to 3 groups according to the resin-based filling materials. An in vitro microbial leakage test (MLT) with a split chamber was used. A mixture of polymicrobial markers (*S. aureus + E. faecalis + P. aeruginosa + B. subtilis + C. albicans*) was placed in the upper chamber and they could only reach the lower chamber containing Brain Heart Infusion broth by way of leakage through the root canal filling. Microbial leakage was verified daily for 60 days. The materials were further evaluated by an agar diffusion test (ADT). Microbial leakage through the root canal filling mass occurred within 6 to > 60 days (minimum of 6, 16 and 22 days and median of 26.8, 42.3 and 46.8 days for Resilon/Epiphany, AH Plus and Sealer 26, respectively). There were no statistically significant differences between Sealer 26 and AH

Plus, and both materials had statistically significant less microbial leakage than Resilon/Epiphany (Table 21.7). AH Plus and Resilon/Epiphany showed an antimicrobial potential in the agar diffusion test. The antimicrobial characteristics of the sealers were not sufficient to prevent the leakage of the bacteria/yeast mixture through the root canal filling mass.

Shipper et al.[415] using *S. mutans* and *E. faecalis* compared bacterial leakage through gutta-percha and Resilon root fillings using two filling techniques: lateral and warm vertical condensation or continuous wave of condensation (System B). The results showed statistically significant differences between the groups. Roots filled with Resilon had minimal leakage, which was significantly less than that observed for roots filled with gutta-percha. All Resilon and Epiphany sealer groups leaked significantly less than all groups in which AH 26 was used as a sealer (gutta-percha and Resilon and AH 26). There was no statistically significant difference in leakage between the Resilon groups. Gesi et al.[138] analyzed the interfacial strengths of Resilon/Epiphany and gutta-percha/AH Plus using a thin-slice push-out test design. The results showed that the interfacial bond strength of Resilon/Epiphany to intraradicular dentin was not higher than that of gutta-percha/AH Plus. Ungor et al.[489] assessed the bond strength of Epiphany/Resilon root canal filling system and compared this with the bond strengths of different pairings of AH Plus, gutta-percha, Epiphany and Resilon. The results showed that within the limits of the push-out test method, the bond strength of the Epiphany sealer/Resilon core combination was not superior to that of the AH Plus sealer/ gutta-percha core combination. Tay et al.[463] examined the susceptibility of Resilon to the action of some hydrolytic enzymes that are present in saliva or secreted by endodontically relevant bacteria. Resilon and polycaprolactone exhibited extensive surface thinning and weight losses after incubation in lipase PS and cholesterol esterase. This study showed that Resilon is biodegradable under the attack of hydrolytic ester bond-cleaving enzymes that may exist as a component of the salivary enzymes.

It is important to report that smear layer removal by EDTA promotes an increase in dentinal permeability, which may influence microbial leakage. Smear layer removal has been shown not to enhance the sealing ability. Pashley et al.[337] considered that the smear layer could favor microorganisms by functioning as a substrate.

**Table 21.7** - Minimum and maximum periods (days) in which microbial microleakage occurred and mean rank of comparisons among the tested sealers

| Materials | N | Minimum (days) | Maximum (days) | Mean rank |
|---|---|---|---|---|
| Sealer 26 | 10 | 22 | > 60 | 20.20 (A) |
| AH Plus | 10 | 16 | > 60 | 17.50 (A) |
| Resilon/Epiphany | 10 | 6 | 42 | 8.80 (B) |

The higher the values in minimum, maximum and mean rank, the less the microbial leakage (Kruskal-Wallis test).

*Different uppercase letters indicate statistically significant difference at $p<0.05$

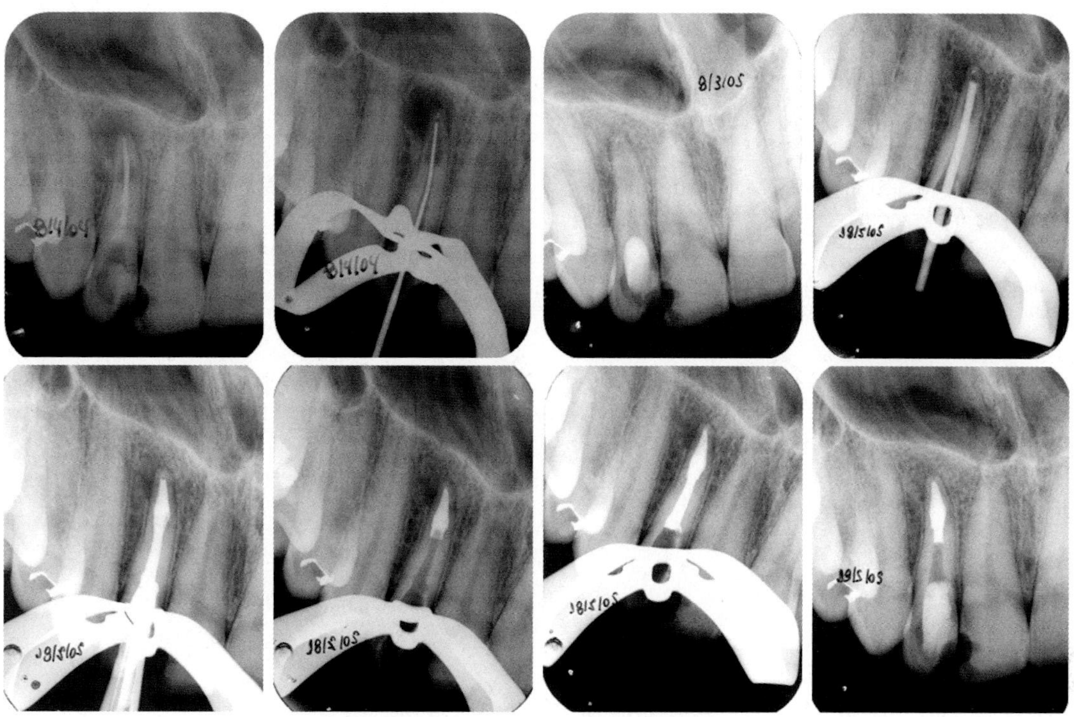

**Figure 21.17A** - Radiographic aspects show root canals filled by the lateral and vertical condensation techniques with gutta-percha.

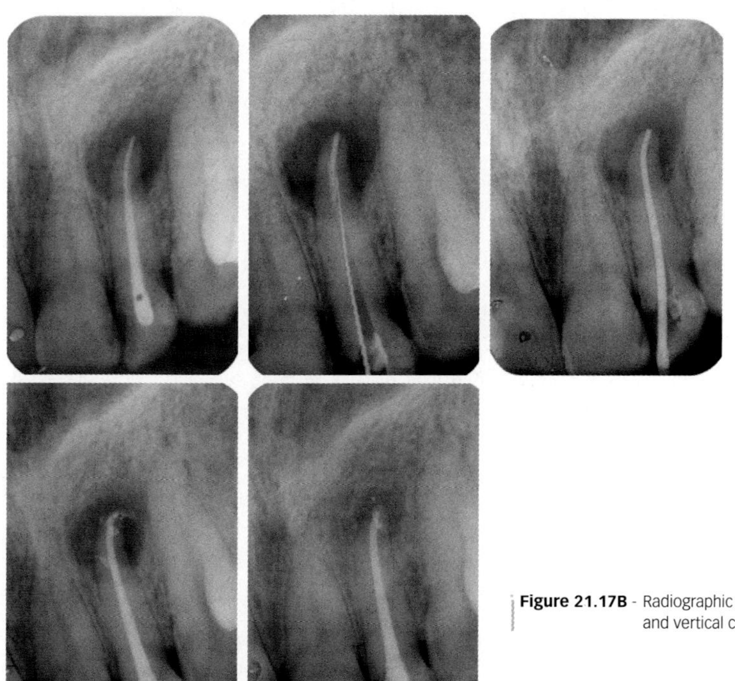

**Figure 21.17B** - Radiographic aspects show root canals filled by the lateral and vertical condensation techniques with gutta-percha.

## REFERENCES


1. Abarca AM, Bustos A, Navia M. A comparison of apical sealing and extrusion between Thermafil and lateral condensation techniques. J Endod 2001;27:670-2.
2. Abdulkader A, Duguid R, Saunders EM. The antimicrobial activity of endodontic sealers to anaerobic bacteria. Int Endod J 1996;29:280-283.
3. Abramovich A, Goldberg F. The relationship of the root canal sealer to the dentine wall. An in vitro study using the Scanning Electron Microscope. J Brit Endod Soc 1976;9:81-6.
4. Abramovitz I, Tagger M, Tamse A, Metsger Z. The effect of immediate vs. delayed post space preparation on the apical seal of a root canal filling: a study in an increased-sensitivity pressure-driven-system. J Endod 2000;26:435-9.
5. Adamo HI, Buruiana R, Schertzer I, Boylan RJ. A Comparison of MTA, super-EBA, composite and amalgam as root-end filling materials using a bacterial microleakage model. Int Endod J 1999;32: 197-203.
6. Adib V, Spratt D, Ng Y-L, Gulabivala K. Cultivable microbial flora associated with persistent periapical disease and coronal leakage after root canal treatment: a preliminary study. Int Endod J 2004;37:542-51.
7. Ahlberg KMF, Assavanop P, Tay WM. A comparison of the apical dye penetration patterns shown by methylene blue and india ink in root-filled teeth. Int Endod J 1995;28:30-34.
8. Alaçam T, Yoldas O, Gülen O. Dentin penetration of 2 calcium hydroxide combinations. Oral Surg Oral Med Oral Pathol 1998;86:469-72.
9. Al-Dewani N, Hayes SJ, Dummer PM. Comparison of laterally condensed and lowtemperature thermoplasticized gutta-percha root fillings. J Endod 2000;26:733-8.
10. Al-Dewani N, Hayes SJ, Dummer PM. Evaluation of the Trifecta obturating technique. Endod Dent Traumatol 2000;16:75-83.
11. Al-Turki M, Akpata ES. Penetrability of dentinal tubules in adhesive-lined cavity walls. Oper Dent 2002;27:124-31.
12. Alves J, Walton R, Drake D. Coronal Leakage: Endodtoxin penetration from mixed bacterial communities through obturated, post-prepared root canals. J Endod 1998;24:587-91.
13. Alves PRV, Aranha N, Alfredo E, Marchesan MA, Brugnera-Jr A, Sousa-Neto MD. Evaluation of hollow fiberoptic tips for the conduction of Er:YAG laser. Photomed Laser Surg 2005;23:410-5.
14. American Dental Association. Council on Dental Materials. Specification no 57 for endodontic filling material, Chicago, 1984. p.147-169.
15. American National Standards Institute Specification No. 57 for endodontic filling materials. J Amer Dent Ass 1984;108:88.
16. Anderson RW, Powell BJ, Pashley DH. Microleakage of three temporary endodontic restorations. J Endod 1998;14:497-501.
17. Antonopoulos KG, Attin T, Hellwig G. Evaluation of the apical seal of root canal fillings with different methods. J Endod 1998;24:655-58.
18. Apicella MJ, Loushine RJ, West LA, Runyan DA. A comparison of root fracture resistance using two root canal sealers. Int Endod J 1999;32:376-80.
19. Aqrabawi JA. Outcome of endodontic treatment of teeth filled using lateral condensation versus vertical compaction. J Contemp Dent Prac 2006;7:17-24.
20. Bakhordar RA, Bui T, Waranabe L. An evaluation of sealing ability of calcium hydroxide sealers. Oral Surg Oral Med Oral Pathol 1989;68:88-92.
21. Balto H. An assessment of microbial coronal leakage of temporary filling materials in endodontically treated teeth. J Endod 2002;28:762-4.
22. Barbosa HG, Holland R, Souza V, Dezan-Junior E, Bernabé PFE, Otoboni-Filho JA, Nery MJ. Healing process of dog teeth after post-space preparation and exposition of the filling material to the oral environment. Braz Dent J 2003;14:103-8.
23. Barbosa SV, Araki K, Spångberg LSW. Citotoxicity of some modified root canal sealers and their leachable components. Oral Surg Oral Med Oral Pathol 1993;75:357-361.
24. Barkhordar RA, Russel T. Effect of doxycycline on the apical seal of retrograde filling materials. J Calif Dent Assoc 1998;26:842-5.
25. Barkhordar RA, Stark MM, Calif SF. Sealing ability of intermediate restorations and cavity design used in endodontics. Oral Surg Oral Med Oral Pathol 1990;69:99-101.
26. Barkins W, Montgomeny S. Evaluation of Thermafil obturation of curved canals prepared by the Canal Master-U System. J Endod 1992;18:285-9.
27. Barkmeier WW, Cooley RL. Laboratory evaluation of adhesive systems. Oper Dent 1992;Suppl 5:50-61.
28. Barkmeier WW, Cooley RL. Shear bond strength, microleakage and SEM study of the XR Bond adhesive system. Am J Dent 1989;2:111-5.
29. Barkmeier WW, Huang CT, Hammesfabr PD, Jefferies SR. In vitro evaluation of two new dentin adhesive systems. J Esthet Dent 1989;1:164-7.
30. Barkmeier WW, Huang CT, Hammesfahr PD, Jefferies SR. Bond strength, microleakage, and scanning electron microscopy examination of the Prisma Universal Bond 2 adhesive system. J Esthet Dent 1990;2:134-9.
31. Barrieshi KM, Walton RE, Johnson WT, Drake DR. Coronal leakage of mixed anaerobic bacteria after obturation and post space preparation. Oral Surg Oral Med Oral Pathol 1997;84:310-4.
32. Barthel CR, Zimmer S, Wussogk R, Roulet JF. Long term bacterial leakage along obturated roots restored with temporary and adesive fillings. J Endod 2001;27:559- 62.
33. Beach CW, Calhoun JC, Bramwell JD, Hutter JW, Miller GA. Clinical evaluation of bacterial leakage of endodontic temporary filling materials. J Endod 1996;22:459-62.
34. Becker TA, Donnelly JC. Thermafil obturation: a literature review. General Dentistry 1997;45:46-55.
35. Begg C, Cho M, Eastwood S, HortonR, Moher D, Olkin I, Pitkin R, Rennie D, Schulz KF, Simel D, Stroup

DF. Improving the quality of reporting of randomized controlled trials. The CONSORT statement. J Amer Dent Ass 1996;276:637-9.
36. Behr M, Rosentritt M, Regnet T, Lang R, Handel G. Marginal adaptation in dentin of a self-adhesive universal resin cement compared with well-tried systems. Dent Mater 2004;20:191-7.
37. Behrend GD, Cutler CW, Gutmann JL. An in-vitro study of smear layer removal and microbial leakage along root-canal fillings. Int Endod J 1996;29:99-107.
38. Bellizi R, Cruse WP. A historic review of endodontics, 1689-1963, part 3. J Endod 1980;6:577- 589.
39. Beltes P, Koulaouzidou E, Kotoula E, Kortsaris AH. In vitro evaluation of the cytotoxicity of calcium hydroxide-based root canal sealers. Endod Dent Traumat 1995;11:245-49.
40. Benatti O, Stolf WL, Ruhnke LA. Verification of the consistency, setting time, and dimensional changes of root canal filling materials. Oral Surg Oral Med Oral Pathol 1978;46:107-13.
41. Berbert A. Comportamento dos tecidos apicais e periapicais após biopulpectomia e obturação do canal com AH-26, hidróxido de cálcio ou mistura de ambos - estudo histológico em dentes de cães. (Livre Docência Thesis). University of São Paulo;1978. 152p.
42. Berutti E. Microleakage of human saliva through dentinal tubules exposure at the cervical level in teeth treated endodontically. J Endod 1996;22:579-82.
43. Beyer-Olsen EM, Ørstavik D. Radiopacity of root canal sealers. Oral Surg Oral Med Oral Pathol 1981;51:320-28.
44. Bhat KS, Walvekar S. Response of subcutaneous connective tissue to materials and drugs: a simplified technique. J Endod 1975;1:202-204.
45. Bing G, Wei R, Li-chao W. Clinical evaluation of root canal obturation with Thermafil technique. J SUN YAT-SEN University 2005;26:470-2.
46. Bobotis HG, Anderson RW, Pashley DH, Pantera EA. A microleakage study of temporary restorative materials used in endodontics. J Endod 1989;15:569-572.
47. Bombana AC. Estudo comparativo da reação tecidual conjuntiva do subcutâneo de ratos, frente a inserção de tubos de polietileno preenchidos com cimento N-Rickert com e sem extravasamento (contribuição ao estudo). (Master´s Thesis). University of São Paulo; 1981.
48. Bovis SC, Harrington E, Wilson HJ. Setting characteristics of composite filling materials. Brit Dent J 1971;131:352-56.
49. Brannström M, Coli P, Blixt M. Effect of tooth storage and cavity cleansing on cervical gap formation in Class II glass-ionomer/composite restorations. Dent Mater 1992;8:327-31.
50. Brayton SM, Davis SR, Goldman M. Gutta-percha root canal fillings, an in vitro analysis. Part I. Oral Surg Oral Med Oral Pathol 1973;35:226-31.
51. Browne RM. Animal tests for biocompatibility of dental materials - advantages and limitations. J Dent Res 1994;22:21-24. Suplement n. 2.
52. Brugnera-Júnior A, Guerisoli DMZ, Marchesan MA, Spanó JCE, Pécora JD. In vitro evaluation of smear layer removal by Er:YAG laser application with five different fiberoptic tip withdrawal techniques. Proceedings of Laser in Dentistry IX 2003;4950:188-94.
53. Bueno MR, Estrela C. Prevalência de tratamento endodôntico e periodontite apical em várias populações do mundo, detectada por radiografias panorâmicas, periapicais e tomografias computadorizadas cone beam. Rev Odontol Brasil Central 2008;17:79-90.
54. Bueno MR, Estrela C, Azevedo BC, Brugnera-Jr. A, Azevedo JR. Tomografia computadorizada Cone Beam: Revolução na odontologia. Rev Ass Paul Cir Dent 2007;61:325-8.
55. Cahn LR. Silver pigmentation of the gums. Arch Clin Oral Pathol 1938;2:41-44.
56. Cailleteau JG, Mullaney TP. Prevalence of teaching apical patency and various instrumentation and obturation techniques in United States dental schools. J Endod 1997;23:394-396.
57. Caliskan MK, Turkun M, Turkun LS. Effect of calcium hydroxide as an intracanal dressing on apical leakage. Int Endod J 1998;31:173-7.
58. Canalda C, Pumarola J. Bacterial growth inhibition produced by root canal sealer cements with a calcium hydroxide base. Oral Surg Oral Med Oral Pathol 1989;68:99-102.
59. Cardoso RJA. Avaliação in vitro da qualidade do vedamento marginal cérvico-apical de alguns agentes cimentantes utilizados na fixação de um retentor intra-radicular pré-fabricado (CYTCO). (Doctoral Thesis). University of São Paulo;1994.
60. Carrascosa A. Efeito antimicrobiano de alguns cimentos endodônticos. (Doctoral Thesis). University of São Paulo;2000. 78p.
61. Carrotte P. Endodontics: part 8. Filling the root canal system. Br Dent J 2004;197:667-72.
62. Carvalho EMOF, Robazza CRC, Antoniazzi JH, Oliveira AM. Avaliação in vitro do selamento marginal apical de diferentes tipos de cimentos à base de óxido de zinco e eugenol frente a vibração intraradicular ultra-sônica. Rev Paul Odont 1995;17:34-35.
63. Carvalho-Jr JR, Correr-Sobrinho L, Correr AB, Sinhoreti MA, Consani S, Sousa-Neto MD. Solubility and dimensional change after setting of root canal sealers: a proposal for smaller dimensions of test samples. J Endod 2007;33:1110-6.
64. Cataldo E, Santis H. Response of the oral tissue to exogenous foreign materials. J Periodontol 1974;45:93-106.
65. Costa CAS, Teixeira HM, Nascimento ABN, Hebling J. Biocompatibility of two current adhesive resins. J Endod 2000;26:512-516.
66. Cergneux M, Ciucchi B, Dietschi JM, Holz J. The influence of the smear layer on the sealing ability of canal obturation. Int Endod J 1987;20:228-32.
67. Chailertvanitkul P, Saunders WP, Mackenzie D, Weetman DA. An in vitro study of the coronal leakage of two root canal sealers using an obligate anaerobe microbial marker. Int Endod J 1996;29:249-55.
68. Chailertvanitkul P, Saunders WP, Mackenzie D. The effect of smear layer on microbial coronal leakage of gutta-percha root fillings. Int Endod J 1996;29: 242-8.
69. Chailertvanitkul P, Saunders WP, Sunders EM, Mackenzie D. An evaluation of microbial coronal leakage in the restored pulp chamber of root-canal treated multirooted teeth. Int Endod J 1997;30:318-22.
70. Chigira H, Yukitani W, Hasegawa T, Manabe A, Itoh K, Hayakawa T, Debari K, Wakumoto S, Hisamitsu H. Self-etching dentin primers containing phenyl-P. J Dent Res 1994;73:1088-95.

71. Chu CH, Lo EC, Cheung GS. Outcome of root canal treatment using Thermafil and cold lateral condensation filling techniques. Int Endod J 2005;38:179-85.
72. Clinton K, Van Himel T. Comparison of a warm gutta-percha obturation technique and lateral condensation. J Endod 2001;27:692-5.
73. Cobankara FK, Üngör M, Belli S. The effect of two different root canal sealers and smear layer on resistance to root fracture. J Endod 2002;28:606-9.
74. Cocleti G. Avaliação da solução Kodak RPX-amat quando utilizada na processadora T4, da Dupont, quanto às densidades ótica e radiográfica, analisadas pelo fotodensitômetro MRA e pelo sistema digital Digora. (Doctoral Thesis). University of São Paulo;1999. 88p.
75. Cohen S, Burns RC. Pathways of the pulp. 8 th ed. Philadelphia: St. Louis: Mosby, 2002. 483p.
76. Coward DD. Partial randomization design in a support group intervention study. West J Nurs Res 2002;24:406-21.
77. Curson I, Kirk EEJ. An assessment of root canal-sealing cements. Oral Surg Oral Med Oral Pathol 1968;26:229-36.
78. Dahl JE. Toxicity of endodontic filling materials. Endod Topic 2005;12:99-43.
79. Davalou S, Gutmann JL, Nunn MH. Assessment of apical and coronal root canal seals using contemporary endodontic obturation and restorative materials and techniques. Int Endod J 1999;32:388-96.
80. Davis JL, Jeansonne BG, Davenport WD, Gardiner D. The effect of irrigation with doxycycline or citric acid on leakage and osseous wound healing. J Endod 2003;29:31-5.
81. Dayan D, Buchner A, Moskona D, Sperling I. Pigmentation of the oral mucosa after root canal filling with AH-26. A light and electron microscopic study. Clin Prevent Dent 1983;5:25-29.
82. De La Macorra JC, Escribano NI. Comparison of two methods to measure permeability of dentin. J Biomed Mater Res 2002;63:531-4.
83. Degee AJ, Wu MK, Wesselink PR. Sealing properties of Ketac-Endo glass ionomer cement and AH26 root canal sealers. Int Endod J 1994;27:239-44.
84. Deveaux E, Hildelbert P, Neut C, Boniface B, Romond C. Bacterial microleakage of Cavit, IRM, and TERM. Oral Surg Oral Med Oral Pathol 1992;74:634-43.
85. Deveaux E, Hildelbert P, Neut C, Romond C. Bacterial microleakage of Cavit, IRM, TERM, and Fermit: a 21-day in vitro study. J Endod 1999;25:653-9.
86. Dirceu RF. Infiltração microbiana em dentes portadores de próteses unitárias provisórias. (Master's Thesis). Federal University of Uberlândia; 2004.
87. Dixon C, Rickert UG. Histological verification of results of root-canal therapy in experimental animals. J Am Dent Assoc 1938;25:1781.
88. Douglas WH, Zakariasen KL. Volumetric assessment of apical leakage utilizing a spectrophptometic, dye recovery method. J Dent Res 1981;60:438. Abstract 512.
89. Douglas WH. Clinical status of dentine bonding agents. J Dent 1989;17:209-15.
90. Drake DR, Wiemann AH, Rivera EM, Walton RE. Bacterial retention in canal walls in vitro: effect of smear layer. J Endod 1994;20:78-82.
91. Duke ES. Adhesion and its application with restorative materials. Dent Clin North Am 1993;37:329-40.
92. Dummer PMH, Lyle L, Rawle J, Kennedy JK. A laboratory study of root fillings in teeth obturated by lateral condensation of gutta-percha or Thermafil obturators. Int Endod J 1994;27:32-8.
93. Dummett CO, Barens G. Pigmentation of the oral tissues: a review of the literature. J Periodontol 1967;38:369.
94. Economides N, Kovatsi VPK, Poulopoulos A, Kolokuris I, Rozos G, Shore R. Experimental study of the biocompatibility of four root canal sealers and their influence on the zinc and calcium content of several tissues. J Endod 1995;21:122-27.
95. Economides N, Liolios E, Kolokuris I, Belteset P. Long-term evaluation of the influence of the smear layer on the sealing ability of different sealers. J Endod 1999;25:123-25.
96. Egger M, Davey Smith G. Meta-analysis: potentials and promise. Brit Med J 1997;315:1371-4.
97. Egger M, Smith GD, Phillips AN. Meta-analysis: principles and procedures. Brit Med J 1997;315:1533-7.
98. Eldeniz AU, Erdemir A, Belli S. Shear bond strength of three resin based sealers to dentin with and without the smear layer. J Endod 2005;31:293-6.
99. Erausquin J, Devoto FCH. Alveolodental ankylosis induced by root canal treatment in rat molars. Oral Surg Oral Med Oral Pathol 1970;30:105-116.
100. Eriksen HM, Kirkevang L-L, Petersson K. Endodontic epidemiology and treatment outcome: general considerations. Endod Topics 2002;2:1-9.
101. Estrela C. Obturação do canal radicular. In: Estrela C. Ciência Endodôntica. Artes Médicas: São Paulo, 2004. p.539-87.
102. Estrela C, Bammann LL, Estrela CRA, Silva RS, Pécora JD. Antimicrobial and chemical study of MTA, Portland cement, calcium hidroxide paste, Sealapex and Dycal. Braz Dent J 2000;11:3-9.
103. Estrela C, Bammann LL, Lopes HP, Moura JA. Análise comparativa da ação antibacteriana de três cimentos obturadores contendo hidróxido de cálcio. Rev Ass Bras Odontol Nac 1995;3:185-187.
104. Estrela C, Bueno MR, Azevedo B, Azevedo JR, Pécora JD. A New Periapical Index Based on Cone Beam Computed Tomography. J Endod 2008;34:1325-31.
105. Estrela C, Bueno MR, Leles CR, Azevedo B, Azevedo JR. Accuracy of cone beam computed tomography and panoramic and periapical radiography for detection of apical periodontitis. J Endod 2008;34:273-9.
106. Estrela C, Camapum FF, Lopes HP. Prevalência de dor nos retratamentos endodônticos. Rev Bras Odontol 1998;55:18-24.
107. Estrela C, Chaves R, Alencar AHG, Guedes AO, Silva JÁ. Influência do ciemtno obturador no sucesso endodôntico. Rev Odontol Brasil Central 2007;16:28-36.
108. Estrela C, Estrela CRA, Bammann LL, Pécora JD. Two methods to evaluate the antimicrobial action of calcium hydroxide paste. J Endod 2001;27:720-3.
109. Estrela C, Moraes ALG, Alencar AHG, Guedes AO, Silva JÁ. Eficácia da condesnsação lateral de guta-percha no selamento endodôntico. Rev Odontol Brasil Central 2008;17:56-64.
110. Estrela C, Leles CR, Hollanda ACB, Moura MS, Pécora JD Prevalence and Risk Factors of Apical

Periodontitis in Endodontically Treated Teeth in a Selected Population of Brazilian Adults. Braz Dent J 2008:19:34-39.
111. Estrela C, Lopes HP, Figueiredo JAP, Resende EV. Análise do selamento apical produzido pelos cimentos Sealapex, Apexit e Sealer 26. Odonto Ciência 1995;10:81-87.
112. Estrela C, Pesce HF, Resende EV, Sydney GB. Évaluation del sellado apical, al comparar las técnicas de obturación condensación lateral e de Nguyen, empleando cemento a base de óxido de zinc y outro conteniendo hidróxido de cálcio. Rev Asoc Odontol Argentina 1993;81:146-149.
113. Estrela C, Pesce HF, Sydney GB, Figueiredo JAP. Apical leakage using various sealers and root canal filling techniques. Braz Dent J 1994;5:59-63.
114. Estrela C, Siqueira RMG, Resende EV, Silva SA, Silva FAC. Influência da substância química, do cimento obturador e do número de sessões na incidência de pericementite traumática. Rev Odontol Brasil Central 1996;06:09-13.
115. Estrela C, Sydney GB, Bammann LL, Felippe Jr O. Mechanism of action of calcium and hydroxyl ions of calcium hydroxide on tissue and bacteria. Braz Dent J 1995;6:85-90.
116. Eurasquin J, Muruzábal M. Root canal fillings with zinc oxide-eugenol cement in the rat molar. Oral Surg Oral Med Oral Pathol 1967;24:547-58.
117. Fauchard P. Le chirurgien-dentiste - traité des dents. TI. 2nd ed. Paris: Chez Pierre Jean Marriete;1745. 182p apud Bellizi R, Cruse WP. A historic review of Endod. 1689-1963, Part 3. J Endod 1980;6:576-589.
118. Ferrari M, Cagidiaco MC, Gesi A, Balleri P. Preliminary report of an experimental design for in vivo testing of bonded restorations applied to a new enamel-dentinal bonding agent. J Prosthet Dent 1993;70:465-7.
119. Ferrari M, Mason PN, Vichi A, Davidson CL. Role of hybridization on marginal leakage and bond strength. Am J Dent 2000;13:329-6.
120. Ferrari M, Tay FR. Technique sensitivity in bonding to vital, acid-etched dentin. Oper Dent 2003;28:3-8.
121. Fidel RAS. Estudo das propriedades físico-químicas de alguns cimentos obturadores dos canais radiculares contendo hidróxido de cálcio. (Doctoral Thesis). University of São Paulo;1993. 169 p.
122. Figueiredo JAP, Figueiredo MAZ. The histological effects of four endodontic sealers implanted in the oral mucosa: submucous injection versus implant in polyethylene tubes. Int Endod J 2001;34:377-385.
123. Figueiredo MAZ, Lorandi CS, Figueiredo JAP. Oral mucosal tattoo induced by endodontic sealers. Braz Endod J 1996;1:11-14.
124. Figueiredo MAZ. Indução à formação de tatuagem em mucosa bucal de coelhos a partir da injeção submucosa de dois cimentos endodônticos: avaliação clínica e histológica. (Doctoral Thesis). Pontifical Catholic University of Rio Grande do Sul;1993. 118p.
125. Filgueiras J, Bevilacqua S, Melo C. Endodontia clínica. Rio de Janeiro: Científica;1962.
126. Finger WJ, Lee KS, Podszun W. Monomers with low oxygen inhibition as enamel/dentin adhesives. Dent Mater 1996;12:256-61.
127. Fisher EJ, Arens DE, Miller CH. Bacterial leakage of mineral trioxide aggregate as compared with zinc-free amalgam, intermediate restorative material, and super-EBA as a root-end filling material. J Endod 1998;24:176-9.
128. Flanders DH. Endodontic patency. How to get it. How to keep it. Why it is so important. N Y State Dent J 2002;68:30-32.
129. Fogel HM, Peikoff MD. Microleakage of root-end filling materials. J Endod 2001;27:456-8.
130. Foster KH. Removal of $Ca(OH)_2$ from the root canal. J Endod 1991;17:187(Abstract).
131. Franco EB, Lopes LG, D'alpino PH, Pereira JC, Mondelli RF, Navarro MF. Evaluation of compatibility between different types of adhesives and dual-cured resin cement. J Adhes Dent 2002;4:271-5.
132. Frank AL, Abou-Rass M, Simon JHS, Glick DH. Endodonzia clinica e chirurgica. Padova, Italy 1988:63-7 cited by Ricucci D. Apical limit of root canal instrumentation and obturation, part 1 literature review. Int Endod J 1998;31:384-93.
133. Friedman S, Komorowski R, Maillet W, Klimaite R, Nguyen SHQ, Torneck CD. In vivo resistance of coronally induced bacterial ingress by an experimental glass ionomer cement root canal sealer. J Endod 2000;26:1-5.
134. Friedman S, Stabholz A, Tom SE. Endodontic retreatment case selections and technique. J Endod 1990;16:543-49.
135. Friend LA, Browne RM. Tissue reactions to some root filling materials. Brit Dent J 1968;125:291- 298.
136. Gaintantzopoulou MD, Willis GP, Kafrawy AH. Pulp reactions to light-cured glass ionomer cements. Am J Dent 1994;7:39-42.
137. Gale MS, Darvell BW. Dentine permeability and tracer tests. J Dent 1999;27:1-11.
138. Gesi A, Raffaelli O, Goracci C, Pashley DH, Tay FR, Ferrari M. Interfacial Strength of Resilon and Gutta-Percha to intraradicular dentin. J Endod 2005;31:809-13.
139. Gettleman BH, Messer HH, El Deeb ME. Adhesion of sealer cements to dentin with and without the smear layer. J Endod 1991;17:15-20.
140. Gettleman, BH, Messer HH, Eldeeb ME. Adhesión de los cementos selladores a la dentina con y sin barro dentinario. Endodoncia 1991;9:83-91.
141. Gilbert S D, Witherspoon DE, Berry CW. Coronal leakage following three obturation techiniques. Int Endod J 2001;34:293-99.
142. Gilhooly RM, Hayes SJ, Bryant ST, Dummer PM. Comparison of cold lateral condensation and a warm multiphase gutta-percha technique for obturating curved root canals. Int Endod J 2000;33:415-20.
143. Gish SP, Drake DR, Walton RE, Wilcox L. Coronal leakage: bacterial penetration through obturated canals following post preparation. J Am Dent Assoc 1994;125:1369-72.
144. Goldberg F, Massone EJ. Patency file and apical transportation: an in vitro study. J Endod 2002;28:510-511.
145. Goldman LB, Goldman K, Kronman JH, Letoumeau JM. Adaptation and porosity of poly-Hema in a model system using two microorganisms. J Endod 1980;6:863-6.
146. Goldman M, Simmonds S, Rush R. The usefulness of dye-penetration studies reexamined. Oral Surg Oral Med Oral Pathol 1989;67:327-32.

147. Goodis HE, White JM, Moskowitz E, Marshall SJ Root canal system preparation: conventional vs laser methods in vitro. J Dent Res 1992;71:162.
148. Goodman A, Schilder H, Aldrich W. The thermomechanical properties of guttapercha. II. The history and molecular chemistry of gutta-percha. Oral Surg Oral Med Oral Pathol 1974;37:954-61.
149. Goodman A, Schilder H, Aldrich W. The thermomechanical properties of guttapercha. IV. A thermal profile of the warm gutta-percha packing procedure. Oral Surg Oral Med Oral Pathol 1981;51:544-51.
150. Goracci C, Tavares AU, Fabianelli A, Monticelli F, Raffaelli O, Cardoso PC, Tay F, Ferrari M. The adhesion between fiber posts and root canal walls: comparison between microtensile and push-out bond strength measurements. Eur J Oral Sci 2004;112:353-61.
151. Gordon TM, Alexander JB. Influence on pH level of two calcium hydroxide root canal sealers in vitro. Oral Surg Oral Med Oral Pathol 1986;60:624-28.
152. Gorduysus MO, Tasman F, Serdar T. et al. Solubilizaing efficiency of different gutta percha solvents: a comparative study. J Nihon University 1997;39:133-35.
153. Greene HA, Wong M, Ingram TA. Comparison of the sealing ability of four obturation techniques. J Endod 1990;16:423-8.
154. Grossman LI. Endodontic Practice. Philadelphia: Lea & febiger, 1978.
155. Grossman LI. An improved root canal cement. J Am Dent Ass 1958;56:381.
156. Grossman LI. Physical properties of root canal cements. J Endod 1976;2:166-75.
157. Grossman LI. Setting time of selected essential oils with a standard root canal cement powder. J Endod 1982;8:277-279.
158. Grossman LI. Solubility of root canal cements. J Dent Res 1978;57:927.
159. Grossman LI. The effect of pH of rosin on setting time of root canal cements. J Endod 1982;8:326-327.
160. Grove CJ. The value of the dentinocemental junction in pulp canal surgery. J Dent Res 1931;11:466-8.
161. Guigand M. In vitro Study of intradentinal calcium diffusion induced by two endodontic biomaterials. J Endod 1997;23:387-90.
162. Gutiérrez JH, Brizuela C, Villota E. Human teeth with periapical pathosis after overinstrumentation and overfilling of the root canals: a scanning electron microscopic study. Int Endod J 1999;32:40-48.
163. Gutknecht N, Franzen M, Schippers M, Lampert F. Bactericidal effect of a 980 nm diode laser in the root canal wall dentin of bovine teeth. J Clin Laser Med Surg 2004;22, 9-13.
164. Gutknecht N, Franzen R, Meister J, Vanweersch L, Mir M. Temperature evolution on human teeth root surface after diode laser assisted endodontic treatment. Lasers Med Sci 2005;20:99-103.
165. Gutmann JL. Adaptation of injected thermoplasticized gutta-percha in the absence of the dentinal smear layer. Int Endod J 1993;26:87.
166. Gutmann JL. Clinical, radiographic and histologic perspectives on success and failure in endodontics. Dent Clin North Amer 1992;36:379-81.
167. Gutmann JL. Preparation of endodontically treated teeth to receive a post-core restoration. J Prosth Dent 1977;38:413-9.
168. Gutusso JL, Witherspoon DE. Obturation of cleaned and shaped root canal system. In: Cohen S, Burns RC. Pathways of the pulp. 8 th ed. Philadelphia: St. Louis: Mosby, 2002. 293-364.
169. Haddix JE, Mattison DG, Shulman AC, Pink EF. Post preparation techniques and their effect on the apical seal. J Prosthet Dent 1990;64:515-9.
170. Haikel Y, Wittenmeyer W, Bateman G, Bentaleb A, Allemann C. A new methodo for the quantitative analysis of endodontic microleakage. J Endod 1999;25:172-77.
171. Hasegawa T, Retief DH, Russell CM, Denys FR. Shear bond strength and quantitative microleakage of a multipurpose dental adhesive system resin bonded to dentin. J Prosthet Dent 1995;73:432-8.
172. Hashieh IA, Pommel L, Camps J. Concentration of eugenol apically released from zinc oxide-eugenol-based sealers. J Endod 1999;25:713-15.
173. Hayashi M, Takahashi Y, Hirai M, Iwami Y, Imazato S, Ebisu S. Effect of endodontic irrigation on bonding of resin cement to radicular dentin. Eur J Oral Sci 2005;113:70-76.
174. Heling I, Gorfil C, Slutzky H, Kopolovic K, Zalkind M, Slutzky-Goldberg I. Endodontic failure caused by inadequate restorative procedures: review and treatment recommendations. J Prosthet Dent 2002;87:674-8.
175. Hermann BW. Calciumhydroxyd als mittel zurn behandel und füllen vonxahnwurzelkanälen. (Doctoral Thesis) Würzburg;1920. 50p.
176. Higginbotham TL. A comparative study of the physical properties of five commonly used root canal sealers. Oral Surg Oral Med Oral Pathol 1967;24:89-101.
177. Higgins JPT, Green S. Cochrane handbook for systematic reviews of interventions 4.2.5. The Cochrane Library. Chichester, UK: John Wiley & Sons, Ltd., 2005.
178. Hiraishi N, Loushine RJ, Vano M, Chieffi N, Weller RN, Ferrari M, Pashley DH, Tay FR. Is an oxygen inhibited layer required for bonding of resin-coated gutta-percha to a methacrylate-based root canal sealer? J Endod 2006;32:429-33.
179. Ho CH, Khoo A, Tan R, Teh J, Lim KC, Sae-Lim V. pH changes in root dentin after intracanal placement of improved calcium hydroxide containing gutta-percha points. J Endod 2003;29:4- 8.
180. Holland GR. Leakage around root canal fillings. Int Endod J 1993;26:15.
181. Holland R, Manne LN, Souza V, Murata SS, Dezan-JR E. Periapical tissue healing after post space preparation with or without use of a protection plug and root canal exposure to the oral environment: study in dogs. Braz Dent J 2007;18:281-288.
182. Holland R, Murata S, Silva MN, Dezan-Jr E, Souza V, Bernabé PFE. Influence of the sealer and a plug in coronal leakage after post space preparation. J Appl Oral Scien 2004;12:223-226.
183. Holland R, Murata SS, Dezan Jr E, Garlipp O. Apical leakage after root canal filling with an experimental calcium hydroxide gutta-percha point. J Endod 1996;22:71-73.
184. Holland R, Murata SS, Dezan-Jr E, Souza V, Bernabé PFE, Otoboni-Filho JA, Nery MJ. Obturação de canal com o cimento Sealer Plus. Análise da infiltração marginal apical linear e volumétrica. Rev Bras Odontol 2001;58:198-200.

185. Holland R, Murata SS, Kissimoto R, Sakagami RS, Saliba O. Infiltração marginal após o emprego do hidróxido de cálcio como curativo de demora. Rev Odont UNESP 1993;22:249-255.
186. Holland R, Murata SS, Saliba O. Efeito a curto e médio prazo dos resíduos de hidróxido de cálcio na qualidade do selamento marginal após a obturação de canal. Rev Paul Odont 1995;17:12-6.
187. Holland R, Murata SS, Souza V, Lopes HP, Saliba O. Análise do selamento marginal obtido com cimentos à base de hidróxido de cálcio. Rev Ass Paul Cir Dent 1996;50:61-64.
188. Holland R, Murata SS. Efeito do hidróxido de cálcio como curativo de demora no selamento marginal após a obturação do canal radicular. Rev Ass Paul Cir Dent 1993;47:1203-7.
189. Holland R, Murata SS. Obturação de canais radiculares com cimentos à base de hidróxido de cálcio. Rev Ass Paul Cir Dent 1995;49:221-24.
190. Holland R, Nery MJ, Bernabé PFE, Mello W. Resposta tecidual à implantação de diferentes marcas de cones de guta-percha. Estudo histopatológico em ratos. Rev Fac Odontol Araçatuba 1975;4:81-89.
191. Holland R, Nery MJ, Souza V, Bernabé PFE, Mello W, Otoboni-Filho JA. The effect of the filling material in the tissue reactions following apical plugging of the root canal with dentin chips. Oral Surg Oral Med Oral Pathol 1983;55:398-401.
192. Holland R, Nery MJ, Souza V, Mello W, Bernabé PFE, Otoboni Filho JA. The effect of corticosteroid-antibiotic dressing on the behaviour of the periapical tissue of dogs' teeth after overinstrumentation. Rev Odontol UNESP 1981;10:21-25.
193. Holland R, Okabe JN, Holland JRC, Souza V, Mello W, Saliba O. Influência do emprego do vácuo na profundidade da infiltração do azul de metileno em dentes com canais obturados. Rev Ass Paul Cir Dent 1990;44:213-16.
194. Holland R, Otoboni Filho JA, Souza V, Nery MJ, Bernabé PFE, Dezan Junior E. Calcium hydroxide and corticosteroid-antibiotic association as dressing in cases of biopulpectomy. A comparative study in dogs' teeth. Braz Dent J 1998;9:67-76.
195. Holland R, Otoboni-Filho JA, Bernabé PFE, Souza V, Nery MJ, Dezan-Jr E. Effect of root canal filling material and level of surgical injury on periodontal healing in dogs. Endod Dental Traumatol 1998;14:199-205.
196. Holland R, Otoboni-Filho JA, Souza V, Mello W, Nery MJ, Bernabé PFE, Dezan-Jr E. Calcium hydroxide and corticosteroid-antibiotic association as dressings in cases of biopulpectomy. A comparative study in dogs teeth. Braz Dent J 1998;9:67-76.
197. Holland R, Otoboni-Filho JA, Souza V, Nery MJ, Bernabé PFE, Dezan-Júnior E. Mineral trioxide aggregate repair of lateral root perforations. Journal of Endodontics 2001;27:281-4.
198. Holland R, Otoboni-Filho JA, Souza V, Nery MJ, Bernabé PFE, Dezan-Jr E. A comparison of one versus two appointment endodontic therapy in dogs' teeth with apical periodontitis. J Endod 2003;29:121-25.
199. Holland R, Otoboni-Filho JA, Souza V, Nery MJ, Bernabé PFE, Dezan-Jr E. Tratamiento endodôntico en una o en dos visitas. Estudio histológico em dientes de perros con lesión periapical. Endodoncia 2003;21:20-27.
200. Holland R, Sant'anna-Jr A, Souza V, Dezan-Jr E, Otoboni-Filho PFE, Nery MJ, Murata SS.. Influence of apical patency and filling material on healing process of dogs' teeth with vital pulp after root canal therapy. Braz Dent J 2005;16:9-16.
201. Holland R, Sakashita MS, Murata SS, Dezan-Jr E. Effect of dentin surface treatment on leakage of root fillings with a glass ionomer sealer. Int Endod J 1995;28:190-93.
202. Holland R, Souza V. Ability of a new calcium hydroxide root canal filling material to induce hard tissue formation. J Endod 1985;11:535-43.
203. Holland R, Souza V, Abdalla T, Russo MC. Sealing properties of some root filling materials evaluated with radioisotope. Aust Dent J 1974;322-325.
204. Holland R, Souza V, Holland-Jr C, Nery JC. Estudo histopatológico do comportamento do tecido conjuntivo subcutâneo do rato ao implante de alguns materiais obturadores de canal radicular. Influência da proporção pó-líquido. Rev Ass Paul Cir Dent 1971;25:101-109.
205. Holland R, Souza V, Mello W, Nery MJ, Bernabé PFE, Otoboni-Filho JA. Manual de Endodontia - Faculdade de Odontologia de Araçatuba – UNESP;1978/1979.
206. Holland R, Souza V, Murata SS, Nery MJ, Bernabé PFE, Otoboni-Filho JA, Dezan-Jr E. Healing process of dog dental pulp after pulpotomy and pulp covering with mineral trioxide aggregate or Portland cement. Braz Dent J 2001;12:109-13.
207. Holland R, Souza V, Nery MJ, Bernabé PFE, Otoboni-Filho JA, Dezan-Júnior E. Reaction of rat connective tissue to implanted dentin tubes filled with a mineral trioxide aggregate or calcium hydroxide. J Endod 1999;25:161-6.
208. Holland R, Souza V, Nery MJ, Bernabé PFE, Otoboni-Filho JA, Dezan-Jr E. Reaction of dog's teeth to root canal filling with Mineral Trioxide Aggregate or a Glass Ionomer Sealer. J Endod 1999;25:728-30.
209. Holland R, Souza V, Nery MJ, Bernabé PFE, Otoboni-Filho JA, Dezan-Jr E, Murata SS. Calcium salts deposition in rat connective tissue after the implantation of calcium hydroxide-containing sealers. J Endod 2002;28:173-76.
210. Holland R, Souza V, Nery MJ, Faraco-Júnior IM, Bernabé PFE, Otoboni-Filho JA, Dezan-Jr E. Reaction of rat connective tissue to implanted dentin tube filled with mineral trioxide aggregate, Portland cement or calcium hydroxide. Braz Dent J 2001;12:3-8.
211. Holland R, Souza V, Nery MJ, Faraco-Júnior IM, Bernabé PFE, Otoboni-Filho JA, Dezan-Jr E. Reaction of rat connective tissue to implanted dentin tubes filled with a white mineral trioxide aggregate. Braz Dent J 2002;13:23-6.
212. Holland R, Souza V, Nery MJ, Mello W, Bernabé PFE, Otoboni Filho JA. Effect of the dressing in root canal treatment with calcium hydroxide. Rev Fac Odontol Araçatuba 1978;7:39-45.
213. Holland R, Souza V, Nery MJ, Mello W, Bernabé PFE, Pannain R. Influência do tempo de estocagem na infiltração marginal do 131 INa em obturações de canal. Rev Bras Odontol 1976;33:164-68.

214. Holland R, Souza V, Otoboni Filho JA, Nery MJ, Bernabé PFE, Dezan Junior E, Garlippe O. Comportamento dos tecidos apicais e periapicais de dentes de cães à obturação de canal com o cimento experimental Sealer Plus. Rev Bras Odontol 2000;57:114-116.
215. Holland R, Souza V, Pannain R, Nery MJ, Mello W, Bernabé PFE. Avaliação da eficiência do selamento marginal de obturações de canal. Influência de variáveis introduzidas no método da condensação lateral. Rev Gaucha Odontol 1975;23:247-253.
216. Holland R, Souza V, Tagliavini RL, Milanezi LA. Healing process of teeth with open apices: histological study. Bull Tokyo Dent Coll 1971;12:333-338.
217. Holland R, Zampieri Jr M, Souza V, Saliba O. Influência de alguns procedimentos clínicos na infiltração marginal de obturações realizadas pela técnica da condensação lateral. Rev Paul Odont 1991;13:29-38.
218. Holland R, Murata SS, Dezan-Jr E, Garllip O. Apical leakage after root canal filling with an experimental calcium hydroxide guta-percha polnt. J Endod 1996;22:71-3.
219. Hollanda ACB, Estrela CRA, Decurcio DA, Silva JÁ, Estrela C. sealing ability of sealer 26, AH Plus and Resilon-Epiphany. General Dentistry 2009; (in press).
220. Hommez GMG, Coppens CRM, DeMoor RJG. Periapical health related to the quality of coronal restorations and root fillings. Int Endod J 2002;35:680-9.
221. Horning TG, Kessier JR. A comparison of three different root canal sealers when used to obturate a moisture-contaminated root canal system. J Endod 1995;21:354-57.
222. Hossain M, Yamada Y, Nakamura Y, Murakami Y, Tamaki Y, Matsumoto K. A study on surface roughness and microleakage test in cavities prepared by Er:YAG laser irradiation and etched bur cavities. Lasers Med Sci 2003;18:25-31.
223. Hovland EJ, Dumsha TC. Leakage evaluation in vitro of the root canal sealer cement Sealapex. Int Endod J 1985;18:179-182.
224. Huang TH, Kao CT. pH measurement of root canal sealers. J Endod 1998;24:236-38.
225. Hülsmann M, Heckendorff M, Lennon A. Chelating agents in root canal treatment: mode of action and indications for their use. Int Endod J 2003 36:810-30.
226. Huang TH, Lii CK, Chai MY, Kao CT. Lactate dehydrogenase leakage of hepatocytes with AH26 and AHplus sealer treatments. J Endod 2000;26:509-11.
227. Huque MF. Experiences with meta-analysis in NDA submissions. Proceedings of the Biopharmaceutical Section of the American Statistical Association 1988;2:28-33.
228. Ibarrola JL, Knowls KJ, Ludlow MO. Retrienability of Thermafil Plastic cores using organic solvents. J Endod 1993;19:417-18.
229. Ingle JI, Beveridge EE, Glick DH, Weichman JA. Modern Endodontic Therapy. In: Endodontics. Ingle JI, Bakland LK. 4th ed. Baltimore: Wilians & Wilkins;1994. p.3-48.
230. Jacobsen EL, Begole EA, Vitkus DD, Daniel JC. An evaluation of two newly formulated calcium hydroxide cements: a leakage study. J Endod 1987;4:164-69.
231. Jacobson S, Von Fraunhofer JA. The investigation of microleakage in root canal therapy. An electrochemical technique. Oral Surg Oral Med Oral Pathol 1976;42:817-23.
232. Jacquot BM, Panighi MM, Steinmertz P, G'Sell C. Microleakage of Cavit, Cavit W, Cavit G e IRM by impedance spectroscopy. Int Endod J 1996;29:256-61.
233. Jacquot BM, Panighi MM, Steinmetz P, G'Seel C. Evaluation of temporary restoration microleakage by means of electrochemical impedance measurements. J Endod 1996;22:586-9.
234. Jadad AR, Moore RA, Carroll D, et al. Assessing the quality of reports of randomized clinical trials: is blinding necessary? Control Clin Trials 1996;17:1-12.
235. Jodaikin A, Austin JC, Cleaton-Jones PE. Pulpal responses to amalgam restorations in cavities with and without smear layer removal. J Oral Pathol 1986;15:415-8.
236. Jodaikin A, Austin JC. The effects of cavity smear layer removal on experimental marginal leakage around amalgam restorations. J Dent Res 1981;60:1861-6.
237. Johnson NT, Zakariasen KL. Spectrophotometric analysis of microleakage in the fine curved canals found in the mesial roots of mandibular molars. Oral Surg Oral Med Oral Pathol 1983;56:305-09.
238. Jordan RE, Suzuki M. The ideal bonding system. J Can Dent Assoc 1992;58:623-5.
239. Jun W, Bin P, Bing F. Evaluation of root canal filling with Thermafil. J Practical Stomatol 2004;20:35-8.
240. Kallus T, Eklund G. Instrumentation for preparation and placement of subcutaneous implants. J Biomed Mat Res 1983;17:735-40.
241. Kaplan AE, Picca M, Gonzales MI, Macchi RL, Molgatini SL. Antimicrobial effect of six endodontic sealers: na in vitro evaluation. Endod Dent Traumatol 1999;2:42-45.
242. Kaplowitz GJ. Evaluation of gutta percha solvents. J Endod 1990;16:939-40.
243. Kaplowitz GJ. Evaluation of the ability of essential oils to dissolve gutta percha. J Endod 1991;17:448- 49.
244. Kapsimalis P, Evans R, Tuckerman MM. Modified autoradiographic technique for marginal penetration studies. Oral Surg Oral Med Oral Pathol 1965;20:494-504.
245. Karadag LS, Bala O, Turkoz E, Mihcioglu T. The effects of water and acetone-based dentin adhesives on apical microleakage. J Contemp Dent Pract 2004;5:93-101.
246. Karapanou V, Vera J, Cabrera P, White RR, Goldman M. Effect of immediate and delayed post preparation on apical dye leakage using two different sealers. J Endod 1996;22:583-5.
247. Kaufman AV, Tagger M, Katz A, Yosef A. Life and AH26 as sealers in thermatically compacted gutapercha root canal fillings: leakage to a dye. J Endod 1989;15:68-71.
248. Kavale KA, Glass GV. Meta-analysis and the integration of research in special education. J Learn Disabil 1981;14:531-8.
249. Kayaoglu G, Erten H, Alacam T, Orstavik D. Short-term antibacterial activity of root canal sealers towards Enterococcus faecalis. Int Endod J 2005;38:483-8.
250. Kazemi RB, Safavi KE, Spangberg LSW, Conn F. Assessment of marginal stability and permeability of an interim restorative endodontic material. Oral Surg Oral Med Oral Pathol 1994;78:788-96.
251. Kazemi RB, Safavi KE, Spangberg LSW. Dimensional changes of endodontic sealers. Oral Surg Oral Med Oral Pathol 1993;76:766-71.

252. Kehoe JC. Intracanal corrosion of a silver cone producing a localized argyria - scanning electron microscope and energy dispersive x-ray analyser analyses. J Endod 1984;10:199-201.
253. Kennedy WA, Walker WA 3rd, Gough RW. Smear layer removal effects on apical leakage. J Endod 1986;12:21-7.
254. Kersten HW, Moorer WR. Particles and molecules in endodontic leakage. Int Endod J 1989;22:118-24.
255. Kersten HW. et al. A standardized leakage test with curved root canals in artificial dentine. Int Endod J 1988;21:191-99.
256. Khayat A, Lee SJ, Torabinejad M. Human saliva penetration of coronally unsealed obturated root canal. J Endod 1993;19:458-81.
257. Kimura Y, Yamazaki R, Goya C, Tomita Y, Yokoyama K, Matsumoto K. A comparative study on the effects of three types of laser irradiation at the apical stop and apical leakage after obturation. J Clin Laser Med Surg 1999;17:261-6.
258. King KT, Andserson RW, Pashley DH, Pantera-Jr EA. Longitudinal evaluation of the seal of endodontic retrofillings. J Endod 1990;16:307-10.
259. Kirkevang LL, Ørstavik D, Hørsted-Bindslev P, Wenzel A. Periapical status and quality of root fillings and coronal restorations in a Danish population. Int Endod J 2000;33:509-15.
260. Kirkevang LL, vaeth M, Hörsted-Bindslev P, Bahrami G, Wenzel A. Risk factors for developing apical periododontitis in a general population. Int Endod J 2007;40:290-299.
261. Koch K, Min PS, Stewart GG. Comparison of apical leakage between Ketac Endo sealer and Grossman Sealer. Oral Surg Oral Med Oral Pathol 1994;78:784-87.
262. Kojima K, Inamoto K, Nagamatsu K, Hara A, Nakata K, Morita I, Nakagaki H, Nakamura H. Success rate of endodontic treatment of teeth with vital and nonvital pulps. A meta-analysis. Oral Surg Oral Med Oral Pathol Oral Radiol Endod 2004;97:95-9.
263. Kolokouris I, Economides N, Beltes P, Viemmas In vivo comparison of the biocompatibility of two root canal sealers implanted into the subcutaneous connective tissue of rats. J Endod 1998;24:82-85.
264. Kopper PMP, Figueiredo JAP, Della Bona A, Vanni JR, Bier CA, Bopp S. Comparative in vivo analysis of the selaing ability of three endodontic sealers in post-prepared root canal. Int Endod J 2003;36:857-63.
265. Kopper PMP, Figueiredo JAP, Só MVR, Juchen LP, Martins PB. Análise comparativa da infiltração apical produzida por três técnicas de obturação em dentes humanos extraídos. Stomatos 1998;6:21-29.
266. Kubo S, Yokota H, Sata Y, Hayashi Y. Microleakage of self-etching primers after thermal and flexural load cycling. Am J Dent 2001;14:163-9.
267. Kuga MC, Moraes IG, Berbert A. Capacidade seladora do cimento sealapex puro ou acrescido de iodofórmio. Rev Odont USP 1988;2:139-42.
268. Kvist T, Rydin E, Reit C. The relative frequency of periapical lesions in teeth with root canal-retained posts. J Endod 1989;15:578-80.
269. Kytridou V, Gutmann JL, Nunn MH. Adaptation and sealability of two contemporary obturation techniques in the absence of the dentinal smear layer. Int Endod J 1999;32:464-74.
270. Lalh MS, Titley KC, Torneck CD, Friedman S. Scanning electron microscopic study of the interface of glass ionomer cement sealers and conditioned bovine dentin. J Endod 1999;25:743-46.
271. Lambrianidis T, Tosounidow E, Tzoanopoulou M. The effect of maintaining apical patency on periapical extrusion. J Endod 2001;27:696-698.
272. Leal JM, Holland R, Esberard RM. Sealapex, CRCS, Fill Canal e N-Rickert, estudo da biocompatibilidade em tecido conjuntivo subcutâneo do rato. Odont Clin 1988;2:7-14.
273. Leduc J, Fishelberg G. Endodontic obturation: a review. General Dentistry 2003;51:232-3.
274. Lee BS, Lin YW, Chia JS, Hsieh TT, Chen MH, Lin CP, Lan WH. Bactericidal effects of diode laser on Streptococcus mutans after irradiation through different thickness of dentin. Lasers in Surg Med 2006;38:62-9.
275. Lee KW, Williams MC, Camps JJ, Pashley DH. Adhesion of endodontic sealers to dentin and gutta-percha. J Endod 2002;28:684-88.
276. Lengheden A. Influence of pH and calcium on growth and attachment of human fibroblasts in vitro. Scand J Dent Res 1994;102:130-36.
277. Leonard JE, Gutmann JL, Guo IY. Apical and coronal seal of roots obturated with a dentine bonding agent and resin. Int Endod J 1996;29:76-83.
278. Lertchirakarn V, Timyam A, Messer HH. Effects of root canal sealers on vertical root fracture resistance of endodontically treated teeth. J Endod 2002;28:217-9.
279. Levitan ME, Himel VT, Luckey JB. The effect of insertion rates on fill length and adaptation of a thermoplasticized gutta-percha technique. J Endod 2003;29:505-8.
280. Lim KC, Tidmarsh BG. The sealing ability of sealapex compared with AH26. J Endod 1986;12:564- 66.
281. Limkangwalmongkol S, Abbot PV, Sandler AB. Apical dye penetration with four root canal sealers and guta-percha using longitudinal sectioning. J Endod 1992;18:535-39.
282. Limkangwalmongkol S, Burtscher P, Abbott PV, Sandler AB, Bishop BM. A comparative study of the apical leakage of four root canal sealers and laterally condensed gutta-percha. J Endod1991;17:495-99.
283. Lipski M. Comparative study on the efficacy of root canal filling with gutta-percha by lateral condensation and Thermafil obturators. Ann Acad Med Stetin 2000;46:317-30.
284. Lloyd A, Thompson J, Gutmann JL, Dummer PMH. Selability of the Trifecta technique in the presence or absence of smear layer. Int Endod J 1995;28:35-40.
285. Lopes-Filho LG, Estrela C. Capacidade seladora do remanescente de obturação do canal radicular frente à infiltração microbiana. Scientific A 2008; (in press).
286. Lovdahl PE. Endodontic Retreatment. The Dental Clinics of North America 1992;36:491-50.
287. Lumley PJ, Walmsley AD, Walton RE, Rippin JW. Effect of precurving endosonic files on the amount of debris and smear layer remaining in curved root canals. J Endod 1992;18:616-9.
288. Lussi A, Imwinkelried S, Stich H. Obturation of root canals with different sealers using non-instrumentation technology. Int Endod J 1999;32:17-23.

289. Madison S, Swason K, Chiles SA. Na evaluation of coronal microleakage in endodontically treated teeth. Part II. Sealer types. J Endod 1987;13:109-12.
290. Madison S, Zakariasen KL. Linear and volumetric analysis of apical leakage in teeth prepared for posts. J Endod 1984;10:422-27.
291. Magura ME, Kafrawi AH, Brown CE, Newton CW. Human saliva coronal microleakage in obturated root canals: an in vitro study. J Endod 1991;17:324-331.
292. Malone KH, Donnelly JC. An in vitro evaluation of coronal microleakage in obturated root canals without coronal restorations. J Endod 1997;23:35-38.
293. Mannocci F, Innocenti M, Bertelli E, Ferrari M. Dye leakage and SEM study of roots obturated with Thermafill and dentin bonding agent. Endod Dent Traumatol 1999;15:60-4.
294. Manson-Hing LR. An investigation of the roentgenographic contrast of enamel, dentine, and aluminum. Oral Surg Oral Med Oral Pathol 1961;11:1456-72.
295. Marciano J, Michailesco PM. Dental guta-percha: chemical composition, x-ray identification, enthalpic studies, and clinical implications. J Endod 1989;15:149-53.
296. Matloff IR, Jensen JR, Singer L, Tabibi A. A comparison of methods used in root canal seal ability studies. Oral Surg Oral Med Oral Pathol 1982;53:203-08.
297. Mayer T, Eickholz P. Microleakage of temporary restorations after thermocycling and mechanical loading. J Endod 1997;23:320-22.
298. McComb D, Smith JC. Comparison of physical properties of polycarboxylate-based and conventional root canal sealers. J Endod 1976;2:228-35.
299. Mcdougall G, Patel V, Santerre P, Friedman. Resistance of experimental glass ionomer cement sealers to bacterial penetration in vitro. J Endod 1999;25:739-42.
300. McElroy DL. Physical properties of root canal filling materials. J Am Dent Ass 1955;50:433-440.
301. McSpadden J. Obturation of the radicular space In: Ingle JI, Bakland LK. Endodontics. 4th.ed. Baltimore: Wilians & Wilkins;1994. p.228-329.
302. Meiers JC, Kresin JC. Cavity disinfectants and dentin bonding. Oper Dent 1996;21:153-9.
303. Mendonça SC, Carvalho-Jr JR, Guerisoli DM, Pécora JD, de Sousa-Neto MD. In vitro study of the effect of aged eugenol on the flow, setting time and adhesion of Grossman root canal sealer. Braz Dent J 2000;11:71-8.
304. Metzger Z, Abramovitz R, Abramovitz I, Tagger M. Correlation between remaining length of root canal fillings after immediate post space preparation and coronal leakage. J Endod 2000;26:724-8.
305. Michanowicz AE, Michanowicz JP, Michanowicz AM, Czonstkowsky M, Zullo TP. Clinical evaluation of low-temperature thermoplasticized injectable gutta-percha: a preliminary report. J Endod 1989;15:602-7.
306. Michelich V, Schuster G, Pashley D. Bacterial penetration of human dentin in vitro. J Dent Res 1980;59:1398-403.
307. Mickel AK, Wright ER. Growth inhibition os Streptococcus anginosus (milleri) by three calcium hydroxide sealers and one zinc oxide-eugenol sealer. J Endod 1999;25:34-37.
308. Miletic I, Prpic-Mehicic G, Marsal T, Tambicandrasevic A, Plesko S, Zarlovic Z, Anic I. Bacterial and fungal microleakage of AH 26 and AH plus root canal sealers. Int Endod J 2002;35:428-32.
309. Mittal M, Chandra S, Chandra S. Comparative tissue toxicity evaluation of four endodontic sealers. J Endod 1995;21:622-24.
310. Mixson JM, Richards ND, Mitchell RJ. Effects of dentin age and bonding on microgap formation. Am J Dent 1993;6:72-6.
311. Moher D, Jones A, Lepage L. Use of the CONSORT statement and quality of reports of randomized trials: a comparative before-and-after evaluation. JAMA 2001;285:1992-5.
312. Moodley D, Grobler SR. Dentine bonding agents: a review of adhesion to dentine. SADJ 2002;57:234-8.
313. Moraes IG. Propriedades físicas de cimentos epóxicos experimentais para obturações de canais radiculares, baseados no AH26. (Doctoral Thesis). University of São Paulo;1984. 149p.
314. Mount GJ. Some physical and biological properties of glass ionomer. Int Endod J 1995;45:135-140.
315. Moura MS, Guedes OA, Alencar AHG, Azevedo BC, Estrela C. Influence of apical limit of root canal obturation on apical periodontitis detected by periapical radiography and cone beam computed tomography. 2008 (submited).
316. Murray PE, Smyth TW, About I, Remusat R, Franquin JC, Smith AJ. The effect of etching on bacterial microleakage of an adhesive composite restoration. J Dent 2002;30:29-36.
317. Nair PNR, Henry S, Cano V, Vera J. Microbial status of apical root canal system of human mandibular first molars with primary apical periodontitis after "one-visit" endodontic treatment. Oral Surg Oral Med Oral Pathol Oral Radiol Endod 2005;99:231-52.
318. Najar AL, Saquy PC, Vansan LP, Sousa Neto MD. Adhesion of a glass-ionomer root canal sealer to human dentine. Aust Endod J 2003;29:20-2.
319. Negm MM. The effect of human blood on sealing ability of root canal sealers: An in vitro study. Oral Surg Oral Med Oral Pathol 1989;67:449-52.
320. Nguyen NT. Obturação dos canais radiculares. In: Cohen S, Burns RC. Caminhos da polpa. Guanabara Koogan, 2nd ed. Rio de janeiro, 1982.p.126-86.
321. Oliver CM, Abbott PV. An in vitro study of apical and coronal microleakage of laterally condensed gutta percha with Ketac-endo and AH26. Aust Dent J 1998;43:262-68.
322. Orfali F, Lilley JD, Molokhia A. The radiopacity of some endodontic sealer cements. J Dent Res 1987;66:876. Abstract 368
323. Ørstavik D, Eriksen HM, Beyer-Olsen EM. Adhesive properties and leakage of root canal sealers in vitro. Int Endod J 1983;16:59-63.
324. Ørstavik D. Materials used for root canal obturation: technical, biological and clinical testing. Endod Topics 2005;12: 25-38.
325. Ørstavik D. Physical properties of root canal sealers: measurements of flow, working time, and compressive strenght. Int Endod J 1983;16:99.
326. Ørstavik D. Physical properties of root canal sealers: measurement of flow, working time, and compressive strength. Int Endod J 1983;16:99-107.
327. Ørstavik D. Seating of gutta percha points: Effect of sealers with varying film thickness. J Endod 1982;8:213.

328. Ørstavik D. Time-course and risk analyses of the development and healing of chronic apical periodontitis in man. Int Endod J 1996;29:150-5.
329. Oynic J. Methods and criteria in evaluation of periapical tissue response. Int Dent J 1970;20:533-538.
330. Ozata F, Onal B, Erdilek N, Turkun SL. A comparative study of apical leakage of Apexit, Ketac Endo, and Diaket root canal sealers. J Endod 1999;25:603-04.
331. Ozok AR, De Gee AJ, Wu MK, Wesselink PR. The influence of resin composite and bonded amalgam restorations on dentine permeability in Class II cavities in vitro. Dent Mater 2001;17:477-84.
332. Ozturk B, Ozer F, Belli S. An in vitro comparison of adhesive systems to seal pulp chamber walls. Int Endod J 2004;37:297-306.
333. Pai S, Yang S, Sue W, Chueh L, Riviera EM. Microleakage between endodontic temporary restorative materials placed at different times. J Endod 1999;25:453-6.
334. Paiva JG, Antoniazzi JH. Endodontia: bases para a prática clínica. 2nd ed. São Paulo: Artes Médicas;1988. p.631-646.
335. Park DS, Yoo HM, Oh TS. Effects of Nd:YAG laser irradiation on the apical leakage of obturated root canals: an electrochemical study. Int Endod J 2001;4:318-21.
336. Pashley DH, Carvalho RM. Dentine permeability and dentine adhesion. J Dent 1997;25:355-72.
337. Pashley DH, Depew DD. Effects of the smear layer, Copalite, and oxalate on microleakage. Oper Dent 1986;11:95-102.
338. Pashley DH, Kalathoor S, Burnham D. The effects of calcium hydroxide on dentin permeability. J Dent Res 1986;65:417-420.
339. Pashley DH, Pashley EL. Dentin permeability and restorative dentistry: a status report for the American Journal of Dentistry. Am J Dent 1991;4:5-9.
340. Pashley DH. Clinical considerations of microleakage. J Endod 1990;16:70-7.
341. Pashley DH. Dentin bonding: overview of the substrate with respect to adhesive material. J Esthet Dent 1991;3:46-50.
342. Pashley DH. Dentin-predentin complex and its permeability: physiologic overview. J Dent Res 1985;64:613-20.
343. Pashley DH. Smear layer: physiological considerations. Oper Dent 1984;3: 13-29.
344. Pashley DH. The effects of acid etching on the pulpodentin complex. Oper Dent 1992;17:229-42.
345. Patierno JM, Rueggeberg FA, Anderson RW, Weller RN, Pashley DH. Push-out strength and SEM evaluation of resin composite bonded to internal cervical dentin. Endod Dent Traumat 1996;12:227-36.
346. Pécora JD, Spanó JCE, Barbin EL.In vitro study of the softening of gutta percha cones in endodontics retreatment. Braz Dent J 1993;4:43-47.
347. Pécora JD. Apresentação de um óleo essencial obtido do Citrus Amantium eficaz na desintegração do cimento de óxido de zinco e eugenol do interior do canal radicular. Odonto 1992;p.130-32.
348. Peng L, Ye L, Tan H, Zhou X. Outcome of Root Canal Obturation by Warm Gutta-Percha versus Cold Lateral Condensation: A Meta-analysis. J Endod 2007;33:106-109
349. Peniche CEC, Sampaio JMP, Collesi RR. Verificação do pH de diversas soluções à base de hidróxido de cálcio. Rev Odont Univ Santo Amaro 1996;1:5-8.
350. Perdigão J, Gomes GK, Lee IL. The effect of silane on the bond strengths of fiber posts. Dent Mater 2006;22:752-8.
351. Perez F, Calas P, Rochd T. Effect of dentin treatment on in vitro root tubule bacterial invasion. Oral Surg Oral Med Oral Pathol Oral Radiol Endod 1996;82:446-51.
352. Peters DD. Two-year in vitro solubility evaluation of four gutta-percha sealer obturation techniques. J Endod 1986;12:139-45.
353. Peters LB, Wesselink PR, Moorer WR. Penetration of bacteria in bovine root dentine in vitro. Int Endod J 2000;33:28-36.
354. Petry AEA, Salles AA, Kilian L, Vidor M, Figueiredo JAP. Evaluation of endodontic sealer radiopacity using digitized imaging equipment. Braz Endod J 1997;2:24-28.
355. Pickenpaugh L, Reader A, Beck M, Meyers WJ, Peterson LJ. Effect of prophylactic amoxicillin on endodontic flare-up in asymptomatic, necrotic teeth. J Endod 2001;27:53-6.
356. Picoli F, Brugnera-Junior A, Saquy PC, Guerisoli DMZ, Pécora JD. Effect of Er:YAG laser and EDTAC on the adhesiveness to dentine of different sealers containing calcium hydroxide. Int Endod J 2003;36:472-5.
357. Pisano DM, Difiore PM, Mcclanahan SB, Lauternschlager BP, Duncan JL. Intraorifice sealing of gutta percha obturated root canals to prevent coronal microleakage. J Endod1998;24:659-62.
358. Pitt-Ford TR. Relation between seal of root filling and tissue response. Oral Surg Oral Med Oral Pathol 1983;55:291-94.
359. Pitt-Ford TR. The leakage of root fillings using glass ionomer cement and other materials. Brit Dent J 1979;146:273-78.
360. Pollard BK, Weller RN, Kulild JC. A standardized technique for linear dye leakage studies: immediate versus delayed immersion times. Int Endod J 1990;23:250-53.
361. Porkaew P, Retief H, Barfield RD, Lacefield WR, Soong SJ. Effects of calcium hydroxide paste as an intracanal medicament on apical seal. J Endodn 1990;16:369-374.
362. Prati C, Nucci C, Toledano M, Garcia-Godoy F, Breschi L, Chersoni S. Microleakage and marginal hybrid layer formation of compomer restorations. Oper Dent 2004;29:35-41.
363. Prati C, Simpson M, Mitchem J, Tao L, Pashley DH. Relationship between bond strength and microleakage measured in the same Class I restorations. Dent Mater 1992;8:37-41.
364. Prati C. What is the clinical relevance of in vitro dentine permeability tests? J Dent 1994;22:83-8.
365. Pulgar R, Segura-Egea JJ, Fernández MF, Serna A, Olea N. The effect os AH26 and AH Plus on MCF-7 breast cancer cell proliferation in vitro. Int Endod J 2002;35:551-556.
366. Pumarola J, Berastegui E, Brau E, Canalda C, Anta MTJ. Antimicrobial activity of seven root canal sealers. Oral Surg Oral Med Oral Pathol 1992;74:216-20.

367. Ramírez-Mejía AM, Garcia RB. Avaliação da infiltração marginal em obturações de canais radiculares: influência de soluções irrigadoras e cimentos obturadores. Rev Odontol USP 1996;10:43-48.
368. Ravanshad S, Torabinejad M, Iran S, Linda L. Coronal dye penetration of the apical filling materials after post space preparation. Oral Surg Oral Med Oral Pathol 1992;74:644-7.
369. Ray HA, Trope M. Periapical status of endodontically treated teeth in relation to the technical quality of the root filling and the coronal restoration. Int Endod J 1995;28:12-8.
370. Retief DH, Mandras RS, Russell CM, Denys FR. Phosphoric acid as a dentin etchant. Am J Dent 1992;5:24-8.
371. Ribeiro FC, Souza-Gabriel AE, Marchesan MA, Alfredo E, Silva-Sousa YT, Sousa-Neto MD. Influence of different endodontic filling materials on root fracture susceptibility. J Dent 2008;36:69-73.
372. Richardson D, Tao L, Pashley DH. Dentin permeability: effects of crown preparation. Int J Prosthod 1991;4:219-25.
373. Rickert UG, Bellizi R, Cruse WP. A historic review of endodontics, 1689-1963, part 3. J Endod 1980;6:576-589.
374. Rickert UG, Dixon CM. The control of root surgery. Transactions 8 Int dental Congress, Section IIIA. n. 9;1981. p.15-22.
375. Roghanizad N, Jones JJ. Evaluation of coronal microlakage after endodontic treatement. J Endod 1996;22:471-73.
376. Rohde TR, Bramwell JD, Hutter JW, Roahen JO. An in vitro evaluation of microleakage of a new root canal sealer. J Endod 1996;26:365- 67.
377. Romanos GE, Henze M, Banihashemi S, Parsanejad HR, Winckler J, Nentwig GH. Removal of ephitelium in periodontal pockets following diode (980 nm) laser application in the animal model: an in vitro study. Photomed Laser Surg 2004;22:177-83.
378. Rothman KJ, Greenland S. Modern epidemiology, 2nd ed. Philadelphia: Lippincott-Raven Publishers, 1998;144.
379. Ruddle CJ. Nonsurgical endodontic retreatment. J Calif Dent Ass 1997;25:769-99.
380. Sacomani GRR, Holland R, Souza V, Garlippe O. Comportamento dos tecidos periapicais de dentes de cães após a obturação de canal com os cimentos Sealer 26 e Sealer 26 modificado. J Bras Endod 2001;2:145-152.
381. Sahli CC, Aguade EB, Vilalta JS, Bruix A. The apical seal of root canal sealing cements using a radionuclide detection technique. Int Endod J 1992;25:250-56.
382. Saleh IM, Ruyter E, Nat R, Philos DR, Haapasalo MP, Ørstavik D. Adhesion of endodontic sealers: scanning electron microscopy and energy dispersive spectroscopy. J Endod 2003;29:595-601.
383. Saleh IM, Ruyter IE, Haapasalo M, Ørstavik D. The effects of dentine pretreatment on the adhesion of root cana sealers. Int Endod J 2002;35:859-66.
384. Sampaio JMP. Contribuição ao estudo do processo reparador do tecido conjuntivo de ratos, quando da introdução de tubos de polietileno contendo dois materiais empregados na obturação de condutos radiculares, nas suas fórmulas originais e acrescidas de delta-hidrocortisona. (Doctoral Thesis). University of São Paulo;1972. 57p.
385. Sampaio JMP. In: Paiva JG, Antoniazzi JH. Endodontia: bases para a prática clínica. 2nd.ed. São Paulo: Artes Médicas;1988. p.659.
386. Santos C, Sousa-Neto MD, Alfredo E, Guerisoli DMZ, Pécora JD, Lia RC. Morphologic evaluation of the radicular dentine irradiated with Nd:YAG laser under different parameters and angles of incidence. Photomed Laser Surg 2005;23:590-5.
387. Sato EFL, Sampaio JMP. Avaliação da adesividade existente entre a dentina e três diferentes cimentos obturadores de canais radiculares. Rev Paul Odont 1985;7:20-32.
388. Saunders EM, Saunders WP. Long-term coronal leakage of JS Quickfill root fillings with Sealapex and Apexit sealers. Endod Dent Traumat 1995;11:181-85.
389. Saunders WP, Saunders EM. Coronal leakage as a cause of failure in root canal therapy: a review. Endod Dent Traum 1994;10:105-8.
390. Saunders WP, Saunders EM. Influence of smear layer on the coronal leakage of Thermafil and laterally condensed gutta-percha root fillings with a glass ionomer sealer. J Endod 1994;20:155-8.
391. Saunders WP, Saunders EM. The root filling and restoration continuum: prevention of long-term endodontic failures. Alpha Omegan 1997;90:40-6.
392. Savioli RN, Silva RG, Pécora JD. Influência de cada componente do cimento de Grossman sobre as propriedades físicas de escoamento. Tempo de endurecimento e espessura do filme. Rev Paul Odont 1994;16:14-16.
393. Savoldi E, Benetti A, Venturi G, Marcoli PA, Bellia M. Pigmentazione della mucosa orale da materiale endodontico. Dent Cadm 1990;58:56-60.
394. Schaffer MA, White RR, Walton RE. Determining the optimal obturation length: a meta-analysis of literature. J Endod 2005;31:271-4.
395. Schafer E, Olthoff G. Effect of three different sealers on the sealing ability of both thermafil obturators and cold laterally compacted gutta-percha. J Endod 2002;28:638 -42.
396. Schäfer E, Zandbiglari T. Solubility of root-canal sealers in water and artificial saliva. Int Endod J 2003;36:660-9.
397. Scherer W, Binder D, David S, Mercurio C, Mello T. Effects of pH on the dentin surface. J Esthet Dent 1992;4:159-63.
398. Schilder H, Goodman A, Aldrich W. The thermomechanical properties of guttapercha. The compressibility of gutta-percha. Oral Surg Oral Med Oral Pathol 1974;37:946-53.
399. Schilder H, Goodman A, Aldrich W. The thermomechanical properties of guttapercha. III. Determination of phase transition temperatures for gutta-percha. Oral Surg Oral Med Oral Pathol 1974;38:109-14.
400. Schilder H, Goodman A, Aldrich W. The thermomechanical properties of guttapercha. V. Volume changes in bulk gutta-percha as a function of temperature and its relationship to molecular phase transformation. Oral Surg Oral Med Oral Pathol 1985;59:285-96.
401. Schilder H. Cleaning and shaping the root canal. Dent Clin N Amer 1974;18:269-296.

402. Schilder H. Filling root canals in three dimensions. Dent Clin N Amer 1967;723-44.
403. Schoop U, Kluger W, Dervisbegovic S, Goharkhay K, Wernisch J, Georgopoulos A, Sperr W, Moritz A. Innovative wave lengths in endodontic treatment. Lasers Surg Med 2006;38:624-8.
404. Schroeder AG. Zum problem der bakteriendichten Wurzelkanalvesorgung. Zahnärztl Welt 1957;58:531-537.
405. Schuurs AHB, Wu MK, Wesselink PR, Duivenvoorden HJ. Endodontic leakage studies reconsidered. Part II. Statistical aspects. Int Endod J 1993;26:44-52.
406. Schwartz RS. Adhesive dentistry and endodontics. Part 2: bonding in the root canal system-the promise and the problems: a review. J Endod 2006;32:1125-34.
407. Seltzer S. Long-term radiographic and histological observations of endodontically treated teeth. J Endod 1999;25:818-822
408. Sen BH, Piskin B, Baran N. The effect of tubular penetration of root canal sealers on dye microleakage. Int Endod J 1996;29:23-28.
409. Sen BH, Buyukyilmaz T. The effect of 4% titanium tetrafluoride solution on root canal walls: a preliminary investigation. J Endod 1998;24:239-43.
410. Sen BH, Piskin B, Baran N. The effect of tubular penetration of root canal sealers on dye microleakage. Int Endod J 1996;29:23-8.
411. Sen BH, Wesselink PR, Turkun M. The smear layer: a phenomenon in root canal therapy. Int Endod J 1995;28:141-8.
412. Sevimay S, Oztan MD, Dalat D. Effects of calcium hydroxide paste medication on coronal leakage. J Oral Rehab 2004;31:240-4.
413. Shahravan A, Haghdoost AA, Adl A, Rahimi H, Shadifar F. Effect of Smear Layer on Sealing Ability of Canal Obturation: A Systematic Review and Meta-analysis. J Endod 2007;33:96-105.
414. Shigetani Y, Tate Y, Okamoto A, Iwaku M, Abu-Bakr N. A study of cavity preparation by Er:YAG laser: effects on the marginal leakage of composite resin restoration. Dent Mater J 2002;21:238-49.
415. Shipper G, Orstavik D, Teixeira FB, Trope M. An evaluation of microbial leakage in roots filled with a thermoplastic synthetic polymer-based root canal filling material (Resilon). J Endod 2004;30:342-7.
416. Shipper G, Teixeira FB, Arnold RR, Trope M. Periapical Inflammation after coronal microbial inoculation of dog roots filled with gutta-percha or Resilon. J Endod 2005;31:91-6.
417. Shipper G, Trope M. In vitro microbial leakage of endodontically treated teeth using new and standard obturation techniques. J Endod 2004;30:154-8.
418. Silva RG, barbin e I, spanó Jce, Savioli RN, Pécora JD. Estudo da adesividade de alguns cimentos obturadores dos canais radiculares. Rev Odontol Bras Cent 1997;6:14-18.
419. Silva RG, Savioli RN, Cruz-Filho AM, Pécora JD. Estudo da estabilidade dimensional, solubilidade e desintegração e radiopacidade de alguns cimentos obturadores dos canais radiculares do tipo Grossman. Rev Ass Bras Odont Nac 1994;2:40-43.
420. Silva RG, Savioli RN, Saquy PC, Pécora JD. Estudo do tempo de endurecimento e da espessura do filme de alguns cimentos obturadores dos canais radiculares do tipo Grossman. Rev Fac Odontol Lins 1993;6:22-26.
421. Sim TP, Sidhu SK. The effect of dentinal conditioning on light-activated glass-ionomer cement. Quintessence Int 1994;25:505-8.
422. Simon JH. The apex: how critical is it? Gen Dent 1994;42:330-4.
423. Simon ST, Bhat KS, Francis R. Effect of four vehicles on the pH of calcium hydroxide and the release of calcium íon. Oral Surg Oral Med Oral Pathol 1995;80:459-64.
424. Sjögren U, Hägglund B, Sundqvist G, Wing K. Factors affecting the long-term results of endodontic treatment. J Endod 1990;16:498-504.
425. Smith MA, Steiman HR. An in vitro evaluation of microleakage of two new and two old root canal sealers. J Endod 1994;20:18-21.
426. Soh G, Sidhu SK. The effect of smear layer removal on marginal contraction gaps. J Oral Rehabil 1994;21:411-7.
427. Sommer RJ, Ostrander D. Clinical Endodontics. Philadelphia: WB Saunder;1956.
428. Sousa-Neto MD, Marchesan MA, Pécora JD, Brugnera-Júnior A, Silva-Sousa YTC, Saquy PC. Effect of Er:YAG laser on adhesion of root canal sealers. J Endod 2002;28:185-7.
429. Sousa-Neto MD, Passarinho-Neto JG, Carvalho-Júnior JR, Cruz-Filho AM, Pécora JD, Saquy PC. Evaluation of the effect of EDTA, EGTA and CDTA on dentin adhesiveness and microleakage with different root canal sealers. Braz Dent J 2002;13:123-28.
430. Sousa-Neto MD, Silva Coelho FI, Marchesan MA, Alfredo E, Silva-Sousa YT. Ex vivo study of the adhesion of an epoxy-based sealer to human dentine submitted to irradiation with Er : YAG and Nd : YAG lasers. Int Endod J 2005;38:866-70.
431. Sousa-Neto MD. Estudo da influência de diferentes tipos de breus e resinas hidrogenadas sobre as propriedades físico-químicas do cimento obturador dos canais radiculares Grossman. (Doctoral Thesis). University of São Paulo;1997. 108p.
432. Souza V, Holland R, Souza RS. Tratamento endodôntico de dentes de cães com polpas vitais em uma ou duas sessões. Influência dos curativos de demora corticosteróide-antibiótico e hidróxido de cálcio. Rev Odontol UNESP 1995;24:47-59.
433. Spångberg L, Langeland K. Biological effects of dental materials. Oral Surg Oral Med Oral Pathol 1973;35:407.
434. Spångberg LSW, Acierno TG, Cha BC. Influence of entrapped air on the accuracy of leakage studies using dye penetration methods. J Endod 1989;15:548-51.
435. Spångberg LSW, Haapasalo M. rationale and efficacy of root canals medicaments and root filling materials with emphasis on tretament outcome. Endod Topics 2002;2:35-58.
436. Spångberg LSW, Pascon EA. The importance of material preparation for the expression of citotoxicity during in vitro evaluation of biomaterials. J Endod 1988;14:247-50.
437. Stabholz A, Khayat A, Weeks DA, Neev J, Torabinejad M. Scanning electron microscopic study of the apical dentine surfaces lased with ND:YAG laser following apicectomy and retrofill. Int Endod J 1992;25:288-91.

438. Stabholz A, Sahar-Helft S, Moshonov J. Lasers in endodontics. Dent Clin North Am 2004;48:809-32.
439. Strindberg LZ. The dependence of the results of pulp therapy on certain factors. An analytical study based on radiographic and clinical follow-up examinations. Acta Odontol Scand 1956;14:1-175.
440. Starkey DL, Anderson RW, Pashley DH. An evaluation of the effect of methylene blue dye pH on apical leakage. J Endod 1993;19:435-39.
441. Stein T. Radiographic "Working length" revisited. Oral Surg Oral Med Oral Path 1992;74:796-9.
442. Sultan M, Pitt Ford TR. Ultrasonic preparation and obturation of root-end cavities. Int Endod J 1995;28:231-8.
443. Suzuki S, Cox CF, White KC. Pulpal response after complete crown preparation, dentinal sealing, and provisional restoration. Quint Int 1994;25:477-85.
444. Swanson K, Madison S. An evaluation of microleakage in endodontically treated teeth. Part I. Time periods. J Endod 1987;13:56-9.
445. Swift EJJr, LeValley BD. Microleakage of etched-dentin composite resin restorations. Quintessence Int 1992;23:505-8.
446. Tagger M, Tagger E, Kfir A. Release of calcium and hydroxyl ions from set endodontic sealers containing calcium hydroxide. J Endod 1988;14:588-91.
447. Tagger M, Tagger E, Tjan AH, Bakland LK. Measurement of adhesion of endodontic sealers to dentin. J Endod 2002;28:351-4.
448. Tagger M, Tagger E. Periapical reactions to calcium hydroxide-containing sealers and AH26 in monkeys. Endod Dent Traumat 1989;5:139-46.
449. Tagger M, Tanse A, Katz A, Korzen BH. Evaluation of the apical seal produced by hybrid rooth canal filling method, combining lateral condensation and thermatic compaction. J Endod 1984;10:299.
450. Takeda FH, Harashima T, Kimura Y, Matsumoto K A comparative study of the removal of smear layer by three endodontic irrigants and two types of laser. Int Endod J 1999;32:32-9.
451. Takeda FH, Harashima T, Kimura Y, Matsumoto K. Efficacy of Er:YAG laser irradiation in removing debris and smear layer on root canal walls. J Endod 1998;24:548-51.
452. Takeuti ML, Rodrigues CRMD, Myaki SI, Rodrigues-Filho LE. Avaliação in vitro da infiltração marginal de um cimento de ionômero de vidro modificado por resina associado ou não a um adesivo fluoretado. Rev Paul Odontol 2000;22:21-25.
453. Tamburic SD, Vuleta GM, Ognjanovic JM. In vitro release of calcium and hydroxyl ions from too types of calcium hydroxide preparation. Int Endod J 1993;26:125-30.
454. Tamse A, Unger U, Rozemberg M. Gutta-percha solvents - a comparative study. J Endod 1986;12:337-39.
455. Tang HM, Torabinejad M, Kettering JD. Leakage evaluation of root end filling materials using endotoxin. J Endod 2002;28:5-7.
456. Tang HM, Torabinejad M, Kettering JD. Leakage evaluation of root end filling materials using endotoxin. J Endod 2002;28:5-7.
457. Tay FR, Gwinnett AJ, Pang KM, Wei SH. Structural evidence of a sealed tissue interface with a total-etch wet-bonding technique in vivo. J Dent Res 1994;73:629-36.
458. Tay FR, King NM, Chan KM, Pashley DH. How can nanoleakage occur in self-etching adhesive systems that demineralize and infiltrate simultaneously? J Adhes Dent 2002;4:255-69.
459. Tay FR, Loushine RJ, Lambrechts P, Weller RN, Pashley DH. Geometric factors affecting dentin bonding in root canals: a theoretical modeling approach. J Endod 2005;31:584-9
460. Tay FR, Loushine RJ, Monticelli F, Weller RN, Breschi L, Ferrari M, Pashley DH. Effectiveness of resin-coated gutta-percha cones and a dual-cured, hydrophilic methacrylate resin-based sealer in obturating root canals. J Endod 2005;31:659-64.
461. Tay FR, Loushine RJ, Weller RN, Kimbrough WF, Pashley DH, Mark YF, Lai CN, Raina R, Willians MC. Ultrastructural evaluation of the apical seal in roots filled with a polycaprolactone-based root canal filling material. J Endod 2005;31:514-9.
462. Tay FR, Pashley DH, Suh BI, Carvalho RM, Itthagarun A. Single-step adhesives are permeable membranes. J Dent 2002;30:371-82.
463. Tay FR, Pashley DH, Yiu CKY, Yau JYY, Yiu-fai M, Loushine RJ, Weller RN, Kimbrough WF, King NM. Susceptibility of a Polycaprolactone-Based Root Canal Filling Material to Degradation. II. Gravimetric Evaluation of Enzymatic Hydrolysis. J Endod 2005;31:737-41.
464. Tay FR, Pashley DH, Yoshiyama M. Two modes of nanoleakage expression in singlestepadhesives. J Dent Res 2002;81:472-6.
465. Taylor JK, Jeansonne BL, Lemon RR. Coronal leakage: effects of smear layer obturation technique, and sealer. J Endod 1997;23:508 - 12.
466. Teixeira FB, Teixeira EC, Thompson J, Leinfelder KF, Trope M. Dentinal bonding reaches the root canal system. J Esthet Restor Dent 2004;16:348-54.
467. Teixeira FB, Teixeira ECN, Thompson JY, Trope M. Fracture Resistance of endodontically treated roots using a new type of resin filling material. J Am Dent Ass 2004;135:646-52.
468. Timpawat S, Amornchat C, Trisuwan W. Bacterial Coronal Leakage After Obturation With Three Root Canal Sealers. J Endod 1994;27:36-39.
469. Timpawat S, Sripanaratanakul S. Apical sealing ability of glass ionomer sealer with and without smear layer. J Endod 1998;24:343-5.
470. Tjan AH, Dunn JR. Microleakage at gingival dentin margins of Class V composite restorations lined with light-cured glass ionomer cement. J Am Dent Assoc 1990;121:706-10.
471. Torabinejad M, Bahjri K. Essential elements of evidenced-based endodontics: steps involved in conducting clinical research. J Endod 2005;31:563-9.
472. Torabinejad M, Handysides R, Khademi AA, Bakland LK. Clinical implications of thesmear layer in endodontics: a review. Oral Surg Oral Med Oral Pathol Oral Radiol Endod 2002;94:658-66.
473. Torabinejad M, Higa RK, Mckendry DJ, Pitt Ford TR. Dye leakage of four root end filling materials: effects of blood contamination. J Endod 1994;20:159-63.
474. Torabinejad M, Hong CU, McDonald F, Pitt-Ford TR. Physical and chemical properties of a new root end filling material. J Endod 1995;21:349-53.

475. Torabinejad M, Hong CU, Pitt Ford TR, Kettering JD. Antibacterial Effects of Some Root End Filling Materials. J Endod 1995a;21:403-7.
476. Torabinejad M, Hong CU, Pitt Ford TR, Kettering JD. Citotoxity of four root-end filling materials. J Endod 1995b;21:489-92.
477. Torabinejad M, Pitt Ford TR, Mckendry DJ, Abedi HR, Miller DA, Kariyawasam SP. Histologic assessment of mineral trioxide aggregate as a root-end filling in monkeys. J Endod 1997; 23:225-8.
478. Torabinejad M, Rastegarr AM, Kettering JD, Pitt Ford TR. Bacterial leakage of mineral trioxide aggregate as a root end filling material. J Endod 1995c;21:109-12.
479. Torabinejad M, Ung B, Kettering JD. In vitro bacterial penetration of coronally unsealed endodontically treated teeth. J Endod 1990;16:566-9.
480. Torabinejad M, Watson TF, Pitt Ford TR. Sealing ability of a mineral trioxide aggregate when used as a root-end filling material. J Endod 1993;19:591-5.
481. Torneck CD. Reactions of rat connective tissue to polyethilene tube implants. Oral Surg Oral Med Oral Pathol 1966;21:379-387.
482. Torneck CD. Reactions of rat conneective tissue to poliethilene tube implants - part II. Oral Surg Oral Med Oral Pathol 1967;24:64-683.
483. Tronstad L, Asbjornsen K, Dorving L, Pedersen I, Eriksen HM. Influence of coronal restorations on the periapical health of endodontically treated teeth. Endod Dent Traumatol 2000;16:218-21.
484. Tronstad L, Barnett F, Flax M. Solubility and biocompatibility of calcium hydroxide-containing root canal sealers. Endod Dent Traumat 1988;4:152-59.
485. Trope M, Chow E, Nissan R. In vitro endotoxin penetration of coronally unsealed endodonontically treated teeth. Endod Dent Traumatol 1995;11:90-94.
486. Trope M, Lost C, Schmitz HJ, Friedman S. Healing of apical periodontitis in dogs after apicoectomy and retrofilling with various filling materials. Oral Surg Oral Med Oral Pathol Oral Radiol Endod 1996:81:221-8.
487. Trope M, Ray Jr HL. Resistance to fracture of endodontically treated roots. Oral Surg Oral Med Oral Pathol 1992;73:99-102.
488. Trowbridge HO. Tooth sensitivity associated with the use of luting cements. Penn Dent J 1995;94:5, 24-6.
489. Ungor M, Onay EO, Orucoglu H. Push-out bond strengths: the epiphany-resilon endodontic obturation system compared with different pairings of Epiphany, Resilon, AH Plus and gutta-percha. Int Endod J 2006;39:643-7.
490. Valdrighi L. Influência dos espaços vazios nos resultados dos tratamentos de canais radiculares. Avaliação radiográfica e histopatológica. Estudo experimental em cães. (Doctoral Thesis). University of Campinas;1976.
491. Valera MC, Anbinder AL, Leonardo M, Parizoto NA, Kleinke UM. Cimentos endodônticos: análise morfológica imediata e após seis meses utilizando microscopia de força atômica. Pesq Odont Bras 2000;14:199-204.
492. Van Noort R, Cardew GE, Howard IC, Noroozi S. The effect of local interfacial geometry on the measurement of the tensile bond strength to dentin. J Dent Res. 1991;70:889-93.
493. Veloso HEP, Estrela CRÀ, Decurcio DA, Alves D, Estrela C. Microbial microleakage in temporary restorative after post space preparation. Odonto Ciência 2008; 23:187-91.
494. Versiani MA, Carvalho-Junior JR, Padilha MIA, Lacey S, Pascon EA, Sousa-Neto MD. A comparative study of physicochemical properties of AH plus and Epiphany root canal sealants. Int Endod J 2006;39:464-71.
495. Vojinovic O, Nyborgh H, Brännström M. Acid treatment of cavities under resin fillings: bacterial growth in dentinal tubules and pulpal reactions. J Dent Res 1973;52:1189-93.
496. Waltimo TM, Boiesen J, Eriksen HM, Ørstavik D. Clinical performance of 3 endodontic sealers. Oral Surg Oral Med Oral Pathol Oral Radiol Endod. 2001;92:89-92.
497. Wang X, Sun Y, Kimura Y, Kinoshita JI, Ishizaki NT, Matsumoto K. Effects of diode lasers irradiation on smear layer removal from root canal walls and apical leakage after obturation. Photomed Laser Surg 2005;23:575-81.
498. Watanabe LG, Marshall Jr GW, Marshall SJ. Variables influence on shear bond strength testing to dentine. In: Tagami J, Toledano M, Prati C, eds. Proceedings of the Granada International Symposium 3-4 December 1999. Como, Italy: Advanced Adhesive Dentistry, pp. 75-90.
499. Watson TF, Billington RW, Williams JA. The interfacial region of the tooth/glass ionomer restoration: a confocal optical microscope study. Am J Dent 1991;4:303-10.
500. Watts A, Paterson RC. Initial biologic testing of root canal sealing materials - a critical review. J Dent 1992;20:259-265.
501. Wayman BE, Kopp WM, Pinero GJ, Lazzari EP. Citric and lactic acids as root canal irrigants in vitro. J Endod 1979;5:258-65.
502. Weisenseel JA, Hicks ML, Peller Jr GB. Calcium hydroxide as an apical barrier. J Endod 1987;13:1-5.
503. Weisman MI. A study of the flow rate of tem root canal sealers. Oral Surg Oral Med Oral Pathol 1970;29:255-61.
504. Wei-xiong X, Zhi-yuan G. A clinical study of Thermafil endodontic obturation in molar root canals. J Stomatol 2004;24:29-30.
505. Wendt SL Jr, Jebeles CA, Leinfelder KF. The effect of two smear layer cleansers on shear bond strength to dentin. Dent Mater 1990;6:1-4.
506. Wennberg A, Ørstavik D. Adhesion of root canal sealers to bovine dentine and gutta-percha. Int Endod J 1990;23:13-9.
507. White JM, Goodis H. In vitro evaluation of an hydroxyapatite root canal system filling material. J Endod 1991;17:561-6.
508. Wieczkowski G Jr, Yu XY, Davis EL, Joynt RB. Microleakage in various dentin bonding agent/composite resin systems. Oper Dent 1992;5:62-7.
509. Wiener BH, Schilder HA comparative study of important physical properties of various root canal sealers. Oral Surg Oral Med Oral Pathol 1972;32:768-77.
510. Wilcox LR, Arnold AD. Coronal microleakage of permanent lingual access restorations in endodontically treated anterior teeth. J Endod 1989;15:584-7.
511. Willershausen B, Marroquin BB, Schafer D, Schulze R. Cytotoxicity of root canal filling materials to three different human cell lines. J Endod 2000;26:703-7.

512. Williams S, Goldman M. Penetrability of the smeared layer by a strain of Proteus vulgaris. J Endod 1985;11:385-8.
513. Wimonchit S, Timpawat S, Vongsavan N. A comparison of techiniques for assessment of coronal dye leakage. J Endod 2002;28:1-4.
514. Wollard RR, Brough SO, Maggio J, Seltzer S. Scanning electron microscopic examination of root canal filling materials. J Endod 1976;2:98-110.
515. Woody TL, Davis RD. The effect of eugenol-containing and eugenol-free temporary cements on microleakage in resin bonded restorations. Oper Dent 1992;17:175-80.
516. Wourms DJ, Campbell D, Hichs ML, Pelleu GB. Alternative solvents to chloroform for gutta-percha removal. J Endod 1990;16:224-26.
517. Wu MK, De Gee AJ, Wesselink PR, Moorer WR. Fluid transport and bacterial penetration along root canal fillings. Int Endod J 1993;26:203-8.
518. Wu MK, De Gee AJ, Wesselink PR. Effect of tubule orientation in the cavity wall on the seal of dental filling materials: an in vitro study. Int Endod J 1998;31:326-32.
519. Wu MK, De Gee AJ, Wesselink PR. Endodontic leakage studies reconsidered. Part I. Methodology, application and relevance. Int Endod J 1993;26:37-43.
520. Wu MK, De Gee AJ, Wesselink PR. Fluid transport and dye penetration along root canal fillings. Int Endod J 1994;27:233-38.
521. Wu MK, De Gee AJ, Wesselink PR. Leakage of AH26 and Ketac Endo used with injected warm gutta-percha. J Endod 1997;23:331-334.
522. Wu MK, De Gee AJ, Wesselink PR. Leakage of four root canal sealers at different thicknesses. Int Endod J 1994;27:304-08.
523. Wu MK, Kontakiotis EG, Wesselink PR. Decoloration of 1% methylene blue solution in contact with dental filling materials. J Dent 1998;26:585- 89.
524. Wu MK, Kontakiotis EG, Wesselink PR. Long-term seal provided by some root-end filling materials. J Endod 1998;24:557-601.
525. Wu MK, Ozok AR, Wesselink PR. Sealer distribution in root canals obturated by three techniques. Int Endod J 2000;33:340-45.
526. Wu MK, Pehlivan Y, Kontakiotis EG, Wesselink PR. Microleakage along apical root fillings and cemented posts. J Prosthet Dent 1998;79:264-9.
527. Wu MK, Wesselink PR, Boersma J. A 1-year follow-up study on leakage os four root canal sealers at different thickness. Int Endod J 1995;28:185-89.
528. Wu MK, Wesselink PR. Diminished leakage along root canal filled with gutta-percha without sealer over time: a laboratory study. Int Endod J 2000;33:121-25.
529. Wu MK, Wesselink PR. Endodontic leakage studies reconsidered. Part I. Methodology, application and relevance. Int Endod J 1993;26:37-43.
530. Wucherpfenning AL, Green DB. Mineral trioxide vs. Portland cement: two biocompatible filling materials. J Endod 1999;25:308 (Abstract PR40).
531. Xun L, Wen-qing C. Comparison of clinical effects about two root canal obturation techniques. J Dental Prevention Treatment 2002;10:287-8.
532. Yamada RS, Armas A, Goldman M, Lin PS. A scanning electron microscopic comparison of a high volume final flush with several irrigating solutions: part 3. J Endod 1983;9:137-42.
533. Yamazaki R, Goya C, Tomita Y, Kimura Y, Matsumoto K. Study on apical leakage of the teeth after argon laser treatment and obturation. J Clin Laser Med Surg 1999;17:121-5.
534. Yap A, Stokes AN, Pearson GJ. An in vitro microleakage study of a new multi-purpose dental adhesive system. J Oral Rehabil 1996;23:302-8.
535. Yap UJ, Stokes AN, Pearson GJ. Concepts of adhesion: a review. N Z Dent J 1994;90:91-7.
536. Yared GM, Dagher FB. Sealing ability of the vertical condensation with different root canal sealers. J Endod 1996;22:06-08.
537. Yesilsoy C, Koren LZ, Morse DR, Kobayashi C. A comparative tissue toxicity evaluation of established and newer root canal sealers. Oral Surg Oral Med Oral Pathol 1988;65:459-67.
538. Yu XY, Davis EL, Joynt RB, Wieczkowski G Jr. Origination and progression of microleakage in a restoration with a smear layer-mediated dentinal bonding agent. Quint Int 1992;23:551-5.
539. Yu XY, Joynt RB, Davis EL, Wieczkowski G Jr. Adhesion to dentin. J Calif Dent Assoc 1993;21:23-9.
540. Yu XY, Joynt RB, Wieczkowski G, Davis EL. Scanning electron microscopic and energy dispersive x-ray evaluation of two smear layer-mediated dentinal bonding agents. Quint Int 1991;22:305-10.
541. Yu-hua Q, Jing-hua Z, Shi-guang H. The comparison of effects between cold lateral condensation and warm vertical gutta-percha compaction in 128 cases. J Jinan University (Medical Edition) 2005;26:559-61.
542. Zakariasen KL, Douglas WH, Stadem P. Comparison of volumetric and linear measurements of root canal leakage. J Dent Res 1981;60:627. Abstract 1273.
543. Zheng QZ, Wang J, Liu LM. Comparison of the clinical effects of three root canal treatments. Shanghai J Stomatol 2004;13:459-61.
544. Zidan O, Ross G, Lee IK, Gomez-Marin O, Yeh SH. The effect of dentin pre-treatment and heat-augmented cure on marginal gap formation of a dentin bonding agent. Dent Mater 1991;7:174-8.
545. Zmener O, Spielberg C, Lamberghini F, Rucci M. Sealing ability properties of a new epoxy resin-based root-canal sealer. Int Endod J 1997;30:332-34.
546. Zmener O. Evaluation of the apical seal obtained with two calcium hydroxide based endodontic sealers. Int Endod J 1987;20:87-90.
547. Zoellner A, Herzberg S, Gaengler P. Histobacteriology and pulp reactions to longterm dental restorations. J Marmara Univ Dent Fac 1996;2:483-90.
548. Zuco LR. Avaliação da infiltração coronária em canais obturados e preparad os para pino. (Master´s Thesis). Luteran University of Brazil;2001. 164p.
549. Zurbriggen T, DelRio CE, Brady JM. Postdebridement retention of endodontic reagents: a quantitative measurement with radioactive isotope. J Endod 1975;1:298-299.

# Diagnosis of Endodontic Failure

**C. Estrela**
*Federal University of Goiás, Goiânia, GO, Brazil*

**O. A. Guedes**
*Federal University of Goiás, Goiânia, GO, Brazil*

**W. Pereira-Júnior**
*Brazilian Dentistry Research and Learning Center, CEPOBRAS, Goiânia, GO, Brazil*

**L. Esponda**
*University of Mexico, Mexico*

**A. G. Cruz**
*University of Guadalajara, Mexico*

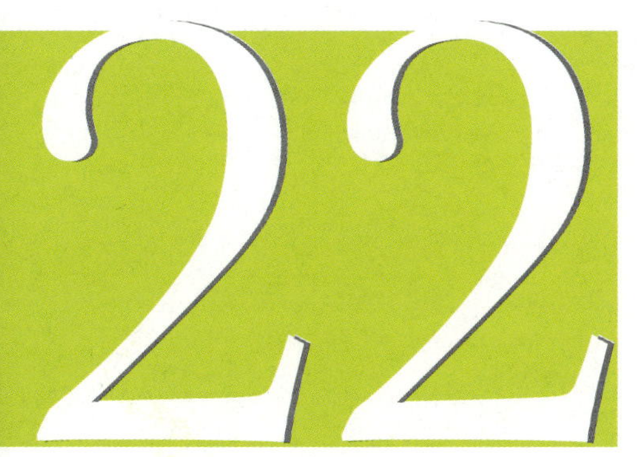

Chapter contents

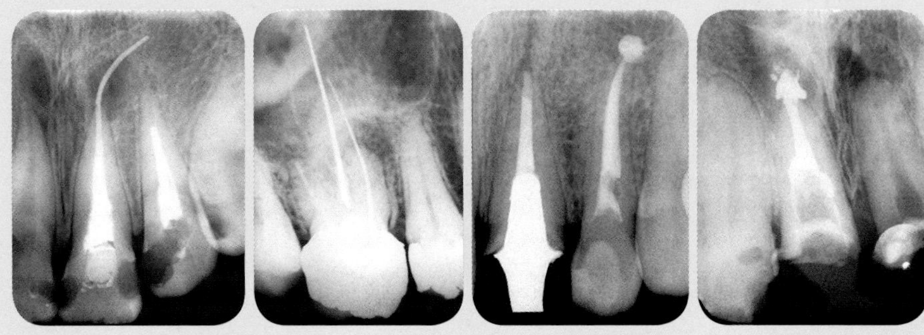

Radiographic images characterizing failure of the treatment.

## 22.1 Introduction

Vestiges of endodontic treatment failure, characterized by the presence of periapical lesion and semiotic post-treatment, are important indicators that further intervention is required. These aspects signal the victory of microorganisms over the body's resistance.

Endodontic failure is generally due to technical (operative) or pathological (present alteration) factors, or is influenced by systemic factors (diseases that complicate the tissue reparation process).

For many years the treatment of choice for endodontic failures was parendodontic surgery or extraction. Endodontic retreatment, as a result of the effectiveness of the sanitization process, shaping and filling of the infected dentinal tubules, has reinforced the importance of microbial control in endodontic infections.

Failures in endodontic diagnosis and treatment methods can be better defined. However, the pathological terms are significant as regards the predictability of success or failure in endodontic treatment.

Success should be determined on the basis of defined criteria, because the conclusions drawn by the available resources that the treatment was well or badly performed (suitable to the process of tissue repair of the pathology found), are based on clinical and radiographic criteria. The histological criteria will be defined in a second moment by microscopic exam, when opportune and necessary.

Prevention of current or future complications resulting from the unsatisfactory endodontic treatment in teeth that will receive metal restorations, fixed prosthesis with or without intracanal retainer, require the removal of the endodontic filling and/or clearance of the root canal, thus justifying the need for endodontic retreatment.

The goal of this chapter is to analyze the etiological factors related to the diagnosis of endodontics failures. With regard to the repair process after endodontic treatment, this chapter discusses the local and systemic factors that can interfere in the reparation process. Among the local factors, the following are mentioned: 1. Infection; 2. Hemorrhage; 3. Tissue destruction; 4. Deficiency in the blood supply; 5. Presence of foreign bodies. The systemic factors include: 1. Nutrition; 2. Stress; 3. State of chronic waste; 4. Hormones and vitamins; 5. Dehydration; 6. Age[105,106].

## 22.2 Endodontic Success

Clinical and radiographic success should be observed after the elapse of an adequate period of time after the treatment. Ingle & Taintor[52] related that although endodontic treatments can demonstrate failures in periods up to 10 years, more often, this is evidenced in the period up to 2 years. Stabholz & Walton[117] pointed out that follow up after treatment should be from 1 to 4 years.

Some aspects for ensuring endodontic success should receive special care, such as suitable restorative treatment. Perfect sealing of the dentinal tubule system implies perfect coronal sealing. Longitudinal control, observing signs and symptoms and radiographic aspects, is a resource used to determine success. As a clinical parameter, considering the initial radiographs to verify the result of endodontic treatment, the period of up to 1 year for vital pulp cases, and 2 years for the cases of endodontic infections can be established. Longitudinal follow up is important, because the condition of the tooth restoration and patient's general health can influence the success.

Bender et al.[6] enumerated some clinical and radiographic criteria representative of successful endodontic treatment: 1. Absence of pain and edema; 2. Absence of drainage and fistula; 3. Tooth in function, with normal physiology; 4. Disappearance of periapical bone rarefaction.

The value of the periapical radiograph is significant in for identifying the quality of endodontic treatment (Fig. 22.1-22.3), however, one should be watchful, because some periapical lesions can be present without showing up clearly in the radiographic exam.

The vestige to suspect of a forgetful root canal, in endodontic treated tooth can be signaled by a persistent pain to thermal test.

Scientific knowledge allied to the clinical symptoms allows the main factors involved in endodontic treatment failure to be mapped.

Holland et al.[45], discussing the influence of the periapical lesions on the success of endodontic treatment, pointed out that a lower percentage of success is observed in endodontic treatments with periapical rarefactions. The authors related the importance of intracanal medication, especially calcium hydroxide in the tissue healing process (Table 22.1).

The essential factors related to endodontic success are summed up as follows: 1. Clinical silence (absence of pain, edema, fistula); 2. Normal periapical bone structure (uniformity of the lamina dura, absence or interruption of radicular resorption); 3. Tooth in function and presence of perfect coronal sealing.

The Figures 22.4 to 22.9 exhibit clinical cases of endodontic treatment suggestive of clinical and radiographic success.

**Table 22.1** - Percentage of success (%) in root canals with and without periapical lesion

| Authors | Success WITHOUT periapical lesion | Success WITH periapical lesion | Total cases (roots) |
|---|---|---|---|
| Strindberg | 88.8 | 67.9 | 479 |
| Grahnen & Hansson | 85.8 | 69.2 | 763 |
| Engstrom et al. | 88.3 | 66.5 | 306 |
| Stroms | 96.1 | 83 | 158 |
| Adeenubi & Rube | 92.2 | 81.6 | 767 |
| Kerekes & Tronstad | 93.6 | 84.3 | 501 |
| Jokinen et al. | 61 | 38 | 2.459 |
| Heling & Tamshe | 79.4 | 52.6 | 213 |
| Grossman et al. | 89.3 | 76.5 | 432 |
| Averbacw | 97.3 | 85 | 211 |
| Buchbinder | 88 | 44 | 162 |
| Castagnola | 73 | 66 | 1.000 |
| Coolidge | 77.6 | 58 | 307 |
| Holst | 83 | 64 | 82 |
| Stein | 76 | 44 | 116 |
| Morse & Yates | 100 | 31.8 | 257 |
| Seltzer et al. | 92.4 | 75.6 | 2.335 |

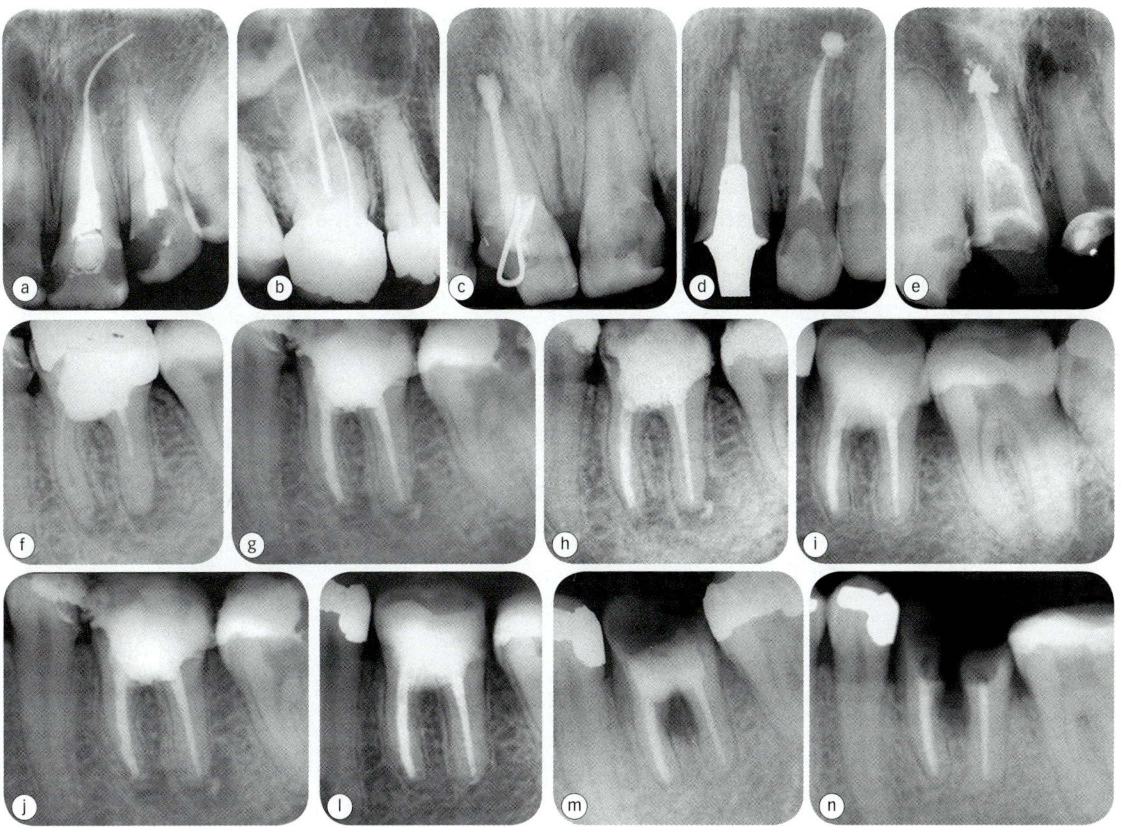

**Figure 22.1** - (**A-N**) Radiographic images characterizing failure of the treatment.

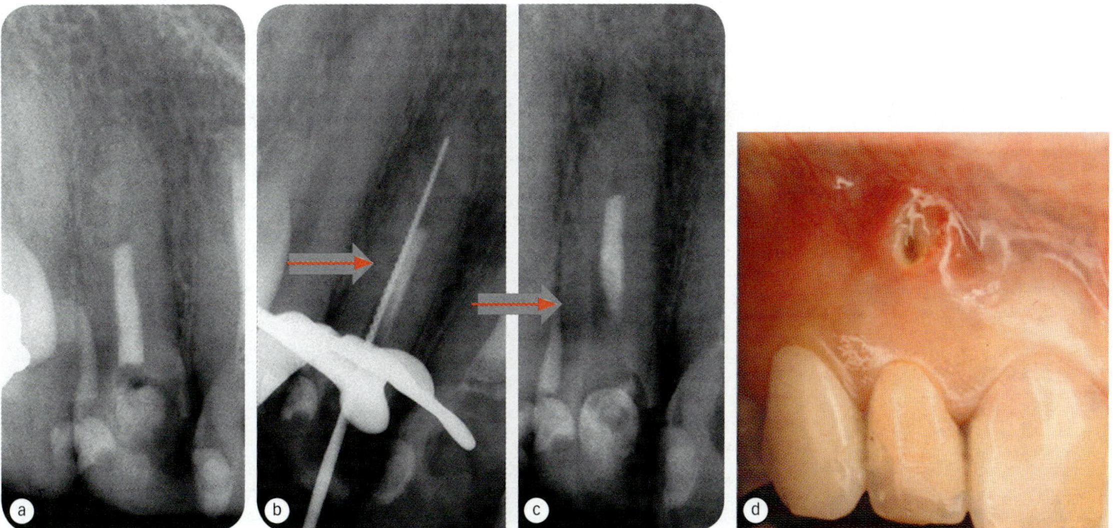

**Figure 22.2** - (**A-D**) Radiographic images characterizing root canal perforation.

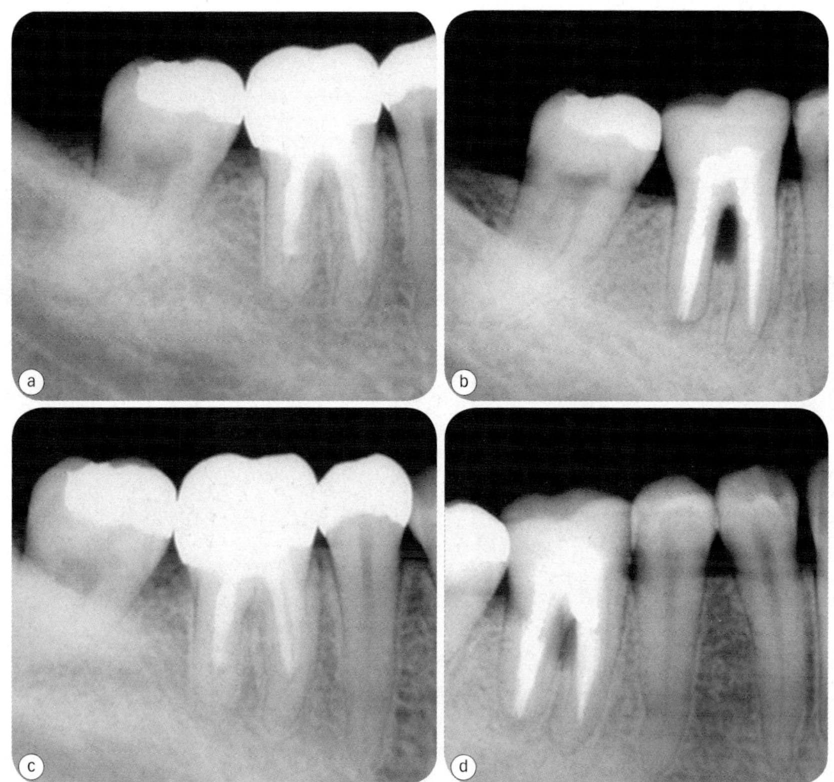

**Figure 22.3** - (**A-D**) Radiographic images characterizing root canal perforation (Courtesy of Prof. Luiz Fernando Naldi Ruiz).

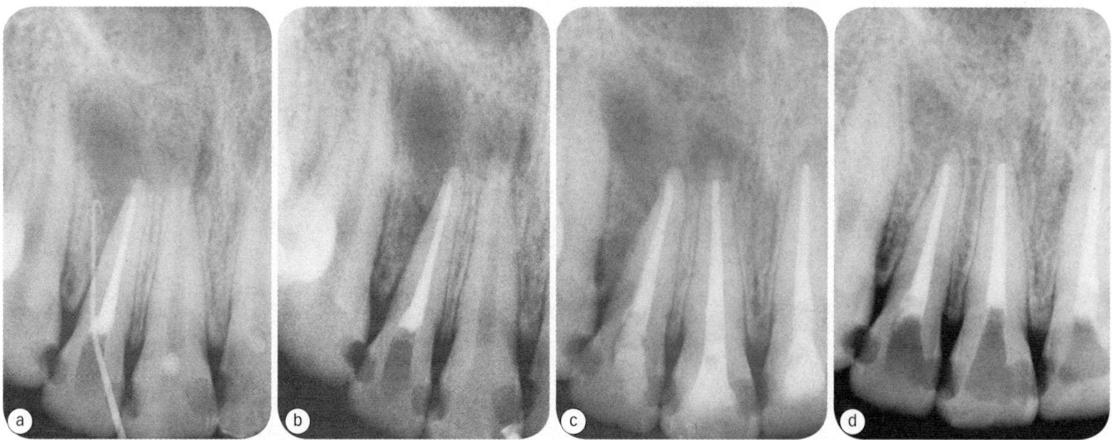

**Figure 22.4** - (**A-B**) Asymptomatic apical periodontitis in tooth #12 with endodontic treatment, characterizing failure of the treatment. (**C-D**). Endodontic retreatment in tooth #12, endodontic treatment in the teeth #11 and #21, clinical and radiographic success after 2 years of control.

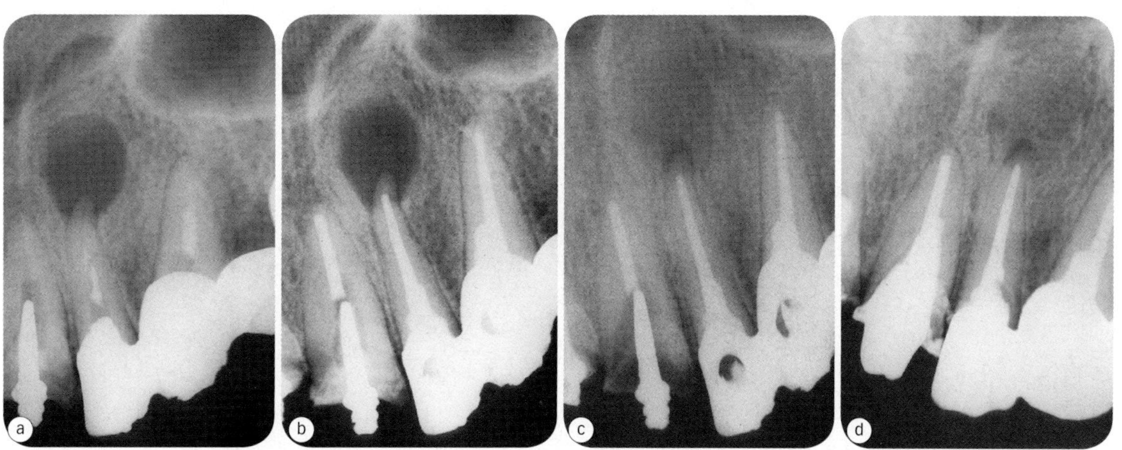


**Figure 22.5** - (**A-B**) Asymptomatic apical periodontitis in tooth #22, characterizing failure of the treatment. Endodontic retreatment in teeth #21, #22 and #23. (**C-D**) Almost total reduction of the periapical bone rarefaction, initially suggesting clinical and radiographic success, after 26 months of control.



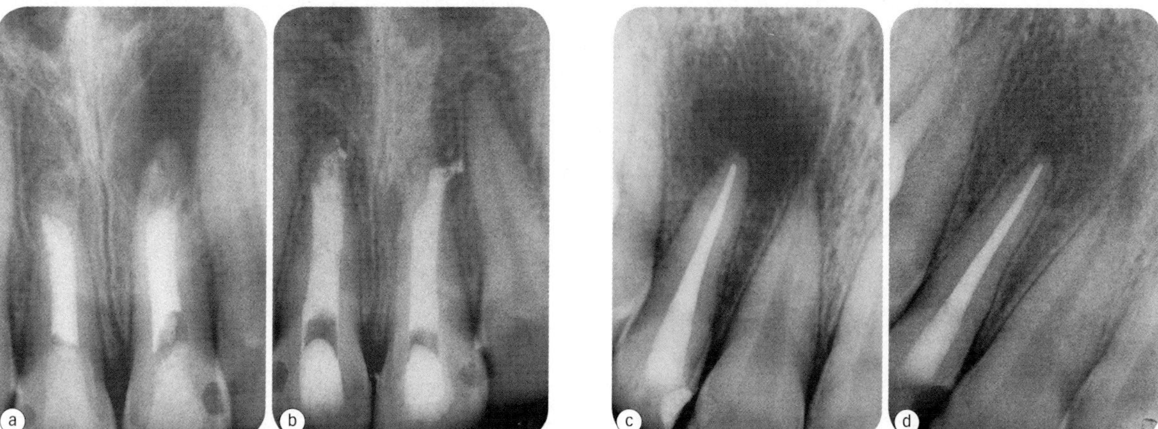


**Figure 22.6** - (**A-B**) Asymptomatic apical periodontitis in tooth #21, characterizing treatment failure. Endodontic retreatment in teeth #11 and #21. clinical and radiographic success, after 2 years of control. (**C-D**) Asymptomatic apical periodontitis in tooth #12. Clinical and radiographic success, after 18 months of control.

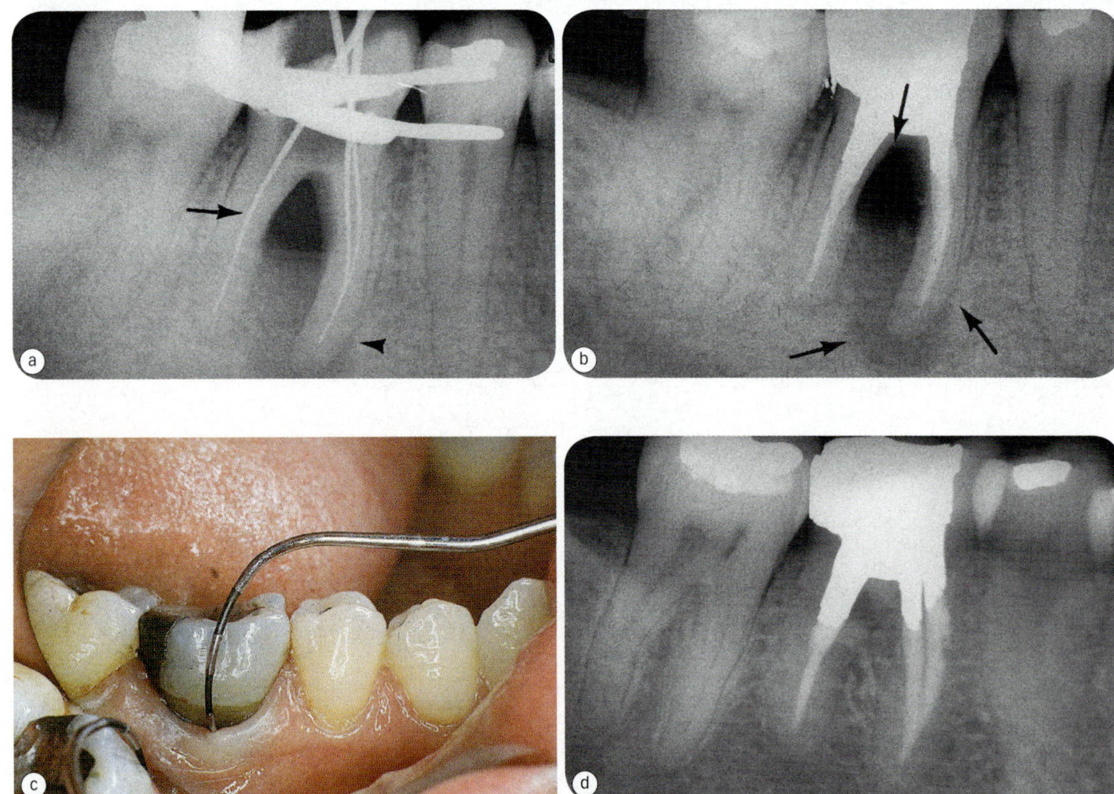

**Figure 22.7** - (**A-D**) Asymptomatic apical periodontitis in tooth #46, associated with periodontal furcation lesion of endodontic origin. Complete reparation after endodontic treatment and restoration, with 2 years of control. (Courtesy of the Prof. Lourdes C. Aguilar de Esponda).

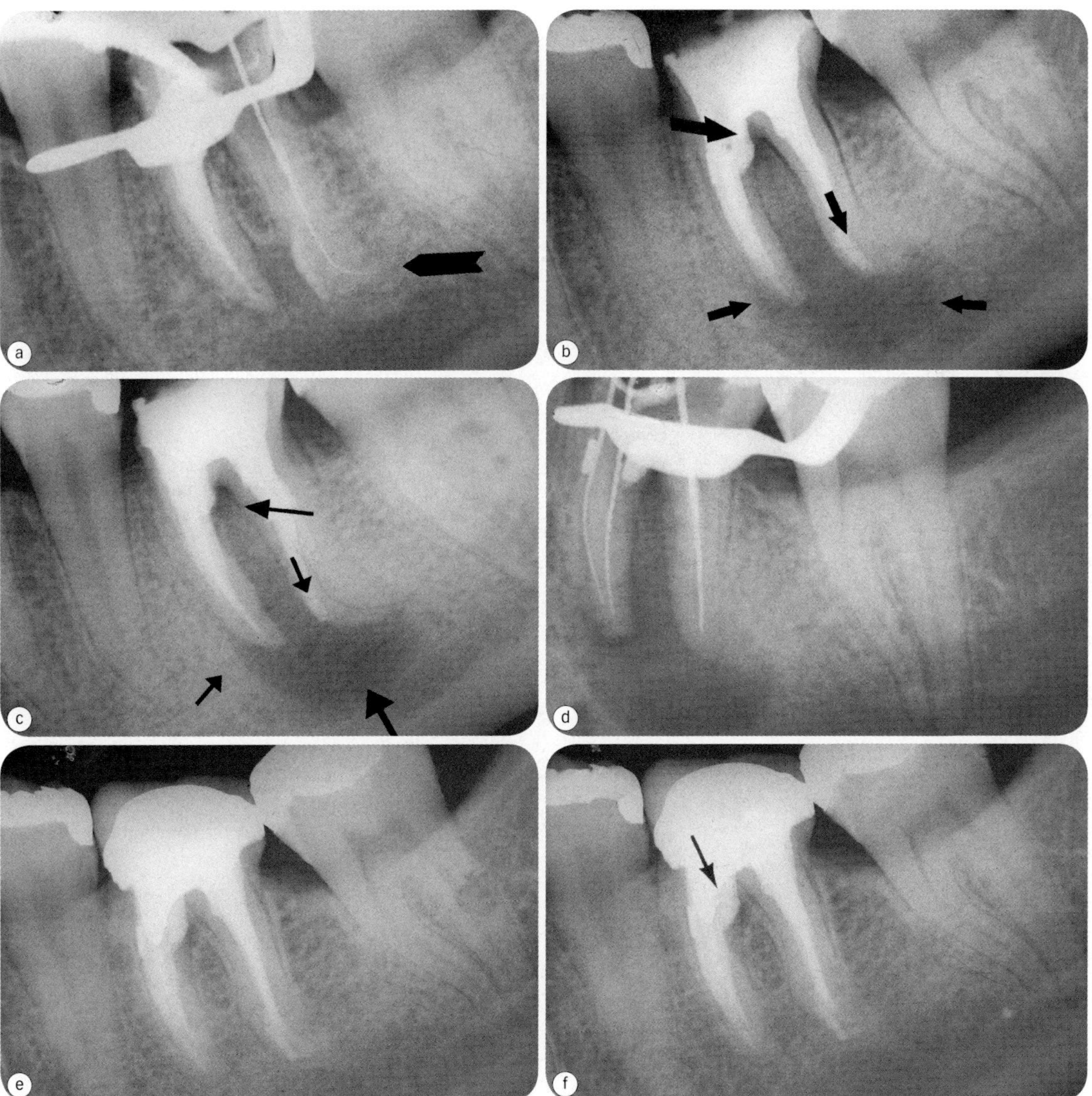


**Figure 22.8** - (**A-F**) Failure of endodontic treatment in tooth #36. Periodontal lesion in furcation area (with drilling), and apical periodontitis. Endodontic retreatment. Complete reparation after endodontic treatment and restoration, with 25 years of radiographic control (Courtesy of the Prof. Lourdes C. Aguilar de Esponda and Dr. Vitor Esponda).

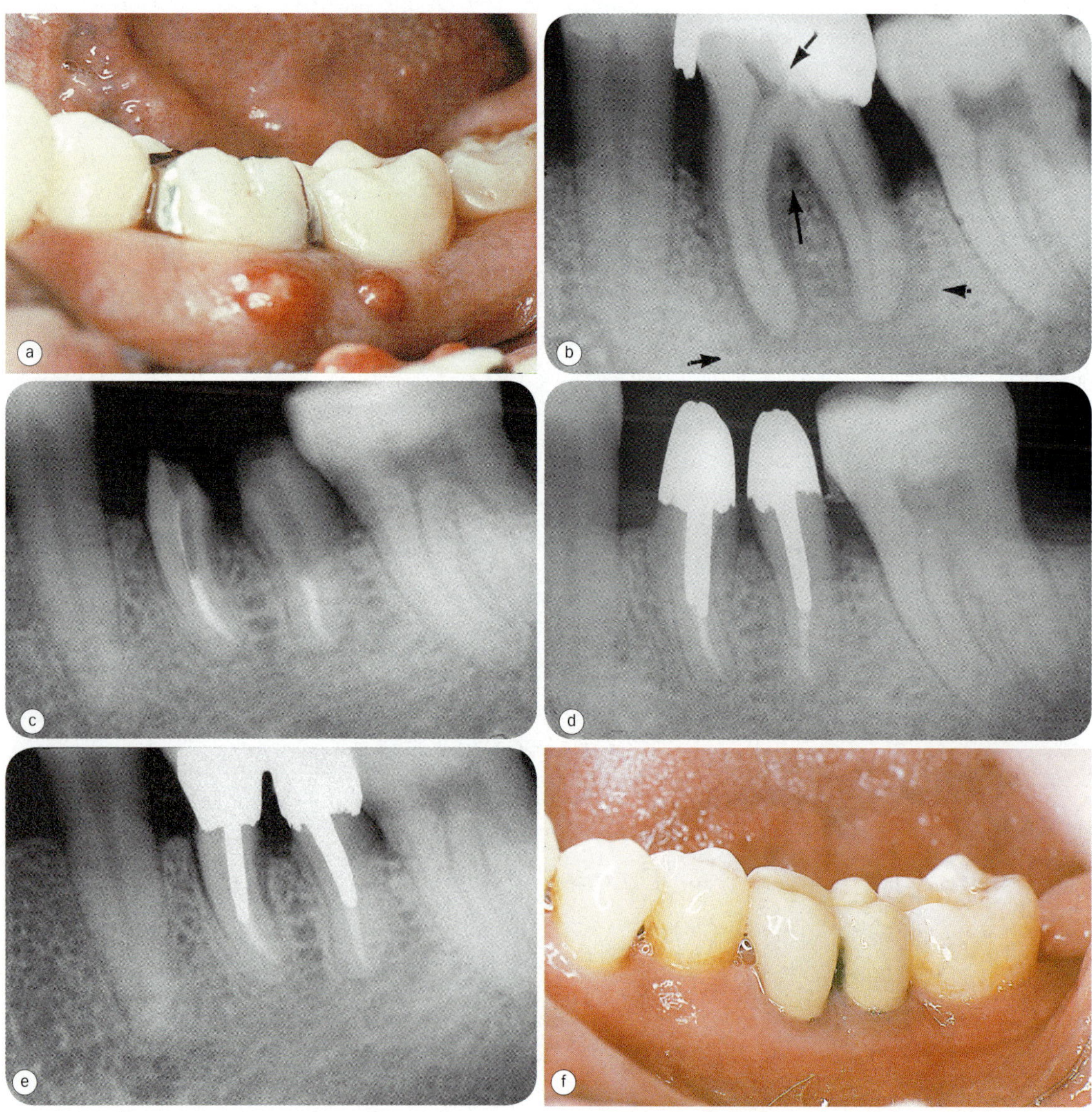


**Figure 22.9** - (**A-F**) Endodontic and periodontal lesion in tooth #46. Endodontic treatment performed and surgical intervention, individualizing the roots, placement of intrar adicular posts, and restoration. Tissue reparation and 3 years of control (Courtesy of Dr. Vitor Esponda and of Prof. Lourdes C. Aguilar de Esponda).

### 22.3 Endodontic Failure

Endodontic failures frequently observed are related to several of the previously mentioned factors. The main causes of factors related to endodontic infections will now be discussed. The maintenance or development of these infections are usually associated with failures in the operative procedures (opening and coronal preparation, sanitization process, modeling, filling and coronal sealing), arising from pathological or current processes of dental trauma.

One of the aspects responsible for adequate microbial control is effective root canal preparation, achieved by adequate emptying and enlargement. The goal of the mechanical action of root canal instrumentation, is removal of the contaminated material from the main root canal. Irrigant solutions are effective, due to their antimicrobial properties, solvent capacity and tissue tolerance, in addition to the depth of their action, surface active volume and capacity – surface tension, and are powerful allies. Associated with this stage, the work of intracanal dressing makes a significant contribution to this antimicrobial process.

Considering the endodontic microbiota present in the different pathological terms, endodontic infections can be divided into: Primary (Infection observed in teeth not submitted to endodontic treatment), secondary (infection present in endodontically treated teeth), and persistent infection (an infectious process that does not respond positively to endodontic treatment)[77,81-86,111-113,119].

Some important studies endeavored to establish the etiology and a standard of clinical conduct when faced with endodontic failures, among which the following are outstanding: Mollander et al.[77], Nair [81,82], Nair et al.[83-86], Sirén et al.[111], Sjögren et al.[112-113], Sundqvist et al.[119].

The distribution of microorganisms in necrotic teeth was demonstrated by Shovelton.[109] The percentage of microorganisms in the cervical region was higher when compared with the middle and the apical thirds of the root. Teeth with chronic processes evidenced a larger proportion of microorganisms than those with acute processes. Following this study, Kakehashi et al.[55] evidenced the potential of pulp reparation in the absence of infection, and the influence of microorganisms on the formation of periapical lesions.

Nair[81] studied the endodontic and periapical microbiota of contaminated human teeth, using transillumination and transmission electronic microscopy in 31 lesions of human teeth without endodontic treatment and with periapical involvement. All the teeth were decayed, with necrotic pulps and periapical bone resorption. Five teeth were symptomatic, and the others were asymptomatic. Out of the 31 lesions, one was radicular cyst. Thirty-one root canals with lesions revealed the presence of a mixed microbiota. Although, in most cases the microbiota was restricted to the root canal, bacteria inside and outside the root canal could be observed inside the body of the 4 granulomas and of the radicular cyst. Structurally, the endodontic microbiota presented loose collections of distinct bacteria, of varied morphology, but not identified – consisting of coccus, short rods and filamentous forms. Most of the microbiota was suspended in the apparent light humidity of the root canal. Less frequently, aggregated bacteria were observed fastened to the dentinal wall of the root canal or free in the middle of a vast number of polymorphonuclear cells in the light of the root canal. Morphologically, the mixed bacterial groups were constituted of coccus, short rods and spirochetes. Four granulomas revealed the presence of bacteria inside the lesion body, and one was a case of actinomycosis. The other three lesions showed the presence of distinct plate bacteria, adhered to the dentinal wall in the apical foramen. In these cases, the microbiota that extended for several depths inside the body of the periapical lesions, caused limited or extensive tissue necrosis and acute response. Characteristically, the microbiota consisted of numerous cocci, short rods, filamentous organisms and many spirochetes. The short rods showed Gram-negative cellular walls. One of the lesions was a radicular cyst that showed a different outline in the light by the stratified scaly epithelium of varied thickness. The cystic cavity contained various erythrocytes, polymorphonuclear and other necrotic cells. Only bacteria and isolated groupings were observed as surplus suspended or interrupted in the light cyst that apparently contained a fluid medium. Transillumination microscopy showed numerous neutrophils containing filamentous organisms in their interior. By electronic microscopy, neutrophils revealed distinct morphological types of phagosomes containing bacteria.

Sjögren et al.[113] studied the factors that affect the result of endodontic treatment, after a period from 8 to 10 years of treatment. Considering the preoperative state of the pulp and of the periapical tissue, they verified a success rate of 96% when there was no periapical lesion, 86% success when it was present, 98% success in the cases of retreatment without periapical lesion and 62% success in retreatment cases that presented periapical lesion. In the teeth with preoperative apical periodontitis, when the instrumentation and filling of the root canal went up to 2 mm of the apex, the prognosis was significantly better than the cases of over filling, or when the filling was more than 2 mm beyond the apex.

Nair et al. [83] investigated extra-radicular infection in human teeth resistant to endodontic therapy, whose radiographic exams, performed from 4 to 10 years after the treatment showed evidences of periapical pathology. The apexes were surgically removed in rectangular blocks that contained the apical portion of the root and the lesion, with a fine sliver of adjacent bone. Analyzed by the light of optic and electronic microscopy after adequate processing, six of the nine specimens revealed the presence of microorganisms in the apical portion, four contained one or more bacterial species, and two revealed the presence of yeasts. Of the four cases in which bacteria could be observed, they were detected by optic microscopy in only 1 biopsy. In the other 3 cases, their presence was confirmed by electronic microscopy. Of the three cases in which the microorganisms were not found, one of them showed histological aspects that suggested the presence of a type of foreign body giant cells. These results suggested that in the majority of the human teeth with periapical lesions resistant to endodontic treatment, microorganisms can persist and have an important role in the treatment success. In cases in which infectious agents are absent, the periapical lesions presented after endodontic treatment can be maintained by immunological factors, resulting from the involvement of a type of foreign body giant cells, as host response, in the periapex of endodontically treated teeth.

Nair et al.[84], analyzing morphologic and not microbial evidences that affect the process of periapex repair after endodontic treatment, pointed out the presence of cholesterol crystals and the true cyst as endogenous factors.

Mollander et al.[77] observed high frequency of enterobacterias isolated in endodontic retreatment, when compared with the teeth treated for the first time.

Sirén et al.[111], investigating the clinical relation procedures and the occurrence of facultative enteric bacteria in radicular infections, noted that *E. faecalis* represented the commoner group of enteric bacteria. In 33% of the cases in which *E. faecalis* was isolated, it appeared as a monoinfection (Table 22.2).

Sjögren et al.[112] investigated the role of infection in the prognosis of endodontic therapy by following up teeth that had their root canals cleaned and filled in a single appointment. Fifty and five single rooted teeth with necrotic pulps and radiographic evidence of periapical bone lesions were endodontically treated. Initial bacterial and post-instrumentation samples were collected of the root canal and transferred to the PYG. All the bacteria in the post-instrumentation samples were identified at species level. The patients re-

**Table 22.2** - Facultative enteric bacteria in radicular infection

| Species | Total | Monoinfection |
|---|---|---|
| *Enterococcus faecalis* | 24 | 8 |
| *Enterobacter cloacae* | 5 | 2 |
| *Enterobacter agglomerans* | 1 | 1 |
| *Enterobacter sakazakii* | 1 | 0 |
| *Klebsiella oxytoga* | 1 | 0 |
| *Acinetobacter sp.* | 1 | 0 |
| *Pseudomonas aeruginosa* | 1 | 1 |

(Sirén et al.[111])

turned annually for clinical and radiographic exam of the filled teeth. In the review consultation, the type of restoration and any sign or symptom associated with the teeth were recorded. Control radiographs were taken. The treatment was considered successful when the outline, width and structure of the periodontal margin were normal or when the periodontal outline was enlarged, mostly as a result of excess filling material. Biopsy specimens of three cases that did not show signs of periapical healing were analyzed by the histological method. Two of these specimens of teeth that were infected at the moment of root canal filling were sent for immunohistochemical analysis. Bacteria of the species *Actinomyces israelii* were isolated from the root canals at the time of filling; the presence of the same bacteria was studied in the surgical tissue. The third specimen was obtained from a case where no bacteria were detected at the time of root canal filling. The tooth was non vital and carious with widespread radiolucence in the periapex before the treatment. Initially, after the endodontic therapy, there was a slight reduction in the size, but the lesion did not show any radiographic sign of improvement after 3 years, so that the tooth was submitted to apical surgery. The tooth remained without symptoms during the entire follow up period. The results showed that bacteria were initially present in the root canals of all the 55 treated teeth. In the final instrumentation, 22 root canals (40%) still contained recoverable bacteria and these were identified by species at the level of 20 out of 22 root canals. The number of species in the root canals with persistent infection varied from 1 to 6, and 93% of these were anaerobic. In most cases there were a low number of bacterial cells in the samples, so that in eight cases, bacteria were only detected after growth enriched in the sample medium and in 9 other cases the number of bacterial cells was $10^2$-$10^3$. Only three samples had more than 104 bacterial cells. Fifty-three teeth (96%) were followed up. Forty-four of the lesions healed completely and 9 cases, all without symptoms, were failures. Seven of the failures were found among the 22 cases in which bacteria had been isolated at the time of root canal filling. Thus, the success rate for teeth with positive samples at the time of filling was 68%. The histological analysis of the cases that failed revealed that filamentous microorganisms that showed positively with the antiserum for *A. israelii*, were present in the periapical tissue. Twenty-nine of the 31 teeth with negative samples at the time of filling healed; a success rate of 94%. One tooth showed no sign of periapical healing after a period 3 years and was therefore, scheduled for surgery. A bacteriological sample extracted from the periapical region in the operation showed growth of *Actinomyces odontolyticus*, *Streptococcus constellatus*, *Propionibacterium acnes* and a type of Campylobacter. Microscopy of the sample revealed aggregated bacteria. Histological analysis of the root tip revealed that the root canal was filled with gutta-percha and that one of the lateral canals in the root tip was obstructed with bacteria. Evaluation of the apical filling level revealed that most of the teeth were filled within 2 mm of the apex. In 10 teeth there was a slight over filling, but in each one of these cases the extent of excess material in the periapical tissue was less than 1 mm. Five of the over filled teeth had positive samples and five had negative samples at the time of filling. The slight over filling seemed not to have any influence on the result, since all the 10 teeth with excessive filling were successful. The size of the periapical lesion apparent in the preoperative period did not have any influence on the result of treatment. These discoveries emphasize the importance of completely eliminating the bacteria from the root canal before filling. This goal cannot be reliably attained in a treatment of one visit because is not possible to eradicate all the infection in the root canal without the support of antimicrobial dressing in several sessions.

Sundqvist et al.[119] determined the microbiota after the failure of endodontic treatment in 54 teeth selected for retreatment. All the teeth presented as asymptomatic, previously treated, and with radiographic evidences of periapical bone lesions. The teeth had a history of endodontic treatment from 4 to 5 years ago; in some cases, the teeth had been regularly followed up for 2 years, and during that time there was no sign of repair. Except in a case with deficient filling, all the teeth had fillings that presented a satisfactory radiographic standard. Five of the teeth had two roots with two canals; the other teeth had only one canal. Radiographic exams were performed to determine the length of the root and to ensure that the gutta-percha had been totally removed. The root canal was then instrumented so that the sample could be collected from the walls. One initial bacteriological sample was collected from the root canal by capturing the fluid on paper tips. The canals were left empty to allow any surviving bacteria to multiply and reach to a detectable level at the next visit. The cavities were filled with zinc and eugenol oxide cement. Seven days elapsed, bacteriological samples were collected, and the root canals were shaped manually and irrigated with 0.5% sodium hypochlorite solution. After the final irrigation, the canals were filled with a calcium hydroxide dressing and a coronal sealing was done. In the third visit, 7 to 14 days later, the dressing was removed and a sample was collected. After this, the canals were filled with gutta-percha using the lateral condensation technique. In 20 cases there was growth of both samples withdrawn in the initial visit and in the second visit. In one case, bacteria (*P. micros* and *F. nucleatum*) grew from the sample withdrawn in the first visit, but not in the samples withdrawn in the second visit. In three cases, microorganisms were recovered from the sample withdrawn in the second visit, after the canal had been left empty, but not in the initial sample. Microorganisms isolated after having left these three root canals were *S. intermedius*, *S. parasanguis*, *L. catenaforme*, and *Candida albicans*. In 19 cases only one species was present, in 4 cases two types of species were present (*S. intermedius* and *L. catenaforme*, *E. alactolyticum* and *P. acnes*, *P. micros* and *S. Mitis*, *P. micros* and *F. nucleatum*), and in one case there was an polymicrobial infection that consisted of 4 species (*S. anginosus*, *E. timidum*, *Propionibacterium propionicum*, and *B. Gracillis*). In all of the 9 cases in which *E. faecalis* was isolated, this was the only microorganism present in the canal. Fifty of the 54 cases treated (93%) were available for another visit. Thirty-seven of the lesions were completely repaired and 13 cases were considered failures: a success rate of 74%.

Eighteen of the 24 teeth (75%) from which bacteria were isolated after removal of the filling, repaired completely, and 19 of the 26 teeth from which there were no microorganisms available repaired: a success rate of 73%. The differences between the results of the 2 groups were not statistically significant. The success rate for the teeth in which *E. faecalis* was isolated after removal of the previous filling was lower (66%) than the average for the whole material entire sample. In samples withdrawn at the time of filling, microorganisms were recovered in 6 root canals. Four of the lesions associated with these teeth did not repair, and 3 of these teeth contained the *E. faecalis* species of bacteria and four canals harbored *A. Israeli*. In the 2 teeth in which there was periapical lesion repair, samples of *E. faecalis* were isolated at the time of filling. Of the teeth with microorganisms not recoverable at the time of filling, 35 of 44 teeth repaired – a success rate of 80%. There was significant difference between the size of the lesions that repaired and those that did not. Of the 50 cases that could be followed up, most of them (37) were filled between 0.5 to 2 mm of the radiographic apex. Another 9 were filled to the level of the apex, and 4 had excess of filling with less than 1 mm (Table 22.3).



**Table 22.3** - Microorganisms recovered from the root canals after the removal of the filling material

| Microbial species | Number of Cases |
|---|---|
| *Enterococcus faecalis* | 9 |
| *Streptococcus anginosus* | 2 |
| *Streptococcus constellatus* | 1 |
| *Streptococcus intermedius* | 1 |
| *Streptococcus mitis* | 1 |
| *Streptococcus parasanguis* | 1 |
| *Peptostreptococcus micros* | 2 |
| *Actinomyces israelii* | 3 |
| *Pseudoramibacter alactolyticus* | 1 |
| *Eubacterium timidum* | 1 |
| *Lactobacillus catenaforme* | 1 |
| *Propionibacterium acnes* | 1 |
| *Propionibacterium propionicum* | 1 |
| *Fusobacterium nucleatum* | 1 |
| *Bacteroides gracilis* | 3 |
| *Candida albicans* | 2 |

(Sundqvist et al.[119])

Nair et al.[85] studied tissue responses to cholesterol and observed that cholesterol crystals can induce and sustain a granulomatous tissue reaction. For so much, they were worth of 24 tubes implanted in 6 India's pigs. To conduct the study, 6 Guinea pigs were used, and 4 tubes were implanted in each of them, totaling 24 tubes. Three of the 4 tubes, were previously filled with a mixture of cholesterol crystals and saline solution and one tube was left empty. Two animals were sacrificed at 2, 4 and 32 weeks, respectively. The histological conditions of the control groups varied according to the studied time. Two weeks after the implant, the conjunctive tissue was observed to be rich in fibroblasts in the external region, with growth entering through the tubes and central cavity. The last group contained a vast number of erythrocytes and necrotic cells. After 4 weeks, the tubes were completely filled with conjunctive tissue and the structures they contained resembled those of the 32 week group. Mushroom-shaped cholesterol crystals presented very circumscribed granulomatous tissue response. After two weeks of observation, rhomboid rifts fissures appeared in the lumen of the tubes peripherally surrounded by conjunctive tissue growth. The size of the fissures seemed to be "nude" inside the central cavity. After 4 and 32 weeks, the fissures formed very circumscribed units completely surrounded by delicate conjunctive tissue, with a healthy appearance. In some cases, collagen fibers addressed filled the fissures, which were surrounded by numerous cells that structurally appeared to be predominantly macrophages. Less frequently, multinucleated giant cells appeared. It is important to emphasize that other cells usually found in inflammation, such as neutrophils, lymphocytes and plasmatic cells were completely absent.

The Table 22.4 shows the causes responsible for failures in endodontic treatment[82].

Considering that *E. faecalis* is an outstanding bacteria in secondary infections, its probable survival mechanism in dentinal tubules, and its resistance to high pH, such as that of calcium hydroxide, has yet to be analyzed.

Love[73] analyzed the probable mechanism that allowed an explanation of how *E. faecalis* can survive and grow inside dentinal tubules and reinfect a filled root canal. Cells of *S. gordonii*, *S. mutans* and *E. faecalis* were cultivated for 56 days, contend several values in human serum. The results evidenced that all three of the species remained viable in the experimental period when cultivated in human serum. Cells of all three of the bacteria were able of invade the dentin and unite to immobilize the collagen. The human serum inhibited the dentinal invasion and the collagen adhesion by *S. gordonii* and *S. mutans*, while the dentinal invasion by *E. faecalis* was reduced in the presence of serum, but not inhibited, and the union to the collagen was intensified. The virulence factor of *E. faecalis* in the failure of endodontically treated teeth, could be related to ability of the *E. faecalis* cells to retain the capacity to invade dentinal tubules and to adhere to collagen in the presence of human serum.

**Table 22.4** - Causes responsible for endodontic failures

| **Causes of Microbial Origin** |
|---|
| 1. Intracanal factor<br>Bacteria<br>Fungi |
| 2. Extracanal factor<br>Actinomycosis |
| **Causes of not Microbial Origin** |
| A. Exogenous Factor (foreign-body-reaction type)<br>Filling material<br>Paper tips |
| B. Endogenous factor<br>Cyst<br>Cholesterol crystals |

(Nair [82])

Evans et al.[29] analyzed the mechanisms involved in the resistance of *Enterococcus faecalis* to the high pH of calcium hydroxide. A JH2-2 culture was exposed to lethal concentrations of calcium hydroxide, with and without pre-treatments. Blocking agents were added to determine the role of protein stress inductor synthesis and the proton pump associated with the cellular wall. *E. faecalis* is well known for supporting elevated pH. At pH of 11.5 or higher, *E. faecalis* does not survive, but it can still survive at a pH below 11.5. Because of the buffering effect of dentin, it is unlikely that the high pH of calcium hydroxide can reach inside the dentinal tubules where *E. faecalis* is capable of, at least in vitro, penetrating deeply. In the root dentin, a pH of only 10.3 can be reached after the intracanal dressing of calcium hydroxide. With the goal of determining the role of proton pumps in sustaining the survival of *E. faecalis* at a very high pH, CCCP was used to close this pump. The results showed that a functioning proton pump, which governs the entry of protons into the cell to acidify the cytoplasm, is critical for the survival of the *E. faecalis* in highly alkaline mediums. Presumably, when the alkalinity of the medium reaches a pH equal to or higher than 11.5 this lifesaving mechanism is suppressed. This study confirmed that *E. faecalis* is resistant to death caused by calcium hydroxide at a pH equal to or lower than 11.1. An adaptive response to alkaline pH and protein synthesis induced by stress seem to have a smaller role in the cellular survival, while a functioning proton pump, which has the capacity to acidify the cytoplasm, was shown to be critical for the survival of these bacteria in mediums with elevated pH. *E. faecalis* is efficiently eliminated by sodium hypochlorite. These discoveries contribute to clarifying the understanding of the *E. faecalis* response to these antimicrobial agents, helping significantly to eradicate the process of these bacteria from infected root canals during modern endodontic treatment. The survival of *E. faecalis* in calcium hydroxide does not seem to be related to protein synthesis, but a functioning proton pump is critical for the survival of *E. faecalis* at high pH.

In view of the above analyses, based on aspects of all the scientific evidences shown in the literature[1-140], one of the most critical and greatest aspects favoring the failure of endodontic treatment is the presence of microorganisms. The importance of establishing an effective protocol for significant microbial control of each type of endodontic infection should be considered. Thus, as presented by Nair[82], the association of factors such as, the agents of microbial virulence (enzymes, toxins, metabolic products, etc.), the type of foreign-body-reaction to dental materials and endogenous agents (cholesterol crystals, cyst) constitute the main causes responsible for endodontic treatment failure. One can also verify that for successful endodontic treatment it is essential to eliminate endodontic infections, perform an adequate sanitization process (filling and shaping of the root canal), use effective antimicrobial substances, such as sodium hypochlorite and calcium hydroxide[24-28]. The need is also emphasized for establishing a longer time for performing the work, so that calcium hydroxide can exercises its functions more effectively. Among the microorganisms present in secondary infections, the high prevalence of *E. faecalis* and its resistance to the treatment with calcium hydroxide is pointed out.

## 22.4 Quality Control of Endodontic Treatment

It is important to establish a standard for the quality control of endodontic treatment, in order to determine endodontic success. The clinical conduct should be monitored by defined protocols, prepared and based on well structured researches.

An important factor to consider is the selection of cases. Clinical diagnosis of the failure of the endodontic treatment performed, by means of anamnesis, clinical and radiographic exam, determines terms that indicate the treatment options. After failure has been verified, retreatment represents the first option to solve the problem.

However, parameters should be established to indicate the new treatment, within the protocols of a selection of cases, thus avoiding failure of the retreatment. [35,36,61,63]

In clinical situations of teeth in which there is doubt regarding the success, the option can be the retreatment. However, the probable challenge facing the new endodontic treatment reverts to the difficulties and inherent complications in removing the root canal filling.

The degree of difficulty depends on the material used (cements, pastes, posts), the anatomy of the pulp cavity (developmental anomalies, dilacerations, calcifications, resorptions) and iatrogenesis (steps, drillings, fractured instruments). In addition to the dental aspects, the status of present pathologies (location) and the systemic status of the patient's general health should be analyzed. Common-sense and the professional's ability are other aspects to consider.

In view of the need for a new coronal restoration with posts or casts, endodontic retreatment should be considered, because failure can occur after the restoration. Apparently successful treatment could fail at any time.

The quality of endodontic treatment has been analyzed in several studies [10,15,16,20,22,24,31,33-37,39,41-44,51,61-63,71,72,75,77,78,81-87,90,92,93,98,99,101-108,110-113,115-119,124,125,127,132,134-137,140]. Perfect coronal sealing is an important determinant of successful endodontic treatment[93,129,132]. The clinical condition of the coronal sealing and the quality of the casts and posts must also be verified.

In this sense, Lopes et al.[68] analyzed the posts, their lengths and the obturation condition of the root canal using 365 radiographies taken in a selection of 500 teeth. The Table 22.5 shows the presence of retainers in the examined teeth. There was predominance in the maxilla, with a percentage of 77%. Another aspect observed is that the teeth with the highest incidence of retainers are the central incisors (29.4%) and the maxillary lateral incisors (26.2%), totaling 55.6%. In Table 22.6, an evaluation was made of the endodontic filling of the teeth with retainers, which presented periapical lesions that could be seen in radiographs. In the total number of teeth evaluated, 59.4% (297) did not present periapical lesion, and 40.6% (203) did present. Of the 203 (40.6%) treatments with periapical lesion, the fillings in 42 (8.4%) cases were apparently normal, in 125 (25%), they were incorrect and in 36 (7.2%) they were absent. In Table 22.7 the retainer lengths are verified. In the total number of cases, the retainers were considered short in 58.4% (292), average in 22.2% (111) and long in only 19.4%.[97] The results obtained were in accordance with the terms under which this evaluation was made, and allowed one to conclude that: 1. In 80.6% of the cases, the retainer lengths were incompatible with the principle of retainer retention ; 2. In 50.4% of the cases, the retainers were placed without taking into consideration the condition of the root canal filling.

**Table 22.5** - Distribution of retainers in the examined teeth

| Maxillary | Tooth | | | | |
|---|---|---|---|---|---|
| | **Central** | **Canine** | **Lateral** | **Pre-molar** | **Total** |
| Maxilla | 147 | 131 | 107 | – | 385 |
| Mandible | 17 | 131 | 10 | 78 | 155 |
| Total | 164 | 141 | 117 | 78 | 500 |

**Table 22.6** - Radiographic evaluation of the endodontic filling of teeth with root posts

| Periapex | Obturation | | | |
|---|---|---|---|---|
| | **Incorrect** | **Absent** | **Correct** | **Total** |
| Normal | 206 | 70 | 21 | 297 |
| Lesion | 42 | 125 | 36 | 203 |
| Total | 248 | 195 | 57 | 500 |

**Table 22.7** - Retainer length; condition of the root canal filling

| Filling | Post length | | | |
|---|---|---|---|---|
| | **Short** | **Medium** | **Long** | **Total** |
| Correct | 157 | 44 | 50 | 248 |
| Incorrect | 107 | 47 | 41 | 195 |
| Absent | 31 | 20 | 6 | 57 |
| Total | 292 | 111 | 97 | 500 |

There are several factors involved in successful retreatment, and before endodontic treatment, the following aspects should be verified: the internal anatomy; effectiveness of the sanitization process; modeling and obturation limit and quality of the root canal; effectiveness of coronal sealing; the pulp, pathological, periodontal and occlusal conditions, presence of operative accidents (loss of working length – step; drilling; fracture of instrument), the individual's general health status and the professional's capacity and ability.

Estrela et al.[27] assessed the prevalence and risk factors of apical periodontitis in endodontically treated teeth in a Brazilian adult subpopulation. A total of 1,372 periapical radiographs were analyzed, based on the quality of root filling, coronal restoration status and presence of posts associated with apical periodontitis (AP). In this cross-section study, based on a full-mouth radiographic survey, randomly selected endodontically treated teeth (except third molars) recorded on patient charts of the Brazilian Dentistry Association (Post-graduation Course in Endodontics, Goiânia, GO, Brazil) were evaluated. The sample consisted of 1,372 periapical radiographs taken using the parallelism technique and all films were developed by a specialized radiological clinic. The inclusion criteria were the following: i) radiographs should be from patients attending the Post-graduation Course in Endodontics for the first time, and ii) endodontic treatments should have been done within the last 10 years. The age of patients ranged from 18 to 60 years. Three independent and skilful endodontists with over 5 years of clinical experience examined the radiographs after thoroughly discussing the interpretation criteria. Endodontic treatment and coronal restorations were rated as adequate in 781 (56.9%) and 881 (64.2%) cases, respectively. Retention with posts was absent in 768 cases (56.0%). The prevalence of AP was analyzed according to radiographic aspects of treatment risk factors. Prevalence of AP was significantly higher in teeth with poor endodontic treatment (66.3%) than in teeth with adequate root canal filling (16.5%). Prevalence of AP was also higher in teeth with poor coronal restoration (52.1%) than in teeth with adequate coronal restoration (30.1%). No significant difference in AP was observed when intracanal posts were either present (35.8%) or absent (39.7%). Poor endodontic treatment increased the risk of AP by almost 10 times (OR=9.96; 95% CI= 7.66–12.95) when compared with adequate endodontic treatment. Likewise, poor coronal restoration was a risk factor for AP (OR=2.53; 95% CI= 2.00–3.20). Poor coronal restorations had a detrimental effect even in teeth with root canal filling considered adequate. In teeth with adequate endodontic treatment, AP prevalence was higher in cases with poor coronal restorations (27.9%) compared with those that were adequately restored (12.1%) (p=0.00). Similar results were observed for teeth with poor endodontic treatment, which presented either poor restoration (AP prevalence of 71.7%) or adequate coronal restoration (AP prevalence of 61.8%). Combined analyses of endodontic treatment and coronal restoration indicated that poor restoration is a risk factor of AP whenever teeth have either adequate (OR=2.80; 95% CI= 1.87–4.22) or poor endodontic treatment (OR=1.57; 95% CI= 1.09–2.25). The prevalence of AP was low when associated with high technical quality of root canal treatment. Adequate root canal filling reduced the risk of AP even in teeth with poor coronal restorations. The presence of intracanal posts had no influence on the risk of AP.

Ray & Trope[93] reported that the technical quality of the coronal restoration was significantly more important than the technical quality of endodontic treatment for apical periodontal health. Tronstad et al.[132] examined the radiographs of 1,001 root-filled teeth and observed a 67.4% success rate. The technical quality of endodontic treatment was found to be more important than the technical quality of the coronal restoration.

In another study, Estrela et al.[24] evaluated the accuracy of imaging methods for the detection of apical periodontitis. Imaging exam records from a consecutive sample of 888 imaging exams of patients with endodontic infection (1,508 teeth), including cone beam computed tomography (CBCT), panoramic and periapical radiographies, were selected. Sensitivity, specificity, predictive values and accuracy of periapical and panoramic radiographies were calculated. Receiver operating characteristic (ROC) analysis was performed to test diagnostic accuracy of panoramic and periapical images. Prevalence of AP was significantly higher using CBCT. It may be concluded that the prevalence of AP was significantly higher using CBCT, comparing periapical and panoramic radiographs. AP was correctly identified in 54.5% using periapical radiographs and in 27.8% with panoramic radiographs. Minor changes in sensitivity were found for different groups of teeth, except for incisors in panoramic radiographs. ROC analysis suggests that AP is correctly identified with conventional methods when it showed severe status. CBCT was shown to be an accurate diagnostic method to identify AP (Fig. 22.10-22.11).

The precision of CBCT for identifying AP by comparing panoramic and periapical radiographs indicated the need for taking care, particularly when one wants to obtain high quality in endodontic treatment planning, with diagnosis and its consequences, such as the prognosis. The probabilities of AP existing and not being discernible by periapical or panoramic radiographs are considerably greater.

Evidently, likewise considering the limitations of periapical radiographs for visualizing AP in view of all the previously mentioned aspects, it will be essential to revise epidemiological studies, considering the quality of periapical aspects offered by CBCT images. Furthermore, it will certainly also reduce the influence on the radiographic interpretation, with less possibility of false negative diagnosis. In the present investigation, the prevalence of AP in endodontically treated teeth, when comparing the panoramic and periapical radiograph and CBCT images was 17.6%, 35.3% and 63.3%, respectively. Considerable discrepancy can be observed between the imaging methods used to identify AP.

Table 22.8 lists several operative factors that can interfere in the success or failure of endodontic treatment.

Recent studies analyzed discussed critically the treatment outcome. Torabinejad & Goodacre[127] analyzed the major factors that can affect the decision regarding whether a tooth receives endodontic treatment or is extracted and replaced by an implant. The decision by the clinician and patient to retain or remove teeth should be based on a thorough assessment of information related to risk factors affecting the long-term prognosis for endodontic and dental implant treatment. The clinician should consider several factors when determining whether to save a tooth through endodontic therapy or extract it and place an implant. These factors pertain to the patient's health status, the condition of the tooth and periodontium, and treatment-related considerations. Patient-related factors include systemic and oral health, as well as patients' comfort and perceptions about treatment. Tooth- and periodontium-related factors include pulpal and periodontal conditions, biological environmental considerations, color characteristics of the teeth, quantity and quality of bone, and soft-tissue anatomy. Treatment-related factors include an assessment of potential procedural complications, required adjunctive procedures and treatment outcomes data.

Cohn[20] discussing the negative treatment outcomes reported that is a significant part of current endodontic practice. Both non-surgical and surgical retreatment procedures share the problem of a significant negative outcome in the presence of apical periodontitis. Intracanal procedures to eliminate infection are technically difficult and perhaps impossible to achieve. There is no evidence that rotary instrumentation is an improvement over traditional methods in this regard. However, recent advances in endodontic microsurgery and bio-inductive materials show more promise in eliminating apical periodontitis. Traditionally, periapical surgery has been considered the 'junior partner' in the revision of a negative outcome. This may need to be reconsidered. Non-surgical retreatment in conjunction with surgery may have a better outcome than either procedure alone because all possible sites of infection are eliminated. This may be important given the pressures to replace 'failed' endodontically treated teeth with implants. Implants represent a challenge to endodontics, created in part by the implant manufacturers. When comparable criteria are applied to outcomes, the survival rates of endodontic treatment and implant placement are the same. Time and cost favor an endodontic procedure. Implant treatment carries the risk of ongoing periodontal and occlusal complications, with particular problems in the esthetic zone. Implants have an 'all or nothing' outcome; that is, if an implant is lost, so is the attached prosthesis. Patients must be provided this information during the treatment planning phase. Accordingly, retreatment procedures should always be carried out first unless the tooth is judged to be untreatable. Endodontists should have some training in the theory and practice of implantology at least to help patients and referring colleagues to make an informed choice regarding all replacement options. Does that mean endodontists should place implants? This will remain an individual decision based on personal preference and the nature of the endodontist's practice.

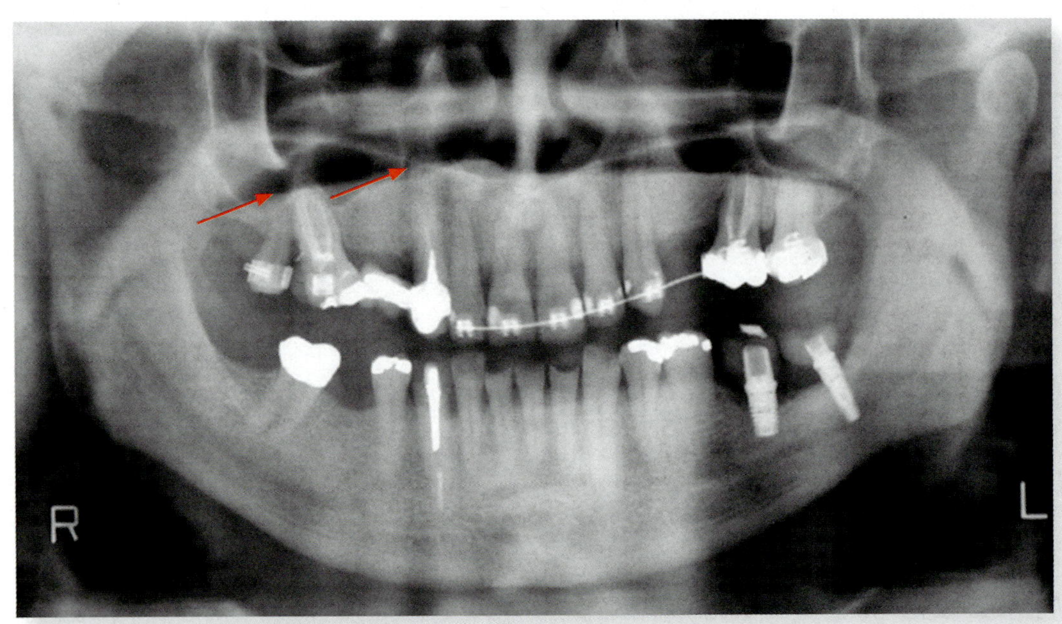


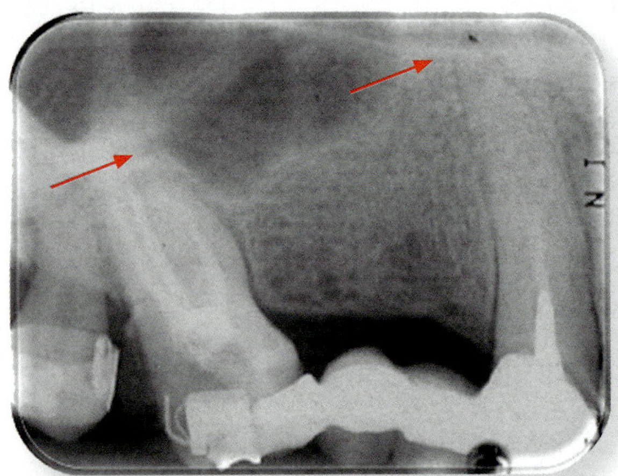

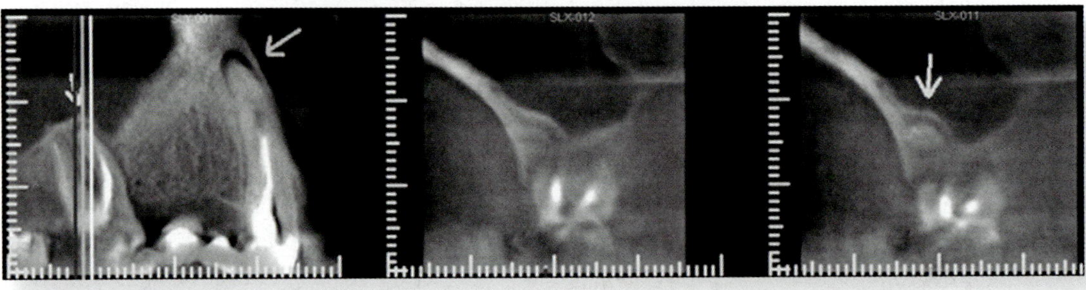

**Figure 22.10** - Radiographic images characterizing failure of the treatment detected by CBCT[24] (IORB, Brasília, DF, Brazil).

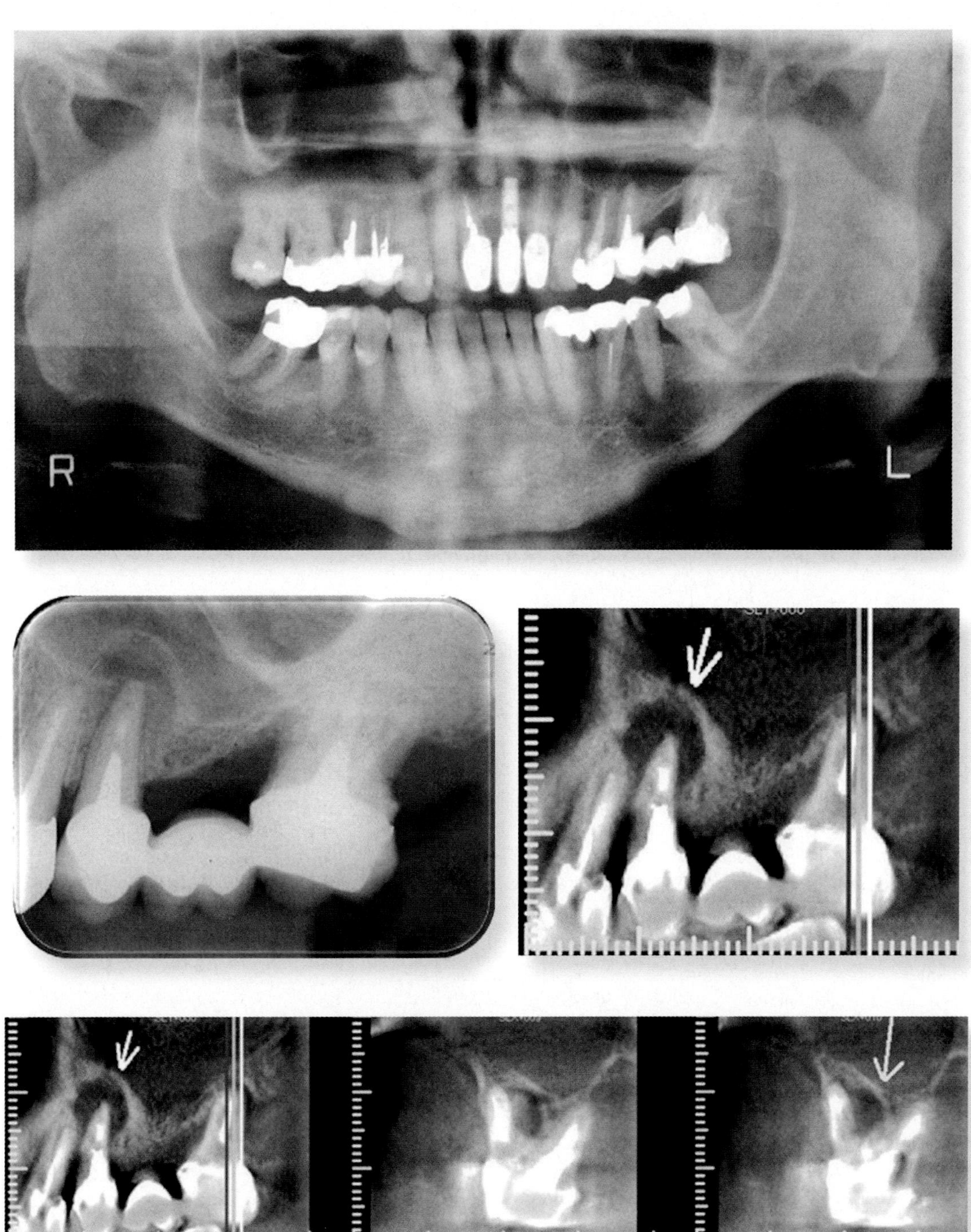


**Figure 22.11** - Radiographic images characterizing failure of the treatment detected by CBCT[24] (IORB, Brasília, DF, Brazil).

**Table 22.8** - Operative factors that can interfere in the sucess or failure of endodontic treatment

| **1. Coronal Opening and Preparation**<br><br>**Technical difficulties**<br>- Inadequate access<br>- Drilling<br>- Instrument fracture<br>- Presence of filling material<br><br>**Anatomical difficulties**<br>- Calcification<br>- Anatomical alterations |
|---|
| **2. Root Canal Shaping**<br><br>**Technical difficulties**<br>- Location of the root canal<br>- Weakness of the dental structure<br>- Presence of additional root canals<br>- Loss of working length - step<br>- Deviation<br>- Foramen transportation<br>- Exaggerated enlargement<br>- Drilling<br>- Endodontic instrument fracture<br>- Over-instrumentation<br>- Root perforation<br><br>**Anatomical difficulties**<br>- Calcified root canal<br>- Lacerated root canal<br>- Tooth out of its normal position |
| **3. Root Canal Filling**<br><br>**Technical difficulties**<br>- Excessive instrumentation<br>- Over or incomplete obturation<br>- Postoperative pain<br>- Reamer fracture (Lentulo, McSpadden)<br>- Cement with fast setting |
| **4. Endodontic Retreatment**<br><br>**Technical difficulties**<br>- Presence of paste<br>- Presence of cement<br>- Gutta-percha and cement<br>- Silver cone and cement<br>- Presence of intracanal retainer |

American Association of Endodontics[92] described some rules to guarantee the quality of endodontic treatment, as shown in Tables 22.9 to 22.11.



**Table 22.9** - Clinical Criteria

| **Clinically Acceptable** |
|---|
| 1. No sensitivity to percussion or palpation |
| 2. Normal mobility |
| 3. Absence of fistula or associated periodontal disease |
| 4. Tooth in function |
| 5. Absence of infection or edema |
| 6. No evidence of subjective discomfort |
| **Clinically Questionable** |
| 1. Sporadic vacant symptoms |
| 2. Sensation of Pressure |
| 3. Low degree of discomfort after percussion, palpation or mastication |
| 4. Discomfort when pressure is applied by the tongue |
| 5. Overlapping symptoms of sinusitis in the region of the treated tooth |
| 6. Occasional need of analgesics to alleviate minimal discomfort |
| **Clinically Unacceptable** |
| 1. Persistent symptoms |
| 2. Fistula or recurring edema |
| 3. Predictable discomfort on percussion or palpation |
| 4. Evidence of irreparable tooth fracture |
| 5. Excessive mobility or progressive periodontal destruction |
| 6. Impossibility of chewing with the tooth |

(Adapted from the American Association of Endodontics[92], rules for quality assurance).

**Table 22.10** - Radiographic Criteria

**Radiographically Acceptable**
1. Space of the periodontal ligament normal to slightly thick (< 1 mm)
2. Disappearance of previous radiotransparent area
3. Normal lamina dura in relation to the adjacent teeth
4. Absence of resorption
5. Dense three-dimensional filling of the visible space of the root canal inside the space limits of the canal 1 mm before the radiographic apex

**Radiographically Questionable**
1. Increased space of the periodontal ligament (< 2 mm)
2. Radiotransparent area of similar extent or slight evidence of repair
3. Lamina dura with irregular thickness in relation to the adjacent teeth
4. Spaces present in the filling
5. Filling material extending beyond the anatomical apex

**Radiographically Unacceptable**
1. Increased space of the periodontal ligament (> 2mm);
2. Absence of bone repair in a periapical rarefaction, or increase in the radiotransparent area;
3. Absence of formation of a new lamina dura;
4. Presence of radiotransparent bone in periapical areas where there was none previously, including lateral radiotransparency;
5. Visible spaces in the root canal that were not filled, or significant emptiness;
6. Excessive overfilling, with visible spaces in the apical third of the tooth
7. Clear evidence of progressive resorption

(Adapted from the American Association of Endodontics[92], rules for quality assurance).

**Table 22.11** - Histological Criteria

**Histologically Acceptable**
1. Absence of inflammation
2. Regeneration of the adjacent periodontal fibers in healthy or inserted cement (Sharpey fibers)
3. Cement formation or repair with new cement in the direction of the apical foramen or through it (rare)
4. Evident bone repair together with healthy osteoblasts surrounding the recently-formed bone
5. Absence of dental resorption; areas that presented resorption previously show cement formation.

**Histologically Questionable**
1. Presence of moderate inflammation
2. Cement areas undergoing resorption and concomitant repair
3. Absence of organization of the periodontal fibers
4. Minimum bone repair, with evidence of osteoclastic activity

**Histologically Unacceptable**
1. Presence of intense inflammation
2. Absence of repair with concomitant resorption of the surrounding bone
3. Active resorption of cement without evidence of repair
4. Presence of bacteria and zones of necrotic tissue
5. Presence of granulation and possible epithelial tissue proliferation

(Adapted from the American Association of Endodontics[92], rules for quality assurance).

The Figures 22.12 to 22.37 show radiographic aspects of endodontic failures.





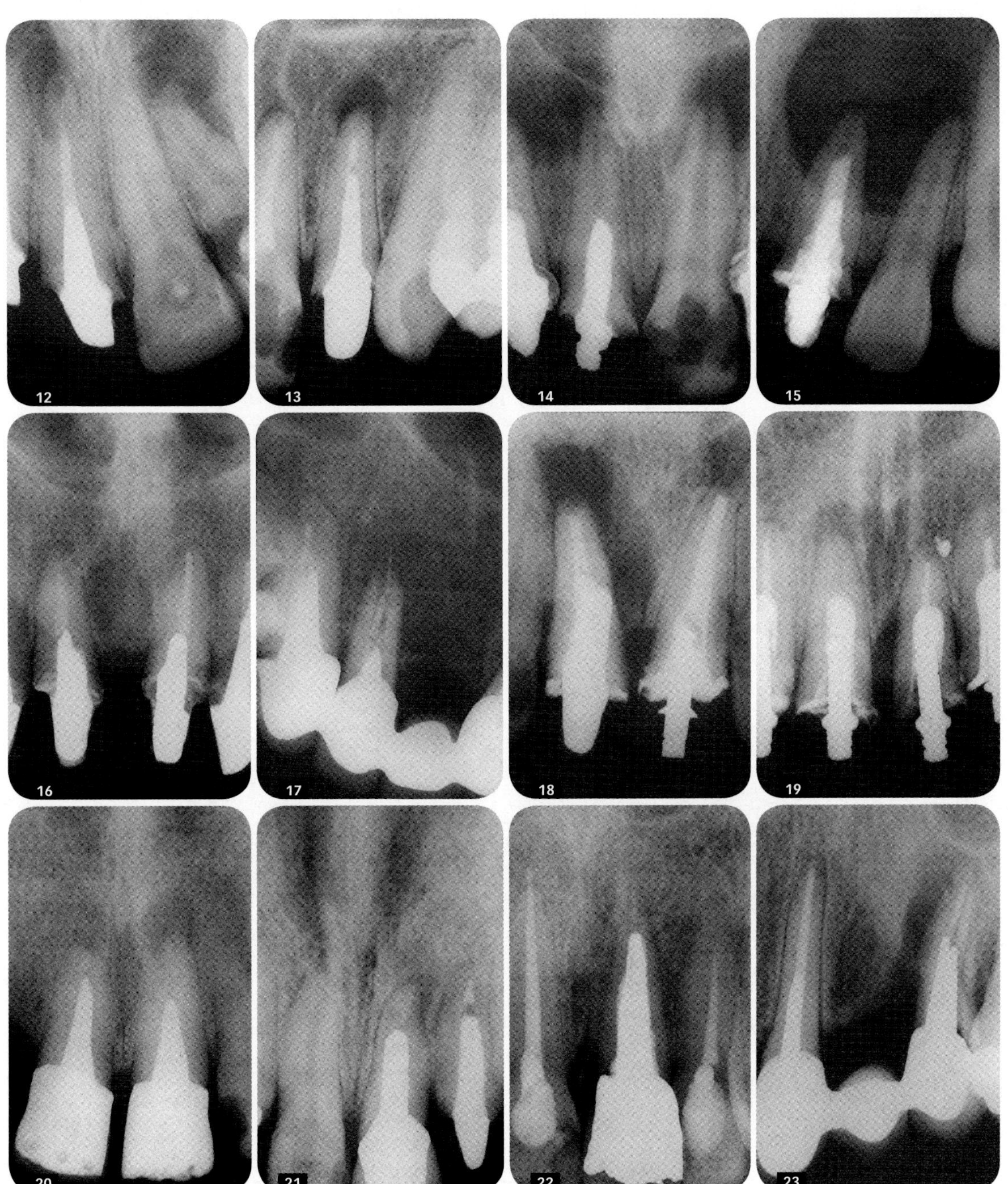


**Figures 22.12 to 22.23** - Radiographic aspects of endodontic failures.

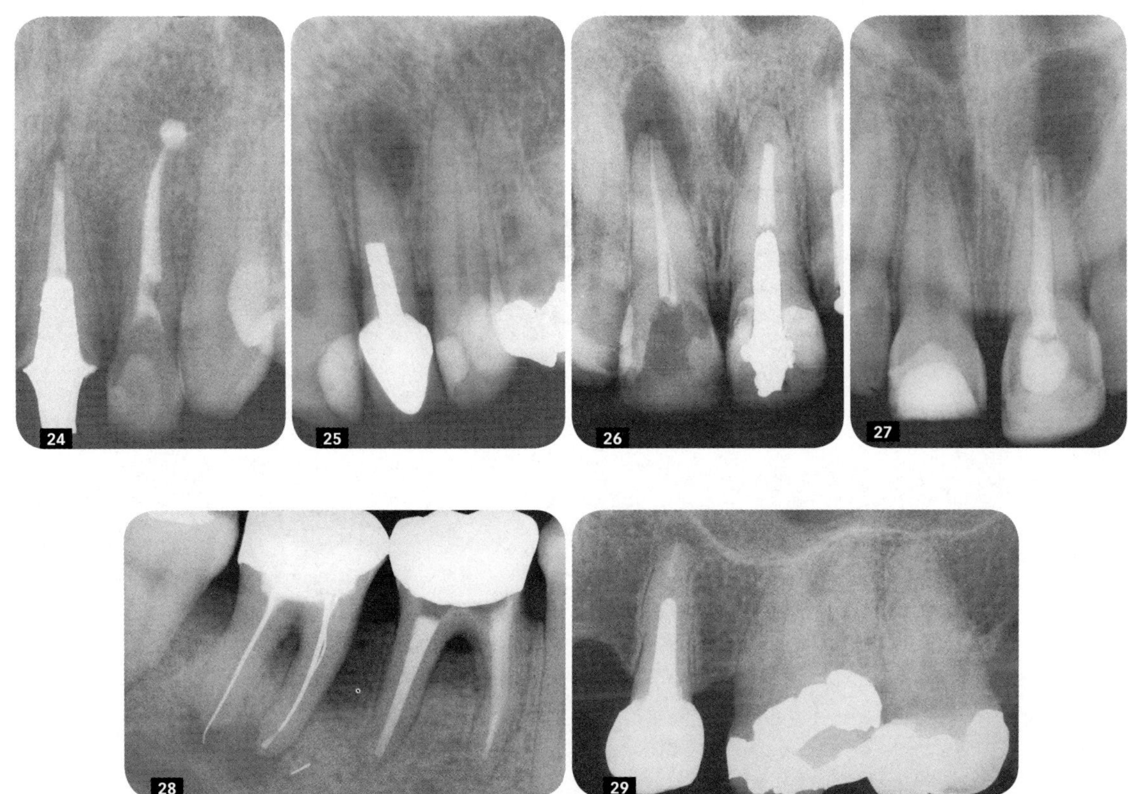

**Figures 22.24 to 22.29** - Radiographic aspects of endodontic failures.

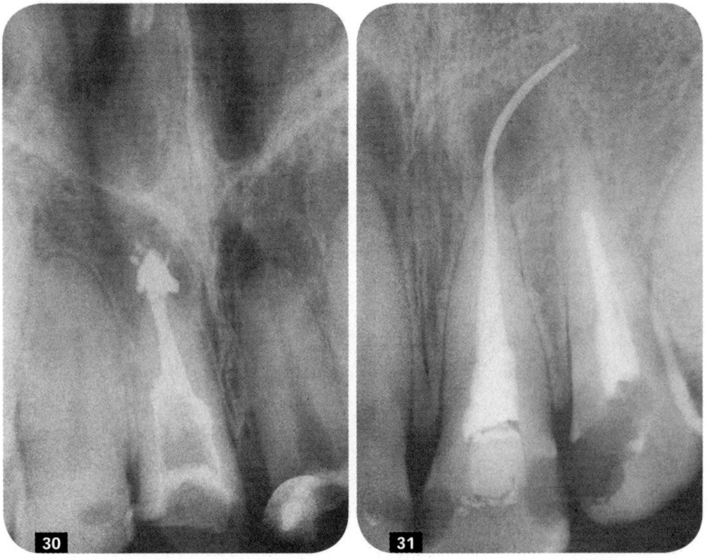

**Figures 22.30 to 22.31** - Radiographic aspects of endodontic failures.

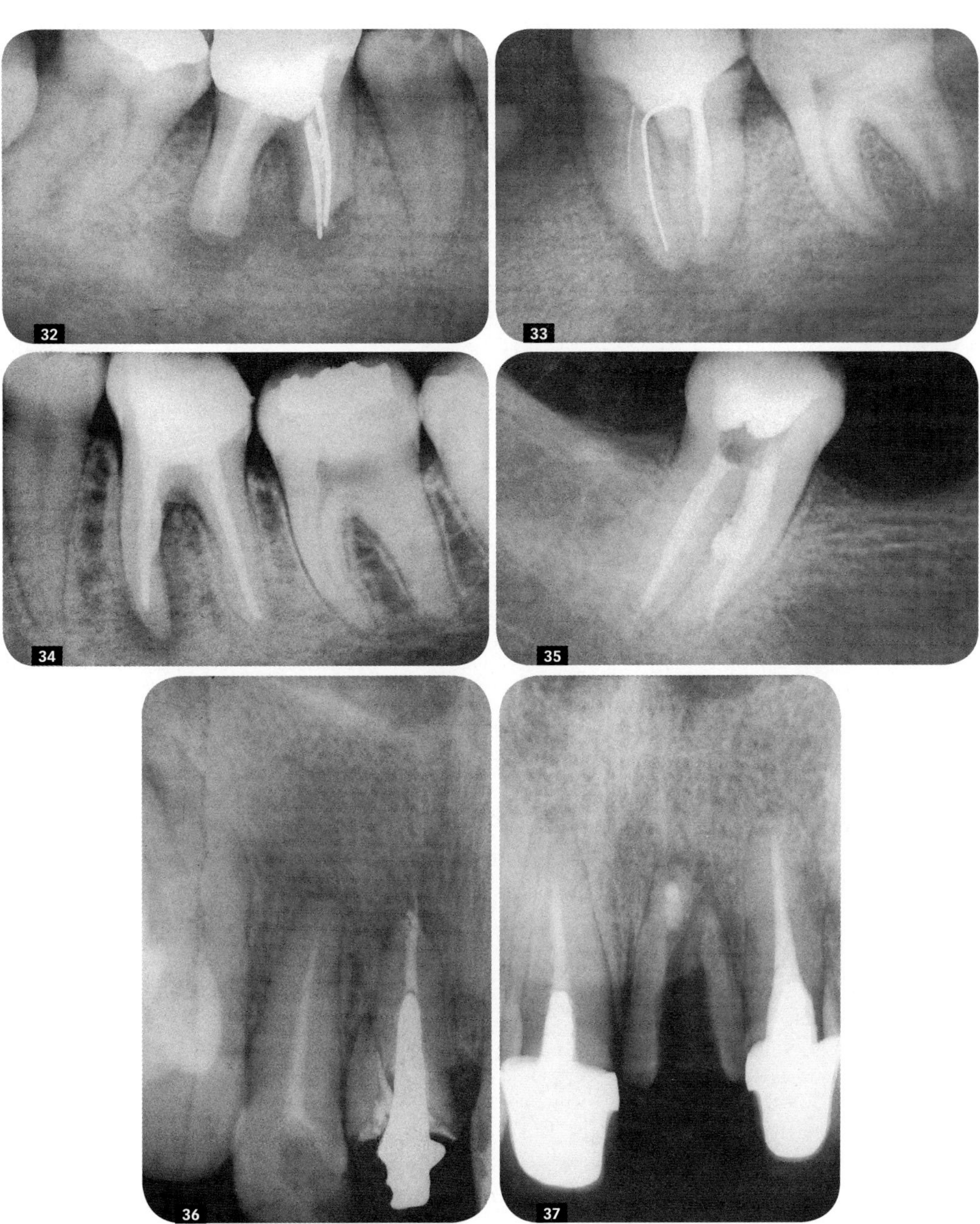


**Figures 22.32 to 22.37** - Radiographic aspects of endodontic failures.

## REFERENCES


1. Alhadainy HA. Root perforations. Oral Surg Oral Med Oral Pathol 1994;78:368-74.
2. Allen RK, Newton CW, Brow-Jr CE. A statistical analysis of surgical and nonsurgical endodontic retreatment cases. J Endod 1989;15:261-6.
3. Arens AE, Torabinejad M. Repair of furcal perforations with mineral trioxide aggregate. Oral Surg Oral Med Oral Pathol 1996;82:84-8.
4. Barbosa SV, Burkard DH, Spangberg LSW. Cytotoxic effects of gutta-percha solvents. J Endod 1994;20:6-8.
5. Baumgartner JC, Falkler WA. Bacteria in the apical 5 mm of infected root canals. J Endod 1991;17:380-3.
6. Bender IB, Seltzer S, Soltanoff W. Endodontic success – a reappraisal of criteria. Oral Surg Oral Med Oral Pathol 1996;22:780-801.
7. Bergenholtz G. Pathogenic mechanisms in pulpal disease. J Endod 1990;16:98-101.
8. Bergenholtz G, lekholm U, Liljenberg B, lindhe J. Morphometric analysis of chronic inflammatory periapical lesions in root-filled teeth. Oral Surg Oral Med Oral Pathol 1983; 55:295-301.
9. Biffi JCG, Souza CJA, Maniglia CAG. Método para a avaliação quantitativa do canal radicular com o auxílio do computador. Rev Ass Paul Cir Dent 1992;46:925-27.
10. Block RM, Bushell A, Grossman LI, Langeland K. Endodontic surgical retreatment – a clinical and histopathologic study. J Endod 1979;3:101-15.
11. Block RM, Pascon EA, Langeland K. Paste technique retreatment study: a clinical, histopathologic, and radiographic evaluation of 50 cases. Oral Surg Oral Med Oral Pathol 1985;60:76-93.
12. Bonetti-Filho I. Avaliação dos tratamentos endodônticos. Rev Gaúcha Odontol 1988;36:309-12.
13. Bramante CM, Berbert A. Acidentes endodônticos – fratura de instrumento. Estomat Cult 1973;7:186-90.
14. Bramante CM, Berbert A. Root perforations dressed with calcium hydroxide or zinc oxide and eugenol. J Endod 1987;13:392-95.
15. Bramante CM, Berbert A, Bernadineli N, Moraes IG, Garcia RB. Acidentes e complicações no tratamento endodôntico. São Paulo: Santos, 2003.
16. Brynolf I. A histologic and roentgenological study of the periapical region of human upper incisor. Odontol Rev 1967;18:1-176.
17. Brystöm A, Sundqvist G. Bacteriologic evaluation of the efficacy of mechanical root canal instrumentation in endodontic therapy. Scand J Dent Res 1981;89:321-28.
18. Bueno CES, Valdrighi L. Efetividade de solventes e de técnicas na desobturação dos canais radiculares. Estudo in vitro. Rev Ass Bras Odontol Nac 2000;8:21-25.
19. Bueno MR, Estrela C. Prevalência de tratamento endodôntico e periodontite apical em várias populações do mundo, detectada por radiografias panorâmicas, periapicais e tomografias computadorizadas cone beam. Rev Odontol Brasil Central 2008;17:79-90.
20. Cohn AS. Treatment choices for negative outcomes with non-surgical root canal treatment: non-surgical retreatment vs. surgical retreatment vs. implants. Endod Topics 2005;11:4–24.
21. Dezan-Jr E. Indução experimental de anacorese no periápice de dentes após obturação dos canais. Estudo em cães em região geográfica endêmica para Leishimaniose. (Doctoral Thesis). Univesity of São Paulo, 2001.
22. Dow PR, Ingle JI. Isotopi determination of root canals failures. Oral Surg Oral Med Oral Pathol 1955;8:1100-04.
23. Estrela C, Bueno MR, Azevedo B, Azevedo JR, Pécora JD. A New Periapical Index Based on Cone Beam Computed Tomography. J Endod 2008;34:1325-31.
24. Estrela C, Bueno MR, Leles CR, Azevedo BC, Azevedo JR. Accuracy of cone beam computed tomography, panoramic and periapical radiographic for the detection of apical periodontitis. J Endod 2008;34:273-79.
25. Estrela C, Camapum FF, Lopes HP. Prevalência de dor nos retratamentos endodônticos. Rev Bras Odontol 1988;55:18-24.
26. Estrela C, César OVS, Sydney GB, Lopes HP, Pesce HF. Prevalência de dor frente ao tratamento da inflamação periapical aguda e crônica. Rev Bras Odontol 1996;53:15-21.
27. Estrela C, Leles CR, Hollanda ACB, Moura MS, Pécora JD. Prevalence and risk factors of apical periodontitis in endodontically treated teeth in a selected population of Brazilian adults. Braz Dent J 2008;19:34-39.
28. Estrela C, Stephan IW. Estudo comparativo do desgaste dentinário na parede distal do canal mésio vestibular do primeiro molar inferior produzido por três técnicas de instrumentação do canal radicular. Rev Odontol Brasil Central 1991;1:11-15.
29. Estrela CRA, Estrela C, Marcomini JL, Loreto-Jr F, Ribeiro RG. Ação antimicrobiana de solventes de guta-percha. Rev Bras Odontol 2001;58:154-57.
30. Evans M, Davies JK, Sundqvist G, Figdor D. Mechanisms involved in the resistance of *Enterococcus faecalis* to calcium hydroxide. Int Endod J 2002;35:221-28.
31. Fachin E, Wenckus C, Aun CE. Retreatment using a modified type instrument. J Endod 1995; 21:425-28.
32. Frank AL. Resorption, perforation and fractures. Dent Clin North Amer 1974;18:465-87.
33. Friedman S. Retreatment of failures. In: Walton RE, Torabinejad M. Principles and practices of endodontics. 2nd ed. Philadelphia: WB Saunders Company. 1996; p. 336-53.
34. Friedman S, Rotstein I, Shar-Lev S. Bypassing gutta-percha root filling with an automated device. J Endod 1989;15:432-37.
35. Friedman S, Stabholz A. Endodontic retreatment – case selection and technique. Part 1: Criteria for case selection. J Endod 1986;12:28-33.
36. Friedman S, Stabholz A, Tamae A. Endodontic retreatment – case selection and technique. Part 3. Retreatment techniques. J Endod 1990;16:543-49.

37. Goldman N, Pearson AH, Darzenta N. Reliability of radiographic interpretations. Oral Surg Oral Med Oral Pathol 1974;38:287-93.
38. Grossman LI. Endodontia prática. Trad. S. Bevilacqua. 8th ed. Rio de Janeiro: Guanabara Koogan. 1976; 190-216.
39. Grossman LI, Shephard LI, Pearson LA. Roentgenologic and clinical evaluation of endodontically treated teeth. Oral Surg Oral Med Oral Pathol 1964;17:368-74.
40. Guldner PHA. Perforaciones accidentales. In: Endodoncia. Diagnóstico y tratamiento. Guldener PHA, Langeland K. Barcelona: Springer. 1995; 396p.
41. Harrison JW, Baumgartner JC, Cvek TA. Prevalence of pain associated with clinical factors during and after root canal therapy. Part 1. Inter appointment pain. J Endod 1983;9:384-87.
42. Harrison JW, Baumgartner JC, Cvek TA. Prevalence of pain associated with clinical factors during and after root canal therapy. Part 2. Pos obturations pain. J Endod 1983;9:434-38.
43. Harrison JW, Baumgartner JC, Zielke DR. Analysis of interappointment pain associated with the combined use of endodontic irrigants and medicaments. J Endod 1981;7:272-76.
44. Hepworth MJ, Friedman S. Retreatment outcome of surgical and non-surgical management of endodontic failure. J Can Dent Ass 1997;63:364-71.
45. Holland R, Valle GF, Taintor JF, Ingle JI. Influence of bony resorption on endodontic treatment. Oral Surg Oral Med Oral Pathol 1983;55:191-203.
46. Holland R, Souza V, Nery MJ, Mello W, Bernabé PFE, Otoboni-Filho CD. Tissue reactions following apical plugging of the root canal with infected dentin chips. A histologic study in dog's teeth. Oral Surg Oral Med Oral Pathol 1980;49:366-69.
47. Hülsmann M. The removal of silver cones and fractured instruments using the Canal Finder System. J Endod 1990;16:596-600.
48. Hülsmann M. Removal of fractured instruments using a combined automated ultrasonic technique. J Endod 1994;20:144-46.
49. Hunter KR, Dobleckl W, Pelleu-Jr GB. Halothane and eucaliptol as alternatives to chloroform for softening gutta-percha. J Endod 1990;16:543-49.
50. Imura N, Zuolo ML. Remoção de retentor intraradicular com aparelho de ultra-som. Rev Ass Paul Cir Dent 1997;51:262-67.
51. Ingle JI. Exitos y fracasos en endodoncia. Rev Ass Odontol Argentina 1962;50:67-74.
52. Ingle JI, Taintor JF. Endodontia. 3rd ed. Rio de Janeiro: Guanabara S.A; 1989.
53. Jeng HW, Eldeeb ME. Removal of hard paste fillings from root canal by ultrasonic instrumentation. J Endod 1987;13:295-98.
54. Johnson WT, Leary JM, Boyer DB. Effect of ultrasonic vibration on post removal in extracted human premolar teeth. J Endod 1996;22:487-88.
55. Kakehashi S, Stanley HR, Fitzgerald RJ. The effects of surgical exposures of dental pulps in germ-free and conventional laboratory rats. Oral Surg Oral Med Oral Pathol 1965;20:340-9.
56. Kaplowitz GJ. Evaluation of gutta-percha solvents. J Endod 1990;16:539-40.
57. Kaplowitz GJ. Using rectified turpentine oil in endodontic retreatment. J Endod 1996;22:621.
58. Krell KV, Fuller MW, Scott GI. The conservative retrieval of silver cones in difficult cases. J Endod 1984;10:269-73.
59. Krell KV, Neo J. The use of ultrasonic endodontic instrumentation in the re-treatment of a paste-filled endodontic tooth. Oral Surg Oral Med Oral Pathol 1985;60:100-02.
60. Kvist T, Rydin E, Reit C. The relative frequency of periapical lesions in teeth with root canal retained posts. J Endod 1989;15:578-80.
61. Lewis RD, Block RM. Management of endodontic failures. Oral Surg Oral Med Oral Pathol 1988;66:711-21.
62. Lin LM, Pascon EA, Skrinbner JE, Gängler P, Langeland K. Clinical, radiographic and histologic study of endodontic treatment failures. Oral Surg Oral Med Oral Pathol 1991;11:603-11.
63. Lin LM, Skribner JE, Gängler P. Factors associated with endodontic treatment failures. J Endod 1992;18:625-27.
64. Lisa R, Wilcox LR. Endodontic retreatment: ultrasonic and chloroform as the final step in reinstrumentation. J Endod 1989;15:125-28.
65. Lopes HP, Araújo-Filho WR. Retratamento endodôntico em dente portador de pino metálico e perfuração radicular. Rev Bras Odontol 1991;48:38-42.
66. Lopes HP, Costa-Filho AS, Loriato D. Remoção de pinos metálicos intra-radiculares de retenção protética. Rev Bras Odontol 1985;42:3-16.
67. Lopes HP, Elias CN, Silveira GEL, Araújo-Filho WR, Siqueira-Jr JF. Extrusão de material do canal via forame apical. Rev Paul Odontol 1997;19:34-36.
68. Lopes HP, Estrela C, Rocha NSM, Costa-Filho AS, Siqueira-Jr JF. Retentores intra-radiculares: análise radiográfica do comprimento do pino e da condição da obturação do canal radicular. Rev Bras Odontol 1997;54:277-80.
69. Lopes HP, Gahyva SMM. Retratamento endodôntico: avaliação da quantidade apical de resíduos de material obturador após a reinstrumentação. Rev Bras Odontol 1992;40:181-84.
70. Lopes HP, Gahyva SMM. Retratamento endodôntico: avaliação do limite apical de esvaziamento, na remoção do material obturador dos canais radiculares. Rev Bras Odontol 1995;52:22-26.
71. Lopes HP, Siqueira-Jr JF, Elias CN. Retratamento endodôntico. In: Endodontia: Biologia e Técnica. Lopes HP, Siqueira-Jr JF. Rio de Janeiro: Medsi. 1999; p. 497-538.
72. Lovdal PE. Endodontic retreatment. Dent Clin North Am 1992; 36:473-90.
73. Love RM. *Enterococcus faecalis* – a mechanism for its role in endodontic failure. Int Endod J 2001;34:399-405.
74. Machtou P, Sarfati P, Cohen AG. Post removal prior to retreatment. J Endod 1989;15:552-54.
75. Mandel E, Friedman S. Endodontic retreatment: A rational approach to root canal instrumentation. J Endod 1992;18:565-69.
76. Metzger Z, Bem-Amar A. Removal of overextended gutta-percha root canal fillings in endodontic failure cases. J Endod 1995;21:287-88.

77. Mollander A, Reit C, Dahlén G, Kvist T. Microbiological status of root-filled teeth with apical periodontitis. Int Endod J 1998;31:1-7.
78. Mor C, Rotstein I, Freidman S. Prevalence of inter appointment emergency associated with endodontic therapy. J Endod 1992;18:509-11.
79. Morse DR, Furst M, Bellot RM, Lefkowitz R, Spritzer I, Sideman B. Infections flare-ups and serious sequel following endodontic treatment: a prospective randomizes trial efficacy of antibiotic prophylaxis in cases of asymptomatic pulpal-periapical lesions. Oral Surg Oral Med Oral Pathol 1987;64:96-109.
80. Mota AS, Biffi JCG, Oliveira MRS, Guimarães CS. Estudo comparativo da força de tração na remoção de pinos pré-fabricados em canais morfologicamente diferentes. Rev Ass Bras Odontol Nac 2000;7:364-71.
81. Nair PNR. Light and electron microscopic studies of root canal flora and periapical lesions. J Endod 1987;13:29-39.
82. Nair PNR. Pathobiology of the periapex. In: Cohen S, Burns RC. Pathways of the pulp. St. Louis: Mosby; 2001.
83. Nair PNR, Sjögren U, Krey G, Sundqvist G. Therapy-resistant foreign body giant cell granuloma at the periapex of a root filled human tooth. J Endod 1990;16:589-95.
84. Nair PNR, Sjögren U, Krey G, Khngerg KE, Sundqvist G. Intra radicular bacteria and fungi in root filled, asymptomatic human teeth with therapy-resistant periapical lesions: a long-term light and electron microscopic follow-up study. J Endod 1990;16:580-88.
85. Nair PNR, Sjögren U, Schumacher E, Sundqvist G. Radicular cyst affecting a root-filled human tooth: a long-term post-treatment follow-up. Int Endod J 1993;26:225-33.
86. Nair PNR, Sjögren U, Sundqvist G. Cholesterol crystals as an etiological factor in non resolving chronic inflammation: an experimental study in guinea pigs. Eur J O Sci 1998;106:644-50.
87. Nori Y, Ehara A, Kawahara T, Takemura N, Ebisu S. Participation of bacterial biofilms in refractory and chronic periapical periodontitis. J Endod 2002; 28:679-83.
88. Oliveira MRS, Biffi JCG, Mota AS, Maniglia CAG. Avaliação da remoção de pinos intra-radiculares pré-fabricados através da técnica ultra-sônica. Rev Ass Paul Cir Dent 1999;53:372-77.
89. Pécora JD, Costa WF, Santos-Filho D, Sarti SJ. Apresentação de um óleo essencial, obtido de *Citrus awiantium*, eficaz na desintegração do cimento de óxido de zinco eugenol do interior do canal radicular. Odonto 1992; 1:130-32.
90. Pesce HF, Bastos-Filho E, Risso VA. Avaliação do índice de ocorrência de retratamentos endodônticos em função da qualidade da obturação, presença ou não de rarefação periapical e sintomatologia. Rev Bras Odontol 1996; 53:29-30.
91. Pitt-Ford TR. Vital pulpectomy – and unpredictable procedure. Int Endod J 1982;15:121-26.
92. Quality Assurance Guidelines, Chicago, 1994 – American Association of Endodontics.
93. Ray HA, Trope M. Periapical status of endodontically treated teeth in relation to the technical quality of the root filling and the coronal restoration. Int Endod J 1995;28:12-18.
94. Reid LC, Kazemi RB, Meiers JC. Effect of fatigue testing on core integrity and post microleakage of teeth restored with different post systems. J Endod 2003; 29:125-31.
95. Reit C. Decision strategies in endodontics: on the design of a recall program. Endod Dent Traumatol 1987;3:233-39.
96. Reit C. The influence of observer calibration on radiographic periapical diagnosis. Int Endod J 1987;20:75-81.
97. Reit C, Gröndahl HC. Endodontic decision – making under uncertainty: a decision analytic approach to management of periapical lesions in endodontically treated teeth. Endod Dent Traumatol 1987;3:15-20.
98. Reit C, Gröndahl HC. Endodontic retreatment decision making among a group of general practitioners. Scand J Dent Res 1988;96:12-18.
99. Reit C, Hollender L. evaluation of endodontic therapy and the influence of observer variation. Scand J Dent Res 1983;91:205-12.
100. Rosenow EC. Studies on elective localization. Focal infection with special reference to oral sepsis. J Dent Res 1919;1:205-68.
101. Rowe AHR, Binnie WH. The incidence and location of microorganisms following endodontic treatment. Br Dent J 1977;142:91-95.
102. Ruddle CJ. Nonsurgical endodontic retreatment. In: Cohen S, Burns RC. Pathways of the pulp. 8th ed. St Louis: Mosby. 2002; 875-929.
103. Santos M. Análise comparativa, in vitro, da eficiência na desobturação dos canais radiculares entre as técnicas manual e sônica – contribuição ao estudo. (Master's Thesis). University of São Paulo. 1990; p.75.
104. Saunders WP, Saunders EM. Coronal leakage as causes of failure in root canal therapy. A review. Endod Dent Traumatol 1994;10:105-08.
105. Seltzer S. Root canal failures. In: Endodontology. Seltzer S. 2nd ed. Philadelphia: Lea & Febiger. 1988; p.439-70.
106. Seltzer S. Repair following root canal therapy. In: Endodontology biologic considerations in endodontic procedures. 2nd ed. Philadelphia: Lea & Febiger; 1988; p.389-438.
107. Seltzer S, Bender IB, Smith J, Freedman I, Nazimor H. Endodontic failures – an analysis based on clinical, roentgenographic and histologic findings. Oral Surg Oral Med Oral Pathol 1967;23:500-30.
108. Seltzer S, Naidorf IS. Flare-ups in Endodontics. I. Etiological factors. J Endod 1985; 11:472-76.
109. Shovelton DS. The presence and distribution of microorganisms within non-vital teeth. Br Dent J 1964; 117:101-07.
110. Siqueira-Jr JF. Aetiology of root canal treatment failure: why well-treated teeth can fail. Int Endod J 2001;34:1-10.
111. Siren EK, Haapasalo MPP, Ranta K, Salmi P, Kerosuo ENJ. Microbiological findings and clinical treatment procedures in endodontic cases selected for microbiological investigation. Int Endod J 1997;30:91-95.
112. Sjögren U, Figdor D, Persson S, Sundqvist G. Influence of infection at the time of root filling on the outcome of endodontic treatment of teeth with apical periodontitis. Int Endod J 1997;30:297-306.

113. Sjögren U, Hägglund B, Sundqvist G. Factors affecting the long-terms results of endodontic treatment. J Endod 1990;16:498-504.
114. Souza V, Holland R, Menezes MR. Comportamento biológico do cimento de óxido de zinco e eugenol após contato com hidróxido de cálcio. Estudo histológico em tecido subcutâneo de ratos. Rev Bras Odontol 1991;1:2-10.
115. Stabholz A, Friedman S. Endodontic retreatment – Case selection and technique. Part 2: Treatment planning for retreatment. J Endod 1988; 14:607-14.
116. Stabholz A, Friedman S, Tanse A. Endodontic failures and retreatment. In: Pathways of the pulp. Cohen S, Burns RC. 6th ed. St Louis: Mosby. 1994; p.690-728.
117. Stabholz A, Walton RE. Avaliação do sucesso e insucesso. In: Walton RE, Torabinejad M. Princípios e prática em endodontia. 1st ed. São Paulo: Santos Livraria e edit. 1997; p.324-335.
118. Stamos DE, Gutmann JL. Survey of endodontic retreatment methods used to remove intra-radicular posts. J Endod 1993;19:366-69.
119. Sundqvist G, Figdor D, Persson S, Sjögren U. Microbiologic analysis of teeth with failed endodontic treatment and the outcome of conservative retreatment. Oral Surg Oral Med Oral Pathol 1998;85:86-93.
120. Swanson K, Madison S. An evaluation of coronal microlekage in endodontically treated teeth. Time periods. J Endod 1987;13:56-59.
121. Sydney GB, Batista A. Retratamento endodôntico. In: Odontologia Integrada. Vanzillotta PS, Gonçalves AR. Rio de Janeiro: Pedro Primeiro. 2002; p. 290-326.
122. Sydney GB, Estrela C. Influence of root canal preparation on anaerobic bacteria in teeth with asymptomatic apical periodontitis. Braz Endod J 1996;1:7-10.
123. Taintor JF, Ingle JI, Fahid A. Retreatment versus further treatment. Clin Prevent Dent 1983;5:8-14.
124. Thoden VVSK, Duivnvoorden HJ, Schuurs AHB. Probalities of success and failure in endodontic treatment: a Bayesian approach. Oral Surg Oral Med Oral Pathol 1981;52:85.
125. Torabinejad M, Cymerman JJ, Frank SM, Lemon RR, Maggio JD, Schilder H. Effectiveness of complete instrumentation. J Endod 1994;20:427-31.
126. Torabinejad M, Dorn SO, Eleazer PD, Frankson M, Jouhari B, Mullin RK, Soluti A. Effectiveness of various medications on post operative pain following root canal obturation. J Endod 1994;20:427-31.
127. Torabinejad M, Goodacre CJ. Endodontic or dental implant therapy – The factors affecting treatment planning. J Amer Dent Ass 2006;137:973-77.
128. Torabinejad M, Lemon RR. Acidentes de procedimentos. In: Princípios e prática em endodontia. Walton RE, Torabinejad M. 1st ed. São Paulo: Santos, 1997; p.306-23.
129. Torabinejad M, Ung B, Kettering JD. In vitro bacterial penetration of coronal unsealed endodontically treated teeth. J Endod 1990;16:566-69.
130. Torneck CD. Reaction of rat connective tissue to polyethylene tube implants, part 2. Oral Surg Oral Med Oral Pathol 1967;24:674-83.
131. Trope E, Chow E, Nissan R. In vitro endotoxin penetration of coronally unsealed endodontically treated teeth. Endod Dent Traumatol 1991;11:90-94.
132. Tronstad L, Asbjornsen K, Dorving L, Pedersen I, Eriksen HM. Influence of coronal restorations on the periapical health of endodontically treated teeth. Endod Dent Traumatol 2000;16:218-21.
133. Vire DE. Failure of endodontically treated teeth. J Endod 1991;17:338-42.
134. Wilcox LR. Endodontic retreatment with halothane versus chloroform solvent. J Endod 1995;21:305-07.
135. Wilcox LR, Krell KV, Madison S, Rittman B. Endodontic retreatment: Evaluation of gutta-percha and sealer removal and canal reinstrumentation. J Endod 1987;13:453-57.
136. Wilcox LR, Surksun RV. Endodontic retreatment in large and small straight canals. J Endod 1991;17:119-22.
137. Wilcox LR, Swift LM. Endodontic retreatment in small and large curved canal J Endod 1991;17:313-15.
138. Wourms DJ, Campbell AD, Hicks ML, Pelleu-Jr GB. Alternative solvents to chloroform for gutta-percha removal. J Endod 1990;16:224-26.
139. Yared GM, Bou-Dagher FE. Influence of apical enlargement on bacterial infection during treatment of apical periodontitis. J Endod 1994;20:535-37.
140. Zakariasen KL, Scott DA, Jensen JR. Endodontic recall radiographs: how reliable is our interpretation of endodontic success of failure and what factors affect our reliability? Oral Surg Oral Med Oral Pathol 1984;57:343-47.

# Treatment of Endodontic Failure

**C. Estrela**

*Federal University of Goiás, Goiânia, GO, Brazil*

**J. C. G. Biffi**

*Federal University of Uberlândia, Uberlândia, MG, Brazil*

**M. S. Moura**

*Brazilian Dentistry Research and Learning Center, CEPOBRAS, Goiânia, GO, Brazil*

**H. P. Lopes**

*Brazilian Endodontic Association, Rio de Janeiro, RJ, Brazil*

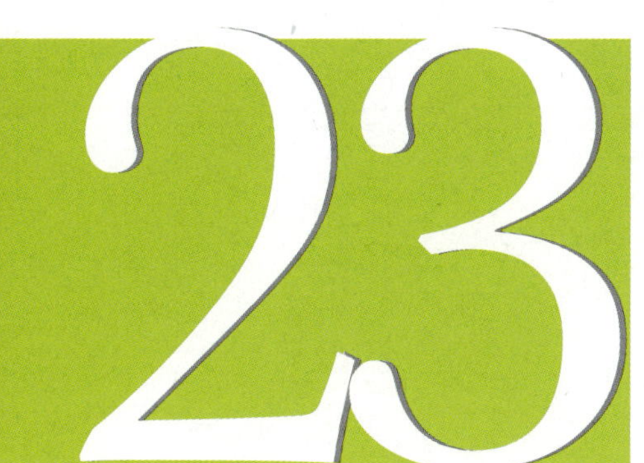


Chapter contents

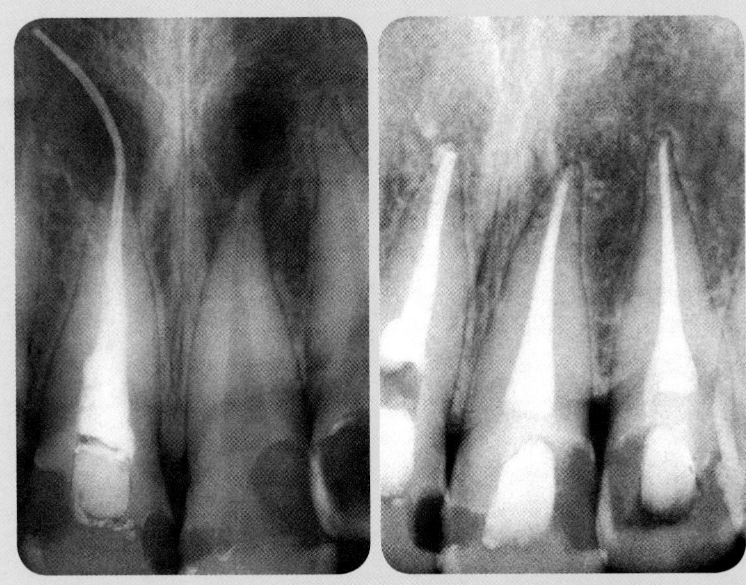

Endodontic retreatment.

## 23.1 Introduction

When failure has been found, structuring new endodontic treatment is a complex process that requires special care. After discussing the factors responsible for the failure, the professional needs to plan the operations required to perform root canal retreatment of the previous unsuccessful treatment. Any reconstruction demands a great deal of attention and selection of know-how.

The new treatment to be performed will consist of almost exactly the same operative phases as those of the initial treatment. Figure 22.8 of the chapter 22 regarding the diagnosis of endodontic failure, points out the technical difficulties found in all the stages of endodontic treatment. The first option for treating the failure is endodontic retreatment, which presents difficulties and complications that make the prognosis doubtful.

Likewise, the clinical and radiographic characteristics of endodontic success should be emphasized. The fundamental aspects related to endodontic success can be summed up as: 1. Clinical silence (absence of pain, edema, fistula); 2. Normal periapical bone structure (uniformity of the lamina dura, normal periodontal space, absence or reduction of bone rarefaction, absence of root resorption or interruption); 3. Tooth in function and presence of perfect coronal sealing. The Figure 23.1 present a clinical case of asymptomatic apical periodontitis with extensive periapical bone destruction; showing clinical and radiographic success after endodontic treatment with calcium hydroxide used as intracanal dressing, 20 months after treatment began.

Redoubled attention should be paid to the careful selection of cases. The professional's care of the patient and case at clinical issue, his/her common-sense, intuition, professional skill and ability are inherent characteristics that must always be valorized.

When indicated, endodontic retreatment should be evaluated from a risks and benefits point of view. A study of the clinical case should be made, in order to allow good planning of the procedures to perform, one capable of defining the most opportune therapeutic options that will certainly avoid embarrassing and unpleasant situations.

The factors responsible for the endodontic failures and the possible treatment options have been discussed a great deal[1-148].

Among local factors capable of causing a possible doubtful prognosis (or that impede use of the correct endodontic technique), the following are emphasized: 1. anatomic-pathological factors (modifications of the internal anatomy; excessive dilacerations; pulp cavity calcifications); 2. current factors of endodontic accidents (working length loss - step; root perforation; endodontic instrument fracture); 3. Endodontic failures (presence of widespread posts; filling only with cements; sealer and gutta-percha; sealer and silver cone; etc). On the other hand, one can also consider factors relative to the patient, such as the characteristics of systemic diseases.

It has been observed that most of the teeth indicated for endodontic retreatment present restorations. The presence of crown and intraradicular retainer obstruct and complicate coronal access. For retreatment, firstly new access to the root canals is required, which is achieved by emptying consisting of clearing or un-obstructing the access.

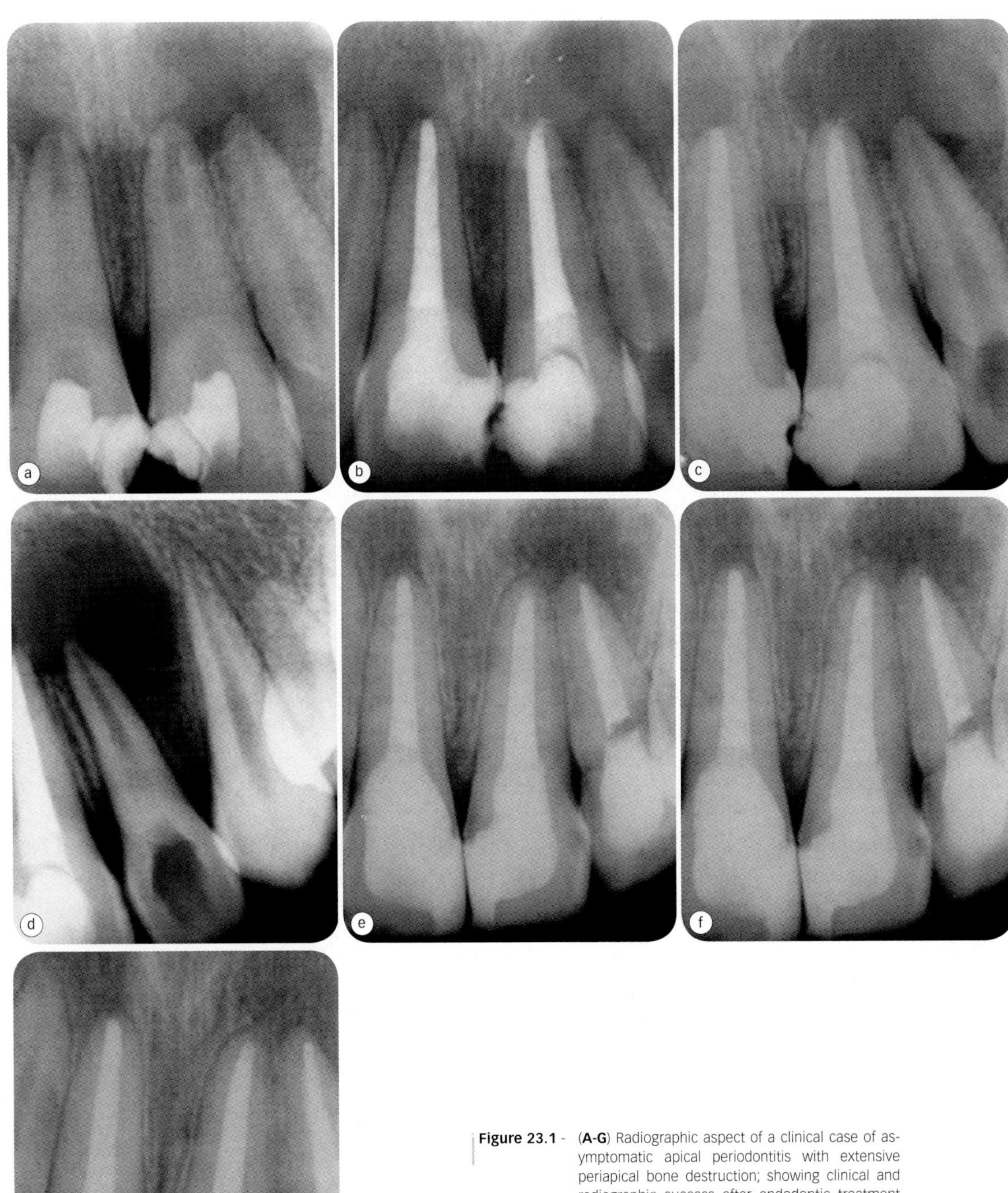


**Figure 23.1** - (**A-G**) Radiographic aspect of a clinical case of asymptomatic apical periodontitis with extensive periapical bone destruction; showing clinical and radiographic success after endodontic treatment with calcium hydroxide used as intracanal dressing; 20 months after treatment began.

Coronal restorations in endodontically treated teeth can be of amalgam, resin composite, cast metal, metal or porcelain crown (with or without intraradicular retainer), or another type of prosthesis. The extensive restorations, crowns and fixed dentures can completely cover the dental crown, which increases the possibilities of accidents during access to the coronal chamber [53,54,119-123]. Every care is required during the procedures to gain new endodontic access because, during the efforts to remove a restoration and/or an intraradicular retainer, there is always a certain risk involved in perforation the tooth [119,120]. Special care should be taken every time a tooth not in its habitual position.

Certainly, the tooth anatomy is better visualized without the presence of the crown. Preparation of the endodontic cavity and removal of the carious dentine should preferentially be performed in teeth without the prosthetic crown. The tooth can be turned and it can be complicated to prepare the access cavity through the crown, and could lead to mistakes, such as deviation or perforation [53,54,119-123].

In endodontic retreatment, the presence of intraradicular posts is common. Their removal can present great difficulties, such as the risk of dental fractures or perforation the root, particularly when there is little remaining dental structure. However, with the recent technical advances in technique and equipment, these sequelae have been minimized.

## 23.2 Emptying of the Root Canal

Several factors that influence the prognosis of success or failure have been discussed, however, there are variables that make the results of studies difficult to interpret. Stabholz et al.[120] related that these difficulties include observer bias in radiographic interpretation, variable levels of patient cooperation, the subjectivity of patient response, variability of the host's response to the treatment, relative validity and reproducibility of the evaluation method, variables the degree of control, as well as the sample size and the differences in the observation periods.

A factor to consider is that the percentage of success is influenced by the preoperative state of the dental pulp, associated with the presence or absence of preoperative periapical lesion.

It is important to verify the residues extruded from periapical region after root canal preparation. The presence of a quantity of apical filling material residues after preparation was observed in 93.34% of the analyzed teeth[69,71]. The residues after a new root canal preparation can change the hermetic seal during the new filling of the root canal and cover it with necrotic remainders or bacteria again, which will probably interfere in the result of the retreatment.

When free access is gained, it allows the entire root canal to be emptied, and is one of the first technical goals after the diagnosis of endodontic treatment failure has been defined. In endodontic retreatment the removal of extensive restorations and intraradicular retainers should be done carefully, otherwise this can be responsible for direct failure or a poor prognosis. In order to avoid or reduce the number of accidents (perforation, dental fractures), adequate treatment planning and a careful selection of cases should always be always considered before beginning the treatment. In the event that the clinical condition makes endodontic retreatment unfeasible, either because it is not worth the risk of a dental fracture, perforation, or of not achieving a better situation than that the one that is presented, the option of periapical surgery can be considered directly.

During the last two decades, there have been different trends in restorative procedures, especially with regard to bonding with adhesive systems or retention with prefabricated intraradicular posts. Particularly with respect to the intraradicular retainers, some aspects have been the target of investigations, such as the type of retainer, length, diameter, root canal preparation to receive the retainer and cements used for fixation.

Conventionally, the posts are cemented, mostly with zinc phosphate cement. However, with the appearance of new resinous materials with excellent bonding capacity, there have been several innovations among the materials for cementation.

The difficulty in establishing new access to the root canal depends on the present material, pulp cavity anatomy, iatrogenesis (loss of working length - steps, perforation, fractured instruments), the presence of intraradicular retainers (type, length, diameter, cement).

The new endodontic treatment seeks to sanitization the root canal, completely remove the material present, establish the new longitudinal and transversal limit of enlargement, obtain an adequate shape and to achieve effective and powerful microbial control over the secondary infection present.

Part of endodontic retreatment planning is adequate diagnosis, associated with judicious selection of cases. The radiographic exam is essential, since it provides a great deal of important information: The probable filling material, the quality and extent of the filling, the presence of under or over filling, mechanical obstructions (cement, fragment of endodontic instrument), cast and post (type, length, and diameter). Knowing these factors, one can foresee the difficulty or easiness of emptying the root canal.

Before endodontic retreatment starts, the probable risks and benefits to the patient must be very well clarified, and written consent must be obtained from the patient to perform the new treatment.

However, as an additional clinical resource for retreatment of a possible failure, one still has the option of performing periapical surgery.

## 23.3 Endodontic Retreatment

In endodontic retreatment, access to the apical region is obtained by means of emptying the root canal, by removing the present filling material. The new modeling of the canal depends on free and direct access to the apical region.

The filling material usually offers resistance to removal. This resistance cannot result in undesirable alterations in the morphology of the root canal, because the goals of endodontic therapy should be maintained[34-37,120-122].

The materials usually found are pastes, cements, gutta-percha, silver points, fragments of broken instruments (file, drill, Lentulo drill). Many techniques have been recommended for removing the filling materials and/or the obstructions from root canals[10,11,13,15,19,20,24,31,34-39,48,53-55,60,61,63,66,67,73,74,76-78,82,90,92,118-120,124,126,128,135,136,138-144].

Among resources available for removing the casts materials, Vani et al.[139] pointed out the use of carbide drills, ultrasound, spring-activated system, post extractor pliers, the small giant device, pneumatically activated system (Coronaflex), and pendulum-activated system (Fig. 23.2).

As follows, the steps usually involved in the process of emptying the root canals with presence of pastes, cements, gutta-percha points, silver points, fractured endodontic instruments will be described.

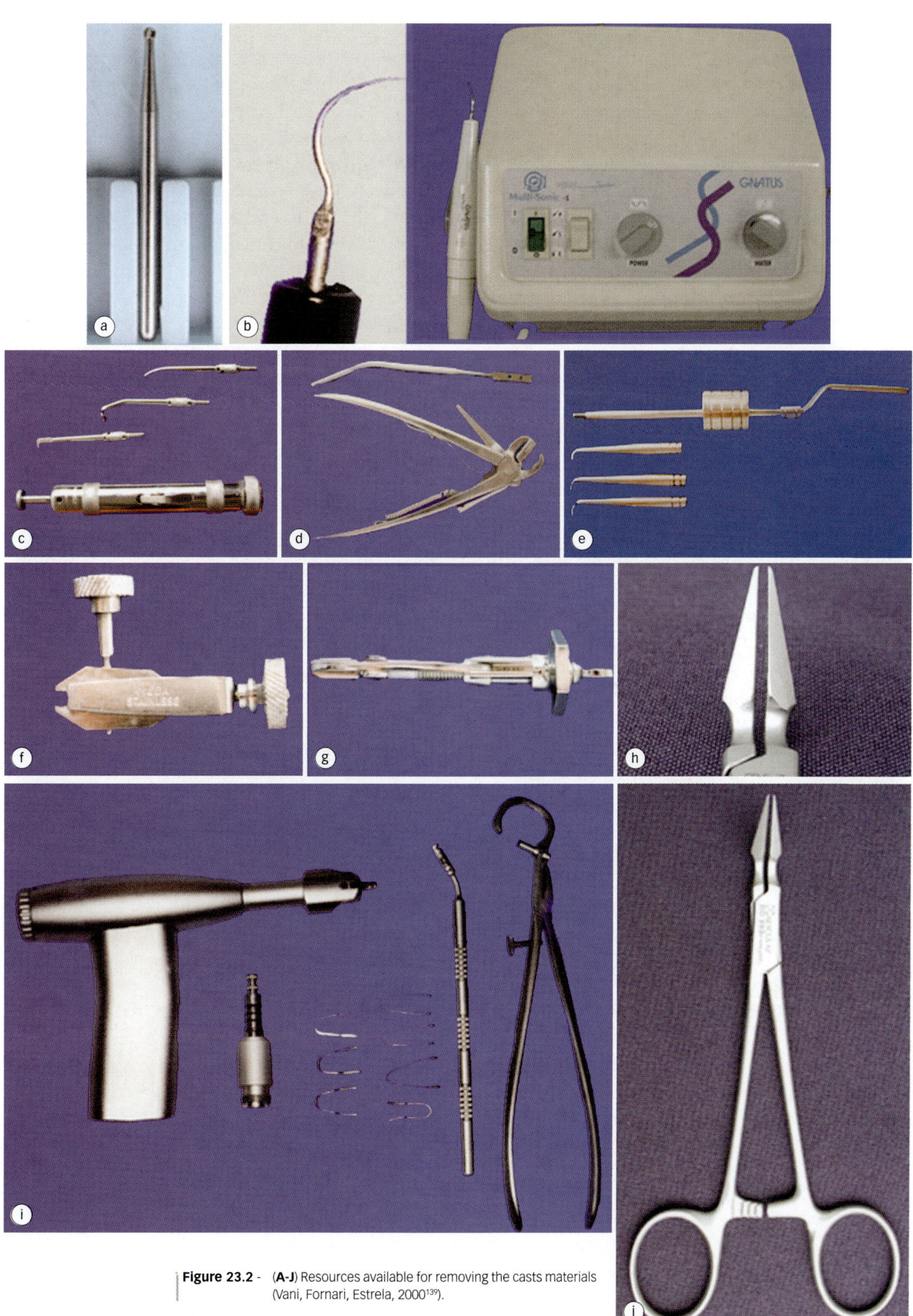


**Figure 23.2** - (**A-J**) Resources available for removing the casts materials (Vani, Fornari, Estrela, 2000[139]).

### 23.3.1 Emptying Root Canal with Pastes and Sealers

The first step is the clinical and radiographic evaluation of the present filling material (paste/ cement), and of the quantity and extent of apical material (presence in the cervical, middle and/or apical regions). In root canals that contain calcium hydroxide pastes, these are not generally difficult to remove. With a K-flex instrument and catheterization, associated with the abundant irrigation-aspiration, the paste is dislocated and removed from inside the root canal. When the root canal is only filled with cement, the clinical case becomes more complex, because in some situations, the cement found is zinc oxide and eugenol-based, zinc phosphate cement, and even some resins. One should pay attention, because various materials have been found obstructing the root canal. The cements are usually of a hard consistency and require a solvent to help to degrade and solubilize them. This material is very difficult to remove. As auxiliary resources to remove cement from inside the root canal, initially it can be worth trying rotary instruments, such as drills LN, modified instruments (instruments prepared exclusively for this purpose), or long carbide drills. The use of these resources demands radiographic follow-up, step-by-step, due to the great risk of perforation. Another resource that helps is ultrasound, as an isolated maneuver or associated with the above-mentioned resources. Completely successful removal is not achieved in all cases treated with cements.

### 23.3.2 Emptying of the Root Canal with Gutta-percha

The initial diagnosis is of significant importance when gutta-percha needs to be removed from the canal. Clinical and radiographic evaluation of the quality of the filling in the three thirds of the root, and of the apical filling limit of the present filling material is essential.

Most cases show filling condensates in the cervical and middle thirds, with failures in the apical third, and lack of adequate filling. After the normal coronal opening procedures, Gates-Glidden's Drills (cervical broaches) are used, especially in the cervical third and beginning of the middle third, which reduces the volume of the filling material. After this, a solvent is sued in the space relative to the cervical third (such as Xylol, or orange oil) and with catheterization and K-flex files, pressure is exerted on the filling remainder that is being influenced by the solvent. Initially, a trepan can be placed under the filling material, because it allows a certain pressure to be exerted.

The hardly condensed gutta-percha cones in root canals can be pushed with small rotary actions. Again, some drops of solvent are placed in the pulp chamber, then with K-flex files (#15, 20, 25), apical pressure and catheterization actions are applied to the material. Afterwards, with the space created by these files, one can try to remove the material with the help of Hedströem files (#20, 25 or 30). In the apical region, mostly in the last 3 mm of filling, the use of solvent should be avoided to prevent possible material overfilling. Gutta-percha extruded into the periapical region can act as a potential irritant.

In curved root canals, care should be redoubled, since there are increased chances of creating steps, occurrence of perforation, foraminal transport, and instrument fractures.

Special care should be taken with Hedströem files, because they can lock into the walls of the canals and fracture. In the cases of under filling, the gutta-percha is removed, as previously mentioned, up to 2 to 3 mm on this side of the apex. To remove the gutta-percha remainder that is kept solid, in other words, without the help of solvent influence, a Hedströem file is used after the use of K-flex. When the obstacle has been overcome, a rasp of the K-flex type is inserted up to 0.5 to 1.0 mm next to the apex. With a controlled clockwise turn, one endeavors to grip the gutta-percha firmly and remove it slowly. One should take care with the under-filling of endodontic cement, because in cases of retreatment, the apical stop is not clearly defined.

### 23.3.3 Emptying of the Root Canal with Silver Points

The access to the root canal in tooth filled with silver points, makes it necessary to first remove the restoration and the filling material present in the coronal chamber. One should take care that the drills do not damage the silver cones. After removing the coronal seal, by the volume of the silver point, one should verify whether it is loose or cemented firmly inside the canal. Careful survey with an endodontic explorer is the first step. If it is not very firm, the silver point should be gripped, using special fine tipped tweezers, and pulled in the coronal direction. If the silver point is cemented and firmly retained inside the canal, ultrasound should be used to disintegrate the cement, when present, in order to facilitate its removal. After the application of ultrasound, one should try to grip the silver point with a fine caliber instrument to remove it. Every care should be taken so that the silver point does not fracture inside the canal, which would complicate the clinical case even further[24].

### 23.3.4 Emptying of the Root Canal with Fractured Instruments

Endodontic instrument fracture is an accident that can be and obstacle to continuing with the treatment, or even jeopardize its success. The principles that govern sanitization and the correct root canal modeling process should be strictly followed, in order to avoid this type of accident.

The commonest causes in instrument fracture are its incorrect handling; unnecessary force in the curvatures and obstacles; Intervening in time; using endodontic instruments outside sequence of increase in caliber; lack of inspection before and after use; excessive work; Inadequate access; and failure in the manufacture of the instrument [13,15,24,34-39,53,118-120].

In the presence of a fractured instrument inside the root canal, the following possible therapeutic options to solve the access problem can be considered: the first attempt is to find the fractured instrument and remove it; the second is find it and embed it in filling material; the third is to close the canal up to the instrument; and the fourth is to opt for endodontic surgery, to solve problem. An important factor during the decision about the solution is with regard to the preoperative state of the dental pulp.

Thus, a metal instrument that cannot be fastened or taken out, should be found to allow its removal during canal preparation, or to conclude the treatment without its removal. The fractured instrument can be overshot using K-flex files, trepan or ultrasonic vibration. When the canal is filled with silver points, the care can follow the same recommendations as for fractured instruments. One uses a small caliber instrument to open space along the walls of the canal and the solid object, and try to overtake the fractured fragment. In the cases of silver points, one tries to break the cement with the ultrasound. Always pre-curve the instruments in the curvatures. As we penetrate inside the canal, abundant irrigation-aspiration should be performed and the course of the instrument guided and followed up by means of X-rays, radiographs to verify possible deviations of the root canal. Once the object has been overtaken or when approaching of the terminal of the root canal, radiographs should be taken to establish the working length. As the root canal preparation proceeds, one can try to use Hedströem files to help to remove the rasp fragment of the #25 K-flex file. This is the first resource to try to overcome this difficult obstacle, considering the other options discussed.

Another device described in the literature is Masserann's Kit. It consists of an excavator device that is applied and closed around the object. A series of cutting drills are used anticlockwise to promote access to the object. As the drills are large and rigid, this technique is restricted to straight lines and wide roots. Its use has to be controlled by frequent radiographs. This technique results in tooth, dentine and root weakness, and considerable sacrifice, in addition to the high risk of perfuration[15,34-37].

If the target goal, removal of the rasp fragment present in the canal is not achieved with any of the previously described methods, endodontic surgery should be opted for as complementary treatment.

The Figures 23.3A-B demonstrate an endodontic retreatment sequence, with emptying the root canal filled with gutta-percha and cement.

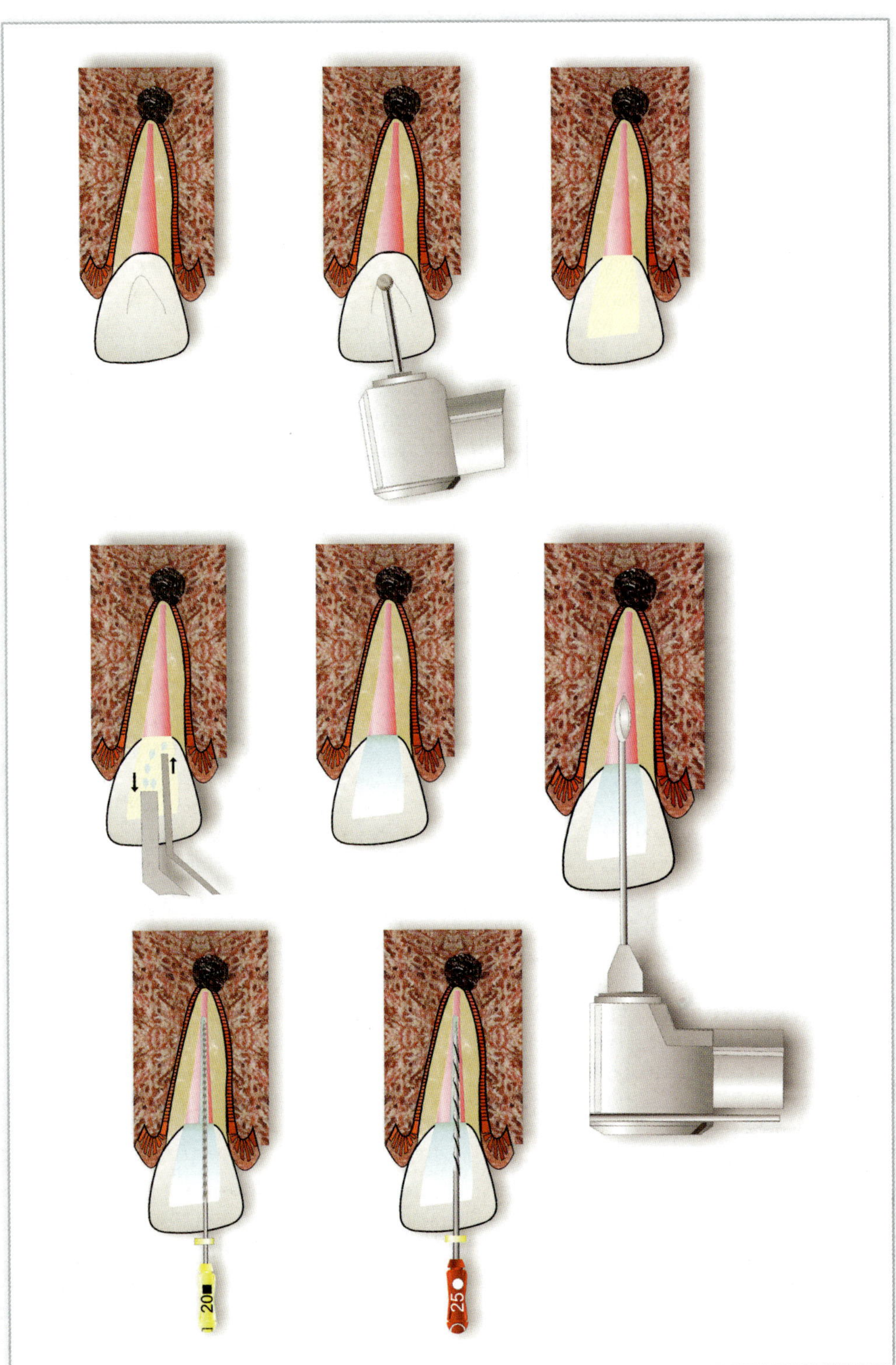


**Figure 23.3A** - Schematic representation of the endodontic retreatment sequence in incisors, with emptying the root canal filled with gutta-percha and cement.

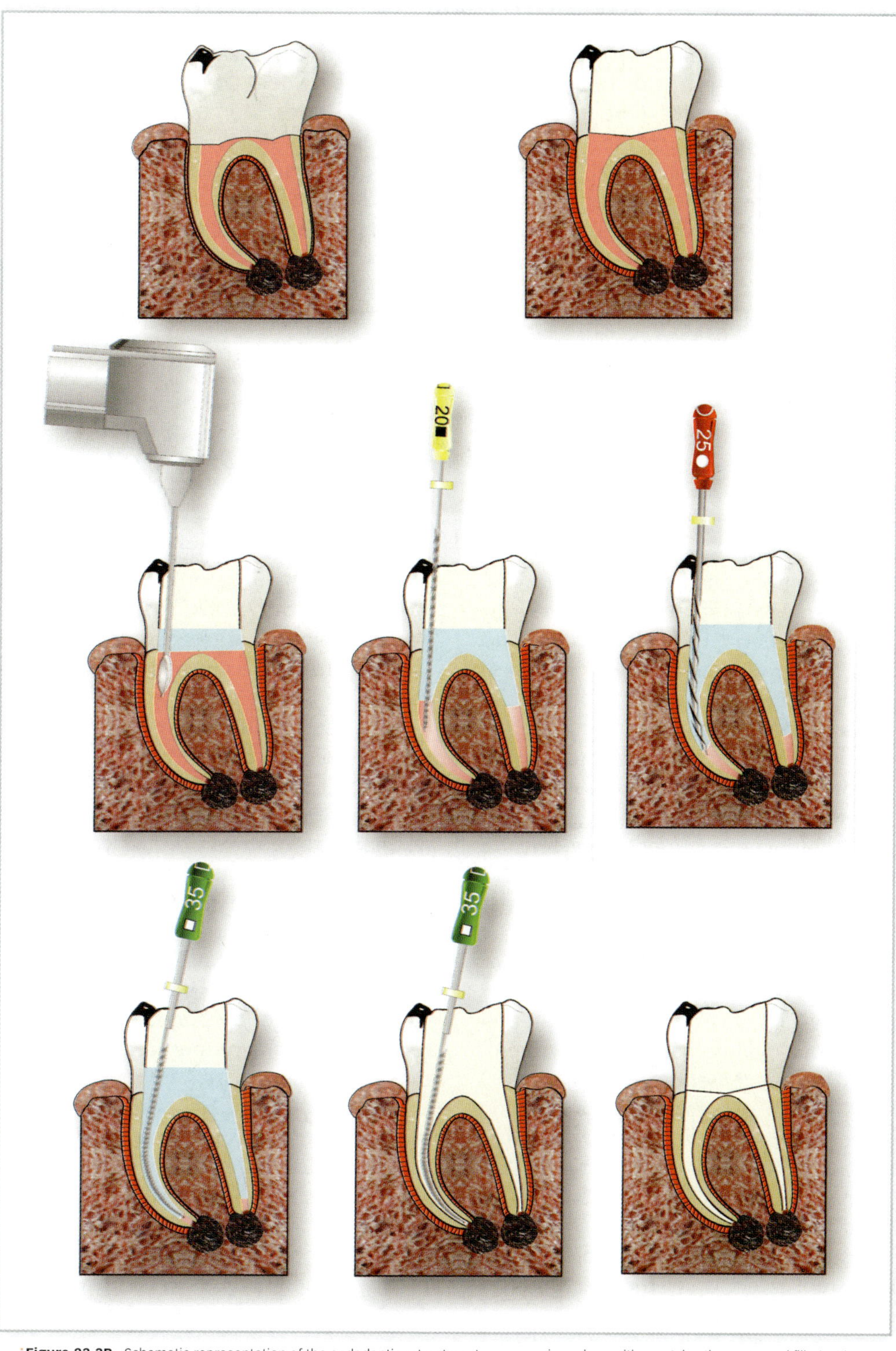


**Figure 23.3B** - Schematic representation of the endodontic retreatment sequence in molars, with emptying the root canal filled with gutta-percha and cement.

### 23.3.5 Emptying the Root Canal with Posts

There is high prevalence of endodontic failure in crowns of teeth with posts. Thus, there are countless devices that favor post removal, allow new access to the root canal and for emptying it. As follows, different resources destined for this purpose are pointed out: the use of the carbide drill, ultrasound, spring-activated system, post extractor pliers, giant small device, pneumatically activated system and pendulum activated system .

### 23.3.6 Post Removal with Ultrasound

In endodontic retreatment, during the removal of the retainers (cast/post), one can come across unpleasant accidents, responsible for leading to direct failure of the treatment or to unfavorable prognosis. Therefore, in order to avoid or decrease operative accidents (perforations and/or dental fractures) adequate planning should be structured for each specific situation. For this purpose, one should know the type of the post involved, and be able to imagine or to identify the cement used. Post removal with the ultrasonic system is performed by means of mechanical energy, with oscillations transmitted to the root retainer, with the goal of fragmenting and disintegrating the cement between the post and dentin. The most used cements are the zinc phosphate, glass ionomer and the resinous cements.

Oliveira et al.[92] evaluated the effectiveness in vitro of ultrasonic vibration for post removal, in 40 single rooted human teeth. They used pre-manufactured posts (Unimetric 215 TR 310L) cemented with zinc phosphate cement. In one group, there was no type of treatment before traction; the other group was submitted to ultrasonic vibration for 3 minutes. The necessary force for the post removal was determined using a universal test machine. At a second stage, the samples were duplicated, using the same groups in inverse procedures, so that each specimen was equally submitted to two different procedures: Post removal without vibration and with previous vibration. The results showed that for the specimens treated with ultrasonic vibration significantly smaller forces were necessary, when compared with the other group. Garrido[38] analyzed the efficiency of ultrasonic vibration, with and without air/water cooling, for removal by traction of molten metal posts cemented with resinous cement, in comparison with posts cemented with zinc phosphate cement. The 42 analyzed human teeth were submitted to traction in the universal test machine. In the groups cemented with resinous cement, the results showed that the ultrasonic vibration without cooling reduced the traction force necessary for removal of the retainers by 71%, statistically different from values obtained in the groups with ultrasonic vibration with cooling and control, which presented similar results to each other. In the groups cemented with zinc phosphate, the ultrasonic vibration with cooling presented the best results, reducing the necessary force required to displace the retainer by 75%. Thus, it was possible note that the presence or absence of cooling interferes in the efficiency of the ultrasonic vibration, depending on the type of cement used to fix the retainers. Silva et al.[114] determined the effect of ultrasonic vibration on the force necessary to remove pre-fabricated and anatomic and cast posts. Two hundred and forty teeth were divided into two groups. In group I, a 0.8-mm metal pre-fabricated post, Unimetric-Maillefer, was utilized; in group II, cast copper-aluminum alloy posts measuring 0.8, 1.0 and 1.2 mm in diameter were used. The root canals were prepared in three different diameters: 0.8, 1.0 and 1.2 mm, with a length of 10 mm. The posts were cemented with glass ionomer cement resulting in 20 specimens for each subgroup. Half of the sample was submitted to ultrasonic vibration for 3 minutes, while the other half did not receive any vibration. The specimens were submitted to traction in a universal testing machine. The application of ultrasonic vibration significantly reduced the retention offered by the glass ionomer cement in the intracanal post fixation. Cementation of well fitting posts to root canals did not necessarily offer a greater retention against displacement provided by a vertical traction force, both in the control and experimental groups. The ultrasonic action was effective both in the pre-fabricated and anatomic and cast posts. The efficacy of ultrasonic vibration was not related to the cement line, or to the post diameter.

Queiroz et al.[97] assessed the influence of the coronal shape of intra-radicular cores on their removal by the use of ultrasound technique. Twenty-four single-rooted bovine teeth were prepared and cast posts were fixed with zinc phosphate cement. The teeth were randomly divided into two groups: group I- received cast cores made without the anatomy of the coronal portion, simulating removal this portion with a bur, and group II- received cores that reproduced the coronal anatomy. Both were treated with an ultrasound appliance in two three-minute cycles (US). The force necessary for post removal was determined using a mechanical test machine. In the second stage of the study, the cores were again cemented and no ultrasound vibration was used on them (C). The force necessary for post removal was determined using a mechanical test machine. It was concluded that the shape of the core without the anatomic coronal portion facilitated removal of intraradicular retention only when associated with the use of ultrasound.

The greater stability of cast intraradicular posts is generated by the base of the coronal portion being seated on the dental remainder, thus providing better accommodation for the core where there is a larger contact area between the two structures. This condition is less favorable to ultrasonic action, as the dissipation of vibratory energy generates less distribution of stress at the cement line, consequently less micro-crack formation, making it difficult to remove. This situation may explain the tensile strength values obtained in the present study with regard to the efficiency of ultrasound in posts without the coronal anatomy reproduced (8.00 Kgf), in comparison with the group with coronal anatomy reproduced (32.36 Kgf). This difference is probably owing to the destabilization of the post because of being less well accommodated in the group without reproduction of the coronal portion, and had a smaller contact area with the dental structure, consequently there was greater concentration of vibratory energy and greater distribution of tension at the cement line, generating greater intensity in the number of micro cracks at the cement line [97].

Gomes et al.[39] reported ultrasound efficacy in the removal of cast posts cemented with zinc phosphate, in a 10 minutes period. The application of ultrasonic vibration significantly reduced the retention required in 39%. The variations in ultrasonic vibration time required to for post removal may be attributed to the differences in post length, as according to Bergeron et al.[8], the extensive depth and greater stability of posts related to the geometry of the coronal root portion, may minimize the action of ultrasonic vibrations and make it difficult to remove the posts. This study confirmed that the application of ultrasound significantly reduced the tensile strength necessary to remove intraradicular posts compared with the groups that did not receive ultrasound application. The groups that did not have ultrasound applied, the retention values were significantly higher and the coronal shape of the post did not influence the traction force necessary to remove it, and the mean values demonstrated that there was no correlation between the diameter of the coronal portion of the post with the force necessary to remove it when the ultrasonic device was not applied.

Ruddle[107] suggested that the ultrasound tip must be applied at the metal/root canal wall interface and wearing around the post in order to expose cementation line, to increase ultrasound efficiency. Alfredo et al.[1] reported the efficiency of reducing the post diameter before applying ultrasound, and the authors' concluded wearing of the post probably increased ultrasound wave efficiency, concentrating vibrations deeply, better reaching the cement that bonds the post to the root canal walls, the mean tension necessary to displace the pots with the reduction post-diameter reduced the necessary tension to remove them by 24% compared with larger posts. The results obtained in the present study confirmed the efficiency of reducing the post diameter before applying ultrasound; tensile strength was 34% for that was anatomically reproduced core and 84% for the core that was not anatomically reproduced.

For the retainer removal, one initially seeks to leave the prosthetic crown. Associated with this procedure, when the post contains cement involving the cervical structure, one performs post wear with a drill LN to reduce it before using ultrasound. When we do not know which cement was used, we can use a cylindrical this case, removal will certainly be facilitated.

For the short and conical post ultrasonic energy is used around the post about for 5 minutes, which in several situations is enough to removes it; If the post is longer and cylindrical shaped it is necessary to apply an ultrasound tip from 5 to 10 minutes.

The following is a suggestion for the technical sequence of the use of ultrasound, according to the Table 23.1 and Figure 23.4-23.5A-E.

**Table 23.1** - Removal of the intraradicular post with ultrasound

| **Technical Sequence of Use of the Ultrasound** |
|---|
| 1. Figure simulating a root with intraradicular post; |
| 2. Initially, with appropriate drills the post is worn away, in other words, the portion of the containment at coronal level, with the purpose of removing its support in the dentine (arrow), leaving it with the same diameter as that of the post at the cervical level; |
| 3. Aspect of the post after wear. Use of ultrasound; |
| 4. Positions recommended for the action of the ultrasound: at the level of lateral and superior cementation line. The time of action of the ultrasound should be limited to one minute per position; |
| 5. Traction of the post with hemostatic tweezers or pliers; in the case of prefabricated post one also can to try rotation in the counterclockwise direction. |
| Observation: If the post has not been removed up to this time, it can be done as described in the following figure |
| 6. With a carbide 1/2 drill, or similar of long neck, the post is worn, opening up a groove in the center of post, taking care to avoid wear of the dentin; |
| 7. The space obtained by the drill will serve as support for the tip of the ultrasound, allowing a closer vibration of the cementation line; |
| 8. Due to groove it is possible to use a sharp probe to cause lateral displacement of part of the post, making a space between the post and the canal wall; |
| 9. Space obtained by displacement of the post; |
| 10. Application of the ultrasound in the lateral space obtained by the displacement of the post. |
| Observation: If the post is not removed with the ultrasonic vibration only, one should alternate the use of the drill with the ultrasonic vibration and traction. |

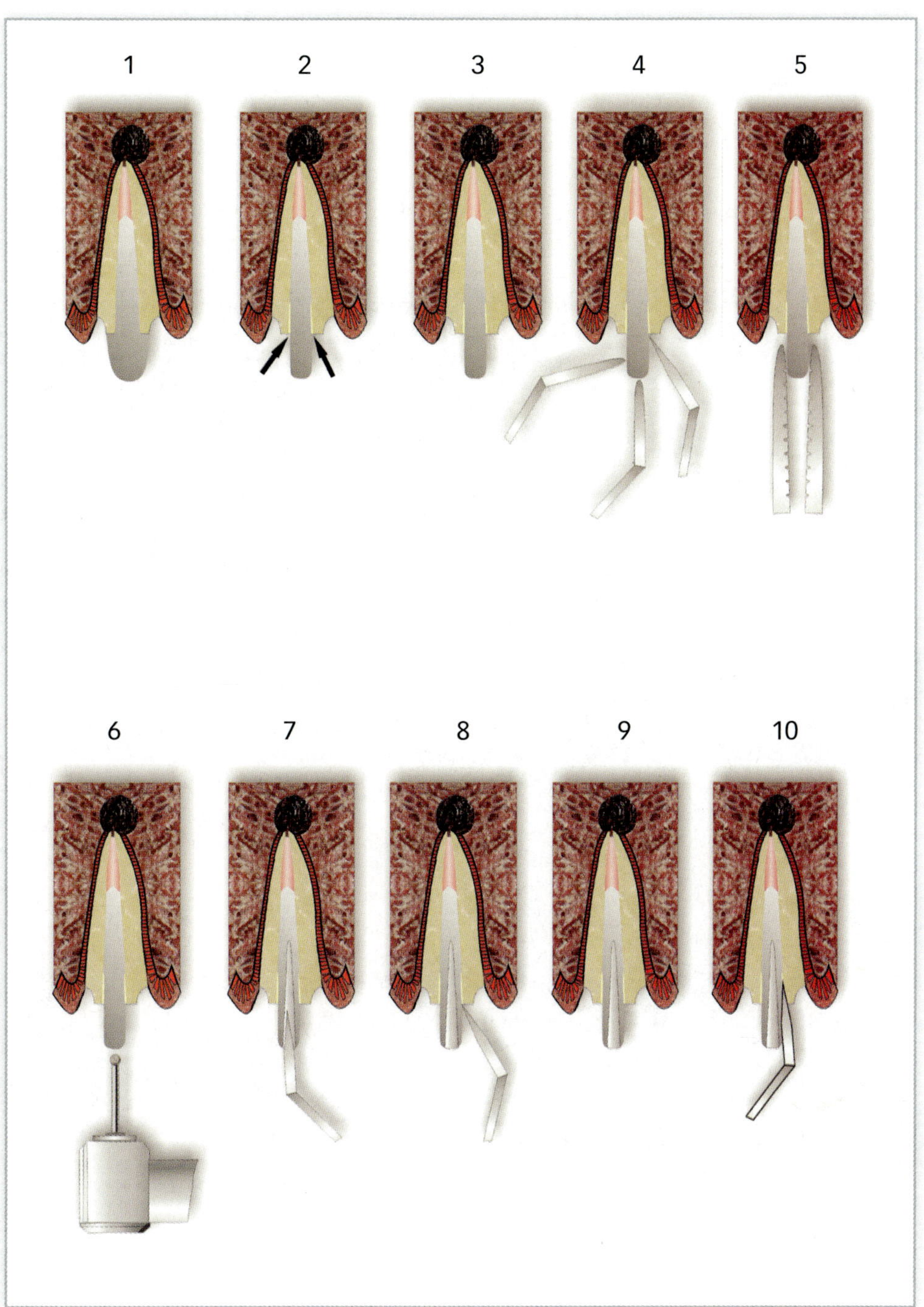


**Figure 23.4** - Schematic representation of the technical sequence of the use of ultrasound to removal the retainers (cast/post).

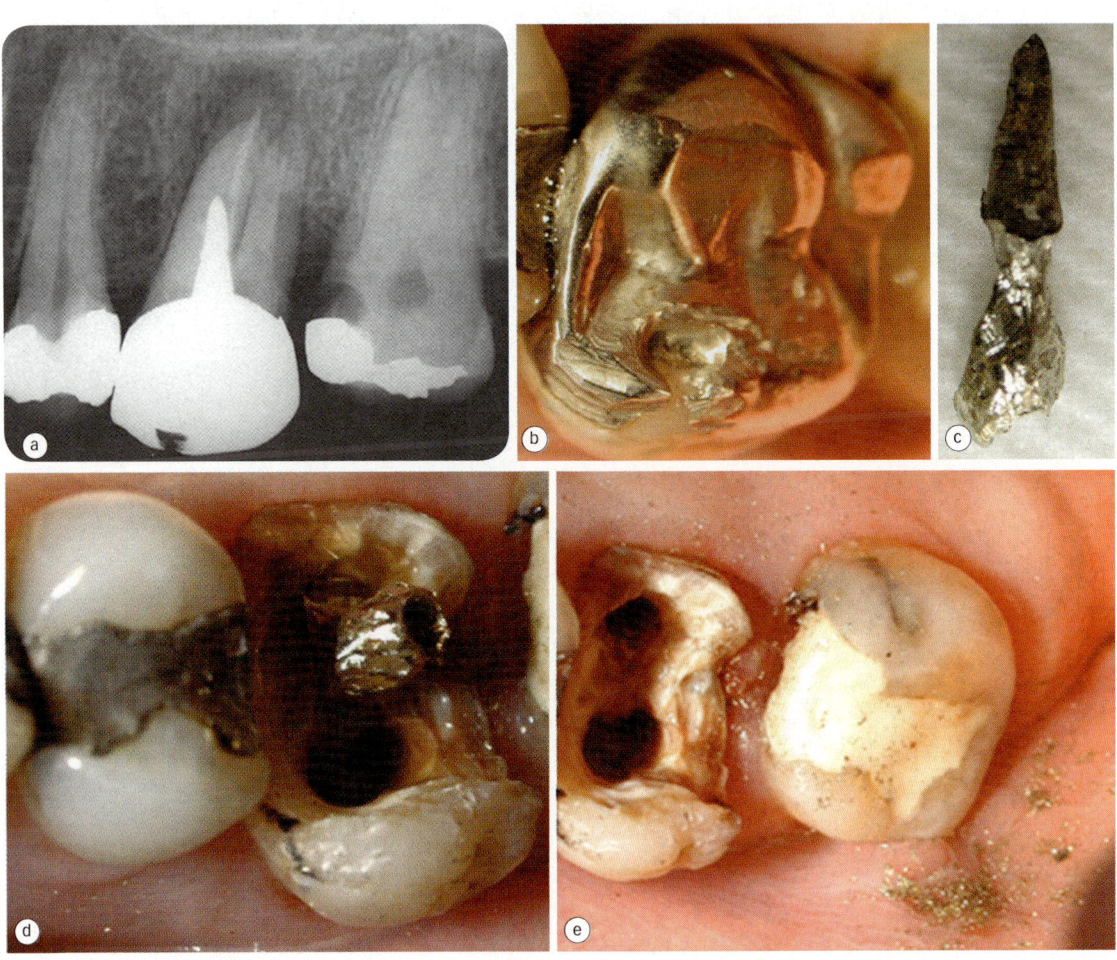

**Figure 23.5** - (**A-E**) Technical sequence of the use of ultrasound to removal the retainers in human molar.

### 23.3.7 Removal with a Spring-activated device

Retainer removal with a spring-activated system is based on a mechanical force of traction. To use it, previous removal of the prosthetic crown is required, as well as the clinical procedures at the metal post surface in order to facilitate fixing the active part of the device. It makes small horizontal grooves about 1 mm deep in the free portion of the metal post, by means of spherical carbide drills of a diameter compatible with the coronal volume of the post, to the point of allowing the adaptation and adjustment of the referred tip traction. This equipment consists of a stem with spring inside it. In the superior portion there is a small table in which the specific removal tip is self-threading; close to the body there is a trigger that releases the spring pressure, and this allows a force of removal of different degrees, depending on the difficulty of each clinical situation, usually varying of 1 or at most 2 degrees. Before the removing part is fixed in the horizontal groove made in the coronal portion of the post, it activates the spring, in order to separate the table from the body of the device, graded by the force required for the case. When the spring pressure has been graded, it adapts the removal tip in the previously made groove, and tries to guide the device along the long axis of the post in the direction of the root. The removal tip will be stabilized close to the post by means of digital pressure and the trigger that is going to liberate and activate the spring, generating the extractive removal force[139].

### 23.3.8 Removal with Carbide Drills

Removing the post by means of wear using carbide steel drills is an accessible and effective method. However, it needs a meticulous radiographic study, which requires radiographs of all three regions of the root canal; analysis of tooth inclination in the arc, a drill direction select control, and good cooling. The ratio between diameter of the root canal and the post, the post length, the drill size, are points that should be analyzed. The drill should have a smaller diameter than the post volume, and at the time of action it should be directed towards the center of the post. Wear should be controlled and slow, and care should be taken to avoid unnecessary wear of root dentin. As we go deeper in the apical direction, millimeter by millimeter, note the direction of the wear. Radiographic follow-up is fundamental to enable control of the direction of wear[139].

This wear method has been used in cases of self-threading metal posts, non-metal posts, and carbon fiber posts.

When there are crowns, the drill has limited access, making post removal more difficult, as it could touch the adjacent crowns. Therefore, this procedure should be carefully planned. The indications are to use long drills (of 28 mm). It should be pointed out that these drills have high cutting power, and frequently dentin wear is completely imperceptible (Fig. 23.6AB). Figures 23.7 to 23.19 present clinical cases of endodontic retreatment showing different materials being removed from inside the root canal.

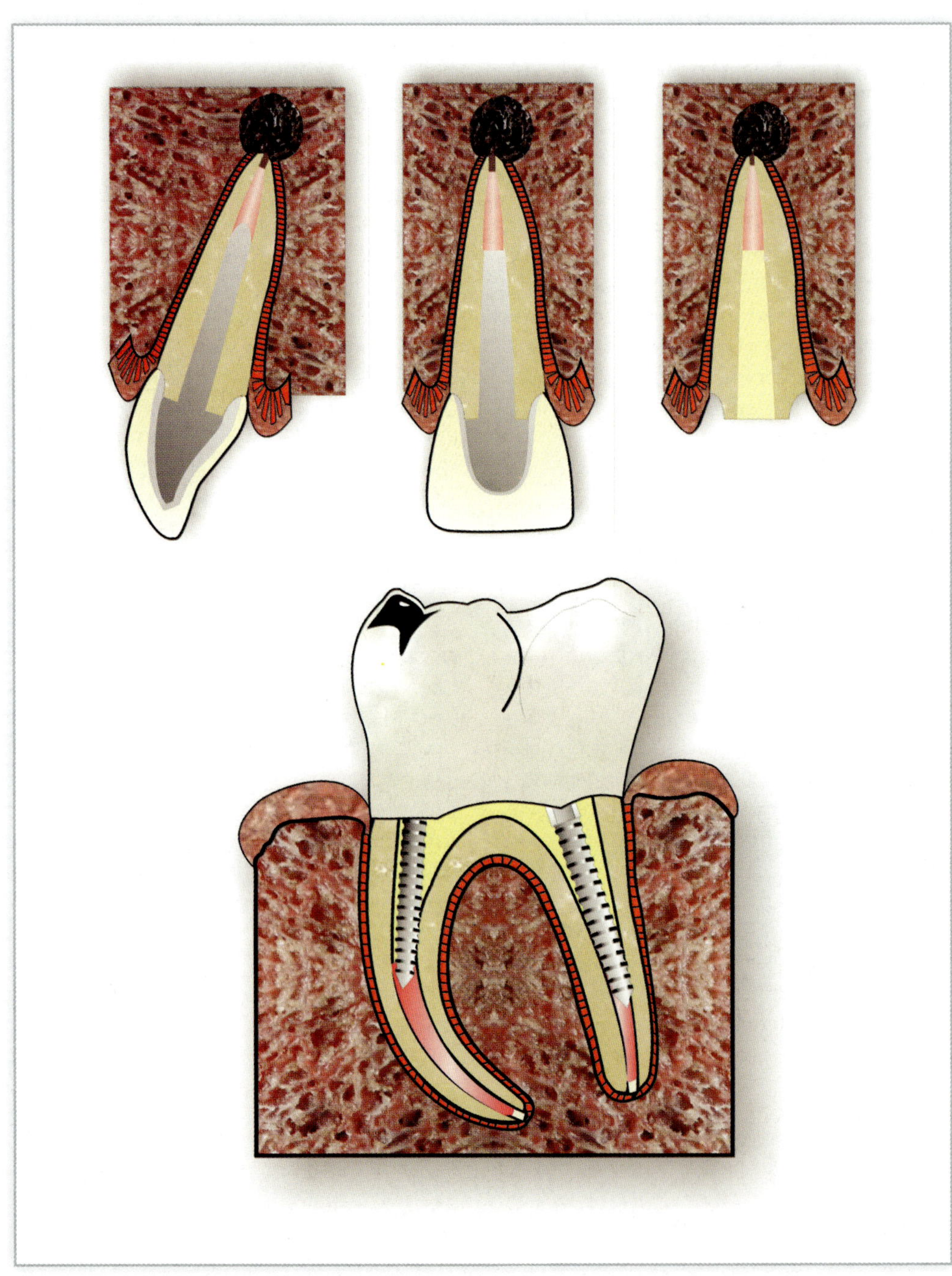

**Figure 23.6A** - Schematic representation of the technical sequence of the use of carbide steel drills to removal the retainers (cast/post).

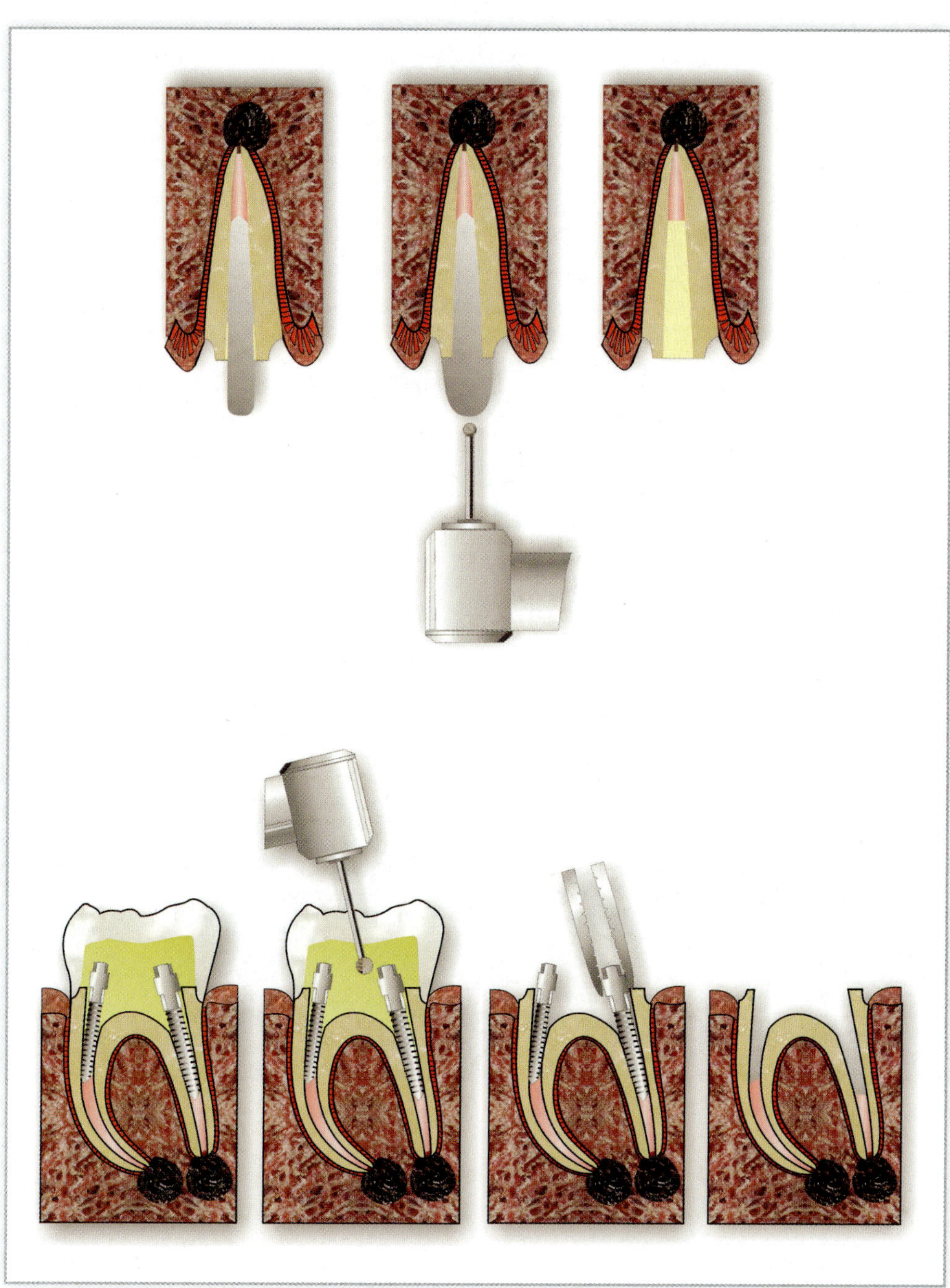

**Figure 23.6B** - Schematic representation of the technical sequence of the use of carbide steel drills to removal the retainers (cast/post).

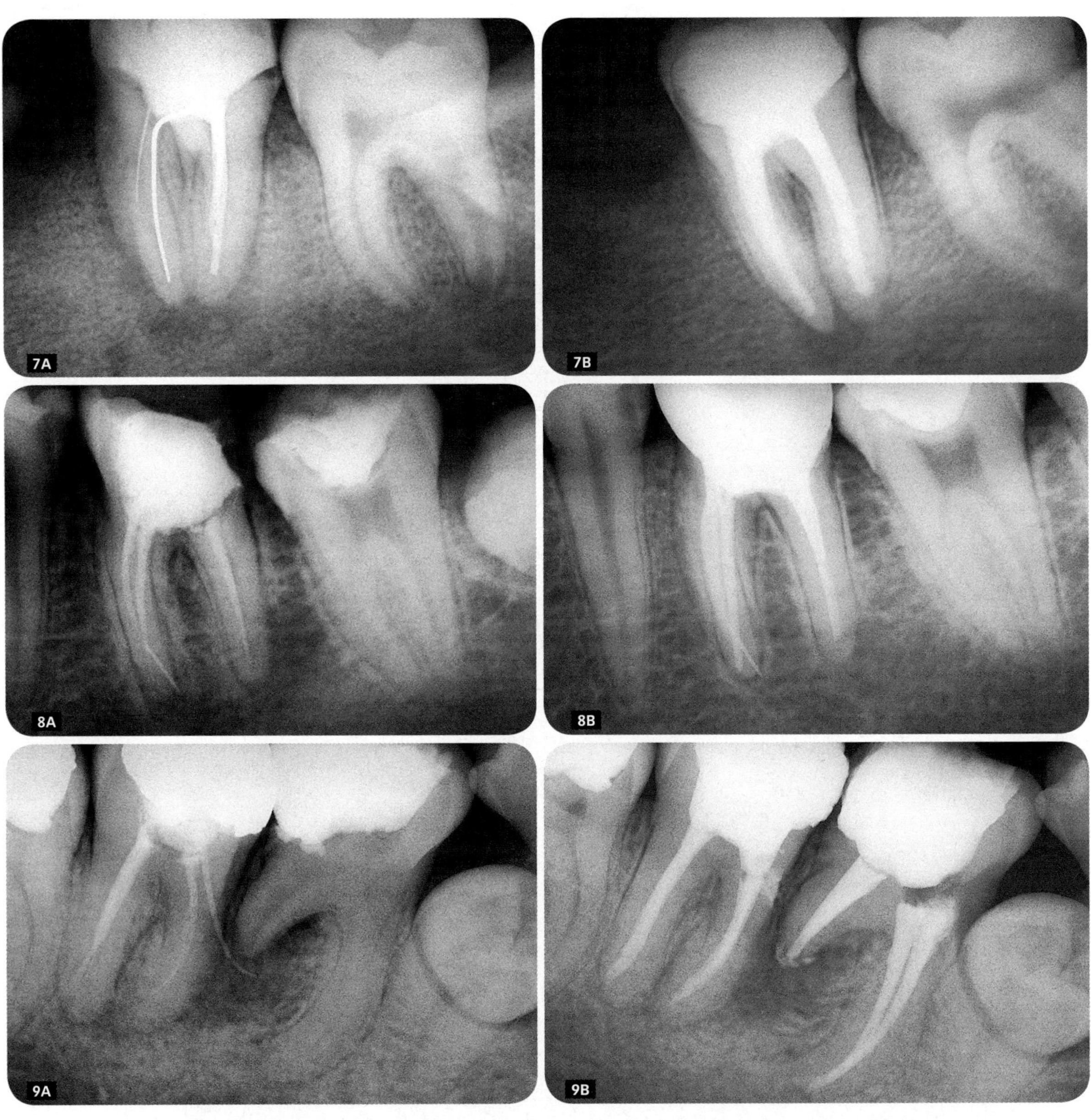


**Figures 23.7A-B to 23.9AB** - Clinical cases of endodontic retreatment showing different materials being removed from inside the root canal.

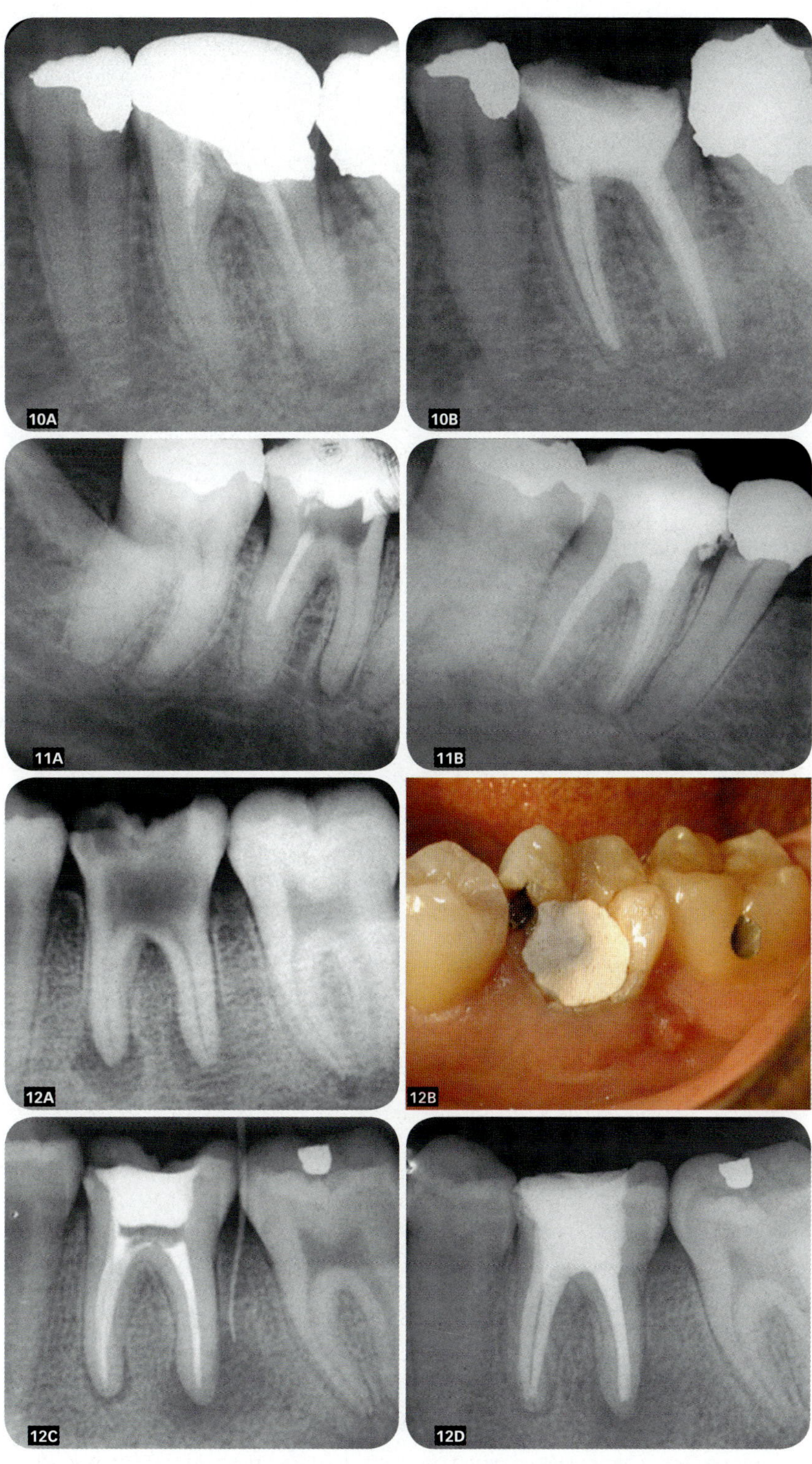


**Figures 23.10A-B to 23.12AD** - Clinical cases of endodontic retreatment showing different materials being removed from inside the root canal.

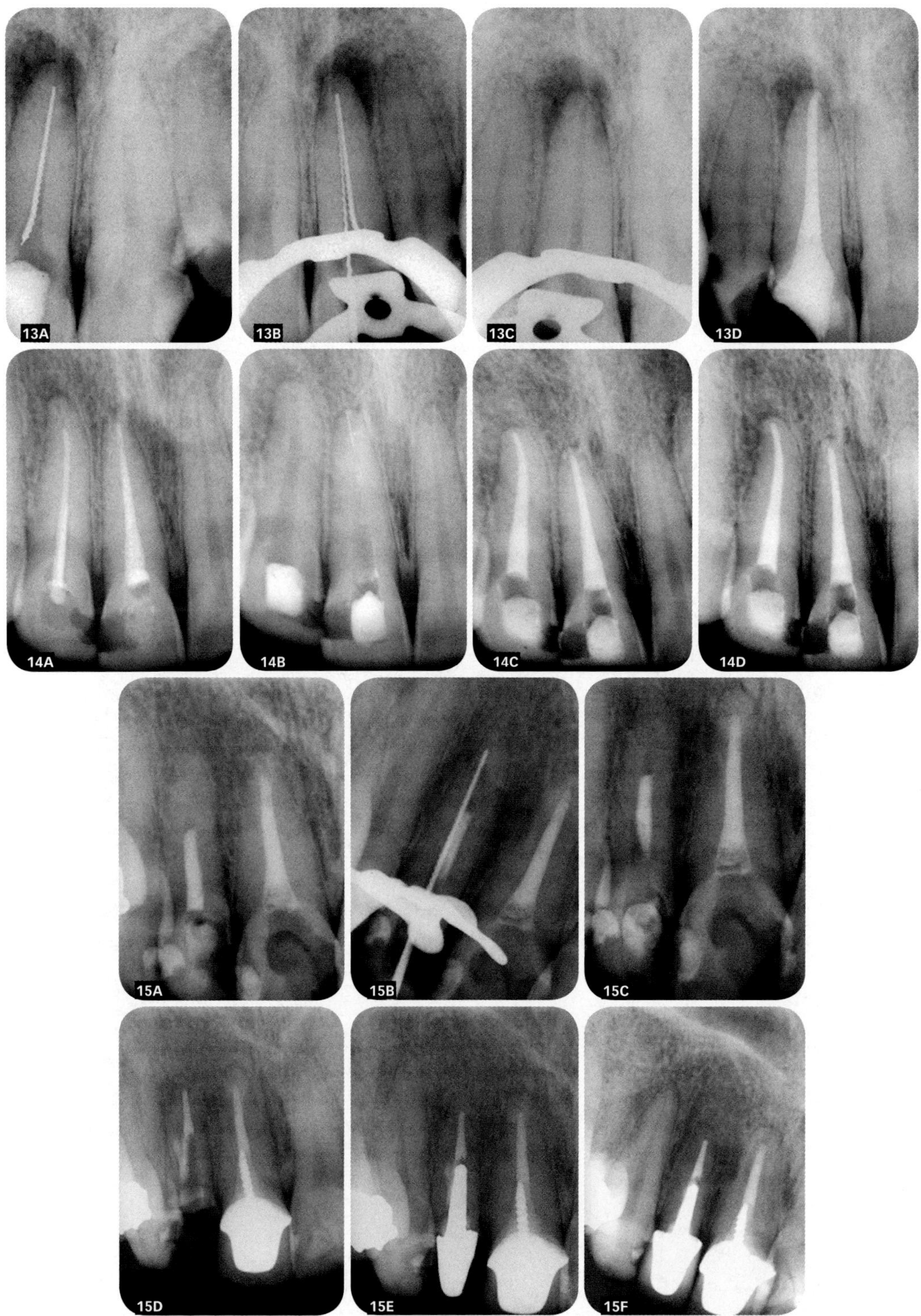


**Figures 23.13A-D to 23.15AF** - Clinical cases of endodontic retreatment showing different materials being removed from inside the root canal.

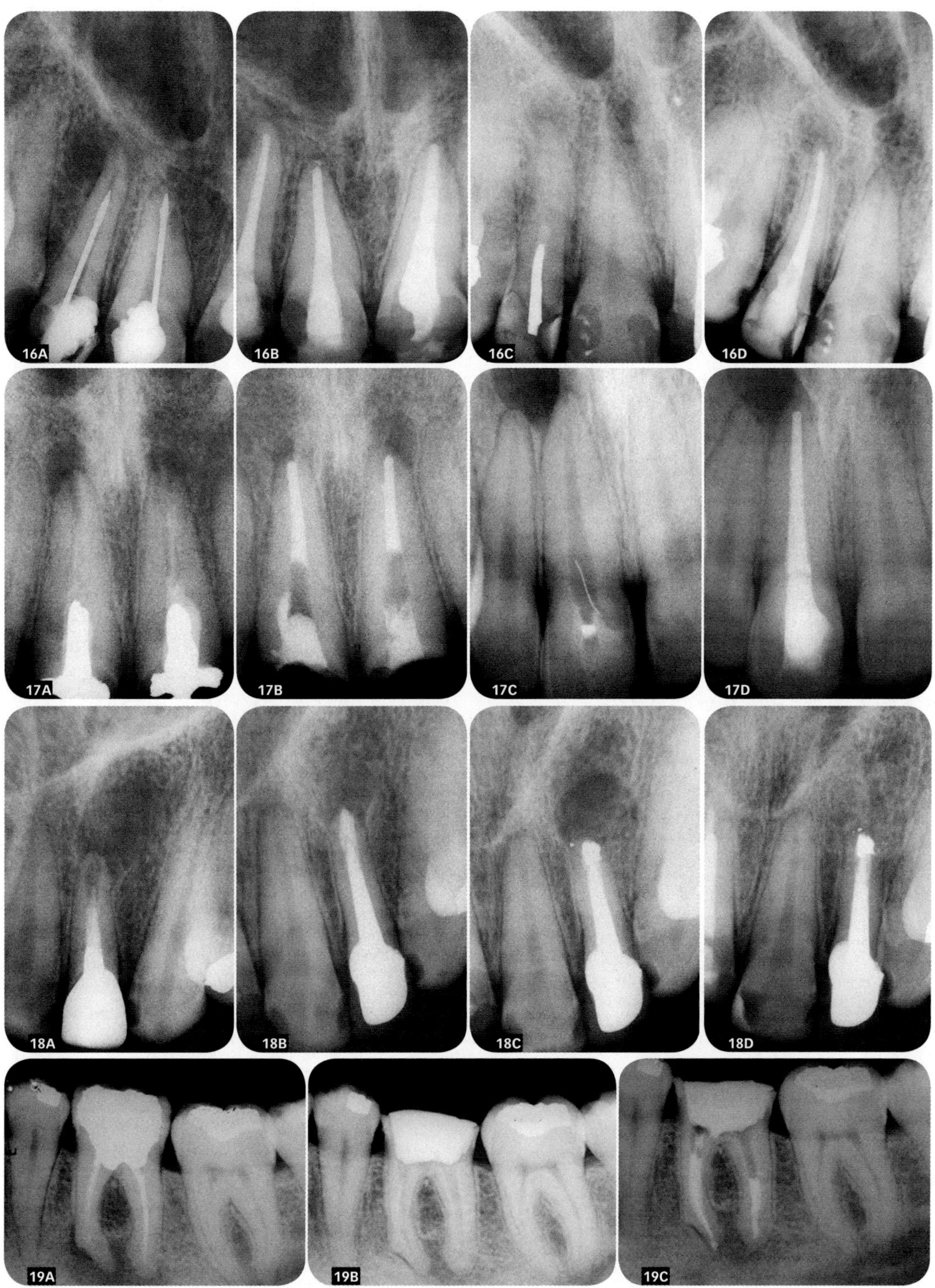


**Figures 23.16A-D to 23.19AC** - Clinical cases of endodontic retreatment showing different materials being removed from inside the root canal.

## 23.4 Solvent

Solvent is a substance used for the purpose dissolving the gutta-percha and/or endodontic cement used for filling the root canal. Softening these materials favors emptying of the root canal.

Different solvents have been indicated for application and use in endodontics, such as chloroform, xylol, eucalyptol, halothane, terebinthina oil, orange oil, among others. Chloroform solubilizes the gutta-percha more quickly than eucalyptol, however, it has been reported to have a possible carcinogenic effect [58,146] and its use in Dentistry has been contraindicated. Usually, professionals mostly use eucalyptol and xylol as solvents. Wourms et al.[146] related that the disadvantage of using eucalyptol is the need to heat it, because cold eucalyptol dissolves the gutta-percha slowly, thus increasing the clinical time required for removing gutta-percha.

As solvent for zinc oxide and eugenol cement, Pécora et al.[94] suggested the use of an essential oil (obtained from the sweet orange tree), which disintegrates it easily.

Some authors studied the dissolution and cytotoxic action of endodontic solvents[4,58,59,93,94]. The antimicrobial property of solvents has not been practically investigated, because it does not constitute an essential property. However, when selecting an ideal solvent, if it should present an antimicrobial effect in addition to being capable of dissolving gutta-percha and cement, it could be of great help in the sanitization process right from the outset of unobstructing the root canal.

Kaplowitz[57] verified that terebinthina oil is weak as a gutta-percha solvent, and requires a longer period of time, as well as heating to a temperature of 71°C to dissolve gutta-percha. Halothane is relatively non-toxic, volatile and non-inflammable, and has been used for inducing anesthesia since 1956. It has sweet smell, is slightly more soluble than ether, and is minimally soluble in the blood. Although it is not a respiratory irritant, it should be handled carefully to minimize its exposure to the environment, due to capacity of producing respiratory depression[146]. Hunter et al. [51] explained that highly volatile halothane can be desirable, because it decreases the quantity of residual solvent that stays in the periapical region and systemic circulation. In spite of claims that halothane is a solvent that dissolves gutta-percha[51,141] it is not yet found on sale for clinical use in endodontics.

Whitworth & Boursin[141] analyzed the dissolution of cements (AH plus, Apexit, Tubli-seal and Ketac endo) by volatile solvents (chloroform and halothane). The authors verified that Ketac endo is indeed insoluble in chloroform and halothane; Tubli-seal presented low solubility in halothane and higher solubility in chloroform; AH plus showed high solubility in chloroform and halothane; chloroform was more effective as endodontic cement solvent than halothane.

Morais et al.[82], evaluating the solvent action on gutta-percha of four chemical substances (chloroform, xylol, eucalyptol and terebinthina oil), verified that chloroform and xylol were the most efficient, and these substances did not completely dissolve gutta-percha, however, promoted its plasticization.

Many difficulties arise in the clinical situations of endodontic retreatment during neutralization of the septic-toxic content present at the time of removing the filling or emptying the root canal, such as the possibility of the extrusion of foraminal residues of the filling material, contaminated smear layer and microorganisms. Therefore, special care must be taken, not only with regard to the endodontic retreatment technique, but also as regards solvent selection.

Estrela et al.[29] studied the antimicrobial action of gutta-percha solvents (halothane, orange oil, eucalyptol and xylol) against microorganisms: *S. aureus*, *E. faecalis*, *P. aeruginosa*, *B. subtilis*, *C. albicans*, and a mixture of these, in periods of 5, 10, 15 and 30 minutes. Halothane showed antimicrobial effectiveness in all the times of analysis for *C. albicans*; starting from 10 minutes for E. faecalis and *P. aeruginosa*; starting from 15 minutes for *S. aureus*; and it was ineffective against *B. subti-*

*lis* and against the mixture. The other solvents were ineffective against all the microorganisms tested, in all observation periods.

After coronal emptying, one introduces 3 to 5 drops of solvent (xylol, orange oil etc.), waits some minutes and then begins the emptying process. As previously mentioned, when the solvent has dissolved the gutta percha, one should take great care that this bad filling mass does not extrude to the periapical region.

## 23.5 Cleaning and Shaping, Intracanal Dressing and Filling

Every time we redo any type of dental treatment, there will certainly always be the possibility of some additional wear, and it is no different when a new preparation of the root canal is performed in endodontic retreatment, when care should be taken with transversal modeling, especially in perforation risk areas. During emptying and new enlargement of the root canal, the main concern is to perform an effective sanitization process, particularly considering a situation of secondary infection. The principles and main points of root canal preparing were discussed in a previously chapter, and are again applicable at this time.

The relative care to take with intracanal dressing in this clinical situation, was also fully discussed in the chapter about calcium hydroxide, as well as in the chapter on diagnosis of endodontic failure. However, the subject of intracanal dressing with calcium hydroxide deserves special attention, with purpose of potentiating the sanitization process previously performed during the modeling phase. Whenever possible, the time of an intracanal dressing with calcium hydroxide should be longer than that proposed in the conventional protocol.

The care taken at the time of filling refers to situations in which there is no longer any apical limit, and there is real risk of this occurring in a filling performed in one session. Therefore, the same protocol should be used for this new filling of the root canal, and the prognosis of the case concerned should be well analyzed.

The success of endodontic treatment requires root canal filling materials to have good sealing quality. The techniques used during and after filling must not impair the ability of these materials to preserve the apical seal. Biffi et al.[9] identified important potential failures in canal cleaning as well as in fillings that had been considered satisfactory radiographically. Some of these factors included empty spaces, areas with only sealer, and remaining pulp tissue in canals to which access was difficult. All of these factors can lead to apical marginal leakage; that is, passage of tissue fluids, proteins, bacteria, and endotoxins through the interface of root canal walls and filling material.

The longevity of an endodontically treated tooth depends on the quality of the coronal restoration. Unsatisfactory endodontic treatment associated with an inadequate coronal restoration may lead to a larger number of periapical inflammatory reactions.

Prado et al.[96] assessed the correlation between leakage from the cervix to the apex and from the apex to the cervix for different post preparation techniques. Sixty roots were filled with gutta-percha by lateral condensation and AH Plus sealer and divided into two groups of 30 roots each. Immediate post preparation was used for one group and delayed preparation was used for the other. Two subgroups of 15 roots each were formed to investigate leakage from cervix-to-apex and from apex-to-cervix. The extent of leakage was determined using a dye, India ink, and a clearing technique that rendered the teeth transparent. Leakage was observed in all samples. The current study revealed that the apical sealing was not affected by either technique – no statistically significant differences were found for the apex-to-cervix leakage group. This finding may be explained by the fact that at least 5.0 mm of filling material was left in place. The results of the current study are remarkably different from those reported in the literature because other studies have assessed only apex-to-cervix leakage, while this study also assessed cervix-to-apex leakage after post preparation. This investigation is justified by the recent attention that has been devoted to procedures conducted after completion of root canal treatment and the impact of these procedures on the prognosis of endodontic therapy. These procedures could result in delayed failure because they may allow microorganisms and their products to migrate to the apical end of the root and later to the alveolar bone, where they may trigger periapical periodontitis. The microorganisms and nutrients can enter the pulp cavity through a permeable restoration, a leaking restoration, or the dental tubules of an unsealed canal.

## 23.6 Complications During the Root Canal Filling

The process of root canal filling diagnosed as an endodontic failure can be a simple procedure, represent a simple conduct, as a good reform, or the beginning of an unpleasant situation in a professional's work. One should always be aware of the unpredictable situations that the treatment of a secondary infection can represent. In this context, situations such as the occurrence of root canal perforation, under filling, dental fracture and pain after retreatment can be expected.

Root canal perforation is a technical accident that results in communication between the crown or the root canals and the periodontal space, capable of affecting the prognosis of endodontic retreatment. Should this accident occur, the patient should be immediately informed of the procedures to be followed, as well as of the treatment options and the effect on the prognosis.

Among factors that affect the prognosis in root canal perforation, some deserve consideration, such as the location in relation to the bony crest (intra-bony or supply-bony); the clinical condition of the dental pulp (vital or necrosis); the extent; the presence or absence of periodontal pocket; time elapsed between perforation and the treatment; the biological compatibility and the sealing capacity of the filling material. The rapidity with which the root perforation is filled favors the prognosis, due to the shorter period of possible microbial contamination. The perforation iatrogenesis can be classified as intra and extra-alveolar, according to the location, depending on the relationship with the alveolar bony crest.

Perforations that occur during crown opening are usually related to lack observation of the dental anatomy. The crown can present with reduced or obstructed volume due to the deposition of reparative dentine, as a result of constant aggressions and/or tissue aging. Total calcification of the coronal crown can also be observed, which complicates the location of and access to the apical region. Failures in the analysis of the initial radiograph favor the accident. Thus, it is opportune to consider the degree of axial inclination of the tooth in relation to the adjacent tooth and the alveolar bone. One should be careful during the coronal opening of badly positioned teeth, mostly second molars, when the first molar has been lost. It is very difficult to visualize the anatomy of the coronal chamber in a tooth with total metal crown, when this is not removed. Frequently the crown could have corrected the turn of the tooth, and the coronal chamber and entrance of the canals are not always located where one might expect them to be. Caries and resorptions also can lead to pulp cavity perforation.

A delicate moment that can lead to a perforation accident in a tooth is while preparing space for a post. This accident is the result of exaggerated or bad dentin removal. In order to prevent this type of accident, it is fundamental to take care during the endodontic procedures, as well as to have adequate knowledge of the internal anatomy and its variations.

Perforation during root canal preparation can occur with certain frequency in curved canals, when one does not observe the precurvature of stainless steel endodontic files which, due to their incapability of bending tend to resume their original position. Another common perforation situation is performing exaggerated wear during preparation, which can be observed on the distal wall of the mesial root of mandibular first molar teeth, on the mesial wall of maxillary premolar teeth, and on the distal wall of the mesiobuccal canal of maxillary first molar teeth[28].

Other common situations that deserve care are the times when passing the step; finding calcified root canals; and removing cement during retreatments. Special care should be taken when of trepan use.

The prevention of perforations during root canal shaping involves intelligent and ideal therapeutic procedures. For curved root canals, the option should be for flexible instruments and a suitable technique. By determining the length of the root canal, one avoids over preparing and foramen displacement.

The options for perforations treatment involve non-surgical and surgical methods, and whenever possible, the first option is the non-surgical method. Perforation can be diagnosed by the sudden appearance of hemorrhage in the root canal, or by persistent hemorrhage after pulp removal; clinical exploration; from the radiographic aspect showing the rasp in the periodontium; by verifying whether there is a lateral lesion and post situated outside the long axis of the root.

The chapter on endodontic surgery discusses the different characteristics of retrofilling materials (amalgam, zinc oxide and eugenol, calcium hydroxide, Rickert cement, super EBA, EBA, glass ionomer and Mineral Trioxide Aggregate).

The ideal restorative material is the one which, in addition to promoting excellent sealing, favors osteogenesis and cementogenesis. There is incessant search to find this material. Calcium hydroxide has shown excellent biological response in tissue healing, however, in the case of sealing perforations, it needs to be associated with the best quality sealers. One of the serious problems observed in the sealing perforations has been the extrusion of filling materials, mostly those that do not present good biological properties, because it could complicate tissue repair (Fig. 23.20).

When the perforation occurs above the bony crest or close to it, in which the junctional epithelium was reached, one of the options would be dental extrusion or to increase the clinical crown. The artificial opening in this case would be dislocated to a region that would enable it to be embodied in the restoration.

In intrabony lateral perforations that occur during instrumentation of the root canal, sealing should be performed immediately, provided that the clinical condition allows this. Perforations that present resorption of adjacent alveolar bone after the sanitization process are treated and modeled, and the intracanal dressing with calcium hydroxide and physiologic solution is kept in place for a period from 30 to 90 days. Should the clinical conditions be favorable, the medication is removed, and a small portion of this material is left in the perforation location; the canal is dried, and the perforated cavity is filled with MTA - Mineral Trioxide Aggregate. After this, the material is protected with glass ionomer cement that will remain as a base for the restoration.

Holland et al.[46] observed that calcium hydroxide in contact with pulp tissue or culture medium produces deposition of calcite crystals. The same crystals observed with calcium hydroxide were reported for MTA[49]. Holland et al.[49] evaluated the healing process of intentional lateral root perforation repaired with mineral trioxide aggregate (MTA). Forty-eight root canals of dog's teeth were instrumented and filled. After partial removal of the filling, an intentional perforation was made with a bur in the lateral area of the root. The perforations were repaired with MTA or Sealapex (control group). Histological analysis was performed 30 and 180 days after treatment. Results showed no inflammation and deposition of cementum over MTA in the majority of the specimens. In the 180-day period, Sealapex exhibited chronic inflammation in all the specimens and slight deposition of cementum over the material in only three cases. In conclusion, MTA exhibited better results than the control group.

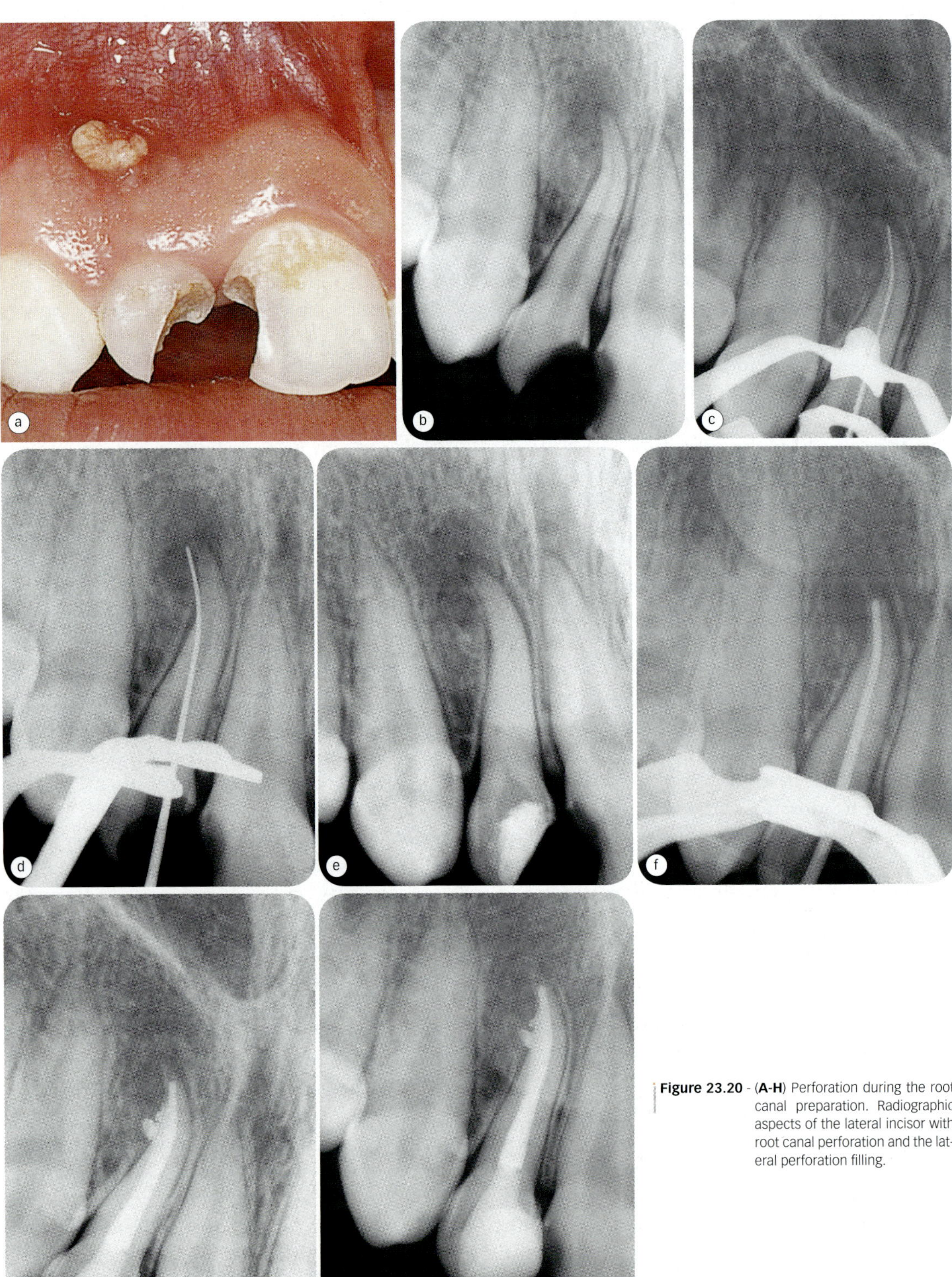


**Figure 23.20** - (**A-H**) Perforation during the root canal preparation. Radiographic aspects of the lateral incisor with root canal perforation and the lateral perforation filling.

When perforation occurs due to over instrumentation with accentuated enlargement of the apical foramen, the treatment consists of determining a new working length, a little on this side of the apex, where the main cone is going to be locked. An apical buffer with calcium hydroxide should be kept, and the remainder of the canal should be closed with calcium hydroxide cement using the lateral condensation technique (Fig. 23.21). If the portion apical to the perforation is not reached by the filling, clinical and radiographic follow-up should be conducted until the success or failure is determined. If failure is verified, the surgical option (periapical surgery) still remains.

Frequently, perforation near the apex presents the best prognosis, and the ones that are smaller in extent are easier to seal. The Table 23.2 show the classification of perforations with regard to location and treatment options.

Each case in particular must be carefully analyzed, to verify the presence or absence of infection; extent of perforation, time elapsed before sealing, the periodontal patient's risk, to see whether the disease interferes directly in the prognosis.

Other possible complication is overfilling. One should understand that the filling material was intended for use inside the root canal, and should not therefore, be allowed to overflow beyond the root apex. If this accident occurs, one should analyze the material used (cement and/or cones) and the quantity that overflowed. In all situations, although some materials have good tissue tolerance, there will be some tissue response, and commonly it is an inflammatory response, whose intensity will depend on several factors (periapical pathological state, overflowed material, quantity, and the individual's systemic state). However, when the overflowed filling material is cement, it can be removed from the root canal. In some cases when the cone overflows, it can be removed. It depends on the clinical case concerned. If the periapical irritation exceeds the tolerance limits, one can still remove it surgically, which does not fail to represent other inconvenience.

Certainly, the most complicated situation to solve is dental fracture while removing a root retainer. Thus, when removing the root retainers, always inform the patient of the risks and benefits.

Another unexpected inconvenience is the pain experienced after endodontic retreatment. Many factors can be responsible for the pain that characterizes periapical inflammation during and after endodontic treatment, such as: the chemical substances, intracanal dressing, instrumentation technique, filling material used and the number of sessions.

Asymptomatic apical periodontitis can be exacerbated due to microorganisms associated with the increase in virulence and the diminished defenses of the body. Extrusion through the apical foramen of microorganisms and their byproducts, contaminated smear layer, medicaments and filling material, all contribute to the induction of postoperative pain.

In addition to these aspects, Seltzer & Naidorf[113] related the following etiologic factors of acute manifestations after endodontic treatment: alteration of the local adaptation syndrome; changes in periapical tissue pressure; microbial factors; effects of chemical mediators; changes in cyclic nucleotides; immunological phenomena; and various psychological factors.

The clinical situations of endodontic retreatment impose many difficulties on the neutralization of the septic-toxic content present, such as the possibility of extrusion of the filling materials, contaminated smear layer and microorganisms to the foramen.

Estrela et al.[25] studied the prevalence of postoperative pain in endodontic retreatment, considering the presence or absence of signs and symptoms, periapical radiographic aspect, patient's age, sex and filling of the root canal. The study involved 184 human teeth that needed endodontic retreatment. The patients were of both genders, aged from 12 to 65 years old. Among the analyzed teeth, 110 were asymptomatic (total absence of pain) and 74 symptomatic (pain, caries, moderate or severe), without apparent edema. The pain was considered slight when the patient did not report the use of analgesics, moderate, not constantly used, severe when constantly used. When failure of the first treatment was detected, the quality of the present filling was evaluated, and was considered incomplete when there was absence of satisfactory filling (radiopaque material partially filling the root canal, this being cement, and/or gutta-percha); and complete, when there was one complete filling of the root canal (presence of radiopaque material throughout the length of the root canal), however, in some cases with radiographic confirmation of maintenance of the periapical area, or characteristic rarefaction, there was clinical evidence of treatment failure. Intervals from 24 to 48 hours elapsed after endodontic retreatment, and all the patients returned for the second appointment, in which we registered the presence or absence of postoperative pain, according to the following criteria: absent, moderate and severe. After the disappearance of signs and symptoms, the intracanal dressing was removed and the tooth was closed definitively. In the teeth with signs and symptoms, presenting moderate pain, analgesic was prescribed; In the case of severe pain, it was managed with paracetamol associated with codeine, and antibiotic (Penicillin or Cephalosporin). The absence of postoperative pain in endodontic retreatment of the asymptomatic teeth was high, 83.3%, 82.8%, 82%, irrespective of the radiographic aspect, absence of periapical bony rarefaction, diffuse bony periapical and circumscribed rarefaction, respectively. In the clinical situations in which the acute periapical inflammatory process[26] was shown to be developing, the absence of postoperative pain was regular, 59%, 50% and 54.5%, respectively corresponding to the radiographic aspects described previously. The percentile of patients with postoperative pain among women patients was higher than in men. As regards the age, the highest prevalence of pain was in patients from 20 to 50 years of age.

Acute exacerbation after or during the endodontic treatment have demonstrated that the prevalence of flare up is low. Several factors of a technical order have been related as being responsible for exacerbating the pain processes during or after endodontic treatment, such as chemical substances, intracanal dressing, instrumentation technique and filling materials. Associated with these factors, are those of a biological nature, which also are representative as stimulators of the painful phenomenon: the microbial condition inherent to the clinical situation, as regards the presence and or absence of periapical lesion, presence of signs and symptoms, systemic diseases, age, gender.

It is opportune to mention that some of the referenced literature is retrospective; presenting different variables that could interfere in the results, in addition to the small universe of studied cases. Thus, the analysis of postoperative pain is a complex and difficult study, because there are various factors responsible for the development or exacerbation of the inflammatory process.

Harrison et al. [43], analyzing the prevalence of pain associated with the clinical factors during and after the endodontic treatment, related that it usually occurs more frequently during the first 24 hours after the filling; that there is no significant relationship with the state of pulp vitality, presence or absence of radiolucent periapical area, number of roots, previous emergency treatment, or the filling level, although fillings 1mm on this side of the radiographic apex had shown a lower rate of postoperative pain.

One notes that in the asymptomatic clinical situations, there is little postoperative pain. This was demonstrated both in cases of endodontic retreatment cases, and in situations of periapical inflammation treatment. For the clinical situations in which there are signs and symptoms present, the rates are higher, both in retreatment and in the treatment of teeth with pulp necrosis with or without periapical bony rarefaction[26].

It should be taken into consideration that several population groups were studied together with the different variables established only by the clinical procedures adopted. Likewise, it is prudent to reaffirm that compliance with the correct operative stages is fundamental for the establishment of success, which frequently starts with pain relief.

**Table 23.2** - Classification of root perforations and treatment alternatives

| **Intraosseous** | | **Extraosseous** | |
|---|---|---|---|
| **Location** | **Treatment Alternatives** | **Location** | **Treatment Alternatives** |
| Coronal chamber floor | $Ca(OH)_2$ paste + MTA + Glass ionomer | Coronal chamber floor | Sealing with glass ionomer and/or composite resin |
| Cervical third | Dental extrusion / increase of clinical crown / $Ca(OH)_2$ paste + MTA + Glass ionomer | Cervical third (Gingival recession after periodontal treatment) | Sealing with glass ionomer and/or composite resin |
| Middle third | $Ca(OH)_2$ paste or MTA + Filling with $Ca(OH)_2$ sealer and gutta-percha points | Middle third (Gingival recession after periodontal treatment) | Sealing with glass ionomer and/or composite resin |
| Apical third | Filling with $Ca(OH)_2$ cement and gutta-percha points | | |

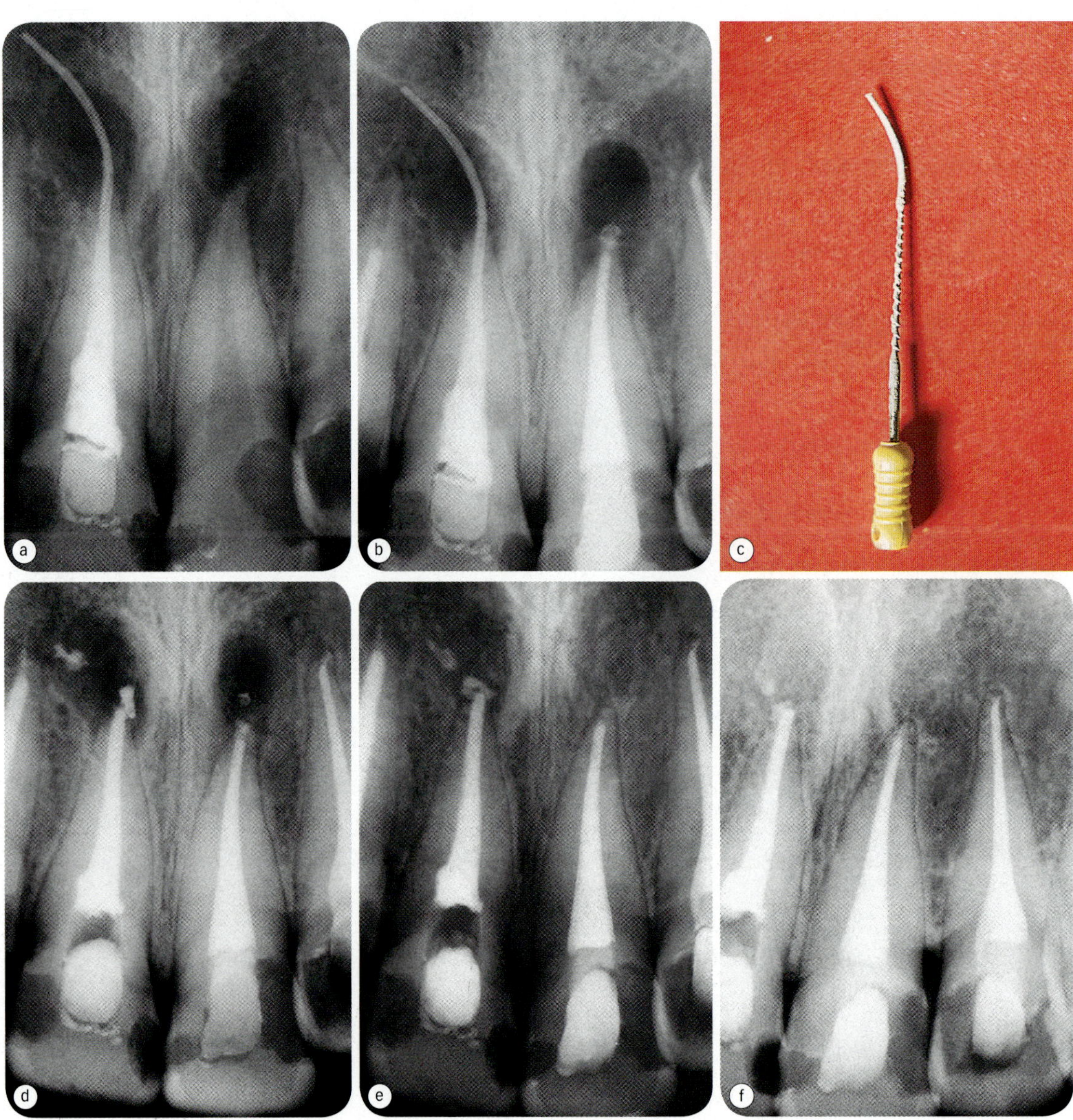

**Figure 23.21** - (**A-F**) Endodontic retreatment – Removal of gutta-percha and cement from an overfilled tooth. Clinical and radiographic follow-up.

1. Alfredo E, Garrido ADB, Souza-Filho CB, Correia-Sobrinho L, Sousa-Neto MD. In vitro evaluation of the effect of core diameter for removing radicular post with Ultraound. J Oral Rehabil 2004;31:590-94.
2. Alhadainy HA. Root perforations. Oral Surg Oral Med Oral Pathol 1994;78:368-74.
3. Allen RK, Newton CW, Brow-Jr CE. A statistical analysis of surgical and nonsurgical endodontic retreatment cases. J Endod 1989;15:261-66.
4. Arens AE, Torabinejad M. Repair of furcal perforations with mineral trioxide aggregate. Oral Surg Oral Med Oral Pathol 1996;82:84-88.
5. Barbosa SV, Burkard DH, Spangberg LSW. Cytotoxic effects of gutta-percha solvents. J Endod 1994;20:6-8.
6. Bender IB, Seltzer S, Soltanoff W. Endodontic success – a reappraisal of criteria. Oral Surg Oral Med Oral Pathol 1996;22:780-801.
7. Bergenholtz G, Lekholm U, Liljenberg B, lindhe J. Morphometric analysis of chronic inflammatory periapical lesions in root-filled teeth. Oral Surg Oral Med Oral Pathol 1983;55:295-301.
8. Bergeron BE, Murchison DF, Schindler WG, Walker WA. Effect of ultrasonic vibration and various sealer and cement combinations on Titanium post removal. J Endod 2001;27:13-17
9. Biffi FCG, Souza CJA, Maniglia CAG. Método para a avaliação quantitativa do canal radicular com o auxílio do computador. Rev Ass Paul Cir Dent 1992;46:925-27.
10. Block RM, Bushell A, Grossman LI, Langeland K. Endodontic surgical retreatment - a clinical and histopathologic study. J Endod 1979;3:101-15.
11. Block RM, Pascon EA, Langeland K. Paste technique retreatment study: a clinical, histopathologic, and radiographic evaluation of 50 cases. Oral Surg Oral Med Oral Pathol 1985;60:76-93.
12. Bonetti-Filho I. Avaliação dos tratamentos endodônticos. Rev Gaúcha Odontol 1988;36:309-12.
13. Bramante CM, Berbert A. Acidentes endodônticos - fratura de instrumento. Estomat Cult 1973;7:186-90.
14. Bramante CM, Berbert A. Root perforations dressed with calcium hydroxide or zinc oxide and eugenol. J Endod 1987;13:392-95.
15. Bramante CM, Berbert A, Bernadineli N, Moraes IG, Garcia RB. Acidentes e complicações no tratamento endodôntico. São Paulo: Santos, 2003. 202p.
16. Brynolf I. A histologic and roentgenological study of the periapical region of human upper incisor. Odontol Rev 1967;18:1-176.
17. Brystöm A, Sundqvist G. Bacteriologic evaluation of the efficacy of mechanical root canal instrumentation in endodontic therapy. Scand J Dent Res 1981;89:321-28.
18. Bueno CES, Valdrighi L. Efetividade de solventes e de técnicas na desobturação dos canais radiculares. Estudo *in vitro*. Rev Ass Bras Odontol Nac 2000;8:21-25.
19. Buoncristiani J, Seto BG, Caputo AA. Evaluation of ultrasonic and sonic instruments for intrarradicular post removal. J Endod 1994;20: 486-89.
20. Costa WF, Antoniazzi JH. Retratamento dos canais radiculares. In: Atualização na clínica odontológica. Bottino MA, Feller C. São Paulo: Artes Médicas. 1992;p.289-325.
21. Dezan-Jr E. Indução experimental de anacorese no periápice de dentes após obturação dos canais. Estudo em cães em região geográfica endêmica para Leishmaniose. (Doctoral Thesis). University of São Paulo, 2001.
22. Dezan-Jr E, Holland R, Lopes HP, Santos CA, Alexandre AC. Retratamento endodôntico: avaliação da quantidade de resíduos após a desobturação com ou sem o uso de solvente. Rev Bras Odontol 1996;53:2-5.
23. Dow PR, Ingle JI. Isotopi determination of root canals failures. Oral Surg Oral Med Oral Pathol 1955;8:1100-1104.
24. Estrela C, Camapum FF, Lopes HP. Insucessos em Endodontia. In: Estrela C, Figueiredo JAP. Endodontia: princípios biológicos e mecânicos. São Paulo: Artes Médicas, 1999. p. 698-730.
25. Estrela C, Camapum FF, Lopes HP. Prevalência de dor nos retratamentos endodônticos. Rev Bras Odontol 1998;55:18-24.
26. Estrela C, César OVS, Sydney GB, Lopes HP, Pesce HF. Prevalência de dor frente ao tratamento da inflamação periapical aguda e crônica. Rev Bras Odontol 1996;53:15-21.
27. Estrela C, Figueiredo JAP, Dorneles J. Aspectos preventivos e terapêuticas das perfurações iatrogênicas em endodontia. Rev Odonto Ciência 1991;9:53-59.
28. Estrela C, Stephan IW. Estudo comparativo do desgaste dentinário na parede distal do canal mésio vestibular do primeiro molar inferior produzido por três técnicas de instrumentação do canal radicular. Rev Odontol Brasil Central 1991;1:11-15.
29. Estrela CRA, Estrela C, Marcomini JL, Loreto-Jr F, Ribeiro RG. Ação antimicrobiana de solventes de guta-percha. Rev Bras Odontol 2001;58:154-57.
30. Evans M, Davies JK, Sundqvist G, Figdor D. Mechanisms involved in the resistance of *Enterococcus faecalis* to calcium hydroxide. Int Endod J 2002;35:221-28.
31. Fachin E, Wenckus C, Aun CE. Retreatment using a modified type instrument. J Endod 1995;21:425-28.
32. Fonseca JA. Problemas e soluções relacionados ao retratamento endodôntico. Rev Bras Odontol 1976;33:276-88.
33. Frank AL. Resorption, perforation and fractures. Dent Clin North Amer 1974;18:465-87.
34. Friedman S. Retreatment of failures. In: Walton RE, Torabinejad M. Principles and practices of endodontics. 2nd ed. Philadelphia: WB Saunders Company. 1996; p. 336-53.
35. Friedman S, Rotstein I, SharLev S. Bypassing gutta-percha root filling with an automated device. J Endod 1989 15:432-37.
36. Friedman S, Stabholz A. Endodontic retreatment - case selection and technique. Part 1: Criteria for case selection. J Endod 1986;12:28-33.

37. Friedman S, Stabholz A, Tamae A. Endodontic retreatment case selection and technique. Part 3. Retreatment techniques. J Endod 1990;16:543-49.
38. Garrido ADB. Análise comparativa da eficiência da vibração ultra-sônica, com e sem refrigeração ar/água, na remoção de pinos fundidos fixados com cimento resinoso e com cimento de fosfato de zinco. (Master's Thesis). University of São Paulo. 2002; p.121.
39. Gomes APM, Kubo CH, santos RAB, santos DR, Padilha RQ. The influence of ultrasound on the retention of cast posts cemented with different agents. Int Endod J 2001;34:93-9.
40. Grossman LI. Endodontia prática. 8th ed. Rio de Janeiro: Guanabara Koogan. 1976;190-216.
41. Grossman LI, Shephard LI, Pearson LA. Roentgenologic and clinical evaluation of endodontically treated teeth. Oral Surg Oral Med Oral Pathol 1964;17:368-74.
42. Guldner PHA. Perforaciones accidentales. In: Endodoncia. Diagnóstico y tratamiento. Guldener PHA, Langeland K. Barcelona: Springer. 1995; 396p.
43. Harrison JW, Baumgartner JC, Cvek TA. Prevalence of pain associated with clinical factors during and after root canal therapy. Part 1. Inter appointment pain. J Endod 1983;9:384-87.
44. Harrison JW, Baumgartner JC, Cvek TA. Prevalence of pain associated with clinical factors during and after root canal therapy. Part 2. Pos-obturation pain. J Endod 1983;9:434-38.
45. Hepworth MJ, Friedman S. Retreatment outcome of surgical and non-surgical management of endodontic failure. Can Dent Ass 1997;63:364-71.
46. Holland R, Valle GF, Taintor JF, Ingle JI. Influence of bony resorption on endodontic treatment. Oral Surg Oral Med Oral Pathol 1983;55:191-203.
47. Holland R, Souza V, Nery MJ, Mello W, Bernabé PFE, Otoboni-Filho CD. Tissue reactions following apical plugging of the root canal with infected dentin chips. A histologic study in dog's teeth. Oral Surg Oral Med Oral Pathol 1980;49:366-69.
48. Holland R, Otoboni-Filho JA, Souza V, Nery MJ, Bernabé PFE, Dezan-Jr E. Mineral trioxide aggregate repair of root perforations. J Endod 2001;27:281-4.
49. Hülsmann M. The removal of silver cones and fractured instruments using the Canal Finder System. J Endod 1990;16:596-600.
50. Hülsmann M. Removal of fractured instruments using a combined automated ultrasonic technique. J Endod 1994;20:144-46.
51. Hunter KR, Dobleckl W, Pelleu-Jr GB. Halothane and eucalyptol as alternatives to chloroform for softening gutta-percha. J Endod 1990;16:543-49.
52. Imura N, Zuolo ML. Remoção de retentor intraradicular com aparelho de ultra-som. Rev Ass Paul Cir Dent 1997;51:262-67.
53. Ingle JI. Exitos y fracasos en endodoncia. Rev Ass Odontol Argentina 1962;50:67-74.
54. Ingle JI, Taintor JF. Endodontia. 3rd ed. Rio de Janeiro: Guanabara S.A; 1989.
55. Jeng HW, Eldeeb ME. Removal of hard paste fillings from root canal by ultrasonic instrumentation. J Endod 1987;13:295-98.
56. Johnson WT, Leary JM, Boyer DB. Effect of ultrasonic vibration on post removal in extracted human premolar teeth. J Endod 1996;22:487-88.
57. Kakehashi S, Stanley HR, Fitzgerald RJ. The effects of surgical exposures of dental pulps in germ-free and conventional laboratory rats. Oral Surg Oral Med Oral Pathol 1965;20:340-349.
58. Kaplowitz GJ. Evaluation of gutta-percha solvents. J Endod 1990;16:539-40.
59. Kaplowitz GJ. Using rectified turpentine oil in endodontic retreatment. J Endod 1996;22:621.
60. Karlovik Z et al. The antibacterial effect of various gutta-percha solvents. Int Endod J 2000;33:153 (Abstract 9th ESSE).
61. Krell KV, Fuller MW, Scott GI. The conservative retrieval of silver cones in difficult cases. J Endod 1984;10:269-73.
62. Krell KV, Neo J. The use of ultrasonic endodontic instrumentation in the retreatment of a paste-filled endodontic tooth. Oral Surg Oral Med Oral Pathol 1985;60:100-02.
63. Kvist T, Rydin E, Reit C. The relative frequency of periapical lesions in teeth with root canal retained posts. J Endod 1989;15:578-80.
64. Lewis RD, Block RM. Management of endodontic failures. Oral Surg Oral Med Oral Pathol 1988;66:711-21.
65. Lin LM, Pascon EA, Skrinbner JE, Gängler P, Langeland K. Clinical, radiographic and histologic study of endodontic treatment failures. Oral Surg Oral Med Oral Pathol 1991;11:603-11.
66. Lin LM, Skribner JE, Gängler P. Factors associated with endodontic treatment failures. J Endod 1992;18:625-27.
67. Lisa R, Wilcox LR. Endodontic retreatment: ultrasonic and chloroform as the final step in reinstrumentation. J Endod 1989;15:125-28.
68. Lopes HP, Araújo-Filho WR. Retratamento endodôntico em dente portador de pino metálico e perfuração radicular. Rev Bras Odontol 1991;48:38-42.
69. Lopes HP, Costa-Filho AS, Loriato D. Remoção de pinos metálicos intra-radiculares de retenção protética. Rev Bras Odontol 1985;42:3-16.
70. Lopes HP, Elias CN, Silveira GEL, Araújo-Filho WR, Siqueira-Jr JF. Extrusão de material do canal via forame apical. Rev Paul Odontol 1997;19:34-36.
71. Lopes HP, Estrela C, Rocha NSM, Costa-Filho AS, Siqueira-Jr JF. Retentores intra-radiculares: análise radiográfica do comprimento do pino e da condição da obturação do canal radicular. Rev Bras Odontol 1997;54:277-80.
72. Lopes HP, Gahyva SMM. Retratamento endodôntico: avaliação da quantidade apical de resíduos de material obturador após a reinstrumentação. Rev Bras Odontol 1992;40:181-84.
73. Lopes HP, Gahyva SMM. Retratamento endodôntico: avaliação do limite apical de esvaziamento, na remoção do material obturador dos canais radiculares. Rev Bras Odontol 1995;52:22-26.
74. Lopes HP, Siqueira-Jr JF, Elias CN. Retratamento endodôntico. In: Endodontia: Biologia e Técnica. Lopes HP, Siqueira-Jr JF. Rio de Janeiro: Medsi. 1999;p. 497-538.
75. Lovdal PE. Endodontic retreatment. Dent Clin North Am 1992;36:473-90.
76. Love RM. Invasion of dentinal tubules by root canal bacteria. Endodontic Topics 2004;9:52-65.
77. Love RM. *Enterococcus faecalis* – a mechanism for its role in endodontic failure. Int Endod J 2001;34:399-405.

78. Machtou P, Sarfati P, Cohen AG. Post removal prior to retreatment. J Endod 1989;15:552-54.
79. Mandel E, Friedman S. Endodontic retreatment: A rational approach to root canal instrumentation. J Endod 1992;18:565-69.
80. Metzger Z, Bem-Amar A. Removal of overextended gutta-percha root canal fillings in endodontic failure cases. J Endod 1995;21:287-88.
81. Mollander A, Reit C, Dahlen G, Kvist T. Microbiological status of root-filled teeth with apical periodontitis. Int Endod J 1998;31:1-7.
82. Morais CAH, Duarte MAH, Moraes IG, Bernadinelli N. Avaliação do poder solvente de guta-percha, de quatro substâncias químicas. Rev Fac Odontol Bauru 1995;3:1-4.
83. Morse DR, Furst M, Bellot RM, Lefkowitz R, Spritzer I, Sideman B. Infections flare-ups and serious sequel following endodontic treatment: a prospective randomizes trial efficacy of antibiotic prophylaxis in cases of asymptomatic pulpal-periapical lesions. Oral Surg Oral Med Oral Pathol 1987;64:96-109.
84. Mota AS, Biffi JCG, Oliveira MRS, Guimarães CS. Estudo comparativo da força de tração na remoção de pinos pré-fabricados em canais morfologicamente diferentes. Rev Ass Bras Odontol Nac 2000;7:364-71.
85. Nair PNR. Light and electron microscopic studies of root canal flora and periapical lesions. J Endod 1987;13:29-39.
86. Nair PNR. Pathobiology of the periapex. In: Cohen S, Burns RC. Pathways of the pulp. 8th ed. St. Louis: Mosby;2001.
87. Nair PNR, Sjögren U, Krey G, Sundqvist G. Therapy-resistant foreign body giant cell granuloma at the periapex of a root- filled human tooth. J Endod 1990;16:589-95.
88. Nair PNR, Sjögren U, Krey G, Khngerg KE, Sundqvist G. Intraradicular bacteria and fungi in root filled, asymptomatic human teeth with therapy-resistant periapical lesions: a long-term light and electron microscopic follow-up study. J Endod 1990;16:580-88.
89. Nair PNR, Sjögren U, Schumacher E, Sundqvist G. Radicular cyst affecting a root-filled human tooth: a long-term post-treatment follow-up. Int Endod J 1993;26:225-33.
90. Nair PNR, Sjögren U, Sundqvist G. Cholesterol crystals as an etiological factor in non resolving chronic inflammation: an experimental study in guinea pigs. Eur J O Sci 1998;106:644-50.
91. Nori Y, Ehara A, Kawahara T, Takemura N, Ebisu S. Participation of bacterial biofilms in refractory and chronic periapical periodontitis. J Endod 2002;28:679-83.
92. Oliveira MRS, Biffi JCG, Mota AS, Maniglia CAG. Avaliação da remoção de pinos intra-radiculares pré-fabricados através da técnica ultra-sônica. Rev Ass Paul Cir Dent 1999;53:372-77.
93. Pascon EA, Spangberg LS. In vitro cytotoxicity of root canal filling materials. 1. Guta-percha. J Endod 1990;16:429-33.
94. Pécora JD, Costa WE, Santos-Filho D, Sarti SJ. Apresentação de um óleo essencial, obtido de *Citrus awiantium*, eficaz na desintegração do cimento de óxido de zinco-eugenol do interior do canal radicular. Odonto 1992;1:130-32.
95. Pesce HF, Bastos-Filho E, Risso VA. Avaliação do índice de ocorrência de retratamentos endodôntico sem função da qualidade da obturação, presença ou não de rarefação periapical e sintomatologia. Rev Bras Odontol 1996;53:29-30.
96. Prado CJ, Estrela C, Panzeri H, Biffi JCG. Permeability of remaining endodontic obturation after post preparation. General Dent 2006;53:41-43.
97. Queiroz EC, Menezes MS, Biffi JCG, Soares CJ. Influence of the shape core on custom cast dowel and core removal by ultrasonic energy. J Oral Rehabil 2007;34:463-67.
98. Ray HA, Trope M. Periapical status of endodontically treated teeth in relation to the technical quality of the root filling and the coronal restoration. Int Endod J 1995;28:12-18.
99. Reid LC, Kazemi RB, Meiers JC. Effect of fatigue testing on core integrity and post microleakage of teeth restored with different post systems. J Endod 2003;29:125-31.
100. Reit C. Decision strategies in endodontics: on the design of a recall program. Endod Dent Traumatol 1987;3:233-39.
101. Reit C. The influence of observer calibration on radiographic periapical diagnosis. Int Endod J 1987;20:75-81.
102. Reit C, Gröndahl HC. Endodontic decision – making under uncertainty: a decision analytic approach to management of periapical lesions in endodontically treated teeth. Endod Dent Traumatol 1987;3:15-20.
103. Reit C, Gröndahl HC. Endodontic retreatment decision making among a group of general practitioners. Scand J Dent Res 1988;96:12-18.
104. Reit C, Hollender L. Evaluation of endodontic therapy and the influence of observer variation. Scand J Dent Res 1983;91:205-12.
105. Rosenow EC. Studies on elective localization. Focal infection with special reference to oral sepsis. J Dent Res 1919;1:205-68.
106. Rowe AHR, Binnie WH. The incidence and location of microorganisms following endodontic treatment. Br Dent J 1977;142:91-95.
107. Ruddle CJ. Nonsurgical endodontic retreatment. In: Cohen S, Burns RC. Pathways of the pulp. 8 ed. St Louis: Mosby. 2002;875-929.
108. Santos M. Análise comparativa, *in vitro*, da eficiência na desobturação dos canais radiculares entre as técnicas manual e sônica – contribuição ao estudo. (Master´s Thesis). University of São Paulo. 1990.
109. Saunders WP, Saunders EM. Coronal leakage as causes of failure in root canal therapy. A review. Endod Dent Traumatol 1994;10:105-08.
110. Seltzer S. Root canal failures. In: Endodontology. Seltzer S. 2nd ed. Philadelphia: Lea & Febiger. 1988;p.439-70.
111. Seltzer S. Repair following root canal therapy. In: Endodontology biologic considerations in endodontic procedures. 2nd ed. Philadelphia: Lea & Fabiger;1988;p.389-438.
112. Seltzer S, Bender IB, Smith J, Freedman I, Nazimor H. Endodontic failures – an analysis based on clinical, roentgenographic and histologic findings. Oral Surg Oral Med Oral Pathol 1967;23:500-30.

113. Seltzer S, Naidorf IS. Flare-ups in Endodontics. I. Etiological factors. J Endod 1985;11:472-76.
114. Silva MR, Biffi JCG, Mota AS, Fernandes-Neto AJ, Neves FD. Evaluation of intracanal post removal using ultrasound. Braz Dent J 2004;15:119-26.
115. Sirén EK, Haapasalo MPP, Ranta K, Salmi P, Kerosuo ENJ. Microbiological findings and clinical treatment procedures in endodontic cases selected for microbiological investigation. Int Endod J 1997;30:91-95.
116. Sjögren V, Figdor D, Spångberg L, Sundqvist G. The antimicrobial effects of calcium hydroxide as a short-term intra-canal dressing. Int Endod J 1991;24:119-25.
117. Sjögren U, Figdor D, Persson S, Sundqvist G. Influence of infection at the time of root filling on the outcome of endodontic treatment of teeth with apical periodontitis. Int Endod J 1997;30:297-306.
118. Sjögren U, Hägglund B, Sundqvist G. Factors affecting the long-terms results of endodontic treatment. J Endod 1990;16:498-504.
119. Souza V, Holland R, Menezes MR. Comportamento biológico do cimento de óxido de zinco e eugenol após contato com hidróxido de cálcio. Estudo histológico em tecido subcutâneo de ratos. Rev Bras Odontol 1991;1:2-10.
120. Stabholz A, Friedman S. Endodontic retreatment - Case selection and technique. Part 2: Treatment planning for retreatment. J Endod 1988;14:607-14.
121. Stabholz A, Friedman S, Tanse A. Endodontic failures and retreatment. In: Pathways of the pulp. Cohen S, Burns RC. 6th ed. St Louis: Mosby. 1994;p.690-728.
122. Stabholz A, Walton RE. Avaliação do sucesso e insucesso. In: Walton RE, Torabinejad M. Princípios e prática em endodontia. São Paulo: Santos. 1997;p.324-335.
123. Stamos DE, Gutmann JL. Survey of endodontic retreatment methods used to remove intra-radicular posts. J Endod 1993;19:366-69.
124. Sundqvist G, Figdor D. Life as an endodontic pathogen. Ecological differences between the untreated and root-filled root canals. Endodontic Topics. 2003;6:3–28.
125. Sundqvist G, Figdor D, Persson S, Sjögren U. Microbiologic analysis of teeth with failed endodontic treatment and the outcome of conservative retreatment. Oral Surg Oral Med Oral Pathol 1998;85:86-93.
126. Swanson K, Madison S. An evaluation of coronal microleakage in endodontically treated teeth. Time periods. J Endod 1987;13:56-59.
127. Sydney GB, Batista A. Retratamento endodôntico. In: Odontologia Integrada. Vanzillotta PS, Gonçalves AR. Rio de Janeiro: Pedro Primeiro. 2002;p. 290-326.
128. Sydney GB, Estrela C. Influence of root canal preparation on anaerobic bacteria in teeth with asymptomatic apical periodontitis. Braz Endod J 1996;1:7-10.
129. Taintor JF, Ingle JI, Fahid A. Retreatment versus further treatment. Clin Prevent Dent 1983;5:8-14.
130. Thoden VVSK, Duivnvoorden HJ, Schuurs AHB. Probalities of success and failure in endodontic treatment: a Bayesian approach. Oral Surg Oral Med Oral Pathol 1981;52:85.
131. Torabinejad M, Bahjri K. Essential elements of evidence-based endodontics: steps involved in conducting clinical research. J Endod 2005:31563-9.
132. Torabinejad M, Cymerman JJ, Frank SM, Lemon RR, Maggio JD, Shilder H. Effectiveness of complete instrumentation. J Endod 1994;20:427-31.
133. Torabinejad M, Dorn SO, Eleazer PD, Frankson M, Jouhari B, Mullin RK, Soluti A. Effectiveness of various medications on post operative pain following root canal obturation. J Endod 1994;20:427-31.
134. Torabinejad M, Kettering JD, McGraw JC, Cummings RR, Dwyer TG, Tobias TG, Tobias TS. Factors associated with endodontic inter appointment emergencies of teeth with necrotic pulps. J Endod 1988;14:261-66.
135. Torabinejad M, Lemon RR. Acidentes de procedimentos. In: Princípios e prática em endodontia. Walton RE, Torabinejad M. São Paulo: Santos. 1997;p.306-23.
136. Torabinejad M, Ung B, Kettering JD. In vitro bacterial penetration of coronal unsealed endodontically treated teeth. J Endod 1990;16:566-69.
137. Torneck CD. Reaction of rat connective tissue to polyethylene tube implants. Part 2. Oral Surg Oral Med Oral Pathol 1967;24:674-83.
138. Trope E, Chow E, Nissan R. In vitro endotoxin penetration of coronally unsealed endodontically treated teeth. Endod Dent Traumatol 1991;11:90-94.
139. Vani JR, Fornari VJ, Estrela C. Métodos de remoção de retentores intraradiculares. J Bras Clin Estética 2000;4-70-74.
140. Vire DE. Failure of endodontically treated teeth. J Endod 1991;17:338-42.
141. Whitworth JM, Boursin EM. Dissolution of root canal sealer cements in volatile solvents. Int Endod J 2000;33:19-24.
142. Wilcox LR. Endodontic retreatment with halothane versus chloroform solvent. J Endod 1995;21:305-07.
143. Wilcox LR, Krell KV, Madison S, Rittman B. Endodontic retreatment: Evaluation of gutta-percha and sealer removal and canal reinstrumentation. J Endod 1987;13:453-57.
144. Wilcox LR, Surksun RV. Endodontic retreatment in large and small straight canals. J Endod 1991;17:119-22.
145. Wilcox LR, Swift LM. Endodontic retreatment in small and large curved canal J Endod 1991;17:313-15.
146. Wourms DJ, Campbell AD, Hicks ML, Pelleu-Jr GB. Alternative solvents to chloroform for gutta-percha removal. J Endod 1990;16:224-26.
147. Yared GM, Bou-Dagher FE. Influence of apical enlargement on bacterial infection during treatment of apical periodontitis. J Endod 1994;20:535-37.
148. Zakariasen KL, Scott DA, Jensen JR. Endodontic recall radiographs: how reliable is our interpretation of endodontic success of failure and what factors affect our reliability? Oral Surg Oral Med Oral Pathol 1984;57:343-47.

# Biological and Clinical Aspects of Traumatic Injuries to the Permanent Teeth

**M. I. S. Côrtes**
*Pontifical Catholic University of Minas Gerais, Belo Horizonte, MG, Brazil*
*Federal University of Minas Gerais, Belo Horizonte, MG, Brazil*

**J. V. Bastos**
*Federal University of Minas Gerais, Belo Horizonte, MG, Brazil*

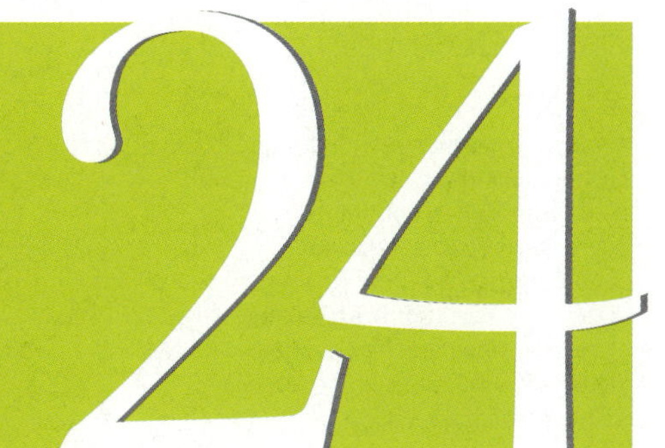

Chapter contents

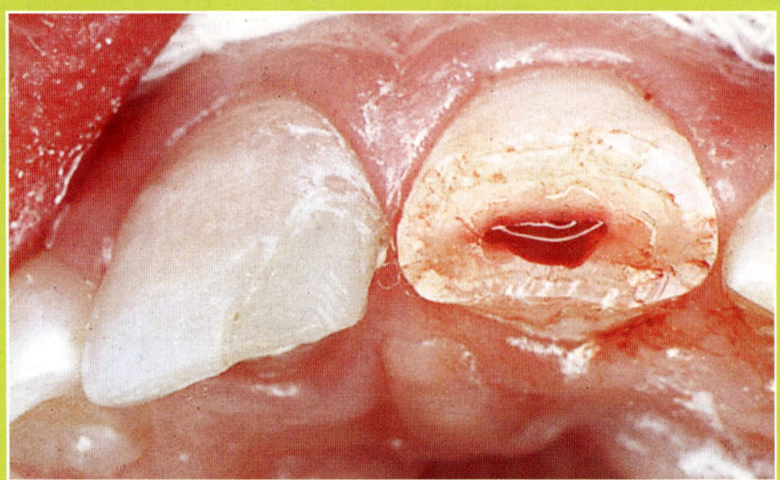

Pulp exposure of tooth #21, submitted to reattachment of the crown fragment without performing conservative treatment of the pulp. The patient complained about intense pain with cold stimulus up to 1 week after reattachment procedure. When the fragment was removed the dark aspect of the bleeding and the absence of normal flow was noticed. Root canal treatment was indicated, because of the irreversible pulp inflammation.

## Chapter contents

## PART 1. Epidemiology, Classification and Socio-Psychological Impact of Traumatic Dental Injuries

### Introduction

Traumatic dental injuries have become the most serious dental public health problem among children and adolescents, due to their high prevalence reported in population studies, severe socio-psychological impact, and the possibility of establishing prevention and control programs, since their causes are widely known[5,69,70,71,84,106]. Moreover, according to Glendor et al.[49] the costs of trauma in permanent dentition are high, because in addition to expenses with the initial treatment, it requires post-treatment control lasting for many years. Borum & Andreasen[20] reported that the treatment of traumatic injuries consumes a great part of the health service resources in Denmark, mainly applied in the treatment of permanent teeth.

Wong & Kolokotsa[109] estimated the total cost, including the direct costs (outpatient costs) and indirect costs (missed working day) of treating children and adolescents with traumatic injuries to their incisors at a Dental Hospital in the United Kingdom. Eighty-one patients (mean age = 9.9, SD = 2.33), who attended the dental trauma clinic at a London teaching hospital between 1990 and 2001 were included in this study. The male:female ratio was 3:2. The median number of visits and median treatment duration were eight visits and 21 months, respectively. The average total cost of treating a patient with one traumatic injury was 856 pounds. It was concluded that the indirect cost was a considerably large proportion (39%) of the total cost. The authors recommended that more specialists in pediatric dentistry can improve access to care locally and contribute to reduce the indirect travelling cost.

A significant decline in the prevalence and severity of dental caries in many countries[10,22,48,92] has drawn attention back to the questions of dental trauma. Nevertheless, there are few epidemiological surveys that include the diagnosis of dental trauma in both developing and industrialized countries, particularly when compared with the innumerable studies of caries and periodontal disease. Dental research in this field has focused on the biological consequences, improvement of new technology for restorative treatment of traumatic dental injuries, and new alternatives to prevent root resorption of replanted teeth[6].

Traumatic injury to the permanent teeth is a neglected oral condition. Over the last few years, however, epidemiologists have been concerned about the need for conducting surveys that allow advances in the direction of preventing the disastrous consequences of dental trauma. In developing countries a great deal still has to be done to control caries. In this case, little importance is being attached to the problem of dental trauma among children and adolescents, although studies published up to now indicate a high prevalence (Table 24.1 to 24.6).

Health education programs have been implemented locally, having some impact on the solution of the problem of dental trauma[11-14,101] (Figure 24.1 to 24.3). The Brazilian Association of Dental Traumatology created a special section on its website, with robust information for the lay community[111].

In addition to the high prevalence, there is the high socio-psychological impact caused by the esthetic implication of fracture of maxillary central incisors, considering the importance of these teeth to the appearance of the face[30]. The socio-psychological trauma that follows fracture is, in many cases underestimated, and sometimes completely ignored. The awareness of "being different", the criticism that the child is exposed to, and the family's disappointment about the child's compromised esthetic appearance are sufficient to cause changes of emotional nature in many children[99].

**Table 24.1** - Population-based studies on the prevalence of traumatic dental injuries in countries of the Regional Office for Africa ("AFRO")

| Country (City) | Author | Age Groups | Sample Size | Prevalence Overall (%) |
|---|---|---|---|---|
| Kenya | Ng'ang'a & Valderhaugh (1988) | 13-15 | 250 | 16.8 |
| Nigeria (Ibadan) | Falomo (1986) | 10-17 | 250 | 16.0 |
| Nigeria (Benin) | Naqvi & Ogidan (1990) | 9-16 | 1102 | 19.1 |

**Table 24.2** - Population-based studies on the prevalence of traumatic dental injuries in countries of the Regional Office for Americas ("AMRO")

| Country (city) | Author | Age Groups | Sample Size | Prevalence Overall (%) |
|---|---|---|---|---|
| Brazil (Bauru) | Bijella FB (1972) | 7-15 | 15675 | 6.0 |
| Brazil (Belo Horizonte) | Côrtes et al. (2001) | 9-14 | 3702 | 12.1 |
| Brazil (Blumenau) | Marcenes et al. (2001) | 12 | 652 | 58.6 |
| Brazil (Cianorte) | Nicolau et al. (2001) | 13 | 764 | 20.4 |
| Brazil (Florianópolis) | Traebert et al. (2003) | 12 | 307 | 18.9 |
| Brazil (Jaraguá do Sul) | Marcenes et al. (1999) | 12 | 476 | 15.3 |
| USA | Macko et al. (1979) | 12-15 | 1314 | 19.1 |
| USA | Oluwole & Leverett (1986) | 11-21 | 5000 | 5.0 |
| USA | Kaste et al. (1996) | 6-20 | 3337 | 18.4 |
| Dom Republic (S. Domingo) | Garcia-Godoy et al. (1981) | 7-14 | 596 | 18.1 |
| Dom Republic (S. Domingo) | Garcia-Godoy et al. (1985) | 6-17 | 1200 | 12.2 |
| Dom Republic (S. Domingo) | Garcia-Godoy et al. (1986) | 7-16 | 596 | 18.9 |

**Table 24.3** - Population-based studies on the prevalence of traumatic dental injuries in countries of the Regional Office for the Eastern Mediterranean ("EMRO")

| Country (city) | Author | Age Groups | Sample Size | Prevalence Overall (%) |
|---|---|---|---|---|
| Iraq | Baghdady et al., (1981) | 6-12 | 6090 | 7.7 |
| Jordan (Amman) | Jamani & Fayyad (1991) | 7-12 | 3041 | 10.5 |
| Jordan (Amman) urban | Hamdan & Rock (1995) | 10-12 | 234 | 19.2 |
| Jordan (Amman) Shouna-rural | Hamdan & Rock (1995) | 10-12 | 225 | 15.5 |
| Sudan | Baghdady et al. (1981) | 6-12 | 3057 | 5.5 |
| Syria (Damascus) | Marcenes et al. (1999) | 9-12 | 1087 | - |

**Table 24.4** - Population-based studies on the prevalence of traumatic dental injuries in countries of the Regional Office for Europe ("EURO")

| Country (city) | Author | Age Groups | Sample Size | Prevalence Overall (%) |
|---|---|---|---|---|
| Denmark | Andreasen & Ravn (1972) | 9-17 | 487 | 22.0 |
| Spain (Mostoles) | Tapias et al. (2003) | 10 | 470 | 17.4 |
| Finland | Jarvinen (1979) | 6-16 | 1614 | 19.8 |
| France | Delattre et al. (1994) | 6-15 | 2020 | 13.6 |
| England | Clarkson et al. (1973) | 11-17 | 756 | 9.8 |
| England/Wales | Todd (1975) | 5-15 | 12952 | - |
| England (Manchester) | Hamilton et al. (1997) | 11-14 | 2022 | 34.4 |
| England (London/Newham) | Marcenes & Murray (2001) | 14 | 2684 | 27.3 |
| England (London/Newham) | Marcenes & Murray (2001) | 14 | 411 | 43.8 |
| Ireland | O'Mullane (1972) | 6-19 | 2792 | 13.0 |
| Ireland | Holland et al. (1988) | 8;12;15 | 7171 | - |
| Ireland | Holland et al. (1994) | 16-24 | 400 | 14.0 |
| Israel | Zadick et al. (1972) | 6-14 | 10903 | 8.7 |
| South Wales | Hunter et al. (1990) | 11-12 | 968 | 15.3 |
| Sweden (urban) | Forsberg & Tedestam (1990) | 7-15 | 1635 | 18.0 |
| Sweden (rural) | Josefsson & Karlander (1994) | 7-17 | 750 | 11.7 |
| Sweden (Vasterbotten) | Borssen & Holm (1997) | 16 | 3007 | 35.0 |
| United Kingdom | Todd & Dodd (1985) | 8-15 | 22375 | - |
| United Kingdom | O'Brien (1994) | 8-15 | 18869 | - |

**Table 24.5** - Population-based studies on the prevalence of traumatic dental injuries in countries of the Regional Office for South East Asia ("SEARO")

| Country | Author | Age Groups | Sample Size | Prevalence Overall (%) |
|---|---|---|---|---|
| India (South Kanara) urban and rural | Gupta et al. (2003) | 8-14 | 2100 | 13.8 |

**Table 24.6** - Population-based studies on the prevalence of traumatic dental injuries in countries of the Regional Office for the Western Pacific ("WPRO")

| Country (city) | Author | Age Groups | Sample Size | Prevalence Overall (%) |
|---|---|---|---|---|
| Malasya | Meon (1986) | 7-12 | 1635 | 3.9 |
| Malasya | Nik-Hussein (2001) | 16 | 4085 | 4.1 |
| Japan | Uji (1988) | 6-18 | 15822 | 21.8 |



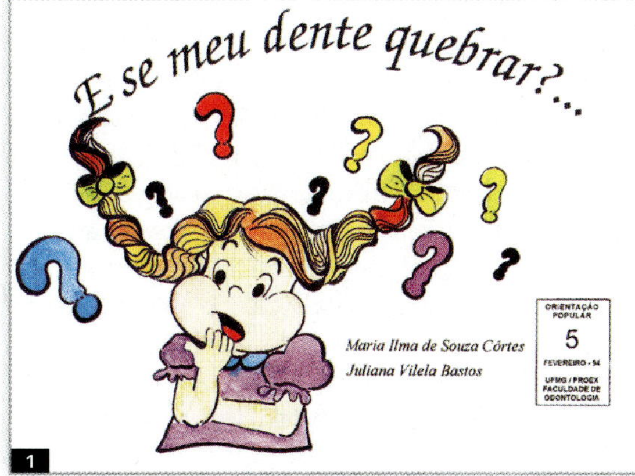


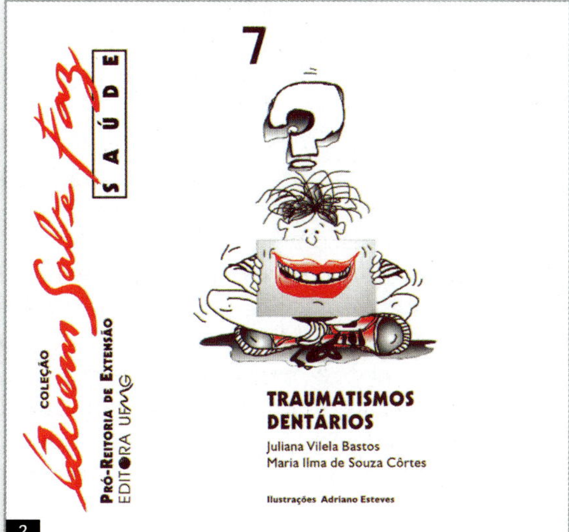


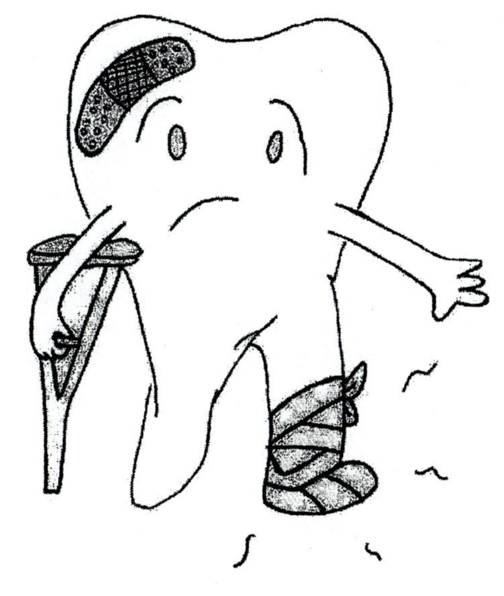


**Figures 24.1 to 24.3** - Educational material for orientation in the schools on the first aid in case of accidents that involve traumatic dental injuries.

## Studies of Prevalence

*"The prevalence of a disease in different populations is to be compared and used to assess dental health status, observe trends within countries or between countries, plan dental health services and preventive programmes and serve as the basis for further research"* [110]. In the field of the oral health of children, substantial advances were made for dental caries. The results of epidemiological surveys on dental caries collected by the oral health programmes of the World Health Organization (WHO) in the last 20 years confirmed a decline of the prevalence and severity of dental caries amongst children and adolescents from developed societies and showed the evidence of an increase in dental caries in some of the developing countries[48,74,75,81]. As some of the data were from national surveys and others from local epidemiological studies, caution is required in making superficial comparisons using only the WHO Country Profile Program. Since the mid 1970s reports from developed countries world-wide showed that the prevalence of dental caries in children and adolescents has declined. However, there continues to have sections of populations for whom caries remains a major problem, mainly in the deprived sections of the society[36,51] who still adopt a cariogenic diet[17].

On the other hand, regarding traumatic injuries to teeth, no comparisons can be made, as no clear trends in the prevalence has become apparent world-wide over the last twenty five years, due to the scarcity of standardized methods for data collection[04]. This comment had already been made by O'Mullane[88], emphasizing that "despite the importance given in literature to dental trauma in children and adolescents, prevalence studies are few and vary considerably in their results and conclusions". Population studies have demonstrated a prevalence varying from 3.9% to 58.6% (Table 24.1 to 24.6). In the last decade a number of studies showed that the prevalence of traumatic injuries in permanent dentition in Europe varied from 8.7% to 43.8% (Table 24.4). Latin American researchers also showed that there was a high prevalence of traumatic dental injuries among schoolchildren, varying from 5.0% to 58.6% (Graphic 24.1). This high variation observed in the studies conducted in various parts of the world could really reflect the cultural differences that include environmental and behavioral differences, or could be the result of the different methodologies applied during data collection. Population-based studies of traumatic dental injuries present limitations, such as absence of standardization of examination procedures and classification adopted for diagnosis of traumatic dental injuries. Moreover, they do not follow a standard for the definition of age, gender, the type of teeth examined, etiology and place of occurrence of the trauma. Many studies of prevalence do not list the methodology of sample selection, generating doubts about its representativeness[8,23,37,46]. As regards the examination methods, artificial light makes it easier to identify correctly the dental structures. Moreover, it is essential for visualizing injuries, such as enamel cracks and discolorations. Studies that adopted natural light during examinations, may have underestimated the prevalence of traumatic dental injuries[8,37,41-44,54,57,60,61].

For the above-mentioned reasons one needs to be careful when endeavoring to establish a world-wide trend by observing published results of dental trauma prevalence[27].

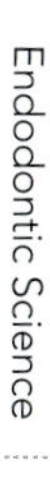


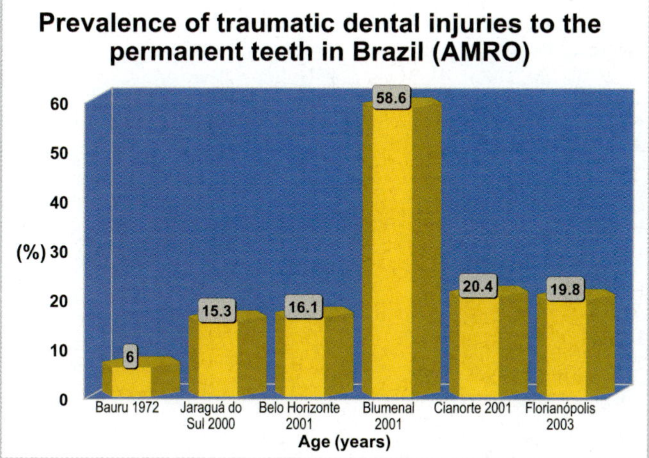


Graphic 24.1

In the survey conducted by Côrtes et al.[29], the prevalence of traumatic injuries varied from 8% (amongst the 9-year olds) up to 16.1% [amongst 14-year olds) (P<0.001) (Graphic 24.2). For all ages the prevalence was higher among boys (P<0.001) (Graphic 24.3). Males were 1.74 times (95% CI=1.41-2.16) more likely to present traumatic dental injury than females. The results of the multiple logistic regression analysis showed that all the variables studied, age, sex, socio-economic status, overjet and lip coverage remained statistically significantly associated after adjustment in the model. Children from high socio-economic status, having an overjet greater than 5.0 mm, with inadequate lip coverage and being male were more likely to have a traumatic dental injury than children from low socio-economic status, having an overjet equal or lower than 5 mm, with adequate lip coverage and being female (Table 24.7). Few reports have included socio-economic indicators. The results of this study showed that schoolchildren from higher socio-economic groups presented a higher prevalence of traumatic dental injuries than those from lower socio-economic groups. The higher risk for adolescents from higher socio-economic status may be due to greater ownership of bicycles, skateboards, roller-skating and access to swimming pools.

Amongst the 448 children who presented some evidence of traumatic dental injury in the permanent dentition, the most frequent was enamel fracture, followed by fracture involving dentin. The results showed that most children who received treatment due to traumatic dental injuries, presented esthetic resin composite restorations (Graphic 24.4). The most affected teeth were the maxillary central incisors, with no difference between the right and left side, and most children presented only one affected tooth (Graphic 24.5 and 24.6). These results are similar to those from other cross-sectional studies.

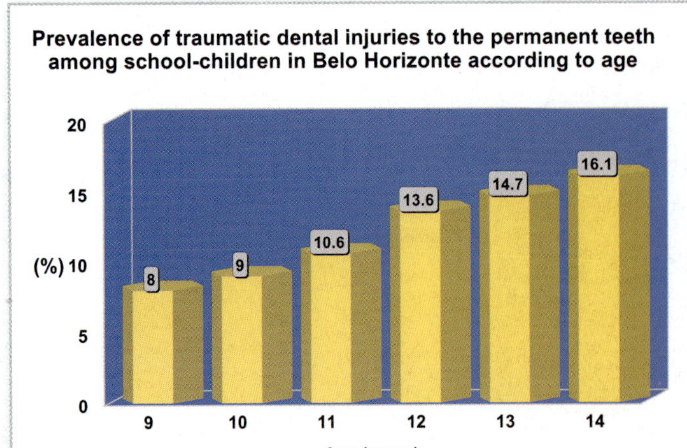


Graphic 24.2

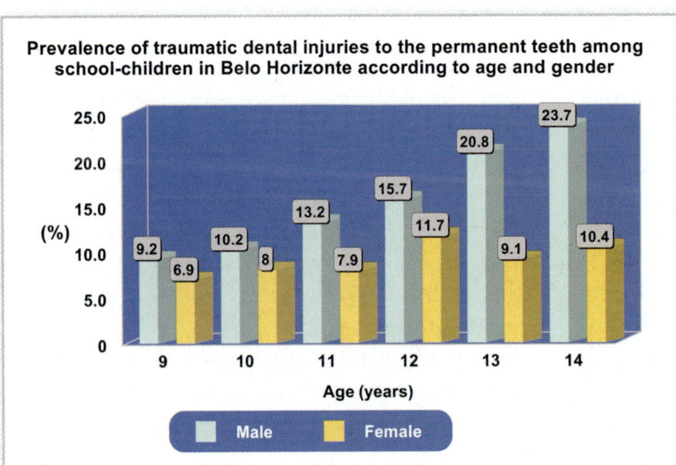


Graphic 24.3

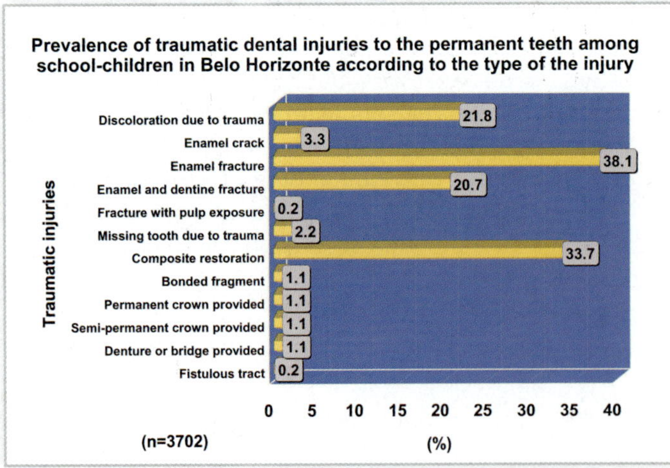


Graphic 24.4

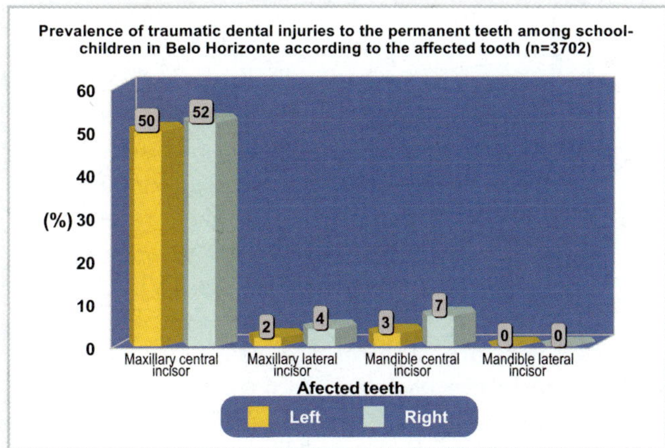


Graphic 24.5

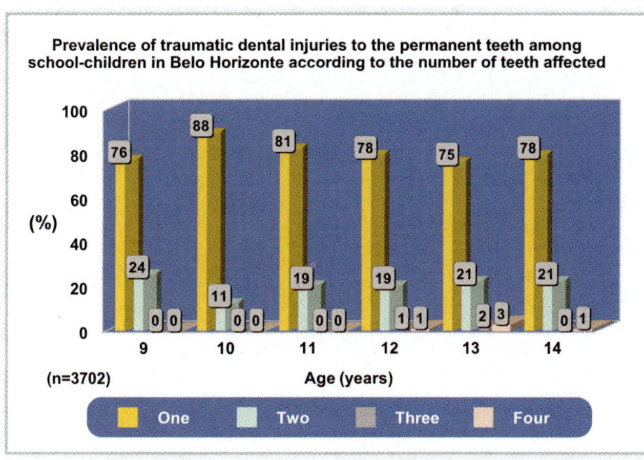


Graphic 24.6

**Table 24.7** - Frequency distribution, simple and multiple logistic regression of socio-economic status, overjet, lip coverage and age on the presence of traumatic dental injuries in schoolchildren of Belo Horizonte Brazil (n = 3461)

| | Traumatic Dental Injury | No Traumatic Dental Injury | Unadjusted Odds Ratio (95% c.i.) | Adjusted Odds Ratio1 (95% c.i.) |
|---|---|---|---|---|
| Socio-economic status | | | | |
| Low | 264 (10.6%) | 2236 (89.4%) | 1 | 1 |
| High | 149 (15.5%) | 812 (84.5%) | 1.55 (1.25-1.92)*** | 1.43 (1.15-1.79)** |
| Overjet | | | | |
| ≤ 5 mm | 281 (10.4%) | 2432 (89.6%) | 1 | 1 |
| > 5 mm | 132 (17.6%) | 616 (82.4%) | 1.85 (1.48-2.39)*** | 1.37 (1.06-1.80)* |
| Lip coverage | | | | |
| Inadequate | 175 (17.9%) | 801 (82.1%) | 1 | 1 |
| Adequate | 238 ( 9.6%) | 2247 (90.4%) | 0.48 (0.39-0.60)*** | 0.56 (0.44-0.72)*** |
| Sex | | | | |
| Female | 167 (8.9%) | 1700 (91.1%) | 1 | 1 |
| Male | 246 (15.4%) | 1348 (84.6%) | 1.85 (1.51-2.29)*** | 1.74 (1.41-2.16)*** |
| Age - 1 year increase | | | 1.16 (1.09-1.24)*** | 1.18 (1.11-1.26)*** |

1 Adjusted for all variables listed above

*** P<0.001; ** P<0.01; * P<0.05

## Classification

Several diagnostic criteria have been used to establish the prevalence of traumatic dental injuries in permanent dentition, leading to a certain difficulty in comparing the clinical and epidemiological results, since each author adopts those of his/her preference according the specific objectives[6,15,27,35,45,64,79,86,104,105].

The classification of Ellis & Davey[35] is based on a numerical system of Classes I to VIII, which describes the anatomical extent of the injuries and uses subjective terms, such as "simple fracture" and "extensive fracture". The system has been widely used in epidemiological surveys. It is not completely appropriate for "field" examinations, because in order to diagnose a Class IV injury, which indicates the absence of pulp vitality, it would be necessary to perform pulp vitality tests and radiographic examinations. Similarly, it is necessary to take a radiograph, preferably, at the time of the accident, to perform the diagnosis of Class VI, root fracture and Class VII, displacement of the tooth. There are no criteria to classify the treatment performed as a result of traumatic injuries or their sequela, such as discoloration, fistula and swelling (Table 24.8).

**Table 24.8** - Diagnostic criteria of traumatic dental injuries - Ellis & Davey[35] (1970)

| Score Criteria | Description |
|---|---|
| Class I | Simple fracture of the crown, involving little or no dentine |
| Class II | Extensive fracture of the crown, involving considerable dentine, but not dental pulp |
| Class III | Extensive fracture of the crown, involving considerable dentine and exposing the dental pulp |
| Class IV | The traumatized tooth which becomes nonvital, with or without loss of crown structure |
| Class V | Tooth loss as a result of trauma |
| Class VI | Fracture of the root, with or without loss of crown structure |
| Class VII | Displacement of the tooth, without fracture of crown or root |
| Class VIII | Fracture of the crown "en masse" and its replacement |

Andreasen & Andreasen[6] have modified the system adopted by the WHO for the International Classification Diseases to Dentistry and Stomatology. This classification is extremely complete and valid for examination and clinical diagnosis of traumatic injuries, including mineralized tissues of the teeth, pulp and periodontium, as well as bone, gingiva and mucosa. However, it is not completely applied to epidemiological research, since some of the assessments can only be made using adequate equipment, appropriate to the examination procedures adopted. Some terms, such as "complicated fracture" and "uncomplicated fracture" are subjective. Moreover, for the diagnosis of some types of injury, such as cementum fracture, root fracture, injuries to periodontal tissues and bone support, radiographic examination is required, which is impracticable in an epidemiological research. Similarly, the classification of Ellis & Davey[35] does not allow the treatment and sequelae of traumatic injuries to be identified. The great value of this classification is that it is the most complete for diagnosis at the time of the examination of the patient with traumatic dental injury, making it possible to trace the adequate treatment plan, and establish the prognosis, based on the injured structures. It is appropriate to use in the dental surgery with diagnostic aids such as radiographic examination, transillumination and sensibility tests. (Tables 24.9 to 24.12)

**Table 24.9** - Diagnostic criteria of traumatic dental injuries - Andreasen & Andreasen (2007): Injuries to the hard tissues and the pulp (codes of the WHO International Classification of Diseases to Dentistry and Stomatology)

| Code | Criteria | Description |
|---|---|---|
| N 502.50 | Enamel infraction | An incomplete fracture (crack) of the enamel without loss of tooth substance |
| N 502.50 | Enamel fracture (uncomplicated crown fracture) | A fracture with loss of tooth substance confined to the enamel |
| N 502.51 | Enamel-dentine fracture (uncomplicated crown fracture) | A fracture with loss of tooth substance confined to the enamel and dentine but not involving the pulp |
| N 502.52 | Complicated crown fracture | A fracture involving enamel and dentine and exposing the pulp |
| N 502.54 | Uncomplicated crown-root fracture | A fracture involving enamel, dentine and cementum but not exposing the pulp |
| N 503.54 | Complicated crown-root fracture | A fracture involving enamel, dentine and cementum and exposing the pulp |
| N 502.53 | Root fracture | A fracture involving dentine, cementum and pulp |

**Table 24.10** - Diagnostic criteria of traumatic dental injuries - Andreasen & Andreasen (2007): Injuries to the periodontal tissues (codes of the WHO International Classification of Diseases to Dentistry and Stomatology)

| Code | Criteria | Description |
|---|---|---|
| N 503.20 | Concussion | An injury to the tooth-supporting structures without abnormal loosening or displacement of the tooth but with marked reaction to percussion |
| N 503.20 | Subluxation (loosening) | An injury to the tooth-supporting structures with abnormal loosening but without displacement of the tooth |
| N 503.20 | Extrusive luxation (peripheral dislocation, partial avulsion) | Partial displacement of the tooth out of its socket |
| N 503.20 | Lateral luxation | Displacement of the tooth in a direction other than axial. This is accompanied by comminution or fracture of the alveolar socket |
| N 503.21 | Intrusive luxation (central dislocation) | Displacement of the tooth into the alveolar bone. This injury is accompanied by comminution or fracture of the alveolar socket |
| N 502.22 | Avulsion (exarticulation) | Complete displacement of the tooth out of its socket |

**Table 24.11** - Diagnostic criteria of traumatic dental injuries - Andreasen & Andreasen (2007): Injuries to the supporting bone (codes of the WHO International Classification of Diseases to Dentistry and Stomatology)

| Code | Criteria | Description |
|---|---|---|
| N 502.60 | Comminution of the mandibular alveolar socket | Crushing and compression of the alveolar socket |
| N 502.40 | Comminution of the maxillary alveolar socket | Crushing and compression of the alveolar socket |
| N 502.60 | Fracture of the mandibular alveolar socket wall | A fracture confined to the facial or oral socket wall |
| N 502.40 | Fracture of the maxillary alveolar socket wall | A fracture confined to the facial or oral socket wall |
| N 502.60 | Fracture of the mandibular alveolar process | A fracture of the alveolar process which may or may not involve the alveolar socket |
| N 502.40 | Fracture of the maxillary alveolar process | A fracture of the alveolar process which may or may not involve the alveolar socket |
| N 502.60 | Fracture of the mandible | A fracture involving the base of the mandible and often the alveolar process |
| N 502.40 | Fracture of the maxilla | A fracture involving the base of the maxilla and often the alveolar process |

**Table 24.12** - Diagnostic criteria of traumatic dental injuries - Andreasen & Andreasen (2007): Injuries to gingiva or oral mucosa (codes of the WHO International Classification of Diseases to Dentistry and Stomatology)

| Code | Criteria | Description |
|---|---|---|
| S 01.50 | Laceration of gingiva or oral mucosa | A shallow or deep wound in the mucosa resulting from a tear, and usually produced by a sharp object |
| S 00.50 | Contusion of the gingiva or oral mucosa | A bruise usually produced by impact with a blunt object and not accompanied by a break in the mucosa, usually causing submucosal haemorrhage |
| S 00.50 | Abrasion of gingiva or oral mucosa | A superficial wound produced buy rubbing of the mucosa leaving a raw, bleeding surface |

In the epidemiological surveys conducted in the United Kingdom, an index was adopted by the Department of Dental Health - University of Birmingham Dental School and Department of Child Dental Health - University of Newcastle Dental School[86,104,105]. After its first use by the National Dental Child Health Survey, in 1973 (Table 24.13) the index was modified, with the exclusion of the "displacement" criteria and inclusion of the criteria "acid-etch composite restoration" and "prosthetics for substitution of teeth lost by trauma", which was then used in the survey of 1983 (Table 24.14). Small modifications were made for its use in 1993 (Table 24.15). The changes made during these three surveys allowed the index to be acceptable for epidemiological research. The exclusion of the criteria "displacement" made it more applicable. This type of injury must be identified with the aid of X-rays, which is impracticable for field screening. To identify tooth displacement, the clinical examination must be carried out at the time of the accident, when signs and symptoms are still present. Adding the criteria for "acid-etch composite restoration" performed due to traumatic injuries, allowed for a larger number of trauma cases to be identified.

**Table 24.13** - Diagnostic criteria of traumatic dental injuries – Todd (1975): *Children's Dental Health in the United Kingdom*

| Code | Criteria | Description |
|---|---|---|
| Code 1 | Discoloration | Self-explanatory |
| Code 2 | Fracture involving enamel | Self-explanatory |
| Code 3 | Fracture involving enamel and dentine | Self-explanatory |
| Code 4 | Fracture involving enamel, dentine and pulp | Self-explanatory |
| Code 5 | Missing due to trauma | Self-explanatory |
| Code 6 | Temporary crown fitted | Refers to items of immediate treatment, such as foil, steel caps, pinch bands, acetate crowns, etc. |
| Code 7 | Permanent or semi-permanent restoration fitted | Includes basket crowns, veneer crowns, post crowns, pinned inlays, etc. |
| Code 8 | Displacement | Self-explanatory |
| Code X | No trauma | Self-explanatory |

**Table 24.14** - Diagnostic criteria of traumatic dental injuries - Todd and Dodd (1985): *Children's Dental Health in the United Kingdom*

| **Code** | **Criteria** | **Description** |
|---|---|---|
| Code 0 | No trauma | |
| Code 1 | Discoloration | |
| Code 2 | Fracture (enamel) | Fracture involving enamel |
| Code 3 | Fracture (enamel and dentine) | Fracture involving enamel and dentine |
| Code 4 | Fracture (involving pulp) | Fracture involving enamel, dentine and pulp |
| Code 5 | Missing due to trauma | Missing due to trauma |
| Code 6 | Acid-etch composite restoration | Acid-etch composite restoration |
| Code 7 | Permanent crown | Including jacket and post crowns, whether porcelain or acrylic |
| Code 8 | Other restorations | Other permanent or semi-permanent restorations. This refers to items of treatment such as stainless steel crowns, pinch bands, cellulose acetate crowns, Directa crowns, pinned inlays, etc. |
| Code 9 | Denture due to trauma | Denture provided due to traumatic loss of the tooth |

**Table 24.15** - Diagnostic criteria of traumatic dental injuries - O'Brien (1995): *Children's Dental Health in the United Kingdom*

| Code | Criteria | Description |
|---|---|---|
| Code 0 | No trauma | |
| Code 1 | Discoloration | |
| Code 2 | Enamel | Fracture involving enamel |
| Code 3 | Enamel and dentine | Fracture involving enamel and dentine |
| Code 4 | Enamel, dentine, pulp | Fracture involving enamel, dentine and pulp |
| Code 5 | Missing due to trauma | Missing due to trauma |
| Code 6 | Acid-etch composite | Acid-etch composite |
| Code 7 | Permanent replacement | Permanent replacement including crown, denture, bridge pontic |
| Code 8 | Temporary restorations | Temporary restorations |
| Code 9 | Assessment cannot be made | Assessment cannot be made |

The classification formulated by Garcia-Godoy et al.[45], which was defined for clinical and epidemiological examination, lacks criteria for the identification of the sequelae of traumatic injuries, as well as treatment performed. Moreover, injuries such as cementum fracture, root fracture, concussion, luxation, lateral luxation, intrusion and extrusion, need radiographic examination to be diagnosed, in addition to a thorough clinical examination, preferably at the time of the accident. Consequently its application is not recommended for epidemiological studies (Table 24.16).

Naqvi & Ogidan[79] proposed a method for the diagnosis of traumatic injuries, to be used in epidemiological surveys, stating that it was simple, fast and did not need sophisticated equipment for diagnosis. Similarly to the classification of Ellis & Davey[35], the numerical system used to describe the anatomical extent of the injury, makes it difficult for the examiner to memorize the 8 classes. The definition of discoloration and/or presence of fistula for the diagnosis of concussion, luxation and displacement are not appropriate, since these sequelae can also occur in other types of injury and not only in those that the authors reported. In this classification the treatment of traumatic injuries was not considered (Table 24.17).

The index applied by the National Institute of Dental Research (NIDR)[15] was used in the first phase of data collection in the oral exam of the National Health & Nutrition Epidemiological Survey (NHANES III) in a sample of 6-50 year old individuals in the United States[64]. In this classification, the so called "pulp repair" criterion requires verification of the presence of lingual restoration as a sign of endodontic treatment, in addition to confirmation of the history of the trauma. The criterion is not applicable, since the correct form of certifying the existence of endodontic treatment would be a radiographic examination. Dark discoloration of the crown was considered as untreated pulp injury, although the correct diagnosis would be accomplished with the aids of pulp sensibility test. Andreasen et al.[03] reported that coronal discoloration in a traumatized tooth could also be due to healing events, such as pulp canal obliteration, which occurs precisely in the presence of vital pulp. Moreover, a transient discoloration can occur as a result of post-traumatic hemorrhage that happens immediately after luxation injury. Thus, any change in color can be considered as a sign of traumatic injury, but not always is indicative of pulp necrosis (Table 24.18).

tablished criteria. From the results, it could be concluded that children with an overjet larger than 3 mm were approximately twice as much at risk of injury to anterior teeth than children with an overjet smaller than 3 mm. In addition, risk of injury of anterior teeth tends to increase with increasing overjet size. The results of Côrtes et al.[29] demonstrated that with an overjet size greater than 5.0 mm were 1.37 times (95% CI=1.06-1.80) more likely to present with a traumatic dental injury than children with an overjet size equal or lower than 5.0mm (Table 24.7 and Graphic 24.7).

With respect to lip protection, the great variety of measures adopted to define the position of the lip and its relation with the anterior teeth, makes comparisons difficult. Forsberg & Tedestam[39] showed that to determine lip protection, one may observe the extension of teeth covered by the upper lip. Children with a short upper lip lacked soft tissue protection over the upper incisors, which would be particularly exposed at the moment of the injury. The majority of authors considered adequate lip protection when children's maxillary teeth were covered by the lips at the rest position[21,29,47,55,69,70,78,89,94]. A significant association was found between lip coverage and the presence of traumatic injury in the survey conducted by Côrtes et al[29]. Children with adequate lip coverage were 0.56 times (95% CI=0.44-0.72) less likely to have a traumatic dental injury when compared to children with inadequate lip coverage (Table 24.7). Differences were observed at all ages (Graphic 24.8). Based on these findings, it is advisable to pay special attention to children with an increased overjet, particularly when lip coverage is inadequate. This may be an indication for orthodontic treatment[102].



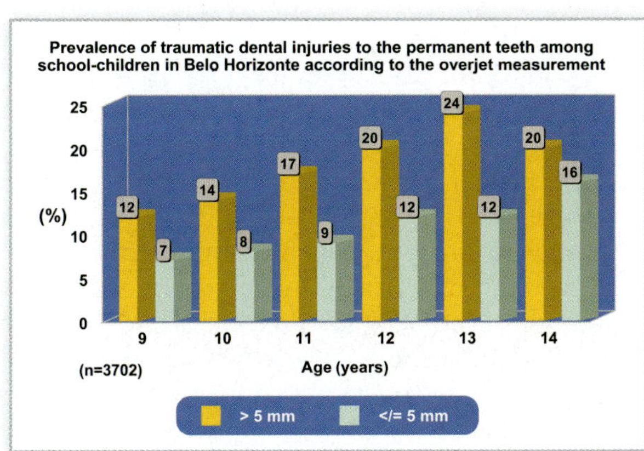


Graphic 24.7

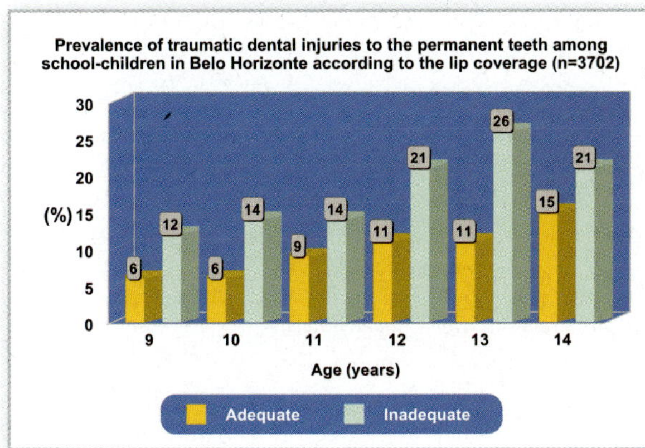


Graphic 24.8

## Socio-economic Status (SSE) and Social Class

The relationship between social class, socio-economic status or purchasing power and the occurrence of traumatic injuries is not clear. Although adopting distinct measures to assess socio-economic background the results of the various studies in different countries showed a relationship with either low or high socio-economic status[29,43,55,60,72]. Environmental, cultural and behavioral factors related to people's socio-economic condition could be the main determinants of the differences found in these studies[43,60]. Few surveys have been performed to demonstrate the environmental and social-cultural impact on the etiology of traumatic injuries.

Petersen[91] described the materialist or structuralism explanation of the relationship between health and inequality that emphasizes the role of the external environment - the conditions under which people live and work. Groups belonging to the lower social classes are exposed to less healthy environments. Health inequalities result from material deprivation. The cultural/behavioral explanation (theory of cultural deprivation or cultural poverty) shows that lower socio-economic groups adopt more dangerous and health-damaging behavior than the higher socio-economic groups. Thus lower socio-economic groups may have fewer opportunities to protect their children by the excessive consumption of harmful commodities or by the under-utilization of preventive health care.

When applying these concepts to dental trauma, one could speculate that groups from low socio-economic status do not know how to protect themselves against accidents and do not adopt adequate preventive measures. This may justify the high prevalence of dental trauma in deprived areas of the UK, such as 34.4% in Bury and Salford[56] and 43.8% in Newham[72]. In most of these countries, safety measures are adopted, and the environment in which the children of high social class live, particularly the one in which they play, is conveniently structured to reduce the risk of accidents. Thus, children from a high social class in industrialized countries may be more protected, than those from a low social class, because not only do they know about adequate protective equipment, but also use it, particularly for practicing sports.

In developing countries, prevention strategies have not yet been implemented, and although the equipment for protection against accidents is known and available, its use is not encouraged. Children from families with high acquisitive power, who own bicycles, skates, roller-skates, and use swimming pools in clubs, are more predisposed to dental trauma than children of low socio-economic status, who do not have access to this type of recreation. Thus, the risk of accidents is higher for children from high socio-economic status, who have access to types of entertainment that offer risks.

In Belo Horizonte, using the ABA-ABIPEME index[2], which establishes the purchasing power of the people, it was shown that children from high socio-economic status were 1.43 times (95% CI=1.15-1.79) more likely to present with a traumatic dental injury than children from low socio-economic status[27] (Table 24.20). Freire[40], based on data collected among 15 year-old schoolchildren in the city of Goiânia, also correlated the occurrence of traumatic injuries with children of high social class. Nevertheless, in a study conducted in another city in the South of Brazil - Jaraguá do Sul - socio-economic status was not significantly associated with the presence of traumatic injuries[70]. Garcia-Godoy et al.,[43] in a study carried out in the Dominican Republic reported a higher prevalence of dental injuries in private than public schools. Children from high and low socio-economic background attended to private and public schools respectively.

### Socio-psychological Impact

The literature pertinent to the socio-psychological aspects of traumatic injuries is replete with speculations, not substantiated by reliable data provided by sound field screenings. Only case reports were separately published[99]. Little is known about the awareness that children have of their fractured incisors and the possible socio-psychological and emotional impact upon their behavior. The aesthetic value of anterior teeth becomes a primary factor in the psychological well being of the individual.

According to Linn[66] the majority of youngsters interviewed in a study reported that the appearance of the teeth was a very important factor in activities, such as finding a job, dating or just making friends. Only 15% did not consider appearance to be anything important in daily life. When adolescents were asked about the reasons for having good oral hygiene, appearance was considered more important than functional or periodontal health.

It is known that health in general, and appearance in particular, are among the main aspects related to the behavior of adolescents[95]. The appearance of the body, especially of the face, plays an important role in human relations[108], the eyes and mouth being the components most commonly associated with physical attraction, acting as key elements in social interactions, and in determining personal success[9].

The meaning of the loss of permanent teeth was illustrated by Richardson[97] through the report of a curious episode. An event reported by Blixen[18] in his book "Out of Africa" told of the serious consequences of a 10 year-old child losing two permanent anterior teeth, as a result of a rock thrown by a child of a different tribe. It is interesting to note that the subject caused such a serious incident that it was discussed by the authorities of the two tribes. The justification for so much concern was the esthetic problem created, which could affect the child's appearance to the point of harming its future, and consequently even the chances of marriage.

In 1955, Slack & Jones[99] stated their personal viewpoint on the psychological trauma, which may follow the fracture of permanent incisors in children. In many cases it was underestimated if not entirely overlooked. They reported severe emotional complications in a nine-year old boy, which were associated with fractured anterior teeth. However, results endorsed by population data were only obtained recently from a case-control study[30].

Baldwin[9] criticized the simplistic and pragmatic manner in which the dentistry class treated facial appearance and esthetics, reflected by the thought that the best oral health is obtained through dental cosmetics. Despite adolescents being concerned about facial esthetics, the role of social, cultural, and psychological aspects is not yet clear. At present, the bio-psycho-social model of oral health is more widely used in Dentistry, with the understanding that it is important to measure the state of oral health and not only the presence or absence of disease itself[100]. The socio-dental indicators, based on social, psychological, cultural and economic effects of oral problems are subjective and inform the oral impact of diseases and conditions, as well as the perceived needs of individuals[31,67,98]. Côrtes et al.[30] evaluated the socio-psychological impact of untreated fractured teeth on the daily living of in a group of Brazilian schoolchildren aged 12-to-14. The index used was the Oral Impact on Daily Performances (OIDP), which was modified and validated to this specific sample. It was concise and easy to manage in a structured interview[1]. The results demonstrated that dental trauma had a great impact on the quality of children's lives, causing limitations in their daily activities. Children with non-restored enamel and dentin fractures were more dissatisfied with the appearance of the anterior teeth, in addition to having difficulty with biting foods and pronouncing certain words. Moreover, by compromising the appearance, the trauma led to emotional problems, limited social contacts, and made the child avoid smiling and showing his/her teeth[30] (Graphic 24.9).

Thus, this survey made a substantial contribution to health service planning. Dental care programs for children and adolescents must prioritize the treatment of traumatic injuries, particularly for having esthetic restorations performed in cases of enamel and dentin crown fractures. Furthermore, it should include health education campaigns with emphasis on first aid in cases of accidents. One can speculate about the possibility of the child developing an inferiority complex, as a result of inadequately restored fractures in anterior teeth, which could be an important factor affecting the child's future success. A group of Brazilian adolescents with restored teeth due to enamel and dentin fractures was compared to adolescents without any traumatic dental injury[96]. The results, using the index of Oral Impacts on Daily Performances, showed that the treatment did not eliminate the impact on their daily living when compared to the results found by Côrtes et al.[30] in a group of children with non-treated enamel and dentin fractured teeth.

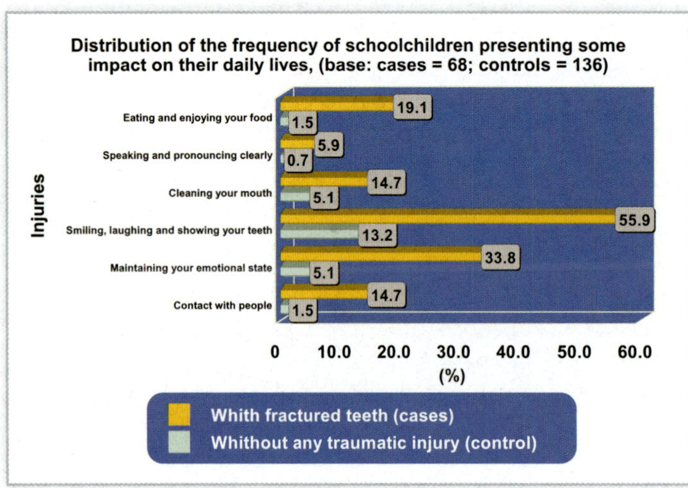


Graphic 24.9

## PART 2. Emergency Procedures in Traumatic Dental Injuries

### General Considerations

Traumatic injuries represent a frequent challenge to the dentists, and due to their acute nature must always be considered as an emergency. Clinical studies have demonstrated that these injuries represent one of the commonest causes of patients seeking medical emergency services[3,60,108,126].

The patient's initial approach plays a decisive role in the success of the treatment of traumatic injuries, a fact that confers a great responsibility to the professional providing this service. Nevertheless, according to Barret & Kenny[25], treatment decisions to resolve the injury are based on rare previous experiences, since the clinicians are not accustomed to emergency situations, in an area that is outside their routine practice. Hamilton et al.[69] concluded that the primary care services available for the treatment of traumatic dental injuries were inadequate and dentists presented insufficient knowledge to deal with emergencies. Since dental trauma represents one situation where dentists are called upon to make unscheduled diagnostic, the professional working in A&E department or public and private surgeries must be aware of the protocols established for the attendance of the emergencies[16].

need for follow-up visits make the patient confident and reassured. Instructions about dental insurance and the need to look for the specific modality claims need to be addressed immediately after the accident. In Brazil, some private schools have special insurance for accidents involving children and adolescents. Some companies provide coverage 365 days a year, inside or outside the school, for all sorts of accidents and can be driven anywhere in the world including a 24 hours assistance. Insurance companies have different plans all over the world, with some personal accident scheme.

Thus, for adequate emergency treatment, the professional must be aware of the epidemiology of dental trauma; the prevalence and distribution as well as clinical and socio-psychological implications. It is also necessary to know the histopathology of traumatic injuries and their sequelae. Finally, although there is no consensus about the aspects involved in emergency protocols, the clinician must be conscious of the development of all the therapeutic resources available. These considerations become particularly important at a time when concern is observed among dental professionals, about the increasing number of libel cases against dentists[100]. Nowadays the scientific development of Dentistry enables better probabilities of therapeutic success. Although there are few systematic reviews in subjects related to the treatment of traumatic dental injuries, a variety of resources exist to help dental professionals to apply Evidence Based Dentistry and keep up to date, to present the best care for the patient[114]. Good therapeutic results depend on multiple factors, for their success. Some of them are the professional's responsibility that must perform the most adequate procedures required. He/she must be skilled, must not perform clinical procedures for which he/she is not technically prepared. This affirmation draws one's attention to the fact that when attending an emergency, the professional plays an essential role in determining the success rate of the treatment. Thus, he/she must have broad knowledge of all areas of Dentistry, in order to make the diagnosis correctly and promptly determine the most adequate treatment plan. According to Dewhurst[56] a correct and immediate diagnosis, in addition to appropriate emergency attendance, will prevent the children and adolescent population from losing their incisors at an early stage of life, due to incorrect diagnosis by the dentist and inadequate emergency treatment.

## Subjective Examination

During the emergency visit, although important, the anamnesis is brief, and directed to obtaining specific information about the accident, history of previous traumatic dental injuries, and a brief medical history. Starting from the obvious questions such as name, age, address and telephone number is valuable to identify possible cerebral involvement. An adequate history shall include answers to WHEN, WHERE and HOW the accident occurred. The interval between the time of the accident (WHEN) and the treatment, significantly influences the prognosis of avulsions, luxations and root fractures with displacement, in addition to pulp exposures (Fig. 24.4A-B). Information about the location of the accident (WHERE), can be important for indicating tetanus prophylaxis, and allow the avulsed tooth, or fragments to be located. Data about the type of accident (HOW), can provide clues about the type, and the anatomical location of the injuries. A classic example is the blow to the chin that may cause fractures of premolars and molars (Fig. 24.5A-B), mandibular symphysis or condylar region (Fig. 24.6A-D).

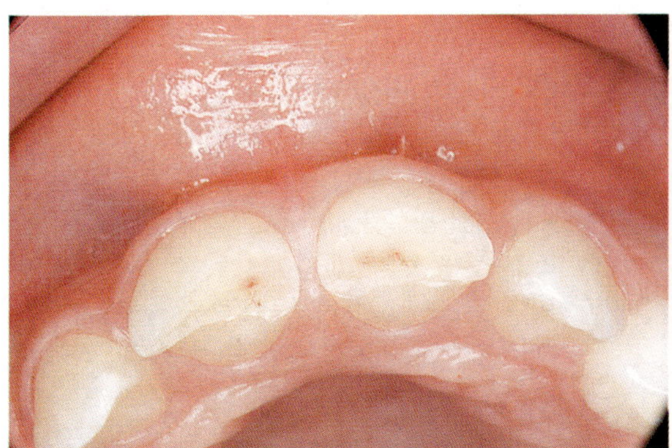

**Figure 24.4** - (**A**) Pulp exposure after short period of time in teeth #11 and #21. There is always the chance of performing conservative treatment.

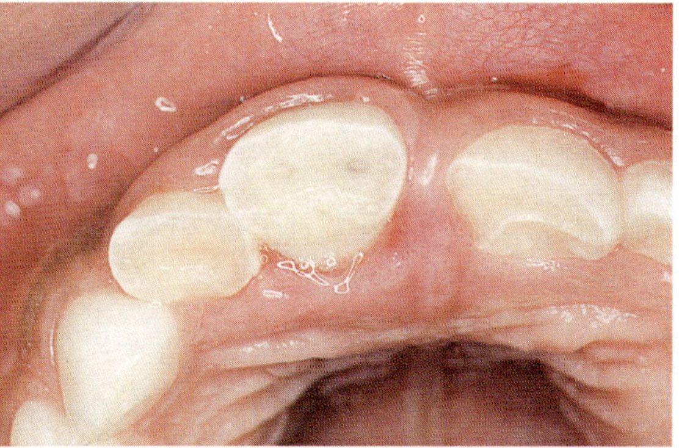

**Figure 24.4** - (**B**) Pulp exposure after long period of time in teeth #11 and 21. Inflammatory pulp alterations are a contraindication for conservative treatment.

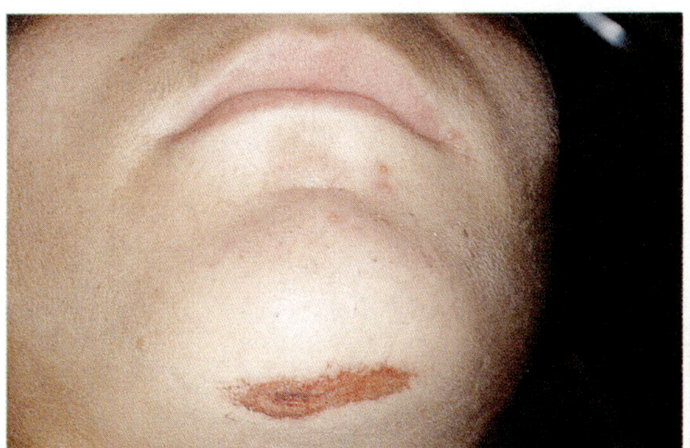

**Figure 24.5** - (**A**) An injury to the chin can result in indirect trauma in other dental or bone structures.

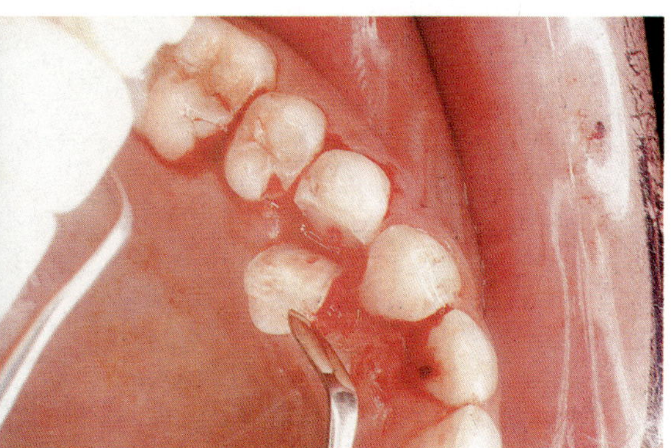

**Figure 24.5** - (**B**) Indirect trauma: crown-root fracture in tooth #14 and fracture of enamel and dentin in teeth #15 and #16, caused by the impact in the chin as demonstrated in Figure 24.5A.

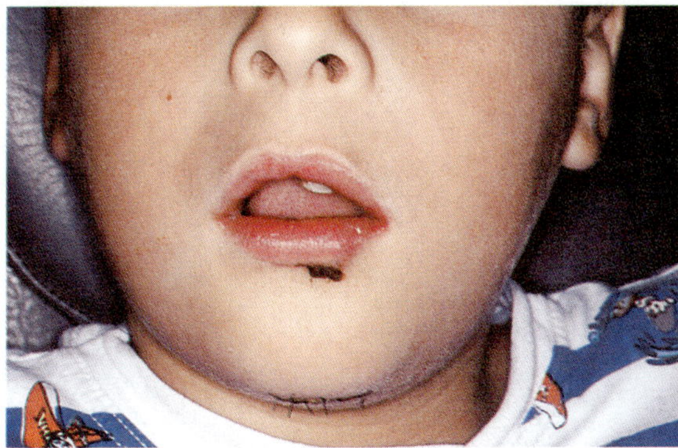

**Figure 24.6** - (**A**) Limitation of mouth opening in a 9 year-old child, after fracture of the two condyles caused by the impact to the chin.

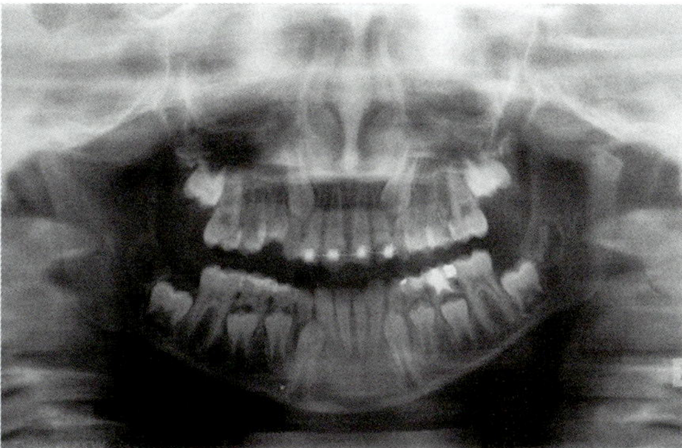

**Figure 24.6** - (**B**) Panoramic radiograph as complementary examination for diagnosis of condyle fracture. The fracture image is observed in the condyle, on the left side.

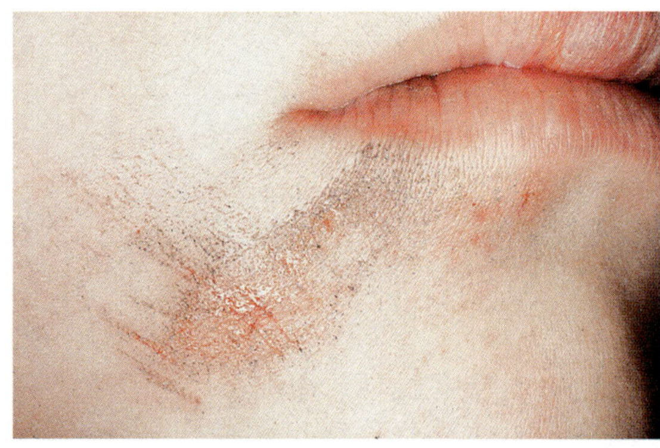

**Figure 24.8** - (**A**) Asphalt concrete particles can be incorporated during the healing process, and when left, they can cause a tattoo phenomenon.

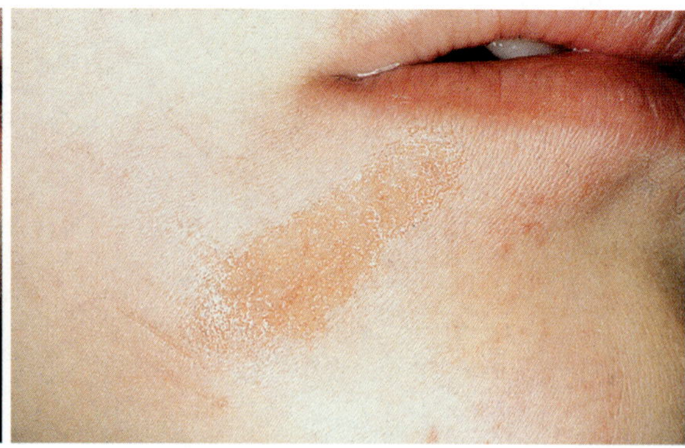

**Figure 24.8** - (**B**) Cleaning of the area with gauze soaked in saline or antiseptic solution.

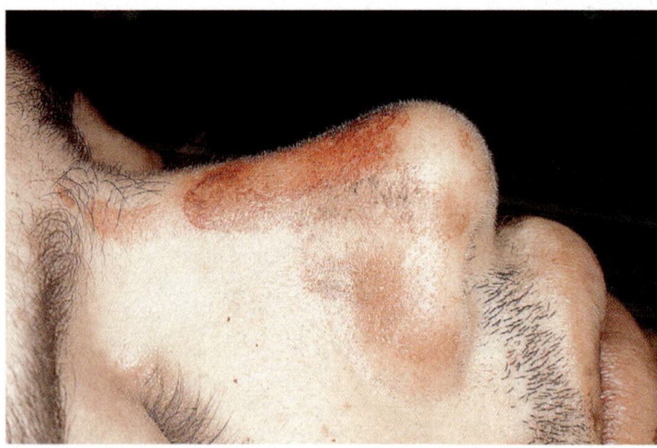

**Figure 24.9** - (**A**) Asphalt concrete particles already incorporated into the healing process.

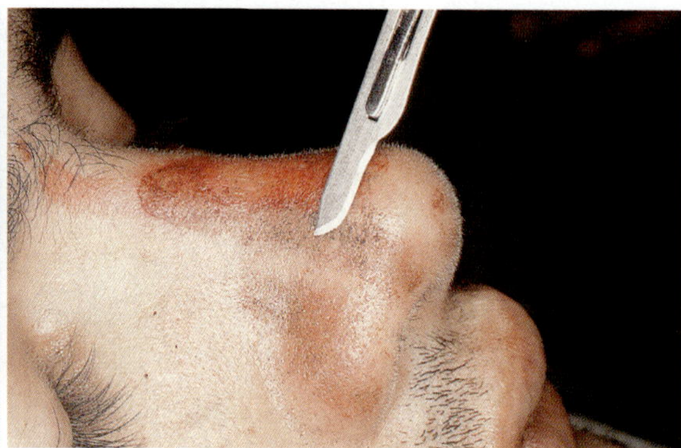

**Figure 24.9** - (**B**) Removal of the asphalt concrete particles through scraping, using a scalpel.

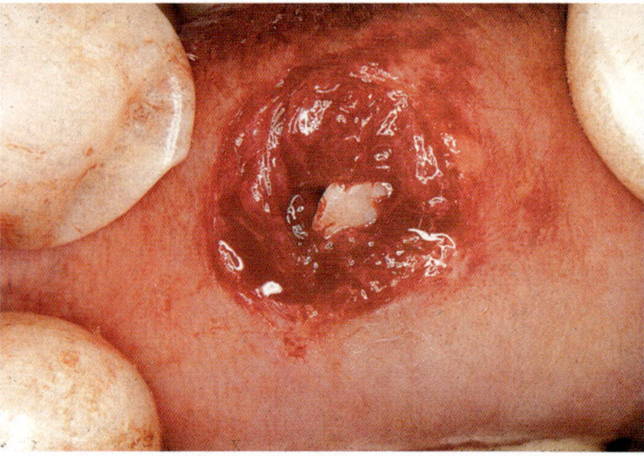

**Figure 24.10** - Tooth fragments identified and located in the lower lip, through visual exam and by palpation.

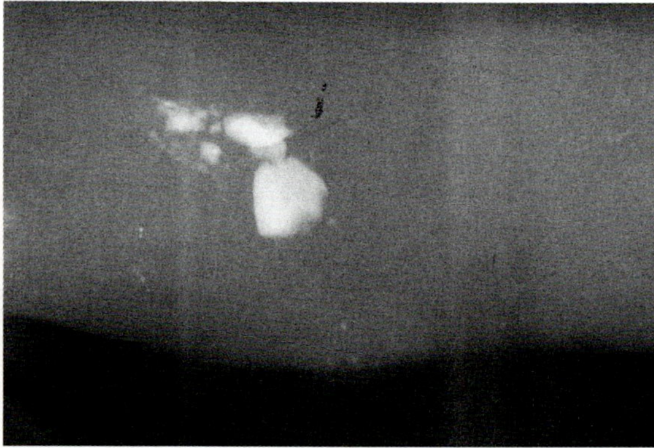

**Figure 24.11** - Observation of fragments of teeth by radiographic exam.

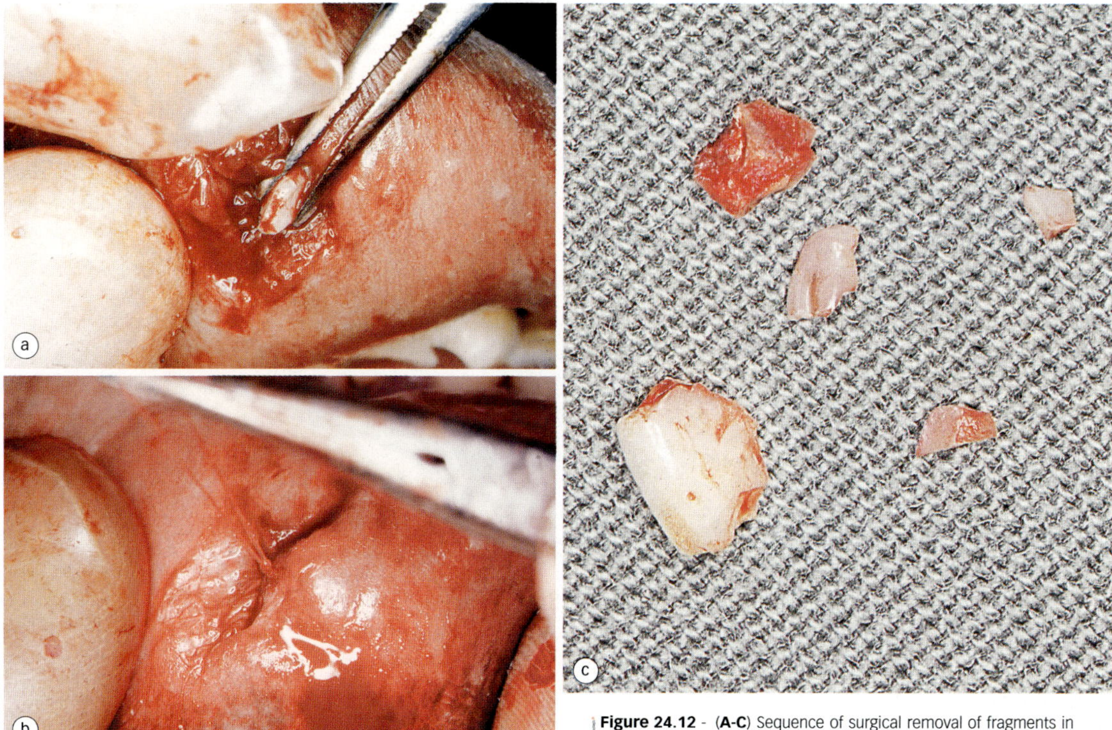


**Figure 24.12** - (**A-C**) Sequence of surgical removal of fragments in the lip.

## Evaluation and Treatment of Supporting Bone Injuries

Supporting bone injuries generally occur due to automobile accidents or violence. Due to their gravity and multiple natures, the patient usually seeks A&E department in hospitals. However, when the clinician is the first professional to be consulted, he/she must be capable of recognizing these injuries, and evaluating the need for referring the patient to a buccomaxillofacial surgeon, depending on the extent of the wounds.

*Fractures of the alveolar socket walls* are a frequent finding related to avulsions and luxations with displacements. Clinically they can be diagnosed by a cracking sound during palpation. Abnormal mobility of the socket wall is simultaneous with the mobility of the teeth. Treatment will be described in the section that deals with luxations.

*Fractures of the alveolar process* are generally situated beyond the apices, but in most cases involve the alveolar walls. They are easily diagnosed during clinical examination due to the simultaneous movement of a group of teeth when performing the mobility test. The treatment consists of a reduction of the fracture, and rigid splinting, maintained for a minimum period of 2 months (Fig. 24.13A-C).

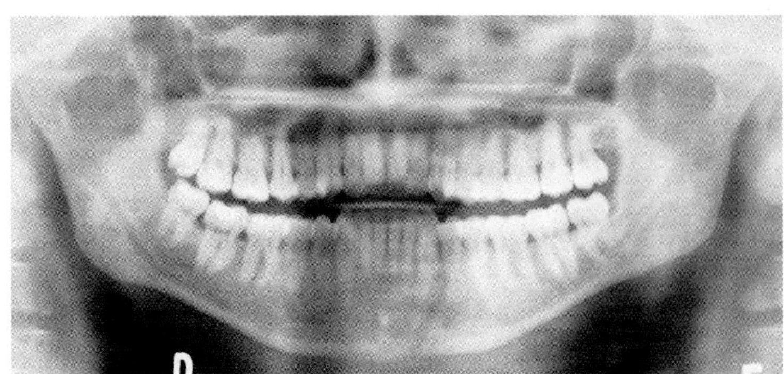

**Figure 24.16** - Panoramic radiograph evidenced the fracture at the chin, between teeth #33 and #34.

## Evaluation and Treatment of Dental Injuries

The clinical examination of affected teeth should be preceded by a careful cleaning of the region, with the intention of removing clots and debris. The presence and extension of the dental fractures and luxations, should be evaluated by visual inspection, palpation, tests of vertical and horizontal percussion and mobility. Sensibility tests should not be performed soon after the injury, because they do not reflect the real pulp condition at that time. Discolorations of the crown should also be considered with care, since they can be transitory. The absence of a tooth must be evaluated with attention, due to the possibility of it having been aspirated or swallowed. Finally, the radiographic exam will provide important data for the diagnosis and prognosis, such as rate of root formation, root fractures, injuries of the supporting structures and tooth displacements. According to Andreasen &; Andreasen[7], determining the presence and the direction of dental displacements and root fractures, depends on taking multiple radiographic exposures with different vertical and horizontal angulations of the central beam.

Not all injuries require immediate intervention during the emergency attendance. Some of them represent a minimum risk of pulp, periodontal and esthetic involvement, such as enamel infractions (Fig. 24.17), enamel fractures (Fig. 24.18) and concussion. However, in partial intrusive luxations (Fig. 24.19), any attempt to replace the tooth immediately will cause more damage to the supporting tissues. This occurs because the re-eruption is possible, particularly in teeth with incomplete root formation. However, clinical and radiographic controls should be performed carefully, so as to determine the exact time for orthodontic extrusion and/or endodontic treatment. In the case of total intrusion, teeth must be evaluated individually, because replacement is sometimes the best option.

The indicated methods for the treatment of injuries that need immediate intervention will be presented further on. It shall be emphasized that the same patient can present a complex set of conditions that require several concomitant procedures.

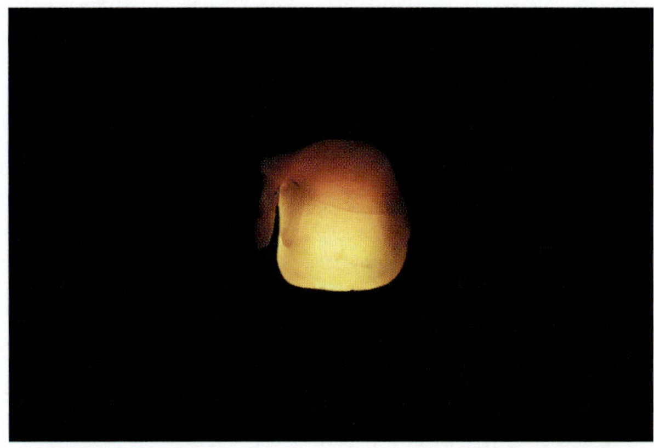

Figure 24.17 - Enamel infraction evidenced by a fiber optic light source.

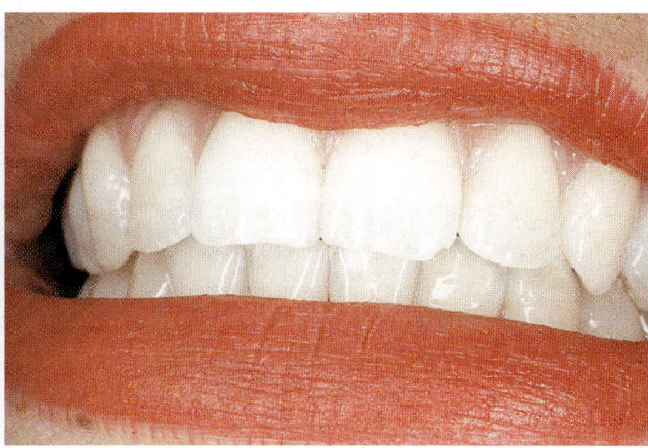

Figure 24.18 - Enamel fracture in the distal angle of tooth #21 that represents a minimum risk for the pulp, periodontal and esthetic involvement.

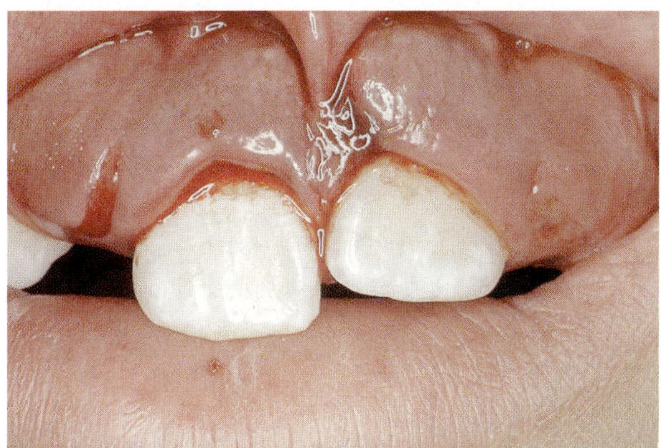

Figure 24.19 - Intrusion of tooth #21 – visualization of the small portion of the crown, in addition to the patient's information about the similarity of the position of the maxillary central incisors before the accident, facilitates the diagnosis.



## Crown Fracture involving Enamel and Dentin

Enamel and dentin crown fractures are characterized by the loss of coronal structure with the exposure of the dentin tubules (Fig. 24.20). Information available at present about pulp alterations has resulted mainly from the classic studies of Brannström[39] in the 1960s, which will be discussed in section 3 of this chapter. The presence of the fracture alone is not a determinant factor for the occurrence of pulp necrosis[26]. Clinically, the pulp exposure can determine dentinal sensitivity when eating, performing oral hygiene and even breathing. There is increased sensitivity in fractures adjacent to the pulp in immature permanent teeth. This is due to a higher number of dentinal tubules with larger diameter[96]. However, from the patient's point of view, the esthetic involvement can be the main reason for the emergency attendance. Thus, the treatment of the crown fracture involving enamel and dentin consists of esthetic restoration as soon as possible. Restoration with a composite resin represents a treatment alternative for these cases. A more feasible alternative, due to the new generation adhesive technology, is reattachment of the original crown fragment. Nothing is comparable with the natural tooth, particularly as regards the finishing and preservation of the shape, as well as the smoothness and brightness of the enamel, leading to better and long lasting esthetic

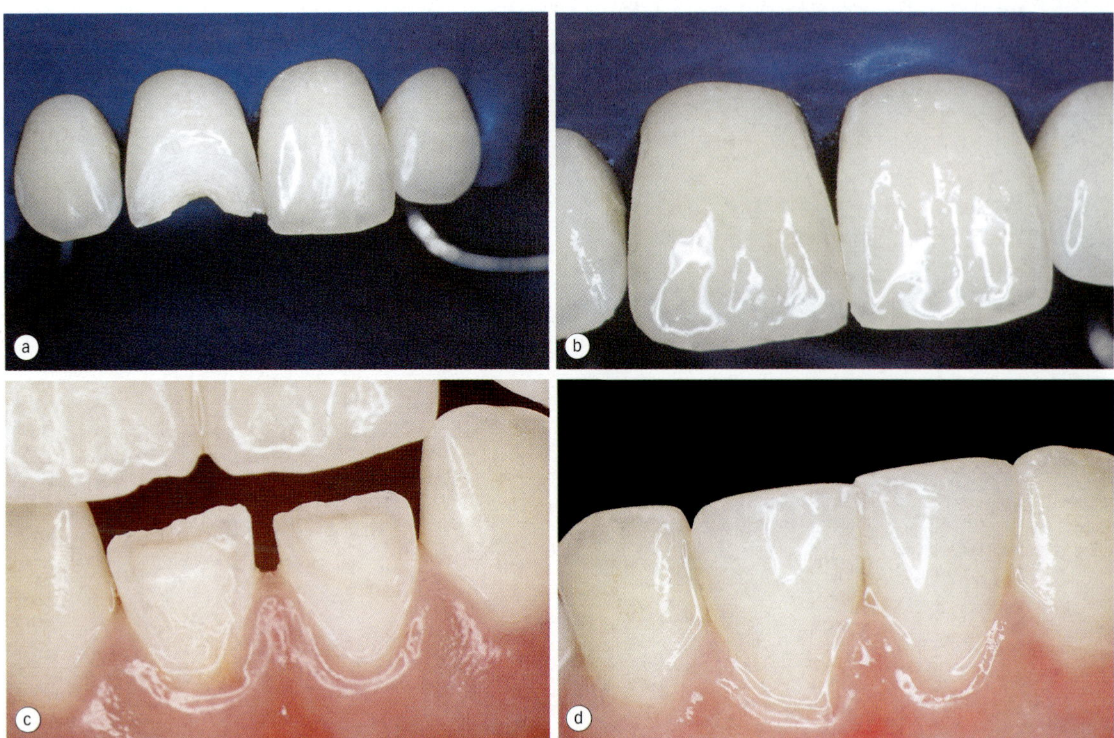


**Figure 24.23** - (**A**) Isolation with rubber dam and preparation of the bevel on a crown fracture involving enamel and dentin in tooth #11. (**B**) Restoration with composite resin. (**C-D**) Restoration with composite resin in fractured teeth #31 and #41. The patient did not take the fractured fragment.

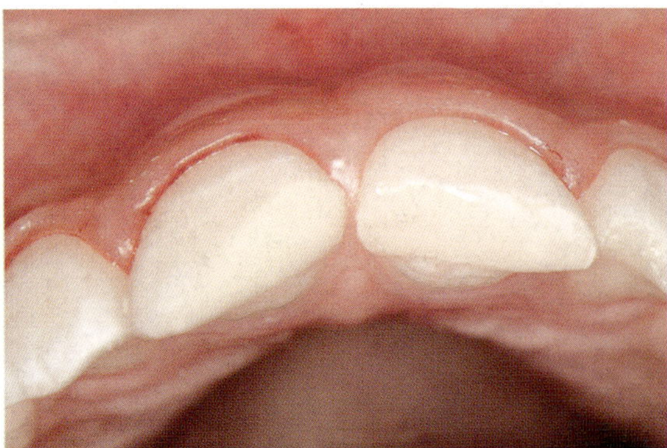

**Figure 24.24** - Crown fracture involving enamel and dentin – exposed dentin is protected with the use of light cured glass ionomer cement.

## Enamel and Dentin Crown Fracture with Pulp Involvement

In crown fractures with pulp involvement, in addition to loss of dental structure, dilaceration of the pulp tissue and its direct exposure to the oral environment occur (Fig. 24.25). In the period right after accidental exposure, the pulp develops an inflammatory response caused by bacterial agents and by-products from the tissue laceration. This process results in the formation of a hyperplasic tissue at the site of the exposure in an attempt to isolate the aggressors, mechanical trauma and microbial irritation[52]. This attempt may succeed, since the accidentally exposed pulp consists of normal tissue. Moreover, this type of fracture allows the inflammatory edema to be drained, minimizing the intra-pulp pressure[74]. Long periods of exposure can lead to a more intense inflammation, extending more deeply into the pulp tissue with formation of micro-abscesses and eventual necrosis. Thus, these injuries must receive treatment as soon as possible, since the main objective is to preserve the vital pulp tissue and provide conditions for forming a biological mineralized tissue barrier. Although the result of the conservative pulp treatment is satisfactory, some factors such as root development, presence of concomitant luxations and the patient's age, should be considered. Moreover, the clinical aspect of bleeding, including the fluidity and color can be decisive in indicating the treatment and must always be considered during the operative procedure (Fig. 24.26A-B; 24.27A-D).

It is well known that traumatic dental injuries occur in schoolchildren, affecting mainly the maxillary central incisors[42]. The stage of root development is a decisive factor in the choice of conservative treatment. At an early stage of development, when the vital pulp is exposed accidentally, any chosen procedure should allow apexogenesis. Thus the coronal affected portion of the pulp should be removed to allow continuity of physiological dentin deposition along the root canal walls, in addition to the completion of root apex closure. All efforts must be made to keep the tissue vital inside the root canal. The objective of the treatment is to eliminate the source of infection, obtain a mineralized tissue barrier at the site of the exposure, and allow root development to continue, with maturation of the dentin by the active odontoblasts[16,40,121]. Conservative treatment is the best alternative for children and adolescents, since removal of the pulp leaves thin root walls, thus increasing the risk of posterior root fractures in the cervical region[40,51,121] (Fig. 24.28A-B; 24.29A-B).

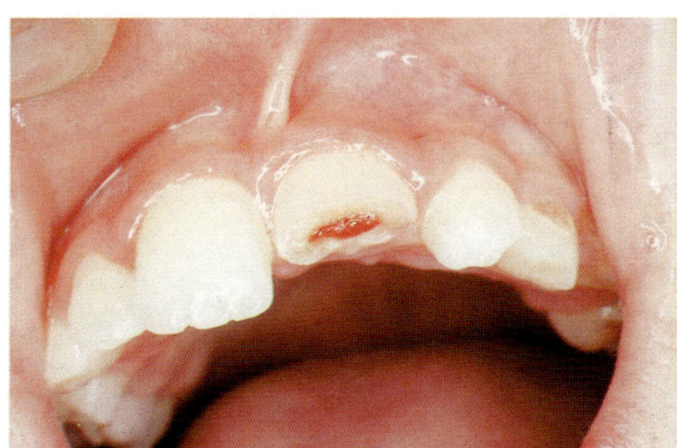

**Figure 24.25** - Crown fracture involving enamel and dentin, with pulp exposure in tooth #11 – in addition to the loss of dental structure, laceration of the tissue and its direct exposure to the oral environment occurred.

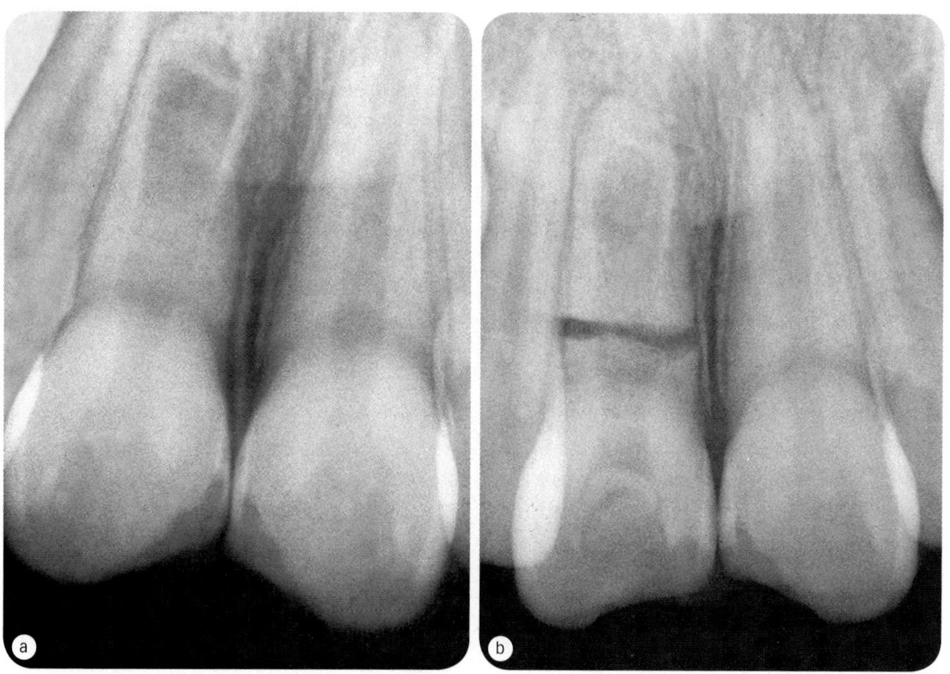


**Figure 24.28** - (**A**) Radiographic observation of mineralized barrier after apexification. (**B**) Root fracture of the cervical third caused by a second injury before filling the root canal system. The bad prognosis is due the position of the fracture.

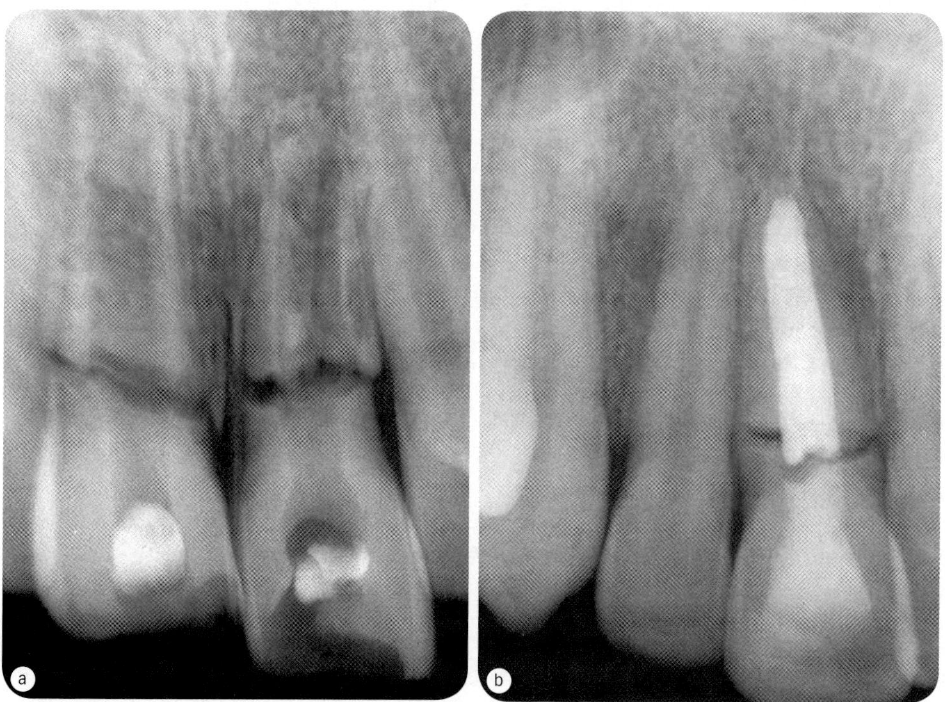


**Figure 24.29** - (**A**) Fracture of the cervical third in teeth #11 and #21, during root canal treatment. (**B**) Fracture occurred after the filling of the root canal system in tooth #21.

Concomitant luxation initially contraindicates conservative treatment, since it affects the apical neurovascular bundle, thereby compromising the pulp blood supply. This involvement, however, determines a different prognosis for teeth with complete root formation and immature teeth. In the latter, the apex is not completely formed, thus presenting a great capacity of maintaining pulp vitality, which favors more conservative procedures. Thus, the choice of treatment depends on the gravity of the lesion to the supporting tissues and on the stage of root formation[11,12,16]. The dimensions of the apical foramen and the high proliferative cellular activity of dental follicle and dental papilla in young permanent teeth allows repair, favoring the maintenance of vitality. However, this re-vascularization of the pulp tissue does not occur in mature teeth with completely closed apical foramen, thus contraindicating conservative treatment.

There are controversies about the age limit for indicating conservative treatment, but it is known that young pulp always presents great reparative capacity due to its abundance of cells and capillaries, in addition to an ample apical foramen that allows a favorable response. The increase in the number of fibers replacing the pulp cells in older individuals, as well as the reduction in pulp stroma by the deposition of mineralized tissue diminishes the regenerative capacity of pulp[32,38,112,116]. Although the safer option for adults is endodontic treatment, the response to conservative treatment can be sometimes favorable if the pulp is normal[62]. The presence of degenerative or inflammatory pulp alterations and periodontal involvement contraindicates these conservative procedures in elderly patients. Laboratory experiments with animals demonstrated a different response to the injury when the pulp of old rats was compared with that of young rats[88,110]. Therefore, the case selection of adult patients needs to be very rational and conscious, by both patient and professional, since results of animal experiments cannot be extrapolated to human beings.

A high rate of healing after conservative treatment has been reported, with a frequency varying from 72 to 96%[34,41,46,50,65,66,68,74,82,102,107]. The criteria for evaluating the success of the treatment are absence of symptoms, positive response to pulp sensibility tests (in cases of pulp capping and curettage), continuity of root development, absence of radiographic signs of periapical lesions and inflammatory root resorption, and radiographic observation of the mineralized tissue barrier[16,50,82] (Fig. 24.30A-C). The importance of post-treatment clinical and radiographic control is evident, in order to observe normality in the long term (minimum of 3-to-4 years).

The great success of conservative treatment is related to the use of calcium hydroxide[16, 17, 40, 49, 50, 66, 68, 73, 82, 108] as it can be verified in Chapter 20. Teuscher & Zander[113] and Zander[125] were the first authors to indicate calcium hydroxide as material for pulpotomy, and the first indication of the technique was presented by Kaiser[79] and Frank[63], later published as "Frank's technique"[64]. Since then, several studies have demonstrated this as the ideal material to promote the formation of a mineralized tissue barrier. Calcium hydroxide on the healthy pulp tissue promotes a superficial necrosis that results in calcification. The pulp cell response to the irritation is the production and secretion of a collagen matrix that later mineralizes, creating the barrier[58].

Some publications defended the possibility of performing restorations with the adhesive system directly on the pulp exposed by traumatic dental injury[22,80,81]; however they lacked a sound basis, as the evaluation of the results lacked evidence based on histopathologic findings for a precise indication of the proposed treatment.

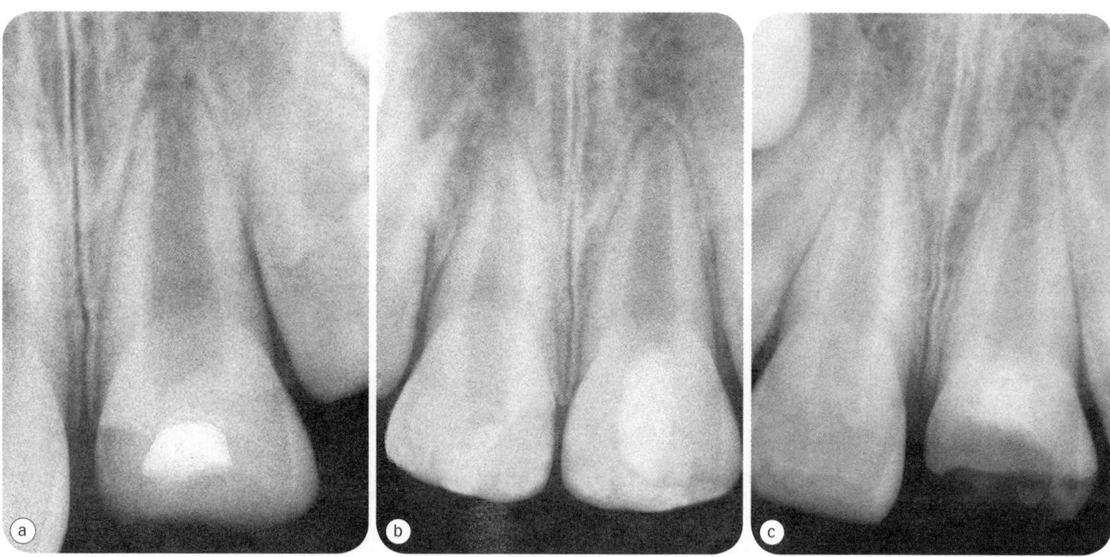


**Figure 24.30** - (**A**) Radiographic view of tooth #21 after pulpotomy due to pulp exposure. The patient was taken for treatment 1 hour after the accident. Note the incomplete root development with open apex. (**B**) Radiographic view 2 months later. Note the continuity of the root development and radiopaque area in the cervical region, showing the formation of the mineralized tissue barrier. (**C**) Radiographic aspect 2 years later. Note the continuity of the root development with apical closure and maturation of the radicular dentin, absence of radiographic signs of periapical alterations and inflammatory root resorptions. At this time, the patient fractured the tooth again.

On the other hand, studies of Hebling[71], Lanza[85] and Pereira et al.[98] demonstrated evident histological differences between the pulp response to capping with calcium hydroxide and adhesive systems. Pulps submitted to calcium hydroxide capping were normal in a period of 45 days, while those submitted to the action of the adhesive system All Bond 2, demonstrated chronic inflammation in periods of 7, 14, 30, 45 and 60 days, suggesting that the resin within the pulp induced a foreign body reaction. Moreover, there was absence of a mineralized tissue barrier in the cases submitted to the action of the adhesive[71].

All these new materials have been tested for use in direct pulp capping, the majority of the results being based on histological findings in laboratory animals. Studies conducted in primate and rat teeth showed pulp healing and the formation of a dentinal bridge. Although these results are favorable as regards the formation of mineralized tissue barrier, further investigations are required before using the materials in human teeth. A recent review showed that adhesive systems are well accepted when applied on human dentin, but not when directly applied on the pulp: they result in inflammation, delay healing, and do not allow the formation of a mineralized tissue barrier. The application of adhesive materials directly on the exposed pulp is very controversial. Again, the results observed in the teeth of animals cannot be extrapolated to the clinical conditions of human teeth. Thus, the authors concluded that adhesive and acid substances are contraindicated for direct application on vital pulp[44].

The studies about MTA (Mineral Trioxide Aggregate) for use directly on the exposed pulp seem promising, because the material allows the formation of the mineralized tissue barrier with little aggression to the pulp[1,2,21,59,61,106,115,118], however the clinical application of the types presented on the market (gray and white Pro-root MTA and MTA Angelus) need better evidence to be used in human teeth in vivo. There is some concern that when used in anterior teeth for the curettage technique (resection of part of the coronal portion of the pulp), pigments inherent to the composition of the material could be released from the mixture and penetrate through the dentinal tubules, resulting in crown discoloration. Up to date the literature is replete of case reports and animal research that do not substantiate the use of MTA. It lacks evidence based research with appropriate methodologies to investigate its benefits in conservative treatment.

Histological substantiation of positive results with the use of the calcium hydroxide on exposed pulps is evident in the literature as observed in Chapter 20. The clinician needs to be aware of the scientific basis presented for indicating new materials for use directly on the pulp tissue. Results based only on clinical applications of a few cases must be considered with strict limitation, because Dentistry based on biological evidence is the great ally of professional success.

### Direct pulp capping

The direct pulp capping can be indicated in small pulp exposures treated a few hours after the trauma. In experimental studies this period was defined as a maximum of 24 hours[47,72,99]. However these results may be analyzed with caution. The treatment starts after rubber dam apposition, preferentially without the use of clamps. The small area of pulp exposure is rubbed with a solution of calcium hydroxide until complete hemostasis, and dried with small cotton balls. Subsequently protection with calcium hydroxide pro-analysis paste (PA) with distilled water vehicle is applied, and then covered with calcium hydroxide cement followed by a layer of light cured glass ionomer cement. It is believed that in small exposures treated after a short period of time, the superficial necrosis caused by the calcium hydroxide is not affected by the presence of the granulation tissue, resulting from the tissue laceration and exposure to the oral environment. Thus, calcium hydroxide acts on the healthy pulp tissue, in addition to eliminating bacteria present at the exposure site. Nevertheless, the indication of direct pulp capping is restricted, because the material interferes with the adaptation, when the chosen technique is reattachment of the crown fragments. It can also compromise the esthetics of composite restorations, depending on the thickness of the material. In cases in which the best indication is pulp capping, a dentinal groove should be prepared to accommodate the material (Fig. 24.31A-C).

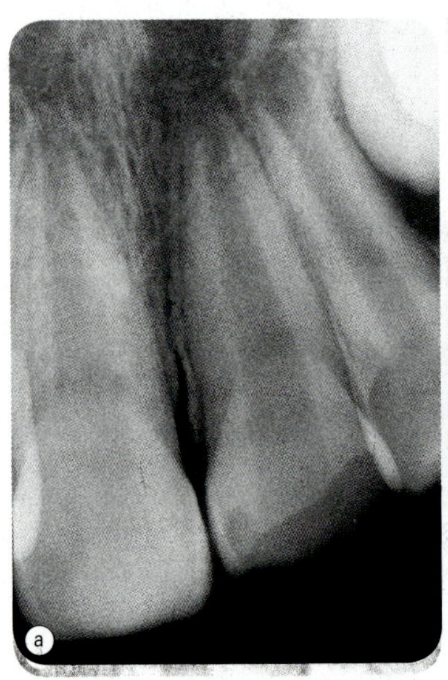

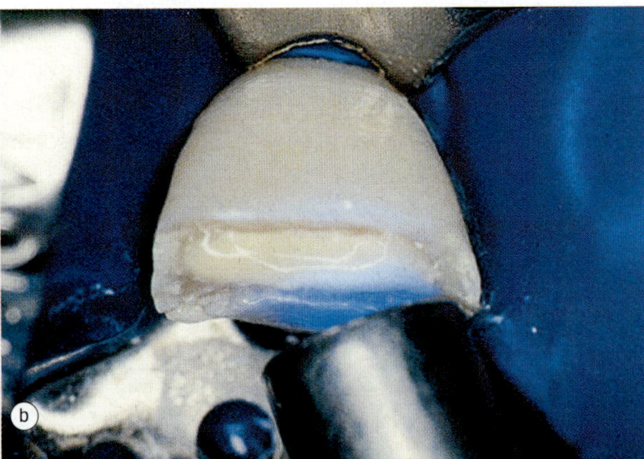

**Figure 24.31** - **(A)** Radiographic aspect of the crown fracture with pulp exposure. **(B)** Direct capping of the small pulp exposure and adjacent dentin with a calcium hydroxide paste and cement, covered by light polymerized glass ionomer cement.

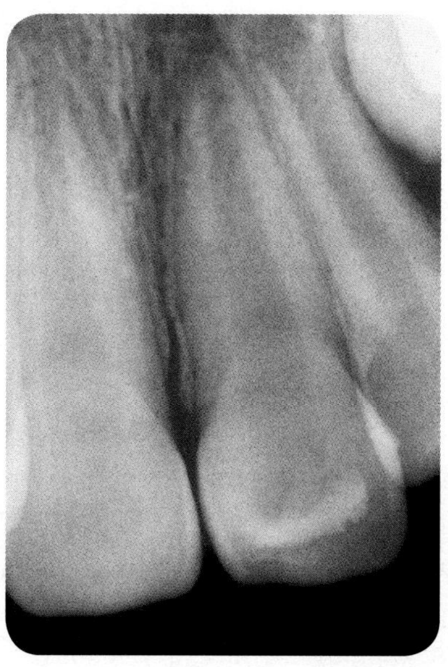

**Figure 24.31C** - Radiographic aspect after the fragment bonding. Note the presence of the radiopaque material in the groove made in the fractured fragment.



**Partial pulpotomy (Pulp curettage)**

Partial pulpotomy (pulp curettage) is indicated in pulp exposures, in which the small extent does not justify performing pulpotomy, but the time elapsed between the time of the accident until treatment, contraindicates direct pulp capping; in other words, the recommended time has passed. It initially consists of enlarging the exposed area with a spherical diamond bur under refrigeration or abundant irrigation with sterile saline solution. Next, the pulp tissue is removed with sharp and small curettes 2 mm below the area of exposure: it is supposed that the pulp is free of infection at this level[49]. After hemostasis by irrigation with sterile saline solution, the irrigation is followed with calcium hydroxide solution and the area is dried with small cotton pellets. The aim of this maneuver is to expose the healthy pulp tissue, and then place the paste of calcium hydroxide PA in a distilled water vehicle, covered with calcium hydroxide cement and a layer of light cured glass ionomer cement, the composite restoration or reattachment of the crown fracture is performed in the same session (Fig. 24.32A-C to 24.35A-B).

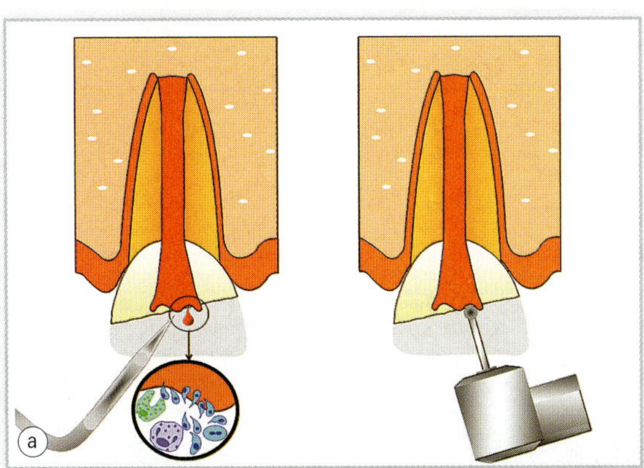


**Figure 24.32** - (**A**) Schematic illustration of the exploration and subsequent magnification of the exposed area with a spherical diamond bur. Adjusted from Andreasen & Andreasen[16]. (**B**) Incisal view of the crown fracture, clinically evidencing a small pulp exposure, treated in a short period of time after the injury. (**C**) Enlargement of the exposure with a spherical diamond bur to allow the curette to penetrate.

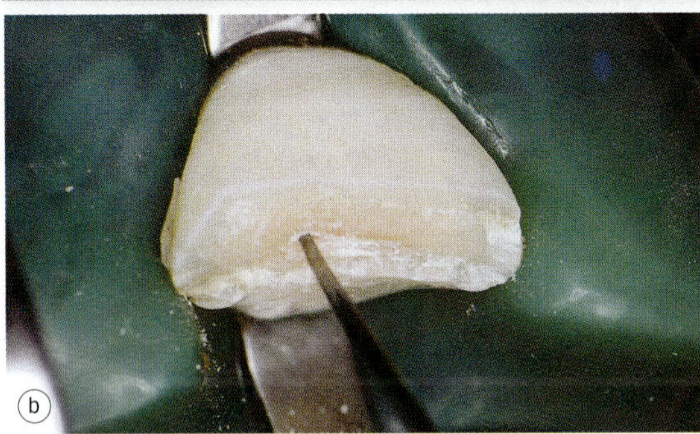


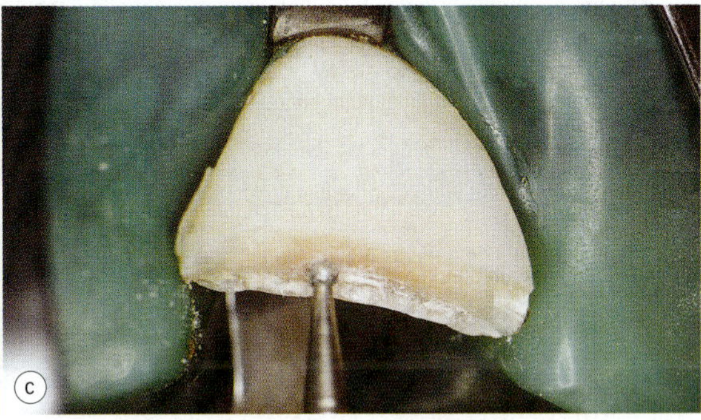


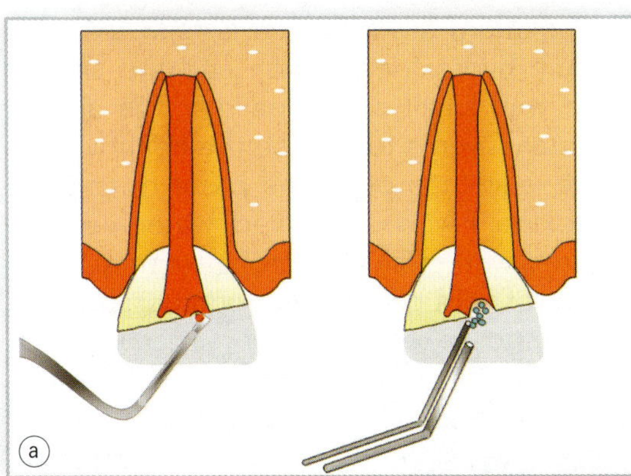


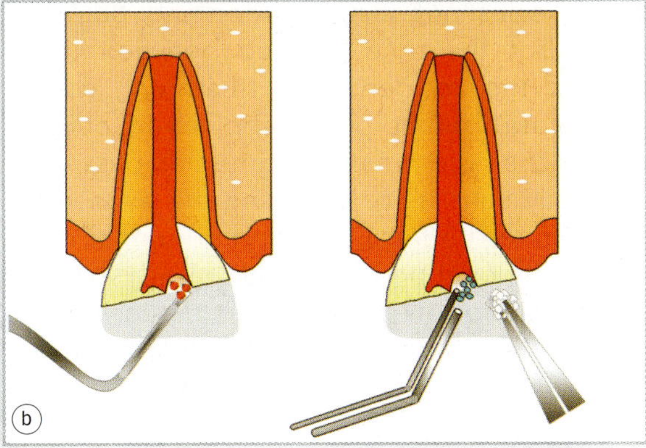


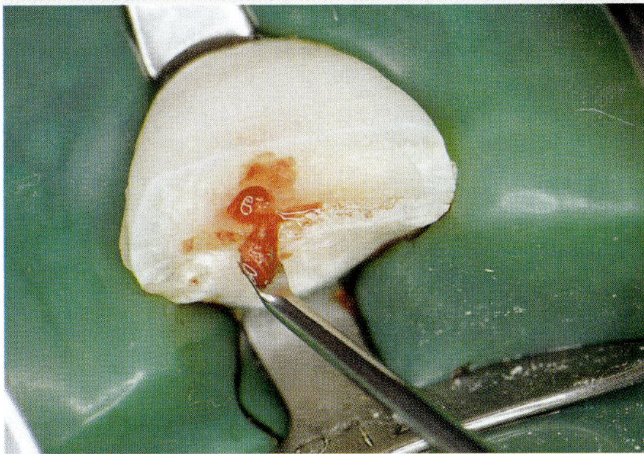

**Figure 24.33** - (**A-B**) Schematic illustration of pulp curettage, deepening the area of exposure by 2mm. After initial irrigation with sterile saline solution, followed by a calcium hydroxide solution, the pulp tissue should be dried with sterilized cotton pellets. (**C**) Visualization of the pulp tissue, after incision with a sharp curette.

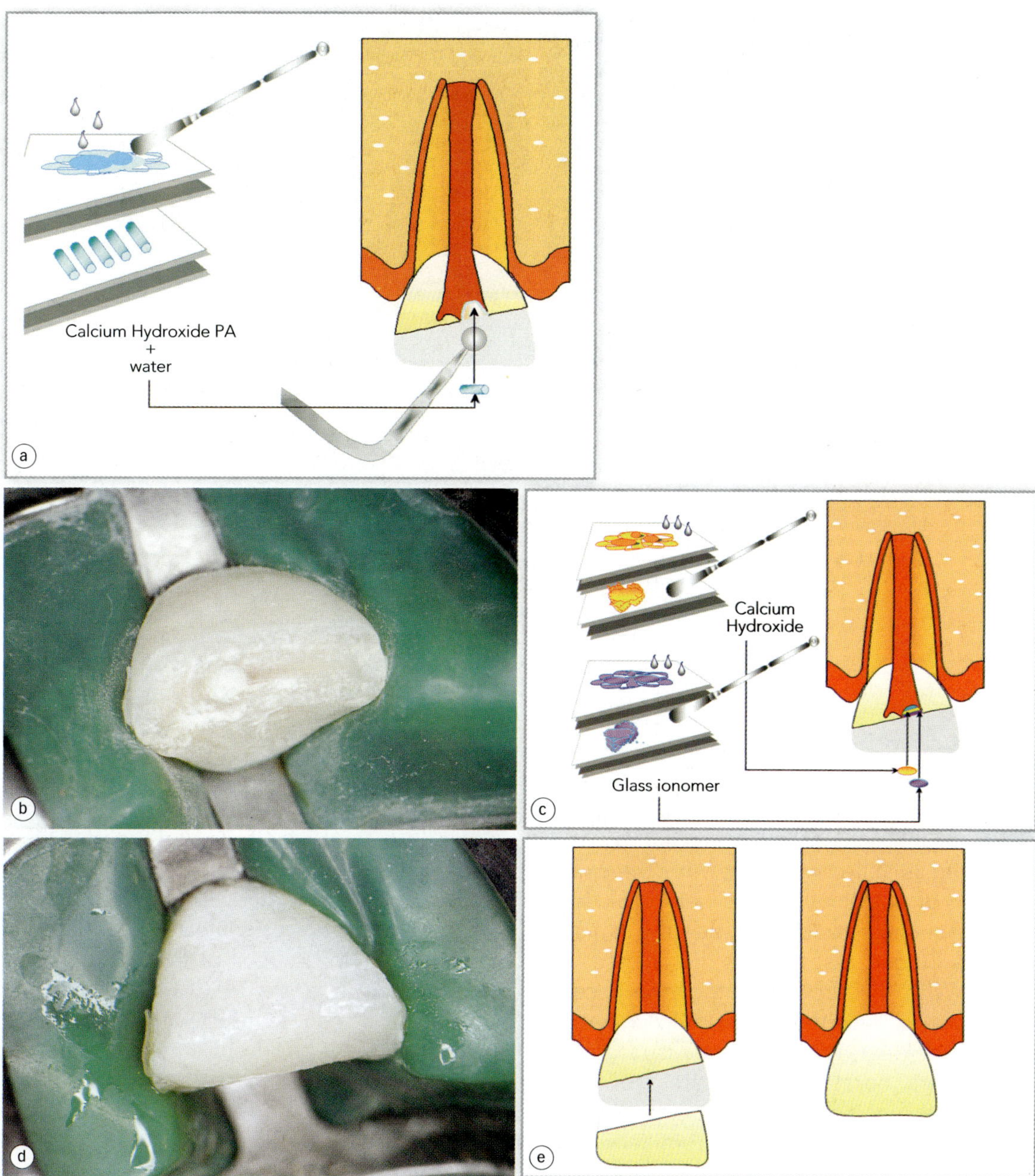


**Figure 24.34 -** (**A**) Schematic illustration of calcium hydroxide PA placement over the pulp tissue. All excess should be removed to avoid influencing the adaptation of the restorative material. (**B**) A layer of calcium hydroxide paste PA. is located on the pulp tissue. After this, apply a layer of calcium hydroxide cement to improve the seal and protection of the exposed area. (**C**) Schematic illustration of calcium hydroxide cement and light cured glass ionomer cement placement. (**D**) Temporary restoration with light cured glass ionomer cement. (**E**) Schematic illustration of the restoration performed immediately after the conservative treatment.

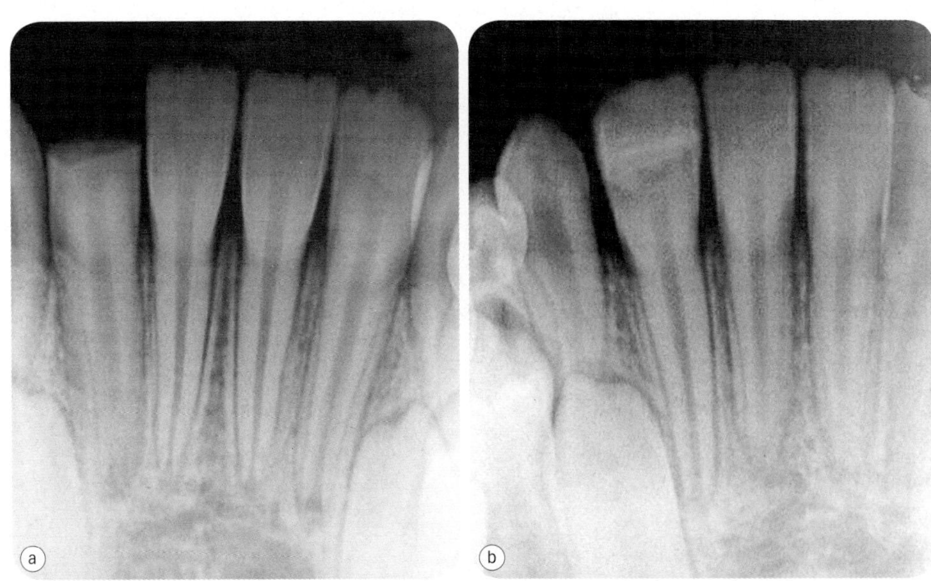

**Figure 24.35** - (**A**) Radiographic aspect of the crown fracture with pulp exposure in tooth #41. (**B**) Radiographic image of tooth #41 after pulp curettage and fragment bonding.

## Pulpotomy

Pulpotomy is indicated in cases in which large exposure of the pulp tissue occurs, and the time elapsed until the time of the treatment is still compatible with the preservation of pulp health. This period of time must be as short as possible, bearing in mind that the longer it is, the less the chances of repair. With the tooth isolated, the access is performed, and the whole pulp chamber is cleaned. Next, the pulp tissue is removed using sharp curettes, which are designed to allow a precise cut approximately 1mm below the cervical level. Anatomically, the incisors do not present a defined delimitation between the pulp chamber and root canal. Thus a great deal of precision is required when cutting the pulp to avoid its displacement in the apical foramen. This would result in a lesion to the apical neurovascular supply, thereby compromising circulation, which would lead to an inadequate response to conservative treatment. This procedure should be followed by abundant irrigation with saline solution until homeostasis is achieved, followed by drying with small sterilized cotton pellets. After that, the remaining pulp tissue is protected with calcium hydroxide paste PA, in a distilled water vehicle, and then covered with calcium hydroxide cement and light cured glass ionomer cement, filling approximately half of the pulp chamber. In the same way as with partial pulpotomy, the restorative procedure must preferably be performed in the same session (Fig. 24.36A-K).

Figures 24.37A-C show the radiographic aspect of the mineralized tissue barrier formed after conservative treatment. Strict radiographic control must be maintained for 3-to-4 years (Fig. 24.38A-C to 24.40A-C).

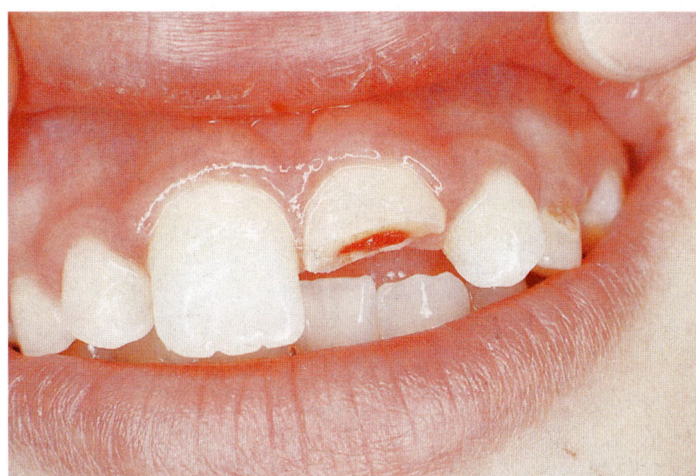

**Figure 24.36A** - Buccal view of the crown fracture, with exposed and hyperplasic pulp. The extent of the exposed tissue and the time elapsed after the trauma indicates the pulpotomy.



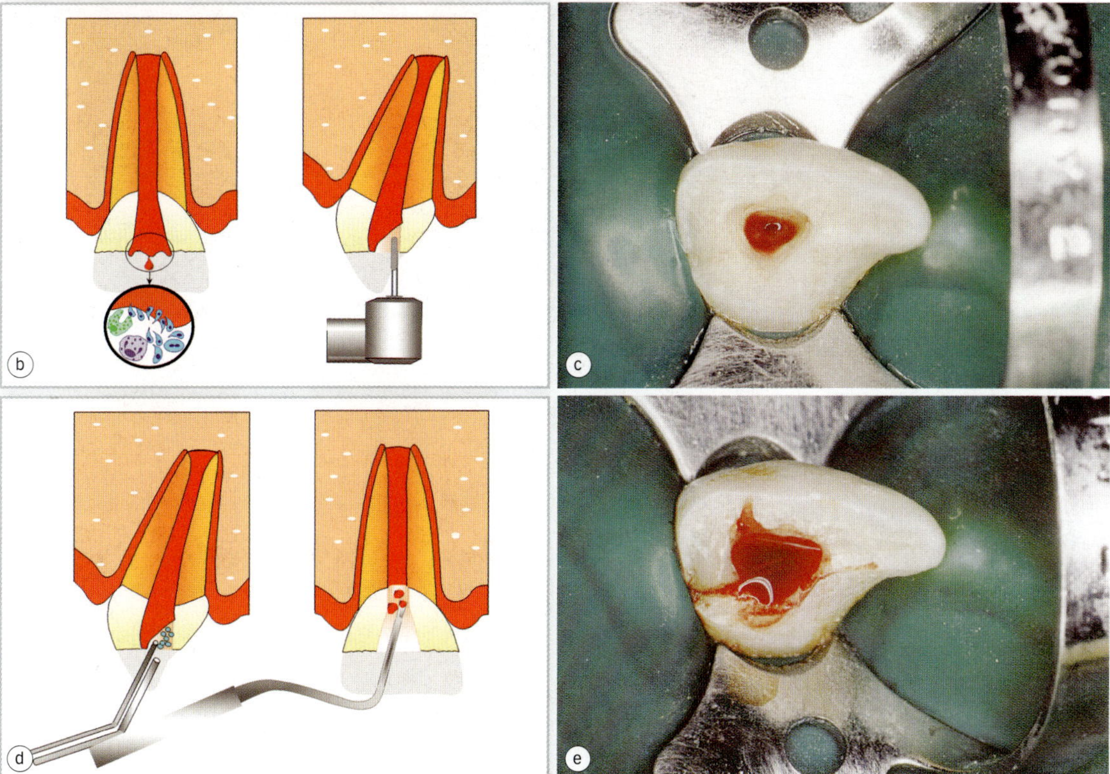


**Figure 24.36** - (**B**) Schematic illustration of the coronal access for pulpotomy (Adjusted from Andreasen & Andreasen[16]). (**C**) Access to the pulp chamber, removing every diverticulum in a tooth with an extensive pulp exposure. (**D**) Schematic illustration of the amputation of the pulp tissue up to the cervical limit and concomitant irrigation to avoid blood inside the pulp chamber. (**E**) Amputation of the pulp tissue below the cervical limit using a specific, sharp curette. At this time "healthy" bleeding can be noted.

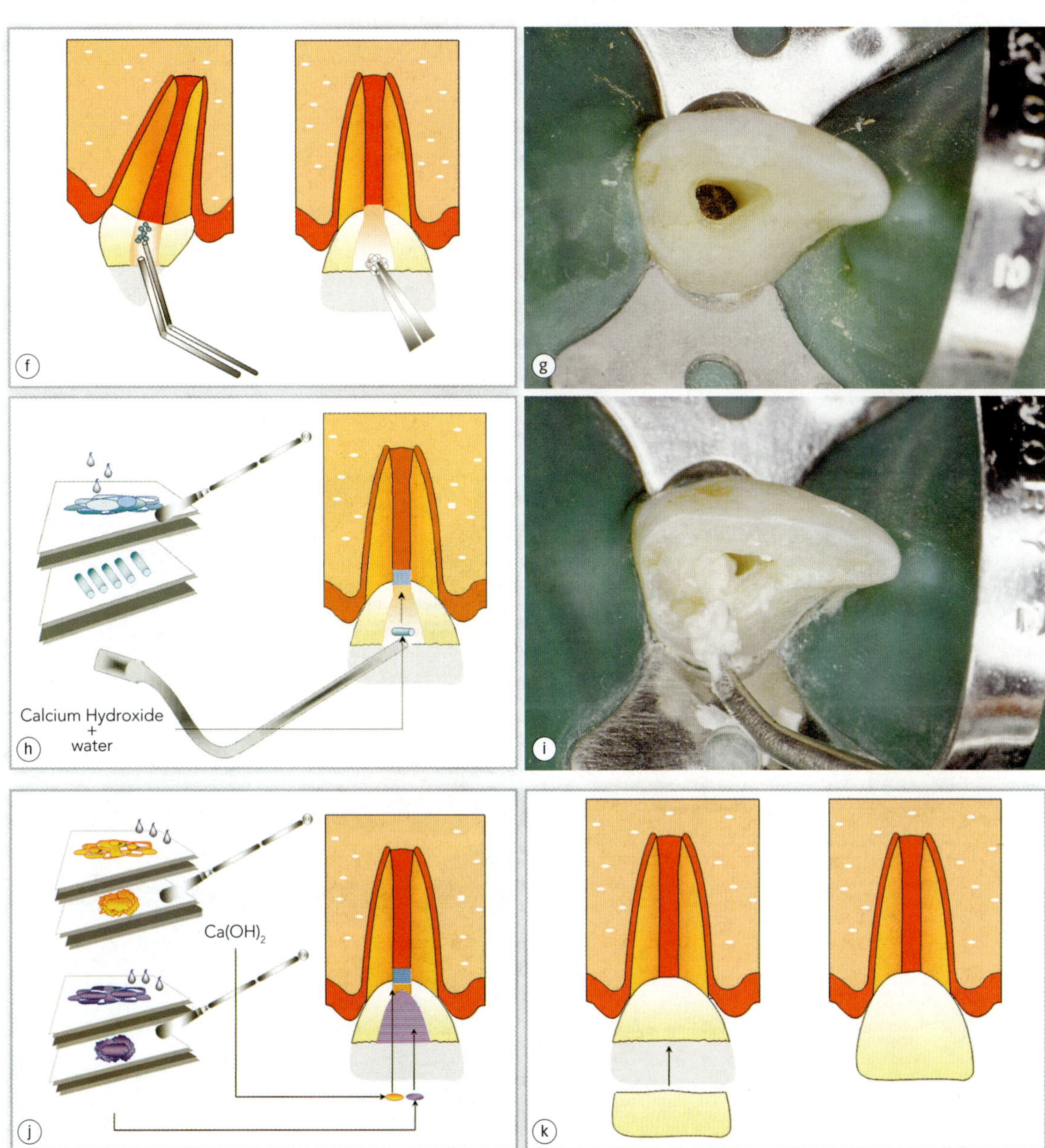


**Figure 24.36** - (**F**) Schematic illustration of hemostasis obtained with abundant irrigation and compression with sterilized cotton pellets. (**G**) Aspect of the pulp tissue after hemostasis. (**H**) Schematic illustration of placing the calcium hydroxide paste in a sterilized water vehicle, on the pulp tissue. (**I**) Protection of the remaining tissue with calcium hydroxide PA paste with distilled water vehicle, covered with a layer of the calcium hydroxide cement, followed by light cured glass ionomer cement. (**J**) Schematic illustration showing a layer of calcium hydroxide cement followed by the filling of the pulp chamber with light cured glass ionomer cement. (**K**) The restoration should preferably be performed during the same session.

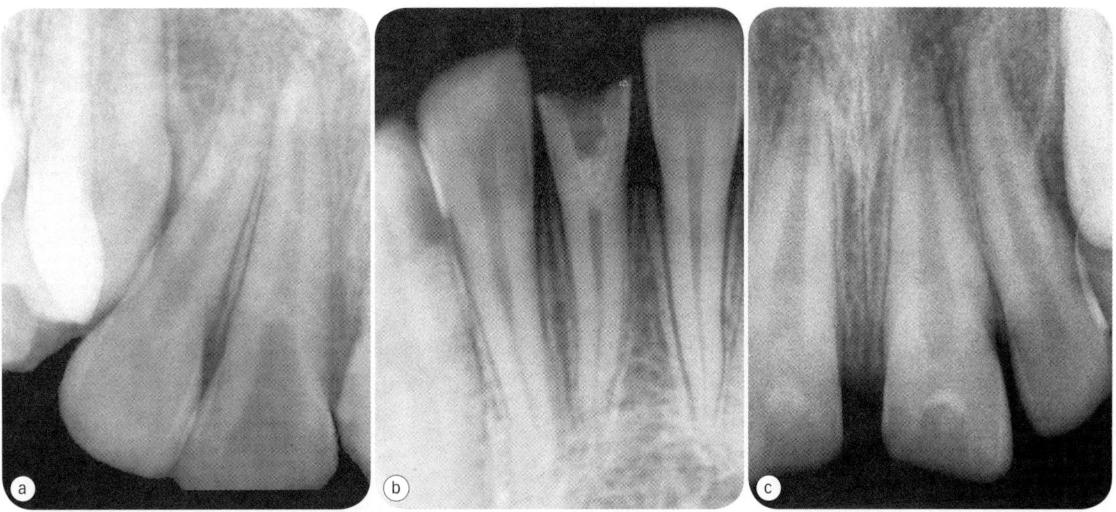

**Figure 24.37** - (**A-C**) Radiographic images of the mineralized barrier formed 2 months after conservative treatment.

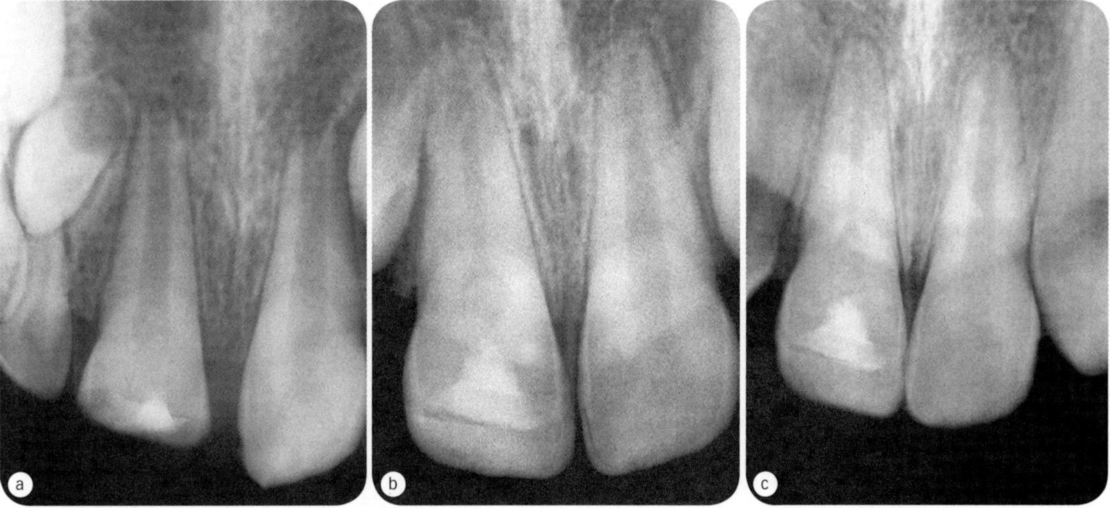

**Figure 24.38** - (**A-C**) Sequence of a radiographic follow-up 7 years after conservative treatment. Note the obliteration of the root canal, without compromising the success of the treatment.

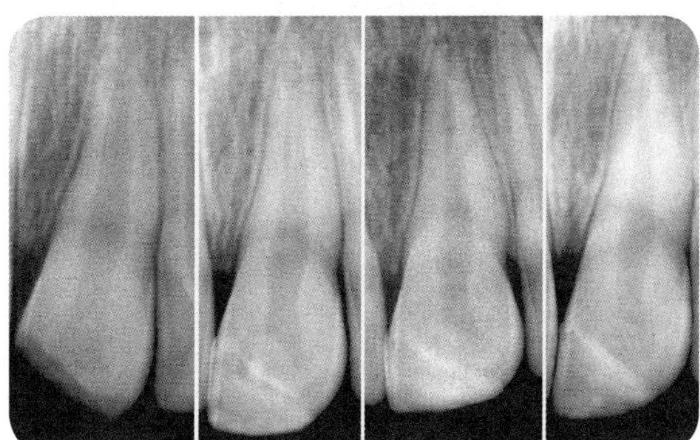

**Figure 24.39** - Sequence of a radiographic follow-up 4 years after the conservative treatment.

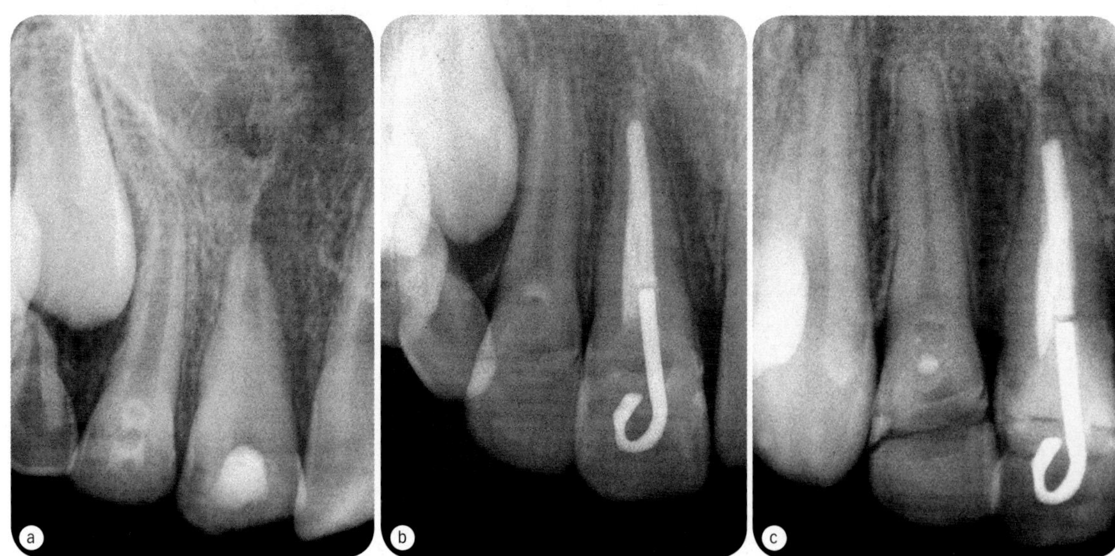

**Figure 24.40** - (**A-C**) Sequence of radiographic control up to 15 years after the conservative treatment.

### Restorative treatment

The restoration alternatives for this type of injury follow the same standards as those mentioned for enamel and dentin fractures, and must be performed immediately after the pulp therapy. Only an adequate seal will guarantee the success of the conservative treatment[90]. If there are impediments such as: lack of time, bleeding due to injuries to soft or supporting tissues, stress and unfavorable psychological conditions, the professional will perform a temporary restoration, using a specific material that produces excellent marginal sealing. In these situations, it is important for the success of the treatment to protect the exposed dentin with calcium hydroxide and light cured glass ionomer cement, since it avoids marginal leakage of bacteria and the diffusion of their toxins[31,48,95].

### Crown-root Fractures

Crown-root fractures involve enamel, dentin and periodontal ligament tissues, and may be associated or not to a pulp exposure. They start in the crown, and extends longitudinally through the pulp chamber to the subgingival area and the alveolar bone crest. They are characterized by the invasion of the biologic width. They occur more frequently in anterior teeth and buccal or oral cusps of premolars and molars in cases of indirect traumatic injury. The coronal fragment is sustained by the periodontal ligament fibers presenting displacement and mobility (Fig. 24.41A-B). When there is pulp exposure, pain is a characteristic symptom associated with fragment mobility. In these cases, the treatment consists of immediate pulpectomy followed by temporary reattachment of the fragment with composite resin (Fig. 24.42A-B). The endodontic treatment is performed in one visit. If there is no pulp exposure, intervention is limited to immobilization of the fragment. The aim is to improve the initial condition preventing the entry of granulation tissue into the fracture line, to adequately plan the best alternative for future restorative procedures. The greatest difficulty in treating these injuries, is to restore the biologic width, which frequently requires different treatment alternatives: gingival and osseous surgery to expose adequate amount of tooth structure for a crown margin; orthodontic or surgical extrusion of the root, exposing the fracture site sufficient for restoring the tooth; combine orthodontic extrusion and periodontal gingival and osseous surgery; reattachment of the fragment even with invasion of biological width; removing the crown, replacement of a fixed bridge across the space and retain the submerged root with its vital pulp[16,24].



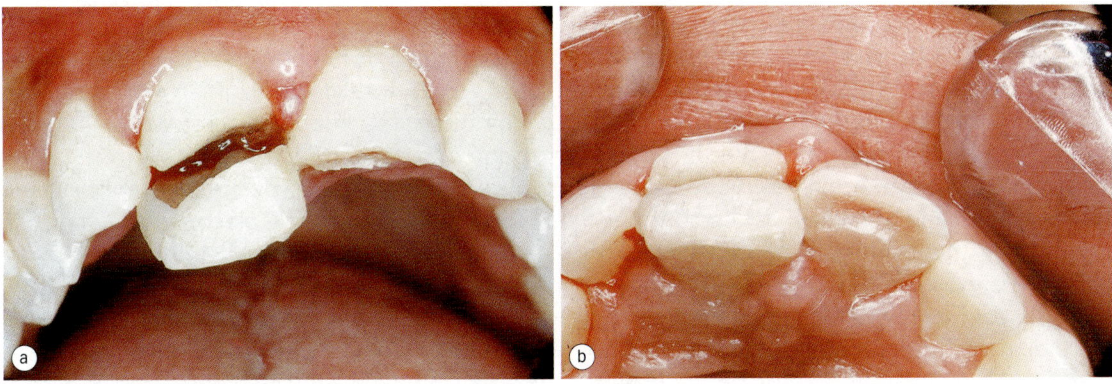

**Figure 24.41** - (**A**) Buccal view of the crown-root fracture in tooth #11 – Note the presence of the pulp exposure and profuse bleeding. (**B**) Incisal view of the fracture – note that despite the displacement, the fragment of the crown is still in place, maintained by the periodontal ligament fibers on the palatine side.

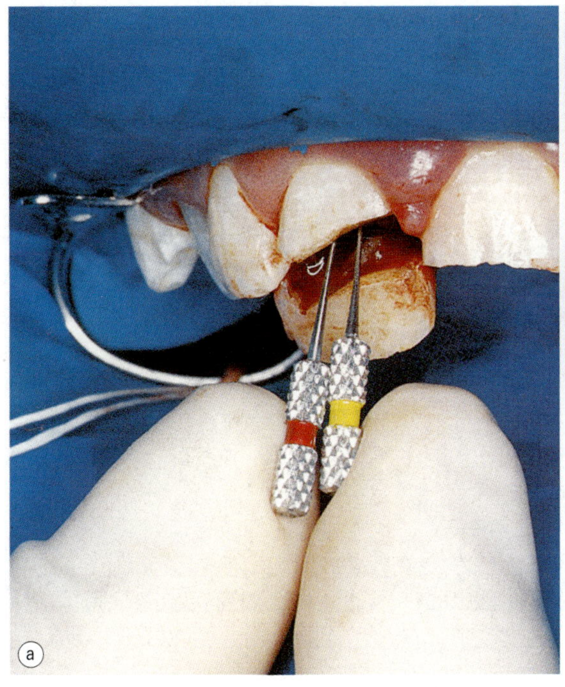

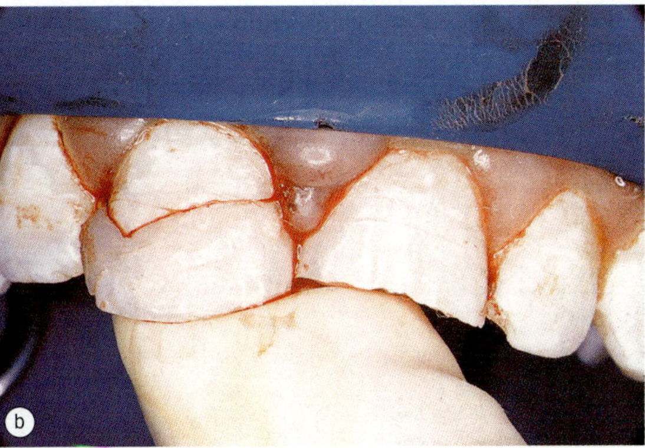

**Figure 24.42** - (**A**) Immediate pulpectomy, since pain is a typical symptom associated with mobility of the fragment. (**B**) Temporary reattachment of the fragment with composite resin.

## Root Fractures

Root fractures cause injuries to mineralized tissues (dentin and cementum), periodontal ligament fibers and pulp structures. They can be classified according to their direction, as horizontal, vertical and oblique; their number, as simple or multiple; and their location, as fractures of the apical, medium and cervical third[16]. Root fractures are essentially diagnosed radiographically, since they can present clinical characteristics similar to extrusive and lateral luxations: slight extrusion, displacement in the lingual direction and mobility of the coronal fragment. Although radiographic diagnosis is facilitated by the generally oblique direction of the fracture line, it may not be identified right after the traumatic injury, even with multiple exposures. Radiographs taken later may be able to reveal the fracture area due to the incisal displacement of the coronal fragment because of hemorrhage, edema or presence of granulation tissue. When interpreting the radiographs, it should also be considered that variations of the vertical angle of the central beam can produce an ellipsoid image simulating multiple fractures (Fig. 24.43A-C).

Due to the large number of tissues involved, root fractures present complex healing patterns. In the past they were considered difficult or impossible to heal. Nowadays, it is well known about their positive prognosis as regards healing, either through mineralized tissue deposition, or by connective tissue interposition. Many studies have demonstrated that root fracture healing depends on certain factors related to the traumatic injury such as degree of mobility and coronal fragment displacement. The procedures adopted during immediate treatment, can also influence healing: whether or not there was replacement and immobilization, as well as the type of splinting. Irrespective of the location, treatment of root fractures consists of replacing coronal fragment by holding it with firm digital pressure.

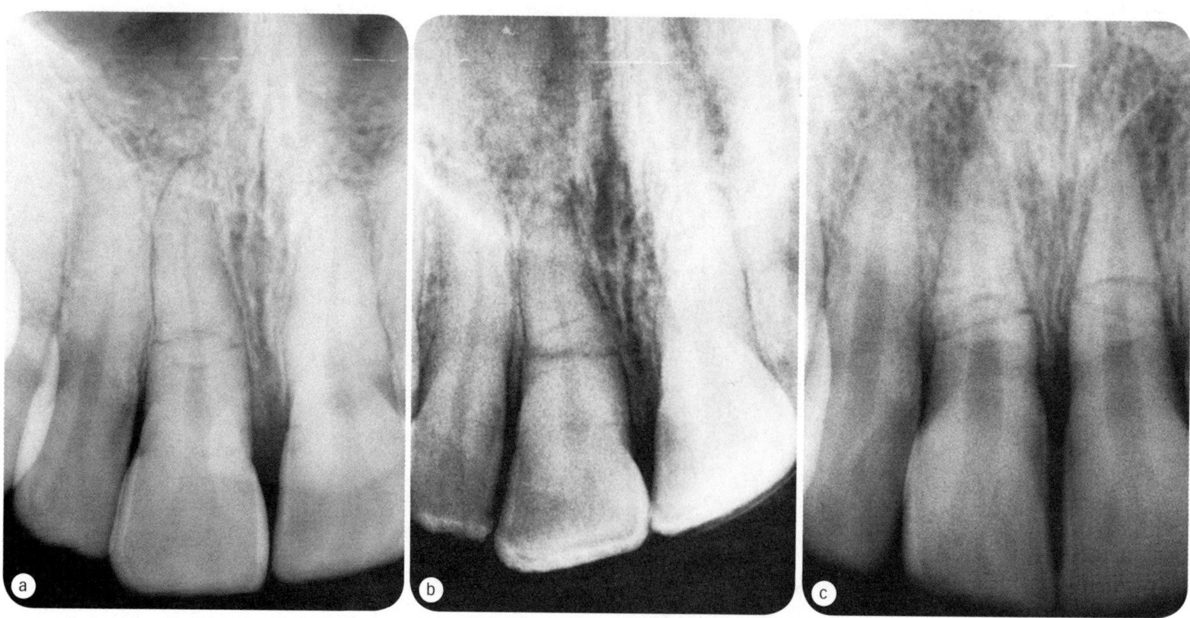


**Figure 24.43** - (**A**) Ellipsoid image of a single of root fracture. (**B**) Changes in the vertical angle of incidence display a single line of an oblique root fracture. (**C**) Irregular radiographic image of multiple root fractures.

After the radiographic confirmation of the correct reduction of the fracture, the tooth must be immobilized. The Ribbond (Dental fiber reinforcement, USA), a combination of ultra-high strength fibers with enhanced bondability is recommended due to its better esthetic results (Fig. 24.44A-G). Nevetheless, ligature wire 0.20 mm fixed with composite resin are less expensive and similar results will be achieved (Fig. 24.45A-B). The occlusion must be checked and adjusted to correct premature contacts. The minimum time of immobilization is 4 weeks, varying in accordance with the fracture location. Cervical fractures may need to be immobilized for longer periods of time (Fig. 24.46A-B and 24.47A-B). During this period, clinical and radiographic control is performed to evaluate the pulp condition and whether or not healing is taking place. All and any endodontic and/or surgical intervention is delayed until the diagnosis of pulp necrosis is defined[6,8,9,19,77,78].

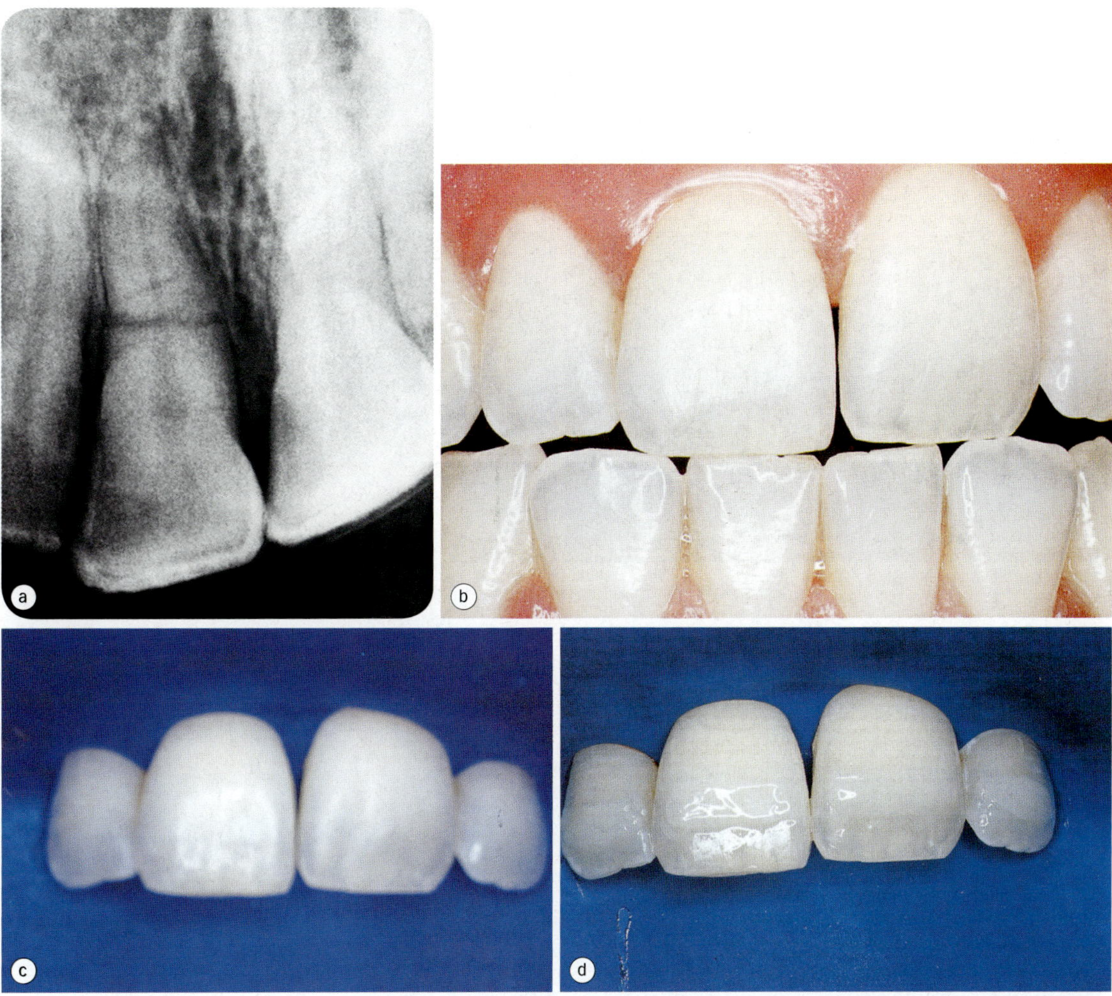


**Figure 24.44** - **(A)** Periapical radiograph for diagnosis of root fracture in the middle third in tooth #11 – Note the absence of displacement. **(B)** Tooth #11 with root fracture in the middle third without displacement. **(C)** Rubber dam isolation for splinting with Ribbond (Dental fiber reinforcement, USA). **(D)** Placement of a layer of composite resin after acid etching and application of the adhesive.

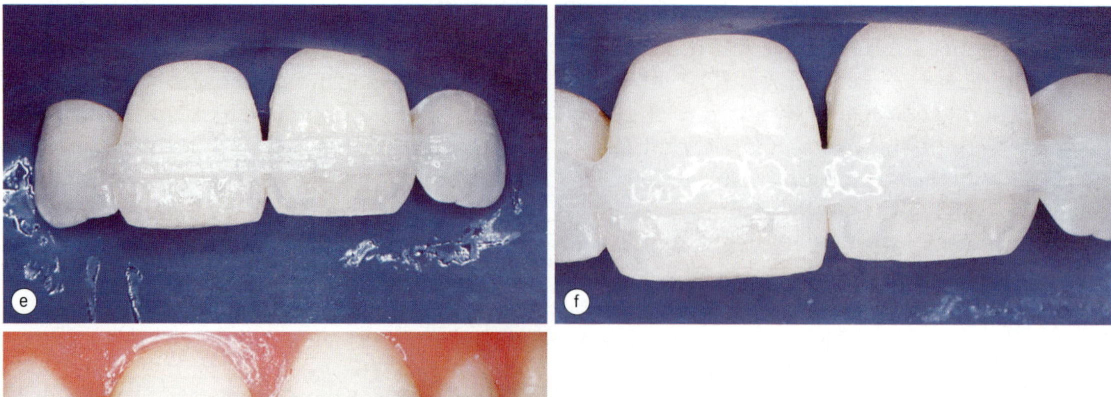

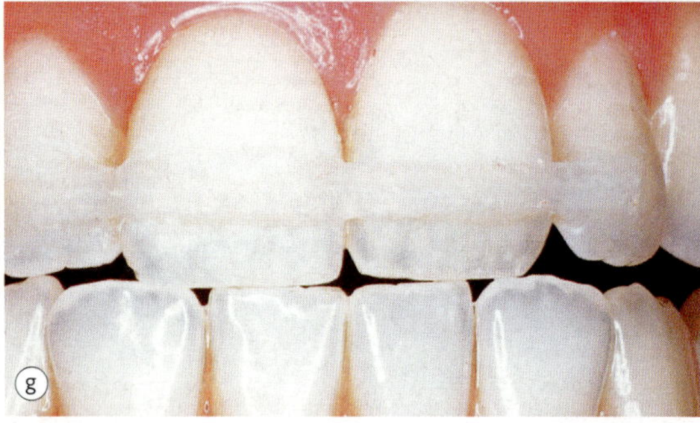

**Figure 24.44** - (**E**) Placement of the Ribbond - Light curing is performed after Ribbond has been adapted. (**F**) Placement of a layer of a light-cured composite resin over the Ribbond. (**G**) After fixture, the presence of premature contacts during the protrusion movement is verified.

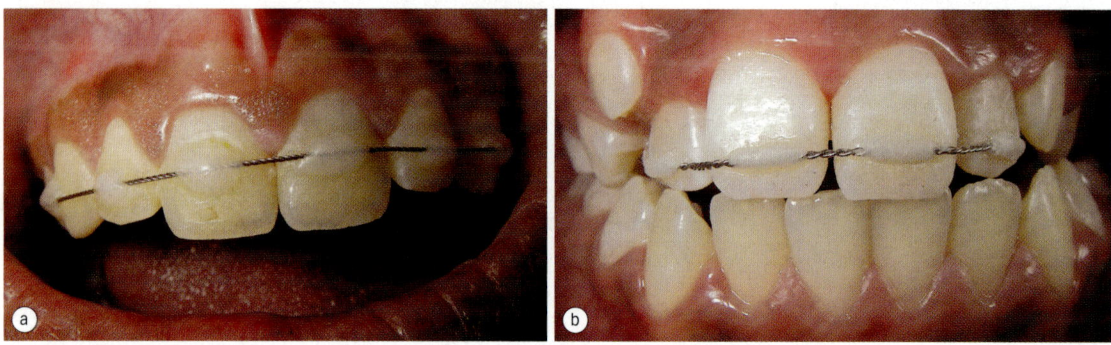

**Figure 24.45** - (**A-B**) Splinting using ligature wire and composite resin.

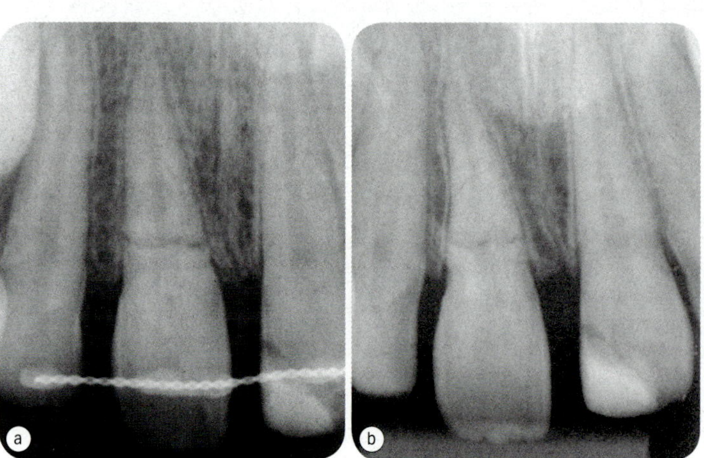

**Figure 24.46** - (**A**) Cervical root fracture in a 10-year-old boy, splinted during 6 months with ligature wire and composite resin. (**B**) Follow-up 2 years after removing splint.

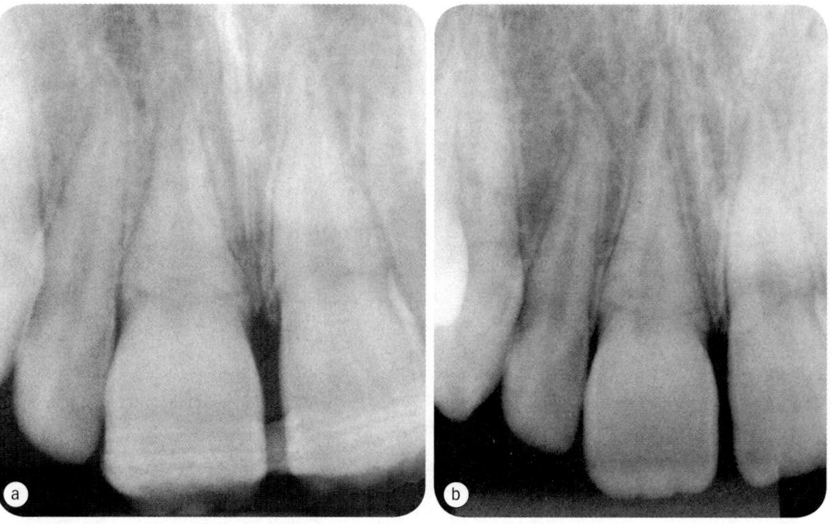


**Figure 24.47** - (**A**) Cervical root fracture in a 10-year-old girl, splinted for 6 months with Ribbond. (**B**) Follow-up 1 year and 9 months after removing splint.

## Concussion and Subluxation

At the time of clinical examination the patient with the diagnosis of concussion informs a marked reaction to percussion in vertical and horizontal direction. However there is no bleeding form the gingival sulcus and no abnormal mobility. Sensitivity tests may reveal a positive response.

Subluxations are injuries that affect either the supporting tissues or the pulp structures. They are characterized by laceration of periodontal ligament fibers, with consequent bleeding and edema. Although there is rupture of a great number of fibers, it is not sufficient to cause displacement of the tooth[11,16]. Pulp involvement occurs due to the stretching, or more rarely, rupture of the apical neurovascular bundle at the time of the traumatic injury. Moreover, the edema in the region of the periodontal ligament can affect the blood supply due to compression of vessels[6,12,13].

Clinically great mobility, sensitivity to vertical percussion and generally, intense bleeding in the region of the gingival sulcus (Fig. 27.48) is observed. Although response to sensibility tests may be negative the pulp may not be necrotic. Eventually, a slight increase of the periodontal ligament space in the apical region can be observed in the radiographic exam (Fig. 24.49).

In young patients, subluxations possibly will present higher mobility and a flexible immobilization may be necessary for a maximum period of 14 days (Fig. 24.50). The aim of this treatment is to stabilize the tooth, to enable regeneration of periodontal fibers, in addition to providing greater comfort to the patient during this phase. Occlusal interferences must be checked. When it is not necessary to immobilize the t ooth, the patient is recommended to have a soft diet at least for two weeks.

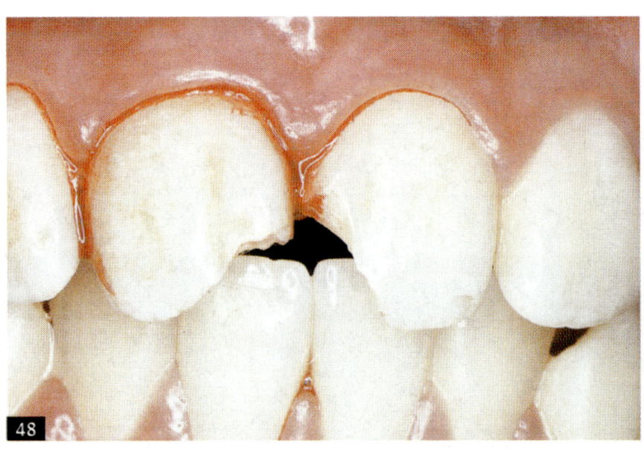

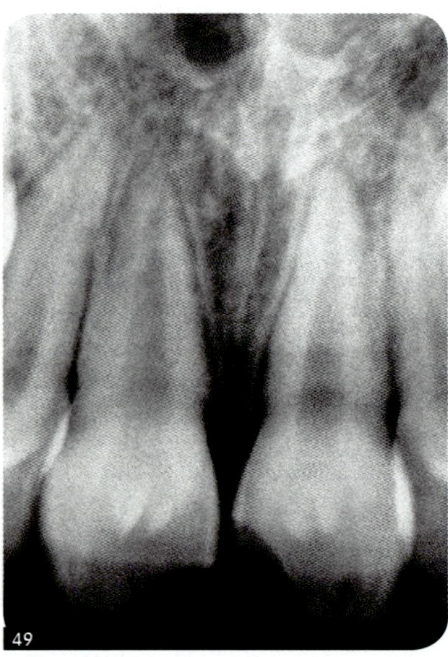

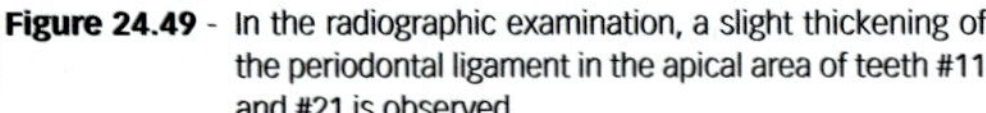

**Figure 24.48** - Clinical aspect of the subluxation in teeth #11 and #21. Note the typical sign of bleeding in the gingival sulcus.

**Figure 24.49** - In the radiographic examination, a slight thickening of the periodontal ligament in the apical area of teeth #11 and #21 is observed.

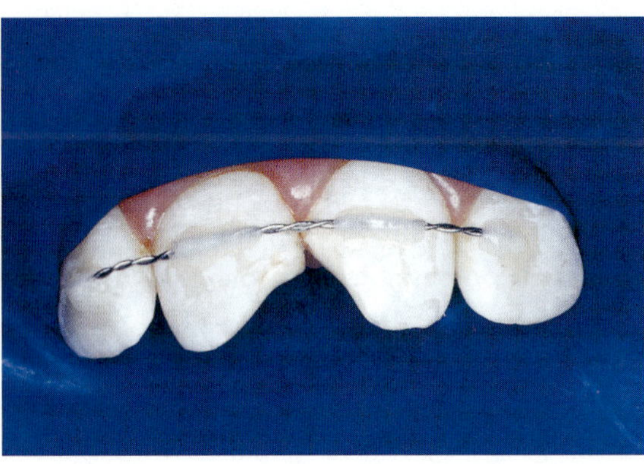

**Figure 24.50** - Flexible splinting of teeth #11 and #21 with subluxation, using ligature wire.

## Extrusive Luxation

The extrusive luxations are characterized by the rupture of periodontal ligament fibers, lesion of sparse points of the root surface and rupture, or stretching of the neurovascular supply at the level of the root apex[6,11-13].

Clinically, partial extrusion of the tooth in the occlusal direction is observed, with eventual displacement of the crown in the lingual direction (Fig. 24.51). Moreover, the tooth presents great horizontal and vertical mobility, sensitivity to percussion tests, and intense bleeding in the cervical region. The tooth may not respond positively to the sensibility tests, although it is not an indicative of pulp necrosis. The radiographic finding of this type of injury is an increase in the periodontal ligament space in the apical region.

The patient him/herself can take the initial care by following the instructions given by the dentist during the first contact at the telephone: reposition the tooth with light digital pressure, and keep it in position by biting on a piece of gauze, cotton or clean cloth until attended by a dentist. This step greatly improves the prognosis when taken immediately after the trauma. In this situation, the procedure to be followed by the clinician is a radiographic and clinical evaluation of the position of the tooth, make the necessary corrections, and perform the flexible immobilization. When the replacement is performed by the professional, this should be atraumatic, by digital pressure, delicate and continuous, in the apical direction, with the goal of gradually displacing the clot formed between the root apex and the apical part of the alveolus. After radiographic verification of the correct position of the tooth, flexible splinting is performed and maintained for two weeks. In all cases the occlusal interferences must be relieved. When attendance is delayed, correct replacement is practically impossible. It is recommended to keep the tooth in its new position, then perform the replacement by orthodontic appliances. The best option is to perform occlusal adjustment, allowing healing to occur.

## Lateral Luxation

The lateral luxations represent complex injuries that involve rupture and laceration of periodontal ligament fibers, lesion of extensive areas of the root surface, and of the alveolar bone. At the level of the apical foramen, strangulation and rupture of the neurovascular supply occurs[6,11-13].

Clinically, the eccentric displacement in the occlusal and lingual direction is observed (Fig. 24.52A), generally associated with the fracture of the buccal wall of the alveolus. In these cases, the crown is positioned in the lingual direction, and the root slides over the buccal surface of the alveolar wall in the apical direction, keeping the tooth firmly imprisoned in its new position. Pain on vertical and horizontal percussion is not a frequent finding, but palpation in the vestibule is generally painful, and allows fracture of the alveolar process and the buccal position of the root apex. A characteristic radiographic finding of this type of injury is the shortened image of the tooth involved, showing higher radiopacity, when compared with the images of the normal adjacent teeth (Fig. 24.52.B). The change in the direction of the long axis of the tooth with lateral displacement, results in an alteration of the vertical angle of incidence of the radiation beam. Moreover, an increase in the space of the periodontal ligament is evidenced when an occlusal radiograph is taken.

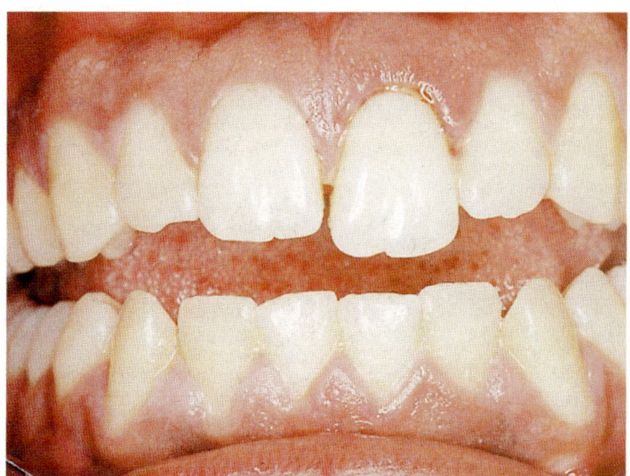

**Figure 24.51** - Extrusive luxation – Clinically, partial extrusion of the tooth in the occlusal direction, is observed.

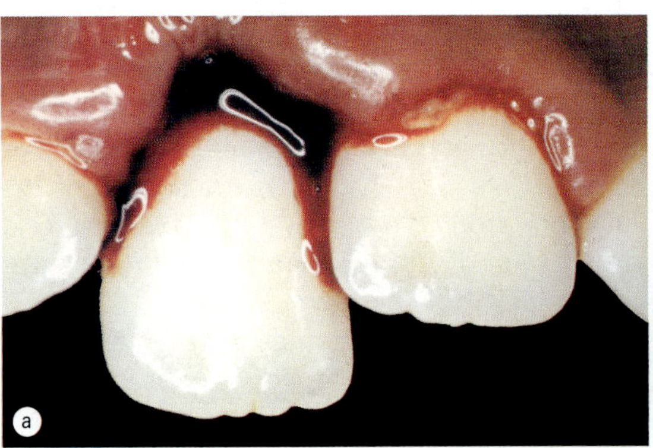

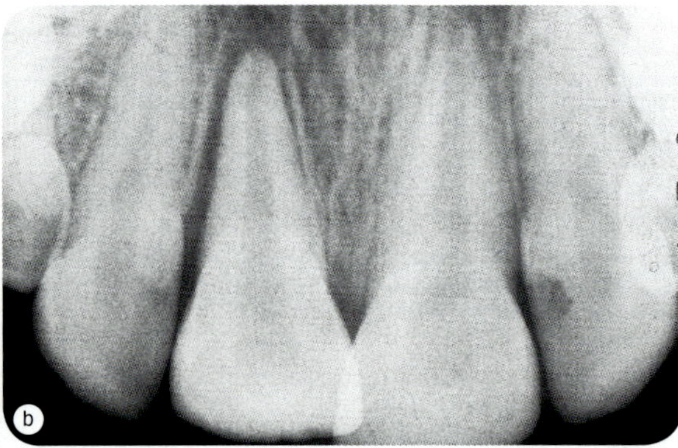

**Figure 24.52** - (**A**) Clinical aspect of tooth #11, with diagnosis of lateral luxation – the displacement in the incisal-palatine direction, probably associated with the fracture of the buccal wall of the alveolus is observed. The crown is positioned in the lingual direction. (**B**) Occlusal radiograph of tooth #11, showing increase in the space of the periodontal ligament – a shortened image of the tooth involved, with higher radiopacity, is observed when compared with tooth #21.

The patient him/herself can take the initial care by following the instructions given by the dentist during the first telephonic contact, as described for extrusive luxations. However, the immediate replacement of the lateral luxation can be very traumatic, due to fracture of the alveolar process, generally requiring professional care. Firm digital pressure must initially be applied at the root apex in the incisal direction, in order to place the root apex back into the alveolus. After this, the tooth must be pressed in the apical direction, until the exact position is reached (Fig. 24.52C). In extreme situations, forceps can be used to retract the tooth slightly, and then replace it to its alveolus. After replacement, a buccal and lingual compression should be applied to ensure that the tooth is completely accommodated in the alveolus and to facilitate periodontal tissue healing. After that, the correct position of the tooth must be verified radiographically, and it must be immobilized with rigid splinting for a period of 3 weeks. In case of fracture to the marginal bone, the period of immobilization can be extended to 6-8 weeks (Fig. 24.52D-G). In all cases, the occlusal interferences must be adjusted. When attendance is delayed, correct replacement is practically impossible. In these cases, the best option is to perform the occlusal adjustment, allow healing to occur and keep the tooth in its new position. Future replacement with orthodontic appliance is reccomended (Fig. 24.53A-I).

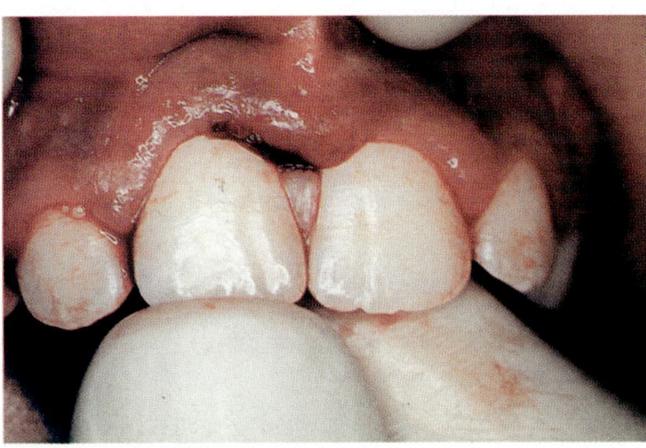

**Figure 24.52C** - The tooth is carefully pressed in apical direction until the exact position is reached.

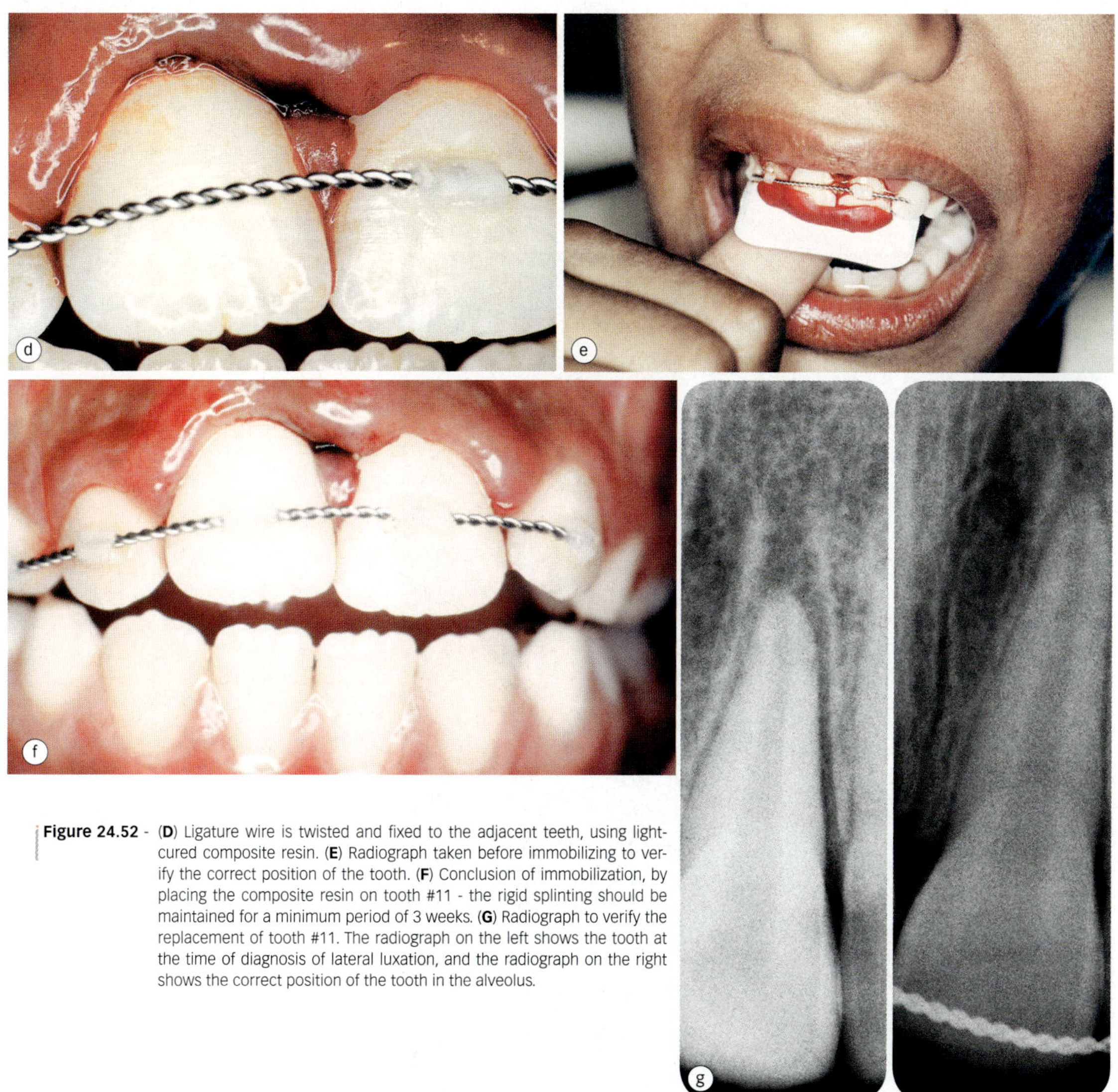

**Figure 24.52** - (**D**) Ligature wire is twisted and fixed to the adjacent teeth, using light-cured composite resin. (**E**) Radiograph taken before immobilizing to verify the correct position of the tooth. (**F**) Conclusion of immobilization, by placing the composite resin on tooth #11 - the rigid splinting should be maintained for a minimum period of 3 weeks. (**G**) Radiograph to verify the replacement of tooth #11. The radiograph on the left shows the tooth at the time of diagnosis of lateral luxation, and the radiograph on the right shows the correct position of the tooth in the alveolus.

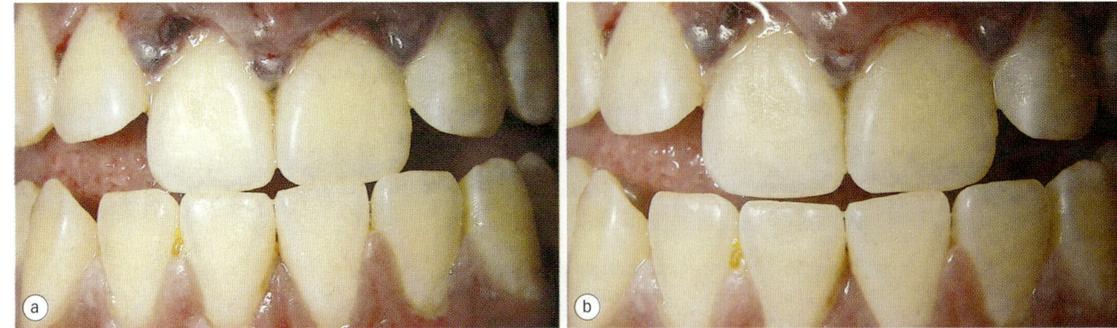


**Figure 24.53** - (**A-B**) Lateral luxation of teeth #11 and #21 in a 15-year-old male after a bicycle accident. Changes in occlusion due to palatal displacement of both teeth.

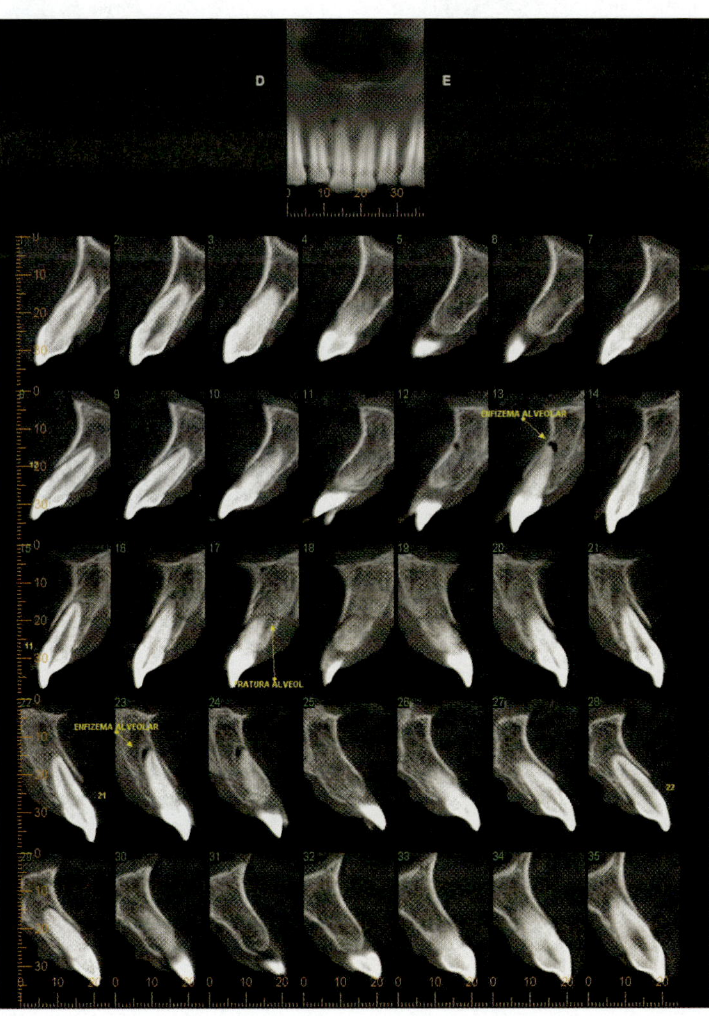


**Figure 24.53C** - Cone Beam Computed Tomography showed: the presence space at the apex, meaning tooth displacement (images 13 and 14 for tooth #11 and images 23 and 24 for tooth #21); presence of fracture in the alveolar bone at the palatal side (images 14 to 17).

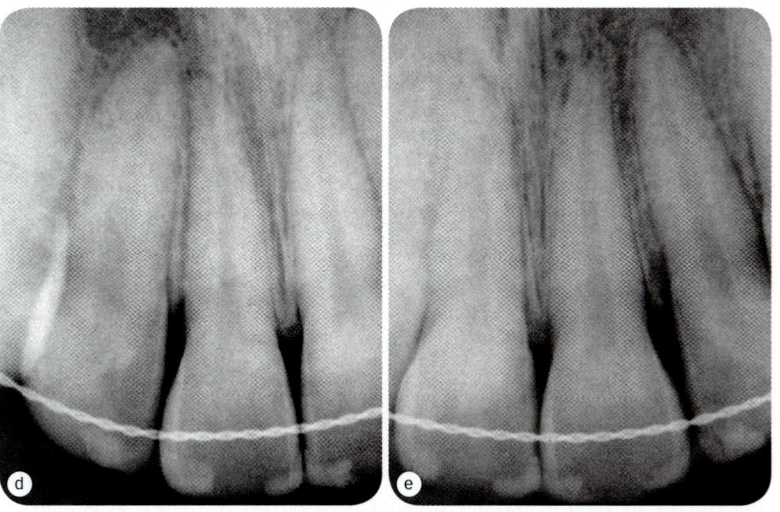

Figure 24.53 - (D-E) Radiographs were taken to confirm teeth position before bonding the ligature wire to the crowns. The teeth needed to be fixed with resin composite in the incisal edges (notice radiopaque images).



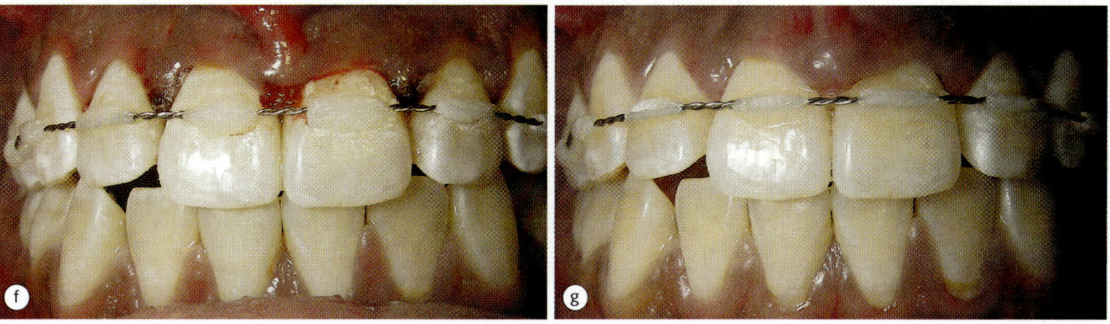

Figure 24.53 - (F) Ligature wire was attached to the teeth after confirming the right position into the alveolar socket. The occlusion was reestablished. (G) Clinical aspect 2 weeks later.

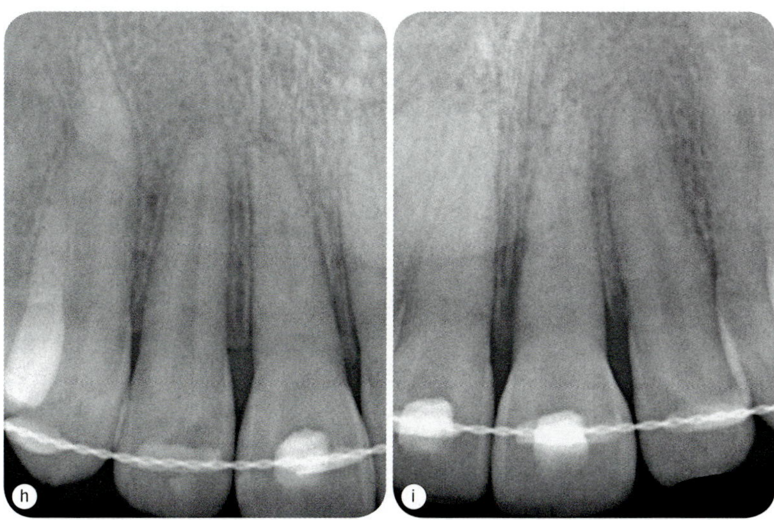

Figure 24.53 - (H-I) Radiographs were taken 2 weeks later after starting endodontic treatment. Notice the radiopaque aspect of root canal space, filled with a calcium hydroxide dressing.

## Avulsion

Avulsion is characterized by the complete displacement of the tooth from its alveolus, causing total rupture of the neurovascular bundle and periodontal ligament fibers, in addition to lesion to the cementoblast layer. Interruption of the blood supply results in necrosis, since revascularization of the pulp to its full extent is a possible, but improbable phenomenon. For this to occur, optimum conditions during the extra-oral period and very specific anatomical factors with regard to the degree of root development, are necessary[54]. Thus, this type of healing should only be expected in immature teeth that were replanted after being maintained under ideal conditions during the extra-oral period.

When a tooth is avulsed the periodontal ligament is ruptured, some of the fibers remain adhered to the alveolar walls, and some of them are attached to the root surface. The part that remains in the alveolus continues to be viable without any additional treatment, as it is nourished by the adjacent alveolar bone. The fibers that remain on the root surface stay viable for minimal extra-oral periods, or under adequate storage conditions. Periodontal ligament healing depends on maintaining the vitality of these remaining fibers on the root surface[14,57,76,87]. The loss of integrity of the ligament, results in fast bone formation in the alveolus, favoring the occurrence of external root resorption.

Thus, it is verified that immediate replantation is the best treatment option after avulsions, particularly when considering the age of the most affected population. Despite the literature being unanimous about the advantages of immediate replantation, daily observations have demonstrated that this is an exception. Most of the time the avulsed teeth are not found, or are kept outside of the alveolus for excessive periods, and in an inadequate media.

In order for replantation to occur as quickly as possible, it must preferably be done by the patient him/herself, or another person at the place of the accident. Therefore, it is fundamental for the professional to give full instructions about performing replantation during the first telephone contact. This information should include full instructions about the entire procedure, starting with washing the tooth, if necessary, with saline solution or under running water, while holding it by the crown; not scrubbing the root or using any type of product; immediately replacing the tooth in its alveolus; biting on a piece of gauze, cotton or clean cloth and going to the dentist's office. If person responsible for the replantation is prevented from acting for technical or emotional reasons, the tooth must be kept in a suitable storage medium until the patient can be attended by a professional[29,30]. A special storage medium such as HBSS, Eagle Medium, Viaspan and Conditioned Medium are ideal for maintaining or revitalizing the periodontal ligament cells and therefore, would have to be available in places where the accidents generally occur: schools, gyms, ambulances, hospitals and accidents & emergency departments[37,75,76,117]. It must be recognized, however, that milk is an excellent storage medium, provided that replantation is performed within six hours. Milk has physiological properties, including pH (6.5-7.2) and osmolarity similar to that of extra-cellular fluid (250-270 mOsm kg-l), it is easily available and relatively free of bacteria, justifying its use as an ideal medium for avulsed teeth[35-37]. Although storage in saline solution has shown to be better than dry storage, it must only be used when there is absolute absence of the above-mentioned storage media[14]. The use of saliva as storage medium, by placing the avulsed tooth under the tongue, or in the patient's or his/her parents' buccal vestibule, is contraindicated due to the risk of the child swallowing the tooth and cross infection, when using other person's mouth. Moreover, the presence of microorganisms and their low osmolarity affect the viability of the periodontal ligament cells, diminishing their clonogenic activity[35,83,86,87].

In cases in which the patient has already performed the replantation, the professional should evaluate the position of the tooth radiographically and clinically, make the necessary corrections, perform the flexible splint.

**Treatment of the root surface**

When the patient arrives at the dental office with the tooth out of the alveolus, the professional must immediately put it into a medium that will not only maintain the vitality of the periodontal ligament cells, but will be capable of replacing the lost cellular nutrients. This storage must only persist for a period as long as necessary for preparing the patient. Hank's balanced saline solution (HBSS) is recommended, for its relatively low cost, in addition to being valid for approximately two years when kept at ambient temperature. The surface of the root must be examined to verify the existence of root fractures and presence of particles of dirt or adhered bone fragments. The tooth must then be rinsed with saline solution until it is completely clean. Although any procedure that involves the manipulation of the root surface is contraindicated, if the rinse is not efficient, gauze humidified in saline solution must be used. The bone fragments must be detached with the aid of a Holemback instrument. In cases of delayed replantation, there have been attempts to treat the root surface with fluoridated solutions, enzymes and acids. The goal of this procedure is to remove remaining portions of necrotic periodontal ligament and to modify the root surface, rendering it more resistant to resorption and facilitating collagen fiber adhesion. Although the association of fluorides and antibiotics have presented the best results[33,109], current researches are not conclusive. Thus, this procedure is not indicated, as additional studies are necessary to substantiate its clinical use. In these cases, only thorough cleaning with gauze dampened with saline solution is recommended, with the intention of removing necrotic periodontal ligament fibers (Fig. 24.54A).

**Treatment of the alveolus**

Preparing the patient for replantation starts with a careful examination of the mouth and the alveolus, followed by periapical radiographs to evaluate the presence of foreign bodies or fractures (Fig. 24.54B-C). It has been suggested that blood clots should be removed before the tooth is replaced, with the delicate use of curettes and irrigation with physiological saline solution (Fig. 24.54D). This procedure will reduce the risk of inflammation as result of foreign bodies in the alveolus, and it helps to produce close contact between the tooth and the alveolar bone[16]. The alveolus should then be inspected, and if the presence of fractures is verified it is fundamental to replace of the fractured bone, modeling it with the aid of an instrument, counterbalanced by digital pressure exerted in the buccal area. In these cases, it could be necessary to replace and suture the gingival lacerations.

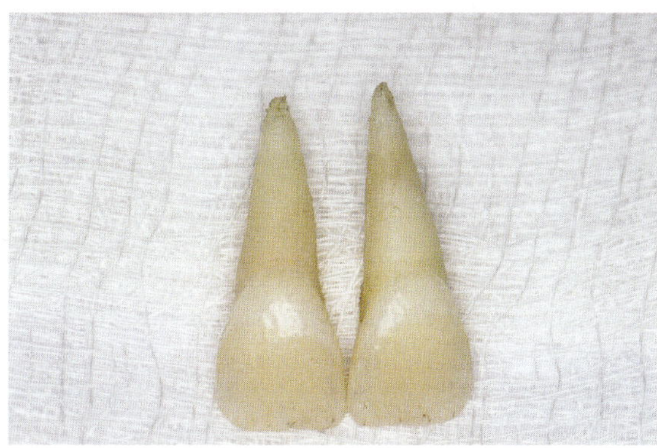

**Figure 24.54A** - Avulsed teeth seen before late replantation (12 hours after avulsion). A gauze soaked in saline solution was used to clean the root surface.

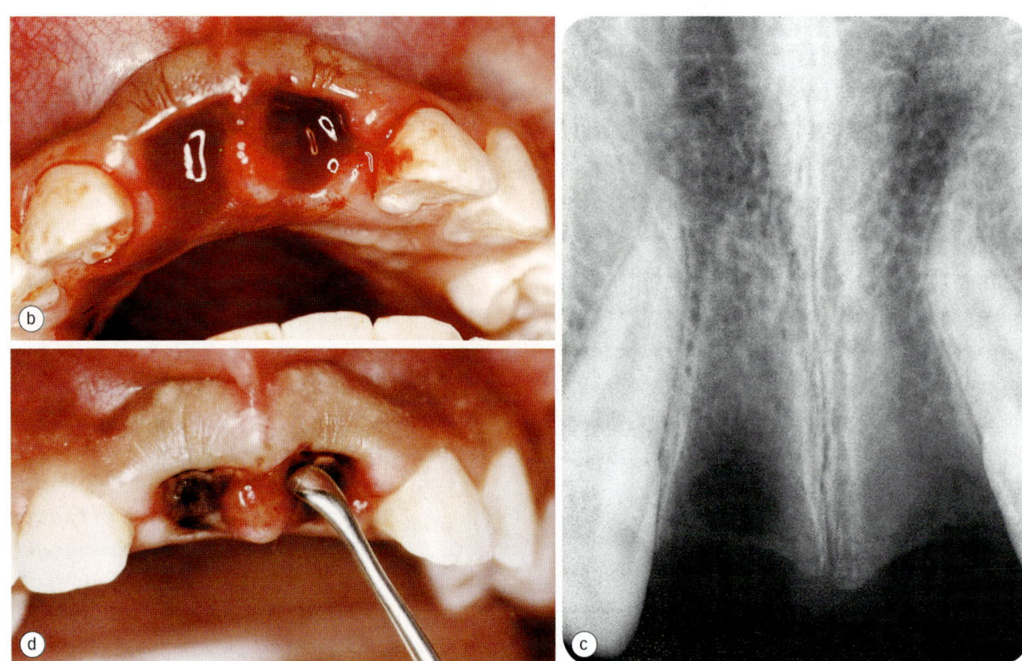

**Figure 24.54** - (**B**) Situation of the alveolus after the avulsion of teeth #11 and #21. Careful inspection is necessary, with the purpose of detecting possible fractures of the alveolar process or foreign bodies. (**C**) The periapical radiograph is also helpful for inspecting the alveolus for possible fractures or presence of foreign bodies. (**D**) Blood clots must be removed before the replacement, delicately using curettes and irrigating the alveolus with saline solution. This procedure reduces the risk of inflammation resulting from the presence of foreign bodies and helps to produce close contact between the tooth and the alveolar bone.

## Repositioning

After the initial preparation, the tooth should be held by the crown and repositioned by slow and gradual digital pressure, until it is introduced into the alveolus to its full extent (Fig. 24.54E). This pressure should be delicate to allow tactile perception of possible remainders inside the alveolus. If resistance is encountered the tooth should be put back into the storage medium again, while the alveolus is reexamined. If any bone fragment is dislodged, it should be repositioned. At the end of the procedure, buccal and lingual compression ensures complete adaptation and guarantees a flow of blood throughout the entire root surface (Fig. 24.54F).

## Splinting

Splinting of replanted teeth should be performed right after repositioning, with the objective of providing stability during the initial period of periodontal ligament healing. Thus, except in cases in which there is associated bone fracture, flexible splinting is recommended, which maintains the tooth in its original position, without occlusal interferences, but allows its physiologic movement, preventing ankylosis from becoming permanent[93]. After correct repositioning has been verified radiographically, the tooth should be splinted, using a double ligature wire (0.08" or 0.20mm), slightly twisted and fixed with composite resin (Fig. 24.54G-K and 24.55) Experimental studies have demonstrated that shorter immobilization periods, 15 to 21 days, favor periodontal ligament healing since they reduce the risk of ankylosis[89,92,119]. In cases of associated fracture of the alveolar process, the splinting should be rigid and it should stay for longer periods, from 40 to 60 days[93].

The Figures 24.56A-H illustrate a case of late replantation in a 7 year-old patient.

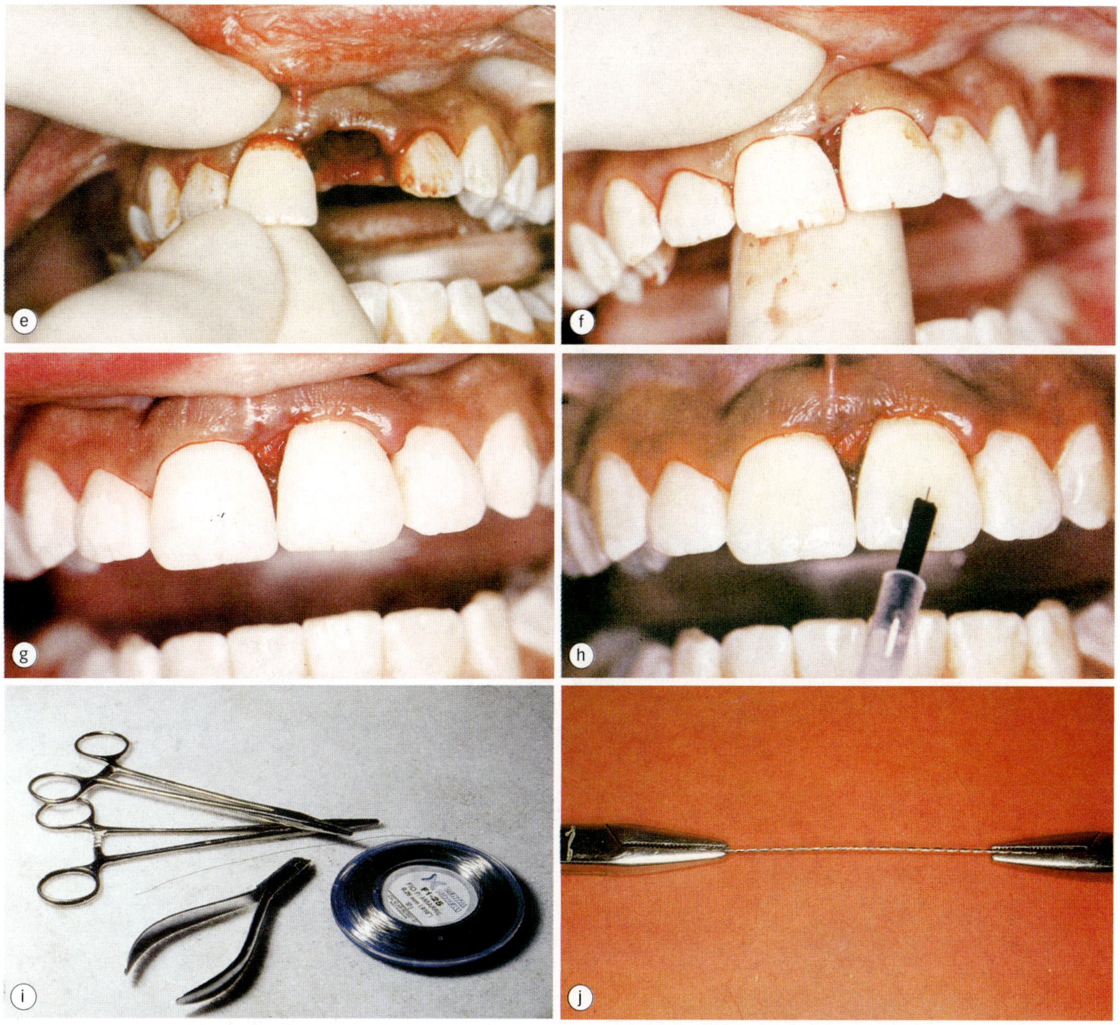

**Figure 24.54** - (**E**) Delicate insertion of tooth #11, using only enough pressure to accommodate it in the alveolus. (**F**) A buccal and lingual compression should be performed in the entire area after repositioning, with the intention of ensuring complete adaptation of the tooth in the alveolus. (**G**) View of the buccal surface after acid etching of the enamel. (**H**) Application of the adhesive on the etched surfaces. (**I**) Material used for the splint: 2 needle holders for suturing; ligature wire 0.08"; cutting pliers. (**J**) The wire should be double, held by the extremities with the needle holders and twisted, but remaining flexible.

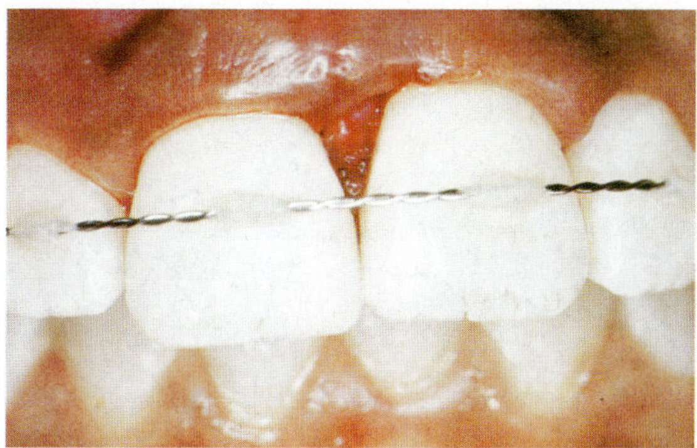

**Figure 24.54K** - Case concluded after placement of resin. In this case, the pulpectomy was performed in the same session, because the teeth had complete root development. The root canals were irrigated abundantly with a solution of sodium hypochlorite, dried with absorbent paper points and temporarily sealed. Continuation of the treatment with calcium hydroxide should be performed 1 week later.

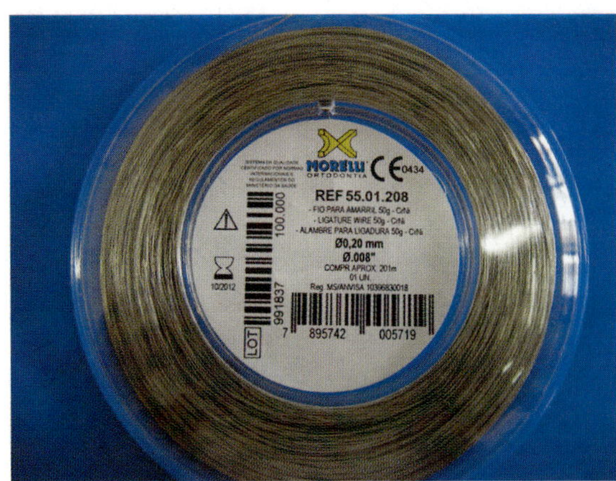


**Figure 24.55** - Ligature wire sold by Dental Morelli – Brazil.

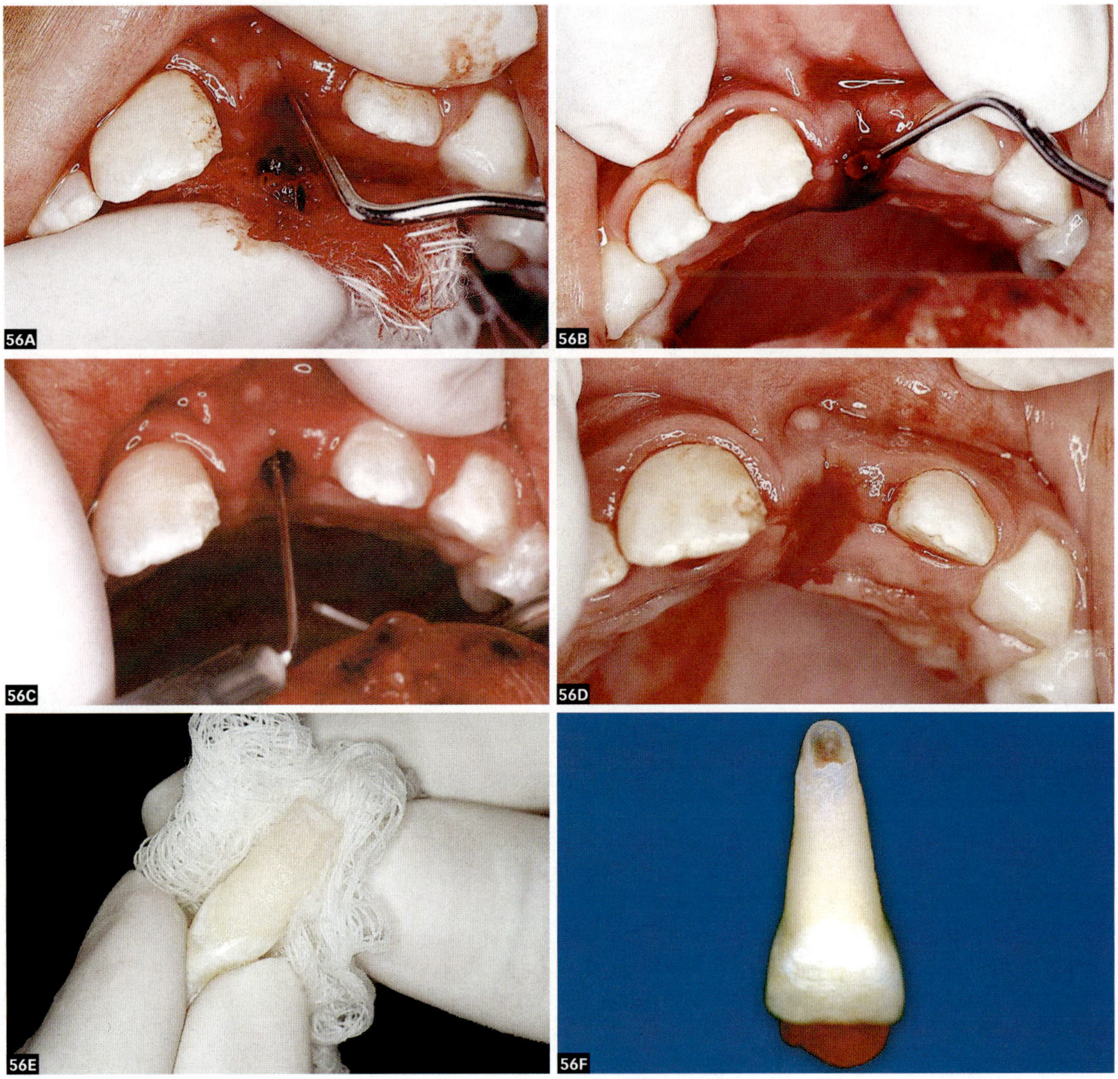

56A

56B

56C

56D

56E

56F

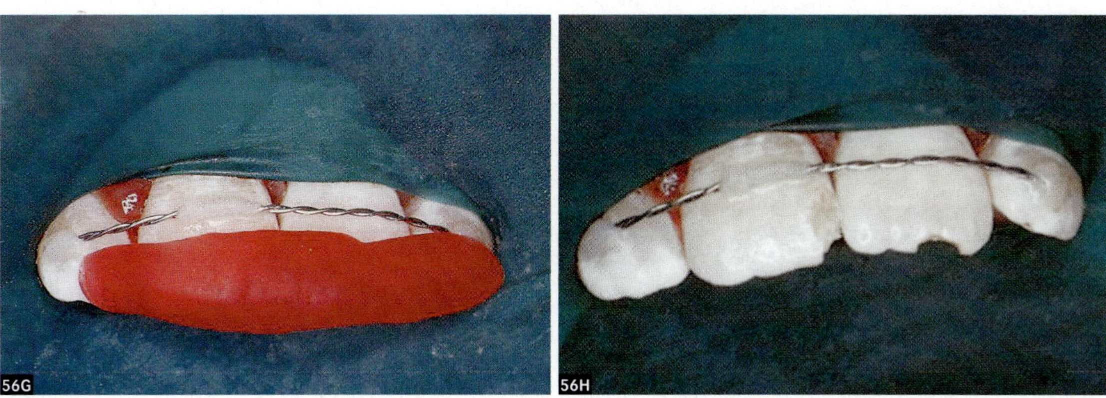

**Figure 24.56** - (**A-H**) Case of late replantation in a 7 year-old patient.

## Root canal treatment

The clinical survey performed by Andreasen & Hjorting-Hansen[20] represented a milestone in the understanding of the phenomena related to healing, after the replantation of avulsed teeth. The authors were the first to correlate the processes of root resorption with the extra-oral period in replanted teeth. Their findings demonstrated that replantation performed within a period of up to thirty minutes, presented a better success rate than those performed after a longer extra-oral period. The authors revolutionized the treatment of avulsed teeth, recommending immediate replantation and subsequent root canal treatment, which up to then, had been performed with the tooth out of the mouth. The procedure recommended by them was widely adopted. Two other aspects deserve special attention: the right time to perform the pulpectomy, and the moment of placing the calcium hydroxide intracanal dressing. The removal of the pulp and the subsequent root canal treatment, right after replantation are decisive factors in the prognosis of replanted teeth. Knowing that complete revascularization of the pulp is improbable, particularly in mature teeth root canal treatment could only be postponed in immature teeth, replanted under ideal conditions of extra-oral period[53,54]. Thus, the time root canal treatment begins is critical for the prevention and treatment of inflammatory root resorption, and should be performed within two to three weeks after replantation. Nevertheless, if on the one hand pulpectomy is of fundamental importance to avoid the propagation of toxic products from the necrotic pulp to the adjacent tissues, the use of calcium hydroxide at this time should be avoided. The overflow of the material through the apical foramen would be detrimental to healing, since calcium hydroxide is cytotoxic to the periodontal ligament cells that are replenishing the root surface[15]. Special care should be taken in teeth with incomplete root development and open apex (Fig. 24.56E-F). Thus, it is recommended that whenever possible, pulpectomy should be performed right after replantation. The root canal should be irrigated with sodium hypochlorite (mature tooh), or saline solution (immature tooth) and dried with absorbent paper points. Next, a sterilized cotton pellet shall be put inside the pulp chamber, and the temporary seal performed with zinc oxide cement and eugenol. Each case should be evaluated individually, but the calcium hydroxide dressing can be performed after one to two weeks.

## Systemic Medication Associated with the Emergency Treatment in Dental Trauma

The systemic medication therapy most frequently used in emergency treatment of the traumatic injuries consists of administering antibiotics, analgesics and anti-inflammatory drugs, in addition to anti tetanus prophylaxis.

Although the use of the systemic antibiotics is widely indicated after replantation of avulsed teeth, this procedure lacks scientific evidence, particularly with regard to the choice of drug and length of treatment. Little is known about the effective value of antibiotics in periodontal and pulp healing[18,53,54,104,105]. The only positive results came from the experimental studies of Hammarström et al.[70], but they cannot be applied to the treatment of patients, due to the pathway and period of drug administration used by the author. Considering the few scientific evidences available at present, the benefits of the systemic use of antibiotics is questionable in the treatment of traumatic injuries, even in cases of replantation. Similarly, it is surprising how scarce studies are in the literature about the effect of systemic antibiotics on healing injuries in soft tissues. In general, it is believed that all these wounds are contaminated, which is the reason why the prophylactic use of antibiotics has been indicated for handling such injuries. However, it has not been proved whether this therapy is of any benefit in the treatment of cutaneous, or mucosal lesions. Moreover, the results with reference to deeper lesions are contradictory.

According to Andreasen[16] the antibiotic chosen for the treatment of soft tissue lesions is Penicillin followed by Erythromycin, and it should be restricted to the following situations:

- highly contaminated lesions, in which cleaning cannot be performed satisfactorily;
- excessive delay in cleaning the wound (more than 24 hours);
- when surgical reduction of bone fractures is necessary;
- cases of systemic debility or compromised immunological status;
- wounds caused by human or animal bites.

The anti-tetanus prophylaxis should always be indicated in cases of soft tissue injuries or contaminated avulsed teeth. In this context, the information about where the accident happened, as well as data about the patient's previous immunization is of fundamental importance. In situations of risk of infection, one dose of vaccine for patients whose immunization is up to date is sufficient. Patients who are not immunized, or who are in the course of the vaccination scheme should first receive passive immunization, and afterwards the conventional vaccine[16].

The indiscriminate use of anti-inflammatory medication after traumatic injuries is also not justified, since the few available experimental studies revealed that it is ineffective for controlling root resorptions[120]. Furthermore, acute inflammatory pulp or periapical status is not frequently found in the development of the pulp condition after the trauma.

Dental trauma is characterized by multiple nature, since it may affect the pulp, mineralized tissues of the teeth and their supporting structures simultaneously. The frequency with which they occur, the distribution according to age group and the etiology, outline a complex problem of treatment

A major difficulty in dealing with traumatized teeth is related to the diagnosis of pulpal changes that occur after the injury, that is: when the endodontic treatment is actually indicated? This increases the responsibility of facing an early or late indication of radical intervention, every two extremely harmful in the context of the age group most affected, 7 to 14 years. If we can not delay this diagnosis, given the speed with which the external inflammatory root resorptions progress in these young teeth, nor is justified an early indication, or "preventive" root canal treatment, in an age where the tooth needs its young and active pulp to complete its root development and obtain root walls thick and strong enough to allow its normal function.

Although studies have demonstrated optimistic success rates of 79% to 96% after root canal treatment in immature permanent teeth, when considering the regression of periapical lesions and the formation of apical barrier of mineralized tissue[59,98,100,120], the long term prognosis is not so favorable. The interruption of the physiologic dentin apposition after removing the pulp tissue, results in extremely thin dentinal walls/root surface of the immature tooth, which increases the risk of cervical root fractures. These fractures can also be directly related to the endodontic treatment, performed in teeth in which root development was in the initial stages or in teeth that have defects resulting from the healing of external inflammatory root resorptions[59] (Fig. 24.57). Therefore, pulp diagnosis after traumatic dental injuries become a challenge for which, unfortunately, most professionals are not prepared.

To overcome this challenge we must be aware of the possibilities of repair of the pulp in young teeth with incomplete root formation. Its vascular supply consists of multiple arterioles, venules and veins passing through the apical foramen, which facilitate and regulate blood flow[101,102]. The fact that the majority of our patients be represented by children and adolescents is a good point that favors pulpal healing. At this stage of development, the pulp presents a good response to injury due to its high capacity of proliferation of mesenchimal cells and formation of new blood vessels which differ from those caused by decay and its sequels. Finally, the professional should be aware of the limitations of diagnostic tools currently available. These detect changes in the activity of sensory nerves in the pulp, not sufficiently sensitive to identify other circulatory alterations, resulting from trauma.

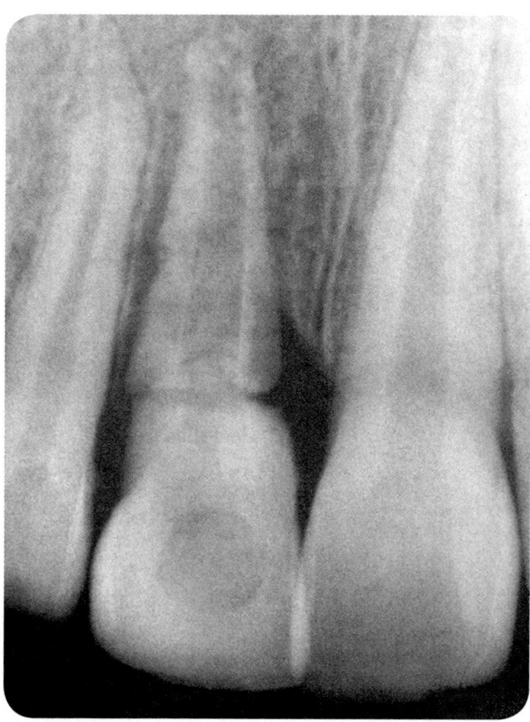

**Figure 24.57** - Radiographic aspect of cervical fracture that occurred in the defective area of the root, resulting from the external inflammatory root resorption.

### Physiopathology of Pulp Alterations

In the context of traumatic dental injuries, pulp alterations are often due to the severed vascular supply at the apical region or the complete arrest of pulpal circulation supply. Therefore, maintaining pulp vitality depends on the occurrence of damage to the structure and its ability to revascularization, which is a function of the extent of damage to the apical nerves and vessels, root development status, and the presence of infection.

### Pulp Response after Crown Fractures Involving Enamel and Dentin

The pulp alterations that follow fractures involving exposure of dentin were described in the classic studies of Brännström[50,51].

The author showed inflammatory changes associated with aggression to the odontoblasts underlying the exposed areas of dentin, with eventual aspiration of the cells or their remnants, into the dentinal tubules. A few days after exposure of dentin surface, it would present covered by a thin layer of plaque resulting from a poor cleaning due to the sensitivity of the exposed dentin. Original bacteria from this plaque and particularly their components would invade the tubules, leading to the loss of the odontoblastic layer. There would then be a diffusion of antibodies, leukocytes and other cells, as well as plasma proteins through the dentinal fluid toward the opening of the tubules. Finally, cells of the central layer of the pulp would differentiate into new odontoblasts, and start the deposition of reparative dentin.

These favorable findings with regard to the resolution of pulp inflammation due to dentin exposure and contamination by saliva would, however, depend on an intact vascular supply and the inhibition of additional microbial invasion. Therefore, enamel and dentin fractures present little risk of complications to the pulp, since the flow of the dentinal fluid is a barrier against bacterial invasion, diluting the bacterial toxins and distributing elements of defense[38,92,134,144,146,163]. On the other hand, the occurrence of concomitant luxation injury compromises the maintenance of pulp vitality. The disturbance of the blood supply to the pulp makes their first defense mechanisms unfeasible, in addition to eliminating the barrier represented by the hydrostatic pressure of the flow of the dentinal fluid. Moreover, the rupture of the pulp tissues at the time of the injury, would lead to localized areas of necrosis, which would facilitate microbial invasion[136,138,174,175].

### Pulp Response After Enamel and Dentin Fracture with Pulp Involvement

When the enamel and dentin fractures with pulp involvement occur, in addition to the aggression represented by direct exposure to the oral environment, there is laceration of the pulp tissue at the fracture site. The alterations that follow are local hemorrhage and inflammation, caused by the breakdown products of lacerated tissue and bacterial toxins. Again, the maintenance of the pulp vascular supply will play a decisive role in the pulp response. If there is no involvement of the periapical neurovascular supply, the pulp response is proliferative and benign, and is characterized by the formation of a granulation tissue underlying the area of exposure, irrespective of its size (Fig. 24.58). Experimental studies[63] in pulps of monkey incisors showed that two days after exposure, the pulp tissue was covered with fibrin and a limited pulp proliferation, with moderate inflammatory cells extending not more than 2mm from the exposed site. One week after exposure, a larger hyperplasia of pulp tissue was observed being projected through the fracture, but the inflammatory infiltrate maintained superficial levels. Impaction of contaminated food debris caused abscesses in the underlying pulp. Thus, although the process of healing does not happen spontaneously, the superficial proliferative response noticed two days after pulp exposure allows partial excision of the hyperplasic tissue, preserving healthy pulp tissue by means of conservative techniques.

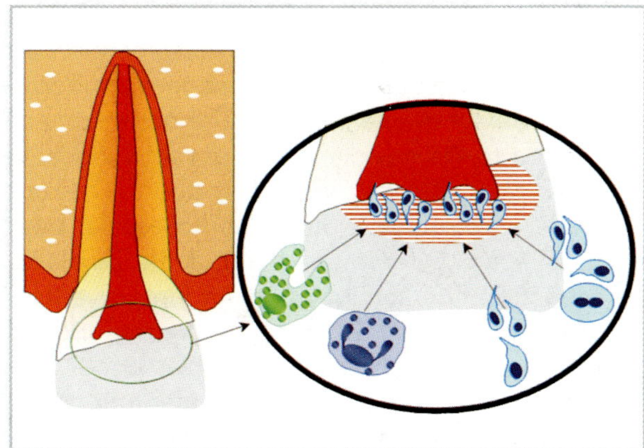

**Figure 24.58** - Schematic illustration of the pulp response after traumatic exposure, characterized by the presence of inflammatory infiltrate up to 2 mm below the exposure site and proliferation of granulation tissue. (Adjusted from Andreasen & Andreasen[22]).



## Pulp Response After Luxation

In luxation injuries, pulp necrosis occur in response to the injury to the apical neurovascular supply, in which nerves and vessels can be compressed, lacerated or ruptured. It and may lead to ischemic necrosis of the pulp tissue, due to the abrupt and complete interruption of the circulation. The regenerative phenomena that follow in some cases consist of replacement of the damaged pulp tissue by defense cells and undifferentiated mesenchymal cells. In addition there is an attempt to recompose the blood supply and achieve nervous regeneration. The revascularization of the ischemic pulp tissue takes place by the ingrowth of new vessels to the interior of the pulp tissue combined with "end-to-end" anastomosis between the existent and the ingrowing vessels. The process of new vascular formation is known as angiogenesis, and involves the direct migration of endothelial cells, their proliferation and the formation of vascular lumen. Experimental studies have demonstrated that the new capillaries are formed from the stimulus of angiogenic factors, released during the inflammatory response, leading to proliferation of endothelial cells in the wall of venules. These cells release enzymes that degrade the underlying basal membrane, creating a path of migration towards the angiogenic stimuli. This proliferation continues moving forward to find other endothelial sprouts or marginal vessels with which join to form new capillary loops, or anastomosis with the adjacent tissue. When these connections are established, the endothelial cells divide and differentiate, forming the vascular lumen and allowing blood circulation, although there is still a great loss of blood cells to the extra-vascular medium, due to the absence of the basal membrane. A new basal membrane will only be deposited as the cells of the new vessels mature and become capable of secreting the components of the extra-cellular matrix. This process depends on the fibroblastic activity and it only advances in the presence of collagen support. The fast anastomosis that are established in the apical area play a key role in the revascularization process during pulp healing[159]. Confinement within mineralized walls limits the diffusion of nutrients derived from neighboring tissues. It also prevents the new vascular formation, whose speed in the pulp is approximately 0.5 mm/day, from reaching the coronal portions in due time to avoid definitive cell degeneration. Thus, the success of pulp revascularization after luxation injuries depends on the conditions that allow anastomosis to occur between the pulp vessels and those of the apical periodontal tissue.

These conditions are determined by the type of injury, stage of root development, and the presence of infection.

The *type of injury* determines not only the degree of involvement of the neurovascular pulp supply, but also of the supporting tissues that supply vessels, cells and other defense elements, responsible for pulp healing. The degree of growing complexity expressed in the classification proposed by Andreasen[13] is a good indicator of the pulp prognosis, since it is based on the extent of the injury. In concussion (Fig. 24.59), and subluxation (Fig. 24.60) the lesion is limited to the periodontal ligament fibers, not being sufficient to displace the tooth. Thus, lesion to the neurovascular bundle is minimal, frequently resulting from the edema that is formed in the space of the ruptured periodontal ligament. In extrusive luxation (Fig. 24.61) there is partial displacement of the tooth in the occlusal direction, due to the rupture of a larger number of periodontal fibers, however, without the occurrence of lesion to the alveolar bone, or root surface. In this case pulp involvement is due to the rupture, or stretching of the neurovascular bundle, at apical foramen, during dental displacement. In lateral (Fig. 24.62) and intrusive (Fig. 24.63) luxations, the lesion to the periodontal ligament extends to the alveolar bone , laterally or apical, and to the cementum of the root, contributing to greater damage to the apical neurovascular bundle which, in addition to being ruptured, is smashed, due to the direction of the dental displacement. As regards the occurrence of pulp necrosis, the literature is unanimous in pointing out displacement as the main determining factor[9,38,58,67,126,127,134,149].

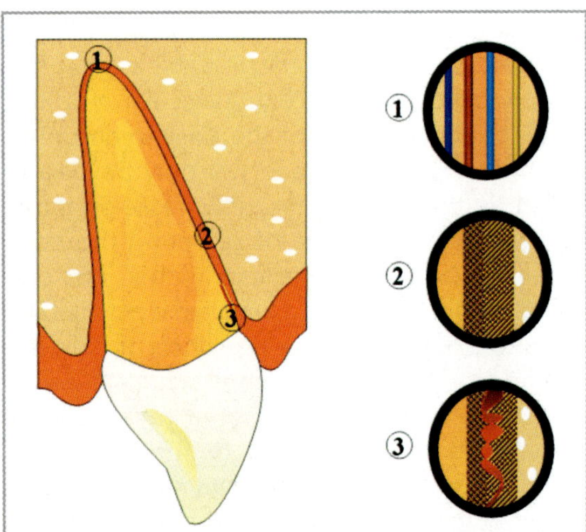


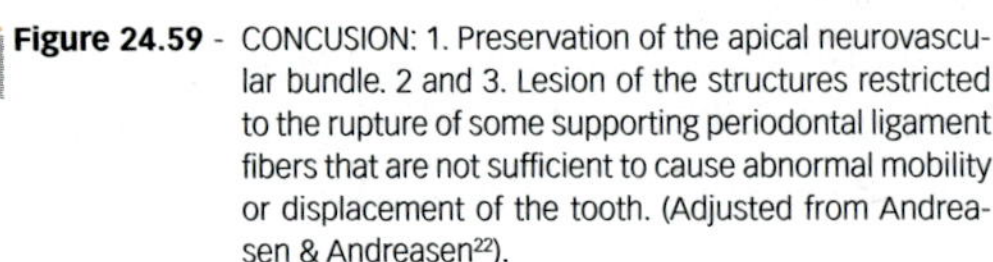

**Figure 24.59** - CONCUSION: 1. Preservation of the apical neurovascular bundle. 2 and 3. Lesion of the structures restricted to the rupture of some supporting periodontal ligament fibers that are not sufficient to cause abnormal mobility or displacement of the tooth. (Adjusted from Andreasen & Andreasen[22]).

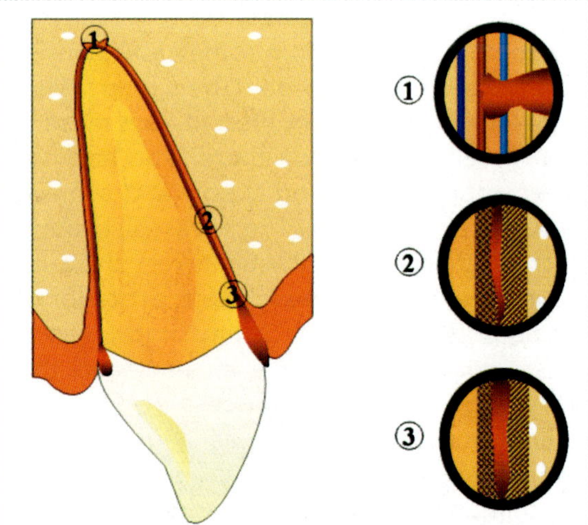


**Figure 24.60** - SUBLUXATION: 1. Stretching and/or compression of the apical neurovascular bundle, caused by the edema formed in the space of the periodontal ligament. 2. Rupture of periodontal ligament fiber bundles leading to the abnormal mobility. 3. Bleeding through the gingival sulcus. (Adjusted from Andreasen & Andreasen[22]).

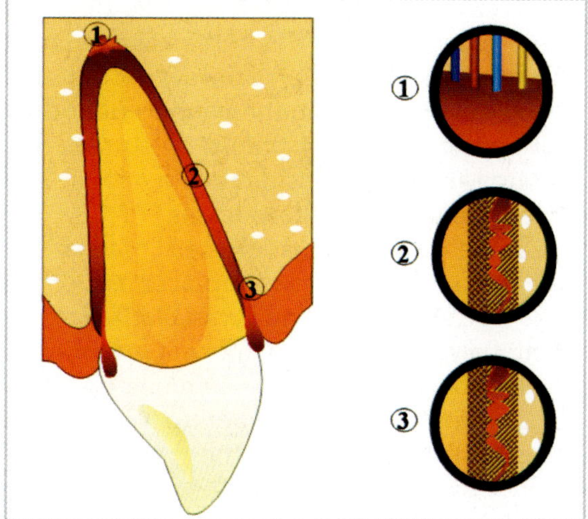


**Figure 24.61** - EXTRUSIVE LUXATION: 1. Stretching and/or total rupture of the apical neurovascular bundle. 2. Rupture of bundles of fibers along the entire periodontal ligament due to the partial displacement of the tooth in the incisal direction. 3. Bleeding through the gingival sulcus. (Adjusted from Andreasen & Andreasen[22]).

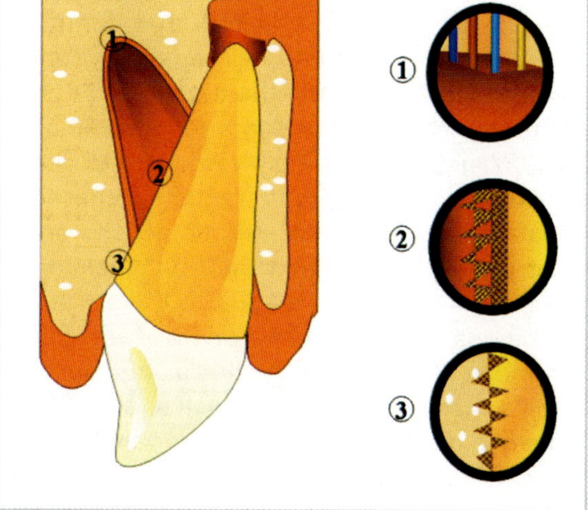


**Figure 24.62** - LATERAL LUXATION: 1. Rupture of the apical neurovascular bundle. 2. Rupture of bundles of fibers along the entire periodontal ligament. 3. Removal of the cementoblastic layer in some points of the root surface due to the eccentric displacement of the tooth. (Adjusted from Andreasen & Andreasen[22]).

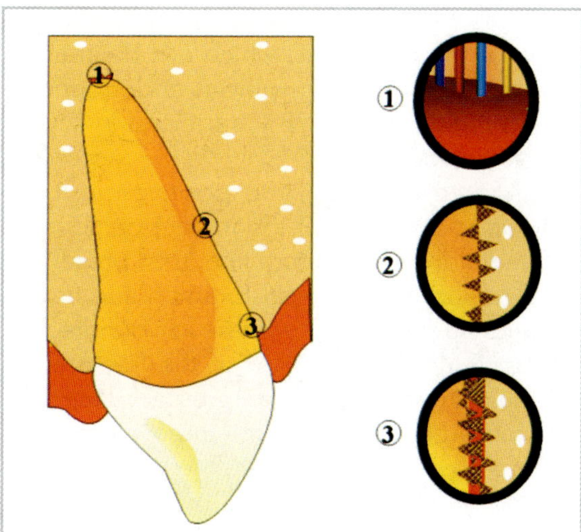


**Figure 24.63** - INTRUSIVE LUXATION: 1. Rupture of the periapical neurovascular bundle. 2. Removal of the cementoblastic layer along the root surface due to the axial displacement of the tooth. 3. Laceration of the fibers along the entire periodontal ligament. (Adjusted from Andreasen & Andreasen[22]).

The *stage of root development* is a determinant factor of the pulp prognosis after luxation injuries, and as regards pulp response, young permanent teeth present high rates of healing. Among the factors that contribute to the great potential for repair in young teeth, one can mention the nature and constitution of the apical odontogenic complex, that consists of the highly vascularized dental papilla, rich in undifferentiated mesenchymal cells, with great mitotic activity and histo-differentiation, and the epithelial root sheath, known to be resistant to the adverse conditions of an inflammatory process. Furthermore, the mucosal nature of the dental papilla in the apical area, as well as the presence of a dense net of arterioles and venules, gives a resilient characteristic to the odontogenic complex, responsible for reducing the impact of traumatic injury, which would avoid a total collapse of the tissue and would minimize the effects of displacements in young teeth. The presence of these structures gives extraordinary regenerative capacity to the young permanent teeth. From the anatomical point of view, young teeth present two characteristics that favor the revascularization of pulp tissue after an injury to the apical neurovascular bundle: the large diameter of the apical foramen, which allows greater interface with the periodontal tissue, enabling the occurrence of rapid anastomosis with the ruptured pulp vessels, known to be the most important mechanism in re-establishing the pulp blood supply; another determining factor is the shorter length of the root that facilitates access of the revascularization process to the most coronal portions of the root canal, and of undifferentiated mesenchymal cells, responsible for replacing necrotic pulp tissue before its infection.

The *presence of infection* can definitively affect the revascularization process, and regeneration of the ischemic pulp tissue after luxation injuries. In the case of associated crown fractures, it has been well established that dentinal tubules represent the main access pathway for invasion by bacteria and/or their toxins. The effect of this invasion on pulp tissue depends on the presence and speed of the flow of dentinal fluid, thickness of the dentinal layer, and condition of the subjacent pulp tissue[50,51,136,138,174,175]. In the case of intact crowns, the probable pathways would anachoresis, and through the harmed periodontal ligament - demonstrated by studies that found similar floras inside the root canal, and in adjacent periodontal pockets[76,99,164].

If the pulp tissue is infected in a state of ischemia, the process of replacement of the necrotic pulp tissue and revascularization are definitely compromised. Once it is formed, a leukocyte infiltrate, and an immune response is structured in an attempt to contain the bacterial invasion.

### Healing of Root Fracture

Root fractures involve both the supporting structures of the tooth (periodontal ligament, root surface and alveolar bone) and its pulp and mineralized tissues (dentin and cementum).

Although involving patterns of healing rather complex due to the large number of structures involved, root fractures have a favorable prognosis as regards the consolidation of the fragments, which can be seen by high rates of healing without endodontic intervention - 56% to 78%, reported in several clinical surveys[5,8,26,42,52,95,125,180,181]. According to Andreasen et al.[8], this positive prognosis is due to the force of the impact being dissipated along the fracture line, thus preserving the region of the apical foramen and consequently the apical neurovascular bundle. The pulp tissue in the region of the fracture can remain intact, or be compressed, lacerated or ruptured, since root fractures can present some type of luxation of the coronal fragment. The research done by Andreasen & Hjørting-Hansen[26] represented a milestone in understanding the phenomena involved in root fractures repair process. Based on the classification proposed by Schindler[155] and on radiographic and histological observations, the authors proposed four classic modalities of healing after root fractures: healing with mineralized tissue, interposition of connective tissue, interposition of bone and connective tissue and the interposition of granulation tissue that means the absence of healing.

In cases in which there is no luxation of the coronal fragment or it is a minimal displacement, the pulp tissue remains intact and its healing takes place in a manner similar to that observed in coronal fractures. Defense cells and undifferentiated mesenchymal cells, progenitors of the odontoblasts, migrate to the site of the fracture where they deposit a mineralized tissue bridge that unites the apical and the coronal fragment. This bridge forms an initial callus that stabilizes the fracture, and is followed by the invagination of periodontal tissue, responsible for the deposition of the cementum that fills the fracture line. This type of healing depends on the maintenance of pulp vitality in both fragments[8] and it corresponds to healing, with the interposition of mineralized tissue[26] (Fig. 24.64A-B).

Radiographic aspect of the consolidation of fracture in the root tooth 11 through the interposition of mineral tissue. In tooth 21 points not to fracture due to the consolidation of the pulp necrosis of the fragment and coronary intervention of granulation tissue.

In cases in which luxation of the coronal fragment involves displacement and consequent compromise of the blood supply, there is an inflammatory response in the region of the fracture line that aims at promoting revascularization and replacement of the ischemic pulp tissue. As in the case of luxations, the success of this process basically depends on the fast anastomosis between the ruptured pulp vessels, and those from the adjacent periodontal ligament, to set up immediately after the injury. Nevertheless, two particularities favor the occurrence of the revascularization process after root fractures: the presence of the fracture line itself, and the fact that only the coronal fragment needs to be revascularized.



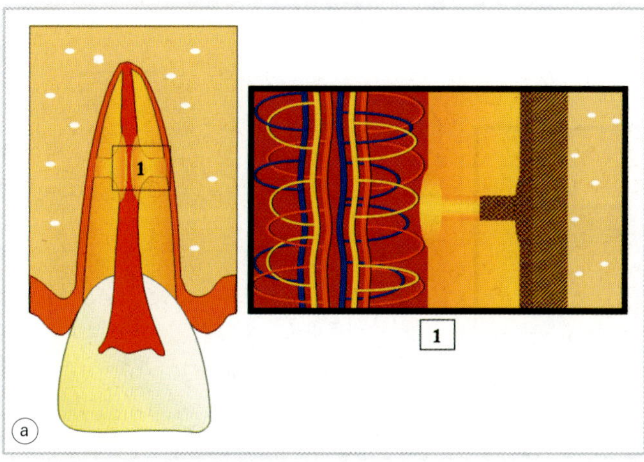


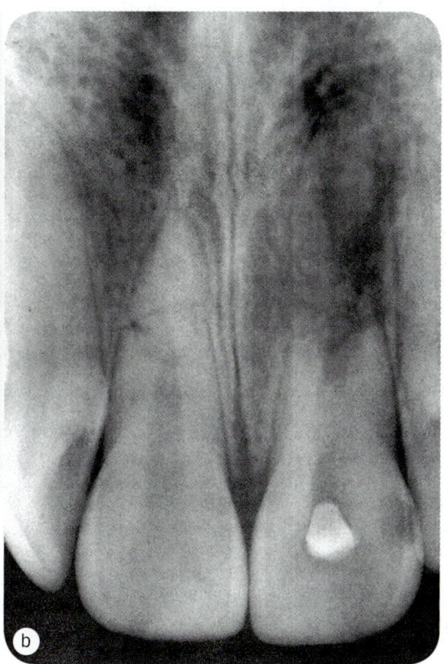


**Figure 24.64** - (**A**) Schematic illustration of the radiographic aspect of root fracture healing with mineralized tissue: although the fracture line is perceptible, the fragments are in close contact and there is no radioluscence the fracture line. Continuity of the lamina dura between the two fragments and rounding of the borders of the fracture are observed. Detail 1. Schematic illustration of the histological aspect: the formation of a dentinal callus is observed in the internal part of the fracture line and the cementum deposition on the external part. (Adjusted from Andreasen & Andreasen[22]). (**B**) Radiographic aspect of root fracture consolidation in tooth 11: healing with mineralized tissue. In tooth #21, non-consolidation of the fracture is observed, due to the pulp necrosis of the coronal fragment and interposition of granulation tissue is noticed.

The fracture line represents a pathway to drain the edema formed, decompressing the region and minimizing the pressure exerted on the pulp vessels, in addition to promoting a large pulp/periodontium interface, a favorable environment for the initial anastomosis. Because the coronal fragment is the only one to be revascularized, its shorter length allows for a faster revascularization. While pulp regeneration is in progress, cellular groups originating from the adjacent periodontal ligament populate the surface of the fracture. This promotes fracture consolidation by deposition of cementum on the surface of the fragments, and interposition of collagen fibers (Fig. 24.65A-B). This type of healing corresponds to interposition of connective tissue mentioned by Andreasen & Hjørting-Hansen[26]. This process results in the nutritional independence of the coronal fragment. Revascularization occurs with the participation of the vessels of the periodontal ligament and the formation of secondary dentin in the fracture line creates a new "apical foramen".

When the injury occurs in youngsters whose alveolar bone growth is not yet complete, the coronal fragment continues to erupt, while the apical fragment remains stationary in the jaw. In these cases, the interposition of bone tissue occurs between the two fragments that have normal periodontal ligaments, and are independent of each other (Fig. 24.66A-B). This type of healing was classified as interposition of bone tissue associated with connective tissue. Total pulp canal obliteration in both fragments is a common finding.

When large displacements of the coronal fragment allow the fracture line to be contaminated, the revascularization process is interrupted. There is pulp necrosis of the coronal portion of the pulp, while the apical fragment is usually vital. In this case, the consolidation process is compromised since a granulation tissue is formed between the fragments in an attempt to contain the bacterial invasion and in response to the aggressor agents released by the necrotic pulp tissue. These events correspond to the category non-healing proposed by Andreasen & Hjørting-Hansen[26], named as interposition of granulation tissue (Fig. 24.67A-B).

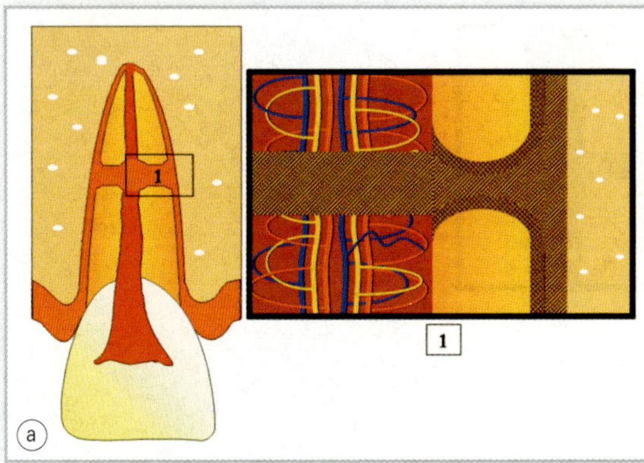


**Figure 24.65** - (**A**) Schematic illustration of the radiographic aspect of root fracture consolidation by the interposition of connective tissue: line of perceptible fracture with a narrow strip of radiolucency separating the segments. Continuity of the lamina dura between the two fragments and rounding of the borders of the fracture is observed. Detail 1. Schematic illustration of the histological aspect. Fractured root surfaces covered by cementum, with connective tissue fibers parallel to the surface of the fracture, or from one fragment to the other. (Adjusted from Andreasen & Andreasen[22]). (**B**) Radiographic aspect of root fracture consolidation in tooth #21 by the interposition of connective tissue.

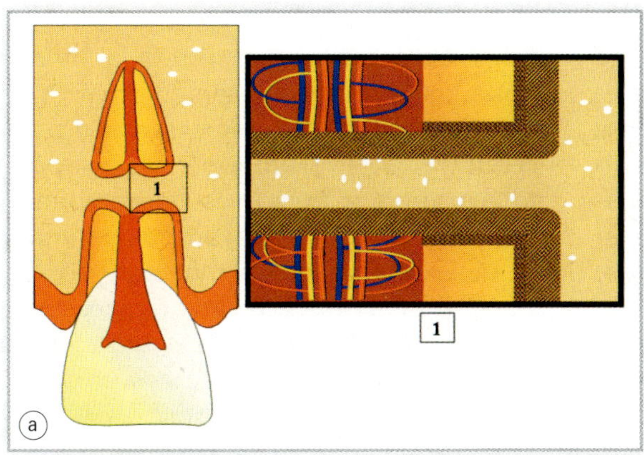


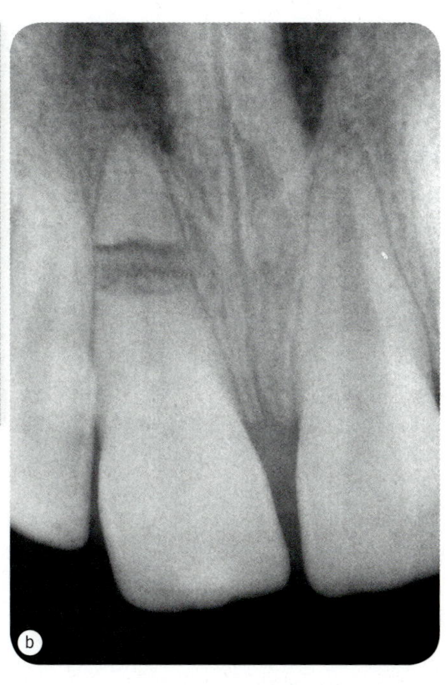


**Figure 24.66** - (**A**) Schematic illustration of the radiographic aspect of root fracture consolidation by the interposition of bone tissue: the bone tissue is seen between fragments; however the periodontal ligament space is normal in continuity with the parts of the periodontal membrane, of each fragment separately. Rounding of the borders of the fracture is observed, and in some cases the bone extends inside the root canal of coronal and apical fragments. Detail 1. Scheme of the histological aspect – Fractured root surfaces covered by cementum with connective tissue fibers linking the surface of the fracture to the alveolar bone interposed between the fragments. (Adjusted from Andreasen & Andreasen[22]). (**B**) Radiographic aspect of root fracture consolidation in tooth #11 by the interposition of bone tissue.

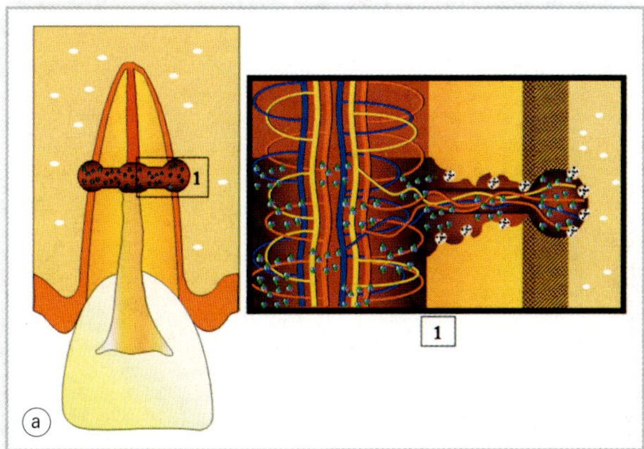


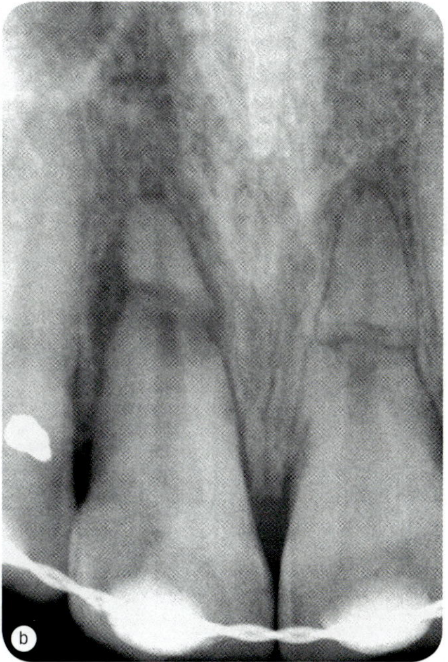


**Figure 24.67** - (**A**) Schematic illustration of the radiographic aspect of the absence of root fracture healing, due to the pulp necrosis in the coronal fragment and interposition of granulation tissue: it is characterized by the distancing of the fragments and presence of extensive radiolucent area in the fracture line, extending to the adjacent alveolar bone. Detail 1. Schematic illustration of the histological aspect, demonstrating granulation tissue interposed between the fragments, as a result of infection of the root canal, usually in the coronal fragment. (Adjusted from Andreasen & Andreasen[22]). (**B**) Radiographic aspect of the absence of root fracture consolidation in tooth #11 due to pulp necrosis of the coronal fragment and formation of granulation tissue between the fragments and in the adjacent alveolar bone. In tooth #21, healing is observed with interposition of bone tissue.

## Pulp Response After Avulsion

Dental avulsion causes the immediate rupture of all of the periodontal ligament fibers, blood and lymphatic vessels, and nerve bundles at the apical foramen resulting in an abrupt and complete interruption of circulation, neurovascular blocking and degeneration of all of the cell populations in the pulp, mainly in the coronal portion (Fig. 24.68). It implies the total displacement of the tooth out of its socket. Similarly to what happens in other luxation injuries, the pulp repair processes also begin apically after an immediate replantation. It comprises the proliferation of capillaries, defense cells and undifferentiated mesenchymal cells, which gradually replace the necrotic pulp tissue.

Experimental studies conducted in animals demonstrated that this process can result in different types of pulp healing, histologically described as: reparative dentin with a normal tubular pattern, reparative dentin with an irregular or absent tubular pattern, reparative dentin with cellular inclusions or osteodentine, irregular immature bone, mature bone or cementum with lamellar pattern, internal resorption and pulp necrosis[61,62,111,159,160]. Although it is not possible to extrapolate these results completely to humans, clinical surveys and experimental studies demonstrated that pulp healing is possible in teeth with incomplete root development. However it is a rare event after replantation of mature teeth, with apical diameter smaller than 1 mm[14,23,24,27,30,61,62,103,10]. Two healing patterns of the pulp tissue of replanted teeth were described radiographically. The first is the deposition of mineralized tissue internally, on the root canal walls leading to a decrease in the lumen of the root canal, and continuity of root development (Fig. 24.69A-D and 24.70A-B). In the other pattern described, the teeth presented arrested root development, and deposition of mineralized tissue in the pulp cavity, however separated from the dentin walls, and in continuity with the periapical alveolar bone (Fig. 24.71A-B).

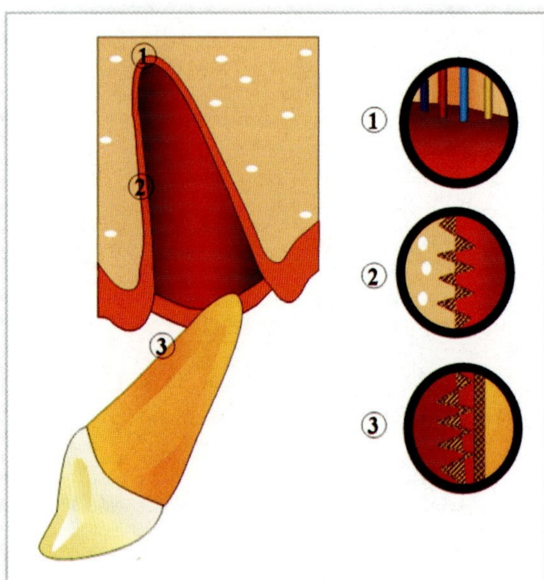


**Figure 24.68** - AVULSION 1. Rupture of the apical neurovascular bundle. 2. Rupture of the fibers along the entire periodontal ligament. The portion that is adhered to the alveolus remains viable because it receives nutrients from the alveolar bone vessels. 3. The portion of the fibers that remain adhered to the surface of the root after the avulsion, are deprived of blood supply and soon consume their stored metabolites leading to necrosis of the periodontal ligament. (Adjusted from Andreasen & Andreasen[22]).

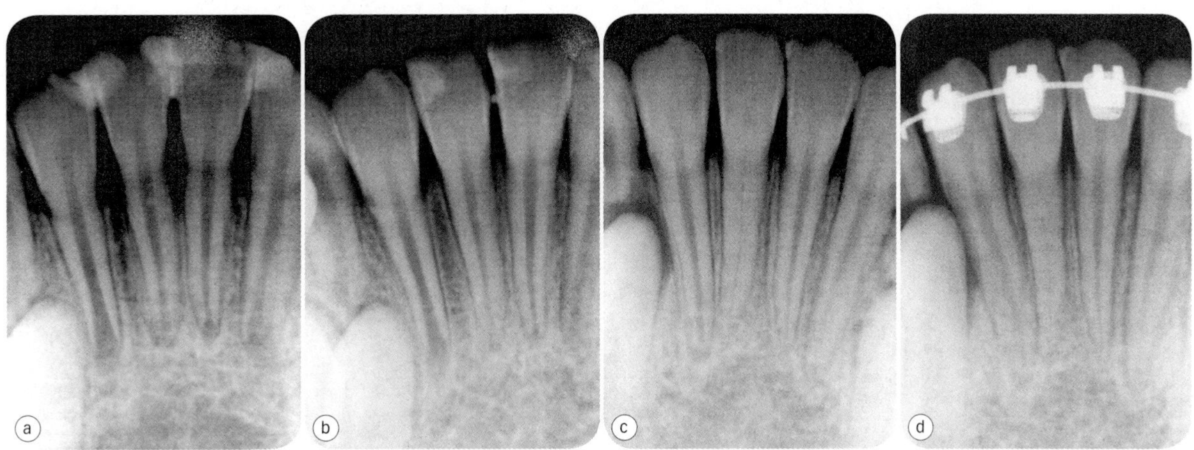

**Figure 24.69** - (**A**) Sequence of pulp healing after avulsion of tooth #31. Replantation performed after 15min; storage medium: milk. (**B**) Radiographically continuity of root development and deposition of mineralized tissue internally in the root canal walls are observed. (**C**) Radiographically continuity of root development and deposition of mineralized tissue internally in the root canal walls are observed. 1 year after replantation, complete root development and pulp canal obliteration are observed. (**D**) Radiographically continuity of root development and deposition of mineralized tissue internally in the root canal walls are observed. 1 year after replantation, complete root development and pulp canal obliteration are observed. Follow-up 3 years after the accident, demonstrating normality of the periapical region. The patient was allowed to have orthodontic appliances after diagnosis of periodontal ligament healing and absence of root resorption.

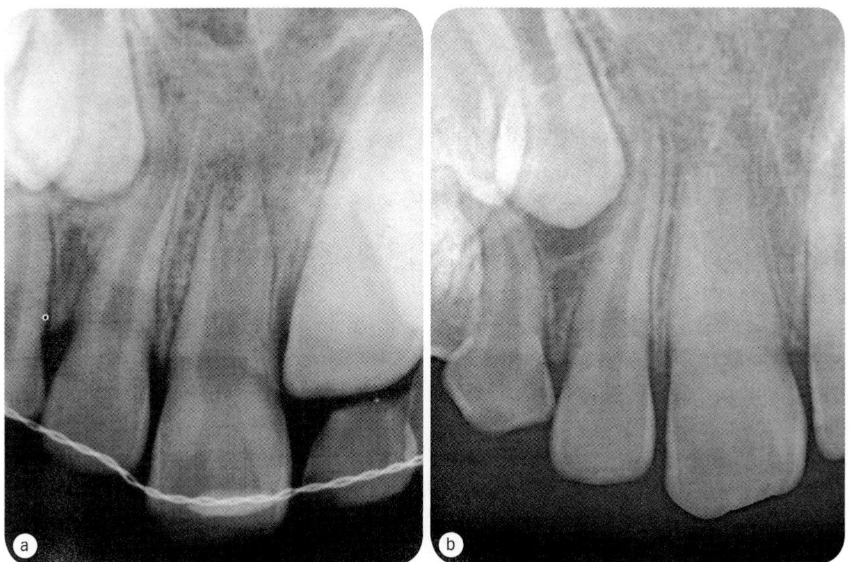

**Figure 24.70** - (**A**) Avulsion in a 7-year-old boy. The tooth was kept in milk for 20 minutes. After replantation a flexible splinting was performed, using ligature wire and composite resin. (**B**) Follow-up after 2 years shows healing with deposition of mineralized tissue internally, on the root canal walls.

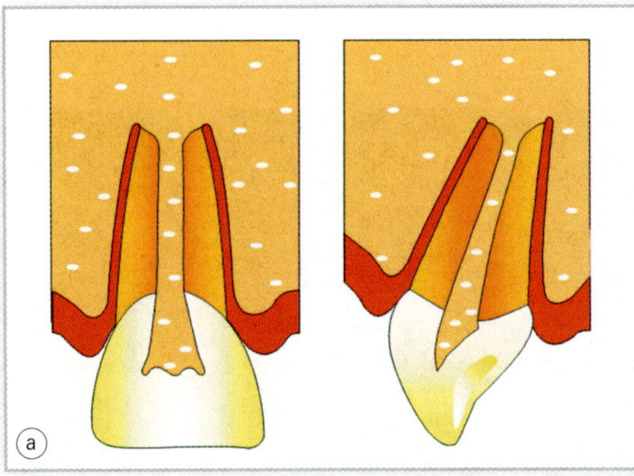

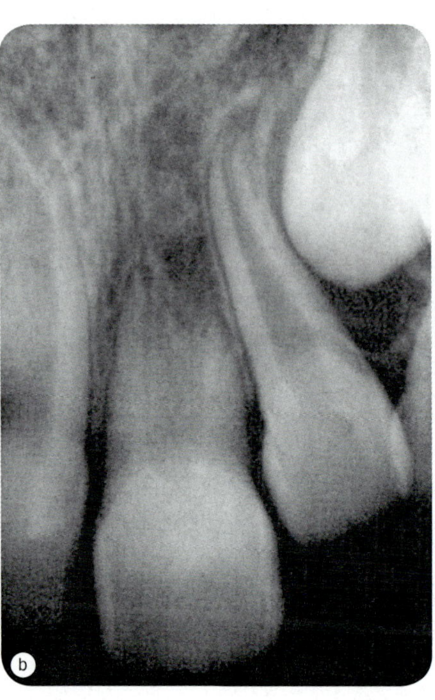

**Figure 24.71** - (**A**) Pulp healing after avulsion - Schematic illustration representing the deposition of mineralized tissue in the pulp cavity in continuity with the alveolar bone and separated from the dentinal walls of the root canal. Adjusted from Andreasen & Andreasen[22]. (**B**) Pulp healing after avulsion of tooth 21. Radiographic aspect of the deposition of the mineralized tissue in the pulp cavity in continuity with the alveolar bone and separated from the dentinal walls of the root canal by a radiolucent line, suggesting the presence of periodontal membrane.

Once again, the capacity of revascularization by anastomosis and new vascular formation will be decisive for the success of pulp healing. Thus, the wide apical foramen of immature teeth explains the higher chances of pulp healing. The larger pulp/ periodontium interface allows a fast process of anastomosis to be established between the blood vessels of the two tissues, guaranteeing that the immune system cells have immediate access to the ischemic pulp tissue[107,159,160]. Experimental studies in mice demonstrated that in replanted molars the defense cells resist to ischemic conditions, differently from what occurs with the odontoblasts and other pulp cells. They quickly respond to control bacterial invasion, remove tissue remnants and promote pulp repair[150]. These initial infection control mechanisms assume a fundamental importance, when one considers the deleterious effects of the presence of microorganisms on the success of the pulp revascularization process[18,61,62]. Experimental studies demonstrated that the presence of microorganisms in the root canal lead to the formation of micro-abscesses between the ischemic pulp tissue and the healing process originated in the apical region, thus compromising the revascularization[61].

Even teeth with incomplete root development, present discrepancies in the rates of pulpal healing, when clinical surveys are compared with experimental studies, the latter presenting the best results. Evidence suggests that in immature permanent teeth, other aspects such as the length of the root, and factors related to the storage period and media also play a role in the development of pulpal healing after replantation[24].

The length of pulp tissue is a strong determinant of the occurrence of revascularization after replantation[24] and auto-transplant[30]. Pulpal healing is the result of the competition between the healing process that starts in the apical region, and the bacterial invasion in the surface of the contaminated root. This happens via anachoresis, or throughout the damaged cervical region.

In teeth with complete root development bacterial invasion is favored, due to the distance in the long root and relative slowness of the revascularization process[11,24].

While the effect of the storage period and media on periodontal ligament healing after replantation of avulsed teeth is well demonstrated by extensive clinical[2,25,27,28,37,68,104,121,130,152] and experimental[14,17,44,45,66,73,88,90,112,135,141,170] literature, the few studies that evaluated the role of these factors in pulp tissue revascularization did not present consensual results[24,103]. Storage in a dry media seems to affect mainly the most peripheral part in the apical region of the pulp, since the remaining pulp tissue is relatively protected by the root walls. As the apical structures are fundamental in the early stages of the revascularization process, dryness of these structures brings immediate complications to the healing of the entire pulp tissue.

The means of wet storage can encourage bacterial survival and jeopardize the healing process.

Thus, humid storage would protect the most apical region of the pulp tissue from drying, and consequently, the revascularization process. Nevertheless, unlike what happens with the periodontal ligament, this beneficial effect is independent of the type of humid storage media, and is limited by the storage period. If this region is contaminated by bacteria from the storage media, or from the oral environment, the humid storage media can favor bacterial survival compromising the healing process.

### Post-traumatic Neural Regeneration

Another important aspect to consider in pulpal healing after injuries with displacement, which involve the rupture of the apical neurovascular bundle, is the regeneration of the nerve fibers. Experimental studies in cats and mice demonstrated that pulp reinnervation after dental replantation always occurs where there is revascularization and regeneration of the pulp tissue, although it is known that nerve density never returns to normal levels[110,111,148]. Again, similar to that which occurs in revascularization, pulp tissue can be re-innerved by healing of the original fibers that were ruptured during the dental displacement, or by the proliferation of collateral axons, originated from fibers in the region adjacent to the apical foramen[148]. The nerve regeneration phenomenon is dependent on revascularization of the pulp tissue and influences its healing. Experimental studies have demonstrated that the regenerated nerve fibers had neuropeptides such as SP and CGRP which, among other properties, promote tissue healing, since they are vessel-active and work as growth factors for endothelial cells. On the other hand, the amount and distribution of the healed nerve fibers depends on the predominant cell type in which the healed tissue replaces the ischemic pulp. The highest nerve density was observed when there was new odontoblast formation, capable of depositing dentin on the root canal walls[110,111]. This interaction between nervous activity and tissue remodeling, known as neurotropism, was demonstrated in active dentinogenesis areas and explains the extensive occurrence of post-traumatic pulp canal obliteration as a result of pulpal healing, after injuries that involve the apical neurovascular bundle.

### Pulp Canal Obliteration – PCO

The deposition of mineralized tissue on the root canal walls is a physiologic process of ageing, or defense of the vital pulp. During root development, the rate of apposition of dentin is 6.0 μm/day and for secondary dentin it may occur at a slower pace. Tertiary dentin is deposited locally in response to an aggressor stimulus at a rate of 3.5 μm / day. This response can be considerably accelerated after traumatic dental injuries, auto-transplants[96,106] and orthodontic treatment[65].

Although there are references to this occurrence in the literature, and to the benign nature of this hard tissue apposition after traumatic injuries [41,42,89,94,119,140,149], Andreasen et al.[10] were responsible for the description of the progressive hard tissue formation along the root canal walls as relatively common after luxation injuries. The post-traumatic pulp canal obliteration (PCO) seems to happen as a consequence of pulp repair after the injury of the apical neurovascular bundle, (Fig. 24.72). The occurrence of PCO has been reported after traumatic injuries in permanent teeth, with frequencies ranging from 3.0 to 24%[10,38,52,58,70,84,147,180]. This accelerated dentin apposition may be due to failures in the neurological regulation of secretory activity of the odontoblasts during revascularization and re-innervation that follows traumatic injury. The presence of parasympathetic innervation in the pulp was described following the trigeminous path. It may inhibit the activity of stimulating the secretory function of odontoblasts - the deposition of dentin[34,53,54]. This regulation could also be performed at distance by elements present in the blood[69,167]. Since the parasympathetic fiber follows the path of the trigeminal sensory fibers and acts antagonistically to the sympathetic fiber, regulating the secretory activity of the odontoblasts[53,54], an injury to the apical nerve bundle, would result in: 1) loss of pulp sensitivity resulting from the lesion of the trigeminal fibers; 2) loss of inhibition of the dentin synthesizer activity by the odontoblasts, with consequent pulp canal obliteration. Depending on the mechanism by which the parasympathetic fiber acts, its inhibitory effect on the secretory activity of the odontoblasts could only be restored after the complete re-innervation or revascularization of the pulp. The result of this uncontrolled situation would be a rapid decrease in the lumen of the root canal, observed radiographically, within a period of one year after the injury, leading to obliteration of the pulp chamber, which may be partial – PPCO – with the lumen of the root canal remarkably decreased, but radiographically visible (Fig. 24.73), or complete – CPCO – when the lumen of the root canal is not observed radiographically (Fig. 24.74). In addition to this obliteration, there can be dystrophic calcification, stimulated by the immune response due to the presence of bacteria, as well as mineralization of thrombus and clots resulting from the post-traumatic hemorrhage. However, irrespective of the radiographic aspect, the space is occupied by the pulp tissue that can be identified histologically.

The occurrence of PCO is related to several factors, such as the type of traumatic injury and the degree of root development at the time of the accident. According to data obtained in clinical surveys, PCO is common after luxation injuries that affect the neurovascular bundle, but that allow it to be revascularized[40,94,145,149,163]. As regards the stage of root development, there is consensus in the literature that PCO is predominant in children 11-years-old and younger, mainly in those teeth with incomplete root development[10,40,58,94]. Moreover, Andreasen et al.[10] also

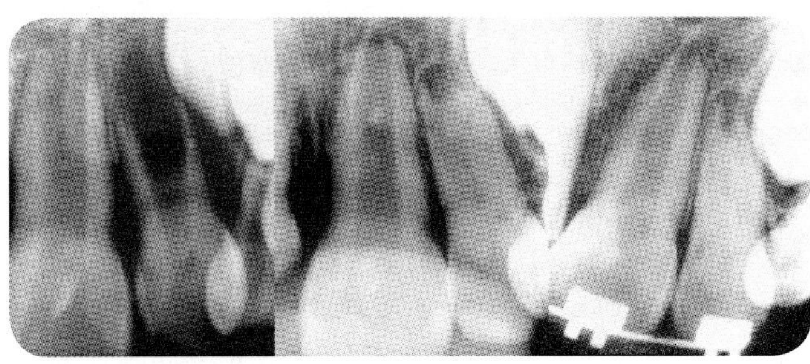

**Figure 24.72** - Development of pulp canal obliteration, observed radiographically 6 months after subluxation of tooth #22.

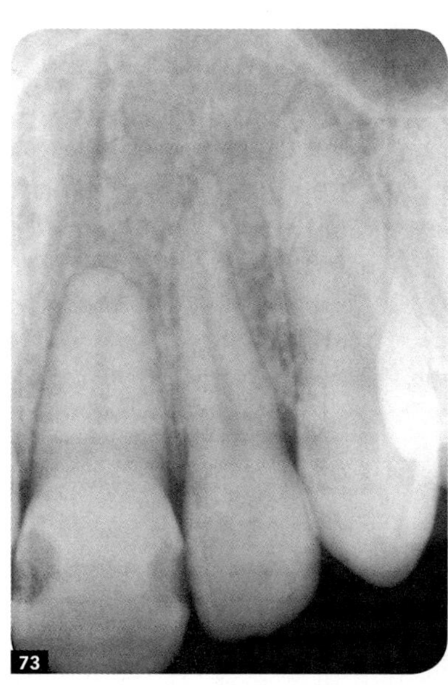

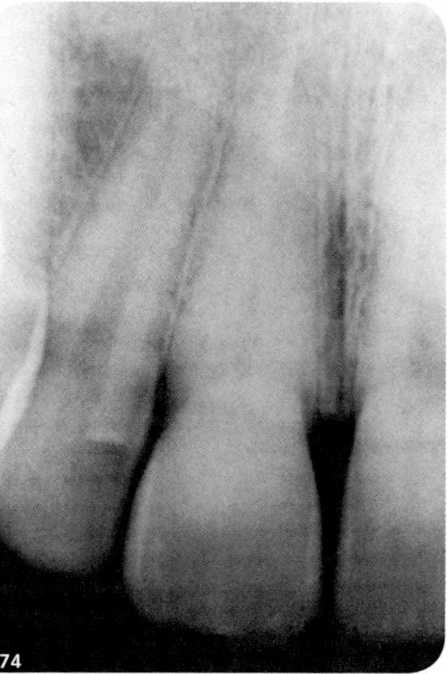

**Figure 24.73** - Partial pulp canal obliteration – in spite of being remarkably decreased, the lumen of the root canal of tooth #21 is still visible radiographically.

**Figure 24.74** - Total pulp canal obliteration – the lumen of the root canal of tooth #11 is not visible radiographically.



reported the type of splint and the degree of replacement of the dislocated tooth as decisive factors. The authors were based on the observation of the higher frequency of PCO after splinting with orthodontic appliances when compared with the acid etching and composite resin technique. As regards to repositioning procedure, the complete replacement of the tooth in its socket may result in an increase of the frequency of PCO in comparison with the absence or incomplete replacement.

Clinically, the teeth with PCO can present a discoloration, explained by the increased thickness of the dentin layer leading to greater reflection of light to external surface[168]. The response to the thermal test is usually negative. The response to the electric pulp testing is positive, although it presents higher thresholds, mainly in cases of total PCO after long periods of observation[10,40,94].

For many years the mere radiographic observation of the decreased lumen of the root canal has been an indication for endodontic treatment. This indication was based on the premise that pulp alterations were responsible for the obliteration and would lead to the pulp necrosis. There are no scientific evidences, clinical or experimental, that sustain the premise. The histological analysis of pulps removed from teeth with PCO, in which prophylactic root canal treatment was performed, demonstrated an increase of collagen content and a decrease in the number of cells. These findings are not sufficient to justify endodontic intervention[119]. There are different opinions on the indication of prophylactic endodontic treatment in the presence of pulp canal obliteration[89,140].

Clinical surveys of teeth with PCO, conducted for periods of up to 20 years, reported periapical alterations at rates ranging from 7 to 16%[10,16,40,94,147], demonstrating that although pulp necrosis is a late complication of PCO, its relatively low frequency does not justify performing prophylactic root canal treatment, particularly when considering the group at higher risk of PCO: moderate luxations in teeth with incomplete root development. Total pulp canal obliteration represents a challenge for endodontic therapy since the future access to the root canal may be unfeasible, in case endodontic intervention is necessary[1,161]. Studies demonstrated that although the phase of access to the root canal is difficult and requires ability and experience, it did not make it difficult to achieve successful endodontic treatment, since 80% of periapical healing was observed after root canal treatment in teeth with PCO and periapical lesion[60,154]. In view of the above-mentioned considerations, the endodontic treatment of teeth with PCO is not justified and is not able to solve the problem of discoloration as a result of the thicker dentin layer that is formed in the pulp chamber. Nevertheless, when obliteration is diagnosed at the beginning of the follow-up process, the decision about whether or not to perform root canal treatment should consider restorative treatment in the case of fractured teeth. However, as the pulp canal obliteration is more common in teeth with incomplete root development, we do not recommend prophylactic endodontic treatment. It is important that the patient (parents/guardian) be aware of the risks of discoloration and/or the possible difficulties in future endodontic treatment, as well as the strict follow-up procedures.

## Diagnosis of the Post-traumatic Pulp Alterations

### Pulp sensibility testing

Stimulation of teeth by thermal tests has been advocated in Dentistry for many years and the most frequently used are heated gutta-percha, ice, ethyl chloride ice, carbon dioxide snow and dichlorodifluoromethane. Similarly, the electric pulp testing (EPT), based on stimulation of sensory nerves, has been used in dental practice worldwide and is available for more than a century.

It is difficult to define the post-traumatic pulpal vitality condition, particularly with regard to the limitations of the examination and diagnostic techniques available, since they are indirect and reflect only some of the parameters of the repair processes. These deficiencies become critical immediately after the traumatic dental injury, when there is an urgency to reestablish the esthetics and function of the teeth involved. However, it is precisely at this stage that the pulp presents intermediate signs, whose clinical and radiographic characteristics are confused with those of necrotic teeth. Absence of response to pulp sensibility tests is a classic example, and has frequently been reported[4,6,9,35,38,41,58,84,92,93,134,142,145,158,165,182]. This loss of sensitivity described in the literature as a "state of shock of the pulp" after the injury, even if permanent, cannot be associated with pulp necrosis, as demonstrated in the study conducted by Bastos & Côrtes[39]. Results from the prospective study of the response to pulp sensibility test after injuries in permanent teeth, confirmed the temporary loss of sensibility as an intermediate phenomenon during pulpal healing, mainly after luxation injuries with displacement. Comparing the initial diagnosis established at the 30$^{th}$ day after the injury, with the final diagnosis, set from two to sixty-nine months after the trauma, it was demonstrated that there was a change in the pulp condition during the follow-up period, when considering the response to the pulp sensibility tests. If on the one hand, the positive initial response was a good indicator of maintaining vitality pulp (positive predictive value = 91.7%) (Fig. 24.75A), the absence of sensitivity in the period immediately after injury may not be related to development of necrosis (negative predictive value = 39.1%) (Fig. 24.75B).

The explanation for this phenomenon is that pulp sensibility tests indicate the situation of the sensorial components of the pulp, and not of its blood supply, which is ultimately responsible for the nutrition and metabolism of the pulp. As revascularization is a faster and more efficient process after the injury, than recovery of the apical nerve bundles, the result is a vital, but insensitive tooth, thus preventing the evaluation of the real pulp condition[4,5,9,39,92]. Another important factor to be considered when interpreting the responses obtained from the pulp sensibility tests, is that the majority of traumatic injuries affect teeth with incomplete root development, known to present insufficient response to these tests[49,72].

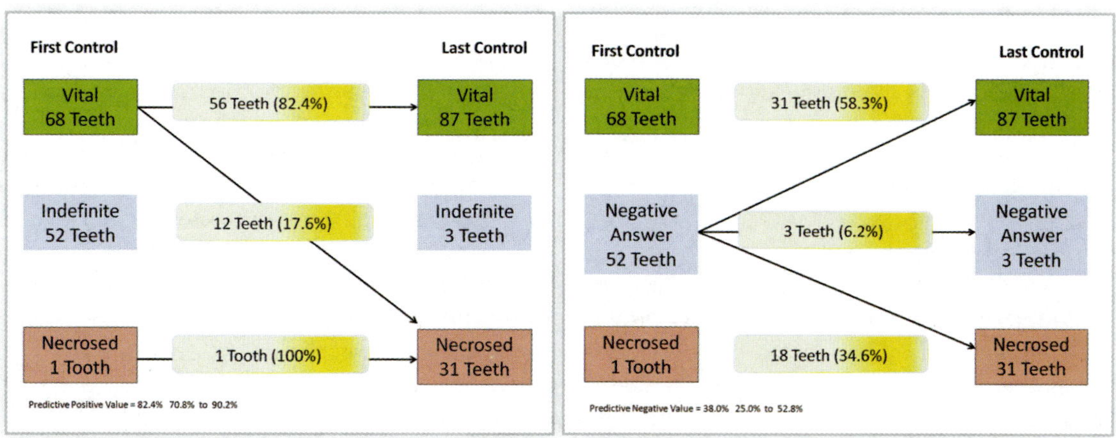


**Figure 24.75** - (**A**) The presence of pulp sensitivity in the period immediately after the injury, is a good indication of maintaining the pulp vitality at a long term basis, since most of the cases that presented positive response at the first examination maintained this response throughout follow-up. Source: Bastos & Côrtes, 2008. (**B**) The loss of pulp sensitivity in the period immediately after the injury can be an intermediate sign of the healing process and may not be associated with the development of pulp necrosis. It is observed that most of the cases that initially did not respond to the pulp sensibility test, responded positively throughout follow-up. Source: Bastos & Côrtes, 2008.

## Laser Doppler flowmetry (LDF)

As discussed above, although pulp prognosis is determined by factors noticed at the time of the injury and immediately afterwards, the definition of the condition pulp can only be achieved in the medium and long term. Explicit signs of necrosis - periapical alterations and inflammatory root resorptions - require a minimum period to be observed radiographically. Nevertheless, waiting for more evident signs of pulp necrosis may endanger the very maintenance of the immature permanent teeth due to the fragility of their root walls making them more susceptible to inflammatory root resorptions.

The search for a more objective assessment of the condition of blood circulation of the pulp resulted in the development of techniques that proposed to measure the pulp blood flow. The use the technology of laser beams - Laser Doppler Flowmetry - has been studied extensively as an alternative for recording the blood flow in healthy teeth and to observe the process of revascularization of traumatized teeth[74,123,124,137]. This technique uses a helium-neon laser light beam that undergoes a change of frequency, according to the Doppler principle, when reflected by the circulating red cells. That fraction of the light, which returns with distortion, is processed to produce a signal that reflects the flow of red blood cells and its average speed. This record is then used as a measure of the blood flow, the value being expressed as a percentage of the complete scale of deflection. Studies tested the clinical applicability of this technique for monitoring the pulp vitality of traumatized teeth, and demonstrated that the signal obtained, provides data about the situation of the pulp blood circulation allowing vital teeth to be distinguished from teeth with pulp necrosis at an early stage. From these conclusions the Laser Doppler Flowmetry was indicated as a promising technique for determining pulp vitality, when compared with other indirect methods available.

The main advantages of this technique would be the fact that it is not invasive, be relatively simple to use and provide an accurate and reproducible record of the pulp blood flow[74,123,137]. Nevertheless, two disadvantages are pointed out, which complicate its clinical use: the equipment is expensive, and the presence of blood pigment within the discolored crown may interfere with laser light transmission[85,132]. Thus, until new methods for assessing pulp blood flow are available, the radiographic and visual symptomatic approach remain the main means of diagnosis of post-traumatic pulp alterations.

## Tooth discoloration

Crown discolorations are frequent after traumatic dental injuries, but they are not always related to the diagnosis of necrosis, since they can be transitory. Transitory discolorations result from moderate luxations that are not sufficiently severe to cause complete rupture of the neurovascular bundle, but they cause pulp ischemia that leads to greater vascular permeability in an attempt to restore the blood supply of the ischemic tissue. Another factor to consider is that during the initial phases of angiogenesis, newly formed immature vessels do not have a basal membrane causing a great overflow of blood cells into adjacent tissues. Either due to post-traumatic intra-pulp hemorrhage, or due to the erythrocytes lost from newly formed vessels, the presence of blood in the pulp tissue is seen through the enamel and the dentin, giving the crown a rosy hue (Fig. 24.76). Once normal circulation has been reestablished, the crown returns to its normal color. This phenomenon can be concomitant with the temporary loss of pulp sensibility, and transitory radiographic alterations signifying each of these clinical manifestations, phases of the process of pulp healing in the absence of infection. On the other hand, invasion of the ischemic pulp tissue by bacteria and their by-products can lead to definitive color alterations of the crown, due to impregnation of the dentinal tubules by necrotic pulp tissue and by-products of its autolysis. In this case, the dental crown becomes darkened and has a purple, brownish, grayish or even bluish shade (Fig. 24.77). Another discoloration that should not be confused with that caused by pulp necrosis is a yellow shade, due to pulp canal obliteration (Fig. 24.78).

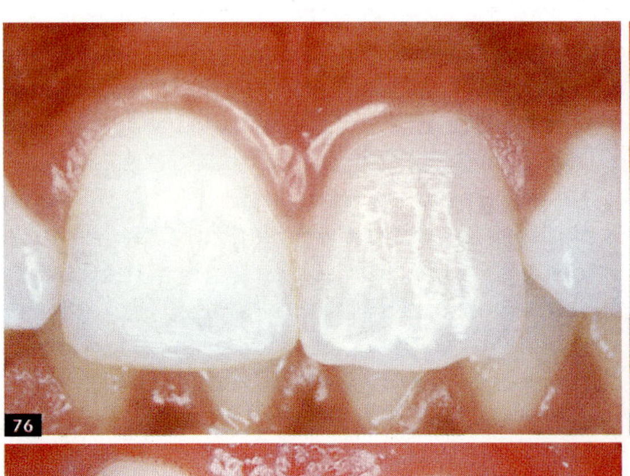
76

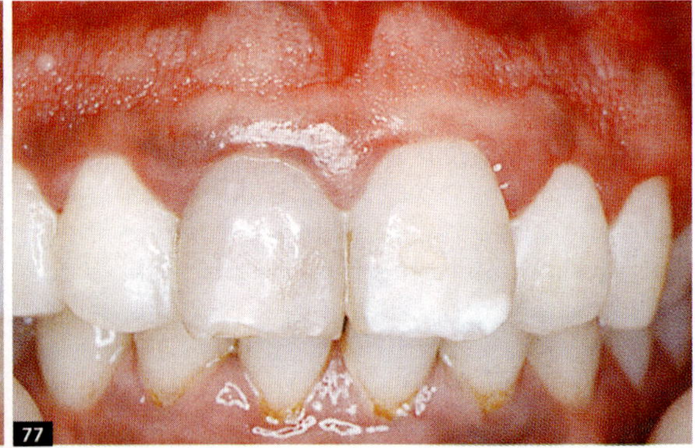
77

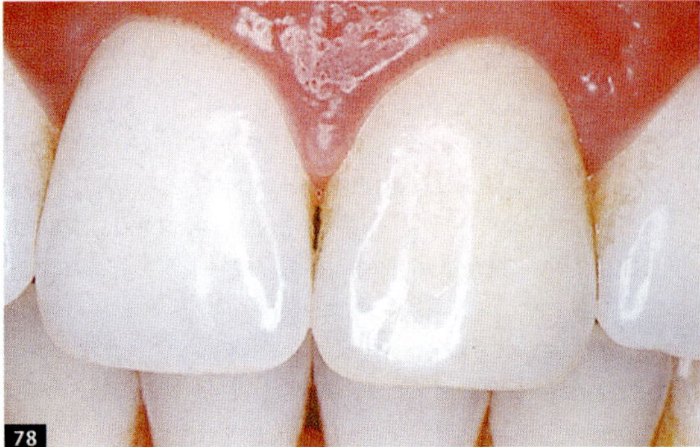
78

**Figure 24.76** - Rosy shade of the crown of tooth #21 resulting from post-traumatic pulp hemorrhage. Once the circulation is reestablished, the crown returns to its normal color.

**Figure 24.77** - Progressive and permanent darkening of tooth #11 resulting from the impregnation of dentinal tubules by necrotic pulp tissue, and by-products of its autolysis.

**Figure 24.78** - Yellow shade of the crown of tooth #21 characteristic of post-traumatic pulp canal obliteration. This color alteration is due to the thicker dentin layer inside the pulp chamber.

## Radiographic examination

The radiographic alterations traditionally associated with the diagnosis of pulp necrosis are: presence of periapical bone rarefaction (Fig. 24.79), presence of inflammatory external root resorptions (Fig. 24.80) and arrested root development (Fig. 24.81). Nevertheless, radiolucent periapical regions can also represent transitory manifestations associated with the process of pulp repair after luxations in teeth with complete root development[6,38,48]. This phenomenon was first described by Andreasen[6] who termed it Transient Apical Breakdown (TAB). Evidences obtained in clinical surveys[5,6,21,56] and experimental studies[178,179]. indicate that this process is related to pulp and periapical repair after lesion of the neurovascular bundle in young permanent teeth, with completely formed apex. It seems that it is a result of displacement of the root after luxation or of the coronal fragment of a fractured root. The collapse of periapical tissue triggers a local inflammatory response in which mediators stimulate the release of osteoclast activating factors. This stimulus can also result from the reaction to a transitory infection in the apical region. Radiographically, this phase would be identified by a radiolucent periapical area and in the apical portion of the root canal. Once repair has reached the remodeling phase, the resorption process resolves. This phase corresponds to radiographic normalization within the root canal and restoration of the periodontal ligament space. Since the radiographic exam shows the final result of the osteoblastic and osteoclastic activity adjacent to the root surface, but not the context in which they occur, these could be erroneously associated with the pulp necrosis. Notice in Figure 24.82A-D a 1 year follow-up of a central incisor that developed TAB. It might be questioned that the delay in treatment after the appearance of the apical radiolucent area could make difficult the prognosis. However there is evidence that the success rate of endodontic treatment is similar for teeth with and without radiolucent apical zone, mainly when treated with calcium hydroxide dressings prior to the root filling.

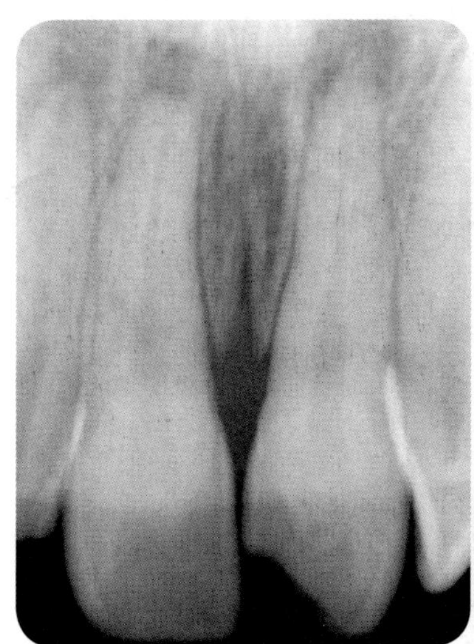

**Figure 24.79** - Radiographic aspect of periapical bone resorption in teeth #12, #11 and #21 characteristic of pulp necrosis.

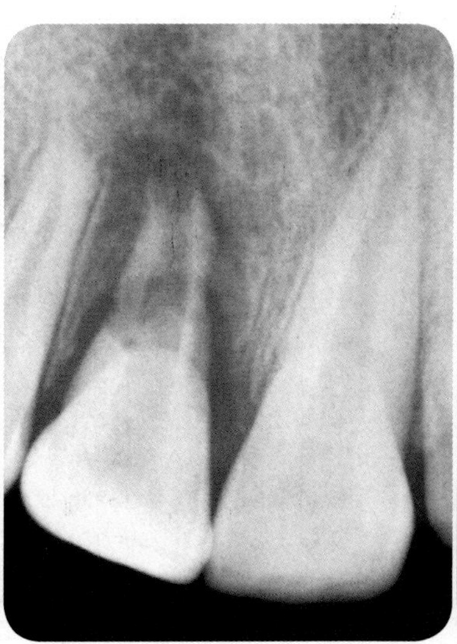

**Figure 24.80** - Radiographic aspect of the progressive external inflammatory root resorption related to the presence of infection of the root canal in tooth #11.

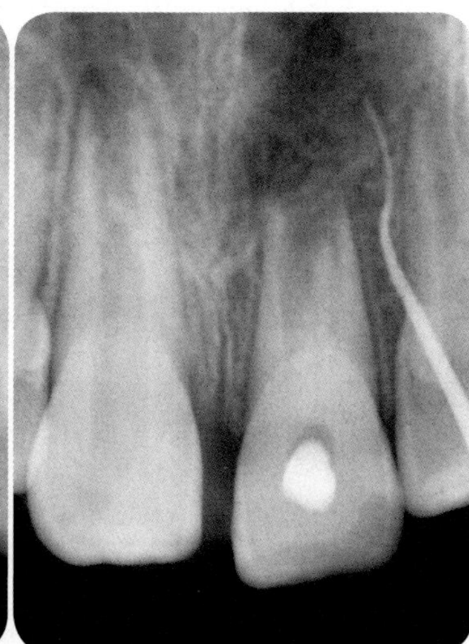

**Figure 24.81** - Arrested root development of tooth #21 due to pulp necrosis.

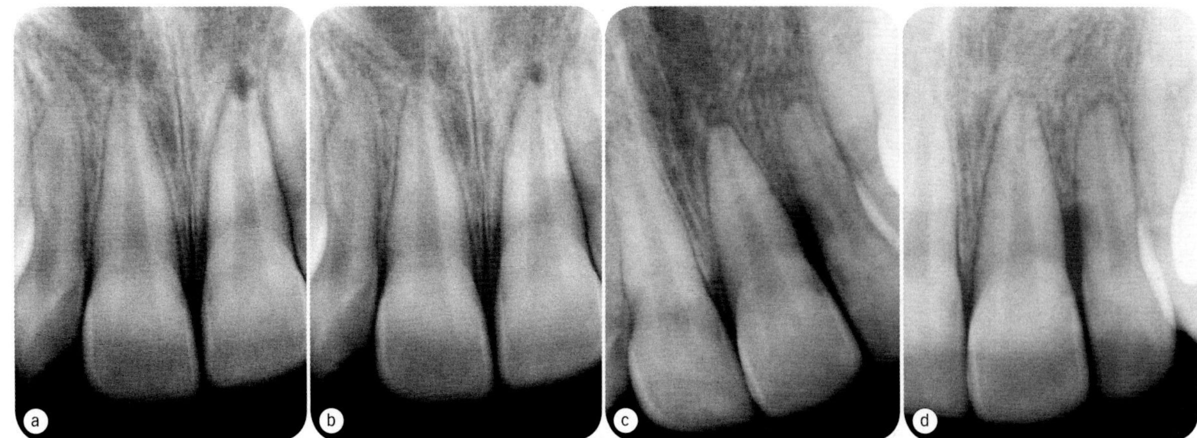


**Figure 24.82** - (**A**) Sequence of Transient Apical Breakdown - TAB after extrusive dislocation of tooth #11: appearance of small radiolucent periapical area 3 months after the injury. (**B**) Radiographic control 6 months after the injury revealing that there was no increase of the radiolucent area. (**C**) 9 months after the injury, healing of the apical region begins, without any endodontic intervention. (**D**) Complete healing of the apical region, 1 year after the injury.

Internal root resorptions, or root canal resorptions were described by Andreasen & Andreasen[21] as a rare finding after traumatic injuries in permanent teeth, being observed at a frequency of 2.0% after luxation injuries. They were classified as replacement and inflammatory root resorption. Both depend on the loss of the odontoblastic layer and pre-dentin, so that the clastic cells have access to the mineralized surface of the dentin. However, they differ with regard to the nature of the stimulus, responsible for maintaining the resorption activity. Since the osteoclasts require continuous stimulation during phagocytosis, and that offered by the exposed dentin is not enough to sustain the process for more than two or three weeks, the presence of a factor to maintain its progression is necessary. In the absence of this factor, resorption is transient and is followed by repair.

In the case of progressive internal inflammatory resorptions, the activity is nourished by the infection present in areas of partial necrosis, located in the more coronal portions of the pulp, subjacent to an area of chronic pulp inflammation[169,178]. Radiographically, it is characterized by an oval-shaped or round form observed within the pulp chamber[21,22] (Fig. 24.83).

Internal replacement resorption occurs from a metaplasia of cells of the pulp tissue in bone cells resulting in the substitution of the internal dentin root wall of the root canal by osteodentine. This resorption process becomes arrested after some time and complete pulp canal obliteration takes place. It should just be observed since it is not progressive. Radiographically, an irregular increase in the size of the pulp chamber is initially observed, followed by the total obliteration of the root canal space (Fig. 24.84A-D).

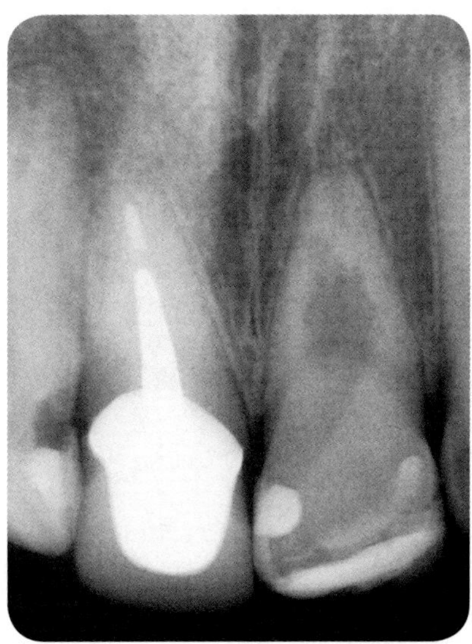

**Figure 24.83** - Radiographic aspect of progressive internal inflammatory resorption. Deformation of the root canal of tooth #21 is observed in the middle third.



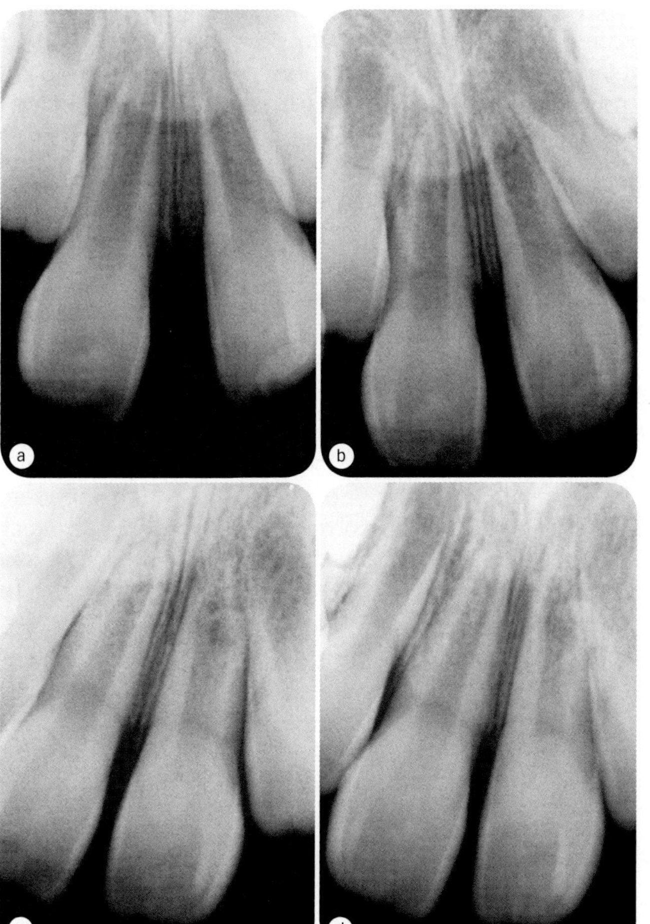

**Figure 24.84** - (**A-D**) Sequence of internal replacement resorption. Deposition of mineralized tissue is observed inside the pulp tissue of tooth #11 after an extrusive luxation.

## Post-traumatic Periodontal Involvement

Injury to the supporting structures, concomitant with the lesion of the apical neurovascular bundle is characteristic of luxation injuries. This compromise can either be restricted to rupture of the periodontal ligament fibers, as in concussions and subluxations, or it can be extended to the surface of the root and alveolar bone, as in luxations with partial or total displacement (avulsion) of the tooth. Thus, the quality of periodontal healing of luxation injuries will depend on the nature and extent of the injury to each of the components of the dental supporting structures.

The *periodontal ligament* is a thin layer (200mm) of connective tissue that surrounds the dental root, forming a protective barrier between the cementum and the alveolar bone. It consists of fibroblasts and a dense network of collagen fibers responsible for the anchorage of the tooth in the alveolar bone. Dispersed in this network of fibers there are numerous blood vessels, nerve fibers, and epithelial rests of the epithelial rests of Malassez that also form a network around the root. Under normal conditions, bone tissue does not invade the periodontal ligament space, although both are quite dynamic and are constantly being remodeled. There are no definitive theories to explain how this harmonious coexistence occurs, but it is known that when the periodontal ligament, or parts of it, are absent, an extremely favorable condition is established for the appearance of dental resorptions[82].

The *dental cementum* is a tissue, very similar to bone, which covers the roots and function as the insertion for the periodontal ligament fibers. It has an organic matrix essentially constituted of collagen and amorphous fundamental substance, and it is 50% mineralized with hydroxyapatite. Its collagen fibers, are secreted by the cementoblasts themselves, in addition to extrinsic fibers, known as Sharpey's fibres, that are formed by fibroblasts of the periodontal ligament, and included in the collagen matrix during root development. Since the cementum does not have remodeling capacity, the Sharpey's fibres do not recover during healing and remodeling of the periodontal ligament. Moreover, unlike the bone and the periodontal ligament, the cementum is not vascular, and it is usually more resistant to resorption. Two structures can be related to this lower susceptibility to resorption: the most external layer constituted of cementoblasts that do not respond to *parathormone* - PTH, a potent mediator of bone resorption[116], and the highly mineralized innermost layer, about 10 mm thick, described as intermediate cementum. A study suggests that it is neither dentin nor cementum; unlike an enamel form secreted by the cells of the epithelial root sheath, and its function would be to bond cementum to dentin[82]. The integrity of this layer plays a central role in the prevention of inflammatory resorptions, since it acts as an effective barrier, sealing the opening of the dentinal tubules externally, on its contact with the cementoblastic layer. In addition to the characteristics described above, experimental studies have identified a protease inhibitor, which could originate from the periodontal ligament and/or in the cementoblastic layer[117].

The *alveolar process* is the thickened ridge of *bone* that contains the *tooth* sockets also referred to as the *alveolar bone*, constituted of the external cortical plates of a central spongy bone and the alveolar bone. The alveolar bone corresponds to the lamina dura observed radiographically, and consists of a perforated bone lamina, in which the periodontal fibers are inserted and through which the blood supply of the periodontal ligament is carried. The cortical plates are superficial layers of lamellar bone, with thin fibers sustained by compact bone. The spongy bone that occupies the central part of the alveolar process is a membranous bone disposed in trabecula, externally covered by a thin layer of connective cells termed endosteum, and occupied internally by bone marrow that has an important role in hematopoiesis and odontogenesis. It is important to emphasize that the alveolar bone has great plasticity and it is in a constant state of remodeling.

## External root resorption

External root resorption represent one of the main complications of the repair process of tooth supporting structures and can frequently lead to the loss of the tooth[3,7,9,15,17,21,27,37,58,80,84,134]. Post-traumatic external resorption can be classified into two main groups: inflammatory and replacement resorption. The initial factor that establishes favorable conditions for activity of the clasts on the root surface is the same in both types: an injury of the cementoblastic layer. Depending on the presence of a maintenance factor that stimulates the clast cells continuously, both resorptions can be either progressive or transitory.

In mild luxations, in which the damage is restricted to the periodontal ligament, compression, stretching or rupture of the periodontal fibers leads to a hemorrhagic state, formation of edema and structuring of an inflammatory response. After the removal of the lacerated tissue, it culminates with the restoration of the normal periodontal ligament. The inflammatory reactions in the periodontal ligament cause the release of chemical mediators of inflammation that act by stimulating the clastic activity at cementoblastic and pre-cementum layers. The *surface resorption* (repair-related resorption) is associated with an injury to the cementoblastic layer, associated with small areas of necrosis in the periodontal ligament, which are not sufficient to maintain the continuity of the resorption process. Without continuous stimulus, osteoclastic activity ceases. Another possibility would be that with little stimulus, the clastic cells would not stand up to the resorption inhibitory factor present in the dentin[177]. Although the denomination surface resorption is well established in the literature (Fig. 24.85), it is important to emphasize that it is a self-limiting inflammatory process not associated with other clastic activity maintenance factors. For this reason, it was also called transitory inflammatory resorption[169] and root resorption associated with minimal necrosis[81].

In more severe luxations, such as extrusive and lateral luxation, the rupture of the neurovascular bundle leads to pulp necrosis and there is a severe injury to the supporting structures: periodontal ligament, root surface and eventually of the adjacent alveolar bone. The attrition generated by the displacement of the tooth inside its alveolus is responsible for the mechanical removal of large portions of the cementoblastic layer, leading to the exposure of dentinal tubules. The access for bacteria and their toxins originates from the infected root canal environment and reaches the external surface of the root. It is responsible for the maintenance of an inflammatory state that results in loss of bone and root structure, called inflammatory resorption[80,169] (Fig. 24.86A-B). It is believed that the main mechanism of inflammatory root resorption is related to the capacity of the endotoxins to trigger the release of activator factors of osteoclastic activity[129] although very little is known about the response of the cementoblasts to the pro-inflammatory cytokines and other possible local factors involved in the modulation of root resorption[82].

When large areas of the periodontal ligament are removed or damaged, healing involves different processes that compete among one another. They originate in the periodontal ligament and adjacent alveolar bone, and their purpose is to populate the root surface. The insufficiency of viable periodontal ligament cells available for this healing, leads to the fusion between mineralized tissues of the root and alveolar bone, promoting a gradual substitution of the dental tissues by bone[78] (Fig. 24.87A-B). *Replacement resorption* was first described by Andreasen & Hjørting-Hansen[27,28]. Starting from a clinical-radiographic and histological evaluation of replanted teeth, the authors described this type of resorption as being a direct union of the bone and the surface of the root, followed by resorption and substitution of the root structure by bone tissue. Subsequent experimental studies[14,17,29,77,131] reinforced this mechanism, demonstrating the role of an extensive lesion to the periodontal ligament in the development of this resorption.

The concepts of ankylosis and replacement resorption were then used as synonyms. However, subsequent studies[78,118] demonstrated that preservation of the cementoblastic layer was a decisive factor in preventing replacement resorption originating from fusion between the medullar bone and the dentinal structure of the root. Thus, these concepts should be considered separately, since ankylosis is the result of loss of periodontal ligament, and replacement resorption depends on the loss of the cementoblastic layer.

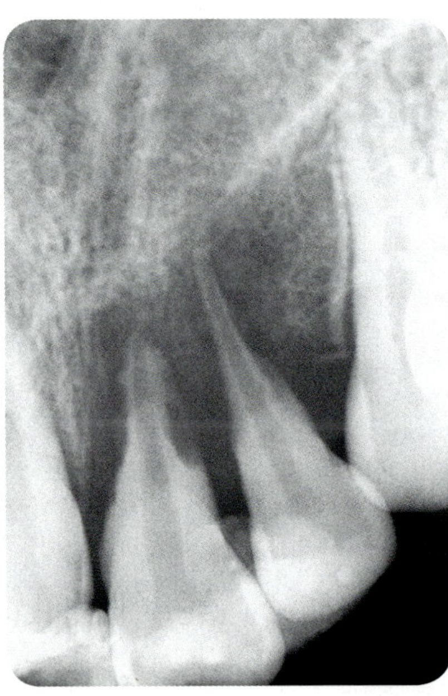

**Figure 24.85** - External surface resorption. Radiographically, one observes healing of a defect resulting from the clastic activity on the surface of the root of tooth #21.

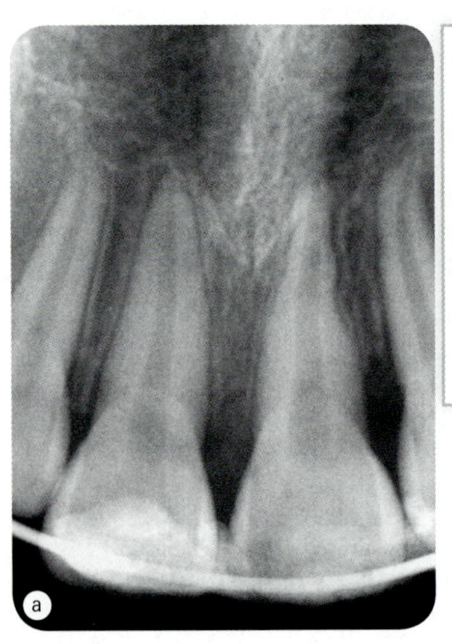

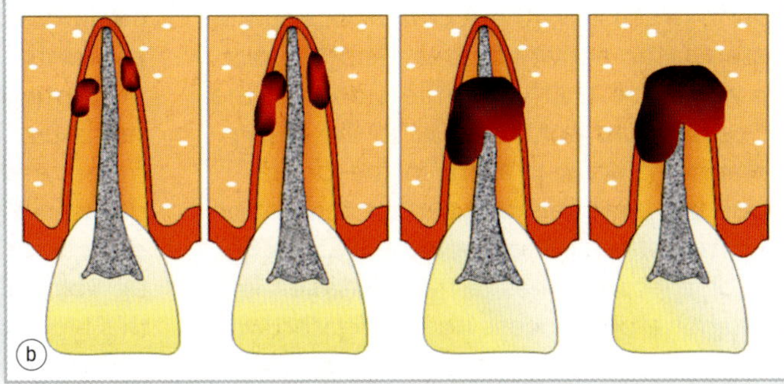

**Figure 24.86** - (**A**) Progressive, inflammatory external root resorption. Radiographically, irregular radiolucent areas are observed on the external surface of the root of teeth 21 and 22 . These areas correspond to the loss of root and bone structure, due to the presence of granulation tissue resulting from the presence of infection on the lumen of the root canal. (**B**) Schematic illustration of the development of the progressive inflammatory external root resorption. (Adjusted from Andreasen & Andreasen[22]).

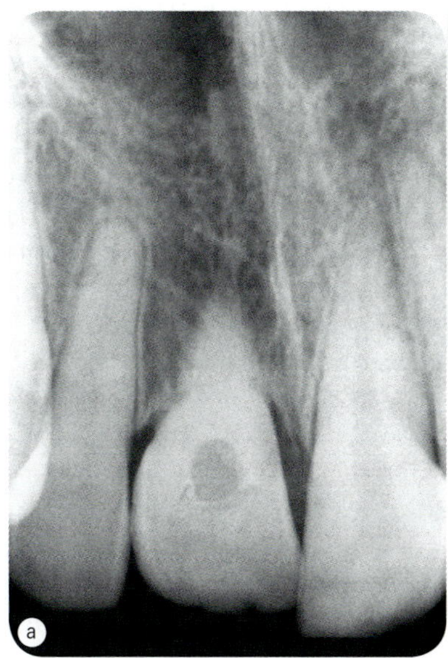

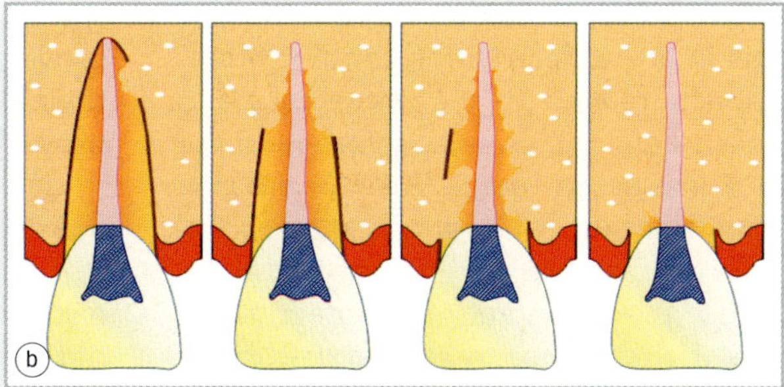

**Figure 24.87** - (**A**) External root replacement resorption. Radiographically, one observes gradual substitution of the dental tissues of the root of tooth #11 by bone tissue. (**B**) Schematic illustration of the development of the external root replacement resorption. (Adjusted from Andreasen & Andreasen[22]).

The factors that maintain replacement resorption are not yet known in detail. It is believed that when the cementoblastic layer is lost, the dentinal surface of the root is colonized by osteoblasts and osteoclasts that usually cover the medullar bone. In response to the stimulus of PTH and of PGEs, the osteoblasts assume an elongated form and increase their inter-cellular spaces, exposing the dentinal matrix for fixation of the osteoclasts and and triggering the process of eliminating the dentin structure, similar to that which occurs during the physiological remodeling of bone tissue. This type of resorption was also called endosseous root resorption[78].

Some studies have suggested that there is an immunopathological mechanism in root resorptions, due to a possible immunogenic potential of the dentin[86,87]. The dentinal proteins are confined and isolated, since odontogenesis [32,166].

This fact can characterize them as "kidnapped" antigens, or in other words, antigens that are not presented to the immunological system by special location or late formation during the development of the natural tolerance. When exposed to the immunological system already in activity, they initiate immunopathological responses, as in the cases of lens and sperm cells. When exposed by the injury of the cementoblastic layer, the dentin would act as a "kidnapped" antigen, inducing an immunopathological reaction responsible for the root resorption. This matter is controversial because there are very few studies in the literature. Other experimental studies are needed in order to investigate the role of immunological mechanisms of root resorption.

### Determinant factors in periodontal healing after replantation

Although external root resorption represent sequelae of the periodontal healing of any lesion, in which the supporting structures of the tooth are compromised, their occurrence is especially relevant after replantation. They are the most frequent consequences ranging from 74 and 96%, and are the main cause of loss of the tooth after replantation. In dental avulsions, in addition to the total rupture of the periodontal ligament and damage to the cementoblastic layer, factors related to the extra-oral period and storage medium can also cause additional damage to the remaining fibers in the surface of the tooth[17]. Moreover, aspects related to the immediate and sequential treatment, can also interfere in the healing of replanted teeth. Since Andreasen & Hjørting-Hansen[27,28] correlated the resorption processes and the duration of the extra-oral period, the immediate replantation and subsequent root canal treatment has been extensively used. Several experimental studies[14,113,162] and clinical surveys[2,23,24,36,37,55,75,153] confirmed the relationship between long, dry extra-alveolar periods, and the frequency of occurrence of root resorption. Thus, the best place to store an avulsed tooth is in its own alveolus. After the avulsion, the remaining cells of the periodontal ligament attached to the surface of the root are deprived of their blood supply, and loose their metabolites. This is due to the high permeability of the animal cells to water, so that they behave like *osmometers*, distending in a hypotonic medium and decreasing in a hypertonic medium, according to the osmotic movement of the water and either the increase or decrease in liquid are critical. To maintain the physiologic cellular metabolism and protect the cells against additional injuries resulting from a long extra-alveolar period, these nutrients should be restored by means of immediate replantation or biological storage as quickly as possible[14,31,47]. Several storage media have been proposed to restore cellular metabolites and favor a physiological pH and osmotic pressure. Theoretically, the immersion of the tooth in an enriched medium before replantation would allow the necrotic cells and the debris to be washed away, minimizing inflammatory root resorption. Moreover, it would revitalize the surviving cells, reducing the incidence and severity of the replacement resorption, since cells with adhesion potential could be present to repopulate the naked root surface before the invasion of bone cells[141].

The first storage media suggested in the literature for maintaining the avulsed tooth were water, saliva and physiological saline solution. Although this would be better than allowing the root to dry[14,47,64], the benefit provided by these media is limited, due to their low osmolarity[47,112,113], and has not been proved in longitudinal clinical surveys[23,25].

The use of a plastic wrapping to protect the avulsed tooth from dehydration as a result of the extra-alveolar period tested in an experimental situation[45], resulted in levels of periodontal healing, similar to those of immediate replantation. These results, however, were not confirmed clinically[25].

In the search of other storage medium superior to water, saliva and sterile saline solution, the use cow's milk was proposed for storing an avulsed tooth, due to its physiological properties - pH (6.5-7.2) and osmolarity similar to that of extra-cellular fluid (250-270 mOsm $Kg^{-1}$). Milk is easy to obtain at the place of the accident, and to is relatively free of bacteria. Nevertheless, the benefits of milk depend on relatively fast storage (within 15 minutes). Although it maintains the osmolarity and the production of proteins for the periodontal ligament cells, thus preventing its cellular death[44,73,113,135,143,170] milk is unable to restore the lost metabolites and cell viability. Thus, the cells lack energy and ions to "repopulate" the periodontal ligament, since its normal morphology is not restored and its capacity to differentiate and undergo mitosis is not recovered[44,57,73,113,170].

Among the solutions capable of restoring the vitality of the periodontal ligament cells suggested in the literature as storage media for avulsed teeth, are cell culture mediums, such as Hank's balanced salt solution. HBSS[44,66,88,105,139,141,170], Eagle's minimal essential medium[31,44] and ViaSpan[88,112,170], in addition to a medium rich in growth factors, obtained from the supernatant of a culture of human periodontal fibroblasts[90,141]. The results of experimental studies confirm that these storage media are ideal for the maintenance or revitalization of periodontal ligament cells.

Several attempts to treat the root surface with destroyed or necrotic periodontal ligament have been verified in the literature, with the objective of reducing the risk of root resorption. There have been proposals to treat the root surface with several types of fluoride solutions[43,55,156,157], antibiotics[43,62,156], ATP Solution[71,183] and acids[184] to remove the remainders of necrotic periodontal ligament from the root surface, and to facilitate the adhesion of the collagen fibers. Alendronate was used in combination with HBSS in an experimental study in dog roots. The results showed that it had statistically significantly more healing than the roots treated with HBSS without alendronate[115]. Iqbal and Bamaas[91] in a study using beagle dogs showed that the percentage of healed periodontal ligament found in the experimental EMDOGAIN treated group was significantly higher than that found in the control group. Similarly, the incidence of replacement resorption was significantly less in the experimental group than in the control group[91]. Another experimental study in dogs suggested that Emdogain, in this particular model, had no effect on cell migration into the. blood clot (and coagulum) and on the re-population of cells on the instrumented root surface[33]. Other therapies have endeavored to substitute the periodontal ligament by bio-compatible materials[83] or autogenous grafts[97]. The best results were obtained with the association of fluorides and antibiotics[43,156]. None of the studies published showed consistent evidence for root surface treatment, the value of the solutions recommended being questionable.

The involvement of the alveolar parts of the periodontal ligament in the healing of replanted teeth is controversial, since the few data obtained from studies in animals are conflicting[19,122]. It can be concluded that the treatment of the alveolus does not interfere in the prognosis of replantation[171].

Until the 1970s, dental splinting followed the same principles as the maxillary fixtures, although a tendency to shorter immobilization periods has existed since 1930. Nowadays it is known that rigid immobilization, necessary for a good consolidation of the bone fractures, can lead to complications when applied to displaced or avulsed teeth. Experimental studies have demonstrated that physiological movement accelerates and improves periodontal ligament healing, reducing the chance of dental ankylosis[20,108]. Another important item is the duration of the period of the immobilization. Minimum periods reduce the occurrence of ankylosis, and they are long enough to produce the necessary stability for the avulsed tooth during the initial period of periodontal ligament healing[128,133,176].

Treatment with systemic antibiotics has been suggested after replantation of avulsed teeth, with the objective of avoiding contamination of the root surface, and reducing the activity of inflammatory resorption. Another effect of the antibiotic would be to control the bacterial population in the alveolus, which is important with respect to the healing pattern of replanted teeth, mainly after an extensive extra-oral period. A single experimental study observed that the administration of parenteral penicillin before extraction, and immediately after tooth replantation, resulted in a smaller occurrence of inflammatory resorption, due to the decrease in bacterial contamination on the root surface and in the pulp[79]. Subsequent studies using doxiciclin[61] and tetracycline[151,152] however, observed that the systemic administration of these antibiotics contributed little to preventing root resorption. The results of clinical surveys also did not confirm the effect of the systemic antibiotics on periodontal healing[25]. Thus the use of systemic antibiotics is questionable and must be avoided to solely contribute to pulp and periodontal healing after tooth replantation.

It is critical to remove the pulp after replantation, in order to prevent and treat external inflammatory root resorption. This resorption is a result of the association of the presence of bacteria inside the root canal/dentinal tubules, and the lesion to the periodontium and surface of the root. Thus, endodontic treatment should begin within one week after replantation of teeth with complete root development (with closed apical foramen) to avoid the propagation of products from necrotic pulp to neighboring periodontal tissues[12,173].

It is recommended that the initial session of the endodontic treatment be performed while the tooth is still splinted. The use of calcium hydroxide-based intracanal dressing has been recommended, due to its antibacterial properties, important in the prevention of inflammatory resorptions, and for its performance in the control and healing of inflammatory resorption[12,46,80,114,172]. In immature teeth, where the apical foramen is wide open and replantation occur within 3 hours after injury, revascularization can be expected[23,103]. Radiographic evaluation should be made 2 to 3 weeks after replantation since periapical radiolucent area or external inflammatory root resorption can be noticed at this time. Endodontic therapy must be initiated immediately with calcium hydroxide therapy, in case of necrotic pulp.

## PART 4. Endodontic Treatment of Immature Traumatized Permanent Teeth

Endodontic treatment of teeth with traumatic injuries is indicated in cases in which conservative treatment was unsuccessful and/or when pulp necrosis occurs[5,10,11,12,16,27]. This is one of the most frequent complications in teeth with a diagnosis of luxation, particularly those presenting complete root development[1,4,22]. Special attention should be given to the signs and symptoms, in order make a correct decision about the treatment and promptly establish it. Several factors that have already been thoroughly discussed in previous sections are determinant for the diagnosis and prognosis, and are directly related to the type and severity of the injury, as well as the stage of root development.

In this chapter, the treatment of teeth with incomplete root development will be emphasized. The diagnosis of pulp necrosis is particularly delicate, due to the difficulty of response to pulp sensibility tests in immature teeth. The nervous structures of the pulp are still not completely developed. Factors that aid diagnosis are discoloration of the crown and, mainly cessation of the former function of the epithelial root sheath, as well as the arrest of dentin deposition on the root canal walls, observed in the x-ray (Fig. 24.88A-B). The radiographic examination is of great importance and care should be taken, not to confuse the image of the pericoronal sac with the presence of apical resorptions. When arrested root development occurs, the foramen remains open and the root canal walls are divergent in the apical region. These characteristics make root canal treatment by the conventional methods unfeasible, complicating the cleaning, shaping and filling of the root canal[10,26]. Moreover, the treatment time is very long, mainly in the case of younger patients.

For many years, the indication for immature teeth requiring root canal treatment was immediate surgery with retrograde filling. This procedure is contraindicated, however, as it results in lesion to the adjacent vital structure, in addition to causing an emotional problem for the child[37].

It is known that pulp revascularization is a probable phenomenon after luxation in immature teeth, which contraindicates immediate root canal treatment[1,2,3,4,7]. It is prudent go through a period of careful observation after the traumatic dental injury occurs. Radiographic follow-up may take place at 3, 6 and 8 weeks after the injury, changing to every three months, for one year which, in most cases is enough to define the diagnosis[7]. The radiographic data of arrested root development and the presence of radiolucent areas indicative of external inflammatory resorption are of fundamental importance to define the presence of pulp necrosis (Fig. 24.89A-B). Replanted immature teeth shall not be treated endodontically until the initial signs of periapical lesion or inflammatory external root resorption are observed. When suitable, endodontic treatment should begin as quickly as possible, because once inflammatory root resorption has become established in immature teeth, its progression is fast due to the frailty of the dentinal walls, and it could lead to their destruction in short period of time (Fig. 24.90)

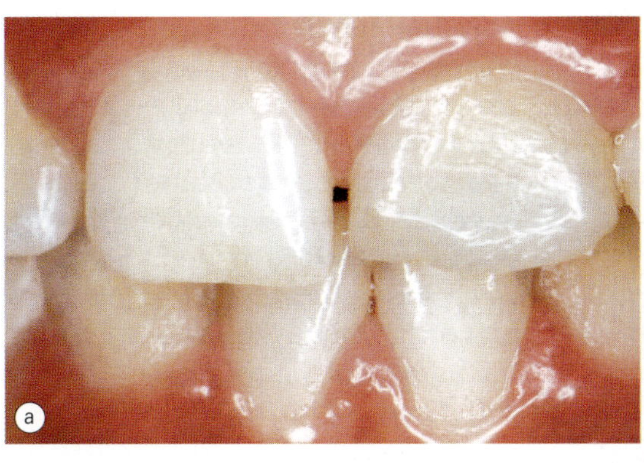

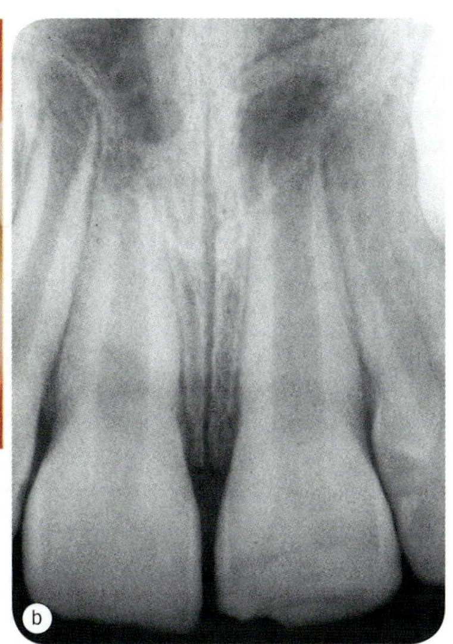

**Figure 24.88** - (**A**) Tooth #21 presents discoloration of the crown 3 months after enamel and dentin fracture, associated with subluxation. (**B**) The radiographic image reveals arrested root development. The diameter of the root canal and apical foramen of tooth #21 present differences, in comparison with tooth #11 that has a vital pulp. Periapical bone rarefaction is also noted in tooth #21.

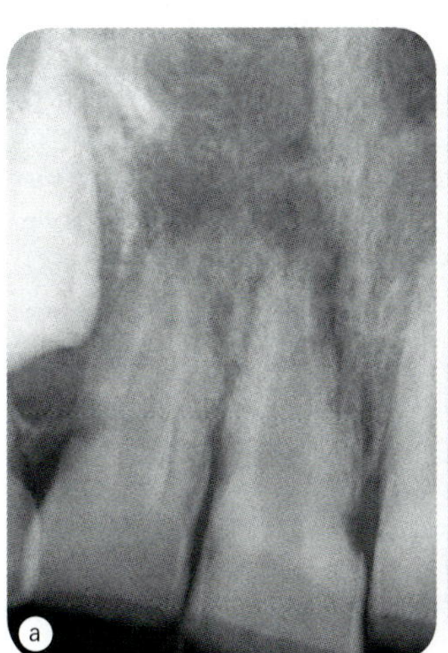

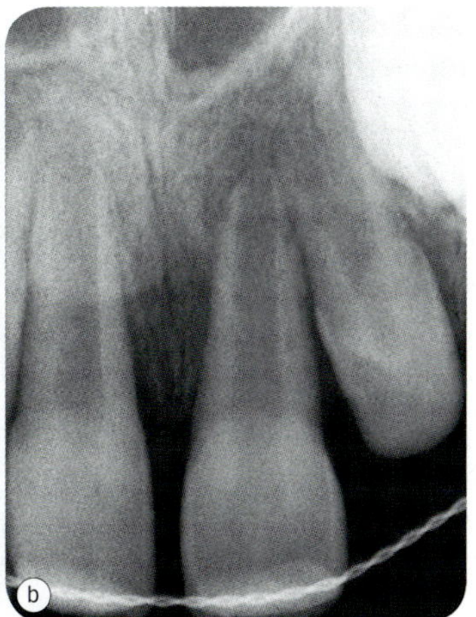

**Figure 24.89** - (**A**) Radiographic image of teeth #11 and #12 with diagnosis of crown fracture involving enamel and dentin and subluxation, examined 2 months after the accident. Radiolucent areas are observed on the surface of the roots, indicative of inflammatory resorption and pulp necrosis. (**B**) Radiographic control taken 15 days after replantation of the 21, maintained dry for 20 minutes after the avulsion. Radiolucent areas are observed on the external surface of the apical region, indicative of inflammatory resorption and pulp necrosis.

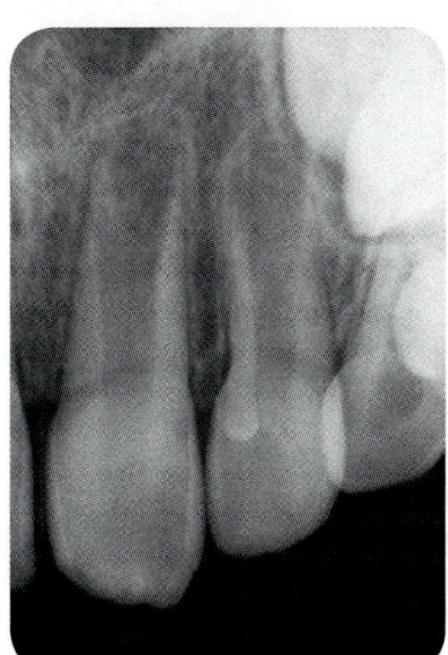

**Figure 24.90** - Radiographic control of tooth #21 after subluxation. The thin root walls are more susceptible to the inflammatory resorption.

The goal of treatment methods recommended for young permanent teeth is to promote apical closure by the formation of a mineralized tissue barrier that makes it possible to fill the canal by conventional methods[8,9,21,32,38,18,19,37]. This barrier can be synthesized as the cellular production of an organic matrix, susceptible to mineralization, requiring alkaline phosphatase activity, as well as an appropriate blood supply. The mineralized barrier resulting from apexification can be formed by tissue similar to cementum[16,29], osteodentine[13,34] or the mixture of connective tissue, bone and particles of calcium hydroxide with the new root portion formed by normal tissue: pulp, odontoblasts, pre-dentin, cementum and apical foramen[36]. In addition, calcium hydroxide has proved to be efficient against most bacteria in the root canal. This is an important property for the treatment of immature teeth, since the thin dentinal walls do not support intensive reaming.

Root canal treatment of teeth with incomplete root development requires special methods that will that will be described. Coronal access should obey the extent of the pulp chamber, as it is known that in immature teeth, pulpal horns are in a more incisal position. The pulp chamber shall be meticulously cleaned in order to avoid discoloration of the crown caused by pulp residues. Therefore, the coronal access tends to be more extensive than in the developed teeth, and one needs to be especially careful with removal of the diverticula (Fig. 24.91A-B). Isolation with rubber dam should be performed, preferentially without the use of clamps, due to the fragility of the root structures, particularly in the cervical region. In addition, in children wearing appliances, in splinted and partially erupted teeth, adaptation of rubber dam can be difficult. Many materials are available to help the apposition of rubber dam for complete isolation of the tooth. The non-eugenol periodontal dressing materials can be positioned to cover the gingival and the incisive papillae. (Fig. 24.92A-E) A new dental material was recently recommended: Top Dam (FGM) is a light cured resin that can be used to complete the isolation with the rubber dam. It has adequate viscosity to allow easy coverage of soft tissues, without undesirable flow; excellent power for sealing; minimum and perfect grip on the gums; do not loose the gum unless forced; gets out in full at the time it is removed (Fig. 24.93A-F).

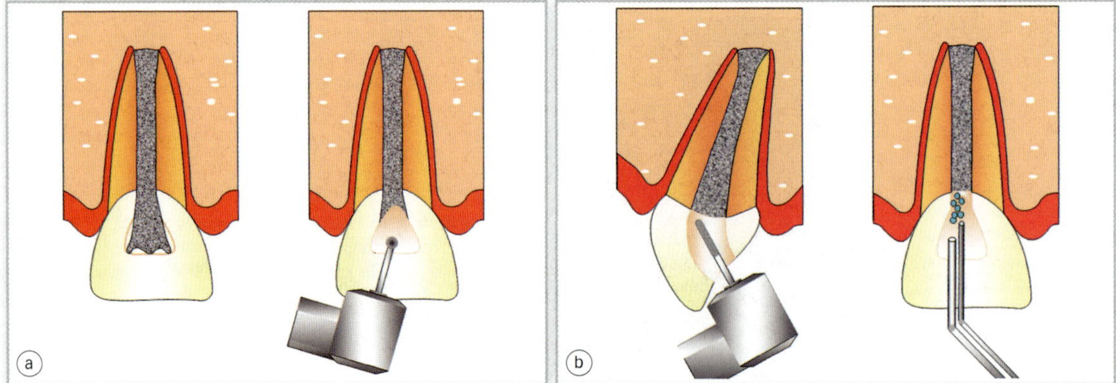


**Figure 24.91** - (**A**) Coronal access should follow the full extent of the pulp chamber. (**B**) Special attention should be given to the removal of the diverticula, present in the pulp chamber, which should be carefully cleaned to avoid crown discoloration.

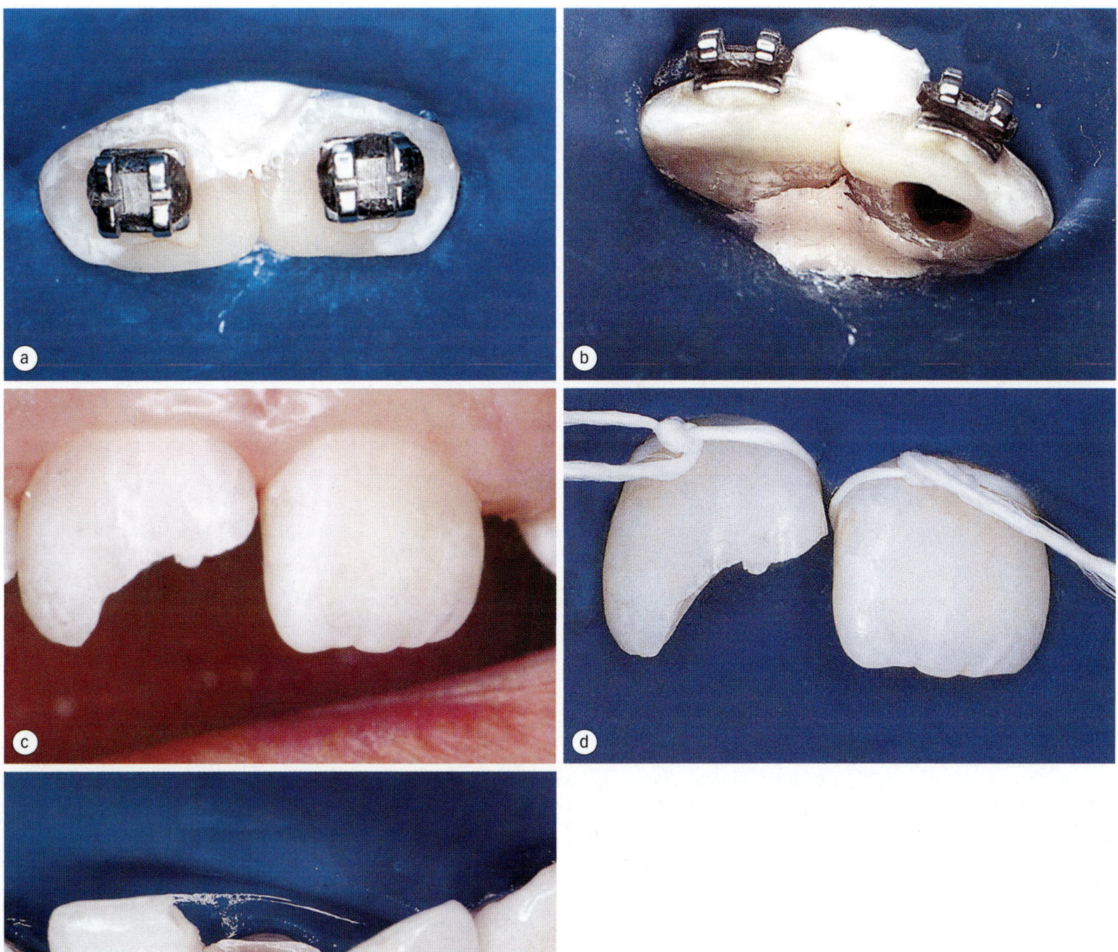

**Figure 24.92** - (**A-B**) Isolation with rubber dam should be performed without the use of clamps. The gingival and incisive papillae are protected with a non-eugenol periodontal dressing material. (**C-D**) Stabilization of the rubber dam, using dental floss, due to expulsive crown of immature, not completely erupted teeth. (**E**) Example of stabilization of isolation with rubber dam, without the use of clamps.

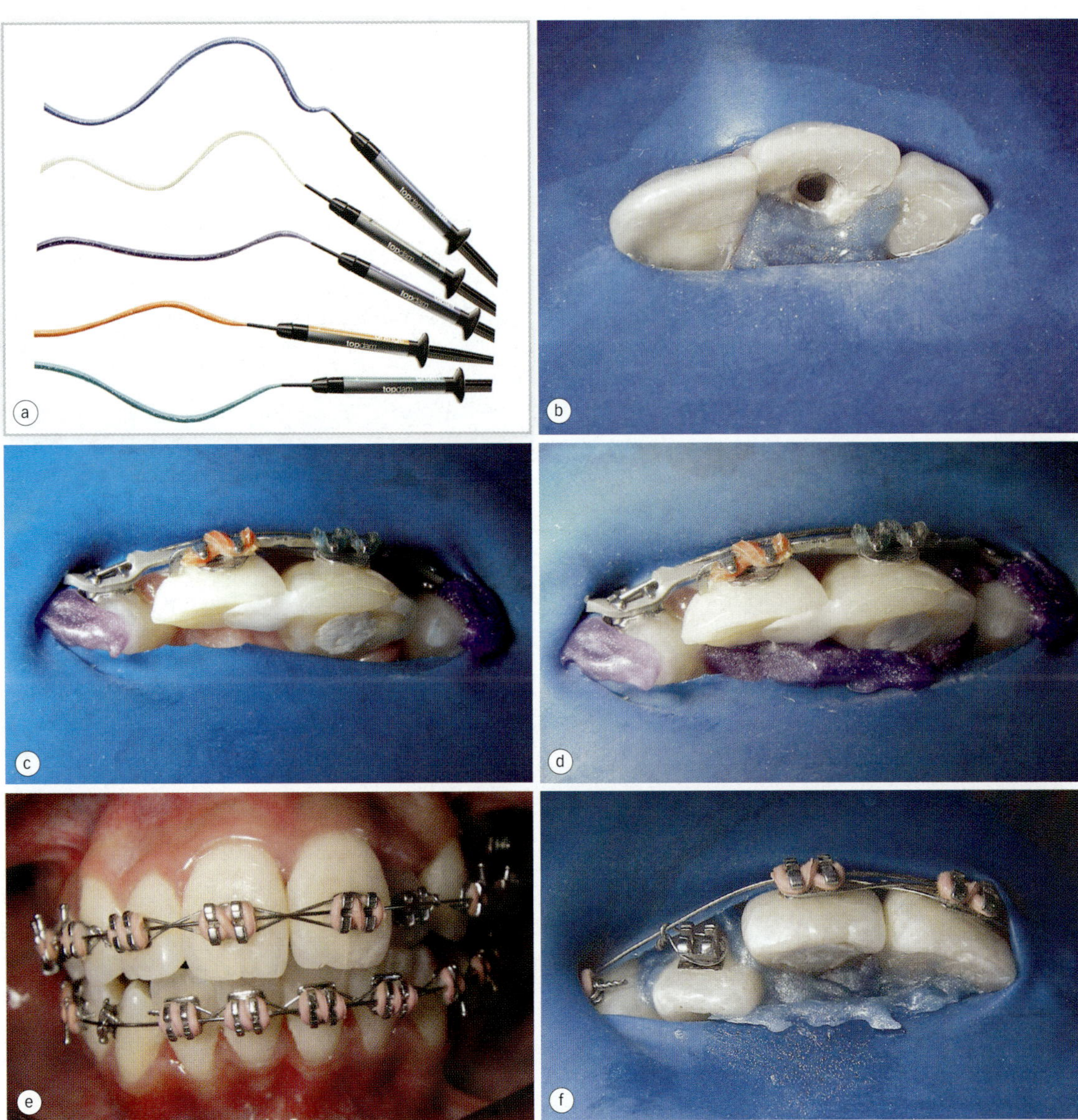


**Figure 24.93** - (**A**) Top Dam (product from FGM – Brazil). (**B**) The use of Top Dam as an aid to apposition of rubber dam in incompletely erupted tooth, to avoid the use of a clamp. (**C-D**) Use of Top Dam in a patient wearing orthodontic appliances. Avulsion of teeth #12, #11, #21 and #22 in an 8-year-old patient. Only the tooth 21 was replanted and endodontically treated. Notice the presence of a provisional fixed bridge to substitute tooth #11. (**E-F**) Use of Top Dam in a patient wearing orthodontic appliances. Endodontic treatment of tooth #11. Notice temporary restoration at the palatal portion of the crown.

The pulp of teeth with incomplete root development is voluminous; presents a less solid aspect and should be removed with a Hedströem file (Fig. 24.94A-B). After pulpectomy, the root canal should be flushed with a sodium hypochlorite at low concentration (0.5 to 1%). The solution should not cross the middle third of the root canal, because the divergent walls of the apical region and the open apex expose periradicular tissue to direct contact. Care should be taken with the depth of penetration of the irrigation needle, and the pressure on the plunger of the syringe during the irrigation. Maintenance of vital tissue in the apical region can improve the quality and speed of apical mineralized tissue deposition[12]. When the pulp is necrotic, concomitant with irrigation careful filling of the dentinal walls can be performed with Kerr type files, using lateral pressure and vertical movements, until the temporary working length is reached (Fig. 24.95A-C).

After taking the radiograph to determine the working length, this should obey a limit of 1 mm below the radiographic apex, with the intention of not damaging the periapical tissue that is in direct continuity with the root canal in immature teeth (Fig. 24.96A-C). It is known that the radiographic limit is not reliable for measuring the length of the root canal, particularly in immature teeth, in which visualization is complicated by the thinness of the mineralized dental structures at the root apex. Baggett et al.[6], with the aim at determining the working length in immature teeth, suggested using absorbent paper points, appropriate to the canal diameter, to define the working length. The paper point is inserted into the root canal until resistance. It is possible to determine the resistance offered by the periapical tissue through careful tactile probing, thus not running the risk of passing the desired limit. The technique was considered valid and reliable, because in 95% of the 35 teeth used, there was coincidence between the estimated length and the radiographic measurement, when observed by two examiners. Although the alternative presented is feasible, confirmation by radiograph is always indispensable.

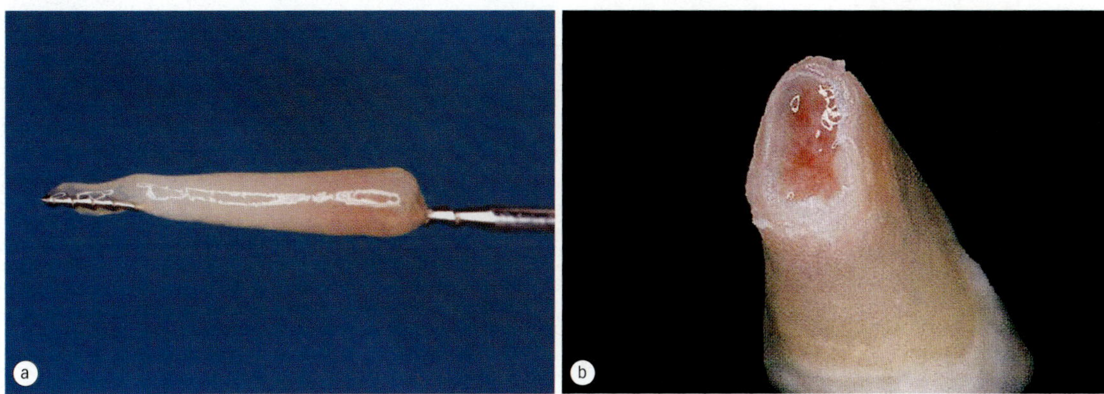


**Figure 24.94** - (**A**) Pulp of an immature tooth removed with the aid of a Hedströem file. (**B**) Aspect of fragility of the root walls in the apical region of teeth with incomplete root development.

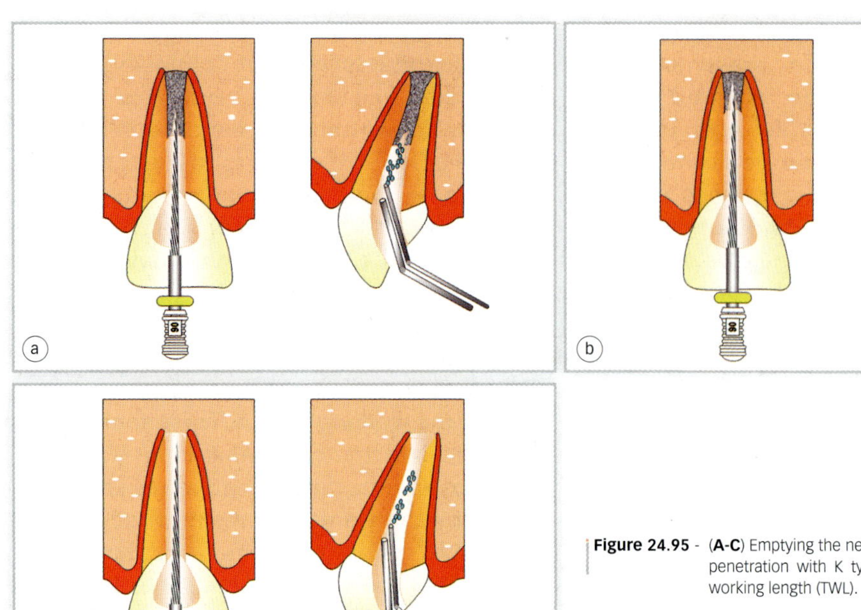
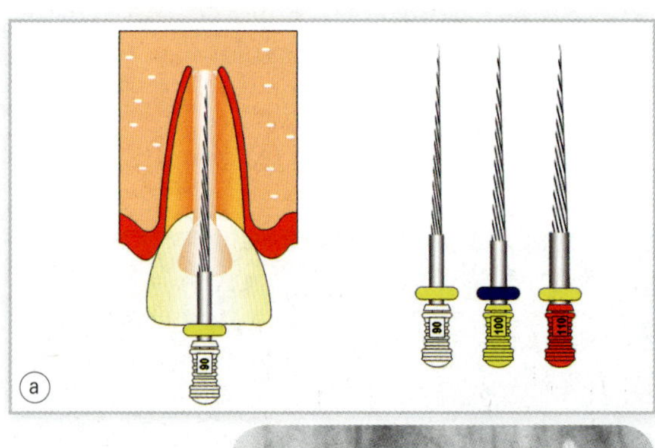

**Figure 24.95** - (**A-C**) Emptying the necrotic content by progressive penetration with K type file up to the temporary working length (TWL).

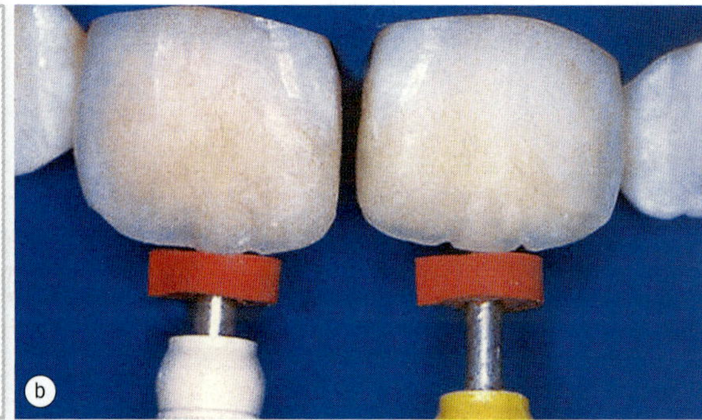
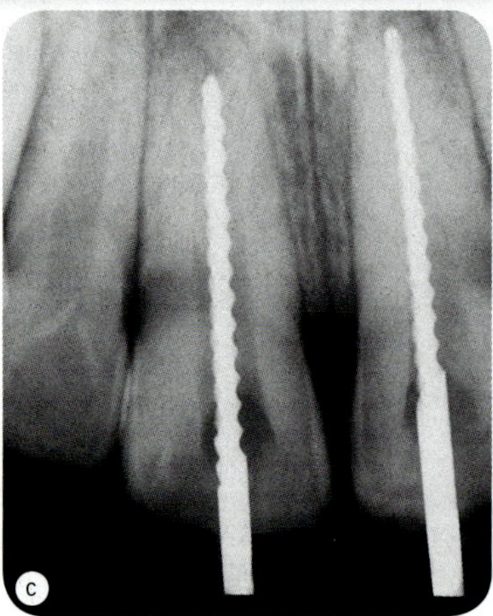

**Figure 24.96** - (**A**) Determining the working length in the teeth with incomplete root development. (**B**) Radiographic determination of the working length in teeth with incomplete root development, 1 mm below the apical limit of the root. (**C**) Radiographic determination of the working length in teeth with incomplete root development, 1 mm below the apical limit of the root.

For appropriate sanitization of the root canal, it is essential to eliminate all the infected dentin, with the adjacent necrotic residues, this being the preponderant factor for apical closure[20,34]. Due to the thin walls that surround a very wide root canal[12,23,34] it is not possible to use conventional techniques, because the instruments do not adapt to the dentinal walls, as occurs in completely formed teeth. In immature teeth, the dentinal tubules do not yet present an appropriate deposition of intertubular dentin and the peritubular dentin has not yet developed completely, offering little or no resistance to the action of the instruments. Thus, circumferential instrumentation is recommended, using the K-type files (Fig. 24.97), with delicate movements of filing, with the aim of not weakening the thin dentinal walls, mainly in the periapical region. Concomitant instrumentation and irrigation should be performed initially with a sodium hypochlorite solution at low concentration (0.5 to 1.0%), with the same care mentioned above, so that the flushing solution does not reach the apical region. Subsequently the canal shall be flushed with a concentrated solution of calcium hydroxide, obtained by the mixture of saline solution and PA calcium hydroxide. Drying should be performed with absorbent paper points of compatible diameter, previously measured at working length, with the intention of not crossing the apex; sometimes they are inverted to adapt to the diameter of the root canal (Fig. 24.98).

Because of the studies of Hermann[17] in the 1920s, calcium hydroxide (Calxyl) was introduced in Dentistry as a substance biologically compatible with pulp and periapical tissues. Thus, the material of choice for the intra-canal dressing is calcium hydroxide, and several vehicles are recommended in the literature, with variations of the time of action and consequently renewal of the dressing, as described in Chapter 20. The use of distilled water is recommended, and the medication must be slightly compressed towards the apex in order to ensure close contact with vital periapical tissues. The mixture should be prepared on a glass plate for a firmer consistency that allows appropriate vertical condensation, with the minimum drainage towards the crown of the tooth (Fig. 24.99A-B). Some of the properties of calcium hydroxide are particularly favorable for apical closure, such as the accentuated antimicrobial effect, due to its extremely alkaline pH, with induction of the formation of a mineralized barrier (Chapter 20). Various techniques are recommended for filling the root canal with calcium hydroxide, and it is at the professional's discretion to choose the one which he/she adapts best, provided that it densely fills the full extent of the root canal. Endodontic files, Lentulo spiral, and special syringes can be used to fill the root canal with calcium hydroxide. The use of Schilder condensers or similar[25] is recommended; the diameter should be chosen according to the canal, so that the material is led directly to the apex and condensed to completely fill the root canal up to the cervical region (Fig. 24.100).

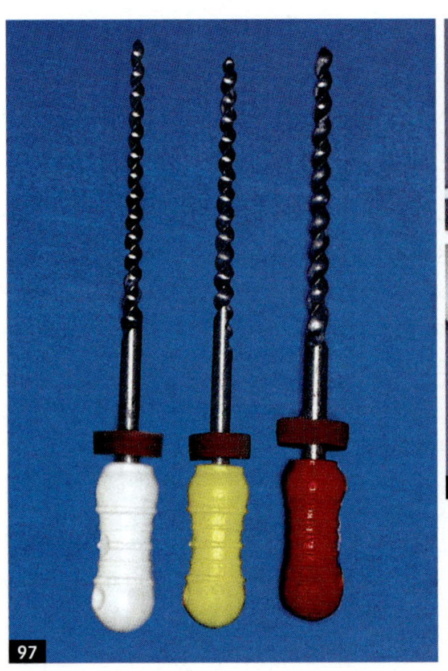

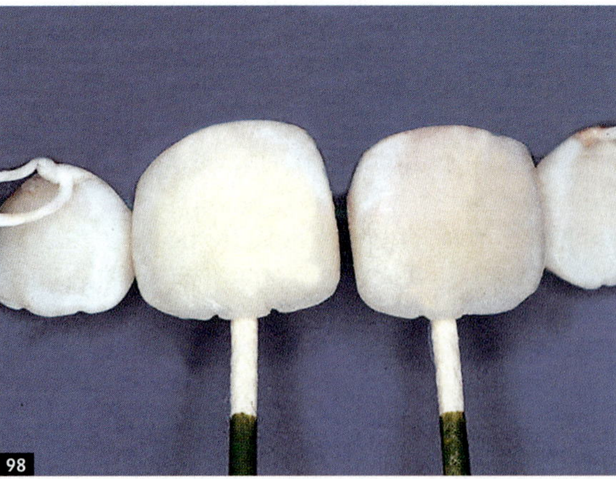

Figure 24.97 - K file 3rd series used for instrumentation of young permanent teeth.

Figure 24.98 - Absorbent paper points with diameter compatible with the root canal are used for the drying, before placement of the calcium hydroxide.

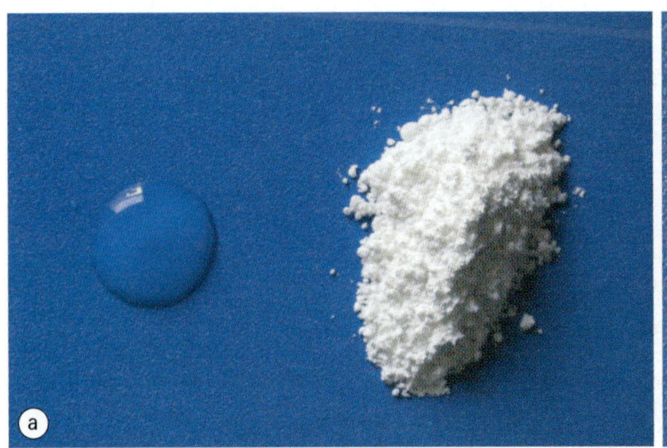

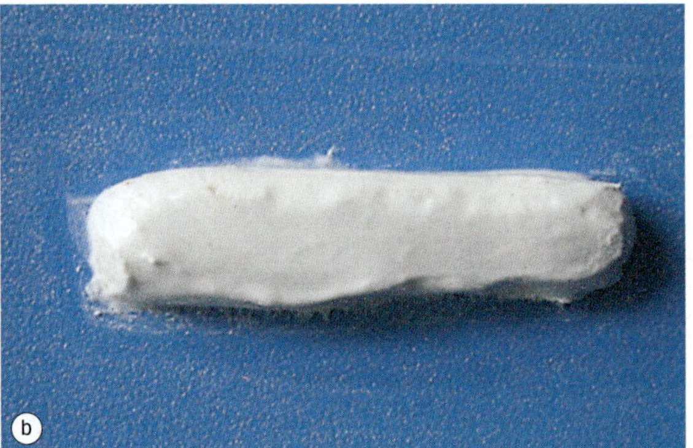

Figure 24.99 - (A-B) Paste of PA calcium hydroxide in distilled water to be used as intracanal dressing.

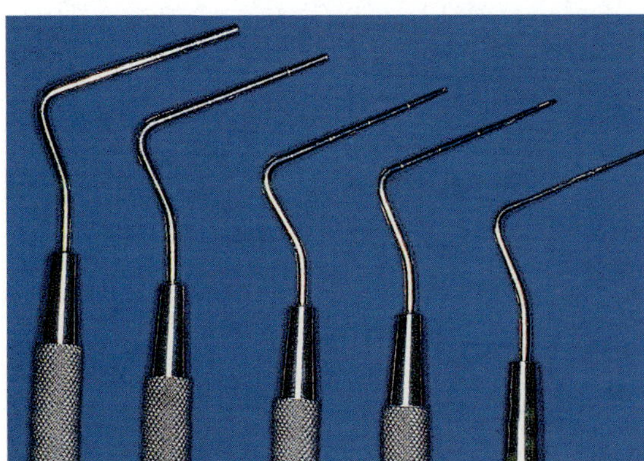

Figure 24.100 - Schilder Type condensers used for placing the calcium hydroxide paste inside the root canal.

The condensers should be previously selected according to the diameter of the different portions of the root canal to be filled, and the first should practically occupy the lumen of the root canal at an approximate distance of 2 to 3 mm below the working length. Slight vertical condensation should take place, without forcing the condenser against the root canal walls, in order to prevent fracture of the fragile root walls. The condensation pressure should be controlled with the intention of preventing the material from being pressed through the apical foramen (Fig. 24.101A-C). In teeth that present purulent exudate, the recommendation is not to condense the calcium hydroxide in the first sessions, until there is control of the drainage. Taking a radiograph is recommended before the temporary seal, to certify the appropriate filling of the root canal to its full extent, from the apical to the cervical region. The image of correct filling resembles that of pulp canal obliteration, since calcium hydroxide presents a radiographic density similar to that of dentin (Fig. 24.102A-B). The pulp chamber should be well cleaned with dentin excavators and cotton balls to completely remove the calcium hydroxide paste which, if left, will interfere in the adaptation of the temporary sealing material. After this, the pulp chamber will be filled with a sterilized cotton ball, and the temporary seal will be performed with the chosen material, at a minimum thickness of 4 mm, to prevent microleakage. Several materials are used, such as zinc oxide eugenol cement, zinc phosphate, glass-ionomer type II cement and light-cured glass-ionomer cement. Because of the long time before the patient returns for the next appointment, glass-ionomer type II cement (restorative) and light-cured glass-ionomer cement are recommended, as these materials present a good marginal seal, and has a adhesive bond to dentin, low solubility, in addition to releasing fluoride to the adjacent structures (Fig. 24.103A-B).



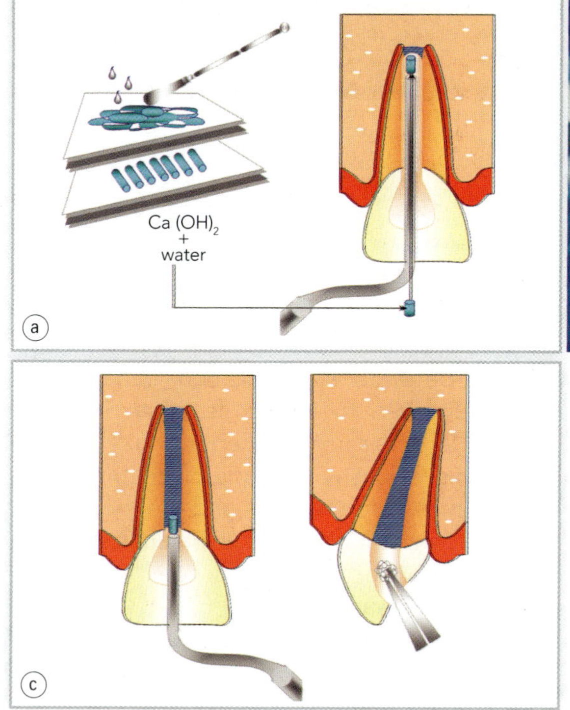


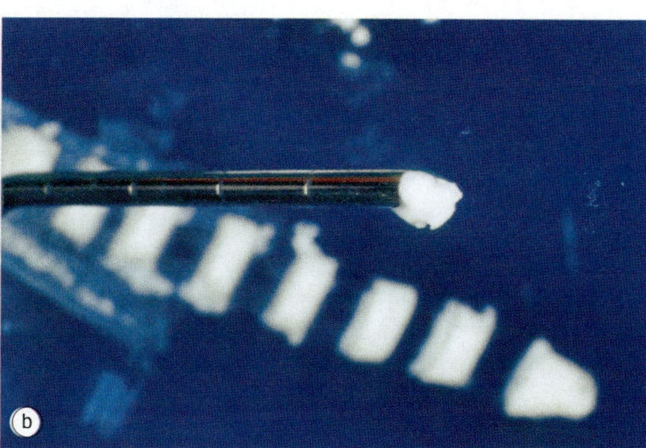


**Figure 24.101** - **(A-C)** Schematic sequence of filling the root canal with calcium hydroxide, using a condenser of diameter compatible with the root canal in its several segments. The first increment will be placed in close contact with the periapical tissue without crossing the apical limit.

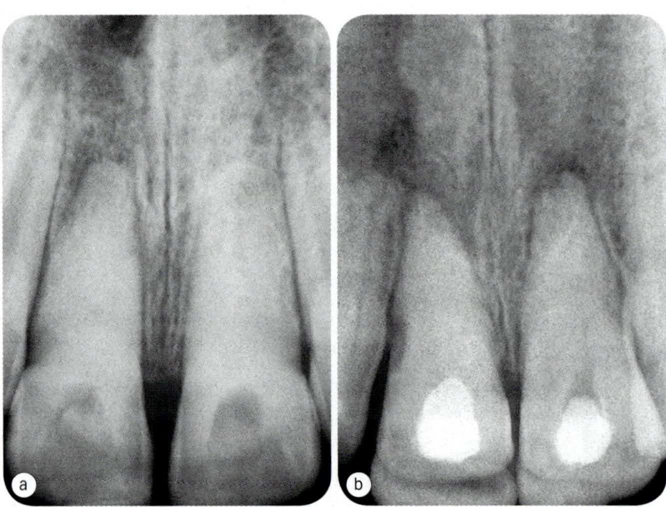

**Figure 24.102** - (**A-B**) Radiographic image of the filling with calcium hydroxide that presents radiographic density similar to that of dentin.

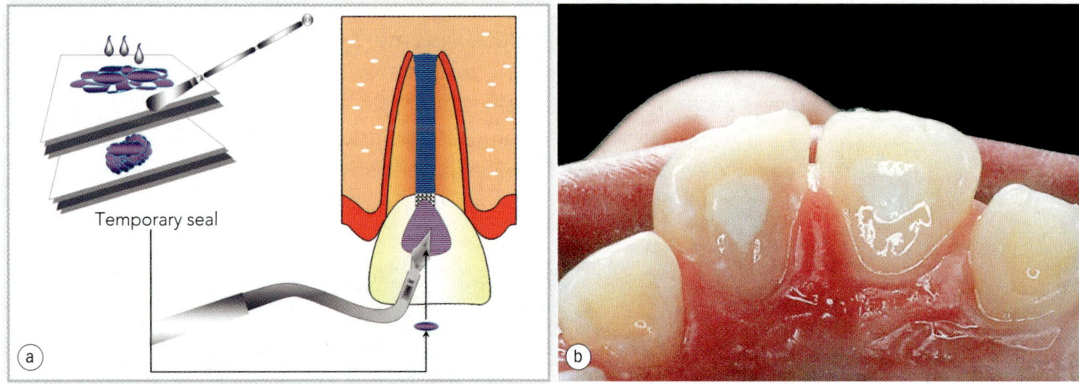


**Figure 24.103** - (**A-B**) Temporary seal with glass-ionomer cement.

Clinical and radiographic control should take place at intervals of 60 days, to verify the presence of calcium hydroxide inside the root canal, integrity of the temporary seal, and condition of the tissues in the periapical region. The intracanal dressing can be changed after 45 and 90 days, or whenever the radiograph demonstrates absence of calcium hydroxide, mainly in the apical region, whenever the presence of fistula and/or swelling is observed. For this, isolation with rubber dam should be performed, preferentially without clamps. The calcium hydroxide should be removed with K-type files with appropriate diameter and irrigation with saline solution or sodium hypochlorite 0.5 to 1.0%. First, the file should be introduced in the center of the calcium hydroxide paste, and then the walls should be scraped with soft filing movements. Subsequently, the root canal should be dried with absorbent paper points and new calcium hydroxide paste inserted, following the same procedures already described previously. The time of treatment varies according to the case, and the medication should be changed until the mineralized tissue barrier is formed and initially confirmed by radiograph. Figures 24.104A-E and 24.105A-E show the radiographic follow-up of root canal treatment in young permanent teeth with traumatic injury and pulp necrosis.

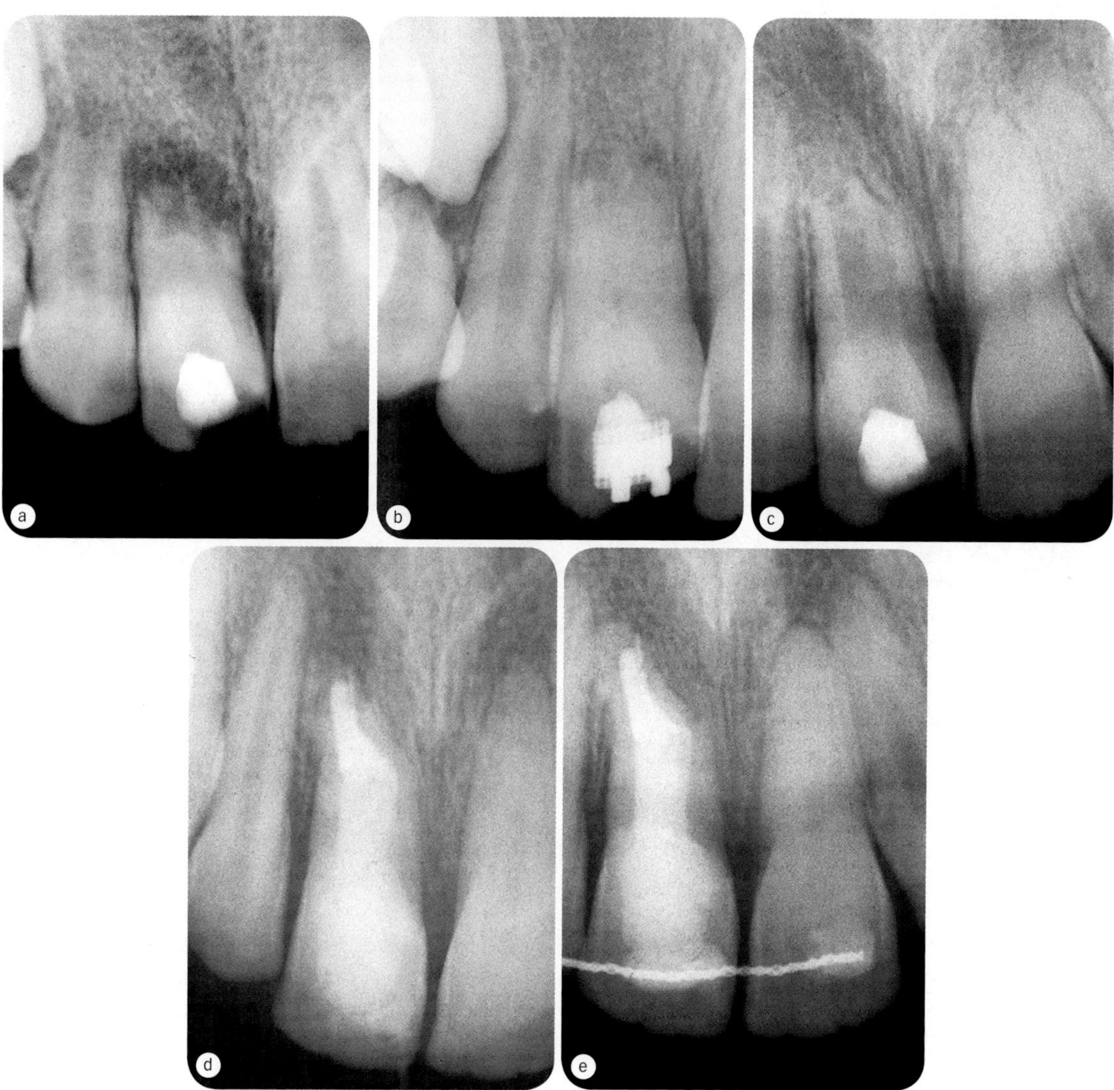


**Figure 24.104A** - (**A**) Radiographic aspect of tooth #11 after orthodontic extrusion, subsequent to the intrusive luxation and extensive crown fracture – in a 7-year-old child. (**B**) Radiograph showing regression of the radiolucent periapical area and continuity of the root development, after 3 months. (**C**) Apical bridging after 1 year. (**D**) Root canal filled by the molded gutta-percha point and vertical condensation technique with Schilder's vertical condensation technique. (**E**) After new accident there was crown fracture accompanied by subluxation. Reattachment of the fragment and flexible splinting was performed.

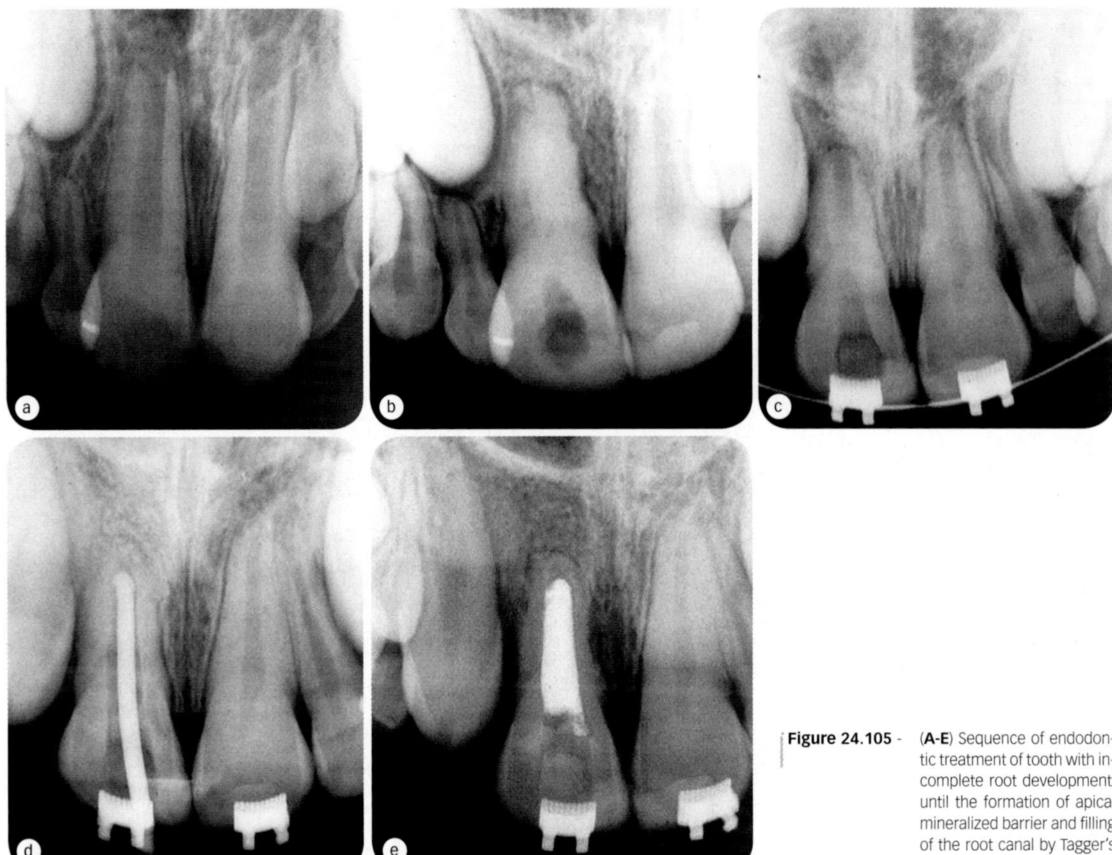

**Figure 24.105** - **(A-E)** Sequence of endodontic treatment of tooth with incomplete root development, until the formation of apical mineralized barrier and filling of the root canal by Tagger's Hybrid Technique.

Despite the classic indication of apexification with the use of calcium hydroxide, there are inherent difficulties in the technique that requires a long time for treatment, and the risk of cervical root fractures that can lead to failure. The introduction of the Mineral Trioxide Aggregate (MTA) in Dentistry, has brought new possibilities, as its mode of action is similar to that of calcium hydroxide[14,28,35]. Thus, the use of MTA for the apical seal of teeth with incomplete root development, makes it possible to perform treatment in a single session that also induces repair. Moreover, the filling of these teeth in a shorter period of time allows immediate restoration, through reinforcement with intra-radicular posts, protecting them against fractures[30]. Some authors report successful treatment in apexification using this new material[24,33,38], however, more research is required, to establish scientific evidence that MTA should replace calcium hydroxide in the treatment of teeth with incomplete root development. Hachmeister et al.[15] observed that the thickness of the layer of MTA placed in contact with the apical region is important for the success of the treatment: the 4mm layer showed greater resistance than the 1 mm. Thus, until the most appropriate protocol is established and based on sound scientific evidence, caution is necessary when working with MTA.

Root canal filling of teeth with incomplete root development should be performed after confirming the presence of the apical bridging, clinically and radiographically. Therefore, after complete removal of the calcium hydroxide paste, an instrument of small caliber should be put into the canal, 1 to 2 mm shorter than the working length, with the purpose of reaching the apical mineralized portion. The presence of the barrier should be confirmed by periapical radiograph immediately afterwards. The largest apical diameter and irregularities of the walls of root canal frequently allows for the adaptation of a wider caliber cone. Thus, the technique of molding the cone by plasticization of its tip, using a warm spatula is recommended (Fig. 24.106A-D). After being slightly warmed, the cone shall be inserted gently but firmly into the root canal and pressed against the apical barrier, which is moistened with saline solution. The gutta-percha cone is allowed to cool for a few seconds. A radiograph should confirm the adaptation of the cone to the full extent of the apical mineralized barrier (Fig. 24.107). As regards the filling technique, Schilder technique of vertical compaction of warm gutta-percha[25], hybrid of Tagger[31] or the lateral condensation are recommended (Fig. 24.108). The first two are more appropriate for very wide and divergent root canals that present very fragile dentinal walls. For all techniques, however, complete control of the pressure exerted on the condensation of the gutta-percha is recommended, in order to avoid rupture of the barrier and/or root fractures. Care must be taken because the force of the finger spreader in the lateral condensation technique can fracture the root. When the barrier formed offers safety, mainly as regards its thickness and resistance, it is better to use thermo-plasticized gutta-percha injection techniques such as Obtura II (Obtura Corporation). In any filling technique used, one should always pay attention to the fragility of the root of teeth with incomplete root development, taking all the necessary care to preserve the tooth. Figure 24.109A presents a filling performed by the lateral condensation technique, and Figure 24.109B shows the Schilder technique of vertical compaction of warm gutta-percha, and reinforcement with glass fiber intra-radicular posts and restoration with composite resin.

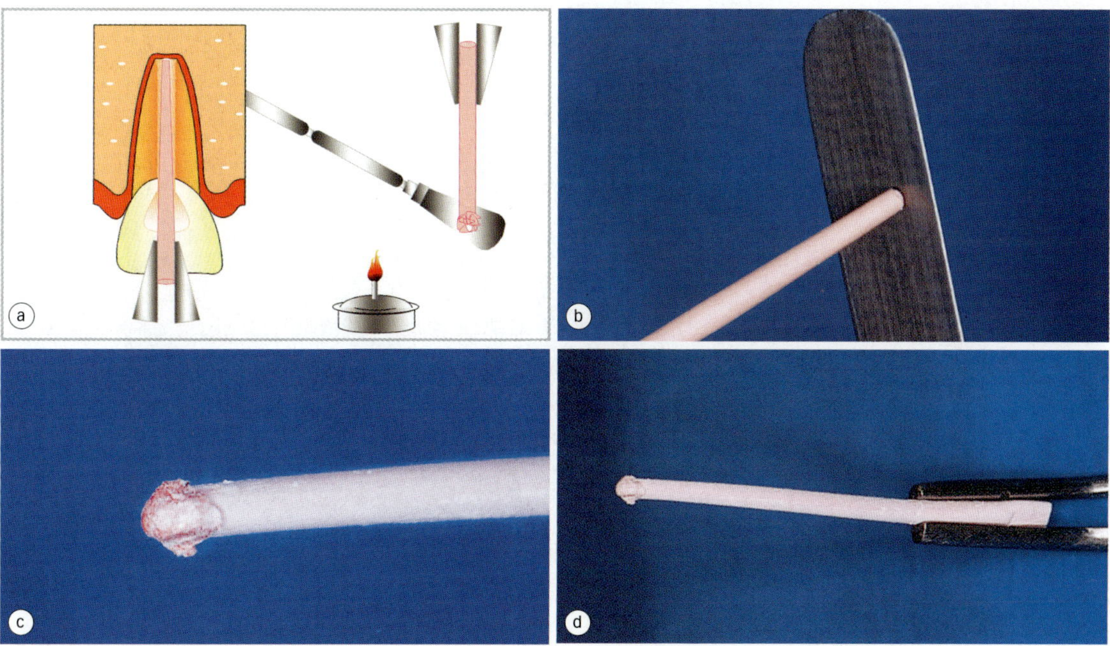


**Figure 24.106** - (**A-B**) Plasticization of the tip of the gutta-percha cone for molding the apical region of the root canal after bridging. (**C**) Aspect of the tip of the gutta-percha cone after molding the apical area. (**D**) At the time of the filling the cone should be introduced with the aid of pliers, in the same position in which it was molded.

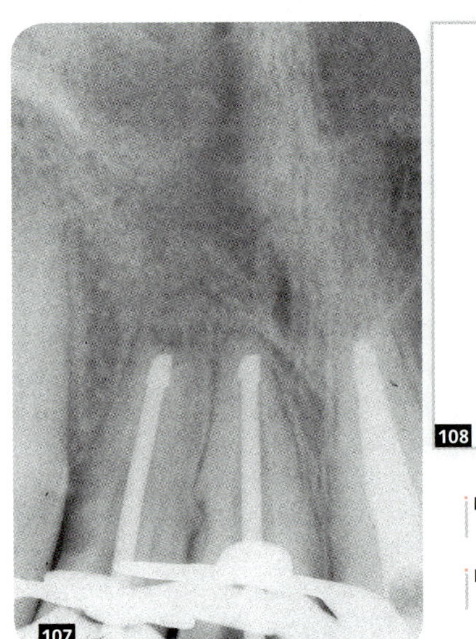

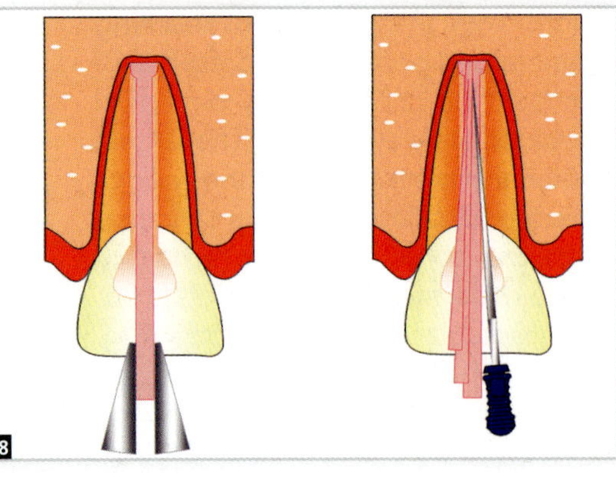

**Figure 24.107** - Radiographic observation of the apical adaptation after cone molding.

**Figure 24.108** - After preparation of the cone, filling can be performed by the conventional lateral condensation technique.

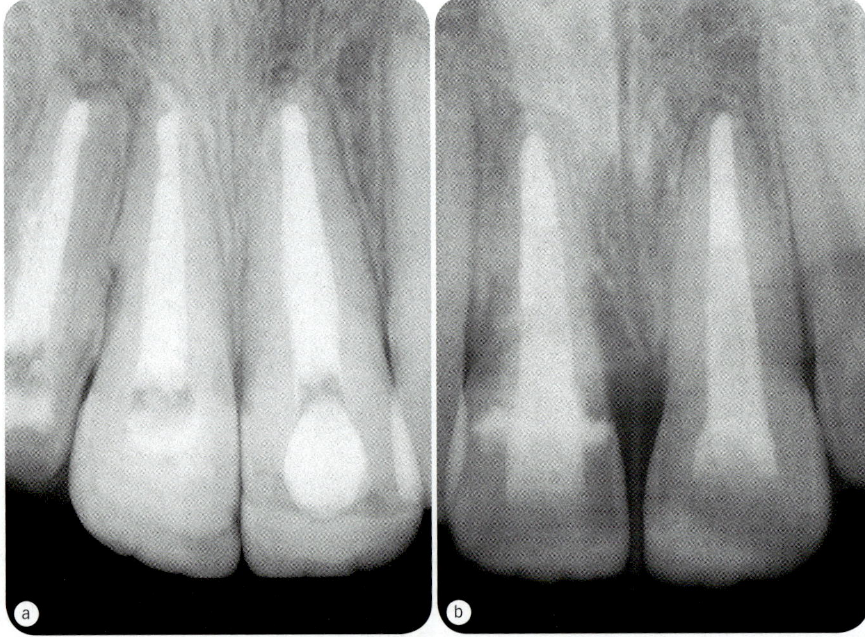

**Figure 24.109A** - (**A**) Radiographic aspect after filling, by the lateral condensation technique. (**B**) Radiographic aspect after filling by Schilder technique of vertical compaction of warm gutta-percha. Restoration with glass fiber intra-radicular post and composite resin.

The temporary seal should preferably be performed with light-cured glass-ionomer cement (Fig. 24.110).

At the end of the apexification process, when the apex is almost completely closed, and the root presents convergent apical dentinal walls, we recommend the use of Mineral Trioxide Aggregate (MTA). It is an alternative to anticipate the end of calcium hydroxide treatment before the closure of the apex. The placement of an apical plug of MTA and its maintenance inside the limits of the root can be achieved in a better technical condition, than in the initial phase of the apexification process, when dentinal walls are divergent at the apex. It is not necessary to wait for the hard tissue barrier formation, since MTA provides the necessary apical stop for root canal fillings and promotes the stimulation for hard tissue deposition Figures 24.111A-C show a case treated with calcium hydroxide and finished with apical plug of MTA before root canal filling.

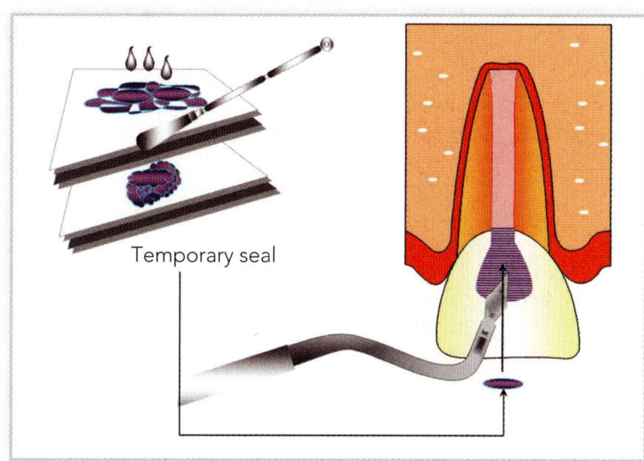


**Figure 24.110** - Schematic representation of Temporary seal with glass-ionomer cement after root canal filling.

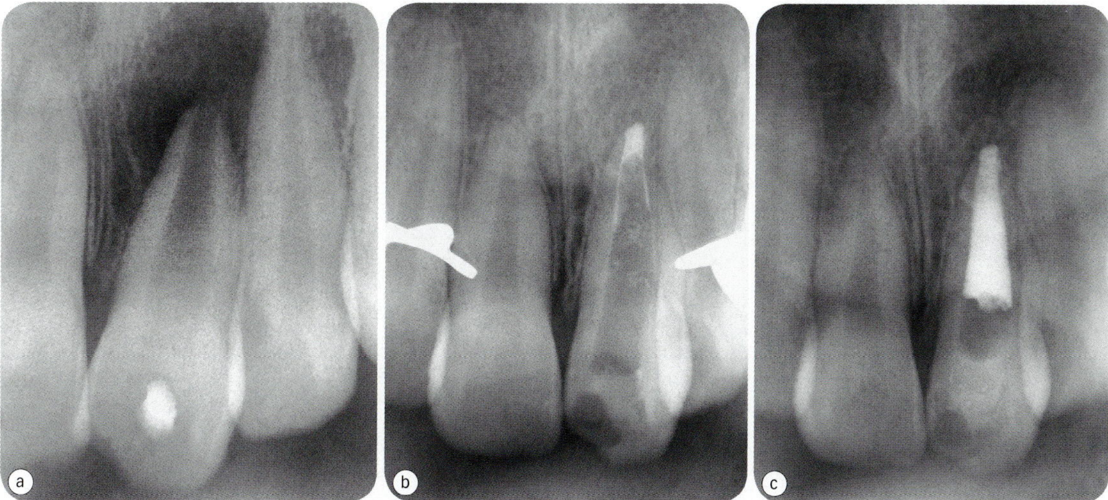


**Figures 24.111** - (**A-B**) Pulp necrosis after enamel and dentin fracture with subluxation in a 10-year-old boy. (**A**) Notice the radiolucency in the apical area of tooth #12; (**B**) Apical plug with MTA one year after treated with calcium hydroxide. Notice that the apex was almost completely closed; (**C**) Root canal filling was completed with gutta-percha points and zinc oxide eugenol sealer.

# References

## PART 1. EPIDEMIOLOGY, CLASSIFICATION AND SOCIO-PSYCHOLOGICAL IMPACT OF THE TRAUMATIC LESIONS


1. Adulyanon S, Sheiham A. Oral Impacts on Daily Performances. In: Measuring Oral Health and Quality of Life. Slade GD. Chapel Hill: University of North Carolina, Dental Ecology; 1997. p.151-60.
2. Almeida PM, Wickerhouser H. Finding a better socio-economic status classification system for Brazil. J Europ Soc Op Mark Res 1991;19:240-50.
3. Andreasen FM, Zhijie Y, Thomsen BL, Andersen PK. Occurrence of pulp canal obliteration after luxation injuries in the permanent dentition. Endod Dent Traumatol 1987;3:103-15.
4. Andreasen JO, Andreasen FM. Dental trauma. In: Pine CM. Community Oral Health. Great Britain: Wright; 1997. p.94-99.
5. Andreasen JO, Andreasen FM. Dental traumatology: quo vadis. Endod Dent Traumatol 1990;6:78-80.
6. Andreasen JO, Andreasen FM, Andersson L. Text book and color atlas of traumatic injuries to teeth. 4th ed. Oxford: Blackwell Publishing Ltd; 2007. 912p
7. Andreasen JO, Ravn JJ. Epidemiology of traumatic dental injuries to primary and permanent teeth in a Danish population sample. Int J Oral Surg 1972;1:235-9.
8. Baghdady VS, Ghose LJ, Enke H. Traumatized anterior teeth in Iraq and Sudanese children - A comparative study. J Dent Res 1981;60:677-80.
9. Baldwin DC. Appearance and aesthetics in oral health. Community Dent Oral Epidemiol 1980;8:244-56.
10. Barmes DE. Epidemiology of dental disease. J Clin Periodontol 1979;4:80-93.
11. Bastos JV, Côrtes MIS. Care and guidance in dental trauma - an approach to the lay community (Abstract). Proceedings of the IV International Conference on Dental Trauma. London. 1993.
12. Bastos JV, Côrtes MIS. Cuidados e orientação em traumatismos dentários: manual para professores e outros agentes multiplicadores. Belo Horizonte: Imprensa Universitária da Universidade Federal de Minas Gerais (UFMG); 1994.
13. Bastos JV, Côrtes MIS. Cuidados e orientação em traumatismos dentários: manual para professores e outros agentes multiplicadores. 2nd ed. Belo Horizonte: Imprensa Universitária da Universidade Federal de Minas Gerais (UFMG); 1997.
14. Bastos JV, Côrtes MIS. E se meu dente quebrar? 2nd ed. Belo Horizonte: Imprensa Universitária da Universidade Federal de Minas Gerais (UFMG); 1997.
15. Bhat M, Swango PA, Musselman RJ, Schneider PE. A new approach for determining prevalence and risk factors for traumatised anterior teeth. J Public Health Dent 1989; 49:105 (Abstract).
16. Bijela MFTB. Estudo de traumatismo em incisivos permanentes de escolares brasileiros de Bauru, Estado de São Paulo (Prevalência, causa e atendimento odontológico). (Doctoral Thesis). São Paulo University; 1972.
17. Blinkhorn AS, Davies RM. Caries prevention. A continued need worldwide. Int Dent J 1996;46:119-25.
18. Blixen K. Out of Africa. London: Putnam; 1937 apud: Richardson ME. Dental accidents diseases and disasters. Brit Dent J 1999;187:291-4.
19. Borssen E, Holm AK. Traumatic dental injuries in a cohort of 16-year-olds in northern Sweden. Endod Dent Traumatol 1997;13:276-80.
20. Borum M K, Andreasen JO. Therapeutic and economic implications of traumatic dental injuries in Denmark: an estimate based on 7549 patients treated at a major trauma centre. Int J Paediatr Dent 2001;11:249-58.
21. Burden DJ. An investigation of the association between overjet size, lip coverage and traumatic injury to maxillary incisors. Eur Ortho Soc 1995;17:513-7.
22. Burt AB. The future of the caries decline. J Public Health Dent 1985;45:261-9.
23. Burton J, Pryke L, Rob M, Lawson JS. Traumatized anterior teeth amongst high school students in northern Sydney. Aust Dent J 1985;30:346-8.
24. Clarkson BH, Longhurst P, Sheiham A. The prevalence of injured anterior teeth in English schoolchildren and adult. J Int Assoc Dent Child 1973;4:21-4.
25. Coelho EAM. Epidemiologia das lesões traumáticas na dentição permanente de crianças e adolescentes nas tribos Maxakali e Krenak. (Master's Thesis). Federal University of Minas Gerais; 2000. 158p.
26. Coelho EAM, Côrtes MIS, Bastos JV, Silva MJB. Epidemiologia das lesões traumáticas da dentição permanente em crianças e adolescentes nas tribos Maxakali e Krenak. In: 19a Reunião da Sociedade Brasileira de Pesquisa Odontológica. São Paulo: Universidade de São Paulo; 2002. p.231.
27. Côrtes MIS. Epidemiology of traumatic injuries to permanent teeth and the impact on the daily living of Brazilian schoolchildren. (Doctoral Thesis). Londres: Department of Epidemiology and Public Health, University College London; 2000. 247p.
28. Côrtes MIS, Bastos JV. Levantamento estatístico dos pacientes atendidos na Clínica de Traumatismos dentários da Faculdade de Odontologia da UFMG nos últimos 12 anos. Relatório técnico – PROEX/UFMG; 2008.
29. Côrtes MIS, Marcenes W, Sheiham A. Prevalence and correlates of traumatic injuries to the permanent teeth of school children aged 9-14 in Belo Horizonte. Endod Dent Traumatol 2001;17:22-6.
30. Côrtes MIS, Sheiham A, Marcenes W. Impact of traumatic injuries to the permanent teeth on oral health related quality of life of 12 to 14 year old Brazilian school-children. Community Dent Oral Epidemiol 2002;30:193-8.
31. Cushing AM, Sheiham A, Maizels J. Developing socio-dental indicators the social impact of dental disease. Community Dent Health 1986;3:3-17.
32. Davies GN, Kruger BG, Homan BT. Dental survey of children in country districts of Queensland. Aust Dent J 1969;14:153-61.

33. Delattre JP, Resmond Richard F, Allanche C, Perrin M, Michel JF, Le Berre A. Dental injuries among schoolchildren aged from 6 to 15, in Rennes (France). Endod Dent Traumatol 1994;11:186-88.
34. Eichenbaum IW. A correlation of traumatized anterior teeth to occlusion. ASDC J Dent Child 1963;4:229-37.
35. Ellis RG, Davey KW. The classification and treatment of injuries to teeth of children. 5th ed. Chicago: Year Book Publishers Inc; 1970.
36. Ellwood RP, O'Mullane DM. The association between area deprivation and dental caries in groups with and without fluoride in their drinking water. Community Dent Health 1995;12:18-22.
37. Falomo B. Fractured permanent incisors among Nigerian school children. ASDC J Dent Child 1986;53:119-21.
38. Forsberg CM, Tedestam G. Traumatic injuries to teeth in Swedish children living in an urban area. Swed Dent J 1990;14:115-22.
39. Forsberg CM, Tedestam G. Traumatic injuries to teeth in Swedish children living in an urban area –Etiological and predisposing factors related to traumatic injuries to permanent teeth. Swed Dent J 1993; 17:183-90.
40. Freire MCM. Oral health and sense of coherence –a study of Brazilian adolescents and their mothers. (Doctoral thesis). London: University of London; 1998.
41. Garcia-Godoy F. A classification for traumatic injuries to primary and permanent teeth. J Pedod 1981;5:295-7.
42. Garcia-Godoy F. Prevalence and distribution of traumatic injuries to the permanent teeth of Dominican children from private schools. Community Dent Oral Epidemiol 1984;12:136-9.
43. Garcia-Godoy F, Dipres FM, Lora IM, Vidal ED. Traumatic dental injuries in children from private and public schools. Community Dent Oral Epidemiol 1986;14:287-90.
44. Garcia-Godoy F, Morban-Laucer F, Corominas LR, Franjul RA, Noyola M. Traumatic dental injuries in schoolchildren from Santo Domingo. Community Dent Oral Epidemiol 1985;13:177-9.
45. Garcia-Godoy F, Sanchez R, Sanchez JR. Traumatic dental injuries in a sample of Dominican schoolchildren. Community Dent Oral Epidemiol 1981;9:193-7.
46. Gauba ML. A correlation of fractured anterior teeth to their proclination. J Ind Dent Assoc 1967;30:105-12.
47. Ghose LJ, Baghdady VS, Enke H. Relation of traumatized permanent anterior teeth to occlusion and lip condition. Community Dent Oral Epidemiol 1980;8:381-4.
48. Glass RL. The first international conference on the declining prevalence of dental caries. J Dent Res 1982;61:1301-83.
49. Glendor U, Jonsson D, Halling A, Lindqvist K. Direct and indirect costs of dental trauma in Sweden: a 2-year prospective study of children and adolescents. Community Dent Oral Epidemiol 2001;29:150-60.
50. Glendor U, Marcenes W, Andreasen JO. Classification, etiology and epidemiology, In: Andreasen JO, Andreasen FM, Andersson L. Text book and color atlas of traumatic injuries to teeth. 4th ed. Oxford: Blackwell Publishing Ltd.; 2007. 217 p.
51. Gratrix D, Holloway PJ. Factors of deprivation associated with dental caries in young children. Community Dent Health 1994;11:66-70.
52. Gupta, K, Tandon, S, Prabhu, D. Traumatic injuries to the incisors in children of South Kanara District. A prevalence study. J Indian Soc Pedod Prev Dent 2002;20:107-13.
53. Gutmann JL, Gutmann MSE. Cause, incidence and prevention of trauma to teeth. Dent Clin North Am 1985;39:1-13.
54. Hamdan MA, Rock WP. A study comparing the prevalence and distribution of traumatic dental injuries among 10-12-year old children in an urban and in a rural area of Jordan. Int J Paediatr Dent 1995;5:237-41.
55. Hamilton FA. An investigation into treatment services for traumatic injuries to the teeth of adolescents. (Doctoral Thesis). University of Manchester; 1994.
56. Hamilton FA, Hill FJ, Holloway PJ. An investigation of dento-alveolar trauma and its treatment in an adolescent population. Part 1: The prevalence and incidence of injuries and the extent and adequacy of treatment received. Br Dent J 1997;182:91-5.
57. Hargreaves JA, Matejka JM, Cleaton-Jones PE, Williams S. Anterior tooth trauma in eleven-year old South African children. ASDC J Dent Child 1995;62:353-5.
58. Holland T, O'Mullane D, Clarkson J, O'Hickey S, Whelton H. Trauma to permanent teeth of children, aged 8, 12 and 15 years, in Ireland. J Paediatr Dent 1988;4:13-6.
59. Hunter ML, Hunter B, Kingdon A, Addy M, Dummer PM, Shaw WC. Traumatic injury to maxillary incisor teeth in a group of South Wales school children. Endod Dent Traumatol 1990;6:260-4.
60. Jamani KD, Fayyad MA. Prevalence of traumatized permanent incisors in Jordanian children according to age, sex and socio-economic class. Odontostomatol Trop 1991;14:17-20.
61. Jarvinen S. Fractured and avulsed permanent incisors in Finish children. A retrospective study. Acta Odontologica Scand 1979;37:47-50.
62. Jarvinen S. Incisal overjet and traumatic injuries to upper permanent incisors. Acta Odontologica Scand 1978;36:359-62.
63. Josefsson E, Karlander EL. Traumatic injuries to permanent teeth among Swedish school children living in a rural area. Swed Dent J 1994;18:87-94.
64. Kaste LM, Gift HC, Bhat M, Swango PA. Prevalence of incisor trauma in persons 6-50 years of age: United States, 1988-1991. J Dent Res 1996;75:696-705.
65. Liew VP, Daly CG. Anterior dental trauma treated after-hours in Newcastle, Australia. Community Dent Oral Epidemiol 1986;14:362-6.
66. Linn EL. Social meanings of dental appearance. J Health Hum Behav 1966; 7:289-95.
67. Locker D, Jokovic A. Using subjective oral health status indicators to screen for dental care needs in older adults. Community Dent Oral Epidemiol 1996;24:398-402.
68. Macko DJ, Grasso JE, Powell EA, Doherty NJ. A study of fractured anterior teeth in a school population. ASDC J Dent Child 1979;46:38-41.
69. Marcenes W, Al-Beiruti N, Tayfour D, Issa S. Epidemiology of traumatic injuries to the permanent incisors of 9-12- year-old schoolchildren in Damascus, Syria. Endod Dent Traumatol 1999;15:117-23.

70. Marcenes W, Alessi ON, Traebert J. Causes and prevalence of traumatic injuries to the permanent incisors of school children aged 12 years in Jaragua do Sul, Brazil. Int Dent J 2000;50:87-92.
71. Marcenes W, Bonecker M. Epidemiologia das doenças bucais In: Buischi YP. Promoção de saúde bucal na clínica odontológica. São Paulo: Artes Médicas; 2000. 336p.
72. Marcenes W, Murray S. Changes in prevalence and treatment need for traumatic dental injuries among 14-year-old children in Newham, London: a deprived area. Community Dent Health 2002;19:104-08.
73. Marcenes, W Zabot, N E, Traebert J. Socio-economic correlates of traumatic injuries to the permanent incisors in schoolchildren aged 12 years in Blumenau, Brazil. Dent Traumatol 2001;17:222-6.
74. Marthaler TM. Caries status in Europe and future trends. Caries Res 1990;24:381-96.
75. Marthaler TM, O'Mullane DM, Vrbic V. The prevalence of dental caries in Europe 1990-1995. ORCA Saturday afternoon symposium 1995. Caries Res 1996;30:237-55.
76. Martin IG, Daly CG, Liew VP. After-hours treatment of anterior dental trauma in Newcastle and western Sydney: a four-year study. Aust Dent J 1990; 35:27-31.
77. Meon R. A study of traumatised permanent anterior teeth in a school population. Singapore Dent J 1986; 11:19-21.
78. Murray S. Dental trauma: a socio-political issue? (Master's Thesis). St. Bartholomew's and the Royal London School of Medicine and Dentistry: University of London; 1996.
79. Naqvi A, Ogidan O. Classification for traumatic injuries to teeth for epidemiological purposes. Odontostomatol Trop 1990;13:115-6.
80. Naqvi A, Ogidan O. Traumatic injuries of anterior teeth in first year secondary school children in Benin-City, Nigeria. Afr Dent J 1990;4:11-5.
81. Naylor NM. Second International Conference on declining caries. Int Dent J 1994;363-458.
82. Ng'ang'a PM, Valderhaug J. The prevalence of fractured permanent incisors in 13 to 15-year- old school children in Nairobi. Afr Dent J 1988;2:76-9.
83. Nguyen QV, Bezemer PD, Habets L, Prahl-Andersen B. A systematic review of the relationship between overjet size and traumatic dental injuries. Eur J Orthod 1999;21:503-15.
84. Nicolau B, Marcenes W, Sheiham, A Prevalence, causes and correlates of traumatic dental injuries among 13-year-olds in Brazil. Dent Traumatol 2001; 17:213-7.
85. Nik-Hussein NN. Traumatic injuries to anterior teeth among schoolchildren in Malaysia Dent Traumatol 2001;17:149-52.
86. O'Brien M. Children's dental health in the United Kingdom 1993. London: H.M.S.O; 1995.
87. Oluwole TO, Leverett DH. Clinical and epidemiological survey of adolescents with crown fractures of permanent anterior teeth. Ped Dent 1986;8:221-5.
88. O'Mullane DM. Injured permanent incisor teeth: an epidemiological study. J Ir Dent Assoc 1972;18:160-73.
89. O'Mullane DM. Some factors predisposing to injuries of permanent incisors in school children. Br Dent J 1973;134:328-32.
90. Otuyemi OD. Traumatic anterior dental injuries related to incisor overjet and lip competence in 12-year-old Nigerian children. Int J Pediatr Dent 1994;4:81-5.
91. Petersen PE. Society and oral health. In: Community Oral Health. Cynthia MP. Great Britain: Wright; 1997. p.20-39.
92. Petersson HG, Bratthall D. The caries decline: a review of reviews. Eur J Oral Sci 1996;104:436-43.
93. Petti S, Tarsitani G. Traumatic injuries to anterior teeth in Italian schoolchildren: prevalence and risk factors. Endod Dent Traumatol 1996;12:294-7.
94. Petti S, Tarsitani G, Arcadi P, Tomassini E, Romagnoli L. The prevalence of anterior tooth trauma in children 6 to 11 years old. Minerva Stomatol 1996;45:213-8.
95. Powell EA. Social and psychological considerations. In: Dentistry for the adolescent. Castaldi CR, Brass GA. 1.ed. London: Saunders; 1980. p.60-67.
96. Ramos-Jorge ML, Bosco VL, Peres MA, Nunes ACGP. The impact of treatment of dental trauma on the quality of life of adolescents - a case-control study in southern Brazil. Dent Traumatol 2007;23:114-9.
97. Richardson ME. Dental accidents diseases and disasters. Brit Dent J 1999; 187:291-94.
98. Sheiham A, Spencer J. Health needs assessment. In: Community Oral Health. Pine CM. Oxford: Wright; 1997. p.39-54.
99. Slack GL, Jones JM. Psycological effect of fractured incisors. Brit Dent J 1955; 6:338.
100. Slade GD. Derivation and validation of a short form oral health impact profile. Community Dent Oral Epidemiol 1997;25:284-90.
101. Soares I, Goldberg F. Endodontia: técnica e fundamentos. Porto Alegre: Artes Médicas; 2001. 376p.
102. Solow B. Orthodontic screening and third party financial. Eur J Orthod 1995;17:79-83.
103. Tapias MA, Jimenez-Garcia R, Lamas F, Gil AA. Prevalence of traumatic crown fractures to permanent incisors in a childhood population: Mostoles, Spain. Dent Traumatol 2003;19:119-22.
104. Todd JE. Children's Dental Health in England and Wales 1973. London: H.M.S.O; 1975.
105. Todd JE, Dodd T. Children's dental health in the United Kingdom 1983. London: H.M.S.O; 1985.
106. Traebert J, Peres MA, Blank V, Boell RS, Pietruza JA. Prevalence of traumatic dental injury and associated factors among 12-year-old school children in Florianopolis, Brazil. Dent Traumatol 2003;19:15-8.
107. Uji T, Teramoto T. Occurrence of traumatic injuries in the oromaxillary region of children in a Japanese prefecture. Endod Dent Traumatol 1988;4:63-6.
108. Vallittu PK, Vallittu AS, Lassila VP. Dental aesthetics - a survey of attitudes in different groups of patients. J Dent 1996; 24:335-8.
109. Wong FS, Kolokotsa K. The cost of treating children and adolescents with injuries to their permanent incisors at a dental hospital in the United Kingdom. Dent Traumatol. 2004;20:327-33.
110. World Health Organization. Standardisation of reporting of dental disease and condition. Technical Report Series 1962; n.242, 23p.
111. www.sbtd.org.br – Brazilian Society of Dental Injury. Accessed in 18th September 2008
112. .Zadik D, Chosack A, Eidelman E. A Survey of traumatized incisors in Jerusalem school children. J Dent Child 1972;8:327-30.
113. Zaragoza AA, Catala M, Colmena ML, Valdemoro C. Dental trauma in schoolchildren six to twelve years of age. ASDC J Dent Child 1998;65:492-4.
114. Zerman N, Cavalleri G. Traumatic injuries to permanent incisors. Endod Dent Traumatol 1993;9:61-4.

1. Abedi HR, Ingle JI. Mineral trioxide aggregate: a review of a new cement. J Calif Dent Assoc 1995;23:36-9.
2. Aeinehchi M, Eslami B, Ghanbariha M, Saffar AS. Mineral trioxide aggregate (MTA) and calcium hydroxide as pulp-capping agentsin human teeth: a preliminary report. Int Endod J 2003;36:225-31.
3. Anaya-Alva S, Loyola-Rodrigues JP. Análise retrospectiva de 787 urgências estomatológicas. ADM 1984;41:75-9.
4. Anderson L, Bodin I. Avulsed human teeth replanted within 15 minutes: a long-term clinical follow-up study. Endod Dent Traumatol 1990;6:37-42.
5. Anderson L, Bodin I, Sörensen S. Progression of root resorption following replantation of human teeth after extended extraoral storage. Endod Dent Traumatol 1989;5:38-47.
6. Andreasen FM. Pulpal healing after luxation injuries and root fracture in the permanet dentition. Endod Dent Traumatol 1989;5:111-131.
7. Andreasen FM, Andreasen JO. Diagnosis of luxation injuries. The importance of standardized clinical, radiographic and photographic techniques in clinical investigations. Endod Dent Traumatol 1985;1:160-9.
8. Andreasen FM, Andreasen JO. Resorption and mineralization processes following root fractures of permanente incisor. Endod Dent Traumatol 1988;4:202-14.
9. Andreasen FM, Andreasen JO, Bayer T. Prognosis of root-fractured permanent incisors-prediction of healing modalities. Endod Dent Traumatol 1989;5:11-22.
10. Andreasen FM, Daugaard-Jensen J. Treatment of traumatic dental injuries in children. Curto Opinion Dent 1991;1:535-50.
11. Andreasen FM, Vestergaard-Pedersen B. Prognosis of luxated permanent teeth - the development of pulp necrosis. Endod Dent Traumatol 1985;1:207-20.
12. Andreasen FM, Zhijie Y, Thomsen BL. Relationship between pulp dimensions and development at pulp necrosis after luxation injuries in lhe permanent dentition. Endod Dent Traumatol 1986;2:90-8.
13. Andreasen FM, Zhijie Y, Thomsen BL, Andersen PK. Occurrence of pulp canal obliteration after luxation injuries in lhe permanent dentition. Endod Dent Traumatol 1987;3:103-15.
14. Andreasen JO. Effect of extra-alveolar period and storage media upon periodontal and pulpal healing after replantation af mature permanent incisors in monkeys. Int J Oral Surg 1981;10:43-53.
15. Andreasen JO. The effect of pulp extirpation of root canal treatment on periodontal healing after replantation af permanent incisors in monkeys. J Endod 1981;7:245-52.
16. Andreasen JO, Andreasen FM. Text book and color atlas of traumatic injuries to teeth. 4th.ed. Oxford Blackwell Publishing; 2007. 897p.
17. Andreasen JO, Andreasen FM. Traumatismos Dentários - Soluções Clínicas. São Paulo: Panamericana;1991. 168p.
18. Andreasen JO, Borum MK, Jacobsen HL, Andreasen FM. Replantation of 400 avulsed permanent incisors: 1. Diagnosis of healing complications. Endod Dent Traumatol 1995;11:76-89.
19. Andreasen JO, Hjorting-Hansen E. Intraalveolar root fractures: radiographic and histologic study at 50 cases. J Oral Surg 1967;25:414-26.
20. Andreasen JO, Hjorting-Hansen E. Replantation of teeth: Radiographic and clinical study of 110 human teeth replanted after accidental loss. Acta Odont Scand 1966;24:263-86.
21. Bakland LK. Management of traumatically injured pulps in immature teeth using MTA. J Calif Dent Assoc 2000;28:855-8.
22. Baratieri LN. Estética – restaurações adesivas diretas em dentes anteriores fraturados. São Paulo: Ed. Santos;1995. p.135-205.
23. Baratieri LN. Odontologia restauradora – Fundamentos e possibilidades. São Paulo: Ed. Santos;2001. 779 p.
24. Baratieri LN, Monteiro S Jr, Caldeira de Andrada MA et al. Tooth fragment reattachment. In: Baratieri LN, Monteiro S Jr, Caldeira de Andrada MA et al. Direct adhesive restorations on fractured anterior teeth. Translated from the 2nd Brazilian ed. São Paulo: Quintessence Books, 1998: p. 134–205.
25. Barret EJ, Kenny DJ. Avulsed permanent teeth: a review of the literature and treatment guidelines. Endod Dent Traumatol 1997;13:153-63.
26. Bastos JV. Prognóstico pulpar após lesões traumáticas na dentição permanente: Avaliação clínico-radiográfca. (Master's Thesis). Federal University of Minas Gerais;1996. 129p.
27. Bastos JV, Côrtes MIS. Care and guidance in dental trauma - an approach to the lay community (Abstract). Proceedings of the IV International Conference on Dental Trauma. London;1993.
28. Bastos JV, Côrtes MIS. Cuidados e orientação em traumatismos dentários: manual para professores e outros agentes multiplicadores. Belo Horizonte: Imprensa Universitária da Universidade Federal de Minas Gerais (UFMG);1994.
29. Bastos JV, Côrtes MIS. Cuidados e orientação em traumatismos dentários: manual para professores e outros agentes multiplicadores. 2nd.ed. Belo Horizonte: Imprensa Universitária da Universidade Federal de Minas Gerais (UFMG). 1997. 26p.
30. Bastos JV, Côrtes MIS. E se meu dente quebrar? 2nd. ed. Belo Horizonte: Imprensa Universitária da Universidade Federal de Minas Gerais (UFMG). 1997. 8p.
31. Bergenholtz G, Cox CP, Loeshe WJ, Syed SA. Bacterial leakage around dental restorations: its effect on the dental pulp. J Oral Pathol 1982;11:439-50.
32. Bernick S, Nedelman C. Effect of aging on the human pulp. J Endod 1975;1:88-94.
33. Bjorvatn K, Selvig KA, Klinge B. Effect of tetracycline and SnF2 on root resorption in replanted incisors in dogs. Scand J Dent Res 1989;97:477-82.
34. Blanco LP. Treatment of crown fractures with pulp exposure. Oral Surg Oral Med Oral Pathol Oral Radiol Endod 1996;82:564-8.
35. Blomlof L. Milk and saliva as possible storage media for traumatically exarticulated teeth prior to replantation. (Doctoral Thesis). Stockholm: Karolinska Institutet, 1981. 26p.
36. Blomlöf L, Andersson L, Linskog S, Hedström K-G, Hammarström L. Periodontal healing of replanted monkey teeth prevented from drying. Acta Odontol Scand 1983;41:117-23.

37. Blomlof L, Otteskog P, Hammarstrom L. Effect of storage in media with different íon strengths and osmolarities on human periodontal ligament cells. Scand J Dent Res 1981;89:180-7.
38. Brännström M. Dentin and pulp in restorative dentistry. Nacka: Sweden Dental therapeutics;1981. 127p.
39. Brânnstrom M. Observations on exposed dentine and the corresponding pulp tissue. Odont Rev 1962;13:235-45.
40. Camp JH. Pulp therapy for primary and young permanent teeth. Dent Clin North Am 1984;28:651-8.
41. Cavalleri G, Zerman N. Traumatic crown fractures in permanent incisors with immature roots: a follow-up study. Endod Dent Traumatol 1995;11:294-6.
42. Cortes MIS. Epidemiology of traumatic injuries to permanent teeth and the impact on the daily living of Brazilian school children. (Doctoral Thesis). Londres: Department of Epidemiology and Public Health, University College London, 2000. 247 p.
43. Côrtes MIS, Bastos JV. E se meu dente quebrar? Belo Horizonte. Imprensa Universitária da Universidade Federal de Minas Gerais (UFMG);1994.
44. Costa CAS, Hebling J, Hanks CT. Current status of pulp capping with dentin adhesive systems: a review. Dent Mater 2000;1:188-97.
45. Courts FJ, Mueller WA, Tabeling JA. Milk as interim storage medium for avulsed tooth. Pediatr Dent 1983;5:183-6.
46. Cox CF, Bergenholtz G, Fitzgerald M, Heys DR, Avery JK, Baker JA. Capping of the dental pulp mechanically exposed to the oral microflora - a 5 week observation of wound healing in monkey. J Oral Pathol 1982;11:327-39.
47. Cox CF, Bergenholtz G, Heys DR, Syed SA, Fitzgerald M, Heys RJ. Pulp capping of dental pulp mechanically exposed to oral microflora: a 1-2 real observation of wound healing in the monkey. J Oral Pathol 1985;14:156-68.
48. Cox CF, Keall HJ, Ostro E, Bergenholtz G. Biocompatibility of surface-sealed dental materials against pulps. Prosthet Dent 1987;57:1-8.
49. Cvek M. A Clinical report on partial pulpotomy and capping with calcium hydroxide in permanent incisors with complicated crown fractured. J Endod 1978;4:232-37.
50. Cvek M. Calcium hydroxide in treatment of traumatized tooth. Eastman Institute – Stockholm: Scania Dental AB;1989.
51. Cvek M. Endodontic management of traumatized teeth. In: Textbook and color atlas of traumatic injuries to the teeth. Andreasen JO, Andreasen FM. 3rd. ed. Copenhagen: Munksgaard, 1994. p.517-86.
52. Cvek M, Cleaton-Jones P, Austin JC, Andreasen JO. Pulp reactions to exposure after experimental crown fractures or grinding in adults monkeys. J Endod 1982;8:391-7.
53. Cvek M, Cleaton-Jones P, Austin J, Lownie J, Kling M, Fatti P. Effect of topical application of doxycycline on pulp revascularization and periodontal healing in reimplanted monkey incisors. Endod Dent Traumatol 1990;6:170-6.
54. Cvek M, Cleaton-Jones P, Austin J, Lownie J, Kling M, Fatti P. Pulp revascularization in reimplanted immature monkey incisors - predictability and effect of antibiotic systemic prophylaxis. Endod Dent Traumatol 1990;6:157-69.
55. Cvek M, Granath LE, Hollender L. Treatment of nonvital permanent incisors with calcium hydroxide. III Variation of occurrence of ankylosis of reimplanted teeth with duration of extra-alveolar period and storage environment. Odont Rev 1974;25:43-56.
56. Dewhurst SN *et al.* Emergency treatment of orodental injuries: a review. Br J Oral Maxillofac Surg 1998;36:165-75.
57. Doyle DL, Dumsha TC, Sydiskis RJ. Effect of soaking in Hank's balanced salt solution or milk on PDL cell viability of dry stored human teeth. Endod Dent Traumatol 1998;14:221-4.
58. Dylewski JJ, Mich AA. Apical closure of nonvital teeth. Oral Surg Oral Med Oral Pathol 1971;32:82-89.
59. Faraco-Jr IM, Holland R. Response of the pulp of dogs to capping with mineral trioxide aggregate or a calcium hydroxide cement. Dent Traumatol 2001;17:163-6.
60. Fleming P, Gregg TA, Saunders IDE. Analysis of an emergency dental service provided at a children's hospital. Inter J Pediat Dent 1991;1:25-30.
61. Ford TR, Torabinejad M, Abedi HR, Bakland LK, Kariyawasam SP. Using mineral trioxide aggregate as a pulp-capping material. J Am Dent Assoc 1996;127:1491-4.
62. Francischone CE. Avaliação clínica e radiográfica, feita a curto e longo prazo, de uma pulpotomia em função da idade do paciente, do grupo de dentes e da propedêutica. (Doctoral Thesis). São Paulo University;1978. 212p.
63. Frank AL. Table clinic. 21st Annual Meeting of American Association of Endodontists. Washington DC, 1964. In: Webber RT. Apexogenesis versus Apexification. Dent Clin North Am 1984;28:669-97.
64. Frank AL. Therapy for the divergent pulpless tooth by continued apical formation. J Am Dent Assoc 1966;72:87-93.
65. Fuks AB, Bielak S, Chosak A. Clinical and radiographic assessment of direct pulp capping and pulpotomy in young permanent teeth. Pediatr Dent 1982;4:240-44.
66. Fuks AB, Chosack A, Klein H, Eidelman E. Partial pulpotomy as a treatment alternative for exposed pulps in crown - fractured permanent incisors Endod Dent Traumatol 1987;3:100-2.
67. Galea H. An investigation of dental injuries treated in an acute cate general hospital. J Am Dent Assoc 1984;109:434-8.
68. Hallet GEM, Porteus JR. Fractureds Incisors Treated by Vital Pulpotomy. Brit Dent J 1963;115:279-87.
69. Hamilton EA, Hill EJ, Holloway PJ. An investigation of dento-alveolar trauma and its treatment in an adolescent population. Part 1: The prevalence and incidence of injuries and the extent and adequacy of treatment received. Br Dent J 1997;182:91-5.
70. Hammarstrom L, Blomlof L, Feiglin B, Anderson L, Lindskog S. Replantion of teeth and antibiotic treatment. Endod Dent Traumatol 1986;2:51-7.
71. Hebling H. Resposta do complexo dentino-pulpar à aplicação de um sistema adesivo em cavidades profundas com ou sem exposição da polpa. (Doctoral ThesisTese de doutorado). São Paulo University;1997. 191p.
72. Heide S, Kerekes K. Delayed direct pulp capping in permanent incisors of monkeys. Int Endod J 1987;20:65-74.

73. Heide S, Kerekes K. Delayed partial pulpotomy in permanent incisors of monkeys. Int Endod J 1986;19:78-89.
74. Heide S, Mjor JA. Pulp reactions to experimental exposures in young permanent monkey teeth. Int Endod J 1983;16:11-9.
75. Hiltz J, Trope M. Vitality of human lip fibroblasts in milk, Hanks balanced salt solution and Viaspan storage media. Endod Dent Traumatol 1991;7:69-72.
76. Hupp JG, Mesaros SV, Aukhil I, Trope M. Periodontal ligament vitality and histologic healing of teeth stored for extended periods before transplantation. Endod Dent Traumatol 1998;14:79-83.
77. Jacobsen I, Kerekes K. Diagnosis and treatment of pulp necrosis in permanent anterior teeth with root fracture. Scand J Dent Res 1980;88:370-6.
78. Jacobsen I, Zachrisson B. Repair characteristics of root fractures in permanent teeth. Scand J Dent Res 1975;83:355-64.
79. Kaiser HJ. Scientific Session. 21st Annual Meeting of American Association of Endodontists. Washington DC, 1964. In: Webber RT. Apexogenesis versus Apexification. Dent Clin North Am 1984;28:669-97.
80. Kanca J. Replacement of a fractured incisor fragment over pulpal exposure: a case report. Quint Int 1993;24:81-4.
81. Kashiwada T, Takashi M. New restorations and direct pulp capping systems using adhesive composite resin. Bull Tokyo Med Dent Univ 1991;38:45-52.
82. Klein H, Fuks A, Eidelman E, Chosack A. Partial pulpotomy following complicated crown fractured in permanent incisors: A clinical and radiographical study. J Pedod 1985;9:142-7.
83. Krasner PR, Rankow HJ. New philosophy for the treatment of avulsed teeth. Oral Surg Oral Med Oral Pathol 1995;79:616-23.
84. Krasner PR. Treatment of tooth avulsion in the emergency department: appropriate storage and transport media. Am J Emerg Med 1990;8:351-5.
85. Lanza LD. Avaliação clínica e microscópica de um sistema adesivo aplicado em proteções pulpares diretas de dentes humanos. (Doctoral Thesis). São Paulo University;1997. 142p.
86. Lekic PC, Kenny DJ, Barrett EJ. The influence of storage conditions on the clonogenic capacity of periodontal ligament cells: implications for tooth replantation. Int Endod J 1998;31:137-40.
87. Lekic P, Kenny D, Moe HK, Barrett E, McCulloch C. Relationship of clonogenic capacity to plating efficiency and vital dye staining of human periodontal ligament cells: implications for tooth replantation. J Periodontol Res 1996;31:294-300.
88. Luostarinen V, Pohoto M, Sheinin A. Dynamics of repair in the pulp. J Dent Res 1966;45:324-30.
89. McDonald N, Strassler HE. Evaluation for tooth stabilization and treatment of traumatized teeth. Dent Clin North Am 1999;43:135-49.
90. Mondelli J. Proteção do complexo dentino-pulpar. São Paulo: Artes Médicas;1998. 316p.
91. Naidoo S. A profile of the oral-facial injuries in child physical abuse at a children's hospital. Child Abuse & Neglect 2000;24:521-34.
92. Nasjleti CE, Castelli WA, Cafesse RG. The effects of different splinting times on replantation of teeth in monkeys. Oral Surg Oral Med Oral Pathol 1982;53:557-66.
93. Oikarinen KS. Tooth splinting: a review of the literature and consideration of the versatility of a wire-composite splint. Endod Dent Traumatol 1990;6:237-50.
94. O'Neil DW, Clark MW, Lowe JW, Harrington MS. Oral trauma in children: A hospital surver. Oral Surg Oral Med Oral Pathol 1989;68:691-6.
95. Pashley DH. Clinical considerations of microleakage. J Endod 1990;16:70-7.
96. Pashley DH, Andringahj-Derkson GD, Derkson ME, Kalathoor SR. Regional variability in the permeability of human dentine. Arch Oral Biol 1987;32:519-23.
97. Patil S, Dumsha TC, Sydiskis RJ. Determining periodontal ligament (PDL) cell vitality from exarticulated teeth stored in saline or milk using fluoresceindiacetate. Int Endod J 1994;27:1-5.
98. Pereira JC, Segala D, Costa CAS. Human pulp response to direct pulp capping with an adhesive system histhologic study. J Dent Res 1997;36:180.
99. Pitt-Ford TR, Roberts GJ. Immediate and delayed direct pulp capping with the use of a new visible light-cured calcium hydroxide preparation. Oral Surg Oral Med Oral Pathol 1991;71:338-42.
100. Ramos DLP. A proteção do profissional. In: Atualização na clínica odontológica: cursos antagônicos. Feller C, Gorab R. 1st ed. São Paulo: Artes Médicas, 2000. p.579-91.
101. Ravn JJ. Follow-up study of permanent incisors with enamel-dentin fractures after acute trauma. Scand J Dent Res 1981;89:355-65.
102. Ravn JJ. Follow up study of permanent incisors with complicated crown fractures after acute trauma. Scand J Dent Res 1982;90:363-72.
103. Robertson A, Robertson S, Noren JG. A retrospective evaluation of traumatized permanent teeth. Int J Paediatr Dent 1997;7:217-26.
104. Sae-Lim V, Wang CY, Choi GW, Trope M. The effect of systemic tetracycline on resorption of dried replanted dogs' teeth. Endod Dent Traumatol 1998;14:127-32.
105. Sae-Lim V, Wang CY, Trope M. Effect of systemic tetracycline and amoxicilin on inflammatory root resorption of replanted dogs' teeth. Endod Dent Traumatol 1998;14:216-20.
106. Schmitt D, Lee J, Bogen G. Multifaceted use of ProRoot MTA root canal repair material. Pediatr Dent 2001;23:326-30.
107. Schröder U. Evaluation of healing following experimental pulpotomy of intact human teeth and capping with calcium hydroxide. Odont Revy 1972;23:329-40.
108. Schwartz S. A one-year statistical analysis of dental emergencies in a pediatric hospital. J Can Dent Assoc 1994;60:966-8.
109. Selvig KA, Bjorvatn K, Bogle GC, Wikesjo UM. Effect of stannous fluoride and tetracycline on periodontal repair after delayed tooth replantation in dogs. Scand J Dent Res 1992;100:200-3.
110. Sheinin A, Pohoto M, Luostarinen V. Defence reactions of the pulp with special reference to circulation. An experimental study in rats. Int Dent J 1967;17:461-75.
111. Soares I, Goldberg F. Endodontia: técnica e fundamentos. Porto Alegre: Artes Médicas Sul;2001.376p.
112. Stanley HR. Management of the aging patient and the aging pulp. J Calif Dent Assoc 1978;57:25-8.

113. Teuscher GW, Zander HA. A preliminary report on pulpotomy. Northwestern University. Q Bull 1938;39:44. In: Webber RT. Apexogenesis versus Apexification. Dent Clin North Am 1984;28:669-97.
114. The Cochrane Collaboration - http://www.cochrane.org/. Acessed in 18th September 2008.
115. Torabinejad M, Chivian N. Clinical applications of mineral trioxide aggregate. J Endod 1999;25:197-205.
116. Toto PD, Staffileno H, Weine FS, Das S. Age change effects on the pulp in periodontitis. Ann Dent 1977;36:13-20.
117. Trope M, Friedman S. Periodontal healing of replanted dog teeth stored in Viaspan, milk and Hank's balanced salt solution. Endod Dent Traumatol 1992;8:183-8.
118. Tziafas D, Pantelidou O, Alvanou A, Belibasakis G, Papadimitriou S. The dentinogenic effect of mineral trioxide aggregate (MTA) in short-termcapping experiments. Int Endod J 2002;35:245-54.
119. Wallace JA, Vergona K. Epithelial rest's function in replantation: is splinting necessary in replantation? Oral Surg Oral Med Oral Pathol 1990;70:644-9.
120. Walsh JS, Fey MR, Omnell LM. The effect of indomethacinon resorption and ankylosis in replanted teeth. ASDC J Dent Child 1987;54:261.
121. Webber RT. Apexogenesis versus Apexification. Dent Clin North Am 1984;28:669-97.
122. WELBURY R.R. Child Physical abuse. In: Textbook and color atlas of traumatic injuries to teeth. Andreasen JO, Andreasen FM, Andersson L. 4.ed. Oxford: Blackwell Publishing; 2007. p.207-16).
123. www.sbtd.org.br - Brazilian Society of Dental Injury. Accessed in 18th September 2008
124. Zanetta-Barbosa D, Carvalho AC. Effect of brief storage in ATP solution on periodontal healing after replantation of teeth in rats. Endod Dent Traumatol 1990;6:193-9.
125. Zander HA. Reaction of the dental pulp to calcium hydroxide. J Dent Res 1939;18:373. In: Webber RT. Apexogenesis versus Apexification. Dent Clin North Am 1984;28:669-97.
126. Zeng Y, Sheller B, Milgrom P. Epidemiology of dental emergency visits to an urban children's hospital. Pediatric Dent 1994;16:419-23.
127. Zervas P, Lambrianidis T, Karabouta-Vulgaropoulou I. The effect of citric acid treatment on periodontal healing after replantation of permanent teeth. Int Endod J 1991;24:317-25.


## PARTE 3. PHYSIOPATHOLOGY OF TRAUMATIC INJURIES


1. Amir FA, Gutmann JL, Witherspoon DE. Calcific methamorphosis: a challenge in endodontic diagnosis and treatment. Quint Int 2001;32:447-55.
2. Anderson L, Bodin I. Avulsed human teeth replanted within 15 minutes: a long-term clinical followup study. Endod Dent Traumatol 1990;6:37-42.
3. Anderson L, Bodin I, Sörensen S. Progression of root resorption following replantation of human teeth after extended extraoral storage. Endod Dent Traumatol 1989;5:38-47.
4. Andreasen FM. Pulpal healing after luxation injuries and root fractures in the permanent dentition. (Doctoral Thesis). Copenhagen: Faculty of Health Sciences, Copenhagen University; 1995. 51p.
5. Andreasen FM. Pulpal healing after luxation injuries and root fractures in the permanent dentition. Endod Dent Traumatol 1989;5:111-31.
6. Andreasen FM. Transient apical breakdown and its relation to color and sensibility changes after luxation injuries to teeth. Endod Dent Traumatol 1986;2:9-19.
7. Andreasen FM, Andreasen JO. Resorption and mineralization processes following root fractures of permanente incisor. Endod Dent Traumatol 1988;4:202-14.
8. Andreasen FM, Andreasen JO, Bayer T. Prognosis of root-fractured permanent incisors - prediction of healing modalities. Endod Dent Traumatol 1989;5:11-22.
9. Andreasen FM, Vestergaard Pedersen B. Prognosis of luxated permanent teeth - the development of pulp necrosis. Endod Dent Traumatol 1985;1:207-20.
10. Andreasen FM, Zhijie Y, Thomsen BL, Andersen PK. Occurrence of pulp canal obliteration after luxation injuries in the permanent dentition. Endod Dent Traumatol 1987;3:103-15.
11. Andreasen FM, Zhijie Y, Thomsen BL. Relationship between pulp dimensions and development of pulp necroses after luxation injuries in the permanent dentition. Endod Dent Traumatol 1986;2:90-8.
12. Andreasen JO. Analysis of topography of surface and inflamatory root resorption after replantation of permanent incisors in monkeys. Swed Dent J 1980;4:135-44.
13. Andreasen JO. Challenges in clinical dental traumatology. Endod Dent Traumatol 1985; 1:45-55.
14. Andreasen JO. Effect of extra-alveolar period and storage media upon periodontal and pulpal healing after replantation of mature permanent incisors in monkeys. Int J Oral Surg 1981;10:43-53.
15. Andreasen JO. External root resorption: its implication in dental traumatology, paedodontics, periodontics, orthodontics and endodontics. Int Endod J 1985;18:109-18.
16. Andreasen JO. Luxation of permanent teeth due to trauma - A clinical and radiographic follow-up study of 189 injured teeth. Scand J Dent Res 1970;78:273-86.
17. Andreasen JO. Periodontal healing after replantation and autotransplantation of incisors in monkeys. Int J Oral Surg 1981;10:54-61.
18. Andreasen JO. The effect of pulp extirpation or root canal treatment on periodontal healing after replantation of permanent incisors in monkeys. J Endod 1981;7:245-52.
19. Andreasen JO. The effect of removal of the coagulum in the alveolus before replantation upon pulpal and periodontal healing of mature permanent incisors in monkeys. Int J Oral Surg 1980;9:458-61.

20. Andreasen JO. The effect of splinting after replantation of permanent incisors in monkeys. Acta Odontol Scand 1975; 33:313-25.
21. Andreasen JO, Andreasen FM. Root resorption following traumatic dental injuries. Proc. Finn. Dent Soc 1992;88:95-114.
22. Andreasen JO, Andreasen FM. Text book and color atlas of traumatic injuries to teeth. 4th.ed. Oxford Blackwell Publishing; 2007. 897p.
23. Andreasen JO, Borum MK, Jacobsen HL, Andreasen FM. Replantation of 400 avulsed permanent incisors: Diagnosis of healing complications. Endod Dent Traumatol 1995;11:51-8.
24. Andreasen JO, Borum MK, Jacobsen HL, Andreasen FM. Replantation of 400 avulsed permanent incisors: Factors related to pulpal healing. Endod Dent Traumatol 1995; 11:59-68.
25. Andreasen JO, Borum MK, Jacobsen HL, Andreasen FM. Replantation of 400 avulsed permanent incisors. Factors related to periodontal ligament healing. Endod Dent Traumatol 1995;11:76-89.
26. Andreasen JO, Hjørting–Hansen E. Intraalveolar root fractures: radiographic and histologic study of 50 cases. J O Surg 1967;25:414-26.
27. Andreasen JO, Hjørting-Hansen E. Replantation of teeth: I Radiographic and clinical study of 110 human teeth replanted after accidental loss. Acta Odont Scand 1966;24:263-86.
28. Andreasen JO, Hjørting-Hansen E. Replantation of teeth: II. Histological study of 22 replanted anterior teeth in humans. Acta Odont Scand 1966;24:287-306.
29. Andreasen JO, Kristersen L. The effect of extraalveolar root filling with calcium hydroxide upon periodontal healing after reimplantation of mature permanent incisors in monkeys. J Endod 1981;7:349-54.
30. Andreasen JO, Paulsen HU, Yu Z, Bayer T, Schwartz O. A long term study of 370 autotransplanted premolars. Part II. Tooth survival and pulp healing subsequent to transplantation. Eur J Orthod 1990;12:14-24.
31. Andreasen JO, Reinholdt J, Riis I, Dybdahl R, Söder P-Ö, Otteskog P. Periodontal and pulpal healing of monkey incisors preserved in tissue culture before replantation. Int J Oral Surg 1978;7:104-12.
32. Arana-Chavez VE. Odontogênese. Revista da APCD 1997; 51:361-6.
33. Araújo M, Hayacibara R, Sonohara M, Cardaropoli G, Lindhe J: Effect of enamel matrix proteins (Emdogain) on healing after re-implantation of "periodontally compromised" roots. An experimental study in the dog. J Clin Periodontol 2003;30:855–61.
34. Avery J. Repair potential of the pulp. J Endod 1981;7:205-12.
35. Barkin PR. Time as a factor in predicting the vitality of traumatized teeth. ASDC J Dent Child 1973;40:188-92.
36. Barrett EJ, Kenny DJ. Avulsed permanent teeth: a review of the literature and treatment guidelines. Endod Dent Traumatol 1997;13:153-63.
37. Barrett EJ, Kenny DJ. Survival of avulsed permanent maxillary incisors in children following delayed replantation. Endod Dent Traumatol 1997;13:269-75.
38. Bastos JV. Prognóstico pulpar após lesões traumáticas na dentição permanente: avaliação clínico-radiográfica. (Master's Thesis). Federal University of Minas Gerais – Faculdade de Odontologia. 1996; 129p.
39. Bastos JV, Côrtes MIS. Estudo prospectivo da resposta às provas de vitalidade pulpar após lesões traumáticas. Pesq Odontol Bras 2000;14:130.
40. Bastos JV, Côrtes MIS. Pulp prognosis of permanent teeth presenting pulp canal obliteration after traumatic dental injuries. 2008. In preparation
41. Bhaskar S, Rappaport H. Dental vitality tests and pulp status. JADA 1973; 86:409-11.
42. Birch R, Rock WP. The incidence of compications following root fracture in permanent anterior teeth. Bristish Dental Journal 1986;160:119-22.
43. Bjorvatn K, Selvig KA, Klinge B. Effect of tetracycline and SnF2 on root resorption in replanted incisors in dogs. Scand J Dent Res 1989;97:477-82.
44. Blomlöf L. Milk and saliva as possible storage media for traumatically exarticulated teeth prior to replantation. (Doctoral Thesis). Stockholm: Karolinska Institutet; 1981. 26p.
45. Blomlöf L, Andersson L, Linskog S, Hedström K-G, Hammarström L. Periodontal healing of replanted monkey teeth prevented from drying. Acta Odontol Scand 1983;41:117-23.
46. Blomlöf L, Lengheden A, Lindskog S. Endodontic infection and calcium hydroxide – treatment. Effects on periodontal healing in mature and immature replanted monkey teeth. J Clin Periodontol 1992;199:652-58.
47. Blomlöf L, Otteskög P, Hammarström L. Effect of storage in media with different ion strengths and osmolalities on human periodontal ligament cells. Scand J Dent Res 1981;89:180-7.
48. Boyd KS. Transient breakdown after following subluxation injury: A case report. Endod Dent Traumatol 1995;11:37-40.
49. Brandt K, Kortegaard U, Poulsen S. Longitudinal study of eletrometric sensitivity of young permanent incisors. Scand J Dent Res 1988;96:334-38.
50. Brännström M. Observations on exposed dentine and the corresponding pulp tissue. Odont Rev 1962;13:235-45.
51. Brännström M. The treatment of dentinal and pulpal exposures. In: Dentin and Pulp in Restorative Dentistry. Stockholm: Nacka Dental Therapeutics AB; 1981. p.111-22.
52. Caliskan MK, Pehlivan Y. Prognosis of root – fractured permanent incisors. Endod Dent Traumatol 1996;12:129-36.
53. Chiego DJ, Avery JK, Klein RM. Neuroregulation of protein synthesis in odontoblasts of the first molar of the rat after wounding. Cell Tissue Res 1987;248:119-23.
54. Chiego DJ, Fisher MA, Avery JK, Klein RM. Effects of denervation on 3H-fucose incorporation by odontoblasts in the mouse incisor. Cell Tissue Res 1983;230:197-203.
55. Coccia CT. A clinical investigation of root resorption rates in reimplanted young permanent incisors: a five-year study. J Endod 1980;6:413-20.
56. Cohenca N, Karni S, Rotstein I. Transient apical breakdown following tooth luxation. Dent Traumatol 2003;19:289-91.
57. Courts FJ, Mueller WA, Tabeling JA. Milk as interim storage medium for avulsed tooth. Pediatr Dent 1983;5:183-6.

58. Crona-Larsson G, Bjarhason S, Norén JG. Effect of luxation injuries on permanent teeth. Endod Dent Traumatol 1991;7:199-206.
59. Cvek M. Prognosis of luxated non-vital maxillary incisors treated with calcium hidroxide and filled with gutta-percha. A retrospective clinical study. Endod Dent Traumatol 1992;8:45-55.
60. Cvek M, Cleaton-Jones P, Austin J, Andreasen JO. Pulp reactions to exposure after experimental crown fractures or griding in adults monkeys. J Endod 1982;8:391-7.
61. Cvek M, Cleaton-Jones P, Austin J, Lownie J, Kling M, Fatti P. Pulp revascularization in reimplanted immature monkey incisors- predictability and effect of antibiotic systemic prophylaxis. Endod Dent Traumatol 1990;6:157-69.
62. Cvek M, Cleaton-Jones P, Austin J, Lownie J, Kling, M, Fatti P. Effect of topical application of doxycycline on pulp revascularization and periodontal healing in reimplanted monkey incisors. Endod Dent Traumatol 1990;6:157-69.
63. Cvek M, Granath L, Lundberg M. Failures and healing in endodontically treated non-vital anterior teeth with post-traumatically reduced pulpal lumen. Acta Odontol Scand 1982;40:171-81.
64. Cvek M, Granath LE, Hollender L. Treatment of non-vital permanent incisors with calcium hydroxide. III Variation of occurrence of ankylosis of reimplanted teeth with duration of extra-alveolar period and storage environment. Odont Rev 1974;25:43-56.
65. Delivanis HP, Sauer GJR. Incidence of canal calcification in the orthodontic patient. Am J Orthod 1982;82:58-61.
66. Doyle DL, Dumsha TC, Sydiskis RJ. Effect of soaking in Hank's balanced salt solution or milk on PDL cell viability of dry stored human teeth. Endod Dent Traumatol 1998;14:221-4.
67. Dumsha T, Hovland EJ. Pulpal prognosis following extrusive luxation injuries in permanent teeth with closed apexes. J Endod 1982;8:410-12.
68. Ebeleseder KA, Friehs S, Ruda C, Pertl C, Glockner K, Hulla H. A study of replanted permanent teeth in different age groups. Endod Dent Traumatol 1998;14:274-8.
69. Edwall L. Regulation of pulpal blood flow. J Endod 1980;6:434-7.
70. Feiglin B. Dental pulp response to traumatic injuries a retrospective analysis with case reports. Endod Dent Traumatol 1996;12:1-8.
71. Francischone CE, Bramante CM, Mondelli J. Reimplante dental: uso do CaATP como agente condicionador da raiz. Rev Bras Odontol 1988;45:2-10.
72. Fulling H-J, Andreasen JO. Influence of maturation status and tooth type of permanent teeth upon eletrometric and termal pulp testing. Scand J Dent Res 1976;84:286-4.
73. Gamsen E, Dumsha TC, Sydiskis R. The effect of drying time on human periodontal ligament cell viability. J Endod 1992;18:189.
74. Gazelius B, Olgart L, Edwall B. Restored vitality in luxated teeth assessed by laser doppler flowmeter. Endod Dent Traumatol 1988;4:265-8.
75. Gonda F, Nagase M, Chen RB, Yakata H, Nakajima T. Replantation: an analysis of 29 teeth. Oral Surg Oral Med Oral Pathol 1990;70:650-5.
76. Grossman LI. Origin of microorganisms in traumatized, pulpless, sound teeth. J Dent Res 1967;46:551-3.
77. Gunday M, Sazak H, Turkmen C. A scanning electron microscopic study of external root resorption in replanted dog teeth. J Endod 1995;21:269-71.
78. Hammarström L, Blomlöf L, Lindskog S. Dynamics of dentoalveolar ankylosis. Endod Dent Traumatol 1989;5:163-75.
79. Hammarström L, Blomlöf LB, Feiglin B, Andersson L, Lindskog S. Replantation of teeth and antibiotic treatment. Endod Dent Traumatol 1986;2:51-7.
80. Hammarström L, Blomlöf LB, Feiglin B, Lindskog S. Effect of calcium hydroxide treatment on periodontal repair and root resorption. Endod Dent Traumatol 1986;2:184-9.
81. Hammarström L, Lindskog S. Factors regulating and modifying dental root resorption. Proc Finn Dent Soc 1992;88:115-23.
82. Hammarström L, Lindskog S. General morphological aspects of resorption of teeth and alveolar bone. Int Endod J 1985;18:93-108.
83. Hardy LB, O'Neal RB, Del Rio CE. Effect of polyactic acid on replanted teeth in dogs. Oral Surg Oral Med Oral Pathol 1981;51:86-92.
84. Häyrinen-Immonen R, Sane J, Perkki K, Malmström M. A six-year follow-up study of sports-related dental injuries in children and adolescents. Endod Dent Traumatol 1990;6:208-12.
85. Heithersay GS, Hirsch RS. Tooth discoloration and resolution following a luxation injuriy : Significance of blood pigment in dentin to laser Doppler flowmetry readings. Quint Int 1993;24:669-76.
86. Hidalgo MM. Estudo sobre o potencial imunogênico da dentina;contribuição para a etiopatogenia da reabsorção dentária. (Doctoral Thesis). São Paulo University – USP;2001.104p.
87. Hidalgo MM, Itano EN, Consolaro A. Recognition of human dentin extract fractions by sera of immunized rabbit and patients showing radicular resorption. J Dent Res 2001;80:1035 (Abstract n.291).
88. Hiltz J, Trope M. Vitality of human lip fibroblasts in milk, Hanks balanced salt solution and ViaSpan storage media. Endod Dent Traumatol 1991;7:69-72.
89. Holcomb JB, Gregory WB. Calcific metamorphosis of the pulp: its incidence and treatment. Oral Surg Oral Med Oral Pathol 1967;24:825-30.
90. Hupp JG, Mesaros SV, Aukhil I, Trope M. Periodontal ligament vitality and histologic healing of teeth stored for extended periods before transplantation. Endod Dent Traumatol 1998;14:79-83.
91. Iqbal MK, Bamaas NS. Effect of enamel matrix derivative (EMDOGAIN) upon periodontal healing after replantation of permanent incisors in Beagle dogs. Dent Traumatol 2001;17: 36-45.
92. Jacobsen I. Criteria for diagnosis of pulp necrosis in traumatized permanent incisors. Scand J Dent Res 1980;88:306-12.
93. Jacobsen I, Kerekes K. Diagnosis and treatment of pulp necrosis in permanent anterior teeth with root fracture. Scand J Dent Res 1980;88:370-6.
94. Jacobsen I, Kerekes K. Long-term prognosis of traumatized permanent anterior teeth showing calcifying processes in the pulp cavity. Scand J Dent Res 1977;85:588-98.

95. Jacobsen I, Zachrisson B. Repair characteristics of root fractures in permanent teeth. Scand J Dent Res 1975;83:355-64.
96. Kallioniemi H, Oksala E. Significance of open apex or fracture of the root tip for the prognosis of vital maxillary canine autotransplantation. Proc Finn Dent Soc 1977;73:126-32.
97. Keller EB, Hayward JR, Nasjleti CE, Castelli WA. Venous tissue replanted on roots of teeth in monkeys. Oral Surg Oral Med Oral Pathol 1972;34:352-63.
98. Kerekes K, Heyde S, Jacobsen I. Follow-up examination of endodontic treatment em traumatized juvenile incisors. J Endod 1980;6:744-8.
99. Kerekes K, Olsen I. Similarities in the microfloras of root canals and deep periodontal pockets. Endod Dent Traumatol 1990;6:1-5.
100. Kleier DJ, Barr ES. A study of endodontically apexified teeth. Endod Dent Traumatol 1991;7:112-17.
101. Kim S. Microcirculation of the dental pulp in health and disease. J. Endod 1985;11:465-71
102. Kim S. Regulation of pulpal blood flow J Dent Res 1985;64:590-6.
103. Kling M, Cvek M, Mejáre I. Rate and predictability of pulp revasculariuzation in therapeutically reimplanted permanent incisors. Endod Dent Traumatol 1986;2:83-9.
104. Krasner PR. Treatment of tooth avulsion in the emergency department: appropriate storage and transport media. Am J Emerg Med 1990;8:351-5.
105. Krasner PR, Person P. Preserving avulsed teeth for replantation. J Am Dent Assoc 1992;123:80-8.
106. Kristerson L. Autotransplantation of human premolars a clinical and radiographic study of 100 teeth. Int J Oral Surg 1985;14:200-13.
107. Kristerson L, Andreasen JO. Influence of root development on periodontal and pulpal healing after replantion of incisors in monkeys. Int J Oral Surg 1984;13:313-23.
108. Kristerson L, Andreasen JO. The effect of splinting upon periodontal and pulpal healing after autotransplantation of mature and immature permanent incisors in monkeys. Int J Oral Surg 1983;12:239-49.
109. Kvinnsland I, Heyeraas, KJ. Dentin and osteodentin matrix formation in apicoectomized replanted incisors in cats. Acta Odontol Scand 1989;47:41-52.
110. Kvinnsland I, Heyeraas KJ, Byers MR. Effects of dental trauma on pulpal and periodontal nerve morphology. Proc Finn Dent Soc 1992;88:125-32.
111. Kvinnsland I, Heyeraas KJ, Byers MR. Regeneration of calcitonin gene-related peptide immunoreactive nerves in replanted rat molars and their supporting tissues. Arch O Biol 1991;36:815-26.
112. Lekic PC, Kenny DJ, Barrett EJ. The influence of storage conditions on the clonogenic capacity of periodontal ligament cells: implications for tooth replantation. Int Endod J 1998;31:137-40.
113. Lekic PC, Kenny DJ, Moe HK, Barrett E, Mc Culloch C. Relationship of clonogenic capacity to plating efficiency and vital dye staining of human periodontal ligament cells: implications for tooth replantation. J Periodont Res 1996;31:294-300.
114. Lengheden A, Blomlöf L, Lindskog S. Effect of delayed calcium hydroxide treatment on periodontal healing in contaminated replanted teeth. Scand J Dent Res 1991;99:147-53.
115. Levin L, Bryson EC, Caplan D, Trope M. Effect of topical alendronate on root resorption of dried replanted dog teeth. Dent Traumatol 2001;17:120-6.
116. Lindskog S, Blomlöf L, Hammarström L. Comparative effects of parathyroid hormone on osteoblasts and cementoblasts. J Cl Periodontol 1987;14:386-9.
117. Lindskog S, HammarstÖm L. Evidence in favor of an anti-invasion factor en cementum or periodontal membrane of human teeth. Scad J Dent Res 1980;88:161-3.
118. Lindskog S, Pierce AM, Blomlöf L, Hammarstöm, L. The role of necrotic periodontal membrane in cementum resorption and ankylosis. Endod Dent Traumatol 1985;1:96-101.
119. Lundberg M, Cvek M. A light microscopy study of pulps from traumatized permanent incisors with reduced pulpal lumen. Acta Odontol Scand 1980;38:89-94.
120. Mackie IC, Bentley EM, Worthington HV. The closure of open apices in non-vital immature incisor teeth. Br Dent J 1988;165:169-73.
121. Mackie IC, Worthington HV. An investigation of replantation of traumatically avulsed permanent incisor teeth. Br Dent J 1992;172:17-20.
122. Matsson L, Klinge B, Hallström H. Effect on periodontal healing of saline irrigation of the tooth socket before replantation. Endod Dent Traumatol 1987;3:64-7.
123. Matthews B, Vongsavan N. Advantages and limitations of laser Doppler flow meters. Int Endod J 1993;26:9-10.
124. Mesaros SV, Trope M. Revascularization of traumatized teeth assessed by laser Doppler flowmetry: case report. Endod Dent Traumatol 1997;13:24-30.
125. Michanowicz AE, Michanowicz JP, Abou–Rass M. Cementogenic repair of root fractures. J Am Dent Ass 1971;82:569–79.
126. Myashin M, Kato J, Takagi Y. Experimental luxation injuries in immature rat teeth. Endod Dent Traumatol 1990;6:121-8.
127. Myashin M, Kato J, Takagi Y. Tissue reactions after experimental luxation injuries in immature rat teeth. Endod Dent Traumatol 1991;7:26-35.
128. Nasjleti CE, Castelli WA, Cafesse RG. The effects of different splinting times on replantation of teeth in monkeys. Oral Surg Oral Med Oral Pathol 1982;53:557-66.
129. Ne RF, Witherspoon DE, Gutmann JL. Tooth resorption. Quintessence Int 1999;30:9-25.
130. Nguyen NH, Miller M, Landry RG. Factors influencing repair and regeneration following replantation. J Can Dent Assoc 1992;58:407-11.
131. Nishioka M, Shiiva T, Ueno K, Suda H. Tooth replantation in germ-free and conventional rats. Endod Dent Traumatol 1998;14:163-73.
132. Nissan R, Trope M, Zhang C, Change B. Dual wavelength spectrophotometry as a diagnostic test of the pulp chamber contents. Oral Surg Oral Med Oral Pathol 1992;74:508-14.
133. Oikarinen KS. Tooth splinting: a review of the literature and consideration of the versatility of a wire-composite splint. Endod Dent Traumatol 1990;6:237-50.
134. Oikarinen K, Gundlach KKH, Pfeifer G. Late complications of luxation injuries to teeth. Endod Dent Traumatol 1987;3:296-303.

135. Oikarinen KS, Seppä ST. Effect of preservation media on proliferation and collagen biosynthesis of periodontal ligament fibroblasts. Endod Dent Traumatol 1987;3:95-9.
136. Olgart L, Brannström M, Johnson G. Invasion of bacteria into dentinal tubules. Experiments in vivo and vitro. Acta Odontol Scand 1974;32:61-70.
137. Olgart L, Gazelius B, Lindh-StrÖmberg U. Laser Doppler flowmetry in assessing vitality in luxated permanent teeth. Int Endod J 1988;21:300-6.
138. Pashley DH. Dentin-predentin complex and its permeability: physiologic overview. J Dent Res 1985;64:613-20.
139. Patil S, Dumsha TC, Sydiskis RJ. Determining periodontal ligament (PDL) cell vitality from exarticulated teeth stored in saline or milk using fluorescein diacetate. Int Endod J 1994;27:1-5.
140. Patterson SS, Mitchell DF. Calcifc metamorphosis of the dental pulp. Oral Surg Oral Med Oral Pathol 1965;20:94-101.
141. Pettiette M, Hupp J, Mesaros S, Trope M. Periodontal healing of extracted dogs' teeth air-dried for extended periods and soaked in various media. Endod Dent Traumatol 1997;13:113-8.
142. Pilleggi R, Dumsha TC, Myslinksi NR. The reliability of eletric pulp test after concussion injury. Endod Dent Traumatol 1996;12:16-9.
143. Pongsiri S, Schlegel D, Zimmermann M. Ueberlebensrate desmodontaler Zellen nach extraoraler Langerung in verschiedenen Medien. Dtsch. Z. Mund Kiefer Gesichtschir, Munchen 1990;14:364-368. Apud: Oikarinen KS. Dental tissues involved in exarticulation, root resorption and factors influencing prognosis in relation to reimplanted teeth. A review. Proc Finn Dent Soc 1993;89:29-44.
144. Ravn JJ. Follow-up study of permanent incisors with enamel dentin fractures after acute trauma. Scand Dent Res 1981;89:355-65.
145. Robertson A. A retrospective evaluation of patients with uncomplicated crown fractures and luxation injuries. Endod Dent Traumatol 1998;14:245-56.
146. Robertson A, Andreasen FM, Andreasen JO, Norén JG. Long-term prognosis of crown-fractured permanent incisors. The effect of stage of root development and associated luxation injury. Int J Paed Dent 2000;10:191-9.
147. Robertson A, Andreasen FM, Bergenholtz G, Andreasen JO, Norén JG. Incidence of pulp necrosis subsequent to pulp canal obliteration from trauma of permanent incisors. J Endod 1996;22:557-60.
148. Robinson PP. An eletrophysiological study of the reinnervation of replanted and auto-transplanted teeth in the cat. Archs O Biol 1983;28:1139-47.
149. Rock NP, Grundy MC. The effect of luxation and subluxation upon the prognosis of traumatized incisor teeth. J Dent Bristol 1981;9:224-30.
150. Rungvechvuttivittaya S, Takashi O, Suda H. Responses of macrophage-associated antigen-expressing cells in the dental pulp of rat molars to experimental tooth replantation. Archs O Biol 1998;43:701-10.
151. Sae-Lim V, Wang CY, Choi GW, Trope M. The effect of systemic tetracycline on reorption of dried replanted dogs' teeth. Endod Dent Traumatol 1998;14:127-32.
152. Sae-Lim V, Wang CY, Trope M. Effect of systemic tetracycline and amoxicilin on inflammatory root resorption of replanted dogs' teeth. Endod Dent Traumatol 1998;14:216-20.
153. Schatz JP, Hausherr C, Joho JP. A retrospective clinical and radiologic study of teeth reimplanted following traumatic avulsion. Endod Dent Traumatol 1995;11:235-9.
154. Schindler WG, Gullickson DC. Rationale for the management of calcific metamorphosis secondary to traumatic injuries. J Endod 1988;14:408-12.
155. Schindler J. Kasuistischerbeitrag zum problem der heilung von zahnwurzelfrakturen mit erhaltung der vitalität der pulpa. Schweiz Mschr Zahnheilk 1941;51:474. Apud: Andreasen JO, Hjørting–Hansen E. Intraalveolar root fractures: radiographic and histologic study of 50 cases. J Oral Surg 1967;25:414-26.
156. Selvig KA, Bjorvatn K, Bogle GC, Wikesjo UM. Effect of stannous fluoride and tetracycline on periodontal repair after delayed tooth replantation in dogs. Scand J Dent Res 1992;100:200-3.
157. Shulman LB, Gedalia I, Feingold RM. Fluoride concentration in root surfaces and alveolar bone of fluoride-immersed monkey incisors three weeks after replantation. J Dent Res 1973;52:1314-6.
158. Skieller V. The prognosis for young teeth loosened after mechanical injuries. Acta Odontol Scand 1960;18:171-81.
159. Skoglund A, Tronstad L. Pulpal changes in replanted and autotransplanted immature teeth of dogs. J Endod 1981;7:309-16.
160. Skoglund A, Tronstad L, Wallenius K. A microangiographic study of vascular changes in replanted and autotransplanted teeth of young dogs. Oral Surg Oral Med Oral Pathol 1978;45:17-28.
161. Smith JW. Calcific methamorphosis: a treatment dilemma. Oral Surg Oral Med Oral Pathol 1982;54:441-4.
162. Söder PÖ, Otteskog P, Andreasen JO, Emodéer T. The effect of drying on the viability of periodontal membrane. Scand. J Dent Res 1977;85:164-8.
163. Stålhane I, Hedegård B. Traumatized permanent teeth in children - I5 years. Part II. Swed Dent J 1975;68:157-69.
164. Sundqvist G. Bacteriological studies of necrotic dental pulps. (Doctoral Thesis). Umeå : University of Umeå, Sweden;1976. 94p.
165. Teitler D, Zadick DT, Eidelman E, Chosack A. A clinical evaluation of vitality tests in anterior teeth following fracture of enamel and dentin. Oral Surg Oral Med Oral Pathol 1972;34:649-52.
166. Ten Cate AR. Histologia Bucal - desenvolvimento, estrutura e função. Rio de Janeiro: Guanabara;2000. 395p
167. Tander KJH. Blood flow and vascular pressure in the dental pulp. Acta Odontol Scand 1980;38:135-44.
168. Torneck CD. The clinical significance and management of calcific pulp obliteration. AO Scientific1990;83.
169. Tronstad L. Root resorption- etiology, terminology and clinical manifestations. Endod Dent Traumatol 1988;4:241-52.
170. Trope M, Friedman S. Periodontal healing of replanted dog teeth stored in Viaspan, milk and Hank's balanced salt solution. Endod Dent Traumatol 1992;8:183-8.

171. Trope M, Hupp JG, Mesaros SV. The role of the socket in the periodontal healing of replanted dog's teeth stored in ViaSpan for extended periods. Endod Dent Traumatol 1997;13:171-5.
172. Trope M, Moshonov J, Nissan R, Buxt P, Yesilsoy C. Short vs. long-term calcium hydroxide treatment of established inflammatory root resorption in replanted dog teeth. Endod Dent Traumatol 1995;11:124-8.
173. Trope M, Yesilsoy C, Koren L, Moshonov J, Friedman S. Effect of different endodontic treatment protocols on periodontal repair and root resorption of replanted dog teeth. J Endod 1992;18:492-6.
174. Vongsavan N, Mathews B. Changes in pulpal blood flow and in fluid flow through dentine produced by autonomic and sensory nerve stimulation in the cat. Proc Finn Dent Soc 1992;88:491-7.
175. Vongsavan N, Mathews B. The permeability of cat dentine in vitro and in vivo. Arch O Biol 1991;36:641-6.
176. Wallace JA, Vergona K. Epithelial rests' function in replantation: is splinting necessary in replantation? Oral Surg Oral Med Oral Pathol 1990;70:644-9.
177. Wedenberg C, Lindskog S. Evidence for a resorption inhibitor in dentin, Scand J Dent Res 1987;95:205-11.
178. Wedenberg C, Lindskog S. Experimental internal resorption in monkey teeth. Endod Dent Traumatol 1985;1:221-7.
179. Wedenberg C, Zetterqvist L. Internal resorption in human teeth - a histological scanning electron microscopic, and enzime histochemical study. J Endod 1987;13:255-9.
180. Yates JA. Root fractures in permanent teeth: a clinical review. Int Endod J 1992;25:150-7.
181. Zachrisson & Jacobsen I. Long term prognosis of 66 permanent anterior teeth with root fracture. Scand J Dent Res 1975;83:345-54.
182. Zadik D, Chosack A, Eidelman E. The prognosis of traumatized permanent anterior teeth with fracture of the enamel and dentin. Oral Surg Oral Med Oral Patol 1979;47:173-5.
183. Zanetta-Barbosa D, Carvalho AC. Effect of brief storage in ATP solution on periodontal healing after replantation of teeth in rats. Endod Dent Traumatol 1990;6:193-9.
184. Zervas P, Lambrianidis T, Karabouta-Vulgaropoulou The effect of citric acid treatment on periodontal healing after replantation of permanent teeth. Int Endod J 1991;24:317-25.


#### PART 4. ROOT CANAL TREATMENT OF TEETH WITH TRAUMATIC INJURY


1. Andreasen FM. Biology of dental trauma: pulpal considerations. Proceedings of Second International Conference on Dental Trauma 1989, Stockholm.
2. Andreasen FM. Pulpal healing after luxation injuries and root fractures in the permanent dentition. (PhD Thesis). Copenhagen: Faculty of Health Sciences, Copenhagen University; 1995. 51 p.
3. Andreasen FM. Transient apical breakdown and its relation to color and sensibility changes after luxation injuries to teeth. Endod Dent Traumatol 1986;2:9-19.
4. Andreasen FM, Vestergaard Pedersen B. Prognosis of luxated permanent teeth - the development of pulp necrosis. Endod Dent Traumatol 1985;1:207-20.
5. Andreasen JO, Andreasen FM. Lesiones Traumáticas de los dientes. 3rd ed. Barcelona: Labor;1984.
6. Baggett FJ, Mackie IC, Worthington HV. An investigation into the measurement of the working length of immature incisor teeth requiring endodontic treatment in children. Brit Dent J 1996;181:96-8.
7. Bastos JV. Prognóstico pulpar após lesões traumáticas na dentição permanente: avaliação clínico-radiográfica. (Master's Thesis). Federal University of Minas Gerais, 1996;129p.
8. Barnett F. The role of endodontics in the treatment of luxated permanent teeth. Dent Traumatol 2002;18:47-56.
9. Bishop BG, Woollard GW. Modern endodontic therapy for na incompletely developed tooth. Gen Dent 2002;50:252-6.
10. Camp JH. Pulp therapy for primary and young permanent teeth. Dent Clin North Am 1984;28:651-68.
11. Cvek M. Calcium hydroxide in treatment of traumatized tooth. Eastman Institute – Stockholm: Scania Dental AB;1989.
12. Cvek M. Treatment of non-vital permanent incisors with calcium hydroxide. Odont Revy 1972;23:27-33.
13. Dylewski JJ, Mich AA. Apical closure of nonvital teeth. Oral Surg Oral Pathol Oral Med 1971;32:82-9.
14. Faraco-Jr IM, Holland R. Response of the pulp of dogs to capping with mineral trioxide aggregate or calcium hydroxide cement. Dent Traumatol 2001;17:163-6.
15. Hachmeister DR, Schindler WG, Walker WA 3rd,Thomas DD. The sealing ability and retention charachteristics of mineral trioxide aggregate in a model of apexification. J Endod 2002;28:386-90.
16. Heithersay GS. Stimulation of root formation in incompletely developed pulpless teeth. Oral Surg Oral Med Oral Pathol 1970;29:620-30.
17. Hermann BW. Detinobliteration der Wurzerlkanale nach der Behandlung mit Kalcium. Zahnartzl. Rudschau 1930;39:888. IN: Webber RT. Apexogenesis versus Apexification. Dent Clin North Am 1984;28:669-97.
18. Holland R, Souza W, Russo MC. Healing processafter root canal therapy in immature human teeth. Rev Fac Odont Araçatuba 1973;2:269-78.
19. Holland R, Souza W, Tagliavini RL, Milanezi LA. Healing Process of teeth with open apices: Histological study. Bull Tokio Dent Coll 1974;12:333-8.
20. Holland R, Nery MJ, Mello W, Souza V, Bernabé PF, Otoboni-Filho JA. Root canal treatment with calcium hydroxide. III-Effects of debris and pressure filling. Oral Surg Oral Med Oral Pathol 1979;47:185-8.
21. Holland R, Souza V, Nery MJ, Bernabe PF, Mello W, Otoboni Filho JA Apical hard- tissue depositionin adult teeth of monkeys with use calcium hydroxide. Aust Dent J 1980;25:189-92.
22. Jacobsen I. Criteria for diagnosis of pulp necrosis in traumatized permanent incisors. Scand J Dent Res 1980;88:306-12.

23. Kerekes K, Heide S, Jacobsen I. Follow-up examination of endodontic treatment in traumatized juvenile incisors. J Endod 1980;6:744-8.
24. Maroto M, Barberia E, Planells P, Vera V. Treatment of a non-vital immature incisor with mineral trioxide aggregate (MTA). Dent Traumatol 2003;19:165-9.
25. Schilder H. Vertical compaction of warm gutta-percha. IN: Gerstein H. Techniques in Clinical Endodontics. Filling root canals in three dimensions. Dent Clin North Am 1983;11:723-44.
26. Sheehy EC, Roberts GJ. Use of calcium hydroxide for apical barrier formation and healing in nonvital immature permanent teeth: a review. Br Dent J 1997;183:241-6.
27. Skieller V. The prognosis for young teeth loosened after mechanical injuries. Acta Odont Scand 1960;18:171-81.
28. Scmitt D, Lee J, Bogen G. Multifaceted use of ProRoot MTA root canal repair material. Pediatr Dent 2001;23:326-30.
29. Steiner JC, Van Hassel HJ. Experimental root apexification in primates. Oral Surg Oral Med Oral Pathol 1971;31:409-15.
30. Steinig TH, Regan JD, Gutman JL. The use and predictable placement of Mineral Trioxide Aggregate in one-visit apexification cases. Aust Dent J 2003;29:34-42.
31. Tagger M, Tamse A, Katz A, Korzen BH. Evaluation of the apical seal produced by a hybrid root canal filling method, combining lateral condensation and thermatic compaction. J Endod 1984;10:200-303.
32. Thater M, Marechaux SC. Induced root apexification traumatic injuries of the pulp in children: follow-up study. ASDC J Dent Child 1988;55: 190-5.
33. Torabinejad M, Chivian N. Clinical applications of mineral trioxide aggregate J Endod 1999;25:197-205.
34. Torneck CD, Smith JS, Grindall P. Biological effects of endodontic procedures on developing incisor teeth. Part IV. Effect of debridement procedures and calcium hydroxide-CMCP paste in the treatment of experimentally induced pulp and periapical pathosis. Oral Surg Oral Med Oral Pathol 1973;35:541-4.
35. Tziafas D, Pantelidou O, alvanou A, Belibazakis G, Papadimitriou S. The dentinogenic effect of mineral trioxide aggregate (MTA) in short-term capping experiments. Int Endod J 2002;35:245-54.
36. Yang SF, Yang ZP, Chang KW. Continuing root formation following apexification treatment. Endod Dent Traumatol. 1990;6:232-5.
37. Webber RT. Apexogenesis versus Apexification. Dent Clin North Am 1984;28:669-97.
38. Whitherspoon DE, Ham K. One-visit apexification: technique for inducing root-end barrier formationin apical closures. Pract Proced Aesthet Dent 2001;13:455-60
39. Whittle M. Apexification of an infected untreated immature tooth. J Endod 26:245-7.

# Endodontic Surgery

**P. F. E. Bernabé**

*São Paulo State University, Araçatuba, SP, Brazil*

**R. Holland**

*São Paulo State University, Araçatuba, SP, Brazil*

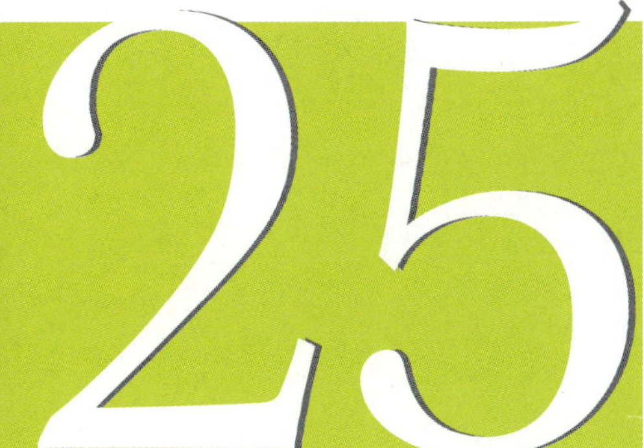

Chapter contents

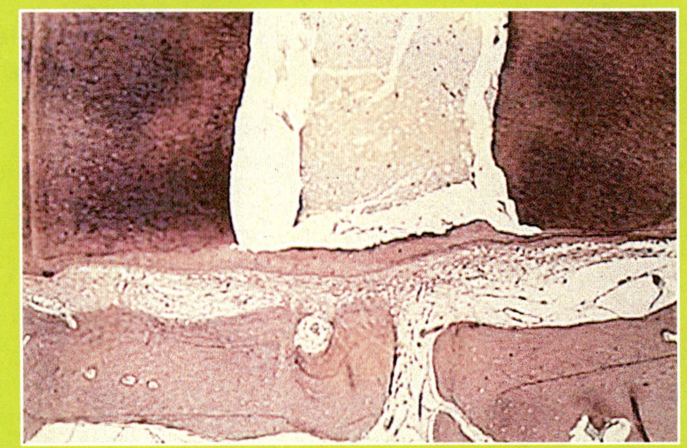

Biological sealing after retrofilling with MTA (H.E. X40).

## 25.1 Introduction

The objective of endodontic treatment is to eliminate microorganisms from the root canal system and to fill the intracanal space with proper materials to prevent new bacterial colonization. The aim of establishing adequate endodontic sealing is to prevent microorganisms and/or endotoxins from reaching the apical and periapical tissues, which is one of the main factors determining the success of this therapy.

The development of materials with excellent physical and biological properties, associated with well performed techniques, have also been essential contributory factors to obtaining high success rates, and significantly reducing the indication of complementary surgical procedures.

Nevertheless, teeth with individual or extensive prosthetic restorations containing intraradicular posts, create situations that cause concern and frequently lead to contraindicating conventional endodontic treatment. Conventional endodontic re-treatment has been successful without requiring surgical therapy. All the possible routine endodontic resources should be explored before resorting to invasive procedures, such as surgery. Several factors inherent to endodontic procedures, such as perforations, instrument breakage, calcifications and anatomic anomalies can lead to treatment failure, and in some cases, conventional endodontic treatment is not sufficient to solve the problem, and surgical endodontic intervention is required. It essential to consider that endodontic surgery is a conservative modality for retaining the tooth in the mouth. Therefore, the risks or benefits of indicating endodontic surgery or implants must be carefully considered, taking into account the patient's oral health and not the tooth or the present circumstances.

In spite all these efforts, there will always be situations in which conventional endodontic treatment becomes impracticable for achieving its objectives. Root canals needing emptying, and complete root fillings can be inaccessible through coronal access, because of several factors of a local, general, or even iatrogenic nature. Under these conditions, the best way to solve the problem is to indicate endodontic surgery.

## 25.2 Surgical Modalities

### Periapical curettage

Among the surgical modalities, periapical curettage is a surgical procedure with the purpose of removing pathological tissue from the alveolar bone, apical or lateral region of teeth with necrosis; as well as removing foreign bodies, whether their etiology is iatrogenic or not, and from teeth with or without periapical lesions; teeth have undergone endodontic treatment, either in cases of pulpitis or necrosis, but that remain symptomatic, even after all the conventional endodontic treatment resources and systemic medications have been exhausted.

Indeed, the lack of histopathologic studies about the factors that can influence tissue repair after periapical curettage, has led to many surgeons failing when using surgical approaches. Thus, even after adequate endodontic treatment, and careful curettage of the periapical lesion, they are frustrated by the relapse of the periapical lesion. Although this is not rare, many insist on repeating the surgery, often adopting the same therapeutic conduct as before (only periapical curettage), in spite of the doubtful and uncertain prognosis.

In an experimental study in dog teeth, periapical curettage was performed in teeth with or without periapical lesion[332-333]. The specimens that had periapical lesions presented worse results than those specimens that had interventions performed in teeth with vital pulp, in other words, without periapical lesions. This result was very significant and of great clinical importance, since the group in which the periapical curettage of the periapical lesions of non-vital teeth was performed without apicoectomy, in spite of completely removing the lesions, there was a recurrence of lesions, concentrating a chronic inflammatory infiltrate, mainly attached to the canal foramens of the apical delta (Fig. 25.1). Why? To answer this question and the previous one, it is necessary to consider that in practice, it is common to observe that some periapical lesions persist after the root canal treatment, which are called refractory lesions[458]. In these situations the bacteria are located deep in the ramifications of the main canal and are mainly anaerobic bacteria, which can survive outside the canal, on the surface of the apex of the tooth, in close contact with the periapical lesion[25,229,459,461,462]. In cases such as these, despite performing careful and thorough periapical curettage, failure to remove the apical portion of the root, which has contaminated ramifications, deltas and cementum craters that favor the relapse of the periapical lesion, this practically becomes an irreversible condition (Fig. 25.2). In these situations it is important to perform not only periradicular curettage, but also apicoectomy. With these procedures, not only the periapical lesion, but also the apical portion with its undesirable content, are eliminated. This was demonstrated in the studies conducted by Otoboni-Filho[332-333], in which they compared teeth, with and without periapical surgery.

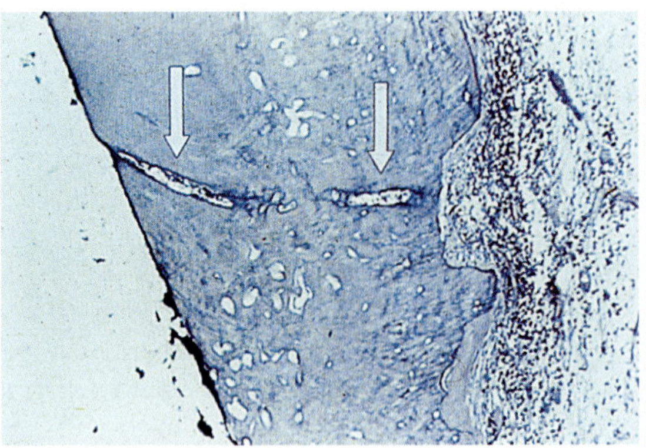

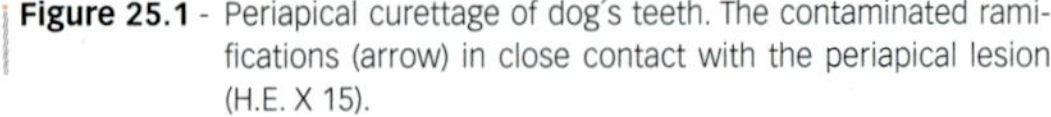

**Figure 25.1** - Periapical curettage of dog's teeth. The contaminated ramifications (arrow) in close contact with the periapical lesion (H.E. X 15).

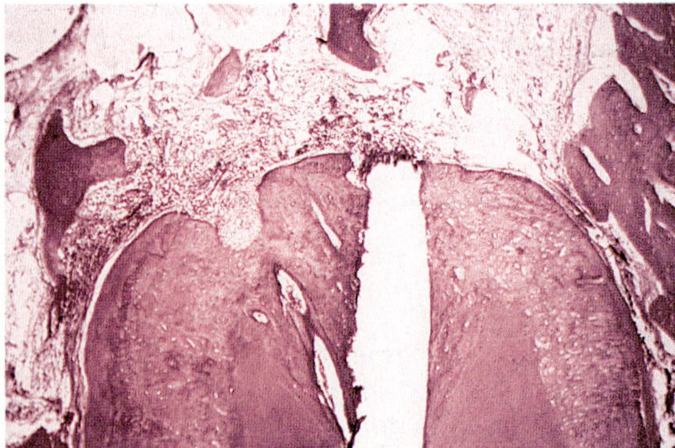

**Figure 25.2** - Periapical curettage of dog's teeth. Refractory lesions in close contact with deltas and cementum craters (H.E. X 15).

When filling the root canals of vital teeth, the filling material can be overextended into the interior of the periodontal ligament, resulting in intense postoperative painful symptomatology, particularly when these materials are zinc oxide and eugenol-based. This same symptom can also be found after endodontic intervention in vital teeth, when there is onset of symptomatic apical periodontitis resulting from various etiologies. In both situations this symptomatology can not be controlled with systemic medication and would urgently need complementary endodontic surgery, after all conservative therapeutic resources have been exhausted. Once surgical treatment has been instituted in such a situation, even if there is no periapical lesion, the professional should proceed as previously mentioned: perform not only curettage of the foreign material, or clean the periapical region in the case of the periodontitis, but also perform root resection or apicoectomy. In these situations the teeth have apical deltas with vital content, which would not explain the reason for the apicoectomy. However, because of the surgical procedures performed at the site, loss of vitality of the tissues contained inside these apical deltas could occur, favoring the onset of a periapical lesion in the future. Therefore apicoectomy, a truly preventive procedure, will prevent the need for further surgical intervention in the future, unless other factors, which will be studied in sequence, also disturb the repair process.

As can be seen, periradicular curettage is an essential, and exceptional technical procedure, performed in conjunction with all the other periradicular modalities, irrespective of whether or not the teeth have periapical lesions. Curettage should never be performed separately, even if the radiograph shows that the root canals are well filled.

The clinical procedures for performing this surgery are simple. Basically,starting with preparation of the patient and other related activities, surgical access to the periapical region through to the conclusion of the periapical curettage itself, the surgical steps are the same, irrespective of the type of surgery performed.

Thus, after antiseptic care, anesthesia, incision and dissection of the mucoperiosteal flap, the buccal plate of the bone may or may not intact. When the buccal bone tissue is compact, with no dehiscence, it is necessary to adopt clinical procedures that make it practical and safe to locate it, without requiring excessive removal of this tissue. One of the classical methods for this type of approach is to perform a small and superficial bone cavity, based on previous determination of the working length, position of radiopaque material (small portion of gutta percha) on the bone depression and radiographic image of the region. On the radiograph, the location of the radiopaque image of the gutta-percha, in relation to the image of the root apex will guide the professional during ostectomy and exposure of the root apex. This procedure is of primordial importance, because the entire apical portion of the root should be exposed, making it easier to see and perform curettage of the related structures.

Ostectomy to expose the root apex can be performed by different methods. The use of manual chisels is safe, particularly when the buccal bone cortical is intact. In these cases, the use of manual chisels instead of burs is important, because it prevents the unnecessary wear of burs on the dental surface, such as the removal of cementum tissue and dentin exposure, which favor dentinal resorption, as will be discussed later.

In cases in which there is no periapical lesion, once the buccal bone cortical has been removed, part of the cancellous bone tissue can be removed to expose the entire root apex using surgical or periodontal curettes of different sizes and gauges. During these procedures, it is necessary to avoid excessive or crude curettage so as not to damage the dental structures and neighboring structures, such as the nervous plexus, maxillary sinus, nasal mucosa etc.

When curetting foreign material from the apex, particularly overfilled material, frequent irrigation and aspiration should be done to help remove the debris.

The aim of periapical curettage, as a complementary surgical procedure performed in conjunction with other periradicular procedures is to remove the periapical lesion completely, enabling not only the root apex to be exposed, but also contributing to enhancing hemostasis of the operative field. Furthermore, it is essential not to discard the periapical lesions that are removed; they should be stored in solutions suitable for tissue conservation and sent for histopathologic exam, to enable definitive diagnosis of the lesion.

When the periapical curettage has been concluded, the bone cavity must be carefully cleaned by frequent irrigation with saline solution and aspiration, to prepare for the operative procedures that follow. When all the planned procedures have been concluded, the bone cavity must be filled with blood coagulum, and then the flap must be sutured with interrupted stitches, using silk 4-0, 5-0, vicryl 910 4-0 or nylon 5-0 threads.

Remember to give the patient basic advice, such getting sufficient rest, taking care with diet, applying compresses, performing oral hygiene, and using the prescribed medications correctly.

**Apicoectomy**

Classically, apicoectomy has been indicated for several clinical situations, such as: cases of root dilacerations that impede adequate conventional treatment; when there is rectification and/or perforation of the root in the apical third; the presence of non-filled apical ramifications; fractured endodontic instruments; root fractures that involve the apical third whether or not accompanied by periapical lesion and presence of apical external root resorptions, in which the problem could not be solved by treatments through the root canal.

Aware of these factors, several authors recommend the surgical procedure of root resection or apicoectomy [288,292,434], not only to make it easier to locate the root canal, but also to eliminate the apical deltas, not always visible on the radiograph, and susceptible to being contaminated, or retaining necrotic material[16,113, 288,292,434]. Many authors have shown that these ramifications of the main are an important cause of failures after endodontic treatment[210,211].

They harbor bacteria which, if not destroyed by the endodontic therapeutic procedures, are capable of maintaining the presence of lesions[30,424,461]. This subject has been extensively investigated at present, and cause great concern due to the possibility that modern endodontic therapies have not been successful against these bacteria located in the depth of the root canal system. Therefore, the data with regard to the percentage of success after the treatment of necrotic teeth with periapical lesion is alarming. Holland et al.[199] and Souza et al.[413] admit that the persistence of contamination, because of bacteria present in these ramifications and apical craters, is one of the most severe factors responsible for the high percentage of failure after the root canal treatment of teeth with periapical lesions. Hess & Keller[174] demonstrated that on an average, these ramifications are present in 42% of human permanent teeth. It can therefore be concluded that in teeth with periapical lesions, these ramifications are generally replete with necrotic and contaminated tissue, capable of negatively influencing repair (Fig. 25.1-25.2).

Reporting the histopathologic results obtained by Otoboni-Filho[333], the best were noted in the group in which the teeth were submitted only to apicoectomy, or by conventional retrograde filling performed after apicoectomy, when compared with the specimens that underwent only curettage of the periapical lesion. In teeth subjected to apicoectomy, the contaminated apical deltas were surgically removed, thus eliminating the contaminating factor. In these situations, it seems clear that the surgical techniques that involve a larger amount of dental tissue (apicoectomy), produce more favorable results (Fig. 25.3) than those that are less wasteful (periapical curettage).

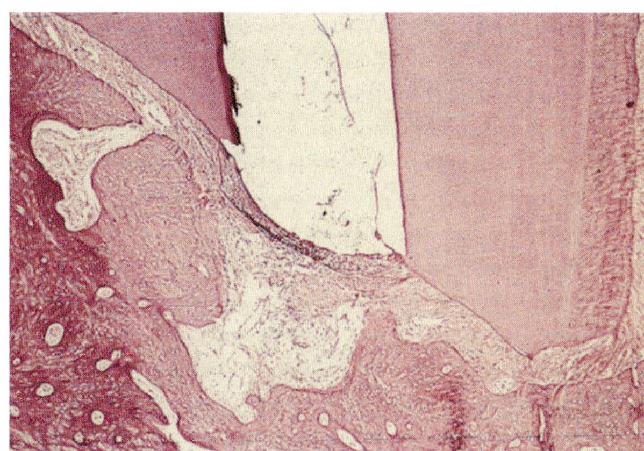

**Figure 25.3** - Apicoectomy of teeth with periapical lesion. Surgical remotion of the contaminated apical deltas producing more favorable results.



Considering that generally the teeth referred for endodontic surgery are cases of previous endodontic treatment failures; and that this is related to several other factors, particularly the presence of contaminated apical ramifications of the main root canal, therefore, in the presence of teeth with periapical lesions, it is recommended to always perform apicoectomy and not only flattening or rounding off of the root apex (apical plasty), a detail that will be touched on further ahead.

After carefully curetting the periapical lesion and amply exposing the apical portion of the root, apicoectomy is performed with a Zekrya #151 bur (Dentsply/Maillefer).

A widely discussed question is whether or not to bevel the apicoectomized root surface. This allows the entire root surface to be exposed, facilitating operative procedures. Today, the tendency is to avoid beveling this surface. It is preferable to perform this cut perpendicular to the long axis of the root, varying only when anatomic situations do not allow adequate visualization and prevent the instituted operative technique from being developed. Gilheany et al[150]. in a study in vitro, sectioned the root with 0° (horizontal cut), 30° or 45° (inclined cuts). The authors observed that the increase in root beveling contributed significantly to the increase in the rates of marginal leakage, including the exposed dentinal surface. In their opinion, the resection performed at angles of 30° or 45°, exposed many more dentinal tubules than the horizontal or 0° cut. Another interesting observation the authors made is that the more the apicoectomized surface is beveled, the deeper the retrofilling should be.

In view of these observations, it can be deduced that beveling can be performed, provided that the type of retrofilling technique that will be used is considered. The technique of conventional retrograde filling performed with burs, or even with ultrasound, does not penetrate deeply. With ultrasound, because of the design of the tips for retrograde preparation, the maximum depth achieved is around 3mm; with burs, Bernabé et al.[50], in 1990, in a un-published work, verified that the average depth of the apical cavities did not pass 1.39 mm. In both situations, beveling of the apicoectomized surfaces should be avoided, because there is a risk of contaminating the periodontal tissues through dentinal tubules. Particularly in root-end cavities prepared with burs, and in the presence of beveling of the dentinal surface, the unsealed dentinal tubules under the retrofilling establish communication between the interior of the root canals, probably contaminated, and the periapical tissues. Under clinical conditions, irrespective of the type of retrofilling material used, this favors a higher probability of relapse of the periapical lesion occurring.

When retrofilling technique is the retrograde endodontic treatment, however, beveling can be performed without severe restrictions. In these cases, retrograde root canal preparation and retrofilling are performed deeper, allowing better cleaning and more extensive filling, preventing the occurrence of contamination through this pathway, consequently not allowing relapse of the lesion.

Another question related to apicoectomy is the possibility that this probable permeability, maintained through the dentinal tubules, is influenced by the presence of a smear layer over the apicoectomized surface. Some admit that the presence of a smear layer can reduce this permeability, and that with its removal, there would be an increase in marginal leakage [441]. This was contested by Peters & Harrison[345], admitting that the use of citric acid on the dentinal surface exposed by surgery, did not affect the level of marginal leakage. On the other hand, Craig & Harrison[98], after a short post-operative period, observed that the removal of the smear layer favored the premature deposition and quantitative increase in cementum on the exposed dentinal surface.

To try to clarify this question, Bernabé et al.[47] conducted an experimental study in dog teeth, in which the root canals were submitted to retrograde endodontic treatment, when they were retro-instrumented and retrofilled with consistent zinc oxide and eugenol sealer, 1mm beneath the cut surface, according to the recommendations of Bernabé[38], in 1994. Later, in two thirds of the studied samples, they applied citric acid (1/3) or trisodium EDTA (1/3) on the dentinal surface exposed during root resection. The authors observed that the process of dental-alveolar repair, beyond the experimental period of 180 days, was not disturbed, irrespective of whether the smear layer was removed or not, either using EDTA, or citric acid (Fig. 25.4). Contrary to these observations, Bernabé et al.[47] believe that the use of this procedure should be better evaluated. Considering these first good results, however, if the option is to remove the smear layer, Bernabé et al.[45] recommended the application of trisodium EDTA for 3 minutes. This application should be limited to the exposed dentinal surface only, avoiding the periodontal and bone tissues, and performed with the assistance of an autoclaved microbrush, or brush for primer, used in operative dentistry. Next, irrigate abundantly with saline solution assisted by aspiration, for removing the medication residues. This procedure is not particularly professed to be routine, and is done only in cases of surgical retreatment, when the presence of contamination of the previously apicoectomized root surface should be considered. With this procedure, it is possible that the exposure of the dentinal tubules would favor the action of calcium hydroxide placed on this surface and retrofilling material, as professed by Bernabé & Holland[52].

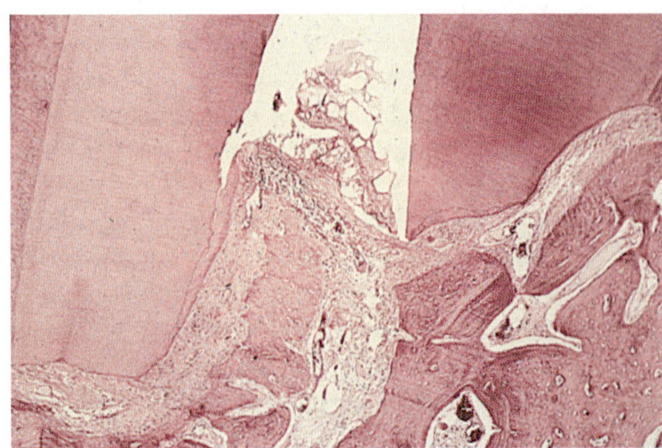

**Figure 25.4** - Retrograde endodontic treatment. Retro-instrumented and retrofilled with consistent zinc oxide and eugenol sealer, 1mm beneath the cut surface. Process of dental-alveolar repair using EDTA to remove the smear layer (H.E. X 40).

Further to resection of the root apex performed with a Zekrya bur # 151 (Dentsply-Maillefer), the following should be considered: these steel burs, driven by high speed handpieces, are chosen because of their cutting efficacy, adequate length and the experience acquired with their use since the release of this bur. Moreover, the studies of Cruz Gonzalez[44] (Guadalajara – Mexico), after sectioning the root portion with this type of bur, observed by scanning electronic microscopy that the dentinal surface was smooth and regular. On the other hand, when diamond or pierced steel burs were used, the same surface presented many grooves or ruts throughout its extent. During this procedure, it is important to concomitantly perform abundant irrigation with saline solution, using a Luer syringe. At the same time, special care should be taken to avoid accidents such as perforation of the maxillary sinus, cutting the nervous plexus, and even inappropriate wear of neighboring dental structures.

Another advantage with regard to apicoectomy is that it facilitates access to the areas of the root portion that usually present difficulties when curetting the periapical lesion, by improving the field of vision and other surgical procedures.

It is important to remember that the apicoectomy and periapical curettage techniques, when indicated separately, should be performed only on teeth that present adequately performed hermetic root canal filling, without failures, and details not always visible on the radiograph. When in doubt, the root canal should be retreated, because the success of this procedure, in addition to other important factors, is dependent on the efficient marginal sealing produced by the filling material.

Another fundamentally important factor related to resection of the apical portion of the root is the possibility of performing an incomplete or irregular apicoectomy. In cases of surgical retreatment, one frequently observes root apexes that underwent badly performed apicoectomies with accentuated bevel, leading to excessive wear of the buccal//oral surface of the root, in comparison with the lingual wall. When this apicoectomy does not attain or involve all the apical areas that may possibly contain ramifications, this could occur because of difficulties during the operation, often determined by the lack of access, anatomic complexity and even the operator's incompetence. As already pointed out, the apical portion of human teeth can have ramifications or apical deltas[174] which, when contaminated, can disturb the repair process and be related to the persistence of periapical lesions. Almeida et al.[10] analyzing histomorphological aspects of apexes of teeth that presented refractory lesions to endodontic treatment, verified that 70% were related to the presence of apical ramifications of the root canal. As mentioned previously, complete removal of the apical portion becomes necessary during surgery. In human beings, this apicoectomy should be 3 mm below the apex, which then frees the periapical environment of the presence of these ramifications. According to Kim et al.[237] root resections performed 1 mm below the root apex reduce 52% of the ramifications and 40% of the lateral canals. Below 2 mm there is a reduction of 78% and 86%, respectively, of these events. When apicoectomy is performed 3 mm below the root apex, there is evidence of a reduction of 93% of the lateral canals, and 98% of the apical ramifications are eliminated. A curious datum shown by the authors was that if the resections are larger (4mm) there is no significant reduction in the incidence of the related data.

Bernabé et al.[48] observed that in some specimens of dog teeth with apical lesions subjected to periapical surgery, root resorption occurred and there was presence of inflammatory infiltrate in the periapical tissues. This unfavorable repair scenario was related to the presence of contaminated apical deltas that were not completely removed during apicoectomy, in addition to the presence of contaminated cementum in contact with the periapical tissues. Note that these occurrences are not detected in the clinical and radiographic exams, making it complicated to establish the causes of failure, particularly if the clinician does not know about these problems. This leads to incorrect procedures being performed, which fail to eliminate the factors that interfere negatively in the repair of the dental alveolar of these teeth and result in the failure of the surgical treatment, or retreatment instituted.

Contaminated apical deltas remaining in the dental apex and disturbing the dental-alveolar repair, indicate the possible influence of the operator's work on the result of the treatment. An identical problem was detected in other studies developed by Bernabé et al.[55,57] in which these contaminated deltas were found, and showed evidence of their significant influenced on the final results of the experiment. This is closely related to insufficient apicoectomy being performed, and failing to remove the deltas completely. Characteristically, they are visible mainly on the lingual portion of the root, probably because of the more accentuated cutting slope. This could explain the presence of Gram-negative bacteria, not only in the apical deltas, but also in the dentinal tubules. Because of deficient apicoectomies, these ramifications can continue to be present without contamination, allowing better repair.

Many of the failures reported in the literature with regard to teeth with periapical lesions subjected to endodontic surgery, are probably also related to the presence of greater contamination that could be present in the apical deltas and ramifications of the apical third of the main root canal, which was not removed, as already discussed. These details serve to alert professionals to take care to perform apicoectomy correctly and ensure complete removal of root portions that can contain apical deltas. A reminder, once again, that when the periapical tissues are exposed to contaminated cementum, which is unfortunately not detected in the clinical and radiographic exams, this can have a negative influence on the success rates, differently from what we studied and reported.

The need for remodeling or trimming the remaining edges of the dentinal surface after an apicoectomy has frequently been discussed. With this procedure, abrasive wear performed with manual or diamond files (System Eva, Kavo) or even burs, would be recommended to reduce or eliminate the dentinal resorption that could occur because of the presence of these edges, all around the circumference of the root. This wear was disseminated among professionals, particularly in Brazil, due to the results of the histological studies conducted by Bernabé[37] in 1981, and his comments about it. At that time, the author reported the hypothesis that faced with the presence of these edges, the body promotes resorptions of these areas to remodel and leave a rounded root, with the approximate anatomy of the root prior to apicoectomy. With more recent scientific knowledge about these resorptions, the same author today understands that this procedure is unnecessary, and has no scientific support. Indeed, wearing the edges or apical plasty will expose a larger area of dentin, accentuating the resorption process even more. Nowadays it is known that these dentinal resorptions would be related to the phenomena, characteristic of auto-immunity and not to the presence of edges, or apical anatomical deformation. There are probably several molecules among the dentinal proteins that can be considered true abducted antigens[94,97,176,367,467] and when they are exposed, a resorption process begins. Considering these concepts, it is understood that there is no sense in exposing a new amount of dentin on the periapical tissues in addition to that which has already occurred during apicoectomy. The wear, performed during apical plasty, beveling all the external edge of the apicoectomized surface, would remove larger portions of cementum that protect the dentin from contact with the periodontium, thus aggravating dentinal apical resorption. Depending on the intensity which which this phenomenon occurs, there can be a larger lateral exposure of the retrofilling material, consequently breaking the efficacy of the intended marginal sealing, in addition to the possibility of exposing the contaminated dentinal tubules, maintaining a source of irritants at the site. When these phenomena occur, particularly simultanously, it can lead to treatment failure. The inflammatory phenomena that have been established, in addition the the infection present in these cases, create local conditions for maintaining the resorptions that are often not detected by the professionals in clinical and radiographic exams, and pass unnoticed or ignored.

Up to now the clinical posture of not wearing these edges during apical plasty, is due to scientific support obtained as a result of more critical evaluations made in several specimens and processed through the years in different studies, conducted by Bernabé et al.[39,43,47,48,59], in addition to the the new knowledge, as already pointed out, as regards the possible causes of these resorptions. It is noted that the edges that remained after the apicoectomy are found intact, with no evidence of resorption, even after the post-operative period of 180 days, by which time the repair has practically been defined. We are aware, however, that further studies on the subject should be conducted, to compare these variables by optic microscopy, which would definitively clear the remaining doubts.

Apicoectomy, as an isolated periapical procedure, can be indicated in some special situations. In cases of persistent exudate, or frequent acute situations, when conventional root canal filling becomes problematic. Therefore, after root canal preparation, filling can be performed during surgery, and the apicoectomy performed before or after the root canal is filled. Provided that it is possible, the professional can also perform the root canal filling in a session before the surgery, thus reducing the surgical time. In these cases, the root apex would be surgically exposed and the apicoectomy performed in the following session.

In this type of surgical treatment, in which the apicoectomy is being performed without having done retrograde filling, it is fundamental to have coronal access, and to fill the root canals adequately and flawlessly. One should be warned, that if the root canals were filled by another professional, and there are doubts about the efficacy of this filling, it is essential for the root canals be refilled. Considering that flaws could occur after root canal fillings, and that they are not always detected by the radiographic exams; even considering that these fillings were performed without incidents, particularly if conventional retrograde filling was indicated and performed after the apicoectomy, thus complementing the instituted treatment safely and effectively. Nevertheless, in some situations, this retrograde filling is not performed, particularly when the professional trusts the good quality of the existent filling, and therefore indicates the apicoectomy only. In this case, using the apicoectomized dentinal surface as reference, remove about 1mm of filling via the apex, using the # 5 condenser of the Bernabe Kit (Fig. 25.5), specially designed for micro-surgery. This condenser has a 1 mm mark at the end, and after being slightly heated, is introduced in a retrograde manner to remove part of the root canal filling (1 mm). Another procedure would be to perform the retrograde discharge with ultrasonic inserts initially (Fig. 25.6), then conclude finishing with the Bernabe Kit condenser. This limit is recommended, because Bernabe[38] demonstrated by histopathologic exams that the prognosis of repair is more favorable when the retrofillings are performed 1 mm below the sectioned dentinal surface (Fig. 25.7-25.8). It is pointed out that apart from the clinical situation described above, this type of procedure can only be used when the retrofillings are very deep, as in the case of retrograde endodontic treatment (Fig. 25.9). Otherwise, as occurs in conventional retrograde fillings in which the depth is limited, removal of 1 mm of this retrofilling decreases its extent inside the root canal, compromising the apical marginal sealing in the space of 1 mm, which was recommended by Bernabé & Holland[52], as well as over the apicoectomized surface Later, the bone cavity must be filled with coagulated blood, the mucoperiosteal flap repositioned, and sutured. In accordance with our protocol, the suture is removed seven days after the operation. Performed the apicoectomy, as the other surgical procedures, and after the cleaning of the bone cavity, follows the collocation of a calcium hydroxide cap (Fig. 25.10).

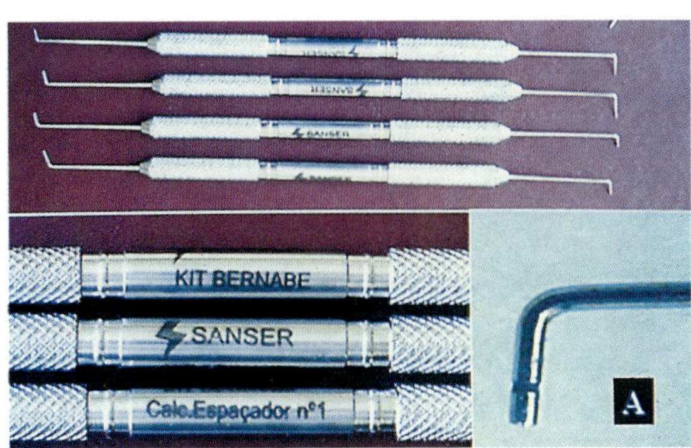


Figure 25.5 - Bernabe Kit.

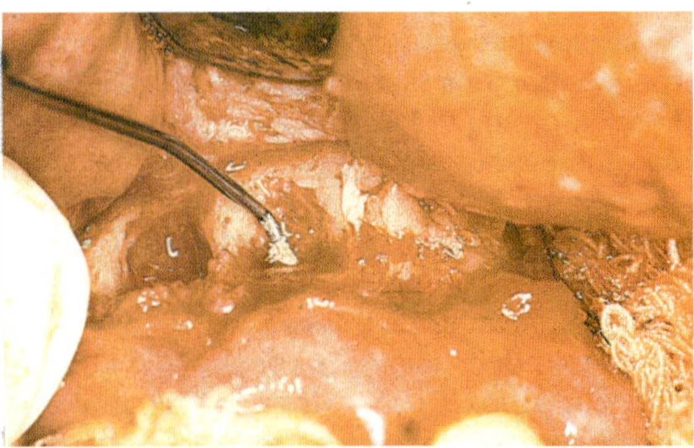

Figure 25.6 - The retrograde discharge with ultrasonic inserts.

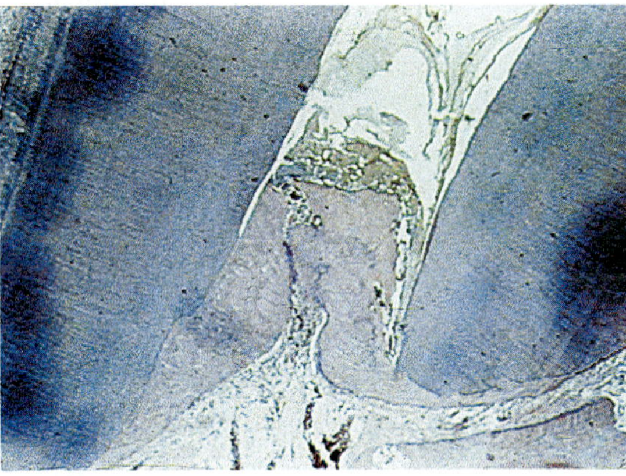

Figure 25.7 - Retrofillings performed 1 mm below the sectioned dentinal surface with consistent zinc oxide and eugenol sealer. Partial biologic sealing.

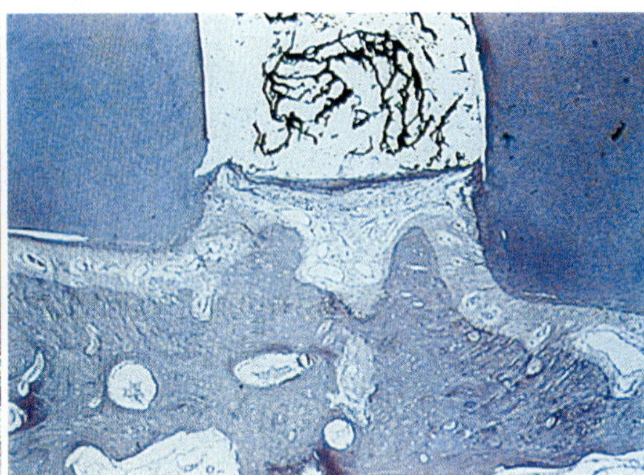

Figure 25.8 - Retrofillings performed 1 mm below the sectioned dentinal surface with gutta-percha. Absence of inflammatory process.

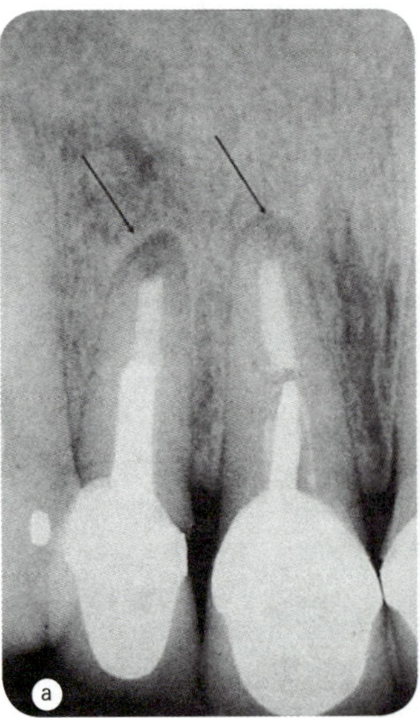


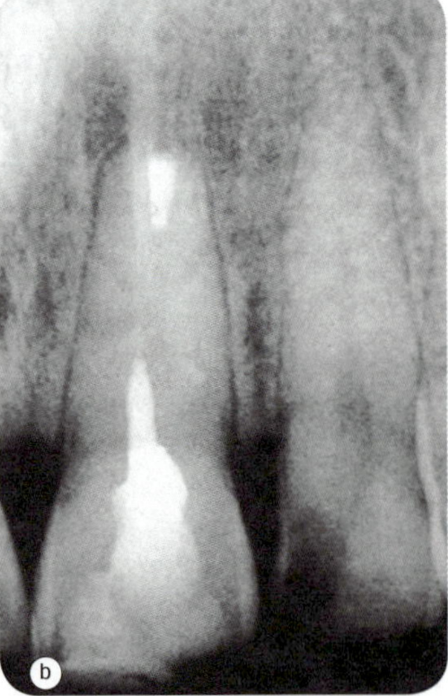


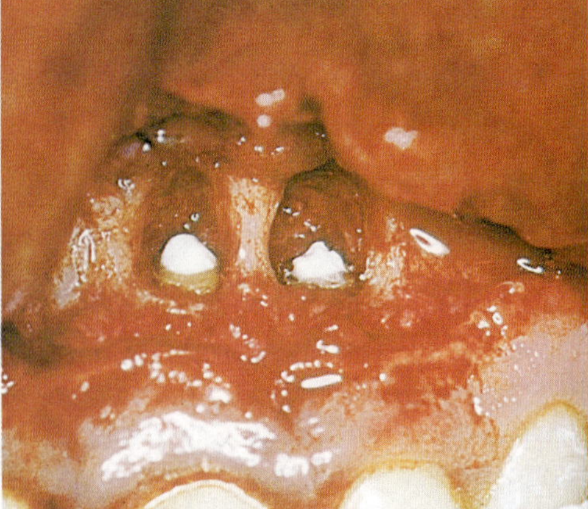

Figure 25.9 - (**A-B**) Apical marginal sealing in the retrofillings performed 1 mm below the apicoectomized surface.

Figure 25.10 - Calcium hydroxide "cap".

## 25.3 Conventional Retrograde Filling

When none of the conventional endodontic procedures allow hermetic sealing, despite the presence of the root canal filling, it is imperative to perform retrograde sealing, or filling. This procedure is therefore considered as an extreme resource, so it should be applied only when conventional treatment fails.

Retrograde fillings are indicated in cases where canals are not accessible via the coronal approach, due to the presence of a metal core, instrument fragment, calcifications, filling material, malformations, internal resorption or defective instrumentation, factors that impede access to the root canal and compromise the result of simpler endodontic surgeries, such as periapical curettage or apicoectomy.

According to Nichols[317], retrograde fillings can be classified either as conventional or modified. Of these, conventional retrograde filling is preferable; this includes a Class 1 preparation in an apical segment of the canal and filling it with adequate material in a restricted space.

Holland et al.[204] conducted an *in vitro* study to verify the efficacy of marginal sealing produced by the two techniques. They verified that in the conventional retrograde filling technique, the level of marginal leakage was much lower, when compared with modified retrograde filling techniques, in which the retrofilling material is placed perpendicularly to the root canal, after the buccal surface of the root is perforated with a bur, until the root canal is reached. After this, the filling material is condensed horizontally until it fills the entire perforation. Only after these procedures the apicoectomy is performed. The more extensive leakage with this modified technique probably results from the worse conditions it produces for retrofilling material condensation, in addition to displacement of the material during root resection.

### Preparation of retrocavities

#### Retrocavities prepared with burs and ultrasound

Retrocavities have been prepared with conventional burs driven by high or low speed handpieces, or by ultrasonic tips or inserts. In this context it should be noted that one of the fundamental factors is related to the depth of the apical cavities. Indeed, with the use of burs, they are relatively shallow, not exceeding 2mm deep[15,16,26,34,60]. Bernabé et al.[50] conducted an in vitro study preparing retrocavities with burs on a mannequin, specially designed to simulate all the difficulties found in the clinic during an operating procedure. They verified that under these conditions, the depth of the apical cavities did not exceed 1.39 mm, which is too shallow, considering that the marginal leakage means recorded with most retrofilling materials are much higher. This study demonstrated that if the retrofilling material is placed in a shallow cavity, it does not produce adequate marginal sealing, thereby facilitating bacteria and endotoxin penetration into the periapical tissues and impeding satisfactory repair. In the clinic, this depth rarely is extended, mainly for essentially technical reasons. The tips of conventional high and low speed equipment are bulky in comparison with the surgical cavities, and it is difficult to place the bur inside these bone cavities. That is why the cavities are always prepared at an angle to the long axis of the root canal, capable of being contoured with the use of a miniature handpiece. Nevertheless, considering the regions of easy access, it is difficult to prepare these cavities in the direction of the long axis, because the contra angle, although it is small, does not always fit into the bone cavity. This contra-angle, developed by Kavo specifically for use in endodontic surgery, is provided with an inverted tapered trunk, or spherical burs.

As already outlined, when burs are used to prepare apical cavities, they are not placed along the long axis of the root canal, and therefore produce inclined retrocavities, due to technical difficulties of access to the apical region. Because of access in the buccal to lingual direction, the inclination of the apical cavities also occurs in the direction towards the lingual wall of retrocavities. This can cause accidents, such as perforation, exposing the periodontal ligament, as demonstrated in studies conducted by Bernabé[48] in dog teeth, comparing retrocavities prepared with burs or ultrasonic tips. Even if this inclined preparation does not induce exposure of the periodontal ligament, the tissues can be damaged. When preparing retrocavities with burs, Bernabé[48] observed an extensive resorption of the cementum and the lingual wall of the retrocavity, almost forming a micro exposure, probably due to the heat generated by the bur, even when adequate cooling is used. In this case, repair probably takes place because a biocompatible material like MTA is used. These details lead one to deduce that the type of retrofilling material used is very important, because if it does not have good biological properties, repair can compromised and failure will be inevitable. It should be pointed out that occurrences of this type, detected at histopathologic level, are rarely recorded in a routine radiographic exam, even if there is an established inflammatory process, because these alterations are masked by the radiopaque retrofilling materials and dental structure. Moreover, in these situations, it is common to observe clinical silence. In addition, this visual observation, even with the assistance of a dental microscope, can also be compromised by the condensation of debris, very common in these cases and regions.

As was shown by Bernabé[37] in a histopathologic study, the use of burs should be avoided, using them only in special situations. During the course of surgery, technical problems such as, electrical or mechanic defects may occur with the use of ultrasound, preventing its use. Under these circumstances, the solution will be to prepare the retrocavities with burs, and the patient should be alerted about the prognosis of the treatment. Thus, the recommended high or low speed bur is the spherical #1 or the inverted tapered trunk #33½, remembering that the Kavo miniature handpiece could offer a better opportunity for preparing cavities that are less inclined in relation to the long axis of the root canal. To avoid excessive dentin wear with this type of procedure, we recommend that special care should be taken to prepare apical cavities with the same shape at that of the original root canal, thus preventing the occurrence of trepanations on the lingual surface of the cavity preparation. Bernabé et al.[43] showed that when retrocavity preparations with burs are made by looking through a dental microscope, there is less wear of the dentinal structure than when these cavities are prepared with the naked eye, without aid of the microscope. Furthermore, from this study it was clear that retrocavities prepared with ultrasound, irrespective of whether or not a dental microscope was used, resulted in less wear, prevented dentinal structure loss, and produced more centered apical preparations in relation to the long axis of the root canal, when compared with the use of burs (Fig. 25.11).

Further to the possible effects of the small depth and inclination of apical cavities, Gilheany et al.[150], considering the level of marginal leakage, established a possible correlation between the depth of the apical box prepared to receive a retrograde filling and the angle of root beveling. They concluded that the bigger the resection angle, the deeper the apical cavity should be. They also verified that by increasing the retrograde filling depth in relation to the axis of the root canal, the index of marginal leakage around the filling material was significantly decreased.

Nevertheless, as regards the problems that can occur with the conventional retrograde fillings, it is necessary to point out that in the presence of lateral canals that were not removed by apicoectomy, or not reached by the preparation of the apical box, communication can occur between the periodontal tissues and the necrotic residues present inside the unfilled root canals or those with deficient fillings. Thus bacteria or toxins can stimulate the development or maintenance of periapical lesions.

In a recent study of periapical tissues conducted in dog's teeth, Bernabé[38] compared retrocavities prepared with burs and ultrasound, and found the presence of debris in both experimental groups. In some of the specimens, it could be noted that these dentinal scrapings or debris were accompanied by an inflammatory process. It is probable that bacteria related to this debris inside the dentinal tubules, could proliferate and contaminate this debris and cause these reactions. What most surprised the author was that debris was also found in the groups in which ultrasound was used, despite the abundant irrigation used and the known cleaning action produced by the ultrasonic system.

According to Bernabé[39], this debris not only contributed to poor adaptation of the retrofillings, but also created a corridor that favored bacterial proliferation, thus affecting the periapical tissues and causing undesired inflammatory reactions. The presence of debris was considered one of the factors responsible for the failures, in spite of the use of several retrofilling materials considered to be biocompatible.

As far back as 1981, in their studies Bernabé[37] analyzed the use of a common optic microscope light, and described other factors occuring in vivo, capable of interfering in the repair process. One of these factors that had not yet been reported in the literature was the occurrence of post-operative external dentinal resorptions on the sectioned dentinal surface and lateral surface of the root. In some specimens, the author found that in spite of placing the retrofilling material (silver amalgam or gutta-percha) on the same plane as the dentin cut, after six months these materials were projected in the direction of the periapical tissues (Fig. 25.12). Although the hypothesis is that this phenomenon occurred due to the expansion of the material, it is believed that resorption occurring near the filling material caused it staying the material projected into the periodontal ligament. According to Bernabé, when this resorption occurred, particularly around or near these cavities, in addition to the shallowness of the material, it was possible that the intended marginal sealing was compromised even further by the retrofilling material. In this case, it would expose the periapical tissues to irritant agents contained inside the root canal, which would be responsible for the frequent failures after conventional retrograde fillings.

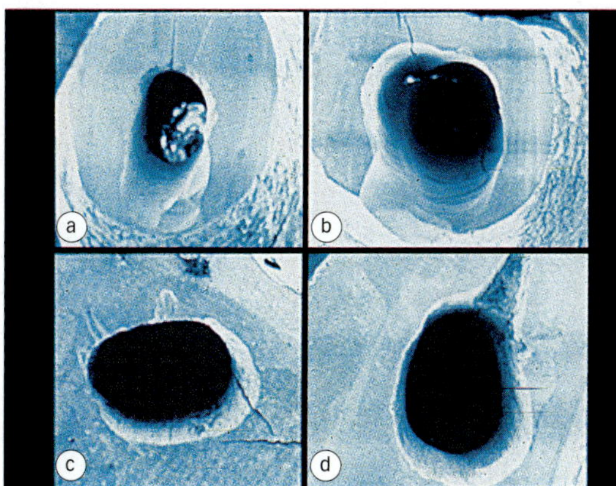


**Figure 25.11** - Retrocavity preparations with burs (**A** and **B**). Retrocavities prepared with ultrasound (**C** and **D**) prevent dentinal structure loss, and produce more centered apical preparations

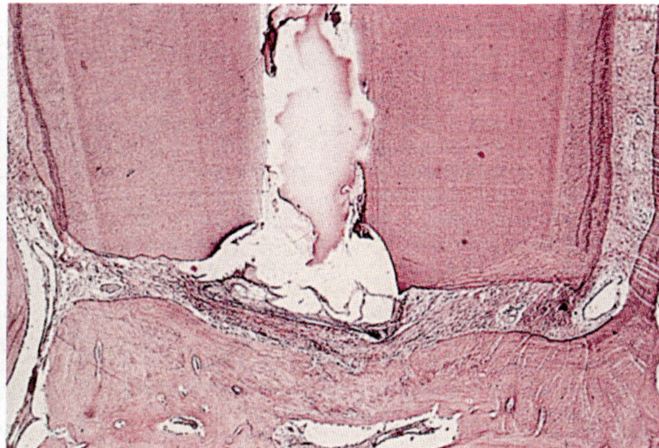

**Figure 25.12** - Projection of the retrofilling material in the direction of the periapical tissues.

These resorptions, were observed in different intensities in almost all experiments conducted by Bernabé et al.[37,38,43,48,53,57,59]. Nevertheless, as previously mentioned, one must not forget that resorption can also be related to phenomena characteristic of autoimmunity. Consolaro[94] admits that the continuation of resorption processes in root subjected to endodontic surgeries after some weeks or months, could indicate the presence of bacteria and their products in the operated area. We agree with the above-mentioned author, because endodontic surgeries are generally performed in infected teeth. Considering the degree or intensity in which resorption can occur and in the presence of shallow retrograde fillings, serious problems can occur after endodontic surgery, although many professionals disbelieve or disregard this.

Considering that these resorption are hardly detected in radiographic exams, particulary in view of the variations in angle used by the professional when taking radiographs, almost always without standardization. This makes it difficult to diagnose the causes of failures after endodontic surgery. It is very important to know that it happens, which process is involved and how to prevent it, or at least use procedures that decrease its incidence, such as, for example, the use of calcium hydroxide over the apicoectomized surface and retrofilling material, as recommended by Bernabé & Holland[52].

The presence of a narrow connection between two canals that contains vital or necrotic tissue, called the isthmus[237], is another factor that can interfere in the repair process, when not adequately identified and conveniently prepared. It is considered to be an integral part of the root canal system, and should be identified as such (Fig. 25.13), and it should be completely involved during the preparation of retrocavities, in other words, it should be cleaned, adequately prepared and finally filled (Fig. 25.14). It can be difficult to see by conventional methods, and frequently it requires the use of a dye, such as methylene blue or trepan blue, making it easier to identify and better define its anatomy. When there is contamination, as occurs in the majority of treated cases, and the presence of isthmus goes unnoticed, or the procedures to prepare it do not achieve the proposed goals, most probably the preparation will be compromised. In this particular situation, the dental microscope is an essential and extremely value tool that makes it easier to locate the isthmus and treat it afterwards, preventing unnecessary and dangerous wear. Since the isthmus is normally situated in an area of strangulation of the root, its preparation involves making a groove to join the two canals (Fig. 25.14). The ideal instrument for this purpose is the use of ultrasonic tips, because have smaller diameters than burs. If no dental microscope is available, the professional can use a magnifying glass head set to magnify the location to be treated, making the procedure more efficient than if it were performed relying on the naked eye.

When preparing the apical box to hold the retrofilling material, a careful clinical exam is necessary to detect the number of canals present in each root, as well as the shape of the root canal and whether it is conical or flattened. Any preparation that does not involve all the canals or all of its extensions, can irreversibly compromise the repair.

Several authors[116,136,157,165,411,422,483] have been concerned about the practice of using ultrasound during endodontic surgical procedures, and have developed in vitro studies, with the purpose of better establishing its advantages. Although several studies have been conducted to clear existent doubts about the subject, ultrasound has indeed been completely incorporated into endodontic surgical practice. When adopting the conventional retrograde filling technique, which involves the preparation of an apical box on the apicoectomized surface, at present its preparation without ultra sound is not admitted.

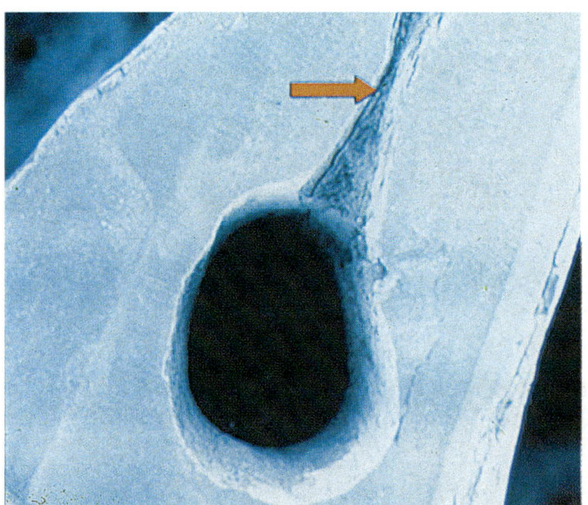

**Figure 25.13** - Isthmus (arrow).

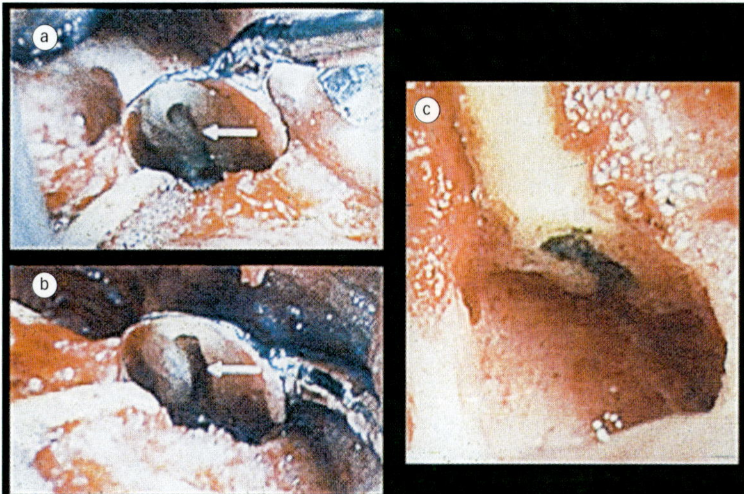


**Figure 25.14** - Isthmus (**A**). Its retropreparation (**B**). Retrofilling with MTA (**C**).

Among the several advantages of the use of ultrasound in endodontic surgery, in spite of anatomic difficulties is possible in most cases to place the ultrasonic tips parallel to the long axis of the root canal (Fig. 25.15), making more parallel preparations, allowing less wear of the dentinal walls, resulting in more conservative preparations with more voluminous or thicker walls. In addition, when apical cavities are made with ultrasound, a deeper preparation is achieved than when conventional burs are used (Fig. 25.16). In an experimental *in vitro* study, Bramante et al.[77] also observed that the preparation of retrocavities with ultrasound following the long axis, make possible more centered and regular apical cavities to be obtained. Ultrasound allows access to the root canal with reduced or even no root beveling, removal of less bone tissue from the surgical site, in addition to producing less debris. According to Sousa et al.[411] ultrasound favors better cleaning of the retrocavities.

A previously mentioned advantage in the preparation of retrocavities with ultrasound is that the bone sites can be smaller than those traditionally recommended. These tips are 3.0 to 3.5mm long, so they do not require unnecessary loss of bone structure, only sufficient for the tips be placed parallel to the long axis of the root canals (Fig. 25.17). There are, however, situations in which periapical lesions are already voluminous or extensive, also exhibiting extensive bone sites, therefore not requiring compensatory wear to lodge these tips.

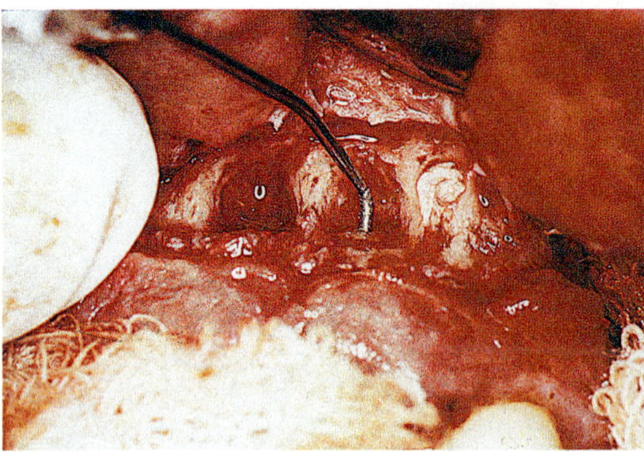

**Figure 25.15** - Retrocavity prepared with ultrasonic tips.

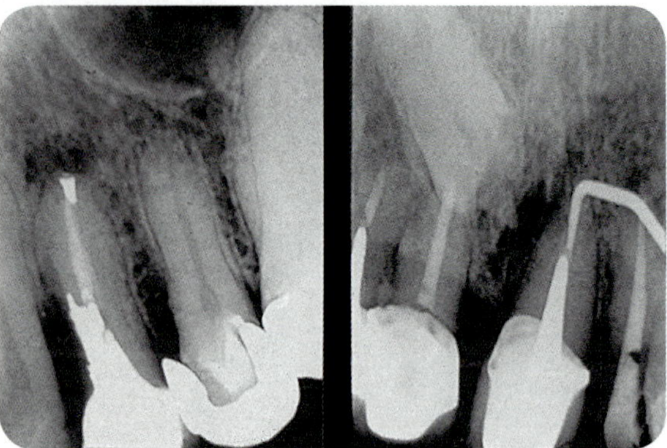

**Figure 25.16** - Apical cavities made with burs (A). Note the apical cavities made with ultrasound tips are deeper than those made with burs.

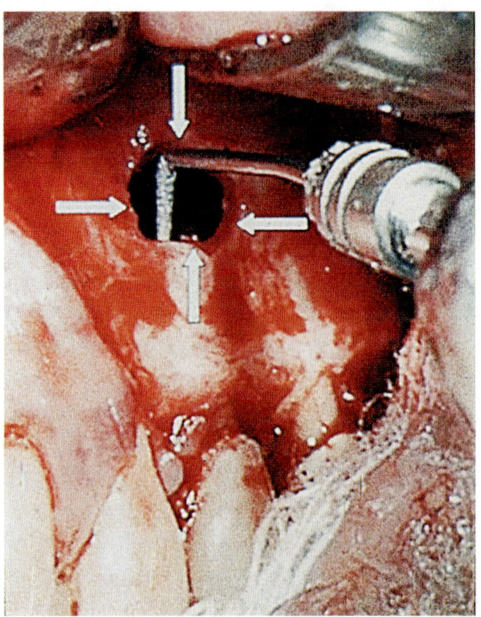

**Figure 25.17** - Few loss of bone structure, only sufficient for the tips be placed parallel to the long axis of the root canals.

Another relevant consideration when using ultrasonic tips is that they produce deeper retrocavity preparations than burs do (Fig. 25.16), in other words, around 3 to 3.5 mm, being the length of the tips most used in endodontic surgeries. In our opinion, despite this greater depth in comparison with the depth reached with burs, this is not at all safe. Considering that apical resorptions occurring in the apical region of apicoectomized surfaces, as previously discussed, are a common event in vivo[37,38,44,47,48,55,56,57,59] as a result of several factors also already mentioned. Although ultrasound prepares deeper apical cavities, one must consider that depending on the intensity and extent of these resorptions around the retrofillings, they can compromise the intended marginal sealing, a factor also influenced by the type of retrofilling material used. One is reminded that these resorptions are not observed in vitro, which limits interpretation of the results in this type of work. In some situations, one must onsider that the 3.0 mm depth achieved in preparations with ultrasound is very close to, or even small, when compared with indexes of marginal leakage found in some retrofillings. Thus, with the manufacture of these longer tips or inserts, approximately 4 to 5 mm, and certainly with the greater depth achieved by the apical preparation and insertion of the retrofilling material, it will be safer with regard to the marginal sealing favored by the material, even in the presence of apical dentinal resorptions[37].

An interesting detail was noted while analyzing retrocavities prepared with ultrasound, under the light of SEM: the presence of furrows or small grooves was seen on the dentinal walls due to the action of ultrasonic diamond tips (Fig. 25.18). In theory, this could even help the mechanic attachment of the retrofilling material to the walls of the apical cavities.

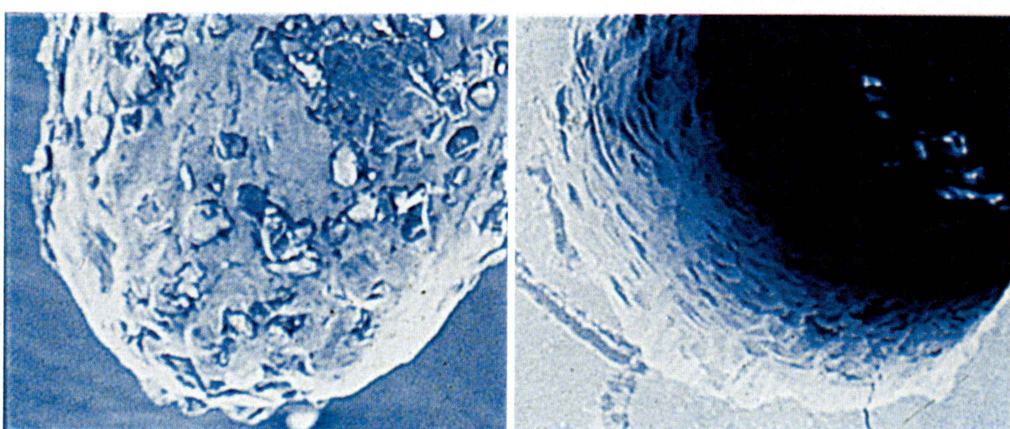

**Figure 25.18** - The presence of furrows or small grooves seen on the dentinal walls due the action of ultrasonic diamond tips.

Some investigations have been conducted to evaluate the efficacy of the use of ultrasound in the preparation of apical cavities. Some[116,157,165] of them performed these preparations with the use of the ultrasound in comparison with the use of conventional burs, and admitted that the residual quantity of smear layer or debris was smaller with ultrasound. Further to the use of ultrasound, it has been recommended by Sumi et al.[423] because of the ease with which these pieces are introduced via the apex; the possibility of conserving a larger amountof dental tissue, and allowing easy cleaning and enlargement of the apical portion of the root canal.

Despite the benefits of ultrasound use when performing endodontic surgeries, many studies have associated ultrasonic apical preparation with the appearance of microfractures on the sectioned dentinal surface[4,31,110,254,273,296,358].

According to Saunder et al.[375], the first authors to report the development of cleavages on dentinal surfaces after cavity preparations with ultrasound, indicated that it could increase the chances of apical marginal leakage. Min et al.[296] understands that these microfractures could serve as a means of communication for the bacteria that remain inside the root canals, with the periodontal tissues. Moreover, these cracks would provide a niche for bacterial development and accumulation of their toxic metabolites. These same authors[296] however, revealed that the fractures tend to be restricted only to the surroundings of the root canal walls, and rarely extend from this wall to the external surface of the root. In the case of fractures described as total, or communicating, Rainwater et al.[258] reported that their incidence would be associated with the presence of remaining dentinal walls that are too thin, and would not resist the stress of ultrasonic energy, thus enabling a favorable pathway to be established for these microleakages to occur.

Saunder et al.[375] believe that these microfractures are of unknown origin, but probably appeared as result of the energy generated by the ultrasonic instruments, when used with equipment working at maximum power. Frank et al.[141], Waplington et al.[473], Min et al.[296] and Calzonetti et al.[82] demonstrated that the power level of the equipment is directly related to the formation of microfractures. Authors, such as Layton et al.[254] also reported the time used for the preparation of these cavities as being one of the factors responsible for the incidence of fractures. They recommend using the ultrasonic tips for a maximum of two minutes. Studies performed by Frank et al.[141] and Gondim-Jr.[156] however, demonstrated that the use of equipment that generated less vibration, such as the sonic system, that uses lower frequencies in comparison with the ultrasonic system, can also produce the development of cracks. Gondim-Jr[156]. had the opportunity to study the incidence of these fractures after the use of ultrasound, considering the size of the roots and different groups of teeth, and concluded that there were no statistically significant differences when considering the mentioned studied factors.

According to Gondim-Jr.[156] the appearance of these cracks or microfractures, could be related to several factors. Among them he mentions the different laboratory processes that dental pieces are subjected to during the in vitro study, and the excessive manipulation of the roots, including the removal of the enamel with sharp instruments, which could contribute to the formation of some of these microfractures. They could also occur when the teeth were extracted or sterilized in autoclaves, due to the thermal expansion and contraction, as well as the stress the teeth undergo during extraction, the effects of dehydration and the storage medium[296,306]. The technique of preparing the roots for the scanning electronic microscopy exam should be considered, due to dehydration and low vacuum conditions, which eventually promote these cracks[273]. Another factor that could influence the appearance of these microfractures would be the technique used for sectioning the root apexes, during specimen preparation to receive the retropreparations[156]. According to reports described by Holcomb et al.[180], Lindauer et al.[270] and Onnink et al.[328], the cracks or the vertical fracture of the root could happen at any stage of root canal filling, during the lateral condensation performed in some types of teeth, or when being subjected to excessive forces.

Indeed, what is actually observed is that there are controversies related to the presence of these cracks or microfractures, because most of the studies have been performed in extracted teeth, thus not discarding the hypothesis of really having occurred due to technique artifacts. This has led to some authors questioning the results obtained, and asking whether they can be extrapolated to the clinic. Thus, in order to avoid these interferences during experiments performed in vitro in extracted teeth that studies have recently been conducted in the teeth of cadavers, because in the opinion of the authors[82,158] the results obtained under these conditions would be more relevant from the clinical point of view.

The sonic system has less vibration in the tips, in comparison with the ultrasonic system, which has also shown to be capable of producing microfractures. The authors[273] observed that the incidence of fractures occurring with the sonic system did not differ significantly when compared with those noted with the use of a spherical low speed bur, despite this group having presented only one case.

Scratches or marginal chipping (Fig. 25.19) can also occur on the dentinal surface as a result apical preparation, particularly when ultrasound is used. Lloyd et al.[273] were the first to report this on the margins of retrograde cavities, after preparing them with a sonic system for this purpose, and comparing it with the use of spherical burs, with and without beveling. Other authors[158,473] also demonstrated presence of these scratches. Gondim-Jr[152]. observed that their incidence seemed to be a constant, because they appeared in the majority of studied teeth in which the preparations had been performed with ultrasound.

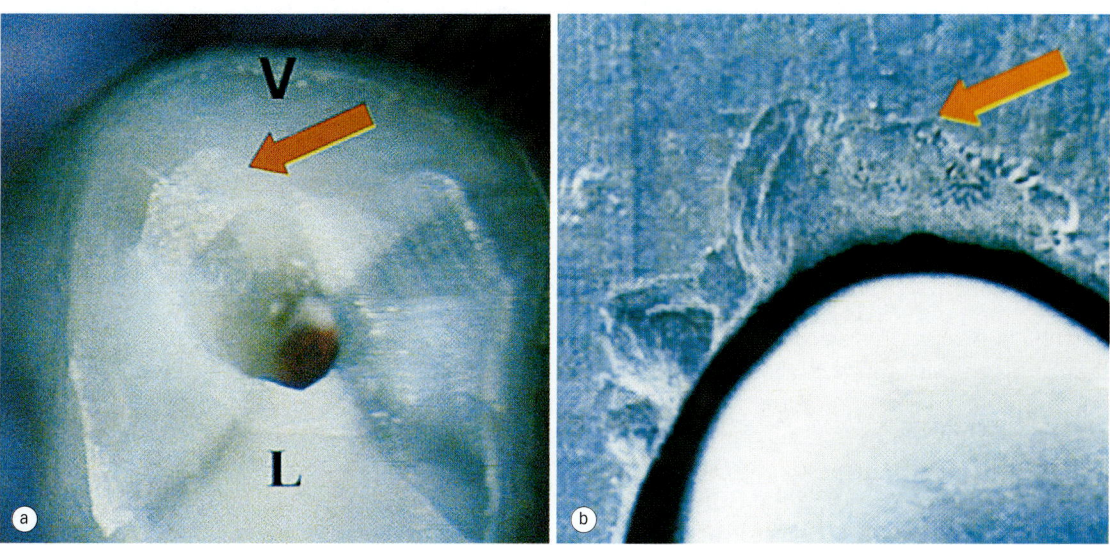


**Figure 25.19** - (**A-B**) Scratches or marginal chipping on the dentinal surface after apical preparation with ultrasound.

Nevertheless, as regards the presence or absence of fractures after the use of ultrasound, as already pointed out, Bernabé[48] working with dog teeth observed no differences in the results, whether using burs or ultrasound for the preparation of retrocavities. One must consider that the studies demonstrating the presence of scratches or marginal chipping and microfractures were performed in vitro, whereas Bernabé's study[48] was conducted in vivo, without using any type of analysis to identify these occurrences, since the study was not carried out for this purpose. Nevertheless, in view of his results, the author believes that there probably were no fractures or cracks; on the contrary, they did not influence the results. It is also probable that the hypothesis of Min et al.[296] about the possible role played by the periodontal ligament in damping the stresses generated during the ultrasonic tip vibration, thus preventing the presence of fractures and heat generation, could possibly have occurred in the experiment developed by Bernabé[48]. This argument is supported by the finding that among the 21 histopathologic issues evaluated by the author, many of them did not present significant differences, considering the two types of apical preparations. It can be mentioned, for example, that irrespective of the procedures performed (bur or ultrasound) neither presented significant differences related to the aspect of the periodontal ligament, which was shown to be organized and of adequate thickness. No differences were found with regard to the intensity of dentinal resorption, bone resorptions, and the intensity and extent of the inflammatory process were equal. These are evidences that very probably indicate why the clinical procedures adopted by Bernabé[48] did not agree with the abnormalities, such as the scratches or microfractures affecting the results, and the authors consider damaging events for achieving the expected success.

Another interesting finding Gondim-Jr.[152] demonstrated was that microfractures or cracks can occur near the margins of the apical cavity, close to the borders of the root canal, and that they are small in extent (Fig. 25.20). On the other hand it is known that root resorptions are common, and occur on the apicoectomized dentinal surface, also involving the borders of the apical cavities, as demonstrated by Bernabé[37,39]. Considering Bernabé's[37,39] and Gondim-Jr's data[156] it is possible to admit that microfractures and scratches occurring close to the cavity borders, could be involved in the resorption process and thus be eliminated without compromising the adaptation of the retrofilling material, or even preventing possible marginal leakage. Doubts remain about the fractures that could occur throughout the entire extent of the dentinal surface, creating communication between the interior of the root canal and the periodontium; the so-called microfractures[358]. It should be emphasized that there are studies, such as the one of Beling et al.[31], demonstrating that in most cases these microfractures are of the intra-dentinal type, and microfractures extending from the borders of the retrograde cavity up to the root cementum are rarely observed (complete fractures). This subject, however, is still surrounded by many doubts and has to be better investigated to eliminate the existent uncertainties.

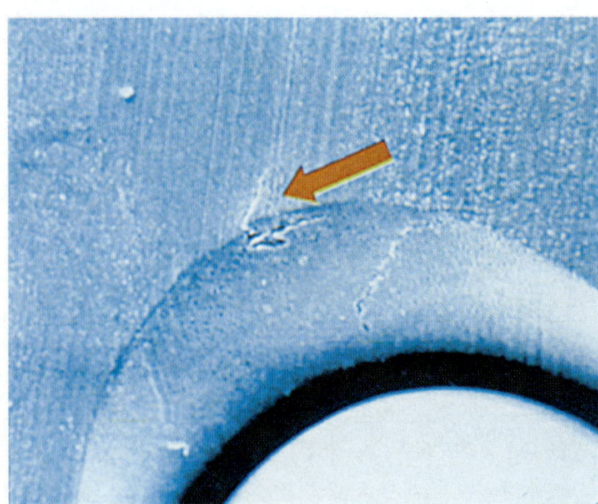

**Figure 25.20** - Microfractures or cracks close to the margin of the apical cavity. Gondim-Jr.[152], 1999. MEV X150.

After the apical cavity has been prepared, abundant and frequent irrigations with saline solution are performed. Anesthetic solutions are also used as irrigants, and are applied with an independent carpule syringe with disposable thin pre-curved needles without bevels. This procedure assists haemostasis, due to the permanent presence of the anesthetic solution in the area. Notwithstanding the efficacy of the irrigations performed, with ultrasound it is advisable to use complementary irrigations. This procedure will more surely prevent the presence of debris or dentinal scraps on the cavity walls, as described by Bernabé[37]. After this, proceed with aspiration and final drying with the aid of absorbent paper points. The absence of humidity inside the retrocavities is of fundamental importance, and depending on the type of retrofilling material used, a more efficient and safer bond to the dentinal walls will be achieved. After the the retrofilling is concluded, a calcium hydroxide "cap" put in place, as recommended by Bernabé & Holland[52], irrespective of the type of retrofilling material used. This calcium hydroxide "cap" must cover the retrofilling material and the entire apicoectomized dentinal surface, and it must not be placed on the periodontal ligament.

As Bernabé[38] demonstrated, there are several local factors responsible for the failures that occur after conventional retrograde fillings are performed. Two of them are fundamental: the lack of depth of the apical box and consequently of the retrofilling material. This, added to the problems that can occur with dentinal resorptions around the retrofillings, despite the use of biocompatible materials, make conventional retrograde fillings a technique with a doubtful prognosis and limited indication, particularly when performed with burs. It should be admitted that conventional retrograde fillings with ultrasound represented a great advance, and in this context could overcome several of the problems that arose with the use of burs. But one cannot forgot that although it is actually a safer procedure, it can fail to achieve its objectives, depending on the intensity of the unfavorable events that can occur in view of its depth. Against this background, we think that the ideal retrofilling technique to select is the one that fills the majority, if not all of the physical and biological requirements to favor the repair process.

Among the surgical techniques that were studied under the light of optic microscopy, it was observed that those enabling the retrofilling material to be placed at a greater depth favored the repair process. Thus, retrograde endodontic treatment deserves attention and due to its results, when compared with other surgical modalities, it has been recommended as the first treatment option, when endeavoring to solve the problems of teeth with refractory periapical lesions, rather than conventional endodontic treatment.

## 25.4 Retrograde Endodontic Treatment

Retrograde endodontic treatment pushes the filling material in deeper, and seems to provide better results than those achieved by conventional retrograde treatment, in which the retrofilling depth does not exceed 3.0 to 3.5 mm.

Although the retrograde endodontic treatment technique, or retro-instrumentation with retrofilling, as some wish to say, has been reported for more than seven decades by Duclos[112], it has not been extensively explored, particulary in histological experimental studies, which are scarce, to demonstrate its efficacy, Anton & Matsas[16] consider it inefficient. Therefore, to verify this type of treatment in a congruous and experimentally standardized manner, the first histological study in the literature, was performed by Bernabé & Nunes[59] who made a comparative analysis between the retrograde endodontic treatment technique and conventional retrograde filling, at that time performed with burs. Through the histopathologic results obtained, these authors verified that in dog's teeth with periapical lesions, retrograde endodontic treatment technique was superior to the retrograde filling technique with class I cavity preparation. In addition, in cases of endodontic treatment via apex, it could be observed at a histological level that filling material placement was deeper and associated with more favorable histopathologic findings (Fig. 25.21). Therefore, even in the presence of root resorption, and more rarely, debris between the filling material and the dentinal wall, it was observed that such factors were insufficient to significantly alter repair. In the cases of retrograde fillings with the preparation of a conventional apical box, however, when these same factors occurred, more unfavorable histopathologic findings were noted (Fig. 25.22), probably related to the apical cavities being shallow, impeding adequate marginal sealing. From the histopathologic point of view, the work developed by Bernabé & Nunes[59] demonstrated that the performance of disinfection and deeper retrofillings, offered greater safety than techniques such as conventional retrograde treatment, with less cleaning and retrofilling.

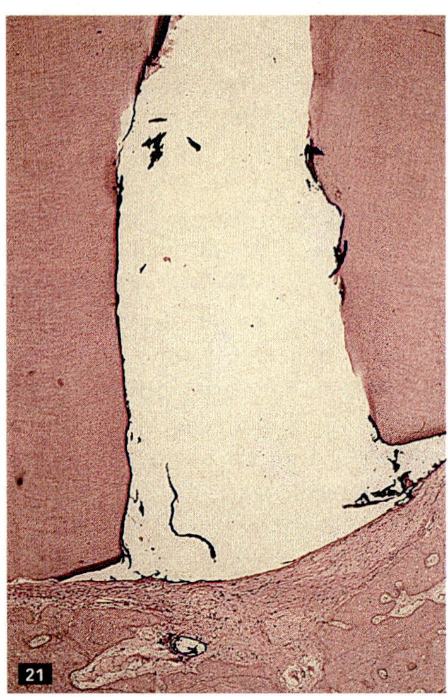


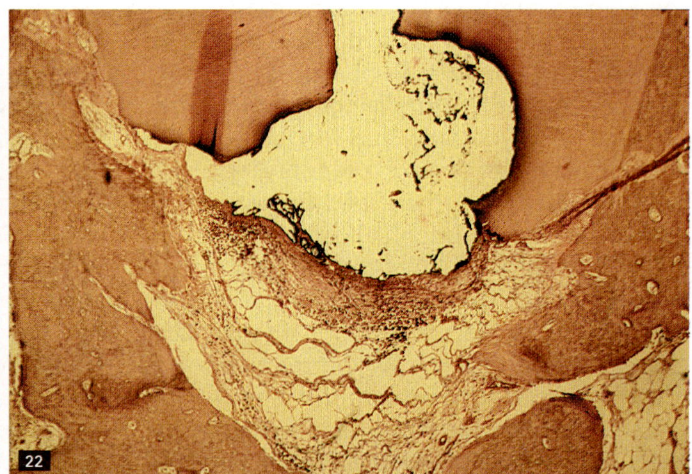


**Figures 25.21 and 25.22** - Endodontic treatment via apex.

In teeth indicated for conventional retrograde filling, it is common to find root canals with inadequate filling, generally associated with incomplete cleaning, which reduces the chances of the therapy being successfull. Nevertheless, with retrograde root canal treatment, careful retro-instrumentation will allow the contaminated necrotic content deep in the canal to be removed, thus favoring a better quality retrofilling and therefore, more extensive and deep apical sealing of the apical portion of the root canal. Weine[476] in a clinical and radiographic study, observed that many of the failures after endodontic surgeries, were immediate or occurred up to five years after the operation. Thus, instead of traditional retrograde filling, in which he stated that adequate apical sealing was generally not achieved, he began to choose root canal preparation and filling the canal through the apical access. In the same way, Nygaard-Ostby[321] proposes filling the canal via the apex, instead of conventional retrograde filling, because he believes that retrograde endodontic treatment favors more efficient cleaning of the irritants located inside the canals, as well as a more satisfactory apical marginal sealing. Reit & Hirsch[361] after clinically evaluating thirty five cases of retrograde root canal treatment, highlighted the potential for success obtained with this type of treatment, combining periapical curettage with surgical cleaning and root canal filling. Wu et al.[482] verified that the quality of the apical sealing produced by retrofillings performed to a depth of 7mm with thermo plasticized gutta-percha, was significantly more efficient than conventional retrograde fillings performed with silver amalgam and inserted in apical cavities only 2 mm deep. On the other hand, Kuga & Keine[247] and Tanomaru-Filho[433] in vitro studies, found no significant differences between the two surgical techniques, or that retrograde root canal filling showed equivalent marginal leakage indexes, in comparison with conventional retrograde fillings.

Note that endodontic procedures used in this surgical technique are performed in accordance with the same basic principles used in conventional orthograde root canal treatment. Furthermore, it is understood that more in depth and specific studies should be conducted to suit the environment in which they are performed. Thus,there would be a more promising scenario for teeth with survival placed at serious risk after being subjected to endodontic surgery. One emphasizes that it is indicated as the first choice technique, based on data reported by Bernabé[37] and on results obtained throughout the experimentation of Bernabé & Nunes[59] and Bernabé[38]. These studies under optic microscopic light analyses revealed excellent results, announcing great advantages in comparison with other endodontic surgical techniques. Indeed, from the good results obtained, retrograde root canal treatment would be contra-indicated only in when there are limitations on access that prevent the technique from being adequately performed.

Authors have no doubts[147,266,382,384,478] that efficient root canal cleaning, followed by adequate filling, is one of the most important requirements for successful endodontic treatment. These are fundamentally important principles and should not be ignored when performing retrograde root canal treatment[136,155]. Several clinical procedures need to be observed, including some adaptations that should be introduced, particularly when there are unusual environmental characteristics.

It is important to consider some of the care authors have taken since the technique was first indicated. Since 1934, when Duclos[112] described retrograde root canal treatment as an alternative for solving cases in which root canal treatment could not be performed via conventional or coronal approaches, there has been great concern about the bacterial state of the root apex. Therefore Duclos[112] recommended "chemical disinfection" of the apical portion of the root, immediately after it was surgically exposed, but reported that its efficacy would be doubtful deeper in the canal. In the 1940s, Sommer[410] recommended the use of a phenol-based substance as a way to "sterilize" the canal after retro-instrumentation. He neutralized the action of this drug with sodium bicarbonate, later using a filling sealer also with anti-septic properties. In 1946, Sommer[410], in addition to the habitual procedures he recommended, suggested trying to disinfect the canal via the retrograde approach and also recommended the application of silver nitrate over the sectioned dentinal surface after retrofilling, followed by the application of a layer of eugenol. According to this author, since the canals were filled with silver cones, the eugenol would precipitate free silver molecules into the dentinal tubules exposed by the apicoectomy, creating a favorable environment for the deposition of cementum and periodontal ligament repair. From then on, the retrograde root canal treatment technique started following the same routine procedures performed during conventional root canal treatment. There were no more references in the literature, to authors that used drugs with recognized antibacterial power and deleterious effects on the apical tissues, and applied them externally on the apicoectomized apical portion with the intention of "sterilization".

It is important to record that all the surgical steps described, starting with curettage of the periapical lesion and proceeding through to apicoectomy are the same, and must be observed in the retrograde root canal treatment technique. After resection of the root, complementary complete removal of the periapical lesion is necessary to prevent a possible occurrence of hemorrhage. Incomplete removal of the periapical lesion can facilitate slight but continuous bleeding that can significantly compromise the following operative procedures. Microscopic portions of blood clot rests that remain adhered to the internal walls of the root canal, via the retrograde approach can disturb adaptation of the retrofilling material, and consequently compromise marginal sealing. Studies conducted by Negm[312] showed that the depth of marginal leakage of dye around the filling sealers was more extensive when contact occurred with human blood, than when specimens were submerged in saliva, or kept dry.

After removal of the periapical lesion and with the operative field free of blood, the following procedures are started:

#### Retrograde determination of the working length

The next procedure is retrograde determination of the working length. This allows the depth of the root canal preparation to be standardized throughout the stage of enlarging the root canal, seeking to reach its entire space until the point where there is an obstruction, such as an intra-radicular post, fractured instrument, or rests of filling sealer etc. This file is put into the canal, via the retrograde technique, with the assistance of thin tipped hemostatic tweezers. This instrument not only achieves fixation of the file, but also works to limit penetration, placing it close to the sectioned dentinal surface. A radiograph is taken later. This retrograde determination of the working length is obtained by measuring the file, from its extremity (tip) up to the junction with the tip of the hemostatic tweezers, thus obtaining the file length that penetrated the root canal, via the retrograde technique. If necessary, after radiographic evaluation, the root canal can be measured and explored again. These procedures seek to facilitate the choice of the main cone, guiding the professional to assure that the full extent of the prepared canal is occupied by this cone, to avoid any empty spaces remaining.

#### Preparation of the root canal via apex

Once the length of the root canal has been determined, via the apex, the retrograde preparation stage, also denominated retro-instrumentation, begins. This stage follows the same instrumentation sequence as that performed during orthograde root canal preparation.

Retro-instrumentation can be performed manually, with the use of conventional K-file, by sonic, or ultrasonic instrumentation, also using K-type endodontic instruments, or a combination of the two techniques.

### Manual retro-instrumentation

With regard to the manual retro-instrumentation, most professionals prefer the K files. During this maneuver, these instruments can be used either by maintaining the cable[38,59,154,387] or not[14,75,136], and can be bent, or pre-curved to facilitate their introduction into the root canal, via retrograde access.

During the movements necessary for enlarging the root canal diameter, the endodontic instruments can be held with hemostatic forceps[16,37,59,74,95,136,361,471], preferably with a thin tip, because this makes it easier to insert them at any angle and not only in a predetermined direction.

In spite of the apicectomy, it can be difficult to introduce the endodontic instruments via the apex. Serota & Krakow[387] propose that instead of excessively reducing the root length, the height of the most apical bone level of the bone cavity should be reduced by a larger amount. Reith & Hirsch[361] understand that retrograde root canal preparation, compared with conventional surgical procedures, sometimes requires more extensive removal of bone tissue. They believe that retrograde root canal treatment is more appropriate for regions where the roots are situated closer to the buccal bone cortical.

The depth reached by the instruments inside the canal has been a concern, because the deeper the action of the instruments, the less the chance of contaminated tissues remaining lodged, which can later continue to irritate the periapical tissues. Whenever possible, the instruments must be taken up to the existent blockage, which in most cases is an intra-radicular post.

During the retro-instrumentation stage, it is necessary for all the dentinal walls of the root canal to be reached by the action of the instruments, so that in the end, the original anatomy of the canal is maintained (Fig. 25.23), without excessive wear. Otherwise, there is a possibility that one portion of dentinal wall is worn more than another (Fig. 25.24-25.25). This is more likely to happen on the lingual wall of the root canal when files with a smooth pre-curvature are used, but not with files pre-curved to a straight angle. Clinically, if these dentinal walls of the root canal remain very thin and are associated with the presence of intra-radicular posts, there is a greater possibility of post-operative root fractures to occur.

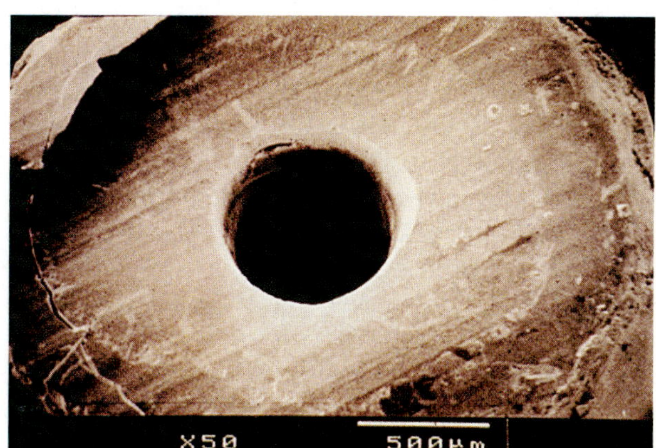


**Figure 25.23** - Original anatomy of the canal maintained after retro-instrumentation. SEM, X50 – Cortesy Prof. Cruz-Gonzales.

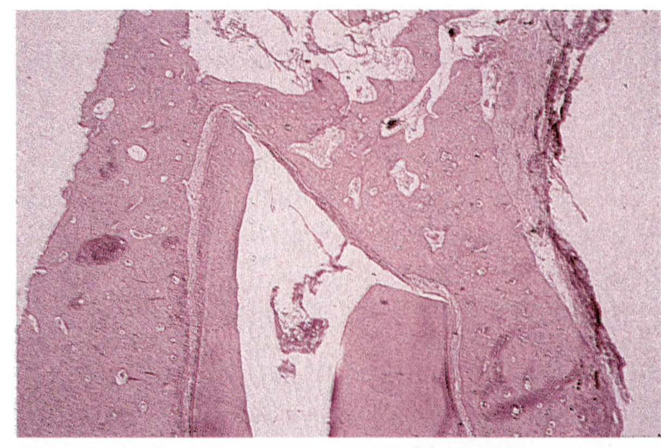

**Figure 25.24** - Portion of dentinal wall worn (H.E X15).

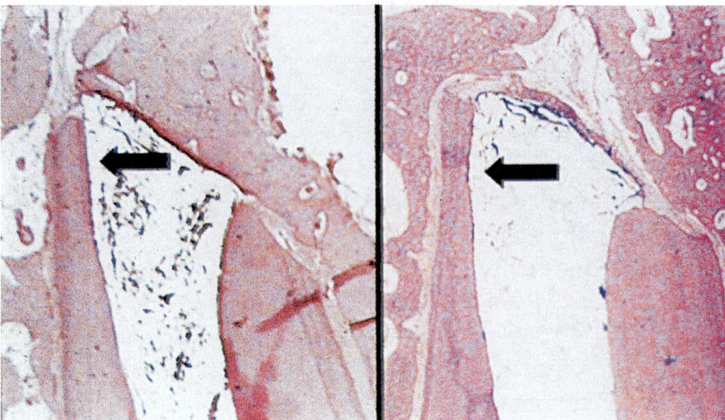

**Figure 25.25** - Portion of dentinal wall worn (arrow).

After a tooth is subjected to retro-instrumentation, the root canal can present a different anatomy to that which it has when preparation is performed via coronal access. According to Bernabé[38] the final geometric shape of the root canal after the conventional root canal preparation techniques is usually an elongated cone with base to the crown and vertex turned towards the root apex. In retrograde root canal treatment, after retro-instrumentation, depending on the volume of the dental root, two cones juxtaposed by vertexes can sometimes be observed. An apical cone, whose base is turned towards the apical opening of the canal, and the vertex, turned towards the crown. Corresponding to the middle portion of the canal, the configuration can involve another cone whose vertex is juxtaposed to the vertex of the apical cone and its base is turned toward the dental crown. When this geometric conformation is present, it is important to determine its size, because it can mean that special care should be taken, depending on the filling technique to be used via the apex. During the entire root canal preparation stage, particularly between the use of one file and another, abundant irrigation must be performed. According to Reith & Hirsch[361] every effort should be made to maintain the irrigating agent inside the root canal. The retrograde irrigation stage of the root canal should be carefully performed, because there is always the risk of the infected necrotic material spreading into the periapical tissues, particularly considering that it is in an open surgical field and with ample possibilities of disseminating the infection.

Several irrigating solutions are indicated for use during the retro-instrumentation stage. Among them are: 3% oxygenated water[321], filtered water[136], sterilized water[102], hydrogen peroxide[14,226], anesthetic[421], heated saline solution[476], sterilized saline solution[136,155], 1% clorazene[294], 0.5% or 3% sodium hypochlorite[361] and saline solution[38,59,74,154,155,]. Although it is preferable to use substances with bactericide power, such as sodium hypochlorite, in cases of contaminated canals one should not forget that they are also potentially toxic[23,313,386]. When the choice is sodium hypochlorite (0.5% or 1%), some special care must be taken to restrict them exclusively to the interior of the root canal. In addition to saline solution, chalk water can also be used, because they are non aggressive substances that have excellent biological properties[225,376]. Remember that the largest contaminating portion, the apical ramifications, was eliminated by resection of the dental apex, and that the irrigating solution acts more as a mechanic device for the elimination of debris. To perform retrograde irrigation of the root canals, different procedures can be used to introduce the irrigant deep into the full extent of the retrograde preparation, making this procedure very efficient.. After abundant irrigation with the purpose of eliminating debris and dentinal scraps originating from the root canal preparation, another important stage is to dry the root canals. If this is not done extremely carefully and correctly, it will allow another variable, humidity to disturb the bonding, or adaptation of the filling material to the dentinal walls, especially when using thermoplasticized gutta-perchas. During this procedure, an absorbent paper point with high-powered absorbency should be chosen, otherwise humidity could remain on the dentinal walls. Moreover, successive changes of low absorption paper points during this phase can slow the process down, and so increase the surgical time even further, which becomes inconvenient for the patient.

**Ultrasonic retro-instrumentation**

Another form of retrograde root canal preparation is the use of sonic and ultrasonic retro-instrumentation. Using the CaviEndo and the Endostar 5, Flath & Hicks[136] demonstrated clinically that retro-instrumentation with files enabled excellent cleaning and root canal preparation to receive a retrofilling. The authors demonstrated that although the files are commonly used in non-surgical endodontic therapy, by adapting the instruments and pre-curving them, excellent access to the apical portion of the root canal can be achieved. As already mentioned, at present there are special instruments (Retrotips), which were developed to enhance and simplify apical cavity preparations in conventional retrograde treatment. Most of them, however, have an active apical extremity that is too short, which does not allow very deep penetration inside the canal, despite its efficacy as regards dentinal wear. Wu et al.[482] proposed the use of Endocursor[62], of Australian origin, to perform retrograde root canal preparation mechanically. Sonic instrumentation has also been used for this purpose. Fong[138] described the use of an instrument (Tips) developed for use in a MM 1500 handpiece, a sonic system from Micro Mega.

Depending on the case, and local conditions, ultrasonic retro-instrumentation, performed in different ways is particularly recommended. One of them is retro-instrumentation by the mixed technique, in other words, the use of type K endodontic files, moved by ultrasound in conjunction with manual instrumentation. When the canals are made accessible via the retrograde approach, the root canal entrance can be enlarged using diamond tips or inserts (Retrotips), and the same applies to the preparation of retrocavities (Power 3 and Scaling position). Immediately after this, retrograde root canal begins with type Kerr endodontic files # 25 or 30, pre-curved adapted for ultrasound, endeavoring to introduce them up to the intracanal obstacle (i.e. an intraradicular post). In these procedures, ultrasound equipment in the Endo scale and power of 3 to 5 is used. Later, the preparation can even be complemented by manual instrumentation, always observing the volume of the apical portion of the root, to avoid excessive wear. While considering canals with easy apical access, retro-instrumentation can also be started and concluded using only type K endodontic files # 25 or 30, driven by ultrasound, and modeling the canal exaggerated wear, thus preventing the occurrence of cracks or fractures.

When root canals are found to be atresic via the retrograde approach, initial exploration can be performed with thin Barnabé Kit spacers. If necessary, one can resort to methylene blue or Tripan blue to locate and mark the correct position of the canal. Later, initially using thin type K files that penetrate the canal, proceed with root canal preparation ending with type K files # 25 or 30, with or without the help of ultrasound. After locating the root canal, another technical option used in cases of canals with difficult access would be to start enlargement using diamond Ultrasonic tips or inserts. Once this initial apical preparation has been performed, retro-instrumentation of the remainder of the root canal is concluded with the use of type K endodontic files driven by ultrasound, manually or a combination of the two.

## 25.5 Retrograde Root Canal Filling

After retro-instrumentation, one of the most important steps is retrofilling of the root canals. Retrograde root canal filling techniques are basically classified as follows:

- Retrofilling technique by vertical condensation:
  - Only with filling sealer.
  - Only with heated gutta-percha.
  - Gutta-percha associated with a filling sealer
- Retrofilling technique by active lateral condensation.
- Retrofilling technique with thermoplasticized gutta-percha.
- Combined or mixed retrofilling technique.

From this classification, one notes that the clinician has the option of different retrofilling techniques. Duclos[112], in 1934, when retrograde root canal preparation was reported for the first time, made reference to the use of a filling sealer with a pasty consistency during the retrofillings. From then on, a common point between most of the authors was the adoption of a filling sealer, either in association with or without a solid material, which could be gutta-percha or a silver cone. However, as it can be noted, there are also retrofilling techniques in which the filling sealer is not used.

### Retrofilling by the vertical condensation technique

#### Retrofilling with only a filling sealer

Among professionals that perform endodontic surgery, most of them prefer the ZOE or zinc oxide and eugenol-based sealer. Nevertheless, another good option is to use calcium hydroxide-based sealers, considering their biological properties.

After choosing the sealer, either the ZOE or calcium hydroxide based, it should prepared by manipulating it to the consistency of glazier's putty. With ZOE-based sealers, a larger ratio of zinc oxide powder to eugenol should be used. Whereas with calcium hydroxide-based sealers, such as Sealapex, after preparing the paste/sealer paste, a certain amount of zinc oxide powder is added until a consistency similar to that of window putty is obtained. To insert the sealer via the apex, small portions are placed in the opening of the root canal and compacted, using the special condensers of the Bernabé Kit. In the beginning, thinner and longer instruments are used to diminish bubble formation. Instruments of larger caliber are used, as increasing amounts of sealer are placed, continuing this vertical condensation, until in the end a compact mass of retrofilling material is obtained.

The level of retrofillings with this technique, as in the other techniques described, should be 1 mm below the apicectomized surface. To do this, end the vertical condensation of the retrofilling material at a small mark at the tip of one of the Bernabé Kit condensers, situated exactly 1 mm from its extremity, coinciding with the apicectomized dentinal surface. This has been recommended, as a result of the findings based on studies conducted by Bernabé[38], in 1994. Among several variables studied in this work, was the level of the retrofillings. The results obtained allowed the author to conclude that retrofillings performed 1 mm below the apicectomized dentinal surfaces, in comparison with those performed at the level of this surface, provide more favorable conditions for repair. This retraction of the retrofilling should be considered a fundamentally important detail in endodontic surgeries, with significant influence on the apical and periapical repair process. Since then, the author has recommended these procedures in all types of endodontic surgical interventions, except conventional retrograde fillings, performed with burs or ultrasound, when retrofillings do not exceed 3 mm. Under these conditions, in addition to the resorptions that can affect the adaptation of the filling material, this retraction could contribute to the definitive rupture of the marginal sealing established by retrofilling, since there would be too little retrofilling material, which could compromise repair.

When retrofilling has been concluded, the apicectomized surface must be properly cleaned with sharp curettes, to eliminate possible rests of filling material. After this, perform a radiographic exam to evaluate the quality of the retrofilling, followed by flatting the surface of the material with a Duflex # 5A or similar polisher.

Next, as recommended by Bernabé & Holland[52], place a calcium hydroxide cap. In this technique the 1 mm space left empty at the time of retrofilling is filled with a calcium hydroxide paste, in other words, a mixture of calcium hydroxide powder and saline solution. This paste is also applied on the full extent of the dentinal surface that was left exposed by the apicectomy, and resembles a cap or hood. During this procedure, contact of the paste with the periodontal ligament must be avoided as far as possible.

The technique of calcium hydroxide cap placement on the apicectomized dental apexes during endodontic surgical procedures, was recommended by Bernabé & Holland[52], but has been practiced by the authors since the 1980s, and is scientifically based on a pioneering experimental study conducted by Bernabé et al.[44]. The authors designed a study in dog's teeth, in which calcium hydroxide was applied on the retrofilling material and apicectomized dentinal surface for a period of only 10 minutes. It was then removed by abundant irrigation and saline solution. Compared with the specimens in which this application was not performed, the authors[57] observed that there was a slight tendency of the resorptions related by Bernabé[37] to occur with less intensity in the group in which the calcium hydroxide was applied. To better analyze this procedure, Bernabé et al.[57] conducted another experimental study, this time applying two types of calcium hydroxide, one hydrosoluble and other not hydrosoluble, as opposed to the previous study[44]. In this study the authors[57] left this calcium hydroxide paste permanently covering the dentinal surfaces and retrofilling material, and later filled the surgical sites with blood clots. They observed that there was a trend towards a more favorable result in the group in which the hydrosoluble calcium hydroxide "cap" was used, than in Group without the hydrosoluble cap. Other relevant data was that the use of the calcium hydroxide "cap" established better conditions for a higher incidence of total biologic sealing and even partial sealing to occur in comparison with the groups in which no calcium hydroxide paste was applied (Fig. 25.26). In addition to confirming the findings of Bernabé et al.[44], as regards the decreased incidence of apical dentinal resorptions, these results demonstrated that in the group in which the hydrosoluble calcium hydroxide (calcium hydroxide powder with saline solution) was used, there was a significant reduction in the frequency of occurrence of microorganisms. Most probably, the time this paste remains in the location before being reabsorbed, is long enough to eliminate the bacteria present in cementoblasts as well, which are responsible for many failures after endodontic surgeries.



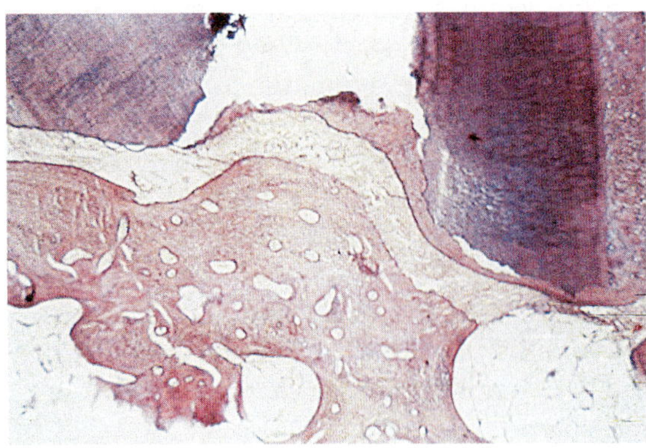
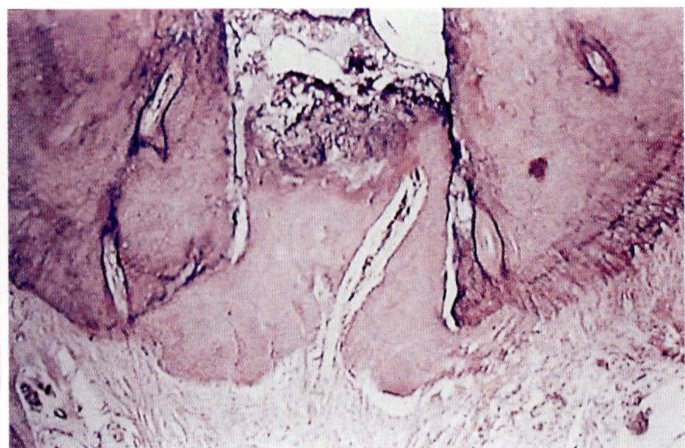

**Figure 25.26** - (**A**) Total biologic sealing (H.E. X 40); (**B**) Root cancal filling with MTA, biologic sealing (H.E. X100).

After the surgical procedures, placing the calcium hydroxide cap, and allowing it to remain permanently at the site, the bone cavity is filled with blood clots, obtained after gentle curettage of the bone cavity walls, followed by suturing the flap with silk or polyglactine 910.

**Retrofilling with heated gutta-percha only**

In this technique, after retrograde root canal preparation, the root canals are retrofilled exclusively with gutta-percha, using a method similar to that used by Marlin & Shilder[284] for conventional endodontic fillings. After first softening the gutta-percha cone by heating it with an alcohol lamp, place a portion of the cone at the entrance of the root canal, via the retrograde approach, using a Hollemback spatula. Immediately afterwards, perform vertical condensation with the Bernabé Kit cold condenser of suitable diameter, especially made for this purpose. Then, place a new portion of gutta-percha, also slightly plasticized by the heat of the flame, and immediately introduce it into the canal, uniting it to the previously inserted layer of gutta-percha. Next, with Bernabé Kit spacers, slightly heated at a short distance from an alcohol lamp flame, plasticize the entire mass of gutta-percha. Now insert another portion of heated gutta-percha, which has been vertically condensed with the cold apical condensers of the Bernabé Kit. Thus, these procedures are repeated successively until the retrofilling has been concluded, resulting in a single, compact mass of gutta-percha. Placement and condensation of the plasticized gutta-percha stop when this filling is 1 mm below the cut surface, as shown on the marked tip of the condenser (Bernabé Kit). On completion of the vertical condensation, the gutta-percha surface is polished with a cold instrument. As mentioned above, radiographs must be taken to verify the quality of the retrofilling, and then placement of the calcium hydroxide "cap", without removing it from the site, as recommended by Bernabé & Holland[52]. The following surgical steps are the same as those that have already been reported. It should be emphasized that this technique has not been used very much, because at present, there are materials that offer greater safety with regard to marginal sealing.

### Retrofilling with gutta-percha associated with a filling sealer

The recommended clinical procedures are similar to those in the previous technique, with the difference that before starting vertical condensation of the heated gutta-percha, an endodontic sealer must first be spread on the canal walls. Using a type Kerr endodontic file, or a Bernabé kit spacer, the filling sealer paste, preferably calcium hydroxide-based (Sealapex), is swabbed on all the internal dentinal surfaces of the root canal. The next step, performed in the same way as before, is vertical condensation of the heated gutta–percha, stopping at 1mm below the apicectomized surface, according to Bernabé.[38] After radiographic analysis of the quality of the retrofilling, the hydrosoluble calcium hydroxide[52] cap is placed on the filling, the surgical cavity is filled with blood clots, and finally the flap is sutured. This technique is preferable to the previous one, because it has the advantage of using a filling sealer that fills up the spaces better, helps adaptation of the gutta-percha and thus enhances the intended marginal sealing.

### Retrofilling technique by active lateral condensation

In similar way to the conventional root canal filling technique, this retrofilling system also uses a solid material and a paste. Among solid materials, the preference is gutta-percha, master cones and accessories.

In our opinion, the recommended filling sealer for this type of procedure is calcium hydroxide-based, Sealapex paste, whose biological properties are well known, and it has excellent biologic behavior when used in conventional root canal treatment. Bernabé et al.[35], in 1994 evaluated the results of an experiment performed in dog's teeth with periapical lesions, after retrograde root canal treatment, using Sealapex as retrofilling material, in paste form, at the level of apicectomized surfaces and demonstrated very encouraging results. Although one recognizes that Sealapex sealer should be better evaluated and studied at 1 mm below the dentinal surfaces exposed by sectioning, the above-mentioned results seem to favor its use instead of zinc oxide and eugenol-based sealers in paste form, particularly if we consider the results obtained by Bernabé[38], in 1994. In this study in dog teeth, the author evaluated the results of several retrofilling techniques, among them, the active lateral condensation technique, via the retrograde approach, using gutta-percha cones and ZOE paste sealer, in other words, the same consistency recommended for orthograde root canal fillings. The results demonstrated that when used under these conditions, ZOE cement in paste form contains a higher quantity of eugenol. This favors greater release of free eugenol[236] leading to more unfavorable histopathologic events in comparison with the other techniques used (Fig. 25.27).

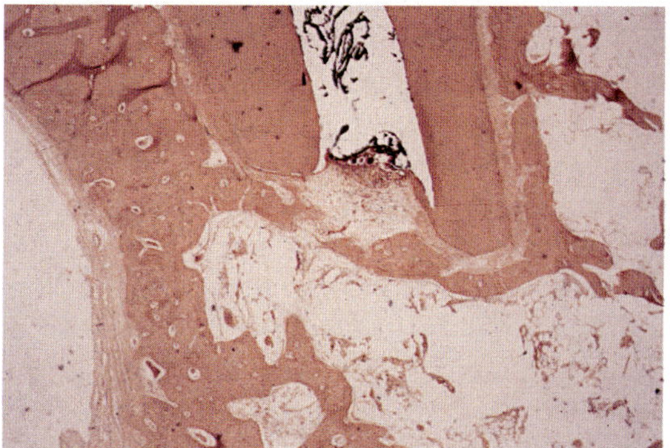

**Figure 25.27** - Chronic inflammatory infiltrate (H.E. X15).

Retrofilling, using the active lateral condensation technique, as proposed by Bernabé[38] is the performed as follows: when retrograde root canal preparation has been concluded, a master gutta-percha cone is selected, with equal diameter to, or one number above that of the last file used in retro-instrumentation. When adapting this cone, it should not fit too tightly or present resistance to removal. There should be some space for the placement of secondary cones in the filling sequence. A radiographic evaluation should be performed to verify cone penetration.

When the master cone has been selected, the root canal should be filled via the retrograde approach, using the classical active lateral condensation technique. Before beginning the retrofilling, a small amount of filling sealer can first be placed inside the root canal, using endodontic files, because of the peculiar anatomy of the canal after retro-instrumentation. The objective of this procedure is to safely insert the filling sealer in the deepest portion of the root canal and on root canal walls, via the retrograde approach. After this, the gutta-percha master cone enveloped in sealer is inserted into the canal in small pumping movements in the apex/crown direction. It is necessary to use the Bernabé Kit apical spacers for lateral condensation of the accessory gutta-percha cones. As these spacers have reduced dimensions, they allow cone tip to reach in deeper at the beginning of condensation, penetrating on the more coronary portion of the root canal, thus endeavoring to meet the requirements of good lateral condensation.[9] The same pumping movements used with the master cone must also be used with the accessory cones. Accessory cones are also used with sealer and active lateral condensation ends the moment the Bernabé Kit spacer does not penetrate the most apical portion of the root, thus ending the placement of secondary cones.

When the retrofilling is concluded, radiographs of the teeth should be taken, and if necessary, any failures of the filling should be corrected. The excess of gutta-percha cones at the dental apex are eliminated by cutting with the aid of a Bernabé Kit apical condenser slightly heated in an alcohol lamp flame. Next, using Bernabé kit condenser with a marked tip, also slightly heated, the retrofilling is removed to a depth of 1 mm below the cut surface[38]. Finally, the filling material is condensed, using a Bernabé kit apical presser, or a pediatric calcium hydroxide applicator to better accommodate the material on the surface (Golgran). After the hydrosoluble calcium hydroxide "cap" has been placed on the root apex[57], the other procedures are repeated, as explained in previous descriptions.

Nevertheless, it is emphasized that before the $Ca(OH)_2$ cap is placed by any chosen technique, all the filling sealer residue that remains on the exposed dentinal surface, or dentinal walls of the intra-canal space (1 mm), should be eliminated with the aid of curettes, Bernabé Kit apical spacers, K-files, or Cramer sterilized gauze (which does not release threads).

**Retrofilling technique set up with thermoplasticized gutta-percha**

Gutta-percha has undoubtedly been one of the most used materials in root canal filling, because of its excellent biological properties. There are several studies promoting the use of heat plasticized gutta-percha[162,283,304,377,486]. However, in 1984, Michanowickz & Czonstkowsky[295] reported the first studies using the low temperature (70° C) thermoplasticized gutta-percha technique, with the Ultrafil System (Hygienic Corporation, Akron, Ohio), developed by the School of Oral Medicine of the University of Pittsburg. Their results were encouraging, evidencing that they had established excellent marginal sealing. Since then, several authors[102,120,136,154,155,199] demonstrating excellent results in their reports, have also indicated thermoplasticized gutta-percha for retrofillings, which suggests that this procedure would be possible and practical.

In the Ultrafil system, one of the most used, gutta-percha is packed inside special needles, and plasticized with the aid of a portable electrical heater, to a temperature of 70° C. The system uses three types of gutta-percha, the Ultrafil Regular Set, the Ultrafil Firm Set and the Ultrafil Endo Set. The insertion of The gutta-percha is inserted into the root canal via the retrograde approach with an Ultrafil Kit metal syringe, with the needles attached to its extremity. Once the tip of the needle is positioned inside the canal (Fig. 25.28), the plasticized gutta-percha is injected inside the root canal (Fig. 25.29) by the pressure provided by a metal plunger that is pushed when the metal syringe trigger is activated. Finally, after the root canal has been filled with the thermoplasticized gutta-percha to 1 mm below the apicectomized surface, a vigorous vertical condensation of the gutta-percha is performed with the aid of a Bernabé Kit apical condenser. Next the calcium hydroxide cap is placed[52].



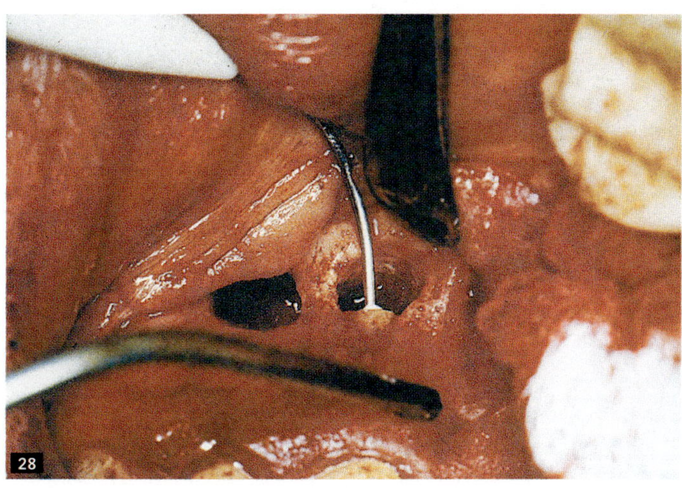

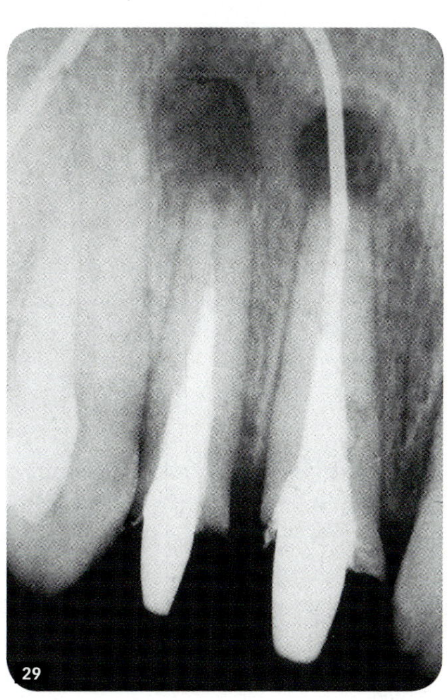

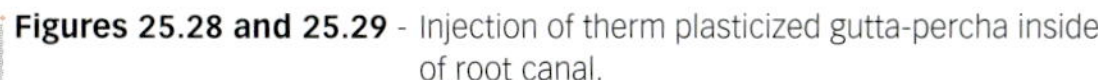

**Figures 25.28 and 25.29** - Injection of therm plasticized gutta-percha inside of root canal.

Bernabé et al.[56] conducted experimental studies in dog's teeth with periapical lesions, with retro-instrumentation of the root canals and retrofillings with thermoplasticized gutta-percha (type Endo-Set), using the Ultrafil system, placing it 1 mm below the apicectomized surface. A great number of the analyzed specimens evidenced the formation of complete biological sealing by cementum tissue deposition (Fig. 25.30 and 25.31), in addition to evident dental-alveolar repair.

Another device for injecting thermoplasticized gutta-percha is the Obtura system, which differs from the Ultrafil system, because it requires higher temperatures for plasticization. Because of this detail, as well as the initial results obtained with the Ultrafil system, and the facility of acquiring and replacing the different types of gutta-percha, at the moment, we prefer the Ultrafil system.

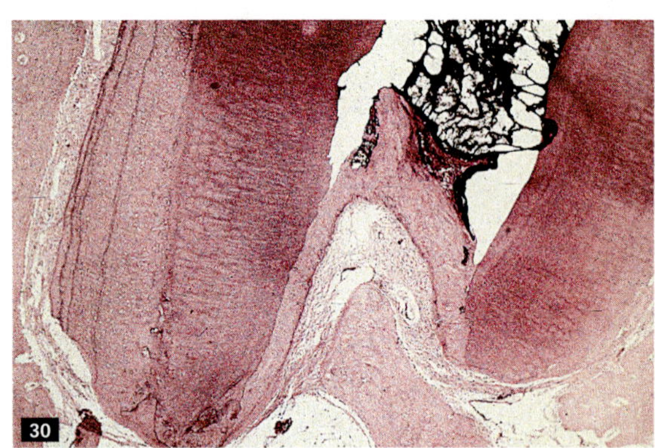


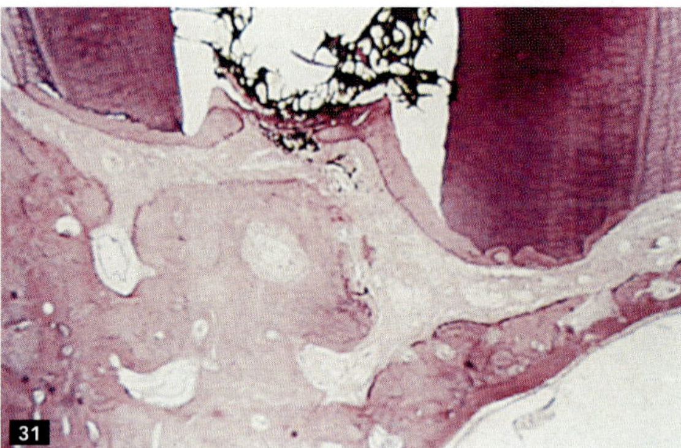


**Figures 25.30 and 25.31** - Biological sealing by cementum tissue deposition (H.E. X40).

**The combined or mixed surgical technique: retro-instrumentation and retrofilling combined with conventional retrograde filling**

Krakow[246] in a chapter of Endodontic Surgery edited in 1976, presented a variation of the retrograde root canal treatment technique. After retro-instrumentation and retrofilling the root canal with filling sealer, the author prepared a Class I cavity at the entrance of the root canal, and then performed the conventional retrograde filling with silver amalgam. During this same year, Wine & Gerstein[475] indicated root canal retrofilling with a filling sealer and gutta-percha cones. If there was any doubt about apical sealing, they recommended preparing a cavity in the apical extremity and later performing retrograde filling.

Another author[74,136,387,421] then recommended performing conventional retrograde filling after re-instrumentation and retrofilling. Bramante et al.[75] are of the opinion that conventional retrograde filling seeks definitive marginal sealing of the root apex. They consider that canal sealing depends on the adaptation of a single cone and the characteristics of the filling sealer, factors that would lead to post-operative failures. In their opinion, therefore, by performing retro-instrumentation and retrofilling, complemented with retrograde filling, good sealing of the canal can be established, thus contributing to the success of the treatment.

In ending this chapter about the indication and performance of some surgical modalities, it would be fitting to emphasize, that although there has been great scientific advancement with the experimental studies conducted, many issues remain to be better explained.

The development of new investigations in the field of endodontic surgery is essential to allow the endodontic surgical procedures used at present to be upgraded.

## 25.6 Retrofilling Material

From our point of view, another fundamentally important factor in the field of endodontic surgery, concerns the choice of retrofilling material which, in addition to the essential property of being capable of marginal sealing, it must mainly be biologically compatible. Otherwise, despite excellent sealing capacity, several unfavorable histopathologic events can occur, which could lead to failure. Following this line of thought, it is worth considering that even if the chosen retrofilling material promotes excellent apical sealing, the external apical root resorptions that can happen, irrespective of the type of material used[37,38], definitively compromise this property. It should be remembered that when the retrofilling material is placed in the retrocavities, it will come into contact with hard, and soft tissues, and remain at this site indefinitely. Therefore it is of fundamental important for it to be non-toxic, and compatible with live tissue. According to Gartner & Dorn[148], the ideal retrofilling material should prevent infiltration of microorganisms and their products into the periapical tissues. It should also be non-toxic, non-carcinogenic, biocompatible with the tissues with which they come into contact, as well as being insoluble in the tissue fluids and dimensionally stable. Furthermore, according to the author, the presence of humidity should not affect sealing ability, in addition to being easy to manipulate and sufficiently radiopaque to facilitate radiographic identification.

In the literature one notes that hundreds of filling materials have been the object of these studies, however, the following are among the most studied: silver amalgam with or without zinc, different types of gutta-percha, zinc polycarboxylate cements (Boston, PCA), zinc phosphate cement, Cavit, zinc oxide and eugenol cement, zinc oxide and eugenol-based cements (IRM, Super EBA, Kalzinol, Rickert, and N-Rickert), glass ionomer, composite resins, dentinal adhesives, calcium hydroxide-based cements (Sealapex, Sealer 26), MTA, and other materials, such as cohesive gold, silver cones, cyanoacrylate, Teflon, hydron, polyHEMA, titanium or ceramic screwing posts.

Of all these materials, we will refer only to those which have scientific support and that have been the object of studies in Endodontics Course at the Dental School of Araçatuba. They are studies developed in vitro, or experimental studies developed in vivo specifically in dog's teeth, using the following materials: silver amalgam, gutta-percha, paste and consistent ZOE cement, consistent Sealapex sealer, IRM cement, Super EBA cement and MTA.

### Silver amalgam

Among the various materials indicated for use in conventional retrograde fillings, silver amalgam was undoubtedly the preference of most clinicians at the time.

Silver amalgam was indicated for retrograde fillings due to the presupposed facts that it easily adapted to any cavity shape by force of condensation; offered less danger of dislodging into the periapical tissues[169,242]; was easy to place in the apical portion[169]; it had bacteriostatic action during the hardening phase[242]; favored good marginal sealing[27,105], and was a biologically compatible material[281,286].

Considering the vast literature about the use of silver amalgam until 1981, there was no in vivo experimental work that provided histopathologic details about its use, only descriptions of clinical and radiographic studies demonstrating its efficacy as retrofilling material[272,277,292,359].

Thus, Bernabé[37] in 1981, performed conventional retrograde fillings in a pioneering experimental study in dog's teeth, with and without periapical lesions, analyzing the behavior of the periapical tissues after retrofillings with silver amalgam without zinc, comparing it with the cold polished gutta-percha. In this study, for each material used, there were two groups of teeth: one with filled canals and another with contaminated empty canals. In the latter, clinical cases were simulated, in which the teeth presented incomplete fillings, canals that were usually contaminated and had periapical lesions. A great number of analyzed specimens in which dental-alveolar repair did not take place with the silver amalgam, as occurred with gutta-percha. The majority of them presented cementum resorptions of different intensities; partial cementum repair on the dentinal surfaces exposed by apicectomy; increased thickening of the periodontal ligament; even more accentuated when in contact with silver amalgam (Fig. 25.32). Another peculiarity in many cases, was the absence of a distinct fibrous capsule in contact with the amalgam which, when present, was of variable thickness, exhibiting inflammatory infiltrate of different intensities (Fig. 25.33). Few were the cases analyzed, in which the periodontal fibers reestablished the periodontal ligament functionally. Inflammatory infiltrate of the lymphohistio-plasmocytic type was present in most specimens, and was of variable intensity and extent. According to Bernabé, at that time, these results demonstrated that the use of silver amalgam should be re-evaluated, and if possible, replaced by other material that had better biological behavior. Only in 1995, Torabinejad et al.[448] developed an in vivo study on dog's teeth, and observed that the use of the amalgam as retrofilling material produced intense Inflammatory infiltrate, inducing a partial repair when compared with the other material, MTA, thus corroborating the results of Bernabé[37] as regards silver amalgam.

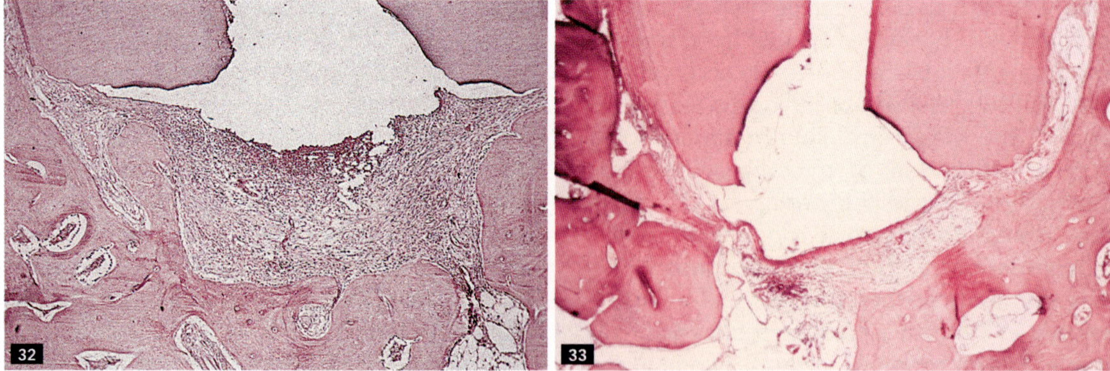


**Figures 25.32 and 25.33** - Retrofilling with silver amalgam. Chronic inflammatory infiltrate (H.E. X40).

Weine[476], reviewing cases of retrograde fillings performed over a period of 19 years, mainly with silver amalgam, and most of them controlled for extensive periods, observed a high rate of failures. The successful cases were related to teeth in which the canals had been filled with gutta-percha, moments before performing the surgical treatment with apical resection at the level of the well condensed portion of the filling. In the face of such observations, the author also believed that this type of treatment should be re-evaluated.

Several disadvantages were related to the use of amalgam, such as silver amalgam being difficult to manipulate, and that contraction and oxidation of the tin and mercury could occur while it was being mixed[401]. These authors, however, admitted that the presence of zinc would eliminate the problem of oxidation.

Jorgensen[230] admitted that zinc free silver amalgam tended to corrode faster than when it contained zinc. Messing[292], on the other hand, explained the need for using silver amalgam with a low amount of zinc, to decrease the expansion and porosity, in case the amalgam was contaminated with blood while retrograde filling was being performed.

According to Liggett et al.[267], adverse tissue reactions, in the long term, could be attributed to the products of silver amalgam corrosion, when placed in direct contact with the tissue fluids. Delivanis & Tabibi[105], six months after performing retrograde fillings with silver amalgam, observed a thin whitened coat over on its surface, as a result of the precipitation of the corrosion products. Bernabé[37] suggested that this phenomenon could have happened in his study. He observed that in teeth with aseptic filled canals retrofilled with silver amalgam, the bone tissue repaired the surgical cavity near the portion corresponding to the sectioned dentinal surface. However, in the portion that was in contact with the silver amalgam, he observed a larger distance from the bone tissue, increasing the periodontal space and inflammatory reaction (Fig. 25.32).

Another factor that could explain the negative results obtained, according to Bernabé[37], would be the marginal sealing obtained after the use of the silver amalgam.

Successful retrograde filling with silver amalgam would be directly related to the effectiveness of the apical sealing. It was demonstrated in vitro, that it did not impede the occurrence of a certain degree of marginal leakage, therefore it did not provide reliable marginal sealing [26,152,153,204,308]. It is known that recently prepared silver amalgam is more susceptible to marginal leakage[26,32] and that it diminishes or stops completely after 3 to 6 months have elapsed[334]. Barry et al.[26] and Russo[369] admitted that this leakage decreased intensely after 48 hours. According to some authors[20,105,217,242], this better sealing of the amalgam, with the passage of time, would be related to the corrosion that the material undergoes in contact with humidity or tissue fluids. It would also be connected with the tendency of the amalgam to expand after hardening, thus contributing to better adaptation of the amalgam to the cavity walls[20,242,247].

Rud & Andreasen[368] however, suggested that such alterations could cause loss of amalgam adherence to the walls of the apical cavity. They affirmed that the sealing property of silver amalgam was altered, due to problems that occur in the structure of the material, when in contact with live tissues. This was confirmed by Moodnik et al.[301] and Tanzilli et al.[434] who observed lack of adaptation of the amalgam to the cavity wall, which caused great concern, because the size of the gap was larger than the diameter of bacteria.

In the opinion of Bernabé[37], these observations were important, and explained part of his results. According to the author, even considering that the sealing properties of silver amalgam could improve with the passage of time, he believed that these factors did not lead to good results, as in the case of conventional retrograde fillings. Once this was exposed, and particularly due to the unprecedented results of the histological point of view related by Bernabé[37] in 1981, the use of the silver amalgam was suspended, and an option of a material that was biologically compatible was sought, which at that time was gutta-percha.

## Gutta-percha

Gutta-percha, one of the most used and studied materials in endodontics, has been shown to be a non-irritant material, with good tolerance by the subcutaneous connective tissue[36,202,297,318,480] or bone tissue[131,224,415] of rats and the periapical tissues of human teeth[71,95].

Although gutta-percha is one of the materials most indicated for retrograde filling[281,319,320], few histological studies have analyzed it under these conditions. Marcotte et al.[281], after filling root canals with gutta-percha and performing apicectomy in dog's teeth, was able to verify its good tissue behavior. In one of the first experimental studies that we developed on this subject[36], among other materials indicated for retrofillings, histopathologic analysis of the reaction of rat subcutaneous connective tissue was performed, when confronted with the implant of a stick gutta-percha from S.S. White. In this study, gutta-percha, together with silver amalgam, pointed out as being one the materials better tolerated by the rat subcutaneous connective tissue, which encouraged us to study it even further.

Thus, we performed a histological study in dog's teeth, with and without periapical lesions[37], as previously mentioned, when retrograde fillings with silver amalgam and gutta-percha were performed. In this study, Bernabé[37] verified that the retrograde fillings performed with cold polished gutta-percha presented more favorable results, with specimens exhibiting excellent histopathologic scenarios (Fig. 25.12 and 25.34) when compared with those presented by silver amalgam (Fig. 25.32-25.33). A common observation in this experiment was the presence of a fibrous capsule in direct contact with the gutta-percha, whose thickness was variable for each case analyzed, which attested the degree of tolerance of gutta-percha by periapical tissues, in agreement with the observations made in experiments conducted by Lantz & Persson[253], Marcotte et al.[281] and Smith[405]. Otoboni Filho[332,333] also using only gutta-percha as apical cavity filling material in his experiment, prepared on the apicectomized dentinal surface, and presenting results similar to those obtained by Bernabé[37], thus proving the already known good biological behavior of gutta-percha, when in contact with connective tissue[36,71,95,202,480]. It is evident that the results using only gutta-percha as retrofilling material has caused amazement, because of the studies always classifying it as a poor marginal sealer, despite proof to the contrary[178,179,203,429]. These divergent results are related to several factors, such as possible differences in the gutta-percha composition. Moreover, some marginal leakage studies did not adequately simulate the clinical conditions of the use of gutta-percha.

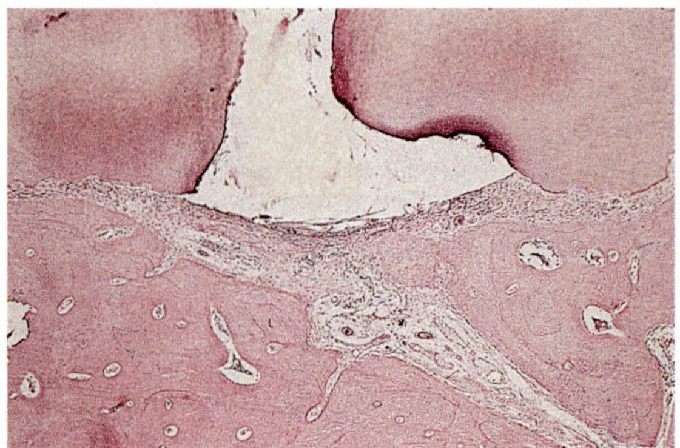

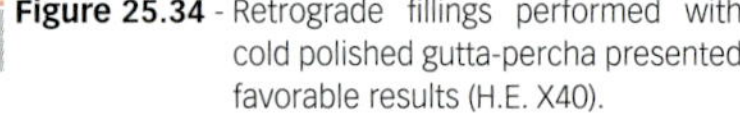

**Figure 25.34** - Retrograde fillings performed with cold polished gutta-percha presented favorable results (H.E. X40).

Another detail to consider is that gutta-percha has frequently been tested under different conditions to those proposed in endodontic surgery. It is imagined that its use is restricted to temporary sealing of cavities exposed to the oral environment, between appointments. Under these conditions, gutta-percha suffers not only the action of temperature alterations, but particularly of masticatory effort, factors that strongly contribute to the occurrence of material dislodgment. There are conditions under which its inability to seal a cavity adequate can be noted. Evidently this does not occur in a conventional retrograde filling.

The use of the gutta-percha in retrofillings lasted a long time. Nevertheless, because of strong criticism as regards its sealing ability, controversial results, as well as the difficulties with adaptation and manipulation in a humid environment, as occurs in endodontic surgery, many professionals stopped indicating it. A factor that possibly contributed to the criticism of gutta-percha use as retrofilling material, was the result of the experiment developed by Holland et al.[209] The authors, studying a certain type of gutta-percha, demonstrated the occurrence of an accentuated inflammatory process, accompanied by an extensive foreign body reaction. Afterwards it was demonstrated that such reaction was due to the presence of talcum that had been incorporated into its mass during the tissue reation of the gutta-percha cones. Although this was isolated occurrence observed in only one specific brand of gutta-percha, the question was whether this could occur with other types and brands of gutta-percha. At that time this information was considered irrelevant for contra-indicating it, because this feature was not observed with other brands of gutta-percha. The type of finishing performed on the gutta-percha surface after its insertion in the retrocavites was another matter that cast doubt on its efficiency in these situations. Tanzilli et al.[434] demonstrated that heat promoted dislodgment of the gutta-percha bond to the dentinal walls and the formation of bubbles or empty spaces on these walls, thus compromising its marginal sealing. Peter & Cunninghan[346] also reported that it underwent dimensional alterations, depending on the way it was manipulated. When compressed, it offered better marginal sealing than when tensioned. It should be considered that when gutta-percha was inserted into the retrograde cavities, it was placed and compressed by vertical condensation, which favored its adaptation and better marginal sealing.

The results observed in the experiments of Bernabé[37] and Otoboni Filho[332,333], are considered very significant to enable one to understand the use of gutta-percha as a retrofilling material. The inflammatory reactions observed close to the retrofillings the authors performed with gutta-percha, could really be related to the marginal leakage and root resorptions, because they prepared the retrocavities with burs, therefore with little depth, which makes them susceptible to problems, as already mentioned. This hypothesis attests to the studies of Bernabé & Nunes[59] and Bernabé[37], who also used gutta-percha in one of the experimental groups. They performed retrograde root canal treatment and retrofilling with this material in deep apical preparations. The good results achieved with the type of material used were encouraging, and were probably related to the depth reached by the gutta-percha, favoring more adequate marginal sealing, in addition to it being biologically compatible (Fig. 25.35-25.38).

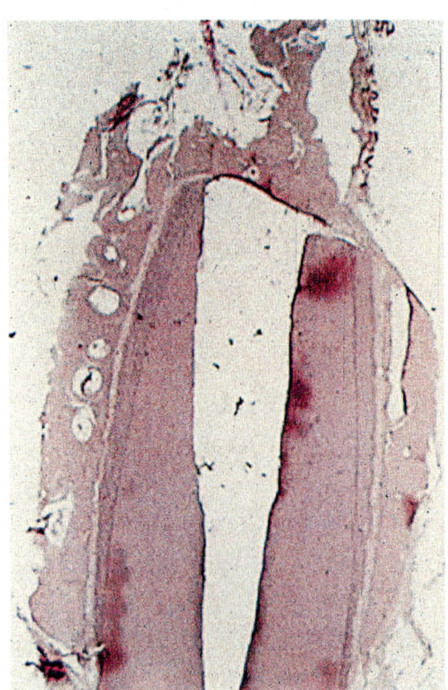

**Figure 25.35** - Adequate marginal sealing.

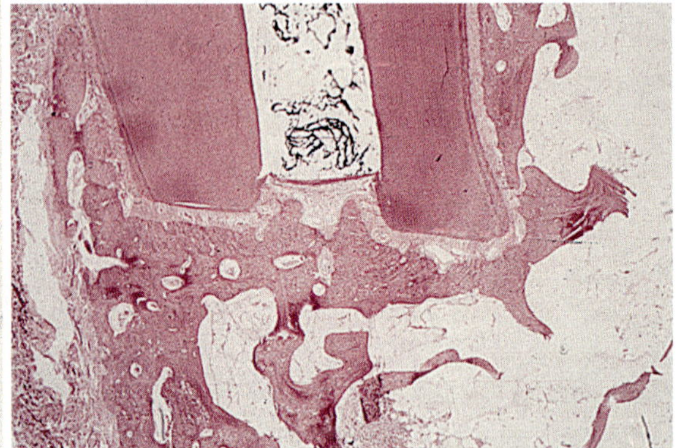

**Figure 25.36** - Adequate marginal sealing.

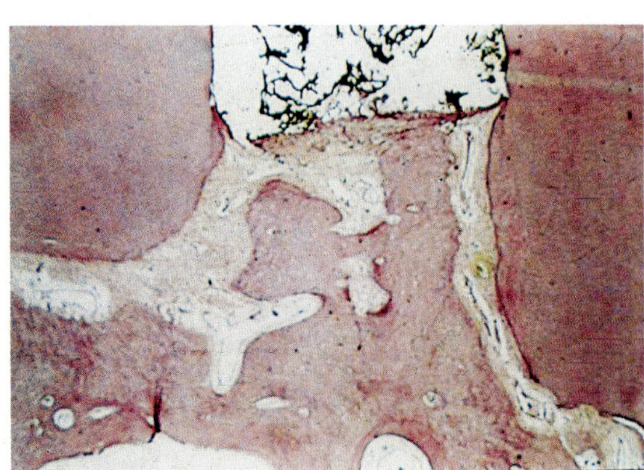

**Figure 25.37** - Adequate marginal sealing.

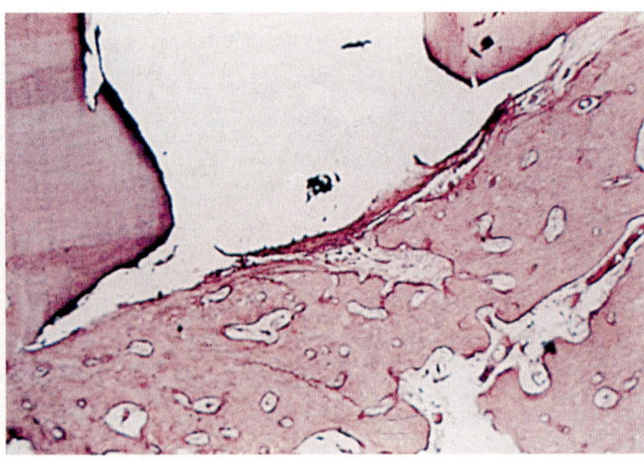

**Figure 25.38** - Adequate marginal sealing.

Indeed, at present gutta-percha is not the only material used for retrofilling, because there are other materials with excellent properties that better meet the biological criteria adopted. Moreover, some of them participate directly in the repair process, which is essential to adequate dental-alveolar repair.

Nowadays, the list of materials indicated for retrofillings is more extensive, a few of which are mentioned as follows: consistent zinc oxide and eugenol cement; ZOE-based sealers such as Super EBA and IRM; composite resins; light polymerized resin composites; dentinal adhesives; glass ionomer sealers; calcium hydroxide-based sealers (Sealapex and Sealer 26); Rickert sealer; N-Rickert sealer; and recently, MTA.

## Sealers containing Zinc Oxide and Eugenol (ZOE)

### Zinc oxide and eugenol sealer

Among all the retrofilling materials used, sealers composed of zinc oxide and eugenol are undoubtedly the most used in endodontic surgery. As we know, this is because most professionals choose the same retrofilling material that is used for conventional root canal fillings.

The zinc oxide and eugenol (ZOE) sealers are widely used in dentistry and especially in endodontics, mainly as root canal filling material. Leal et al.[258] and Simões-Filho[398] analyzing research data, noted that the original ZOE sealer and some sealers that had eugenol and zinc oxide in their compositions, were the most used for root canal fillings. Nevertheless, according to Leal[259] the zinc oxide and eugenol sealer has a number of physical-chemical features, such as impermeability, constant volume, solubility, disintegration, consistency, low cost, simplicity and efficacy. In Leal's opinion[259] these are features that have made it one of the most used sealers in dentistry up to now.

These properties led to it being indicated for retrofillings by Nicholls[317] principally because of good clinical-radiographic results obtained, and because it does not require great skill to insert it in retrocavities. Weine & Gerstein[475] preferred to use it instead of silver amalgam in retrograde fillings or for sealing perforations. Berbert et al.[33] also reported it as being an easy to use, electrically insulating and impermeable material.

The use of the zinc oxide and eugenol sealer in endodontic surgery has also been indicated by Bernabé[37], but with a thicker consistency than that used in conventional root canal treatment, or in other words, with less eugenol. Thus, larger amount of zinc oxide powder is added to the paste of this cement, giving it a consistency similar to that of "glazier's putty". To better define the subject, this author conducted the first experimental study, using zinc oxide and eugenol cement of a pasty consistency from S.S. White, after retrograde root canal treatment, up to the level of the dentinal apicectomized surface, or 1 mm below this surface. In most of the specimens, complete dental-alveolar repair occurred, characterized by the new bone formation filling the entire cavity that had been occupied by the periapical lesion, insertion of new periodontal fibers, cementum tissue deposition over the dentin exposed by the apicectomy, as well as the formation of a fiber capsule in direct contact with the retrofilling material, free of inflammatory process (Fig. 25.39-25.40). The group in which zinc oxide and eugenol cement of a pasty consistency had been placed up to 1 mm below the apicectomized surface, the presence of biological sealing by new cementum tissue deposition was observed, obliterating the retrograde entrance of the root canal, a detail that had not yet been recorded in the literature at that time (Fig. 25.41-25.42).In his experiment Bernabé[37] also evidenced that zinc oxide and eugenol cement of a pasty consistency behaved better, from a biological point of view (Fig. 25.43), than gutta-percha (Fig. 25.36) or gutta-percha associated with the pasty zinc oxide and eugenol cement (Fig. 25.27), particularly when the retrofillings were performed 1 mm below of the cut surface.

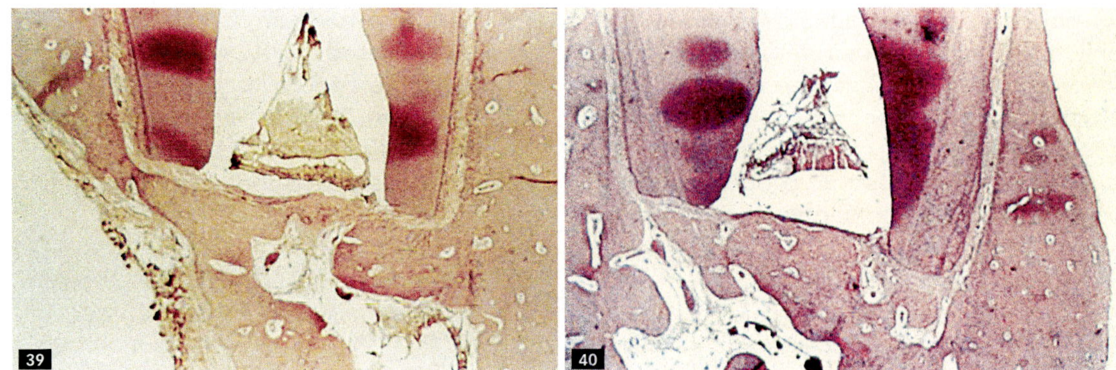

**Figures 25.39 and 25.40** - Formation of a fiber capsule in direct contact with the retrofilling material, free of inflammatory process (H.E. X15).

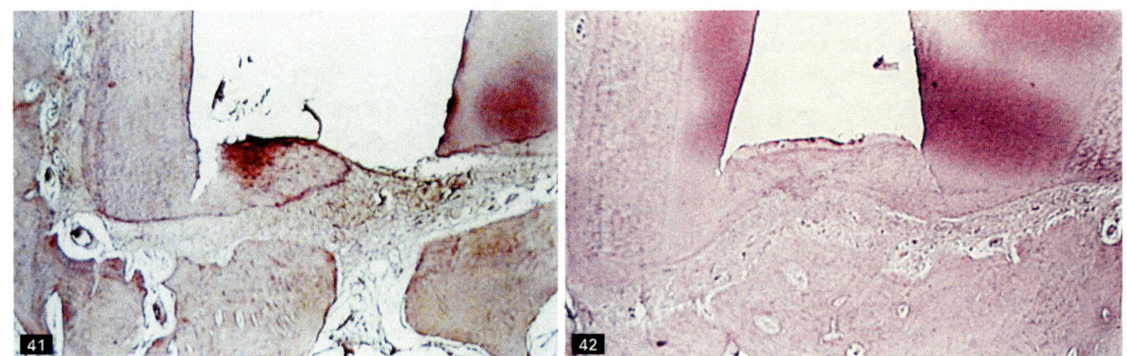

**Figures 25.41 and 25.42** - Biological sealing by new cementum tissue deposition, obliterating the retrograde entrance of the root canal (H.E. X40).

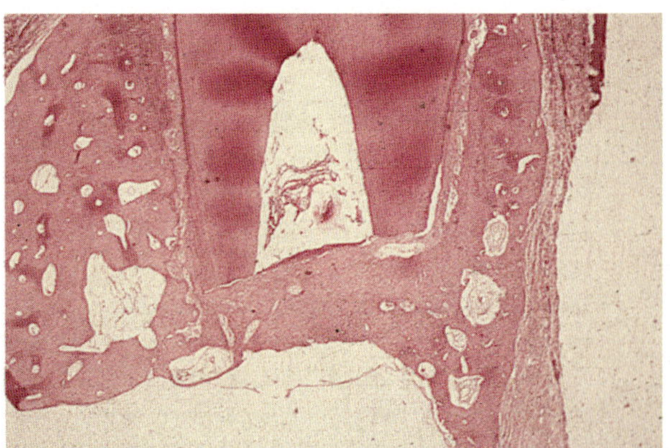

**Figure 25.43** - Formation of a fiber capsule in direct contact with the retrofilling material, free of inflammatory process (H.E. X15).

Other experimental studies conducted in dog's teeth, and developed in lectures on Endodontics at Araçatuba – UNESP (non-published data) used the ZOE cement of a pasty consistency in different retrograde endodontic techniques[44,47,55,57], such as during retrograde endodontic treatment and also after conventional retrograde filling performed with the bur or ultrasound[48,58]. Similarly, as was shown by Bernabé[38] in 1994, the above-mentioned experiments confirmed the good biological compatibility of the ZOE cement of a pasty consistency (Fig. 25.44-25.49).



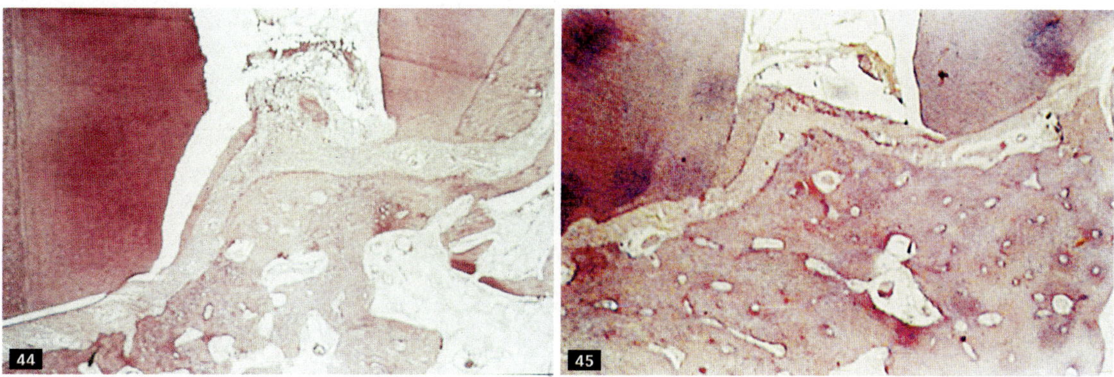


**Figures 25.44 and 25.45** - Biological sealing. Absence of inflammatory process (H.E. X40).

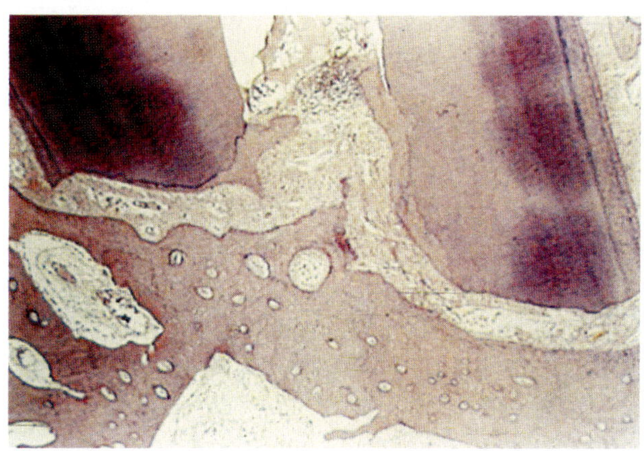

**Figure 25.46** - Partial biological sealing. Presence of discreet inflammatory process (H.E. X15).

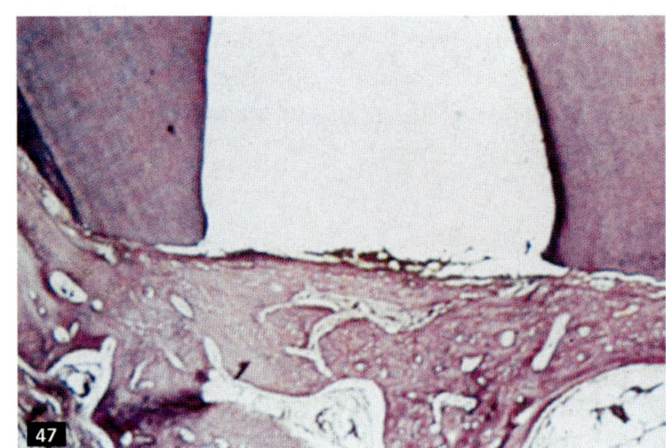

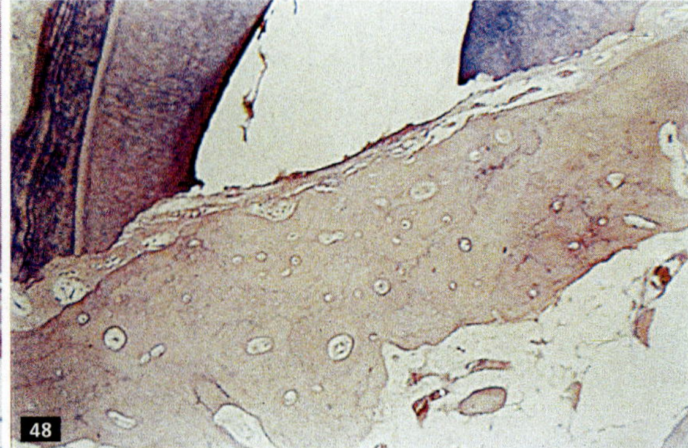

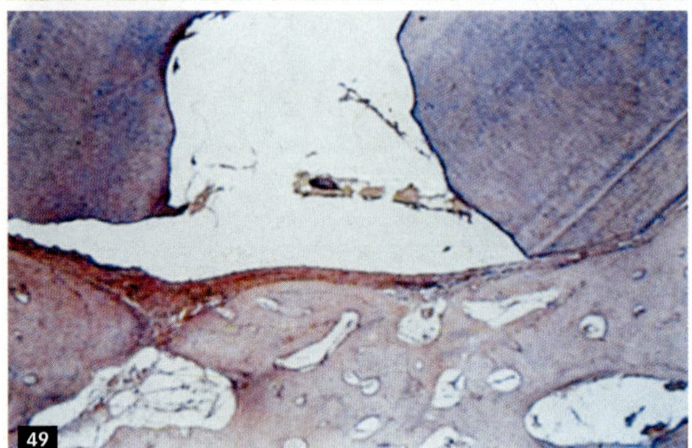

**Figures 25.47 to 25.49** - Fiber capsule in direct contact with the retrofilling material, free of inflammatory process (H.E. X40).

Performing also three inedited studies about the subject[44,55,57] the authors obtained excellent results with the consistent cement of ZOE, using it on the retrograde root canal treatment (data not published). The authors, who performed three unprecedented studies on the subject[44,55,57], obtained excellent results with the pasty ZOE cement used in retrograde root canal treatment (data not published). In one of the experimental groups of each of the aforementioned studies, after retro-instrumentation and placement of the ZOE cement with a pasty consistency, this material as well as the dentinal surface exposed by the apicectomy were capped with calcium hydroxide. In the specimens that were capped with calcium hydroxide, there was an accentuated improvement in the biological behavior of the pasty ZOE cement (Fig. 25.50) when compared with the specimens of the groups without this cap (Fig. 25.51), because in the capped group, there was an increase in the incidence of biological sealing. This better repair was classified this way, because the deposition of a cementum-like tissue occurred, which covered the entire cement and the dentinal surface exposed by the apicectomy, in addition to decreasing the bacterial presence in the region.

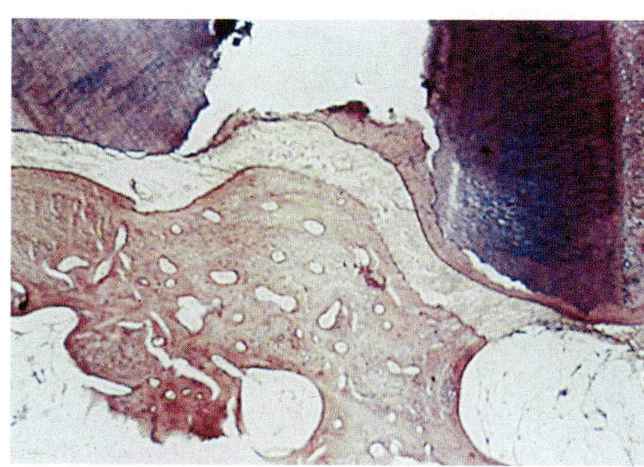

Figure 25.50 - Biological sealing. Absence of inflammatory process (H.E. X40).

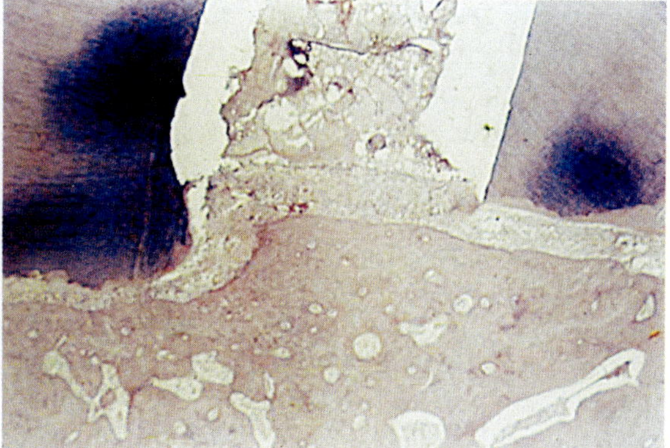

Figure 25.51 - Absence of inflammatory process (H.E. X40).

It is pointed out once again that hard tissue deposition on the ZOE cement of a pasty consistency, characterized as a biological sealing, only occurred in a few of the specimens, in which the retrofillings with this cement were located 1 mm below the apicectomized surface[38,55,57]. Nevertheless, this phenomenon occurred in most cases in which the calcium hydroxide cap was placed over the ZOE cement of a pasty consistency [55,57].

In Bernabé's opinion[37], this repair seems to be in disagreement with the studies that use zinc oxide and eugenol in conventional root canal treatment. The zinc oxide and eugenol cement, as well as the endodontic sealers that contain it, demonstrated high irritant power in experiments performed on rat subepithelial connective tissue[205,297] or in dog's teeth[76,190,198,201,208], rat's teeth[117], cat's teeth[365], human teeth[265,487] and cell cultures[271,364]. On the other hand, some authors have achieved good histopathological results after conventional root canal filling of human teeth with zinc oxide and eugenol cement, such as the case of Baume et al.[29] and Lambjerg-Hansen[251]. One of the factors that may have contributed to this observation, in the case of Lambjerg-Hansen[251], was the presence of dentinal scraps between the live tissue and the filling sealer, in all cases.

In this context, Bernabé[37] considered it fundamental to emphasize that in biological evaluations of conventional root canal treatment, the authors generally used creamy textured fluid ZOE sealers. Even with the creamy consistency, considered clinically ideal, making it easier to use in root canal filling, it has a higher proportion of eugenol in relation to zinc oxide. Most authors that analyzed the sealer are unanimous in affirming that the toxicity of the sealer is mainly related to the presence of eugenol[206,222,271,300,303,307,428]. Its pharmacological effect is complex, and probably depends on the concentration of its free fraction that will be exposed to the tissues. Beneficial pharmacological responses occur when the tissue is exposed to low concentrations of eugenol[282].

Considering the excellent results obtained in his experiment using the zinc oxide and eugenol sealer of a pasty consistency after retrograde root canal treatment, Bernabé[37] attributed this to the powder-liquid ratio used (1.0 g of zinc oxide to 0.2 mL of eugenol). The root canals were retrofilled with a very thick paste, with a consistency similar to that of glazier's putty, practically impossible to use in conventional root canal fillings. Under these conditions, there was a much lower amount of eugenol than is normally used, thus favoring the obtainment of more satisfactory biological results. Holland et al.[215,212], implanting the zinc oxide and eugenol sealer in rat subcutaneous connective tissues, reported that the inflammatory reaction was more intense in specimens that received the sealer prepared with a larger quantity of liquid. In cases of indirect dental pulp protection[166], or in dental pulp capping of pulp that had been exposed experimentally[96,291], it was observed that the results were better when the powder-liquid ratio of the sealer used contained less eugenol.

Therefore, when the zinc oxide and eugenol sealer or ZOE-based sealer is used in the clinic, it should be handled with the least possible amount of eugenol, and a larger amount of zinc oxide powder, to obtain a thicker or pastier consistency, as was used by Bernabé in all the studies reported here. In practice, this ideal ZOE sealer consistency is obtained when it has a thick consistency similar to that of glazier's putty when finally mixed. This can be checked by using a stainless steel spatula to roll the sealer on a glass plate: it must not adhere or leave excessive oily traces on the plate. Thus, one produces several small portions, or filaments of sealer that are easy to insert in the retrocavities.

Furthermore, according to Bernabé's report[37], it shows effective marginal sealing[73,119,257,325,342] and well known bactericidal properties[159,175,329]. An unfavorable factor related to ZOE sealer is that it is very fragile, brittle, takes a long time to harden, and is soluble in oral tissue fluids[335]. The latter property, however, was not reported in Bernabé's study[38]. On the contrary, the author showed the material present in the entire apical extent of the root canal, and always at the level of the dentinal apicectomized surface, probably a sign of its non-solubility. The absence of this solubilization has been considered as one of the ideal characteristics of retrofilling materials. Since they are exposed to the tissue fluids of the periapical region, it is important for these materials to be resistant to dissolution or decomposition by tissue fluids[164].

*Super EBA cement/IRM cement*

The descriptions of the mentioned cements have been placed together, as it makes it easier to discuss the studies in which they are compared with ZOE cement and MTA.

Due to disadvantages that were shown with the use of silver amalgam as retrofilling material[1,107,456], and the problems caused as regards the possibility of resorption of other indicated materials, such as Cavit[135], ZOE[335], and the so-called reinforced modified ZOE cement, alternatives for use in retrofillings have been suggested, namely IRM and Suprer-EBA.

IRM is a dental material widely used as a temporary seal[232]. Gartner & Dorn[148] demonstrated the use of IRM (Intermediate Restorative Material) in retrograde fillings, emphasizing that it is a cement composed of zinc oxide (80%), reinforced with 20% polymethylmethacrylate fibers, to eliminate the problem of resorption and to make it more resistant. The liquid is composed of a minimum part of acetic acid (1%) added to eugenol (99%). Dorn & Gartner, in a clinical study with follow-up of up to 10 years, verified 91% success after use of IRM in retrofillings.

According to Owadally et al.[335], the introduction of IRM into endodontic surgery was also due to the need for substituting silver amalgam, because of toxicity-related problems, corrosion, and other physical and even biological inconveniences. This biological incompatibility of silver amalgam as a retrofilling material was demonstrated in a histopathological study conducted by Bernabé[37] in dog's teeth, comparing it with gutta-percha, in cases of aseptic or contaminated canals. At no time was any result observed that encourage the use of this material, thus showing the need for replacing it with a more biocompatible material, as reported by Owadally et al[335].

Just as in retrofillings, the materials are mixed to a more solid consistency, to make it easier to insert them in retrocavities. In the case of IRM, Civjan et al.[91] found that by increasing the powder-liquid ratio, the compressive strength of the material increased, and the hardening time as well as its solubility diminished. Crooks et al.[99] conducted a study with IRM, to evaluate marginal leakage after its use in retrofillings, and when mixed in different powder-liquid ratios. They observed that no significant marginal leakage occurred, when comparing the different proportions used. These data suggested that use of IRM, with higher proportion of powder to liquid is acceptable, does not affect the sealing property of the material, and has numerous advantages in comparison with the proportions recommended by the manufacturers. According to the authors, it is easier and more practical to insert in retrocavities, also less toxic, less soluble and its hardening time is shorter.

The other alternative, or reinforced zinc oxide and eugenol-based material used in retrofillings is Super-EBA cement, reinforced with the aluminum oxide (alumina). It was initially launched by Staines in England, as Stailine Super-EBA, without aluminum oxide.

Super-EBA cement, known for its use for the definitive cementation of prosthesis, and as a temporary restorative material has been used by Hendra[172] as retrofilling material since 1970. It was developed to improve the physical properties of the ZOE-based cements, such as shortening the hardening time and making it less soluble[335]. In its original presentation it contained one flask of liquid and two of powder, one fast hardening, and the other normal hardening speed. In Staines's (England) commercial formula, the Super-EBA powder is constituted of 60% zinc oxide, 34% silicon dioxide and 6% natural resin. The liquid is composed of 62.5% ortho-ethoxybenzoic acid (EBA) and 37.5% eugenol. In 1985, Szeremeta-Browar et al.[425] reported a modification of the Stailine Super-EBA formula, made by Bosworth Co., by replacing the silicon dioxide with aluminum oxide (alumina), in the same proportion, which commercially corresponds to Super EBA Cement of Bosworth Co., available on the American market and used by us. According to Szeremeta-Browar et al.[425], these two types of Super EBA cements (Stailine and Bosworth) can be considered equivalent, based on declarations by the Council of the American Association of Dental Products and Equipment.

According to Oynic & Oynick[337], Super EBA is easy to manipulate, adheres to the cavitary walls, thus does not need retentive retrocavities, and can even be used in cases in which a completely dry field is not obtained. Due to its plasticity, it can easily be placed even when the mixture is pasty. The hardening time allows it to be used in adequate and sufficient time, and when in contact with the tissues it has a fast hardening property. This facility, however, is contested by Szeremeta-Browar et al.[425] who consider Super EBA extremely difficult to manipulate, as it needs large amounts of powder and liquid to obtain an ideal consistency, is very difficult to place in retrocavities and it hardens too fast. It adheres firmly to the dentinal walls, and this complicates condensation and makes it difficult to remove the excess afterwards. Bondra et al.[69] report that temperature and humidity variations drastically alter the working time of IRM and Super EBA, especially the latter.

According to Oynick & Oynick[337] and Szeremeta-Browar et al.[425], the addition of other components to zinc oxide and eugenol to reinforce them, gives this material properties such as being capable of bearing high compression forces, and enduring great stresses, having neutral pH and presenting low solubility. Oynick & Oynick[337] reported over 14 years of clinical experience with using Super EBA as retrofilling material, and recording approximately 200 cases of this material being used in human teeth.

Retrofilling materials are exposed to tissue fluids in the periapical region and depending on the type of material considered, it would be important for these materials to be resistant to dissolution or decomposition by tissue fluids[164].

According to ANSI;/ADA[19] specification number 30, a cement can loose up to 1.5% in weight after immersion for 24 hours in distilled water. The disintegration of Super EBA cement varies from 0% to 0.2%. According to the results reported by Torabinejad et al.[446], neither the Super EBA nor the MTA showed signs of solubilization after 21 days immersed in water, differently from IRM. According to Arnold et al.[19], when placing retrofilling materials, disintegration can be influenced by alterations in pH and osmolarity of the medium, and by the time taken for manipulation and subsequent contact with the tissue fluids.

The authors affirmed that these fluids and the periapical tissues are physiologically altered. Even in the absence of abscess, retrofilling material is exposed to an acid pH environment for a certain period of time, due to the acute stage of inflammation that precedes repair. Arnold et al.[19] reported that initial contact of the material with the blood clot or humidity can have an adverse effect on its solubility. According to these authors, the cements immersed in water 10 minutes after mixture presented very high infiltration, when compared with cement samples that were immersed one hour after they were mixed. However, they demonstrated that with Super EBA there were no significant differences in levels of solubility (loss of weight of the material) when the above-mentioned comparison was made. They also noted that disintegration was related to the pH of the solution: the lower the pH, the higher the disintegration.

Owadally & Pitt-Ford[336], using scanning electronic microscopy, observed no signs of Super EBA deterioration after storing it in a phosphate buffer for six months. From a clinical point of view, another important factor to consider is that when the materials are placed in retrocavities, they are initially covered by blood clots, and later by fibrous tissue. Thus the tissue fluids have a low capacity to attack, because even under favorable conditions, the material can still be covered by new cementum tissue[19]. In re-implanted monkey's teeth retrofilled with different materials, among them zinc oxide and eugenol cement, IRM and Super EBA, Pitt-Ford et al.[353] detected no sign of material dissolution by phagocytes. Analysis by Bernabé et al.[58] after retrofillings in dog's teeth with cements composed of zinc oxide and eugenol, demonstrated total absence of solubilization. Nevertheless, specimens retrofilled with ZOE cement only, evidenced a large number of giant cells on the surface, and in some specimens, a higher amount of material inside the macrophages, when compared with other ZOE-based cements, such as IRM and Super EBA.

Bernabé et al.[58] conducted a histopathological study on dog teeth with periapical lesions (data not published) in which they evaluated the results obtained after retrofillings performed with IRM, Super EBA, ZOE cement and MTA. The retrocavities were prepared with burs, and after an experimental period of 180 days, the statistical analysis showed that MTA, IRM (Fig. 25.52) and Super EBA (Fig. 25.53) presented similar results, there being no statistically significant differences among them; but significant only as regards the results presented by the pasty ZOE cement. The authors believed that the differences between the IRM and Super EBA groups could be attributed to the intense presence of dentinal debris detected in the latter group, and they were statistically significant, in comparison with the others. The harmful effects this debris in the retrocavities interfere in the marginal sealing of the material and consequently, repair. This is probably the main factor responsible for the differences between the materials, considering that debris are often associated with contamination, and also taking into consideration that this study was performed in contaminated root canals. Nevertheless, it should be considered that Pitt-Ford et al.[353] retrofilled monkey teeth with several different retrofilling materials, among them IRM associated with demineralized human dentinal scraps. Close to this material, they observed a few inflammatory cells confined to a small area, where these scraps had already been resorbed.

The findings demonstrated that there were no statistically significant differences, when comparing the histopathological occurrences among IRM associated with these dentinal scraps, Super EBA, Cavit or IRM alone without dentinal scraps. It should be considered that these scraps were not contaminated, differing from what commonly happens when preparing retrocavities whose canal walls (dentinal tubules) are generally contaminated.

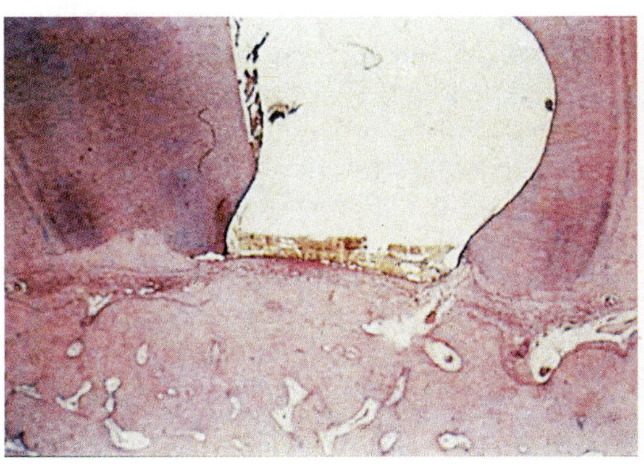

**Figure 25.52** - Retrofilling with IRM cement. Absence of inflammatory process (H.E. X40).

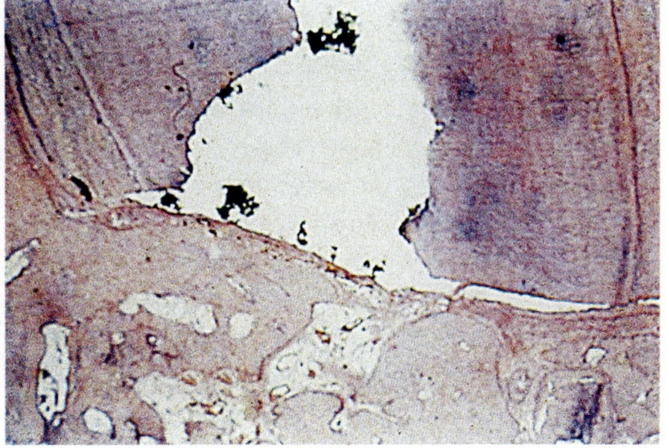

**Figure 25.53** - Retrofilling with Super EBA cement. Absence of inflammatory process (H.E. X40).

Trope et al.[465] demonstrated histopathological results obtained with IRM and Super EBA cements, similar to those obtained by Bernabé et al.[58]. After preparing retrocavities in dog' teeth and retrofilling them with several materials, the authors found that the best results were obtained with the Super EBA and the IRM after 180 days, compared with silver amalgam, glass ionomer and composite resin. Super EBA cement presented the best histopathological results, and differed statistically from other materials. When compared with IRM, however, this difference was not statistically significant, although the Super EBA specimens presented a lower number of inflammatory cells.

In two identical studies, Pitt-Ford et al.[351,352] studied the effects of re-implanting monkey mandibular molars after being retrofilled with IRM or Super EBA. They concluded that the histopathological events exhibited by Super EBA were clearly similar to those of IRM, and that the biological responses were significantly better, less severe and less extensive than with silver amalgam. A similar procedure was performed by Pitt-Ford et al.[354], re-implanting monkey's teeth retrofilled with IRM or ZOE cements, associated with gutta-percha. After eight weeks, the results demonstrated that both presented excellent behavior in this situation, greatly superior to silver amalgam. IRM was also the material used by Dean et al.[104] to fill root perforations performed in dog's teeth, either associated with tissue regeneration barriers, or not. The specimens that were evaluated after 24 weeks, exhibited small areas of Inflammatory infiltrate adjacent to the material. Nevertheless, this did not disturb the formation of new bone tissue. After preparing retrocavities, using round burs with the aid of a micro contra-angle, Harrison & Johnson[167] retrofilled them with either IRM cement, or silver amalgam. They made their observations 10 and 45 days after they performed the experiment. The specimens at 45 days already demonstrated accentuated dental-alveolar repair and significant bone repair. The Inflammatory infiltrate was considered small, even absent, in many cases. No cases presented acute inflammatory cells. Nevertheless, chronic cells occurred occasionally and not very concentrated, without disturbing the repair process. New cementum tissue covered the entire sectioned dentinal surface. There was a dense branch of collagen fibers in contact with the IRM, characterizing encapsulation, to which fibers ran parallel to the material surface. According to the authors, the results the specimens retrofilled with silver amalgam presented, were exactly identical to those presented by IRM. Contrary to what has been observed, the authors reported that the presence of eugenol and other chemical components with irritant potential, present in IRM cement, were not significant factors to alter the healing process in the initial periods. These results also contradict those verified by in vitro studies that demonstrated a certain degree of cytotoxicity of IRM in short-term evaluations[241,450].

Trope et al.[465] analyzed the behavior of the periapical tissues in dog's teeth submitted to retrograde fillings, and demonstrated the presence of a basophilic line in close contact with Super EBA. They reported that this could be interpreted as a possible resorption of material by the tissue, although they reported no macrophages in the area phagocyting the material. They believed that this histological discovery could be the first indication of hard tissue formation, in this case cementum, which would be deposited over the material. Similarly to these authors, a basophilic line was also described by Schröder & Granath[379], in cases of calcium hydroxide capping, as a histological sign of the beginning of hard tissue formation. Histopathological exams performed by Bernabé et al.[58] in specimens retrofilled with Super EBA, at no time revealed anything similar to the basophilous line.

Bernabé et al.[38,58] attributed the good results to solid ZOE cement, due to factors such as the powder-liquid ratio used. The author indicated that a quite thick, solid mass, practically impossible to use in root canal fillings by conventional methods was used in the retrofillings, as already discussed. It is emphasized that the powder-liquid ratio used in the study by Bernabé et al.[58], as regards IRM and Super EBA cements, complied with the manufacturer's specifications. Therefore nothing was done to make it thicker or more solid, as happened with solid ZOE cement. This could even be unnecessary, considering reports of Fitzpatrick & Steiman[134], when they remind us that Super EBA is an aluminum oxide-reinforced (alumina) ZOE cement and also contains ortho-ethoxybenzoic acid. According to them, the addition of this acid would help to reduce the amount of eugenol used, making it better tolerated when in contact with periapical tissues. Chong et al.[90] also studying the behavior of ZOE-based cements, affirmed that the eugenol present in IRM, as an organic composition, could be similar to polymethylmethacrylate, one of the components, and thus, limit its release. They also believed that the cytotoxicity of Super EBA and IRM cements would be related to the presence of eugenol in their formulas. By implanting polyethylene tubes filled with silver amalgam, IRM and Super EBA in mouse shinbones, Olsen et al.[327] could attest that in the initial periods of observation, the inflammatory responses were more intense, but after 100 postoperative days, the bone repair process was appropriate. In some specimens retrofilled with IRM, they observed that the bone tissue was deposited in direct contact with the material. In the authors' opinion, the decrease in inflammatory response, either with IRM or Super EBA, was due to a chemical process, in which the free eugenol (a phenolic compound) or the ethoxybenzoic acid, were sequestered by the serum and extracellular proteins. Fujiwasa & Masuhara[143] demonstrated the great affinity of these compounds to bovine serum, in comparison with other organic compounds. This connection would be an electrostatic interaction of the ortho-ethoxybenzoic acid and eugenol with cationic or anionic groups of albumin protein. They believe that the danger represented by prolonged eugenol release into the tissues decreases, due to this type of connection, associated with cleansing of the location, caused by the blood flow. According to the reports of Hume[221,223], when recent preparations of ZOE cement initially come into contact with fluids, fast and intense eugenol release occurs, decreasing, as the material hardens. Olsen et al.[327] reported that fibrous tissue formation acting as a stabilizing barrier and maintaining a buffer area, would reduce the toxicity that initially exists after the use of ZOE-based cements. The initial inflammatory responses to Super EBA are attributed to the ortho-ethoxybenzoic acid, or some of its components.

Similarly, Torabinejad et al.[450] believe that the toxicity of the ZOE-based, Super EBA and IRM cements could be due to the presence of free eugenol in the mass of these compositions. They could verify that as opposed to what happened with Super EBA, the samples of hardened IRM were more cytotoxic when in contact with cells cultivated in Petri plates, than the fresh or recently prepared samples. In the case of EBA, it was observed that samples of the already hardened cement were less toxic than recently prepared samples. They attribute these differences to the possible disintegration of IRM cement, with eugenol release within it. Moreover, in the same study, the toxicity was observed by comparing cellular lysis through the release of radioactive chrome. The data of this release showed that the toxicity ranged from slight to moderate when compared with hardened or recently prepared samples after 4 hours of incubation. After 24 hours of incubation, however, the degree of cytotoxicity decreased, the best result being obtained with MTA, followed by silver amalgam, Super EBA and IRM. Either hardened or recently prepared, IRM was more toxic. These results corroborate those of Bruce et al.[79], who verified that retrofilling cements, among them Super EBA, when exposed to certain types of cells cultures, in vitro, became less toxic with the passage of time.

Furthermore, several other researchers have investigated the in vitro toxicity of these retrofilling materials. Thus, Spångberg[416], in studies on HeLa cells, analyzed the cytotoxic effect of some retrofilling materials, and found that fresh or recently prepared samples of IRM produced total lysis of these cells. On the other hand, when he tested samples hardened for 1 to 4 weeks, the toxicity decreased significantly. A similar result was obtained by Weinberg & Hasselgren[477] demonstrating that the cytotoxicity of IRM and ZOE decreased with time. Bruce et al.[79] analyzing the effects of Super EBA after 24 hours and 30 days, in monkey kidney cell cultures, observed that the toxicity of the material decreased after seven days of incubation, and remained this way until the end of the experiment. Tronstad & Wennberg[463], verified that samples of pasty ZOE cement were moderately toxic. In 1994, Chong et al[90]. determined the effects of IRM and Super EBA on cell cultures, in vitro, using recently prepared or aged samples, after they were stored in distilled water for 72 hours,. The recently prepared IRM samples were the most toxic, being statistically significant in comparison with all the other tested materials, except for Kalzinol. According to the authors, Super EBA, which demonstrated a response similar to that of glass ionomer, is recommended as retrofilling material, as it causes low toxicity. Torabinejad et al.[450], using cell cultures of mice, determined the in vitro toxicity of silver amalgam, IRM, Super EBA and MTA, using fresh or hardened samples. They observed that recently prepared or already hardened MTA samples were less toxic than those of Super EBA and IRM. Recently prepared Super EBA Samples, however, were less irritating than IRM, under the same conditions. Furthermore, by the radioactive chrome release method, depending on the degree of toxicity of the material, they were able to verify that the samples recently prepared are more toxic than the hardened ones. After 24 hours of incubation, toxicity decreased, with the best result being obtained with MTA, and the worst with IRM. Osório et al.[330], using a culture of human gum fibroblasts, determined the cytotoxic effects of Super EBA, CRCS and MTA, among other materials. The results demonstrated that MTA present no signs of irritation, and Super EBA exhibited high toxicity levels. Based on their results, the authors concluded that MTA and CRCS were the less irritating retrofilling materials.

Retrofilling materials have also been examined by implants made in subcutaneous connective tissue, or bone tissue of small animals. Thus, Blackman et al.[65] implanting IRM in bone and subcutaneous connective tissue of mice, observed the presence of a small fibroses on the tissues around the material at 80 days. In 1990, Mcarre & Ellender[38] comparing the biocompatibility of Super EBA, and ZOE cement, 100 days after implants in subcutaneous connective tissue of mice, observed presence of a moderate inflammatory response. Later, the implants were encapsulated by a fibrous connective tissue. Implanting IRM in pig's jaws for a period of 4 to 12 weeks, Bhambhani & Bolanos[62] noticed the formation of a fine fibrous capsule, in which inflammation was absent, or if present, was very slight. Olsen et al.[327] evaluated the reaction of the bone tissue of mouse shinbones to Teflon tube implants containing IRM and Super EBA, after periods of between 7 and 100 days. After 56 days had elapsed they observed complete repair around the tubes that contained IRM. Around the tubes filled with Super EBA, they observed presence of a moderate inflammation. Nevertheless, after 100 days, they observed presence of complete repair around of the tubes containing the Super EBA. According to the authors, the biocompatibility demonstrated by IRM and Super EBA, reinforce the need for replacing silver amalgam by the two studied materials. Torabinejad et al.[447] implanted Teflon tubes containing Super EBA and MTA, in pig jaws. The results analyzed two months later, allowed them to conclude that both are biocompatible, although the histopathological results with MTA were slightly superior to those of Super EBA. In 1997, Tassery et al.[435] performed intra-bone implants of Super EBA and Vitremer in rabbits. Over the longest period of 12 weeks, the results showed similar histopathological results between the two materials. Pertot et al.[344] performed a similar study, implanting Super EBA in rabbit bone tissues, and compared it with glass ionomer. They observed that Super EBA showed excellent biological behavior, and found a fibrous and thick connective tissue frequently interposed between the material and the newly formed bone tissue. Kearney[233], implanting IRM in the subcutaneous connective tissue of mice, observed that it caused practically no inflammation, or only slight inflammation after 90 days of observation. In 1998, Steinbrunner et al.[419] determined the biocompatibility and osteogenic potential of Super EBA, after implants in the subcutaneous connective tissue of mice. The reactions studied microscopically after 15, 30 and 60 days demonstrated that Super EBA was well tolerated by the tissues, but was unable to produce osteogenic calcification or stimulate dystrophic calcification. In that same year, Torabinejad et al.[452], performed intra-osseous implants of Teflon tubes filled with MTA, Super EBA, IRM and silver amalgam in pig jaws and shinbones. The implants in the jaws were placed 10 days after the implants had been placed in the shinbone, and the animals were sacrificed at 80 days. Of all the materials, MTA presented the most favorable results. In both types of implants, MTA was the only one that presented no Inflammatory infiltrate in the tissues adjacent to the material, in addition to showing the bone tissue in close contact with it in several specimens. Between IRM and Super EBA, the events showed no statistically significant differences. Fibrous connective tissue was often observed in close contact with these two materials.

The marginal sealing provided by retrofilling material is also important, because it is capable of either impeding contact or not, with the periapical tissues within the contaminated root canal. Bernabé et al.[49] conducted an in vitro study to evaluate the marginal sealing provided by five retrofilling materials, MTA, IRM, Super EBA, glass ionomer and silver amalgam with varnish (Copalite) in retrocavities prepared in human teeth. The specimens were dipped in 2% methylene blue and submitted to vacuum for fifteen minutes, and then remained in the dye for a further 24 hours. The analysis of the results showed a significant difference among the materials, and MTA (Fig. 25.54) presented the lowest leakage index. Glass ionomer (Fig. 25.55), silver amalgam (Fig. 25.56) and Super EBA (Fig. 25.57) presented similar results among them, and IRM showed the highest leakage index (Fig. 25.58).

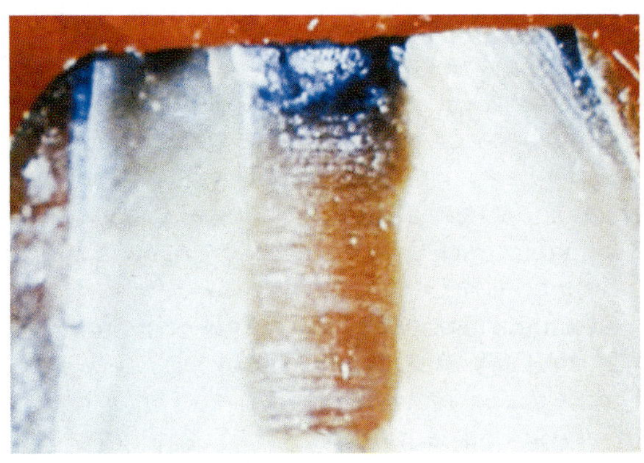

Figure 25.54 - Evaluation of the leakage of 2% methylene blue provided by MTA. X100.

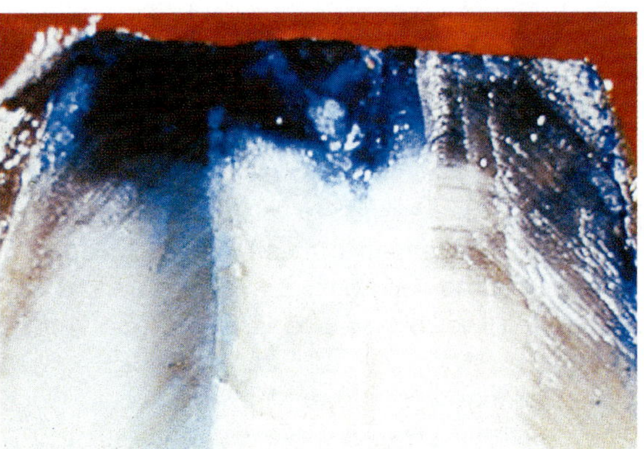

Figure 25.55 - Evaluation of the leakage of 2% methylene blue provided by glass ionomer. X100.

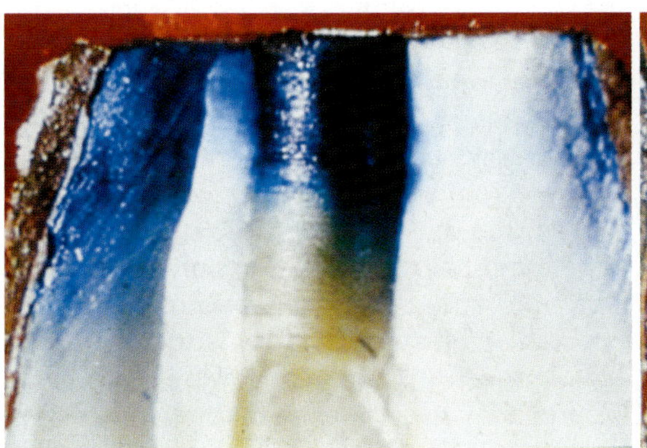

Figure 25.56 - Evaluation of the leakage of 2% methylene blue provided by silver amalgam with varnish (Copalite). X100.

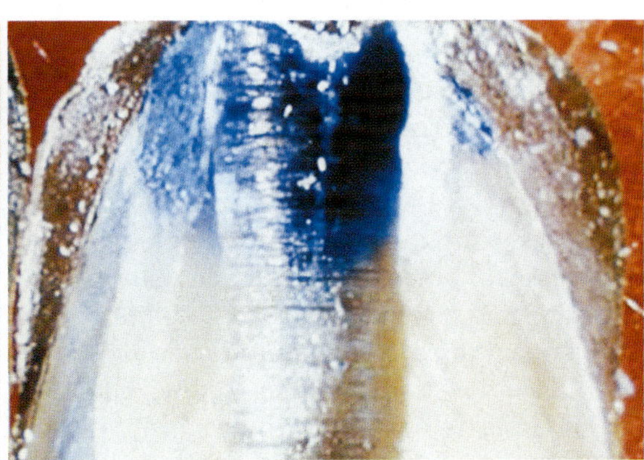

Figure 25.57 - Evaluation of the leakage of 2% methylene blue provided by Super EBA. X100.

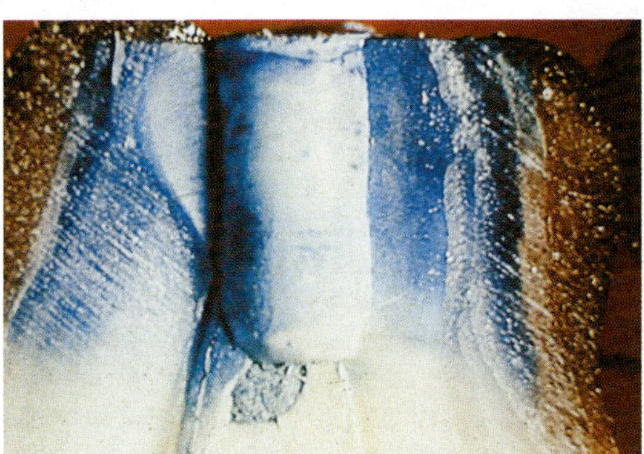

Figure 25.58 - Evaluation of the leakage of 2% methylene blue provided by IRM. X100.

With the same goal of evaluating the marginal sealing of retrofilling materials, Bondra et al.[69] verified that after the use of IRM and Super EBA, the dye penetration at the material / dentinal wall interface was significantly less than that found with silver amalgam, and there were no differences between them. Similar data were obtained by Higa et al.[177], and in the in vitro studies by Smee et al.[404] who also verified the superiority of IRM and Super EBA, in comparison with silver amalgam. In a study in which several retrofilling materials were used, Inoue et al.[228] evaluated the marginal leakage indexes, both in the coronal and apical directions, after 24 weeks. They observed that the leakage levels in specimens of IRM and glass ionomer groups, were similar among them and superior to silver amalgam in the initial periods. A longer period of observation revealed that there were no differences among them. Nevertheless, in studies conducted by Thirawat & Edmunds[438] to evaluate the sealing capacity of several retrofilling materials, they observed that Super EBA had worse behavior than glass ionomer cements, resin composite plus bonding agent, or bonding agents only. Results contrary to this were reported by King et al.[238] demonstrating better results with the use of Super EBA, when compared with glass ionomer and other retrofilling materials.

The Inoue et al.[228] studies demonstrated the presence of crystals on the surface of IRM, similar to foliage, or leaves of a plant, which could suggest possible solubility of the material. They believed that in vivo, fluids circulating around the apical retrofillings were able to solubilize IRM. When this happens, it could probably be responsible for irritations and interfere in the repair process. This was also observed in IRM by Fitzpatrick & Steiman[134] who attributed the phenomenon to an artifact of technique, in other words: the polisher was wrapped with IRM powder to prevent it from adhering to the instrument. In the specimens in which the retrofilling material surfaces were polished with aid of drills, this did not happen. In this author's opinion, the clinical significance of these crystals is still unknown.

Using the fluorescent Rodamina B marker, Torabinejad et al.[456] verified that apical cavities retrofilled with MTA presented the least leakage when compared with silver amalgam and Super EBA, and of the latter two silver amalgam was shown to have the higher leakage index.

Szeremeta-Browar et al.[425] used autoradiographs to evaluate in vitro, the marginal leakage after performing different procedures in the root apex. In one group apical cavities were prepared with a high speed inverted tapered trunk carbide drill #33½, and retrofilled with silver amalgam and Super EBA. In another group, the root canals were filled by the lateral condensation technique only, or submitted to the apicectomy, without cavity preparations. This study demonstrated that lateral condensation produced the best sealing when compared with the others retrofilling techniques, however without being statistically significant in comparison with Super EBA. The latter was statistically superior to the groups that only had the root apexes apicectomized.

King et al.[238], studying the marginal leakage index of Super EBA compared with glass ionomer and other retrofilling materials, reported interesting data. In addition to the good sealing provided by Super EBA, they found that this material tends not to deteriorate over a period of up to three months. Owadally & Pitt-Ford[336], studying the physical properties of IRM and Super EBA, found that even when placed in contact with bovine serum for a period of up to 6 months, they showed no significant signs of disintegration. When a certain amount of hydroxyapatite was added to the IRM, however, the material disintegrated. In a previous study, Owadally et al.[335] also studied the sealing capacity of IRM whether or not aggregated to hydroxyapatite, and compared it with Super EBA, silver amalgam and Kalzinol. They observed that irrespective of the percentage of hydroxyapatite added to IRM, there was no difference in the leakage indexes between IRM and Super EBA. The leakage means, however, were lower only for IRM cement, compared with silver amalgam and Kalzinol.

MacDonald et al.[278], using dye infiltration and fluid filtration techniques, conducted a study with some materials indicated for retrofillings, among them the silver amalgam and Super EBA cement. The Super EBA group was divided into two groups: one used dry apical cavities, the other humid cavities. Compared with silver amalgam, Super EBA showed lower marginal leakage indexes. According to the authors' evaluation, there were no statistically significant differences between the two groups of Super EBA (dry or humid cavities), in any analyzed period. In dry cavities, considering the initial periods of evaluation, the mean marginal leakage was substantially higher.

Whereas, MacDonald et al.[278] affirmed that water is essential for accelerating the hardening reaction of ZOE-based cements. In both groups, Super EBA cement was immediately exposed to 100% humidity after being placed in the retrocavities. Its hardening time after mixture is about 7 to 8 minutes. For the authors, it seems unlikely that an accelerated hardening could have any effect on the leakage observed 6 to 24 hours later. The water present in the cavities reduced the surface tension and might have allowed better adaptation of Super EBA. According to MacDonald et al.[278], this could explain why the marginal leakages that occurred in the initial periods were smaller in the group in which retrofillings were performed in humid apical cavities. But it does not explain what might have happened in specimens that had significantly reduced marginal leakages after one month. Moreover, according to these authors, the specimens with Super EBA presented larger amounts of leakage with an irregular pattern. They believed that was due to the hydrolysis of the cement matrix, resulting in its disintegration or fragmentation, causing a larger accumulation of debris, and consequently facilitating the leakage. Nevertheless, they reported that in the beginning it is normal for Super EBA to present minimum marginal leakage, which decreases after 7 days, and then remains relatively constant.

The effective marginal sealing provided by Super EBA was also demonstrated in a series of other studies, such as those of Saunders et al.[375]; O'Connor et al.[322]; Biggs et al.[63]; Reeh & Combe[360]; Bohsali et al.[68]; Chailertvanitkul et al.[89], and Gagliani et al.[146]

Through the scanning electronic microscopy (SEM), Bramante et al.[78] verified that N-Rickert cement and Super EBA were the retrofilling materials that presented the best adaptations near the apical cavity walls. Pasty zinc oxide and eugenol, IRM and silver amalgam presented slightly superior adaptation to that presented by gutta-percha and glass ionomer, but were shown to have very irregular surfaces. The authors observed that no complete marginal adaptation was observed in specimens retrofilled with IRM. Bernardinelli[60], evaluating maladjustments of several retrofilling materials, verified that Super EBA cement was the third best material in adapting to cavity walls, being superior to glass ionomer cement. Abdal et al.[1] observed a zero maladjustment index, and greatly reduced leakage with glass ionomer, these data being significantly superior to those of Super EBA cement and IRM, as regards the two appraised features. However, they verified that the maladjustments in adaptation, as well as the marginal leakage indexes, were higher in IRM specimens, when compared with those of Super EBA. Fitzpatrick & Steiman[134] conducted a study to evaluate the adaptation of IRM and Super EBA by SEM, in retrofillings when using different techniques for finishing the retrofilling material at the end. The specimens that received retrofilling material surface polishing performed after the material hardened, using special carbide burs for polishing, presented the best adaptations near the cavity walls, in specimens retrofilled with either IRM or with Super EBA, showing no significant differences between them. The specimens that were polished by instruments, or with humid cotton balls presented the most irregular adaptations. Recently, Forte et al.[139] evaluated the sealing capacity of Super EBA, when finishing the retrofilling material surface with burs, or final polishing with an appropriate (round polisher) instrument. The surfaces of the retrofillings that received final finishing with the bur initially presented significantly greater marginal leakage than when the surface was only polished. Nevertheless, this difference disappeared as the observation period lengthened. Inoue et al.[228], using scanning electronic microscopy, evaluated the adaptation of several retrofilling materials, among them IRM. The exams detected gaps near the dentinal walls in the adaptation of all the materials, in which the spaces varied from 5 to 10 micrometers.

Oynick & Oynick[337] who were pioneers in the use of Super EBA for retrograde fillings, performed dozens of clinical treatments, and by radiographic exams, they verified that it presented excellent behavior, superior to that obtained with silver amalgam. These results were attested by an analysis made with aid of the scanning electronic microscopy and histopathologic evaluation. Other clinical / radiographic studies were performed, such as the study by Dorn & Gartner[107], to verify the percentage of success attained after conventional retrograde fillings performed with IRM, Super EBA and silver amalgam. Over 488 cases were analyzed, with up to 10 years of follow-up. They verified that the percentage of success reached with Super EBA was around 95% and with IRM, 91%, vastly superior to the 75% reached by silver amalgam. Based on their discoveries, they concluded that either IRM or Super EBA presented favorable conditions for use as apical sealing materials. Pantschev et al.[339] analyzed over 100 patients who had been submitted to surgical treatment, and whose teeth received Super EBA or silver amalgam as retrofilling materials. The clinical – radiographic evaluation results demonstrated that around 56% success was attained with Super EBA, and 51.9% with silver amalgam, there being no statistically significant differences between them. Bogaerts[67] also reported excellent clinical results after the use of Super EBA, in cases of root perforations that occurred during root canal treatment. Wiscovitch & Wiscovitch[479] described a retrofilling technique in which the chosen material was Super EBA, the results of which showed it to be a promising material.

**Consistent Sealapex Sealer**

The first calcium hydroxide-based sealers for root canal filling sold were CRCS and Sealapex, in the 1980s. They were followed by Sealer 26 and Apexit. A series of experimental studies were carried out to analyze the physical and biological properties of these materials[70,93,181,199,213,220]. One of the most studied sealers, Sealapex has the property of stimulating biological sealing[213], as well as being a good marginal sealer, and it is equal to or better than the other known filling sealers.[220,268]

In 1985, Holland & Souza[213], conducted a pioneer study in dog's and monkey's teeth to verify the capacity of Sealapex sealer to induce hard tissue formation. After 180 days, they observed that it had induced mineralized tissue deposition at apical level in 33.30% of the cases of over-instrumentation, and in 70% of the specimens, in which the manipulation and filling limit was CDC. They noted that when the filling material was confined inside the root canal, there was no inflammatory reaction of the periodontal ligament, thus showing good tissue tolerance.

These data were also proven by Silva[395] who studied the biological compatibility of calcium hydroxide based sealers, and observed that Sealapex was the one that allowed the best mineralized tissue deposition, being the only shown to completely seal the radicular apex in 37.5% of the cases. Tagger & Tagger[427], using monkey's teeth, under similar experimental conditions, observed that with Sealapex, complete apical sealing occurred in 50% of the cases, and noted the absence of inflammatory infiltrate in the periodontal ligament, in the apical foramen area.

Specifically for Sealapex sealer, some studies demonstrated that it produced better marginal sealing when compared with zinc oxide and eugenol- based [7,181,256,280] and resin sealers[268]. Probably the better sealing quality of Sealapex is because it has calcium oxide in its formulation. In contact with humidity, the calcium oxide reacts with the water to form calcium hydroxide. As this reaction results in increased volume[81], this would help better adaptation of the material to the canal walls.

Furthermore, Guigand et al.[161] points out another advantage of calcium oxide. According to them, it seems to produce an ultrastructural transformation in the dentinal matrix that has not been mineralized. Thus, on the dentinal surfaces of the root canal untouched by instrumentation, the calcium oxide would eliminate the extracellular matrix, reducing the dentin/filling material interface to a minimum, producing a more efficient sealing. The authors' observations show penetration into the dentinal tubules of a mineralized substance in the teeth filled with calcium oxide, whereas, in the teeth filled with calcium hydroxide, this penetration did not occur.

Other studies in the literature have demonstrated the sealing effectiveness of Sealapex, compared with other calcium hydroxide-based sealers, such as Sealer 26 and modified Sealer 26, although generally speaking, these cements are good marginal sealers. Sacomani[370] reported the same results as regards the apical sealing efficiency provided by Sealapex and Modified Sealer 26. Favinha[130] observed better apical sealing with Sealapex than with Modified Sealer 26. Valera et al.[469] noted the same marginal leakage between Sealapex and Sealer 26. Better sealing with AH 26, than with Sealapex[269,400], or the opposite, better sealing with Sealapex than with AH 26[85,268] has also been observed. Evidently, differences in experimental methodology might have contributed to these divergences of results, nevertheless indicating Sealapex, Modified Sealer 26, Sealer 26 and AH 26 as recommendable sealers.

Sealapex has antibacterial potential, another property that could contribute obtaining good results, which would act to inactivate bacteria that resist root canal preparation. The literature, however, has shown that zinc oxide and eugenol-based sealers produce more significant results than calcium hydroxide-based sealers. Zinc oxide and eugenol-based sealers have been shown to produce a good halo of inhibition of bacterial growth[106,324,356,420]. Al-Khatib et al.[8] also analyzed the antibacterial potential of several filling sealers against some bacterial species. After several incubation periods, the readouts showed greater antimicrobial activity for zinc oxide and eugenol-based sealers, when compared with sealers containing calcium hydroxide. Nevertheless, Canalda & Pumarola[84] comparing the behavior of calcium hydroxide-based sealers (C.R.C.S. and Sealapex) with some zinc oxide and eugenol based (Tubliseal and Endomethasone) or resin-based (AH 26) sealers against some bacterial species, observed that the inhibition halos caused by them were similar.

Nevertheless, it should be mentioned that tests are frequently conducted by direct contact of the test specimens with the bacteria seeded in the culture. Moreover, the incubation periods are always short. It is known that in zinc oxide and eugenol-based sealers, antibacterial activity is performed mainly by the liquid[323]. It is also known that after mixing the zinc oxide with eugenol, a residue of free eugenol remains. Thus, the antibacterial action of the material probably begins soon after its adaptation in the plate containing the inoculated culture medium, and effectively persists until the free eugenol is totally inactivated.

On the other hand, the antimicrobial activity of calcium hydroxide-based materials mainly depends on the performance of the hydroxyl ions[121,239,367]. As the ionization is slow and prolonged[395,426,464], it is expected that Sealapex has a slight, but persistent, inhibitory action. This hypothesis was apparently proved by Panzarini et al.[340] while treating dog's teeth with experimentally induced chronic periapical lesions, detected less presence of bacteria in the apical ramifications of the canal in the cases in which Sealapex filling sealer was used, than those in which zinc oxide and eugenol was used.

The above-mentioned hypothesis was confirmed in the in vitro study of Shalhaf et al.[393], who tested the antimicrobial activity of the Roth, C.R.C.S. and Sealapex sealers against Streptococcus faecalis. The analysis of the bacterial growth curves showed that one hour after preparation, the Roth and C.R.C.S. sealers presented a significantly better antimicrobial effect than Sealapex sealer. Twenty-four hours after preparation, the zinc oxide and eugenol-based sealers (Roth) presented better activity than the calcium hydroxide-based sealers (CRCS and Sealapex). Nevertheless, seven days after the sealers were prepared, Sealapex provided a significantly better anti-bacterial effect than the other two tested cements. The authors concluded that the antimicrobial activity of the sealers changed according to the time interval between the mixture of their components and the contact period with the bacteria.

The increase in antibacterial activity of Sealapex, with time, was also verified by Heling & Chandler[171]. The tests were made in tubes of bovine tooth dentin, previously contaminated with Streptococcus faecalis. The authors observed that the sealer presented greater activity seven days after the application, than after 24 hours.

As mentioned, the products that contain or form calcium hydroxide act efficiently on the bacteria through the hydroxyl ions liberated by the decomposition of its molecule. According to Estrela[121], the high pH caused by the liberated ions has two important enzymatic properties: it inactivates bacterial enzymes, which has an antibacterial effect, and activates tissue enzymes, which has a mineralizing effect. The above-mentioned author points out that the action mechanism of hydroxyl ions in the control of the bacterial enzymatic activity can probably be explained, as starting from the existence of a pH gradient in the cytoplasmic membrane, which would alter the transport of nutrients and organic components into the cell.

Furthermore, the antibacterial activity of calcium hydroxide acts not only on the bacteria, but also on bacterial endotoxins. This is important, because it has been admitted that these substances have fundamental participation in the synthesis and release of cytosine, mainly in osteoclast activation. It was that through hydroxyl ions, calcium hydroxide is capable of degrading endotoxins, with beneficial effects on the treatment performed[372,373].

Finally, the antibacterial activity of calcium hydroxide is complemented indirectly by its capacity to absorb carbon dioxide[92,338]. The reduction of this gas within the root canal and in the periapical atmosphere would hinder the survival of many anaerobic bacteria. This possibility was demonstrated experimentally by Kontakiotis et al.[243], after they verified that the number of optional or strict anaerobic bacteria was significantly smaller after the microorganisms had been incubated in chambers containing calcium hydroxide, than in those without it.

Some authors also admitted in addition to their antibacterial activity, hydroxyl ions resulting from calcium hydroxide stimulate alkaline phosphatase deposition[64,88,458,464]. It is known that this enzyme, found in mineralization areas with a pH of 8.6 to 10.3[309,439] is capable to of inducing calcium phosphate precipitation in the organic matrix, which reacts with the calcium ions to form hydroxyapatite crystals[383].

Therefore, if on the one hand the hydroxyl ions released by calcium hydroxide (one of the components of Sealapex), in the calcium oxide reaction with humidity, are important in modifying the periapical atmosphere of teeth with chronic periapical lesions, on the other hand, the participation of calcium ions in the formation of mineralized tissue is equally as important.

Several studies have demonstrated that no bactericidal power was detected for Sealapex and Sealer 26[123]. Duarte et al.[110] comparing Sealer 26 with Sealapex, observed that Sealer 26 had bactericidal power, which had not been noted with Sealapex. Pumarola et al.[355] noted little bactericidal action by Sealapex. Kontakiotis et al.[243] informed that Sealapex had weak bactericidal power. Siqueira-Jr. & Gonçalves[399] observed extensive areas of bacterial growth inhibition with Sealer 26, while Sealapex showed low activity.

Furthermore, Otoboni-Filho[264] reported that AH 26, the predecessor of Sealer 26, liberates formaldehyde after hardening. In his opinion, considering similarity to the formulation of Sealer 26, the same release can be admitted. It is probable that the bactericidal property of Sealer 26 is more related to the release of formaldehyde than to hydroxyl and calcium ion release, because after hardening, the material is not very soluble. Thus, Silva et al.[395], at 30 days observed a pH 11.37 for Sealapex and 9.64 for Sealer 26; with the amount of calcium released by Sealapex being larger. Among the four calcium hydroxide-based cements, the same authors observed that Sealapex showed the highest pH in all the studied periods.

Alkalinization of the root canal system by the calcium hydroxide-based sealers is evidently more problematic, mainly because of the previously mentioned buffer action of dentin that imposes resistance to pH changes. Esberard et al.[118] observed no external alkalinization of the dentin with Sealapex and Sealer 26. Staehle et al.[417] observed alkalinization only inside the canal. Fuss et al.[145], in an in vitro study, observed that the antibacterial action of Sealapex, in 1 to 7 days, was shown to be significantly greater at 7 days. Moreover, in vitro experiments conducted by Shalhav et al.[393] analyzed the antibacterial activity of the Roth, CRCS and Sealapex sealers against *Streptococcus faecalis*. The sealers were prepared, and after the periods of 1 hour, 24 hours and 7 days after mixture, a suspension of bacteria was put in contact with the filling sealers. Bacterial growth was evaluated every 30 minutes, for 16 hours. At the times of 1 hour and 24 hours, Sealapex sealer exhibited antibacterial activity inferior to that of the other two sealers. However, at 7 days, it provided an antibacterial effect significantly superior to that of the other studied sealers. The increase in antibacterial activity in the course of time was also demonstrated in experiments with dentin tubes contaminated with S. faecalis. Thus, at seven days, there was greater antibacterial activity had been observed at 24 hours[171].

It should be pointed out that Sealapex is more soluble than Sealer 26 and it has a higher pH. In its formulation Sealapex has calcium oxide which, when in contact with tissue fluids, changes into calcium hydroxide that releases calcium and hydroxyl ions that would be diffused by the root canal system. Thus, from the theoretical point of view, when this sealer comes into contact with tissue fluids, this would release the above-mentioned ions for an undetermined period, given its solubility. With Sealer 26 being less soluble, this would not happen. Furthermore, it is not known whether Sealer 26 would have long term bactericidal action through formaldehyde release at a distance. Remember that along with the hydroxyl ions, calcium ions are released, which compete not only to reduce the local carbon gas, but also participate in the repair with the formation of calcite granulations.

In practice, considering the various factors involved in calcium hydroxide-based sealers found on the market, there is good reason for choosing Sealapex paste or solid, depending on the retrofilling technique used.

Thus, based on the excellent results obtained by Holland & Souza[213], Sealapex has been used for some years, in retrograde root canal treatment, of the same pasty consistency as that used in conventional root canal treatment[40,51]. In these publications the authors discussed a pilot study in which pasty Sealapex sealer showed good biological behavior, excellent dento-alveolar repair, which encouraged its indication for retrofillings, mainly in cases of retrograde root canal treatment.

Sealapex sealer can also be used in retrofillings in a thicker form[46,51,255,432], i.e., containing a larger amount of zinc oxide powder that would facilitate its insertion in apical cavities.

Solid Sealapex sealer aggregated to zinc oxide powder, in addition to providing excellent results at histopathological[40,46,51] and clinical-radiographic[255] levels, have also shown to be an excellent marginal sealer. Bernabé et al.,[50] in 1990, in an unpublished in vitro study, performed retrograde fillings with several materials, among them, Sealapex cement, in the pasty or solid form. They observed that specimens with Sealapex in the solid form, with larger amount of zinc oxide powder, showed the lowest marginal leakage indexes. The table shows that the level of marginal leakage was almost zero (last horizontal bar), compared with pasty Sealapex, which also showed little marginal leakage when compared with other studied retrofilling materials. Tanomaru-Filho et al.[431,432], with the aim of evaluating the apical sealing capacity provided by different retrofilling materials, also observed that solid Sealapex and Sealer 26 presented better marginal sealing in comparison with ZOE sealers.

Bernabé et al.[46] studying retrofillings performed with solid Sealapex sealer in dog teeth, made the interesting observation that there was partial deposition of new cementum in contact with the sealer (Fig. 25.59-25.61), and no case of complete biological apical sealing was observed. The absence of the total biological sealing is probably related to a small proportion of calcium oxide remaining in the mass of the sealer after the addition of larger amount of zinc oxide powder. Sealapex sealer actually contains calcium oxide in the proportion of 54% in its formulation, and not calcium hydroxide. When the calcium oxide in Sealapex comes into contact with the humidity of the root canal walls and periapical tissues, and absorbs this water, it will create calcium hydroxide under expansion. Theoretically, this expansion would contribute to enhancing the sealing quality of the cement. By increasing the concentration of zinc oxide in the mass of the cement, there would probably be a proportional decrease in the amount of calcium oxide, consequently originating a smaller amount of calcium hydroxide. It is known that the property of calcium hydroxide of inducing hard tissue deposition is linked to the capacity of calcium and hydroxyl ion release [216,380,388]. Thus, it is probable that the calcium ions, directly involved in the mineralization process, would be released in very small amounts, affecting the quality of the intended apical sealing[46].

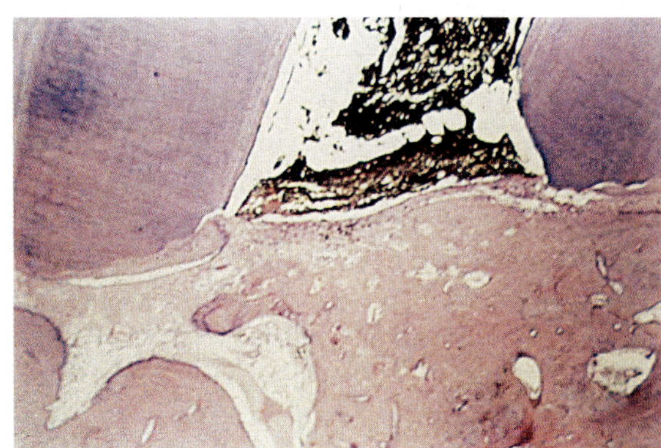

**Figure 25.59** - Fiber capsule in direct contact with the retrofilling material (H.E. X40).

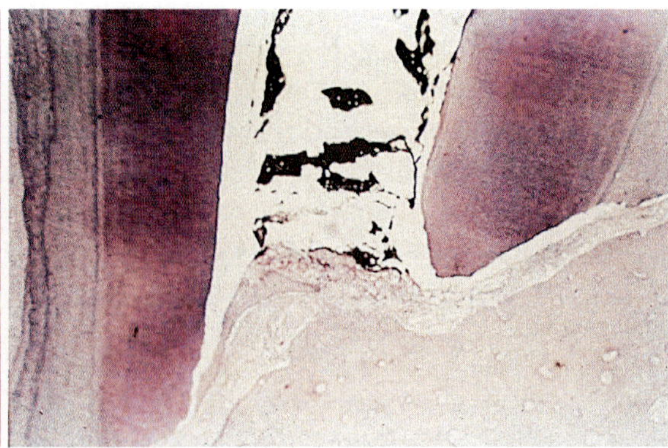

**Figure 25.60** - Partial deposition of new cementum covering the denude dentin (H.E. X15).

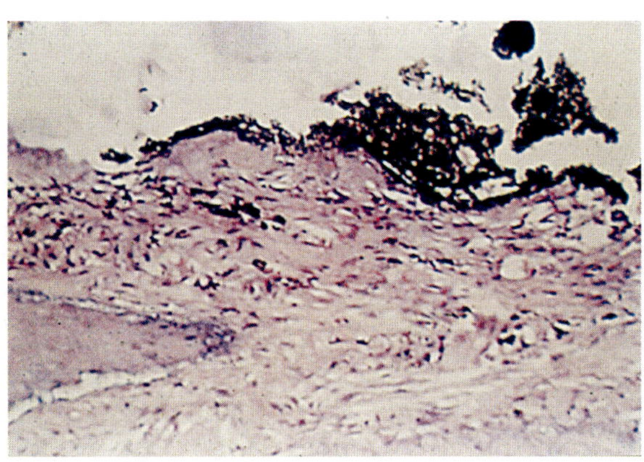

**Figure 25.61** - Partial biological sealing. Fiber capsule in direct contact with the retrofilling material. Macrophages within retrofilling material particles (H.E. X200).



Despite the divergences, some studies[395,489] have reported that calcium hydroxide-based sealers present a certain amount of disintegration, and are materials considered as possibly capable of being reabsorbed as well. This property still has to be confirmed, and further studies are required, particularly because of the divergent results probably due to differences in study methodologies.

Furthermore, among the calcium hydroxide sealers, Sealapex has been the most criticized, especially because of its solubility and reabsorption, factors that would affect the efficiency of the intended marginal sealing. Thus, Zmener et al.[489], in a study involving the subcutaneous connective tissue of mice, noted intense macrophage reaction, while Tronstad et al.[460] in a study of intra-bony implants of Sealapex sealer contained in Teflon pieces in dog's jaws, noted reabsorption and dissolution of part of the implanted material. Moreover, Sealapex was partially solubilized, and in most of the cases, was replaced by connective tissue. Tronstad et al.[460] observed that the mentioned specimens presented a histopathological condition of severe macrophage reaction and slight inflammatory reaction. Several authors who conducted studies on the biocompatibility of Sealapex[70,213,395] also observed the presence of macrophages near the location where cement had overflowed containing dark granulated material inside their cytoplasms.

These reabsorptions occurred with Sealapex, nevertheless, they were not observed histologically in root canal fillings performed in dog's and monkey's teeth [70,196,213], when the cement remained inside the canal, and no appreciable alterations in marginal sealing were noted when the filled specimens were submerged in water for 75 days. According to Holland et al.[195], in long term control, no radiographic data was observed that could suggest resorptions of the material inside the canal. This was also reported by Gutman & Fava[163].

In a histopathological study conducted by Bernabé et al.[46] in dog's teeth, no evidence of reabsorption of the material that could affect the results was observed. As previously mentioned, Sealapex has been used with or without the aggregation of zinc oxide powder for over fifteen years, and radiographically nothing has been observed that confirms the resorption of this. Long term radiographic follow up of human teeth, in which Sealapex was used as a retrofilling material, still shows evidence of the retrofilling material in place, (radiopacity) without signs of being resorbed (Fig. 25.62-25.63). Furthermore, in another study developed by Holland et al.[197], the authors demonstrated that there was no resorption, despite the postoperative time of one year and ample contact between the mentioned material and the periapical tissues.

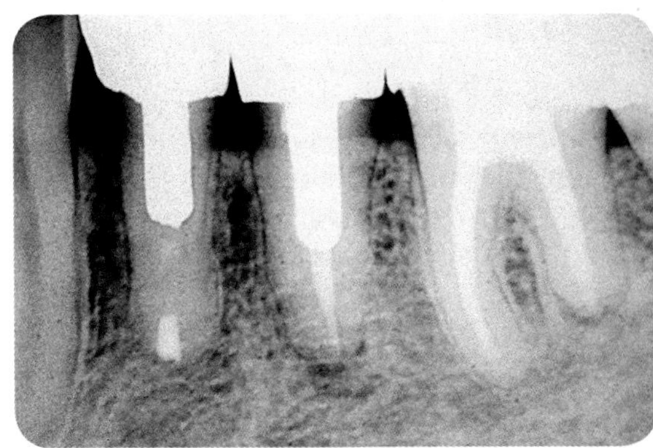

Figure 25.62 - Retrofilling with Sealapex at 15 years ago. No radiographic evidence of reabsorption of the material.

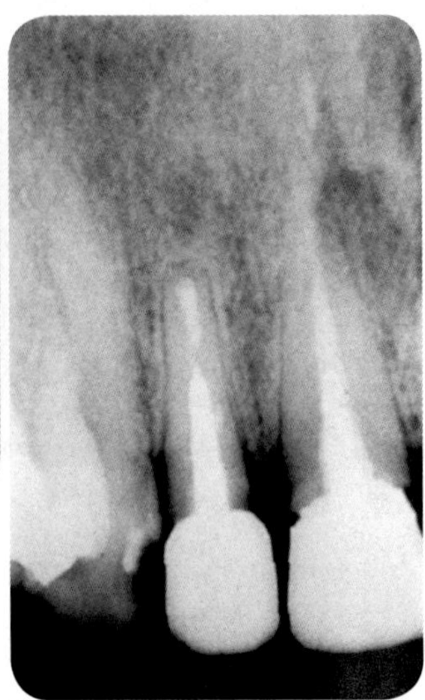

Figure 25.63 - Retrofilling with Sealapex at 8 years ago. No radiographic evidence of reabsorption of the material.

Holland & Souza[213] observed that in cases in which Sealapex sealer had overflowed into the periapical tissues, the histopathological results were different. In some specimens, there was presence of chronic inflammatory reaction around the material, with a high frequency of macrophages, and with particles of filling material inside the cytoplasm, suggesting that the material was being resorbed. Nevertheless, in other specimens, the overfilled material was encapsulated by a hard tissue, and in addition to the particles of material, new formed cementum tissue was also visualized enclosed in it, and apparently not resorbed. These results were confirmed in another experiment performed by Holland et al.[197], who observed hard tissue deposition in cases in which Sealapex was contained inside the canal or even when discreetly near the apical foramen. In 1985, Holland & Souza[213], in a study in dog and monkey teeth, assessed Sealapex capacity to induce hard tissue formation, the authors observed that in cases of overfilling the sealer, there was formation of an osteoid tissue or resorption of the material in the affected area.

In 1989, Tagger & Tagger[427] also verified that Sealapex had apparently been solubilized and substituted by a new mineralized tissue. These authors believed this solubilization of Sealapex to be beneficial, because when the sealer was replaced by cementum tissue, it would prevent leakage through the apical foramen, because of obliteration by mineralized material.

Gutmann & Fava[163] reported a clinical case in which there was overfilling of the sealer Sealapex after they filled the root canals of a central and lateral incisor. After 4 months, complete dissolution of the Sealapex and decrease in periapical radiolucent areas was observed radiographically.

In 1991, Sleder et al.[402], after in vitro filling of human teeth, analyzed the solubility of a calcium hydroxide-based sealer, Sealapex, compared with the Tubli-Seal, after leaving them submerged in saline solution. The solutions were changed weekly, to allow continuous dissolution of the cements, and to prevent a balance from being established between the solution and the sealer. The results showed that Sealapex was not more soluble than Tubli-Seal, suggesting that Sealapex could resist exposure to tissue fluids, without significant leakage, which could allow more time for the biochemical action of calcium hydroxide.

As regards Sealapex resorption, Silva[395] verified the formation of mineralized tissue in the overfilled material, suggesting that possible solubilization of the material had been replaced by mineralized tissue. This solubilization of Sealapex, which Barnett et al.[24] interpreted as a disadvantage, in Silva's opinion[395] should be rethought, since he understands that studies with the "usage test", as regards apical sealing are scarce, and its correlation with secondary tests is difficult to extrapolate. In cases of contaminated canals with periapical lesions, relative solubilization would still be more desirable considering the antibacterial activity and neutralization of the acidic pH of the area.

In a study using polyethylene tubes filled with several filling materials, among them Sealapex, implanted in mouse subcutaneous connective tissues for the period of 14 and 90 days, Valera[470] verified that the Sealapex caused an inflammatory reaction with prevalence of macrophage cells. These cells interacted intensely and directly with the material and their cytoplasms were shown to be loaded with black particles, probably proceeding from the filling material. Similar reactions were observed by Loyal et al.[256]; Molloy et al.[299], while Holland & Souza[213] only observed this reaction, when the sealer overflowed into the periapical tissues in root canal fillings of dog teeth. Valera[470] verified that this sealer remained inside the tubes, where only the phagocytized particles were carried by the macrophages. The author observed, a larger concentration of macrophages around this sealer, loaded with particles of the material, enlarging the inflammatory area, but not hindering the fibroses and fibroblastic proliferation, as observed in the postoperative period of 90 days.

According to Valera[470], the responses obtained are probably explained by the great interaction between the macrophages and Sealapex sealer. In agreement with Berbert & Consolaro[35], the polymorphonuclear contact with the Sealapex sealer releases enzymes to the extracellular environment, destroying the structural proteins of the tissue. It is possible that this tissue lyses can attract macrophages to this area. According to Camargo[83], this sealer interacts with the macrophages, favoring constant cellular renewal, required and stimulated by the cellular death that occurs.

In this same study, using Atomic Force Microscopy, Valera[470] observed that Sealapex sealer presented extensive disintegration, seen after six months. This Sealapex sealer property involves release of the products of this disintegration. Similar results were obtained by Tagger et al.[426], who reported solubilization of this cement and its capacity to disintegrate. They also observed calcium and hydroxyl ions release sixty minutes after it was mixed. Furthermore, they found an increase in pH in the course of time. Leonardo et al.[263] agreed with the results of Tagger et al.[426] when they observed that the release of ions from Sealapex is high and very fast. Also in agreement with the studies of Valera[470], the alterations observed on the surface of Sealapex sealer are related to its disintegration, when extensive structural alterations were detected in the course of time. However, after six months, the surface of the material reached a more uniform characteristic suggesting that the disintegration the sealer underwent might have decreased or even halted.

Fidel et al.[132] conducted an in vitro study of the solubility and disintegration of calcium hydroxide-based endodontic sealers, CRCS, Apexit, Sealer 26 and Sealapex. For each sealer six test specimens were made using Teflon molds. After a period three times longer than the normal time taken for the sealer to harden, the test specimens were taken out of the mold, weighed, put in plastic containers containing distilled deionized water, and kept in the incubator for seven days. After this period, the samples were washed, dehumidified for 24 hours, then submitted to a second weighing. The loss of mass of each sample was recorded and the numerical value considered as being the solubility and the disintegration of the material. The results were based on ADA specification #57, in which the Apexit and Sealer 26 sealers presented low solubility and disintegration indexes; but Sealapex presented a higher index. As regards CRCS, the solubility and disintegration reached the maximum limit indicated by the ADA specification.

In an in vitro study conducted by Silva[395], analyzing the concentration of ionic calcium in four calcium hydroxide-based sealers (Sealapex, CRCS, Apexit and Sealer 26), it could be inferred that Sealapex showed the highest solubility. In subcutaneous tissue, this solubility, releasing $Ca^{+2}$ ions to the tissues, with subsequent elimination of the material by macrophage activity, played an important role in cellular differentiation and fibroplasias. The author believes that the amount of calcium hydroxide contained in the calcium hydroxide-based cements resulted in a larger or smaller amount of free or conjugated calcium, however, the amount of ionic calcium was exponentially different, possibly because of its greater solubilization.

This is of clinical relevance, in view of the statement that solubility is an inconvenient property of sealers. In the case of Sealapex, however, it would be beneficial from the physiochemical and biological point of view. Greater calcium ion release would lead to the beginning of the mineralization process, by the immediate formation of calcium carbonate, also observed by Holland et al.[187], soon after the application of calcium hydroxide on the pulp tissue of dog teeth. Furthermore, according to Silva, the continuity of ionization of calcium hydroxide will depend on the composition and solubility of the material, and should have a great deal of influence on the final mineralization of the tissue. Today, it is known that when the root canal is filled with a calcium hydroxide-based sealer, the dissociation of calcium and hydroxyl ions, which stimulates the process of biological apical sealing, is desirable.

Another material that deserves more emphasis at present, however, is MTA (Mineral Trioxide Aggregate), developed in Loma Linda University - California, United States.

**Mineral Trioxide Aggregate, MTA**

An important discovery appeared in the area of endodontics and resulted in a great revolution in Dentistry. In 1993, Lee et al.[261] published the first scientific work using a new material: MTA. Through an in vitro study, the authors tested this new material experimentally in cases of lateral radicular perforation in human molars. In this experiment, the authors still used IRM and silver amalgam. The analysis, performed with aid of optical microscopy, after immersion of the specimens in methylene blue for 48 hours, demonstrated that the MTA group presented the lowest rates of marginal leakage, being statistically superior to the other materials. In that same year, Torabinejad et al.[456] using human teeth, compared the sealing ability of MTA with silver amalgam and IRM, by means of marginal leakage of fluorescent Rodamina B. They also observed that MTA presented hermetic marginal sealing, being superior to Super EBA, which presented less infiltration compared with silver amalgam.

The Mineral Trioxide Aggregate (MTA) appeared in the early 1990s, as an experimental material developed by Prof. Mahmoud Torabinejad. It was prepared at the Loma Linda University - California, United States, with the goal of eliminating communication between the interior and exterior of the tooth. According to Lee et al.[261], it was originally indicated as a retrofilling material, after the performance of endodontic surgeries, and in cases of intra-radicular and furcation perforations.

MTA has also been researched and is suitable under different clinical conditions however: in perforations resulting from communication between internal and external resorptions, in the conservative treatment of dental pulp (pulpotomy and pulp capping), and as stimulating material for apexification. Moreover, it has been used as an intra-coronal barrier before dental bleaching and as apical plug in cases of difficulties with fixing the main gutta-percha cone. More daring indications include its use as endodontic sealer in the treatment of deciduous and permanent teeth. In reality, MTA can be used in a humid environment, as occurs in most of the mentioned indications, due to its composition and mainly because of its biocompatibility.

According to Lee et al.[261], MTA hardens in the presence of humidity. It is supplied as a powder (Fig. 25.64) of fine hydrophilic particles that harden after hydration. The powder is composed mainly of tricalcic silicate, tricalcic aluminate, tricalcic oxide and silicate oxide, in addition to a small amount of other mineral oxides, and the addition of bismuth oxide, mainly responsible for the radiopacity of the material[446].



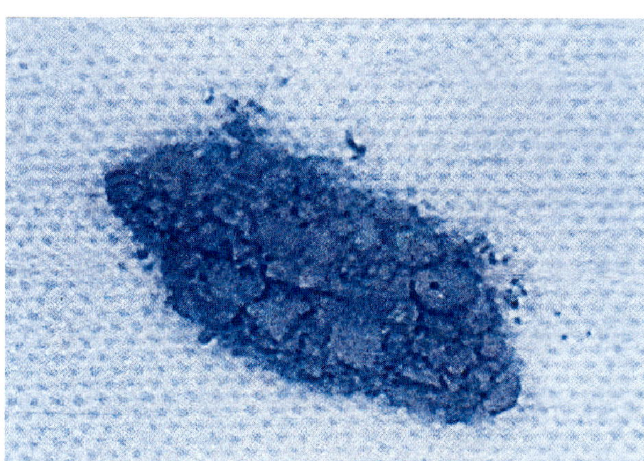

**Figure 25.64** - Macroscopic aspect of powder of gray MTA.

In 1998, MTA was evaluated and approved by American FDA (U.S. FOOD AND DRUGS ADMINISTRATION) and released commercially in 1999, as ProRoot MTA® (Dentsply Dental Tulsa, Oklahoma - USA). From what can be seen, the related publications always refer to its composition, introducing some small modifications, perhaps because it was not intended to reveal the true identity of the product.

According to study of Torabinejad et al.[446], the main molecules present in MTA are calcium and phosphorus ions. According to these authors, since these ions are also the main components of dental tissues, they confer excellent biocompatibility on MTA, when in contact with cells and tissue. The analysis performed demonstrated that after hardening, MTA is constituted of calcium oxide in the form of discreet crystals, and calcium phosphate with an amorphous structure, and a granular aspect. The average composition of the prisms is made up of 87% calcium, 2.47% silica, and the rest is oxygen. The areas of the amorphous structure contain 33% calcium, 49% phosphate, 2% carbon, 3% chloride and 6% silica. Through chemical trials and X-ray diffraction, Herzog-Flores et al.[173] analyzed the physical-chemical composition of MTA reporting that 18% of it is insoluble in water, 0.36% would correspond to MgO and 90% to CaO, its structure being 80% crystalline. Through atomic absorption spectrophotometry they quantified the release of calcium ions from MTA in 24 hours (8.8 ppm), 7 days (10.08 ppm) and 15 days (10.10).

More recently, (early 2001), the manufacturer of ProRoot MTA® modified some of the information contained in original MSDS (Material Safety Data Sheet), adding that the material is composed of 75% Portland cement, 20% bismuth oxide and 5% dehydrated calcium sulfate. That fact was omitted in experimental studies and original descriptive leaflets until then, as could be attested via the Internet, when we accessed the site of Dentsply - Tulsa Dental, in March, 1999.

Truly, the original composition of MTA always caused curiosity in those who were interested in the material. This mystery started to be solved when Wucherpfening & Green[484] published an abstract about the mentioned material. In this short summary, the authors affirmed that this material was almost identical macroscopically, microscopically and by the diffraction of x-rays to Portland cement (cement used in constructions). The authors added that these two materials had similar behavior in cell cultures and also when applied to the pulp of rat teeth. Curiously, these observations have not yet been published, being limited to this abstract.

Estrela et al.[122] however, studied the chemical and antibacterial properties of some materials, including Portland cement (Cimento Portland Itaú – Minas Gerais, Brazil) and MTA. They observed that Portland cement contained the same chemical elements as MTA, except bismuth (Note: bismuth oxide is added to the product to confer adequate radiopacity). The authors also observed that Portland cement had antibacterial activity and pH, similar to that of MTA.

At the same time, Holland et al.[192] studied Portland cement (Cimento Itaú – Minas Gerais, Brazil), MTA and chemically pure calcium hydroxide, filling dentin tubes and implanting them in rat's subcutaneous rat tissues, as done with the latter two materials[191]. The results between MTA and Portland cement were similar, or in other words, calcite granulations were observed in contact with the studied materials, and also inside the dentinal tubules. Moreover, a Von Kossa positive bridge of hard tissue was also observed. According to the results obtained, the authors suggest that the action mechanism of the 3 materials is similar. With the objective of confirming these data, other experimental projects were developed.

Holland et al.[182] performed fillings of 20 root canals in dog teeth, 10 with MTA and 10 with Portland cement. After the root canal preparation, the cements were prepared with saline solution and put into the root canal with the aid of a Lentulo drill, followed by filling with the lateral condensation technique. Ninety days after the filling, the pieces were removed and processed for histomorphological analysis. Eight cases of biological sealing with new cementum were observed with MTA, at different levels and with absence of inflammatory infiltrate (Fig. 25.65). The other two specimens exhibited partial sealing and/or absence of sealing with little overfilling and little chronic inflammatory infiltrate in both cases. With Portland cement seven cases of complete biological sealing at the level of the apical foramen occurred (Fig. 25.66) and one inside the canal. The last two cases had partial biological sealing, one at the foramen and the other intracanal, both exhibiting little chronic inflammatory infiltrate. The result of this study confirmed the data obtained in two other experiments performed in rat's subcutaneous tissues[192], and the pulp of dog's teeth[185] (Fig. 25.67-25.68). Saidon et al.[374] performing implants of Pro-Root MTA and Portland Cement in rat jaws, after 2 and 12 months verified bone repair, with minimal inflammatory process, occurred adjacent to both materials, proving that they are well tolerated when implanted.



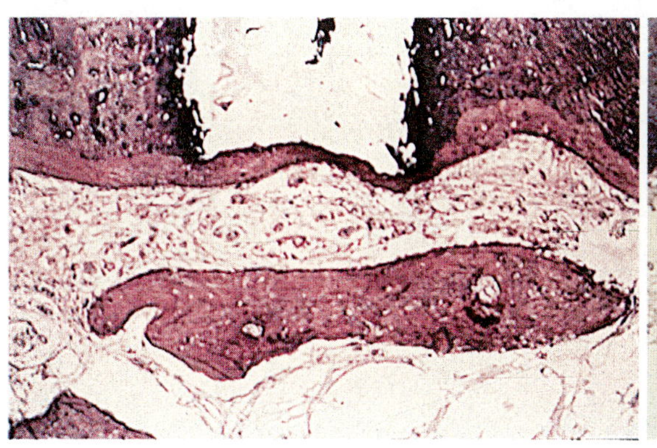

**Figure 25.65** - Filling with MTA (90 days). Biological sealing with new cementum. Absence of inflammatory process (H.E. X100).

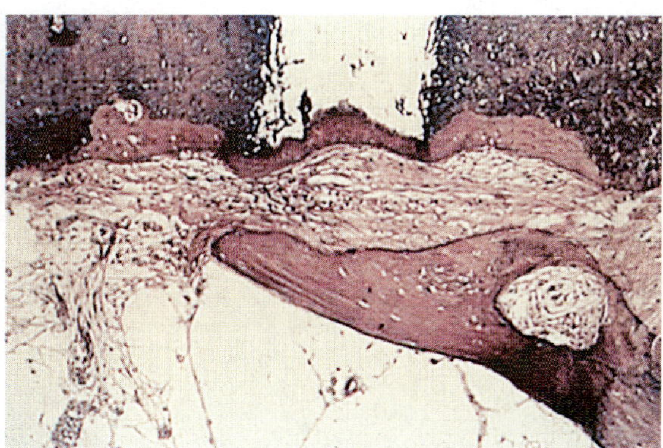

**Figure 25.66** - Filling with Portland cement (90 days). Biological sealing with new cementum. Absence of inflammatory process (H.E. X100).

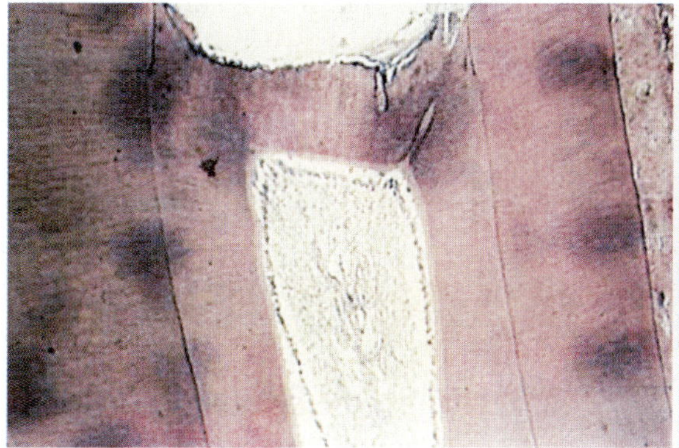

**Figure 25.67** - Pulpotomy in dog's teeth with MTA (60 days) (H.E. X40).

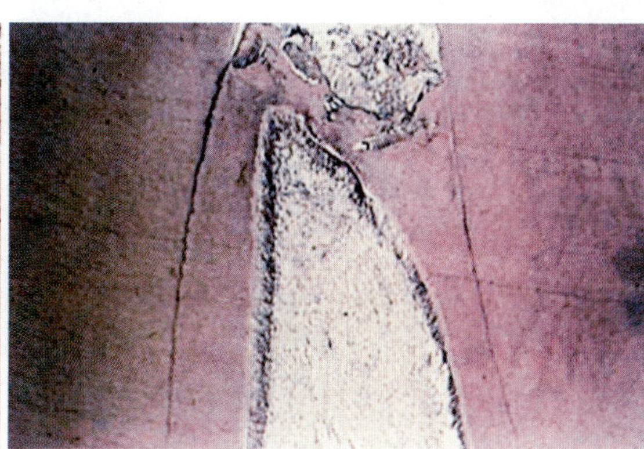

**Figure 25.68** - Pulpotomy in dog's teeth with Portland cement (60 days) (H.E. X40).

Bernabé et al.[42], using the contaminated root canals of dog's teeth performed retrofillings with MTA and Portland Cement. After the period of 180 days, they observed similar results between the two products, in which many of the specimens analyzed, histopathological analysis showed the deposition of cementum tissue in direct contact to the retrofilling material, characterizing biological sealing (Fig. 25.69-25.70). Similar results had been observed by Bernabé et al.[58] under the same experimental conditions, using MTA in comparison with IRM, Super EBA and consistent ZOE (Fig. 25.71-25.72).

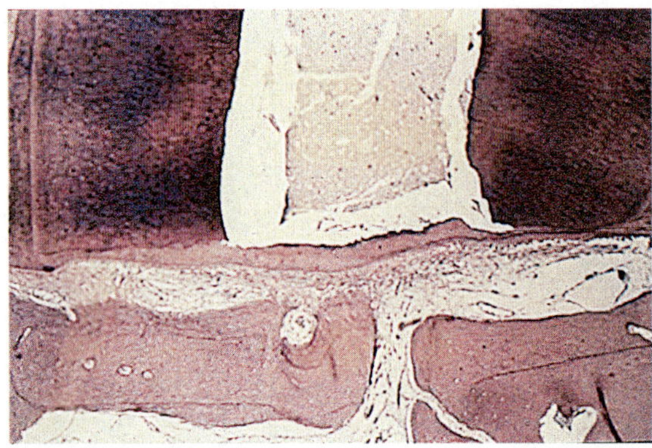

**Figure 25.69** - Biological sealing after retrofilling with MTA (H.E. X40).

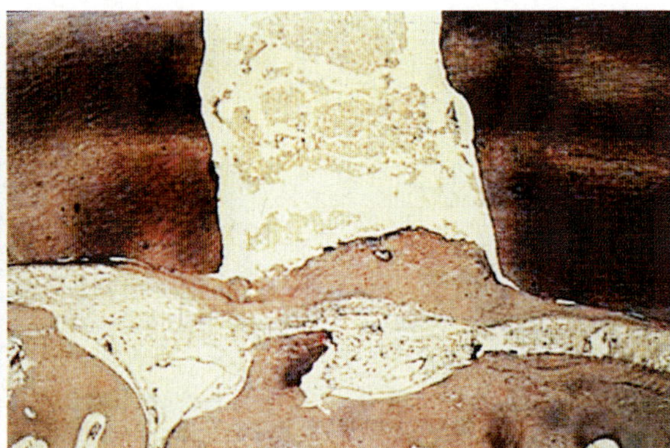

**Figure 25.70** - Biological sealing after retrofilling with Portland cement (H.E. X40).

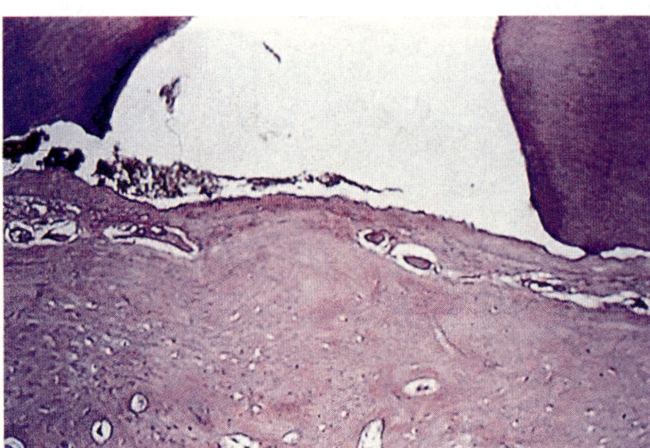

**Figure 25.71** - New cementum covering denude dentin and retrofilling material (H.E. X100).

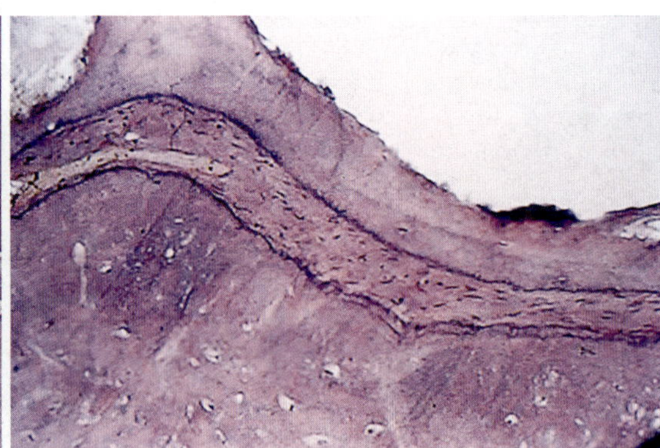

**Figure 25.72** - Total biological sealing. New cementum covering retrofilling material (H.E. X200).

From the above description, it is observed that all the experiments mentioned, support the results reported by Wucherpfening & Green[484] and Estrela et al.[122] that suggest that MTA and Portland cement are similar materials.

The studies of Safavi & Nichols[371] comparing the effects of MTA and Portland cement on the secretion of PGE2 of monocytes should also be mentioned. These authors demonstrated that the soluble products of MTA and Portland cement presented a similar inhibitory effect on the secretion of PGE2 of monocytes. Franco[140] studied the reaction of the filter area tissue of 10 rats to the implant of polyethylene tubes filled with MTA (ProRoot MTA®) and Portland cement (Cimento Zebu). The results demonstrated that the tissue response in 2 weeks was similar for both materials, being characterized by acute inflammatory reaction, milder sensitivity to ProRoot MTA® with predominance of fibrous tissue, fibrin and congested vessels, lymphocytes and giant cells in some samples of Portland cement. Moraes et al.[302] implanting polyethylene tubes filled with Portland cement in rat's subcutaneous connective tissue for the periods of 7, 12 and 60 days, observed the latter was biocompatible. With the object of finding an alternative to the study of MTA, Abdullah et al.[2] developed experiments in cell cultures with a new type of Portland Cement with an accelerated hardening time, in comparison with a glass ionomer cement, MTA and unmodified Portland Cement. The results after 12, 24, 48 and 72 hours, demonstrated that both variations of Portland Cement were not toxic and had the potential to produce bone repair. They verified that the addition of calcium chloride (10 and 15%, as accelerating agent, did not produce any adverse effect, enhancing the biocompatibility of the material. These studies open perspectives to enable the production of a material for dental restoration and also for orthopedic use.

Based on the series of studies conducted with MTA, as well as the studies that compared MTA with Portland Cement, the company Angelus®, in Londrina – Paraná, Brazil, performed a series of analysis until they achieved Brazilian formula for MTA, and released it on the market registered as MTA-Angelus®, in competition with ProRoot MTA® of Dentsply. Holland et al.[193] implanted MTA-Angelus® in rat subcutaneous connective tissues after being introduced into dentinal tubules, with the purpose of observing whether the tissue behavior was similar to Pro-Root MTA®. With the aid of polarized light and Von Kossa reaction it was demonstrated that the tissue behavior analysis was identical to that related for Dentsply ProRoot MTA® cement. Thus, calcite granulations were observed close to the material (Fig. 25.73) and inside the dentinal tubules (Fig. 25.74). Near the material on the lumen of the tube, the formation of a Von Kossa positive hard tissue bridge was observed, as well as calcite granulations (Fig. 25.75).

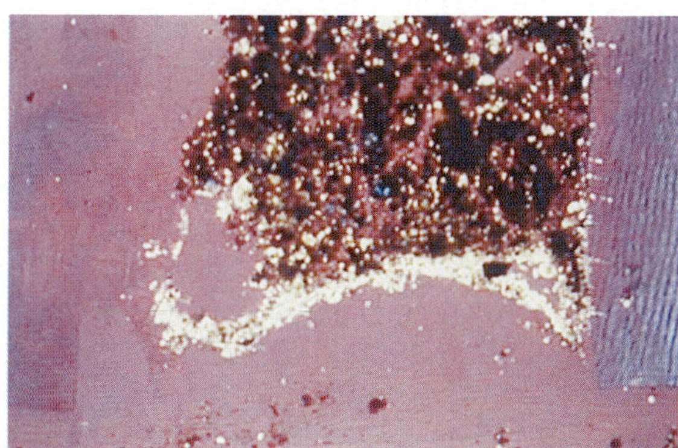

**Figure 25.73** - MTA-Ângelus® - 30 days implanted in rat subcutaneous connective tissues. Calcite granulations close to the material (Polarized light, X40).

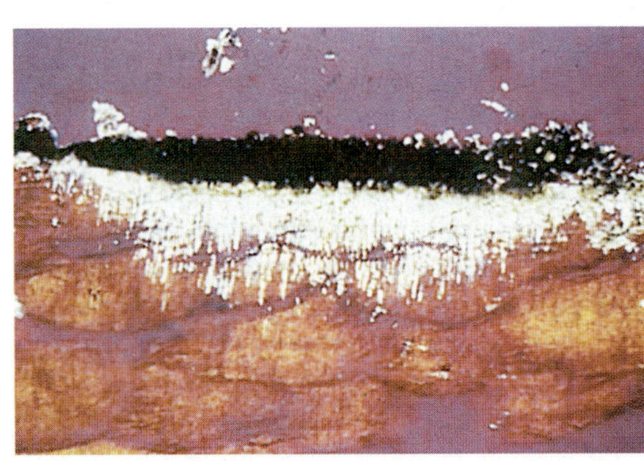

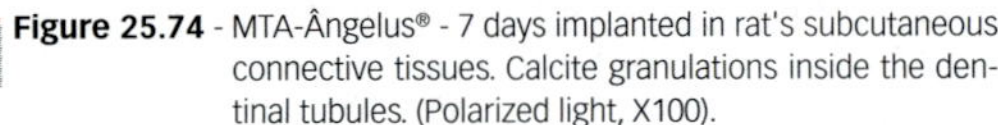

**Figure 25.74** - MTA-Ângelus® - 7 days implanted in rat's subcutaneous connective tissues. Calcite granulations inside the dentinal tubules. (Polarized light, X100).

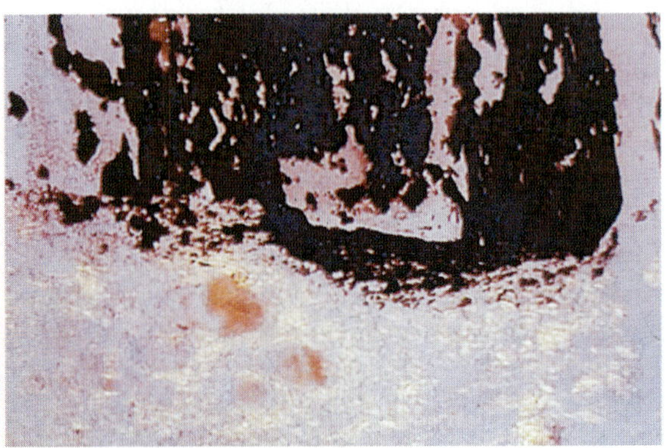

**Figure 25.75** - MTA-Ângelus® - 7 days implanted in rat's subcutaneous connective tissues. Formation of a Von Kossa positive hard tissue bridge near the MTA on the lumen of the tube. (X100).

In view of the results of the aforementioned studies, MTA and Portland cement behaved similarly. Considerations about Portland cement (construction cement) being the basis of the commercial products ProRoot MTA and the MTA Angelus®, released in Brazil, will be made. Such considerations are important to gain better knowledge of this material that revolutionized the dentistry field, and from this knowledge, understand its behavior and propose improvements in its potential, either as regards its physical or biological properties.

Studies about the marginal sealing ability of MTA, compared with other materials, after the use of dye or even bacteria penetration, has shown that it is the most effective sealant.

### Biologic properties of MTA and Portland cement

Among the properties that a filling material should have, is the bactericidal or bacteriostatic effect. Some studies have demonstrated the antimicrobial potential of MTA[219,453] and Portland cement[122], showing a high alkaline pH and concentration of hydroxyl ions. The antimicrobial activity of MTA is lower than that of calcium hydroxide[122], however, probably due to the decrease in ionic diffusion of hydrated products over the course of time. Torabinejad et al.[449] compared the antimicrobial effect of silver amalgam, zinc oxide and eugenol, Super EBA and MTA. None of the studied materials demonstrated antimicrobial activity against strict anaerobic microorganisms. With MTA, however, some effect on 5 of 9 types of facultative bacteria studied could be observed. Hong et al.[219] showed the antimicrobial effect of MTA against some bacteria, having a larger effect against *Lactobacillus sp, Streptococcus mitis, Streptococcus mutans* and *Streptococcus salivarius* and a lower antimicrobial effect against *Streptococcus faecalis*.

Kettering & Torabinejad[235] using the AMES test, conducted a study to evaluate the mutagenic potential of MTA, Super EBA®, IRM®. The results demonstrated that these materials do not have carcinogenic potential.

As regards the toxicity of MTA, which has been investigated by several researchers, either in in vitro experiments (cell cultures) or in vivo (implants in bone tissue of different animals, in rat's subcutaneous connective tissues, dog's teeth, monkeys etc.), all demonstrating that it has excellent biological behavior[444,447]. Pitt-Ford et al.[349] and Torabinejad et al.[443] reported that MTA has shown the ability to stimulate the release of cytokines from osteoblasts, indicating that it actively promotes hard tissue formation, and participates directly in this process, being much more than a simple inert material. Koh et al.[241], in a cytomorphological study in the presence of human osteoblasts, also reported that MTA favored stimulation of cytokine production, allowing cell adhesion to the material. Exams with scanning electronic microscopy revealed the presence of healthy cells in contact with MTA in the periods of 1 and 3 days, as well as the presence of elevated levels of interleukin and osteocalcin. Thompson et al.[440] evaluated the capacity of a culture of cementoblasts to differentiate on the surface of MTA, by observing the production of prosthetic markers of mineralization. The results demonstrated that MTA promoted the production of osteocalcin, thus stimulating the production of a mineralized matrix by the cementoblasts. The increase in the release of interleukin was also proved by Mitchell et al.[298] The participation of MTA in stimulating the activation of cell response, according to Koh et al.[240] is due to the calcium phosphate phase. This phase seems to cause a change in cellular behavior, stimulating the adhesion of the osteoblasts near the MTA. The cytotoxicity of MTA was also the object of a study by Osorio et al.[330], in several materials indicated for retrofillings, when it was observed that MTA had the lowest level of cytotoxicity. This property of MTA was also investigated by Zhu et al.[448], who inserted MTA in a cell culture, and observed by SEM that osteoblasts adhered to and spread over its surface. Keiser et al.[234], also studying the cytotoxicity of MTA in cell cultures of the human periodontal ligament, observed that it was biocompatible, favoring its indication for retrofillings. Moretton et al.[305], based on the results with MTA, after intra-osseous implants in rat's subcutaneous connective tissues, reported that this material would be an osteoconductor and not osteoinductive. Recently, Abdullah et al.[2] studying MTA, Portland Cement and two variations of Portland cement with the addition of calcium chloride (10% and 15%), to accelerate its hardening, could verify high levels of cytokine and osteocalcin release. With MTA, they observed that the indexes of cytokine and osteocalcin release remained in progression for up to 48 hours, after which a reduction of these levels occurred. With modified Portland Cement (with calcium chloride), however, they noted that the concentrations of cytokine and osteocalcin continued to remain elevated for up to 72 hours. There was significant cellular growth on the surface of these materials, covering it totally, demonstrating its biocompatibility. In the author's opinion, the cells found on the surface of modified Portland cement (with calcium chloride) suggests that the surface of the material is not irritant and does not affect the structural integrity of the cell, keeping its cytoplasmic extensions, which is important, because this configuration allows a tridimensional integration with the bone tissue.

**Action Mechanism of MTA**

Comparing the tissue response to MTA with that obtained when using calcium hydroxide, some similarities between the materials[53] are observed. Both seem to stimulate hard tissue formation (dentin and cementum). Lee et al.[261] informed that the main components of MTA would be tricalcic silicate, tricalcic aluminate, tricalcic oxide and silicate oxide. In addition to the trioxides there were other mineral oxides that would be responsible for the chemical and physical properties of this aggregate. Furthermore, according to these authors, MTA powder is constituted of fine thin hydrophilic particles that harden in the presence of water. Two years later, Torabinejad et al.[446] studied the physical and chemical properties of MTA. They observed that all MTA was divided into two specific phases, constituted of calcium oxide and calcium phosphate. They verified that calcium oxide presented discreet crystals and calcium phosphate, an amorphous structure. Since calcium oxide is one of components of MTA, it would theoretically explain the similarity of MTA and calcium hydroxide action.

With the purpose of better analyzing the subject, Holland et al.[191] implanted tubes of dentin filled with calcium hydroxide or MTA in rat subcutaneous tissues. The pieces were removed after 7 or 30 days and processed without being decalcified. Thus, cuts of hard tissue obtained with a microtome were analyzed for calcium salts, with the aid of polarized light and Von Kossa staining. They noted that with calcium hydroxide, there was formation of calcite granulations, birefringent to the polarized light, near the lumen of the tube (Fig. 25.76). Under these granulations a Von Kossa positive hard tissue bridge was formed (Fig. 25.77). Moreover, the presence of calcite granulations, birefringent to the polarized light, was also observed inside the dentinal tubules (Fig. 25.78). With MTA, the same was observed, only the number of calcite granulations was a little smaller than the number observed with calcium hydroxide, and these granulations were in contact with the studied material, which did not occur with calcium hydroxide (Fig. 25.79-25.81).

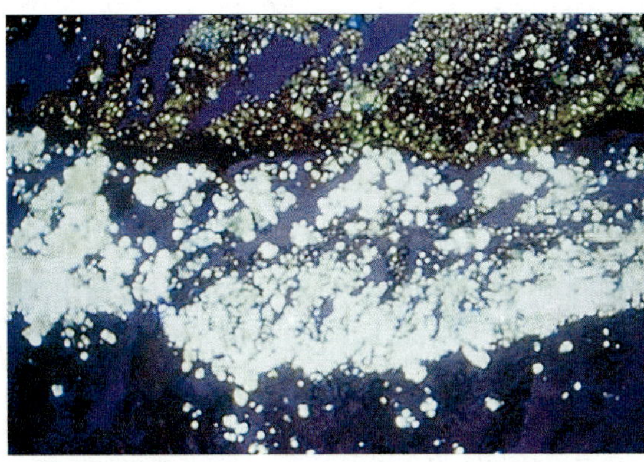

**Figure 25.76** - Calcium hydroxide (7 days). Calcite granulations, birefringent to the polarized light, near the lumen of the tube. X100.

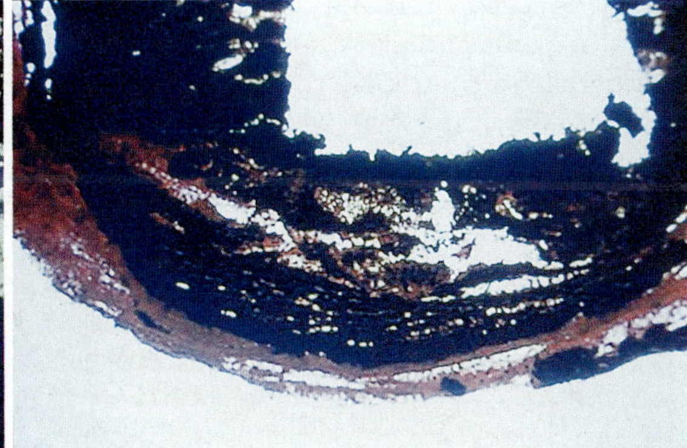

**Figure 25.77** - Calcium hydroxide (7 days). Von Kossa positive granulations, near the lumen of the tube. X40.

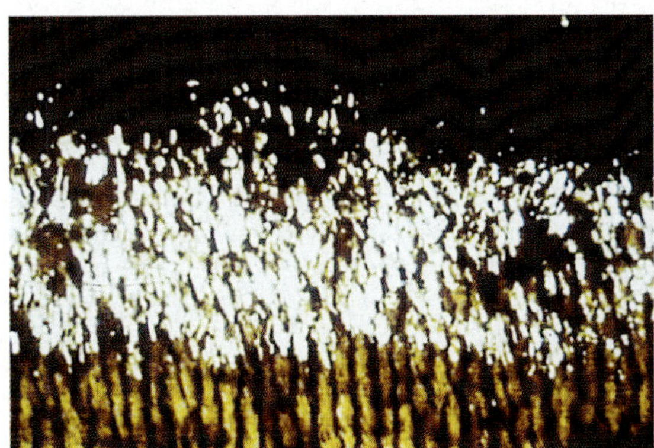

**Figure 25.78** - Calcium hydroxide (7 days). Calcite granulations, birefringent to the polarized light, inside the dentinal tubules. X100.

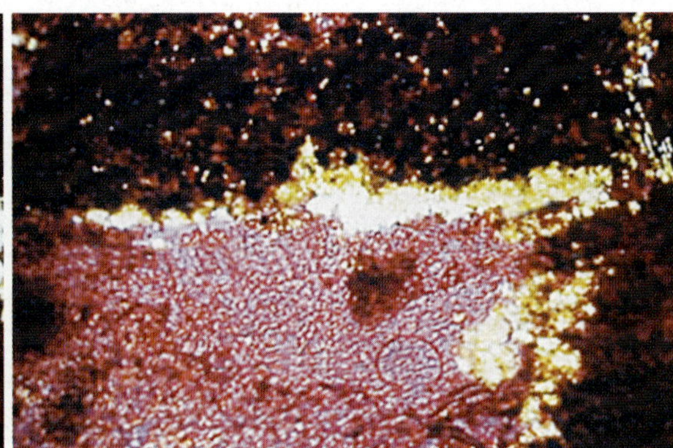

**Figure 25.79** - MTA (30 days). Calcite granulations, birefringent to the polarized light, in contact with the material. X100.

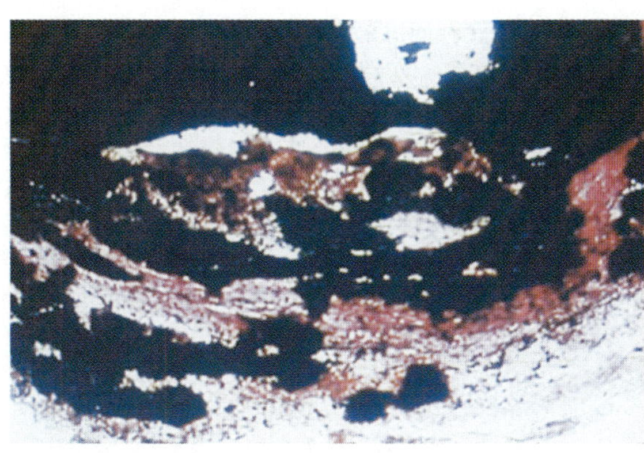

**Figure 25.80** - MTA (7 days). Von Kossa positive irregular tissue, near the lumen of the tube. X40.

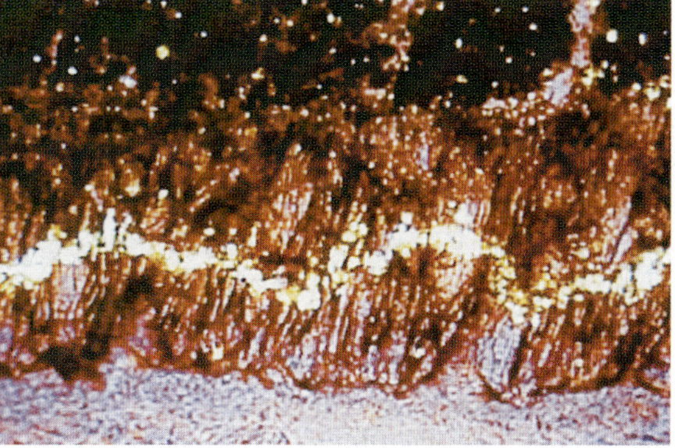

**Figure 25.81** - MTA (7 days). Calcite granulations, birefringent to the polarized light, inside the dentinal tubules. X100.

Several studies that analyzed calcium hydroxide, showed presence of calcite granulations in subcutaneous connective tissue[412], dental pulp[187,215] and periapical tissues[190,207]. According to Holland[215], these granulations are formed by the reaction of calcium hydroxide with the carbonic gas of the tissue. These same granulations were described by Seux et al.[388] in an in vitro experiment. Furthermore, the authors noted an accumulation of fibronectin, a glycoprotein, in close contact with these calcite crystals, in a culture medium without cells. When pulp cells were placed in contact with this environment, there was the formation of cells with the morphological aspect of odontoblasts. In the absence of calcite granulations, there was only proliferation of fibroblasts. Seux et al.[388] concluded that these findings constituted strong evidence of the role of the calcite granulations and of fibronectin, as the beginning of hard tissue barrier formation.

The study of Holland et al.[191], in rat subcutaneous tissues, showed a similarity of results between calcium hydroxide and MTA. Both materials determined the formation of calcite granulations and a subjacent hard tissue bridge. Therefore, the action mechanism of MTA would be the same as that of calcium hydroxide. When preparing the paste with water, the calcium oxide in MTA powder would be converted in calcium hydroxide. This, in contact with the tissue fluids would dissociate into calcium and hydroxyl ions. The calcium ions, reacting with carbonic gas of the tissues, would originate calcite granulations. Near these granulations there is an accumulation of fibronectin, which allows cellular adhesion and differentiation. There would then be formation of a hard tissue bridge.

A similar tissue reaction to that of MTA can be observed with the filling sealer, Sealapex. This sealer contains calcium oxide in its formulation. When implanting Sealapex contained in a dentin tube in rat's subcutaneous tissues, the same results described for MTA[192] were observed; that is, formation of calcite granulations and hard tissue bridge[183] occurred. This observation with Sealapex reinforces the validity of the action mechanism described for MTA.

Following up this question, one could emphasize that after MTA is hydrated, the solution becomes saturated with calcium ions ($Ca^{2+}$) and hydroxyl ions ($OH^-$) that combine with sulphate ions, silicate and aluminate, forming hydrated calcium silicates (50 to 60%), calcium hydroxide (20 to 25%) and calcium sulphoaluminates (15 to 20%), the main compounds of the hydrated paste[290].

Depending on the constant changes in ionic saturation, the calcium hydroxide formed can further solubilize and dissociate into calcium ions ($Ca^{2+}$) and hydroxyl ($OH^-$), which are mainly responsible for the action mechanism of the material[215].

Carbon dioxide ($CO_2$) produced as result of catabolism of our cells solubilizes, diffusing to the interstitial liquids and from these to the blood, being conducted in the bloodstream to the lungs, where is transformed into the gaseous state, being finally exhaled. The carbon dioxide ($CO_2$) in an aqueous solution, as in interstitial liquids or blood plasma, acts as a biological buffer, undergoing a series of reactions, including the participation of the carbonic anhydrase enzyme, with the purpose of regulating the pH of the environment where it is located, being found in several forms: $CO_2$ (carbon dioxide), $H_2CO_3$ (carbonic acid), $HCO_3$ (bicarbonate ion), $CO_3$ (carbonate ion)[114,391,392]. The pH of the pulp and periapical tissues will be influenced by its inflammatory stage; that is, under normal conditions the pH is neutral or slightly alkaline (7.2 to 7.4). In acute inflammations the pH decreases, becoming acidic (6.5 or less) due to the lactic acid from the anaerobic glycolysis of the inflammatory cells, and also due to the accumulation of $CO_2$ at the site, derived from blood stasis. In chronic inflammations, however, the pH returns to neutral (7.0 to 7.2), due to the increase of tissue vascularity[289]. Moreover, it should be emphasized that the use of topical substances and medications can also the pH of tissues.

Thus, when using a material with an alkaline pH, such as calcium hydroxide, MTA or Portland cement, on the pulp or in contact with the periapical tissues, the pH of the local tissues will be increased due to the saturated solution of hydroxyl ions ($OH^-$). As a way to balance the pH of the environment, carbon dioxide ($CO_2$), carbonic acid ($H_2CO_3$) or bicarbonate ions ($HCO_3^-$), present in the medium, will react with the hydroxyl ions, increasing the concentration of carbonate ions considerably ($CO_3^{2-}$) These will react with the calcium ions in the solution ($Ca^{2+}$) forming granulations of calcium carbonate as a form of calcite ($CaCO_3$) on the tissue[215].

These calcite granulations are characterized by presenting high birefringence, easily identified under polarized light. According to Leinz & Campos[262], the birefringence of calcite is 0.172. These granulations also can be identified by the histochemical method of Von Kossa that identifies the calcium by its black coloration. According to Carr et al.[86], the Von Kossa dye is truly a dye of substitution that demonstrates the presence of anions of insoluble calcium salts, such as $PO_4^{3-}$ and $CO_3^{2-}$, more than the calcium itself.

As already mentioned, Seux et al.[388] demonstrated, in vitro, that fibronectin presents high affinity for calcium carbonate granulations, shown by the high concentration of fibronectin around the calcite crystals.

Fibronectin belongs to a group of molecules of substratum adhesion, responsible for cellular migration, adhesion and differentiation, being produced by fibroblasts, macrophages and endothelial cells[466].

Thus, fibronectin would be responsible for the migration and adhesion of pulp and periodontal cells that would synthesize and deposit collagen type I, forming extracellular organic matrix. Moreover, fibronectin would induce the differentiation of pulp cells into odontoblasts, or cells of the periodontium into cementoblasts, mainly responsible for the deposition of minerals[388].

The liquid phase, saturated with hydroxyl ions, also seems to be responsible for the slight layer of superficial pulp necrosis, situated between the mineralized tissue bridge and the material, and found in a few specimens, submitted to pulpotomy with MTA[407] or Portland cement[185]. These observations are a little different from those noted with several calcium hydroxide pastes submitted to the same conditions[201,407]. It is emphasized that this superficial necrosis is mostly absent, and when present, it is much thinner than that observed with the chemically pure calcium hydroxide.

Holland et al.[188] developed an experimental study in dog's teeth, making experimental perforations on the lateral portion of the root, and therefore, not on the furcation as did Pitt-Ford et al.[350] These perforations were sealed with Sealapex or MTA, the results being analyzed histologically, after 30 and 180 days. The best results were observed with the use of MTA, with many cases of sealing occurring by deposition of newly formed cementum, allied to the absence of inflammation in the periodontal ligament. Small areas of alkalosis also were observed, however only at 30 days. With Sealapex, the presence of chronic inflammation was noted in all the specimens, and a small deposition of newly formed cementum on the material, in only three cases. Thus, the results were much better with the use of MTA.

In some cases, perforations were also experimentally performed at the furcation level, (data not published), and results similar to those of the lateral perforations were observed; that is, newly formed cementum in contact with MTA, sealing the perforation.

Among all cases analyzed by Holland et al.[188] the worse results were found in cases of overfilling, and a larger amount of overfilling was observed with the use of Sealapex, which was attributed to the larger outflow of this material. The worst results observed with Sealapex in perforations, when compared with the situation observed in root canal fillings, might be related to the larger area of contact with the periodontal tissues in the case of perforation[188,213]. Considering that the best results with MTA were obtained when the material was kept inside the perforation cavity, one understands the clinical importance of avoiding overfilling.

The clinical use of MTA in lateral perforations or furcation has contributed to the excellent results obtained by professionals who have used it. In addition to the disappearance of clinical symptomatology, repair of the damaged area has been observed in radiographs. The literature has shown that professionals use MTA in different clinical procedures, even without correct scientific basis.

**Use of MTA in Endodontic Surgeries**

Studies conducted by Pitt-Ford et al.[348] in dog's teeth, using silver amalgam and MTA, demonstrated that there was hard tissue formation on MTA, as well as higher deposition of osseous tissue adjacent to it, after periods of 10 and 18 weeks. Torabinejad et al.[448] also studied the biological response of periapical tissues of dog's teeth, after apicoectomy and retrograde filling with MTA. They noted that the newly formed cementum was deposited not only on the dentin exposed by the apical sectioning, but also on the studied material, presenting a satisfactory result. Results considered efficient were also obtained by Torabinejad et al.[443], who examined the response of periapical tissues of monkey's teeth to MTA and silver amalgam. After the period of 5 months, the authors noted that of the six specimens with MTA analyzed, five presented connective tissue adjacent to material free of inflammatory process, and a complete barrier of cementum deposited on it. These results contrasted with silver amalgam, because there was no sealing and in all specimens, there was the presence of an inflammatory process.

Bernabé et al.[58], using dog's teeth with contaminated canals, performed retrograde fillings with consistent ZOE, IRM, Super EBA and MTA. After 180 days had elapsed, the histopathological analysis showed similar results between the studied materials, except consistent ZOE sealer, which presented the worst results, which were attributed to the fact that this group presented a higher incidence of debris. In this study it could be observed that MTA was the only retrofilling material used, which stimulated the deposition of cementum tissue in close contact, favoring "biological sealing" (Fig. 25.71-25.72), similar to that reported by Torabinejad et al.[443,448].

With the purpose of studying the behavior of the periapical tissues of dog teeth submitted to the conventional retrograde filling, Bernabé et al.[41] investigated the influence of the type of apical preparation (retrocavities type Class 1) performed, with the aid of a rotary bur or Ultrasonic tip for retrosurgery.

These apical cavities were retrofilled with MTA and consistent ZOE sealer. The results were analyzed 180 days later, once again showing the superiority of MTA as retrofilling material, from the biological point of view. It was observed that it was the only material that stimulated cementum tissue deposition in close contact with the filling material, irrespective of whether the retrocavities had been prepared with burs or ultra sound (Fig. 25.82-25.83). Considering the general results, the authors ranked the materials from best to worst, as follows: retrocavities with ultrasound and retrofilled with MTA; retrocavities with bur and retrofilled with MTA; retrocavities with ultrasound and retrofilled with consistent ZOE; retrocavities with burs and retrofilled with consistent ZOE.

Recently an experiment was developed by Bernabé et al.[42], in which the authors performed a comparative study between MTA and Portland cement, using them in retrocavities prepared with ultrasound. Similar results between the two types of materials could be observed, also characterized by the deposition of cementum tissue, in addition to presenting complete dental-alveolar repair (Fig. 25.84-25.85), in most of the specimens analyzed.

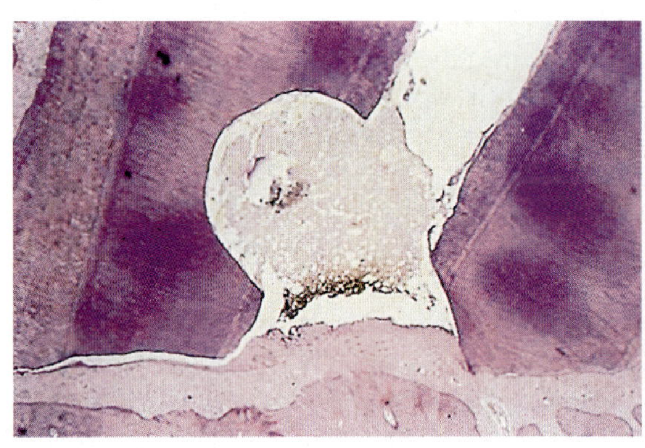

**Figure 25.82** - Retrocavity prepared with burn. Retrofilled with MTA (180 days). Formation the new cementum in contact with material (H.E. X40).

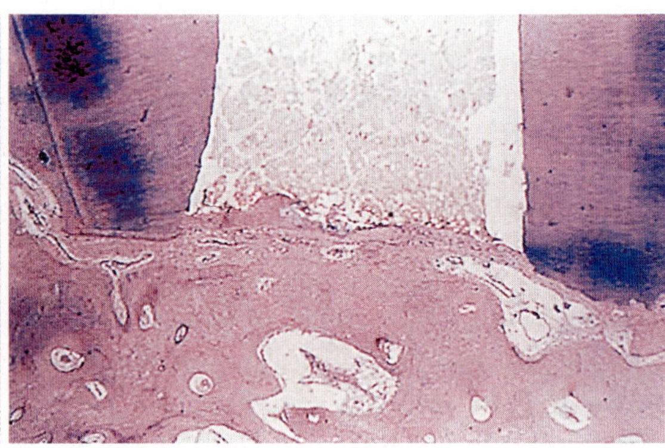

**Figure 25.83** - Retrocavity prepared with ultrasound. Retrofilled with MTA (180 days). Formation the new cementum in contact with material (H.E. X40).

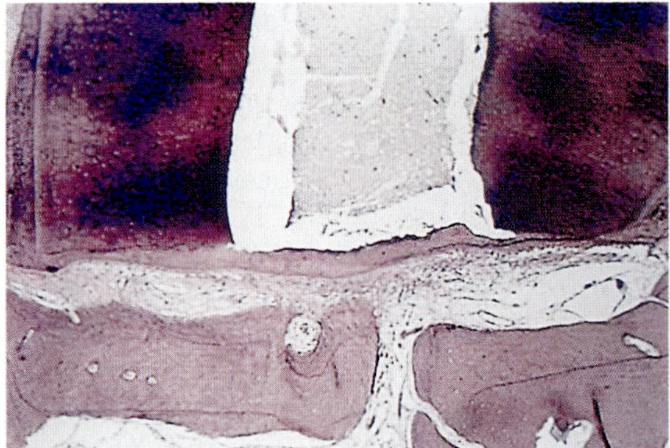

**Figure 25.84** - Retrofilling with MTA (180 days). Complete dental-alveolar repair and deposition of new cementum in contact with retrofilling material (H.E. X40).

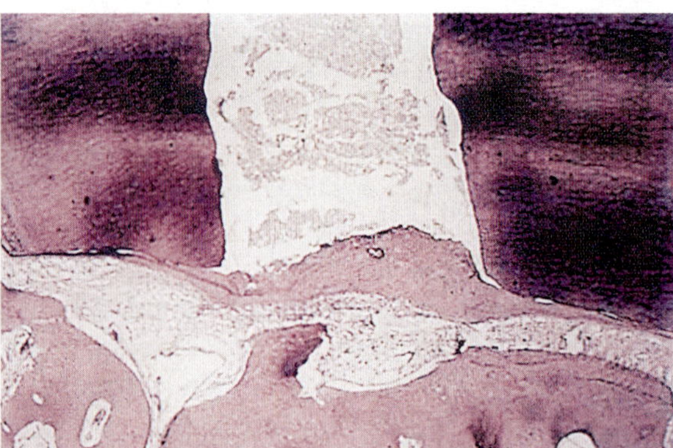

**Figure 25.85** - Retrofilling with Portland cement (180 days). Complete dental-alveolar repair and deposition of new cementum in contact with retrofilling material (H.E. X40).

## Clinical Application

After containing the hemorrhage and drying of the apical cavities with paper points, MTA is placed. It should preferably be inserted with suitable instruments such as the MAP SYSTEM (Fig. 25.86). With the tip of this instrument near the entrance of the retrocavities, MTA is gently inserted and condensed with special Bernabé Kit pressers. Practically, and to avoid bubbles during MTA insertion, this operation should performed in stages, in other words, placement of small portions and condensation, initially with thin pressers, and later using larger pressers. At the end, the material surface is lightly polished with the tip of a Dycal applier or pediatric polisher, exerting slight vertical and lateral pressure to encounter the apical cavity walls. Ultrasound can also be used to help the condensation of the material, as mentioned before. The cavity should not be irrigated at this time, due to the risks of removing the material. After this the calcium hydroxide "cap" is placed, covering the dentinal surface and the retrofilling sealer (Fig. 25.87). This cap is used to decrease the dentinal resorption that usually occurs after apicoectomies. The bone cavity is filled at the end by causing a hemorrhage or, when indicated, the placement of an implant or bone graft associated with the use of membrane or barrier.

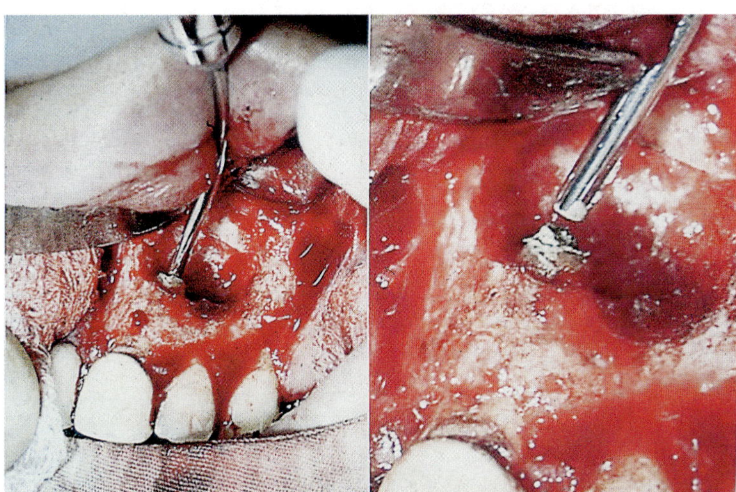

**Figure 25.86** - Insertion of MTA with MAP SYSTEM®.

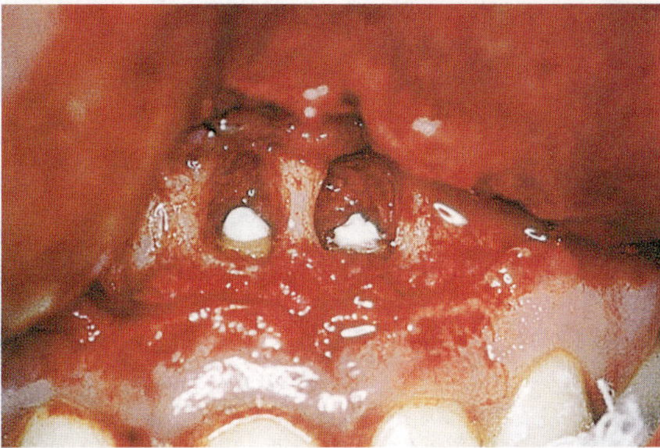

**Figure 25.87** - Calcium hydroxide "cap" covering the dentinal surface and the retrofilling material.

Final radiographic evaluation is required immediately after the sealer and cap are placed, as well as later follow up, to prove the efficiency of the operation, and long term success (Fig. 25.88-25.93).

Due to the difficulties of handling the material and to facilitate the placement of MTA in the retrocavities, Lee[260] developed an original system that consists of using a bur to make grooves on the surface of a resin block. After the MTA has been prepared with a spatula, it is immediately placed in these grooves. The excess material should be removed with a damp cotton swab. The MTA placed in the groove is then removed with the tip of a Hollenback spatula and deposited directly into the retrocavity and condensed. According to the author, depending on the amplitude of the retrocavity and the size of the portions of MTA placed in each groove, it may be necessary to use of 3 to 5 portions of the material.

In conclusion, we believe that the introduction of MTA to Dentistry has led to huge advances, particularly in solving the distressing problems of root perforations, and the perspectives of its use in pediatric dentistry. The other applications, such as fillings the canals of teeth, with or without incomplete rhizogenesis, direct protection of the dental pulp (capping and pulpotomy) and even retrofillings, constitute clinical situations that are being well solved with other materials. The success obtained with these other materials in the pulp and periapical tissues, however, was not being reproduced in the case of root perforations. MTA, therefore, fills this space, in addition to having other applications, as already demonstrated and discussed.

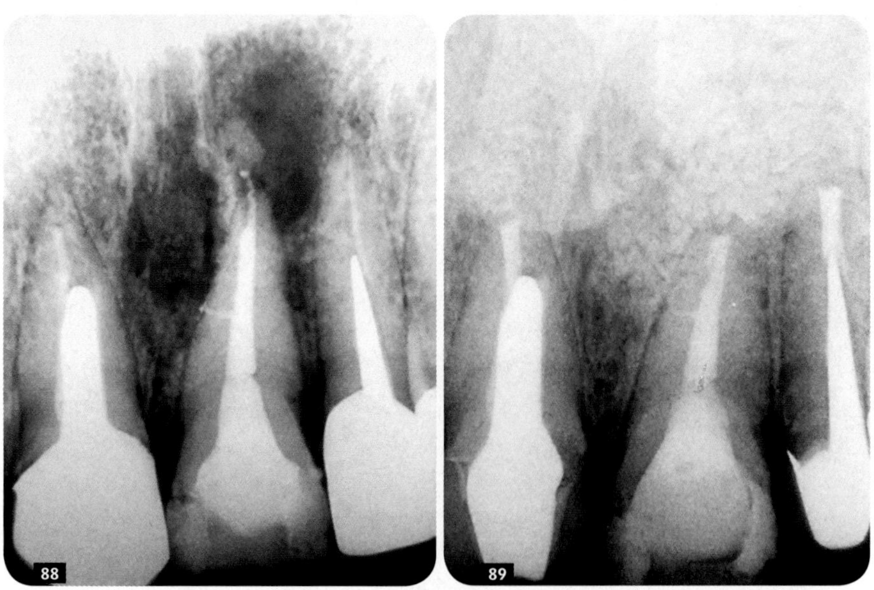


**Figures 25.88 and 25.89** - Radiographic evaluation. Evidence of repair after 3 years.

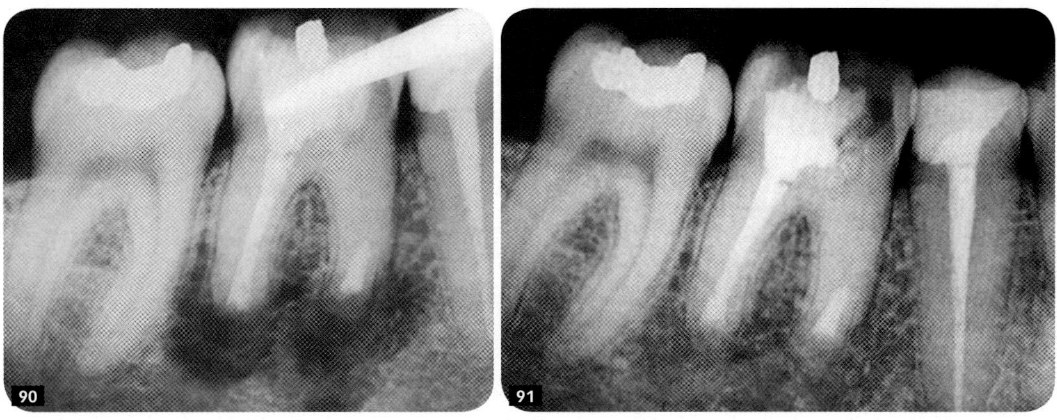


Figures 25.90 and 25.91 - Radiographic evaluation. Evidence of repair after 5 months.



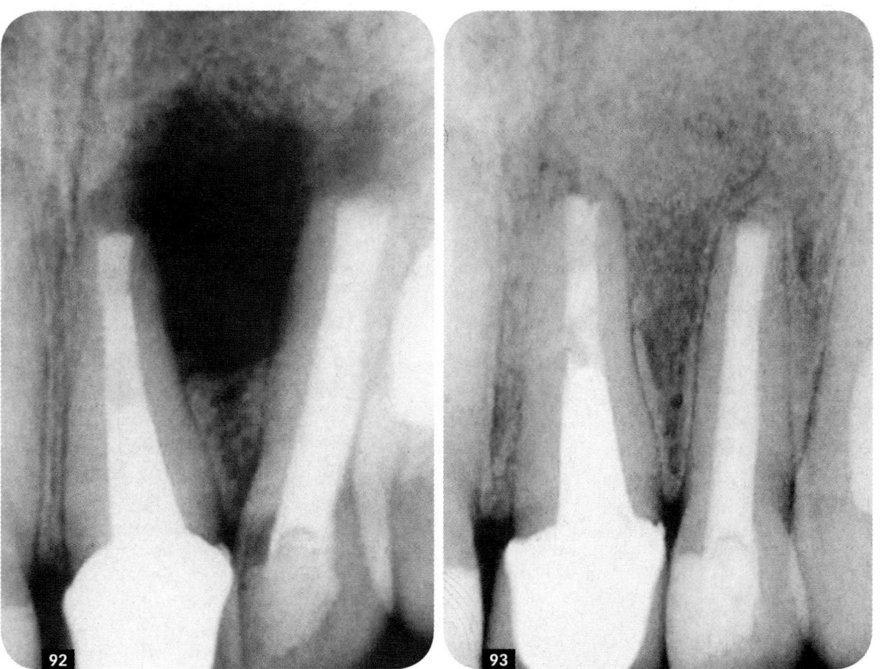


Figures 25.92 and 25.93 - Radiographic evaluation. Evidence of repair after 1 year and 6 months.

1. Abdal AK, Retief DH, Jamison HC. The apical seal via the retrosurgical approach. Part II. An evaluation of retrofilling materials. Oral Surg Oral Med Oral Pathol 1982; 54:213-18.
2. Abdullah D et al. An evaluation of accelerated Portland cement as a restorative material. Biomat 2000; 23:4001-10.
3. Abedi HR et al. The use of mineral trioxide aggregate (MTA) as a direct pulp capping agent. J Endod 1996; 22:199. (Abstracts).
4. Abedi HR, Van Mierlo BL, Wilder-Smith P, Torabinejad M. Effect of ultrasonic root-end cavity preparation on the root apex. Oral Surg Oral Med Oral Pathol Oral Radiol Oral Endod 1995; 80:207-13.
5. Adamo HL et al. A comparison of MTA, Super EBA, composite and amalgam as root-end filling materials using a bacterial microleakage model. Int Endod J 1999;32:197-203.
6. Ainamo J, Löe H. A stereomicroscopic investigation of the anatomy of the root apices of 910 maxillary and mandibular teeth. Odontol Tidskr 1968; 76:417-26.
7. Alexander JB, Gordon TM. A comparison of the apical seal produced by two calcium hydroxide sealers and a Grossman-type sealer when used with laterally condensed gutta-percha. Quintessence Int 1985; 16:615-21.
8. Al-Khatib ZZ, Baum RH, Morse DR, Yelsilsoy C, Furst L. The antimicrobial effect of various endodontic sealers. Oral Surg Oral Med Oral Pathol 1990;70:784-90.
9. Allison DA, Michelich RJ, Walton RE. The influence of master cone adaptation on the quality of the apical seal. J Endod 1981; 7:61-5.
10. Almeida JFA, Wada M, Takase T, Nakamura K, Arisue K, Nagahama F, Yamasaki M. Clinical study of refractory apical periodontitis treated by apicoectomy. Part 1. Root canal morphology of resected apex. Int Endod J 1998; 31:53-6.
11. Almeida-Filho RMR. MTA x Cimento Portland: análise comparativa de algumas de suas propriedades químicas, físicas e biológicas. (Monografy). Araçatuba: Faculdade de Odontologia de Araçatuba – UNESP; 2002.
12. Alves JD. Cimento. In: Manual de tecnologia do concreto. Alves JD. 2nd ed. Goiânia: UFG; 198. p.223-42.
13. Alvord WR. Prognosis and treatment of pulpless decíduos teeth. J Am Dent Assoc 1929;16:93-7.
14. Amagasa T, Nagase M, Sato T, Shioda S. Apicoectomy with retrograde gutta-percha root filling. Oral Surg Oral Med Oral Pathol 1989; 68:339-42.
15. Anton RG, Matsas MN. Retrofilling in endodontic therapy. J Dist Columbia Dent Soc 1971; 45:20-21.
16. Anton RG, Matsas MN. Retrofilling technic in endodontic therapy. Dent Surv 1971; 47:21-23.
17. Aqrabawi J. Sealing ability of amalgam, super EBA cement, and MTA when used as retrograde filling materials. Br Dent J 2000; 188:266-28.
18. Arens DE, Torablnejad M. Repair of furca perforations with mineral trioxide aggregate: two cases reports. Oral Surg Oral Med Oral Pathol 1996; 82:84-88.
19. Arnold JW, Rueggeberg FA, Anderson RW, Weller RN, Borke JL, Pashley DH. The dissintegration of super EBA cement in solutions with adjusted pH and osmolarity. J Endod 1997; 23:663-68.
20. Arwill T, Persson G, Thilander H. The microscopic appearence of the periapical tissue in cases classified as "uncertain" or "unsuccessful" after apicectomy. Odontol Revy 1974; 25:27-42.
21. Associação Brasileira de Cimento Portland. Gerência de Tecnologia. Manual de ensaios físicos do cimento. 3.ed. São Paulo: ABCP; 2000. 94p. (MT-3).
22. Associação Brasileira de Cimento Portland. Guia básico de utilização do cimento Portland. 5th ed. São Paulo: ABCP; 1999. 28p. (BT-106).
23. Attalla MN, Calvert JM. Irritational properties of root canal medicaments. J Can Dent Ass 1969; 35:76-82.
24. Barnett F et al. In vivo sealing ability of calcium hidroxide: containing root canal sealers. Endod Dent Traumatol 1989; 5;23-26.
25. Barnett F, Stevens R, Tronstad L. Demonstration of Bacteroides intermedius in periapical tissue using indirect immunofluorescence microscopy. Endod Dent Traumatol 1990; 6:153-56.
26. Barry GN, Heyman RA, Elias A. Comparison of apical sealing methods. A preliminary report. Oral Surg Oral Med Oral Pathol 1975; 39:806-11.
27. Barry GN, Selbst AG, D'anton EM, Madden RM. Sealing quality of polycarboxylate cements when compared to amalgam as retrofilling material. Oral Surg Oral Med Oral Pathol 1976; 42:109-16.
28. Bates CF et al. Longitudinal sealing ability of mineral trioxide aggregate as a root-end filling material. J Endod 1996; 22:575-78.
29. Baume LJ, Hoz J, Risk LB. Radicular pulpotomy of category 3 pulps. Part III. Histologic evaluation. J Prosthet Dent 1971; 26:649-57.
30. Baumgartner JC, Falkler-Júnior WA. Bacteria in the apical 5 mm of infected root canals. J Endod 1991; 17:380-83.
31. Beling KL, Marshall JG, Morgan LA, Baumgartner JC. Evaluation for cracks associated with ultrasonic root-end preparation of gutta-percha filled canals. J Endod 1997; 23:323-26.
32. Ben-Amar A, Kaffe I, Gorfil C. Marginal leakage in amalgam restorations and its prevention. Israel J Dent Med 1978; 27:25-29.
33. Berbert A. Comportamento dos tecidos apicais e periapicais após pulpectomia e obturação do canal com AH26, hidróxido de cálcio ou mistura de ambos: estudo histológico em dentes de cães. (Thesis). University of São Paulo; 1978. 174p.
34. Berbert A, Bramante CM, Passanezi E, Barroso JS. Cirurgias parendodônticas. In: Endodontia. Considerações biológicas e aplicação clínica. Hizatugu R, Valdrighi L. Piracicaba: Ed. Aloisi Ltda; 1974. p.252-301.
35. Berbert CCV, Consolaro A. Influência de cimentos endodônticos na migração neutrofílica pelo teste de "Skin Window". Rev Fac Odontol Bauru 1994; 2:81-87.

36. Bernabé PFE. Estudo histológico da reação do tecido conjuntivo subcutâneo do rato ao implante de alguns materiais utilizados nas obturações retrógradas dos canais radiculares. (Master's Thesis). University of São Paulo; 1977. 55p.
37. Bernabé PFE. Comportamento dos tecidos periapicais após apicectomia e obturação retrógrada. Influência do material obturador e das condições do canal radicular. Estudo histológico em dentes de cães. (Doctoral Thesis). University of São Paulo; 1981. 124p.
38. Bernabé PFE. Estudo histopatológico realizado em dentes de cães com lesão periapical após apicectomia e tratamento endodôntico via retrógrada. Influência do nível da obturação e do material obturador. (Thesis). University of São Paulo; 1994. 352p.
39. Bernabé PFE. Influência da smear layer sobre a superfície dentinária exposta após apicectomia e tratamento endodôntico via retrógrada. Estudo histopatológico em dentes de cães. 1994.
40. Bernabé PFE. Procedimentos clínicos que podem favorecer a reparação após a realização de cirurgias parendodônticas. In: Conceitos e procedimentos para uma nova odontologia. Dotto CA, Antoniazzi JH. São Paulo: VM Comunicações Ltda; 2002. p.68-81.
41. Bernabé PFE et al. Evaluation of root end preparations and retrofilling materials in pulpless dog' s teeth. (in press).
42. Bernabé PFE et al. Healing process of root end treatment using ultrasonic instrument and MTA or Portland cement. (in press).
43. Bernabé PFE, Barbosa HG, Silva RS, Cintra LTA, Gomes-Filho JE, Bernabé DG. Avaliação in vitro de retrocavidades preparadas com brocas ou ultra-som realizadas com ou sem o auxílio do microscópio odontológico. 1999.
44. Bernabé PFE, Cruz-Gonzalez A, Holland R, Dezan-Júnior E. Aplicação tópica de hidróxido de cálcio sobre o cimento de óxido de zinco e eugenol empregado no tratamento endodôntico via retrógrada. Estudo histopatológico em dentes de cães. 1994. (Projeto FAPESP, Processo n° 300727/93).
45. Bernabé PFE, Holland R, Kröling AE, Zardo M, Dezan-Jr E, Souza V, Nery MJ, Otoboni-Filho JA. Influência do smear layer sobre a superfície dentinária exposta após a realização da apicectomia: Removê-lo ou não? Rev Bras Odontol 1999; 56:120-25.
46. Bernabé PFE, Holland R, Kröling AE, Zardo M, Dezan-Jr E. Comportamento dos tecidos periapicais de dentes de cães, com lesões periapicais, submetidos à obturação retrógrada convencional com auxílio do ultra-som. Avaliação do processo de reparo considerando-se o tipo de material retrobturador e a utilização ou não do microscópio clínico odontológico. 2002.
47. Bernabé PFE, Holland R, Kröling AE, Zardo M, Dezan-Jr E. Influência da smear layer sobre a superfície dentinária exposta após apicectomia e tratamento endodôntico via retrógrada. Estudo histopatológico em dentes de cães. 1998.
48. Bernabé PFE, Holland R, Kröling AE, Zardo M. Comportamento dos tecidos periapicais de dentes de cães, com lesão periapical, após obturação retrógrada convencional. Influência do tipo de preparo da cavidade e do material retrobturador. 2000.
49. Bernabé PFE, Holland R, Queiroz AC, Souza V, Nery MJ, Otoboni-Filho JA, Dezan-Jr E, Gomes-Filho JE. Avaliação da capacidade seladora de alguns materiais retrobturadores. Rev Odontol Bras Central 2002; 11:68-71.
50. Bernabé PFE, et al. Histological evaluation of MTA as a root-end filling material. Int Endod J 2007;40:758-65.
51. Bernabé PFE, Holland R. Cirurgia parendodôntica: quando indicar e quando realizar. In: Atualização na Clínica Odontológica. Gonçalves EAN, Feller C. São Paulo: Ed. Artes Médicas; 1998. p.217-54.
52. Bernabé PFE, Holland R. O emprego do hidróxido de cálcio nas cirurgias parendodônticas. Rev Assoc Paul Cir Dent 1998; 52:460-65.
53. Bernabé PFE, Holland R. O emprego do MTA na cirurgia parendodôntica. Endonews 1999; 2:2-5.
54. Bernabé PFE, Holland R. O emprego do MTA. Tratamento de perfurações (furca e raiz) e cirurgia parendodôntica. Arq Dent Gaúcho 2002; 9:20-23.
55. Bernabé PFE, Kröling AE, Holland R, Zardo M, Dezan-Jr E. Tratamento endodôntico via retrógrada realizado em dentes de cães com lesões periapicais. Avaliação histomorfológica da ação do EDTA e do hidróxido de cálcio aplicados sobre a superfície dentinária apicectomizada e material retrobturador. 2000.
56. Bernabé PFE, Kröling AE, Holland R, Zardo M. Tratamento endodôntico via retrógrada. Estudo histopatológico dos tecidos periapicais de dentes de cães após o emprego da guta-percha termo-plastificada (Sistema Ultrafil). 1997.
57. Bernabé PFE, Kröling AE, Zardo M, Holland R, Dezan-Júnior E. Estudo histopatológico dos tecidos periapicais de dentes de cães após apicectomia e tratamento endodôntico via retrógrada. Influência da aplicação tópica de hidróxido de cálcio com veículos hidrossolúvel e não hidrossolúvel sobre o material retrobturador e superfície dentinária. 1996.
58. Bernabé PFE, Morandi R, Holland R, Souza V, Nery MJ, Otoboni-Filho JA, Dezan-Jr E, Gomes-Filho JE. Comparative study of MTA with other materials in retrofilling of pulpless dog's teeth. Braz Dent J 2005;16:149-55.
59. Bernabé PFE, Nunes RC. Comportamento dos tecidos periapicais de dentes de cães após obturação retrógrada. Estudo da influência do preparo de cavidades sobre a superfície apical apicectomizada comparativamente com o tratamento endodôntico via retrógrada. 1986.
60. Bernardineli N. Obturação retrógrada - Avaliação da adaptação às paredes das cavidades e infiltração marginal, em função dos materiais obturadores e de agentes de limpeza. (Thesis). University of São Paulo; 1993. 168p.
61. Bertrand G. Use of ultrasound in apicoectomy. Quint Int 1976; 4:9-12.
62. Bhambhani SM, Bolanos OR. Tissue reactions to endodontic mateials implanted in the mandible of guinea pigs. Oral Surg Oral Med Oral Pathol 1993; 76:493-501.
63. Biggs JT, Benenati FW, Powell SE. Ten-year in vitro assesment of the surface status of three retrofilling materials. J Endod 1995; 21:521-25.

64. Binnie WH, Mitchell DF. Induced calcification in the subdermal tissues of the rat. J Dent Res 1973; 52:1087-91.
65. Blackman R, Gross M, Seltzer S. An evaluation of the biocompatibility of a glass ionomer-silver cement in rat connective tissue. J Endod 1989; 15:76-79.
66. Block RM, Lewis RD. Surgical treatment of iatrogenic canal blockages. Oral Surg Oral Med Oral Pathol 1987; 63:722-32.
67. Bogaerts P. Treatment if root perforations with calcium hidroxide and Super EBA cement: a clinical report. Int Endod J 1997; 30:210-19.
68. Bohsali K, Pertot WJ, Hosseini B, Camps J. Sealing ability of super EBA and Dyract as root-end fillings: a study in vitro. Int Endod J 1998; 31:338-42.
69. Bondra DL, Hartwell GR, MacPherson MG, Portell FR. Leakage in vitro with IRM, high copper amalgam, and EBA cement as retrofillings materials. J Endod 1989; 15:157-60.
70. Bonetti-Filho I. Avaliação da biocompatibilidade de quatro técnicas de obturação de canais radiculares: estudo em dentes de cães. (Doctoral Thesis). São Paulo State University; 1990. 110p.
71. Boulger EP. The foreign body reaction of rat tissue and human tissue to gutta-percha. J Amer Dent Ass 1933; 20:1473-81.
72. Bramante CM, Berbert A, Bernardineli N, Moraes IG. Retroinstrumentação com retrobturação. Rev Bras Odontol 1986; 43:6-12.
73. Bramante CM, Berbert A, Bernardineli N. Materiais seladores provisórios: avaliação da propriedade seladora com $^{131}$INa. Rev Assoc Paul Cir Dent 1977; 31:10-3.
74. Bramante CM, Berbert A, Bernardineli N. Retroinstrumentação e retro obturação. Técnica cirúrgica combinada com obturação retrógrada. Rev Bras Odontol 1992; 40:38-40.
75. Bramante CM, Berbert A, Bernardineli N. Técnica cirúrgica combinada de retroinstrumentação e retrobturação com obturação retrógrada. Rev Bras Odontol 1993; 41:95-96.
76. Bramante CM, Berbert A. Root perforations dressed with calcium hydroxide or zinc oxide and eugenol. J Endod 1987; 13:392-95.
77. Bramante CM, Bramante A, Bernardineli N. Característica do preparo apical para obturação retrógrada realizada com ultra-som. Rev Assoc Paul Cir Dent 1998; 52:221-3.
78. Bramante CM, Pinto SAH, Berbert A, Bernadineli N. Análise, através da microscopia eletrônica de varredura, de alguns materiais utilizados em obturação retrógrada. Rev Bras Odontol 1990; 77:29-34.
79. Bruce GR, McDonald NJ, Sydiskis R J. Citotoxity of retrofill materials. J Endod 1993; 19:288-92.
80. Caicedo R et al. Sealing capacity of super EBA, Pro-Root MTA, Diaket in the repair of root perforations. J Endod 2000; 26:553. (Abstracts).
81. Caicedo R, Von-Fraunhofer JA. The properties of endodontic sealer cements. J Endod 1988; 14:527-34.
82. Calzonetti KJ, Iwanowski T, Komorowski R, Friedman S. Ultrasonic root end cavity preparation assessed by an in situ impression technique. Oral Surg Oral Med Oral Pathol Oral Radiol Oral Endod 1998; 85:210-15.
83. Camargo WR. Interação dos cimentos sealapex e CRSC com os macrófagos: estudo morfológico dos efeitos citotóxicos. (Master's Thesis). University of São Paulo. 1993; 93p.
84. Canalda C, Pumarola J. Bacterial growth inhibition produced by root canal sealer cements with a calcium hydroxide base. Oral Surg Oral Med Oral Pathol 1989; 68:99-102.
85. Canalda-Sahli C, Brau-Aguade E, Sentis-Vilalta J, Aguade-Bruix S. The apical seal root canal sealing cements using a radionuclide detection technique. Int Endod J 1992, 25:250-56.
86. Carr LB et al. A method of demonstrating calcium in the tissue sections using chloranilic acid. J Histochem Cytochem 1961; 9:415-17.
87. Casaes HMD. Avaliação do agregado de trióxido mineral (MTA), sob duas formulações diferentes, em capeamento pulpar direto de ratos. (Monografy) Feira de Santana: Universidade Estadual de Feira de Santana; 2001. 63p.
88. Catanzaro-Guimarães SA, Alle N. Estudo histoquímico da reação tecidual ao hidróxido de cálcio. Rev Estomatol Cult 1974; 8:79-82.
89. Chailertvanitkul P, Saunders W P, Saunders EM, Mackenzie D. Polymicrobial coronal leakage of super EBA root-end fillings following two methods of root-end preparation. Int Endod J 1998; 31:348-53.
90. Chong BS, Owadally ID, Pitt-Ford TR, Wilson RF. Antibacterial activity of potential retrograde root filling materials. Endod Dent Traumatol 1994; 10:66-70.
91. Civjan S, Huget EF, Wolfhard G, Waddell LS. Characterization of zinc oxide-eugenol cements reinforced with acrylic resin. J Dent Res 1972; 51:107-14.
92. Cohen S, Lasfargues JJ. Quantitative chemical study of root canal preparations with calcium hydroxide. Endod Dent Traumatol 1988; 4:108-13.
93. Cohen T, Gutmann JL, Wagner M. An assessment in vitro of the sealing properties of calcibiotic root canal sealer. Int Endod J 1985; 18:172-78.
94. Consolaro A. Reabsorções Dentárias nas Especialidades Clínicas. Dent Press – Maringá, 2002. 448p.
95. Coolidge ED. Root resection as a cure for chronic periapical infection: A histologic report of a case showing complete repair. J Am Dent Ass 1930; 17:239-49.
96. Costa CAS, Benatti-Neto C, Comelli Lia RC, Oliveira MRB, Costa JH, Gonzaga HFS. Pulp-capping studies with zinc oxide-eugenol, varying the age of materials, correlated with fluidity. Rev Odontol UNESP 1993; 22:223-30.
97. Cotran R, Kumar V, Ins SL. Robbins pathologic basis of disease. 4th ed. Philadelphia: Saunders; 1989. p.163-267.
98. Craig KR, Harrison JW. Wound healing following demineralization of resected root ends in periradicular surgery. J Endod 1993; 19:339-47.
99. Crooks WG, Anderson RW, Powell BJ, Kimbrough WF. Longitudinal evaluation of the seal of IRM root end fillings. J Endod 1994; 20:250-52.
100. Cummings GR, Torablnejad M. Mineral trioxide aggregate (MTA) as an isolating barrier for internal bleaching. J Endod 1995; 21:228. (Abstracts).
101. Dalçoqulo C et al. Selamento apical após retrobturações com MTA, IRM, ionômero de vidro e cianocrilato. Rev Assoc Paul Cir Dent; 55:194-98.
102. Dawood AJ, Pitt-Ford TR. Surgical approach to the obturation of apically flared root canais with thermoplasticized gutta-percha. Int Endod J 1989; 22:138-41.

103. Deal BF et al. Chemical and physical properties of MTA, Portland Cement and a new experimental material, fast-set MTA. J Endod 2002; 28:252. (Abstracts).
104. Dean JW, Lenox RA, Lucas FL, Culley WL, Himel UT. Evaluation of a combined surgical repair and guided tissue regeneration technique to treat recent root canal perforations. J Endod 1997; 23:525-32.
105. Delivanis P, Tabibi A. A comparative sealability study of different retrofilling materiais. Oral Surg Oral Med Oral Pathol 1978; 45:273-81.
106. Delivanis PD, Mattison GD, Mendel RW. The survivability of $F_{43}$ strain of *Streptococcus sanguis* in root canals filled with gutta-percha and Procosol cement. J Endod 1983; 9:407-10.
107. Dorn SO, Gartner AH. Retrograde filling materials: a retrospective success-failure study of amalgam, EBA, and IRM. J Endod 1990; 16:391-93.
108. Duarte MAH et al. Avaliação da contaminação do MTA Ângelus e do Cimento Portland. J Bras Cir 2002; 6:155-57.
109. Duarte MAH et al. pH and calcium íon release of 2 root-end filling materials. Oral Surg Oral Med Oral Pathol Oral Radiol Endod 2003;93:345-47.
110. Duarte MAH, Leite SCS, Kuga MC, Ogata M, Pedroso JA. Fraturas apicais associadas a métodos de retropreparação cavitária. Rev Fac Odontol Lins 1997; 10:6-9.
111. Duarte MAH, Weckwerth PH, Moraes IG. Análise da ação antimicrobiana de cimentos e pastas empregados na prática endodôntica. Rev Odontol Un São Paulo 1997; 11:299-305.
112. Duclos JI. Indications et technique des diverses methodes d'obturation des canaux par voie apicale. Rev Stomatol 1934; 36:767-68.
113. Edmunds DH, Thirawat J. Sealing ability of amalgam used as a retrograde root filling in endodontic surgery. Int Endod J 1989; 22:290-94.
114. Eichhorn GL. Inorganic Biochemistry. NewYork: El sevier; 1973:536-43.
115. Eidelman E et al. Mineral trioxide aggregate vs. formocresol in pulpotomized primary molars: a preliminary report. Pediatr Dent 2001; 23:15-18.
116. Engel TK, Steiman HR. Preliminary investigation of ultrasonic root end preparation. J Endod 1995; 21:443-45.
117. Erausquin J, Devoto FC. Alveolodental ankylosis induced by root canal treatment in rat molars. Oral Surg Oral Med Oral Pathol 1970; 30:105-16.
118. Esberard RM, Carnes-Jr DL, Del Rio CE. pH changes at the surface of root dentin when using root canal sealers containing calcium hydroxide. J Endod 1996; 22:399-401.
119. Esberard RM, Leal JM, Simões-Filho AP, Bonetti-Filho I, Leonardo MR, Lofredo LCM. Avaliação da infiltração marginal dos principais materiais seladores provisórios frente à Rodamina B a 0,2%: estudo in vitro. Odontol Clin 1986: 1:21-5.
120. Escobar C, Michanowicz AE, Czonstkowsky M, Miklos FL. A comparative study between injectable low-temperature (70°) gutta-percha and silver amalgam as a retrosed. Oral Surg Oral Med Oral Pathol 1986; 61:504-07.
121. Estrela C. Análise química de pastas de hidróxido de álcio, frente a liberação de íons cálcio, de íons hidróxila e formação de carbonato de cálcio, na presença de tecido conjuntivo de cão. (Doctoral Thesis). São Paulo: Faculdade de Odontologia, Universidade de São Paulo. 1994. 140p.
122. Estrela C, Bammann LL, Estrela CRA, Silva RS, Pécora JD. Antimicrobial and chemical study of MTA, Portland cement, calcium hydroxide paste, Sealapex and Dycal. Braz Dent J 2000; 11:3-9.
123. Estrela C, Bammann LL, Lopes HP, Moura JA. Análise da ação antibacteriana de três cimentos obturadores contendo hidróxido de cálcio. Rev Ass Bras Odontol Nac 1995; 3:185-87.
124. Estrela C, Sydney GB, Bammann LL, Felippe-Júnior O. Estudo do efeito biológico do pH na atividade enzimática de bactérias anaeróbias. Rev Fac Odontol Bauru 1994; 2:31-38.
125. Estrela C, Sydney GB, Bammann LL, Felippe-Júnior O. Mechanism of action of calcium and hydroxyl íons of calcium hydroxide on tissue and bacteria. Braz Dent J 1995; 6:85-90.
126. Evers N, Smith W. The analysis of drugs and chemicals. London: Charles Griffin; 1955. p.495-97.
127. Faraco-Jr IM. Avaliação histomorfológica da resposta da polpa de dentes de cães submetida ao capeamento com sistema adesivo, cimento de hidróxido de cálcio e dois tipos de agregado de trióxido mineral. (Tese de Doutorado). São Paulo State University; 1999. 251p.
128. Faraco-Jr IM, Holland R. Comportamento da polpa dentária diante do capeamento com sistema adesivo Single Bond. Rev Ass Paul Cir Dent 2000; 54:282-87.
129. Faraco-Jr IM, Holland R. Response of the pulp of dogs to capping with mineral trioxide aggregate or a calcium hydroxide cement. Dent Traumatol 2001; 17:163-66.
130. Favinha SNG. Estudo do comportamento biológico em dentes de cães e da capacidade seladora marginal de cimentos experimentais à base de resina plástica ou com diferentes proporções de hidróxido de cálcio. (Master's Thesis). University of Marília; 1999. 179p.
131. Feldmann G, Nyborg H. Tissue reaction to root filling materials. I – Comparison between gutta-percha and silver amalgam implanted in rabbit. Odont Revy 1962; 13:1-14.
132. Fidel RAS et al. Estudo in vitro sobre a solubilidade e a desintegração de alguns cimentos endodônticos que contém hidróxido de cálcio. Rev Odontol Univ São Paulo 1994; 8:217-20.
133. Fischer EJ et al. Bacterial leakage of mineral trioxide aggregate as compared with zinc-free amalgam, intermediate restorative material, and super-EBA as a root-end filling material. J Endod 1998; 24:176-79.
134. Fitzpatrick EL, Steiman HR. Scanning electron microscopic evaluation of finishing techniques on IRM and EBA retrofillings. J Endod 1997; 23:423-27.
135. Flanders DH, James GA, Burch B, Dockum N. Comparative histopathologic study of zincfree amalgam and cavit in connective tissue of the rat. J Endod 1975; 1:56-59.
136. Flath RK, Hicks ML. Retrograde instrumentation and obturation with new devices. J Endod 1987; 13:546-49.
137. Fogel HM, Peikoff MD. Microleakage of root-end filling materials. J Endod 2001; 27:456-58.

138. Fong CD. A sonic instrument for retrograde preparation. J Endod 1993; 19:374-75.
139. Forte SG, Hauser MJ, Hahm C, Hartwell GR. Microleakage of Super EBA with and without finishing as determined by fluid filtration method. J Endod 1998; 24:799-801.
140. Franco KPB. Estudo histológico comparativo entre o MTA e o cimento de portland. (Monografia). Feira de Santana: Faculdade de Odontologia da Universidade Estadual de Feira de Santana; 2001. 57p.
141. Frank RJ, Antrim DD, Bakland LK. The effect of cavity preparations on root apexes. Endod Dent Traumatol 1996; 12:100-03.
142. Friedman S. Retrograde approaches in endodontics therapy. Endod Dent Traumatol 1991; 7:97-107.
143. Fujiwasa S, Masuhara S. Binding of eugenol and ethoxybenzoic acid to bovine serum albumin. J Dent Res 1981; 60:860-64.
144. Funteas UR et al. A comparative analysis of Mineral Trioxide Aggregate and Portland cement. J Endod 2002; 28:259. (Abstracts).
145. Fuss Z, Weiss EI, Shalhav M. Antibacterial activity of calcium hydroxide containing endodontic sealers on *Enterococcus faecalis* in vitro. Int Endod J 1997; 30:397-402.
146. Gagliani M, Taschieri S, Molinari R. Ultrasonic root-end preparation: influence of cutting angle on the apical seal. J Endod 1998; 24:726-29.
147. Garberoglio R, Brannström M. Scanning electron microscopic investigation of human dentinal tubules. Arch Oral Biol 1976; 21:355-63.
148. Gartner AH, Dorn SO. Advances in endodontic surgery. Dent Clin North Am 1992; 38:357-78.
149. Giammusso SE. Manual do concreto. Rev São Paulo 1992; 164.
150. Gilheany PA, Figdor D, Tyas MJ. Apical dentin permeability and microleakage associated with root end resection and retrograde filling. J Endod 1994; 20:22-26.
151. Glickman GN, Koch K. 21sT - Century endodontics. J Am Dent Assoc 2000; 131:39S-46S.
152. Goldberg F, Frajlich S. Análise in vitro del sellado apical com amalgama por medio del Iodo 131. Rev Ass Odontol Argentina 1970; 58:101-16.
153. Goldberg F, Frajlich S. Análisis de la capacidad de sellado. Diferentes materiales y técnicas de obturación de conductos. Rev Ass Odontol Argentina 1980; 68:13-16.
154. Goldberg F, Torres MD, Bottero C, Alvarez AF. Uso de la guta-percha termoplastizada como material para la obturación retrograda. Rev Assoc Odontol Argentina 1991; 79:142-46.
155. Goldberg F, Torres, MD, Bottero C. Thermo-plasticized gutta-percha in endodontic surgical procedures. Endod Dent Traumatol 1990; 6:109-13.
156. Gondim-Jr E. Estudos dos efeitos do preparo sônico e ultra-sônico de cavidades retrógradas em dentes recém extraídos: análise de réplicas com microscópio eletrônico de varredura. (Master's Thesis). University of Campinas; 1999. 165p.
157. Gorman MC, Steiman HR, Gartner AH. Scanning electron microscopic evaluation of root-end preparations. J Endod 1995; 21:113-17.
158. Gray GJ, Hatton JF, Holtzmann DJ, Jenkins DB, Nielsen CJ. Quality of root-end preparations using ultrasonic and rotary instrumentation in cadavers. J Endod 2000; 26:281-83.
159. Grossman L. Antimicrobial effect of root canal cements. J Endod 1980; 6:594-97.
160. Guerini V. A history of Dentistry. Philadelphia: Lea & Febiger; 1909. p.117-18. apud Ingle JI, Beveridge EE. Endodontia. 2nd ed. Rio de Janeiro: Interamericana; 1979; 546-629.
161. Guigand M, Vulcain JM, Dautel-Morazin A, Bonnaure-Mallet M. An ultrastructural study of some root canal walls in contact with endodontic biomaterials. J Endod 1997; 23:327-30.
162. Gutmann JL, Creel DC, Bowles WH. Evaluation of heat transfer during root canal obturation with termoplasticized gutta-percha. Part I. In vitro heat levels during extrusion. J Endod 1987; 13:378-83.
163. Gutmann JL, Fava LRG. Perspectives on periradicular healing using Sealapex: a case report. Int Endod J 1991; 24:135-38.
164. Gutmann JL, Harrison JW. Surgical endodontics. Boston: Blackwell Scientific, 1991. 468p.
165. Gutmann JL, Saunders WP, Nguyen L, Guo IY, Saunders EM. Ultrasonic root end preparation. Part 1. SEM analysis. Int Endod J 1994; 27:318-24.
166. Harran E, Comelli Lia RC, Martin E, Benatti-Neto C. Analisis comparativo entre el óxido de cinc y eugenol fluido y solido utilizados en protecciones pulpares indirectas: estudio histomorfológico en perros. Rev Esp Endod 1985; 3:45-51.
167. Harrison JW, Johnson SA. Excisional wound healing following the use of IRM as a root-end filling material. J Endod 1997; 23:19-27.
168. Hartwell GR, England MC. Healing of furcation perforations in primate teeth after repair with decalcified freeze-dried bone: a longitudinal study. J Endod 1993; 19:357-61.
169. Harty FJ, Parkins BJ, Wengraf AM. Success rate in root canal therapy. A retrospective study of convencional cases. Br Dent J 1970; 128:65-70.
170. Helene PRL. Cimento portland: algumas características de interesse à patologia dos concretos. Engenharia 1981; 429:31-38.
171. Heling I, Chandler NP. The antimicrobial effect within dentinal tubules of four root canal sealers. J Endod 1996; 22:257-59.
172. Hendra JP. EBA cement: a practical system for all cementations. J Br Endod Soc 1970; 4:28-32.
173. Herzog-Flores DS et al. Análisis fisicoquímico del mineral trioxido agregado (MTA) por difracción de raios X, calorimetria e microscopía electrónica de barrido. Rev ADM 2000; 57:125-31.
174. Hess W, Keller O. Le tavole anatomiche di W. Hess i O. Keller. Pistoia: Edizioni Scientifiche Oral B. 1988. 128p.
175. Heys RJ, Fitzgerald M. Microleakage of three cement bases. J Dent Res 1991; 70:55-58.
176. Hidalgo MM. Estudo sobre o potencial imunogênico da dentina - contribuição para a etiopatogenia da reabsorção dentária. (Doctoral Thesis). University of São Paulo, 2001. 103p.
177. Higa RK, Torabinejad M, McKendry DJ, McMillan PJ. The effect of storage time on the degree of dye leakage of root-end filling materials. Int Endod J 1994; 27:252-56.

178. Hirsch L, Weinreb MM. Marginal fit of direct acrylic restorations. J Am Dent Ass 1958; 56:13-21.
179. Hobson P. An investigation into the bacteriological control of infected root canals. Br Dent J 1959; 20:63-70.
180. Holcomb JQ, Pitts DL, Nicholls JI. Further investigation of spreader loads required to cause vertical root fracture during lateral condensation. J Endod 1987; 13:277-84.
181. Holland et al. Infiltração marginal dos cimentos endodônticos. Rev Gaúcha Odontol 1991; 39:413-16.
182. Holland R et al. Agregado de trioxido mineral y cemento Portland em la obturación de conductos radiculares de perro. Endodoncia 2001; 19:275-80.
183. Holland R et al. Calcium salts deposition in rat connective tissue after the implantation of calcium hydroxide-containing sealers. J Endod 2002; 28:173-76.
184. Holland R et al. Comportamento da polpa dental do cão diante da exposição pulpar ou pulpotomia e proteção direta com o sistema All Bond 2. Rev Cienc Odontol 1998; 1:75-80.
185. Holland R et al. Healing process of dog dental pulp after pulpotomy and pulp covering with mineral trioxide aggregate or Portland cement. Braz Dent J 2001; 12:109-13.
186. Holland R et al. Healing process of dogs' dental pulp after pulpotomy and protection with calcium hydroxide or Dycal. Rev Odontol UNESP 1979/1980; 8/9:67-73.
187. Holland R et al. Histochemical analysis of the dogs' dental pulp after pulp capping with calcium, barium, and strontium hydroxides. J Endod 1982; 8:444-47.
188. Holland R et al. Mineral trioxide aggregate repair of lateral root perforations. J Endod 2001; 27:281-84.
189. Holland R et al. Reaction of dogs' teeth to root canal filling with mineral trioxide aggregate or a glass ionomer sealer. J Endod 1999; 25:728-30.
190. Holland R et al. Reaction of human periapical tissue to pulp extirpation and immediate root canal filling with calcium hydroxide. J Endod 1977; 3:63-67.
191. Holland R et al. Reaction of rat connective tissue to implanted dentin tubes filled with mineral trioxide aggregate or calcium hydroxide. J Endod 1999; 25:161-66.
192. Holland R et al. Reaction of rat connective tissue to implanted dentin tube filled with mineral trioxide aggregate, Portland cement or calcium hydroxide. Braz Dent J 2001; 12:3-8.
193. Holland R et al. Reaction of rat connective tissue to implanted dentin tubes filled with a white mineral trioxide aggregate. Braz Dent J 2002; 13:23-26.
194. Holland R et al. Recambio del hidróxido de calcio después de la pulpotomia y su influencia en la reparación: estudio histológico en dientes de monos. Endodoncia 1999; 17:35-45.
195. Holland R et al. Análise do selamento marginal obtido com cimentos à base de hidróxido de cálcio. Rev Ass Paul Cir Dent 1996; 50:61-64.
196. Holland R et al. Comportamento dos tecidos periapicais de dentes de cães após a obturação de canal com Sealapex acrescido ou não de iodofórmio. Rev Odontol UNESP 1990; 19:97-104.
197. Holland R et al. Comportamento dos tecidos periapicais de dentes de cães com rizogênese incompleta após obturação de canal com diferentes materiais obturadores. Rev Bras Odontol 1992; 49:49-53.
198. Holland R et al. Healing process after pulpotomy and covering with calcium hydroxide, Dycal or MPC: histological study in dogs teeth. Rev Fac Odontol Araçatuba 1978; 7:185-91.
199. Holland R, Bernabé PFE, Murata SS, Nakasako MT, Dezan-Júnior E. Qualidade seladora de guta-perchas de diferentes procedências. Rev Gaúcha Odont 1995; 43:252-54.
200. Holland R, Crivelini MC, Zampieri-Jr M, Souza V, Saliba O. Qualidade do selamento marginal obtido com diferentes cimentos à base de hidróxido de cálcio. Rev Paul Odontol 1991; 13:27-35.
201. Holland R, Mello W, Nery MJ, Souza V, Bernabé PF, Otoboni-Filho JA. Healing process of dog's dental pulp after pulpotomy and pulp covering with calcium hydroxide in powder or paste form. Acta Odontol Ped 1981; 2:47-51.
202. Holland R, Nery MJ, Mello W. Resposta do tecido conjuntivo subcutâneo do rato ao implante de alguns materiais obturadores de canal. Rev Fac Odontol Araçatuba 1973; 2:217-25.
203. Holland R, Nery MJ, Souza V, Bernabé PFE, Mello W, Pannain R. Propriedade seladora de alguns materiais obturadores temporários. Rev Ass Paul Cir Dent 1976; 30:175-78.
204. Holland R, Pannain R, Nery MJ, Bernabé PFE, Mello W. Estudo in vitro da infiltração marginal após obturação retrógrada ou apicectomia. Rev Fac Odontol Araçatuba 1974; 3:23-31.
205. Holland R, Souza V, Holland-Jr C, Nery MJ. Estudo histológico do comportamento do tecido conjuntivo subcutâneo do rato ao implante de alguns materiais obturadores de canal radicular: influência da proporção pó-líquido. Rev Ass Paul Cir Dent 1971; 25:101-10.
206. Holland R, Souza V, Mello W, Russo MC. Healing process of the pulp stump and periapical tissues in dog teeth. II. Histopathological findings following root filling with zinc oxide-eugenol. Rev Fac Odontol Araçatuba 1977; 6:59-67.
207. Holland R, Souza V, Mello W, Russo MC. Healing process os the pulp stump and periapical tissue in dog teeth. III. Histopathological findings following root filling with calcium hydroxide. Rev Fac Odontol Araçatuba 1978; 7:25-37.
208. Holland R, Souza V, Milanezi LA. Resposta do coto pulpar e tecidos periapicais a algumas pastas empregadas na obturação dos canais radiculares. Arq Cent Estud Fac Odontol UFMG 1971; 8:189-97.
209. Holland R, Souza V, Nery MJ, Bernabé PFE, Mello W. Resposta tecidual à implantação de diferentes marcas de cones de guta-percha. Estudo histológico em ratos. Rev Fac Odont Araçatuba 1975; 4:81-89.
210. Holland R, Souza V, Nery MJ, Mello W, Bernabé PFE, Otoboni-Filho JA. A histological study of the effect of calcium hydroxide in the treatment of pulpless teeth of dogs. J Br Endod Soc 1979; 12:15-23.
211. Holland R, Souza V, Nery MJ, Mello W, Bernabé PFE, Otoboni-Filho JA. Root canal treatment of pulpless teeth with calvital or zinc oxide-eugenol, in one or two sittings. Histological study in dog. Rev Fac Odontol Araçatuba 1978; 7:47-53.

212. Holland R, Souza V, Nery MJ, Mello W. Resposta do tecido conjuntivo subcutâneo do rato ao implante de alguns materiais obturadores de canal. Rev Fac Odontol Araçatuba 1973; 2:217-25.
213. Holland R, Souza V. Ability of a new calcium hydroxide root canal filling material to induce hard tissue formation. J Endod 1985; 11:535-43.
214. Holland R, Valle GF, Taintor JF, Ingle JI. Influence of bony resorption on endodontic treatment. Oral Surg Oral Med Oral Pathol 1983; 55:191-203.
215. Holland R. Histochemical response of amputed pulps to calcium hydroxide. Rev Bras Pesq Med Biol 1971; 4:83-95.
216. Holland R. Processo de reparo da polpa dental após pulpotomia e proteção com hidróxido de cálcio. Estudo morfológico e histoquímico efetuado em cães. (Doctoral Thesis). São Paulo State University; 1966. 65p.
217. Holland-Jr C, Komatsu J, Russo M. Estudo comparativo da infiltração marginal de radioisótopos em restaurações de amálgama de prata preparado com limalhas convencional ou esferoidal. Rev Fac Odontol Araçatuba 1975; 4:119-27.
218. Hong CU et al. Healing of furcal lesions repaired by amalgam or mineral trioxide aggregate. J Endod 1994; 20:197. (Abstracts).
219. Hong CU, Torabinejad M, Kettering JD. The effects of three retrofilling materials on selected oral bacteria. J Endod 1993; 19:200.
220. Hovland EJ, Dunsha TC. Leakage evaluation in vitro of the root canal sealer cement Sealapex. Int Endod J 1985; 18:179-82.
221. Hume WR. Effect of eugenol on respiration and division in human pulp, mouse fibroblasts, and liver cells in vitro. J Dent Res 1984; 63:1262-65.
222. Hume WR. In vitro studies on the local pharmacodynamics, pharmacology and toxicology of eugenol and zinc oxide-eugenol. Int Endod J 1988; 21:130-34.
223. Hume WR. The pharmacologic and toxicological properties of zinc oxide-eugenol. J Am Dent Ass 1986; 113:789-91.
224. Hunter HA. The effect of gutta-percha, silver points and Rickert's root sealer on bone healing. J Can Dent Ass 1957; 23:385-88.
225. Ingle JI, Beveridge EE. Endodontia. 2nd ed. Rio de Janeiro: Interamericana, 1979. p.546-629.
226. Ingle JI. Endodontics. Philadelphia: Lea & Febiger, 1965. p.54-77.
227. Ingle JI. Endodontics. Philadelphia: Lea & Febiger, 1974. p.23-230, p.500-65.
228. Inoue S, Yoshimura M, Tinkle JS, Marshall FJ. A 24-week study of the microleakage of four retrofilling materials using a fluid filtration method. J Endod 1991; 17:369-75.
229. Iwu C, MacFarlane TW, MacKenzie D, Stenhouse D. The microbiology of periapical granulomas. Oral Surg Oral Med Oral Pathol 1990; 69:502-55.
230. Jorgensen KD. Amalgams in dentistry. USA, Dept of Commerce, Dental Materials Research, National Bureau of Standards 1972, 33. apud Moodnik RM, Levey MH, Besen MA, Borden BC. Retrograde amalgam filling: a scanning electron microscopic study. J Endod 1975; 1:28-31.
231. Junn DJ et al. Quantitative assessment of dentin bridge formation following pulp capping with mineral trioxide aggregate (MTA). J Endod 1998; 24:278. (Abstracts).
232. Kazemi RB, Safavi K, Spangberg LSW. Assessment of marginal stability and permeability of an interim restorative endodontic material. Oral Surg Oral Med Oral Pathol 1994; 78:788-96.
233. Kearney WW. IRM: a tissue tolerance study. (Thesis). Detroit: University of Detroit MI, USA; 1998.
234. Keiser K et al. Citotoxicity of mineral troxide aggregate using human periodontal ligament fibroblasts. J Endod 2000; 26:288-91.
235. Kettering JD, Torabinejad M. Investigation of mutagenicity of mineral trioxide aggregate and other commonly used root-end filling materials. J Endod 1995; 21:537-39.
236. Kielbassa AM, Attin T, Hellwig E. Diffusion behaviour of eugenol from zinc oxide-eugenol mixtures through human and bovine dentin in vitro. Oper Dent 1997; 22:15-20.
237. Kim S, Pecora G, Rubinstein R, Dörscher-Kim J. Microsurgery in endodontics. W.B. Saunders Company, 2001. 172p.
238. King KT, Anderson RW, Pashley DH, Pantera EA. Longitudinal evaluation of the seal of endodontic retrofillings. J Endod 1990; 16:307-10.
239. Kodukula PS. Role of pH in biological wastewater treatment process. In: Physiological models in microbiology. Bazin MJ, Prosser JI. Flórida: CRC Press; 1988. p.14-34.
240. Koh ET et al. Mineral trioxide aggregate stimulates a biological response in human osteoblasts. J Biomed Mater Res 1997; 37:432-39.
241. Koh ET, McDonald F, Pitt-Ford TR, Torabinejad M. Celular response to Mineral Trioxide Aggregate. J Endod 1998; 24:543-47.
242. Komatsu J, Martins J, Takayama S, Sasaki T, Russo M. Influência da umidade no selamento marginal em restaurações a amálgama de prata. Estudo in vitro com 131INa. Rev Bras Odontol 1969; 26:153-58.
243. Kontakiotis E, Georgopoloulou M, Panopoulos P, Nakoy M. In vitro study of the antibacterial properties of two calcium hydroxide-based root canal sealers. Int Endod J 1996; 29:210. (Abstract).
244. Kontakiotis E, Nakou M, Georgopoulou M. In vitro study of the indirect action of calcium hydroxide on the anaerobic flora of the root canal. Int Endod J 1995; 28:285-89.
245. Krakow AA, Berk H. Efficient endodontic procedures with the use of the pressure syringe. Dent Clin North Am 1965; 9:387-99.
246. Krakow AA. Endodontic surgery. In: Cohen S, Burns R. Pathways of the pulp. Saint Louis: C.V. Mosby Company, 1976. p.479-83.
247. Kuga MC, Keine KC. Selamento apical e qualidade das obturações proporcionadas pela obturação retrógrada e retroinstrumentação com retrobturação. Rev Bras Odontol 1989; 46:41-46.
248. Kutller Y. Endodoncia práctica. México: Ed. «A.L.P.H.A.», 1961. p.292.
249. Kwak KI et al. The effect of obturation timing and thickness of mineral aggregate matrix on sealing ability. J Endod 2000; 26:557. (Abstracts).

250. Laghios CD et al. Comparative radiopacity of tetracalcium phosphate and other root-end filling materiais. Int Endod J 2000; 33:311-15.
251. Lambjerg-Hansen H. Vital and mortal pulpectomy on permanent human teeth: an experimental comparative histologic investigation. Scand J Dent Res 1974; 82:243-32.
252. Langeland K, Rodrigues H, Dowden W. Periodontal disease, bacteria, and pulpal histopathology. Oral Surg Oral Med Oral Pathol 1974; 37:257-70.
253. Lantz B, Persson PA. Periodontal tissue reactions after surgical treatment of root perforation in dog's teeth. A histologic study. Odont Revy 1970, 21:51-62.
254. Layton CA, Marshall G, Morgan LA, Baumgartner JC. Evaluation of cracks associated with ultrasonic root-end preparation. J Endod 1996; 22:157-60.
255. Leal JM, Bampa JU. Cirurgias parendodônticas: indicações, contra-indicações, modalidades cirúrgicas. In: Endodontia: tratamento de canais radiculares. Leonardo MR, Leal JM. 3rd ed. São Paulo: Panamericana. 1998; p.737-801.
256. Leal JM, Holland R, Esberard RM. Sealapex, C.R.C.S., Fill Canal e N-Rickert, estudo da biocompatibilidade em tecido conjuntivo subcutâneo de rato. Odontol Clín 1988; 2:7-14.
257. Leal JM, Simões-Filho AP, Esberard RM, Bonetti-Filho I, Lofredo LCM. Materiais seladores provisórios: avaliação da permeabilidade frente a rodamina B a 2%. Rev Gaúcha Odontol 1984; 32:271-76.
258. Leal JM, Simões-Filho AP, Leonardo MR. Estudo in vitro sobre a infiltração e o comportamento dimensional dos cimentos de uso endodôntico "Fill Canal" e "Trin Canal". Rev Bras Odontol 1975; 32:169-73.
259. Leal JM. Materiais obturadores de canais radiculares. In: Endodontia: tratamento de canais radiculares. Leonardo MR, Leal JM, Simões-Filho AP. São Paulo: Médica Panamericana, 1982. p.264-95.
260. Lee ES. A new mineral trioxide aggregate root-end filling technique. J Endod 2000; 26:764-65.
261. Lee SJ et al. Sealing ability of a mineral trioxide aggregate for repair of lateral root perforations. J Endod 1993; 19:541-44.
262. Leinz V, Campos JES. Guia para determinação de minerais. 10th ed. São Paulo: Nacional, 1986. 92p.
263. Leonardo MR et al. Hidróxido de cálcio em endodontia: avaliação da alteração do pH e da liberação de íons de cálcio em produtos endodônticos à base de hidróxido de cálcio. Rev Gaúcha Odontol 1992; 40:69-72.
264. Leonardo MR, Silva LA, Tanomaru-Filho M, Bonifácio KC, Ito IY. Avaliação in vitro da atividade antimicrobiana de pastas utilizadas em endodontia. Rev Ass Paul Cir Dent 1999; 53:367-70.
265. Leonardo MR. Contribuição para o estudo da reparação apical e periapical pós-tratamento de canais radiculares. (Thesis). São Paulo State University; 1973. 126p.
266. Leonardo MR. Reparação apical e periapical pós-tratamento endodôntico. Proservação. In: Endodontia: tratamento de canais radiculares. Leonardo MR, Leal JM. 2nd ed. São Paulo: Médica Panamericana, 1991. p.460-94.
267. Liggett WR, Brady JM, Tsaknis PJ, Del-Rio CE. Light microscopy, scanning electron microscopy, and microprobe analysis of bone response to zinc and non-zinc amalgam implants. Oral Surg Oral Med Oral Pathol 1980; 49:254-62.
268. Lim KC, Tidmarsh BG. The sealing ability of Sealapex compared with AH 26. J Endod 1986; 12:564-66.
269. Limkangwalmongkol S, Abbott PV, Sandler AB. Apical dye penetration with four root canal sealers and gutta-percha: using longitudinal sectioning. J Endod 1992, 18:535-39.
270. Lindauer PA. Vertical root fractures in curved root under simulated clinical conditions. J Endod 1989; 15:345-49.
271. Lindqvist L, Otteskog P. Eugenol: liberation from dental materials and effect on human diploid fibroblast cells. Scand J Dent Res 1981; 88:552-56.
272. Littman LC. Apical resection with retrograde amalgam technique. Dent Stud 1970; 48:25.
273. Lloyd A, Jaunberzins A, Dummer PMH, Bryant S. Root-end cavity preparation using the MicroMega Sonic Retroprep Tip™. SEM analysis. Int Endod J 1996; 29:295-301.
274. Loxley EC et al. The effect of various intracanal oxidizing agents on the push-out strength of mineral trioxide aggregate (MTA), intermediate repair material (IRM), and super EBA cement used as perforation repair materiais. J Endod 2001; 27:218. (Abstracts).
275. Luebke RG, Glick DH, Ingle JI. Indications and contraindications for endodontic surgery. Oral Surg Oral Med Oral Pathol 1964; 18:97-113.
276. Luiz MR. Avaliação do reparo apical e periapical, em dentes de cães com lesão periapical após obturação retrógrada com diferentes materiais retrobturadores. (Doctoral Thesis). São Paulo State University – UNESP. 2002; 193p.
277. Luks S. Root end amalgam technic in the practice of endodontics. J Am Dent Ass 1956; 53:424-28.
278. MacDonald A, Moore BK, Newton CW, Brown CE. Evaluation of an apatite cement as a root end filling material. J Endod 1994; 20:598-604.
279. MacPherson MG, Hartwell GR, Bondra DL, Weller RN. Leakage in vitro with high-temperature thermoplasticized gutta-percha high cooper amalgam, and warm gutta-percha when used as retrofilling materials. J Endod 1989; 15:212-15.
280. Madison S, Wilcox LR. An evaluation of coronal microleakage in endodontically treated teeth. Part III. in vivo study. J Endod 1988; 14:455-58.
281. Marcotte LR, Dowson J, Rowe NH. Apical healing with retrofilling materials amalgam and gutta-percha. J Endod 1975; 1:63-65.
282. Markowitz K, Moynihan M, Liu M, Kim S. Biologic properties of eugenol and zinc oxide-eugenol: a clinical oriented review. Oral Surg Oral Med Oral Pathol 1992; 73:729-37.
283. Marlin J, Krakow AA, Desilets PR, Gron P. Clinical use of injectioin-molded thermoplasticized gutta-percha for obturation of the root canal system. A preliminary report. J Endod 1981; 7:277-81.
284. Marlin J, Schilder H. Physical properties of gutta-percha when subjected to heat and vertical condensation. Oral Surg Oral Med Oral Pathol 1973; 36:872-79.
285. Martell B, Chandler NP. Electrical and dye leakage comparison of MTA, super EBA and IRM. J Endod 2000; 26:545. (Abstracts).

286. Martin LR, Tidwell F, Tenca JI, Pelleu GB, Longton RW. Histologic response of rat connective tissue to zinc-containing amalgam. J Endod 1976; 2:25-27.
287. Matsumiya S, Kitamura M. Histopathological and histobacteriological studies of the relation between the condition of sterilization of the interior of the root canal and the healing process of periapical tissue in experimentally infected root canal treatment. Bull Tokyo Dent Coll 1960; 1:1-19.
288. Matsura SJ. A simplified root-end filling technic using silver amalgam. J Mich St Dent Assoc 1962; 44:40-41.
289. McCormick JE. Tissue pH of developing periapical lesions in dogs. J Endod 1983; 9:47-51.
290. Mehta PK, Monteiro PJM. Concreto: estrutura, propriedades e materiais. São Paulo: Pini, 1994. 584p.
291. Mello W, Holland R, Souza V. Capeamento pulpar com hidróxido de cálcio ou pasta de óxido de zinco e eugenol: estudo histológico comparativo em dentes de cães. Rev Fac Odontol Araçatuba 1972; 1:33-44.
292. Messing JJ. The use of amalgam in endodontics surgery. J Br Endod Soc 1967; 1:34-36.
293. Messing JJ. Treatment of periapical areas in anterior teeth. Br Dent J 1967; 123:286-90.
294. Metrick L. Obliteration of the apical third of the canal from the apex of the root. J Can Dent Assoc 1956; 22:474.
295. Michanowicz A, Czonstkowsky M. Sealing properties of an injection-thermoplasticized low-temperature (70°C) gutta-percha: a preliminary study. J Endod 1984; 10:563-66.
296. Min MM, Brown-Jr CE, Legan JJ, Kafrawy AH. In vitro evaluation of effects of ultrasonic root-end preparation on resected root surfaces. J Endod 1997; 23:624-28.
297. Mitchell DF. The irritational qualities of dental materials. J Amer Dent Ass 1959; 59:954-66.
298. Mitchell PJ et al. Osteoblast biocompatibility of mineral trioxide aggregate. Biomaterials 1999; 20:167-73.
299. Molloy D et al. Comparative tissue tolerance of a new endodontic sealer. Oral Surg Oral Med Oral Pathol 1992; 73:490-93.
300. Molnar EJ. Residual eugenol from zinc oxide-eugenol compounds. J Dent Res 1967; 46:645-49.
301. Moodnik RM, Levey MH, Besen MA, Borden BC. Retrograde amalgam filling: a scanning electron microscopic study. J Endod 1975; 1:28-31.
302. Moraes SH et al. Reação do tecido conjuntivo subcutâneo de rato ao implante do cimento Portland. J Bras Endod 2001; 2:326-9.
303. Moreira GH, Souza V, Holland R, Saliba O. Effect of zinc acetate on the sealing and irritating properties of the zinc oxide-eugenol cement. Rev Odontol UNESP 1981; 10:35-40.
304. Moreno A. Thermomechanically softened gutta-percha root canal filling. J Endod 1977; 3:186-88.
305. Moretton TR et al. Tissue reactions after subcutaneous and intraosseous implantation of mineral trioxide aggregate and ethoxybenzoic acid cement. J Biomed Mater Res 2000; 52:528-33.
306. Morgan LA, Marshall JG. A scanning electron microscopic study of in vivo ultrasonic root-end preparations. J Endod 1999; 25:567-70.
307. Morse DR, Martell B, Pike CG, Fantasia J, Esposito JV, Furst L. A comparative tissue toxicity evaluation of gutta-percha root canal sealers. Part II. Forty-eight hour findings. J Endod 1984; 10:484-86.
308. Mortensen DW, Boucher-Júnior NE, Ryge G. A method of testing for marginal leakage of dental restorations with bacteria. J Dent Res 1965; 44:58-63.
309. Moura RA. Microbiologia clínica: técnicas de laboratório. 2nd ed. São Paulo: Atheneu. 1982; p.230-56.
310. Myers K et al. The effects of mineral trioxide aggregate on the dog pulp. J Endod 1996; 22:198. (Abstracts).
311. Nakata TT et al. Perforation repair comparing mineral trioxide aggregate and amalgam using an anaerobic bacterial leakage model. J Endod 1998; 24:184-86.
312. Negm MM. The effect of human blood on the sealing ability of root canal sealers: an in vitro study. Oral Surg Oral Med Oral Pathol 1989; 67:449-52.
313. Nery MJ, Souza V, Holland R. Reação do coto pulpar e tecidos periapicais de dentes de cães a algumas substâncias empregadas no preparo do canal radicular dos canais radiculares. Rev Fac Odontol Araçatuba 1974; 3:245-58.
314. Nery RS. Comportamento dos tecidos apicais e periapicais de dentes decíduos de cães, após pulpotomia e obturação dos canais radiculares com Sealapex, Sealer Plus e MTA. (Doctoral Thesis). São Paulo State University; 2000. 311p.
315. Nery RS. Avaliação do comportamento histomorfológico de dentes decíduos de cães, após pulpectomia e obturação dos canais radiculares com diferentes materiais. (Master's Thesis). Araçatuba: Faculdade de Odontologia, Universidade Estadual Paulista. 1999. 253p.
316. Neville AM. Propriedades do concreto. 2nd ed. São Paulo: Pini, 1997. 828p.
317. Nicholls E. Retrograde filling of the root canal. Oral Surg Oral Med Oral Pathol 1962; 15:463-73.
318. Nicholson RJ, Casanova F, Greenspan J, Stark MM. Comparison of tissue response between a synthetic gutta-percha and a natural gutta-percha endodontic filler. Oral Surg Oral Med Oral Pathol 1975; 39:802-25.
319. Nordenram A, Svärdström G. Results of apicectomy. A clinical-radiological examination. Swed Dent J 1970; 63:593-604.
320. Nordenram A. Biobond for retrograde root filling in apicoectomy. Scand J Dent Res 1970; 78:251-55.
321. Nygaard-Ostby B. Apicectomy: introduction to endodontics. Oslo: Universitetsforlaget, 1971. p.73-5.
322. O'Connor RP, Hutter JW, Roahen JO. Leakage of amalgam and Super-EBA root-end fillings using two preparations thecniques and surgical microscopy. J Endod 1995; 21:74-78.
323. Ogata M, Leal JM, Miranda VC, Lofredo LCM. Cimentos endodônticos. Efeito da relação pó-líquido na ação antimicrobiana. Rev Gaúcha Odontol 1984; 32:250-54.
324. Ogata M, Miranda VC, Leal JM. Cimentos de uso endodôntico. Estudo in vitro da ação antimicrobiana. Rev Paul Endod 1982; 3:84-87.
325. Ogawa A, Holland R, Souza V. Influência do selamento cavitário no processo de reparo da polpa dental após pulpotomia e proteção com hidróxido de cálcio. Rev Fac Odontol Araçatuba 1974; 3:51-59.
326. Oliveira HM. Cimento Portland. In: Bauer LAF. Materiais de construção. 3rd ed. Rio de Janeiro: LTC – Livros Técnicos e Científicos, 1987. p.35-62.

327. Olsen FK, Austin BP, Walia N. Osseous reaction to implanted ZOE retrograde filling materials in the tibia of rats. J Endod 1994; 20:389-94.
328. Onnink PA, Davis RD, Wayman BE. An in vitro comparison of incomplete root fractures associated with three obturation techniques. J Endod 1994; 20:32-37.
329. Orstavik D. Antibcterial properties of root canal sealers, cements and pastes. Int Endod J 1981; 14:125-33.
330. Osório RM, Hefti A, Vertucci FJ, Shawley AL. Cytotoxicity of endodontic materials. J Endod 1998; 24:91-96.
331. O'Sullivan SM, Hartwell GR. Obturation of a retained primary mandibular second molar using mineral trioxide aggregate: a case report. J Endod 2001; 27:703-05.
332. Otoboni-Filho JA. Estudo histológico do comportamento dos tecidos periapicais do dente do cão após curetagem periapical, apicectomia e obturação retrógrada. (Master's Thesis). São Paulo State University; 1981. 64p.
333. Otoboni-Filho JA. Estudo histológico comparativo entre o tratamento endodôntico, curetagem periapical, apicectomia e obturação retrógrada em dentes de cães com lesão periapical. (Doctoral Thesis). São Paulo State University; 1987. 100p.
334. Ousley JS, Wagner MJ, Taylor PP. Effect of surface conditioners on amalgam marginal leakage. J Dent Child 1970; 37:62-68.
335. Owadally ID, Chong BS, Pitt-Ford TR, Watson TF. The sealing ability of IRM® with the addition of hydroxyapatite as a retrograde root filling. Endod Dent Traumatol 1993; 9:211-15.
336. Owadally ID, Pitt-Ford TR. Effect of addition of hydroxyapatite on the physical properties of IRM. Int Endod J 1994; 27:227-32.
337. Oynick J, Oynick T. A study of a new material for retrograde fillings. J Endod 1978; 4:203-06.
338. Panopoulos P, Kontakiotis E. Changes in pH and weight of calcium hydroxide pastes. Int Endod J 1990; 23:56. (Abstract).
339. Pantschev A, Carlsson AP, Andersson L. Retrograde root filling with EBA cement or amalgam: a comparative clinical study. Oral Surg Oral Med Oral Pathol 1994; 78:101-04.
340. Panzarini SRB, Souza V, Holland R, Dezan-Jr E. Tratamento de dentes com lesão periapical crônica: influência de diferentes tipos de curativo de demora e do material obturador de canal radicular. Rev Odontol UNESP 1998; 27:509-26.
341. Pashley DH, Michelich V, Kehl T. Dentin permeability: effects of smear layer removal. J Prosthet Dent 1981; 46:531-37.
342. Pécora JD, Roselino RB. Instabilidade dimensional dos materiais utilizados para selamento provisório de cavidades em endodontia. Rev Fac Farm Odontol Ribeirão Preto 1982; 19:69-77.
343. Perez AL, Al-Awadhi S. A comparative assessment of primary osteoblasts and MG-63 Osteosarcoma cells when contact with ProRoot MTA vs white MTA. An SEM study. J Endod 2002; 28:257. (Abstract).
344. Pertot WJ, Stephan G, Tardieu C, Proust JP. Comparison of the intraosseous biocompatibility of Dyract and Super EBA. J Endod 1997; 23:315-19.
345. Peters LB, Harrison JW. A comparison of leakage of filling materials in demineralized and non-demineralized resected root ends under vacuum and non-vacuum conditions. Int Endod J 1992; 25:273-78.
346. Peters MA, Cunningham J. Gutta-percha points at apicoectomy. To push or to pull? Oral Surg Oral Med Oral Pathol 1979; 47:176-78.
347. Phillips R, Gilmore W, Swartz M, Schenker S. Adaptation of restorations in vivo as assessed by 45Ca. J Am Dent Ass 1961; 62:23-34.
348. Pitt-Ford TR et al. Mineral trioxide aggregate as a root-end filling material. J Endod 1994; 20:188. (Abstract n.l).
349. Pitt-Ford TR et al. Using mineral trioxide aggregate as a pulp-capping material. J Am Dent Assoc 1996; 127:1491-94.
350. Pitt-Ford TR et al. Use of mineral trioxide aggregate for repair of furcal perforations. Oral Surg Oral Med Oral Pathol 1995; 79:756-62.
351. Pitt-Ford TR, Andreasen JO, Dorn SO, Kariyawasan SP. Effect of IRM as a root end fillings on healing after replantation. J Endod 1994; 20:381-85.
352. Pitt-Ford TR, Andreasen JO, Dorn SO, Kariyawasan SP. Effect of Super-EBA as a root end filling on healing after replantation. J Endod 1995; 21:13-15.
353. Pitt-Ford TR, Andreasen JO, Dorn SO, Kariyawasan SP. Effect of various zinc oxide materials as root-end fillings on healing after replantation. Int Endod J 1995; 28:273-78.
354. Pitt-Ford TR, Andreasen JO, Dorn SO, Kariyawasan SP. Effect of various sealers with gutta-percha as root-end fillings on healing after replantation. Endod Dent Traumatol 1996; 1:3-7.
355. Pumarola J, Berastegui E, Brau E, Canalda C, Anta MTJ. Antimicrobial activity of seven root canal sealer: results of agar diffusion and agar dilution tests. Oral Surg Oral Med Oral Pathol 1992; 74:216-20.
356. Pupo J, Biral RR, Benatti O, Abe A, Valdrighi L. Antimicrobial effects of endodontic filling cements on microrganisms from root canal. Oral Surg Oral Med Oral Pathol 1983, 55:622-27.
357. Rabinowitch BZ. Pulp management in primary teeth. Oral Surg Oral Med Oral Pathol 1953; 6:542-50.
358. Rainwater A, Jeansonne BG, Sarkar N. Effects of ultrasonic root-end preparation on microcrack formation and leakage. J Endod 2000; 26:72-5.
359. Rakower W. Indication and technique for the root end amalgam seal. N Y St Dent J 1968; 34:609-12.
360. Reeh ES, Combe EC. A new single-step technique for apical retrofilling that significantly reduces microleakage. J Endod 1997; 23:149-51.
361. Reit C, Hirsch J. Surgical endodontic retreatment. Int Endod J 1986; 19:107-12.
362. Richman MJ. The use of ultrasonic in root canal therapy and root resection. J Dent Med 1957; 12:12-8.
363. Rocha MJC et al. O uso do hidróxido de cálcio e do agregado de trióxido mineral (MTA) em pulpotomias de dentes decíduos. UFES Rev Odontol 2000; 2:38-44.
364. Rodrigues H, Spangberg L, Langeland K. Biologic effects of dental materials 9. Effect of zinc-oxide eugenol cements on hela cells in vitro. Estomatol Cult 1975; 9:191-94.
365. Rowe AH. Effect of root filling materials on the periapical tissues. Br Dent J 1967; 122:98-102.

366. Roy CO et al. Effect of an acid environment on leakage of root-end filling materials. J Endod 2001; 27:7-8.
367. Rubim E, Farber JL. Patologia. Rio de Janeiro: Interlivros; 1990.
368. Rud J, Andreasen JO. A study of failures after endodontic surgery by radiographic, histologic and stereomicroscopic methods. Int J O Surg 1972; 1:311-28.
369. Russo M. Infiltração marginal do 131INa em restaurações de amálgama de prata. Arq Cent Est Fac Odontol UFMG 1970; 7:21-36.
370. Sacomani GRR. Estudo in vitro da infiltração marginal apical em dentes humanos e estudo in vivo do comportamento dos tecidos apicais e periapicais de dentes de cães à obturação de canal com os cimentos Sealer 26 e Sealer 26 Modificado. (Master's Thesis). University of Marília; 1999. 138p.
371. Safavi K, Nichols FC. Secretion of PGE2 from monocytos exposed to MTA or Portland cement. J Endod 2000; 26:540. (Abstracts).
372. Safavi KE, Nichols FC. Alteration of biological properties of bacterial lipopolysaccharide by calcium hydroxide treatment. J Endod 1994; 20:127-29.
373. Safavi KE, Nichols FC. Effect of calcium hydroxide on bacterial lipopolysaccharide. J Endod 1993; 19:76-78.
374. Saidon J et al. Tissue reaction to implanted Mineral Trioxide Aggregate or Portland cement. J Endod 2002; 28:247. (Abstracts).
375. Saunders WP, Saunders EM, Gutmann JL. Ultrasonic root-end preparation Part 2. Microleakage of EBA root-end fillings. Int Endod J 1994; 27:325-29.
376. Schilder H, Amsterdam M. Inflammatory potential of root canal medicaments. Oral Surg Oral Med Oral Pathol 1959; 12:211-21.
377. Schilder H. Filling root canals in three dimensions. Dent Clin North Am 1967; 11:723-44.
378. Schmitt D et al. Multifaceted use of ProRoot MTA root canal repair material. Pediatr Dent 2001; 23:326-30.
379. Schröder U, Granath LE. Early reaction of intact human teeth to calcium hydroxide following experimental pulpotomy and its significance to the development of hard tissue barrier. Odontol Revy 1971; 22:379-95.
380. Schröder U. Effects of calcium hydroxide-containing pulp-capping agents on pulp cell migration, proliferation, and differentiation. J Dent Res 1985; 64:541-48.
381. Schwartz RS et al. Mineral trioxide aggregate: a new material for endodontics. J Am Dent Assoc 1999; 130:967-75.
382. Seltzer S, Bender IB, Turkenkopf. Factors affecting successful repair after rooth therapy. J Am Dent Assoc 1963; 67:651-62.
383. Seltzer S, Bender IB. A polpa dental: considerações biológicas na prática dentária. 2nd ed. Rio de Janeiro: Labor. 1979; 499p.
384. Seltzer S, Bender IB. The inter-relationship of pulp and periodontal disease. Oral Surg Oral Med Oral Pathol 1963; 16:1474-90.
385. Seltzer S, Soltanoff W, Bender IB, Ziontz M. Biologic aspects of endodontics. I. Histologic observations of the anatomy and morphology of root apices and surrounding structures. Oral Surg Oral Med Oral Pathol 1966; 22:375-85.
386. Seltzer S. Endodontology: biologic consideration in endodontic procedures. New York: McGraw-Hill, 1971. p.1-32.
387. Serota KS, Krakow AA. Retrograde instrumentation and obturation of the root canal space. J Endod 1983; 9:448-51.
388. Seux D et al. Odontoblast-like cytodifferentiation of human dental pulp cells in vitro in the presence of a calcium hydroxide-containing cement. Arch Oral Biol 1991; 36:117-28.
389. Shabahang S et al. A comparative study of root-end induction using osteogenic protein-1, calcium hydroxide and mineral trioxide aggregate in dogs. J Endod 1999; 25:1-5.
390. Shabahang S, Torabinejad M. Treatment of teeth with open apices using mineral trioxide aggregate. Pract Periodont Aesthet Dent 2000; 13:315-20.
391. Shakhashiri BZ. Chemical demonstrations: a handbook for teachers of chemistry. Madison: Univ. Wisconsin Press, 1983. 344p.
392. Shakhashiri BZ. Chemical demonstrations: a handbook for teachers of chemistry. Madison: Univ. Wisconsin Press, 1985. 312p.
393. Shalhav M, Fuss Z, Weiss E. Antimicrobial activity of calcium hydroxide-containing endodontic sealers on Streptococcus faecalis in vitro. Int Endod J 1996; 29:208. (Abstract).
394. Silva LAB, Leonardo MR, Faccioli LH, Figueredo F. Inflammatory response to calcium hydroxide based root canal sealers. J Endod 1997; 23:86-90.
395. Silva LAB. Cimentos obturadores de canal radicular à base de hidróxido de cálcio. Avaliação histopatológica do reparo apical e periapical em dentes de cães da resposta inflamatória em tecido sucutâneo e da migração celular em cavidade peritoneal de camundogos: análise do pH concentração de cálcio total e condutividade. (Doctoral Thesis). University of São Paulo; 1995. 191p.
396. Silva MR. Aglomerantes. In: Materiais de construção. Silva MR. 2nd ed. São Paulo: Pini, 1991. p.13-43.
397. Silva MR. Água. In: Materiais de construção. Silva MR. 2nd ed. São Paulo: Pini, 1991. p.67-8.
398. Simões-Filho AP. Contribuição para o estudo de materiais obturadores de canais radiculares: verificação da solubilidade e desintegração. (Doctoral Thesis). São Paulo State University; 1969. 108p.
399. Siqueira-Jr JF, Gonçalves AB. Antibacterial activities of root canal sealers against selected anaerobic bacteria. J Endod 1996; 22:79-80.
400. Siqueira-Jr JF, Rocas I N, Lopes HP, Uzeda M. Coronal leakage of two root canal sealers containing calcium hydroxide after exposure to human saliva. J Endod 1999; 25:14-16.
401. Skinner EW, Phillips RW. The science of dental materials. 6.ed. Philadelphia: Saunders, 1967. 298p.
402. Sleder FS, Ludlow MO, Bohacek JR. Long-term sealing ability of a calcium hydroxide sealer. J Endod 1991; 17:541-43.
403. Sluyk SR et al. Evaluation of setting properties and retention characteristics of mineral trioxide aggregate when used as a furcation perforation repair material. J Endod 1998; 24:768-71.

404. Smee G, Bolanos OR, Morse DR, Furst ML, Yesilsoy C. A comparative leakage study of P-30 resin bonded ceramic, teflon, amalgam and IRM as retrofilling seals. J Endod 1987; 13:117-21.
405. Smith N. A histological study of the root end after apicectomy. Aust Dent J 1967; 13:586-90.
406. Snider D et al. Effect of root canal obturation and/or coronal seal on the success of root canal therapy. J Endod 1999; 25:294. (Abstracts).
407. Soares IML. Resposta pulpar ao MTA - Agregado de trióxido mineral - comparada ao hidróxido de cálcio em pulpotomias: histológico em dentes de cães. (Thesis). Florianópolis: Faculdade de Odontologia, Universidade Federal de Santa Catarina; 1996. 74p.
408. Soltanoff W. Apical sealing procedures. J N J Dent Assoc 1974; 44:36-38.
409. Sommer RF, Ostrander FD, Crowley MC. Clinical endodontics: a manual of scientific endodontics, Philadelphia: W.B. Saunders, 1956. p.323-64.
410. Sommer RF. Essentials for successful root resection. Am J Orthod & Oral Surg Oral Med O Pathol 1946; 32:76-100.
411. Sousa SMG, Bramante CM, Bernardineli N. Preparo cavitário apical - comparação entre técnicas. Rev Odontol Univ São Paulo 1995; 9:259-64.
412. Souza V et al. Reaction of rat connective tissue to the implant of calcium hydroxide pastes. Rev Fac Odontol Araçatuba 1977; 6:69-79.
413. Souza V, Bernabe PFE, Holland R, Nery MJ, Mello W. Tratamento não cirúrgico de dentes com lesões periapicais. Rev Bras Odontol 1989; 46:39-46.
414. Spångberg L. Biological effects of root canal filling materials. 7 – Reaction of bony tissue to implanted root canal filling material in guineapigs. Odont Tidskr 1969; 77:133-59.
415. Spångberg L. Comparison between tissue reactions to gutta-percha and polytetrafluorethelene implanted in the mandible of the rat. Svensk Tandläk T 1968; 61:705-15.
416. Spångberg LSW. Biologic effects of root canal filling materials. The effect on bone tissue of two formaldehyde-containing root canal filling pasts: N2 and Riebler's paste. Oral Surg Oral Med Oral Pathol 1974; 38:934-44.
417. Staehle HJ, Spiess V, Heinecke A, Muller HP. Effect of root canal filling materials containing calcium hydroxide on the alkalinity of root dentin. Endod Dent Traumatol 1995; 11:163-68.
418. Starkey PE. Pulpectomy and root canal filling in a primary molar: report of a case. J Dent Child 1973; 40:213-17.
419. Steinbrunner RL, Brown-Jr CE, Legan JJ, Kafrawy AH. Biocompatibility of two apatite cements. J Endod 1998; 24:335-42.
420. Stevens RH, Grossman LI. Antimicrobial effect of root canal cements on an abligate anaerobic organism. J Endod 1981; 7:266-71.
421. Storms JL. Root canal therapy via the apical foramen - radical or conservative? Oral Health 1978; 68:60-65.
422. Sultan M, Pitt-Ford TR. Ultrasonic preparation and obturation of root-end cavities. Int Endod J 1995; 28:231-38.
423. Sumi Y, Hattori H, Hayashi K, Ueda M. Ultrasonic root-end preparation: clinical and radiographic evaluation of results. J Oral Maxillofac Surg 1966; 54:590-93.
424. Sundqvist G. Ecology of the root canal. J Endod 1992; 18:427-30.
425. Szeremeta-Browar TL, Vancura JE, Zaki AE. A comparison of the sealing properties of different retrograde thecniques: an autoradiographic study. Oral Surg Oral Med Oral Pathol 1985; 59:82-87.
426. Tagger M, Tagger E, Kfir A. Release of calcium and hydroxyl ions from set endodontic sealers containing calcium hydroxide. J Endod 1988; 14:588-91.
427. Tagger M, Tagger E. Periapical reactions to calcium hydroxide-containing sealers and AH 26 in monkeys. Endod Dent Traumatol 1989; 5:139-46.
428. Tagliavini RL, Holland R, Milanezi LA. Implante de alguns componentes de fórmulas de cimentos cirúrgicos em tecido conjuntivo subcutâneo de ratos. Estudo histológico. Rev Fac Odontol Araçatuba 1974; 3:261-73.
429. Takayama S, Russo M, Holland R. Permeabilidade e infiltração marginal de radioisótopos em restaurações dentais. Rev Bras Odontol 1968; 25:60-67.
430. Tang HM et al. Endotoxin leakage of four root end filling materials. J Endod 1997; 23:259. (Abstract).
431. Tanomaru-Filho M et al. Capacidade de selamento apical imediata e mediata de materiais retrobturadores. J Bras Endo/Perio 2001; 2:296-99.
432. Tanomaru-Filho M et al. Capacidade seladora de diferentes cimentos endodônticos em obturações retrógradas. Rev Fac Odontol Lins 1998; 11:58-61.
433. Tanomaru-Filho M. Capacidade de selamento das técnicas de obturação retrógrada, retroinstrumentação com retrobturação e associação destas, utilizando-se os cimentos de N-Rickert, CRCS e Sealer 26. (Master's Thesis). University of São Paulo; 1992. 134p.
434. Tanzilli JP, Raphael D, Moodnik RM. A comparison of the marginal adaptation of retrograde techniques: a scanning electron microscopic study. Oral Surg Oral Med Oral Pathol 1980; 50:74-80.
435. Tassery H, Remusat M, Kuobi G, Pertot WJ. Comparison of the intraosseous biocompatibility of Vitremer and Super EBA by implantation into the mandible of rabbits. Oral Surg Oral Med Oral Pathol 1997; 83:602-08.
436. Taylor GN, Bump R. Endodontic considerations associated with periapical surgery. Oral Surg Oral Med Oral Pathol 1984; 58:450-55.
437. Taylor HFW. Cement chemistry. 2nd ed. London: Thomas Telford, 1997. 460p.
438. Thirawat J, Edmunds DH. Sealing ability of materials used as retrograde root fillings in endodontic surgery. Int Endod J 1989; 22:295-98.
439. Thompson SW, Hunt RD. Selected histochemical and histopathological methods. Flórida: Charles C. Thomas. 1966; p.615-46.
440. Thompson TS et al. Osteocalcin expression by cementoblasts attached to mineral trioxide aggregate. J Endod 2001; 27:242. (Abstracts).
441. Tidmarsh BG, Arrowsmith MG. Dentinal tubules at the root ends of apicected teeth: a scanning electron microscopic study. Int Endod J 1989; 22:184-89.
442. Tittle K et al. Apical closure induction using bone growth factors and mineral trioxide aggregate. J Endod 1996; 22:198. (Abstracts).
443. Torabinejad M et al. Histologic assessment of mineral trioxide aggregate as a root-end filling in monkeys. J Endod 1997; 23:225-28.

444. Torabinejad M et al. Tissue reaction to implanted root-end filling materials in the tibia and mandible of guinea pigs. J Endod 1998; 24:468-71.
445. Torabinejad M, Chivian N. Clinical applications of mineral trioxide aggregate. J Endod 1999; 25:197-205.
446. Torabinejad M, Hong CU, McDonald F, Pitt-Ford TR. Physical and chemical properties of a new root-end filling material. J Endod 1995; 21:349-53.
447. Torabinejad M, Hong CU, Pitt-Ford TR, Kariyawasam SP. Tissue reaction to implanted Super-EBA and mineral trioxide aggregate in the mandible of guinea pigs: a preliminary report. J Endod 1995; 21:569-71.
448. Torabinejad M, Hong CU, Lee SJ, Monsef M, Pitt-Ford TR. Investigation of mineral trioxide aggregate for root-end filling in dogs. J Endod 1995; 21:603-08.
449. Torabinejad M, Hong CU, Pitt-Ford TR, Kettering JD. Antibacterial effects of some root end filling materials. J Endod 1995; 21:403-06.
450. Torabinejad M, Hong CU, Pitt-Ford TR, Kettering JD. Citotoxicity of four root end filling material. J Endod 1995; 21:489-92.
451. Torabinejad M, Pitt-Ford TR. Root end filling materials: a review. Endod Dent Traumatol 1996; 12:161-78.
452. Torabinejad M, Pitt-Ford TR, Abedi HR, Kariyawasan SP, Tang HM. Tissue reaction to implanted root-end filling materials in the tibia and mandible of guinea pigs. J Endod 1998; 24:468-71.
453. Torabinejad M, Rastegar AF, Kettering JD, Pitt-Ford TR. Bactericid leakage of mineral trioxide aggregate as a root-end filling material. J Endod 1995; 21:109-12.
454. Torabinejad M, Riga RK, McKendry DJ, Pitt-Ford TR. Dye leakage of four root end filling materials: effects of blood contamination. J Endod 1994; 20:159-63.
455. Torabinejad M, Smith PW, Kettering JD, Pitt-Ford TR. Comparative investigation of marginal adaptation of mineral trioxide aggregate and other commonly used root-end filling materials. J Endod 1995; 21:295-99.
456. Torabinejad M, Watson TF, Pitt-Ford TA. Sealing ability of a mineral trioxide aggregate when used as a root end filling material. J Endod 1993; 19:591-95.
457. Trava-Airoldi VJ, Corat EJ, Pena AFV, Leite NF, Valera MC, Freitas JR, Baranauskas V. Development of chemical vapor deposition diamond burrs using hot filament. Rev Sci Instrum 1996; 67:1-3.
458. Tronstad L, Andreasen JO, Hasselgren G, Kristerson L, Riis I. pH changes in dental tissues after root canal filling with calcium hydroxide. J Endod 1981; 7:17-21.
459. Tronstad L, Barnett F, Cervone F. Periapical bacterial plaque in teeth refractory to endodontic treatment. Endod Dent Traumatol 1990; 6:73-77.
460. Tronstad L, Barnett F, Flax M. Solubility and biocompatibility of calcium hydroxide – containing root canal sealers. Endod Dent Traumatol 1988; 4:152-59.
461. Tronstad L, Barnett F, Riso K, Slots J. Extrarradicular endodontic infections. Endod Dent Traumatol 1987; 3:86-90.
462. Tronstad L, Kreshtool D, Barnett F. Microbiological monitoring and results of treatment of extraradicular endodontic infection. Endod Dent Traumatol 1990; 6:129- 36.
463. Tronstad L, Wennberg A. In vitro assessment of the toxicity of filling materials. Int Endod J 1980; 13:131-38.
464. Tronstad L. Clinical endodontics. New York: Thieme Medical Publishers; 1991. p.98-149.
465. Trope M, Lost C, Schmitz HJ, Friedman S. Healing of apical periodontitis in dogs after apicoectomy and retrofilling with various filling materials. Oral Surg Oral Med Oral Pathol Oral Radiol Oral Endod 1996; 81:221-28.
466. Trowbridge HO, Emling RC. Inflamação: uma revisão do processo. 4th ed. São Paulo: Quintessence, 1996. 174p.
467. Tung K, Menge AC. Sperm and testicular autoimmunity. In: The autoimmune diseases. Rose NR, MacKay IR. Orlando: Academic Press, 1985. p.537-90.
468. Vaidergorin ELL. Características dos cimentos portland: uma abordagem química. In: Instituto de Pesquisas Tecnológicas. Tecnologia de edificações. Publicação IPT 1785, IPT/Ded 016, 1988. p.19-22.
469. Valera MC, Leonardo MK, Bonetti-Filho I. Cimentos endodônticos: selamento marginal apical imediato e após armazenamento de seis meses. Rev Odontol Univ São Paulo 1998; 12:355-60.
470. Valera MC. Estudo da compatibilidade biológica de alguns cimentos endodônticos à base de hidróxido de cálcio e um cimento de ionômero de vidro: avaliação do selamento marginal apical e análise morfológica por microscopia de força atômica. (Doctoral Thesis). São Paulo State University. 1995; 333p.
471. Vasiliu D. Techniquè de l'obturation retrograde du canal radiculaire après la résection apicale. Rev Stomatol Chir Maxillofac 1977; 78:483-89.
472. Verçoza EJ. Aglomerantes hidráulicos. In: Materiais de construção. Verçoza EJ. Porto Alegre: EMMA, 1975. p.110-35.
473. Waplington M, Lumley PJ, Walmsley D. Incidence of root face alteration after ultrasonic retrograde cavity preparation. Oral Surg Oral Med Oral Pathol Oral Radiol Oral Endod 1997; 83:387-92.
474. Weidmann G et al. Structural materials. Oxford: Butterworth Heinemann; 1994. apud Estrela C, Bammann LL, Estrela CRA, Silva RS, Pécora JD. Antimicrobial and chemical study of MTA, Portland cement, calcium hydroxide paste, Sealapex and Dycal. Braz Dent J 2000; 2:3-9.
475. Weine FS, Gerstein H. Periapical surgery. In: Endodontic therapy. Weine FS. 2nd ed. Saint Louis: Mosby; 1976. p.339-42.
476. Weine FS. Preparación y obturación retrograda. Una solución ante problemas quirurgicos periapicales. Rev Esp Endod 1984; 2:69-81.
477. Wennberg A, Hasselgren G. Cytotoxicity evaluation of temporary filling materials. Int Endod J 1981; 14:121-24.
478. Whittaker DK, Kneale MJ. The dentine-predentine interface in human teeth. A scanning electron microscope study. Br Dent J 1979; 146:43-46.
479. Wiscovitch JG, Wiscovitch GJ. Surgical apical repair with Super-EBA cement: a one-visit alternative treatment to apexification. J Endod 1995; 21:43-46.
480. Wolfson EM, Seltzer S. Reactions of rat connective tissue to some gutta-percha formulations. J Endod 1975; 1:395-402.

481. Wu MK et al. Long-term seal provided by some root-end filling materials. J Endod 1998; 24:557-60.
482. Wu MK, Kean SD, Kersten HW. Quantitative micro-leakage study on a new retrograde filling technique. Int Endod J 1990; 23:245-49.
483. Wuchenich G, Meadows D, Torabinejad M. A comparison between two root end preparation techniques in human cadavers. J Endod 1994; 20:279-82.
484. Wucherpfening AL, Green DB. Mineral Trioxide vs Portland cement: two biocompatible filling materials. J Endod 1999; 25:308. (Abstract).
485. Yatsushiro JD et al. Longitudinal study of the microleakage of two root-end filling materials using a fluid conductive system. J Endod 1998; 24:716-19.
486. Yee FS, Marlin J, Krakow AA, Gron P. Three dimensional obturation of the root canal using injection molded, thermoplasticized dental gutta-percha. J Endod 1977; 3:168.
487. Ywabuchi M. Histopathological study: comparison of healing after vital and devitalized pulp extirpations. Bull Oral Pathol 1959; 4:1-5.
488. Zhu Q et al. Adhesion of human osteoblasts on root end filling materials. J Endod 2000; 26:404-06.
489. Zmener O, Guglielmotti MB, Cabrini RL. Biocompatibility of two calcium hydroxide based endodontic sealers: a quantitative study in the subcutaneous connective tissue of the rat. J Endod 1988; 14:229-35.

# Healing Process After Endodontic Treatment

**E. F. Mendonça**
*Federal University of Goiás, Goiânia, GO, Brazil*

**C. Estrela**
*Federal University of Goiás, Goiânia, GO, Brazil*

26

Chapter contents

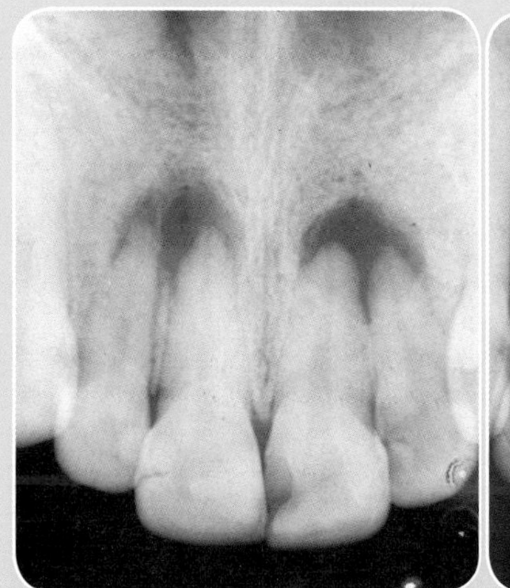
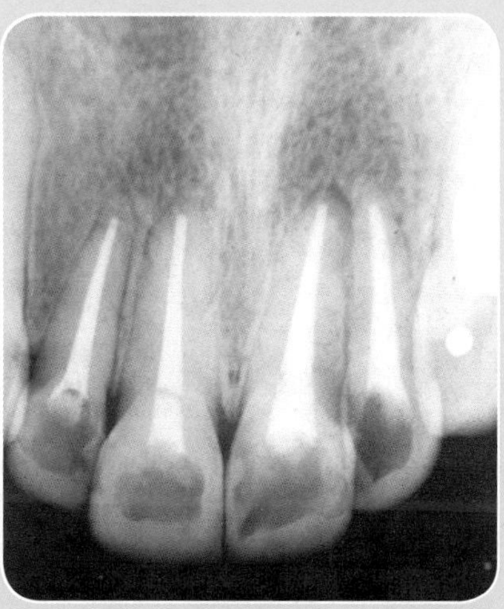

Healing process following endodontic treatment in teeth with apical periodontitis.

## 26.1 Introduction

The healing process is a sequence of events that occur to remove the injurious agents. It starts with the body's basic defense mechanism inflammation. Injurious agents vary, being either infectious, i.e., bacteria, fungi and virus, or non-infectious agents, such as situations occasioned by dentists during dental treatment[23,31,35]. Depending on the aggressor, there will be distinct inflammatory responses, despite the common pathways[20].

Inflammation is characterized by different phases according to the clinical location and/or systemic characteristics, involving semiologic aspects as regards signs and indications, and by the microscopic aspects of the cellular populations located in the developmental phase of a certain reaction. There are acute and chronic phases, with an intermediate sub-acute or sub-chronic phase[35].

The chronic inflammatory phase shows that the stimulating agent that originated the defense process is still in the lesion, maintaining the stimulation activity, and indicating the need for defense cells to arrive at this location in order to identify and eliminate the aggressor[20,29,35].

After the removal of the irritating agents, it is no longer necessary to maintain this stimulation activity, and this chronic process develops towards definitive repair of the lesion.

According to Trowbridge & Emling[35], the healing events occur a little later than the inflammatory events, but they overlap, as the phagocytosis process, which is pivotal for healing, occurs during both acute and chronic inflammation, together with fibroplasias and angiogenesis. Healing only begins with inflammation and ends with the definite removal of the irritant agent that caused the tissue response.

Blood, connective tissue and microcirculation are directly associated with inflammation as they are required to react against the stimulating agents. Antibodies and leukocytes, usually found in blood, need a competent vascular organization to develop the repair against microorganisms and other aggressors[20].

Healing can occur by two processes: regeneration or repair, depending on the regenerative capacity of the affected cells, extent of the lesion and proliferative activity of connective tissue stroma[21,34,35,36].

Regeneration is the process that substitutes the affected tissue by cells with similar characteristics to those previously lost, restoring the shape and function of the tissue. Repair is characterized by the formation of connective tissue with the predominance of fibroblasts.

In the regeneration process, the cells could be classified as labile, stable and permanent, according to the tissue response. The labile cells are reproduced throughout life in some tissues, such as epithelial tissue and blood, and in other tissues they are used as replacement for injured cells, such as fibroblasts, osteoblasts, condroblasts, flat muscular cells and endothelial cells. This is also true for all the mesenchyme-derived cells present in the connective tissue of the periodontium in the apical region.

The permanent cells, such as the neurons, are not capable of mitosis after being differentiated[35].

This chapter deals with the healing process after endodontic treatment, focusing on the events that occur in the periodontal region of dental root apex, with its peculiarities.

The periodontium of the root apex region consists of various tissues, namely cementum, periodontal ligament and alveolar bone.

According to Cawson et al.[2], the cementum is similar to bone, covering the external surface of the roots. There are two types of cementum: acellular and cellular. The first covers the entire root surface and the second, mostly in the apical third, contains cementocytes, which become included in irregularly distributed lacunae, similarly to osteocytes.

The periodontal ligament contains sets of collagen groups that link the tooth to the alveolar process; the collagen fibers of the periodontal ligament insert towards the alveolar bone, providing a perforated chamber that favors circulation.

Between each set of periodontal ligament fibers, connective tissue lacunae are formed, allowing the defense and connective tissue cells, together with the microcirculation, to prevent tissue damage from external aggressions and help the cementum and alveolar process to be renewed and remain in function[20].

The most frequent diseases in the apical periodontium are of an inflammatory nature, stimulated by complete or partial death of the dental pulp tissue, mostly of bacterial etiology caused by the development of dental caries. When not treated, caries compromises both coronal and radicular pulp tissue. The bacterial toxins reach the periapical region promoting substantial alterations in the connective tissue of the periodontal ligament, initiating inflammation[31,32].

Endodontic treatment provides the conditions for the healing process to begin when the biomechanical principles are complied with and sanitization of the root canal is performed accordingly.

Previously, the repair of conjunctive tissue lesions was characterized by microscopic descriptions of fibroplasia, collagen synthesis and neovascularization. However, recent evidences in cellular biology have provided more accurate explanations of the mechanisms, types of cells and chemical agents that control these activities. Amongst the chemical mediators, several growth factors secreted by cells have a role in the healing process[36].

The events involved in the healing process can be grouped in 4 phases: injury, inflammation, proliferation and remodeling. The injury to the periodontal ligament leads to the onset of the inflammatory phase, by an activation cascade of several systems, such as the coagulation, complement and kinines systems. The cascade systems are dynamic processes that are inter-related and promote alterations in the microenvironment, producing vasodilatation of the adjacent vessels that decreases the pH level and the oxygen tension and increases the local concentration of lactates[21,26,27,29,30,32,35].

As a result of these activities, a population of cells invades the injured area and replicate, characterizing the proliferation phase. A great number of inflammatory cells, together with macrophages of the previous inflammatory process and endothelial cells, characteristic of the repair process, constitute the granulation tissue.

The remodeling phase is the biological product of these cells, through differentiations that result in the regenerated tissue according to the extent of the injured area.

Cell specificity during the different stages of repair suggests that there is a specific chemotactic receptor responsible for this specificity, since the production and increase of cellularity seems to be dependent on growth or mitogenic agents. These are recruited during the inflammatory phase. Furthermore, the microenvironment of the lesion is of considerable importance in determining the types and number of cells present.

Lesions of inflammatory nature are characterized by the frequent migration of polymorphonuclear leukocytes, monocytes, lymphocytes, plasma cells, mast cells, osteoblasts and osteoclasts. The last few decades have been marked by great interest in the mediators, responsible for the recruitment and activation of these cells, in the inflammatory and repair processes, particularly the cytokines or chemokines. They link to specific receptors in the cells that initiate the transduction of signals, generating an amplitude of cellular responses, including chemotaxis and activation of the inflammatory cells and bony tissue[33].

The events that comprise the different stages of periapical lesion healing are: primary response to the tissue injury; inflammatory reaction and complement system activation; vascular response with the coagulation system activation (reaction in cascade); the creation of a new micro-environment in the periodontal region; cell recruitment under the influence of several chemical mediators and growth factors that can be mitogenic or chemotactic agents; cell replication; and the sprouting of a new vascular system promoted by angiogenesis stimulated within the connective tissue stimulated by the inflammatory cell infiltrate.

The repair process of a periapical lesion involves several aspects. The first is with regard to cases of pulpectomy, since the presence of dental pulp suggests the presence of a structured connective tissue which, when removed, may result in areas of plasmatic exudation with little bone destruction. The second involves cases of pulp necrosis in lesions of chronic development where there is already evidence of bony lyses. In such cases, the endodontic treatment suppresses the irritating agents, and the healing process will provide the objective conditions for inflammation to develop towards repair through sequential phases.

Chronic lesions, for example non-suppurative asymptomatic apical periodontitis, commonly described as radicular granuloma, are extremely slow developing lesions. Once the source of infection within the root canal has ceased, healing begins with the preexisting granulation tissue in the periapex.

The healing process after endodontic treatment of lesions radiographically diagnosed as radicular inflammatory cyst, have been discussed by Nair[22]. The author considers two types of cysts, in agreement with Simon's report [34] of a periapical cyst in the apical region, presenting lining epithelium that opens towards the foramen. There is another variant of radicular cyst consisting of the epithelial lining without direct communication with the root canal. Nair[22] denominated the aspect described by Simon[34] as a "pocket cyst". According to Nair[22], only teeth that present this type of apical pocket cyst are capable of healing completely after endodontic treatment.

There are strong evidences that foreign-body reaction, with the presence of multinuclear giant cells, occurs when the filling material overflows into the periodontal space, resulting in the development of asymptomatic periapical lesions that can remain refractory to endodontic therapy for a long period of time[22-25].

Figures 26.1 to 26.6 exhibit the radiographic and histopathologic aspects of a clinical case of persistent periapical lesion, containing the overfilling material.

To summarize, it is important to consider the diagnosis of the pathological condition to be treated; the therapeutic procedure, whether to perform pulpectomy or disinfection of the necrotic tissue, and the phases involved in the inflammatory process from acute to chronic, with cellular infiltration, connective tissue, and chemical and mitogenic mediators related to cells that constitute the repair process: injury – inflammation – proliferation – remodeling[21,31,32,35,36].

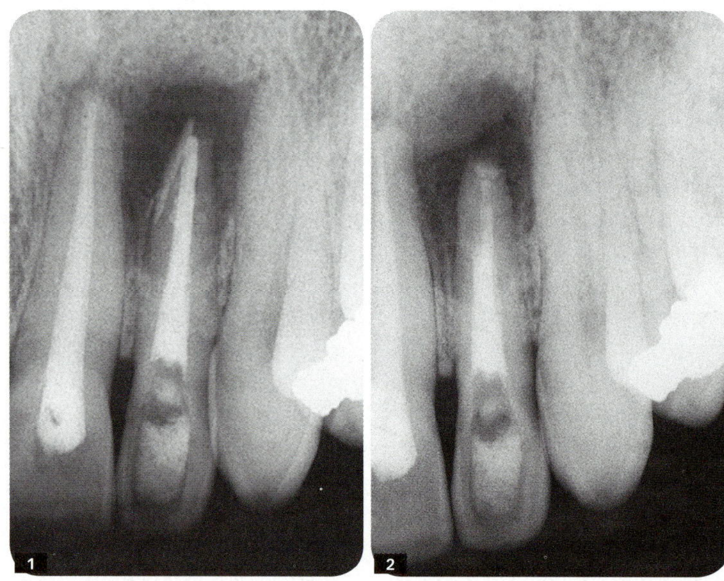

**Figures 26.1 and 26.2** - Radiographic aspect of asymptomatic periapical lesion in maxillary lateral incisor, with and without overfilling.

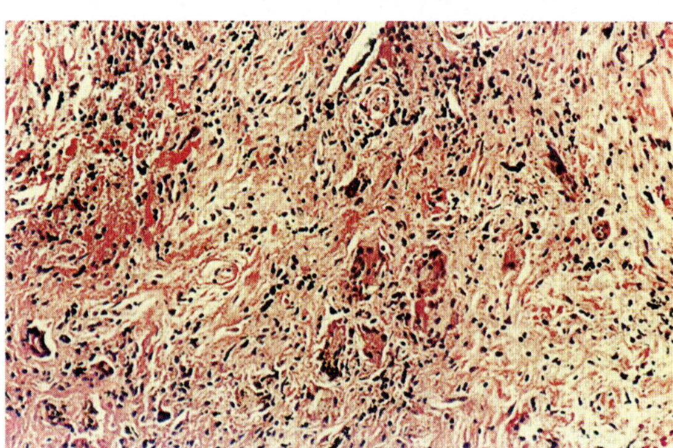

**Figure 26.3** - Mild inflammatory chronic cell infiltration with multinucleated giant cells in a connective fibrous stroma (repair process with failure) (H.E.)

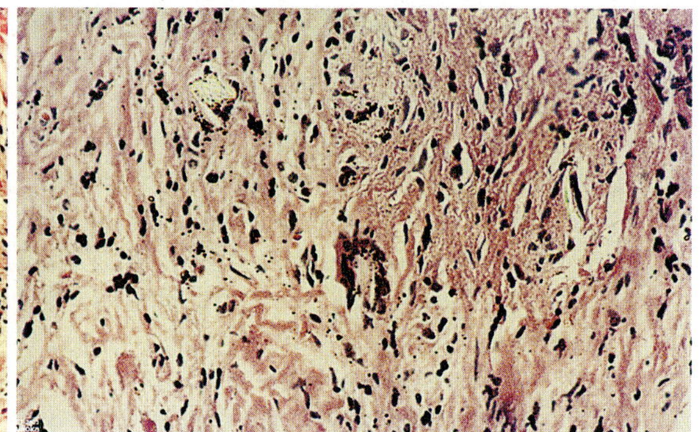

**Figure 26.4** - Higher magnification of Figure 26.3 (H.E.).

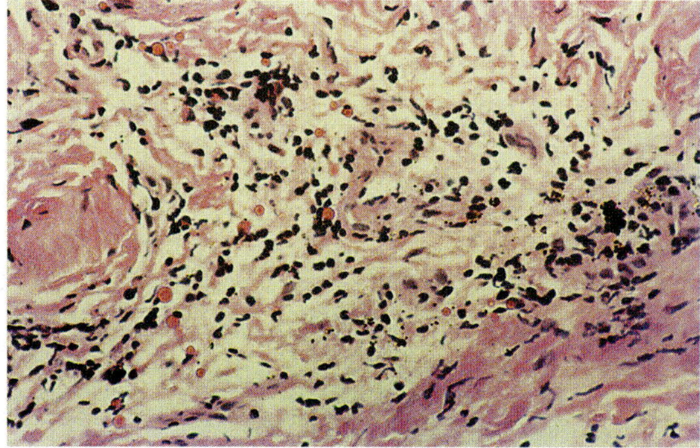

**Figure 26.5** - Infiltration of mononuclear cells with Russell bodies, which are the hyaline corpuscles (H.E.).

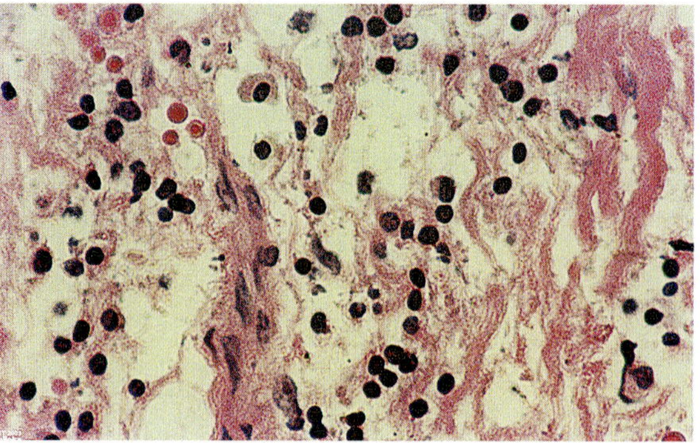

**Figure 26.6** - Higher magnification of Figure 26.5 (H.E.).

## 26.2 Apical Periodontal Inflammation

After periapical lesion, inflammatory response begins as a means of defense, with local and systemic manifestations, depending on the extent of the injury. Its initial phase is characterized by the formation of tissue exsudate which recruits the cells capable of producing the necessary chemical mediators for the reconstruction of the injured periodontal tissue. This inflammatory exsudate allows the bacterial toxins to be diluted, and ultimately proceeds with the removal of the remaining irritants. Tissue destruction results in the release of a substance similar to histamine, which promotes dilation of the capillaries and arterioles. Vasodilatation is also promoted by the biological products of the activation of the complement and kinine systems (Fig. 26.7).

The complement system involves 20 or more proteins that circulate in the blood in an inactive form. With injury in the periodontal region and plasma exsudation, the complement system is activated to produce a variety of proteins that are of fundamental importance in the healing process. For example, $C_{5a}$ is chemotactic for neutrophils and macrophages, essential in the phagocytosis of irritants and microbes. These cells also express several growth factors that modulate the repair process. $C_{3a}$ and $C_{4a}$ stimulate mast cells and basophiles to release histamine, very important in the maintenance of vascular permeability and constitution of the inflammatory exsudate. The kinines system is responsible for the transformation of an inactive enzyme, kallikrein, present in the blood and in the tissue, into its active form, bradykinin, which contributes to the production of the inflammatory exsudate by increasing vasodilatation, thus increasing vascular permeability[21,30,31,35,36].

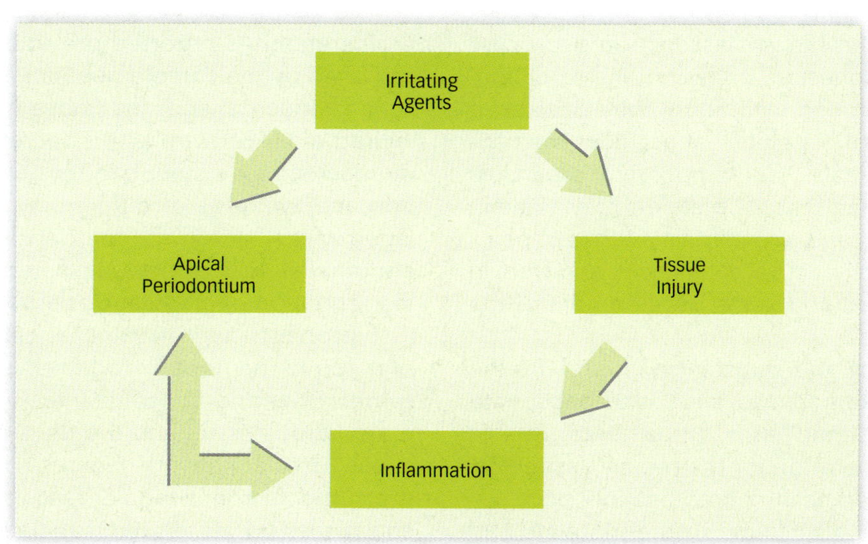


**Figure 26.7** - Tissue response to irritating agent in the apical periodontium.

Associated with bradykinin and other kinines, such as kalydine and leukotaxine and complement system, a set of chemical and enzymatic agents reinforces the increase in the permeability of the endothelial wall, facilitating the exit of the plasma proteins, leukocytes and red cells. Amongst these agents are the globulin factors of permeability, Hageman factor, prostaglandins and cyclic AMP. The leukocyte diapedesis occurs in the presence of chemotactic factors released in the interstitial connective tissue as a result of the injury to the periodontal ligament and alveolar bone.

Vessel lesions can occur when there is over instrumentation during the preparation of the root canal, mostly in cases of pulpectomy. The vascular reaction to the trauma differs according to the size or extent of the area involved. In the periapical region, there are vases that initially contract, stimulated by vasoactive substances that act on the myofilaments of the endothelial walls. These substances include cathecolamines that are released by the platelets and plasma during the inflammatory process. As the intravascular volume is reduced, the blood viscosity is increased and the flow in the injured region is reduced. During this process, individual cells suffer irreversible coalescence in a process involving adhesion, cohesion and coalition. When combined with fibrin, they develop a blood clot of platelets that occludes the capillary terminals. Contemporary researches have revealed that the platelets play a role in hemostasis, and also contain a series of pharmacologically active substances involved in inflammation and in the development of the healing[20,21,41].

Some of the substances found in the platelets are enzymes, such as tri-phosphate adenosine, that has a fundamental role in energy generation for the repair. Vasoactive amines, adrenalin, noradrenaline and histamine, are also found in the platelets and are powerful mediators of the inflammatory reaction. Growth factors released from the platelet degranulation of $\alpha$ granule, such as FCDP, promote the repair, through attraction of fibroblasts, endothelial cells and monocytes[11,12,19,20,29,31,32,35].

Other important component after activation of the coagulation system is blood clot formation. A number of reactions occur for the conversion of fibrin from its precursor fibrinogen. Fibrin production involves the cleavage of an inactive molecule of fibrinogen into an enzyme denominated thrombin using the extrinsic and intrinsic pathways. The extrinsic pathway is a result of tissue injury with the release of a complex denominated thromboplastin and the intrinsic pathway involves vessel injury leading to platelet interaction with the Hageman factor (Factor XII). Both pathways lead to the formation of an activated prothrombin that converts into thrombin[19,20,29,31,35].

The clot formation has a preponderant role in the healing process, mostly in cases of chronic periapical lesions that require surgical removal. After the lesion is removed, the surgical bed fills with blood and the inflammatory process begins with activation of the coagulation system and consequently, clot formation that has the basic function of sustaining the repair[19,20,29,31,35].

The next phase to begin is denominated proliferation. As reported previously, factors activated by the complement act as chemotactic for macrophages that move towards the injured area. Growth factors secreted locally by macrophages stimulate fibroblast migration and synthesis of different types of collagen which, along with the development of endothelial cells of new capillaries, result in the formation of granulation tissue[19,20,29,31,35].

Fibroblasts and endothelial cells are pivotal for tissue repair, together with other events occurring concomitantly, which generate fibrous tissue and the development of a new vascular network. Fibrous tissue needs the nutrients from a regular vascular network, and the blood vessels and capillaries require matrix support and protection for their development and extension.

The connective tissue in the area under repair is generally composed of Type I and

II collagens, cells, vessels and a matrix rich in glycoproteins and proteoglycans. Collagen is secreted by fibroblasts attracted to the area and stimulated by a multiplicity of growth factors, such as PDGF (platelet derived growth factor), TGF-β (transforming growth factor β), FGF (fibroblast growth factor), EGF (epithelial growth factor) and IGF-1 (insulin growth factor). Fibronectin is also a tissue factor that stimulates collagen production by fibroblasts. Collagen formation involves a series of enzymatic reactions and several co-factors that control this progress. The collagen matrix facilitates angiogenesis, acting as structural protection for the new fragile vessels and providing the necessary time for anastomosis to occur. Additional components of the matrix secreted by fibroblasts, denominated adherence factors, control the endothelial cell development promoting the adherence of these cells to the basal membrane of collagen. Laminin is one of the glycoproteins that have this function[19,20,29,31,35].

Angiogenesis occurs as a response to the hypoxia following tissue injury, as well as the release of cell factors. The platelets are primarily responsible for angiogenesis. The activated platelets attract macrophages to the affected area through chemotactic action of PDGF and FGF basic (FGFb). FGFb is a powerful chemotactic and mythogenic agent for endothelial cells. TGF-β is also found in the platelets and has an indirect effect on angiogenesis by promoting the release of the tumoral necrosis factor (TNF-α) and interleukin 1 (IL-1) by the macrophages[19,20,29,31,35].

More recent investigations indicate that angiogenesis results from a balance between positive and negative regulators, or also called angiogenic stimulators. New vessel formation starts with the activation of hydrolytic enzymes, such as those for collagenasis, denominated stromelysin and plasminogen. These enzymes act on the vessel walls dissolving their basal membranes and releasing endothelial cells. These cells then migrate through the injured area under the influence of a chemotactic gradient. In the areas of tissue hypoxia the cells form lumens and fuse into channels to allow a continuous flow of blood. Mesenchymal cells near the new vessels are important, because some become intimately associated with the vascular network and are known as pericytes. These cells play an important role in the growth inhibition of the adjacent endothelial cells, consequently regulating angiogenesis. Mesenchymal cells have also been involved in the differentiation into osteoblasts under the influence of the morphogenic proteins of the bone promoting osteogenesis. After tissue oxygenation and consequent homeostasis, there is a reduction in cells such as macrophages, and of the factors released by platelet activation[19,20,29,31,35].

The different collagens, "along with glycosamineglycanes, hyaluronidases and adhesion factors such as fibronectin and integrins are components of the extracellular matrix. The role of the matrix includes the adhesion and direction of the cellular migration as well as the cell polarity and orientation. Another characteristic of the proliferation stage includes elevated water content and an increased number of vessels"[36].

With regards to bony tissue healing, in this proliferation phase, the mesenchymal cells can differentiate into osteoblasts that will produce bony matrix. Most of the time, the bony tissue of embryonic origin, as well as the growth and chemocin factors, are biologically active substances involved in this process, as has been mentioned previously. According to Goldbring & Golching[12] cytokines are defined as soluble products released by a cell, which can modulate the activity of other cells and its own multiple biological activities. Chemocins have common functional properties, for example, the interleukins, monocins or lymphocins. Chemocins can also be considered as regulators of cell growth and differentiation in the immune and hematopoietic systems.

The growth factors involved in the bony repair are described as follows: the transforming growth factor beta (TGF-β) includes 25 molecular factors, such as the morphogenetic bony proteins. TGF-β is released in the sites of degranulation of platelets, macrophages and extracellular matrix. It is activated by the acidic environment of the injured area and has the function of stimulating osteoblastic activity and intraosseous regeneration.

PDGF is released from the platelet α granules and is a powerful mytogen, especially for fibroblasts. It is a competent factor that allows the cells to respond to other biological mediators and also acts to modulate the blood flow, therefore having a significant role in the repair. Other important factors are FGF and IGF.

Following bone injury, there is onset of the inflammatory process with complement activation, vessel ruptures, clot formation, as in cases of endodontic surgery. The sum of these events produces a microenvironment that is specific for cells with the function of promoting the cleaning of necrotic areas and promoting tissue healing. In its initial phase, this is not fully characterized. However, oxygen and pH gradient are decreased. These terms are fundamental for the activation of leukocytes, lymphocytes, macrophages and condrocytes[19,20,29,31,35].

The blood exsudate that occurs following the removal of lesion consists of hematogenic components such as erythrocytes, fibrin and platelets. The platelets are a source of biologically active healing factors, released from their α-granules that contain PDGF, FGF and TGF-β, which are chemotactic and cell activity regulators. The presence of these factors attracts cells to the affected area functions to exert their reparative functions. For example, the passage of the mesenchymal cells from phase $G_0$ to phase $G_1$ is promoted by PDGF, consequently transforming them into competent cells. Competence is the stage when a cell becomes responsible for the factor modulation for additional growth. TGF-β stimulates the progression of cells from $G_1$ to phase S, stimulating the cells to divide. Other current components of the clot can include undifferentiated mesenchymal cells, macrophages, polymorphonuclear leukocytes, lymphocytes and mast cells. In addition to the cellular components, the characteristic of this stage is to break off the vascular channels for bony nutrition. This traumatic event will lead to the osteoclasts removing the necrotic margins and organizing the bony surface. Macrophages and osteoclasts act in the removal of non-vital tissue, characterizing the demolition phase. In addition to their phagocytosis and cleaning activity of the area, the macrophages express important regulatory factors, including IL-1 necessary for angiogenesis and activation of fibroblasts and osteoprogenitor cells[19,20,29,31,35].

By the third and fifth day after the lesion, coagulum cells and products condense. Endothelial cell derivatives of the adjacent vessels migrate, proliferate and they form new capillaries that penetrate the clot. A stimulus for the new vessel formation, seems to be the local hypoxia; the direction in which angiogenesis occurs is guided by the chemical gradients. The gradients are established between the central area with low oxygen concentration and the peripheral areas, as well as chemotactic actions of PDGF and FGF. The pH of the area is acidic and this period also is characterized by migration of fibroblasts towards the coagulum. Fibroblasts together with the proliferated vessels form a network of connective tissue denominated granulation tissue. The connective tissue matrix protects the development of new vessels and provides space for endothelial cell adhesion.

The osteoprogenitor cells appear on the third day and are of two types: predetermined and induced. The osteoprogenitor cells are derivatives of the periosteum and cells of medullae. With participation of TGF-β, these cells can express an osteoblast phenotype. The induced cells migrate to the lesion by the blood vessels and are referred to as pericytes. Undifferentiated mesenchymal cells can also be considered as osteoprogenitor cells induced by BMP (bone morphogenetic protein) and can be converted into osteoblasts[21].

### 26.3 Remodeling

In this phase, according to the injured area and the granulation tissue formed, osteogenesis starts followed by the mineralization process.

### 26.4 Osteogenesis and Mineralization

Bone formation by the osteoblasts includes the synthesis and intracellular processing of Type I collagen. This collagen is expressed by the osteoblasts that are extracellularly modified, forming tropocollagen molecules that are united to form collagen fibrils. Hydroxyapatite crystal deposition begins ten days after the healing process has started. This stage has been associated with pH elevation, probably because of the alkaline phosphatase enzyme. It has been speculated that this enzyme promotes calcium phosphate precipitation, starting the mineralization process. Mineral deposition occurs along the collagen fibers, perhaps at the expense of alkaline phosphatase. The mineralization is limited by the available physical space found among collagen fibrils lengthwise. Osteoid is the term used to describe the organic matrix produced by osteoblasts before mineralization.

In the healing process, it is essential to have a proper blood supply, therefore the Havers system plays an important role. This system consists of organized concentrical rings of lamellar bone surrounding a central canal that contains lymphatic and blood vessels. The osteocytes depend on this system for the metabolic needs and viability of the bony matrix. When the blood supply is interrupted, osteocytes die, resulting in bone resorption and necrosis.

Cementum repair results from the differentiation of cementoblasts from the undifferentiated cells of the granulation tissue or of cells of the periodontal ligament.

According to Seltzer[31], the apical periodontal repair process could briefly be explained in the following way:

1. In addition to the bony tissue, cementum is formed and deposited in the resorbed apical cementum area;
2. New bone is formed in the trabeculae periphery to replace the affected bony tissue;
3. Inflammatory and capillary cells are reduced;
4. Granulation tissue collagen fibers are substituted by new trabecular bone;
5. Periodontal space is consequently reduced.

The Figure 26.8 illustrates the main phases in the repair process of the periodontium.

Nowadays substances that stimulate the repair process have been used. Guided tissue regeneration (GTR) is a new option that became available for the correction of apical defects. Several factors related to the tooth can influence the prognosis of endodontic surgery, such as the loss of bone quantity and location. Some studies indicated that the prognosis is substantially reduced in teeth with a total loss of local marginal bone. In this technique, a resorbable collagen membrane and mineral inorganic bone of bovine origin is used. However, there is the need for further studies to demonstrate the real effectiveness of these techniques[3].

In a previous study developed by Garret et al.[11], in which the use of a bioresorptive membrane as guide for the repair of periapical lesions was compared with a control group that did not use this procedure, they verified that there was no beneficial effect whatever when using this technique.

### 26.5 Factors that interfere in the healing process

The repair of periapical lesions, after endodontic procedures is also dependent on the influence of systemic and local factors, in other words, the success of the repair process will depend on the existence of factors that influence repair[29,31,32,35].

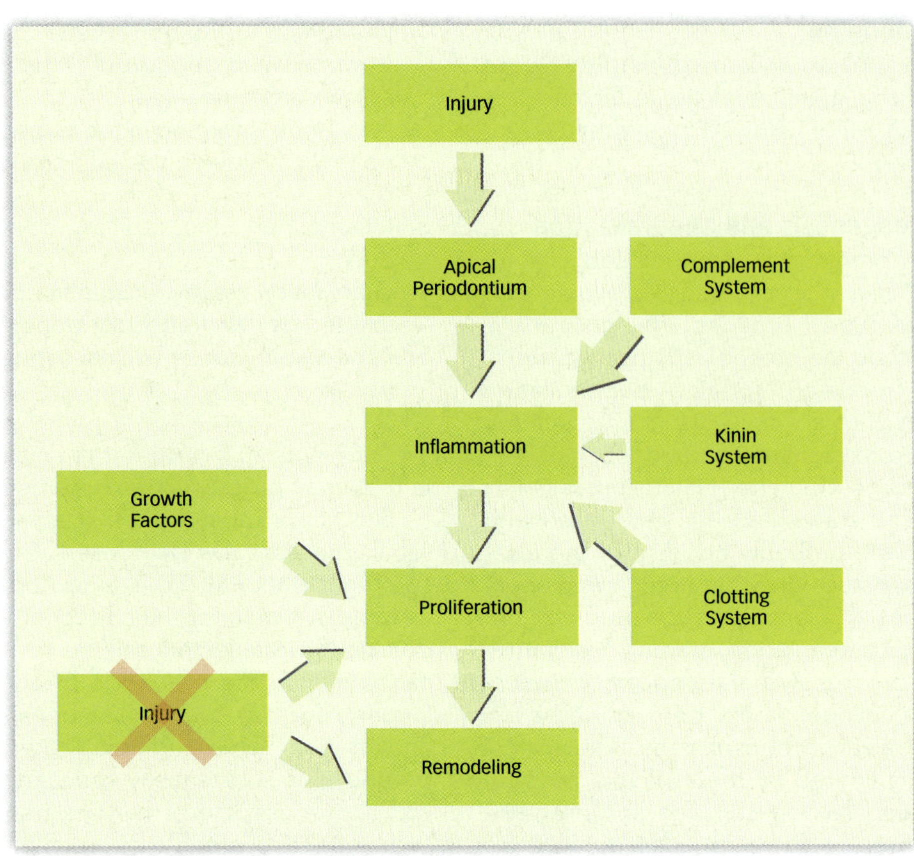


**Figure 26.8** - Main phases in the repair process of the periodontium.

**Local factors:**

1. Infection;
2. Hemorrhage;
3. Tissue injury;
4. Interference with the blood supply;
5. Foreign bodies

**Systemic factors:**

1. Nutrition;
2. Stress;
3. State of chronic debilitation;
4. Hormones and vitamins;
5. Dehydration and age.

## 26.6 Local Factors

### Infection

Infection in the periapical region or inside the root canals, as a result of the presence of microorganisms, is one of the factors that prevent granulation tissue formation and interferes with the healing process. The presence of the phlogogenous agents in the lesion induces the transformation of the inflammation into an infectious process of a chronic nature, with possible exacerbations. In some cases, with the purpose of assisting the repair process, drainage or debridement of the injured area is essential, with the purpose of reducing or eliminating microorganisms, enabling the granulation tissue to develop. In addition to these surgical procedures it is sometimes necessary to use an antimicrobial or antifungal agent depending on identifying the agent.

**Hemorrhage**

Hemorrhage and clot formation are essential for the healing process, through activation of the coagulation and plasminogen–plasmin systems, which trigger the development of the inflammatory process. However, excessive bleeding causes periodontitis in the periapical region by the compression of the local structures. Furthermore, the blood clot from iatrogenic procedures in the apical limit delays the beginning of the repair process, because it is necessary for the coagulum to be resorbed first.

In addition to hemorrhage due to over-instrumentation, there is also the risk of bacterial contamination of the periodontal area, with possible bacteremia.

**Tissue injury**

The extent and severity of the injury are also factors that prevent repair. Therefore, the less intense the trauma, the faster will be the onset of the repair process. Tissue injury with cellular necrosis favors colonization by microorganisms, which could generate an infectious process in the location.

The tissue destruction or injury is common during the dental pulp tissue extirpation procedures and during instrumentation of the root canal, mostly in cases of overfilling beyond the apical limit. It is important for the endodontist to perform the procedures within the root canal limits.

In cases of dental pulp necrosis with apical bone rarefaction it is important that the procedures are performed only inside the root canals. There are authors who recommend that the instrumentation should reach the granulation tissue, but not exceed the limits of the granulation area. It is important to consider that in cases of tissue necrosis in the alveolar process, the repair process will only become effective with the liquefaction of the necrotic tissue by complete emptying of the area. Subsequently, fibronectin bonds to the collagen and to the cellular membranes to facilitate phagocytosis. Fibronectin and the cellular remains are chemotactic for macrophages and fibroblasts. The presence of macrophages in the injured area signals the beginning of the repair process.

In cases of overfilling materials in the rarefaction areas, the repair is generally impeded until the material is resorbed, or in the case of inert particles, the process will result in a chronic process, characterized by the presence of macrophages, however, with low cellular renewal, and preventing the effective repair[13].

**Interference with the blood supply**

The more vascularized, the better the inflammatory reaction for healing purposes. Therefore, tissues with ischemic areas, or with arteriosclerosis, tend to become infected more frequently, and with greater tissue injury. Therefore, the establishment of granulation tissue is essential for the repair process. Angiogenesis allows oxygen and nutrition to enter the cells. This process is self-regulated during the repair process. The endothelial cells of quiescent capillaries are activated by the release of cytokines and growth factors such as the FGF and VEGF[13].

An important factor to consider is that in the young individuals the repair process develops more easily than in older individuals.

**Foreign objects**

As was previously reported, overfilling of materials in the periodontal space, such as gutta-percha cones, filling cements, cotton pellets or even chemical products, prevents repair from developing. Sometimes, the repercussion of these iatrogenic events can appear several years after the endodontic treatment, or remain as chronic inflammatory lesions.

Irritations of chemical and mechanical origin can interfere in the healing process. Cases of overfilling with foreign bodies lead to repair with encapsulation of the foreign object by fibrous connective tissue. With reference to the phagocytic cells of the inflammatory process, Nyborg &Tullin[26] declared that the macrophages have difficulty in removing the excess of gutta-percha and that it is rare that cement becomes deposited over the gutta-percha or silver cones, the latter being rarely used in the endodontic routine nowadays. It is common to observe external apical radicular resorptions and these intact filling materials in routine radiographic exams.

Apical periodontitis is initially caused by microorganisms that reside in the infected root canals. There are convincing evidences that other independent factors can adversely affect the success of conventional endodontic therapy. In a morphologic study evidence was presented to confirm the potential of two endogenous factors that can interfere with the periapical healing after endodontic treatment. The specimens consisted of surgical biopsies of asymptomatic periapical lesions that persisted after a 44 month follow up. The biopsies were examined by optic and electronic microscopy. The lesion was characterized by the presence of a great central area delineated by stratified scaly epithelium. The most interesting aspect in the lesion was the presence of a vast number of cholesterol crystals congregated in the connective tissue that surrounded the cystic sac. An optic microscopy and extensive electronic investigation of the apical region of the root canals, and of the failed lesion, was performed in an attempt to reveal the presence of microorganisms. These discoveries suggest that intrinsic factors, such as the products of degenerating tissues and cholesterol crystals, and the cystic condition of the lesion of themselves can adversely affect the periapical repair process after endodontic treatment. Consequently, apical lesions can remain refractory to the conventional endodontic therapy for long periods of time[24].

The presence of cholesterol crystals can be a factor that interferes in the periapical repair after conventional endodontic treatment. Nair et al. [25] observed the role of cholesterol crystals in healing, which were implanted in animals. The pure cholesterol crystals were implanted in the subcutaneous tissue of Guinea pigs. The samples were observed for 2, 4 and 32 weeks after the implant, and prepared for optic and electronic microscopy. The samples revealed connective tissue penetrating through the drillings. The crystals were surrounded by numerous macrophages and multinucleated giant cells forming a very circumscribed area of tissue reaction. The cells, however, were unable to eliminate the crystals during the observation period of 8 months. The congregation of macrophages and giant cells, known as apical inflammation and mediators of the main factors of bony resorption, suggest that congestion of cholesterol crystals can be a factor in the failure of some periapical lesions after conventional endodontic treatment[25].

## 26.7 Systemic Factors

The systemic factors that can interfere in the repair process are related as follows: age, nutrition, protein depletion, fats and carbohydrates, chronic diseases, consumption, diabetes, renal diseases, blood dyscrasias, hormonal alterations, vitamin depletion, dehydration.

The endodontic treatment prognosis in older people is poorer when compared with young individuals. There is a correlation between age and nutritional factors. In general the susceptibility to infectious agents is relatively higher in elderly individuals, which is also related to immune system deficiency. Therefore, the association between age, nutritional status and immune system, interfere substantially in the healing process.

Therefore, people suffering from anorexia, or surgical trauma that results in a negative nitrogen balance, are susceptible to complement suppression, decreasing the resistance to diseases and healing. Furthermore, lysozime, IgG and secretor IgA are decreased.

Protein deficiency is also one of the factors that interfere in the repair process. In addition to protein deficiency in the body, when there is a deficiency of Vitamin C, fibroplasia is also retarded. Other authors report that stress associated with the above-mentioned factors also interferes in the repair process[31,32].

Carbohydrates and lipids are the providers of energy for the repair process. When the body lacks carbohydrates, there is interference in the repair process. Fatty acids are the precursors of prostaglandins, chemical mediators of inflammation, and important in the clot formation.

Chronic diseases, such as tuberculosis, diabetes and other diseases have a debilitating effect, similarly interfering with the development of repair.

In tuberculosis patients, the blood oxygenation is not adequate, therefore, there is deficiency in tissue oxygenation and consequently, a deficient repair process.

When diabetic patients are controlled, they can be submitted to endodontic treatment.

Individuals with renal disturbances also require special attention during endodontic procedures, particularly chronic renal patients that require hemodialysis. The lymphocytes T are reduced in number in the blood and severe bleeding can occur. This bleeding can be caused by an abnormal platelet function, thrombocytopenia or even by the use of anticoagulants. Therefore, when endodontic treatment is needed in these patients, preventive measures have to be taken, especially in cases of surgery.

In blood dyscrasia, patients with anemia or leukemia require attention. In cases of anemia, there is inadequate repair due to deficiency in the blood supply of the affected region. The leukemia patients have a higher probability of infection, mostly in cases with granulocytopenia. In this situation the use of prophylactic antibiotics is necessary. In patients under chemotherapy treatment, endodontic procedures are not indicated. First hematologic control is necessary, because there is low resistance to microorganisms, due to suppression of the immune response.

In individuals that present defects of coagulation, thrombocytopenia and anemia, the repair process is generally affected. Cases of local thrombosis lead to the decrease in platelet activation, thus reducing the growth factors and limiting the repair cascade. The tissue oxygen decrease that also accompanies serious anemia interferes in the repair process. Long term corticosteroid use also retards the repair process because they inhibit collagen synthesis by acting as antiphlogistic. Therefore, before any endodontic procedure, it is essential to investigate the patients' systemic health by thorough anamnesis[13].

Patients with malignant neoplasia under radiotherapy treatment in high doses require special care in cases of endodontic treatment particularly endodontic surgery, because the blood supply in the irradiated areas is deficient and similarly contribute to failure of the repair process.

Hepatic diseases interfere in protein synthesis and other basic processes of metabolism and mineralization, therefore the repair of periapical lesions is adversely affected. Patients with hepatic cirrhosis or hepatitis, have low levels of vitamin K, very important in the clot formation process.

Amongst the bleeding disorders, hemophilia and Willebrand Disease are the most representative. Endodontic therapy that can induce bleeding, such as surgeries should not be done without the previous indication of blood, plasma, plasmapheresis, or antifibrinolytic agents, followed by the application of hemostatic products to control hemorrhage.

The hormonal alterations can affect the healing of periapical lesions, in view of their effects on the bone metabolism. Osteoporosis is one of these effects, characterized by a disturbance in the formation of the bony matrix. Cushing's Syndrome consists of an excessive decrease in the thickness of the cortical bone, and trabecular bone spaces are substantially reduced. The number of osteoblasts is reduced and areas of newly formed bone demonstrate a reduction in osteoblastic activity.

Another factor that should be considered is stress that promotes a series of alterations in the individual's body. Stress can originate from infection, exhaustion, hormonal disturbances and emotional disturbances. Countless studies related in the literature demonstrate that individuals under stress have greater susceptibility to infections, and that the healing process is more difficult.

Vitamin C deficiency, mostly in intra-bony lesions, interferes in repair. This vitamin is necessary for collagen formation of all fibrous tissue structures, in other words of the bony matrix, dentin and cartilage.

Ascorbic acid deficiency prevents the normal development of connective tissue. Both collagen and glycosaminoglycans formation are affected, and so are fibroblasts, resulting in the formation of defective fibers. Finally, the lack of Vitamin C leads to a decrease in bony matrix formation, leading to osteoporosis.

Vitamin K deficiencies interfere in clot formation, and lack of Vitamin D in the mineralization process, therefore these are important situations in tissue healing. It is also important to relate dehydration as one of the factors that affect the development, because the loss of water from the blood increases its viscosity and consequent stagnation in the capillaries, preventing nutrient exchanges and causing phlogistic activity in the region.

The patient's medical and dental history, or a health good inventory is essential to establish a good prognosis, thus predicting successful treatment that will ultimately lead to a good healing process.

## 26.8 Influence of intracanal dressing on healing process

Modern thinking has moved towards the use of an intracanal dressing, with a potentially effective action against different types of respiratory bacteria (aerobic, anaerobic and microaerophiles) which act by inhibiting the action of osteoclasts present in the area of dental resorption and favor the repair process of altered periapical tissue[7]. Estrela & Holland[7] discussed the biological and antimicrobial role of calcium hydroxide, and reported that the characteristics of calcium hydroxide come from its dissociation into calcium and hydroxyl ions. The action of these ions on tissues and bacteria explains the biological and antimicrobial properties of this substance - 1. Dentin is considered the best pulp protective, and calcium hydroxide has proved, through numerous studies, to be capable of inducing the formation of a mineralized bridge over pulp tissue. 2. It is necessary, whenever possible, to allow time for the calcium hydroxide paste to manifest its potential of action against the microorganisms present in endodontic infections. The maintenance of a high concentration of hydroxyl ions can change bacteria enzymatic activity and promote its inactivation. 3. The site of action of hydroxyl ions of calcium hydroxide includes the enzymes in the cytoplasmic membrane. This medication has a broad scope of action, and therefore is effective against a wide range of microorganisms, regardless of their metabolic capability. In the microbial world, cytoplasmic membranes are similar, irrespective of the morphological, tinctorial and respiratory characteristics of microorganisms, which mean that this medication has a similar effect on aerobic, anaerobic, Gram-positive and Gram-negative bacteria. 4. Calcium hydroxide as a temporary dressing, used between appointments, promotes better results in the periapical healing process than the treatment performed in one appointment.

Its capacity to stimulate tissue repair through the induction of mineralization, confirms the biological action of calcium hydroxide[1,4-10,13-18].

Establishing the strategies for microbial control of root canal requires knowledge of the relations between the bacteria, anatomy and host response. These are obstacles that the endodontist needs to overcome. Knowledge about microbiological phenomena and ultra-structural anatomy are important for achieving success in the treatment of endodontic infection. It is relevant and necessary to understand that it is the host that monitors the biological process to favor healing. The choice of intracanal dressing correlates with two relevant aspects, namely: antimicrobial potential and tissue tolerance. In most clinical cases, these substances are in contact with only non vital tissue in the root canal and little contact with the periapical tissue. Their real function is to control microorganisms only in the root canal[7].

Intracanal dressing continues to be the target of discussions concerning several of its aspects. Considerations about the real necessity of its use in pulp necrosis and apical periodontitis, the selection of the substance to be used, the time it should remain in the radicular canal, its effect on different microorganisms found in endodontic infections, and its influence on tissue healing process are justifications for new researches structured within adequate critical analysis and well established methodologies[4-10].

The selection of the intracanal dressing is based on important referential parameters – firstly, depending on its antimicrobial potential; secondly, histocompatibility and lastly, the capacity of favoring the tissue healing process. Thus, it is necessary to consider knowledge of the endodontic microbiota (primary or secondary infection); the mechanism of action of calcium hydroxide; antimicrobial efficacy of intracanal dressing - the time it takes to act in dentinal tubules, microbial resistance and tissue tolerance[6].

Heithersay[13] admits that calcium ions may be of importance when calcium hydroxide is used in the treatment of pathologies associated with pulpless teeth. These ions can reduce capillary permeability in the mass of new capillaries in granulation tissue associated with these pulpless teeth. One particular enzyme involved in most productive energy-using processes, is pyrophosphatase, which is also calcium ion dependent. This enzyme is a member of phosphatase enzymes, important in the mineralization process.

Holland et al.[17]observed the healing process in dog teeth with apical periodontitis after root canal treatment in one or two appointments. Premolars and anterior dog teeth had their root canals opened to the oral environment for 6 months before being treated. After root canal negotiation they were filled by the lateral condensation technique with gutta-percha points and Sealapex in one appointment or after a dressing with calcium hydroxide for 7 and 15 days. Six months after the treatment the animals were sacrificed and the tissues prepared for histomorphological analysis. Scores attributed to the different histomorphological events were submitted to statistical analysis, which resulted in ranking the experimental groups from the best to the worst in the following order: (a) calcium hydroxide 14 days; (b) calcium hydroxide 7 days; and (c) one appointment. It was concluded that the use of a calcium hydroxide dressing helps to achieve better results than the treatment in one appointment. The healing process observed in this experiment with the one appointment treatment was interesting. One believes that the results could partly be attributed to the Sealapex alkalinity. In another study, Holland et al.[18] based their research on the same parameters to study Sealer 26. The results showed the better status of periapical tissue (with mineralized barrier) when the treatment performed in two appointments with use the intracanal dressing (calcium hydroxide paste).

The main cause of apical periodontitis is endodontic infection (caused by bacteria and their byproducts). Thus, good therapeutic strategy is to resolve the cause of the problem (microorganisms in the root canal) and naturally their consequences (pathological alterations) are better solved.

The Figures 26.9 to 26.15 showed healing process following endodontic treatment in teeth with apical periodontitis.

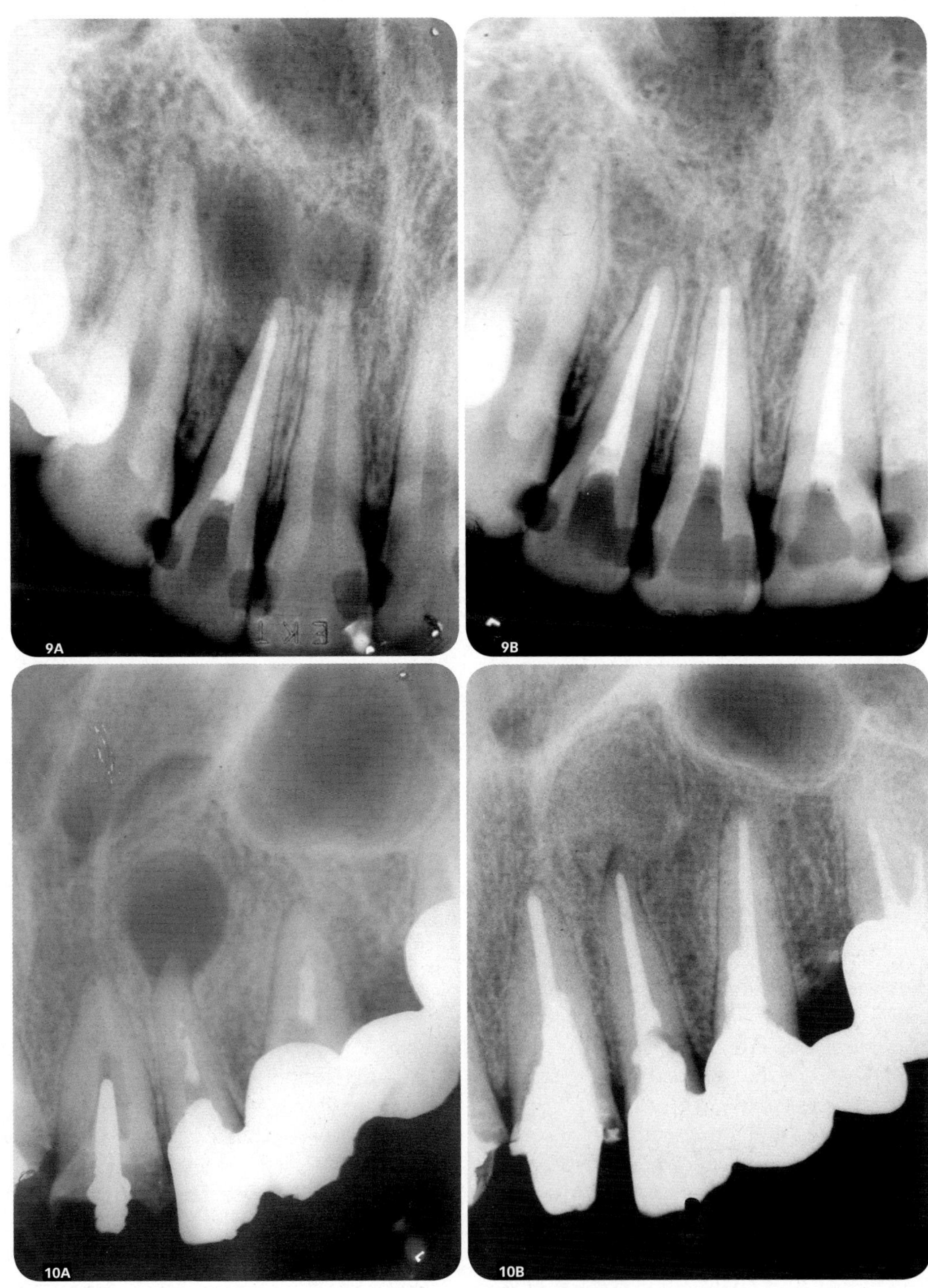


**Figures 26.9 and 26.10** - (**A,B**) Healing process following endodontic treatment in teeth with apical periodontitis.

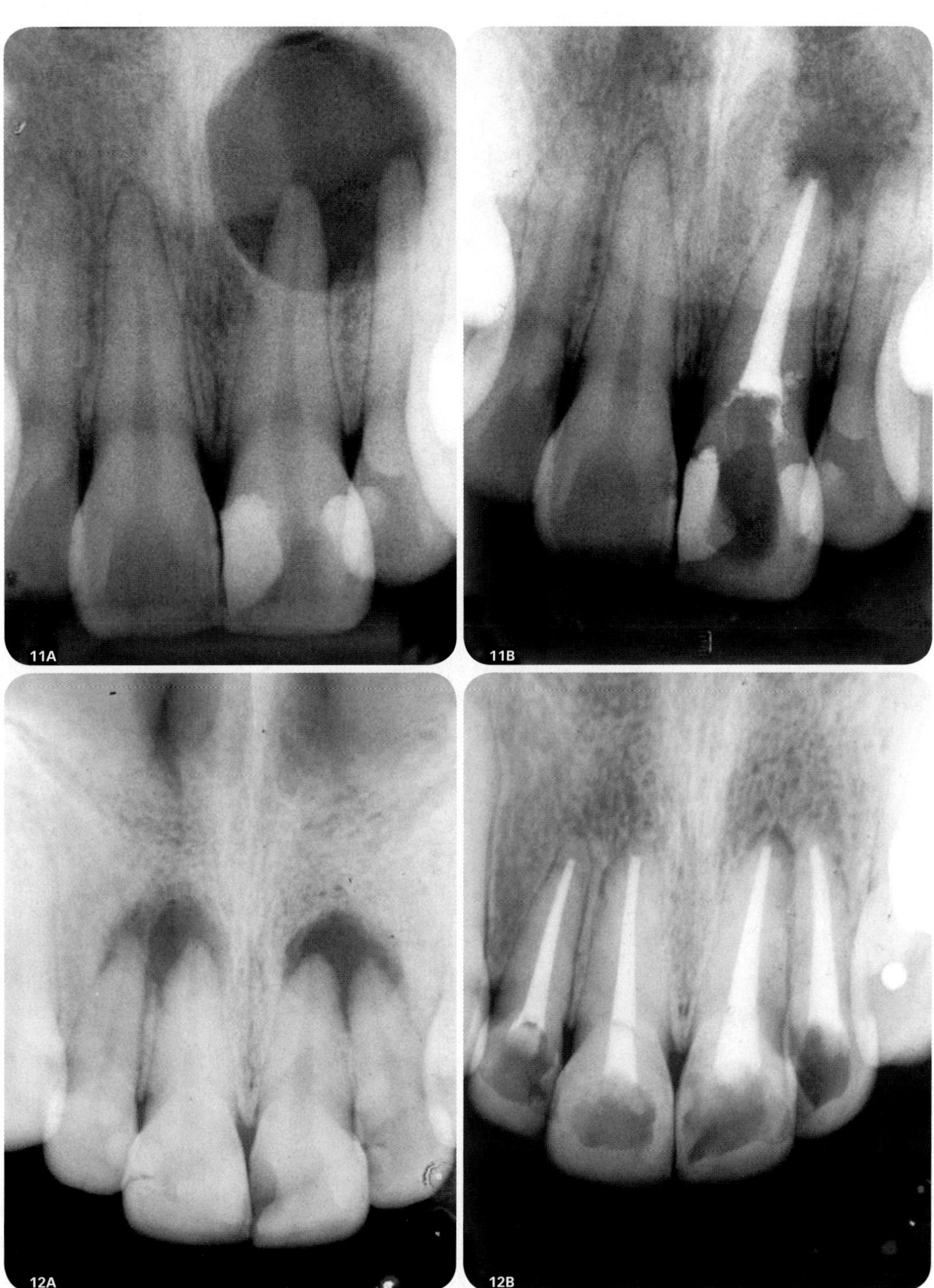


**Figures 26.11 and 26.12** - (**A,B**) Healing process following endodontic treatment in teeth with apical periodontitis.

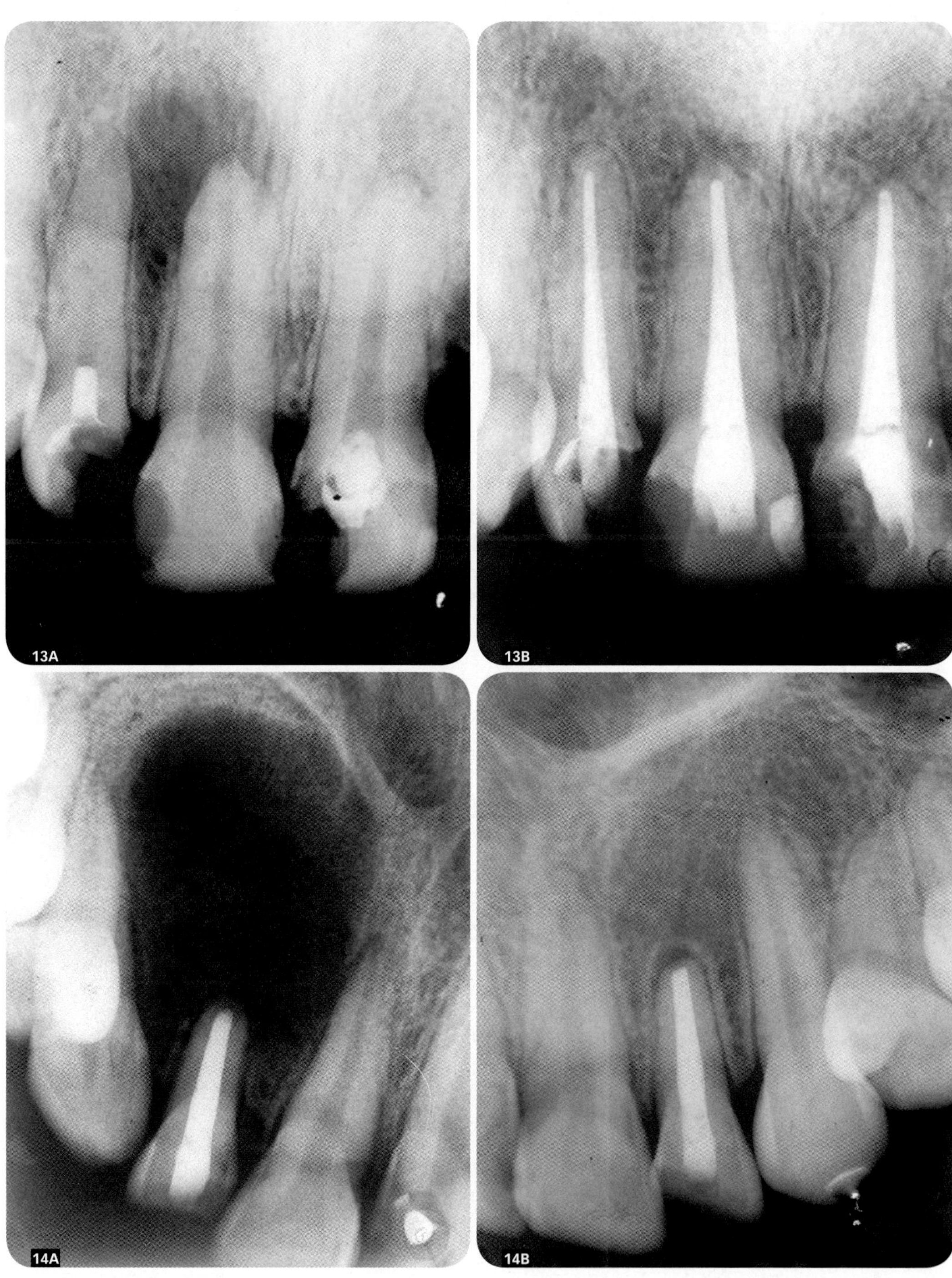


**Figures 26.13 and 26.14** - (**A,B**) Healing process following endodontic treatment in teeth with apical periodontitis.

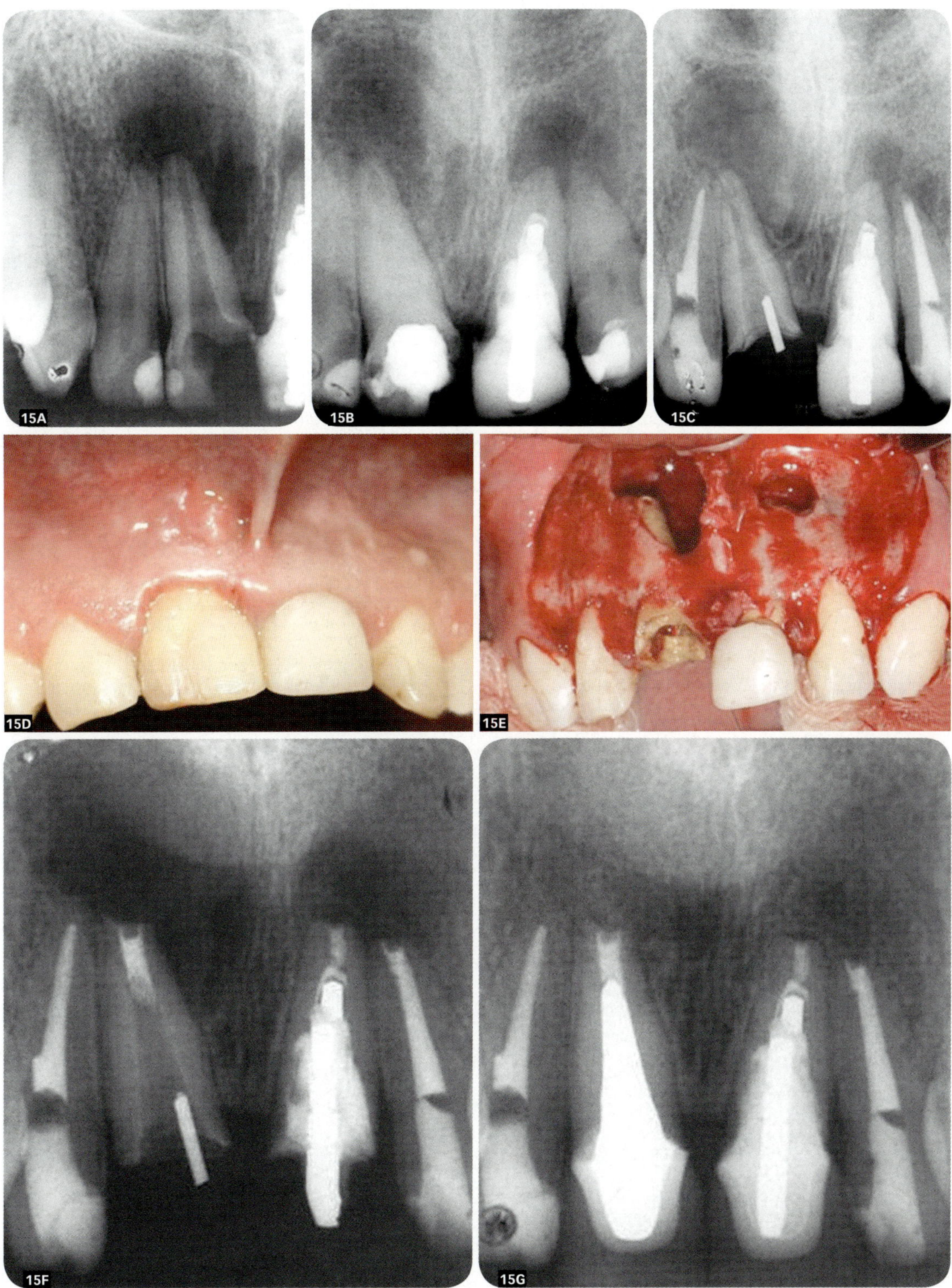


Figure 26.15 - (A-G) Healing process following endodontic treatment in teeth with apical periodontitis.

1. Binnie WH, Mitchel DF. Induced calcification in the subdermal tissues of the rat. J Dent Res 1973;52:1087-91.
2. Cawson RA, Binnie WH, Eveson JW. Atlas colorido de enfermidades da boca – Correlações Clínico Patológicas. 2nd ed. São Paulo: Artes Médicas; 1995.
3. Dietrich T, Zunker P, Dietrich D, Bernimoulin JP. Periapical and periodontal healing after osseous grafting and guided tissue regeneration treatment of apicomarginal defects in periradicular surgery: results after 12 mounts. Oral Surg Oral Med Oral Pathol 2003;95:474-82.
4. Estrela C. Análise química de pastas de hidróxido de cálcio frente a liberação de íons cálcio, de íons hidroxila e a formação de carbonato de cálcio, na presença de tecido conjuntivo de cão. (Doctoral Thesis) University of São Paulo.
5. Estrela C, Bammann LL, Estrela CRA, Silva RS, Pécora JD. Antimicrobial and chemical study of MTA, Portland cement, calcium hydroxide paste, Sealapex and Dycal. Braz Dent J 2000;11:3-9.
6. Estrela C, Bammann LL, Pimenta FC, Pécora JD. Control of microorganism in vitro by calcium hydroxide pastes. Int Endod J 2001;34:416-418.
7. Estrela C, Holland R. Calcium hydroxide: study based on scientific evidences. J Applied Oral Science 2003;11:269-282.
8. Estrela C, Pimenta FC, Ito IY, Bammann LL. Antimicrobial evaluation of calcium hydroxide in infected dentinal tubules. J Endod 1999;26:416-418.
9. Estrela C, Pimenta FC, Ito IY, Bammann LL. In vitro determination of direct antimicrobial effect of calcium hydroxide. J Endod 1998;24:15-17.
10. Estrela C, Sydney GB, Bammann LL, Felippe-Júnior O. Mechanism of the action of calcium and hydroxyl ions of calcium hydroxide on tissue and bacteria. Braz Dent J 1995;6:85-90.
11. Garret K, Kerr M, Hartewell G, O'Sullivan S, Mayer P. The effect of a bioresorbable matrix barrier in endodontic surgery on the rate of periapical healing: an in vivo study. J Endod 2002;28:503-6.
12. Goldring MB, Golching SR. Skeletal tissue response to cytokines. Clin Orthop Rel Res 1990;58:245-78.
13. Heithersay GS. Calcium hydroxide in the treatment of pulpless teeth with associated pathology. J Brit Endod Soc 1975;8:74-93.
14. Hermann BW. Calciumhydroxyd als mittel zurn behandel und füllen vonxahnwurzelkanälen. Thesis in Natural Science. Würzburg; 1920. 50p.
15. Holland R. Histochemical response of amputed pulps to calcium hydroxide. Rev Bras Pesq Med Biol 1971;4:83-95.
16. Holland R. Processo de reparo do coto pulpar e dos tecidos periapicais após biopulpectomia e obturação de canal com hidróxido de cálcio ou óxido de zinco e eugenol. Estudo histológico em dentes de cães. (Livre-Docência Thesis). Araçatuba: São Paulo State University;1975.
17. Holland R, Otoboni-Filho JA, Souza V, Nery MJ, Bernabé PFE, Dezan-Jr E.Tratamiento endodôntico em una o en dos visitas. Estudio histológico en dientes de perros con lesión periapical. Endodoncia 2003;21:20-7.
18. Holland R, Otoboni-Filho JA, Souza V, Nery MJ, Bernabé PFE, Dezan-Jr E. A comparison of one versus two appointment endodontic therapy in dogs' teeth with apical periodontitis. J Endod 2003;29:121-5.
19. Hollinger J, Wong M. The integrated processes of hard tissue regeneration with special enphasis on fracture healing. Oral Surg Oral Med Oral Pathol 1996;82:594-606.
20. Kumar V, Abbas AK, Fausto N. Acute and chronic inflammation. In: Kumar, V.; Abbas, A.K.; Fausto, N. Eds. Robbins and Cotran pathologic basis of disease. 7th. Philadelphia: Elsevier, 2005. p.47-86.
21. Mitchell OF, Shankawalker G.B. Osteogenic potencial of calcium hydroxide and other materials in soft tissue and bone wounds. J Dent Res 1958;37:1157-63.
22. Nair PNR. Review - New perspectives on radicular cysts: do they heal? Int Endod J 1998;31:155-60.
23. Nair PNR, Sjögren U, Krey G, Kahnberg KE, Sundqvist G. Therapy-resistant Foreign Body Giant Cell Granuloma at he periapex of a Root-filled Human tooth. J Endod 1990;16:589-95.
24. Nair PNR, Sjögren U, Schumacher E, Sundqvist G. Radicular cyst affecting a root-filled human tooth: a long-term post-treatment follow-up. Int Endod J 1993;26:225-33.
25. Nair PNR, Sjögren U, Sundqvist G. Cholesterol crystals as an etiological factor in non-resolving chronic inflammation: an experimental study in guines pigs. Eur J Oral Sci 1998;106:644-50.
26. Nyborg H, Tullin B. Healing process after pulp extirpation. An experimental study of 17 teeth. Odont Tids 1965;73:430.
27. Osborn JW, Ten Cate AR. Histologia Dental Avançada. 4.ed. São Paulo: Quintessence Books; 1988. p.81-95.
28. Rasmussen P, Mjor IA. Calcium hydroxide as ectopic bone inductor in rats. Scand J Dent Res 1971; 79:24-30.
29. Rubin E, Gorstein F, Rubin R, Schwarting R, Strayer D. Rubin Patologia – Bases clinicopatológicas de medicina. 4th ed. Rio de Janeiro: Guanabara Koogan, 2006.
30. Safavi KE, Nichols FC. Alteration of biological properties of bacterial lipopolysaccharide by calcium hydroxide treatment. J Endod 1994; 20:127-129.
31. Seltzer S. Repair folowing root canal therapy. In: Endodontology biologic considerations in endodontic procedures. 2nd ed. Philadelphia: Lea Fabinger; 1988. p.389-438.
32. Seltzer S, Bender IB. A polpa dental. 2nd ed. Rio de Janeiro: Labor; 1979. 499 p.
33. Silva TA, Garlet GP, Fukada SY, Silva JS, Cunha FQ. Chemokines in Oral Inflammatory Diseases: Apical Periodontitis and Periodontal Disease. J Dent Res 2007; 86:306-19.
34. Simon JHS. Incidence of periapical cysts in relation to root canal. J Endod 1980; 6:845-48.
35. Trowbridge HO, Emling RC. Inflammation. A review of the process. 4th ed. Chicago: Quintessense books; 1993. 172p.
36. Wong M, Hollinger J, Pinero G. Integrated processes responsible for soft tissue healing. Oral Surg Oral Med Oral Pathol 1996;82:475-92.

# Intraradicular Posts for Endodontically Treated Teeth

**C. R. Leles**
*Federal University of Goiás, Goiânia, GO, Brazil*

**S. S. Rocha**
*Federal University of Goiás, Goiânia, GO, Brazil*

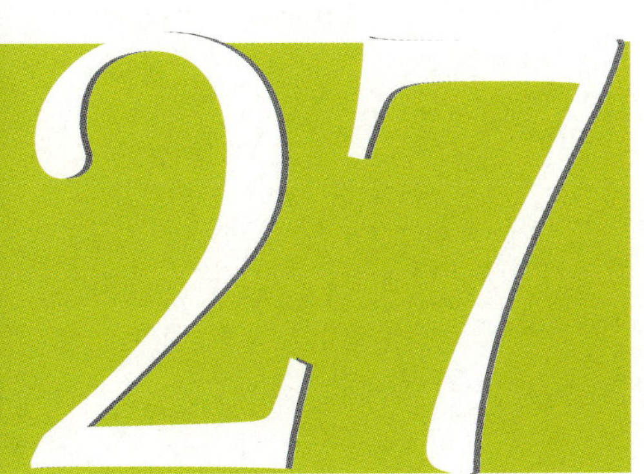

**J. B. Souza**
*Federal University of Goiás, Goiânia, GO, Brazil*

**A. L. S. Busato**
*Luteran University of Canoas, RS, Brazil*

Chapter contents

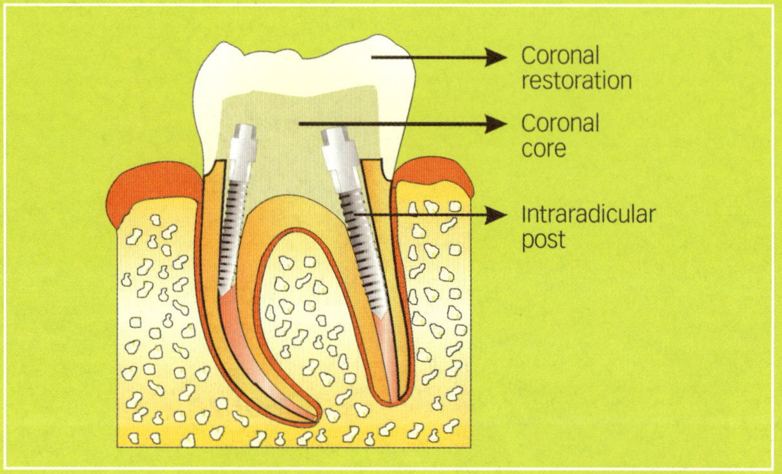


Components of a prefabricated post system.

## 27.1 Introduction

The endodontic treatment makes it possible to re-establish the function of teeth harmed by uncountable pathological alterations, with pulp and/or periapical involvement, and maintain the viability of teeth which, in the past, would have had to be extracted. However, the endodontically treated tooth is only definitively recovered at the end of the restorative treatment.

The restoration of these teeth can frequently be complex because most of the crown, or all of it is lost, due to decay, traumatic injuries or the presence of previous extensive restorations.

There is an important relationship between the amount of lost dental structure and the capacity of the tooth to resist occlusal forces. The larger the amount of lost dental structure, the less the structural resistance of the tooth and the greater the risk of fracture[71]. The endodontic procedure reduces the resistance of the tooth by about 5%, because of the structure lost due to the endodontic access. The association with a MOD preparation reduces the fracture strength of the cusps up to 60%[94]. Therefore, loss of marginal crests is the most important contributory factor to the loss of structural resistance of the tooth.

The loss of additional dental structure during endodontic therapy, associated with dental reduction produced by prosthetic or restorative preparations commonly results in insufficient support for the restoration. These factors determine the need for coronal reconstitution to return the structural resistance of the tooth and to favor appropriate retention of the future restoration.

Frequently, core filling of the dental remainder performed with direct restorative materials, such as resin composite, glass ionomer cement or amalgam, is enough to reconstitute the coronal part that will serve as support for a crown (Fig. 27.1). But in the cases in which there is considerable loss of coronal structure, there is no possibility of providing enough retention and resistance to complete the coronal core. Under these conditions, intraradicular forms of retention may be required.

The endodontically treated tooth that needs intraradicular retention should receive a restoration structurally composed of components with specific functions (Fig. 27.1). In a direct relationship of functional dependence, the coronal restoration is retained by the coronal core, which is retained by the intraradicular post.

Therefore, the final restoration is a complementary unit made on core, divided into two portions: coronal and radicular. The radicular portion, called intraradicular post, can form a single structure that extends up to the coronal portion in the form of cast core, or can be a distinct prefabricated structure, united to the coronal portion by complementary material applied directly on the post-remaining dental structure set.

For a long time the structure formed by the crown and intraradicular core in a single piece, known as "Richmond's crown", was used. This structure, however, was replaced by the intraradicular and coronal core separately from the artificial crown, which has the advantages of improving the marginal adaptation, not limiting the direction of inserting the crown to the one allowed by the long axis of the tooth; and making it possible to replace unsatisfactory crowns without necessarily demanding removal of the core[45,106].

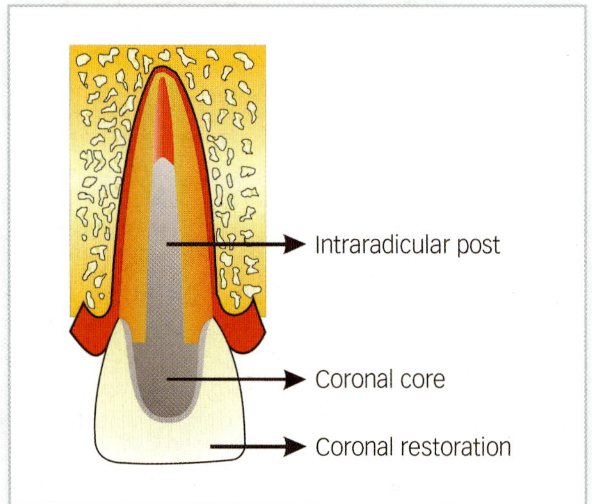


**Figure 27.1** - Parts of an intraradicular retention system.

## 27.2 Intraradicular Retention Systems - Selection criteria

The two basic forms of intraradicular posts - cast and prefabricated - present innumerable variations, according to the material, fabrication technique, morphologic and biomechanical characteristics and clinical applications.

### Intraradicular cast posts

For a long time, intraradicular cast posts were considered the standard treatment for teeth with reduced coronal structure. Their use has long history of proven clinical success[12].

Cast posts are very versatile and are widely used, allowing them to be used in virtually all cases. One of their advantages is that they have better adaption to the root canal, since the cores is built to adapt completely to the endodontic space. Therefore, it is the treatment choice for elliptic or excessively expulsive root canals, in which the circular prefabricated post does not adapt firmly to the root canal walls, resulting in greater thickness of the cement layer. These characteristics result in high rigidity, decreased cement thickness and anti-rotational characteristics. Moreover, as the coronal portion of the core is fixed to the intraradicular post, there is no failure problem in the union between the coronal and radicular parts[105].

However, as disadvantages, they require two clinical sessions in order to obtain the mold or casting pattern, and to cement the core, in addition to involving laboratory costs[73]. In vitro studies have suggested that there is a larger risk of root fracture, because the conical form of the post has the potential of exercising a wedge effect on the root[112], although this effect has not been definitively proven in controlled clinical studies[72,74].

A cast post is indicated in cases in which the alignment of the future crown is very different from the inclination of the long axis of the root canal, which is commonly observed in anterior teeth. Its conformation also allows the direction of insertion of preparations of the coronal part of the core to be corrected, in cases of multiple pillar teeth of a fixed denture.

It is emphasized that in most anterior teeth and in some premolars with no coronal structure (Fig. 27.2A-B), there is not enough space to allow an appropriate volume of completion material to form a solid structural unit, restricting the indication of prefabricated posts associated with direct core. In these cases, the cast metal core is the most appropriate treatment option. Whereas, in the molars there usually is enough space to accommodate a completion material and the angulation of the root canal is not considered a significant problem. In this case, the use of prefabricated posts results in more conservative preparations, less costs and the restoration is easier and simpler to perform. Furthermore, metal post-and-core foundations can negatively affect the esthetic qualities of all-ceramic restorations by altering light transmission[31,128].

When cast cores are used, type IV gold alloys are the most suitable, as they present appropriate mechanical resistance and low corrosion[66,105]. As a result, the probability of a significantly higher survival rate than for posts fabricated from the semi-precious alloy is mentioned[10]. The base metal alloys, as Ni-Cr and Cr-Al, although widely used, should be avoided. Ni-Cr alloys have an excessively high modulus of elasticity (around 200 GPa), which can induce root fracture, and also hinder the intra-oral preparation of the coronal part of the core. Although Cr-Al alloys have a more favorable modulus of elasticity, their low resistance to corrosion can compromise root coloration, in addition to causing dentinal cracks. The silver-palladium alloys represent a viable alternative because they present similar characteristics to the gold alloys and relatively less cost[23,73].

The patterns for casting can be obtained directly in the mouth, through molding with self-curing acrylic resin, or indirectly in the laboratory starting from a model obtained with an elastomeric molding material. The technique of obtaining the cast core follows the traditional casting procedures[104].

The cementation can be performed with zinc phosphate cement, glass ionomer or resinous cement. The decision about the type of cementation is essentially dependent on the preference of the professional[105,113]. However, conventional cementation with zinc phosphate presents long-term proven clinical success[16,] and provided that the dimensions and adaptation of the post are appropriate, there are no evidences about differences in the clinical performance of different cements for cast core fixation[66].



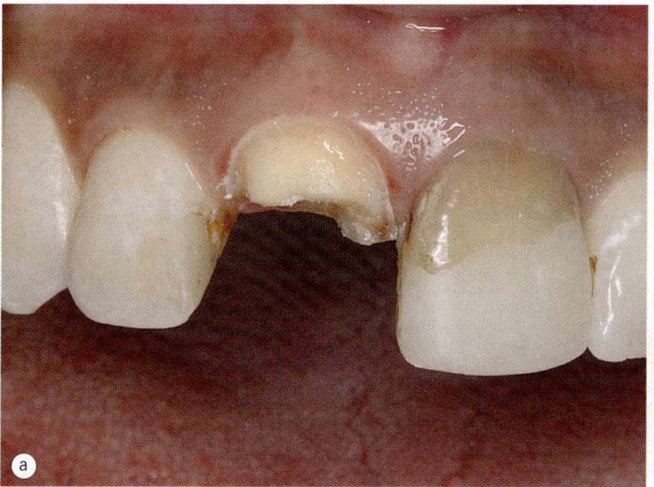

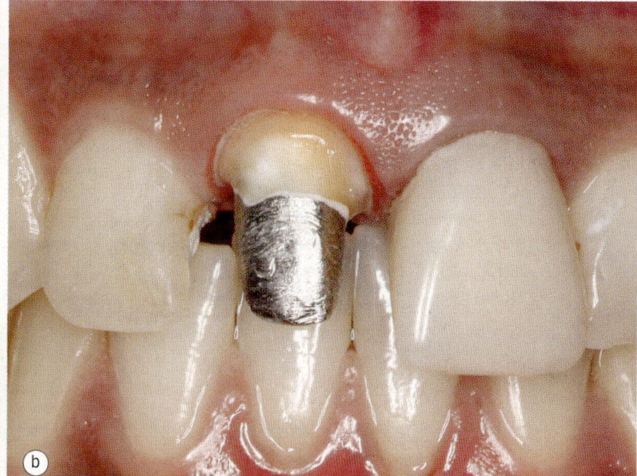

**Figure 27.2** - (**A-B**) Incisor with indication for cast metal core.

## Intraradicular prefabricated posts

To use a prefabricated post it is necessary to have sufficient preparation to accommodate the post dimensions. Unlike the cast core, they are better suited to and present better adaptation in circular and small diameter root canals.

The prefabricated post systems are constituted by three components: (1) the prefabricated post, (2) the cementation material and (3) the material of the coronal core (Fig. 27.3). The large number of combinations of the several types of post system components and cores available on the market increase the complexity of the process of selecting the most appropriate system for each specific clinical situation. As there is no system that can be applied in all clinical situations, and as most of the possible combinations are supported only by in vitro evaluations, without direct clinical correlation, a careful biomechanical evaluation is necessary to establish the best clinical performance of the treatment[106].

Table 27.1 summarizes the most relevant properties of the main prefabricated post systems in combination with the core and cementation materials.

## Prefabricated post materials

The main types of prefabricated posts can be classified as metal (stainless steel, commercially pure titanium and titanium-aluminum-vanadium alloy) and non-metal (carbon fiber, ceramic and fiberglass) (Fig. 27.4). Metal posts are more commonly used and they present favorable clinical reports, although the number of available systems on the market has increased due to patients' esthetic demands.

**Table 27.1.** Comparative properties of the main systems of prefabricated posts, materials for coronal cores and cementation of posts.

| Type of post material | Mechanical resistance | Resistance to corrosion | Esthetic | Radiopacity |
|---|---|---|---|---|
| **Metal** | | | | |
| • Stainless steel | High | Medium | No | Very High |
| • Titanium | Medium | High | No | Medium |
| • Titanium-aluminum-Vanadium | Medium | High | No | Medium |
| **Non-metal** | | | | |
| • Carbon Fibers | Low | High | No | Low |
| • Ceramic | High | High | High | High |
| • Fiberglass | Low | High | High | Low |

| Type of coronal core material | Adhesion | Resistance | Time of reaction | Dimensional stability | Microleakage | Easy to Use |
|---|---|---|---|---|---|---|
| Resin composite | Yes | High | Fast | Medium/High | Medium | Easy |
| Amalgam | no | High | Slow | High | Low | Medium |
| Glass Ionomer | Yes | Low/Medium | Medium | High | Low | Easy |

| Type of cementation material | Adhesion | Resistance | Film thickness | Solubility | Microleakage | Easy to Use |
|---|---|---|---|---|---|---|
| Resinous | High | High | Thicken | Low | Medium | Difficult |
| Phosphate of zinc | Has none | Acceptable | Appropriate | High | High | Easy |
| Glass Ionomer | High | Low | | High | Low | Medium |

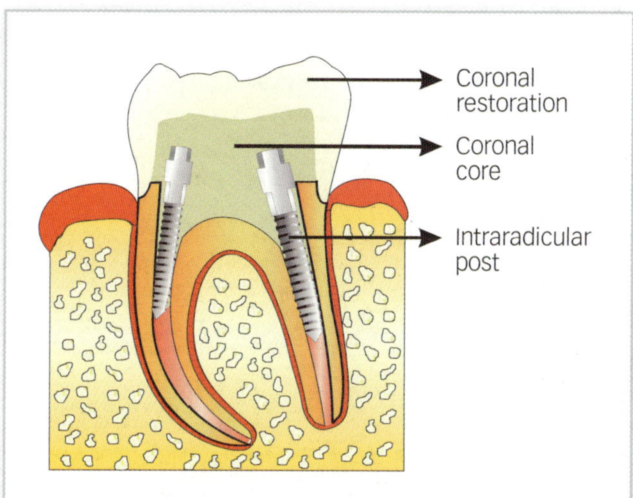


**Figure 27.3** - Components of a prefabricated post system.

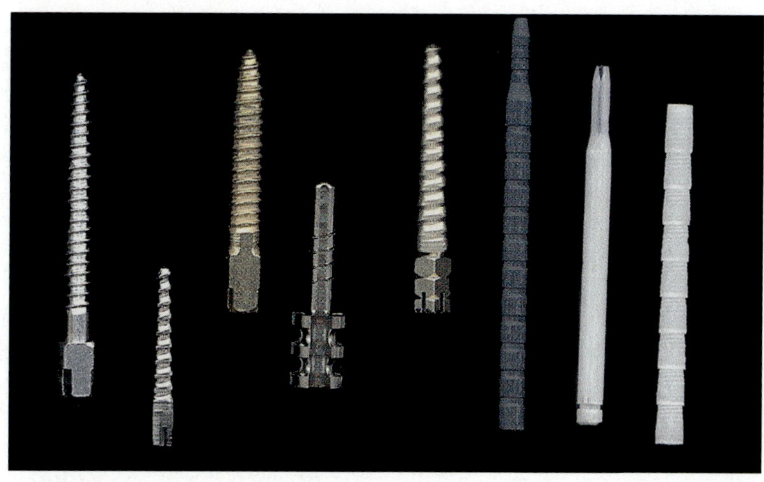

**Figure 27.4** - Types of metal and non-metal posts.

For a satisfactory clinical performance, the prefabricated post should combine biomechanical properties such as, high resistance, good retention and stress distribution, resistance to corrosion and the possibility of being inserted with minimum risk of perforation and smallest amount of preparation.

The material that composes the prefabricated post influences the resistance to root fracture, because there are posts with different rigidity levels (modulus of elasticity) in relation to the root dentin, which alters the form as the forces are distributed along the root (Table 27.2). Carbon fiber posts present smaller modulus of elasticity, similar to that of dentin, while the metal posts present higher rigidity[4,90]. Another advantage of the carbon fiber posts is the ease of adjusting the length of the posts and of removal in the case of endodontic retreatment.

**Table 27.2.** Modulus of elasticity of the dental structure and post materials

| Structure | Modulus of Elasticity (GPa) |
|---|---|
| Enamel | 50-58 |
| Dentin | ±32 |
| Cu-Al | 110 |
| Titanium | 117 |
| Zirconium | 200 |
| Stainless steel | 200 |
| Polyethylene fiber | 17 |
| Carbon fiber | 45 |
| Fiberglass | 33 |

Experimental studies have shown that teeth restored with carbon fiber posts present larger resistance to fracture in comparison with teeth that receive prefabricated or cast metal posts[25,30,48,92]. The effect resulting from the lower rigidity of the post is probably a smaller stress concentration that leads to the root fracture, in other words, when a system with components of different rigidity is submitted to load (dentin and post), the component with greater rigidity is capable of resisting to greater force without distortion. The component with lower rigidity fails and releases the applied stress[30]. This effect can be observed in vitro tests, when teeth with different types of intraradicular core are submitted to fracture by load application. The majority of the fractured teeth restored with cast metal posts were not reparable. In contrast, the majority of fractures in the fiber post group were limited to the cervical portion of the root including the core-dentin interface, since the stress was concentrated in the cervical area and the outer root surface. This type of fracture is easier to repair repeatedly[42,63].

The ceramic posts (zirconium) and the fiberglass posts provide optical properties similar to the metal free ceramic crowns, which provide them with esthetic properties superior to those of metal posts. Zirconium posts are biocompatible, radiopaque, present high mechanical resistance and they are suitable for anterior and premolar teeth where esthetic appearance is an essential factor[47,53]. They are more rigid, however less retentive than the posts with similar shape and made of stainless steel.[91] Different methods of laboratory processing of zirconium posts are available, through pressing methods that make it possible to obtain a post and core system in one piece[51,53]. As a result of the high modulus of elasticity of the zirconium posts, much higher than that of dentin (Table 27.2), their use has been discouraged.

The fiberglass post consist of cylindrical or conical posts involved in a resinous matrix with load, with biomechanical properties similar to those of carbon fiber posts, such as a modulus of elasticity similar to that of dentin, producing a stress field similar to that of natural teeth[85], but with ideal esthetic superiority for use associated with metal-free restorations[14,30]. However, controlled clinical studies are necessary to confirm the clinical success with different levels of dentinal remainder[25].

Both fiberglass and carbon fiber posts have the disadvantage of being radiolucent, although some systems have been developed with a smaller degree of radiolucence. Titanium posts have a radiopacity similar to that of gutta-percha.

## 27.3 Material for the Coronal Core

The coronal part of the core provides retention and stability to the final restoration. The load distribution capacity of root posts is influenced by the coronal core material, whose ideal characteristics should include easy technique for use, fast reaction time, high resistance, dimensional stability with minimum risk of leakage and an effective bonding mechanism. Resin composite, amalgam and glass ionomer cement are the materials of choice for the coronal core of prefabricated posts.

Resin composite and amalgam can be considered the materials that better distribute loads around the surface of the core, significantly reducing cervical stress[125]. However, glass ionomer has lower resistance in comparison with amalgam and resin, and its bond to dentin is considered weak[66]. Due to its low mechanical properties, glass ionomer has few advantages that justify its indication as core material, its use being limited to blocking small retentive areas[19,20,66].

Although amalgam has high resistance to compression and low risk of leakage, it has a retarded time of crystallization and absence of adhesive properties. Moreover, cores with small thickness are highly subject to fractures. It is possible to increase their fracture strength with the use of adhesive techniques to amalgam[28], but its use is not very advisable for making cores due to the temporary nature of the bond and time and additional cost of the procedure[66].

Resin composite offers appropriate clinical strength, although its maximum limit of resistance is inferior to that of amalgam. It undergoes significant polymerization shrinkage; its resistance to microleakage is almost completely dependent on the cementation agent, and it is questionable whether the adhesive agent is capable of impeding microleakage in the long term[66].The satisfactory strength, reduction in clinical time when using it and its bonding capacity are properties that have made resin composite the material most used for cores, in conjunction with most of the prefabricated post systems[19,54,80].

Because of presenting similar mechanical properties to those of dentin, resin composites are also widely used for root reinforcement in teeth with very thin roots, improving structural strength by decreasing excessively wide root canals.

For the core build-up procedure, a large variety of composite resin materials are available to the clinician, ranging from packable to microhybrid to flowable composites[76]. There are specific resins for cores, such as the Ti-Core (Essential Dental Systems), hybrid resin with 75% of inorganic load, which is chemically polymerized and releases fluoride, and Bis-Core (Bisco), with similar physicochemical characteristics, however being dual setting. Goracci et al.[38,] mentioned results obtained by Monticelli et al.[76], when they evaluated the structural integrity of the core material and its adaptation to the post surface by SEM observations of post-and-core units prepared in vitro. They found that flowable composites exhibited better results than hybrid composites and composites marketed as core materials. The same authors also validated the use of flowable composites as core materials, as a result of the findings of an in vivo trial, in which post-and-core restorations exhibited satisfactory clinical service over a 2-year follow-up period. If they confirm this result in additional studies, the flowable composites present the advantages of generating smaller polymerization stresses, providing greater longevity of the bond to the dental structure as well as to the prefabricated post.

With the introduction of prefabricated FRC posts, continuous efforts have been made to improve the bonding potential of current adhesive systems inside root canals[3,32,33,34,75,81].

The use of fiber posts to restore endodontically treated teeth is mainly advantageous for preventing root fractures. However, for a successful build-up of a subsequent resin core, it is necessary to establish a effective bond between the resin and the post as well as between the resin and the dentin.[1] The retention of the core portion to the post depends on the strength of the chemical and micromechanical interaction between a fiber-reinforced material and a composite resin. Furthermore, this bond has to rapidly reach levels of sufficiently high strength to resist the stress transmitted during core trimming and adaptation of the provisional crown[37].

In the search for an effective bond between fiber-reinforced material and composite resin, studies have shown that the interfacial bond strength was significantly enhanced if the post surface had been preliminary coated with a silane coupling agent[1,37,38]. The authors concluded that although adhesion to intraradicular dentin is more challenging to achieve than bonding to crown tissues, the post-retention achieved with current luting systems and techniques is adequate to ensure the clinical success of adhesive post-retained restorations. This is indispensable, since the fracture strength of the restored endodontically treated tooth is a function of the strength of the root/remaining coronal tooth structure and the post/core, as well as the bond strength between them[79].

## 27.4 Cementation Material

The purpose of the intraradicular post cementation material is to help retention, allow sealing along the root canal and to promote a layer of cushioning that contributes to the uniform distribution of stress between the post and the root canal wall[27,112]. A cement with good characteristics should have high resistance, small coating thickness, low solubility, adhesion capacity, easy manipulation and marginal sealing that blocks microleakage[27,58,73,106].

Zinc phosphate, glass ionomer (conventional and modified) and resinous (resin composite, resin without load and dentinal adhesive agent) cements are the most used for prefabricated post cementation[73]. There are advantages and disadvantages inherent to each these cements, and none has all of the ideal properties required for prefabricated post cementation.

Zinc phosphate cement has disadvantages like high solubility and lack of adhesion[106], but the long history of success in clinical use makes it suitable for cementation of cast or prefabricated posts with good adaptation[27].

Glass ionomer cement has weak adhesion to dentin, is highly susceptible to humidity and the benefits resulting from its capacity to inhibit decay in dentin due to fluoride release has not yet been clinically proved[73,106]. Post retention provided by glass ionomer is not superior to that of the other conventional cements[55]. Similarly, there is no definitive information on the effectiveness of the resin modified ionomer for intraradicular post cementation, and the risk of expansion after setting can be a risk factor for root fracture[73,106,117]. In a 10-year retrospective longitudinal study Balkenhol et al.[10] evaluated the survival time of custom-fabricated cast post and core. With respect to luting materials, they found that the post and cores inserted with glass ionomer cement had a higher risk of failure.

The adhesive resins are relatively insoluble and promote better retention, in comparison with conventional cements[119]. The retention provided by resinous cement is less influenced by greater cement thickness when the post does not completely adapt to the root canal, which can happen with the use of prefabricated posts[7]. These factors made the use of resinous cements for intraradicular post fixation quite common.

However, there are two potential problems with resinous cements they are more sensitive to the manipulation technique and more adversely affected by inadequate preparation of the root canal surface[67,117]. In addition to the problems of bonding to dentin in general, there are difficulties associated with the use of adhesive systems in root canals[82,117]. There are structural differences between root dentin and coronal dentin, as well as problems with the presence of provisional cements, endodontic sealers, and irrigant solutions in a canal with limited access. It was suggested that the cement bonding to dentin could be inhibited by the presence of phenolic components, such as the eugenol present in most of the endodontic cements[67,111], but no difference has been verified in the retention of posts cemented with zinc phosphate or resin composite in root canals filled with cements with and without eugenol[102].

The bond strength between various posts and luting agents, as well as the effect of post surface treatments on bond strength and retention of posts in root canals have been investigated extensively[35,52,56,57,68,69,83,84,87,97-100,116,118,124,127]. Studies have shown the prevalence of adhesive failures in intracanal posts[15,89]. These findings indicate that failure after testing mostly occurred at the interface between the luting agent and radicular dentin. Irrespective of the failure type, post surface treatment with a silane coupling agent is advisable to enhance the adhesion of the resin cement used for luting[97]. With respect to glass fiber posts, in addition to silanization, airborne particle abrasion of posts and the combination of this with silane coating were also found to significantly increase the bond strength of resin cements to these posts[97].

Considering the resinous cements, the 4-META-based cements have shown the highest resistance to removal and provide the greatest resistance to root fracture[68,111]. However, the increase in retention with the use of adhesive resinous cements, proved in in vitro tests, does not assure a reduced risk of displacement of the post under normal clinical conditions[73].

Special attention should be given to the post cementation procedure, since the most common failures have been the loss of post retention[10], while root fracture is still the most serious type of failure[121].

Recent studies have emphasized the advantages of glass ionomer cements for the cementation of posts in root canals. Yan et al.[126] evaluating the response to thermal stimuli of glass ionomer cements, concluded that under wet conditions glass ionomers maintain their original dimensions when heated, and this type of behavior may be considered 'smart' behavior.

When performing tensile bond strength tests of glass fiber posts luted with different cements, Bonfante et al.[13] showed that resin cements and glass ionomer cements are able to provide clinically sufficient retention of glass fiber posts. Furthermore, they emphasized that glass ionomer cements may be especially indicated when the application of the adhesive technique is difficult.

Figures 27.5 to 27.17, show the cementation of a glass fiber post in a maxillary left central incisor (21) using the adhesive technique (Silano, Adesivo Prime&Bond 2.1 and Enforce cement, Dentisply, USA). The tooth presents an extensive resin composite restoration and great color alteration, and it will be restored with a complete crown of pure porcelain. The fiberglass post (FGM, BRAZIL) was selected together with the resin composite filling (Z100, 3M ESPE) to increase the strength of the coronal structure and not to compromise the esthetic result of the metal-free restoration.

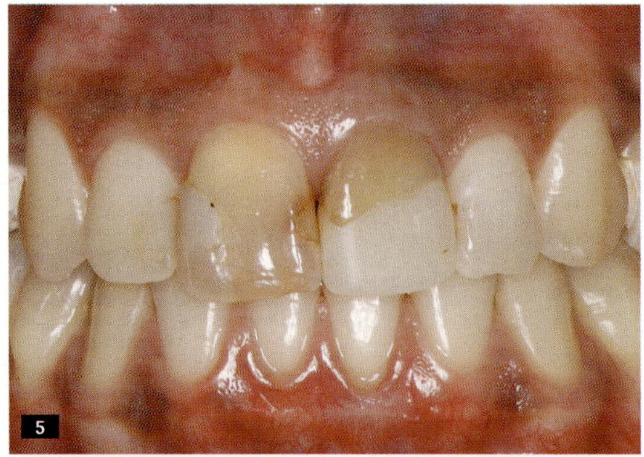


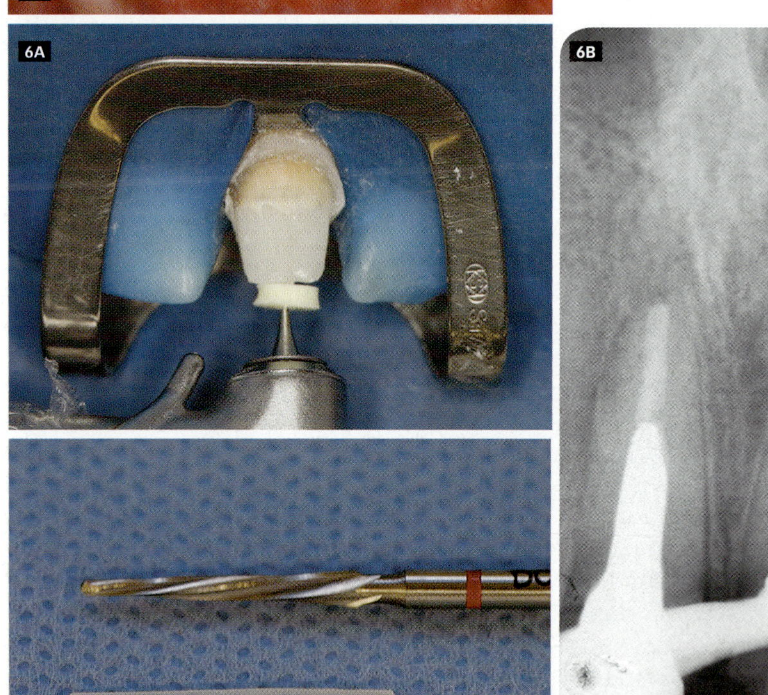


**Figure 27.5** - Maxillary left central incisor with an extensive resin composite restoration
**Figure 27.6** - (**A-B**) Removal of 2/3 of the endodontic filling.
**Figure 27.7** - Selected fiberglass post and the drill for root canal preparation.

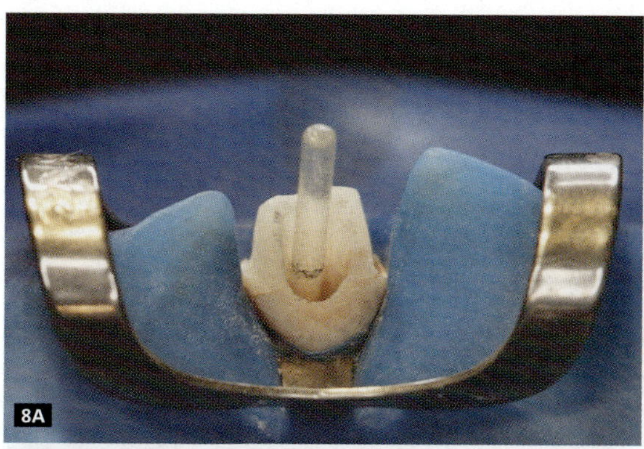


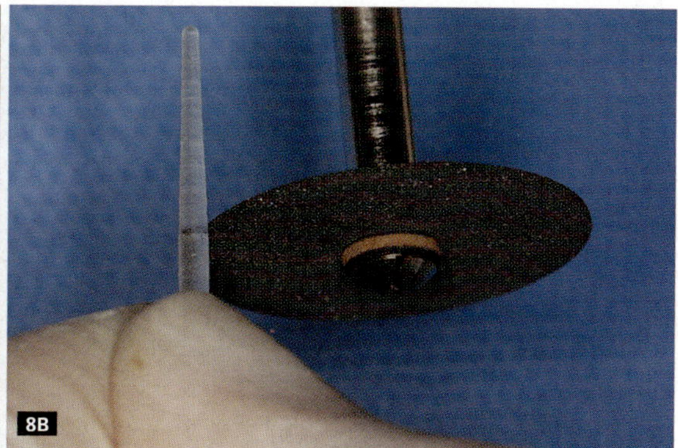


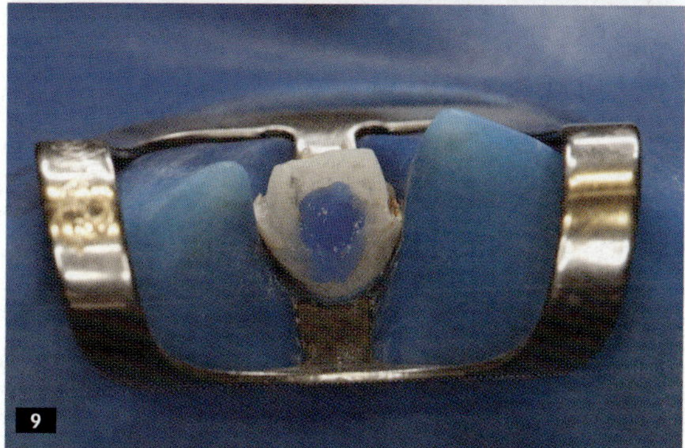


**Figure 27.8** - (**A-B**) Demarcation and cutting of the post with carborundum disk.
**Figure 27.9** - Etching of the root canal with 37% phosphoric acid.
**Figure 27.10** - Drying of the root canal with paper points after removing the phosphoric acid with water.
**Figure 27.11** - (**A-B**) Application and removal of the adhesive excess.

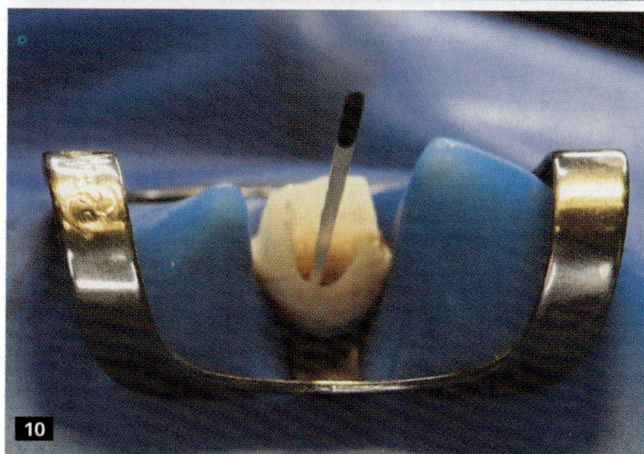


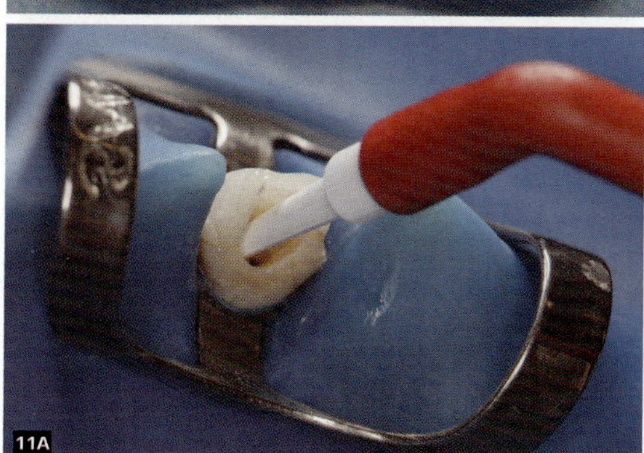


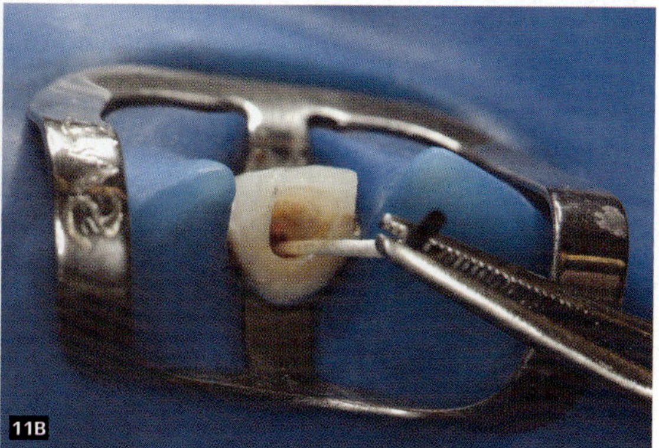

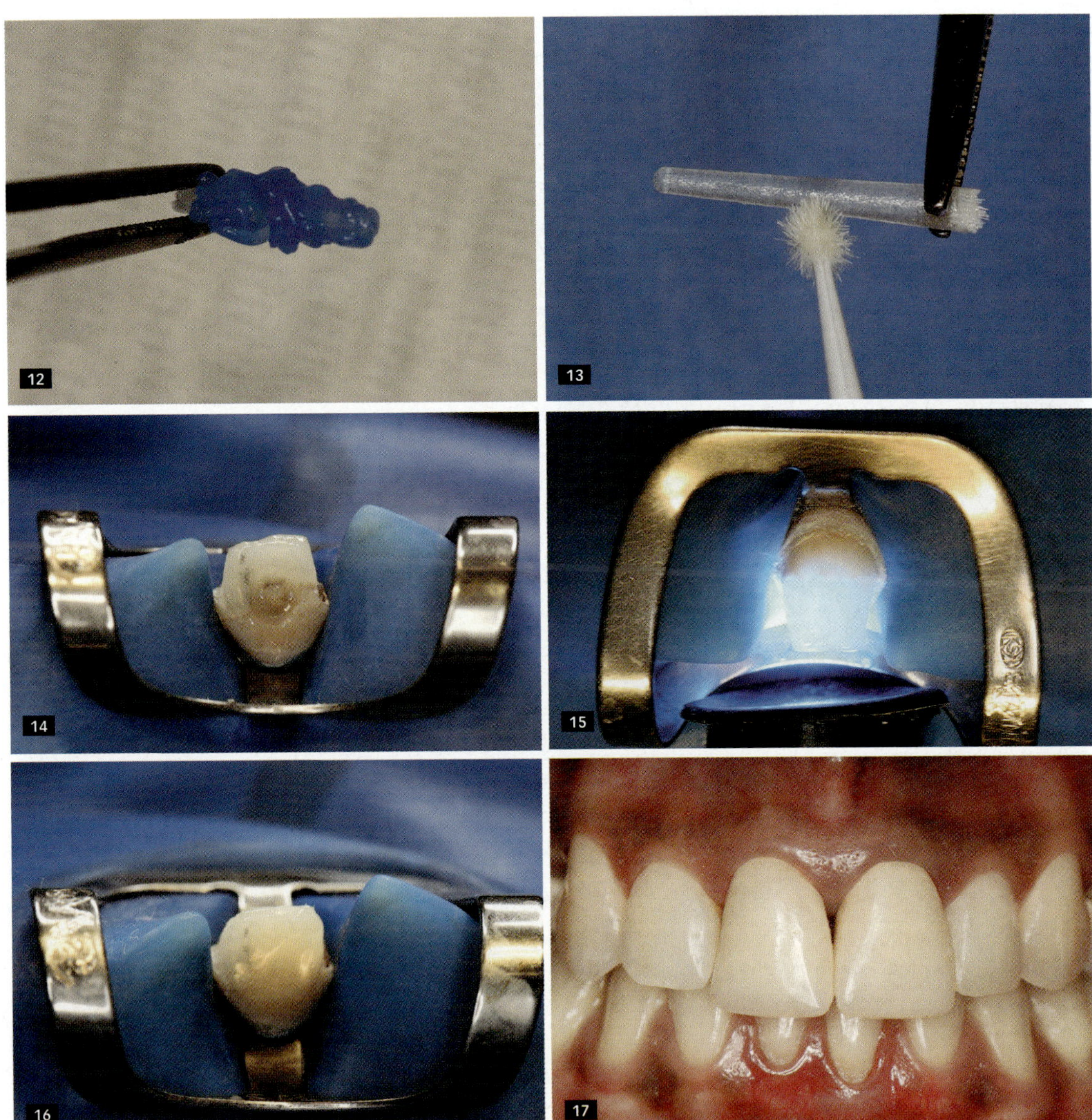


**Figure 27.12** - Cleaning the fiberglass post with phosphoric acid.
**Figure 27.13** - Application of silane to the fiberglass post.
**Figure 27.14** - Resinous cement applied in the root canal.
**Figure 27.15** - Light polymerization of the post positioned inside the root canal.
**Figure 27.16** - Palatine view of the tooth after filling with resin composite.
**Figure 27.17** - Frontal view of the maxillary left central incisor with temporary acrylic resin restoration.

## 27.5 Mechanical Aspects of Intraradicular Retention

The retention of intraradicular post systems is affected by a series of variables that include the length, diameter and superficial configuration of the post, root canal shapes, type and cementation method and location of the tooth in the arch[117].

### Intraradicular post length

The length of the post has significant influence on intraradicular retention. Disregarding other factors, the longer the post, the greater the retention. In other words, the post should be as long as possible, without harming the apical seal of the root canal filling. Posts that are much too short have a high risk of failure of retention and cause higher risk of root fracture.

There are no rigid rules, but several clinical criteria were recommended to help to determine the ideal length of an intraradicular post. These criteria include the following parameters (Fig. 27.18):

1. The post length should be longer, or at least equal to the occlusocervical or incisocervical dimension of the crown of the restored tooth;
2. The post should comprise at least two thirds of the total length of the root;
3. The post should reach at least half of the distance between the alveolar bony crest and the root apex;
4. The post should be as long as possible, maintaining a minimum remainder of root canal filling of 4 to 5 millimeters.

Although the greatest post length increases the retention, on the other hand it increases the risk of root perforation during the preparation of the root canal. The maximum length, therefore, is usually limited by the need for maintaining approximately 4 millimeters of apical filling.

In cases of prefabricated posts, a length from 7 to 11 millimeters is usually enough to provide appropriate retention[37-50]. But the maximum length of the post can, in certain cases, be restricted due to clinical factors, such as the presence of curvature of the roots, calcifications, dilacerations and ramifications of root canals[129].

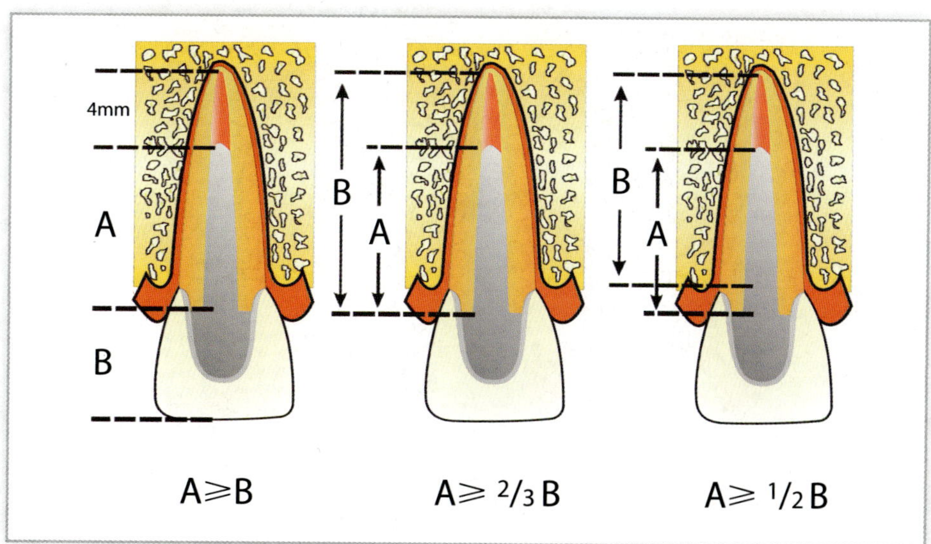


**Figure 27.18** - Clinical parameters for determining the length of the intraradicular post.

## Post diameter

Increase in the diameter does not significantly increase the retention of the post,[113] thus, the increase in length is more important than the increase in diameter to obtain greater resistance to removal[64,78]. The increase in the resistance of the post occurs at the cost of reduction in root fracture strength as a consequence of the decrease in dentinal remainder[23].

Definition of the post diameter should be compatible with the preservation of root dentin, reduction in the risk of fracture and root perforation. The following guidelines are recommended (Fig. 27.19):

1. The diameter of the post should not exceed a third of the total diameter of the root in its entire length;
2. The post diameter should be a maximum of 1 millimeter at its most apical extremity, maintaining of a wall of surrounding dentin of at least 1mm;
3. Do not increase the space for a post beyond the diameter of the original endodontic preparation.

## Configuration of the post surface and retention form

The format of the intracanal post is usually dictated by the format of the root canal because the adaptation of the post to the root canal walls is an important factor for retention. An individualized cast post should be used for ovoid and elliptic root canals, and a prefabricated intracanal post for straight and parallel root canals.

Modifications were incorporated into prefabricated posts to increase the retention and resistance, and at the same time, reduce the stress generated in the remaining structure[117].

Prefabricated posts can be classified according to their configuration or retention form. Their configuration can be conical, parallel or a combination of parallel-conical. As regards the retention form, they are classified as active or passive[30].

Conical posts present larger stress concentration in the coronal portion and low concentration in the apical area[24,112]. The lower stress concentration induced in the apical area is due to the absence of the angulated

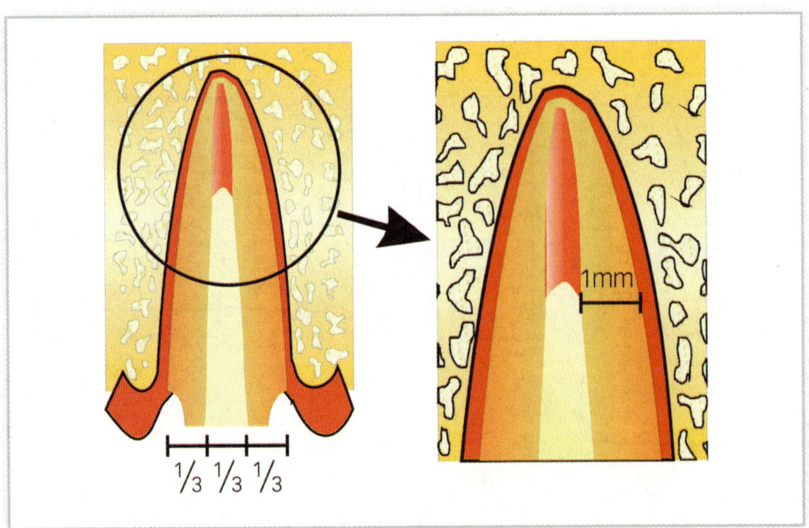


**Figure 27.19** - Clinical parameters for determining the diameter of the intraradicular post.

form and to the conservation of the dental structure[30]. The conical configuration can favor the wedge effect transmitted to the remaining structure[107].

Parallel posts disperse the stress evenly along their length, except in the apical area, where there is a concentration of stress[95]. This has led to the development of the angulated form of the post apex, allowing better seating and consequently less reduction of the dental structure in this area[30].

Active posts are characterized by being threaded during insertion. The threads penetrate into the dentin walls of the root canal preparation, aiding post retention[21,39,112]. The use of posts with a large space between the threads presents smaller risk than posts with a larger number of threads and a small space between them, which is an important factor to observe, since it also generates risks, such as an increase in stress[26]. To minimize the stress induced in the walls during active post insertion, the creation of threads in the dentin is indicated before post insertion, as well as selecting posts with smaller diameter and smaller number of threads, and unscrewing a fourth of turn, after the post has been inserted[26,96]. Active posts are suitable for short roots, in cases of anatomical defects or due to accidental causes that provide little depth for the placement of a post. In these cases is necessary to obtain the maximum possible retention. However, active posts can induce more tension in the preparation walls than passive posts. The threaded posts are more retentive, but they develop more stress when actively inserted[36,48,77].

A passive post does not adapt completely and it does not present active retention in the dentin during the trial or the insert, being maintained in position by the cementation agent. Posts with smooth surfaces develop minimum stress, but they provide the least retention. In certain parallel post systems, the extremities are conical, which can be beneficial if the root apex is conical. Therefore, the extremity of every passive post with parallel sides can be thin during the clinical procedure. Active posts are the most retentive, followed by the passive parallel and passive conical posts.[113] Ideally, the professional should have available a passive post system for most of the clinical situations and an active post system for short roots.

## 27.6 Clinical Performance of Teeth with Intraradicular Retention

The ample availability of clinical solutions has considerably increased the possibilities of success, but it can generate confusion for the clinician and result in inadequate use of the technique. Similarly, the decision of whether or not to provide intraradicular retention for a endodontically treated tooth is not simple.

Although there is a large volume of published information, there are no absolute guidelines for most clinical situations. In vitro studies are usually conducted to evaluate the different retention systems and technical variations related to the clinical approach[30]. But the results of laboratory researches are frequently conflicting and not always clinically applied[44,73]. The majority of clinical studies found in the literature are retrospective, but they are also insufficient for defining safe clinical approaches with proven effectiveness[44].

In 1993, Creugers et al.[22] conducted a systematic review to evaluate the success of treatment with post systems, but no randomized controlled clinical trial was identified in the literature at that time. Moreover, this lack of clear definition of success and failure criteria makes it difficult to compare evaluations among the different clinical studies[22].

A longitudinal study of Torbjörner et al.[121] revealed that failure of retention is the most common problem in teeth with both cast and prefabricated intraradicular posts, while root fracture was the most severe failure. Indeed, a systematic review conducted by Goodacre et al.[36] which included clinical studies concerning the evaluation of complications subsequent to the use of intraradicular posts (Table 27.3), found an incidence of 10% of cases with problems associated with the displacement of the post (5%), root fractures (3%), dental decay (2%) and periodontal involvement (2%).

**Table 27.3** - Frequency of more common complications associated with the use of intraradicular post.

| Complication | Number of included studies | Number of cases evaluated | Frequency of complications | |
|---|---|---|---|---|
| | | | N | % |
| Post Displacement | 11 | 2596 | 135 | 5.20 |
| Root Fracture | 13 | 3043 | 95 | 3.12 |
| Dental decay | 4 | 1047 | 16 | 1.53 |
| Periodontal involvement | 3 | 283 | 6 | 2.12 |

(Goodacre et al.[36])

A systematic review with meta-analysis was conducted by Heydecke & Peters[44] for comparison of the clinical and in vitro performance of cast and prefabricated post in the restoration of anterior teeth. Starting with a search and bibliographical evaluation with pre-defined inclusion criteria, a total of ten in vitro studies and six in vivo studies were included in the meta-analysis. The comparison of the resistance and the type of fracture in vitro did not reveal differences among the two post systems. The evaluation of the clinical performance of teeth treated with direct post in 3 selected studies presented a longevity estimated between 86 and 88%, after 6 years[44].

A prospective clinical study conducted by Ellner et al.[29] in 2003, compared the effectiveness of four different cast and prefabricated intraradicular post systems for a period of up to 10 years. The total percentage of failures was 6% and no significant difference was found among the systems.

There is little clinical evidence available, starting with treatments using different core systems performed under the usual clinical conditions. In addition with the contradictory results of published studies, makes any definitive inference in favor or against the use of cast or prefabricated core inconsistent. Both treatment options are recommended, provided they are applied in accordance with their indications and with clinical care while they are being performed[44].

Another important limitation of the retrospective clinical studies refers to the control of clinical variables related to the treatment methods, usually subject to bias. For example, the clinical decision to perform treatment with the cast core is based primarily on the amount of coronal remainder, in other words, it is preferable to restore teeth with little or no remaining coronal structure with cast posts, while teeth with a substantial amount of coronal structure receive prefabricated posts or only a coronal filling core. Consequently, knowing that the prognosis of the tooth is intimately related to the amount of remaining dentin, by following this protocol, teeth restored with cast posts present a higher risk of failure, not because of problems inherent to the treatment itself, but because the professional indicates its use for teeth with extensive loss of coronal structure and little remaining dentin, which consequently have a higher potential of failure and a worse prognosis with regard to fracture[73].

Fortunately, cast posts involve longer clinical time, comparatively higher costs, and under similar clinical conditions, the direct posts significantly reduce the treatment time and the costs to the patient. However, controlled clinical studies are still scarce and they are not conclusive with regard to the selection of the best treatment alternative for different degrees of dentinal structure loss.

## 27.7 Clinical Criteria for the Indication of Intraradicular Retention

Two factors are essential for selecting the most appropriate system for each clinical situation: maximization of retention and minimization of the risk of root fracture[50]. The advent of non-metal post systems and the continuous development of the adhesion processes and materials for cores have led to conceptual and practical changes in the use of posts and cores over the last few years.

However, the amount of remaining dentin can be considered the most important factor for maintaining the structural resistance of the tooth and reducing the risk of root fracture[62,72]. When there is appropriate preservation of dental structure, the selection of the post has little or no influence on the resistance to root fracture[70].

Unlike the concept that the intraradicular post would be always necessary to reinforcei the tooth after the endodontic treatment[42,61], experimental evidences show that intraradicular cores do not increase the resistance of the tooth to fracture[6,41,109,123].

Dentin is the tissue that makes the tooth strong; it supports and transmits the functional loads to the periodontium and bony base. Thus, the intracanal post does not increase the resistance of the root, and can even weaken it, due to inadequate preparation, because the preparation for enlarging the root canal to receive the post results in additional loss of dentin that reduces the structural resistance of the tooth, and this also happens as regards the coronal portion[5]. Therefore, it is essential to provide conservative preparations to avoid needless weakening of the dental structure[5,40].

In addition to the dentinal wear to prepare the root canal to receive the post, which can increase the risk of root fracture, other potential problems can be linked to intraradicular retention, such as the need for endodontic retreatment or replacement of the prosthesis associated with the removal of the cores, root fractures, risk of perforation of the root during the preparation or removal of the retainer and displacement of the retainer due to retention failure.

Factors that influence the selection of the intraradicular retention system are related to practical clinical matters, such as reducing the time of clinical work, simplifying the technique and decreasing costs. Most of the prefabricated post systems present clear advantages as regards these aspects and their growing use has simplified clinical solutions[17,18]. However, the indication of prefabricated posts in teeth with absence of coronal remainder should be considered with caution.

Clinically, cast cores are usually indicated for anterior teeth with moderate or severe loss of coronal structure. Whereas, in molars, the use of intraradicular cores is frequently unnecessary due to the larger amount of remaining dentin and because they are primarily submitted to axial loads. Molars with minimum loss of coronal structure can be appropriately restored with amalgam or other direct restorative materials[8]. Molars with significant coronal loss usually allow satisfactory retention with the use of direct filling cores with retention in the pulp chamber and the more coronal portion of the root canals, either associated or not with one or more prefabricated intraradicular posts. Premolars with little or no remaining coronal structure can be restored with both cast and prefabricated posts[73]. Thus, for teeth that are primarily submitted to lateral forces, such as the incisors and canines, there is greater possibility of indicating intraradicular retention, since the amount of remaining coronal structure is significantly reduced. Single rooted teeth (especially the incisors) are submitted to non-axial loads, therefore resulting in greater stress when functional loads are applied.

Other complicating factors should also be considered, as regards situations in which excessive additional load can be placed on the tooth. Teeth involved occlusal guidance, abutment teeth of fixed or removable prosthesis, or teeth subjected to parafunctional loads can demand more cautious restorative approaches when preparing the treatment plan.

Table 27.4 guides the clinical conduct as regards whether or not to indicate intraradicular retention, considering the amount of coronal structure loss in the tooth after the endodontic treatment. It is important to emphasize that there are conflicting evidences and several inconclusive points in the literature. Therefore, these parameters should be considered after a cautious critical judgment and each case should be evaluated individually. In addition to the clinical guidelines, another six general principles should be considered as safe approaches for the restoration of endodontically treated teeth, with or without the need of intraradicular retention[103]:

1. Covering the cusp or extra-coronal restorations (for example, complete crowns) should be suitable for all the posterior teeth;
2. Anterior teeth with intact marginal crests and conservative endodontic access should be restored with direct materials restricted to the cavitary preparation;
3. When a direct restoration is the option for posterior teeth with substantial amount of coronal remainder, resin composite and adhesive techniques should be indicated for the dentin;
4. Intraradicular posts should only be used when there is not enough remaining dental structure to retain the coronal cores;
5. Intraradicular posts are more frequently required in anterior teeth than in posterior teeth;
6. The definitive restoration should be performed, at the most, a few weeks after the end of the endodontic treatment to reduce the potential microbial leakage resulting from a break in the coronal sealing of the temporary restoration.

**Table 27.4** - Clinical conduct considering the amount of coronal structure loss of the tooth after the endodontic treatment

| Amount of coronary structure loss | Need for intraradicular Retention | Preparation type | Need for Restoration |
|---|---|---|---|
| Minimum loss of coronal structure | Does not need | Maintenance of the endodontic filling up to the bony level. The dental preparation is limited to the preparation for endodontic treatment. | Restoration of the preparation for endodontic access (GI, RMGI, RC, Am) |
| Loss of up to half of the coronal structure | It does not usually need, unless the tooth is submitted to significant lateral stresses (anterior teeth). Premolar and molars rarely need it. | Maintenance of the endodontic filling up to the bony level. The dental preparation is limited to the preparation for endodontic treatment and to promote retention of the core. | Restoration of the preparation for endodontic access and recomposition of the tooth (GI, RMGI, RC, Am), or of the coronal filling core (RMGI, RC) and indirect restoration (inlay/onlay or complete crowns) |
| Loss of more than half of the coronal structure | It usually needs intraradicular retention. | Removal of root canal filling material and intraradicular preparation, and maintenance of the largest possible amount of remaining coronal structure. | Cast or prefabricated core. Maintenance of the coronal remainder promotes an anti-rotational effect of the core and favors retention of the post-core set. |
| Complete loss of coronal structure | It always needs intraradicular retention. | Removal of root canal filling material and intraradicular preparation | Cast Core |

GI-glass ionomer; RMGI -resin modified glass ionomer; RC-resin composite; Am-amalgam

## 27.8 Characteristics of the Final Restoration

### The splint effect

The splint effect is defined as a metal collar that encompasses the coronal structure in 360 degrees around the parallel walls of dentin that extend coronally at the end of the preparation of the tooth, increasing resistance to the root fracture[104,107,114].

The bracing action is promoted by a total crown restoration that reduces the tendency of the post and cores to transfer the occlusal forces to the root, causing a wedge effect and predisposing the root to the vertical fracture[11,107]. A definitive restoration that extends for at least 1.5 to 2 millimeters apically to the junction between the coronal cores and the remaining dental structure is enough to produce the splint effect, reduce the risk of root fracture [65,73,107] and of the coronal core materials[86,88] (Figure 27.20). When a carbon fiber post is used in teeth with absence of the splint effect, occlusal loads can cause micromovement of the crown, breaking the marginal seal of the restoration and resulting in marginal leakage[73].

Additionally, a minimum thickness of coronal structure, between the internal wall of the root canal and the external surface of the crown preparation is clinically desirable[107,120]. The larger the thickness of the remaining coronal dentin, the less the probability of failure by root fracture, in the event of the post being displaced[46,65].

Preservation of the coronal structure to the greatest possible extent during the dental preparation for total crown potentiates the splint effect to the maximum and significantly enhances the prognosis of tooth[72]. In extensively destroyed teeth, surgery to augment the clinical crown and/or orthodontic extrusion can be suitable to expose healthy dental structure necessary for obtaining the possibility of cervical bracing. In these situations, when it is impracticable to obtain the splint effect, the prognosis of the survival of the tooth should be considered with extreme caution[73]. Finally, in teeth with severely compromised coronal-radicular structure, taking into consideration the prognosis of the treatment, extraction of the tooth and replacing it with a conventional or implant-supported prosthesis can be considered a more feasible and predictable long-term approach[72].



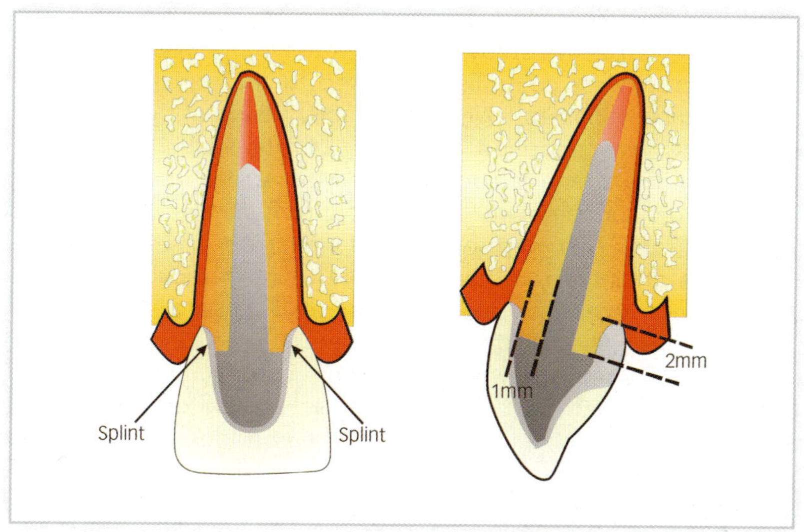


**Figure 27.20** - Splint effect produced by the restoration completely bracing the circumference of the coronal remainder.

A proposal for improving the prognosis of roots with thin remaining walls is intraradicular reinforcement by increasing the internal thickness of the root with an adhesive resin restoration associated with the use of light transmitting posts for internal polymerization, and consequent reduction of the root canal diameter[59]. An in vitro evaluation showed that this procedure promotes a significant increase in resistance to root fracture and it minimizes the negative effect of the absence of the splint effect.[101] However, long term longitudinal studies are necessary to verify the effectiveness of this type of treatment option.

**The type of final restoration**

Clinical studies have proved that the placement of an intraradicular post does not have a significant effect on the survival of endodontically treated teeth, but they suggested that the type of the final restoration influences the clinical success of the treatment[108-110]. This concept has been generalized to the point where complete coronal covering has become the most usual procedure for reducing fracture risk, both in anterior and posterior teeth[9].

A strong association between the type of final restoration and the survival of endodontically treated teeth was observed by Aquiline & Caplan[2] in a cohort retrospective study, in which other clinical factors were controlled. Among the studied clinical variables, significantly inferior prognosis was observed for teeth with dental decay at the time of endodontic access, second molars, teeth without intraradicular post and teeth that were prepared less than 8 days after the root canal filling. Teeth that did not receive complete crowns presented a 6 times higher failure rate than teeth restored with complete crowns[2].

Other restoration forms with or without occlusal covering, such as direct and indirect resin[60], porcelain inlays[16] and complex amalgam restorations[8,115] were also tested at several levels of coronal remainder of posterior teeth. However, there are no safe data to prove effectiveness comparable with that of covering with complete crowns[2].

Although there is a positive association between the complete coronal covering and the survival of endodontically treated teeth, there is no established relationship of cause and effect, which could only be verified through randomized controlled clinical trials[2]. Moreover, prospective studies that include analyses of cost-effectiveness are necessary. Therefore, treatment recommendations should be made on an individual bases, and although it is not indispensable in all cases, the use of complete crowns is considered a positive factor for maintaining long term clinical success[2].

**Quality of the restoration**

From the point of view of endodontic success, the quality of the final restoration is a factor that should not be overlooked. Special attention should be given to the potential of possible leakage of the final restoration causing failure of the initially acceptable endodontic treatment[61,93,122]. Microbial infiltration along the root canal filling when coronal sealing is not effective compromises the long term success.

## 27.9 Other Clinical Procedures Related to the intraradicular posts

Determining the length of the preparation for the intraradicular retainer is especially related to the remaining coronal dentin, root length, height of the bony crest and the number of root canals.

Methods for removing the filling material from root canals that need further endodontic treatment or that it will be prepared to receive intraradicular retainer have been previously discussed. However, it must be considered that during removal of the root canal filling material, the tooth has to be prepared immediately after the filling. Ideally, as soon as the endodontist concludes the root canal filling, he/she should take advantage of the opportunity and makes the preparation. At this time, the filling material can be debased by heating with a vertical condenser, or even with rotating instruments, such as Gates-Glidden drills. When the material is removed after filling, it is not always effective to remove the filling material by means of a heating system, which makes it necessary to use drills.

The arsenal of endodontic instruments consists of several models of instruments (or rotating systems), capable of preparing a root canal efficiently, in shorter period of time and with little stress. The appearance of flexible instruments, such as the nickel-titanium unit driven by an electric motor with continuous rotation, and with variable tappers, favors cervical preparation. Enlargement in the cervical-apical direction, which is accepted as consensus all over the world, allows the apical shape to be maintained, and also previously defines the preparation to receive an intraradicular retainer. The different instruments suitable for the cervical preparation have already been discussed, and among them, the orifice shaper, coronal shaper, orifice opener, Line-angle access, Gates-Glidden and largo drills can be listed. These rotating instruments, designed for cervical preparation during endodontic treatment, leave this area prepared to receive the intraradicular retainer. The refinement and the conclusion of intraradicular preparation after endodontic treatment will be defined later, with planning of the restoration type (and consequently, the type of intraradicular post) to be selected as the best option.

Several factors always deserve care during the preparation for the retainer, such as:

1. The inclination of the teeth in the arch;
2. The volume of the roots (root structures with little thickness, or thin, with presence of risk areas);
3. The longitudinal depth of the preparation, with consequent removal of the filling material, more than acceptable for a perfect endodontic sealing;
4. The traverse preparation of the root canal, with exaggerated wear, compromising the tooth (susceptibility to perforation and root fracture);
5. The format of the preparation, altering the morphology of the root canal and the stability of the retainer, depreciating the continuous conical-funneled format.

The measures for maintaining the aseptic technique during preparation to receive the intraradicular post should be valued at all times. After the removal of the cervical portion of the filling material, the root canal presents different conditions for the development of microorganisms that can stay in the dentinal tubules or penetrate in the root canal during the preparation for the post, through restorations with leakage[43]. These microorganisms should be eliminated with the use of antimicrobial agents. Sodium hypochlorite is a potent antimicrobial agent, irrigation being necessary during preparation with a view to microbial control. When preparation has been concluded, EDTA can be used to eliminate the dentinal smear layer, which favors a better mechanical bonding of the cement to the dentinal walls. Other substances used as intracanal medication during the endodontic treatment, such as calcium hydroxide, can also be used, although in order for it to be effective, the time it stays in place is a decisive factor.

It is important to use intracanal medication between the sessions, in order to control the contamination of the tubules and ramifications. The majority of lateral root canals are not filled during endodontic treatment. Therefore, it is essential that the intraradicular post and/or cement fills the entire space emptied during preparation. An empty space favors communication with the periodontium through the lateral root canals, and can consequently originate periapical pathologies.

Similarly, the presence of a temporary restoration with intraradicular retention is essential to maintain the interdental, proximal and occlusal relationship, and to reestablish the function and esthetics of the tooth until the definitive restoration is made.

## References


1. Aksorrnmuang J, Foxton RM, Nakajima M, Tagami J. Microtensile bond strength of a dual-cure resin core material to glass and quartz fibre posts. J Dent 2004;32:443-450.
2. Aquilino SA, Caplan DJ. Relationship between crown placement and the survival of endodontically treated teeth. J Prosthet Dent 2002;87:256-263.
3. Ari H, Yasar E, Belli S. Effects of NaOCl on bond strength of resin cement to root canal dentin. J Endod 2003;29:248-251.
4. Asmussen E, Peutzfeldt A, Heitmann T. Stiffness, elastic limit,and strength of newer types of endodontic posts. J Dent 1999;27:275-278.
5. Assif D, Gorfil C. Biomechanical considerations in restoring endodontically treated teeth. J Prosthet Dent 1994;71:565-567.
6. Assif D, Bitenski A, Pilo R, Oren E. Effect of post design on resistance to fracture of endodontically treated teeth with complete crowns. J Prosthet Dent 1993;69:36-40.
7. Assif D, Nevo E, Aviv I, Himmel R. Retention of endodontic posts with a composite resin luting agent: effect of cement thickness. Quintessence Int 1988;19:643-646.
8. Assif D, Nissan J, Gafni Y, Gordon M. Assessment of the resistance of fracture of endodontically treated molars restored with amalgam. J Prosthet Dent 2003;89:462-465.
9. Bader JD, Shugars DA, Roberson TM. Using crowns to prevent tooth fracture. Community Dent Oral Epidemiol 1996;24:47-51.
10. Balkenhol M, Wostmann, Rein C, Ferger P. Survival time of cast post and cores: A 10-year retrospective study. J Dent 2007;35:50-58.
11. Barkhordar RA, Radke R, Abbasi J. Effect of metal collars on resistance of endodontically treated teeth to root fracture. J Prosthet Dent 1989;61:676-678.
12. Bergman B, Lundquist P, Sjögren U, Sundquist G. Restorative and endodontic results after treatment with cast posts and cores. J Prosthet Dent 1989;61:10-15.
13. Bonfante G, Kaizer OB, Pegoraro LF, do Valle AL. Tensile bond strength of glass fiber posts luted with different cements. Braz Oral Res 2007;21:159-164.
14. Boudrias P, Sakkal S, Petrova Y. Anatomical post design meets quartz fiber techneology: rationale and case report. Compendium 2001;22:337-348.
15. Braga NMA, Paulino SM, Alfredo E, Sousa-Neto MD, Vansan LP. Removal resistance of glass-fiber and metallic cast posts with different lengths. J Oral Sci 2006;48:15-20.
16. Caputo AA, Standlee JP. Pins and posts-why, when and how. Dent Clin North Am 1976;20:299-311.
17. Christensen GJ. Posts: necessary or unnecessary. JADA 1996;127:1522-1526.
18. Christensen GJ. Posts and cores: state of the art. JADA 1998;129:96-97.
19. Cohen BI, Pagnillo MK, Condos S, Deutsch AS. Four different core materials measured for fracture strength in combination with five different designs of endodontics posts. J Prosthet Dent 1996;76:487-495.
20. Cohen BI, Pagnillo MK, Newman I, Musikant BL, Deutsch AS. Retention of a core material supported by three post head designs. J Prosthet Dent 2000;83:624-628.
21. Cooney JP, Caputo AA, Trabert KC. Retention and stress distribution of tapered-end endodontic posts. J Prosthet Dent 1986;55:504-506.
22. Creugers NHJ, Mentink AGB, Kayser AF. An analysis of durability data on post and core restorations. J Dent 1993;21:281-284.
23. Dale JW, Moser J. A clinical evaluation of semiprecious alloys for dowels and cores. J Prosthet Dent 1977;38:161-164.
24. Davy DT, Dilley GL, Krejci RF. Determination of stress patterns in root-filled teeth incorporation various dowel designs. J Dent Res 1981;60:1301-1310.
25. Dean JP, Jeansonne BG, Sarkar N. In vitro evalution of a carbon fiber post. J Endod 1998;24:807-810.
26. Deutsch AS, Musikant BL, Cavallari J. Retentive properties of a new post and core system. J Prosthet Dent 1985;53:12-14.
27. Diaz-Arnold AM, Vargas MA, Haselton DR. Current status of luting agents for fixed prosthodontics. J Prosthet Dent 1999;81:135-141.
28. Donald HL, Jeansonne BG, Gardiner DM, Sarkar NK. Influence of dentinal adhesives and a prefabricated post on fracture resistance of silver amalgam cores. J Prosthet Dent 1997;77:17-22.
29. Ellner S, Bergendal T, Bergman B. Four post-and-core combinations as abutments for fixed single crowns: a prospective up to 10-year study. Int J Prosthodont 2003;16:249-254.
30. Fernandes AS, Dessai GS. Factors affecting the fracture resistance of post-core reconstructed teeth: a review. Int J Prosthodont 2001;14:355-363.
31. Fernandes AS, Shetty S, Coutinho I. Factors determining post selection: a literature review. J Prosthet Dent 2003;90:556-562.
32. Ferrari M, Vichi A, Grandini S. Efficacy of different adhesive techniques on bonding to root canal walls: an SEM investigation. Dent Mater 2001;17:422-429.
33. Ferrari M, Vichi A, Grandini S, Goracci C. Efficacy of a self-curing adhesive-resin cement system on luting glass-fiber post sinto root canals: na SEM investigation. Int J Prosthod 2001;14:543-549.
34. Ferrari M, Grandini S, Simonetti M, Monticelli F, Goracci C. Influence of a microbrush on bonding fiber posts into root canals under clinical conditions, Oral Surg oral Med Oral Pathol Oral Radiol Endod 2002;94:627-631.
35. Fujishima A, Fujishima Y, Ferracane JL. Shear bond strength of tour comercial bonding systems to cpTi. Dent Mater 1995;11:82-86.
36. Goodacre CJ, Bernal G, Rungcharassaeng K, Kan JYK. Clinical complications in fixed prosthodontics. J Prosthet Dent 2003;90:31-41.

37. Goracci C, Raffaelli O, Monticelli F, Balleri B, Bertelli E, Ferrari M. The adhesion between prefabricated FRC posts and composite resin cores: microtensile bond strength with and without post-silanization. Dent Mater 2005;21:437-444.
38. Goracci C, Grandini S, Bossù M, Bertelli E, Ferrari M. Laboratory assessment of the retentive potential of adhesive posts: A review. J Dent 2007:35;827-835.
39. Greenfeld RS, Roydhouse RH, Marshall FJ, Schoner BA. Comparison of two post systems under applied compressive shear loads. J Prosthet Dent 1989;61:17-24.
40. Gutmann JL. The dentin-root complex: anatomic and biologic considerations in restoring endodontically treated teeth. J Prosthet Dent 1992;67:458-467.
41. Guzy G E, Nicholls J I. In vitro comparison of intact endodontically treated teeth with and without endo-post reinforcement. J Prosthet Dent 1979;42:39-44.
42. Hayashi M, Takahashi Y, Imazato S, Ebisu S. Fracture resistente of pulpless teeth restored with post-cores and crowns. Dent Mater 2006;22:477-485.
43. Heling I, Gorfil C, Slutzky H, Kopolovic K, Zalkind M, Slutzky-Goldberg I. Endodontic failure caused by inadequate restorative procedures: review and treatment recommendations. J Prosthet Dent 2002;87:674-678.
44. Heydecke G, Peters MC. The restoration of endodontically treated, single-rooted teeth with cast or direct posts and cores: a systematic review. J Prosthet Dent 2002;87:380-386.
45. Hudis SI, Goldstein GR. Restoration of endodontically treated teeth: a review of the literature. J Prosthet Dent 1986;55:33-38.
46. Hunter AJ, Feiglin B, Williams JF. Effects of post placement on endodontically treated teeth. J Prosthet Dent 1989;62:166-172.
47. Ichikawa Y, Akagawa Y, Nikai H, Tsuru H. Tissue compatibility and stability of a new zirconia ceramic in vivo. J Prosthet Dent 1992;68:322-326.
48. Isidor F, Odman P, Brondum K. Intermittent loading of teeth restored using prefabricated carbon fiber posts. Int J Prosthodont 1996;9:131-136.
49. Jacobi R, Shillingburg H. Pins, dowels and other retentive devices in posterior teeth. Dent Clin North Am 1993;37:367-390.
50. Kahn FH. Selecting a post system. J Amer Den Ass 1991;122:70-71.
51. Kakehashi Y, Lüthy H, Naef R, Wohlwend A, Schärer P. A new all-ceramic post and core system: clinical, technical, and in vitro results. Int J Periodont Rest Dent 1998;18:587-593.
52. Kern M, Wegner SM. Bonding to zirconia ceramic: adhesion methods and their durability. Dent Mater 1998;14:64-71.
53. Koutayas SO, Kern M. All-ceramic posts and cores: the state of the art. Quintessence Int 1999;30:383-392.
54. Kovarik RE, Breeding LC, Caughman WF. Fatigue life of three core materials under simulated chewing conditions. J Prosthet Dent 1992;68:584-590.
55. Krupp JD, Caputo AA, Trabert KC, Standlee J P. Dowel retention with glass-ionomer cement. J Prosthet Dent 1979;41:163-166.
56. Lau VMS. The reinforcement of endodontically treated teeth. Dent Clin North Am 1976;20:313-327.
57. Le Bel AM, Lassila LVJ, Kangasniemi K, Vallittu PK. Bonding of fibre-reinforced composite post to root canal dentin. J Dent 2005;33:533-539.
58. Li ZC, White SN. Mechanical properties of dental luting cements. J. Prosthet Dent 1999;81:597-609.
59. Lui JL. Composite resin reinforcement of flared canals using light-transmitting plastic posts. Quintessence Int 1994;25:313-319.
60. Mannocci F, Bertelli E, Sherriff M, Watson TF, Ford TRP. Three-year clinical comparison of survival of endodontically treated teeth restored with either full cast coverage or with direct composite restoration. J Prosthet Dent 2002;88:297-301.
61. Mannocci F, Ferrari M, Watson TF. Microleakage of endodontically treated teeth restored with fiber posts and composite cores after cyclic loading: a confocal microscopic study. J Prosthet Dent 2001;85:284-290.
62. Marchi GM, Paulillo AMS, Pimenta LAF, Lima FAP. Effect of different filling materials in combination with intraradicular posts on the resistance to fracture of weakened roots. J Oral Rehabil 2003;30:623-629.
63. Martinez-Insua A, Da Silva L, Rilo B, Santana U. Comparison of the fracture resistances of pulpless teeth restored with a cast post and core or carbon-fiber post with a composite core. J Prosthet Dent 1998;80:527-532.
64. Mattison G D. Photoelastic stress analysis of cast-gold. J Prosthet Dent 1982;48:407-411.
65. McLean A. Criteria for the predictably restorable endodontically treated tooth. J Can Dent Assoc 1998;64:652-656.
66. McLean A. Predictably restoring endodontically treated teeth. J Can Dent Assoc 1998;64:782- 787.
67. Mendoza DB, Eakle S. Retention of posts cemented with various dentinal bonding cements. J Prosthet Dent 1994;72:591-594.
68. Mendoza DB, Eakle S, Kahl EA, Ho R. Root reinforcement with a resin-bonded preformed post. J Prosthet Dent 1997;78:10-14.
69. Miller BH, Nakajima H, Powers JM, Nunn ME. Bond strength between cements and metals used for endodontic posts. Dent Mater 1998;14:312-320.
70. Milot P, Stein RS. Root fracture in endodontically treated teeth related to post selection and crown design. J Prosthet Dent 1992;68:428-435.
71. Mondelli J, Steagal IL, Ishikiriama A, Navarro MF, Soares FB. Fracture strength of human teeth with cavity preparation. J Prosthet Dent 1980;43:419-422.
72. Morgano S M. Restoration of pulpless teeth: application of traditional principles in present and future contexts. J Prosthet Dent 1996;75:375-80.
73. Morgano SM, Brackett SE. Foundation restorations in fixed prosthodontics: current knowledge and future needs. J Prosthet Dent 1999;82:643-57.
74. Morgano SM, Milot P. Clinical success of cast metal posts and cores. J. Prosthet Dent 1993;70:11-16.
75. Morris MD, Lee K-W, Agee KA, Bouillaguet S, Pashley DH. Effects of sodium hypochlorite and RC-prep on bond strengths of resin cement to endodontic surfaces. J Endod 2001;27:753-757.
76. Monticelli F, Goracci C, Ferrari M. Micromorphology of the fiber post-resin core unit: a scanning electron microscopy evaluation. Dent Mater 2004;20:176-183.

77. Naumann M, Kiessling S, Seemann R. treatment concepts for restoration of endodontically treated teeth: A nationwide survey of dentists in Germany. J Prosthet Dent 2006;96:332-338.
78. Nergiz I, Schmage P, Ozcan M, Platzer U. Effect of length and diameter of tapered posts on the retention. J Oral Rehabilitation 2002;29:28-34.
79. NG CCH, Dumbrigue H, Al-Bayat MI, Griggs JA, Wakefield CW. Influence of remaining coronal tooth structure location on the fracture resistance of restored endodontically treated anterior teeth. J Prosthet Dent 2006;95:290-296.
80. Newburg RE, Pameijer CH. Retentive properties of post and core systems. J Prosthet Dent 1976;36:636-643.
81. Ngoh EC, Pashley DH, Loushine RJ, Weller N, Kimbrough F. effects of eugenol on resin bond strengths to root canal dentin. J Endod 2001;27:411-414.
82. Nothdurft FP, Oisouech OR. Clinical evaluation of pulpless teeth with conventionally cemented zirconia posts: A pilot study. J Prosthet Dent 2006;95:311-314.
83. OíKeefe KL, Powers JM, McGuckin RS, Pierpont HP. In vitro bond strength of silica-coated metal posts in roots of teeth. Int J Prosthodont 1992;5:373-376.
84. OíKeefe KL, Miller BH, Powers JM. In vitro tensile bond strength of adhesive cements to new post materials. Int J Prosthodont 2000;13:47-51.
85. Pegoretti A, Fambri L, Zappini G, Bianchetti M. Finite element analysis of a glass fibre reinforced composite endodontic post. Biomaterials 2002;23:2667-2682.
86. Pereira JR, Ornelas F, Conti PCR, Valle AL. Effect of a crown ferrule resistance of endodontically treated teeth restored with prefabricated posts. J Prosthet Dent 2006;95:50-54.
87. Perel ML, Muroff FI. Clinical criteria for posts and cores. J Prosthet Dent 1972;28:405-411.
88. Pilo R, Cardash HS, Levin E, Assif D. Effect of core stiffness on the in vitro fracture of crowned, endodontically treated teeth. J Prosthet Dent 2002;88:302-306.
89. Pithan S, Vieira RS, Chain MC. Tensile bond strength of intracanal posts in primary anterior teeth: an in vitro study. J Clin Pediatr Dent 2002;27:35-39.
90. Purton DG, Love RM. Rigidity and retention of carbon fiber versus stainless steel root canal posts. Int Endod J 1996;29:262-265.
91. Purton DG, Love RM, Chandler NP. Rigidity and retention of ceramic root canal posts. Operative Dentistry 2000;25:223-227.
92. Purton DG, Payne JA. Comparison of carbon fiber and stainless steel root canal posts. Quintessence International 1996;27:93-97.
93. Ray HA, Trope M. Periapical status of endodontically treated teeth in relation to the technical quality of the root filling and the coronal restoration. Int Endod J 1995;28:12-18.
94. Reeh ES, Messer HH, Douglas W H. Reduction in tooth stiffness as a result of endodontic and restorative procedures. J Endod 1989;15:512-517.
95. Reinhardt RA, Krejici RF, Pao YC, Stannard JG. Dentin stresses in post-reconstructed teeth with diminishing bone support. J Dent Res 1983;62:1002-1008.
96. Ross RS, Nicholls JL, Harrington GW. Comparison of strain generated during placement of five endodontic posts. J Endod 1991;17:450-456.
97. Sahafi A, Peutzfeldt A, Asmussen E, Gotfredsen K. Bond strength of resin cement to dentin and to surface-treated posts of titanium alloy, galss fiber, and zirconia. J Adhes Dent 2003;5:153-162.
98. Sahafi A, Peutzfeldt A, Asmussen E, Gotfredsen K. Effect of surface treatment of prefabricated posts on bonding of resin cement. Oper Dent 2004;29:60-68.
99. Sahafi A, Peutzfeldt A, Asmussen E, Gotfredsen K. Retention and failure morphology of prefabricated posts. Int J Prosthodont 2004;17:307-312.
100. Sahafi A, Peutzfeldt A, Ravnholt G, Asmussen E. Resistance to cyclic loading of teeth restored with posts. Clin Oral Invest 2005;9:84-90.
101. Saupe WA, Gluskin AH, Radke RA. A comparative study of fracture resistance between morphologic dowel and cores and a resin-reinforced dowel system in the intraradicular restoration of structurally compromised roots. Quintessence Int 1996;27:483-491.
102. Schwartz RS, Murchison DF, Walker WA. Effects of eugenol and noneugenol endodontic sealer cements on post retention. J Endod 1998;24:564-567.
103. Scurria MS, Shugars DA, Hayden WJ, Felton DA. General dentistsí patterns of restoring endodontically treated teeth. J Am Dent Assoc 1995;126:775-779.
104. Shillingburg HT, Kessler JC. Restauração de dentes tratados endodonticamente. São Paulo: Quintessence Publishing Co., Inc., 1991:14.
105. Sivers JE, Johnson WT. Restoration of endodontically treated teeth. Dent Clin North Am 1992;36:631-649.
106. Smith CT, Schuman NJ, Wasson W. Biomechanical criteria for evaluating prefabricated post-and-core systems: a guide for the restorative dentist. Quintessence Int 1998;29:305-312.
107. Sorensen JA, Engelman MJ. Ferrule design and fracture resistance of endodontically treated teeth. J Prosthet Dent 1990;63:529-536.
108. Sorensen JA, Martinoff JT. Intracoronal reinforcement and coronal coverage: a study of endodontically treated teeth. J Prosthet Dent 1984;51:780-784.
109. Sorensen JA, Martinoff JT. Clinically significant factors in dowel design. J Prosthet Dent 1984;52:28-35.
110. Sorensen JA, Martinoff JT. Endodontically treated teeth as abutments. J Prosthet Dent 1985;53:631-636.
111. Standlee JP, Caputo AA. Endodontic dowel retention with resinous cements. J Prosthet Dent 1992;68:913-917.
112. Standlee JP, Caputo AA, Collard EW, Pollack MH. Analysis of stress distribution by endodontic posts. Oral Surg 1972;33:952-959.
113. Standlee JP, Caputo AA, Hanson EC. Retention of endodontic dowels: effects of cement, dowel length, diameter, and design. J Prosthet Dent 1978;39:401-405.
114. Stankiewicz NR, Wilson PR. The ferrule effect: a literature review. Int End J 2002;35:575-581.
115. Starr CB. Amalgam crown restorations for posterior pulpless teeth. J Prosthet Dent 1990;63:614-619.

116. St-Georges AJ, Sturdevant JR, Swift Jr EJ, Thompson JY. Fracture resistance of prepared teeth with bonded inlay restorations. J Prosthet Dent 2003;89:551-557.
117. Stockton LW. Factors affecting retention of post systems: a literature review. J Prosthet Dent 1999;81:380-385.
118. Taira Y, Yanagida H, Matsumura H, Yoshida K, Atsuta M, Suzuki S. Adhesive bonding of titanium with a thione-phosphate dual funcitional primer and self-curing luting agents. Eur J Oral Sci 2000;108:456-460.
119. Tjan AHL, Tjan AH, Greive JH. Effects of various cementation methods on the retention of prefabricated posts. J Prosthet Dent 1987;58:309-313.
120. Tjan AHL, Whang SB. Resistance to root fracture of dowel channels with various thicknesses of buccal dentin walls. J Prosthet Dent 1985;53:496-500.
121. Torbjörner A, Karlsson S, Ödman PA. Survival rate and failure characteristics for two post designs. J Prosthet Dent 1995;73:439-444.
122. Tronstad L, Asbjornsen K, Doving L, Pedersen I, Eriksen HM. Influence of coronal restorations on the periapical health of endodontically treated teeth. Endod Dent Traumatol 2000;16:218-221.
123. Trope M, Maltz D, Tronstad L. Resistance to fracture of restored endodontically treated teeth. Endod Dent Traumatol 1985;1:108-111.
124. Wegner SM, Dern M. Long-term resin bond strength to zirconia ceramic. J Adhes Dent 2000;2:139-147.
125. Yaman P, Thorsteinsson TS. Effect of core materials on stress distribution of posts. J Prosthet Dent 1992;68:416-420.
126. Yan Z, Sidhu SK, Carrick TE, McCabe JF. Response to thermal stimuli of glass ionomer cements. Dent Mater 2007;23:597-600.
127. Yanagia H, Matsumura H, Taira Y, Atsuta M, Shimoe S. Ashesive bonding of composite material to cast titanium with varying surface preparations. J Oral Rehabil 2002;29:121-126.
128. Zalkind M, Hochmann N. Esthetic considerations in restoring endodontically treated teeth with posts and cores. J Prosthet Dent 1998;79:702-705.
129. Zillich RM, Corcoran JF. Average maximum post lengths in endodontically treated teeth. J Prosthet Dent 1984;52:489-491.